Comprehensive Online Resources Available!
http://go.jblearning.com/respiratorycare

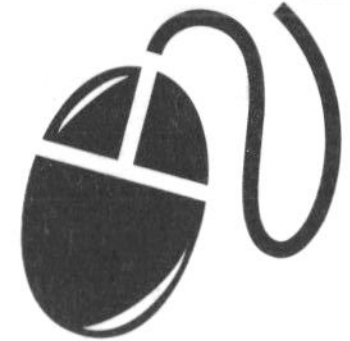

A companion Web site where students will find complete, interactive materials to support *Respiratory Care: Principles and Practice, Second Edition*

Features

- **Self-Assessment Questions**
  Multiple choice and matching questions for each chapter help reinforce the material learned in the text. Assessments are automatically graded, and results can be submitted to the course instructor.
- **Animated Flash Cards**
  This study tool provides a definition and asks the student to give the appropriate key term. The student then can compare his or her answer to the correct one.
- **Crossword Puzzles**
  The puzzle clues and answers are based on the key terms used in the text, reinforcing each term's importance.
- **Interactive Glossary**
  Searchable by chapter and by term, this glossary makes it even easier to locate and study key terms.

Also Available for Instructors

- Instructor's Manual
- PowerPoint Presentations
- TestBank

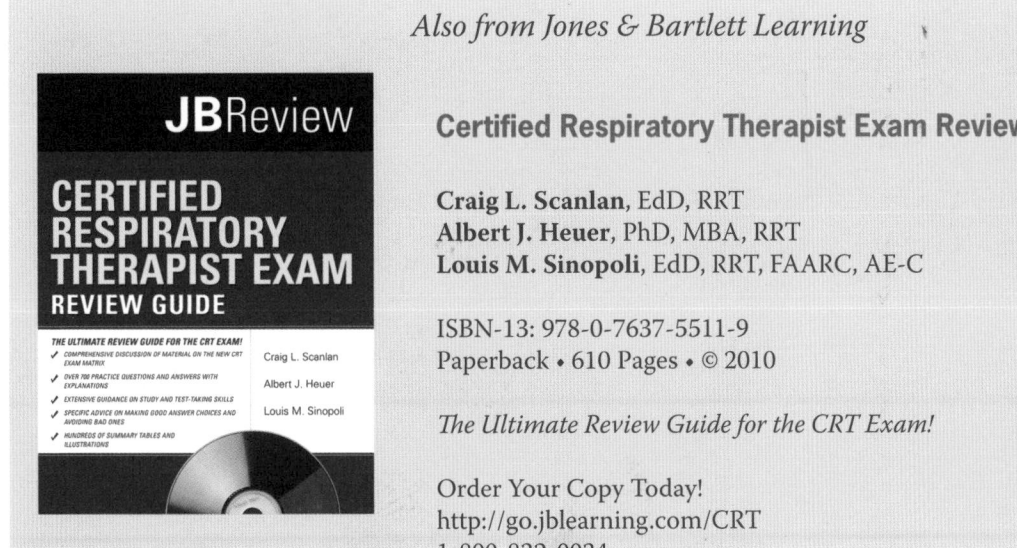

Respiratory Care

Principles and Practice

Second Edition

Dean R. Hess, PhD, RRT, FAARC
Assistant Director of Respiratory Care
Massachusetts General Hospital
Associate Professor of Anesthesia
Harvard Medical School
Editor-in-Chief
Respiratory Care

Neil R. MacIntyre, MD, FAARC
Professor of Medicine
Medical Director of Respiratory Care Services
Duke University Medical Center

Shelley C. Mishoe, PhD, RRT, FAARC
Associate Provost and Professor of
Respiratory Therapy and Graduate Studies
Georgia Health Science University

William F. Galvin, MSEd, RRT, CPFT, AE-C, FAARC
Assistant Professor
School of Allied Health Professions
Director of Respiratory Care Program
Administrative and Teaching Faculty
TIPS Program
Gwynedd-Mercy College

Alexander B. Adams, MPH, RRT, FAARC
Research Associate in Pulmonary/Critical
Care Medicine
Regions Hospital
Assistant Professor of Medicine
University of Minnesota Medical School

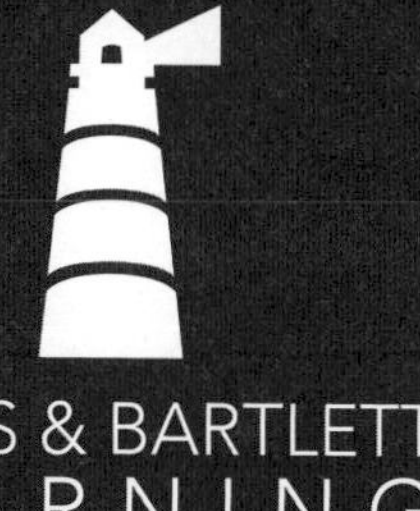

JONES & BARTLETT
LEARNING

World Headquarters
Jones & Bartlett Learning
40 Tall Pine Drive
Sudbury, MA 01776
978-443-5000
info@jblearning.com
www.jblearning.com

Jones & Bartlett Learning books and products are available through most bookstores and online booksellers. To contact Jones & Bartlett Learning directly, call 800-832-0034, fax 978-443-8000, or visit our website, www.jblearning.com.

Substantial discounts on bulk quantities of Jones & Bartlett Learning publications are available to corporations, professional associations, and other qualified organizations. For details and specific discount information, contact the special sales department at Jones & Bartlett Learning via the above contact information or send an email to specialsales@jblearning.com.

Production Credits
Chief Executive Officer: Ty Field
President: James Homer
SVP, Chief Operating Officer: Don Jones, Jr.
SVP, Chief Technology Officer: Dean Fossella
SVP, Chief Marketing Officer: Alison M. Pendergast
SVP, Chief Financial Officer: Ruth Siporin
SVP, Editor-in-Chief: Michael Johnson
Publisher: David D. Cella
Associate Editor: Maro Gartside
Editorial Assistant: Teresa Reilly
Production Manager: Julie Champagne Bolduc
Production Editor: Jessica Steele Newfell
Marketing Manager: Grace Richards
Manufacturing and Inventory Control Supervisor: Amy Bacus
Composition: Shepherd Incorporated
Cover Design: Kristin E. Parker
Photo Research and Permissions Supervisor: Christine Myaskovsky
Associate Photo Researcher: Sarah Cebulski
Cover and Title Page Image: © Barauskaite/ShutterStock, Inc.
Printing and Binding: Courier Corporation
Cover Printing: Courier Corporation

Library of Congress Cataloging-in-Publication Data
Hess, Dean R.
Respiratory care : principles and practice / Dean R. Hess . . . [et al.]. —2nd ed.
p. ; cm.
Includes bibliographical references and index.
ISBN-13: 978-0-7637-6003-8 (alk. paper)
ISBN-10: 0-7637-6003-X (alk. paper)
1. Respiratory therapy. I. Hess, Dean.
[DNLM: 1. Respiratory Therapy. WF 145]
RC735.I5R4755 2011
616.2'0046—dc22

2010031899

6048

Printed in United States of America
15 14 13 12 11 10 9 8 7 6 5 4 3 2

Contents

Preface

Ten years is a long time. A lot can happen in 10 years. In the 10 years since the publication of the *First Edition* of this book, the New England Patriots won the Super Bowl 3 times, the Boston Red Sox won the World Series twice, the Boston Celtics won an NBA championship, and the Boston Bruins won the Stanley Cup. Some might have thought that impossible, just as some might have thought a second edition of this book impossible. But we are back, better than ever, in champion form, with the *Second Edition* of *Respiratory Care: Principles and Practice.*

As you will see, the *Second Edition* is completely reorganized. Patient assessment has been moved to the beginning of the book, which recognizes the important role of patient assessment in everyday respiratory care practice. This is followed by respiratory therapeutics, respiratory diseases, applied sciences, and, finally, the professional aspects of respiratory care. Many topics important to contemporary practice have been added. These include geriatrics, patient safety, disaster management, home care, and expanded coverage of neonatal/pediatrics. Nearly all of the art has been updated or replaced in this edition. Full color photographs and illustrations are used to embellish the text. Many new authors have been added to breathe new life into the material, more than half of whom are practicing respiratory therapists. Because the book has been so thoroughly rewritten and reworked, it appears more like a third or fourth edition than a second edition.

All of the successful pedagogical features of the *First Edition* have been retained for this edition. These features include the use of the clinical practice guidelines of the American Association for Respiratory Care (AARC), glossary terms, key points, and respiratory recaps. In addition to the text itself, online features are available to support students and faculty. For students, there are chapter quizzes, case studies, and additional interactive activities. For faculty, we provide PowerPoint presentations, an ImageBank, a TestBank, and more. A companion website is available for this text at http://go.jblearning.com/respiratorycare.

The focus of the text is respiratory therapy practice in the 21st century. The modern respiratory therapist must be a technologist, physiologist, and clinician. The respiratory therapist of today is expected to be a clinical leader, which includes input into the development of multidisciplinary care plans and implementation of respiratory care protocols. Moreover, contemporary practice is evidence based. Each of these important aspects of modern respiratory care practice was carefully considered in the preparation of this book.

The primary audience of this book is respiratory therapy students. We have written this book for students, having considered the examination matrix of the National Board for Respiratory Care (NBRC) to ensure that all of the topics on the board exams (and more) are included. In the online TestBank, questions are keyed to the examination matrix. But this is more than a book designed to assure success on the board exams. *Respiratory Care, Second Edition* includes many topics beyond the NBRC exam matrix that are intended to help students become well-rounded members of the patient care team.

We strived to make this text readable and the content within reach of students. We included boxes, tables, and illustrations to assist learning. We carefully edited the book for consistency in writing style throughout. However, we have not watered down the content. The material may be challenging at places, but the intent was not to make it difficult. Rather, it is written to help students maximize their contributions when interacting with physicians and other members of the healthcare team. An important aspect of professional interactions is the ability to use the language that others use at the bedside; whether a respiratory therapist, physician, or other healthcare professional, the language should always be the same.

Although this text is intended primarily for students, it will be useful for others as a reference book. For the respiratory therapist who graduated from school some time ago, this book should serve as a refresher and update. For those who are not respiratory therapists, the content should provide insight into respiratory therapy practice and could serve as a reference text.

There are innumerable persons to be thanked for their contributions to the success of this project. First, I thank my co-editors. They embraced the vision and worked hard to make this book the best that it can be. Second, I thank all of the chapter authors who dealt with our prodding to complete their chapters to our expectations. Finally, I owe a mountain of gratitude to everyone at Jones & Bartlett Learning who poured their talents into this project and unselfishly went out of their way, without complaint, to make this book second to none.

It is my hope that the *Second Edition* of *Respiratory Care: Principles and Practice* will assist students as they master the art and science of respiratory care, that it contributes to an improvement in the stature of the respiratory care profession, and most importantly that it improves the care of patients with respiratory disorders.

Dean R. Hess, PhD, RRT, FAARC

Contributing Authors

Bekele Afessa, MD
Associate Professor of Medicine
Mayo Clinic College of Medicine

Allan G. Andrews, MS, RRT
Clinical Specialist in Metabolics
University Hospital Respiratory Care
University of Michigan Health System

Sherry Barnhart, RRT-NPS, FAARC
Coordinator of Discharge Planning
Arkansas Children's Hospital

Will Beachey, PhD, RRT, FAARC
Professor and Director, Respiratory Therapy Program
St. Alexius Medical Center

Laura H. Beveridge, MEd, RRT
Assistant Professor, Department of Respiratory Therapy
Georgia Health Science University

Rhonda Bevis, EdD, RRT
Director of Clinical Education
Armstrong Atlantic State University

Rajesh Bhagat, MD
Assistant Professor, Staff Physician
Division of Pulmonary, Critical Care, and Sleep Medicine
University of Mississippi Medical Center

Peter Bliss, BSME
Phillips Healthcare

John Boatright, PhD, RRT
Chair, Associate Professor
Henrietta Schmoll School of Health
Respiratory Care Department
St. Catherine University

Pamela L. Bortner, MBA, RRT, FAARC
Clinical Specialist
Department of Respiratory Care
The Toledo Hospital

Richard D. Branson, MSc, RRT, FAARC
Professor of Surgery
University of Cincinnati

Melissa K. Brown, BS, RRT-NPS, RCP
Instructor, Respiratory Therapy Program
Grossmont Community College
Clinical Research Facilitator, Chest Medicine and Critical Care Medical Group
Sharp Memorial Hospital

Joseph Buhain, MBA, RRT, NREMTB
Program Director, Respiratory Care and Simulation Studies
St. Paul College
Course Director for Pulmonary Sciences
Concordia University

Ellen Cannefax, RRT, RPFT, AE-C
Scottsdale Healthcare

Robert L. Chatburn, MHHS, RRT-NPS, FAARC
Clinical Research Manager, Respiratory Institute Cleveland Clinic
Adjunct Associate Professor, Department of Medicine
Lerner College of Medicine of Case Western Reserve University

Bashir A. Chaudhary, MD, MD, FAASM, FACCP
Assistant Dean for Clinical Affairs
School of Allied Health Sciences
Director, Sleep Institute of Augusta
Medical College of Georgia

Francis C. Cordova, MD
Associate Professor of Medicine
Division of Pulmonary and Critical Care Medicine
Temple University School of Medicine

Christopher E. Cox, MD, MPH
Assistant Professor of Medicine
Duke University

Gerald J. Criner, MD
Florence P. Bernheimer Distinguished Service Chair
Director of Pulmonary and Critical Care Medicine and Temple Lung Center
Temple University School of Medicine

John D. Davies, MA, RRT, FAARC
Clinical Research Coordinator
Department of Pulmonary Medicine
Duke University Medical Center

Scott H. Donaldson, MD
Associate Professor of Medicine
University of North Carolina at Chapel Hill

Kristin Engebretsen, PharmD, DABAT
Clinical Toxicologist, Emergency Medicine Department
Regions Hospital

Paul Enright, MD
Professor of Medicine
The University of Arizona

Maha Farhat, MD
Harvard Pulmonary and Critical Care Combined Fellowship Program
Harvard Medical School

Daniel F. Fisher, MS, RRT
Assistant Director, Respiratory Care Services
Massachusetts General Hospital

Paolo Formenti, MD
Dipartimento di Anestesiologia
Terapia Intensiva e Scienze Dermatologiche
Università degli Studi
Milan, Italy

Donna D. Gardner, MSHP, RRT
Director of Clinical Education and Assistant Professor
Department of Respiratory Care
School of Allied Health Sciences
University of Texas Health Science Center at San Antonio

Michael A. Gentile, RRT, FAARC, FCCM
Associate in Research
Duke University Medical Center

Andrew J. Ghio, MD
Assistant Consulting Professor
Division of Pulmonary and Critical Care Medicine
Department of Medicine
Duke University Medical Center

Lynda T. Goodfellow, EdD, RRT, AE-C, FAARC
Associate Professor and Director
School of Health Professions, College of Health and Human Sciences
Georgia State University

Joseph A. Govert, MD
Associate Professor
Duke University Medical Center

Carl F. Haas, MLS, RRT, FAARC
Educational Coordinator
University Hospital Respiratory Care
University of Michigan Health System

Charles William Hargett III, MD
Assistant Professor of Medicine
Division of Pulmonary, Allergy, and Critical Care Medicine
Duke University Medical Center

John E. Heffner, MD
Garnjobst Chair, Department of Medicine
Providence Portland Medical Center
Professor of Medicine
Oregon Health and Science University

Kathleen M. Hernlen, MBA, RRT
Assistant Professor, Respiratory Therapy School of Allied Health Sciences
Medical College of Georgia

Yuh-Chin T. Huang, MD, MHS, FCCP
Professor of Medicine
Division of Pulmonary, Allergy, and Critical Care Medicine
Duke University Medical Center

Angela King, RRT
Senior Director
Clinical Ventilation–Americas, ResMed

Erika Lease, MD
Duke University Medical Center

Thomas Malinowski, BS, RRT, FAARC
Director, Respiratory Services, Neurodiagnostics
Community Asthma Action Program
Mary Washington Healthcare

Douglas E. Masini, EdD, RPFT, RRT-NPS, AE-C, FAARC
Director, Respiratory Therapy Department
Armstrong Atlantic State University

Steven C. Mason, RRT/NPS
Massachusetts General Hospital

Robert A. May, MD
Medical Director, Respiratory Care Program
University of Toledo

Charles D. McArthur, BA, RRT, RPFT
Consultant
Core Respiratory Services

Robert McCoy, RRT
Managing Director
Valley Inspired Products, Inc.

Benjamin D. Medoff, MD
Chief, Pulmonary and Critical Care Unit
Massachusetts General Hospital

Rafat O. Mohammed, MD
Fellow, Division of Pulmonary, Critical Care, and Sleep Medicine
University of Mississippi Medical Center

Christine J. Moore, MEd, RRT-NPS, CPFT
Lecturer and Laboratory Coordinator
Armstrong Atlantic State University

John Mullarkey, BA, RRT, AE-C
Clinical Manager, Respiratory Care Department
Temple University Hospital

Timothy R. Myers, BS, RRT-NPS
Director, Woman's and Children's Respiratory Care and Procedural Services
Pediatric Heart Center
Rainbow Babies and Children's Hospital and MacDonald's Hospital for Women
Adjunct Assistant Professor of Pediatrics
Case Western Reserve University School of Medicine

Avi Nahum, MD, PhD
Pulmonary/Critical Care Medicine
Healthpartners—Regions Hospital

Catherine O'Malley, RRT
Cystic Fibrosis Specialist
Children's Memorial Hospital

Timothy Op't Holt, EdD, RRT, AE-C, FAARC
Professor of Cardiorespiratory Care
University of South Alabama

Marcos I. Restrepo, MD, MSc
South Texas Veterans Health Care System
The University of Texas Health Sciences Center at San Antonio

Ruben D. Restrepo, MD, RRT, FAARC
Associate Professor, Department of Respiratory Care
The University of Texas Health Sciences Center at San Antonio

Bryce R. H. Robinson, MD
Assistant Professor of Surgery
University of Cincinnati

Bruce K. Rubin, MEngr, MD, MBA, FRCPC
Jessie Ball duPont Professor and Chairman, Department of Pediatrics
Professor of Biomedical Engineering
Virginia Commonwealth University School of Medicine

Robert L. Sheridan, MD
Trauma, Emergency Surgery, and Critical Care
Massachusetts General Hospital and Shriners Hospital for Children

Scott L. Shofer, MD, PhD
Assistant Professor, Division of Pulmonary, Allergy, and Critical Care
Duke University Medical Center

Kathleen A. Short, RRT, RN
Director, Respiratory Care Department
University of North Carolina Hospitals

Mark Simmons, MS, RRT
Program Director, Respiratory Care
York College of Pennsylvania

Priscilla Simmons, MSN, EdD, APRN, BC
Professor of Nursing
Eastern Mennonite University

Jaspal Singh, MD, MHS, FCCP
Associate Clinical Professor of Medicine
University of North Carolina at Chapel Hill

Kelly Sioris, PharmD
Senior Clinical Toxicologist
SafetyCall International, PLLC

Helen M. Sorenson, MS, RRT, FAARC
Associate Professor, Department of Respiratory Care
University of Texas Health Sciences Center

Karen Stewart, MSc, RRT, FAARC
Associate Administrator
Charleston Area Medical Center

William S. Stigler, MD
Fellow, Harvard Pulmonary and Critical Care Program
Harvard Medical School

Arthur Taft, PhD, RRT, FAARC
Associate Professor and Program Director, Department of Respiratory Therapy
Medical College of Georgia

Victor F. Tapson, MD
Department of Pulmonary, Allergy, and Critical Care Medicine
Duke University Medical Center

Vinko F. Tomicic, MD
Director of Intensive Care Unit
Clínica Las Lilas
Santiago, Chile

Amy E. Treece, MD
Pulmonary and Critical Care
Duke University Medical Center

Teresa A. Volsko, MHHS, RRT, FAARC
Program Director
Youngstown State University

Momen M. Wahidi, MD, MBA
Director, Interventional Pulmonology and Bronchoscopy
Associate Professor of Medicine
Duke University Medical Center

Jeffrey J. Ward, MEd, RRT, FAARC
Assistant Professor of Anesthesiology
University of Minnesota, College of Medicine
Mayo Clinic Program in Respiratory Care
Mayo Clinic College of Medicine Medical Simulation Center

Susan Whiddon, MS, RRT
Instructor, Director of Clinical Education, Respiratory Therapy
School of Allied Health Sciences
Medical College of Georgia

James R. Yankaskas, MD, MS
Professor of Medicine
University of North Carolina at Chapel Hill

Reviewers

Brent Blevins, RN, RRT, BSN
Director Clinical Education, Professor
Cooperative Respiratory Care Program
St. Mary's and Marshall University

Amy Ceconi, PhD, RRT, RPFT, NPS
Program Director
Bergen Community College

Lea Endress, BS, RRT, RPFT, RCP
Respiratory Therapy Instructor
Respiratory Therapy Program
San Joaquin Valley College

David Fry, BS, RRT, CPFT
Director of Clinical Education
Department of Respiratory Care
Temple College

Wesley M. Granger, PhD, RRT
Associate Professor, Program Director
Department of Clinical and Diagnostic Sciences
Respiratory Therapy Program
The University of Alabama Birmingham

Jennifer Gresham, MA, RRT-NPS
Assistant Professor
Department of Respiratory Care
Midwestern State University

Michael Haines, MPH, RRT-NPS, AE-C
Respiratory Therapy Instructor
San Joaquin Valley College

Suezette Hicks, BA, RRT-CPFT
Director Respiratory Care Program
Black River Technical College

Lisa Johnson, MS, RRT-NPS
Clinical Assistant Professor
Director of Clinical Education
Respiratory Care Program
Stony Brook University

Robert L. Joyner Jr., PhD, RRT, FAARC
Director, Respiratory Therapy Program
Associate Professor and Chair
Department of Health Sciences
Salisbury University

Traci Marin, MPH, RRT
Program Director
Victor Valley College

Cynthia McKinley, RRT
Assistant Professor
Director of Clinical Education, Respiratory Care Program
Lamar Institute of Technology

Larry McMullin, MM, RRT, RPFT
Clinical Coordinator, Assistant Professor
Respiratory Care Program
Ferris State University

Kim J. Morris-Garcia, MEd, RRT, NPS
Associate Master Technical Instructor
Director of Clinical Education
Respiratory Therapy and BAT Programs
University of Texas at Brownsville and Texas Southmost College

Jennifer M. Purdue, MA, RRT-NPS, AE-C, RN
Associate Professor, Program Chair
Department of Respiratory Care
Ivy Tech Community College

Christopher Rowse, MS, RRT, RPFT, RPSGT
Professor
Northern Essex Community College

Georgianna Sergakis, PhD, RRT
Assistant Professor, Clinical Program Director
Respiratory Therapy Division
The Ohio State University

Frank Sinsheimer, RCP, RRT, EdD
Professor Emeritus, Respiratory Therapy
Los Angeles Valley College

Stephen G. Smith, MPA, RT, RRT
Chair, New York State Board for Respiratory Therapy
Clinical Assistant Professor
Stony Brook University

Don Steinert, MA, RRT, MT, CLS
Associate Professor
University of the District of Columbia

Chris Trotter, BS, RRT
Assistant Professor
Cooperative Respiratory Care Program
Saint Mary's and Marshall University

LaVerne Yousey, RRT, MSTE
Professor of Respiratory Care, Emeritus
University of Akron

Rick Zahodnic, PhD, RRT-NPS, RPFT, AE-C
Clinical Coordinator
Respiratory Therapy Program
Macomb Community College

SECTION I

Respiratory Assessment

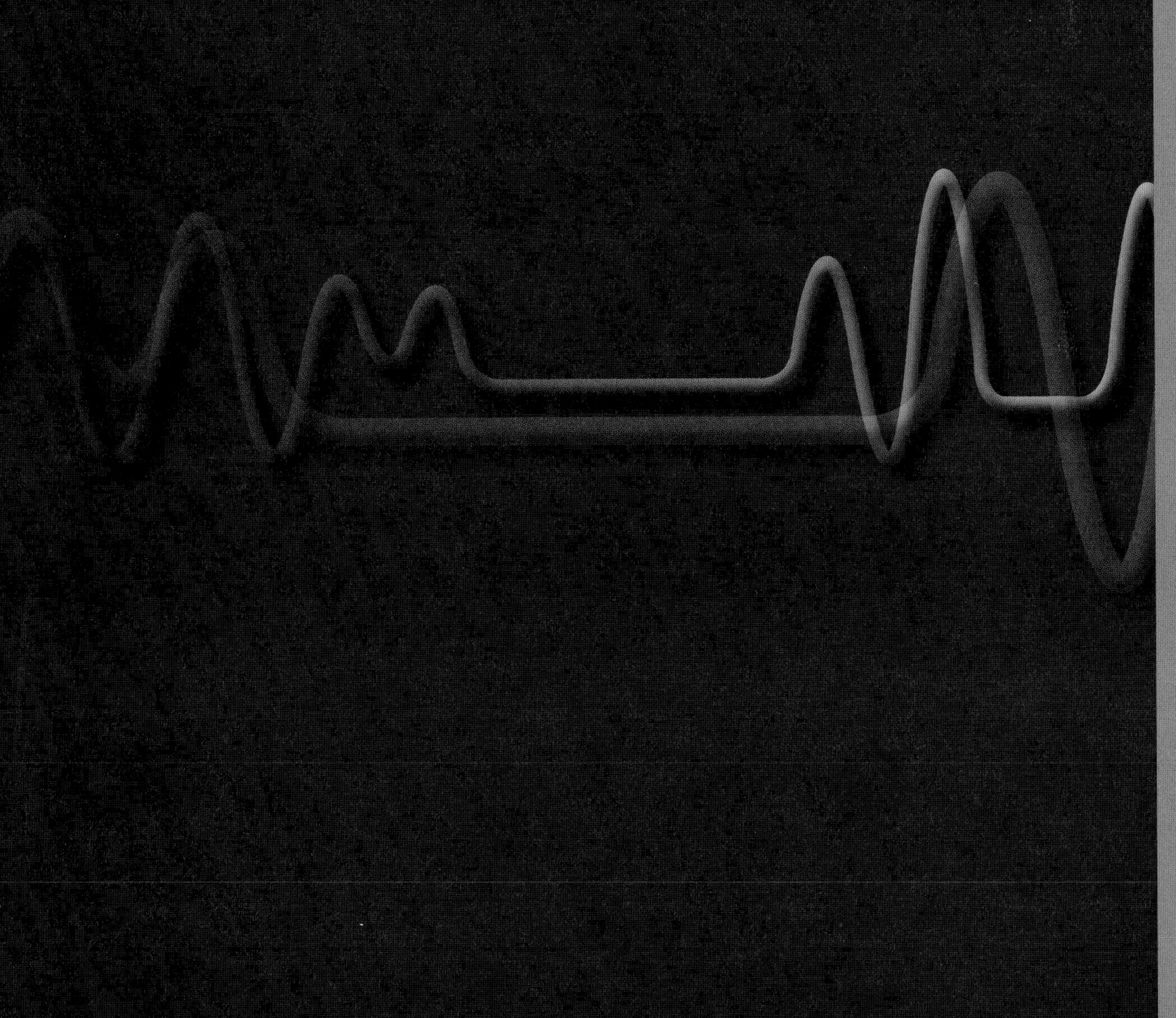

CHAPTER 1

History and Physical Examination

Priscilla Simmons

OUTLINE

Creating a Therapeutic Climate
Components of the Health History
Vital Signs
Techniques of Assessment
Physical Examination of the Lungs and Thorax
Assessment of Other Body Systems

OBJECTIVES

1. Discuss the factors essential in the creation of a therapeutic climate.
2. Explain three considerations of an effective health history.
3. Explain the relevance of cultural diversity in the history-taking process.
4. List the major components of a health history.
5. Identify the four major examination techniques.
6. Define common terms used in assessment of the respiratory system.
7. Explain the technique for auscultation of the chest.
8. Define terms associated with normal and abnormal breath sounds.
9. List the signs associated with respiratory distress.
10. Identify common pathologic processes of the respiratory system and pertinent physical findings that extend to other body systems.
11. Identify the significance of various chest landmarks.
12. Explain the significance of sounds heard during cardiac auscultation.
13. Explain the significance of jugular venous distention.
14. Explain common findings associated with an assessment of the neurologic system.

KEY TERMS

auscultation
barrel chest
Biot respirations
bradypnea
bronchial breath sounds
bronchophony
Cheyne-Stokes breathing
clubbing
crackles
cyanosis
dyspnea
egophony
flail chest
grunting
hyperpnea
hyperresonant
hyperventilation
inspection
jaundice
Kussmaul respirations
kyphosis
lordosis
murmur
orthopnea
pack years
pallor
palpation
paradoxical respiration
paroxysmal nocturnal dyspnea
pectus carinatum
pectus excavatum
percussion
platypnea
plethora
pleural friction rub
precordium
resonant
rhonchus
scoliosis
stridor
tachypnea
tactile fremitus
tympanic
vesicular breath sounds
wheezes
whispered pectoriloquy

INTRODUCTION

This chapter provides a guide to essential assessment techniques used by the respiratory therapist. In the hospital, many members of the healthcare team examine the patient. In the community setting, however, fewer members of the healthcare team assess the patient, thereby warranting a more thorough examination by the respiratory therapist. Whatever the setting, no clinician regularly uses all the available assessment techniques. In fact, some techniques are rarely used. The emphasis of this chapter is on the pathophysiology underlying common respiratory abnormalities and the typical assessment findings associated with them.

Creating a Therapeutic Climate

The patient's perception of the respiratory therapist's competence is of prime importance. When any healthcare provider is perceived as uncaring, the patient may remember that attitude most vividly. Even worse, that poor image may come to characterize all the members of the profession for the patient. To ensure a therapeutic, professional relationship, competence and caring must coexist. A clinician can communicate caring through a gentle demeanor and an unhurried, unabrupt manner. Maintaining eye contact is essential. Also appropriate is the judicious use of touch, such as patting or squeezing a patient's hand or shoulder. Respiratory therapists should dress appropriately because a professional appearance communicates respect for the patient. A patient's judgment of a healthcare provider often is based on physical appearance. These measures help establish rapport and a climate of professional caring, a goal in every professional relationship.

> **RESPIRATORY RECAP**
>
> **Variables Supporting a Therapeutic Climate**
> - Caring demeanor
> - Competence
> - Eye contact
> - Judicious use of touch
> - Professional image

Components of the Health History

The health history provides a detailed, chronologic health record of the patient's status. For the purpose of developing an individualized plan of care, the health history elicits information about variables affecting the patient's health. The value of the history should not be underestimated because it guides the selection of appropriate physical examination techniques, helps the respiratory therapist develop an accurate index of suspicion, and ultimately leads to appropriate and effective therapeutic intervention. Because obtaining a comprehensive history is time consuming, many healthcare providers assess primarily the body systems of concern. Clearly, the heart and lungs are the systems of primary interest for respiratory therapists.

> **RESPIRATORY RECAP**
>
> **The Health History**
> - Chief complaint
> - History of present illnesss
> - Occupational and environmental history
> - Geographic exposure
> - Activities of daily living
> - Smoking history
> - Cough and sputum production
> - Family history
> - Medical history
> - Review of systems

Chief Complaint

The chief complaint (CC) is the problem or concern that prompted the patient to seek healthcare. When documenting the CC in the patient record, the examiner should use the patient's own words in quotation marks.

History of Present Illness

The history of present illness (HPI) is the chronologic, narrative account of the patient's health problem. It should describe in detail information relevant to the CC, including a description of the onset of the problem, the date the symptoms occurred and whether they developed gradually or suddenly, and the setting in which they developed. Also included is a description of the signs and symptoms associated with the problem. The mnemonic *OLD CART* can help the examiner gather information accordingly, as follows:

> **RESPIRATORY RECAP**
>
> **History of Present Illness**
> - Onset
> - Location
> - Duration
> - Character
> - Associated Manifestations
> - Relieving factors
> - Treatment

Onset (when the problem started)

Location of pain, shortness of breath, or other symptoms

Duration of pain, shortness of breath, or other symptoms

Character, quantity, and quality of pain; shortness of breath; or other symptoms

Associated manifestations (the setting in which the pain, shortness of breath, or other symptoms developed)

Relieving factors or factors that diminish or aggravate the pain, shortness of breath, or other symptoms

Treatment (any medications or other remedies that relieve or exacerbate shortness of breath)

Occupational and Environmental History

The examiner should inquire as to whether the patient is employed, retired, or laid off. Are there any current or past hazards at work, such as exposure to asbestos, coal dust, silica, molds, dust, or animals? Is the patient under stress at work? Is the patient satisfied with his or her job?

Geographic Exposure

Has the patient traveled to foreign countries? Has the patient been in military service?

Activities of Daily Living

Has the patient experienced difficulty with or change in the ability to provide self-care?

Smoking History

Does the patient smoke cigarettes or done so in the past? How long has the patient smoked cigarettes? This answer is usually expressed in **pack years** and is calculated as follows. A pack a day for 1 year is known as *1 pack year*. Two packs a day for a year is *2 pack years*, and so on. What is the patient's willingness to quit? The examiner should also inquire as to whether the patient smokes a pipe, cigars, or illicit drugs, such as marijuana or crack cocaine.

Cough and Sputum Production

The examiner should ask about the presence of cough and sputum. If the patient has a cough, the timing of the cough (for example, in the morning, at night, after eating) and whether sputum is produced should be noted. If sputum is produced, the examiner should determine its amount, consistency, color, and odor, as well as whether the frequency of the cough and the amount of sputum has increased recently.

Family History

Any family history of genetically transmitted disease (for example, cystic fibrosis, alpha-1 antitrypsin deficiency), cancer, heart disease, tuberculosis (TB), or human immunodeficiency virus (HIV) should be noted.

Medical History

Dates of past health problems, hospitalizations, symptoms, and treatment should be noted in the history, as well as whether the problem is ongoing, resolved, or recurrent. Are immunizations current? Does the patient have any food, drug, insect, or environmental allergies?

Review of Systems

A review of the systems provides the opportunity for the examiner to methodically question the patient about the health of each body system. It differs from the physical examination in that the data are collected verbally. A thorough review of each system is unnecessary, but the examiner should include a detailed review of the systems affected by the present illness. If the patient answers with a negative response, a denial of that specific complaint should be noted. For example, "Patient denies pain with deep inspiration and coughing."

Vital Signs

Pulse, respirations, and blood pressure are considered *vital signs*. These are commonly measured, along with body temperature, as indicators of the patient's health status. The pulse rate and rhythm can be measured by cardiac auscultation or palpation of any artery, with the radial artery being most commonly used for this purpose. The pulse is counted for a minimum of 15 seconds and then mathematically adjusted to the rate per minute. The normal pulse rate for adults is 60 to 100 beats per minute; the rate is more rapid for infants and children. The respiratory rate is measured by inspection of the movement of the chest for 1 minute. The normal respiratory rate for adults is 12 to 20 breaths per minute; it is more rapid for infants and children.

Blood pressure is measured either with a sphygmomanometer or an indwelling arterial catheter. Normal blood pressure for adults is 120/80 mm Hg; measurements are lower for infants and children.

Body temperature can be measured via the oral, rectal, or axillary sites using a traditional thermometer. Infrared sensors are also used for the forehead or tympanic sites. Core temperature monitoring is measured in the distal esophagus or pulmonary artery. Normal body temperature is 37° C (98.6° F). The term *fever* refers to a higher-than-normal body temperature (hyperthermia), whereas hypothermia is a temperature lower than normal.

AGE-SPECIFIC ANGLE

Compared with adults, infants and children have higher respiratory rates, higher pulse rates, and lower blood pressure readings.

Techniques of Assessment

Inspection

As an examination technique, **inspection** ranges from casual observation to visual scrutiny of the patient.

RESPIRATORY RECAP

Respiratory Assessment Techniques

» Inspection
» Palpation
» Percussion
» Auscultation

Palpation

Palpation is the process whereby the examiner uses the hands to feel for body movement, lumps, masses, and skin characteristics. Palpation can be either light or deep.

Percussion

Percussion requires the examiner to place a finger firmly against a body part and strike that finger with a fingertip from the other hand. The technique for the right-handed examiner is as follows:

1. Hyperextend the middle finger of the nondominant hand (pleximeter finger).
2. Press the distal interphalangeal joint firmly on the surface to be percussed. Avoid contact with any other part of the hand because vibrations may be dampened.
3. Hold the forearm of the other arm close to the surface, with the hand turned up at the wrist, and partially flex the middle finger (plexor).
4. Strike the pleximeter with the tip of the plexor with a quick, sharp, and relaxed wrist motion and aim at the distal interphalangeal joint (**Figure 1–1**). Withdraw briskly to avoid dampening the vibrations. Use one to two blows at each location.

The resulting sounds can suggest either normal underlying tissue or typical sounds associated with given abnormalities.

Five percussion tones (**Table 1–1**) are commonly recognized: flat, dull, resonant, hyperresonant, and

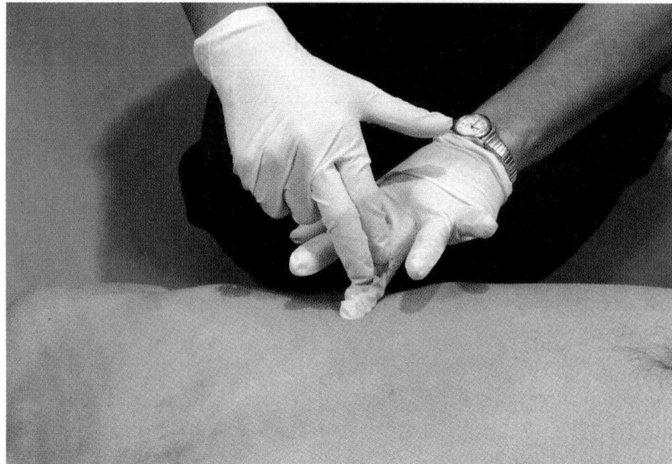

FIGURE 1–1 Percussion technique.

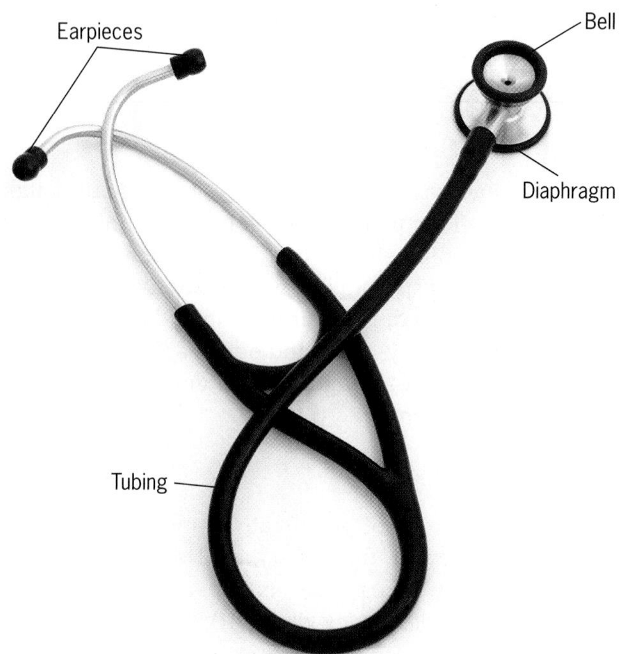

FIGURE 1–2 Stethoscope, illustrating diaphragm and bell.

TABLE 1–1 Characteristics of Percussion Notes

Type of Tone	Intensity	Pitch	Duration	Quality
Flat	Soft	High	Short	Extremely dull
Dull	Medium	Medium-high	Medium	Thudlike
Resonant	Loud	Low	Long	Hollow
Hyperresonant	Very loud	Very low	Longer	Booming
Tympanic	Loud	High	Medium	Drumlike

RESPIRATORY RECAP

Percussion Notes
» Flat
» Dull
» Resonant
» Hyperresonant
» Tympanic

tympanic. A flat percussion note is soft, high pitched, and of short duration. It may be elicited by percussion of the thigh. A dull percussion note is of medium intensity, pitch, and duration. It is heard over the liver or a tumor. A **resonant** note is loud, low in pitch, and of long duration. It may be heard over normal lung tissue. A **hyperresonant** note is very loud, lower in pitch, longer in duration, and commonly heard over an emphysematous lung. A **tympanic** note is loud and drumlike, with a high pitch. It may be heard over a gastric bubble.

Auscultation

After inspection, **auscultation** is the most commonly used physical assessment technique, particularly for assessment of the respiratory system. Auscultation involves listening to body sounds with a stethoscope placed on bare skin. The stethoscope has several important components (**Figure 1–2**). The diaphragm is the larger side of the stethoscope head and is made of rigid plastic. The bell is the smaller cup on the other side of the head and is covered with a plastic or rubber ring. The bell is useful for detection of certain cardiac and vascular sounds. The diaphragm is used more frequently. Note that both adult and pediatric diaphragms and bells exist, with the latter being smaller. Some stethoscopes come with interchangeable parts. The examiner should ensure that the appropriate sizes are being used.

Quality stethoscopes have tubing specifically engineered to conduct sound very well. It is possible to purchase stethoscopes that actually magnify sound. Most stethoscopes, however, simply block out other noise, thereby allowing the examiner to hear body sounds unimpeded. An appropriate tubing length is about 12 inches. Earpieces must fit snugly and comfortably. The earpieces must point toward the nose of the examiner to project sound toward the tympanic membrane of the examiner's ears.

Physical Examination of the Lungs and Thorax

The astute clinician is thoroughly familiar with human anatomy. An in-depth knowledge of structure and function is vital to the interpretation of assessment findings in terms of underlying pathologic processes. **Figure 1–3** illustrates thoracic landmarks and the surface anatomy of the chest.

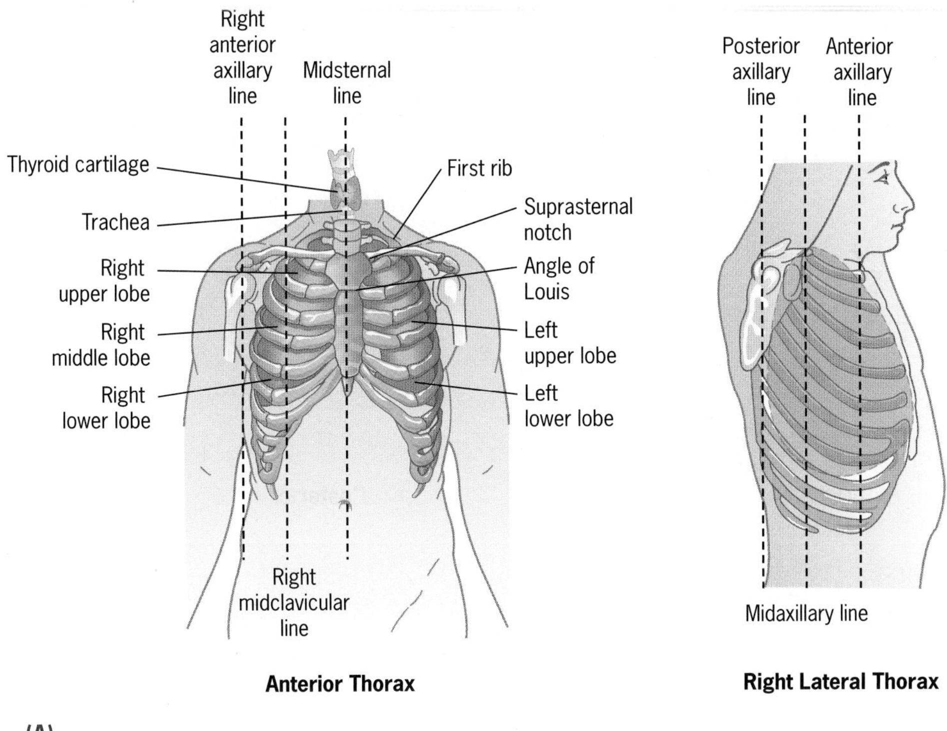

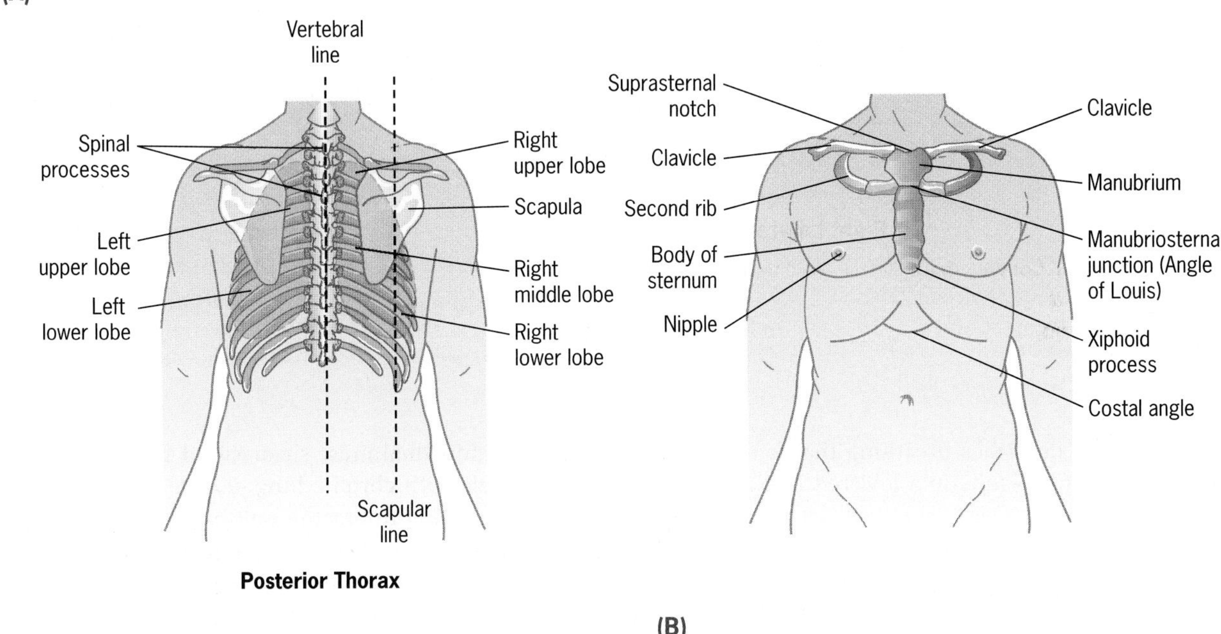

FIGURE 1–3 **(A)** Thoracic landmarks. **(B)** Topographic landmarks of the chest.

(continues)

Inspection

Observing Respirations

The clinician must be familiar with common respiratory patterns (**Figure 1–4**). **Tachypnea** describes a persistent rate of respiration faster than 20 breaths per minute. It may be present in individuals who are hypoxemic and those who have pain in the thoracic region. Similarly, if liver enlargement or abdominal distention compromises diaphragmatic movement, tachypnea may result. At times, however, tachypnea is merely a patient response to the realization that respirations are being observed and counted. Tachypnea also occurs in individuals with fever and in those with restrictive ventilatory defects, such as pulmonary fibrosis or pneumonectomy.

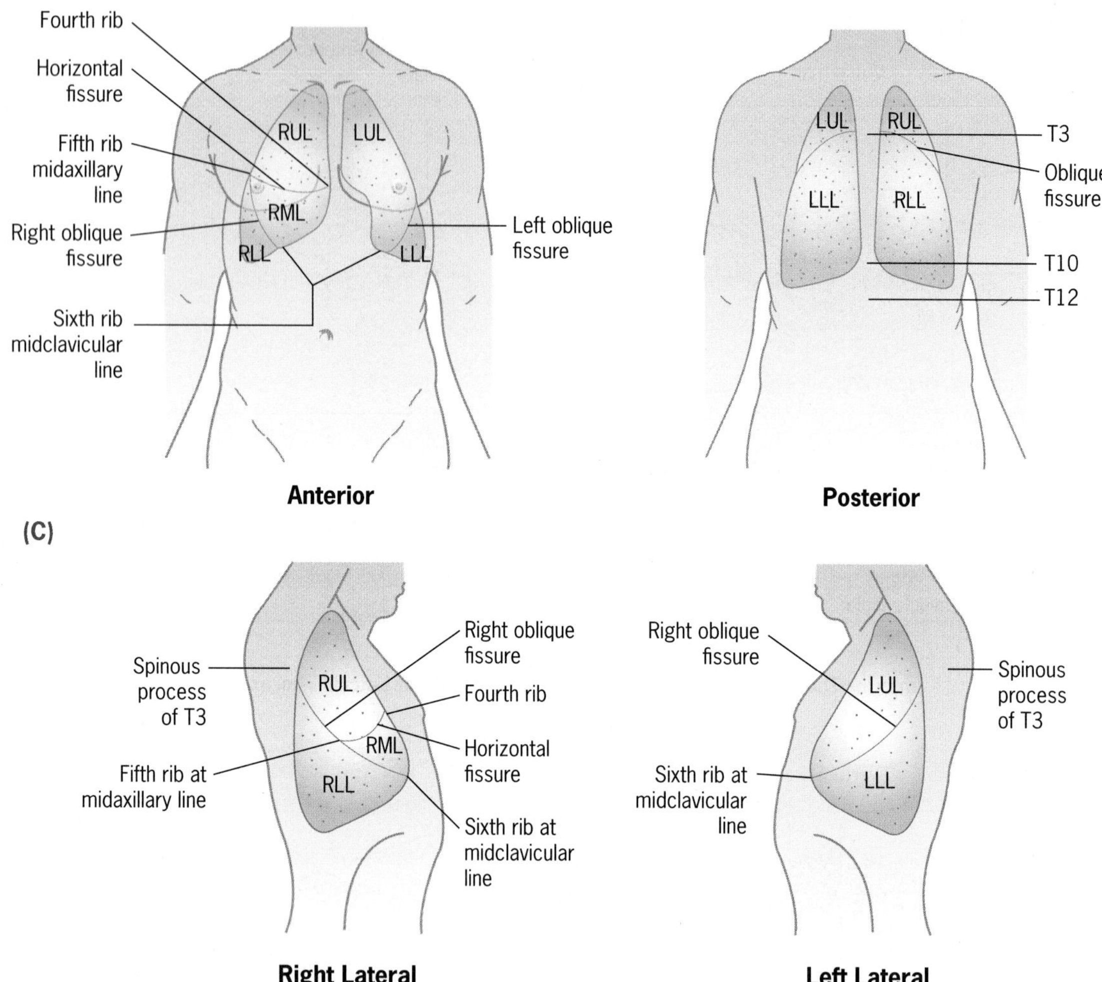

FIGURE 1–3 Continued. (**C**) Surface anatomy of the thorax.

Hyperpnea describes breathing that is rapid, deep, and labored. If it results in a lowered P_{CO_2}, **hyperventilation** is the term that applies. **Kussmaul respirations** describe hyperventilation as a compensatory mechanism for metabolic acidosis, most commonly diabetic ketoacidosis. Conversely, **bradypnea** is a rate slower than 12 breaths per minute. It may suggest neurologic impairment or acid–base disturbance but may be a normal finding in physically fit individuals.

Dyspnea is a term that simply means difficult or labored breathing, with the individual feeling short of breath. **Platypnea** refers to an individual's difficulty in breathing unless lying flat. **Orthopnea** indicates that an individual must sit or stand to breathe. Many individuals with chronic lung disease must assume an upright position to breathe well. Such individuals often find it more comfortable to sleep in a chair. **Paroxysmal nocturnal dyspnea** is characterized by sudden shortness of breath that occurs several hours after the individual lies down. It commonly suggests cardiac dysfunction in that the heart is unable to adequately pump a circulatory volume expanded by fluid reabsorbed from the legs, which became edematous during the day.

Cheyne-Stokes breathing is characterized by episodes of slow, shallow breaths, which rapidly increase in depth and rate. This crescendo-decrescendo pattern is followed by periods of apnea. Such breathing may be a normal variant in young children and the elderly. Otherwise, it occurs in individuals with cerebral disease and congestive heart failure.

Biot respirations are symptomatic of elevated intracranial pressure and meningitis. This breathing pattern is characterized by a short burst of uniform, deep respirations, followed by periods of apnea lasting 10 to 30 seconds.

RESPIRATORY RECAP

Patterns of Respiration

- » Tachypnea
- » Hyperpnea
- » Kussmaul respirations
- » Bradypnea
- » Dyspnea
- » Platypnea
- » Orthopnea
- » Paroxysmal nocturnal dyspnea
- » Cheyne-Stokes respirations
- » Biot respirations

Use of Accessory Muscles

Muscles of the back, neck, and abdomen are known as *accessory muscles* of respiration. Although they play a relatively minor role in normal respiration, their function becomes more prominent during exercise or respiratory distress. Use of accessory muscles implies an increased work of breathing or diaphragm weakness.

Retractions suggest a barrier to inspiration, occurring anywhere along the respiratory tract. To overcome this barrier, the respiratory muscles contract more vigorously, resulting in a more negative intrapleural pressure. Retractions resemble a "sucking in" of structures, such as the intercostal spaces, suprasternal space, and subclavian spaces. In such a situation, the examiner documents that the patient "has retractions," "is retracting," or "is using accessory muscles."

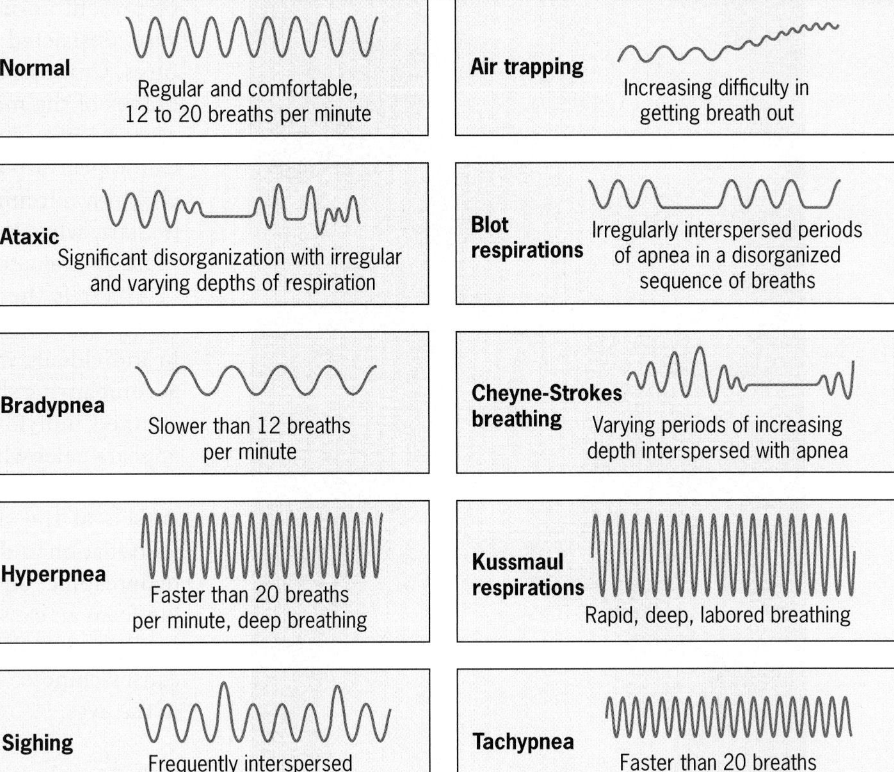

FIGURE 1–4 Patterns of respiration. This article was published in *Mosby's Guide to Physical Examination*. Seidel HM, Ball JW, Dains JE, et al. Copyright Elseiver (Mosby) 1999.

Nasal Flaring and Pursed-Lip Breathing

Individuals in respiratory distress commonly exhibit nasal flaring, presumably in an attempt to decrease the resistance to airflow through the nostrils. Those with emphysema commonly use pursed lips during the expiratory phase to maintain airway patency and better control expiratory flow.

Flail Chest and Paradoxical Respiration

Flail chest is a term describing the appearance of a thorax with multiple rib fractures, causing instability of the chest wall. In this situation the chest wall moves outward on expiration and inward on inspiration. This movement, which is contrary to normal chest movement, is known as **paradoxical respiration**. Flail chest with paradoxical respiration indicates a serious injury and will result in hypoxia if left untreated.

The chest and abdomen also should move in synchrony during the respiratory cycle. Paradoxical inward movement of the abdomen during the inspiratory phase indicates diaphragm weakness or paralysis. Paradoxical inward movement of the chest wall during inspiration indicates paralysis of the chest wall muscles, as may occur with high thoracic spine injury or low cervical spine injury.

Shape of the Chest

The examiner should observe the shape of the patient's chest. Abnormalities of the thorax can be significant factors in lung disease. Typically, a patient with emphysema has a **barrel chest** (**Figure 1–5**). The lateral diameter of the chest is normally twice the anteroposterior diameter. With a barrel-shaped chest configuration, the anteroposterior diameter is equal to the lateral diameter. Although obstructive lung disease causes this characteristic change in chest configuration, certain other abnormalities of thoracic shape result in restrictive lung disease. **Pectus excavatum**, or a funnel-shaped sternum, describes a sternum that is depressed and deviated somewhat like a funnel (**Figure 1–6**). Similarly, **pectus carinatum**, or a pigeon-breasted sternum, describes a chest that bows out at the sternum, similar to that of a pigeon. These abnormalities in thoracic configuration may result in lung disease as the patient ages. **Scoliosis**, for instance, causes lateral curvature of the spine, **kyphosis** causes forward curvature of the spine, and **lordosis** causes backward curvature of the spine (**Figure 1–7**).

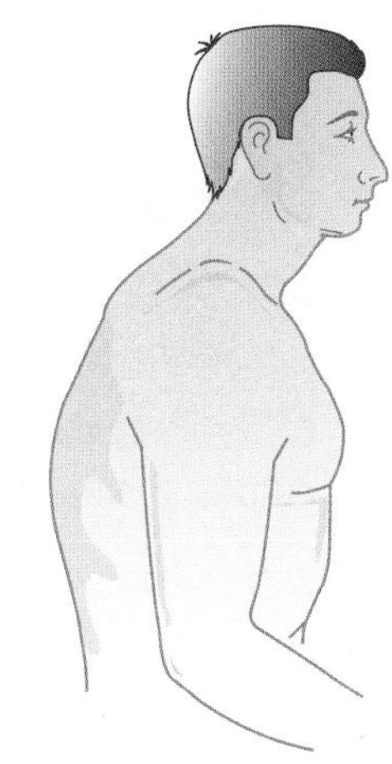

FIGURE 1–5 Barrel chest.

The examiner also should note whether the trachea is midline in the neck. A tension pneumothorax causes

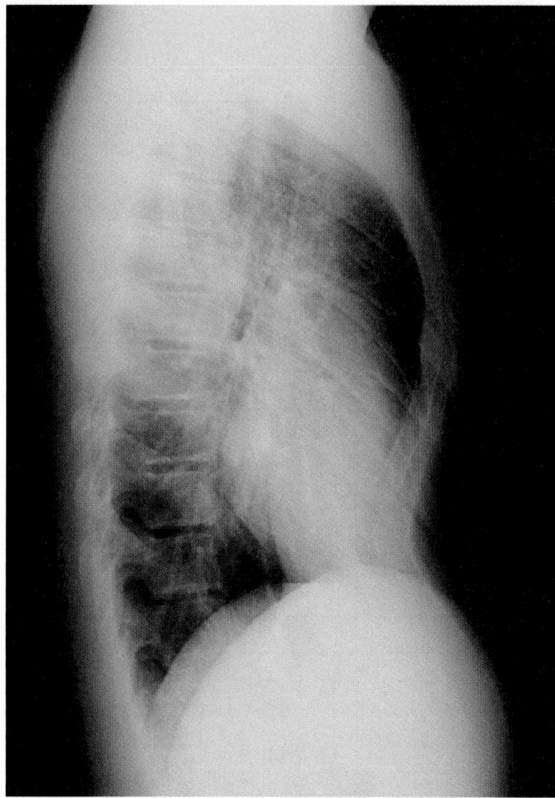

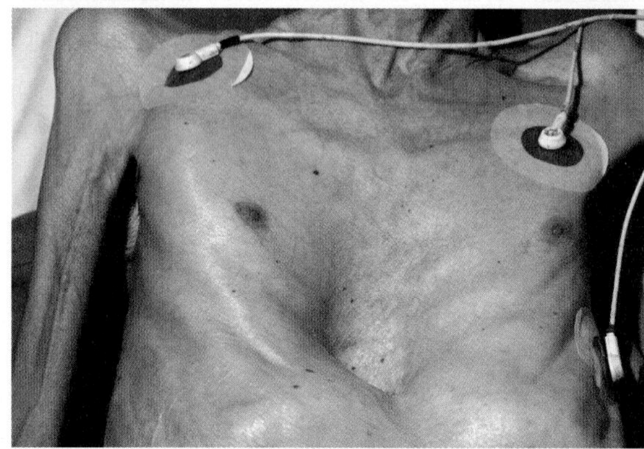

FIGURE 1–6 Pectus excavatum.

tracheal deviation away from the collapsed lung. Atelectasis or lung resection causes the trachea to be deviated toward the affected side.

Skin Color

The color of the patient's skin should be noted. Although several abnormalities in skin color exist, **cyanosis** is of prime significance to the respiratory therapist. When hemoglobin is poorly saturated with oxygen, the skin assumes a bluish hue, which is initially apparent in the nail beds. Cyanosis may be present normally in the nail beds of a person who is vasoconstricted as a result of exposure to cold temperatures. Cyanosis also may be noted in the mucous membranes of the mouth; this site is of particular use in the assessment of individuals with dark skin. Cyanosis also can appear around the mouth (circumoral). In healthy children, circumoral cyanosis is quite common, particularly when they are cold. The significance of cyanosis must be evaluated in light of other clinical findings.

RESPIRATORY RECAP

Skin Color
- » Cyanosis
- » Pallor
- » Plethora
- » Jaundice

Pallor is the term assigned to describe diminished skin color accompanying anemia. It also may be seen in individuals with severe peripheral vasoconstriction accompanying shock. Detecting pallor is easier in lighter-skinned individuals, but the color of darker skin also appears paler when the individual is severely anemic.

Plethora is a term describing the fullness of blood vessels at the skin surface. Plethora may occur with vasodilation and may be present in individuals who are hypercapnic. **Jaundice** is the yellowish skin color arising from an elevated serum bilirubin level. Any disorder resulting in bile being retained in the liver ultimately causes jaundice. Jaundice is first apparent in the sclera of the eyes.

Clubbing of Fingers

Clubbed fingers result from enlargement of the distal phalanges and develop as a compensatory mechanism when an individual has chronic hypoxia, such as with congenital heart defects or chronic lung disease. The appearance of **clubbing** is exactly as the term implies: the finger distal to the base of the nail looks like a small club (**Figure 1–8**). Affected fingertips appear full, fleshy, and vascular. Clubbing is associated with lung tumors, bronchiectasis, cystic fibrosis, congenital heart disease, and liver and gastrointestinal disease; it is hereditary in some cases. However, clubbing does *not* occur in conjunction with chronic obstructive pulmonary disease.

Palpation

Subcutaneous Emphysema

Subcutaneous emphysema is the presence of air in the subcutaneous tissues of the neck, chest, and face. The tissues may be painful and appear swollen. In addition, a crackling or popping sound may be auscultated when a stethoscope is placed over the tissue. An examiner also may detect subcutaneous emphysema by palpating bubbles as the finger pads are rolled over the affected areas.

Respiratory Expansion

The assessment of respiratory expansion is used primarily to determine whether the lungs are expanding symmetrically. Asymmetry of expansion may be present with a pneumothorax, atelectasis, lung resection, or main stem intubation. To perform this examination, the examiner places the thumbs along each costal margin at the back.

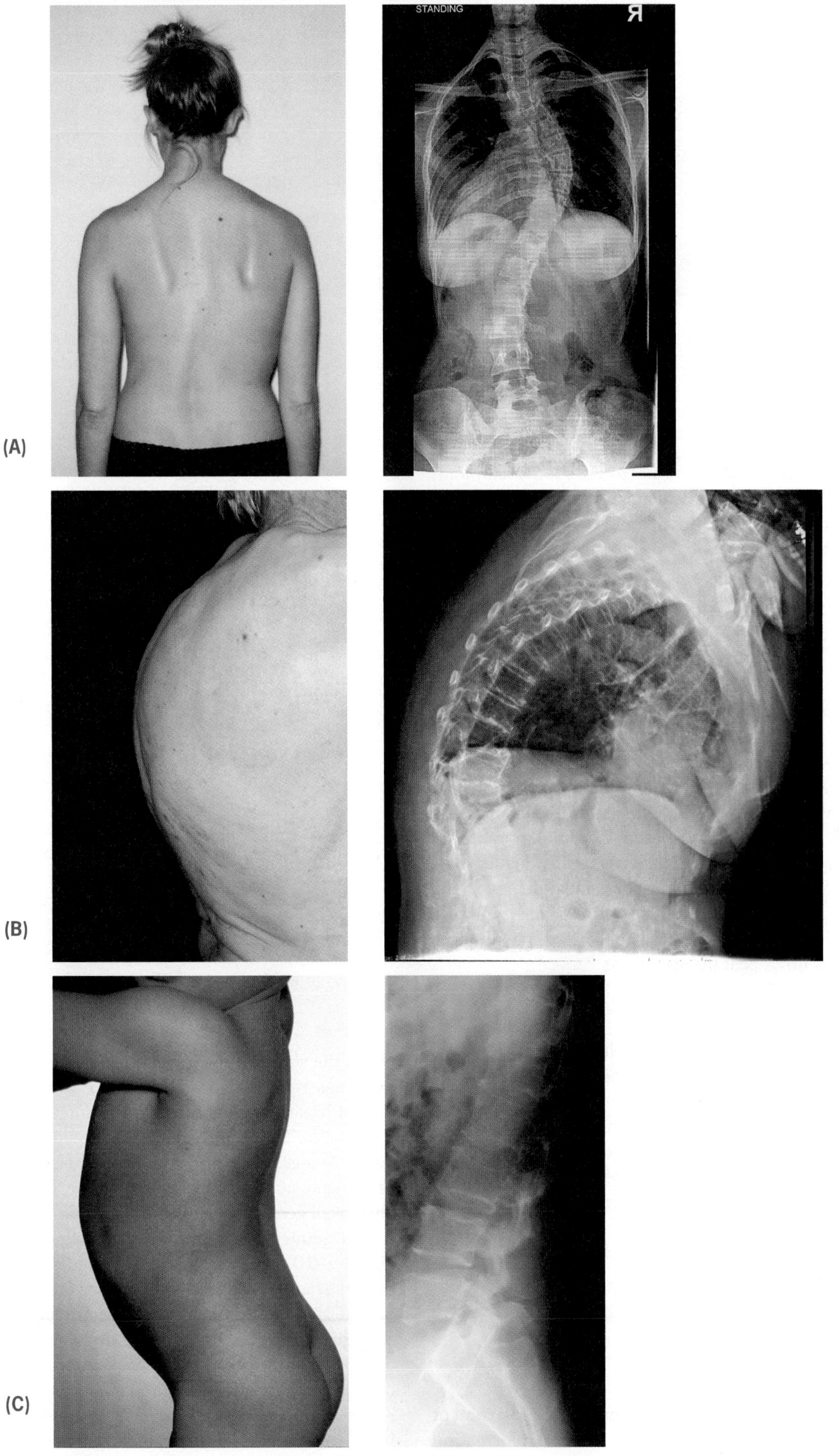

FIGURE 1–7 (**A**) Scoliosis. (**B**) Kyphosis. (**C**) Lordosis.

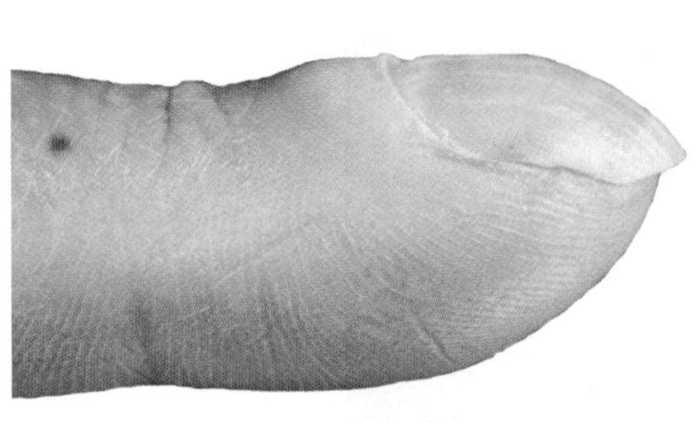

(A)

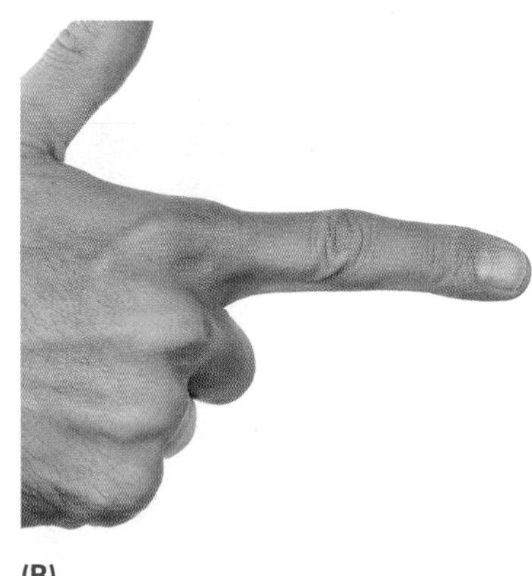

(B)

FIGURE 1–8 (**A**) Clubbing of the finger. (**B**) Normal digit.

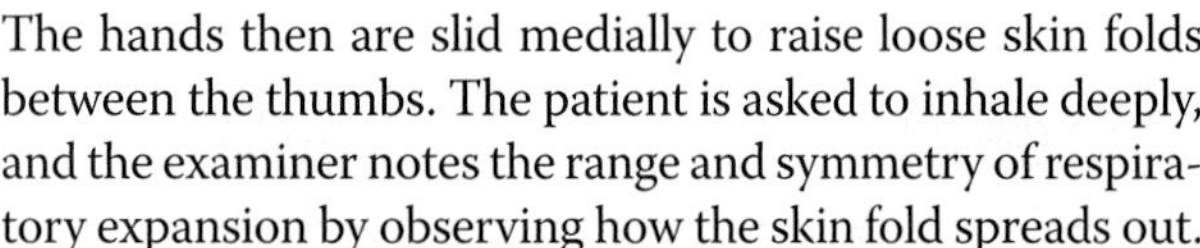

The hands then are slid medially to raise loose skin folds between the thumbs. The patient is asked to inhale deeply, and the examiner notes the range and symmetry of respiratory expansion by observing how the skin fold spreads out.

Tactile Fremitus

Tactile fremitus is defined as the palpation of vibrations of the chest wall as a patient speaks. To elicit these vibrations, the examiner presses the bony part of the palm of the hand against the patient's chest wall. For comparison between lungs, both sides are assessed concurrently. The patient is asked to repeat the words *ninety-nine* or *one-one-one.* When the lungs are healthy, vibrations are barely palpable. When the lung tissue is consolidated, however, vibrations are increased. Consolidation occurs when lung tissue that is normally aerated is "made solid" by filling with fluid, mucus, pus, or cellular debris. In the patient with large amounts of secretions in the airways, palpation of the fremitus that is produced may be possible as gas flows past the secretions.

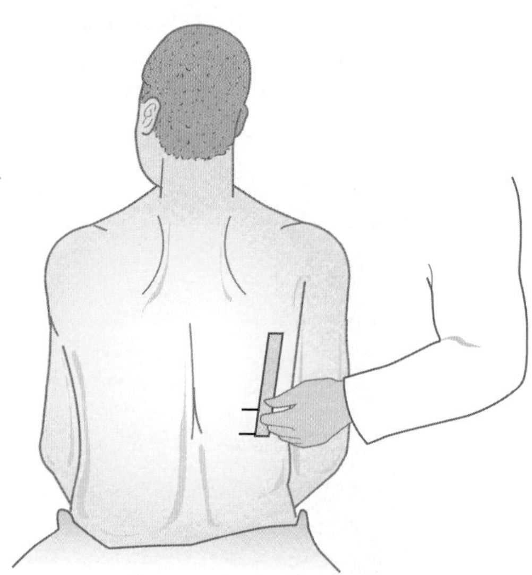

FIGURE 1–9 Measuring diaphragmatic excursion.

Percussion

Chest percussion can be used to elicit several abnormal findings. With a pneumothorax or emphysema, the affected hemithorax produces a hyperresonant or tympanic percussion note. With consolidation, pleural effusion, or atelectasis, the percussion note is dull or flat. A useful application of percussion is to determine diaphragmatic excursion. The difference in posterior, dependent resonance between maximum inhalation and maximum exhalation represents diaphragmatic excursion (**Figure 1–9**). Diaphragmatic excursion is affected by emphysema, pneumothorax, pleural effusion, atelectasis, consolidation, phrenic nerve injury, and diaphragmatic weakness.

Auscultation

The stethoscope is the most frequently used instrument in respiratory assessment and yields valuable information about the status of the lungs. Because the lower lobes of the lungs are posterior in the thorax, complete auscultation of breath sounds through the anterior chest wall is impossible. Therefore, examiners should avoid the temptation to auscultate only the anterior chest wall because of its easy accessibility. Auscultation of the posterior chest wall generally yields more useful information.

The sequence for lung field auscultation is shown in **Figure 1–10**. The examiner first should assess the apex of the lungs as they extend above the scapulae by listening on one side of the thorax and then moving to the corresponding area on the other side. Below the scapulae the examiner continues to move back and forth, listening to corresponding areas on both sides and comparing the sounds. Sounds generated by normal lungs differ according to location in the respiratory system (**Table 1–2**).

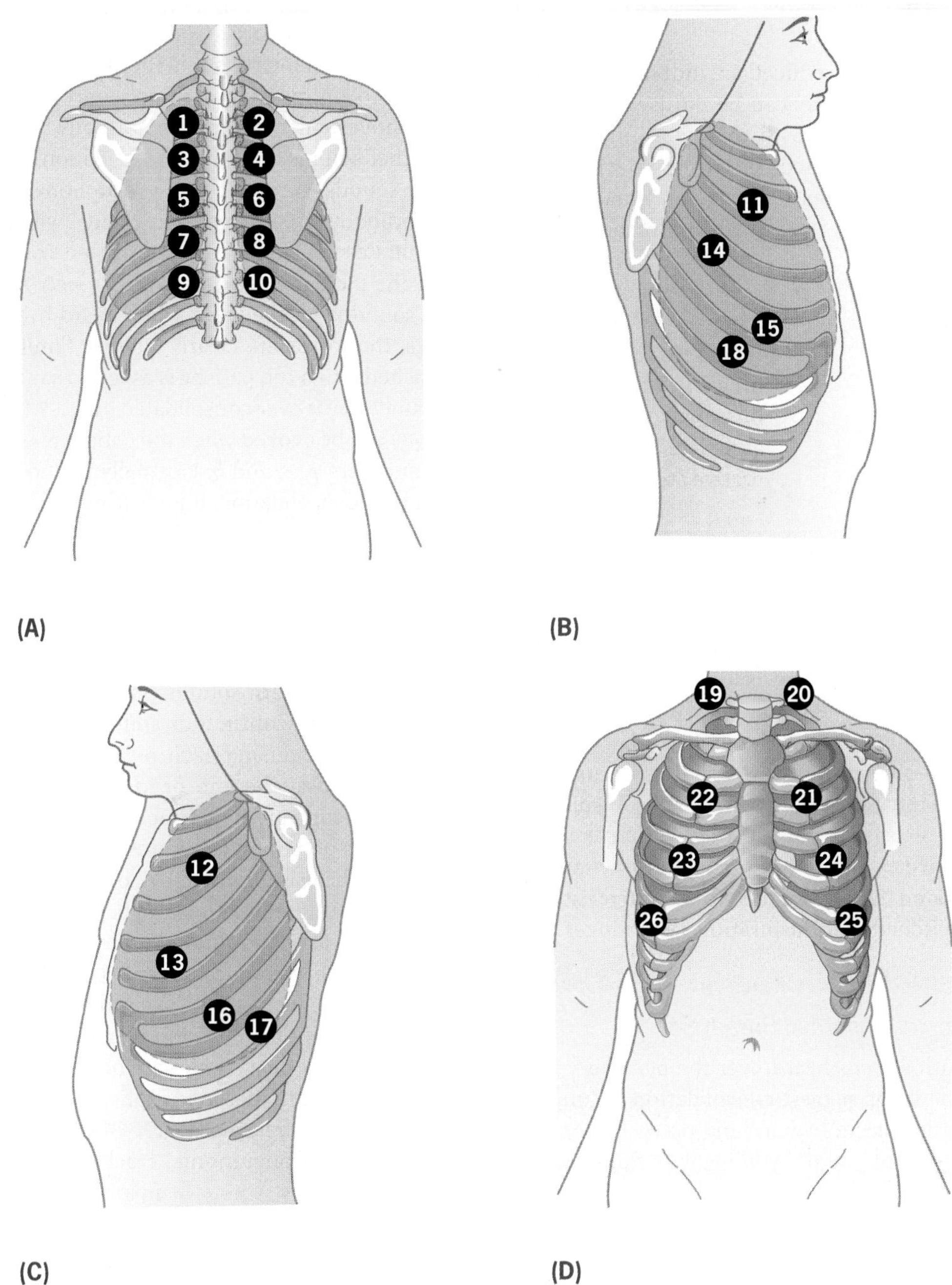

FIGURE 1–10 Suggested sequence for systematic percussion and ausculation of the thorax from the posterior (**A**), right lateral (**B**), left lateral (**C**), and anterior (**D**) views.

TABLE 1–2 Lung Sounds Assessed by Auscultation

Sound	Characteristics
Vesicular	Heard over most lung fields; low pitch; soft and short expirations; accentuated in thin person or child and diminished in overweight or very muscular individuals
Bronchovesicular	Heard over main bronchus area and upper right posterior lung field; medium pitch; expiration equaling inspiration
Bronchial/tracheal (tubular)	Heard only over trachea; high pitch; loud and long expirations, often somewhat longer than inspiration

Intensity of Breath Sounds

Breath sounds may be reduced in individuals with a number of conditions. They can be diffusely decreased with shallow breathing or with the hyperinflation and decreased airflow that occurs with hyperinflation (for example, emphysema or acute asthma). Localized diminished breath sounds occur with airway obstruction, atelectasis, and main stem intubation. Decreased breath sounds at the lung bases are commonly associated with postoperative atelectasis.

> **RESPIRATORY RECAP**
>
> **Auscultation**
>
> » Intensity of breath sounds
>
> » Presence of bronchial breath sounds
>
> » Presence of adventitious breath sounds: crackles, rhonchi, wheezes, stridor, pleural friction rubs

Characteristics of Normal Breath Sounds

Bronchial breath sounds are heard over the trachea, at the manubrium anteriorly, and between the scapulae posteriorly. These breath sounds are louder and higher in pitch. Expiratory sounds are as long as or slightly longer than the inspiratory component. Bronchovesicular breath sounds are heard over the junction between the bronchi and alveoli. Anteriorly, the sounds occur in the first and second interspaces between the ribs. Inspiratory and expiratory phases are equally long. **Vesicular breath sounds** are heard over the lung periphery, where the alveoli are located. These sounds are characteristically soft and low pitched, and inspiration lasts longer than expiration.

Characteristics of Abnormal Breath Sounds

Bronchial breath sounds heard over the periphery or in the bases of the lungs suggest consolidation of lung tissue. Consolidation occurs when lung tissue that is normally aerated is "made solid" by filling with fluid, mucus, pus, or cellular debris. Consequently, sounds generated by air movement through the bronchi resonate more clearly to pulmonary regions where only vesicular or bronchovesicular sounds are normally heard.

Other sounds typical of consolidation are the so-called voice sounds—bronchophony, egophony, and whispered pectoriloquy. **Bronchophony** is elicited when the examiner auscultates over an area of suspected consolidation and asks the patient to say the words *ninety-nine*. Normally, this sound is muffled, but when heard over consolidated lungs, the words are clearly audible. Similarly, **egophony** is elicited when the patient is asked to say the letter *e* and it sounds like *a* over consolidated lungs. **Whispered pectoriloquy** can be evoked when the patient is asked to whisper the numbers *1*, *2*, and *3*. Normally this sound is soft, but with lung consolidation, it is clearly audible.

Crackles

Crackles, or rales (pronounced *rawls*, although many clinicians say *rails*), are commonly heard adventitious, or abnormal, breath sounds (**Figure 1–11**). Crackles are classified as "discontinuous sounds," meaning that they wax and wane during each respiratory cycle. They are usually heard at the end of inspiration and are fine in quality and high pitched. Crackles result when the terminal airways pop open late in inspiration because fluid or secretions have accumulated. Consequently, crackles are heard most often over the lung bases.

Crackles are a common finding in individuals with congestive heart failure. In this condition, fluid accumulates in the interstitial spaces between the capillaries and alveoli. As the condition worsens, the fluid fills the alveoli. Initially the crackles are heard in the bases of the lungs. Crackles that ascend higher up the lung fields are related to an increasing degree of congestive heart failure. In cases of pneumonia, crackles are heard over the involved lobe. In some individuals who have remained supine for long periods, crackles may be auscultated in the dependent areas of the lung.

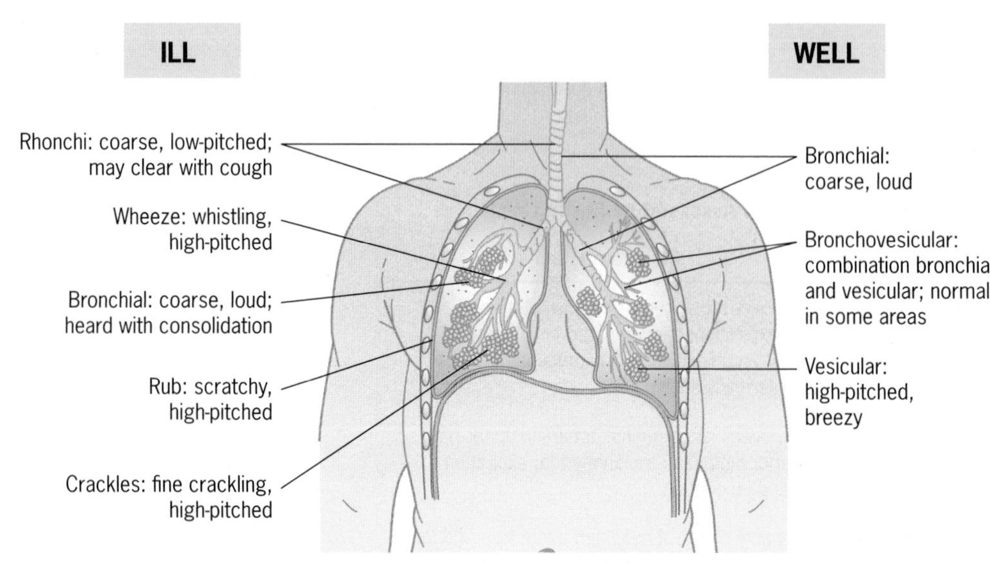

FIGURE 1–11 Breath sounds noted in the ill and well patient.

Rhonchi

The definition of a **rhonchus** (singular) or *rhonchi* (plural) is subject to some debate. To a certain degree the use of the term varies among clinical practice sites. However, the American Thoracic Society (ATS) has defined *rhonchi* as being deeper, rumbling sounds that are more pronounced on expiration. These sounds are likely to be continuous. Generally, they are caused by air passing through an airway partially obstructed by thick secretions, spasm of the airways, or presence of a tumor. Higher-pitched or sibilant rhonchi arise in the smaller bronchi, such as in the case of asthma. Lower-pitched, sonorous, or snoring rhonchi are more commonly heard in association with thick secretions in the larger airways. At times the rumbling may be palpable through the chest wall.

Wheezes

Wheezes may be either high or low in pitch. High-pitched wheezes are often called *sibilant* wheezes. They are musical or whistling in nature, caused by air passing through narrowed airways, such as in the bronchospasm of asthma (reactive airway disease). Most often, sibilant wheezes are heard on expiration, although they may be heard throughout the respiratory cycle. Although wheezes are most often associated with asthma, wheezes also can be present in individuals with other conditions, such as congestive heart failure and foreign body aspiration.

Stridor and Grunting

Stridor is a crowing sound commonly caused by inflammation and edema of the larynx and trachea. It may be heard after extubation, when tracheal damage has occurred with resultant edema. Stridor, however, is most commonly associated with croup in children and frequently is accompanied by a barking cough. Usually, stridor is a nocturnal assessment finding related to the possible development of edema in the upper airway while a child is in a dependent position during sleep. Mouth-breathing related to nasal congestion often causes a thickening of secretions that further compounds the stridor. The constellation of findings includes improvement of symptoms with air humidification. Taking the child outside into the cool night air may be an effective intervention. If the child does not improve, however, the stridor must be evaluated further because of the danger of airway obstruction. **Grunting** is a sound heard in newborns with respiratory distress. It occurs when the glottis is closed in an attempt to maintain lung volume.

> **AGE-SPECIFIC ANGLE**
>
> Stridor is associated with croup in children. Grunting is associated with respiratory distress in the newborn.

Pleural Friction Rubs

A **pleural friction rub** is a continuous grating sound such as is audible when two pieces of leather are rubbed together. Another analogy is that a friction rub sounds as though the palms of both hands are sliding against each other. This sound is produced when the visceral and parietal pleurae become inflamed and no longer glide silently against each other during the respiratory cycle. Consequently, the sound is localized and exists only over the area of pleural irritation. Pleural friction rubs may be intermittent.

Pleural friction rubs may accompany a pleural effusion—the accumulation of fluid in the usually empty pleural cavity. Causes of pleural effusion include malignant seeding of metastatic tumors onto the pleural linings. Pleural friction rubs also may be heard in individuals with infectious processes involving the pleural cavity. After thoracic surgery, residual blood in the pleural cavity eventually becomes sludge and may irritate the pleurae, resulting in a friction rub.

Signs of Respiratory Distress

Table 1–3 lists the common physical findings of respiratory diseases.

TABLE 1–3 Physical Findings of Respiratory Diseases

Condition	Percussion Note	Fremitus	Breath Sounds	Adventitious Sounds
Normal	Resonant	Normal	Vesicular	None
Left heart failure	Resonant	Normal	Vesicular	Crackles or occasionally wheezes
Pleural effusion	Dull or flat	Decreased	Decreased or absent	None or pleural rub
Consolidation	Dull	Increased	Bronchial	Crackles, rhonchi, or egophony
Bronchitis	Resonant	Normal or decreased	Prolonged exhalation	Wheezes, crackles, or rhonchi
Emphysema	Hyperresonant	Decreased	Decreased or absent	None
Pneumothorax	Hyperresonant	Decreased	Decreased or absent	None
Atelectasis	Dull	Decreased	Decreased or bronchial	None or crackles
Asthma	Resonant or hyperresonant	Normal or decreased	Vesicular	Wheezes
Pulmonary fibrosis	Resonant	Normal	Vesicular	Crackles

Assessment of Other Body Systems

The respiratory system interfaces with all other organ systems. Consequently, evaluation of the respiratory system does not occur in an assessment vacuum. The following discussion highlights assessment techniques used to monitor the heart, blood vessels, and brain.

The Heart and Blood Vessels

Location and Significance of Various Chest Landmarks

The chest wall overlying the heart is known as the **precordium**. Each heart valve is auscultated best by placement of the stethoscope in a specific location on the precordium. To do so, the cartilaginous structures, known as *interspaces*, lying between the ribs must be located, first by identification of the clavicle. Note that the space immediately under the clavicle does not count as an interspace. Next, the first rib should be identified. The cartilage under the first rib is the first interspace. Counting the ribs is done by movement of the fingers down from each rib to the corresponding interspace. The second interspace is important for assessment of the semilunar valves.

The accuracy of the counting process may be verified in the following way. Identify the ridge of bone that is the joint between the manubrium and sternum, known as the *sternal angle* or *angle of Louis*. The interspace to either side immediately below the sternal angle is the second interspace. On the posterior thorax the spinous processes of the vertebrae are useful landmarks. The spinous process of the seventh cervical vertebra (C7) is identified when the patient extends the head and neck forward and down. The most prominent spinous process is C7; directly below that is the first thoracic vertebra (T1).

A thorough cardiac auscultation involves systematic movement of the stethoscope over the precordium. First, the base of the heart should be auscultated, namely, the aortic and pulmonic valves. The aortic valve is assessed in the second interspace to the right of the sternal border, where it is heard best because the valve "points" in that direction (**Figure 1–12**). The stethoscope then is moved to the second interspace at the left sternal border, the best location for assessment of pulmonic valve function. All other assessments occur on the left side of the sternum. The tricuspid valve is heard at the fifth interspace at the left sternal border, and the mitral valve is assessed where the fifth interspace intersects the midclavicular line. The mitral valve, or apical area, is not only useful as a landmark for auscultation but also provides other useful information. This relatively small left ventricular apex is the area where the left ventricle protrudes from behind the right ventricle, known as the *point of maximal impulse (PMI)*. The left ventricle taps gently against an area of the thoracic wall no more than 2 cm in diameter (**Figure 1–13**). Left ventricular hypertrophy may be the cause of an enlarged PMI.

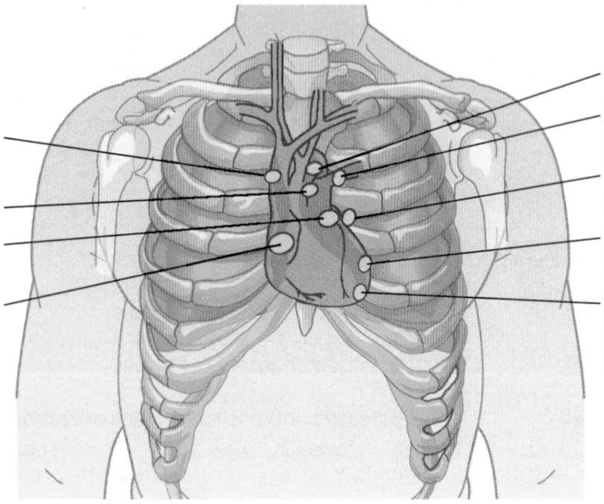

FIGURE 1–12 Areas for auscultation of the heart.

Cardiac Auscultation

Listening to heart sounds involves notations of rate and rhythm, extra heart sounds, and murmurs. Heart rate and rhythm should be observed first. A regular rhythm with a rate between 60 to 100 beats per minute is ideal; however, certain irregularities represent harmless variants. Conversely, other irregularities may herald serious consequences. Auscultation used to determine rate and rhythm is done with the stethoscope at the apex of the heart, a procedure commonly known as *taking an apical rate.*

S_1 and S_2

Normal heart sounds are classified as S_1 and S_2. (*S* originates simply from the word *sound.*) S_1 is the first heart sound and results from closure of the atrioventricular (mitral and tricuspid) valves. S_1 is also described as sounding like *lub*. As the ventricles eject most of their blood, ventricular pressure drops below aortic pressure, resulting in closure of the aortic and pulmonic valves, which in turn produces S_2, or the second heart sound, also known as *dub*.

A normal variant may be auscultated with the stethoscope at the second interspace along the left sternal border. In many individuals, a "split S_2" may be heard here during inspiration, a sound that occurs when pulmonic valve closure happens a few milliseconds after closure of the aortic valve. Typically, this action takes place during inspiration, as increasing intrathoracic pressure causes blood to strike the pulmonic valve with greater force.

S_3 and S_4

S_3 and S_4 are extra sounds generated by certain aberrant blood flow mechanisms. These sounds are best heard at the left fifth intercostal space at the midclavicular line, also known as the *mitral*, or *apical, area.* An S_4 immediately precedes the S_1, and the S_3

follows immediately after the S_2. These rhythms are commonly called *gallops* because of their resemblance to the sound of a horse galloping. To auscultate for either an S_3 or an S_4, the bell of a stethoscope is pressed lightly against the skin. Pressing too firmly obliterates the sounds. The S_3 and S_4 are heard best with the patient in a left side-lying position.

An S_3 results from rapid ventricular filling. When ventricular pump failure occurs, an increased amount of residual blood remains in the heart chambers after a contraction. Consequently, the ventricles fill faster during diastole. This pumping of blood into an already partially filled ventricle causes vibrations heard as an S_3. An S_3 occurs immediately after the S_2. It resembles a split S_2 but differs in location. A split S_2 is heard in the pulmonic area, whereas the S_3 is heard at the apex.

An S_4 is a sound caused most often by a stiff ventricle, such as may be the case in hypertension or after a myocardial infarction. For an S_4 to be present, an atrial contraction must occur. Consequently, this heart sound is often known as an *atrial gallop.* An S_4 cannot exist in the presence of atrial fibrillation, a condition in which the atria do not contract. The vibrations causing an S_4 are thought to be due to atrial contraction occurring in the presence of a stiffened or *noncompliant* ventricle. The S_4 precedes the S_1.

Murmurs

A simple description of a cardiac **murmur** is an extra sound heard in conjunction with S_1 and S_2. Several mechanisms describe the etiology of murmurs. Murmurs occur when blood regurgitates into the chamber from which it came. Sometimes valvular dysfunction develops as a sequela to rheumatic heart disease after infection with β-hemolytic streptococci. This syndrome results in valves that are distorted in shape and calcified.

Other murmurs arise when a large volume of blood flows through a valve, such as occurs during pregnancy, anemia, or hyperthyroidism. Murmurs also result from blood flowing through a narrowed or stenotic valve. A final category of murmurs arises from congenital defects resulting in blood flow through openings not normally present.

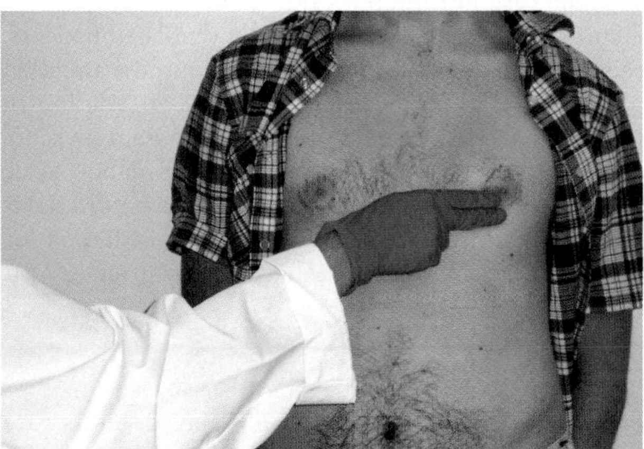

FIGURE 1–13 Palpation of the apical pulse.

Classification of Murmurs

Murmurs are classified as early, middle, or late systolic—that is, occurring between S_1 and S_2. Others are diastolic, coming between S_2 and the next S_1. The intensity of murmurs is graded from I to VI and is recorded in Roman numerals. A grade I murmur is very faint and may not be heard in all positions. Generally, a highly trained ear is required for detection of this sound. Murmurs that are grades II through IV increase progressively in intensity, with a grade V murmur being very loud. A grade VI murmur may be heard without the stethoscope in contact with the chest.

> **RESPIRATORY RECAP**
> **Cardiac Auscultation**
> » Heart rate and rhythm
> » Extra sounds
> » Murmurs

Murmurs differ in quality and are described as blowing, rasping, harsh, coarse, grating, whistling, or musical. In addition, they are classified according to the location at which the sound is loudest. This location corresponds to the area of the precordium where the valve in question is best auscultated, such as the fifth interspace midclavicular line or mitral area.

Murmurs and Infective Endocarditis

Many murmurs are classified as functional, innocent, or physiologic, meaning that they are clinically insignificant. Others are significant in that they suggest a progressive pathologic process that may eventually require surgical intervention. Some murmurs signify a defect that requires prophylaxis against *infective endocarditis.* Formerly known as *subacute bacterial endocarditis,* infective endocarditis develops when bacteria colonize on the heart valves. The immune response causes growth of fibrotic tissue, which consequently results in development of vegetation on valves. Clearly, this interferes with efficient hemodynamics, and a murmur ensues. Another danger exists if the vegetation breaks off and the resulting emboli lodge elsewhere in the body. The bacteria then reproduce in that location. *Prophylaxis against infective endocarditis* is the term given to antibiotic therapy administered before any invasive or surgical procedure, including dental work. Innocent or physiologic murmurs require no such prophylaxis; however, innocence can be determined only by echocardiogram. Diastolic murmurs—those occurring between S_1 and S_2—suggest the need for prophylaxis against infective endocarditis.

Jugular Venous Distention

The inspection component of a cardiac assessment primarily involves observation of the right internal jugular vein, the vessel that reflects pressure changes better than other superficial veins. Oscillations in this vein reflect changing pressures within the right atrium. Similarly, distention of this neck vein suggests a distended right

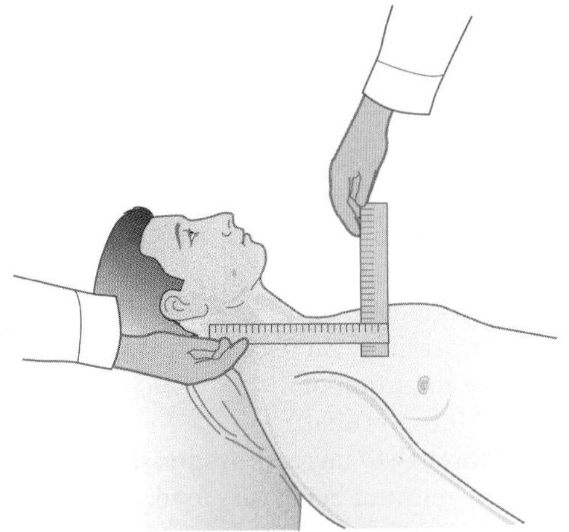

FIGURE 1–14 Technique used to measure jugular venous pressure.

ventricle, which often suggests right ventricular failure. Distended neck veins are normal in an individual in the supine position. Furthermore, neck veins fill temporarily with any activity that raises intrathoracic pressure, such as coughing, conversing, or bearing down (the Valsalva maneuver). To assess for pathologic processes, however, the following technique is used to determine the degree of jugular venous distention. The patient is placed in a supine position, with the head of the bed at a 45-degree angle (**Figure 1–14**). With a centimeter ruler, the vertical distance between the sternal angle and the highest level of jugular vein pulsation then is measured on both sides. Neck veins that fill to a level of 2 cm or less are considered normal. More than this level suggests increased right ventricular pressure and is associated with right-sided heart failure.

TABLE 1–4 Glasgow Coma Scale

Observation	Score
Eye Opening	
Spontaneous	4
In response to voice	3
In response to pain	2
None	1
Verbal Response	
Oriented response	5
Confused response	4
Inappropriate words	3
Incomprehensible words	2
None	1
Motor Response	
Obeys commands	6
Localizes	5
Withdraws	4
Flexes (decorticate)	3
Extends (decerebrate)	2
None	1

TABLE 1–5 Ramsay Sedation Scale

Level	Response
1	Anxious, agitated, restless
2	Cooperative, oriented, tranquil
3	Responding to commands only
4	Asleep, brisk response to stimulus
5	Asleep, sluggish response to stimulus
6	Unarousable

The Neurologic System

Because of the system's complexity, an assessment of the neurologic system can be daunting. This brief summary focuses on the most common neurologic abnormalities.

Level of Consciousness

When a patient experiences an alteration in the level of consciousness because of trauma or some other hypoxic or metabolic event, the Glasgow Coma Scale (**Table 1–4**) is commonly used. This scale uses a numeric scoring method to document eye-opening response, verbal response, and integrated motor response. Scores range from a low of 3 points, which suggests brain death, to a maximum of 15 points, which indicates full consciousness.

Other indications of neurologic integrity are normality and equality of strength in all extremities. Clearly, any less-than-normal finding suggests impairment and warrants full evaluation. Pupils may be evaluated for size, equality, reaction to light, and accommodation. Normal reactivity is documented as *PEARLA*, or *pupils equal and reacting to light and accommodation*. However, although pupillary assessment is commonly performed, abnormalities in size and reaction are a late finding and may indicate significant brain dysfunction.

A decreasing level of consciousness is the first finding to suggest neurologic impairment. However, because sleep is itself a decreased level of consciousness, it is important to distinguish between normal sleep or a state suggesting a serious pathologic condition, such as is the case in carbon dioxide narcosis or respiratory failure. In critically ill, mechanically ventilated patients, sedation and decreased level of consciousness are often pharmacologically induced. The level of sedation in these patients is often assessed with the Ramsay score (**Table 1–5**) or the Richmond Agitation Sedation Scale (**Table 1–6**). Delirium in the intensive care unit (ICU) is measured with the Confusion Assessment Method for Assessing Delirium in the Intensive Care Unit (CAM-ICU) (**Figure 1–15**).

Posturing

Patients with neurologic injury may demonstrate decerebrate or decorticate posturing (**Figure 1–16**). Decerebrate posturing may result from a painful stimulus of a comatose patient with a low-level brain stem

TABLE 1-6 Richmond Agitation Sedation Scale (RASS)

Score	Term	Description
+4	Combative	Overtly combative, violent, immediate danger to staff
+3	Very agitated	Pulls or removes tube(s) or catheter(s), aggressive
+2	Agitated	Frequent nonpurposeful movement, fights ventilator
+1	Restless	Anxious but movements not aggressive or vigorous
0	Alert and calm	
–1	Drowsy	Not fully alert, but has sustained awakening (eye opening/eye contact) to voice (≥10 seconds)
–2	Light sedation	Briefly awakens with eye contact to voice (<10 seconds)
–3	Moderate sedation	Movement or eye opening to voice (but no eye contact)
–4	Deep sedation	No response to voice, but movement or eye opening to physical stimulation
–5	Unarousable	No response to voice or physical stimulation

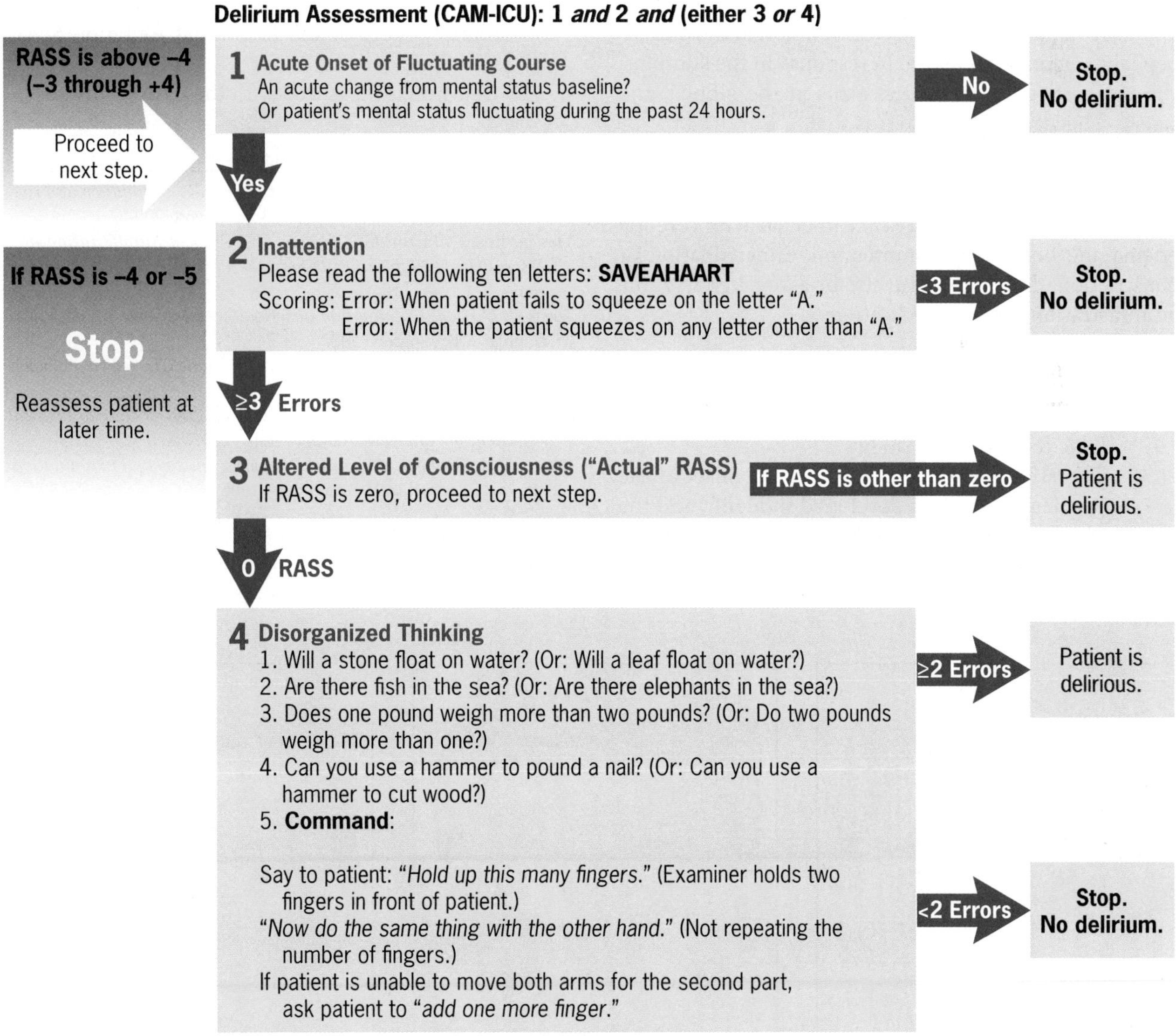

Delirium Assessment (CAM-ICU): 1 *and* 2 *and* (either 3 *or* 4)

RASS is above –4 (–3 through +4)

Proceed to next step.

If RASS is –4 or –5

Stop

Reassess patient at later time.

1 Acute Onset of Fluctuating Course
An acute change from mental status baseline?
Or patient's mental status fluctuating during the past 24 hours.

Stop. No delirium.

Yes

2 Inattention
Please read the following ten letters: **SAVEAHAART**
Scoring: Error: When patient fails to squeeze on the letter "A."
Error: When the patient squeezes on any letter other than "A."

Stop. No delirium.

3 Altered Level of Consciousness ("Actual" RASS)
If RASS is zero, proceed to next step.

If RASS is other than zero

Stop. Patient is delirious.

4 Disorganized Thinking

1. Will a stone float on water? (Or: Will a leaf float on water?)
2. Are there fish in the sea? (Or: Are there elephants in the sea?)
3. Does one pound weigh more than two pounds? (Or: Do two pounds weigh more than one?)
4. Can you use a hammer to pound a nail? (Or: Can you use a hammer to cut wood?)
5. **Command**:

Patient is delirious.

Say to patient: "*Hold up this many fingers.*" (Examiner holds two fingers in front of patient.)
"*Now do the same thing with the other hand.*" (Not repeating the number of fingers.)
If patient is unable to move both arms for the second part, ask patient to "*add one more finger.*"

<2 Errors

Stop. No delirium.

FIGURE 1–15 Confusion Assessment Method for Assessing Delirium in the Intensive Care Unit (CAM-ICU). Reprinted from Guenther U, Popp J, Koecher L, et al. Validity and reliability of the CAM-ICU flowsheet to diagnose delirium in surgical ICU patients. *Crit Care.* 2010; 25:144–156, Figure 1. Copyright 2010, with permission from Elseiver. Available at: http://www.sciencedirect.com/science/journal/08839441.

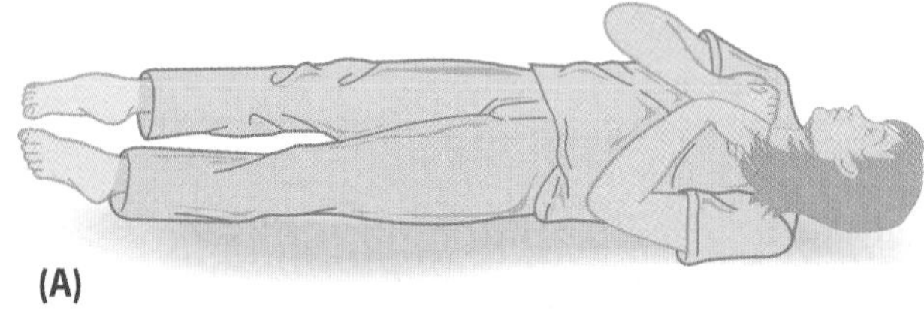

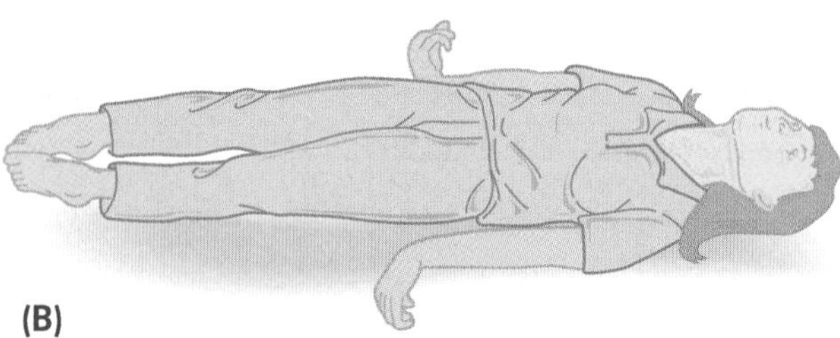

FIGURE 1–16 (**A**) Decorticate posturing. (**B**) Decerebrate posturing.

compression. The patient responds with extension and internal rotation of the arms and extends the legs. Decorticate posturing results when a painful stimulus is applied to a comatose patient with a lesion in the mesencephalic region of the brain. In response to the stimulus, the patient rigidly flexes the arms at the elbows and wrists. The legs may be flexed as well.

Pupillary Dilation

Pupillary dilation (**Figure 1–17**) can occur with cerebral edema and brain stem compression. Either dilation or constriction of the pupils can also be associated with the administration of some medications.

KEY POINTS

- The health history provides a detailed, chronologic record of the patient.
- The HPI offers a description of the onset of the problem, whether it developed suddenly, and the setting in which it developed.
- The four examination techniques commonly used are inspection, palpation, percussion, and auscultation.
- The use of accessory muscles implies an increased work of breathing.
- The assessment of respiratory expansion helps determine whether the lungs are expanding symmetrically.
- Auscultation of the chest allows assessment of diminished breath sounds, bronchial breath sounds, and adventitious breath sounds, such as crackles, rhonchi, wheezing, stridor, and pleural friction rubs.
- Listening to heart sounds involves notations of the rate and rhythm, extra heart sounds, and murmurs.
- The Glasgow Coma Scale is used to assess the level of consciousness.
- The level of sedation in critically ill, mechanically ventilated patients is often assessed with the Ramsay score or the Richmond Agitation Sedation Scale.
- Delirium is measured with the CAM score.

SUGGESTED READING

Bickley LS, Szilagyi PG. *Bates' Guide to Physical Examination and History Taking*. 9th ed. Philadelphia: JB Lippincott; 2007.

Des Jardins T, Burton GG, Phelps TH. *Clinical Manifestation and Assessment of Respiratory Disease*. 5th ed. Philadelphia: Elsevier; 2005.

Jarvis C. *Physical Examination and Health Assessment*. 5th ed. Philadelphia: WB Saunders; 2007.

Lehrer S. *Understanding Lung Sounds with Audio CD*. 3rd ed. Philadelphia: Elsevier; 2008.

Seidel HM, Ball JW, Benedict W, Dains JE. *Mosby's Guide to Physical Examination*. 6th ed. St. Louis: Mosby; 2007.

Swartz MH. *Textbook of Physical Diagnosis: History and Examination*. 5th ed. Philadelphia: WB Saunders; 2006.

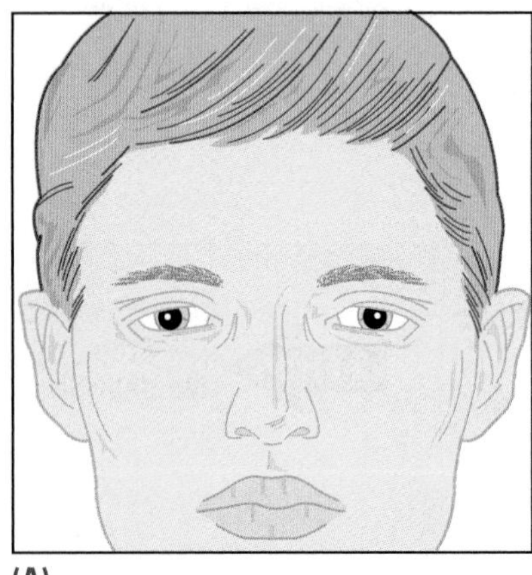

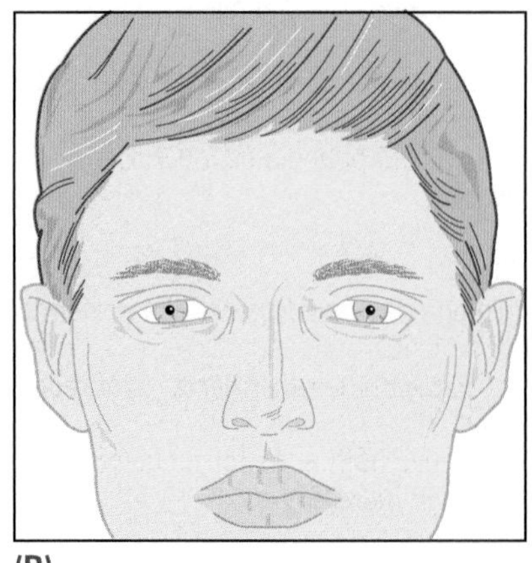

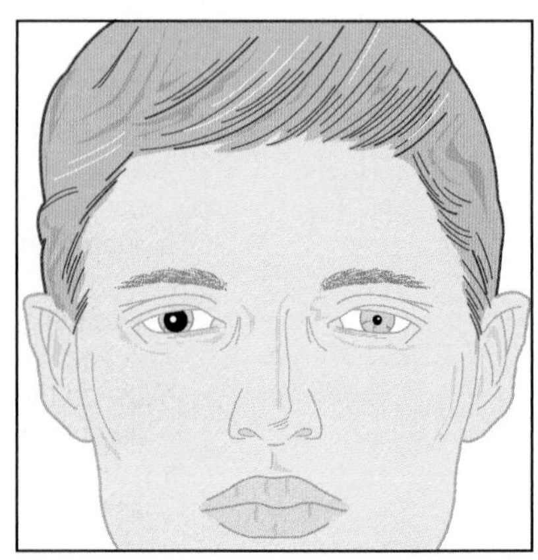

FIGURE 1–17 (**A**) Dilated pupils. (**B**) Constricted pupils. (**C**) Unequal pupils.

CHAPTER 2

Gas Exchange

Yuh-Chin T. Huang
Erika Lease
Will Beachey

OUTLINE

Physiology of Gas Exchange
Assessment of Gas Exchange
Physiologic Mechanisms of Hypercapnia

OBJECTIVES

1. Discuss the physiology of gas exchange.
2. Calculate alveolar Po_2.
3. Describe oxygen and carbon dioxide transport between the lungs and tissues.
4. Compare the oxyhemoglobin equilibrium curve and the carbon dioxide equilibration curve.
5. Distinguish between hypoxemia and hypoxia.
6. Describe the relationship between $Paco_2$, carbon dioxide production, and alveolar ventilation.
7. Calculate dead space fraction.
8. List causes of hypoxemia, hypoxia, and hypercapnia.

KEY TERMS

Bohr effect
fetal hemoglobin
Fick equation
Fick's law
Haldane effect
hemoglobin
hypercapnia
hypoxemia
hypoxia
methemoglobin
multiple inert gas elimination technique (MIGET)
oxygen consumption ($\dot{V}o_2$)
oxyhemoglobin equilibrium curve (OEC)
Pco_2
Po_2

INTRODUCTION

Understanding the physiology of gas exchange is crucial for clinicians as is identifying the methods that can be used to assess its effectiveness. This chapter focuses on the specifics of gas exchange and its assessment.

Physiology of Gas Exchange

Partial Pressure of Gas in the Lung

The gases in the lung are carbon dioxide (CO_2), oxygen (O_2), nitrogen (N_2), and water (H_2O). Each behaves in the alveolus as though it were independent of the others. According to Dalton's law, the partial pressures of all equal the atmospheric pressure (P_{atm}, which will be referred to throughout this chapter as PB, also known as *barometric pressure*) in the lungs, as follows:

$$P_B = P_{CO_2} + P_{O_2} + P_{N_2} + P_{H_2O}$$

where P_{CO_2}, P_{O_2}, P_{N_2}, and P_{H_2O} are partial pressures of CO_2, O_2, N_2, and H_2O, respectively.

The gases in the ambient air are CO_2, O_2, and N_2. The partial pressure of a gas in ambient air is also a function of its atmospheric concentration, and the sum of the partial pressures should equal PB:

$$P_B = P_{CO_2} + P_{O_2} + P_{N_2}$$

The partial pressure of a gas in ambient air is a function of its atmospheric concentration. In dry air the partial pressure of O_2 in the inspired gas (P_{IO_2}) is computed as follows:

$$P_{IO_2} = F_{IO_2} \times P_B$$

where PB is the atmospheric pressure and F_{IO_2} is the fractional concentration of O_2. At sea level, PB is 760 mm Hg and F_{IO_2} is 0.21. Therefore, the P_{IO_2} of dry air is 159.6 mm Hg at sea level. The P_{IO_2} is less in the bronchi, where inspired gas is fully saturated with water vapor at body temperature (i.e., where P_{H_2O} is 47 mm Hg at 37° C [98.6° F]); P_{IO_2} under these conditions is computed as follows:

$$P_{IO_2} = (P_B - P_{H_2O}) \times F_{IO_2} = (760 - 47) \times 0.21 \cong 150 \text{ mm Hg}$$

Alveolar P_{O_2} (P_{AO_2}) is even less than the inspired bronchial P_{O_2} because alveoli contain CO_2 in addition to water vapor. Normal ventilation maintains a relatively constant alveolar P_{CO_2} of about 40 mm Hg. Therefore, since the sum of all alveolar gas pressures must be equal to atmospheric pressure, inspired gas P_{O_2} falls by about 40 mm Hg when it enters the alveoli. If the amount of O_2 diffusing out of the alveoli into the capillary blood were exactly equal to the amount of CO_2 diffusing from the capillary blood into the alveoli, P_{AO_2} would be calculated by simply subtracting P_{ACO_2} from the P_{IO_2} equation above. However, O_2 diffuses out of the alveoli at a greater rate than CO_2 diffuses into the alveoli. At rest, capillary blood removes about 250 mL/min of O_2 from the alveoli, replacing it with only about 200 mL/min of CO_2. The ratio of alveolar CO_2 excretion to blood O_2 uptake is called the *respiratory exchange ratio* (R) and has a resting value of about 0.8 (i.e., R = 200 mL/min ÷ 250 mL/min = 0.8). This uneven exchange has the ultimate effect of amplifying the effect of P_{aCO_2} on P_{AO_2}.

TABLE 2-1 Barometric Pressure, Ambient P_{O_2}, and Alveolar P_{O_2} at Different Altitudes

Altitude (Feet)	PB (mm Hg)	Ambient P_{O_2} (mm Hg)	Alveolar P_{O_2} (mm Hg)
0	760	159	109
3000	682	143	103
5000	630	132	92
8000	564	118	78
10,000	523	110	70
12,000	483	101	61
15,000	412	90	50
18,000	379	80	40
20,000	349	73	33
30,000	226	47	7

The P_{AO_2} is calculated using the alveolar gas equation:

$$P_{AO_2} = (F_{IO_2}) \times (P_B - P_{H_2O}) - \{P_{aCO_2} \times [F_{IO_2} + (1 - F_{IO_2})/R]\}$$

The simplified alveolar gas equation for computing P_{AO_2} when the F_{IO_2} is ≤ 0.6 is as follows:

$$P_{AO_2} = F_{IO_2}\,(P_B - 47) - P_{ACO_2}/R$$

Thus, P_{AO_2} on room air is about 100 mm Hg, computed as follows:

$$P_{AO_2} = 0.21(760 - 47) - 40/0.8 \approx 100 \text{ mm Hg}$$

At high altitudes, where PB is less than 760 mm Hg, P_{IO_2} decreases, although the fractional concentration of O_2 in the air remains at 0.21 (**Table 2-1**). Alveolar P_{O_2} decreases more than the atmospheric P_{O_2} because of excreted CO_2 and the pressure of water vapor. At a temperature of 37° C (98.6° F), the saturated water vapor pressure is 47 mm Hg, regardless of barometric pressure.

Blood Gas Transport

In humans the metabolic processes of the body (e.g., O_2 consumption and CO_2 production) occur through the integrated functions of the heart, lungs, and blood. Atmospheric O_2 brought into the alveoli of the lungs through ventilation diffuses across the alveolocapillary membrane into the blood, and ultimately into the erythrocytes, where it binds reversibly to the hemoglobin molecule. The heart produces blood flow, causing the erythrocytes to travel to the tissue capillaries, where O_2 dissociates from hemoglobin and diffuses down its concentration gradient into the tissue cells to be consumed in the mitochondria. This whole process is frequently referred to as the *oxygen pathway*.

At the same time, CO_2 produced as a by-product of metabolism diffuses down its concentration gradient from the tissues into the blood and flows to the alveolar

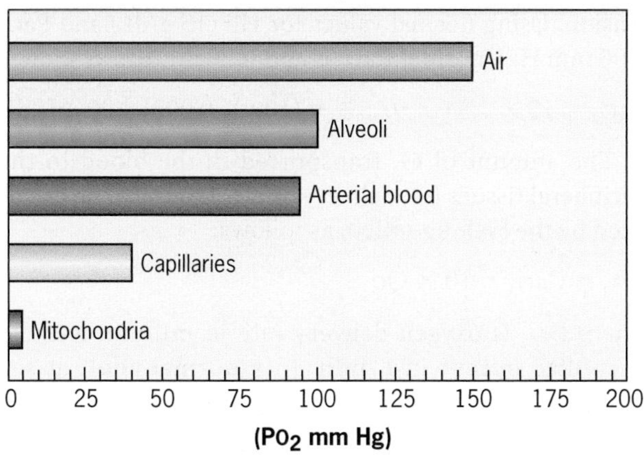

FIGURE 2–1 The oxygen gradient from the alveolar space to the mitochondria. Note the stepwise decrement in PO_2 from 100 mm Hg in the alveolar space to values of a few mm Hg at the mitochondria, where most of the oxygen is consumed. Adapted from Baum GL, et al. *Textbook of Pulmonary Diseases*. 6th ed. Lippincott Williams & Wilkins; 1998.

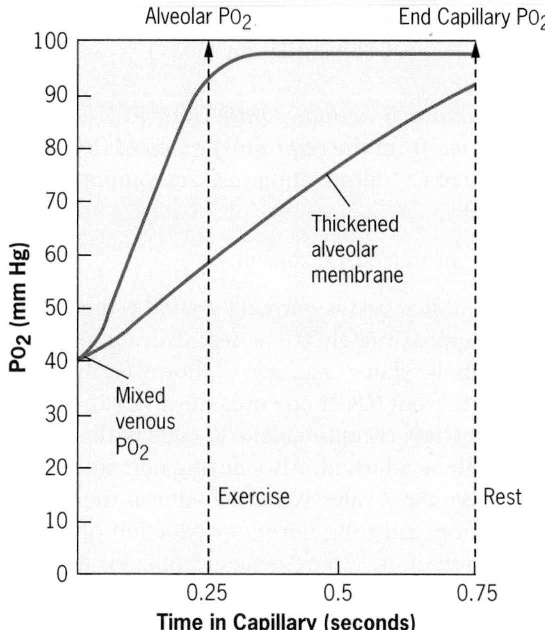

FIGURE 2–2 Typical time courses for the change in PO_2 in the pulmonary capillary. Note that it takes an average of 0.75 second for each erythrocyte to traverse the pulmonary microcirculation. In healthy lungs the hemoglobin becomes virtually completely oxygenated within 0.25 second. In abnormal lungs with significant $\dot{V}A/\dot{Q}$ mismatch and thickened alveolocapillary membrane, the hemoglobin at end-capillary may not be fully saturated. This effect is further accentuated by exercise, which shortens the capillary transit time. Modified from Baum GL, et al. *Textbook of Pulmonary Diseases*. 6th ed. Lippincott Williams & Wilkins; 1998.

capillaries, where it again diffuses down its concentration gradient into the alveoli and is eliminated by ventilation in exhaled gas. These gas-transport mechanisms use the physical processes of diffusion (between lungs and blood and between tissues and blood), chemical reactions (between O_2 or CO_2 and hemoglobin), and bulk gas and blood movement (ventilation and blood flow).

Oxygen Pathway

The O_2 pathway begins in the atmosphere, where PO_2 is about 160 mm Hg at sea level, and ends at the mitochondria, where PO_2 is only a few millimeters of mercury (**Figure 2–1**). The lungs' only blood–air interface is the alveolocapillary membrane; thus, O_2 and CO_2 exchange occurs only in the alveoli. Alveolar ventilation is the only portion of the total minute ventilation that affects arterial blood gases.

Pulmonary capillary blood leaving the alveoli contains the same PO_2 as alveolar gas. However, the PO_2 in *arterial* blood is slightly lower than alveolar PO_2 because local matching of ventilation and perfusion in normal lungs is imperfect; in addition, a small amount of unoxygenated blood is added to pulmonary capillary blood through anatomic shunts connecting the venous bronchial circulation to the pulmonary venous blood. The arterial blood is then pumped to the systemic capillaries, where O_2 diffuses into the tissue cells to support aerobic metabolism. The bulk of molecular O_2 (about 90%) is consumed in the cellular mitochondria.

Oxygen Uptake

O_2 is taken up by the approximately 300 million alveoli, each of which is about 300 μm in diameter. The huge alveolar surface area (approximately 75 m^2) and the thin alveolocapillary membrane (less than 0.5 μm thick) provide an extremely efficient mechanism for O_2 uptake. With each tidal inspiration, approximately 500 mL of air enters the lungs. If anatomic dead space (conducting airway volume) is 150 mL and the respiratory rate is 12 breaths/min, alveolar ventilation is 4.2 L/min [(500 mL – 150 mL) × 12/min].

When alveolar O_2 diffuses into the pulmonary capillaries, it binds with hemoglobin in the erythrocytes. Each erythrocyte traverses the pulmonary capillary in about 0.75 second (pulmonary capillary transit time) (**Figure 2–2**). Within the first third of this brief transit time (0.25 second), the alveolar and capillary PO_2 equilibrate, and hemoglobin is almost oxygenated to capacity. At the same time, CO_2 diffuses into the alveoli and is removed by ventilation. The efficiency of O_2 and CO_2 exchange is determined primarily by the match between ventilation and perfusion, that is, the $\dot{V}A/\dot{Q}$ relationship of the alveoli. Low-$\dot{V}A/\dot{Q}$ units imply poor ($\dot{V}A/\dot{Q} < 0.8$) or absent ($\dot{V}A/\dot{Q} = 0$) ventilation with respect to blood flow, impairing O_2 uptake. High-$\dot{V}A/\dot{Q}$ units imply poor ($\dot{V}A/\dot{Q} > 0.8$) or absent ($\dot{V}A/\dot{Q} = \infty$) blood flow with respect to ventilation, resulting in inefficient elimination of CO_2 from the pulmonary arterial blood. Complete loss of ventilation with respect to blood flow ($\dot{V}A/\dot{Q} = 0$) is called *shunt*, whereas complete loss of pulmonary blood flow with respect to ventilation ($\dot{V}A/\dot{Q} = \infty$) is called *dead space*.

The *respiratory exchange ratio* (R or RER) should be differentiated from the *respiratory quotient* (RQ), which is the ratio of CO_2 production to O_2 consumption at the tissue level:

$$RQ = CO_2 \text{ produced}/O_2 \text{ consumed}$$

The value of R at rest is normally a good estimate of the RQ. It is approximately 0.8 at rest. During exercise or high metabolic states (e.g., sepsis), however, the R value may deviate from 0.8. If one uses the alveolar gas equation under these conditions, the R value in the equation will need to be adjusted. Also, during non-steady-state-like exercise, the R value is not the same as the RQ value due to factors affecting normal production of CO_2 and consumption of O_2. An extreme example for discrepant R and RQ values is seen in a 100-meter dash. A trained athlete often holds his or her breath for prolonged periods during the run. During these periods, R is essentially zero, but tissue gas exchange continues with an RQ greatly exceeding 0.8.

Oxygen Transport

Once O_2 diffuses into the pulmonary capillaries, it binds rapidly to hemoglobin. Oxygen does not *oxidize* hemoglobin; rather, it *oxygenates* hemoglobin, a reversible process. Combined with oxygen, hemoglobin is called *oxyhemoglobin* (HbO_2), whereas unoxygenated hemoglobin is called *deoxyhemoglobin* (Hb). The hemoglobin molecule takes up and releases O_2 molecules in a process known as *cooperative binding*; as O_2 molecules successively bind with hemoglobin, the hemoglobin molecule physically changes its shape, which increases its affinity for the next O_2 molecule. Similarly, the release of the first O_2 molecule facilitates the release of each remaining molecule. The cooperative binding phenomenon is responsible for the sigmoid shape of the **oxyhemoglobin equilibrium curve (OEC)** (**Figure 2–3**), which also is commonly called the oxygen dissociation curve.

Oxygen is carried in the blood in two forms: (1) dissolved O_2 in the plasma and (2) combined with Hb. Each gram of Hb can combine with a maximum of 1.34 mL O_2, whereas 0.003 mL O_2 dissolves in 100 dL plasma for 1 mm Hg plasma PO_2. By convention, arterial blood O_2 content (CaO_2) is expressed in terms of mL O_2 per 100 mL blood, or mL/dL. Similarly, Hb concentration is expressed in g/dL. Thus, the blood's CaO_2 (in mL/dL) is computed as follows:

$$CaO_2 = ([Hb] \times 1.34 \times SaO_2) + (PaO_2 \times 0.003)$$

where CaO_2 is the arterial oxygen content, SaO_2 is the hemoglobin O_2 saturation, and PaO_2 is the arterial oxygen tension. Using normal values for Hb (15 g/dL) and PaO_2 (100 mm Hg), normal CaO_2 is about 20 mL/dL, as shown:

$$CaO_2 = 15 \times 1.34 \times 97.5\% + (100 \times 0.003) \approx 20 \text{ mL/dL}$$

The amount of O_2 transported in the blood to the peripheral tissues (O_2 delivery or DO_2) thus can be calculated by the **Fick equation**, as follows:

$$DO_2 = CaO_2 \times 10 \times \dot{Q}c$$

where DO_2 is oxygen delivery rate in mL/min and $\dot{Q}c$ is cardiac output in L/min. In a normal adult at sea level and at rest, DO_2 is approximately 1000 mL/min (assuming hemoglobin concentration of 15 g/100 mL, 97.5% HbO_2 saturation, and a $\dot{Q}c$ of 5 L/min). Without hemoglobin (i.e., only dissolved O_2 in plasma), one would need a cardiac output of at least 80 L/min to support the normal resting O_2 consumption of about 250 mL/min in adult humans.

Increases in delivery of O_2 to the peripheral tissues are more efficiently accomplished through increases in hemoglobin concentration and cardiac output than by an increased SaO_2 (**Figure 2–4**). When the arterial PO_2 is 60 mm Hg, corresponding with a hemoglobin O_2 saturation of about 90%, the SaO_2 can only rise by an additional 10%, no matter how high the PaO_2 is raised. Once the hemoglobin is 100% saturated, further increases in PaO_2 merely increase the amount of O_2 dissolved in the plasma, which is only a 0.3 mL/dL increase for each 100 mm Hg rise in PO_2.

Oxygen Consumption

The body's **oxygen consumption ($\dot{V}O_2$)** can be described by the Fick principle, as follows:

$$\dot{V}O_2 = \dot{Q}c \times (CaO_2 - C\bar{v}O_2) \times 10$$

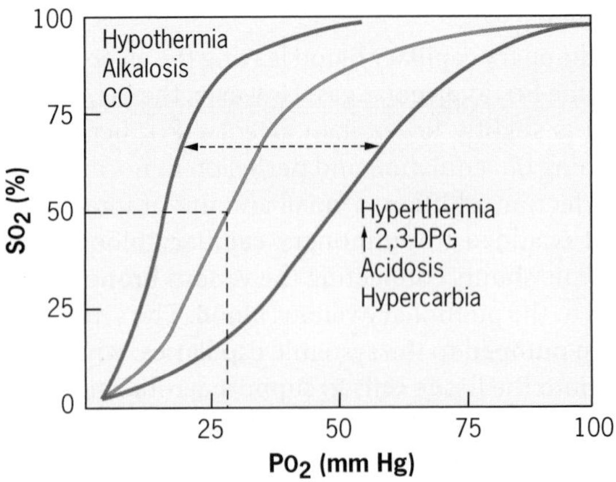

FIGURE 2–3 Oxyhemoglobin equilibrium (or dissociation) curve of hemoglobin. The normal P_{50} value is indicated by the dashed lines. The changes in position of the curve associated with various conditions are indicated by the dashed arrows. Modified from Baum GL, et al. *Textbook of Pulmonary Diseases*. 6th ed. Lippincott Williams & Wilkins; 1998.

where $\dot{Q}c$ is cardiac output, Cao_2 is arterial O_2 content (1.34 × Hb × Sao_2), and $C\bar{v}o_2$ is venous O_2 content (1.34 × Hb × $S\bar{v}o_2$). In a normal adult at rest, Cao_2 is almost 20 mL/dl (see above) and $C\bar{v}o_2$ is about 15 mL/dL (1.34 × 15 × 75%). Thus, the arterial-venous O_2 content difference, or $C(a\text{-}\bar{v})o_2$, is about 5 mL/dL, or 50 mL/L; this means the body tissues extract about 50 mL of O_2 from each liter of blood perfusing them. If the cardiac output is 5 L/min, then $\dot{V}o_2$ is 250 mL/min. Thus, under normal resting conditions, the tissues extract about 25% of O_2 delivered to them. The O_2 extraction fraction can increase under conditions such as exercise (increased tissue O_2 demand), congestive heart failure (decreased cardiac output and O_2 delivery), and severe anemia (reduced Cao_2), leading to a lower $C\bar{v}o_2$. Conversely, the O_2 extraction fraction decreases in disease states that greatly increase cardiac output (e.g., sepsis), leading to a higher $C\bar{v}o_2$. **Table 2–2** shows the resting blood and O_2 supply of various organs. Brain tissue and cardiac muscle extract a much higher percentage of the O_2 delivered to them than do other organs. For this reason, the brain and heart are highly susceptible to O_2 deprivation caused by lack of blood flow (ischemia) and low Cao_2 (hypoxemia).

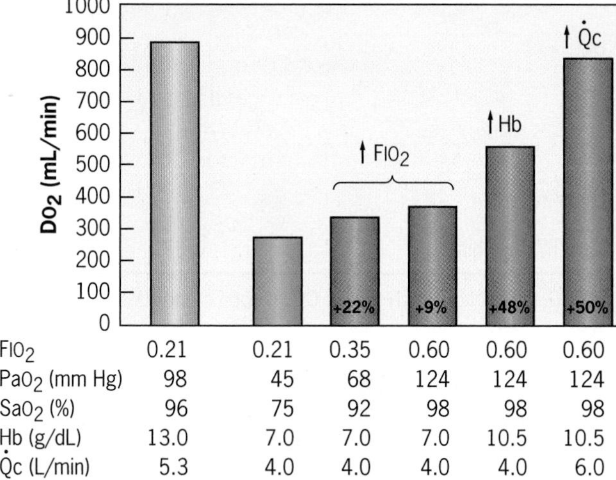

FIGURE 2–4 Relative effects of changes in Pao_2, hemoglobin, and $\dot{Q}c$ on oxygen delivery (Do_2) in a critically ill patient. Do_2 in a normal 75-kg subject at rest is shown in the green bar, and Do_2 in a patient with hypoxemia, anemia, and reduced $\dot{Q}c$ is shown in the blue bar. The red bars show the effect of sequential interventions on Do_2. The numbers in each bar represent the calculated increase in Do_2 compared with the preceding value. Reproduced from Huang Y-C. Monitoring oxygen delivery in the critically ill. *Chest.* 2005;125:554–560.

The majority of O_2 (90%) used by the cell is consumed by the mitochondria. The remainder is used by other subcellular organelles. In mitochondria, molecular O_2 is reduced to water by cytochrome *c* oxidase after accepting electrons from the respiratory chain. High-energy phosphate compounds (such as adenosine triphosphate [ATP]) are generated by the process of oxidative phosphorylation. ATP provides most of the energy required for the biologic function of cells.

Hemoglobin

Hemoglobin is the major protein of erythrocytes, which allows humans to transport molecular O_2 from the lungs to the tissues and CO_2 from the tissues to the lungs. Because hemoglobin exists inside the red blood cell, high concentrations can be carried without affecting the blood's oncotic pressure. *Heme* is an iron-containing pigment, and *globin* is a protein consisting of amino acid or polypeptide chains. Human hemoglobin is a tetramer (four polypeptides) consisting of two α-polypeptides and two β-polypeptides, each containing a heme moiety. The

TABLE 2–2 Oxygen Supply and Consumption of Various Organs

Organ	Blood Flow (mL/min) (% Cardiac Output)	Blood Flow (mL/100 g)	Arterial-Venous O_2 Difference (Volume %)	O_2 Consumption (mL/min)
Heart	210 (4)	70.0	11.4	23.9
Brain	760 (15)	50.0	6.3	47.9
Kidney	1220 (24)	400.0	1.3	15.9
Liver	510 (10)	29.0	4.1	20.9
Gastrointestinal tract	715 (14)	35.0	4.1	29.3
Skeletal muscle	760 (15)	2.5	6.4	60.8
Skin	215 (4)	9.5	1.0	2.15
Other organs (fat, etc.)	715 (14)	—	—	—
Total cardiac output	5100			200.9

Modified from Jain KK, Fischer B. *Oxygen in Physiology and Medicine.* Springfield, IL: Thomas; 1989. Courtesy of Charles C. Thomas Publishers, Ltd.

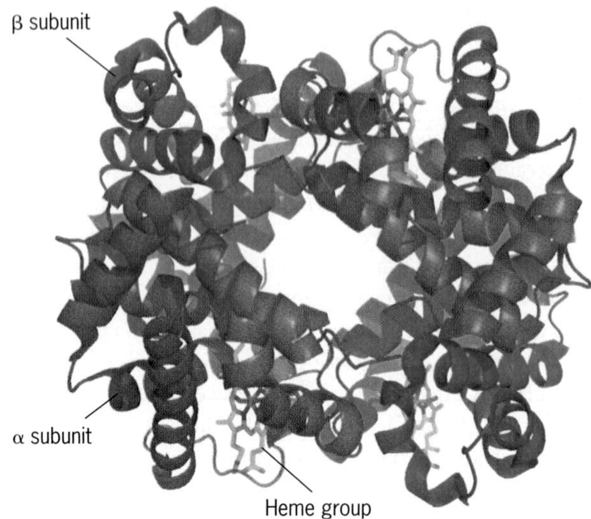

FIGURE 2–5 Structure of human adult hemoglobin.

tetramer consists of 547 amino acids and has a molecular weight of 64,800 daltons. The heme and globin interact with each other in a way that determines the O_2-binding characteristics of hemoglobin. The heme groups to which the O_2 binds are located in the protein parts of the molecule. Heme is the complex of chelated iron in a cyclic tetrapyrrole (porphyrin) ring (**Figure 2–5**). The iron atom is located in the center of the porphyrin ring between four nitrogens. The porphyrin carries side chains that maintain the heme group in the proper orientation within the protein portion of the hemoglobin molecule. There are four sites for oxygen binding for each molecule of hemoglobin.

As oxygen molecules successively bind with heme groups, the hemoglobin molecule physically changes its shape, causing it to reflect and absorb light differently when it is oxygenated than when it is deoxygenated. This phenomenon is responsible for the bright red color of oxygenated hemoglobin and the deep purple color of deoxyhemoglobin. This difference in light absorption and reflection makes it possible to measure the amount of oxygenated hemoglobin present in a blood sample through a process known as *spectrophotometry*, or as it is clinically known, *oximetry*.

Deoxyhemoglobin and oxyhemoglobin are also referred to as being in the *T*, or *tense, state* and the *R*, or *relaxed, state*, respectively.[1] The R state has an O_2 affinity about 150 times greater than the T state. The transition between these conformational states is induced by the shift of the heme iron when O_2 is bound or released. This process is modulated by S-nitrosylation of hemoglobin, or the binding of nitric oxide to the cysteine residues of hemoglobin.[2,3]

Oxyhemoglobin Equilibrium Curve

O_2 affinity to hemoglobin increases during progressive oxygenation, a phenomenon called *cooperativity*. The cooperativity is responsible for the sigmoid shape of the OEC (oxyhemoglobin dissociation curve), which affects how O_2 is loaded and unloaded under physiologic conditions. Its position often is expressed by the P_{50}, or the Po_2 that corresponds with 50% hemoglobin saturation. The normal P_{50} for human hemoglobin is approximately 27 mm Hg. When the O_2 affinity increases, the OEC shifts to the left (reduced P_{50}). When the O_2 affinity decreases, the OEC shifts to the right (increased P_{50}). The actual shape and position of the OEC are influenced by many factors (**Table 2–3**).

TABLE 2–3 Effect of Various Factors on the Affinity of Hemoglobin to Oxygen and P_{50}

Factors	Changes	O_2 Affinity	P_{50}
pH	↑ (Alkalemia)	↑	↓
	↓ (Acidemia)	↓	↑
2,3-DPG	↑	↓	↑
	↓	↑	↓
Temperature	↑	↓	↑
	↓	↑	↓
Pco_2	↑	↓	↑
	↓	↑	↓
CO	↑	↑	↓
Methemoglobin	↑	↑	↓
Fetal hemoglobin	↑	↑	↓

2,3-DPG, 2,3-Diphosphoglycerate; CO, carbon monoxide.

RESPIRATORY RECAP

Oxygen Equilibration Curve (Oxygen Dissociation Curve)

- » The sigmoid curve describes the relationship between oxygen saturation and Po_2
- » A shift to the left causes an increased affinity of hemoglobin for oxygen
- » A shift to the right causes a decreased affinity of hemoglobin for oxygen
- » Numerous physiologic conditions affect the position of the curve

Several factors affect hemoglobin's affinity for O_2, resulting in either a left (increased affinity) or right (decreased affinity) shift in the OEC position, changing the hemoglobin O_2 saturation for a given Pao_2 (refer to Figure 2–3). Increased 2,3-diglycerophosphate (2,3-DPG) in the erythrocyte, acidemia, increased $Paco_2$, and hyperthermia decrease hemoglobin affinity for O_2 (right shift of the curve). In contrast, decreased 2,3-DPG, alkalemia, decreased $Paco_2$, and hypothermia increase hemoglobin affinity for O_2 (left shift of the curve).

The hydrogen ion concentration in erythrocytes is regulated mainly by Pco_2; the effect of CO_2 on hemoglobin's oxygen affinity is called the **Bohr effect**. In the pulmonary capillaries, $[H^+]$ decreases within the red blood cells (RBCs) as CO_2 is eliminated by ventilation, and the

O_2 affinity of hemoglobin increases, which augments O_2 loading. In the peripheral capillaries the process is reversed. CO_2 produced by cellular metabolism diffuses into the RBC, causing $[H^+]$ to rise within the cells, and the O_2 affinity of hemoglobin is decreased, facilitating O_2 unloading. These combined effects are physiologically favorable because they enhance both O_2 uptake in the lungs and O_2 release in the tissues.

The position of the OEC can be altered by organic phosphates, notably ATP and 2,3-DPG. The concentration of 2,3-DPG in RBCs is four times more plentiful than ATP because of the increased glycolytic activity.[4] An increase in 2,3-DPG facilitates release of O_2 by shifting the OEC to the right. Through this important mechanism, RBCs defend against tissue hypoxia after vigorous exercise, after ascent to high altitude, and in numerous diseases associated with reduction in O_2 availability (such as anemia, right-to-left shunt, congestive heart failure, and the chronic hypoxemia of chronic obstructive pulmonary disease). Low levels of 2,3-DPG in the RBCs with corresponding increases in O_2 affinity have been observed in individuals with hypophosphatemia, hexokinase deficiency, and septic shock, and in stored blood used for transfusions.

Changes in temperature alter the conformation of hemoglobin and thus the position of the OEC. Hyperthermia or hypothermia increases or decreases the P_{50} by approximately 2 mm Hg per degree Celsius. CO_2 affects the OEC through the formation of H^+ and carbamino compounds. Increases in carbamino compounds also shift the OEC to the right, similar to increases in $[H^+]$.

When hemoglobin is bound to carbon monoxide (CO), its affinity for O_2 is greatly increased; the binding of CO to one heme site increases O_2 affinity of the other binding sites, causing a leftward shift of the OEC. This effect on hemoglobin O_2 affinity explains why the formation of 50% carboxyhemoglobin causes more severe tissue hypoxia than when various forms of anemia cause the reduction of hemoglobin concentration to half the normal concentration.

Methemoglobin is formed when the ferrous (Fe^{+2}) iron center of the heme molecule is oxidized to the ferric state (Fe^{+3}). Normally the heme iron in deoxyhemoglobin is in the ferrous state (Fe^{+2}). There are six electrons in the outer shell, four of which are unpaired. When oxygen is bound, one of these electrons is partially transferred to the oxygen, and iron is oxidized (i.e., the ferrous state becomes a ferric state). The oxidation, however, is reversible because when the oxygen is released, the electron is transferred back to the heme iron. When an oxidizing agent is present (i.e., an agent that will take away electrons from the heme iron), the electrons on the heme iron are successively removed and thus are not available to bind oxygen. Normal RBCs contain less than 1% methemoglobin. The effects of methemoglobin on peripheral capillary O_2 release and subsequent tissue hypoxia are qualitatively the same but quantitatively less than that produced by equal amounts of carboxyhemoglobin. **Box 2–1** lists clinical conditions associated with increased methemoglobin formation.

BOX 2–1

Conditions Associated with Methemoglobinemia

Hereditary

- M hemoglobins
- Cytochrome b_5 reductase deficiency

Acquired

- Nitrites and nitrates: sodium nitrite, amyl nitrite, nitroglycerin, nitroprusside, silver nitrate, inhaled nitric oxide
- Aniline dyes: aminobenzenes, nitrobenzene
- Acetanilid and phenacetin
- Sulfonamides, sulfasalazine
- Other: lidocaine, chlorate, phenazopyridine, ferrous sulfate, quinones

Fetal hemoglobin (hemoglobin F) has higher affinity for O_2 than adult hemoglobin (hemoglobin A). The increased O_2 affinity of hemoglobin F can be attributed to the replacement of β chains in hemoglobin A by γ chains, which do not bind readily with 2,3-DPG. The high affinity of hemoglobin F for O_2 permits the fetus to extract maximal amounts of O_2 from the maternal venous blood, which has a relatively low O_2 content.

Genetic hemoglobin abnormalities can be associated with increases (such as Chesapeake or Yakima) or decreases (such as Seattle or Kansas) in O_2 affinity. This effect also is believed to be mediated by the altered binding of 2,3-DPG to the abnormal peptide chains.

Carbon Dioxide Equilibrium Curve

The CO_2 hemoglobin equilibrium curve is essentially linear over the physiologic range of $Paco_2$ (**Figure 2–6**), in contrast to the S-shaped oxyhemoglobin equilibrium curve. This means a change in alveolar ventilation is much more effective in changing arterial CO_2 content than O_2 content; for example, a doubling of the alveolar ventilation in the healthy lung cuts the blood CO_2 content in half but changes arterial O_2 content very little because hemoglobin is already nearly 100% saturated with normal ventilation. The steepness of the CO_2 hemoglobin equilibrium curve also permits continued excretion of CO_2 even in the presence of significant mismatching of pulmonary ventilation and blood flow.[5,6] This explains why CO_2 retention is seen only in patients with severe ventilation-perfusion mismatch.

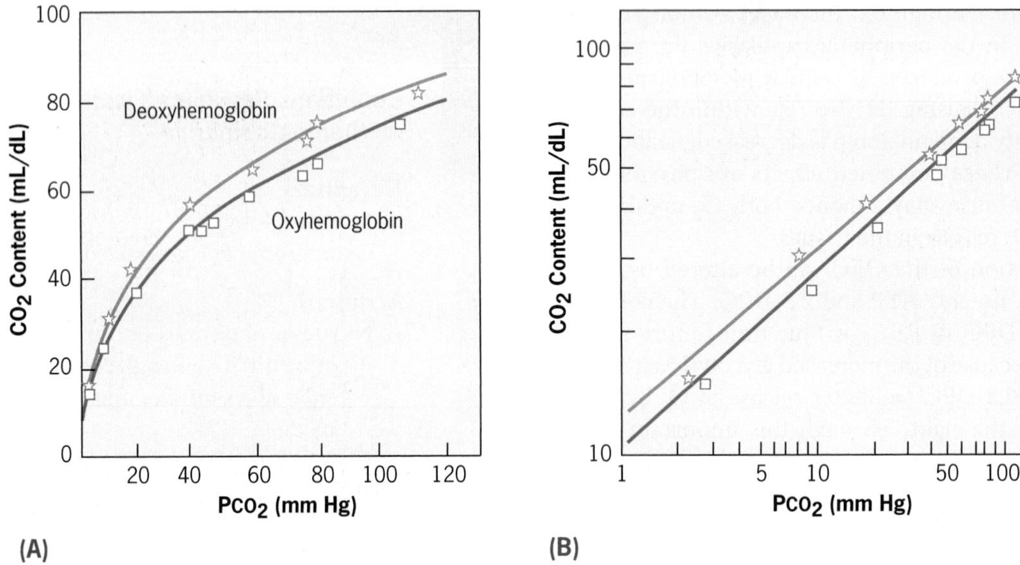

FIGURE 2–6 (**A**) Carbon dioxide curve of blood. (**B**) Logarithmic transformation of the curve that linearizes the relationship between CO_2 content and $P{CO_2}$. Modified from Baum GL, et al. *Textbook of Pulmonary Diseases*. 6th ed. Lippincott Williams & Wilkins; 1998.

The hemoglobin molecule simultaneously carries O_2 and CO_2, but not at the same binding sites. Oxygen combines with the molecule's heme groups, whereas CO_2 combines with the amino groups of the α- and β-polypeptide chains. The presence of O_2 on the heme portions of hemoglobin hinders the combination of amino groups with CO_2 (i.e., it hinders formation of carbaminohemoglobin); thus, the affinity of hemoglobin for CO_2 is greater when it is not combined with oxygen (**Haldane effect**). Conversely, carbaminohemoglobin has a decreased affinity for O_2 (Bohr effect). Thus, oxygenated blood carries less CO_2 for a given $Pa{CO_2}$ than deoxygenated blood (refer to Figure 2–6). It should be appreciated that the Haldane and Bohr effects are mutually enhancing. As O_2 diffuses into the tissue cells, it dissociates from the hemoglobin molecule, enhancing its ability to carry CO_2 (Haldane effect). At the same time, CO_2 diffusion into the blood at the tissue level decreases hemoglobin's affinity for O_2 (Bohr effect), enhancing the release of O_2 to the tissues.

Carbon Dioxide Transport

The transport pathway of CO_2 begins with the diffusion of CO_2 from tissues into the capillary blood. About 90% of the CO_2 that enters the blood diffuses into the RBCs, where it undergoes one of three chemical reactions: (1) it remains as dissolved CO_2, (2) it combines with the NH_2 groups of hemoglobin to form carbaminohemoglobin, or (3) it combines with water to form H_2CO_3, which dissociates into H^+ and $HCO^-{}_3$ (bicarbonate). The remaining 10% of the CO_2 in the plasma exists as dissolved CO_2 and carbamino compounds after reacting with NH_2 groups of plasma proteins.

The amount of CO_2 that dissolves in plasma at 37° C is about 0.03 mmol/L for every mm Hg of $P{CO_2}$; thus, dissolved CO_2 in the blood is calculated by multiplying the $P{CO_2}$ by 0.03 mmol/L. Because the normal $Pa{CO_2}$ is about 40 mm Hg, the normal amount of dissolved CO_2 in arterial blood is 40 × 0.03, or 1.2 mmol/L. Although the amount of dissolved CO_2 is relatively small, it is in equilibrium with the plasma $Pa{CO_2}$, which in turn determines the direction and rate of CO_2 diffusion at body tissue and alveolar levels. In plasma, CO_2 undergoes the following reaction:

$$CO_2 + H_2O \rightarrow H_2CO_3 \rightarrow HCO_3^- + H^+$$

The rate of this reaction is relatively slow in plasma, and the amount of carbonic acid (H_2CO_3) in the plasma is extremely small; even so, plasma H_2CO_3 is a major determinant of the blood's H^+ concentration (i.e., the pH). Because dissolved CO_2 determines the plasma H_2CO_3 concentration, dissolved CO_2 plays a key role in determining the blood pH.

The reaction rate of CO_2 with H_2O in the erythrocyte is about 13,000 times faster than in the plasma due to the influence of carbonic anhydrase, an intracellular catalytic enzyme. As a result H^+ is rapidly generated, but it is immediately buffered by hemoglobin and thus removed from solution. Consequently, the reaction keeps moving to the right, continually drawing more CO_2 into the erythrocyte, generating HCO_3^- in the process. As HCO_3^- accumulates in the erythrocyte, its intracellular concentration rises; HCO_3^- then diffuses down its concentration gradient into the plasma. This mechanism is responsible for nearly all of the HCO_3^- in the plasma.

Before hemoglobin buffers H^+, its negative charges are exactly balanced by the positive ions inside the erythrocyte. As it buffers H^+ ions, the hemoglobin molecule's net negative charge is reduced, but this reduction is exactly matched by newly generated HCO_3^-, and intracellular electroneutrality is maintained. Therefore, when negatively charged HCO_3^- ions diffuse out of the erythrocyte, an electropositive environment develops inside the erythrocyte. In response, Cl^-, the most abundant anion in the plasma, diffuses into the erythrocyte (the so-called *chloride shift*), which maintains intracellular electrical neutrality. The process of bicarbonate–chloride exchange in the RBCs is mediated by the anion exchange protein I (AEI, or band 3 protein) on the RBC membrane.[7,8] Some movement of water inward occurs simultaneously with the chloride shift to maintain osmotic equilibrium, resulting in a slight swelling of erythrocytes in venous blood relative to those in arterial blood.

Carbonic anhydrase can be inhibited by acetazolamide, a drug used in the treatment of glaucoma and acute mountain sickness. Inhibition of carbonic anhydrase in the erythrocyte slows the reaction of CO_2 with H_2O, resulting in continued HCO_3^- formation in the erythrocyte even after the blood has left the peripheral capillaries. When the blood reaches the pulmonary capillaries, the dissolved CO_2 quickly diffuses into alveolar gas, but because of the slowed reaction between CO_2 and H_2O, HCO_3^- in the erythrocyte cannot dehydrate fast enough to unload all of the CO_2 just acquired from the tissues. Thus the Pa_{CO_2} rises as blood flows through the systemic arteries, because the unloading reaction slowly continues. The overall result would be a rise in arterial P_{CO_2} were it not for the stimulatory effect CO_2 has on the brain's medullary chemoreceptors. Acetazolamide also inhibits carbonic anhydrase and thus the CO_2 hydration reaction in the renal tubule cells. This inhibits HCO_3^- reabsorption from the glomerular filtrate and causes HCO_3^- loss in the urine.

Ventilation-Perfusion Distribution

Exchange of O_2 and CO_2 between blood and air occurs continuously in the more than 300,000,000 alveoli. A single alveolus, however, is unlikely to be the basic functional unit of the lung, which is defined as the smallest region within which there is gas exchange homogeneity (i.e., disease that occurs within these units does not affect gas exchange). There are more than 100,000 such functional units, which probably correspond to acini subtended by respiratory bronchioles.[9,10] The adequacy of function of each terminal respiratory unit is determined by local matching between ventilation and perfusion ($\dot{V}_A/\dot{Q}$). In general, inadequate ventilation relative to perfusion (low $\dot{V}_A/\dot{Q}$ and shunt) has the greatest effect on O_2 uptake by the lungs and thus results in **hypoxemia**. On the other hand, excessive ventilation relative to perfusion (high $\dot{V}_A/\dot{Q}$ and dead space) hinders the lungs' ability to eliminate CO_2 and may cause **hypercapnia** in severe cases, especially in individuals with limited ability to increase ventilation.

The effects of $\dot{V}_A/\dot{Q}$ matching on the efficiency of gas exchange in the lungs can be illustrated with the two-compartment lung model (**Figure 2–7**). In an ideal lung consisting of two alveolar units (A and B) with each receiving 2.0 L/min of alveolar ventilation and 2.5 L/min of blood flow, the $\dot{V}_A/\dot{Q}$ ratio is 0.8 for the individual units A and B and thus the entire lung (Figure 2–7A). Assuming no barrier to diffusion of O_2 and a normal P_{O_2} in the pulmonary artery, the P_{O_2} of alveolar gas is the same as the P_{O_2} of end-capillary and arterial blood. An O_2 gradient between alveolus and capillary blood does not exist. In a normal lung a slight degree of $\dot{V}_A/\dot{Q}$ mismatch occurs, primarily because of the greater effects of gravity on the distribution of perfusion than on ventilation (Figure 2–7B). Thus although the $\dot{V}_A/\dot{Q}$ ratio for the whole lung remains at 0.8, the $\dot{V}_A/\dot{Q}$ ratios for the two units A and B are 1.0 and 0.6, respectively, causing the mean P_{O_2} in the blood leaving the lung to decrease slightly and produce a P_{O_2} difference between alveolus and pulmonary capillary of 4.4 mm Hg. Uneven distribution of blood flow also may result in similar effects, especially in the upright lung.

Measurement of $\dot{V}_A/\dot{Q}$ Distribution

It has long been recognized that the lung is not homogeneous; that is, the gas exchange units in the lungs have different $\dot{V}_A/\dot{Q}$ ratios. Various models have been proposed to explain the gas exchange behavior of the lung. One such model divides the lung into three compartments: an ideal compartment in which gas exchange is optimal ($\dot{V}_A/\dot{Q}$ ratios = 1), a second compartment with unperfused alveoli (dead space or $\dot{V}_A/\dot{Q}$ ratios = ∞), and a third compartment with unventilated alveoli (shunt or $\dot{V}_A/\dot{Q}$ ratios = 0). This model had been the gold standard for assessing ventilation-perfusion inequality in patients with lung disease. Major conceptual advances became possible with the introduction of the **multiple inert gas elimination technique (MIGET)**,[11] which allows a more complete description of distributions of $\dot{V}_A/\dot{Q}$ ratios. The MIGET is based on the physical principles governing inert gas elimination by the lungs. When an inert gas in solution is infused into systemic veins, the proportion of gas eliminated by ventilation from a lung unit depends only on the solubility of the gas and the $\dot{V}_A/\dot{Q}$ ratio of that unit. The relationship is given by the following equation:

$$\frac{Pc'}{P\bar{v}} = \frac{\lambda}{(\lambda + \dot{V}_A/\dot{Q})}$$

where Pc' and $P\bar{v}$ are the partial pressures of the gas in end-capillary blood and mixed venous blood, respectively, and λ is the blood-gas partition coefficient. The ratio of Pc' over $P\bar{v}$ is known as the *retention.*

To obtain the $\dot{V}_A/\dot{Q}$ distribution of the lung, a saline solution containing low concentrations of six inert gases of different solubility (sulfur hexafluoride [SF_6], ethane, cyclopropane, isoflurane, diethyl ether, and acetone) is

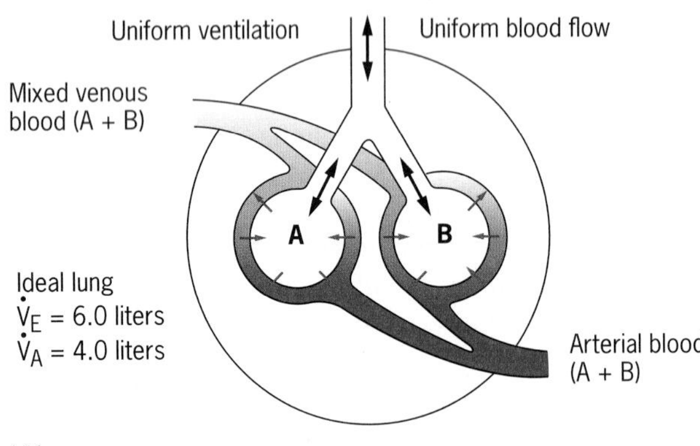

	A	B	(A + B)
Alveolar ventilation (L/min)	2.0	2.0	4.0
Pulmonary blood flow (L/min)	2.5	2.5	5.0
Ventilation/perfusion distribution	0.8	0.8	0.8
Mixed venous PO_2 (mm Hg)	40.0	40.0	40.0
Mixed venous O_2 saturation (%)	75.0	75.0	75.0
Alveolar PO_2 (mm Hg)	101.0	101.0	101.0
Arterial PO_2 (mm Hg)	101.0	101.0	101.0
Arterial O_2 saturation (%)	97.5	97.5	97.5

(A)

Nonuniform ventilation

Uniform blood flow

Mixed venous blood (A + B)

A

B

Normal lung

$\dot{V}_E$ = 6.0 liters

$\dot{V}_A$ = 4.0 liters

Arterial blood (A + B)

	A	B	(A + B)
Alveolar ventilation (L/min)	2.5	1.5	4.0
Pulmonary blood flow (L/min)	2.5	2.5	5.0
Ventilation/perfusion distribution	1.0	0.6	0.8
Mixed venous PO_2 (mm Hg)	40.0	40.0	40.0
Mixed venous O_2 saturation (%)	75.0	75.0	75.0
Alveolar PO_2 (mm Hg)	111.0	94.0	104.6
Arterial PO_2 (%)	111.0	94.0	100.2
Arterial O_2 saturation (%)	97.8	96.4	97.1

(B)

FIGURE 2–7 Ventilation-perfusion relationships of an ideal lung (**A**) and a healthy lung (**B**) are illustrated with a two-compartment model. Note that the ventilation-perfusion maldistribution is responsible for an alveolar-arterial Po_2 difference of about 4.4 mm Hg; the remainder of the normal Po_2 difference is caused by anatomic shunts (ignored in this illustration). Adapted from Forster RE, et al., eds. *The Normal Lung: Physiological Basis of Pulmonary Function Tests*. 3rd ed. Year-Book; 1986.

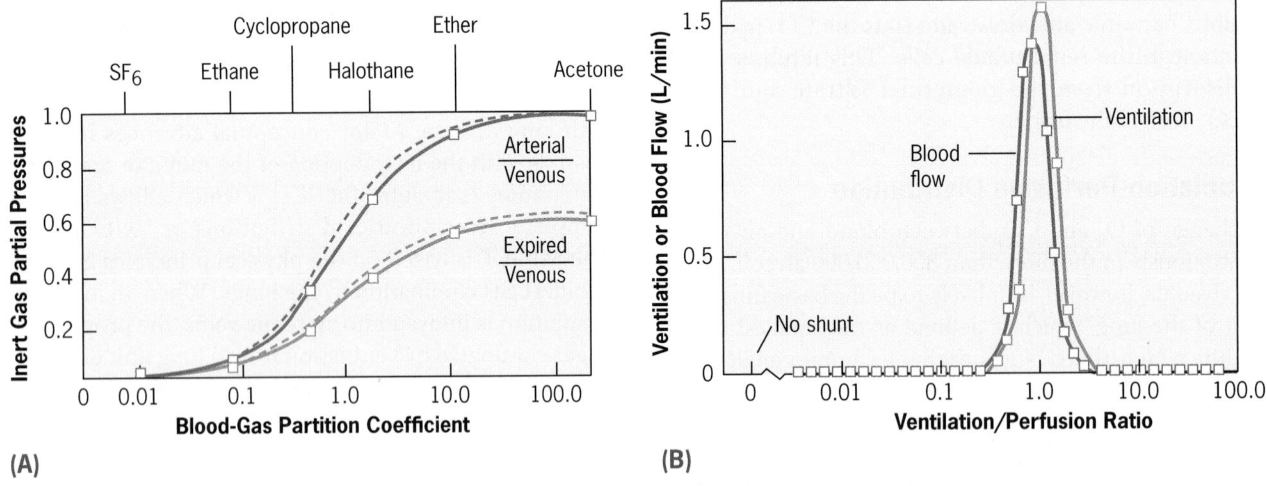

FIGURE 2–8 Distribution of ventilation-perfusion ratios determined by the multiple inert gas elimination technique. Data from a 22-year-old normal subject are illustrated. (**A**) Features data points for inert gas retention (upper curve) and excretion (lower curve). Broken lines join the points. The two solid lines show the values of retention and excretion for a lung with no ventilation-perfusion inequality. (**B**) Illustrates recovered distribution of ventilation-perfusion ratios. Adapted from Wagner PD, et al. Continuous distributions of ventilation-perfusion ratios in normal subjects breathing air and 100% O_2. *J Clin Invest.* 1974;54:53–68.

infused slowly into a peripheral vein until a steady state is reached. The inert gas concentrations in the arterial, mixed venous, and expired gas samples are collected and analyzed (**Figure 2–8**). Retention and excretion values for the inert gases are graphed against their solubility in blood (Figure 2–8A). With a 50-compartment model, the retention-solubility plots can be transformed to obtain the distribution of $\dot{V}A/\dot{Q}$ ratios in the lung (Figure 2–8B). A lung containing shunt units shows increased retention of the least-soluble gas, sulfur hexafluoride (SF_6). Conversely,

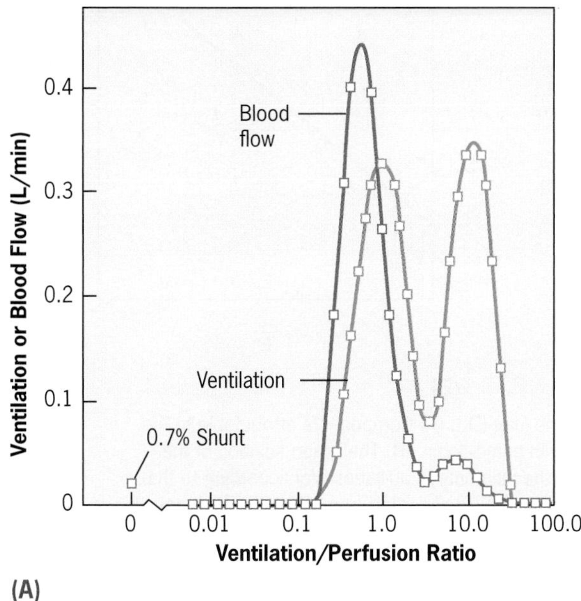

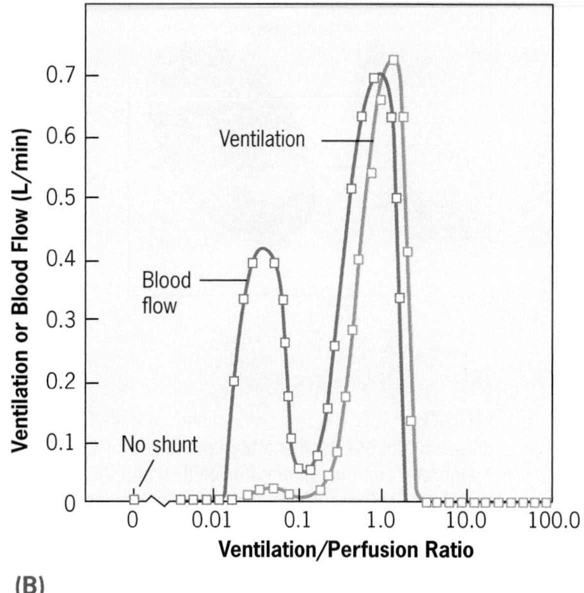

FIGURE 2–9 Examples of the distribution of ventilation-perfusion ratios in individuals with chronic obstructive pulmonary disease. **(A)** Type A (individuals with predominantly emphysema) tend to have areas of very high $\dot{V}_A/\dot{Q}$. **(B)** Type B (patients with predominantly chronic bronchitis) often have areas of very low $\dot{V}_A/\dot{Q}$. Shunt ($\dot{V}_A/\dot{Q} = 0$) is rarely seen in either type. Adapted from Wagner PD, et al. Ventilation-perfusion inequality in chronic obstructive pulmonary disease. *J Clin Invest.* 1977;59:203–216.

a lung having large amounts of ventilation-to-lung units with very high $\dot{V}_A/\dot{Q}$ ratios shows increased retention of the high-solubility gases (such as ether and acetone).

Figure 2–8 shows the distribution of $\dot{V}_A/\dot{Q}$ ratios from a 22-year-old healthy volunteer.[11] The distributions for both ventilation and blood flow (dispersion) are narrow and span only one log of $\dot{V}_A/\dot{Q}$ ratios. Essentially, no ventilation or blood flow occurs outside the range of approximately 0.3 to 3.0 on the $\dot{V}_A/\dot{Q}$ ratio scale, and no significant intrapulmonary shunt is detected. With aging, the dispersion of ventilation and perfusion increases. As much as 10% of the total blood flow may go to lung units with $\dot{V}_A/\dot{Q}$ values of less than 0.1, but still no shunt is detected. The increased low-$\dot{V}_A/\dot{Q}$ regions adequately explain the decreased Pa_{O_2} and increased alveolar-arterial O_2 difference with aging. The cause of such age-related $\dot{V}_A/\dot{Q}$ mismatch often is attributed to degenerative processes in the small airways with aging.

$\dot{V}_A/\dot{Q}$ Distributions in Lung Disease

Various abnormal patterns of $\dot{V}_A/\dot{Q}$ distributions measured by the MIGET method adequately explain gas exchange abnormalities in diseased lungs.[12] For example, **Figure 2–9** shows the distribution of $\dot{V}_A/\dot{Q}$ ratios from an individual with chronic obstructive lung disease. The $\dot{V}_A/\dot{Q}$ distribution is bimodal, and large amounts of ventilation go to lung units with extremely high $\dot{V}_A/\dot{Q}$ ratios (Figure 2–9A). This $\dot{V}_A/\dot{Q}$ pattern can be seen in individuals with predominant emphysema.[13] Presumably the high-$\dot{V}_A/\dot{Q}$ regions represent lung units in which many capillaries have been destroyed by the emphysematous process. The presence of a small shunt (3.1%) and the coexisting low $\dot{V}_A/\dot{Q}$ in which ventilation is inadequate relative to blood flow (note the slight left shift of the main mode of blood flow in Figure 2–9A) can explain the mild arterial hypoxemia found in this individual (Pa_{O_2} 63 mm Hg).

Individuals with chronic obstructive pulmonary disease (COPD) characterized predominantly by chronic bronchitis generally show a different pattern of $\dot{V}_A/\dot{Q}$ distribution (Figure 2–9B). The main abnormality in these individuals is the large number of lung units with very low $\dot{V}_A/\dot{Q}$ ratios (i.e., the small amount of ventilation relative to blood flow); this explains the more severe hypoxemia generally found in this type of COPD patient compared with COPD patients with predominantly emphysema. The low-$\dot{V}_A/\dot{Q}$ units in COPD patients with predominantly chronic bronchitis likely reflect airway obstruction caused by retained secretions and mucous gland hyperplasia.

$\dot{V}_A/\dot{Q}$ Mismatch and Carbon Dioxide Retention

Abnormal $\dot{V}_A/\dot{Q}$ distributions produce hypoxemia, but not necessarily hypercapnia. Even though a low $\dot{V}_A/\dot{Q}$ interferes with the efficiency of CO_2 elimination, it is often associated with a normal or even low Pa_{CO_2}. The reason is that the regulatory chemoreceptors in the medulla of the brain increase the ventilatory drive in response to a rising Pa_{CO_2}; this increases total minute ventilation. However, a significant portion of this increased ventilation is inefficient with respect to CO_2 elimination because it goes to lung units with high $\dot{V}_A/\dot{Q}$ ratios. This regional hyperventilation lowers the P_{CO_2} of these units, balancing out the high P_{CO_2} of low-$\dot{V}_A/\dot{Q}$

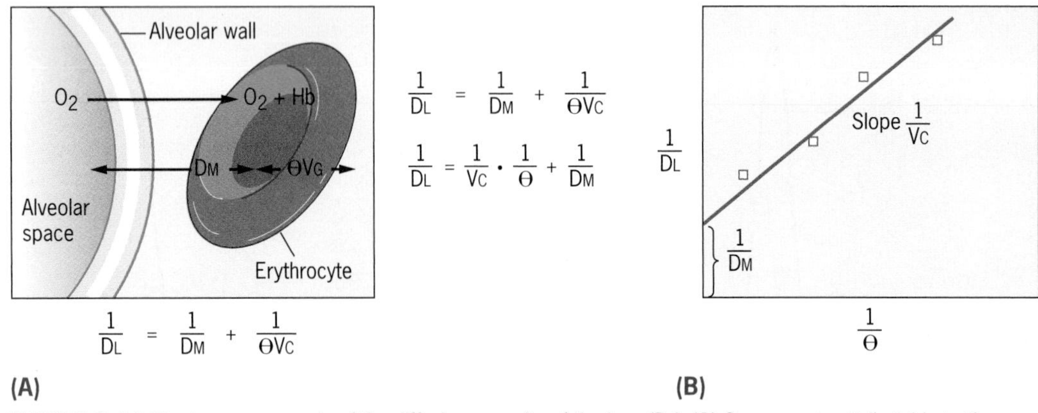

FIGURE 2–10 The two components of the diffusing capacity of the lung (DL). (**A**) Components attributable to the diffusion process itself and the time taken for O_2 (or CO) to react with hemoglobin. (**B**) The graph solution of the membrane component of diffusion (DM) and the volume of blood in the pulmonary capillaries ($\dot{V}$c) according to the Roughton-Forster analysis. DM and $\dot{V}$c are derived by plotting 1/θ against 1/DL. Adapted from West JB. *Textbook of Respiratory Medicine.* 2nd ed. WB Saunders; 1994.

units. Thus, depending on the severity of $\dot{V}A/\dot{Q}$ mismatch (i.e., the relative numbers of high- and low-$\dot{V}A/\dot{Q}$ units), a hypoxemic patient can have low, normal, or high arterial Pco_2. $\dot{V}A/\dot{Q}$ mismatch is the primary mechanism for hypercapnia seen in severe COPD patients. These patients require an increased minute ventilation to achieve a given Pao_2 or $Paco_2$ and thus incur an increased work of breathing.

Regulatory Control of $\dot{V}A/\dot{Q}$ Matching

The alveolar Po_2 appears to be the most important factor involved in regulating the distribution of $\dot{V}A/\dot{Q}$ within the lung. Hypoxemia in the pulmonary vascular system causes vasoconstriction (hypoxic pulmonary vasoconstriction), greatly increasing resistance to blood flow in hypoxic (underventilated or low-$\dot{V}A/\dot{Q}$) regions of the lungs. This phenomenon tends to restore the $\dot{V}A/\dot{Q}$ matching of the regions. For example, in lung units with low $\dot{V}A/\dot{Q}$ ratios (hypoventilated), local alveolar Po_2 decreases, and the resulting constriction of the associated arterioles reduces the local pulmonary blood flow, which tends to restore the local $\dot{V}A/\dot{Q}$ ratio toward its normal value. This effect is more widespread in the lungs of people living in high altitudes, who are chronically exposed to low ambient O_2 concentrations. High-altitude residents have better $\dot{V}A/\dot{Q}$ matching than sea-level residents, as reflected by a smaller $P(A - a)o_2$ difference.[14]

Diffusion

O_2 from the ambient air is carried into the terminal alveolar units of the lungs by two physical processes: (1) bulk gas flow in the conducting airways, and (2) molecular diffusion in the distal alveolar units. From the alveolus, O_2 must diffuse across the alveolocapillary membrane, plasma, and erythrocyte membrane before it can react with hemoglobin. The diffusion gradient between gas and blood for O_2 is the Po_2 difference between alveolar gas and mixed venous blood. In normal individuals this gradient is approximately 60 mm Hg (PAo_2 of 100 mm Hg and $P\bar{v}o_2$ of 40 mm Hg). At rest the diffusion process is virtually complete within the first third (0.25 second) of the mean capillary transit time of 0.75 second (**Figure 2–10**).

Diffusion of gases across the alveolocapillary membrane is described by **Fick's law** of diffusion (**Equation 2–1**). Fick's law states that for a given gas, the amount of gas transferred across a membrane is proportional to the membrane's surface area, a diffusion constant (derived from the gas solubility and molecular weight), and the diffusion pressure gradient. Increased gas solubility and decreased gas density would increase its diffusibility. Gas diffusion rate is inversely proportional to the thickness of the membrane.

Carbon monoxide is the gas of choice to measure the diffusion capacity of the lung. Unlike O_2, the partial pressure of CO in capillary blood is negligible, and equilibration between blood and alveolar gas CO never occurs; in contrast, gas and blood Po_2 equilibrate in the first third of the blood's capillary transit time, which means no diffusion occurs as blood traverses the remaining two-thirds of the capillary distance. O_2 diffusion rate is thus affected by blood flow rate, which interferes with the assessment of the alveolocapillary membrane's ability to transfer O_2. Because CO equilibration between capillary blood and alveolar gas never occurs, the CO diffusion rate is strictly determined by the characteristics of the alveolocapillary membrane itself. The reason blood CO pressure is negligible is that hemoglobin has an extremely high affinity for CO (more than 200 times greater than its affinity for O_2) and instantly removes CO from solution. Diffusion capacity of the lung for CO is measured in mL CO/min/mm Hg of alveolar partial pressure:

$$DLCO = \frac{\dot{V}CO}{PACO}$$

EQUATION 2–1

Fick's Law of Diffusion

$$\dot{V}_{gas} = \frac{A}{T} \times D \times (P_1 - P_2)$$

where

V_{gas} = Amount of gas transferred

A = Surface area for diffusion

T = Thickness of the membrane

D = Diffusion constant

$(P_1 - P_2)$ = Concentration gradient across the membrane

Because the lung is too complex to determine the area and the thickness of the blood–gas barrier, the diffusion equation can be rewritten to combine the factors A, T, and D into one constant, DL, as follows:

$$V_{gas} = D_L \times (P_1 - P_2)$$

Thus, the diffusing capacity for a gas is given by the following equation:

$$D_L = \frac{V_{gas}}{P_A - P_{c'}}$$

where PA and Pc′ are the partial pressures of the gas in alveolar space and capillary blood, respectively, and DL is the diffusing capacity of the lung.

where DLCO is the diffusing capacity of the lung for CO, $\dot{V}$CO is the amount of CO transferred across the alveolocapillary membrane each minute, and PACO is the partial pressure of CO in the alveolar space. This unit is a *conductance* unit (i.e., flow per unit of pressure), which is the reciprocal of a *resistance* unit (pressure generated per unit of flow). Under some circumstances (such as in heavy cigarette smokers), the CO partial pressure in the blood cannot be neglected because carboxyhemoglobin in the blood is sufficiently high to reduce the rate of CO uptake. In this case a correction must be made for so-called back-pressure of CO during the DLCO calculation.

The diffusing capacity for O_2 in the lungs is higher than that for CO and can be estimated by multiplying the diffusing capacity for CO by 1.25. It may seem odd that DLO_2 is greater than DLCO, considering hemoglobin's much greater affinity for CO than O_2. This peculiarity is explained by the fact that O_2 is more *soluble* than CO in the alveolocapillary membrane and the plasma and therefore diffuses more rapidly. The fact that hemoglobin has 210 times greater affinity for CO than O_2 simply means that at a given partial pressure (PCO or PO_2), the hemoglobin carries more CO than O_2. This is unrelated to O_2 and CO *diffusion rate* across the alveolocapillary membrane, which is determined by molecular weight and solubility coefficients.

Anatomically, the diffusing capacity of the lung can be separated into two components: the alveolocapillary membrane plus the erythrocyte cell membrane and the reaction with hemoglobin (Figure 2–10A). These components can be regarded as resistances in series in the transfer of O_2. Based on this model, Roughton and Forster showed that the following relationship exists:

$$\frac{1}{D_L} = \frac{1}{D_M} + \frac{1}{\theta \dot{V}_C}$$

where DM is the diffusing capacity of the membrane (which includes the alveolocapillary membrane, the plasma, and the red cell membrane), θ is the rate of reaction of CO (or O_2) with hemoglobin, and $\dot{V}$c is the volume of blood in the pulmonary capillaries. In the equation, values for DM and $\dot{V}$c can be obtained graphically via measurement of the diffusing capacity for CO at both high and normal alveolar PO_2 values (Figure 2–10B). Increasing the alveolar PO_2 reduces the value of θ for CO because CO has to compete with a higher pressure of O_2 for the hemoglobin. When the values of 1/DL obtained at two different PO_2 values are plotted against 1/θ, as shown in Figure 2–10, the slope of the line is l/ $\dot{V}$c, whereas the intercept on the vertical axis is 1/DM.

Based on this equation, the diffusing capacity can be reduced if DM is decreased (when the thickness is increased or the area is reduced), if θ is reduced (such as in cases of anemia), or if $\dot{V}$c is reduced (as in pulmonary embolism). Mathematically, the term DM is as important as θ $\dot{V}$c in determination of the diffusing capacity of the lung. However, in clinical medicine the more common factor affecting the diffusing capacity is $\dot{V}$c. For example, increasing the pulmonary artery pressure when left atrial pressure is low (thus increasing the perfusion pressure of the pulmonary circulation) can increase DL substantially because higher perfusion pressure recruits and distends pulmonary capillaries and thus increases $\dot{V}$c. The increase in DL during exercise and with changes from the upright to the supine position also can be explained by capillary dilation and recruitment, resulting in an increase in $\dot{V}$c. The reduced diffusing capacity in many cases of lung diseases, including those characterized by increased alveolar septal thickness (such as pulmonary fibrosis), also has been attributed to a decreased $\dot{V}$c caused by loss of pulmonary capillaries from destruction and distortion of lung parenchyma, rather than a decreased DM.

Abnormalities that increase the thickness of the alveolocapillary membrane—that is, the distance for diffusion—rarely prevent the equilibration of PO_2 between the alveolar gas and capillary blood; thus, diffusion impairments due to thickened membranes are generally not responsible for reduced arterial PO_2 *at rest.* The major cause of resting hypoxemia in these patients is a mismatch between ventilation and blood flow. That is, the processes that increase diffusion distance generally decrease lung compliance, which in turn decreases ventilation in these areas. Blood perfusing these underventilated areas tends to be inadequately oxygenated. During exercise, however, blood flow velocity in patients with thickened alveolocapillary membranes may increase enough to prevent equilibration between alveolar gas and capillary blood during the short transit through the lung, causing arterial hemoglobin desaturation. Thus, exercise can unmask diffusion defects that are not apparent at rest. A falling PaO_2 with exercise indicates that diffusion defect may be an important contributing factor for hypoxemia.

Assessment of Gas Exchange

Assessment of Hypoxemia

The effectiveness of gas exchange can be assessed by several methods. The simplest approach is to measure gas tension in arterial blood. More complicated approaches rely on tracer gases and modeling of gas exchange, such as the MIGET, as discussed previously. However, no measurement technique allows an exact description of the complex behavior of gas exchange in the lungs.

Arterial PO_2

The arterial PO_2 provides some information about the degree of $\dot{V}A/\dot{Q}$ matching. The major advantage of the measurement is its simplicity. Normal values of PaO_2 decrease with age. Regression equations have been developed to predict the age-specific PaO_2 in supine and sitting positions.[12,13] Supine PaO_2 is normally lower than upright or seated PaO_2. However, these equations have relatively large standard errors of estimation. The definition of hypoxemia in adults depends on the age of the individual and the altitude (**Table 2–4**). In general, a low PaO_2 while breathing room air indicates the presence of $\dot{V}A/\dot{Q}$ mismatch, shunt, or alveolar hypoventilation, but a normal PaO_2 does not necessarily imply a normal $\dot{V}A/\dot{Q}$ distribution of the lung.

Alveolar-Arterial PO_2 Difference

The alveolar-arterial PO_2 difference ($P[A - a]O_2$) is calculated as the difference between the PAO_2 and the PaO_2. PAO_2 is computed from the alveolar gas equation (**Equation 2–2**). The $P(A - a)O_2$ is more sensitive and specific than the arterial PO_2 alone as an indicator of $\dot{V}A/\dot{Q}$ abnormalities.

The $P(A - a)O_2$ in healthy adults breathing room air increases with age. As a general rule, the $P(A - a)O_2$ for an individual should be no more than half the chronologic age and no more than 25 mm Hg while breathing room air.[15,16] Thus, the upper normal limit of $P(A - a)O_2$

TABLE 2–4 Acceptable PaO_2 Ranges for Adults in Supine Position at Sea Level*

Age (years)	30	40	50	60	70	80	90
PaO_2 (mm Hg)	>90	>85	>80	>75	>70	>65	>60

*Values are calculated with the equation of Sorbini CA, Grassi V, Solinas E, Muiesan G. Arterial oxygen tension in relation to age in healthy subjects. *Respiration.* 1968;25(1):3–13.

EQUATION 2–2

Simplified Alveolar Gas Equation

$$PAO_2 = FIO_2\,(PB - PH_2O) - \frac{PaCO_2}{R}$$

where

PB = Barometric pressure

PH_2O = Water vapor pressure at body temperature (47 mm Hg at 37° C)

FIO_2 = Fractional concentration of oxygen in inspired gas

R = Respiratory exchange ratio

At room air ($FIO_2 = 0.21$) with an R of 0.8, the equation can be simplified as follows:

$$PAO_2 = 0.21\,(713) - 1.25 \times PaCO_2 = 150 - 1.25 \times PaCO_2$$

for a 30-year-old person is 15 mm Hg, whereas the upper normal limit of $P(A - a)O_2$ for a 60-year-old individual is 25 mm Hg. The $P(A - a)O_2$ in normal adults is the result of the combination of mild $\dot{V}A/\dot{Q}$ mismatch and a small anatomic right-to-left shunt. Each of these mechanisms is responsible for about half the total $P(A - a)O_2$. At sea level, none of the $P(A - a)O_2$ difference in normal individuals is caused by diffusion limitation, even during heavy exercise. Diffusion disequilibrium may contribute to increased $P(A - a)O_2$ during exercise and at high altitudes.[17]

The $P(A - a)O_2$ increases with increasing alveolar PO_2. In lungs with severe nonuniform $\dot{V}A/\dot{Q}$ distribution, the $P(A - a)O_2$ reaches a maximum at FIO_2 of 0.6 to 0.7 and then decreases at higher FIO_2 values (**Figure 2–11**). The decline in $P(A - a)O_2$ at higher FIO_2 is caused by more uniform rises in PAO_2, which overcome the nonuniform distribution of $\dot{V}A/\dot{Q}$ ratios. This nonlinear relationship between the $P(A - a)O_2$ and FIO_2 makes reference $P(A - a)O_2$ values obtained with supplemental O_2 difficult to use in critically ill patients, whose FIO_2 values vary frequently.

PaO_2/FIO_2 and PaO_2/PAO_2 Ratio

The PaO_2/FIO_2 ratio is a simple, bedside index of O_2 exchange when $\dot{V}A/\dot{Q}$ mismatch is the primary cause of hypoxemia. However, this ratio loses reliability when hypoventilation contributes to hypoxemia. The PaO_2/PAO_2 ratio is another easily calculated index of oxygenation. It has advantages and disadvantages similar to that of the PaO_2/FIO_2 ratio. In addition, the PaO_2/PAO_2 ratio can be misleading if $P\bar{v}O_2$ fluctuates. For example, when cardiac output decreases, the $P\bar{v}O_2$ falls because the tissues have more time to extract O_2 from the arterial blood. Thus, more profoundly hypoxemic mixed venous blood decreases PaO_2, resulting in lower PaO_2/PAO_2, but the decrease is not because of worsening gas exchange in the lungs but because of low cardiac output. The PaO_2/FIO_2 ratio is affected by $PaCO_2$ (e.g., hypoventilation).

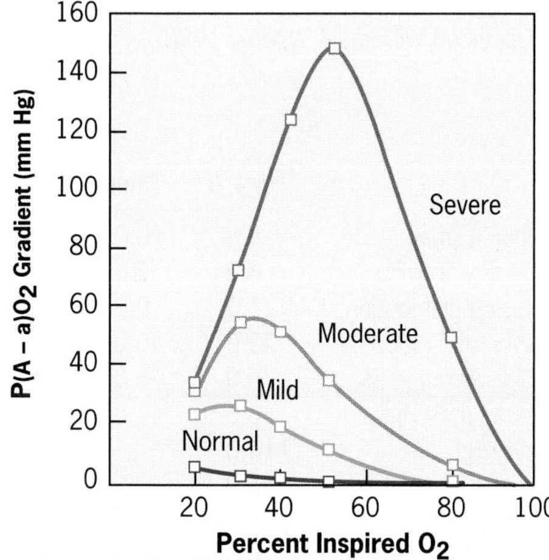

FIGURE 2–11 $P(A - a)O_2$ gradient attributable to ventiliation-perfusion mismatch. Adapted from Dantzker DR. Mechanisms of hypoxemia and hypercapnia. In: Bone RC, ed. *Critical Care: A Comprehensive Approach*. American College of Chest Physicians; 1984.

Shunt

The presence of right-to-left shunt can be differentiated from low-$\dot{V}A/\dot{Q}$ causes of hypoxemia by breathing 100% O_2. While the individual breathes pure O_2, the alveolar PO_2 in different lung units differs according to differences in alveolar PCO_2. Lung units with low $\dot{V}A/\dot{Q}$ ratios increase their PO_2 values maximally with elevation of the inspired PO_2, but shunt does not. The amount of the shunt can be calculated with the following equation:

$$\frac{\dot{Q}s}{\dot{Q}T} = \frac{Cc'O_2 - CaO_2}{Cc'O_2 - C\bar{v}O_2}$$

where $\dot{Q}s/\dot{Q}T$ is the shunt ($\dot{Q}s$) as a fraction of cardiac output ($\dot{Q}T$), $Cc'O_2$ is end-capillary O_2 concentration, CaO_2 is arterial O_2 concentration, and $C\bar{v}O_2$ is mixed venous O_2 concentration. Healthy individuals have a small shunt that amounts to 2% to 5% of the cardiac output. This shunt or venous admixture occurs because some venous blood normally drains into the pulmonary veins, left atrium, or left ventricle from bronchial and myocardial (Thebesian) circulation.

Breathing 100% O_2 increases the arterial PO_2 to greater than 600 mm Hg in normal adults. If PaO_2 only rises to 250 mm Hg during 100% O_2 breathing, the shunt is about one-fourth the cardiac output (25%). This procedure does not determine the anatomic location of a shunt, which may be intracardiac or intrapulmonary, but the calculation can help the clinician focus the differential diagnosis for causes of hypoxemia that develop predominantly by shunt mechanisms. Furthermore, because PaO_2 shows little response to variations in FIO_2 at shunt fractions that exceed 25%, the clinician may be encouraged to reduce toxic and marginally effective concentrations of O_2. However, the shunt calculation frequently overestimates the true shunt because alveoli with very low $\dot{V}A/\dot{Q}$ ratios (<0.1) may collapse completely during O_2 breathing.

Physiologic Mechanisms of Hypoxemia

Hypoventilation decreases the PaO_2 and increases the arterial PCO_2. If $\dot{V}A/\dot{Q}$ distribution remains uniform, no alveolar-arterial difference would develop for either O_2 or CO_2. Although hypoxemia caused by hypoventilation can be corrected with supplemental O_2, the primary treatment should be directed toward support of alveolar ventilation.

$\dot{V}A/\dot{Q}$ mismatch (low-$\dot{V}A/\dot{Q}$ units) is the most common cause of hypoxemia associated with lung diseases. **Figure 2–12** illustrates the way $\dot{V}A/\dot{Q}$ mismatch can

> **RESPIRATORY RECAP**
>
> **Physiologic Mechanisms of Hypoxemia**
>
> » Alveolar hypoventilation
> » Right-to-left shunt (intracardiac or intrapulmonary)
> » Ventilation-perfusion mismatch
> » Diffusion defect
> » Low mixed venous O_2 content
> » Low P_{IO_2} (e.g., at altitude)

cause hypoxemia with a two-compartment lung model. High-$\dot{V}_A/\dot{Q}$ units do not cause hypoxemia directly because the blood perfusing these units is well oxygenated. Hypoxemia associated with asthma, chronic bronchitis, emphysema, pneumonia, and interstitial lung diseases is mostly caused by $\dot{V}_A/\dot{Q}$ mismatch. Hypoxemia caused by $\dot{V}_A/\dot{Q}$ mismatch usually responds well to supplemental O_2.

The effects of a right-to-left shunt on gas exchange are shown schematically in **Figure 2–13**. In this example, 33% of the total blood flow (2.0 L/min) is shunt. Although gas exchange in units A and B is unimpaired, the net result from the mixture of blood from these two units and the shunt pathway is a reduction of Pa_{O_2} and the creation of the alveolar-arterial O_2 difference. This effect on P_{O_2} is similar to that caused by $\dot{V}_A/\dot{Q}$ mismatch. Because of the absence of ventilation in the shunt pathway, hypoxemia resulting from right-to-left shunt cannot be corrected via breathing of 100% O_2. Thus 100% O_2 breathing allows $\dot{V}_A/\dot{Q}$ mismatch to be differentiated from shunt as the cause of hypoxemia. Classic examples of right-to-left shunt include atelectasis, arteriovenous malformation caused by hereditary hemorrhagic telangiectasia (Osler-Weber-Rendu disease), liver cirrhosis, and congenital heart diseases (Eisenmenger syndrome, tetralogy of Fallot).

Diffusion defect may be a cause of hypoxemia under certain circumstances. In healthy individuals resting at sea level, O_2 equilibrates quickly between the blood and gas phases in the alveolar region of the lung, and diffusion limitation does not occur. During exercise at higher altitudes (greater than 10,000 feet), the $P(A - a)_{O_2}$ can increase because of diffusion impairment. Such

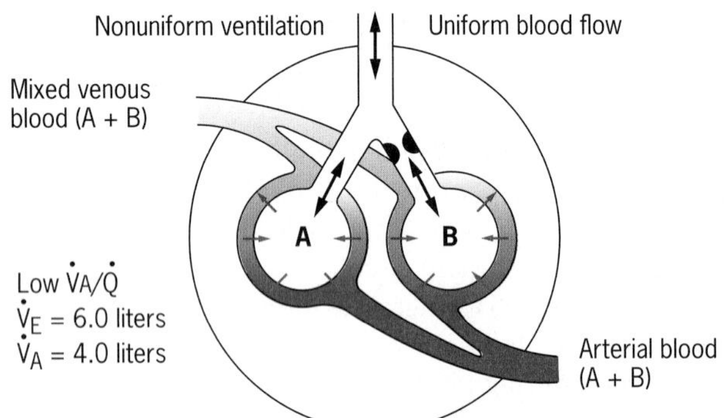

	A	B	(A + B)
Alveolar ventilation (L/min)	3.2	0.8	4.0
Pulmonary blood flow (L/min)	2.5	2.5	5.0
Ventilation/perfusion distribution	1.3	0.3	0.8
Mixed venous P_{O_2} (mm Hg)	40.0	40.0	40.0
Mixed venous O_2 saturation (%)	75.0	75.0	75.0
Alveolar P_{O_2} (mm Hg)	116.0	66.0	106.0
Arterial P_{O_2} (mm Hg)	116.0	66.0	84.0
Arterial O_2 saturation (%)	98.2	91.7	95.0

FIGURE 2–12 Effects of nonuniform distribution of ventilation with uniform blood flow on gas exchange in a two-compartment lung model. If the total ventilation remains at 4 L/min, but unit A receives four times as much ventilation as unit B (3.2 L/min versus 0.8 L/min) and the distribution of perfusion is uniform (2.5 L/min for each unit), the $\dot{V}_A/\dot{Q}$ ratio for unit A becomes 1.3, whereas that for unit B is 0.3. Oxygen tension and saturation must decrease in blood leaving unit B with low $\dot{V}_A/\dot{Q}$; oxygen saturation must rise in blood leaving unit A with high $\dot{V}_A/\dot{Q}$. Because of the sigmoid shape of the oxyhemoglobin equilibrium curve, high P_{O_2} in the blood leaving high-$\dot{V}_A/\dot{Q}$ unit A is not sufficient to compensate for the low P_{O_2} contributed by low-$\dot{V}_A/\dot{Q}$ unit B. The final P_{O_2} in the pulmonary venous blood, which is derived from blood flow–weighted average of oxygen content, decreases. The arterial blood then would have a P_{O_2} of 84 mm Hg instead of 100 mm Hg, as in the healthy lung. Adapted from Baum GL, et al. *Textbook of Pulmonary Diseases*. 6th ed. Lippincott Williams & Wilkins; 1998.

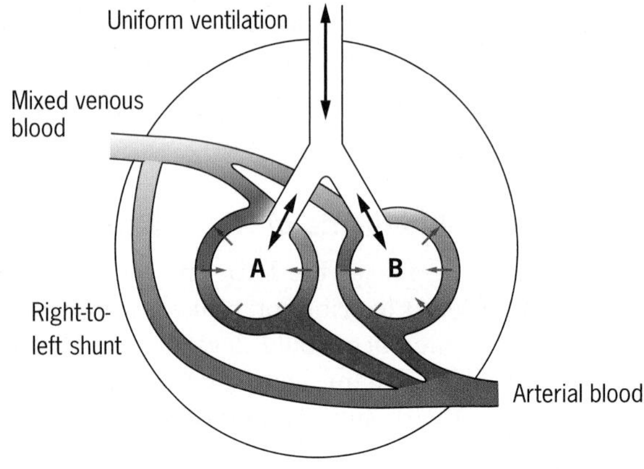

	A + B	Shunt	(A + B + shunt)
Alveolar ventilation (L/min)	4.8	0.0	4.8
Pulmonary blood flow (L/min)	4.0	2.0	6.0
Ventilation/perfusion distribution	1.2	0.0	0.8
Mixed venous P_{O_2} (mm Hg)	40.0	40.0	40.0
Mixed venous O_2 saturation (%)	75.0	75.0	75.0
Mixed venous P_{CO_2} (mm Hg)	46.0	46.0	46.0
Alveolar P_{O_2} (mm Hg)	114.0	—	114.0
Arterial P_{O_2} (mm Hg)	114.0	40.0	59.0
Arterial O_2 saturation (%)	98.2	75.0	90.5
Arterial P_{CO_2} (mm Hg)	36.0	46.0	39.0
$P(A - a)_{O_2}$ difference (mm Hg)	0.0	—	55.0

FIGURE 2–13 Effects of right-to-left shunt on gas exchange in a two-compartment lung model. Adapted from Baum GL, et al. *Textbook of Pulmonary Diseases*. 6th ed. Lippincott Williams & Wilkins; 1998.

TABLE 2–5 Mechanisms of Tissue Hypoxia

Mechanisms	Examples	Response to Oxygen
Hypoxemic	Lung diseases, high altitude	Good in most cases (except in right-to-left shunt)
Anemic	Severe anemia, carbon monoxide poisoning, methemoglobinemia	Generally ineffective in pure anemia; high F_{IO_2} effective in CO poisoning
Stagnant	Cardiac failure, hypovolemia, peripheral vascular diseases, cardiac arrest	Poor
Histotoxic	Cyanide poisoning	Poor

exercise-induced diffusion abnormality at high altitudes is a result of the combined effects of a lower ambient P_{O_2}, which decreases the diffusion gradient, and an increase in the rate of blood flow, which shortens the capillary transit time (refer to Figure 2–10). As discussed previously, in individuals with severe lung diseases who exercise, diffusion impairment also can be an important determinant of hypoxemia because the pulmonary capillary blood volume is decreased, further exacerbating the effect of short capillary transit time during exercise. Similar to $\dot{V}_A/\dot{Q}$ mismatch, hypoxemia caused by diffusion impairment can be corrected by 100% O_2 breathing.

Low mixed venous oxygen content may also contribute to hypoxemia. The O_2 content of pulmonary artery (mixed venous) blood usually has little effect on arterial P_{O_2} in individuals with normal lungs. In the presence of abnormal lungs with a substantial amount of either $\dot{V}_A/\dot{Q}$ abnormalities, a large right-to-left shunt, or both, the O_2 content in the mixed venous blood has a considerable effect on arterial P_{O_2} because the abnormal lung is unable to fully oxygenate the blood when it traverses the pulmonary circulation. For a given $\dot{V}_A/\dot{Q}$ mismatch, the lower the mixed venous O_2 content, the lower the arterial P_{O_2}. This mechanism of hypoxemia is particularly important in critically ill individuals with serious cardiopulmonary diseases. Clearly, the response to supplemental O_2 depends on the relative contributions of $\dot{V}_A/\dot{Q}$ mismatch and right-to-left shunt to hypoxemia if mixed venous oxygen content remains the same. Correcting low mixed venous oxygen content (e.g., by increasing cardiac output) can significantly increase Pa_{O_2}.

Tissue Hypoxia

Complex disturbances of cellular function can be produced by **hypoxia**, primarily because of inadequate production of high-energy phosphate compounds such as ATP. When O_2 is insufficient, glucose is metabolized anaerobically to pyruvate and lactate. Organs that use large amounts of O_2, such as the brain and heart, are more susceptible to hypoxia. When blood Pa_{O_2} is reduced acutely, symptoms and signs of cerebral hypoxia (such as impaired judgment, motor incoordination, or altered mental status) and cardiac hypoxia (such as myocardial ischemia or arrhythmias) tend to manifest first. When hypoxia becomes more severe and prolonged, the respiratory centers of the brain stem are affected and death usually occurs as a result of respiratory failure. Although tissue hypoxia may be associated with a variety of clinical conditions, it is generally divided into four categories (**Table 2–5**).

Hypoxemic hypoxia results from an inadequate amount of O_2 in the blood (reduced Pa_{O_2}) caused by either lung diseases or decreased O_2 in the inspired air (such as at high altitude). Supplemental O_2 corrects tissue hypoxia by raising the Pa_{O_2} in most cases, excepting right-to-left shunt.

Anemic hypoxia results from a reduction in blood O_2 content, which may be caused by severe anemia or the presence of dyshemoglobin states (such as carboxyhemoglobin or methemoglobin). In anemic individuals, Pa_{O_2} is normal but the absolute amount of O_2 transported per unit volume of blood is diminished. Because the hemoglobin is well saturated with O_2, supplemental O_2 provides little benefit in augmenting O_2 delivery to the tissues unless the Pa_{O_2} is raised into the hyperbaric range. CO poisoning not only decreases the O_2-binding capacity of hemoglobin but also shifts the OEC curve to the left, impairing the unloading of O_2 at the peripheral tissues. O_2 is useful in CO poisoning because it displaces CO from hemoglobin and decreases the half-life of carboxyhemoglobin and CO in the tissues. This effect is greatly facilitated by hyperbaric O_2 therapy.

Stagnant hypoxia is a result of poor tissue perfusion, as may be seen in cases of severe cardiac failure, hypovolemic shock, cardiac arrest, and peripheral vascular diseases. The amount of O_2 delivered to the tissues each minute is reduced in these conditions due to low cardiac output or poor tissue perfusion. Poor perfusion may increase tissue edema, increasing the distance through which O_2 has to travel before it reaches the cells. This further enhances tissue hypoxia. Supplemental O_2 usually is not helpful unless tissue perfusion can be restored.

Histotoxic hypoxia is an inability to use O_2 at the cellular level, as with cyanide or sulfide poisoning. These chemical poisons produce cellular hypoxia by inhibiting electron-transfer function by cytochrome oxidase so that O_2 cannot be reduced to water. Because O_2 delivered to the tissues by the blood is not used, the venous

RESPIRATORY RECAP

Mechanisms of Tissue Hypoxia

- Hypoxemic hypoxia
- Anemic hypoxia (including carboxyhemoglobin, methemoglobinemia)
- Stagnant hypoxia (e.g., venous stasis)
- Histotoxic hypoxia (e.g., cyanide)

blood tends to have a high Pa_{O_2}. Supplemental O_2 has little benefit unless the underlying toxic process is reversed.

Mixed Venous P_{O_2}

Mixed venous P_{O_2} ($P\bar{v}_{O_2}$) is the P_{O_2} in blood of the pulmonary artery. It is a measurement that reflects the oxygen concentration of the pooled venous blood returning from the body to the heart. Both $P\bar{v}_{O_2}$ and $S\bar{v}_{O_2}$ are important in the assessment of the body's oxygen delivery (D_{O_2}) and oxygen consumption ($\dot{V}_{O_2}$). Based on Fick's equation, $S\bar{v}_{O_2}$ can be derived as follows:

$$\dot{V}_{O_2} = \dot{Q}c \times (CaO_2 - C\bar{v}O_2)$$

$$= \dot{Q}c \times 1.34 \times [Hb] \times (Sa_{O_2} - S\bar{v}_{O_2})$$

By rearranging the above equation, we have:

$$S\bar{v}_{O_2} = Sa_{O_2} - [\dot{V}_{O_2}/(1.34 \times [Hb] \times \dot{Q}c)]$$

As determined by the equation above, the relationship between Sa_{O_2} and $S\bar{v}_{O_2}$ depends on the term $[\dot{V}_{O_2}/(1.34 \times [Hb] \times \dot{Q}c)]$. Thus it is not possible to predict $S\bar{v}_{O_2}$ from Sa_{O_2} unless we know $\dot{Q}c$ and $\dot{V}_{O_2}$. $S\bar{v}_{O_2}$ should be measured in blood drawn from the distal port of the pulmonary artery catheter, which represents the true mixture of venous blood from the upper body via the superior vena cava (SVC), the lower body via the inferior vena cava (IVC), and from the heart via the coronary sinuses.

At rest, the normal $P\bar{v}_{O_2}$ is 35 to 40 mm Hg and $S\bar{v}_{O_2}$ is approximately 75%. A $P\bar{v}_{O_2}$ below 35 mm Hg in a critically ill individual suggests that O_2 extraction is increased and that tissues may be hypoxic. However, a normal or a higher-than-normal value does not always mean that the tissues have adequate oxygenation. For example, in sepsis, blood may bypass tissues through the peripheral arterial-venous shunting. Therefore, less O_2 is extracted by the tissues, leading to higher-than-normal $P\bar{v}_{O_2}$, but tissue oxygenation is impaired. In the individual with cyanide poisoning, O_2 delivered to the tissues cannot be used because the cytochrome oxidase of the respiratory transport chain is inhibited. $P\bar{v}_{O_2}$ increases despite severe tissue hypoxia. In the absence of impaired oxygen utilization (e.g., cyanide poisoning and sepsis), mixed venous O_2 content is directly related to cardiac output. When cardiac output and thus oxygen delivery decrease, the tissues respond by extracting more O_2 from the blood to maintain tissue oxygenation, causing venous O_2 content to fall. The interpretation of $P\bar{v}_{O_2}$ must take into account the individual's clinical condition.

Because of the declining use of pulmonary artery catheters, many clinicians now measure O_2 saturation in blood withdrawn from a central venous catheter (Scv_{O_2}). Because of its easy accessibility, Scv_{O_2} has been used to guide medical therapy, for example, in assessing the adequacy of fluid resuscitation in septic shock.[18] It is important to remember that this measurement, although frequently called mixed venous measurement, in fact only assesses the SVC venous saturation. Scv_{O_2} does not include venous saturation from coronary sinuses. Scv_{O_2} also may vary depending on the location of the tip of the central venous catheter (i.e., whether the tip is in the SVC, IVC, or the junction). Although $S\bar{v}_{O_2}$ and Scv_{O_2} follow a parallel course in normal individuals, their relationship in critically ill patients is variable.[19] In one study, the differences between $S\bar{v}O_2$ and Scv_{O_2} ranged from −8.1% to 16.5%.[20]

Physiologic Mechanisms of Hypercapnia

A common mechanism for hypercapnia is alveolar hypoventilation. According to the alveolar ventilation equation, Pa_{CO_2} is inversely related to alveolar ventilation. Because alveolar ventilation is the difference between total minute ventilation and dead space ventilation, hypercapnia can be caused by a decrease in total minute ventilation or an increase in physiologic dead space.

Physiologic dead space represents lung units with reduced or absent blood flow, resulting in ineffective CO_2 exchange capacity. The dead space fraction of the tidal volume (V_D/V_T) can be calculated from the Bohr equation:

$$V_D/V_T = \frac{P_{ACO_2} - P\bar{E}_{CO_2}}{P_{ACO_2}}$$

where V_D is physiologic dead space, V_T is tidal volume, $P\bar{E}_{CO_2}$ is mixed expired P_{CO_2}, and P_{ACO_2} is alveolar P_{CO_2}. P_{ACO_2} is assumed to be equal to Pa_{CO_2}. If Pa_{CO_2} is 40 mm Hg and $P\bar{E}_{CO_2}$ is 27 mm Hg, the V_D/V_T ratio is 0.33. The Bohr equation requires a measurement of mixed expired gas. Alternatively, V_D/V_T can be estimated from the $\dot{V}_E$ and Pa_{CO_2} with an isopleth nomogram (**Figure 2–14**).

Physiologic dead space consists of the conducting airways (anatomic dead space) and the abnormally high $\dot{V}_A/\dot{Q}$ (underperfused) units in the gas exchange regions (alveolar dead space). CO_2 exchange between gas and blood does not occur in anatomic dead space. Its volume varies little in disease states but does vary moderately with V_T because airways dilate slightly with inspiration. The volume of anatomic dead space can be measured by the single-breath nitrogen washout technique. However, in clinical practice, measurement of anatomic dead space usually is not necessary because its size can be predicted (anatomic dead space in mL = ideal body weight in pounds). In patients receiving mechanical ventilation, the volume of anatomic dead

RESPIRATORY RECAP

Physiologic Mechanisms of Hypercapnia

- » Alveolar hypoventilation (increased dead space, decreased minute ventilation)
- » Severe $\dot{V}_A/\dot{Q}$ mismatch
- » Increased CO_2 production (only in patients with severe $\dot{V}_A/\dot{Q}$ abnormalities and borderline ventilatory reserve

space may be increased because of mechanical bronchodilation. Positive pressure ventilation also can increase dead space if tubing is added between the Y-adaptor and the artificial airway (mechanical dead space). An endotracheal tube or tracheostomy decreases anatomic dead space.

High-$\dot{V}_A/\dot{Q}$ units (alveolar dead space) are less efficient in CO_2 exchange than units with normal $\dot{V}_A/\dot{Q}$; that is, more overall ventilation is required to produce a given change in Pa_{CO_2}. In the sitting position, V_D/V_T is about 0.3 and varies little with age. It can increase to 0.6 or more in lung disease states characterized by increased number of high-$\dot{V}_A/\dot{Q}$ units, such as emphysema, shock, and pulmonary embolism. During exercise, V_D/V_T normally decreases to below 0.2 primarily because of an increase in V_T.[21] In disease states, V_D/V_T may not decrease to normal levels, and in severe cases it may even increase with exercise.[22]

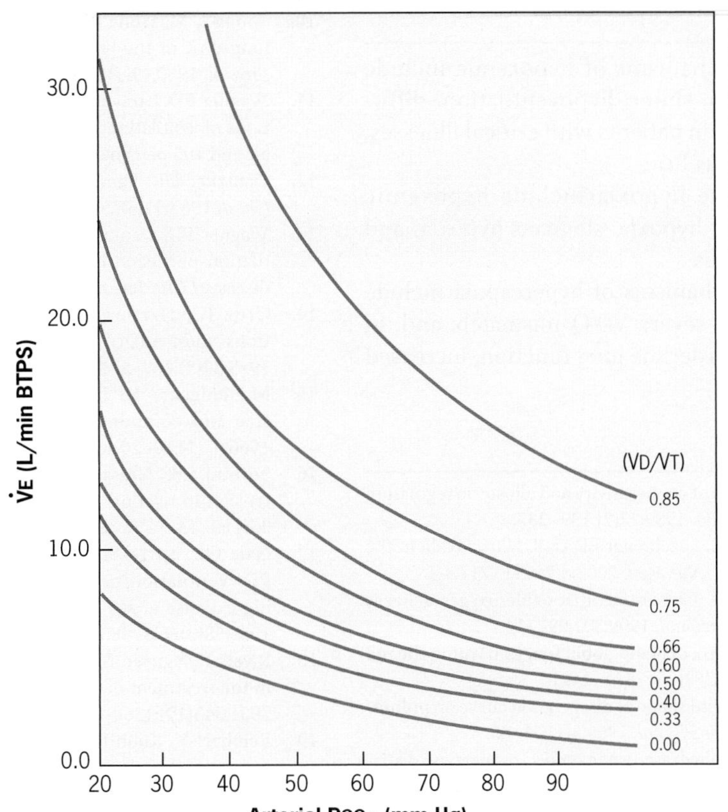

FIGURE 2–14 An isopleth nomogram used to estimate V_D/V_T from minute ventilation ($\dot{V}_E$) and arterial P_{CO_2}. Adapted from Baum GL, et al. *Textbook of Pulmonary Diseases*. 6th ed. Lippincott Williams & Wilkins; 1998.

Maldistribution of ventilation and perfusion usually does not cause hypercapnia, but CO_2 exchange is clearly affected by severe $\dot{V}_A/\dot{Q}$ mismatch. As $\dot{V}_A/\dot{Q}$ falls, local P_{CO_2} rises, reaching the value of the mixed venous P_{CO_2} at a $\dot{V}_A/\dot{Q}$ of 0. The resulting increase in P_{CO_2} is small (40 to 47 mm Hg), but CO_2 content changes considerably because of the steep slope of the CO_2 dissociation curve. Elimination of CO_2 retained in the blood due to high $\dot{V}_A/\dot{Q}$ usually is accomplished by alveoli with better blood flow. However, the poorly perfused alveoli must be ventilated alongside the units with better perfusion, which means total ventilation must increase to maintain a normal Pa_{CO_2}. The increase in ventilation occurs rapidly because of the sensitivity of central chemoreceptors to altered levels of Pa_{CO_2}.

The ventilatory work required for this compensation is usually small, as can be illustrated by the following extreme example. If one-half the cardiac output goes to alveoli that are no longer ventilated, the remaining alveoli would receive twice the normal amount of blood flow and would thus need to double their ventilation to prevent hypercapnia. This increased ventilation represents an increase over normal resting ventilation of about 25% to 30% to maintain a Pa_{CO_2} of about 30 mm Hg, which is only a small fraction of the normal ventilatory reserve. Obviously, this fraction is increased in individuals with limited ventilatory reserve. The ease of this compensation and the magnitude of normal ventilatory reserve account for the low incidence of hypercapnia in individuals with $\dot{V}_A/\dot{Q}$ mismatch. However, as the mismatch becomes greater, compensation becomes more difficult to achieve. In the previous example, if retained CO_2 were excreted in only 10% rather than 50% of the alveoli, a much higher $\dot{V}_A/\dot{Q}$ would be present in the compensating alveoli. In this circumstance a 200% increase in ventilation would be required to maintain normocapnia. Although normal ventilatory reserve is unlikely to be exceeded except in extreme $\dot{V}_A/\dot{Q}$ mismatch, the reserve may be minimal in disease. In addition, the work of breathing can be increased substantially in disease states. CO_2 produced by respiratory muscles may place an additional burden on the lungs when increments in ventilation require high levels of muscular work. Thus, a decreased ventilatory reserve combined with a high work of breathing and severe $\dot{V}_A/\dot{Q}$ mismatch can lead to hypercapnia. Occasionally an increase in CO_2 production (for example, caused by overfeeding) may cause hypercapnia in patients with severe $\dot{V}_A/\dot{Q}$ abnormalities and borderline ventilatory reserve.

KEY POINTS

- Physiologic mechanisms of hypoxemia include $\dot{V}A/\dot{Q}$ mismatch, shunt, hypoventilation, diffusion defect, and, in patients with critical illnesses, low mixed venous Po_2.
- Causes of tissue hypoxia include hypoxemic hypoxia, anemic hypoxia, stagnant hypoxia, and histotoxic hypoxia.
- Physiologic mechanisms of hypercapnia include hypoventilation, severe $\dot{V}A/\dot{Q}$ mismatch, and, in patients with borderline lung function, increased CO_2 production.

REFERENCES

1. Perutz MF. Mechanisms of cooperativity and allosteric regulation in proteins. *Q Rev Biophys.* 1989;22(2):139–237.
2. McMahon TJ, Moon RE, Luschinger BP, et al. Nitric oxide in the human respiratory cycle. *Nat Med.* 2002;8(7):711–717.
3. McMahon TJ, Stamler JS. Concerted nitric oxide/oxygen delivery by hemoglobin. *Meth Enzymol.* 1999;301:99–114.
4. Bunn HF, Jandl JH. Control of hemoglobin function within the red cell. *N Engl J Med.* 1970;282(25):1414–1421.
5. West JB. Effect of slope and shape of dissociation curve on pulmonary gas exchange. *Respir Physiol.* 1969;8(1):66–85.
6. Carter MJ. Carbonic anhydrase: isoenzymes, properties, distribution, and functional significance. *Biol Rev Camb Philos Soc.* 1972;47(4):465–513.
7. Knauf P. Anion transport in erythrocytes. In: Andreoli T, Hoffman J, Fanestil D, eds. *Physiology of Membrane Disorders.* 2nd ed. New York: Plenum Press; 1986.
8. Tanner MJ. Molecular and cellular biology of the erythrocyte anion exchanger (AE1). *Semin Hematol.* 1993;30(1):34–57.
9. Hedenstierna G, Hammond M, Mathieu-Costello O, Wagner PD. Functional lung unit in the pig. *Respir Physiol.* 2000; 120(2):139–149.
10. Young I, Mazzone RW, Wagner PD. Identification of functional lung unit in the dog by graded vascular embolization. *J Appl Physiol.* 1980;49(1):132–141.
11. Wagner PD, Laravuso RB, Uhl RR, West JB. Continuous distributions of ventilation-perfusion ratios in normal subjects breathing air and 100 percent O_2. *J Clin Invest.* 1974;54(1):54–68.
12. Dantzker DR. Ventilation-perfusion inequality in lung disease. *Chest.* 1987;91(5):749–754.
13. Wagner PD, Dantzker DR, Dueck R, Clausen JL, West JB. Ventilation-perfusion inequality in chronic obstructive pulmonary disease. *J Clin Invest.* 1977;59(2):203–216.
14. Cruz JC, Hartley LH, Vogel JA. Effect of altitude relocations upon $AaDo_2$ at rest and during exercise. *J Appl Physiol.* 1975;39(3):469–474.
15. Mellemgaard K. The alveolar-arterial oxygen difference: its size and components in normal man. *Acta Physiol Scand.* 1966;67(1):10–20.
16. Sorbini CA, Grassi V, Solinas E, Muiesan G. Arterial oxygen tension in relation to age in healthy subjects. *Respiration.* 1968; 25(1):3–13.
17. Gale GE, Torre-Bueno JR, Moon RE, Saltzman HA, Wagner PD. Ventilation-perfusion inequality in normal humans during exercise at sea level and simulated altitude. *J Appl Physiol.* 1985;58(3):978–988.
18. Rivers E, Nguyen B, Havstad S, et al. Early goal-directed therapy in the treatment of severe sepsis and septic shock. *N Engl J Med.* 2001;345(19):1368–1377.
19. Reinhart K, Kuhn HJ, Hartog C, Bredle DL. Continuous central venous and pulmonary artery oxygen saturation monitoring in the critically ill. *Intensive Care Med.* 2004;30(8):1572–1578.
20. Varpula M, Karlsson S, Ruokonen E, Pettila V. Mixed venous oxygen saturation cannot be estimated by central venous oxygen saturation in septic shock. *Intensive Care Med.* 2006; 32(9):1336–1343.
21. Murray J. *The Normal Lung.* Philadelphia: WB Saunders; 1986.
22. Jones N. Determinants of breathing patterns in exercise. In: Whipp B, Wasserman K, eds. *Exercise: Pulmonary Physiology and Pathophysiology.* New York: Marcel Dekker; 1991.

CHAPTER 3

Acid–Base Balance

Yuh-Chin T. Huang
Erika Lease
Will Beachey

OUTLINE

Physiology of Acid–Base Balance
Definition of Acid and Base
Concept of pH
Buffer Solutions
Henderson-Hasselbalch Equation
Base Excess
Anion Gap
Strong Ion Difference
Regulation of pH
Erythrocytes and Acid–Base Control
Acid Production and Excretion
Acid–Base Disorders
Interpretive Strategies for Acid–Base Disorders
Case Study

OBJECTIVES

1. Describe the concept of pH.
2. Describe buffer systems that are important physiologically.
3. Describe the Henderson-Hasselbalch equation.
4. Explain the strong ion difference.
5. Calculate the anion gap.
6. Compare the clinical significance of the alpha-stat and pH-stat approaches.
7. List causes of acid–base disorders.
8. Interpret arterial blood gas results in relation to acid–base disorders.

KEY TERMS

acid
alpha-stat hypothesis
anion gap
base
bicarbonate buffer system
buffer
carbonic acid (H_2CO_3)
Henderson-Hasselbalch equation
law of mass action
metabolic acidosis
metabolic alkalosis
pH
pH-stat hypothesis
respiratory acidosis
respiratory alkalosis
strong ion difference (SID)

INTRODUCTION

Acid–base disturbances are common in acutely ill patients. An important part of respiratory care practice is the identification and treatment of acid–base disturbance. This chapter defines acid and base physiology and lists causes of acid–base disorders.

Physiology of Acid–Base Balance

The human body generates various acids derived from metabolism. These acids are mainly **carbonic acid (H_2CO_3)** (200 mmol/kg body wt/24 hr) and acids of phosphate and sulfates (0.3–0.8 mEq/kg/24 hr). Carbonic acid is also called *volatile acid* because it is eliminated by the lungs as CO_2. The acids of phosphate and sulfates are also called *nonvolatile acids*. Nonvolatile acids can only be eliminated by the kidneys. *Acid–base balance* refers to physiologic mechanisms that regulate the hydrogen ion concentration $[H^+]$ of blood and body fluids within a range compatible with life. The lungs and the kidneys are the two primary organs essential in maintaining the acid–base balance.

Definition of Acid and Base

In a reaction that may proceed in either direction, the **law of mass action** may be written as follows:

$$[A] + [B] \leftrightarrow [C] + [D]$$

The reactions have rate constants for both the forward (k_1, $A + B \rightarrow C + D$) and reverse (k_2, $C + D \rightarrow A + B$) directions, which determine the concentrations of reactants until chemical equilibrium is reached, when the following occurs:

$$\frac{k_1}{k_2} = \frac{[C][D]}{[A][B]}$$

The term k_1/k_2 is the equilibrium constant K_{eq}.

An **acid** (HA) is any substance that donates a proton $[H^+]$ to an aqueous solution (proton donor). It dissociates completely or partially into a hydrogen ion, $[H^+]$, and its conjugate base, A^-:

$$HA \leftrightarrow H^+ + A^-$$

The acidity or pH of the solution depends on the concentration of dissociated $[H^+]$. The degree to which an acid dissociates depends on its dissociation constant (K_a):

$$K_a = \frac{[H^+][A^-]}{[HA]}$$

K_a determines the concentration of $[H^+]$. If the acid is strong, K_a is large and $[H^+]$ and [A] are much higher than [HA]. One example of strong acid is hydrochloric acid (HCl), which has a K_a of nearly infinity. In solution, nearly 100% of HCl molecules dissociate to form $[H^+]$ and $[Cl^-]$:

$$HCl \leftrightarrow H^+ + Cl^-$$

A 0.1 N (or 0.1 mEq/L) HCl solution would contain 0.1 mEq/L of $[H^+]$.

In contrast, a weak acid has a small K_a. For example, acetic acid is a weak acid with a K_a of 1.8×10^{-5}. In solution, only a portion of acetic acid molecules dissociate to form $[H^+]$ and $[\text{acetate}^-]$:

$$\text{Acetic acid} \leftrightarrow H^+ + \text{Acetate}$$

A 0.1 N acetic acid solution would contain about 0.0013 mEq/L of $[H^+]$.

A **base** is any substance that accepts a proton $[H^+]$ from an aqueous solution (proton acceptor). It dissociates completely or partially into its component ions, $[OH^-]$ and $[B^+]$:

$$BOH \leftrightarrow OH^- + B^+$$

A solution that contains a base is also frequently referred to as an *alkaline solution*. The strength or alkalinity of a base depends on the degree to which it dissociates in solution. A strong base has a greater affinity to H^+, whereas a weak base has a lesser affinity to H^+. One example of a strong base is sodium hydroxide (NaOH). It dissociates almost completely in solution:

$$NaOH \leftrightarrow Na^+ + OH^-$$

In the body, most of the bases are present as the conjugate base of an acid (i.e., A^- in the earlier equation). Strong acids have weak conjugate bases, so most H^+ is in the free ionized form (weak proton acceptors). On the other hand, weak acids have strong conjugate bases that bind most of the available H^+ so that little remains in the free ionized form (strong proton acceptors).

Concept of pH

The concept of pH was developed by Sørenson in 1909. **pH** is defined as the negative logarithm or exponent (to the base 10) of the $[H^+]$:

$$pH = -\log[H^+]$$

The dissociation of pure water molecules (H_2O or HOH) into H^+ and OH^- helps explain this concept.

$$H_2O \leftrightarrow H^+ + OH^-$$
$$K_a = [H^+] \times [OH^-]/[H_2O]$$

Because water's K_a is exceedingly small, very little $[H^+]$ and $[OH^-]$ are present in the solution. This equation can be rearranged to yield the following:

$$[H^+] \times [OH^-] = [H_2O] \times K_a$$

Because $[H_2O]$ is basically a constant (very little dissociation), $[H_2O] \times K_a$ is also a constant (K_w). The numerical value of K_w is about 10^{-14}. Therefore, at equilibrium, pure water contains 10^{-7} mol/L of H^+ and 10^{-7} mol/L of OH^-. The pH of water, which contains $[H^+]$ of 10^{-7} mol/L (or 100 nmol/L), would be

$$pH = -\log(10^{-7}) = -(-7) = 7$$

The pH scale ranges from 0 to 14 pH units. Because pH is the negative logarithm of $[H^+]$, a decrease in pH indicates an increase in $[H^+]$, and vice versa. **Table 3–1** shows the approximate relationship between pH and $[H^+]$.

In chemistry, when a solution has a pH of 7.0, we call it a *neutral solution* (neither acidic nor basic). A solution with a pH less than 7.0 is called *acidic*; a solution with a

TABLE 3-1 Approximate Relationship Between pH and $[H^+]$

pH	$[H^+]$ nmol/L
6.80	158
6.90	126
7.00	100
7.10	79
7.15	71
7.20	63
7.25	56
7.30	50
7.35	45
7.40	40
7.45	35
7.50	32
7.55	28
7.60	25
7.70	20
7.80	16
8.0	10

Modified from Beachey W. *Respiratory Care Anatomy and Physiology.* 2nd ed. Copyright Elsevier (Mosby) 2007.

pH greater than 7.0 is called *alkaline*. The normal pH of the blood is slightly alkaline (7.4), which corresponds to $[H^+]$ of 40×10^{-9} mol/L, or 40 nmol/L.

Buffer Solutions

A **buffer** is any that contains either a weak acid and its conjugate base or a weak base with its conjugated acid. A buffer solution can resist a big change in $[H^+]$, and therefore in pH, when an acid or a base is added. An example of a buffer solution is the carbonic acid and its conjugate base, HCO_3^-, or bicarbonate. The dissociation of carbonic acid is as follows:

$$H_2CO_3 \leftrightarrow HCO_3^- + H^+$$

If a strong acid, hydrochloric acid (HCl), is added to the carbonic acid/sodium bicarbonate ($NaHCO_3$) buffer solution, bicarbonate ions will react with the added H^+ to form more carbonic acid and a neutral salt (NaCl):

$$HCl + H_2CO_3/Na + HCO_3^- \rightarrow H_2CO_3 + NaCl$$

The strong acidity of HCl is thus converted to the relatively weak acidity of H_2CO_3, preventing a large drop in pH.

TABLE 3-2 Buffer Systems in Different Body Compartments

Site	Buffer System
Interstitial fluid	Bicarbonate Phosphates Proteins
Blood	Bicarbonate Hemoglobin (in red blood cells) Plasma proteins Phosphates
Intracellular fluid	Proteins Phosphates Bicarbonate
Bone	Calcium carbonate

When a strong base, sodium hydroxide (NaOH), is added, it will react with the carbonic acid to form bicarbonate (HCO_3^-) and water:

$$NaOH + H_2CO_3/Na + HCO_3^- \rightarrow NaHCO_3 + H_2O$$

According to this reaction, OH^- from NaOH will react with H^+ to form H_2O; in the process, the strong base, NaOH, is changed to a relatively weak base, $NaHCO_3$, minimizing the large increase in pH that would have otherwise been caused by the addition of NaOH.

RESPIRATORY RECAP

Acids, Bases, and Buffer

- An acid donates a proton in solution.
- A base accepts a proton in solution.
- pH is a measure of hydrogen ion concentration.
- A buffer minimizes the change in pH when a strong acid or strong base is added.

The body has several buffer systems within its extracellular (intravascular and interstitial) and intracellular compartments (**Table 3-2**). The main buffering systems are (1) bicarbonate in plasma, interstitial, and intracellular water and carbonate in bone; (2) intracellular proteins, including hemoglobin in red blood cells; (3) plasma proteins; and (4) intracellular and extracellular phosphates. The extent to which each buffer contributes to the defense of body pH varies with differing kinds of acid–base disturbances. **Table 3-3** shows the individual buffers' contributions to total buffering capacity in whole blood.

Among all the buffering systems, the **bicarbonate buffer system** is the most important because it is present in appreciable quantities in nearly all body fluids and is readily available to stabilize pH. Bicarbonate differs from other body buffers in that the product of its reaction with H^+ is H_2CO_3, an acid that can be converted to CO_2 and eliminated by the lung as a gas. The reaction between H_2CO_3 and $H_2O + CO_2$ is facilitated by an enzyme called carbonic anhydrase. The carbonic acid is sometimes referred to as volatile acid.

$$H^+ + HCO_3^- \rightarrow HCO_3 \rightarrow H_2O + CO_2$$

TABLE 3–3 Individual Buffer Contributions to Whole Blood Buffering

Buffer Type	Percentage of Total Buffering
Bicarbonate	53
Plasma bicarbonate	35
Erythrocyte bicarbonate	18
Nonbicarbonate	47
Hemoglobin	35
Organic phosphates	3
Inorganic phosphates	2
Plasma proteins	7
Total	100

Modified from Beachey W. *Respiratory Care Anatomy and Physiology.* 2nd ed. Copyright Elsevier (Mosby) 2007.

The body also produces nonvolatile acids, which are acids other than carbonic acid. They are produced from an incomplete metabolism of carbohydrates, fats, and proteins. Common nonvolatile acids in humans are lactic acid, phosphoric acid, sulfuric acid, acetoacetic acid, and beta-hydroxybutyric acid. When nonvolatile acids are added to the body, they lower the HCO_3^-. On average, approximately 24,000 mmol/day of H^+ is from volatile acid (carbonic acid) and is eliminated by the lungs. Only about 50 mmol/day of H^+ is from nonvolatile acids and is eliminated by the kidneys.

Henderson-Hasselbalch Equation

In 1909, Lawrence J. Henderson used the law of mass action to express the hydrogen ion equilibrium (**Equation 3–1**). Using the convention in which $[H^+]$ is expressed as pH, Hasselbalch rearranged Henderson's equation and applied it to the carbonic acid buffer system. The **Henderson-Hasselbalch equation** accurately describes the equilibrium relationships among pH, P_{CO_2}, and HCO_3^-. Because the P_{CO_2} of the arterial blood is regulated by alveolar ventilation, it is used to indicate the respiratory component of the acid–base state. The $[HCO_3^-]$ is an estimate of the nonrespiratory, or metabolic, component of the acid–base state. However, the Henderson-Hasselbalch equation does not describe the regulation of acid–base balance in that the bicarbonate buffer system is influenced by the independent and direct effect of P_{CO_2} on $[HCO_3^-]$. Thus, changes in $[HCO_3^-]$ do not indicate metabolic changes alone.

Base Excess

The concept of base excess was introduced by Siggaard-Andersen, from Copenhagen, in the late 1950s. *Base excess* is defined as the amount of strong acid (in mmol/L) that must be added to the blood sample in vitro to return the sample to pH 7.40 after equilibration while maintaining the partial pressure of carbon dioxide at 40 mm Hg. If blood has a pH of 7.40 and a P_{CO_2} of 40 mm Hg, the base excess will be 0 mmol/L. Siggaard-Andersen developed a nomogram to determine base excess in the clinical setting (**Figure 3–1**). This nomogram was later incorporated into blood gas analyzers to allow automatic calculation.

The base excess approach produced the concept of excess $[HCO_3^-]$ in arterial plasma that accounts for changes in the metabolic component of acid–base disorders. However, the concept of base excess did not hold up when applied to whole blood or plasma changes in vivo. First, plasma in vivo is in contiguity with interstitial fluid that has less buffer capacity. The base excess approach deals with this argument by assuming a hemoglobin concentration of 50 g/L, thus reducing the apparent buffer capacity of the blood in vitro. This issue requires standardization of in vitro data to whole blood with a constant hemoglobin concentration. Second, in patients with chronic elevation of P_{CO_2}, the base excess approach would have diagnosed a coexisting alkalinizing metabolic process decreasing the acidity. Despite its deficiencies, base excess is still used in some clinical settings because of its simplicity.

EQUATION 3–1

The Henderson-Hasselbalch Equation

$$pH = pKa + \log\frac{[HCO_3^-]}{[CO_2]}$$

This is the Henderson equation, which can be rearranged as follows:

$$[H^+] = 24 \times \frac{P_{CO_2}}{[HCO_3^-]}$$

where $[H^+]$ is in nEq/L, P_{CO_2} is in mm Hg, and $[HCO_3^-]$ is in mmol/L. This is the Hasselbalch equation.

Because the pKa of carbonic acid is 6.1 and the solubility constant for CO_2 in plasma is 0.0301, the Henderson-Hasselbalch equation is as follows:

$$pH = 6.1 + \log\frac{[HCO_3^-]}{0.0301 \times P_{CO_2}}$$

Anion Gap

The **anion gap** (AG) represents the concentration of all the unmeasured anions in the plasma. AG is calculated from the following formula:

$$\text{Anion gap} = [Na^+] - ([Cl^-] + [HCO_3^-])$$

The normal anion gap is 12 ± 4 mmol/L and is mostly caused by negatively charged plasma proteins, sulfate, and phosphate. An increased anion gap represents additional unmeasured anions, which can be endogenous, such as lactate or ketones, or exogenous, such as salicylate. When excessive acid anions are produced during metabolic acidosis, the H^+ produced reacts with bicarbonate anions (buffering), and the CO_2 produced is excreted via the lungs (respiratory compensation). The net effect is a decrease in the concentration of measured anions (i.e., HCO_3^-) and an increase in the concentration of unmeasured anions (the acid anions), so the anion gap increases.

The anion gap is useful clinically to signal the presence of a metabolic acidosis during the interpretation of acid–base disorder, to help differentiate between causes of a metabolic acidosis (high anion gap versus normal anion gap metabolic acidosis), and to assist in assessing the biochemical severity of the acidosis and follow the response to treatment (e.g., during the treatment of diabetic ketoacidosis). AG can also be lower than normal in myeloma in which immunoglobulin G (IgG) paraproteins increase. These paraproteins act as weak bases because of the basic amino acids, lysine and arginine, which have isoelectric points close to pH = 9.0. They thus have a weak positive charge in the physiologic pH range.

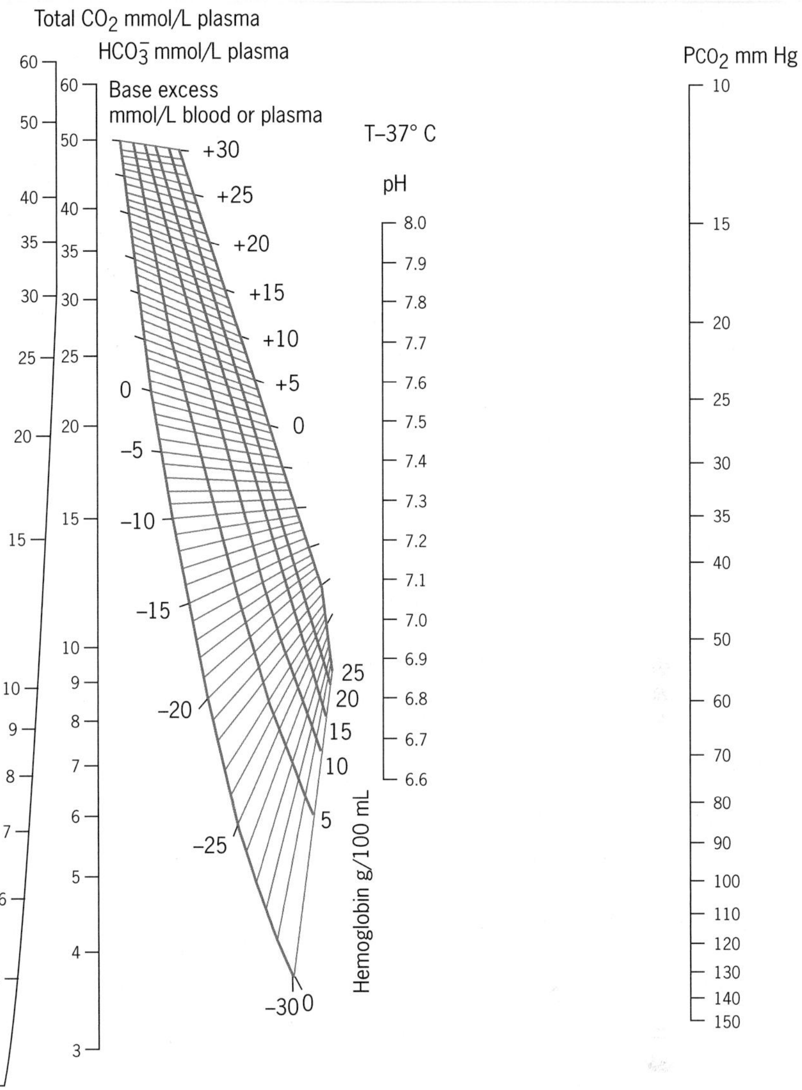

FIGURE 3–1 Siggaard-Andersen alignment nomogram. (1) A line is constructed between pH and P_{CO_2}. (2) Actual plasma is read directly at the intersection of the line. (3) Base excess is hemoglobin dependent and can be read at the intersection of the constructed line and the patient's hemoglobin value. (4) Standard value can be determined via construction of another line through the base excess–hemoglobin point and a P_{CO_2} of 40 mm Hg and by reading of the scale. (5) Buffer base can be computed from the equation BB = 41.7 + (0.42 × Hb) + BE. Modified with permission from Mahoney JJ, Hodgkin J, Van Kessel A. Arterial blood gas analysis. In: Burton G, Hodgkin J, Ward J, eds. *Respiratory Care: A Guide to Clinical Practice.* Lippincott Williams & Wilkins; 1997.

Clinical correlation should always be used to interpret AG. For examples, lactic acidosis with a lactate level of 5 to 10 mmol/L can be associated with sepsis, but the AG may be within the reference range in as many as 50% of these cases.[1] There are several reasons why this may occur. First, the lactate may not be high enough to push the anion gap out of the reference range. Second, administration of large amounts of intravenous saline solution (NaCl) in septic shock may increase the levels of chloride and thus decrease AG. Third, in lactic acidosis, plasma lactate may move intracellularly in exchange for chloride via an antiporter. This contributes to an increase in chloride concentration in the plasma, decreasing the AG. Finally, albumin, the major unmeasured anion contributing to the value of the anion gap, may be low in patients with septic shock and lactic acidosis. Because every gram decrease in albumin will decrease the anion gap by 2.5 to 3 mmol/L, a high anion gap lactic acidosis may appear as a normal anion gap acidosis in a patient with hypoalbuminemia.

Strong Ion Difference

Based on the bicarbonate-centered approach of acid–base balance, it appears that the concentrations of $[H^+]$ and $[HCO_3^-]$ are the main forces regulating acid–base problems. However, such thinking is obviously incorrect. For example, in a strong alkaline solution there are almost no hydrogen ions present; thus, $[H^+]$ cannot be responsible for the behavior of the alkaline solution. In addition, as mentioned earlier, both respiratory and metabolic changes affect the $[HCO_3^-]$; thus, CO_2 and

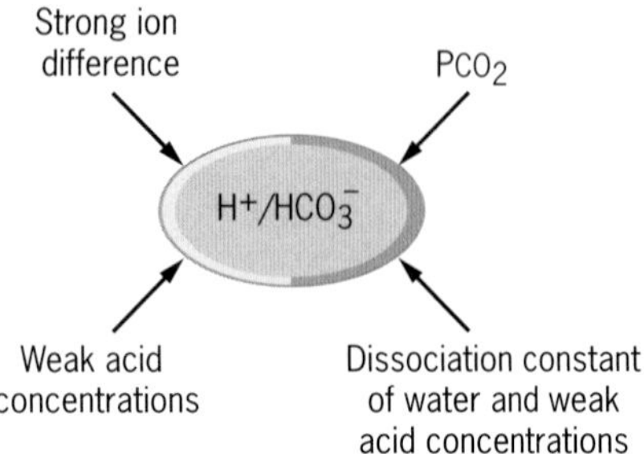

FIGURE 3–2 Important factors in the control of hydrogen and bicarbonate ions using the Stewart approach (strong ion difference). Modified from Story DA, et al. Bench-to-bedside review. A brief history of clinical acid-base. *Crit Care.* 2004;8:253. Reproduced with permission.

bicarbonate in the Henderson-Hasselbalch equation are not independently regulated. Recognizing these deficiencies of the bicarbonate-centered approach, Peter Stewart introduced an alternate approach to acid–base physiology and disorders in the early 1980s based on principles of electroneutrality, conservation of mass, and dissociation of electrolytes. The Stewart model has three independent variables controlling pH: **strong ion difference (SID)**, the total weak acid concentrations, and $P\text{CO}_2$ (**Figure 3–2**).[2,3]

In physiologic fluids the main strong electrolytes are Na^+, K^+, and Cl^-. These strong ions influence $[H^+]$ by the law of electrical neutrality and the dissociation of water, meaning that the net charge must be zero in any system at equilibrium. Thus, in a solution of Na^+, K^+, and Cl^- in water, $[Na^+] + [K^+] + [H^+] - [Cl^-] - [OH^-] = 0$. The effect of strong ions may be lumped into a single term that expresses the net negative or positive charge that they exert. This is the [SID]. In plasma, [SID] is normally calculated as follows:

$$[SID] = [Na^+] + [K^+] - [Cl^-]$$

Strong organic ions, such as lactate or ketones, normally are present in very low concentration and their effects on [SID] are minimal. In metabolic acidosis, these anions can be present in high concentrations and exert more significant effects on [SID]. Other strong inorganic ions are usually ignored because they are present in low concentrations. Therefore, $[SID] + [H^+] - [OH^-] = 0$, where the independent variable is [SID] and the dependent variables are $[H^+]$ and $[OH^-]$. In normal plasma, $[Na^+]$ is 140 mmol/L, $[K^+]$ is 4 mmol/L, and $[Cl^-]$ is 104 mmol/L. Thus, the normal [SID] is approximately 40 mmol/L.

RESPIRATORY RECAP

Anion Gap and Strong Ion Gap

- The anion gap is useful in the interpretation of acid–base disorders.
- Anion gap should be corrected for albumin concentration.
- The Stewart model has three independent variables controlling pH: strong ion difference, the total weak acid concentration, and $P\text{CO}_2$.

Total weak acids (A_{tot}) are all buffers present in a partially dissociated state in the physiologic pH range. Weak acids have dissociation constant (K_a) values between 10^{-4} and 10^{-12}. However, only those with K_a close to 4×10^{-8} (pH = 7.4) are effective buffers. These buffer systems include plasma proteins ($K_a = 3 \times 10^{-7}$), proteins and phosphates in cells ($K_a = 5.5 \times 10^{-7}$), and hemoglobin in red blood cells ($K_a = 2.5 \times 10^{-7}$ for oxyhemoglobin; 6.3×10^{-9} for deoxyhemoglobin). The effectiveness of weak acids as buffers depends not only on the dissociation constant but also on $[A_{tot}]$, which is the sum of the dissociated (A^-) and undissociated (HA) forms:

$$[A_{tot}] \text{ (mmol/L)} = [HA] + [A^-]$$

In this equation, $[A_{tot}]$ is an independent variable and [HA] and $[A^-]$ are dependent variables. In plasma, $[A_{tot}]$ represents the ionic equivalent of the plasma proteins and may be estimated via multiplication of the protein content by 0.24. Thus, at a normal total protein of 70 g/L, $[A_{tot}]$ is 0.24×70, or 17 mmol/L. This value comprises $[A^-]$ of 15 mmol/L and [HA] of 2 mmol/L at pH = 7.4. Even though plasma proteins behave as weak acids, they are mostly dissociated (15/17, or approximately 90%) at normal arterial pH.

The last independent variable in Stewart's model is $P\text{CO}_2$. The variations in $P\text{CO}_2$ and $[H^+]$ alter total CO_2 content, which then governs how the bicarbonate buffer system acts.

Variations in the relative magnitude of the independent variables involved in control of acid–base status produce differing effects in different fluid compartments and tissues. In intracellular fluids, [SID] is large and dominated by a high $[K^+]$. High protein and phosphate concentrations ($[A_{tot}]$) also minimize the effects of reductions in [SID] resulting from falls in $[K^+]$ or accumulation of strong organic ions, such as lactate. In tissues, $P\text{CO}_2$ is high and increases by metabolism, but $[HCO_3^-]$ is low. Changes in $P\text{CO}_2$ influence $[H^+]$ in tissues much less than in plasma. Control of intracellular $[H^+]$ is achieved through buffering and exchange of strong ions with extracellular fluid, thereby changing [SID], and through diffusion of CO_2 from the cell. In interstitial fluid and other ultrafiltrates of plasma, such as lymph or cerebrospinal fluid, $[H^+]$ is influenced only by changes in [SID] and $P\text{CO}_2$ because protein is virtually absent and the weak acid system does not have a role. In plasma, [SID] also tends to regulate the pH, but variations in $P\text{CO}_2$ may bring about large and rapid changes in arterial $[H^+]$.

The SID approach appears to provide more straightforward explanations than the bicarbonate-centered approaches for many acid–base phenomena seen in the critical care setting.[1–4] This includes explanations for metabolic alkalosis associated with decreased plasma albumin concentrations,[5,6] the mechanism of hyperchloremic acidosis,[7] and the role of ammonia in acid–base homeostasis.[3] The SID approach also refines detecting unmeasured ions, or the anion gap. The traditionally defined anion gap does not take into account the large changes in plasma albumin concentration often seen in critically ill patients. Unless a correction factor is used, an increased anion gap may go unrecognized.[4,8] This has led to the concept of albumin-corrected anion gap.[9] Anion gap is reduced by approximately 2.5 mmol/L for every 1 g/dL fall in albumin:

$$\text{Anion gap (corrected)} = \text{Anion gap} + 2.5\,(4.2 - [\text{Albumin}])$$

The SID approach may also provide a better understanding of the various management strategies, including fluid management,[7,10,11] buffer therapy,[12] and renal replacement therapy.[13] Although well supported by clinical evidence, the SID approach is more difficult to use in everyday clinical practice. There is currently no clear strategy to determine which of the modern approaches, the SID approach or the bicarbonate-centered approach, is the better one.

Regulation of pH

It is important to bear in mind that the arterial blood gas measures pH in the blood, a compartment of extracellular fluid (ECF). The normal pH of arterial blood (7.40) is slightly higher than that of capillary and venous blood (about 7.36). The pH of most remaining ECF is virtually identical to that of capillaries and venous blood because H^+ can permeate across the endothelial barrier. The pH of intracellular fluid (ICF) is lower and ranges from 6.8 to 7.2. Extracellular pH is maintained at 0.6 to 0.8 pH units higher than the prevailing intracellular pH at any given temperature, thereby providing a sink for disposal of the acids produced by intracellular metabolism. The control mechanism for this constant pH gradient is called the **alpha-stat hypothesis**.

The alpha-stat hypothesis, first proposed by Rahn and colleagues, states that the degree of ionization (alpha) of the imidazole groups of intracellular proteins remains constant despite change in temperature. The pH of neutrality varies inversely with temperature, increasing from 6.8 at 37° C (98.6° F) and 7.0 at 25° C (77° F) to nearly 7.5 at 0° C (32° F). Rahn and colleagues have proposed that, in living systems, regulatory mechanisms attempt to keep intracellular pH at or very close to the neutrality of water (pH when $[H^+] = [OH^-]$).[3,14]

The importance of the alpha-stat concept can be illustrated by the following example. During exercise on a cold day, an individual's core temperature is 37° C, and intracellular and blood pH are 6.8 and 7.4, respectively. The intracellular Pco_2 is 40 mm Hg. In the exercising muscle, the temperature is 41° C (105.8° F) and Pco_2 is 48 mm Hg (due to increased metabolism), but intracellular and blood pH decrease to 6.7 and 7.35, respectively. In the skin, the temperature is cooled to 25° C and intracellular Pco_2 is 22 mm Hg, but intracellular and blood pH increase to 7.0 and 7.6, respectively. Thus, despite these striking regional variations in pH and Pco_2, the relative alkalinity, or the net charge of imidazole buffer, between cells and blood is maintained throughout the body.

The alpha-stat hypothesis is in contrast to the **pH-stat hypothesis**. The pH-stat hypothesis argues that the pH should be kept constant despite changes in temperature. This is the same as saying that ECF pH should be kept at 7.4 regardless of what the temperature is.

The clinical significance of whether to use the alpha-stat or the pH-stat hypothesis can be illustrated in the problem of whether to temperature correct blood gas results. The pH-stat approach is implicitly the approach used by anyone who corrects blood gas results to the patient's temperature but who interprets the values against the reference range relevant to 37° C. Even though no reference range is available for temperatures other than 37° C, pH-stat proponents assume that the reference range for 37° C is valid at all temperatures. The alpha-stat approach is to never temperature correct blood gas results because the pH and Pco_2 values at 37° C reliably reflect the in vivo acid–base status of the patient. In addition, most acid–base nomograms are valid only at 37° C, and temperature correction does not improve clinical decision making.

Another clinical example of the difference between the alpha-stat and pH-stat hypotheses can be seen in the management of induced hypothermia. A patient is cooled to 20° C (68° F) for cardiac surgery while on cardiac bypass. An arterial blood sample drawn and analyzed at 20° C has pH 7.65 and Pco_2 18 mm Hg. If this same sample is analyzed at 37° C, the values would be pH 7.4 and Pco_2 40 mm Hg. So which values are correct? The values done at 37° C can be interpreted against the known reference values for 37° C and would be considered to be normal. This is the alpha-stat approach. The pH-stat approach would interpret the values for 20° C against the reference values for 37° C. This would lead to the conclusion that this patient has a significant respiratory alkalosis and that some intervention needs to be taken to correct this.

It seems that the alpha-stat theory has gained much wider acceptance than the pH-stat approach. The alpha-stat hypothesis emphasizes the importance of maintaining alpha so that the net charge on all proteins is kept constant despite changes in temperature. This ensures that all proteins, especially enzymes, can function optimally despite temperature changes. Nonetheless, it is still unclear whether patients managed by the alpha-stat approach have major differences in outcome compared with those managed by the pH-stat approach.

Erythrocytes and Acid–Base Control

Erythrocytes contain hemoglobin, which offers large buffering capacity by the imidazole group of the histidine residues, which has a pKa of about 6.8. This is suitable for effective buffering at physiologic pH. Hemoglobin in red blood cells (RBCs) is quantitatively about six times more important than the plasma proteins as a buffer because it is present in about twice the concentration and contains about three times the number of histidine residues per molecule. For example, if blood pH changes from 7.5 to 6.5, hemoglobin would buffer 27.5 mmol/L of H^+, and total plasma protein buffering would account for only 4.2 mmol/L of H^+.

When O_2 dissociates from hemoglobin (deoxygenation), $[H^+]$ inside the erythrocyte decreases. As CO_2 enters the erythrocyte, it reacts with water to form carbonic acid. The carbonic anhydrase in the erythrocyte enables the hydration of CO_2 to proceed rapidly. The carbonic acid then ionizes to form H^+ and HCO_3^-. The H^+ offsets the decrease in H^+ during the deoxygenation process. HCO_3^- formed during the process moves out of the cell and Cl^- moves into the cell, a phenomenon called *chloride shift*. This exchange process is mediated by a transmembrane protein called anion exchange protein I (AEI) or band 3 protein. CO_2 that enters the erythrocytes also binds at the αNH_2 groups of the β chain of hemoglobin, forming carbamates very rapidly. This reaction is also facilitated by deoxygenation of hemoglobin.

Deoxyhemoglobin (T form) is a more effective buffer at physiologic pH than oxyhemoglobin (R form) because of its smaller K_a (1.4×10^{-8} for deoxyhemoglobin and 2.5×10^{-7} for oxyhemoglobin), which allows deoxyhemoglobin to buffer venous acidity more effectively. This phenomenon is called the *isohydric exchange*; that is, the buffer system ($HHbO_2-HbO_2^-$) is converted to another more effective buffer ($HHb-Hb^-$) exactly at the site where an increased buffering capacity is required. By these mechanisms, erythrocytes can buffer sudden changes in ions or P_{CO_2} and help maintain relatively constant conditions in plasma and ECF. Clinically, RBC transfusion not only increases oxygen delivery by increasing hemoglobin but also provides essential buffer for the management of metabolic acidosis.

Acid Production and Excretion

Approximately 24,000 mmol/day of H^+ is generated from volatile acid (carbonic acid) and 50 mmol/day of H^+ from nonvolatile acids. The volatile acid is eliminated by the lungs in the form of CO_2, whereas nonvolatile acid is eliminated by the kidneys. Thus the lungs and the kidneys are the two main organs responsible for acid–base control.

The Lungs and Acid–Base Control

Oxidative metabolism produces CO_2, forming H_2CO_3. Because H_2CO_3 is in equilibrium with dissolved CO_2, the lungs can lower blood H_2CO_3 by eliminating CO_2 through ventilation. Thus, through eliminating CO_2 via the exhaled gas, the lungs can produce rapid changes in pH.

The amount of CO_2 elimination, which is proportional to alveolar ventilation, can be reflected by the Pa_{CO_2} through the alveolar ventilation equation:

$$Pa_{CO_2} = 0.863 \times \dot{V}_{CO_2}/\dot{V}_A$$

This equation is useful because neither metabolic rate nor ventilation needs to be measured to assess the adequacy of breathing in relation to metabolic demand. One can just examine P_{CO_2} in arterial blood, which represents the balance between metabolic CO_2 production and ventilation. In tissues and venous blood, P_{CO_2} reflects primarily the balance between metabolism and blood flow. The extent to which arterial P_{CO_2} reflects the adequacy of ventilation also depends on carbonic anhydrase activity in allowing rapid equilibration of P_{CO_2} between pulmonary capillary blood and alveolar gas. Thus Pa_{CO_2} is increased by drugs that inhibit carbonic anhydrase, such as acetazolamide.

The ventilatory responses to acid–base disorders of nonrespiratory origin are extremely important in the regulation of $[H^+]$ because they change rapidly. The control system for respiratory regulation of acid–base balance can be considered using the model of a simple servo control system. The components of such a simple model are a controlled variable that is monitored by a sensor, a central integrator that interprets the information from the sensor, and an effector mechanism that can alter the controlled variable (**Table 3–4**). In long-term responses to acid–base disturbances, the response of the central medullary chemoreceptors is the most important factor in the ventilatory set point. The central medullary chemoreceptors respond to the $[H^+]$ in cerebrospinal fluid (CSF).

The Kidneys and Acid–Base Control

The kidneys are responsible for excretion of the fixed acids (nonvolatile acids). These acids amount to about 70 to 100 mmol/day. The kidneys also play an important role in the reabsorption of the filtered bicarbonate. Daily

TABLE 3–4 Control System for Respiratory Regulation of Acid–Base Balance

Control Element	Physiologic or Anatomic Correlate	Comments
Controlled variable	Arterial P_{CO_2}	A change in arterial P_{CO_2} alters arterial pH (as calculated by the Henderson-Hasselbalch equation).
Sensors	Central and peripheral chemoreceptors	Both respond to changes in arterial P_{CO_2} (as well as some other factors).
Central integrator	The respiratory center in the medulla	
Effectors	The respiratory muscles	An increase in minute ventilation increases alveolar ventilation and thus decreases arterial P_{CO_2}. The net result is of negative feedback that tends to restore the P_{CO_2} to the set point.

filtered bicarbonate equals the product of the daily glomerular filtration rate (180 L/day) and the plasma bicarbonate concentration (24 mmol/L). This is 180 × 24 = 4320 mmol/day. About 85% to 90% of the filtered bicarbonate is reabsorbed in the proximal tubule, and the rest is reabsorbed by the intercalated cells of the distal tubule and collecting ducts.

Proximal Tubules

The proximal tubules are the main site for bicarbonate reabsorption. The mechanisms for bicarbonate reabsorption are shown in **Figure 3–3**. Four major factors regulate bicarbonate reabsorption: luminal HCO_3^- concentration, luminal flow rate, arterial Pco_2, and angiotensin II (via decrease in cyclic AMP). An increase in any of the following four factors causes an increase in bicarbonate reabsorption: luminal HCO_3^- concentration, luminal flow rate, arterial Pco_2, and angiotensin II (via decrease in cyclic AMP).

Besides reabsorbing bicarbonate, proximal renal tubules also produce ammonium (NH_3). NH_3 is produced from glutamine by the action of the enzyme glutaminase and from glutamate during the conversion to alpha-ketoglutarate. Since the pKa for NH_3 is very high (about 9.2), NH_3 is present entirely in the acid form, ammonium ion, or NH_4^+. NH_4^+ is not measured as part of the titratable acidity. About 75% of the proximally produced ammonium is removed from the tubular fluid in the medulla so that the amount of ammonium entering the distal tubule is small. A low urine pH greatly increases the ammonium excretion. This ammonium excretion is augmented further if an acidosis is present. This augmentation with acidosis helps restore extracellular pH toward normal.

Loop of Henle

HCO_3^- in the thick ascending limb of the loop of Henle is reabsorbed via mechanisms very similar to those in the proximal tubule (i.e., apical Na^+-H^+ antiporter, basolateral $Na^+-HCO_3^-$ co-transporter and Na^+-K+ ATPase exchanger). The cells in this part of the tubule also contain carbonic anhydrase. Bicarbonate reabsorption here is stimulated by the presence of luminal furosemide.

Distal Tubules

Compared with the proximal tubules, the distal renal tubules have a lower capacity for excreting the daily fixed acid load (≈70 mmol/day), although the capacity can increase to as much as 700 mmol/day. The maximal capacity of 700 mmol/day takes about 5 days to reach. The distal tubules can decrease the pH to about 4.5, thus creating a thousandfold (or 3 pH units) gradient for H^+ across the distal tubular cell. The distal tubules excrete H^+ by reabsorbing the remaining bicarbonate and adding ammonium (NH_4^+) to luminal fluid.

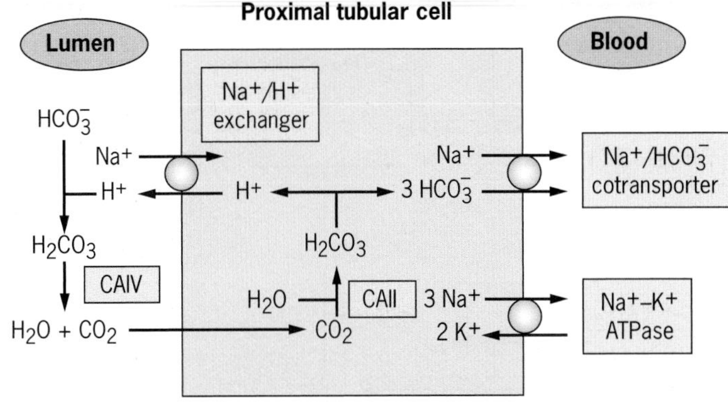

FIGURE 3–3 Schematic representation of the excretion of H^+ in the proximal renal tubules. The Na^+ is reabsorbed in exchange for H^+ via a Na^+–H^+ antiporter. The H^+ reacts with HCO_3^- to form H_2O and CO_2 under the influence of brush border carbonic anhydrase V (CAIV). CO_2, which is lipid soluble, then diffuses into the tubular cell. In the cell, CO_2 combines with H_2O to produce HCO_3^-. This process is also facilitated by carbonic anhydrase II (CAII). The HCO_3^- crosses the basolateral membrane via a Na^+–HCO_3^- co-transporter, which transfers three HCO_3^- for every one Na^+. The basolateral membrane also has an active Na^+–K^+ ATPase (sodium pump), which transports three Na^+ out per two K^+ in. This pump is electrogenic in a direction opposite to that of the Na^+–HCO_3^- cotransporter. The net effect is the reabsorption of one molecule of HCO_3^- and one molecule of Na^+ from the tubular lumen for each molecule of H^+ secreted. This mechanism does not lead to the net excretion of any H^+ from the body because the H^+ is consumed in the reaction with the filtered bicarbonate in the tubular lumen. If the bicarbonate is not reabsorbed, this would be equivalent to an acidifying effect since it would mean that H^+ is accumulating in the cells.

The mechanisms of HCO_3^- reabsorption in the distal tubule are somewhat different from those in the proximal tubule (**Figure 3–4**). H^+ is secreted by the intercalated cells, involving an H^+-ATPase (rather than an Na^+-H^+ antiporter). HCO_3^- transfer across the basolateral membrane involves a $HCO_3^- - Cl^-$ exchanger (rather than an $Na^+-HCO_3^-$ cotransporter). The net effect is the excretion of one H^+ in exchange for one HCO_3^- and one Na^+ to the bloodstream. The distal tubule has only a limited capacity to reabsorb HCO_3^-, so if the filtered HCO_3^- load is high and a large amount is delivered distally, there will be net HCO_3^- excretion in the urine.

Reabsorption of bicarbonate is completed in the intercalated cells of the late distal tubules and collecting ducts. At this site, excess H^+ is actively secreted and combines with phosphate ion and ammonia in the tubules. This process is responsible for reabsorption of the remaining 10% to 15% of the filtered HCO_3^-. This exchange process is achieved by several transporters, including the vacuolar H^+-ATPase (for H^+ secretion across the apical membrane); the Cl^-/HCO_3^- exchanger (for extruding HCO_3^- across the basolateral membrane); and carbonic

> **RESPIRATORY RECAP**
>
> **Two Major Functions of the Kidney in Acid–Base Balance**
>
> » Excretion of the fixed acids (acid anion and associated H^+): about 1 mmol/kg/day
>
> » Reabsorption of filtered bicarbonate: 4000 to 5000 mmol/day

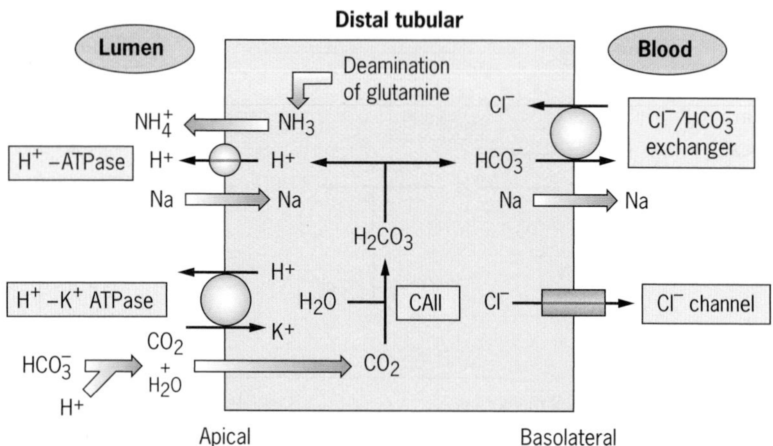

FIGURE 3–4 Schematic representation of the excretion of H^+ in the distal renal tubules. H^+ combines with NH_3 produced by deamination of amino acids to form NH_4^+. This is exchanged for Na^+ that is returned to the bloodstream. H^+ is secreted by the intercalated cells via an H^+–ATPase (rather than a Na^+–H^+ antiporter). Like in the proximal renal cell, HCO_3^- in the distal tubular lumen also combines with H^+ to form H_2O and CO_2. CO_2 then diffuses into the tubular cell, combining with H_2O to produce HCO_3^-. HCO_3^- is transferred across the basolateral membrane via a HCO_3^-–Cl^- exchanger (rather than a Na^+–HCO_3^- co-transporter). The net effect is the excretion of one H^+ in exchange for one HCO_3^- and one Na^+ to the bloodstream. The distal tubule has only a limited capacity to reabsorb HCO_3^-, so if the filtered HCO_3^- load is high and a large amount is delivered distally, there will be net HCO_3^- excretion in the urine. CAII, carbonic anhydrase II.

anhydrase II (for providing both H^+ for luminal secretion and HCO_3^- for basolateral extrusion into the plasma).

As in the proximal tubules, H^+ also combines with ammonium (NH_3) in the distal tubules to form NH_4^+ in the filtrate (refer to Figure 3–4). NH_4^+ excretion in severe acidosis can reach 300 mmol/day in humans. H^+ can also be excreted as phosphate, the major component of titratable acids. The amount of phosphate present in the distal tubule, however, does not vary greatly, and changes in phosphate excretion play a minor role in response to an acid load.

In summary, the following factors regulate renal bicarbonate reabsorption and acid excretion:

1. *Extracellular volume.* When the volume depletion decreases glomerular filtration rate (GFR), the filtered load of bicarbonate is proportionately reduced. The Na^+ retention in response to volume depletion enhances HCO_3^- reabsorption. Conversely, ECF volume expansion results in renal Na^+ excretion and secondary decrease in HCO_3^- reabsorption.
2. *Arterial* P_{CO_2}. An increase in arterial P_{CO_2} (hypercapnia), which increases the production of carbonic acid, increases renal H^+ secretion and HCO_3^- reabsorption. The HCO_3^- retention explains the renal compensation for chronic respiratory acidosis.
3. *Potassium and chloride deficiency.* Hypokalemia (low K^+ levels) increases the secretion of H^+ in the renal tubules, resulting in increases in HCO_3^- reabsorption in the kidney. Low chloride increases reabsorption of more HCO_3^- along with Na^+.
4. *Phosphate excretion.* Because the amount of phosphate present in the distal tubule does not vary greatly, changes in phosphate excretion play a minor role in response to an acid load.
5. *Ammonium.* The kidney responds to an acid load by increasing tubular production and urinary excretion of NH_4^+. Increases in ammonium excretion take several days to reach their maximum. Ammonium excretion increases when urine pH decreases, and this relationship is markedly enhanced with acidosis.
6. *Aldosterone and cortisol (hydrocortisone).* Aldosterone at normal levels has no role in renal regulation of acid–base balance. High aldosterone levels (as in hyperaldosteronism) increase Na^+ reabsorption and urinary excretion of H^+ and K^+, resulting in a metabolic alkalosis. Low aldosteronism alone, on the other hand, rarely is associated with a metabolic acidosis. Low serum cortisol (as in adrenal insufficiency) can cause a mild metabolic acidosis that has a normal anion gap.

Acid–Base Disorders

Metabolic Acidosis

With **metabolic acidosis**, the pH is decreased with decreased HCO_3^-. Processes that increase the production of nonvolatile acids or lead to an excessive loss of bases from the body can produce metabolic acidosis. Both processes increase [H^+] and decrease pH. Acidosis is a potent stimulus to increase ventilation, and as a consequence P_{CO_2} falls. This hyperventilation was first described by Kussmaul in patients with diabetic ketoacidosis in 1874. The compensatory hyperventilation of metabolic acidosis is characterized by deep and labored breathing with normal or reduced frequency, a breathing pattern referred to as Kussmaul respirations. The initial stimulation of the central chemoreceptors is due to small increases in [H^+] in the CSF. The increase in ventilation causes a fall in arterial P_{CO_2}, which inhibits the ventilatory response. The increase in ventilation in response to metabolic acidosis usually starts within minutes and is usually well advanced at 2 hours of onset, but maximal compensation may take 12 to 24 hours to develop.

The effectiveness of the compensatory hyperventilation also depends on the ventilatory capacity, the efficiency of pulmonary gas exchange, and the ventilatory control mechanisms. Patients with lung diseases and central nervous system diseases may not be able to mount an adequate ventilatory compensation response

TABLE 3-5 Common Causes of Metabolic Acidosis

Increased Unmeasured Anions (Increased Anion Gap, Increased Nonvolatile Acids)
Ketoacidosis: diabetic, alcoholic, starvation
Lactic acidosis: hypoxia, circulatory failure, drugs and toxins, enzyme defects
Poisoning: salicylates, ethylene glycol, methanol
Renal failure
Normal Unmeasured Anions (Normal Anion Gap, Loss of Bicarbonate)
Renal tubular acidosis, chronic pyelonephritis, obstructive uropathy
Hypoaldosteronism
Potassium-sparing diuretics (spironolactone)
Diarrhea
Pancreatic or biliary fistulas, ureterosigmoidostomy
Carbonic anhydrase inhibitors: acetazolamide
Excessive intake of ammonium chloride, cationic amino acids

and thus are prone to more severe acidosis. A number of other factors may also attenuate this hyperventilation effect. For example, in diabetic acidosis, severe dehydration may increase $[Na^+]$ and decrease GFR, resulting in increased HCO_3^- reabsorption. The concomitant metabolic alkalosis thus serves to offset some degree of acidosis. In patients with acidosis due to kidney diseases, such as uremia, these adaptive responses may not be available.

Metabolic acidosis is traditionally categorized based on the size of the anion gap into increased anion gap versus normal anion gap acidosis. **Table 3–5** lists common causes of metabolic acidosis.

Metabolic Alkalosis

Metabolic alkalosis is diagnosed by increased pH in association with increased HCO_3^-. Metabolic alkalosis usually occurs when there is a loss of fixed acids or a gain in blood buffer base. Fixed acids can be lost from the renal or gastrointestinal route. In this case, serum Cl^- is usually decreased and metabolic alkalosis can be corrected by replacing intravascular volume with saline (NaCl) (chloride-responsive metabolic alkalosis). High aldosterone and cortisol increase Na^+ reabsorption and urinary excretion of H^+ and K^+. The process increases HCO_3^- reabsorption, resulting in metabolic alkalosis. In these conditions, serum Cl^- is usually unaffected and metabolic alkalosis does not respond to saline replacement (chloride-unresponsive metabolic alkalosis). Ingestion of bicarbonate may also cause metabolic alkalosis, especially when the amount exceeds the bicarbonate-excreting capacity of the kidneys.

Low potassium (hypokalemia) increases H^+ secretion in the renal tubules, resulting in increased reabsorption of HCO_3^-. Severe loss of K^+ may accompany Cl^- in the kidneys, leading to depletion of intracellular $[K^+]$ and a fall in intracellular $[H^+]$—an intracellular acidosis complicating an extracellular alkalosis. This effect may lead to respiratory muscle weakness, as sometimes seen in periodic paralysis. Correction of metabolic alkalosis requires the correction of hypokalemia in this case. **Table 3–6** lists common causes of metabolic alkalosis.

TABLE 3-6 Common Causes of Metabolic Alkalosis

Associated with Chloride (Volume) Depletion (Chloride-Responsive)
Vomiting, gastric drainage
Diuretic therapy
Posthypercapnic alkalosis
Associated with Hyperadrenocorticism (Chloride-Unresponsive)
Cushing syndrome
Primary aldosteronism
Bartter syndrome
Licorice ingestion
Excessive Alkali Intake
Milk-alkali syndrome
Ingestion of sodium bicarbonate
Severe Potassium Depletion

Respiratory Acidosis

Respiratory acidosis is characterized by a low pH and an elevated Pa_{CO_2} (hypercapnia). The two main causes of respiratory acidosis are alveolar hypoventilation and severe $\dot{V}_A/\dot{Q}$ mismatch. **Table 3–7** shows common causes of respiratory acidosis. Chronic obstructive pulmonary disease is the most common cause of chronic respiratory acidosis. When respiratory acidosis (hypercapnia) is uncompensated, this implies the presence of acute ventilatory failure. Renal compensation for respiratory acidosis begins as soon as Pa_{CO_2} rises. Full compensation usually takes days.

Respiratory Alkalosis

Respiratory alkalosis is associated with reduction in Pa_{CO_2} caused by hyperventilation. Reduction in Pa_{CO_2} reduces carbonic acid and thus $[HCO_3^-]$ in plasma. Two compensatory responses tend to minimize the fall in $[H^+]$: (1) retention of Cl^- through a fall in its renal excretion and (2) a small accumulation of lactate resulting from the stimulation of glycolysis in erythrocytes and liver. Retention of Cl^- tends to characterize chronic states of hyperventilation, but increases in the concentration of lactate may occur very rapidly. These compensatory changes are associated with increases in $[H^+]$ and a fall in $[HCO_3^-]$. The reductions in Pa_{CO_2} and $[H^+]$ in hyperventilation are accompanied by a surprisingly large increase in $[CO_3^{-2}]$, predisposing to hypocalcemia and tetany. **Table 3–8** lists conditions that lead to respiratory alkalosis. Note that respiratory alkalosis can also be caused by overly aggressive mechanical ventilation.

Interpretive Strategies for Acid–Base Disorders

Interpretation of acid–base disorders should follow a step-by-step strategy (**Table 3–9**). The strategy begins with clinical assessment, an essential first step that allows

TABLE 3–7 Common Causes of Respiratory Acidosis

Associated with Alveolar Hypoventilation
Drugs: anesthetics, sedatives, hypnotics, narcotics
Neuromuscular diseases: poliomyelitis, myasthenia gravis, Guillain-Barré syndrome, amyotrophic lateral sclerosis
Morbid obesity (Pickwickian syndrome)
Severe kyphoscoliosis
Idiopathic (primary alveolar hypoventilation syndrome)
Associated with Severe Ventilation-Perfusion Mismatch
Chronic obstructive pulmonary disease
Advanced diffuse lung parenchymal diseases (such as sarcoidosis or pulmonary fibrosis)

TABLE 3–8 Common Causes of Respiratory Alkalosis

Associated with Normal Lungs
Anxiety
Fever
Drug overdose: salicylates, respiratory stimulants (such as strychnine)
CNS lesions: encephalitis, meningitis, tumor
Pregnancy
Sepsis
Liver cirrhosis
High altitudes
Associated with Ventilation-Perfusion Mismatch
Acute bronchial asthma
Pneumonia
Pulmonary vascular diseases: pulmonary embolism
Early diffuse lung parenchymal diseases (such as sarcoidosis or pulmonary fibrosis)
Pulmonary edema
Iatrogenic
Overly aggressive mechanical ventilation

TABLE 3–9 Interpretive Strategies for Acid–Base Disorders

Clinical assessment (history, physical examination, interventions)
Acid–base diagnosis
Examine arterial pH, which indicates the primary acid–base disorder
Examine $Paco_2$ and serum bicarbonate
Determine whether condition is acute or chronic (compensation)
Determine whether there are secondary disorders
Overall clinical diagnosis

an acid–base diagnosis based on the available clinical information (history, physical examination, and interventions). Knowledge of the pathophysiology of conditions that cause acid–base disorders is extremely useful in making these initial assessments.

The next step is to systematically evaluate the arterial blood gas results and other laboratory results to make a diagnosis of the acid–base disturbance. To make an acid–base diagnosis, one should look at the arterial pH first. With very rare exceptions, the pH in the arterial blood indicates the primary acid–base disorder. If the pH is decreased (<7.4), an acidosis must be present. On the contrary, if the pH is increased (>7.4), alkalosis must be present. It is also important to note that changes in pH should be assessed relative to the baseline pH, if known. The baseline pH may not be 7.4, especially in patients with chronic acid–base disorders.

One can then determine whether the disorder is of respiratory or metabolic origin by examining the changes in bicarbonate, $Paco_2$, and pH. As a rule of interpretation, the primary disorder is named based on the pH. Remember that HCO_3^- is a base and that CO_2 is a weak acid. Thus, if the pH is acidemic and the $Paco_2$ is elevated, the primary disorder must be respiratory acidosis. If the pH is alkalemic and bicarbonate is elevated, the primary disorder must be metabolic alkalosis. One should also keep in mind that changes in $Paco_2$ or HCO_3^- need to be assessed relative to their respective baseline values, if known, and not necessarily the normal values of 40 mm Hg and 24 mmol/L, respectively.

The next step is to determine whether the compensatory response is present and, if so, whether it is adequate. This can be a major problem in the assessment of acid–base disorders in part because of the nonlinear compensatory response. The uncertainty of time lapse between the onset of the primary acid–base disorder and the clinical evaluation may also be a problem. Remember that it takes time to fully compensate for the primary disorder. Lung compensation for metabolic acid–base disorders occurs fairly quickly (within minutes) and is usually maximal within 24 hours. Renal compensation for respiratory acid–base disorders, however, does not reach its maximum until 3 to 5 days later. Thus, uncertainty about the onset of a respiratory disorder would complicate the interpretation of the adequacy of renal compensatory response. Various equations have been published to describe the expected degree of compensation for an acid–base disorder. Some example equations are shown in **Box 3–1**. Clinically, the equation for respiratory compensation for metabolic acidosis is most accurate because the compensatory response is fairly linear. It is also relatively simple to determine whether or not respiratory acidosis or alkalosis is acute. In acute respiratory acidosis, an increase in $Paco_2$ should produce a decrease in pH by 0.08 (or 0.10 for easy calculation), and vice versa for acute respiratory alkalosis.

The most accurate method, however, is the confidence band technique, as shown in **Figure 3–5**. If the expected and actual values match, there is no evidence of mixed disorder (i.e., changes in $Paco_2$ or HCO_3^- can be fully explained by compensatory response). Note that maximal compensatory response does not return the extracellular pH to normal. This is the main reason why pH indicates the primary disorder. The compensatory response of acid–base data always should be interpreted in the context of clinical evaluation of the patient's condition, including factors of time, therapy, and the integrity of pulmonary and renal function.

BOX 3–1

Expected Compensation for Acid–Base Disturbances*

Renal Compensation for Respiratory Acidosis

Predicted $[HCO_3^-] = 24 + (Pa_{CO_2} - 40) \times 0.1$ (acute)

Predicted $[HCO_3^-] = 24 + (Pa_{CO_2} - 40) \times 0.35$ (chronic)

Renal Compensation for Respiratory Alkalosis

Predicted $[HCO_3^-] = 24 - (40 - Pa_{CO_2}) \times 0.2$ (acute)

Predicted $[HCO_3^-] = 24 - (40 - Pa_{CO_2}) \times 0.5$ (chronic)

Respiratory Compensation for Metabolic Acidosis

Predicted $Pa_{CO_2} = 1.5 \times [HCO_3^-] + 8$

Respiratory Compensation for Metabolic Alkalosis

Predicted $Pa_{CO_2} = 0.73 \times [HCO_3^-] + 20$

*If the acid–base status exceeds the expected level of compensation, a mixed acid–base disturbance is present.

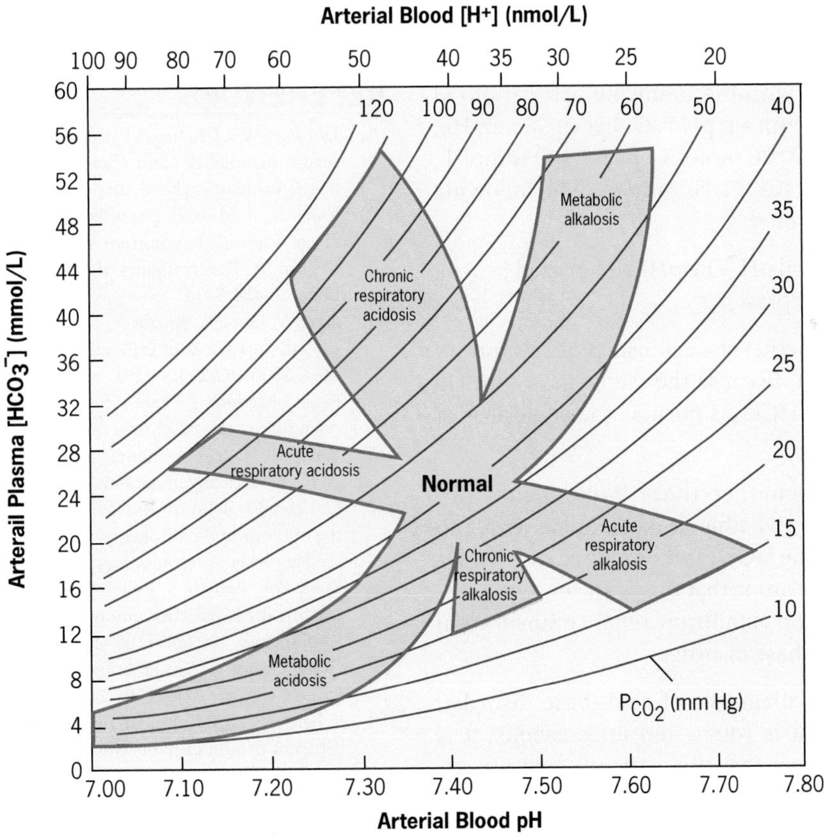

FIGURE 3–5 Davenport diagram for acid–base disorders. Reproduced from *Fluid and Electrolytes: Physiology and Pathophysiology* by Cogan MG (Editor). Copyright 1991 by McGraw-Hill Companies, Inc.—Books. Reproduced with permission of McGraw-Hill Companies, Inc.—Books in the format textbook via Copyright Clearance Center.

If the changes in HCO_3^- or Pa_{CO_2} cannot be adequately explained by the compensatory response alone, the fourth step must determine what kind of second or even third acid–base disorder is present. This process can be facilitated greatly by reviewing other clues, some of which are summarized in **Table 3–10**. Once a diagnosis of acid–base disorder is made, one can then formulate therapies or perform additional tests to determine the causes of the acid–base disorder.

TABLE 3–10 Some Aids to Interpretation of Acid–Base Disorders

Clue	Possible Secondary Acid–Base Disorder
High anion gap	Metabolic acidosis
Ketonuria	Alcoholic ketoacidosis, diabetic ketoacidosis
Hypokalemia and/or hypochloremia	Metabolic alkalosis (vomiting, diuretics)
Hyperchloremia	Normal anion gap acidosis (diarrhea, renal tubular acidosis)
Elevated creatinine and urea	Uremic acidosis or metabolic alkalosis from hypovolemia (prerenal renal failure)
Hyponatremia or hypernatremia	Metabolic alkalosis from volume contraction

CASE STUDY

A 30-year-old unconscious male patient is brought into the emergency room with the following arterial blood gas values breathing room air: pH 7.27, $Paco_2$ 56 mm Hg, Pao_2 70 mm Hg, HCO_3^- 26 mmol/L, $[Na^+]$ 140 mmol/L, $[K^+]$ 4.0 mmol/L, and $[Cl^-]$ 105 mmol/L. The following steps should be performed:

Step 1. Examine arterial pH. The pH is decreased (<7.4). Thus, an acidosis is present.

Step 2. Determine whether the acidosis is of respiratory or metabolic origin. Because the $Paco_2$ is 56 mm Hg (>40 mm Hg) and HCO_3^- is normal, the acidosis is of respiratory origin.

Step 3. Determine whether there is compensatory response, and if so, whether it is adequate. Refer to Box 3–1. Because the HCO_3^- is the value calculated for this $PaCO_2$, we determine that this is an acute respiratory acidosis with no significant renal compensation or secondary acid–base disorder.

Step 4. Final clinical diagnosis of acid–base disorder. Because the patient is young and unconscious, it is reasonable to suspect that this patient's acute respiratory acidosis may be caused by alveolar hypoventilation due to overdose of central nervous system depressants.

KEY POINTS

- An acid is any substance that donates a proton $[H^+]$ to an aqueous solution, and a base is any substance that accepts a proton $[H^+]$ from an aqueous solution.
- A buffer solution minimizes changes in pH when a strong acid or a strong base is added.
- pH is defined as the negative logarithm or exponent (to the base 10) of the $[H^+]$.
- Acid–base disturbances can be described with the Henderson-Hasselbalch equation and the strong ion difference.
- Base excess is the amount of strong acid that must be added to the blood sample to return the sample to pH 7.40 while maintaining the $Paco_2$ at 40 mm Hg.
- The anion gap can be used to determine the cause of metabolic acidosis.
- The Stewart model has three independent variables controlling pH: strong ion difference, total weak acid concentration, and Pco_2.
- The lungs can compensate for metabolic acid–base disturbances, and the kidneys can compensate for respiratory acid–base disturbances.
- The primary acid–base disturbances are respiratory acidosis, respiratory alkalosis, metabolic acidosis, and metabolic alkalosis.

REFERENCES

1. Dorwart WV, Chalmers L. Comparison of methods for calculating serum osmolality from chemical concentrations, and the prognostic value of such calculations. *Clin Chem.* 1975;21:190–194.
2. Jones N. Acid–base physiology. In: Crystal R, West JB, eds. *The Lung: Scientific Foundation.* New York: Raven Press; 1991.
3. Kellum JA. Determinants of blood pH in health and disease. *Crit Care.* 2000;4:6–14.
4. Fencl V, Jabor A, Kazda A, Figge J. Diagnosis of metabolic acid–base disturbances in critically ill patients. *Am J Respir Crit Care Med.* 2000;162:2246–2251.
5. Figge J, Mydosh T, Fencl V. Serum proteins and acid–base equilibria: a follow-up. *J Lab Clin Med.* 1992;120:713–719.
6. Wilkes P. Hypoproteinemia, strong-ion difference, and acid–base status in critically ill patients. *J Appl Physiol.* 1998;84:1740–1748.
7. Liskaser FJ, Bellomo R, Hayhoe M, et al. Role of pump prime in the etiology and pathogenesis of cardiopulmonary bypass-associated acidosis. *Anesthesiology.* 2000;93:1170–1173.
8. Story DA, Poustie S, Bellomo R. Estimating unmeasured anions in critically ill patients: anion gap, base deficit, and strong ion gap. *Anaesthesia.* 2002;57:1109–1114.
9. Figge J, Jabor A, Kazda A, Fencl V. Anion gap and hypoalbuminemia. *Crit Care Med.* 1998;26:1807–1810.
10. Scheingraber S, Rehm M, Sehmisch C, Finsterer U. Rapid saline infusion produces hyperchloremic acidosis in patients undergoing gynecologic surgery. *Anesthesiology.* 1999;90:1265–1270.
11. Constable PD. Hyperchloremic acidosis: the classic example of strong ion acidosis. *Anesth Analg.* 2003;96:919–922.
12. Rehm M, Finsterer U. Treating intraoperative hyperchloremic acidosis with sodium bicarbonate or tris-hydroxymethyl aminomethane: a randomized prospective study. *Anesth Analg.* 2003;96:1201–1208.
13. Rocktaschel J, Morimatsu H, Uchino S, Ronco C, Bellomo R. Impact of continuous veno-venous hemofiltration on acid–base balance. *Int J Artif Organs.* 2003;26:19–25.
14. Rahn H, Reeves RB, Howell BJ. Hydrogen ion regulation, temperature, and evolution. *Am Rev Respir Dis.* 1975;112:165–172.

CHAPTER 4

Arterial Blood Gas Analysis and Sampling

Yuh-Chin T. Huang
Erika Lease
Will Beachey

OUTLINE

OBJECTIVES

1. Compare methods to measure Po_2, Pco_2, pH, and oxygen saturation.
2. Describe the technique used to obtain blood samples by arterial puncture.
3. Describe preanalytic errors in blood gas analysis.
4. Discuss issues related to temperature correction of blood gases.
5. Describe methods of quality control and proficiency testing of blood gases.

KEY TERMS

Allen test
arterial blood gas (ABG)
Clark electrode
Clinical Laboratory Improvement Amendment (CLIA)
oximeter
point-of-care testing (POCT)
Sanz electrode
Severinghaus electrode
tonometry

INTRODUCTION

The analysis of arterial blood gases has become an indispensable tool in clinical practice. The primary measurements (Po_2, Pco_2, and pH) provide important information about oxygenation, ventilation, and acid–base balance. They also guide respiratory and metabolic interventions in critically ill patients. This chapter discusses arterial blood gas measurements and the physiologic basis for the interpretation of arterial blood gas data.

History of Arterial Blood Gas Analysis

Acid–Base Balance

By the 18th century, normal blood was recognized as alkaline. Alkalinity was later found to be related to carbon dioxide (CO_2) content (bicarbonate) in the blood. In 1909, Lawrence J. Henderson applied the law of mass action to describe the relationship of bicarbonate (HCO_3^-) to dissolved CO_2, or carbonic acid (H_2CO_3). This equation, known as the *Henderson equation*, was later transformed by Karl A. Hasselbalch into the logarithmic form known as the *Henderson-Hasselbalch equation* (see Chapter 3).

Measurement of pH

Wilhelm Ostwald first measured the concentration of hydrogen ions in 1896 using a platinum electrode in solutions saturated with hydrogen gas. He discovered that the potential generated by the platinum electrode was a logarithmic function of the strength of the acid. The Ostwald platinum electrode was later modified and used by Hasselbalch in 1912 to measure blood acidity. Phyllis T. Kerridge constructed the first blood pH electrode in 1925. A thermostated blood pH apparatus was invented in 1931 but was not commercially available until the mid-1950s. Manuel Sanz developed the modern ultramicro pH electrode in the late 1950s.

Measurement of PCO_2

CO_2 was discovered in 1754 by Joseph Black and later detected in exhaled air and the blood. Until the mid-1950s, PCO_2 was either derived from the CO_2-combining power, which involved the equilibration between blood and a gas with known CO_2 content, or calculated from the Henderson-Hasselbalch equation after measurement of pH with a glass electrode and CO_2 content by Van Slyke's manometric method.

The polio epidemics of the 1950s, which resulted in large numbers of patients requiring ventilatory support and monitoring, led to the development of the Astrup apparatus to replace the older, more cumbersome methods. The Astrup apparatus measured pH and PCO_2 based on the principle that the relationship between the pH and log PCO_2 of blood was linear in the clinically relevant range. By measuring pH at two different PCO_2 values, a linear plot of the measured pH against log PCO_2 could be generated. The PCO_2 in the unknown sample then could be obtained by extrapolation. The deviation of the measured pH–log PCO_2 line from the normal position defines the metabolic acid–base imbalance of an individual and the concept of standard base excess.

The modern PCO_2 electrode was introduced by Richard Stow in 1957 and later modified by Severinghaus.

Measurement of PO_2

The discovery of oxygen (O_2) is usually credited to Joseph Priestley, who termed this gas *dephlogisticated air*. In 1777, Antoine Lavosier changed the name to *principe acidifiant* or *principe oxygine* in the mistaken belief that all acids contained O_2. The word *oxygen* (*oxys* = acid, *gene* = to produce) became standard even before it was proven that all acids do not contain O_2.

Measurement of PO_2 in the blood was first achieved in the late 19th century by Edward Pfluger and August Krogh, who developed a bubble method that involved equilibration of small gas bubbles with large volumes of blood followed by analysis of gas tensions in the bubbles. In 1942, Francis Roughton and Per Scholander modified this method to measure carbon monoxide (CO) using a syringe with a calibrated capillary for equilibration so that only a small amount of blood was needed. This syringe method was adapted later by Richard Riley for measuring PO_2 in the blood, and it became known as the *Riley bubble method*. The Riley bubble method was widely used, primarily as a research tool to study ventilation-perfusion relationships in the lung. In 1954, Leland Clark constructed the first modern PO_2 electrode, which measured PO_2 based on the polarographic principle. Its miniaturization subsequently allowed the incorporation of the entire electrode into the modern blood gas analyzer.

Gas Exchange Between the Lungs and Blood

Humphrey Davy first demonstrated the presence of both O_2 and CO_2 in blood in 1799. In 1837, Heinrich Gustav Magnus quantified the amount of O_2 and CO_2 in blood. He found that arterial blood contained more O_2, but less CO_2, than venous blood. These findings led to his hypothesis that blood gas exchange took place in the lungs, whereas the oxidation and generation of body heat occurred elsewhere. However, the mechanism of gas exchange in the lungs was hotly debated between two schools of scientists in the 18th century. The secretionists, represented by Carl Ludwig, Christian Bohr, and John Scott Haldane, believed that the lungs actively pumped the respiratory gases into the blood. The diffusionists, led by Edward Pfluger, claimed that all exchange of respiratory gases occurred by simple diffusion. The diffusion theory eventually prevailed after a series of elegant studies by August and Marie Krogh in the early 1890s.

Hemoglobin and the Oxyhemoglobin Equilibrium Curve

The discovery of hemoglobin is usually credited to Felix Hoppe-Seyler, who crystallized it and described its spectrum in 1862. He also found that O_2 molecules form a loose and dissociable compound with hemoglobin, which he termed *oxyhemoglobin*. Carl Gustav von Hufner reported that 1 g of crystalline hemoglobin could combine with 1.34 mL of O_2. The in vivo relationship between Po_2 and O_2 content was demonstrated first by Paul Bert in 1878. This nonlinear relationship constituted the *oxyhemoglobin equilibrium curve* (OEC), also commonly called the *oxyhemoglobin dissociation curve.* The molecular basis for the OEC was not understood until the detailed chemical structure of the hemoglobin molecule was unveiled and the conformational changes of the molecule associated with binding and release of O_2 were defined by Linus Pauling and Max Perutz in the late 1940s.

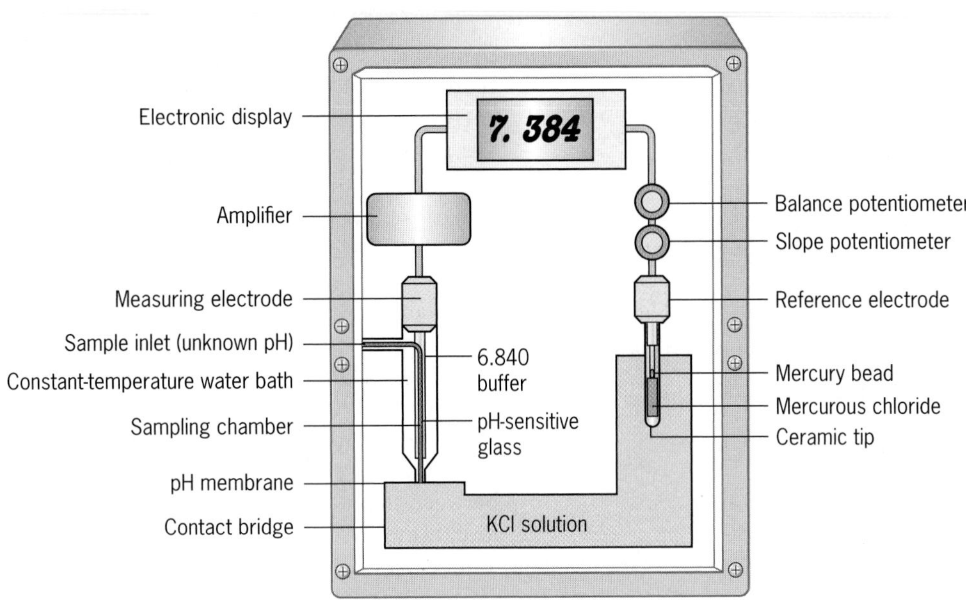

FIGURE 4–1 Schematic illustration of the modern pH electrode. Adapted from Shapiro BA. *Clinical Application of Blood Gases.* 4th ed. Mosby; 1989.

Blood Gas Analyzers

pH Electrode

Measurement of pH is based on the linear relationship between the potential differences and pH variations across a pH-sensitive glass membrane. **Figure 4–1** shows the basic design of the modern pH electrode, which consists of two chemical half-cells separated by a pH-sensitive glass membrane. One half-cell has a reference electrode, usually made of mercury-mercurous chloride (calomel), and the other has a measuring electrode, usually composed of silver-silver chloride. The mercury-mercurous chloride of the reference electrode provides a constant reference voltage at a constant temperature. The silver-silver, chloride-measuring electrode detects the voltage difference across the glass membrane produced by two solutions with different pH levels. The measuring half-cell is embedded within a chamber containing a buffer with a pH of 6.840, which is encased in a constant-temperature water bath. The measuring half-cell is connected to the reference half-cell by a potassium chloride (KCl) contact bridge, which completes the electronic circuit. To prevent contamination, the KCl solution is separated from the unknown blood in the sampling chamber by a membrane.

The modern pH electrode has a small sampling chamber that allows the use of aliquots of blood volume as small as 25 μL. The pH electrode includes a balance potentiometer set to display 6.840 when the 6.840 buffer solution is placed in the measuring half-cell, as well as a slope potentiometer set to display 7.384 when the measuring half-cell is filled with 7.384 buffer solution. Because the potential difference is a linear function of the pH, two-point calibration (for example, pH values of 6.840 and 7.384) is usually sufficient for accurate blood pH measurement. The modern pH electrode is sometimes referred to as the **Sanz electrode**.

> **RESPIRATORY RECAP**
>
> **pH and Blood Gas Electrodes**
>
> » A pH electrode measures the voltage difference across a glass membrane produced by two solutions of different pH.
>
> » A Pco_2 electrode measures pH change caused by CO_2 diffusion from the sample.
>
> » A Po_2 electrode uses the principles of polarography.
>
> » Oximetry uses light absorption at specific wavelengths.

Pco_2 Electrode

The principle of Pco_2 measurement is that changes of pH induced by the diffusion of CO_2 across a permeable membrane are proportional to Pco_2 in contact with the membrane. Thus, the basic design of the Pco_2 electrode consists of a CO_2-permeable, but H^+-impermeable, membrane that separates the blood sample from the measuring half-cell (**Figure 4–2**). The measuring half-cell contains a dilute electrolyte solution (sodium bicarbonate and sodium or potassium chloride). When CO_2 in the blood sample diffuses across the permeable membrane, it undergoes the following reaction: $CO_2 + H_2O \rightarrow H_2CO_3 \rightarrow H^+ + HCO_3^-$. Because H^+ concentration is directly proportional to CO_2 in contact with the membrane, pH measured by a pH electrode can be used as an indirect measure of Pco_2.

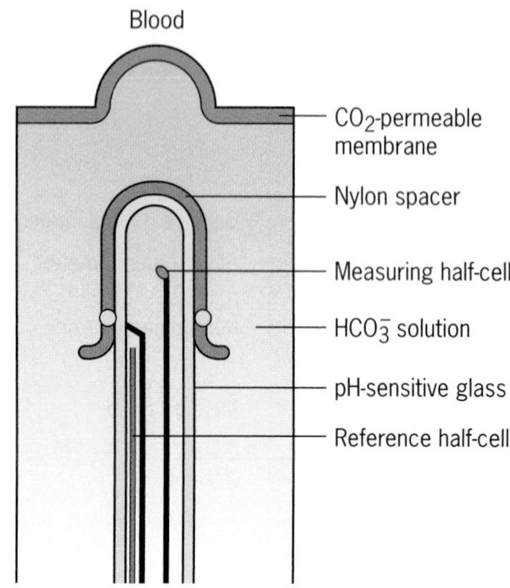

FIGURE 4–2 Schematic illustration of the modern P_{CO_2} electrode.

The design of the P_{CO_2} electrode is slightly different from the pH electrode in that the pH-sensitive glass electrode is separated from the permeable membrane by nylon mesh or other spacers that allow bicarbonate solution to exist between the glass and membrane. The measuring and reference half-cells are silver-silver chloride. The entire pH electrode is bathed in electrolyte solution, which serves as the electronic bridge between the measuring and reference half-cells. The modern P_{CO_2} electrode, commonly referred to as the **Severinghaus electrode**, is a modification of the electrode developed by Stow in the early 1950s. Gas mixtures with a CO_2 concentration of 5% and 10% are commonly used to calibrate the P_{CO_2} electrode.

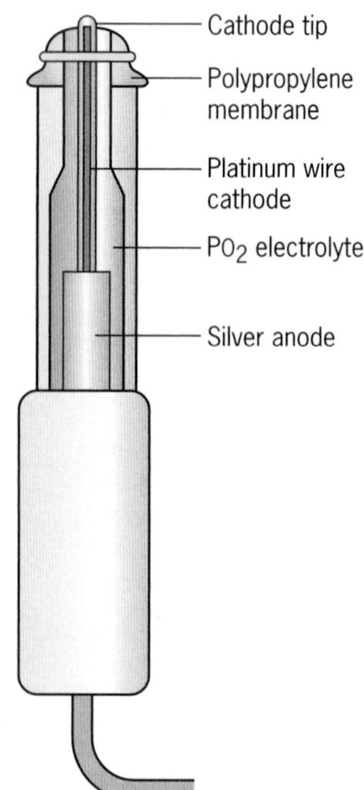

FIGURE 4–3 Schematic illustration of the P_{O_2} electrode. Adapted from Shapiro BA. *Clinical Application of Blood Gases.* 4th ed. Mosby: 1989.

P_{O_2} Electrode

The P_{O_2} electrode, or **Clark electrode**, consists of a platinum cathode and silver anode immersed in a dilute, buffered potassium chloride solution (**Figure 4–3**). The Clark electrode measures P_{O_2} with the principle of polarography. The electric current produced by a cathode (negative electrode) in a solution is directly proportional to the availability of O_2 molecules at the cathode tip. When the O_2 molecules come in contact with the platinum cathode, they are reduced to hydroxide anion, as follows: $O_2 + 2H_2O + 4 \text{ electrons} \rightarrow 4\,OH^-$. The source of electrons comes from oxidation of the silver anode by the chloride anions attracted to the anode, forming silver chloride. Because the amount of O_2 reduced is directly proportional to the number of electrons (or current), P_{O_2} in the solution can be determined by measurement of the change in current between the anode and cathode. The modern P_{O_2} electrode system is usually covered by an O_2-permeable but electrically nonconductive membrane (such as polypropylene or polyethylene), which allows slow diffusion of O_2 from the blood into the electrode while preventing degradation of the electrode by the blood.

Gas mixtures with O_2 concentrations of 0% and 12% or 20% usually are used to calibrate the electrode. For convenience and economy, the calibration gases for the P_{O_2} and P_{CO_2} electrodes usually are combined, with one gas composed of 5% CO_2 and 12% or 20% O_2 balanced with nitrogen and a second gas containing 10% CO_2 and 90% nitrogen. The P_{O_2} electrode also responds to halothane, resulting in inaccurate P_{O_2} measurements in blood drawn from patients anesthetized with this drug.

Oximeter

Hemoglobin content in the blood can be measured by an **oximeter**, a spectrophotometer that uses specific wavelengths in the oxyhemoglobin spectrum. The light at those wavelengths is absorbed at the vibrational frequencies of the molecule of interest (such as oxyhemoglobin) in the solution. The concentration of the molecule in the solution can be determined through quantification of the amount of light absorbed by the solution. Modern oximeters, such as the CO-oximeter, can generate multiple spectra (usually four) that allow distinction among four major hemoglobin species: oxyhemoglobin, reduced hemoglobin (deoxyhemoglobin), carboxyhemoglobin, and methemoglobin (**Figure 4–4**).

Point-of-Care Arterial Systems

Arterial blood gas (ABG) can also be measured by portable analyzers (**Figure 4–5**) that allow testing to be done at the bedside. This is known as **point-of-care testing (POCT)**. Some units just measure pH, P_{O_2}, and P_{CO_2}, whereas others also offer the ability to measure electrolytes, glucose, and hematocrit. Most use single-use disposable cartridges that contain many of the same devices typically found in traditional laboratory arterial blood gas analyzers. The sensors are micro-fabricated thin-film electrodes. Others use multiple-use disposable cartridges with up to 100 uses over 72 hours.

The major advantages of POCT systems are their small sampling volumes and more rapid therapeutic turnaround time of blood gas results, which allows faster decision making.[1,2] Some systems can measure ABG with as little as 0.5 mL of blood. This ability is essential for caring for neonates because the blood volumes needed for traditional ABG analyzers (2.7 to 3.0 mL) may represent as much as 10% of neonates' blood volumes. Different portable blood gas systems, however, may have different accuracies. In one study of a point-of-care testing system, reproducibility (coefficient of variation) was good (<2%) for electrolytes, glucose, urea, and pH; satisfactory (<6.5%) for blood gases and creatinine; but poor (21%) for hematocrit.[3]

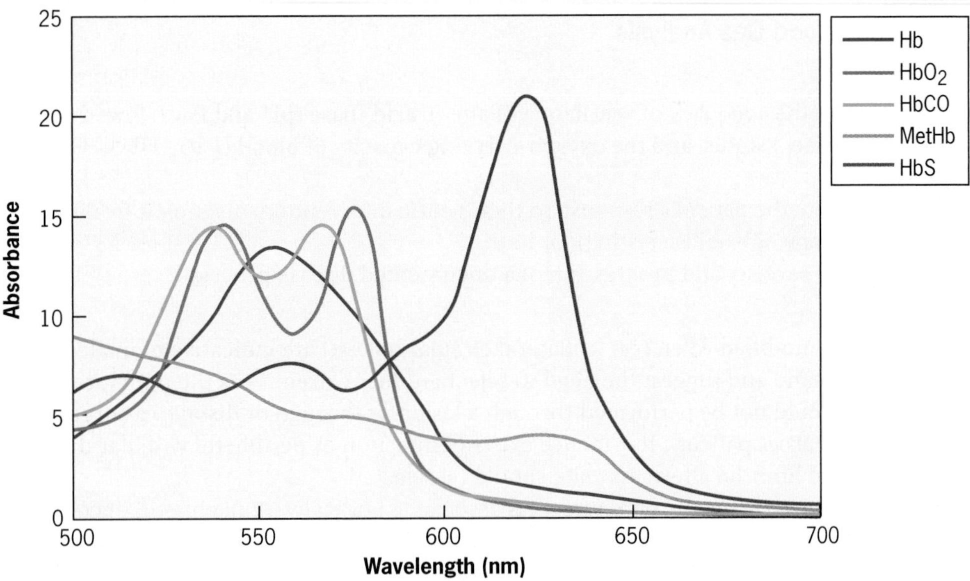

FIGURE 4–4 Absorption spectra for different types of hemoglobin molecules. Adapted from Radiometer Medical. *Blood Gas, Oximetry, and Electrolyte Systems Reference Manual.* Radiometer Medical; 1996.

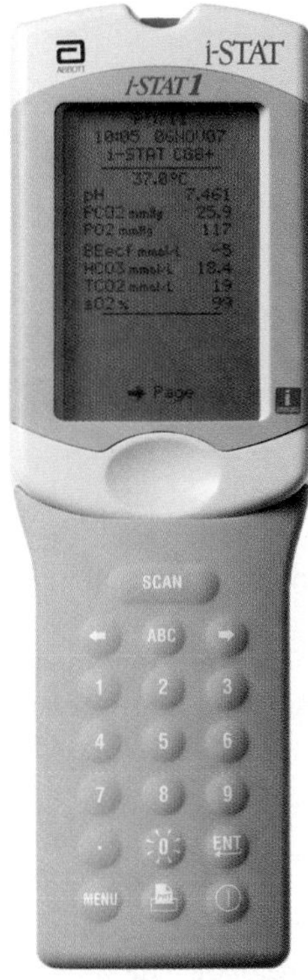

FIGURE 4–5 Point-of-care testing device.

Blood Gas Sampling

Sites of Arterial Puncture

The ideal arterial sampling site should be easily accessible, have collateral blood flow, and be relatively insensitive to pain. Based on these criteria, the radial artery is the preferred site for arterial puncture and cannulation for adult patients (**CPG 4–1**). The brachial artery is a good alternative if the radial arteries are unavailable. Femoral artery punctures should be used only if absolutely necessary because the artery is deep under the skin and the risk of undetected postpuncture bleeding is increased. The limited collateral arterial flow makes the lower limb more susceptible to ischemia if the femoral artery is occluded by clot or hematoma. In addition, the risk of infection is higher because the femoral artery is close to the perineum. Other arteries (axillary, dorsalis pedis) are used infrequently.

Allen Test

Before radial arterial puncture or cannulation is performed, the modified **Allen test** is performed to ascertain that there is adequate ulnar artery perfusion to the hand (**Figure 4–6**). This test was proposed originally in 1929 by Edgar V. Allen as a noninvasive evaluation of the patency of the arterial supply to the hand of individuals with thromboangiitis obliterans. The test was later modified for use as a test of collateral circulation before arterial cannulation.

The patient makes a fist to force blood from the hand, and pressure is applied to compress the ulnar and radial arteries (Figure 4–6A). The patient then relaxes the hand, and obstructing pressure is removed from the ulnar artery while the radial artery remains compressed (Figure 4–6B). If the ulnar artery is patent, the hand should become flushed within 10 seconds, constituting a normal or positive Allen test. If the Allen test is abnormal, ulnar perfusion to the hand should be assumed to be poor, and the radial artery in the contralateral wrist or other alternative site should

CLINICAL PRACTICE GUIDELINE 4–1

Sampling for Arterial Blood Gas Analysis

Indications

- The need to evaluate the adequacy of ventilatory ($Paco_2$), acid–base (pH and $Paco_2$), and oxygenation (Pao_2 and Sao_2) status, and the oxygen-carrying capacity of blood (Pao_2, Hbo_2, Hb, and dyshemoglobins)
- The need to quantitate the patient's response to therapeutic intervention, diagnostic evaluation (such as oxygen therapy or exercise testing), or both
- The need to monitor severity and progression of a documented disease process

Contraindications

- Negative results of a modified Allen test (collateral circulation test) are indicative of inadequate blood supply to the hand and suggest the need to select another extremity as the puncture site.
- Arterial puncture should not be performed through a lesion or through or distal to a surgical shunt (such as in a dialysis patient). If evidence exists of infection or peripheral vascular disease involving the selected limb, an alternative site should be selected.
- Agreement is lacking regarding the puncture sites associated with a lesser likelihood of complications. However, because of the need to monitor the femoral puncture site for an extended period, femoral punctures should not be performed outside the hospital.
- A coagulopathy or medium- to high-dose anticoagulation therapy, such as heparin or Coumadin, streptokinase, or tissue plasminogen activator (but not necessarily aspirin), may be a relative contraindication for arterial puncture.

Hazards and Complications

- Hematoma
- Arteriospasm
- Air or clotted-blood emboli
- Anaphylaxis from local anesthetic
- Introduction of contagion at sampling site and consequent infection in patient; introduction of contagion to sampler by inadvertent needle stick
- Hemorrhage
- Trauma to the vessel
- Arterial occlusion
- Vasovagal response
- Pain

Assessment of Need

- History and physical indicators, such as positive smoking history, recent onset of difficulty in breathing independent of activity level, or trauma
- Presence of other abnormal diagnostic tests or indices, such as abnormal pulse oximetry reading or chest x-ray film
- Initiation of, administration of, or change in therapeutic modalities (for example, initiation, titration, or discontinuance of supplemental oxygen or initiation of, changes in, or discontinuance of mechanical ventilation)
- Projected surgical interventions for patients at risk
- Projected enrollment in a pulmonary rehabilitation program

Assessment of Test Quality

- Sampling of arterial blood for any indication listed is useful for patient management only if the sampling procedure is carried out according to an established, proven protocol. The validity of test results can be voided if any of the following occur:
  - The sample is contaminated by air, improper anticoagulant or inappropriate anticoagulant concentration, flush solution (if sample is drawn from an indwelling catheter), or venous blood.
  - The sample clots because of improper anticoagulation of the collection device, improper mixing, or exposure to air.
  - Analysis is delayed (>15 minutes for samples held at room temperature or >60 minutes for samples held at 4° C [39.2° F).

Modified from AARC clinical practice guideline: sampling for arterial blood gas analysis. *Respir Care*. 1992;37:913–917. Reprinted with permission.

be considered for arterial blood sampling. Although the modified Allen test has significant false-positive and false-negative rates, it remains a simple, useful screening test to assess the adequacy of ulnar collateral perfusion of the hand.

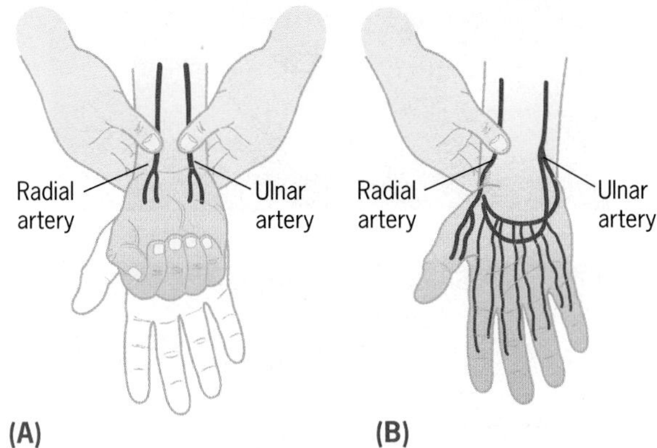

FIGURE 4–6 Allen test. (**A**) The patient is asked to open and close the hand into a fist several time with both radial and ulnar arteries compressed. (**B**) Release the ulnar artery. The entire hand and digits should fill with blood, indicating good collateral flow into the radial artery system.

Radial Arterial Puncture

After collateral circulation has been assessed, the patient is prepared for puncture of the radial artery (**Figure 4–7**). The radial artery is located via palpation for maximal arterial pulsation (Figure 4–7A). A towel is rolled under the wrist, with the hand hyperextended to bring the radial artery closer to the skin surface (Figure 4–7B). The puncture site is cleansed with an alcohol swab, iodophor solution, or other appropriate disinfectant. The arterial puncture can be performed with either a glass syringe lubricated with a minimal amount of liquid heparin or a special vented, preheparinized (100 to 200 IU), self-filling plastic syringe (Figure 4–7C). The blood gas syringe should be fitted with a 1-inch 22- or 23-gauge needle.

With the nondominant hand locating the maximal arterial pulsation and the dominant hand holding the syringe needle at a 45-degree angle pointing in the opposite direction of arterial flow with the needle bevel up, the skin is punctured and the needle advanced. Because the radial nerve lies lateral to the artery, care must be

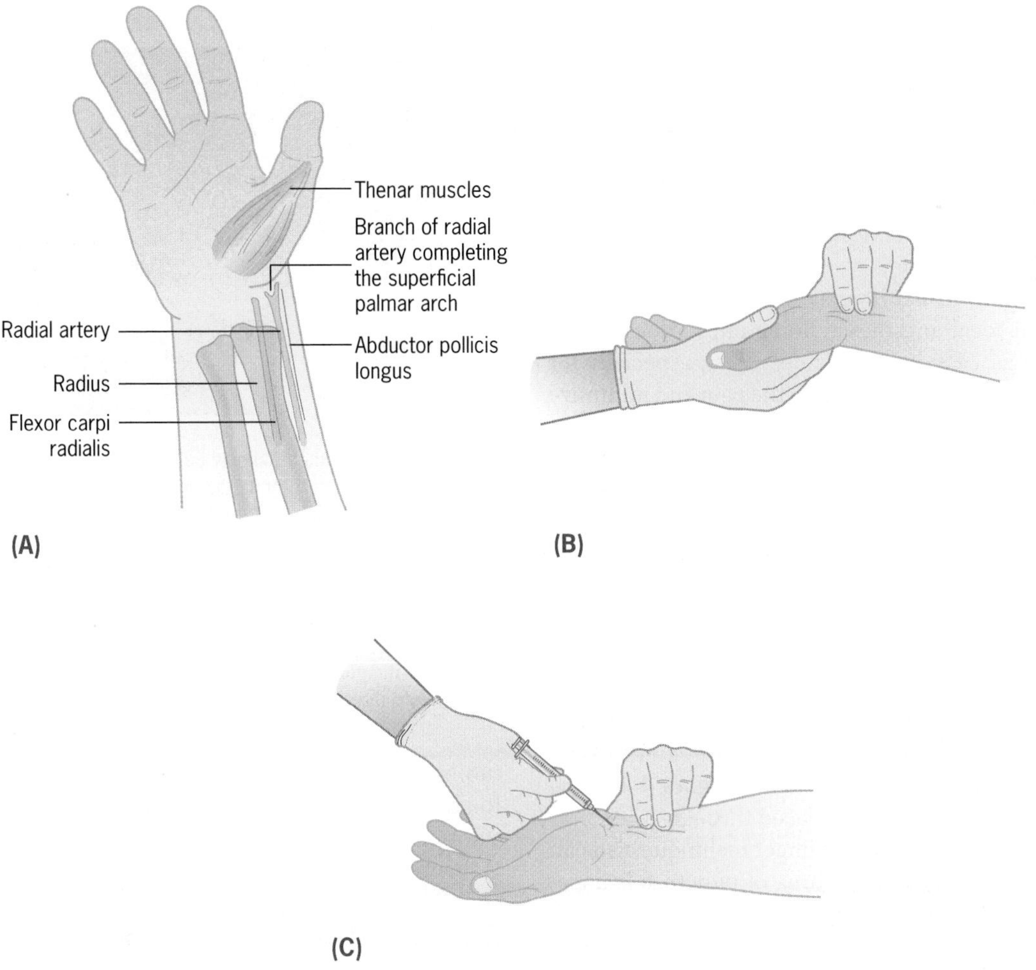

FIGURE 4–7 Radial artery sampling. (**A**) Anatomic location of radial artery. (**B**) Palpation of radial artery to determine the point of puncture. (**C**) Insertion of needle. Adapted from Dudley HAF, Eckersley JRT, Paterson-Brown S. *A Guide to Practical Procedures in Medicine and Surgery*. Butterworth-Heinemann; 1989.

taken not to direct the needle toward the lateral aspect of the wrist. Once the artery is entered, a flash of arterial blood is seen in the needle hub. Approximately 2 to 3 mL of arterial blood is collected as the arterial pressure fills the syringe. Usually, aspiration is unnecessary.

After the desired blood volume has been obtained, the needle is withdrawn from the artery and the site compressed for at least 5 minutes. This compression decreases the possibility of hematoma formation, compartment syndrome, and ecchymosis, which may interfere with future arterial punctures. Longer compression times may be necessary for patients receiving anticoagulants (e.g., heparin, Coumadin) or those with coagulation defects (e.g., thrombocytopenia, chronic renal failure, disseminated intravascular coagulation). After bleeding has stopped, an elastic bandage is applied with moderate pressure. The exposed needle should be disposed of safely in a puncture-resistant container, and air bubbles should be expelled. The syringe is then sealed with a cap and gently mixed for a few seconds, and the blood is analyzed immediately.

Punctures of Other Arterial Sites

For brachial artery puncture, the arm should be hyperextended and the hand pronated to best stabilize the artery. The brachial artery should be palpated on the medial side of the biceps tendon, 1 to 2 cm distal to the antecubital fossa. Care must be taken to not direct the puncture medially because this site is the most frequent location of the median nerve. The femoral artery is entered perpendicularly, with the patient in the supine position. The artery is best palpated and fixed just below the inguinal crease. The femoral nerve lies lateral and the femoral vein medial to the artery.

Most individuals can tolerate a single arterial puncture without local anesthesia. Sometimes a local anesthetic (such as 1% lidocaine) is necessary, especially for arterial cannulation or to decrease the pain and minimize anxiety-induced changes in a patient's blood gas values. Complications associated with arterial puncture include hematoma, arteriospasm, and thrombosis, all of which may result in hand ischemia if perfusion is not restored promptly. The patient's reaction to arterial puncture may range from feelings of uneasiness to vasovagal syncope.

Radial Arterial Cannulation

Arterial cannulation is performed when frequent arterial blood gas measurements are required and when continuous monitoring of arterial blood pressure is necessary. Usually the radial artery is cannulated (**Figure 4–8**). The arterial catheter is commonly placed through a percutaneous puncture, although a Seldinger technique also can be used. Before insertion, the area of puncture is anesthetized with 2% lidocaine (without epinephrine, which increases the risk of arterial spasm). A 20-gauge beveled needle with a clear plastic flash chamber is used. A straight, stiff, Teflon or polyurethane catheter with a hub at its distal end is placed over the needle. After insertion, the catheter is attached to a kit consisting of connective tubing, a stopcock for blood gas sampling, a transducer for blood pressure monitoring, and a continuous flush solution to prevent clotting in the catheter. The catheter is secured in place with tape or sutures.

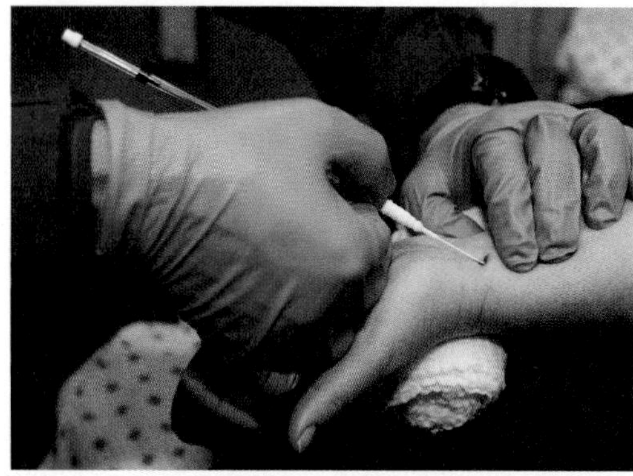

(A)

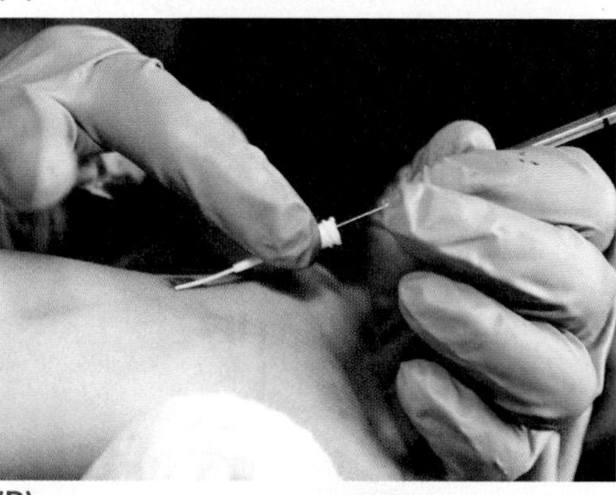

(B)

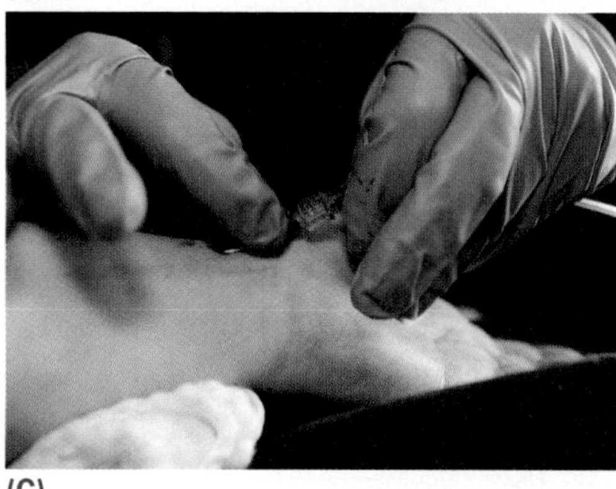

(C)

FIGURE 4–8 The catheter should be inserted using sterile technique. Hyperextend the wrist to bring the artery closer to the surface. Palpate the pulse with two fingers, tracking the course of the vessel. (**A**) Insert the needle over the radial artery. Advance the needle at an approximate 20 to 40 degree angle until there is a flash of pulsating blood as the needle enters the artery. (**B**) Immobilize the needle with your free hand, and advance the guide wire. Then remove the needle, leaving only the guide wire in the artery. Advance the catheter into the artery over the guide wire. (**C**) Remove the guide wire, and connect the tubing to the catheter.

Capillary Blood Gases

Capillary samples may be used to estimate pH and Pco_2 in infants or other individuals when arterial blood gas analysis is indicated but arterial access is difficult (**CPG 4–2**). The site is warmed before the procedure

CLINICAL PRACTICE GUIDELINE 4–2

Capillary Blood Gases

Indications

- Arterial blood gas analysis indicated but arterial access not available
- Noninvasive monitor readings are abnormal: transcutaneous values, end-tidal CO_2, and pulse oximetry
- Assessment of initiation, administration, or change in therapeutic modalities (mechanical ventilation) is indicated
- A change in patient status is detected by history or physical assessment
- Monitoring the severity and progression of a documented disease process is desirable

Contraindications

- Capillary punctures should not be performed at or through the following sites: posterior curvature of the heel (because the device may puncture the bone); the heel of a patient who has begun walking and has callus development; the fingers of infants (to prevent nerve damage); previous puncture sites; inflamed, swollen, or edematous tissues; cyanotic or poorly perfused tissues; localized areas of infection; and peripheral arteries.
- Capillary punctures should not be performed on patients younger than 24 hours because of poor peripheral perfusion.
- Capillary punctures should not be performed when direct analysis of oxygenation is needed.
- Capillary punctures should not be performed when direct analysis of arterial blood is needed.
- Relative contraindications include peripheral vasoconstriction and polycythemia (caused by shorter clotting times); hypotension may be a relative contraindication.

Hazards and Complications

- Infection
- Introduction of contagion at sampling site and consequent infection in patient, including calcaneus osteomyelitis and cellulitis
- Inadvertent puncture or incision and consequent infection in clinician obtaining sample
- Burns
- Hematoma
- Bone calcification
- Nerve damage
- Bruising
- Scarring
- Puncture of posterior medial aspect of heel (possibly resulting in tibial artery laceration)
- Pain
- Bleeding
- Inappropriate patient management (possibly resulting from reliance on capillary P_{O_2} values)

Limitations of Method

- Inadequate warming of the site before a puncture may result in capillary values that correlate poorly with arterial pH and P_{CO_2} values.
- Undue squeezing of the puncture site may result in venous and lymphatic contamination of the sample.
- A second puncture may be necessary to obtain an adequate amount of blood for analysis.
- Variability in capillary P_{O_2} values precludes use of these samples to assess oxygenation status.

Assessment of Need

- Capillary blood gas sampling is an intermittent procedure that should be performed when a documented need exists. Routine or standing orders for capillary puncture are not recommended. The following may assist the clinician in assessing the need for capillary blood gas sampling:
    - History and physical assessment
    - Noninvasive respiratory monitoring values: pulse oximeter transcutaneous values, end-tidal CO_2 values

(continues)

Clinical Practice Guideline 4–2 *(continued)*

- Patient response to initiation, administration, or changes in therapeutic modalities
- Lack of arterial access for blood gas sampling

Assessment of Test Quality

- The validity of the test may be jeopardized if any of the following occur:
  - The sample is contaminated by air.
  - Clots prevent accurate analysis.
  - Quantity of sample is insufficient for analysis.
  - Analysis of sample is delayed (>15 minutes for sample at room temperature, or >60 minutes for samples held at 4° C).

Modified from AARC clinical practice guideline: capillary blood gases. *Respir Care.* 1994;1180–1183. Reprinted with permission.

to arterialize the blood. A puncture or small incision is made with a lancet into the cutaneous layer of the skin in a highly vascular area. Blood is collected in a heparinized glass capillary tube. Capillary punctures should not be performed through previous puncture sites; through inflamed, edematous, cyanotic, or poorly perfused tissues; through areas of infection; through peripheral arteries; through the posterior curvature of the heel, to avoid injuring bone; or in the fingers of neonates, to avoid nerve damage. Excessive squeezing of the puncture site may result in venous or lymphatic contamination of the sample. Capillary sampling should not be performed on infants younger than 24 hours because of poor peripheral perfusion. Relative contraindications include peripheral vasoconstriction, polycythemia (caused by shorter clotting times), and hypotension.

Capillary blood is handled similar to arterial blood samples; it should be free of contamination by air or blood clots and analyzed in an appropriate time frame. Extreme variability in capillary Po_2 values precludes the use of this technique to assess oxygenation.

Quality Control

Sample Procurement

After the arterial blood specimen is obtained, any air bubble larger than 5% of the blood sample should be expelled. Because room air contains a Pco_2 of essentially zero and a Po_2 of approximately 150 mm Hg (at sea level), air bubbles in the blood sample lower the Pco_2 values of the blood sample and cause the Po_2 to approach 150 mm Hg. The syringe must be capped immediately, and the technician in the blood gas laboratory must take great care to ensure that ambient air does not mix with the sample as it is introduced into the blood gas analyzer.

Because sodium heparin has a pH of approximately 7.0, too much heparin may affect the pH. In general, 0.05 to 0.1 mL of heparin per milliliter of blood does not affect the pH value and provides adequate anticoagulation. The volume of the dead space is proportional to the size of the syringe. For example, the dead space of a 5-mL syringe with a needle is about 0.2 mL. Thus 2 to 4 mL of blood should be obtained so that it contains at least 0.05 mL heparin per 1 mL blood but no more than 0.1 mL heparin per 1 mL blood. Thus, before arterial blood is obtained, the syringe should be flushed with heparin and ejected so that the volume of heparin in the syringe is kept at a minimum. The commercially available preheparinized syringes have minimized such a contamination problem because they use dry, lyophilized heparin. If electrolyte measurements are performed with the blood sample, lithium heparin should be used, rather than sodium heparin.

Once the arterial blood gas sample is obtained, the syringe should be promptly transported (within 15 minutes at room temperature) to the arterial blood gas laboratory for analysis. Many intensive care units (ICUs) have a vacuum tube transport system to the laboratory, which is ideal for distances of 200 feet or more. A delay could lead to erroneous values because gas diffusion through the plastic syringe wall or between a bubble and blood increases with time, especially when the blood gas tensions differ significantly from those of room air.

The diffusion rate is also affected by temperature. If the sample cannot be analyzed immediately, it should be collected in a glass syringe (which decreases diffusion across the barrel of the syringe) and placed in ice (slush or chips) to hasten cooling. Putting the sample in ice slush also slows down oxygen consumption by white blood cells (WBCs), which is approximately 0.1 mL of O_2 from 100 mL blood in 10 minutes at body temperature. This effect is exaggerated if the WBC count is very high (leukocyte larceny). The decrease in Po_2 from the delay is more prominent if the hemoglobin saturation of the arterial blood is high. For example, if the sample is not iced, Po_2 drops to below 250 mm Hg in

1 hour if the original PO_2 is 400 mm Hg. However, if PO_2 is 50 mm Hg, the loss of 0.1 mL O_2 per 100 mL blood makes a very small change in PO_2 because the primary change occurs in the hemoglobin saturation.

Plastic syringes are commonly used for convenience. However, they should not be used if there will be a delay until analysis such that the sample must be placed on ice. When the syringe is cooled, the solubility of O_2 and CO_2 in the sample increases, causing more gas to go into solution and thus reducing its partial pressure. Because plastic is relatively permeable to O_2 and CO_2, oxygen diffuses across the plastic into the sample. When the sample is subsequently warmed in the analyzer to 37° C (98.6° F), gas comes out of solution, resulting in a reported PO_2 and PCO_2 greater than what was in the sample drawn from the patient.

All of the above factors cause preanalytic errors, which are errors affecting blood gas results that occur before the sample is introduced into the blood gas analyzer. **Box 4–1** lists common preanalytic errors.

> **BOX 4–1**
>
> **Common Arterial Blood Gas Preanalytic Errors**
>
> Room air contamination of sample
> Heparin dilution of sample
> Blood clots from inadequate heparin
> Hyperventilation during sample collection
> Long delay time between sample collection and analysis
> Excessive sample metabolism (leukocyte larceny with high WBC count)
> Inadequate wait time between change in inspired oxygen or ventilation and collection of blood sample

Sample Analysis

The blood gas sample should be mixed well before analysis. Although mixing has minimal effect on blood gases and pH, it is necessary if hemoglobin or hematocrit is to be measured by a CO-oximeter. As previously mentioned, any air bubbles need to be removed before thorough mixing occurs. Blood clots also should be removed so that the blood gas analyzer does not become plugged. Expelling one or two drops of blood from the syringe tip onto a gauze pad or tissue directly before introduction into the analyzer helps ensure that clots are not present and that air bubbles are not introduced.

Blood gas analyzer calibrations are required in accordance with the manufacturer's instructions, with a frequency determined by volume of use. Calibration reagents are usually standard CO_2 and O_2 gases (for example, 5% CO_2 + 20% O_2 + 75% N_2 and 10% CO_2 + 90% N_2) for PO_2 and PCO_2 sensors, and phosphate buffers (e.g., pH 6.840 and pH 7.384) for pH. The reagents are referenced to the National Institute of Standards and Technology (NIST). Most modern blood gas instruments perform automatic calibration at least every 30 minutes. When a blood gas sample has very high values (for example, a PO_2 value of 600 mm Hg), the operator may need to measure tonometered blood with known values at similar extreme levels to ascertain the instrument's degree of inaccuracy.

Tonometry of Blood

Because of the unique O_2-binding characteristics of hemoglobin and complex viscosity characteristics of normal fresh blood, whole blood must be carefully tonometered so that exact gas tensions can be prepared for analysis by a blood gas instrument. A **tonometry** reference method has been developed and recognized as the internationally accepted standard method. The method requires fresh blood (less than 24 hours old) from asymptomatic donors, which should be nonhemolyzed and without leukocytosis or high blood lipid levels. Gas mixtures, the composition of which has been verified by a mass spectrometer or with a CO_2 and O_2 gas analyzer, can be used to equilibrate the blood. If human blood is not available, bovine hemoglobin solutions (containing both deoxygenated and oxygenated hemoglobin) also can be used. These bovine preparations have been shown to yield data closely resembling those obtained with human blood. These solutions also can be formulated to provide precision data for the pH and electrolytes.

Quality Control and Proficiency Testing

The quality of results is crucial for blood gas analysis. The general aspects of quality control are regulated by the federal government through the **Clinical Laboratory Improvement Amendment (CLIA)**. A properly designed quality control program enables proper function of the blood gas analyzer on a routine basis. Quality control procedures for a blood gas analyzer differ from other analyses performed in the clinical laboratory environment because the patient sample is fresh whole blood.

The optimal technique used to establish the extent of inaccuracy and imprecision of an individual blood gas analyzer is the use of whole blood tonometry with samples of fresh, anticoagulated, whole blood. However, the technical and economic advantages of whole blood tonometry must be balanced by its hazard potential and labor-intensive process. Alternatives to whole blood tonometry are commercially available prepackaged materials such as aqueous buffer solutions,

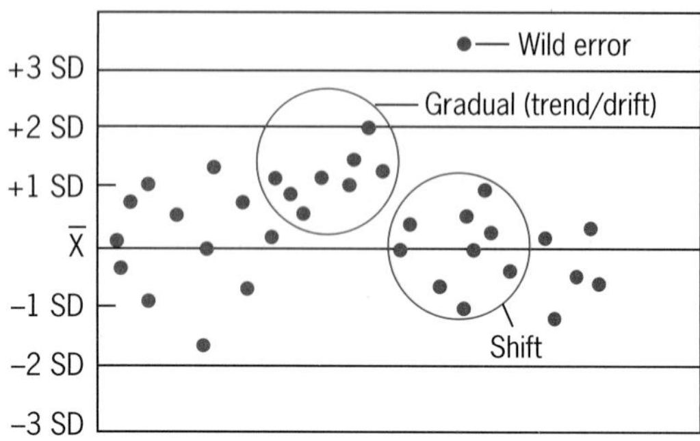

FIGURE 4–9 Three types of analytic errors identified on a Levey-Jennings chart: wild error (outlier), gradual error (trend, drift), and a shift to a new (in this case, lower) mean. SD, standard deviation. Adapted from Branson RD, Hess DR, Chatburn RL. *Respiratory Care Equipment*. 2nd ed. Lippincott Williams & Wilkins; 1999.

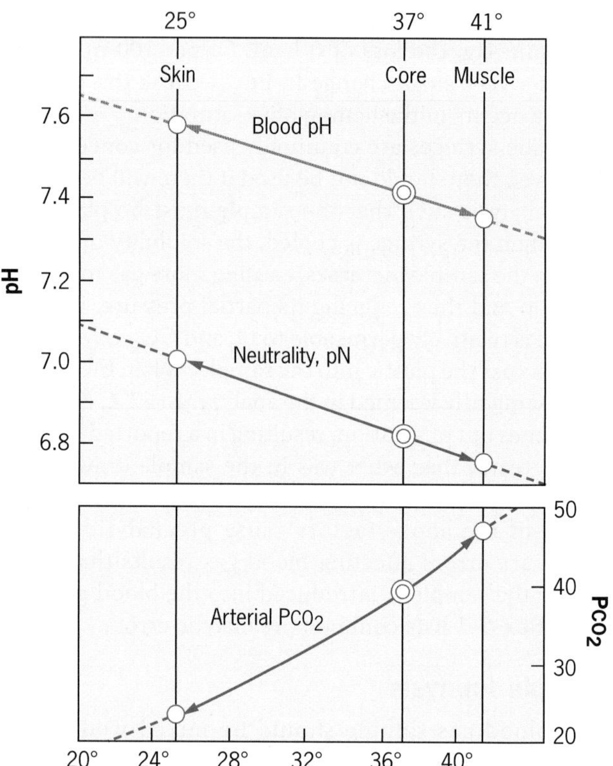

FIGURE 4–10 Expected changes in blood pH and Pco_2 in the arterioles of skin at 25° C and working muscle at 41° C of a healthy man with a core temperature of 37° C. Adapted from Rahn H. Body temperature and acid-base regulation. *Pneumonologie.* 1974;151:87–94.

RESPIRATORY RECAP

Calibration, Quality Control, and Proficiency Testing

- Calibration adjusts the analyzer to reference standards.
- Quality control analyzes materials of known values for pH, Pco_2, and Po_2.
- Proficiency testing analyzes materials from an external source that have values unknown to the tester.

blood-based (hemoglobin containing) materials, and perfluorocarbon-oil emulsions. However, the physical and chemical properties of these controls do not match those of whole blood.

Whichever materials are chosen, the results of the quality control program should be recorded in a manner that allows the operator to easily detect changes in performance of the instrument. This detection is most commonly done with Levey-Jennings charts (**Figure 4–9**). CLIA requires at least two levels of control for pH, Pco_2, and Po_2 on each work shift or every 8 hours of operation. Because internal quality control programs better estimate precision than accuracy, external proficiency testing programs are used. These programs are available from sources such as the College of American Pathologists (CAP) and the American Thoracic Society (ATS).

Temperature Correction

Controversy exists regarding whether blood gas values should be corrected for the actual individual's body temperature in clinical practice. The argument for temperature correction (such as during hypothermia) is that blood gas values measured at 37° C (98.6° F) may not accurately reflect the true oxygenation and acid–base status of the body. Although Po_2 changes with temperature (7% per degree Celsius), O_2 capacity, O_2 content, and hemoglobin saturation do not. Thus, the Po_2 of the arterial blood in a cold extremity may be only 40 mm Hg, but the saturation value is 96%. If such a temperature-corrected value of Po_2 is reported, the Po_2 may seem dangerously low to the clinician whereas in fact the hypothermic patient is adequately oxygenated. The same argument also applies to the acid–base status. Pco_2 and pH change with temperature (4% per degree Celsius for Pco_2; 0.0146 units per degree Celsius for pH), but the bicarbonate and intracellular neutrality do not.

The argument for not correcting for body temperature is best illustrated with the example of heavy exercise (**Figure 4–10**).[4] Blood at the core temperature of 37° C (98.6° F) has a pH of 7.4, which is alkaline relative to the intracellular fluid (ICF) with a pH of 6.8. Blood in the exercising muscles, which have a temperature of 41° C, (105.8° F) has a lower pH of 7.35 and a higher Pco_2 of 48 mm Hg. Blood in the cooler skin (25° C [77° F]) has a higher pH of 7.6 and a lower Pco_2 of 22 mm Hg. Despite these striking regional variations in pH and Pco_2, the CO_2 content and the relative alkalinity between blood and ICF remain constant. Thus the pH and Pco_2 values at 37° C (98.6° F) reliably reflect the in vivo acid–base status of the patient. In addition, most acid–base nomograms are valid only at 37° C (98.6° F), and temperature correction does not improve clinical decision making.

Based on these arguments, routine blood gas measurements have been recommended to be consistently reported at 37° C (98.6° F) without correction for actual body temperature.[5,6] On rare occasions the temperature-corrected values for arterial (and alveolar) values may be more appropriate, such as for the calculation of the alveolar-arterial O_2 gradient or arterial-alveolar end-tidal CO_2 gradient in patients with abnormal temperatures. The Po_2 or Pco_2 values of the arterial blood and alveolar gas should be expressed at body temperature.

KEY POINTS

- Arterial blood samples are used to analyze Po_2, Pco_2, pH, hemoglobin O_2 saturation, carboxyhemoglobin, and methemoglobin.
- Common preanalytic errors include sample contamination with air or heparin and a prolonged time between sample procurement and analysis.
- Calibration, quality control, and proficiency testing are used to ensure correct blood gas analyzer function.
- Temperature correction of blood gases usually is unnecessary.

REFERENCES

1. Castro HJ, Oropello JM, Halpern N. Point-of-care testing in the intensive care unit: the intensive care physician's perspective. *Am J Clin Pathol.* 1995;104(4 suppl 1):S95–S99.
2. Kendall J, Reeves B, Clancy M. Point of care testing: randomised controlled trial of clinical outcome. *BMJ.* 1998;316(7137):1052–1057.
3. Papadea C, Foster J, Grant S, et al. Evaluation of the i-STAT Portable Clinical Analyzer for point-of-care blood testing in the intensive care unit of a university children's hospital. *Ann Clin Lab Sci.* 2002;32(3):231–243.
4. Rahn H. Body temperature and acid-base regulation. *Pneumonologie.* 1974;151(2):87–94.
5. Mahoney J, Hodgkin J, Van Kessel A. Arterial blood gas analysis. In: Burton G, Hodgkin J, Ward J, eds. *Respiratory Care: A Guide to Clinical Practice.* 4th ed. Philadelphia: Lippincott; 1997.
6. Hansen JE. Arterial blood gases. *Clin Chest Med.* 1989; 10(2):227–237.

CHAPTER 5

Respiratory Monitoring

Dean R. Hess

OUTLINE

Pulse Oximetry
Capnography
Transcutaneous Blood Gas Monitoring
Respiratory Rate and Pattern

OBJECTIVES

1. Explain how pulse oximetry estimates arterial oxygen saturation.
2. Discuss the limitations of pulse oximetry.
3. Describe techniques to address errors caused by motion and low pe rfusion.
4. Explain how the pulse oximeter plethysmographic waveform can be used to assess peripheral perfusion.
5. Describe methods used to measure carbon dioxide in the exhaled gas.
6. Compare sidestream and mainstream capnography.
7. Compare time-based and volume-based capnography.
8. Discuss the physiologic issues related to end-tidal P_{CO_2} and how they affect the relationship between end-tidal and arterial P_{CO_2}.
9. Explain how volume-based capnography can be used to measure carbon dioxide production and cardiac output.
10. Discuss the principle of operation of transcutaneous blood gas monitors.
11. Discuss the limitations of transcutaneous blood gas monitoring.
12. Describe techniques that can be used to measure respiratory rate.

KEY TERMS

Beer-Lambert law
capnogram
capnography
capnometry
electrical impedance tomography (EIT)
end-tidal P_{CO_2}
fiberoptic plethysmography
impedance pneumography
mass spectrometer
penumbra effect
perfusion index (PI)
piezoelectric plethysmography
plethysmographic variability index (PVI)
pulse oximetry
pulsus paradoxus
Raman spectroscopy
respiratory inductance plethysmography (RIP)
spectrophotometry
thermistor
thermocouple
transcutaneous monitoring

INTRODUCTION

Monitoring is a continuous, or nearly continuous, evaluation of the physiologic function of a patient in real time to guide management decisions, including when to make therapeutic interventions and assessment of those interventions. Monitoring often is used to assure patient safety. Monitoring also is used to assess patient response to clinical interventions. In this chapter, respiratory monitoring of oxygenation, ventilation, and respiratory rate is discussed.

Pulse Oximetry

Pulse oximetry noninvasively estimates the hemoglobin oxygen saturation of arterial blood (**CPG 5–1**).[1–3] It is based on **spectrophotometry**, the process by which substances are identified by their absorption (also called *extinction*) of specific wavelengths in the electromagnetic spectrum. The various hemoglobin molecules absorb wavelengths between 500 and 1000 nm in the infrared and visible light regions. The **Beer-Lambert law** defines the relationship between the concentration of a substance and the amount of light absorbed:

$$A = L \times C \times \varepsilon$$

where L is the optical path length, C is the concentration of the substance, and ε is the absorption of the particular wavelength used. A separate wavelength is required for each substance to be identified. Most pulse oximeters use two wavelengths, red (660 nm) and infrared (940 nm), at which oxyhemoglobin (HbO_2) and deoxyhemoglobin (Hb) have different absorption characteristics.

> **RESPIRATORY RECAP**
>
> **Pulse Oximetry**
>
> » Pulse oximetry measures oxygen saturation with a variation of the Beer-Lambert law.
>
> » Accuracy is ±4% and can be affected by abnormal hemoglobins, motion, and low perfusion.
>
> » Some newer pulse oximeters measure carboxyhemoglobin and methemoglobin.
>
> » Some newer-generation pulse oximeters display the perfusion index (PI) and plethysmogram variability index (PVI).

Red and infrared light-emitting diodes (LEDs) in the oximeter probe serve as light sources (**Figure 5–1**). Because HbO_2 and Hb differ in light absorption at each wavelength, the amount of red and infrared light transmitted is related to oxygen saturation (**Figure 5–2**). A photodiode positioned on the opposite side of the probe serves as the photodetector. To identify the oxygen saturation of arterial blood only, the device relies on the pulsatile nature of arterial flow. During systole, a new volume of blood enters the arteriolar bed, and light absorption increases. During diastole, absorption decreases to a minimal level (**Figure 5–3**). Measuring pulsatile absorption eliminates the effects of nonpulsatile components such as tissue, bone, and venous blood.

Oxygen saturation (Spo_2) is related to the ratio of minimum and maximum absorption at each wavelength (**Figure 5–4**). A calibration curve is plotted for the pulse-added absorption at the two wavelengths and stored in a software algorithm. Devices vary by manufacturer in the type of LED, photodiode, and microprocessor used. Because the Spo_2 calculation is based on a constantly updated signal ratio, no calibration is required.

Most pulse oximeter probes (**Figure 5–5**) use *transmittance spectrophotometry*, sending light through the arterial bed to a photo detector on the opposite side.

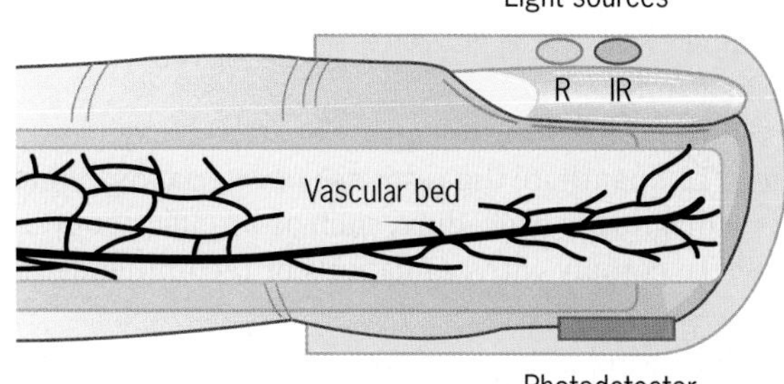

FIGURE 5–1 Pulse oximeter probe fitted over finger, showing position of light sources and detector.

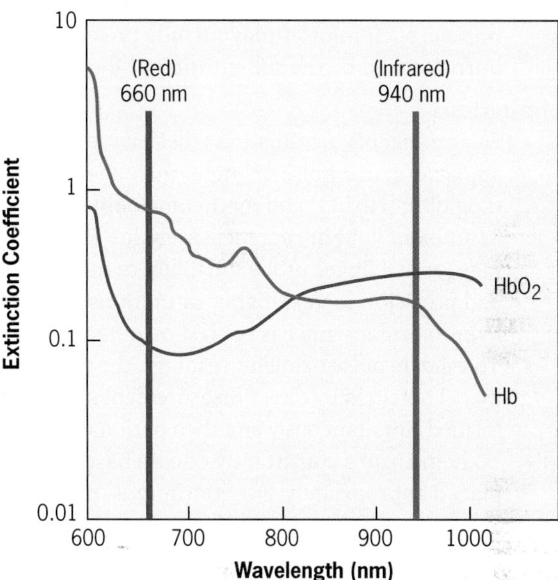

FIGURE 5–2 Absorption spectra for oxyhemoglobin and deoxyhemoglobin for the range of wavelengths relevant to pulse oximetry.

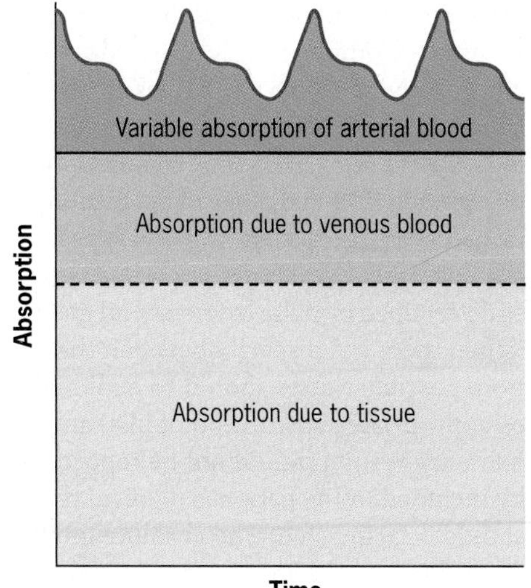

FIGURE 5–3 Dynamic and static light absorption during pulse oximetry. Used with permission of Philips Respironics, Murraysville, Penn.

CLINICAL PRACTICE GUIDELINE 5–1

Pulse Oximetry

Indications

- To monitor the adequacy of arterial oxyhemoglobin saturation
- To quantitate the response of arterial oxyhemoglobin saturation to therapeutic intervention or to a diagnostic procedure, such as bronchoscopy
- To comply with regulations or recommendations

Contraindications

- A need for continuous measurement of pH, partial pressure of arterial carbon dioxide ($Paco_2$), total hemoglobin, or abnormal hemoglobins may be a relative contraindication to pulse oximetry.

Hazards and Complications

- Pulse oximetry (Spo_2) is considered a safe procedure. However, because of device limitations, false-negative results for hypoxemia or false-positive results for normoxemia or hyperoxemia may lead to inappropriate treatment. Also, tissue injury may occur at the measuring site as a result of probe misuse; such injuries may include pressure sores from prolonged application or electrical shock and burns caused by the substitution of incompatible probes between instruments.

Limitations

- Factors, agents, or situations that may affect readings, limit precision, or limit the performance or application of a pulse oximeter include motion artifact, abnormal hemoglobins (primarily carboxyhemoglobin [HbCO] and methemoglobin [Hbmet]), intravascular dyes, exposure of the measuring probe to ambient light during measurement, low perfusion states, skin pigmentation, nail polish or nail coverings (with a finger probe), inability to detect saturations below 83% with the same degree of accuracy and precision seen at higher saturations, and inability to quantitate the degree of hyperoxemia present; hyperbilirubinemia has been shown *not* to affect the accuracy of Spo_2 readings.
- To validate pulse oximeter readings, the correlation between Spo_2 and arterial oxyhemoglobin saturation (Sao_2) obtained by direct measurement should be assessed; these measurements initially should be performed simultaneously and then periodically reevaluated in relation to the patient's clinical state.
- To help ensure consistency of care based on Spo_2 readings, the proper probe must be selected and placed appropriately. For continuous, prolonged monitoring, the high- and low-limit alarms are set appropriately; the specific manufacturer's recommendations are followed; the device is applied and adjusted correctly to monitor response time and electrocardiographic coupling; the strength of the plethysmograph waveform or the pulse amplitude is assessed; and the device is checked to ensure that it is detecting an adequate pulse.
- Spo_2 results should be documented in the patient's medical record and should detail the conditions under which the readings were obtained: date, time of measurement, and pulse oximeter reading; the patient's position, activity level, and location during monitoring (the physician's order determines the patient's activity level); the inspired oxygen concentration or supplemental oxygen flow, specifying the type of oxygen delivery device; the type of probe and the placement site; the model of the device (if more than one type is available for use); the simultaneously obtained arterial pH, partial pressure of arterial oxygen (Pao_2), and $Paco_2$ values and directly measured saturations of HbCO, Hbmet, and oxyhemoglobin (if direct measurement was not simultaneously performed, an additional, one-time statement must be made explaining that the Spo_2 reading has not been validated by comparison to directly measured values); the stability of readings (length of observation time and range of fluctuation; for continuous or prolonged studies, review of the recording may be necessary); the patient's clinical appearance, a subjective assessment of perfusion at the measuring site (for example, signs of cyanosis or lowered skin temperature); and the correlation between the patient's heart rate as determined by pulse oximeter and that obtained by palpation and use of an oscilloscope.
- When there is a disparity between the Spo_2 and Sao_2 readings and the patient's clinical presentation, possible causes should be explored before results are reported. Monitoring at alternative sites or appropriate substitution of instruments or probes may resolve the discrepancies. If not, the pulse oximetry results should not be reported; rather, a statement describing the corrective action should be included in the patient's medical record, and direct measurement of arterial blood gas values should be requested. The absolute limits that constitute unacceptable disparity vary with the patient's condition and the specific device. Clinical judgment must be exercised.

Modified from AARC clinical practice guideline: pulse oximetry. *Respir Care.* 1991;36:1406–1409. Reprinted with permission.

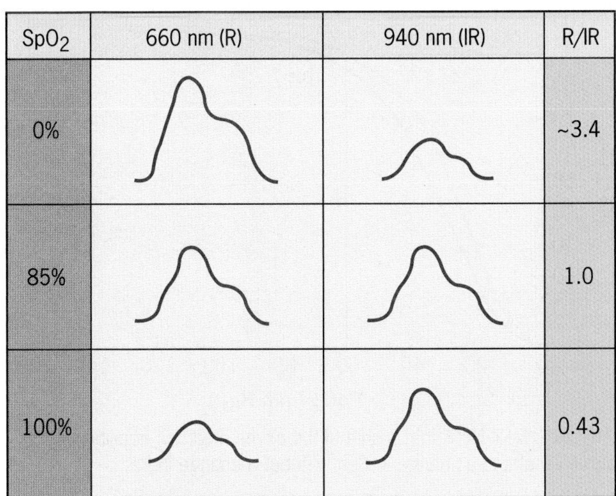

SpO2
660 nm (R)
940 nm (IR)
R/IR
0%
~3.4
85%
1.0
100%
0.43

FIGURE 5–4 Relationship between red and infrared light absorption for different oxygen saturations.

With *reflectance spectrophotometry*, pulse oximeter sensors place the light source and detector on the same side of the arterial bed.

In general, pulse oximeter measurements have an accuracy of ±4% at Spo_2 greater than 80%. They are less accurate at Spo_2 less than 80%, but the clinical importance of this is questionable. The calibration curves are developed from studies on healthy volunteers and vary by manufacturer depending on the range of concentrations achieved by the volunteers and the accuracy of the gold standard, usually a co-oximeter. Not only do manufacturer-derived calibration curves vary from manufacturer to manufacturer, but also the output of the LEDs can vary from probe to probe. Ideally, the same pulse oximeter and probe should be used for repeated measurements in the same patient.

To appreciate the implications of the accuracy of pulse oximetry, one must consider the oxyhemoglobin equilibration (or dissociation) curve. If the pulse oximeter

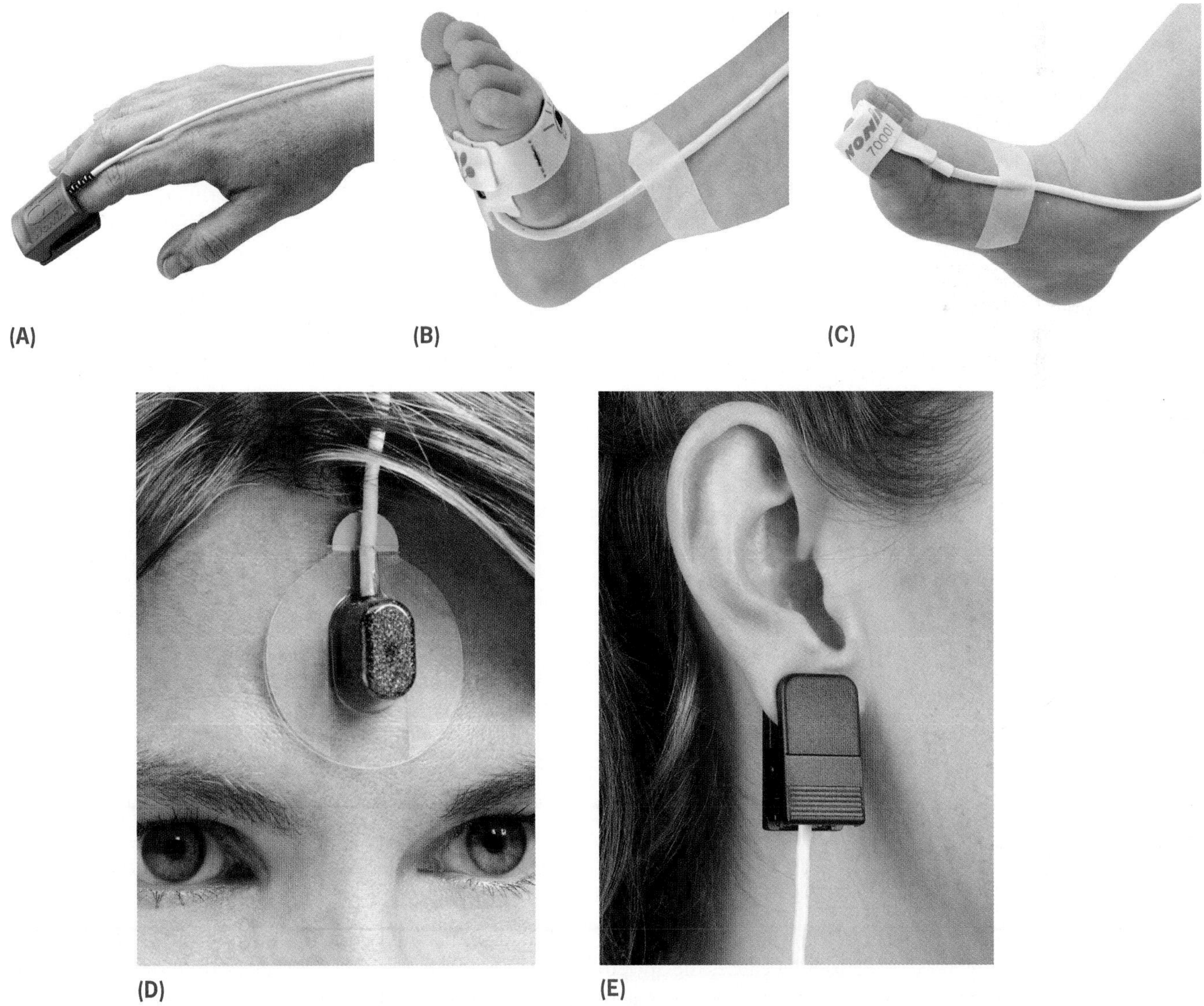

(A) (B) (C)

(D) (E)

FIGURE 5–5 Examples of pulse oximetry probes. (**A**) Finger probe. (**B**) Foot probe. (**C**) Toe probe. (**D**) Forehead probe. (**E**) Ear probe.

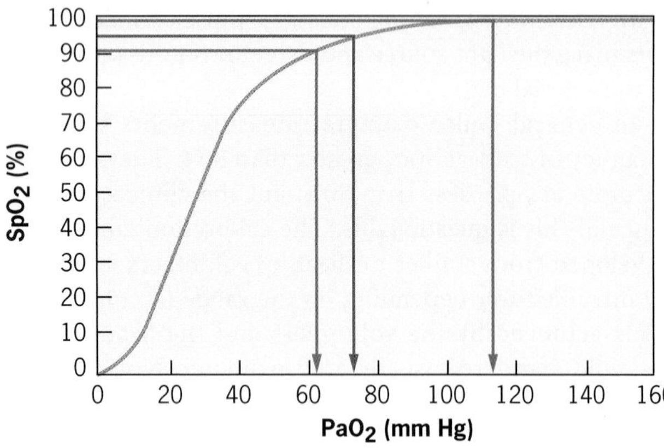

FIGURE 5–6 If the pulse oximeter displays Spo_2 95%, the arterial oxygen saturation could be as low as 91% or as high as 99%. Note that this translates to a wide range of Pao_2.

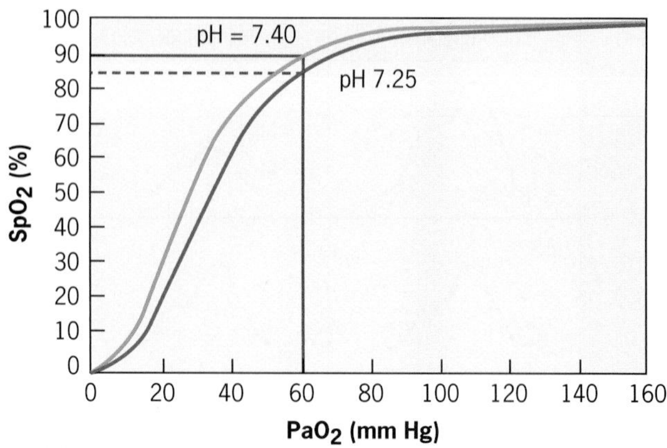

FIGURE 5–7 Note that a shift in the oxyhemoglobin equilibration curve results in a change in Spo_2 without a change in Pao_2.

displays a Spo_2 of 95%, the true saturation could be as low as 91% or as high as 99% (**Figure 5–6**). If the true saturation is 91%, the Pao_2 will be about 60 to 70 mm Hg. If the true saturation is 99%, however, the Pao_2 might be very high. A shift of the oxyhemoglobin equilibration curve can change the Spo_2, although no change in Pao_2 has occurred (**Figure 5–7**). For example, a respiratory acidosis will cause the curve to shift to the right, resulting in a decrease in Spo_2 even with no change in Pao_2.

In the intensive care unit (ICU), pulse oximetry is monitored on a continuous basis. Outside the ICU, the availability of portable, battery-powered units has resulted in the common practice of spot-checking hospitalized patients during clinical care or oxygen therapy. Although this practice may enhance appropriate oxygen therapy, allowing weaning or discontinuation of unnecessary prescriptions, it has some potential problems. It provides no direct information about the $Paco_2$ and may not accurately reflect the Pao_2 because of changes in the shape and position of the oxyhemoglobin dissociation curve.

Limitations

Most pulse oximeters only measure the percentage of HbO_2 relative to the sum of HbO_2 and Hb (functional saturation):

$$Spo_2 = \frac{HbO_2}{(HbO_2 + Hb)} \times 100\%$$

Refer to **Figure 5–8**. Because of the light absorption characteristics of carboxyhemoglobin (HbCO) relative to HbO_2 (Figure 5–8A), the oximeter overestimates HbO_2 saturation by an amount roughly equal to the HbCO level.[4] For methemoglobin (Hbmet), the light absorption for red and infrared light is nearly identical, resulting in a Spo_2 estimate of 85% (Figure 5–8B).[4] Thus, Hbmet causes the Spo_2 to be inaccurately low for an arterial oxygen saturation greater than 85% and it causes the Spo_2 to be inaccurately high for an oxygen saturation less than 85%. Fetal hemoglobin[5] and sickle cell anemia[6] do not affect the accuracy of pulse oximetry.

Care must be taken to ensure that the pulse oximeter probe is fitted correctly. If the pulse oximeter probe does not fit correctly, light can be shunted from the LEDs directly to the photodetector. This will cause a falsely low Spo_2 if Sao_2 is greater than 85%, and a falsely elevated Spo_2 if Sao_2 is less than 85%. This is called the **penumbra effect**.

Several studies have found that the accuracy and performance of pulse oximeters are affected by deeply pigmented skin.[7] Although one study suggests that nail polish may have less effect on the accuracy of pulse oximetry than previously thought, it is prudent to remove nail polish before pulse oximetry is initiated.[8] Intravascular dyes (methylene blue and indocyanine green) also cause an underestimation of Spo_2. Hyperbilirubinemia has no effect on accuracy because the absorption peak for bilirubin (460 nm) is below that used in pulse oximetry. Xenon and fluorescent lighting affect some probes, a problem that can be prevented by shielding.

Pulse oximeters require a pulsating vascular bed. Under conditions of low flow, pulse oximetry becomes unreliable. Under these conditions, an ear probe may be more reliable than a finger probe. Although pulse oximeters are generally reliable over a wide range of hemoglobin levels, they become less accurate and reliable with conditions of severe anemia (hematocrit < 24 g/dL at low saturations, and hematocrit $< 10\%$ at all saturations). Venous pulses and a large dicrotic notch may affect the accuracy of pulse oximetry.

Pulse oximetry is usually a safe procedure. Tissue injury may result from incorrect probe application or electrical shock and burns from substitution of incompatible probes between instruments.

Approaches to Deal with Errors Caused by Motion and Low Perfusion

Pulse oximetry is accurate when all hemoglobin is either oxyhemoglobin or deoxyhemoglobin, when there are no other absorbers between the LEDs and the detector other than those present during the empirical calibration, and when all the blood that pulsates is

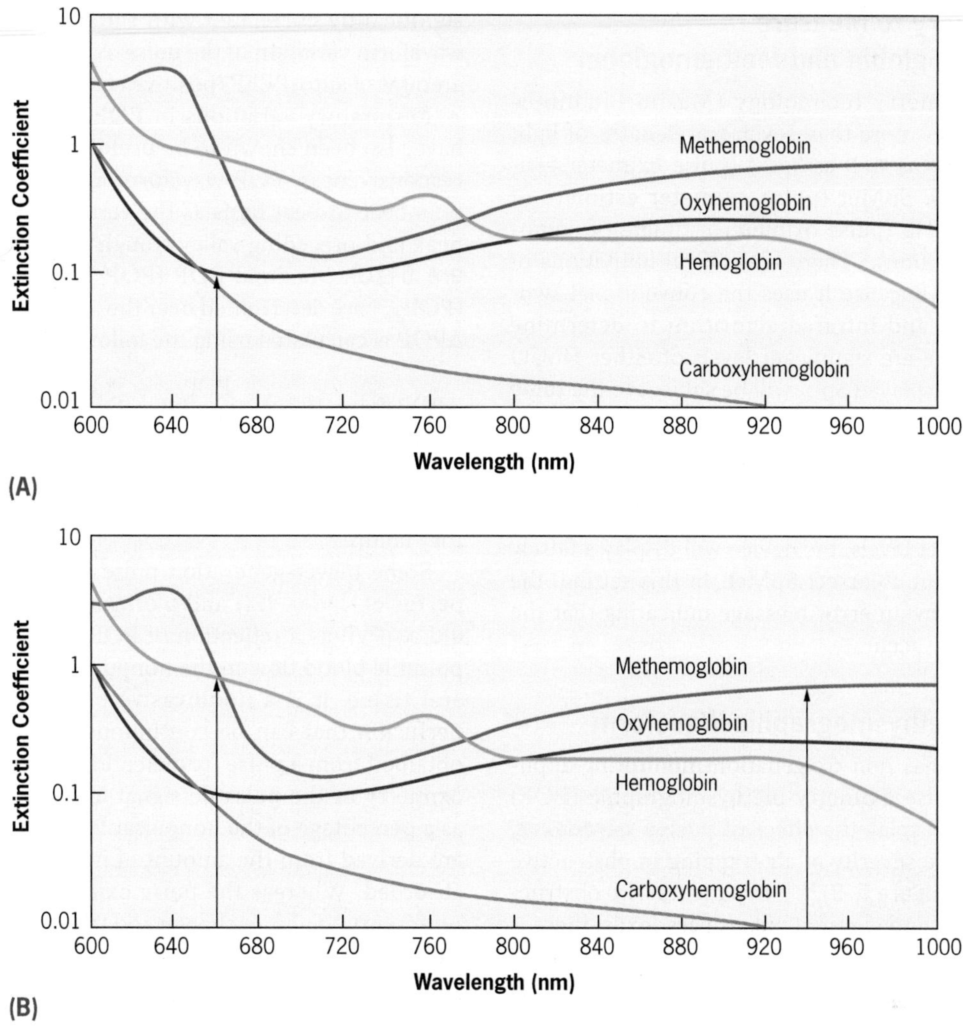

FIGURE 5–8 **(A)** At 660 nm, note that the absorptions for oxyhemoglobin and for carboxyhemoglobin are nearly identical. **(B)** Note that the absorption for methemoglobin is nearly identical at 660 nm and 940 nm.

arterial blood. Motion and low perfusion can induce considerable errors into pulse oximetry accuracy.[9] With low perfusion, there is an increase in the ratio of venous blood to arterial blood at the measuring site. Moreover, lower perfusion is associated with lower pulse amplitude, so the noise of motion has a greater effect when combined with a low signal. Strategies to address issues related to motion and low perfusion include averaging the saturation data over a longer period of time and suspending the reporting of data until clean data are available.

Manufacturers of pulse oximeters have developed motion-resistant technologies and sophisticated algorithms, some using parallel processing with multiple algorithms, in an attempt to eliminate motion artifacts from the pulse signal. Three approaches are Fourier artifact-suppression technology (FAST; Philips Medical Systems, Andover, Mass.), discrete saturation transform (DST; Masimo, Irvine, Calif.), and variable cardiac gated averaging (Nellcor, Pleasanton, Calif.).[10] Because these algorithms are proprietary, the details on how each manufacturer's technology identifies and processes the incoming signals are not available. The DST comprises a reference signal generator, an adaptive filter, and a peak picker, which work in concert to determine the most likely Spo_2 value based on the incoming signals. The FAST algorithm identifies the frequency components of the pulse rate and compares those to the frequency components of the incoming signal to select the component that is at the pulse rate for both the red and infrared wavelengths. The OxiMax N-600 from Nellcor uses the variable cardiac gated averaging algorithm, which attenuates incoming signals that do not occur synchronously with the average rhythm of the pulse rate and allows the parts of the waveform that are synchronous with the heart rate to remain unattenuated and thus contribute more to the calculated Spo_2.

The clinical performance of new-generation pulse oximeters is better than that of earlier devices, although there is no strong and convincing evidence that the performance of any single new-generation device is superior to that of any of the others.

Pulse Oximetry to Measure Carboxyhemoglobin and Methemoglobin

New pulse oximetry technology (Masimo Rainbow Technology) uses more than seven wavelengths of light to measure Spo_2 as well as Spco (pulse oximeter estimate of HbCO), SpMet (pulse oximeter estimate of Hbmet), and SpHb (pulse oximeter estimate of hemoglobin concentration).[4] There are several limitations of this technology. Because it uses the conventional two-wavelength red and infrared algorithm to determine Spo_2, when there are significant levels of either HbCO or Hbmet, the displayed Spo_2 will be subject to the same errors described earlier. However, the presence of a high Spco or SpMet display would alert the user to this error. Another limitation is the crosstalk between the Hbmet and HbCO measurement channels. In the presence of significant Hbmet levels, the device will display a falsely elevated Spco but a correct SpMet. In this setting, the device will display an error message indicating that the Spco may not be accurate.

Use of the Plethysmographic Waveform

Pulse oximetry has non-oxygenation-monitoring applications. The pulse oximetry plethysmographic (POP) waveform may display the effect of **pulsus paradoxus**, and therefore the severity of air trapping in obstructive airway disease (**Figure 5–9**).[11–14] In patients with obstructive lung disease and elevated pulsus paradoxus, there is an altered pulse oximetry baseline tracing manifested as the respiratory waveform variation. Pulsus paradoxus is significantly correlated with the degree of respiratory waveform variation of the pulse oximetry tracing and the amount of auto-PEEP (positive end-expiratory pressure).

Respiratory variations in POP waveform amplitude have also been shown to be useful in prediction of fluid responsiveness. POP waveform amplitude is measured on a beat-to-beat basis as the vertical distance between peak and preceding valley trough in the waveform (**Figure 5–10**). Maximal POP (POP_{max}) and minimal POP (POP_{min}) are determined over the same respiratory cycle. ΔPOP is calculated using the following formula:

$$\Delta POP\,(\%) = 100 \times \frac{POP_{max} - POP_{min}}{(POP_{max} + POP_{min})/2}$$

A ΔPOP greater than 15% is predictive of fluid responsiveness in mechanically ventilated patients with circulatory failure.[15]

Some newer-generation pulse oximeters display the **perfusion index (PI)** and **plethysmographic variability index (PVI)** as a reflection of POP. PI is the ratio of the pulsatile blood flow to the nonpulsatile blood in peripheral tissue. It is a noninvasive measure of peripheral perfusion that can be continuously and noninvasively obtained from a pulse oximeter. PI is calculated by pulse oximetry as the pulsatile signal (during arterial inflow) as a percentage of the nonpulsatile signal, both of which are derived from the amount of infrared (940-nm) light absorbed. Whereas the pulse oximeter plethysmogram represents a volume change and the arterial blood pressure represents a pressure change, cyclical shifts in the plethysmogram reflect similar cyclic changes in blood

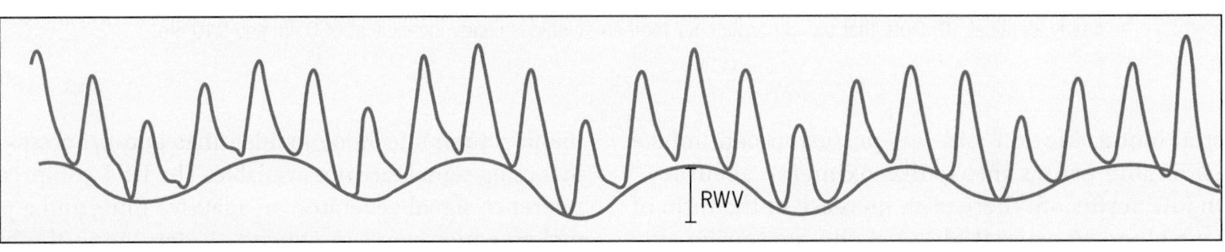

(A)

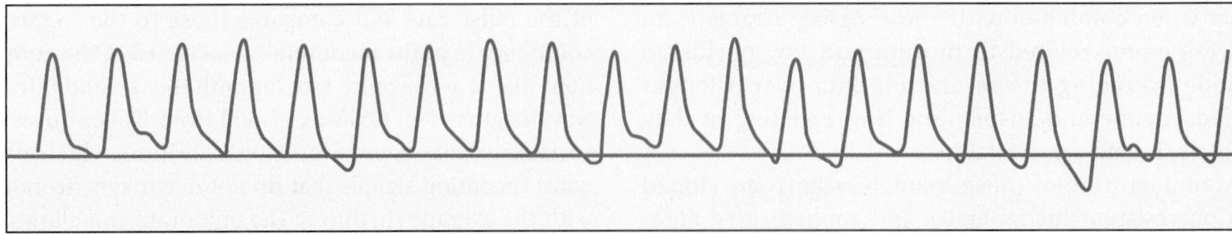

(B)

FIGURE 5–9 Pulse oximeter tracings from a 60-year-old woman with an exacerbation of chronic obstructive pulmonary disease who was admitted to the ICU in ventilatory failure. (**A**) The patient's pulse oximetry tracing at the time of admission, revealing the respiratory variability in the pulse oximeter plethysmography tracing. Her measured pulsus paradoxus at this time was 16 mm Hg. (**B**) The patient's pulse oximetry tracing after 12 hours of aggressive therapy. Her pulsus paradoxus at this time was 8 mm Hg. Note the absence of respiratory waveform variation (RWV) in the baseline of the oximeter tracing after the clinical improvement in airflow and the resolution of elevated pulsus paradoxus. Reproduced from Hartert TV, et al. Use of pulse oximetry to recognize severity of airflow obstruction in obstructive airway disease: correlation with pulsus paradoxus. *Chest.* 1999;115:475–481.

pressure. These changes reflect an intrathoracic pressure relative to the intravascular volume. PVI is a measure of the dynamic changes in the PI that occur during the respiratory cycle:

$$\text{PVI (\%)} = 100 \times (PI_{max} - PI_{min})/PI_{max}$$

Similar to ΔPOP, the greater the PVI, the greater variability there is in the waveform variability over a respiratory cycle.

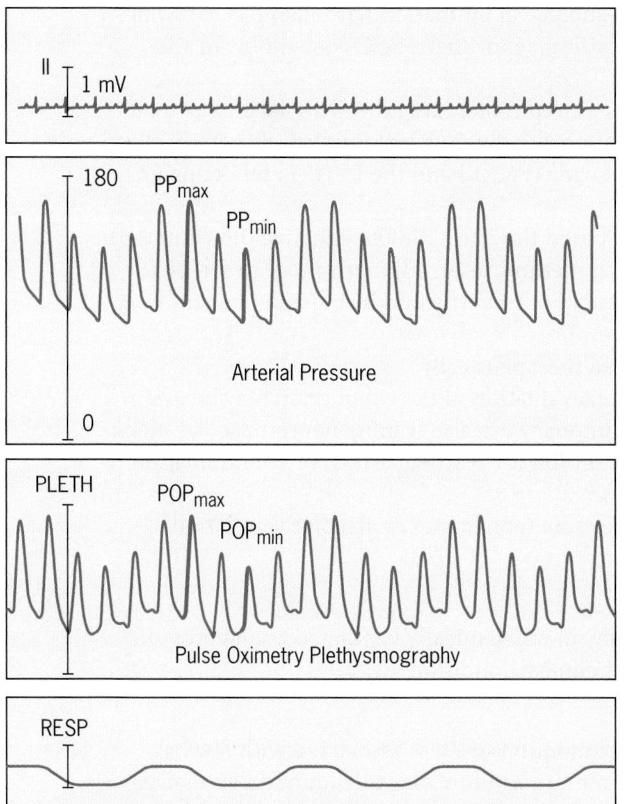

FIGURE 5–10 Comparison between invasive arterial pressure and pulse oximeter plethysmography recordings. Simultaneous recording of electrocardiographic lead (II), systemic arterial pressure, pulse oximetry plethysmography (PLETH), and respiratory signal (RESP) in one illustrative patient. POP, pulse oximetry plethysmographic; PP, pulse pressure. Reproduced from Cannesson M, Besnard C, Durand PG, Bohé J, Jacques D. Relation between respiratory variations in pulse oximetry plethysmographic waveform amplitude and arterial pulse pressure in ventilated patients. *Crit Care.* 2005;9:R562–R568.

Capnography

Capnometry and capnography are noninvasive techniques that measure the carbon dioxide levels in expired gas (**CPG 5–2**).[16] **Capnometry** refers to the numeric display of CO_2 measurements taken from the airway. When the CO_2 is plotted against time and displayed graphically as a waveform, it is called **capnography**. Most capnometers measure CO_2 by infrared absorption, although mass spectrometry and Raman spectrometry can also be used.

Two airway sampling systems are used in capnometry: *mainstream* sensors and *sidestream* sensors (**Figure 5–11**). There are advantages and disadvantages of each approach (**Table 5–1**). The mainstream capnometer is placed directly into the breathing circuit, usually directly at the airway. Infrared light is passed across the airstream to a photodetector. Improvements in analyzer technology and miniaturization have resulted in the development of low-dead-space, lightweight, and durable mainstream sensors. Because they are positioned on the airway, they may be adversely affected by the accumulation of moisture, secretions, and debris. Mainstream designs are best suited to patients with artificial airways.

The sidestream capnometer uses small-bore tubing to aspirate gas from or adjacent to the airway. The tubing aspirates the respiratory gases to a remote measuring chamber for analysis. Moisture and secretions must be removed from the tubing with traps, filters, purging, or reverse flow maneuvers before the sample enters the analysis cell. Some tubing is designed to be water vapor permeable, allowing moisture to escape by diffusion and evaporation. There is always an analysis delay when sidestream monitors are used because of the time required to move the sample from the airway to the sensor. The delay depends on the length of the tubing, its diameter, and the rate at which the gas is aspirated. Sidestream capnometers can be incorporated into nasal cannula designs for nonintubated patients (**Figure 5–12**).

The CO_2 infrared absorption peak (4.26 μm) lies between two peaks for water and very close to a peak for nitrous oxide (**Figure 5–13**). The latter poses an interference problem during the administration of nitrous oxide (N_2O) as an anesthesia gas. Correction factors and

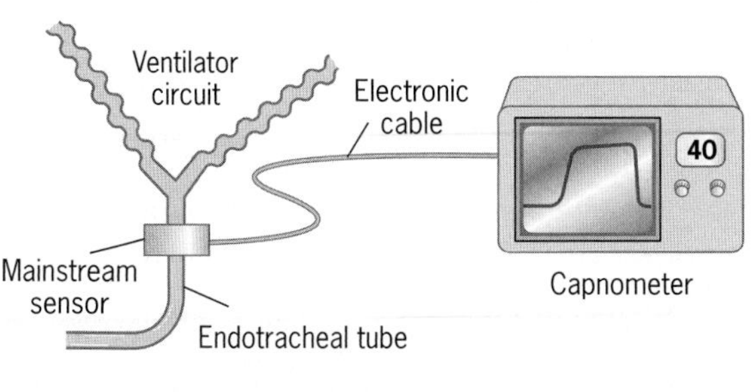

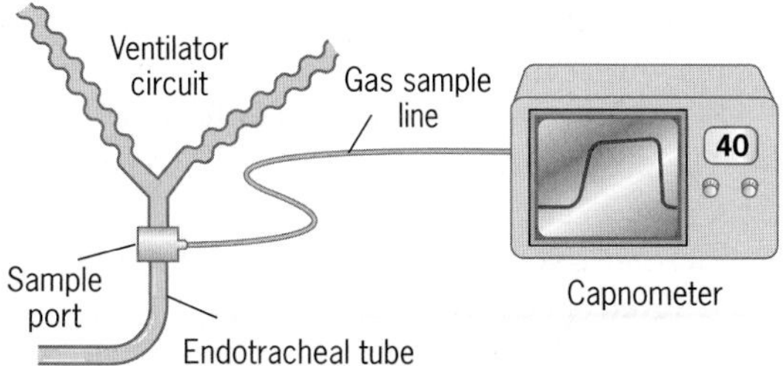

FIGURE 5–11 (**A**) Mainstream capnometry. (**B**) Sidestream capnometry.

CLINICAL PRACTICE GUIDELINE 5–2

Capnometry and Capnography During Mechanical Ventilation

Indications

- To evaluate exhaled CO_2, especially end-tidal CO_2, which is the maximum partial pressure of CO_2 exhaled during a tidal breath (just before the beginning of inspiration) and is designated P_{ETCO_2}
- To monitor the severity of pulmonary disease and evaluate the response to therapy, especially therapy intended to improve the ratio of dead space to tidal volume (V_D/V_T) and the matching of ventilation to perfusion ($\dot{V}/\dot{Q}$), and possibly to increase coronary blood flow
- As an adjunct to determine that tracheal rather than esophageal intubation has taken place (low or absent cardiac output may negate its use for this indication); colorimetric CO_2 detectors are adequate devices for this purpose
- To continuously monitor the integrity of the ventilatory circuit, including the artificial airway
- To evaluate the efficiency of mechanical ventilatory support through determination of the difference between the arterial partial pressure of carbon dioxide (Pa_{CO_2}) and the P_{ETCO_2}, reflecting CO_2 elimination
- To monitor the adequacy of pulmonary and coronary blood flow; to estimate effective (nonshunted) pulmonary capillary blood flow by a partial rebreathing method; as an adjunctive tool to screen for pulmonary embolism; to monitor the matching of ventilation to perfusion during independent lung ventilation for unilateral pulmonary contusion
- To monitor inspired CO_2 when CO_2 gas is administered therapeutically
- To graphically evaluate the ventilator–patient interface; evaluation of the capnogram may be useful in the detection of rebreathing of CO_2, obstructive pulmonary disease, waning neuromuscular blockade (curare cleft), cardiogenic oscillations, esophageal intubation, cardiac arrest, or contamination of the monitor or sampling line with secretions or mucus
- Measurement of the volume of CO_2 elimination to assess metabolic rate or alveolar ventilation, or both

Contraindications

- There are no absolute contraindications to capnography in mechanically ventilated adults provided the data obtained are evaluated in light of the patient's clinical condition.

Hazards and Complications

- Capnography with a clinically approved device is a safe, noninvasive test associated with few hazards. With mainstream analyzers, use of too large a sampling window may introduce an excessive amount of dead space into the ventilator circuit. Care must be taken to minimize the amount of additional weight placed on the artificial airway by the sampling window or, in the case of a sidestream analyzer, by the sampling line.

Limitations

- The composition of the respiratory gas mixture may affect the capnogram, depending on the measurement technology used; the infrared spectrum of CO_2 has some similarities to the spectra of oxygen and nitrous oxide; the reporting algorithm of some devices (primarily mass spectrometers) assumes that the only gases present in the sample are those that the device is capable of measuring—when a gas that the mass spectrometer cannot detect (such as helium) is present, the reported values of CO_2 are incorrectly elevated in proportion to the concentration of the undetectable gas present.
- The breathing frequency may affect the capnograph. High breathing frequencies may exceed the response capabilities of the capnograph. In addition, a breathing frequency above 10 breaths/min has been shown to affect devices differently.
- The presence of Freon (used as a propellant in metered dose inhalers) in the respiratory gas has been shown to artificially increase the CO_2 reading of mass spectrometers (that is, to show an apparent increase in the CO_2 concentration). A similar effect has not yet been demonstrated with Raman or infrared spectrometers.
- Contamination of the monitor or sampling system by secretions or condensate, use of a sample tube that is too long, a sampling rate that is too high, or obstruction of the sampling chamber can lead to unreliable results.

(continues)

Clinical Practice Guideline 5–2 *(continued)*

- Use of filters between the patient airway and the sampling line of the capnograph may lead to lowered P_{ETCO_2} readings.
- Low cardiac output may cause a false-negative result when attempting to verify endotracheal tube position in the trachea. False-positive results have been reported with endotracheal tube position in the pharynx and when antacids or carbonated beverages, or both, are present in the stomach.
- Decreased tidal volume delivery is possible during volume modes, some dual control modes, and time-cycled pressure limited ventilation with low continuous flow rates if the sampling flow rate of a sidestream analyzer is too high, especially in neonates and pediatrics.
- Inaccurate measurement of expired CO_2 may be caused by leaks of gas from the patient/ventilator system preventing collection of expired gases.

Modified from AARC clinical practice guideline: capnometry and capnography during mechanical ventilation—2003 revision and update. *Respir Care.* 2003;48:534–537. Reprinted with permission.

TABLE 5–1 Mainstream and Sidestream Capnometers

Advantages	Disadvantages
Mainstream Capnometer Sensor at patient airway Fast response (crisp waveform) Short lag time (real-time readings) No sample flow to reduce tidal volume	Secretions and humidity block sensor Sensor heated to prevent condensation Bulky sensor at patient airway Does not measure N_2O Difficult to use with nonintubated patients Cleaning and sterilization of reusable sensor
Sidestream Capnometer No bulky sensors or heaters at airway Ability to measure N_2O Disposable sample line Can be used with nonintubated patients	Secretions block sample tubing Water trap required Slow response to CO_2 changes Sample flow may decrease tidal volume

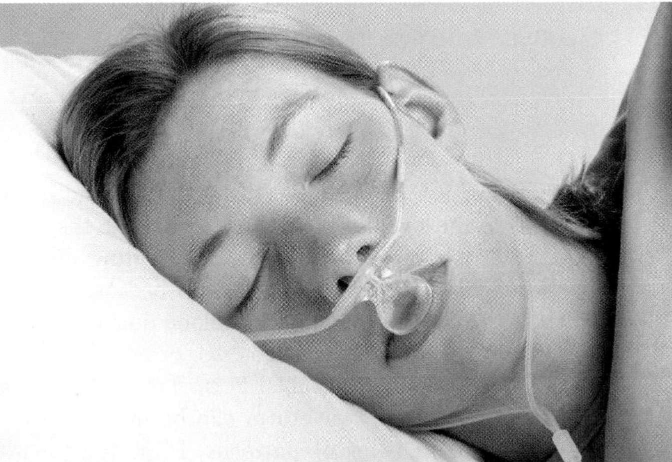

FIGURE 5–12 Nasal cannula designed for CO_2 sampling and oxygen administration (Smart CapnoLine, Oridion). The cannula samples CO_2 from both the nares and the mouth while oxygen is delivered through pinholes directed toward both the nose and mouth.

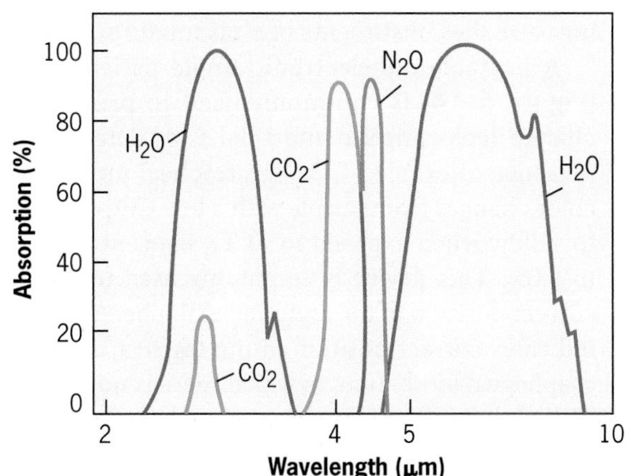

FIGURE 5–13 Carbon dioxide absorption spectra. Adapted from Decker M, Strohl K. *Pulse Oximetry. Biophysical Measurement Series: Respiration*. SpaceLabs Medical; 1994.

filters can be used to address this problem. Conventional sidestream infrared analyzers must be calibrated on a regular basis. Room air (zero) and 5% CO_2 are used to perform a two-point calibration. Newer commercially available capnometers allow self-zeroing and calibration features. Until recently, the infrared radiation technique used for capnography was nondispersive blackbody technology. Molecular correlation spectroscopy is also available, which uses a radiation source that emits only CO_2-specific radiation and uses a small sample cell (15 μL) and a low flow rate.

The **mass spectrometer** is used to measure respiratory and anesthetic gases. Multichannel units are available to monitor several patients simultaneously. A mass spectrometer aspirates sample gas into a vacuum chamber, where it is ionized by an electron beam. The charged molecules are accelerated through a magnetic field and disperse according to their mass and charge. This dispersion allows them to be separated before they reach a panel of detectors. Because even molecules of similar mass (N_2O and CO_2) ionize to different species (N_2O^+ and CO_2^+), this technique allows accurate measurement of several gases. Mass spectrometers have the advantage of being able to measure all respiratory gases breath by breath and are the most accurate analyzers in clinical use. However, they generally are too expensive and cumbersome for use outside the operating room or research settings.

Another method that can be used to measure CO_2 in capnographs is **Raman spectroscopy**. When ultraviolet or visible light strikes gas molecules, energy is absorbed and reemitted at the same wavelength and direction. A small fraction of the absorbed energy is reemitted at new wavelengths in a phenomenon known as *Raman scattering*. Raman scattering results in reemission at a longer wavelength to produce a red-shifted spectrum. The wavelength shift and amount of scattering can be used to measure the constituents of a gas mixture.

A portable nonelectronic single-patient-use device (**Figure 5–14**) is commonly used to produce a color change (colorimetric end-tidal CO_2 detection) in the presence of exhaled CO_2 (i.e., tracheal intubation). The color changes from purple with a low CO_2 concentration to yellow when exposed to a CO_2 concentration of 2.0% to 5.0%. This device is commonly used to confirm the correct position of the endotracheal tube. A color change indicates correct position in the trachea, as opposed to esophageal intubation, in which there is no color change. This technique can also be used to detect accidental tracheal placement of a nasogastric tube (**Figure 5–15**). In this case, a color change indicates incorrect placement of the tube in the trachea.[17]

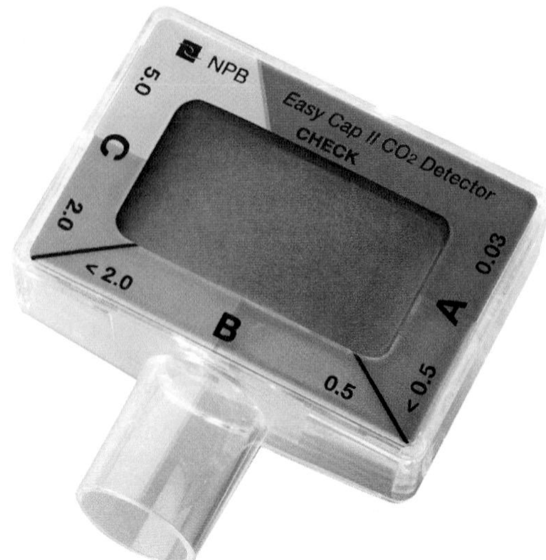

FIGURE 5–14 Colorimetric CO_2 sensor designed to confirm endotracheal intubation. It fits between the endotracheal tube and the manual bag-valve O_2 device.

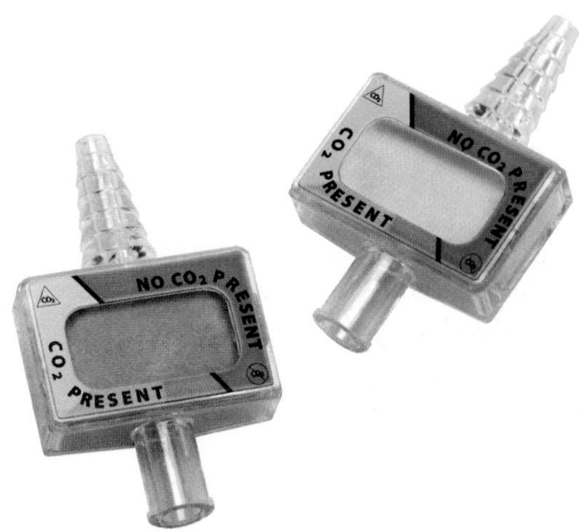

FIGURE 5–15 Colorimetric CO_2 sensor designed to confirm nasogastric tube placement.

Time-Based Capnography

The traditional **capnogram** plots P_{CO_2} on the vertical axis and time on the horizontal axis. During inhalation, P_{CO_2} at the airway equals zero. At the beginning of exhalation, it remains low as the anatomic dead space empties. As the alveolar gas begins to mix with the dead space, CO_2 rises rapidly. A plateau, representing alveolar gas, develops, rising gently, presumably because of CO_2 added to the alveoli from capillary blood during exhalation (**Figure 5–16**). Peak exhaled P_{CO_2} or **end-tidal P_{CO_2}** (P_{ETCO_2}) represents the alveolar P_{CO_2}.

The capnographic waveform can be inspected for specific abnormalities or patterns. In patients with airways obstruction, the slope of the alveolar plateau increases because of inhomogeneous alveolar emptying (**Figure 5–17**). Regions of the lung with delayed emptying caused by increased resistance (long time constants) continue to add CO_2 to expired gas during the latter part of exhalation.

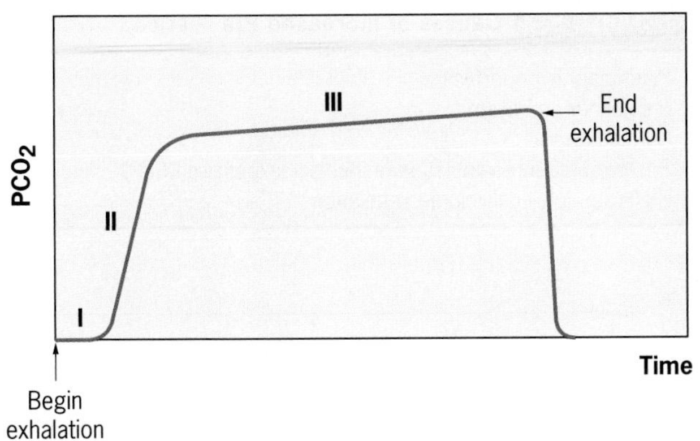

FIGURE 5–16 Time-based capnogram. I, anatomic dead space; II, the transition from anatomic dead space to the alveolar plateau; III, the alveolar plateau.

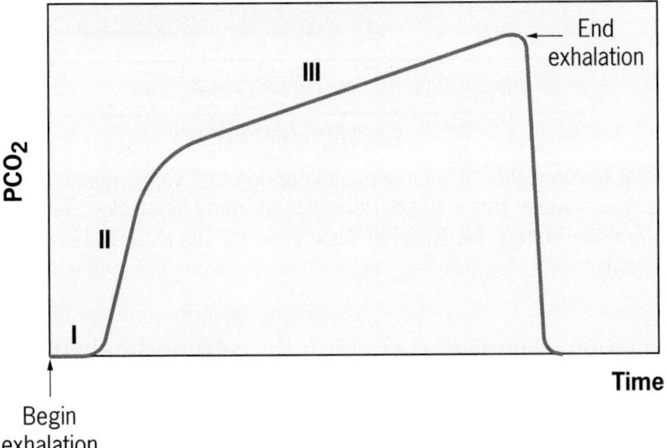

FIGURE 5–17 Capnogram produced with airflow obstruction.

TABLE 5–2 Causes of Increased and Decreased P_{ETCO_2}

Increased P_{ETCO_2}	Decreased P_{ETCO_2}
Increased CO_2 production and delivery to the lungs: Fever, sepsis, bicarbonate administration, increased metabolic rate, seizures	*Decreased CO_2 production and delivery to the lungs:* Hypothermia, pulmonary hypoperfusion, cardiac arrest, pulmonary embolism, hemorrhage, hypotension
Decreased alveolar ventilation: Respiratory center depression, muscular paralysis, hypoventilation, COPD	*Increased alveolar ventilation:* Hyperventilation
Equipment malfunction: Rebreathing, exhausted CO_2 absorber, leak in ventilator circuit	*Equipment malfunction:* Ventilator disconnect, esophageal intubation, complete airway obstruction, poor sampling, leak around endotracheal tube cuff

End-Tidal P_{CO_2}

End-tidal P_{CO_2} is determined by the production of CO_2, its subsequent delivery to the lungs by cardiac output, alveolar ventilation, and proper sampling and equipment performance. **Table 5–2** lists causes of an increase or decrease in the P_{ETCO_2}. P_{ETCO_2} is used clinically to ensure that the tracheal tube or mask ventilates the lungs, to estimate the Pa_{CO_2}, to detect changes in pulmonary blood flow or dead space ventilation, and to detect the addition of excess CO_2 to the systemic circulation.

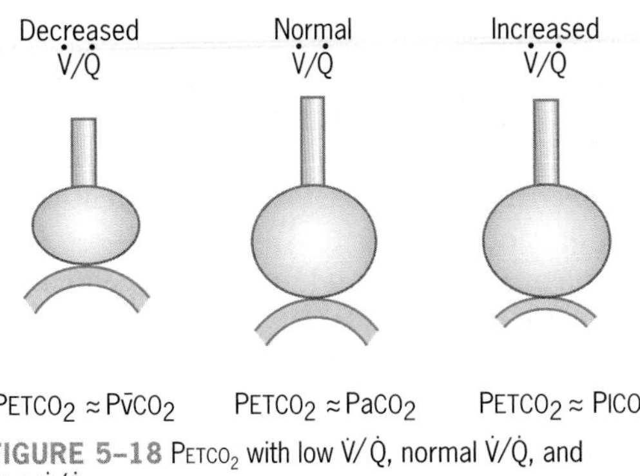

FIGURE 5–18 P_{ETCO_2} with low $\dot{V}/\dot{Q}$, normal $\dot{V}/\dot{Q}$, and high $\dot{V}/\dot{Q}$.

> **RESPIRATORY RECAP**
>
> **Capnography**
>
> » Capnography uses either mainstream or sidestream sampling.
>
> » The CO_2 level is measured by infrared absorption, mass spectrometry, or colorimetric techniques.
>
> » End-tidal P_{CO_2} often is an imprecise reflection of Pa_{CO_2}.
>
> » Capnography is useful in the detection of esophageal intubation.
>
> » Volumetric capnography can be used to measure carbon dioxide production and cardiac output.

The P_{CO_2} of an individual lung unit depends on $\dot{V}/\dot{Q}$ (**Figure 5–18**). Without perfusion (pure dead space; $\dot{V}/\dot{Q} = \infty$), the P_{ACO_2} is similar to the inspired P_{CO_2} (i.e., zero). With a normal $\dot{V}/\dot{Q}$ unit, the P_{ACO_2} is the same as the arterial P_{CO_2} (i.e., 40 mm Hg). With a low $\dot{V}/\dot{Q}$ unit, the P_{ACO_2} increases toward the $P\bar{v}_{CO_2}$ (i.e., 45 mm Hg). The P_{ACO_2}, and thus the end-tidal P_{CO_2}, must always remain between zero and the $P\bar{v}_{CO_2}$. P_{ETCO_2} is normally several mm Hg less than the Pa_{CO_2}. However, the relationship between the Pa_{CO_2} and P_{ETCO_2} will vary depending on the relative contributions of various $\dot{V}/\dot{Q}$ units comprising the lungs.

The presence of CO_2 in exhaled gas usually indicates tracheal intubation. Exhaled CO_2 does not always ensure proper endotracheal tube placement, however, because the tube could be in the main stem bronchus or in the pharynx. Although esophageal intubation generally results in a very low P_{ETCO_2}, falsely elevated readings may occur if the patient ingested antacids or carbonated beverages. The elevated value should diminish with subsequent breaths. Even with proper endotracheal tube placement, the P_{ETCO_2} may remain deceptively low with cardiogenic shock. P_{ETCO_2} is also used to detect tracheal placement of a nasogastric tube. A P_{ETCO_2} near zero suggests that the gastric tube is *not* in the trachea.[17]

Even though P_{ETCO_2} approximates Pa_{CO_2} in normal individuals, capnometry cannot routinely be used as a substitute to measure arterial P_{CO_2}. Most critically ill patients have ventilation-perfusion abnormalities, particularly an increased ratio of dead space to tidal volume

(VD/VT), resulting in a significant Pa_{CO_2} − P_{ETCO_2} difference ($P[a - ET]CO_2$) (**Table 5–3**). Even patients whose $P(a - ET)CO_2$ is calibrated by simultaneous arterial blood gas and capnometry measurements do not remain stable enough over time to render the measurement a reliable estimate of Pa_{CO_2}.

With no pulmonary blood flow, P_{ETCO_2} equals zero. Because the end-tidal CO_2 is partly determined by the amount of blood flow returning to the lungs from the systemic circulation, it has been used to verify the effectiveness of cardiopulmonary resuscitation (CPR). Adequate CPR is associated with increasing P_{ETCO_2} levels. It has been suggested that if end-tidal CO_2 does not rise above 10 mm Hg after 20 minutes of pulseless resuscitation, the prognosis is poor.

Pulmonary embolism is associated with an increased VD/VT. The $P(a - ET)CO_2$ is increased with pulmonary embolism. Because many conditions increase VD/VT, an increased $P(a - ET)CO_2$ is not specific to pulmonary embolism.

Capnometry has also been proposed as a means to determine optimum PEEP during mechanical ventilation and as an adjunct to weaning. In patients with acute respiratory distress syndrome (ARDS), for example, excessive levels of PEEP increase VD/VT and $P(a - ET)CO_2$. This approach has not proved reliable enough for routine use in ICU patients. As a noninvasive monitor during the ventilator discontinuation process, capnometric measurements of the respiratory rate and elevated P_{ETCO_2} have also been unreliable.

TABLE 5–3 Causes of Increased $P(a - ET)CO_2$

Pulmonary hypoperfusion
Pulmonary embolism
Cardiac arrest
Positive pressure ventilation (especially excessive PEEP)
High-rate, low-tidal-volume ventilation

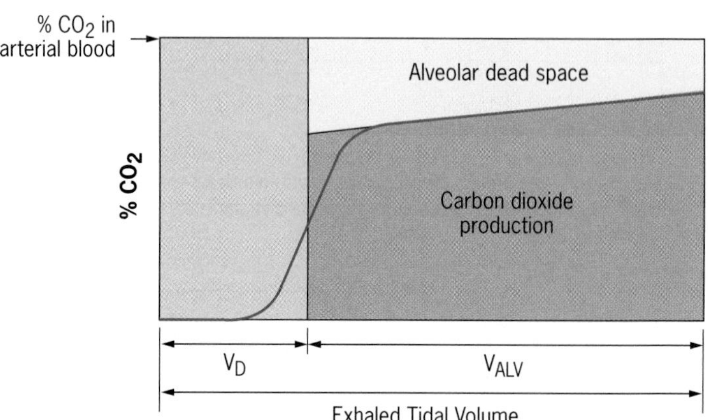

FIGURE 5–19 Components of volume-based capnogram. VD, anatomic dead space; VALV, alveolar gas volume. Reproduced from Longnecker David, et al. 2008. *Anesthesiology*. McGraw-Hill, New York. (© The McGraw-Hill Companies, Inc.)

Volume-Based Capnography

A normal volume-based capnogram is shown in **Figure 5–19**. It is displayed with the P_{CO_2} on the vertical axis and the volume on the horizontal axis.[18–20] At the beginning of exhalation, the P_{CO_2} remains zero as gas from the anatomic dead space leaves the airway (phase I). The capnogram rises sharply as alveolar gas mixes with dead space gas (phase II). The capnogram then forms a plateau during most of exhalation (phase III). Phase III represents gas flow from the alveoli and therefore is called the *alveolar plateau*. The P_{CO_2} at end-exhalation is the P_{ETCO_2}. Anatomic dead space, alveolar dead space volume, and the volume of exhaled CO_2 ($\dot{V}_{CO_2}$) can be determined from the volume-based capnogram.

Because $\dot{V}_{CO_2}$ is determined by metabolic rate, this can be used to estimate resting energy expenditure (REE):

$$REE = \dot{V}_{CO_2}(L/min) \times 5.52\ kcal/L \times 1{,}440\ min/day$$

Normal $\dot{V}_{CO_2}$ is approximately 200 mL/min (2.8 mL/kg/min).

Using volume-based capnography, it is possible to noninvasively measure cardiac output with the partial CO_2 rebreathing technique (**Figure 5–20**).[21–26] $\dot{V}_{CO_2}$ is calculated on a breath-by-breath basis, and the Fick equation is applied to establish the relationship between $\dot{V}_{CO_2}$ and cardiac output ($\dot{Q}$):

$$\dot{V}_{CO_2} = \dot{Q} \times (C\bar{v}_{CO_2} - Ca_{CO_2})$$

where $C\bar{v}_{CO_2}$ represents the CO_2 content of mixed venous blood and Ca_{CO_2} represents the CO_2 content of arterial blood. CO_2 rebreathing is performed for 35 seconds every 3 minutes. Assuming that $\dot{Q}$ remains constant during the rebreathing procedure yields the following:

$$\Delta\dot{V}_{CO_2} = \dot{Q} \times (\Delta C\bar{v}_{CO_2} - \Delta Ca_{CO_2})$$

where $\Delta\dot{V}_{CO_2}$ is the change in $\dot{V}_{CO_2}$ between normal breathing and rebreathing, $\Delta C\bar{v}_{CO_2}$ is the change in mixed venous carbon dioxide content, and ΔCa_{CO_2} is the change in arterial carbon dioxide content. If $C\bar{v}_{CO_2}$ remains constant during rebreathing, the following equation is used:

$$\Delta\dot{V}_{CO_2} = \dot{Q} \times (-\Delta Ca_{CO_2})$$

When end-capillary content (Cc'_{CO_2}) is used in place of Ca_{CO_2}, pulmonary capillary blood flow (PCBF), the blood flow that participates in alveolar gas exchange, is measured rather than $\dot{Q}$, and the following equation is used:

$$\Delta\dot{V}_{CO_2} = PCBF \times (-Cc'_{CO_2})$$

Assuming that $-Cc'_{CO_2}$ is proportional to ΔP_{ETCO_2}, the following equation can be used:

$$PCBF = \Delta\dot{V}_{CO_2} / (S \times \Delta P_{ETCO_2})$$

where ΔP_{ETCO_2} is the change in P_{ETCO_2} between normal breathing and rebreathing, and S is the slope of the

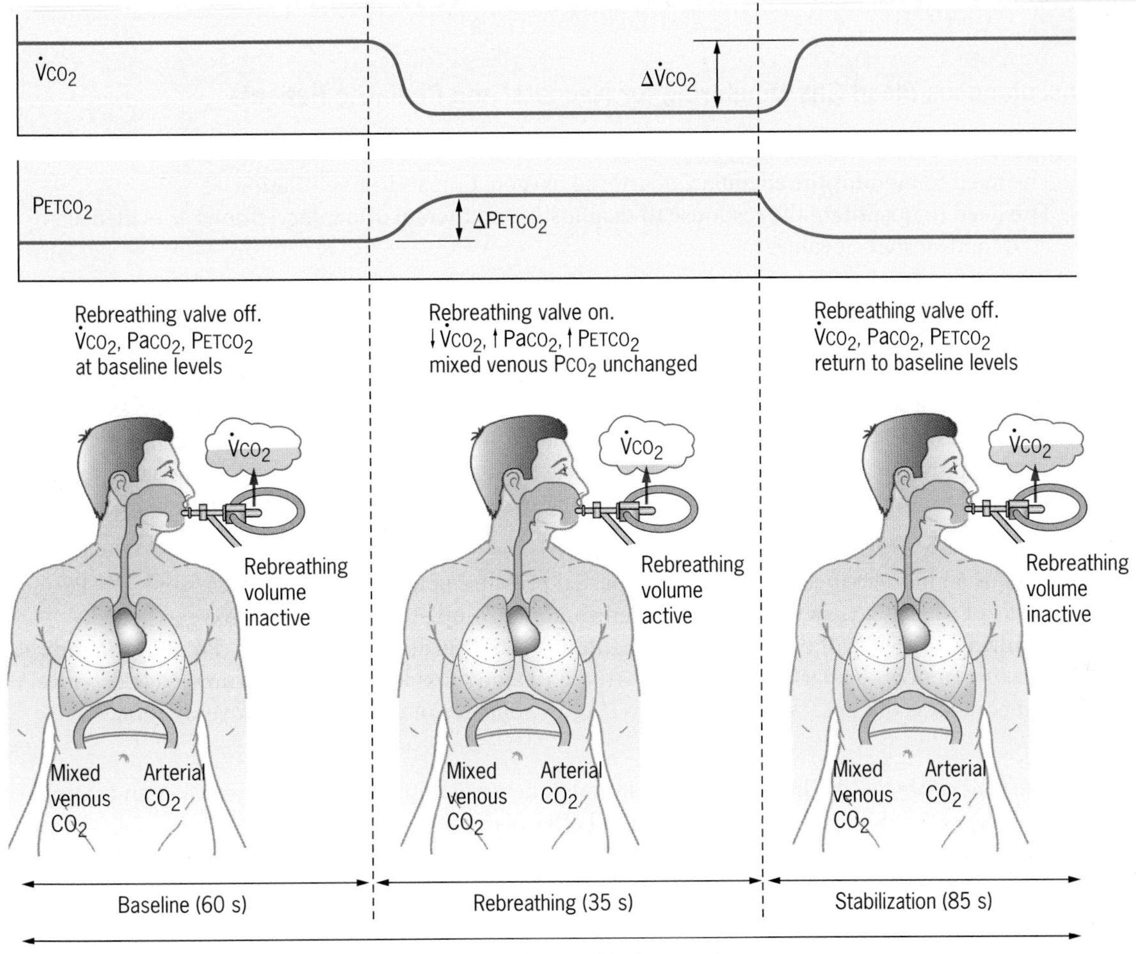

FIGURE 5–20 Rebreathing cycle used by to measure cardiac output using the partial CO_2 rebreathing technique. Modified from Longnecker David, et al. 2008. *Anesthesiology*. McGraw-Hill, New York. (© The McGraw-Hill Companies, Inc.)

carbon dioxide dissociation curve from hemoglobin. Because cardiac output is the sum of PCBF and intrapulmonary shunt flow,

$$\dot{Q} = PCBF/(1 - Q_S/Q_T)$$

The noninvasive method for estimating Q_S/Q_T is adapted from Nunn's iso-shunt plots, which are a series of continuous curves indicating the relation between arterial oxygen pressure (PaO_2) and FIO_2 at different levels of right-to-left shunt. PaO_2 is noninvasively estimated using a pulse oximeter.

There are several potential limitations of partial rebreathing for the measurement of cardiac output. In nonparalyzed patients, rebreathing increases the respiratory rate, which reduces the magnitude of the signal and limits the ability to detect changes in $PETCO_2$ and $\dot{V}CO_2$. Noise is increased by respiratory pattern irregularities that produce an unstable $PETCO_2$ and $\dot{V}CO_2$, and these may impair accuracy. Additional cardiac output not calculated due to shunt fraction is estimated from SpO_2 and FIO_2, and these may also introduce errors.

Transcutaneous Blood Gas Monitoring

Transcutaneous monitoring of O_2 and CO_2 ($PtcO_2$ and $PtcCO_2$) uses measurements at the skin surface to provide estimates of PaO_2 and $PaCO_2$ (**CPG 5–3**).[27] This type of monitoring has been used with neonates, infants, small children, and patients with peripheral vascular disease. The devices warm the skin to induce hyperemia, then electrochemically measure oxygen and carbon dioxide partial pressures at the skin surface, providing a noninvasive means of continuously monitoring arterial oxygenation and ventilation. They have been particularly

RESPIRATORY RECAP

Transcutaneous Blood Gas Monitors

- Warmed electrodes are placed on the skin to measure the $PtcO_2$ and $PtcCO_2$, which are used to estimate the PaO_2 and $PaCO_2$.
- The electrodes operate on the same principles as blood gas electrodes.
- A miniaturized single sensor combines the measurement of pulse oximetry (SpO_2) and $PtcCO_2$.

CLINICAL PRACTICE GUIDELINE 5–3

Transcutaneous Blood Gas Monitoring for Neonatal and Pediatric Patients

Indications

- The need to monitor the adequacy of arterial oxygenation and/or ventilation
- The need to quantitate the response to diagnostic and therapeutic interventions as evidenced by $Ptco_2$ and/or $Ptcco_2$ values

Contraindications

- In patients with poor skin integrity or adhesive allergy, or both, transcutaneous monitoring may be relatively contraindicated.

Hazards and Complications

- $Ptco_2$ and $Ptcco_2$ monitoring are considered safe procedures, but because of device limitations, false-negative and false-positive results may lead to inappropriate treatment of the patient. In addition, tissue injury may occur at the measuring site (e.g., erythema, blisters, burns, skin tears).

Limitations

- $Ptco_2$ is an indirect measurement of the partial pressure of arterial oxygen (Pao_2) and, like Pao_2, does not reflect oxygen delivery or oxygen content. Complete assessment of oxygen delivery requires knowledge of the hemoglobin, saturation, and cardiac output values. $Ptcco_2$ is an indirect measurement of the partial pressure of arterial carbon dioxide ($Paco_2$), but knowledge of delivery and content is not necessary to use $Ptcco_2$ as an indicator of the adequacy of ventilation.

Technical

- The procedure may be labor intensive, although newer designs have made it quicker and simpler.
- A prolonged stabilization period is required after placement.
- Manufacturers state that electrodes must be heated to produce valid results; however, clinical studies suggest that valid results may be obtained with $Ptcco_2$ electrodes operated at lower-than-recommended temperatures or with no heat.
- The theoretic basis for mandatory heating of the $Ptco_2$ electrode has not been established.
- Improper calibration, trapped air bubbles, and damaged membranes are possible and may be difficult to detect.

Clinical

- Hyperoxemia (Pao_2 over 100 mm Hg)
- Hypoperfused state (shock, acidosis)
- Improper electrode placement or application
- Use of vasoactive drugs
- Nature of the patient's skin and subcutaneous tissue (skinfold thickness, edema)

Modified from AARC clinical practice guideline: transcutaneous blood gas monitoring for neonatal and pediatric patients—2004 revision and update. *Respir Care.* 2004;49:1069–1072. Reprinted with permission.

useful in neonates and infants, in whom arterial sampling is technically difficult. Also, because intact circulation is a prerequisite for successful hyperbaric oxygen therapy, candidates with peripheral vascular disease are screened with transcutaneous O_2 monitors. Because $Ptco_2$ is affected by perfusion, it may reflect the quantity of oxygen delivered to the skin under the electrode (the product of cardiac output and arterial oxygen content). $Ptco_2$ has been used in adults to monitor the results of vascular surgery, the intent being to evaluate perfusion rather than Pao_2 per se.

The transcutaneous oxygen electrode uses the polarographic technique. The anode is surrounded by heating coils, and the platinum cathode is centered inside the anode ring. The heating coil induces local hyperemia to arterialize the skin surface. A flat membrane separates the electrode from the skin. Oxygen diffuses from the blood vessels to the skin surface and through the membrane into the electrode.

Transcutaneous carbon dioxide electrodes use a flat glass membrane permeable to CO_2. A pH electrode is positioned behind the membrane in a bicarbonate buffer.

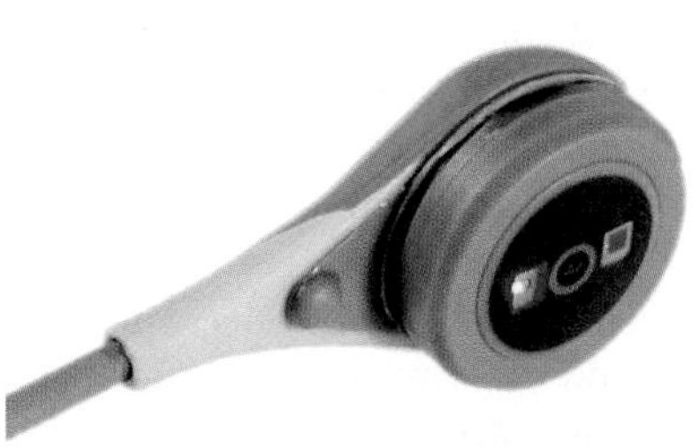

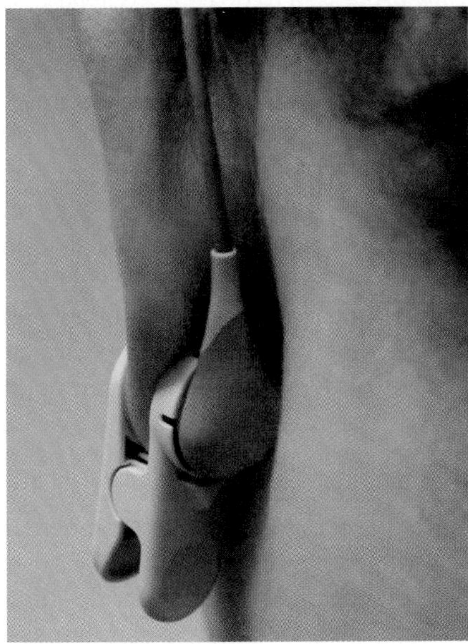

FIGURE 5–21 A sensor for noninvasive monitoring of transcutaneous carbon dioxide and oxygen saturation.

Carbon dioxide diffuses from the skin through the membrane and reacts with the buffer to produce a change in [H^+]. Similar to the PCO_2 blood gas electrode, the $PtcCO_2$ electrode detects changes in [H^+] but is calibrated to display PCO_2. Unlike the $PtcO_2$ electrode, a reasonably good correlation with $PaCO_2$ can be obtained at a temperature of 37° C (98.6° F). Because $PtcCO_2$ is consistently greater than $PaCO_2$, manufacturers incorporate a correction factor so that the $PtcCO_2$ that is displayed approximates the $PaCO_2$. Like $PtcO_2$, the proximity with which $PtcCO_2$ approximates $PaCO_2$ is the result of a complex set of physiologic events, and thus it is incorrect to believe that $PtcCO_2$ is the $PaCO_2$. For example, decreased tissue perfusion causes the $PtcCO_2$ to increase.

A miniaturized single sensor combines the measurement of pulse oximetry (SpO_2) and $PtcCO_2$ (**Figure 5–21**).[28–31] It uses a heated Severinghaus electrode combined with a pulse oximetry sensor, and is attached to the earlobe with a clip. The sensor is calibrated using a one-point dry gas calibration with 7% CO_2 when the sensor is placed in its calibration chamber. The sensor is heated to 42° C to induce local vasodilation and enhance skin permeability for CO_2 to improve gas diffusion at the site of measurement. A drop of contact gel is applied in the center of the attachment clip before the sensor is applied. The sensor is removed after 8 hours, recalibrated, and fixed on the other ear lobe.

A limitation in the use of transcutaneous blood gas monitoring is the need for a heated electrode. This carries the risk of skin burns and requires that the sensor be rotated among monitoring sites on a regular basis. The reliability of transcutaneous monitoring for accurately estimating arterial blood gases is often questioned, which has led to limited use of this technology.

Respiratory Rate and Pattern

The respiratory rate is one of the four vital signs. It is a core component of monitoring, because respiratory rate slowing (*bradypnea* or *apnea*) or increasing (*tachypnea*) may warn of clinical deterioration or impending respiratory arrest. In sleep laboratories, sophisticated respiratory rate and pattern monitoring are required during polysomnography. Respiratory (apnea) monitors are also used for infant studies in the home.

The respiratory rate is easily measured at the bedside by counting chest excursions for 30 seconds (and multiplying by 2 to obtain breaths/min) or for 60 seconds. However, this method may be inaccurate, perhaps because clinicians underestimate the importance of this vital sign. A number of other methods are available to monitor this important parameter accurately.[32]

With **impedance pneumography**, the respiratory rate and excursion can be measured by use of two electrodes placed on the chest wall. A high-frequency (20 to 100 Hz) and low-ampere AC current (less than 100 μA) is passed between the electrodes on the chest surface (this is, of course, a current too small to be felt by the patient). The strength of the current when it reaches the receiving electrode varies according to the *impedance,* or effective resistance of the tissue between the electrodes. During chest expansion, as the distance between the electrodes increases, impedance increases, causing the current to decrease. The change in current is electronically processed to calculate the respiratory rate (**Figure 5–22**). During normal tidal breathing, the signal can also be calibrated to measure tidal volume. However, volume measurements deteriorate with patient movement or a change in position. Moreover,

RESPIRATORY RECAP

Techniques to Measure the Respiratory Rate

- » Counting by inspection at the bedside
- » Impedance pneumography
- » Respiratory inductance plethysmography
- » Fiberoptic plethysmography
- » Nasal temperature- and pressure-sensing devices
- » Piezoelectric plethysmography

an obstructive apnea cannot be detected with this method, because the chest wall continues to move despite cessation of airflow. These systems usually are configured as a plug-in module for bedside monitoring of the respiratory rate in the ICU. They use the same electrodes that generally are applied to the patient for cardiac rhythm monitoring. Infant home apnea monitors are based on this technology.

Electrical impedance tomography (EIT) is an imaging technique in which an image of the conductivity is inferred from surface electrical measurements. EIT adhesive electrodes are applied to the skin, and an electric current, typically a few milliamperes of alternating current at a frequency of 10 to 100 kHz, is applied across two or more electrodes. The resulting electrical potentials are measured, and the process repeated for numerous different configurations of applied current. The lungs become less conductive as the alveoli become filled with air, and more conductive if alveoli become airless (collapsed, edematous, or consolidated). There is interest in the potential use of EIT to determine appropriate setting of PEEP.

The most accurate method for indirect measurement of tidal volume is **respiratory inductance plethysmography (RIP)**. Inductance sensors use a circuit of coiled wire woven into an elastic band and excited by an AC current. *Inductance* results from alternating electrical currents that create magnetic fields around themselves and the changes in those magnetic fields that alter other electrical currents they encounter. During tidal breathing, the bands stretch and relax. As the belt is displaced during chest expansion, changes in the magnetic fields around the wire coils result in changes in the excitation current. Variations in the excitation current caused by the expansion and contraction of the belt are electronically processed to provide a display of the ventilatory pattern, rate, and change in volume.

When rib cage and abdominal bands are used simultaneously, respiratory motion is described more completely, resulting in tidal volume measurements that correlate well with spirometry (±10%). RIP is stable and comfortable despite patient movement, which makes it suitable for use in sleep laboratories. This noninvasive technique has also been used in the ICU to monitor noninvasive ventilation and to conduct studies of the effect of PEEP on the functional residual capacity. Because it is more expensive than impedance pneumography, its use in the ICU usually is reserved for cases in which noninvasive measurements of tidal volume or changes in functional residual capacity are desired.

A modification of inductance plethysmography, **fiberoptic plethysmography**, uses optical fibers woven into elastic belts. Light is passed through the fibers into a photodetector. When rib cage or abdominal displacements stretch the elastic belt, large changes in light transmission through the fibers result. The change in light transmission is electronically processed to provide data similar to RIP. This technique has the advantage of being free of electrical interference and electrically safe for patients. It also is more sensitive than conventional RIP to small changes in lung volume. Clinical experience with this device is limited.

Temperature and pressure probes can be used to measure the rate and pattern of airflow. Disordered breathing, hypopneas, and apneas are characterized in this way. **Thermistors** and **thermocouples** detect bidirectional airflow at the nose and mouth by sensing the temperature

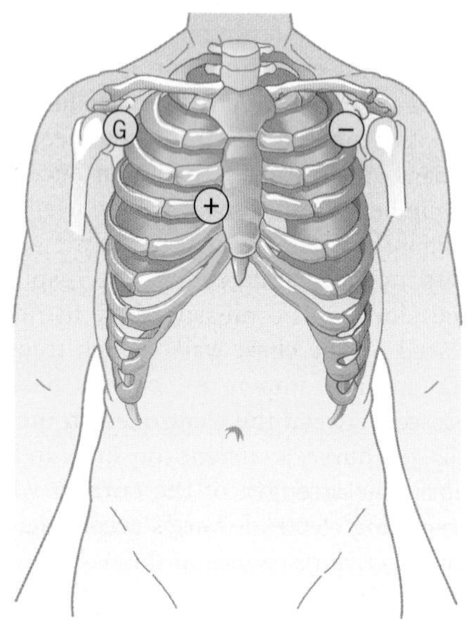

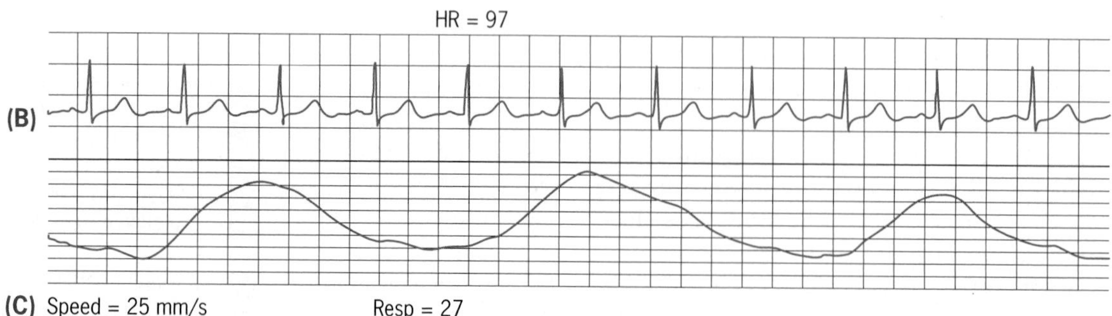

FIGURE 5–22 **(A)** Electrode placement for three-lead array. **(B)** Cardiac rate and rhythm recorded from a single ECG lead. **(C)** Respiratory impedance pneumography tracing obtained from the same electrode array.

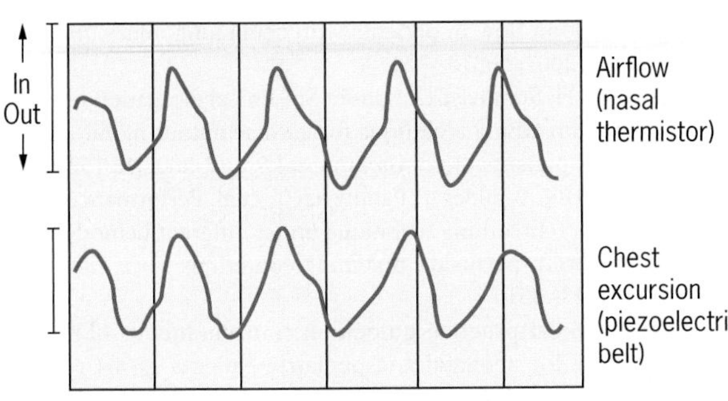

FIGURE 5–23 Airflow and chest and abdominal excursion waveforms are used to monitor respiratory rate and pattern during sleep studies. Adapted from materials from Pro-Tech Services, Woodinville, Wash.

difference between inspired room air and exhaled air that has been warmed to body temperature (**Figure 5–23**). The ability of these devices to detect airflow diminishes if the room air temperature approaches body temperature. Likewise, if the sensor touches skin and rises to body temperature, airflow cannot be detected. Other limitations of thermally based sensors are that they cannot be calibrated in terms of airflow and provide only qualitative information, that moisture condensing on the probe compromises temperature-sensing capabilities, and that loss of signal may occur if the sensor becomes dislodged from the airstream.

To simplify the plethysmography apparatus, the wire coils have been removed from the elastic belts and replaced by a piezoelectric buckle (**piezoelectric plethysmography**). This reduces the cost and allows for belts that can be adjusted to different-size patients. The buckle encloses a sensor, which generates a voltage in response to stretch passed through the ends of the belts. The sensor is not calibrated, however, and provides only a qualitative record of chest or abdominal movement, hence the term *effort belts* (refer to Figure 5–22). Effort belts based on piezoelectric sensors do not require a battery. As with all belt-type transducers, the quality and interpretability of the respiratory signal are affected if the belt loosens or slips out of the original position.

Rib cage and abdominal belts with mercury strain gauges have been phased out because of the hazard of mercury exposure. Most modern mechanical ventilators have integrated airflow transducers designed to monitor and display the respiratory rate. End-tidal CO_2 monitors also display respiratory rate.

KEY POINTS

- Pulse oximetry measures oxygen saturation by passing two wavelengths of light through a pulsating vascular bed.
- The accuracy of pulse oximetry is ±4%.
- A number of factors can affect the accuracy and performance of pulse oximetry.
- Capnometry measures the concentration of carbon dioxide exhaled from the lungs.
- Capnography can be useful for detection of esophageal intubation.
- End-tidal P_{CO_2} may not be an accurate reflection of Pa_{CO_2}.
- Volumetric capnography can be used to measure carbon dioxide production and cardiac output.
- Transcutaneous P_{O_2} and P_{CO_2} are measured with a heated electrode placed on the skin.
- The respiratory rate and pattern can be monitored through observation of chest wall motion, monitoring of nasal airflow, and measurement of chest wall motion.

REFERENCES

1. AARC clinical practice guideline: pulse oximetry. *Respir Care.* 1991;36:1406–1409.
2. Mannheimer PD. The light–tissue interaction of pulse oximetry. *Anesth Analg.* 2007;105:S10–S17.
3. McMorrow RCN, Mythen MG. Pulse oximetry. *Curr Opin Crit Care.* 2006;12:269–271.
4. Barker SJ, Badal JJ. The measurement of dyshemoglobins and total hemoglobin by pulse oximetry. *Curr Opin Anaesthesiol.* 2008;21:805–810.
5. Rajadurai VS, Walker AM, Yu VY, Oates A. Effect of fetal haemoglobin on the accuracy of pulse oximetry in preterm infants. *J Paediatr Child Health.* 1992;28:43–46.
6. Kress JP, Pohlman AS, Hall JB. Determinants of hemoglobin saturation in patients with acute sickle chest syndrome. A comparison of arterial blood gases and pulse oximetry. *Chest.* 1999;115:1316–1320.
7. Feiner JR, Severinghaus JW, Bickler PE. Dark skin decreases the accuracy of pulse oximeters at low oxygen saturation: the effects of oximeter probe type and gender. *Anesth Analg.* 2007;105:S18–S23.
8. Yamamoto LG, Yamamoto JA, Yamamoto JB, Yamamoto BE, Yamamoto PP. Nail polish does not significantly affect pulse oximetry measurements in mildly hypoxic subjects. *Respir Care.* 2008;53:1470–1474.
9. Petterson MT, Begnoche VL, Graybeal JM. The effect of motion on pulse oximetry and its clinical significance. *Anesth Analg.* 2007;105:S78–S84.
10. Gehring H, Nornberger C, Matz H, et al. The effects of motion artifact and low perfusion on the performance of a new generation of pulse oximeters in volunteers undergoing hypoxemia. *Respir Care.* 2002;47:48–60.
11. Bendjelid K. The pulse oximetry plethysmographic curve revisited. *Curr Opin Crit Care.* 2008;14:348–353.
12. Cannesson M, Desebbe O, Rosamel P, et al. Pleth variability index to monitor the respiratory variations in the pulse oximeter plethysmographic waveform amplitude and predict fluid responsiveness in the operating theatre. *Br J Anaesth.* 2008;101:200–206.
13. Shelley KH. Photoplethysmography: beyond the calculation of arterial oxygen saturation and heart rate. *Anesth Analg.* 2007;105:S31–S36.
14. Desebbe O, Cannesson M. Using ventilation-induced plethysmographic variations to optimize patient fluid status. *Curr Opin Anaesthesiol.* 2008;21:772–778.
15. Hartert TV, Wheeler AP, Sheller JR. Use of pulse oximetry to recognize severity of airflow obstruction in obstructive airway disease: correlation with pulsus paradoxus. *Chest.* 1999;115:475–481.
16. AARC clinical practice guideline: capnometry and capnography during mechanical ventilation—2003 revision and update. *Respir Care.* 2003;48:534–537.

17. Araujo-Preza CE, Melhado ME, Gutierrez FJ, et al. Use of capnometry to verify feeding tube placement. *Crit Care Med.* 2002;30:2255–2259.
18. Riou Y, Leclerc F, Neve V, et al. Reproducibility of the respiratory dead space measurements in mechanically ventilated children using the CO2SMO monitor. *Intensive Care Med.* 2004;30:1461–1467.
19. Kallet RH, Daniel BM, Garcia O, et al. Accuracy of physiologic dead space measurements in patients with acute respiratory distress syndrome using volumetric capnography: comparison with the metabolic monitor method. *Respir Care.* 2005;50:462–467.
20. Blanch L, Romero PV, Lucangelo U. Volumetric capnography in the mechanically ventilated patient. *Minerva Anesthesiol.* 2006;72:577–585.
21. Tachibana K, Imanaka H, Takeuchi M, et al. Noninvasive cardiac output measurement using partial carbon dioxide rebreathing is less accurate at settings of reduced minute ventilation and when spontaneous breathing is present. *Anesthesiology.* 2003;98:830–837.
22. Tachibana K, Imanaka H, Miyano H, et al. Effect of ventilatory settings on accuracy of cardiac output measurement using partial CO_2 rebreathing. *Anesthesiology.* 2002;96:96–102.
23. Yem JS, Tang Y, Turner MJ, et al. Sources of error in noninvasive pulmonary blood flow measurements by partial rebreathing. A computer model study. *Anesthesiology.* 2003;98:881–887.
24. de Abreu MG, Geiger S, Winkler T, et al. Evaluation of a new device for noninvasive measurement of nonshunted pulmonary capillary blood flow in patients with acute lung injury. *Intensive Care Med.* 2002;28:318–323.
25. Odenstedt H, Stenqvist O, Lundin S. Clinical evaluation of a partial CO_2 rebreathing technique for cardiac output monitoring in critically ill patients. *Acta Anaesthesiol Scand.* 2002;46:152–159.
26. de Abreu MG, Winkler T, Pahlitzsch T, et al. Performance of the partial CO_2 rebreathing technique under different hemodynamic and ventilation/perfusion matching conditions. *Crit Care Med.* 2003; 31:543–551.
27. AARC clinical practice guideline: transcutaneous blood gas monitoring for neonatal and pediatric patients—2004 revision and update. *Respir Care.* 2004;49:1069–1072.
28. Bernet-Buettiker V, Ugarte MJ, Frey B, et al. Evaluation of a new combined transcutaneous measurement of PCO_2/pulse oximetry oxygen saturation ear sensor in newborn patients. *Pediatrics.* 2005;115:e64–68.
29. Senn O, Clarenbach CF, Kaplan V, et al. Monitoring carbon dioxide tension and arterial oxygen saturation by a single earlobe sensor in patients with critical illness or sleep apnea. *Chest.* 2005;128:1291–1296.
30. Rodriguez P, Lellouche F, Aboab J, et al. Transcutaneous arterial carbon dioxide pressure monitoring in critically ill adult patients. *Intensive Care Med.* 2006;32:309–312.
31. Kocher S, Rohling R, Tschupp A. Performance of a digital PCO_2/SpO_2 ear sensor. *J Clin Monit Comput.* 2004;18:75–79.
32. Curley FJ, Smyrnios NA. Routine monitoring of critically ill patients. *J Intensive Care Med.* 1990;5:153–174.

CHAPTER 6

Hemodynamic Monitoring

Joseph A. Govert
Dean R. Hess

OUTLINE

OBJECTIVES

1. Discuss the clinical importance of monitoring heart rate and rhythm.
2. Compare noninvasive and invasive techniques used to monitor arterial blood pressure.
3. Describe the clinical significance of systolic pressure variation and pulse pressure variation.
4. Discuss the roles of arterial blood pressure, central venous pressure, and pulmonary artery pressure in hemodynamic monitoring.
5. Describe the pulmonary artery catheter.
6. Identify waveforms from the pulmonary artery catheter.
7. Discuss pitfalls related to measurements of cardiac output.
8. Compare methods used to measure cardiac output.
9. Calculate systemic vascular resistance and pulmonary vascular resistance.

KEY TERMS

arterial blood pressure
a wave
cardiac arrhythmia
central venous pressure (CVP)
diastolic
Fick equation
heart rate
pulmonary artery (PA) catheter
pulmonary artery wedge pressure (PAWP)
pulmonary vascular resistance (PVR)
pulse contour waveform analysis
pulse pressure variation (PPV)
systemic vascular resistance (SVR)
systolic
thermodilution
v wave
Wood units

INTRODUCTION

Hemodynamic monitors measure cardiovascular parameters in a continuous or nearly continuous fashion. As shown in **Table 6–1**, there are many different measurable hemodynamic measurements. Some measurements require invasive devices, whereas others can be made by simple observation. This chapter covers invasive and noninvasive hemodynamic monitors, with particular attention to the role of hemodynamic monitoring of the patient with respiratory disease.

Cardiac Rate and Rhythm

As one of the vital signs, **heart rate** provides a readily accessible bedside measure of cardiovascular status. With electrocardiographic (ECG) techniques, cardiac rhythms can be displayed at the bedside and/or transmitted to a central monitoring area, where the cardiac rhythms of many patients can be monitored by one individual and, if needed, printed and stored for later review.

The heart rate is controlled by electrical impulses that arise regularly at the sinus node in the right atrium. The normal resting heart rate is 60 to 100 beats/min. It accelerates during exercise and slows during sleep as a result of the direct influence of the autonomic nervous system on the sinus node. During exercise, or with pain or anxiety, the sympathetic nerves act on the sinus node to increase the heart rate. Parasympathetic, or vagal, effects slow the rate. **Cardiac arrhythmias** (excessively fast or slow rates and irregular rhythms) frequently occur during the course of critical illness, especially during cardiopulmonary failure, serious infections, myocardial infarction, and toxic overdose.

> **RESPIRATORY RECAP**
>
> **Cardiac Monitoring**
>
> » Bedside ICU monitors measure the heart rate and detect arrhythmias.
>
> » Telemetry is used for cardiac monitoring outside the ICU.

Heart rate can be measured at the bedside by counting the peripheral pulse. The radial pulse is most commonly used for this purpose. It is counted for 15 to 30 seconds and multiplied to calculate beats per minute. However, obtaining an accurate pulse in critically ill patients can be difficult. In hypotensive patients, the only palpable pulses may be over the carotid or femoral arteries. In patients with cardiac arrhythmias, peripheral pulses may vary in intensity because of poor transmission of the irregular beats. In these cases the apical heartbeat should be auscultated at the chest to obtain an accurate measurement.

With ECG electrodes, cardiac electrical activity can be detected at the skin surface and processed to display the heart rate and waveforms. The electrodes are applied to the chest and extremities in standardized arrays, and the electrode array is connected directly to the bedside monitor or ECG machine or is plugged into a radio transmitter that sends the signals to a central telemetry console.

For almost every patient in the intensive care unit (ICU), the heart rate and rhythm are displayed on a bedside monitor. These systems accurately measure the heart rate; identify dangerous arrhythmias, such as ventricular tachycardia and fibrillation; and recognize episodes of myocardial ischemia. They are equipped with audio and visual alarms that can trigger the printing of a rhythm strip or freeze the monitor screen for immediate review. Patients on hospital telemetry units wear small electronic boxes to transmit the ECG to central monitoring stations; this has allowed early transfer of otherwise stable patients from the ICU to the comfort and convenience of private rooms. The patient's electrodes are connected by wires to a small radio transmitter at the bedside that encodes the ECG signals into radio frequency waves and transmits them to strategically placed antennas, then on to the receiving unit, where they are decoded for display and analysis.

TABLE 6-1 Normal Ranges for Certain Hemodynamic Measurements

Variable	Units	Normal Range
Systolic blood pressure (SBP)	mm Hg	90–140
Diastolic blood pressure (DBP)	mm Hg	60–90
Mean arterial pressure (MAP)	mm Hg	65–105
Pulmonary artery systolic pressure (PASP)	mm Hg	15–30
Pulmonary artery diastolic pressure (PADP)	mm Hg	4–12
Mean pulmonary artery pressure (MPAP)	mm Hg	9–16
Right ventricular systolic pressure (RVSP)	mm Hg	15–30
Right ventricular end-diastolic pressure (RVEDP)	mm Hg	0–8
Central venous pressure (CVP)	mm Hg	0–8
Pulmonary artery wedge pressure (PAWP)	mm Hg	2–12
Cardiac output (CO)	L/min	Varies with size of patient
Cardiac index (CI)	L/min/m^2	2.5–3.5

Reprinted from Nelson LD. The new pulmonary artery catheters: right ventricular ejection fraction and continuous cardiac output. *Crit Care Clin.* 1996;12:795. Copyright 1996, with permission of Elsevier. Available at: http://www.sciencedirect.com/science/journal/07490704.

Arterial Blood Pressure

The **arterial blood pressure** is one of the vital signs. Monitoring techniques for blood pressure include intermittent manual determinations with sphygmomanometry; automated, noninvasive devices; and indwelling arterial cannulas that provide continuous pressure measurements and waveform graphics.

Intravascular pressure is determined by blood flow and vascular resistance:

$$\text{Pressure} = \text{Flow} \times \text{Resistance}$$

Flow is determined by cardiac output, and resistance is determined by vascular tone. The arterial waveform consists of peak, or **systolic**, blood pressure corresponding to cardiac contraction; an anacrotic and dicrotic notch; and a nadir, or **diastolic**, blood pressure (**Figure 6–1**). The anacrotic notch is a reflected pressure wave that rebounds from the peripheral vessels. The dicrotic notch represents closure of the aortic valve. In the peripheral vessels a normal increase in elasticity and resistance results in a peaked and narrower waveform. Systolic pressure in the radial artery, therefore, is about 6 mm Hg higher than a simultaneous measurement in the brachial artery. This difference diminishes in patients with inelastic arteries, such as the elderly or those with vascular disease.[1,2]

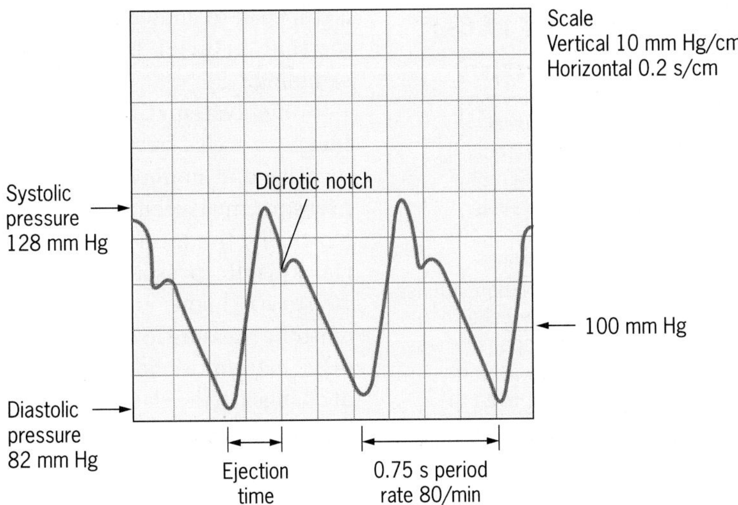

FIGURE 6–1 Arterial blood pressure waveform.

Noninvasive methods used to measure blood pressure generally use a blood pressure cuff, which is gradually inflated around an extremity to a pressure above the systolic pressure and then slowly deflated while the artery is auscultated for Korotkoff sounds. Automated noninvasive blood pressure monitors program inflation and deflation of the cuff at selected intervals. Most of these systems are based on oscillometry and use a sensitive transducer to measure not only total cuff pressure but also the minute oscillations in the cuff caused by the pulsating vessel. The systolic and diastolic pressures are recognized by changes in oscillation intensity (**Figure 6–2**). These devices are available with programmable blood pressure intervals, memory, display, and print features. Portable units are available for use on hospital wards, and plug-in modules for multifunctional critical care monitors. Manual and automated cuff measurements correlate well with simultaneous intra-arterial values. However, in adults, the first Korotkoff sound generally does not appear until 4 to 15 mm Hg below the intravascular systolic pressure, and the last sound disappears 3 to 6 mm Hg above the intravascular diastolic pressure.[1]

Noninvasive systems have limitations and complications. Poor-fitting cuffs may lead to measurement errors. Larger cuffs must be used with obese patients, because undersized cuffs can result in an overestimation of arterial pressure. In hypotensive, edematous, or vasoconstricted patients, automated systems may not be able to detect weakly transmitted blood pressure sounds. Programmable noninvasive systems have also been associated with ulnar palsies, skin injury at the site of inflation, and extremity ischemia when used with frequent inflation-deflation cycles.

Intra-arterial monitoring is indicated for critically ill patients with extremes of blood pressure requiring aggressive resuscitation efforts or titration of potent vasoactive agents. Small catheters, usually 18- or 20-gauge, are inserted into the radial, femoral, axillary, dorsalis pedis, or brachial artery based on ease of access and relative frequency of complications. The cannula is connected to a bedside pressure transducer, usually with

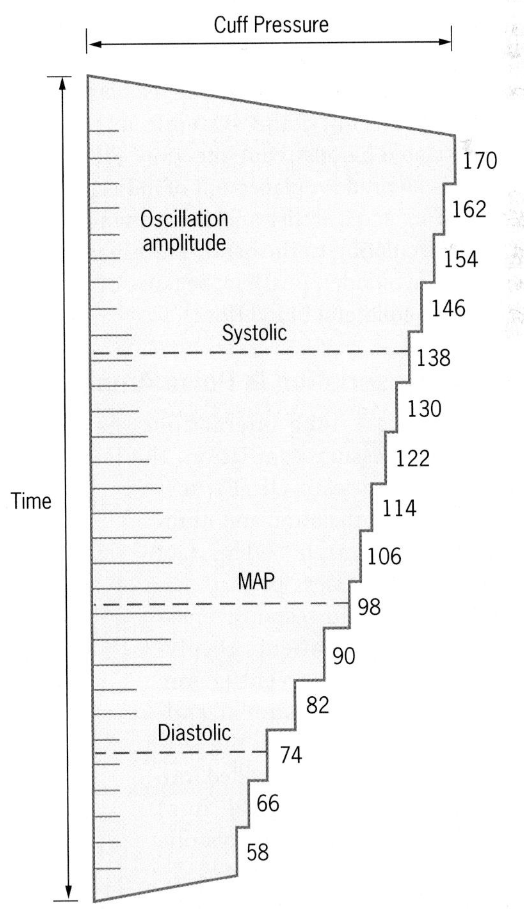

FIGURE 6–2 Noninvasive blood pressure measurements are derived from analysis of oscillation amplitude during a programmed cuff inflation-deflation cycle. Modified from materials courtesy of Critikon LLC, Tampa, Fla. (GE Heathcare Monitoring Solutions)

RESPIRATORY RECAP

Arterial Blood Pressure

- » Automated noninvasive systems are based on oscillometry or photoplethysmography.
- » Invasive systems use transducers attached to an intra-arterial catheter.
- » Respiratory variation in pulse pressure can be used to assess fluid responsiveness.
- » Pulse contour waveform analysis can be used to assess cardiac output.

a stopcock to allow intermittent arterial blood sampling.[3]

Some systematic differences exist between invasive and noninvasive pressure measurements. Normally, the intra-arterial systolic pressure is 10% to 20% higher and the diastolic pressure lower in distal extremities because of changes in the elasticity and caliber of the arteries. This effect, known as *distal pulse amplification*, causes a widened pulse pressure without affecting mean arterial pressure. For patients who are rewarming after cardiopulmonary bypass or receiving vasopressors for septic shock, measurements obtained from the radial artery have been shown to underestimate central (femoral artery) pressures. Failure to recognize this phenomenon may lead to the inappropriate use of vasoactive agents.[4]

Intra-arterial monitoring is associated with several well-recognized complications, including injury to the artery or adjacent nerves, bleeding, ischemia and infection of the extremity, and systemic infection due to catheter-related bloodstream infection. The radial artery generally is favored for placement of indwelling cannulas because of its accessibility and the presence of vascular collateral circulation to the hand. The ulnar and brachial arteries are avoided, if possible, because of their tenuous and variable collateral blood flow.[3]

Respiratory Variation in Pulse Amplitude

Due to the heart–lung interactions that occur during positive pressure ventilation, the left ventricular stroke volume varies cyclically; it is maximal during inhalation and minimal during exhalation.[5–7] This fact has been used to assess preload status and predict fluid responsiveness in deeply sedated patients receiving positive pressure ventilation. Using the systolic pressure at end-exhalation as the baseline, the systolic pressure variation is divided into two components: an increase (Δup) and a decrease (Δdown) in systolic pressure from baseline (**Figure 6–3**). Volume expansion decreases systolic pressure variation and Δdown. The respiratory changes in systolic pressure result not only from changes in transmural pressure (mainly related to changes in left ventricular stroke volume) but also from changes in extramural pressure (i.e., from changes in pleural pressure). Thus, respiratory changes in systolic pressure may be observed despite lack of variation in left ventricular stroke volume.

Pulse pressure, the difference between the systolic and the diastolic pressure, is proportional to left ventricular stroke volume. Respiratory changes in left ventricular stroke volume are reflected by changes in peripheral pulse pressure during the respiratory cycle. Therefore, it has been proposed that fluid responsiveness may be assessed by calculating the respiratory **pulse pressure variation (PPV)** as follows:

$$PPV\ (\%) = 100 \times (PP_{max} - PP_{min})/PP_{mean}$$

where PP_{max} is the maximal pulse pressure, PP_{min} is the minimal pulse pressure, and PP_{mean} is the average pulse pressure (**Figure 6–4**). PPV can be used to assess the hemodynamic effects of volume expansion. PPV greater than 15% allows discrimination between responders and nonresponders to a fluid challenge.[5–8]

Pulse Contour Waveform Analysis

Pulse contour waveform analysis uses a variety of techniques to allow data describing either cardiac output or stroke volume to be derived from the arterial pressure waveform.[9,10] This method uses an arterial catheter to provide a continuous measure of cardiac output. In order to translate a pressure waveform into a volume waveform, some measure of arterial compliance is required. There are two calibrated pulse contour waveform analysis devices available. The LiDCOplus system requires an independent calibration with a lithium dilution technique to account for arterial compliance. The PiCCO system is a pulse contour analysis device that employs transpulmonary **thermodilution**. The Vigileo monitor is a noncalibrated device that uses an arterial pressure transducer that samples at a frequency of 100 Hz to

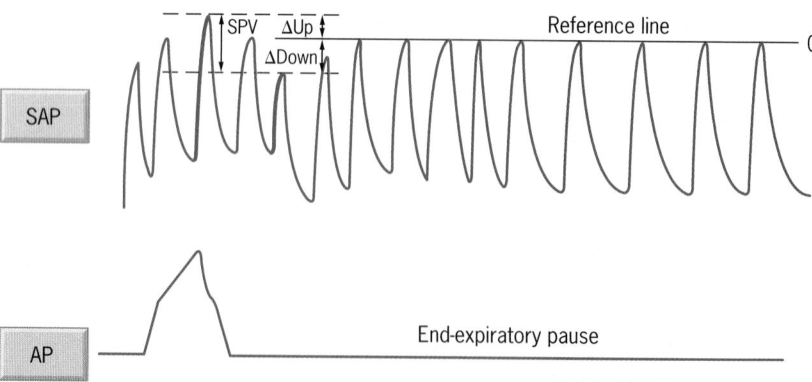

FIGURE 6–3 Systolic pressure variation (SPV) after one positive pressure breath followed by an end-expiratory pause. Reference line permits the measurement of Δup and Δdown. Bold indicates maximal and minimal pulse pressure. AP, airway pressure; SAP, systolic arterial pressure. With kind permission from Springer Science+Business Media: *Intensive Care Med*, Fluid responsiveness in mechanically ventilated patients. 2003;26:352–360. Bendjelid K, Romand J. Reproduced with permission.

characterize the pulse waveform. These, along with the patient's demographics, are analyzed to estimate stroke volume and cardiac output.

Central Venous Pressure Monitoring

Central venous pressure (CVP), which is measured in the superior vena cava, is the filling pressure in the right atrium. Single-lumen or multilumen catheters are positioned in the superior vena cava via the subclavian (**Figure 6–5**) or internal or external jugular vein to permit CVP monitoring, intravenous access for medication infusions, and venous blood sampling. The femoral vein also is a commonly used access site, especially during emergencies. Femoral catheters positioned in the common iliac vein or inferior vena cava have been shown to provide a reasonable estimate of CVP, at least in the absence of increased abdominal pressure or vena caval injury.[11] When CVP measurements are necessary, the femoral site is usually avoided.

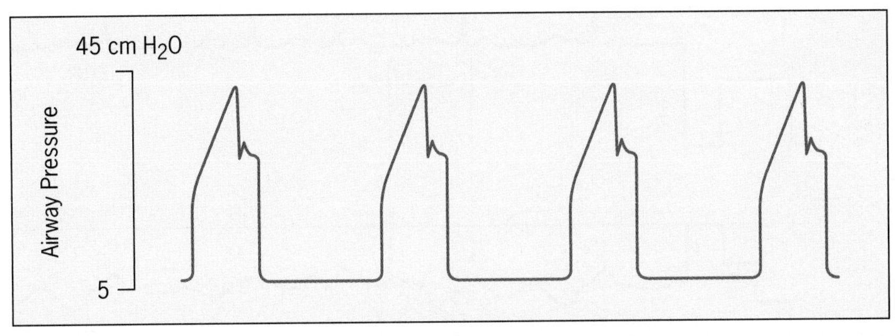

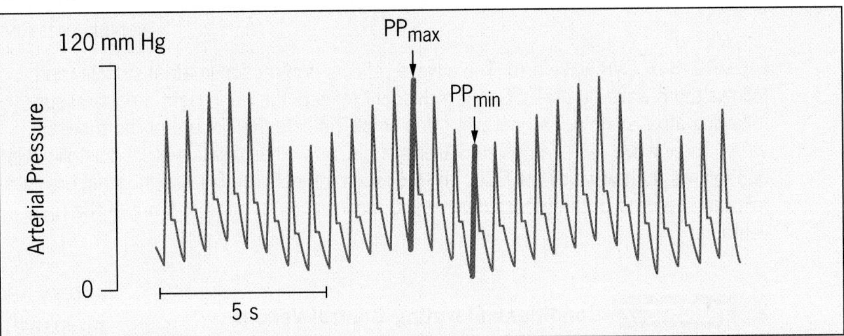

FIGURE 6–4 Respiratory changes in airway and arterial pressures in a mechanically ventilated patient. The pulse pressure (systolic minus diastolic pressure) is maximal (PP_{max}) at the end of the inspiratory period and minimal (PP_{min}) three heart beats later (i.e., during the expiratory period). The respiratory changes in pulse pressure are calculated as the difference between PP_{max} and PP_{min}, divided by the mean of the two values, and expressed as a percentage. From Michard F, Teboul J. Using heart-lung interactions to assess fluid responsiveness during mechanical ventilation. *Crit Care.* 2000;4:282–289. Reproduced with permission from BioMed Central.

In adults, central venous catheters usually measure 7 Fr (about 2.3 mm) in diameter and 16 to 20 cm in length. They are constructed of biocompatible plastics, most commonly polyethylene, Teflon, and polyurethane. All intravascular catheters are designed with certain important properties, including flexibility, a smooth surface, thromboresistance, lack of kink memory, and chemical stability.

In the presence of a competent tricuspid valve, the CVP waveform reflects both venous return to the right atrium (during ventricular systole) and right ventricular end-diastolic pressure. There are normally three positive components and two negative deflections in the right atrial (RA) waveform (**Figure 6–6**). Electrocardiographic correlation is required for correct identification of these events. In the right atrium, there is an 80- to 100-ms delay in the detection of mechanical events from their appearance on the ECG as a result of the length of tubing in the system. Normal right atrial pressures vary from 0 to 7 mm Hg. Elevations in RA pressure are seen in a number of conditions (**Table 6–2**).

A number of cardiac rhythm disturbances can produce characteristic abnormalities in the CVP waveform. Atrial fibrillation is associated with lack of organized atrial activity and therefore loss of the normal **a wave**. Atrial flutter may produce characteristic sawtooth f waves in the CVP tracing (as well as on the ECG) at a rate of 240 to 340 beats per minute. Atrioventricular dissociation (ventricular pacing, complete heart block,

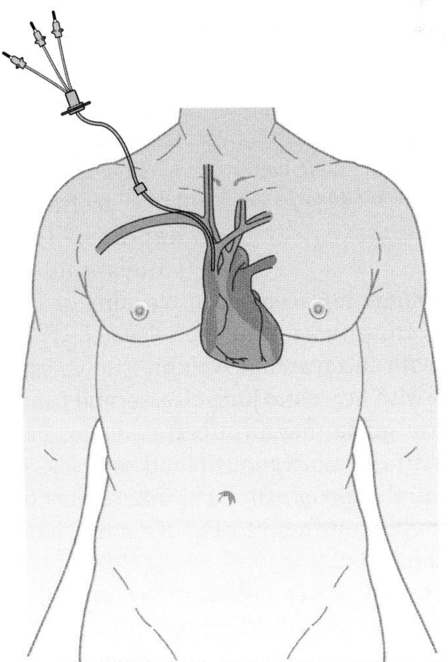

FIGURE 6–5 Placement of triple-lumen central venous catheter. Adapted from Taylor C, et al. *Fundamentals of Nursing.* 5th ed (Figure 16-10). Lippincott Williams & Wilkins; 2005.

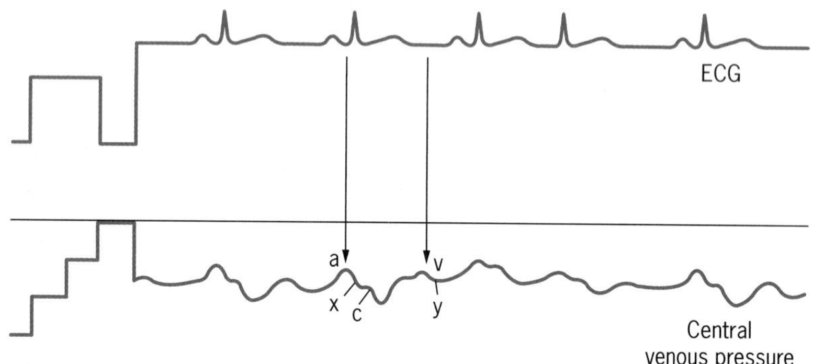

FIGURE 6–6 CVP waveform. The a wave reflects contraction in atrial systole, and follows the p wave on the ECG. The x descent reflects the fall in right atrial pressure following atrial systole. The c wave, often small, reflects the closure of the tricuspid valve. The v wave represents ventricular systole, as well as passive atrial diastolic filling and follows the t wave of the ECG. The y descent reflects the fall in right atrial pressure following opening of the tricuspid valve and the initiation of passive filling of the right ventricle.

TABLE 6–2 Conditions Elevating Central Venous Pressure

Volume overload
Impaired right ventricular contractile function
Pulmonary hypertension
Right ventricular infarction
Pulmonic stenosis
Tricuspid valvular disease
Left-to-right shunts

RESPIRATORY RECAP

Central Venous Pressure

- » CVP is measured in the superior vena cava.
- » CVP is used to estimate intravascular volume status.
- » Central venous catheters can be used to obtain blood samples for laboratory analysis.

ventricular tachycardia) may manifest cannon a waves (or giant a waves) due to the simultaneous contraction of atrium and ventricle while the tricuspid valve is closed.

The CVP is particularly useful in volume-depleted states. Low values guide fluid and blood volume replacement in bleeding or hypovolemic patients. However, a normal or elevated CVP correlates poorly with intravascular volume status, especially for patients with heart and lung disease, and cannot be used reliably to guide therapy. Central venous catheters are also used to obtain venous blood samples. A relatively new central venous oximetry catheter has the capability for continuous monitoring of central venous oxygen saturation ($Scvo_2$).

Central venous catheterization has well-recognized complications. Mechanical complications related to insertion of the catheter include pneumothorax, bleeding, and injury to nerves, vessels, or the thoracic duct. Fewer complications are seen when the operator is skilled and ultrasound is used to identify the venous anatomy.[12] Malpositioned catheters can cause cardiac arrhythmias, valvular injury, chamber perforation, and cardiac tamponade. Infection can develop at the insertion site, sometimes resulting in bacteremia with prolonged use. Antimicrobial-coated catheters have been developed to reduce the incidence of infectious complications.

Pulmonary Artery Catheters

Flow-directed **pulmonary artery (PA) catheters** (also known as Swan-Ganz catheters) have the ability to measure pressures and sample blood from the right atrium, right ventricle, and pulmonary artery.[13] PA catheters also enable left atrial pressure to be estimated from the pulmonary artery occlusion pressure (also called pulmonary artery wedge pressure or pulmonary capillary wedge pressure) and enable the clinician to measure the cardiac output.

The catheter has a balloon at the tip that is inflated with air, which allows blood flow to direct the catheter through the right ventricle into the pulmonary artery. The right internal jugular vein or the left subclavian vein may be the easiest site to use in difficult access conditions, such as pulmonary hypertension. These approaches take advantage of the predesigned curve of the catheter. Fluoroscopy may be necessary when the cephalic or femoral site is used because of the tortuous vascular pathway to the pulmonary artery. The standard adult thermodilution PA catheter is usually 7 to 7.5 Fr and approximately 110 cm long, with a balloon capacity of 1.5 mL. Smaller catheters are available for pediatric patients. From the internal jugular or subclavian vein in adults, the catheter generally is properly positioned at 45 to 60 cm.

Pulmonary artery catheters have three or four ports for pressure measurements, thermodilution injections, and medication infusion (**Figure 6–7**). A proximal port 30 cm from the tip resides in the right atrium–superior vena cava, and a distal port is positioned at the tip in the pulmonary artery. The catheter tip balloon can be inflated intermittently to allow wedging in the distal pulmonary artery. The **pulmonary artery wedge pressure (PAWP)** provides an estimate of left atrial and left ventricular end-diastolic or filling pressure

RESPIRATORY RECAP

Pulmonary Artery Catheters

- » Measures the pulmonary artery pressure and pulmonary artery wedge pressure.
- » Thermodilution catheters measure cardiac output.
- » Oximetric catheters measure the mixed venous oxygen saturation.
- » Blood samples from pulmonary artery catheters are used to measure mixed venous blood gases.

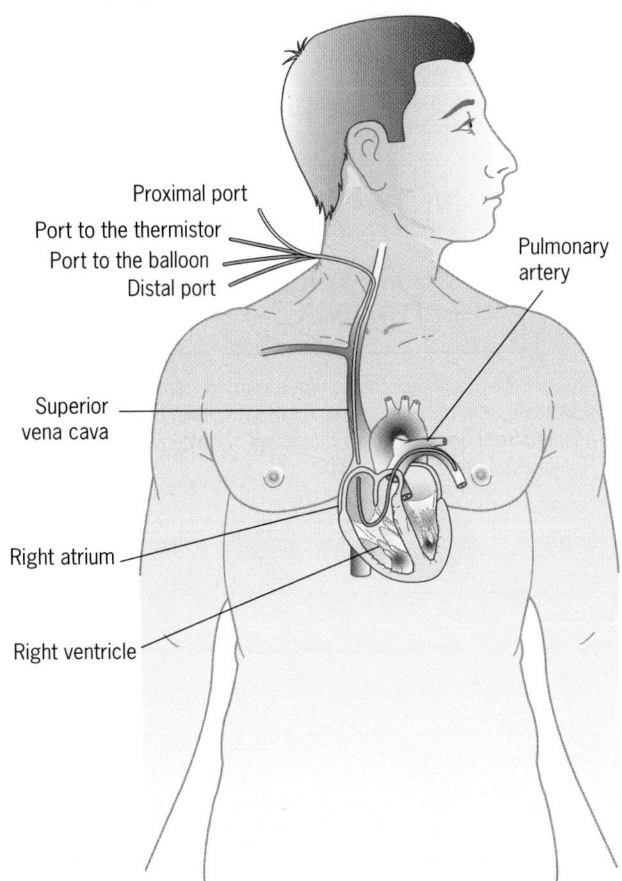

FIGURE 6–7 Monitoring ports on the pulmonary artery catheter. Adapted from Schulte am Esch J. *Atlas of Anaesthesia*. 3rd ed. Thieme Medical Publishers; 2006.

(LVEDP). Each anatomic position produces a characteristic waveform (**Figure 6–8**).

Careful observation of pressure waveforms permits evaluation of mechanical events within the atria and ventricles and offers important diagnostic information in a wide variety of cardiopulmonary disease states. Consequently, information from the PA catheter can provide diagnostic and potentially therapeutic information (**Table 6–3**). However, appropriate use of the PA catheter requires very careful data gathering and interpretation.

Catheter Setup

The catheter must be appropriately zeroed and referenced for accurate diagnostic information to be obtained. Although zeroing and referencing are done in one step, they represent two separate processes. *Zeroing* is performed by opening the system to air to establish atmospheric pressure as zero. *Referencing* (or *leveling*) is accomplished by placing the air–fluid interface of the catheter (or the transducer) at the level of the right atrium to negate the effects of the weight of the catheter tubing and fluid column.[14] It is important to note that the phlebostatic level changes with differences in the position of the patient.

The pulmonary artery catheter is positioned using pressure waveform or fluoroscopic guidance. Fluoroscopic guidance often helps in obtaining accurate catheter placement in patients with marked right atrial or

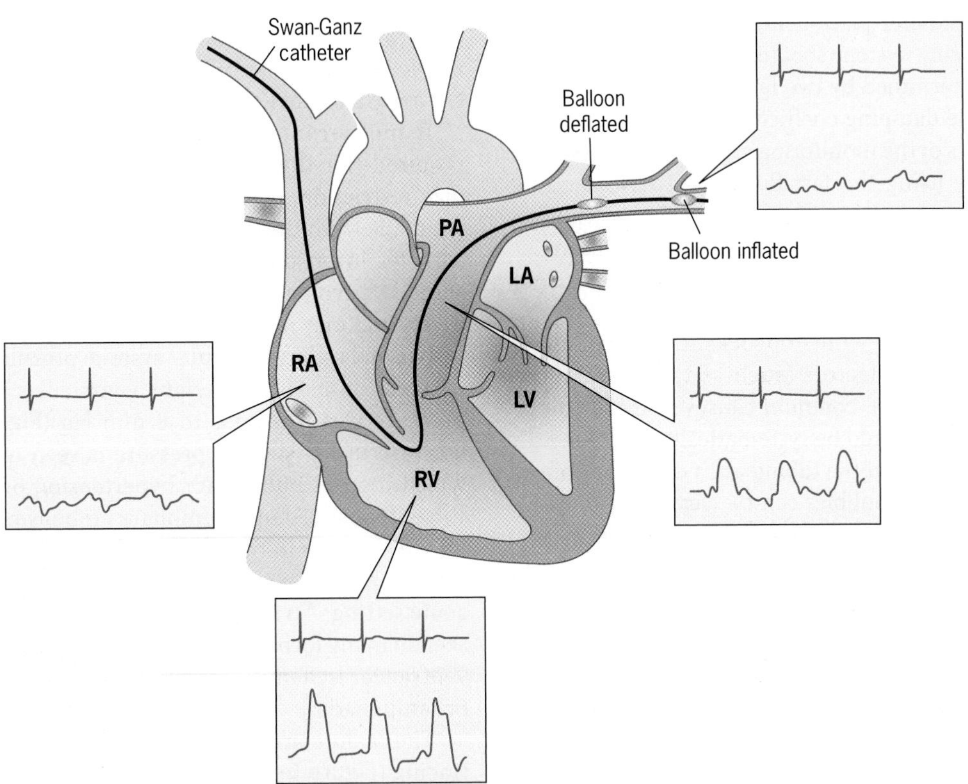

FIGURE 6–8 Waveforms from various sites on the pulmonary artery catheter. Modified from Longnecher D, Brown D, Newman M, Zapol W. 2007. *Anesthesiology*. McGraw-Hill, New York. (© The McGraw-Hill Companies, Inc.)

TABLE 6–3 Indications for Pulmonary Artery Catheterization

Measure cardiac output
Assess pulmonary hypertension
Assess intravascular volume
Differentiate among shock states (hypovolemic versus heart failure)
Differentiate diffuse pulmonary infiltrates (cardiac versus pulmonary)
Differentiate pericardial constriction, restrictive cardiomyopathy, and tamponade
Assess severity of valvular heart disease
Assess cardiomyopathy
Define intracardiac shunts (e.g., atrial or ventricular septal defects)

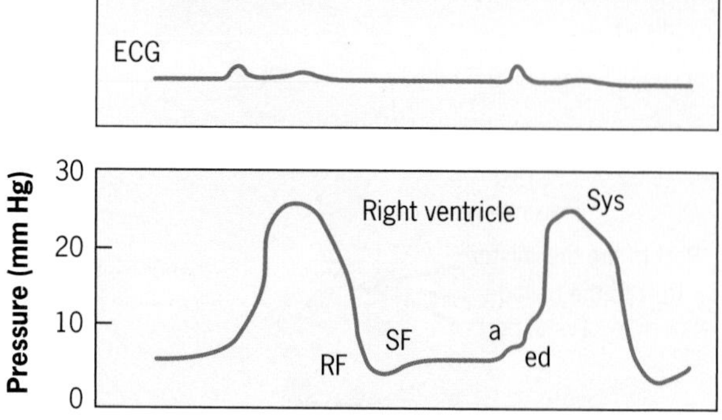

FIGURE 6–9 Right ventricular waveform. RF, rapid filling; SF, slow filling; a, atrial contraction; ed, end-diastole; Sys, systole. Adapted from Gore JM, et al. *Handbook of Hemodynamic Monitoring*. Little, Brown; 1985.

ventricular dilatation, severe tricuspid regurgitation, or left bundle branch block.

Once in position, the catheter allows simultaneous recording of pressure waveforms from the right atrium and pulmonary artery or pulmonary artery wedge pressure. Pulmonary artery wedge pressure measurements are made by inflating the balloon at the distal tip of the catheter with approximately 1.0 to 1.5 mL of air. Once the balloon is full of air, it floats or is flow directed until it occludes a segment of the pulmonary artery. The waveform noted following occlusion of the pulmonary artery reflects the transmitted pressure of the left atrium. It does not reflect true left ventricular ventricular end-diastolic volume, nor does it reflect capillary hydrostatic pressures[15] or transmural pressures.[16–19]

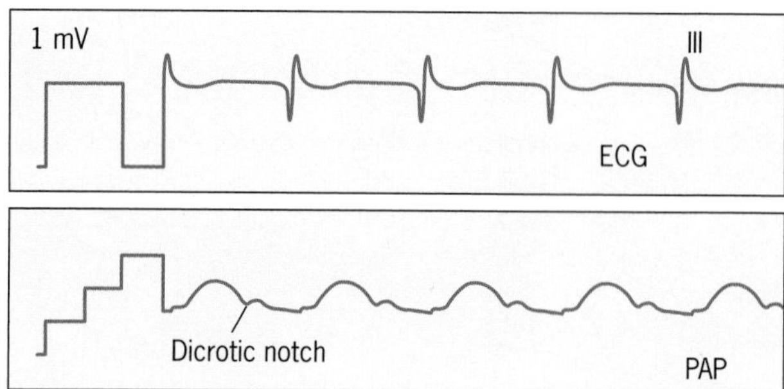

FIGURE 6–10 Pulmonary artery waveform.

Following catheter placement, the dynamic response of the monitoring system should be assessed. Dynamic response is determined by two factors: the resonant frequency and the damping coefficient of the system. Both of these aspects of the monitoring system can be assessed at the bedside using the fast-flush test, performed by briefly opening and closing the valve in the continuous flush device.[20] This produces a square wave displacement on the oscilloscope, followed by ringing and a return to baseline.

Connecting tubing with stopcocks, excessive tubing lengths, and patient factors (such as tachycardia and high output states) are common causes of underdamping. These factors should be systematically addressed. In contrast, air bubbles in the tubing are a common source of overdamping; the bubbles can be cleared by flushing the system through the stopcock.

Pressure Waveforms

CVP measurements are obtained from the proximal port of the PA catheter. Two pressures are typically measured in the right ventricle (RV): the peak right ventricular systolic pressure and the right ventricular end-diastolic pressure. Ventricular diastole is made up of an early rapid filling phase (during which approximately 60% of filling occurs), a slow phase (during which another 25% of filling occurs), and an atrial systolic phase (which produces the a wave in the RV tracing).

If measurement of RV end-diastolic pressure is required (for the diagnosis of cardiac tamponade, cardiac restriction, or pericardial constriction), recordings are made from the distal tip of the catheter during initial catheter insertion. Routine monitoring of RV pressure should be avoided because it is usually not clinically necessary and may induce arrhythmia.

Normal right ventricular systolic pressure varies from 15 to 30 mm Hg, and right ventricular end-diastolic pressure varies from 0 to 8 mm Hg (**Figure 6–9**). An increase in RV systolic pressure is seen in disorders in which there is pulmonary hypertension or in pulmonic valve stenosis. Acute pulmonary embolism can also produce elevations in the RV systolic pressure, although RV systolic pressures rarely exceed 40 to 50 mm Hg in the acute setting. An increase in RV end-diastolic pressure is seen in many forms of cardiomyopathy, as well as in right ventricular ischemia, infarction, and cardiac constriction or tamponade.

The main components of the pulmonary artery (PA) tracing (**Figure 6–10**) are the systolic and diastolic pressures and the dicrotic notch, which represents closure of

TABLE 6–4 Conditions Causing Pulmonary Hypertension

Left heart failure of any cause
Primary lung disease
Mitral valvular disease
Pulmonary embolism
Hypoxemia with pulmonary vasoconstriction
Idiopathic pulmonary arterial hypertension
Left-to-right shunts

TABLE 6–5 Causes of Elevated Pulmonary Artery Wedge Pressure

Left ventricular volume overload
Left ventricular systolic dysfunction
Primary left ventricular diastolic dysfunction
Myocardial ischemia or infarction with decreased left ventricular compliance
Mitral stenosis

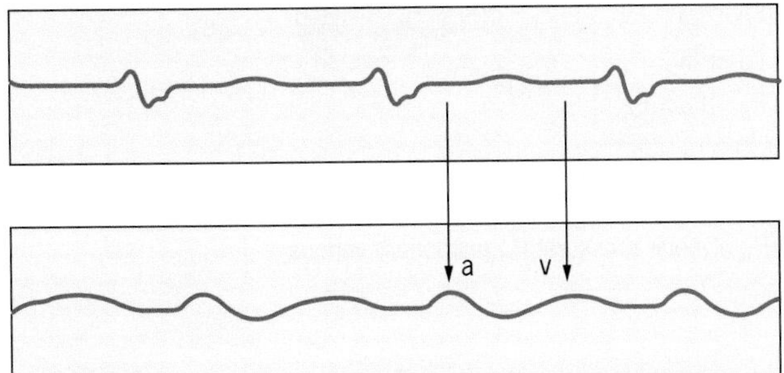

FIGURE 6–11 Pulmonary artery wedge pressure. The a wave reflects contraction in atrial systole. The c wave, reflecting the closure of the mitral valve, is often not seen. The v wave represents both ventricular systole and passive atrial diastolic filling.

the pulmonic valve. Normal pulmonary artery systolic pressures vary from 15 to 30 mm Hg, whereas pulmonary artery diastolic pressures vary from 4 to 12 mm Hg. Elevations in PA pressures are seen with volume overload or with a variety of conditions in which pulmonary vascular resistance is elevated (**Table 6–4**).

The pulmonary artery occlusion pressure tracing is obtained by inflating a balloon at the distal tip of the catheter to obstruct forward blood flow through that particular branch of the pulmonary artery. This creates a static column of blood between the catheter tip and the left atrium, allowing the pressure at both ends of the column to equilibrate. The pressure at the distal end of the catheter is then equal to that of the left atrium, and is termed the pulmonary artery (or pulmonary capillary) wedge pressure (PAWP). As is seen in **Figure 6–11**, the PAWP tracing is similar in general configuration to that seen in the right atrium.

The electrical and mechanical correlation between ECG and PAWP tracings is similar to that seen in the right atrium, but the electromechanical delay is longer because of the time necessary for left atrial mechanical events to be transmitted through the pulmonary vasculature to the distal tip of the catheter. Elevations in the a wave of the PAWP tracing can be seen with increased resistance to left ventricular filling of any cause (**Table 6–5**). Elevations in the **v wave** of the PAWP tracing represent either mitral regurgitation or an acute volume load to the left atrium. Severe mitral regurgitation is often associated with large v waves in the PAWP tracing, but they are neither sensitive nor specific for this condition.[21] The PAWP generally reflects the left ventricular end-diastolic pressure as long as there is no obstruction to flow between the left atrium and left ventricle.[22,23] Often the PAWP is used as a surrogate for left ventricular preload (or what is often referred to as volume status). It is very important to note that the PAWP is only a reliable index of left ventricular preload when ventricular compliance is normal or unchanging. Positive pressure ventilation, myocardial ischemia or infarction, cardiac tamponade, and a variety of drugs can profoundly decrease ventricular compliance, thereby interfering with accurate estimation of left ventricular preload via the PAWP.

In patients with pulmonary disease and respiratory failure, the PAWP can exceed the left ventricular end-diastolic pressure secondary to constriction of small veins in hypoxic lung segments, again making the PAWP a poor surrogate for left ventricular preload.

Pitfalls in Interpreting Waveforms

The accuracy of the PAWP is dependent on a continuous fluid column between the left atrium and the distal catheter tip. If the pressure in the surrounding alveoli exceeds capillary pressures and compresses the capillaries, the pressure at the catheter tip will reflect alveolar pressure and not left atrial pressure. This concept (**Figure 6–12**) has been used to divide the lungs into three physiologic zones of blood flow, which are based on the relationship between alveolar pressure, mean pulmonary artery pressure, and pulmonary capillary pressure.[24]

The PAWP is an accurate estimate of left atrial pressure only when the pulmonary capillary pressure exceeds the mean alveolar pressure (zone 3). This zone is located in the most dependent portion of the lung, where vascular pressures are the highest (due to gravity). Indicators of non–zone-3 catheter site placement include abnormal position on lateral chest radiographs, marked respiratory variation in the PAWP tracing, and increases in PAWP of more than 50% of the amount of PEEP applied.

During normal spontaneous breathing, alveolar pressure (relative to atmospheric pressure) decreases during inspiration and increases during expiration. During

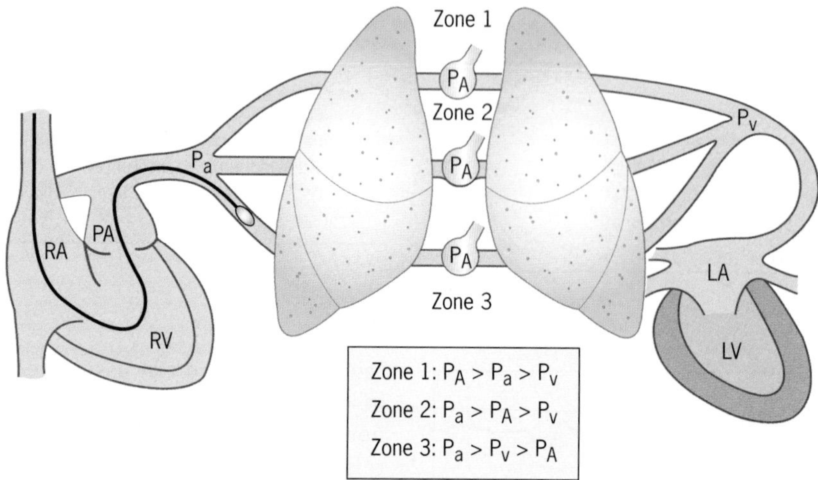

FIGURE 6–12 West zones of the lungs, determined by the relationship between alveolar pressure and pulmonary vascular pressures. RA, right atrium; RV, right ventricle; PA, pulmonary artery; P_a, pulmonary arterial pressure; P_A, alveolar pressure; P_V, pulmonary venous pressure; LA, left atrium; LV, left ventricle.

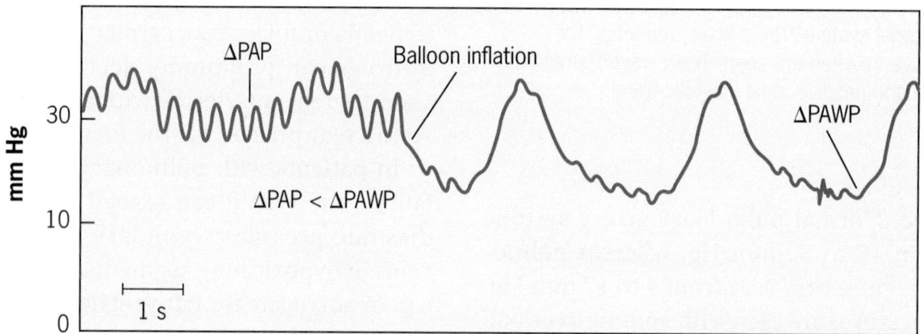

FIGURE 6–13 Pressure trace recorded during positive pressure mechanical ventilation from a pulmonary artery catheter located in West lung zone 1. Pressure swings in the pulmonary artery occlusion pressure (ΔPAWP) reflect changes in airway pressure and are significantly higher than swings in pulmonary artery pressure (ΔPa), which result from changes in pleural pressure. Modified with permission from Longnecker D, Brown D, Newman M, Zapol W. *Anesthesiology*. McGraw-Hill; 2007. (© The McGraw-Hill Companies, Inc.)

positive pressure ventilation, alveolar pressure increases during inhalation and decreases during exhalation. The changes in alveolar pressure are transmitted to the cardiac structures and are reflected by changes in central venous, pulmonary artery, and PAWP measurements during inspiration and expiration. At end-expiration, pleural and intrathoracic pressures are equal to atmospheric pressures, regardless of the mode of ventilation. Thus, the true transmural pressure, and therefore the PAWP, should be measured at end-expiration.

Alveolar pressure will not return to atmospheric pressure at end-expiration in the presence of positive end-expiratory pressure, a change that can affect the measurement of intravascular pressures. PEEP can be applied therapeutically or may result from incomplete expiration of alveolar gas leading to air trapping (auto-PEEP). The effects of either form of PEEP on the PAWP are variable and depend largely on the compliance of the lungs and the chest wall. The effects of PEEP are generally felt not to be important, with notable exceptions. One exception may be in the situation in which the catheter is not in zone 3. By definition, in zone 3 no airway pressure should be transmitted to the vasculature. If the respiratory variation seen in the PAWP tracing exceeds that seen in the pulmonary artery tracing, then the PAWP may be unreliable due to non-zone-3 conditions (**Figure 6–13**).[25]

Even though there may be a small effect of PEEP on intravascular pressure measurements, it is not advisable to eliminate (turn off) PEEP temporarily while pressure measurements are being made, because this may induce hemodynamic instability due to changes in venous return or may cause alveolar derecruitment with subsequent severe hypoxemia.

The effect of PEEP on vascular pressures in the thorax is determined by the relationship between lung compliance and chest wall compliance:[26]

$$\Delta Ppl/\Delta Paw = C_L/(C_L + Ccw)$$

where Ppl is pleural pressure, Paw is airway pressure, C_L is lung compliance, and Ccw is chest wall compliance. A general estimate of the true transmural filling pressures can be made in the presence of PEEP by subtracting one-half of the PEEP level from the PAWP if lung and chest wall compliance are normal, 25% of the PEEP if lung compliance is reduced and chest wall compliance is normal, and 75% of the PEEP if chest wall compliance is reduced and lung compliance is normal. The effects of PEEP on PAWP are usually small and rarely affect clinical management.

Cardiac Output Measurement

In addition to providing pressure measurements, the pulmonary artery catheter facilitates measurement of cardiac output via the **Fick equation**:

$$\dot{Q}c = \dot{V}o_2/(Cao_2 - C\bar{v}o_2)$$

where $\dot{Q}c$ is cardiac output, Cao_2 is arterial O_2 content ($1.34 \times Hb \times Sao_2$), and $C\bar{v}o_2$ is mixed venous O_2 content ($1.34 \times Hb \times S\bar{v}o_2$). If arterial blood gases, mixed venous blood gases, and oxygen consumption are measured, cardiac output can be calculated. Mixed venous blood gas samples are obtained from the distal port of the pulmonary artery catheter, and oxygen consumption is measured by indirect calorimetry.

The indicator dilution principle predicts that when an indicator substance is added to a stream of flowing blood, the flow rate will be inversely proportional to the mean concentration of the indicator at a downstream site. In the case of a PA catheter, the indicator used is a known volume of either dextrose or saline that is colder than blood. The indicator is injected as a bolus through the proximal port of the pulmonary artery catheter and mixes with blood in the right ventricle. This mixing lowers the temperature of intraventricular blood, which flows past the distal temperature sensor. The temperature sensor records the temperature change over time, and the monitor can electronically display a temperature–time curve. The area under this curve is inversely proportional to the flow rate in the pulmonary artery. This flow rate should be equal to cardiac output in the absence of an intracardiac shunt.

The thermodilution method has been well validated when compared with calculation of cardiac output using the Fick method. There are, however, several important sources of error. Tricuspid regurgitation leads to an attenuated peak and a prolonged washout phase of the temperature–time curve. This is due to cold injectate refluxing into the vena cava, with resultant decreased pulmonary artery cooling (lowered peak) and delayed appearance of injectate that has moved retrograde into the vena cava and is then recirculated (prolonged washout). The net effect is an underestimation of cardiac output. Both right-to-left and left-to-right intracardiac shunts can produce falsely elevated cardiac output measurements by the thermodilution technique. Right-to-left intracardiac shunts produce shunting of cold injectate into the left heart, which reduces pulmonary artery cooling, lowers the peak of the temperature–time curve, and overestimates cardiac output. Left-to-right shunting results in increased right heart volumes and dilution of the injectate, thereby attenuating the height of the temperature–time curve and resulting in an overestimation of cardiac output.

Continuous thermodilution catheters are available and correlate reasonably well with bolus thermodilution methods.[27,28] This type of catheter is equipped with a 10-cm thermal filament located about 20 cm from the catheter tip. The filament is intermittently warmed to about 44° C. The resulting change in blood temperature is detected at the catheter tip and used to generate a thermodilution curve for determining cardiac output. Although the output is called continuous cardiac output, the measurement is an average cardiac output that is updated every 30 seconds and averaged over 3 to 6 minutes.

Continuous Oximetric Monitoring

Some pulmonary artery catheter designs incorporate continuous oximetric monitoring of pulmonary artery oxygen saturation using fiberoptic reflectance spectrophotometry. These devices employ reflectance spectrophotometry, in which light is transmitted through a fiberoptic bundle, the light is reflected from the blood, and the amount of light absorbed by hemoglobin is determined. Oxygen saturation is then determined based on the differential absorption of light by oxyhemoglobin and deoxyhemoglobin. This technology has reasonable correlation with measured mixed venous oxygen saturation determined using co-oximetry, but is prone to drift.

The mixed venous oxygen level provides a global indication of the level of tissue oxygenation. Normal mixed venous Po_2 is 35 to 45 mm Hg, and normal mixed venous So_2 is 65% to 75%. Factors affecting mixed venous oxygen level can be illustrated by the following equation, which is a rearrangement of the Fick equation:

$$S\bar{v}o_2 = Sao_2 - \dot{V}o_2/\dot{Q}c \times Hb \times 1.34$$

Note that a decrease in cardiac output results in a decreased $S\bar{v}o_2$. The primary interest in continuous monitoring of $S\bar{v}o_2$ is to detect changes in cardiac output.

Other less commonly used applications of pulmonary artery catheters include measurement of right

TABLE 6–6 Characteristic Hemodynamic Profiles of Certain Cardiopulmonary Disorders

Condition	CVP/RA	PAP	PAWP	CO	SVR	PVR	BP
Hypovolemic shock	↓	↓	↓	↓	↑	Normal	↓
Cardiogenic shock	↑	↑	↑	↓	↑	Normal	↓
Septic shock	Normal or ↓	Normal or ↓	Normal or ↓	Normal or ↑	↓	Normal or ↓	↓
Pulmonary embolism	↑	↑	Normal or ↓	Normal or ↓	↑	↑	Normal or ↓

CVP/RA, central venous and right atrial pressures; PAP, pulmonary artery pressure; PAWP, pulmonary artery wedge pressure; CO, cardiac output; SVR, systemic vascular resistance; PVR, pulmonary vascular resistance; BP, systemic arterial blood pressure.

ventricular ejection fraction and extravascular lung water measurements. Pulmonary artery catheters are also available for cardiac pacing.

Vascular Resistance

In addition to calculating cardiac output, the PA catheter facilitates estimation of **systemic vascular resistance (SVR)** and **pulmonary vascular resistance (PVR)**:

$$SVR = (MAP - CVP)/\dot{Q}c$$
$$PVR = (\text{Mean PAP} - PAWP)/\dot{Q}c$$

Normal SVR is 900 to 1400 dyne × s × cm^{-5}, and normal PVR is 150 to 250 dyne × s × cm^{-5}. **Wood units** are a simplified system for measuring pulmonary vascular resistance that uses pressure in mm Hg and cardiac output in L/min. To convert to dyne × s × cm^{-5}, multiply by 80. These calculations are derived from Ohm's law, which states that resistance in a circuit is equal to the pressure drop across the circuit divided by flow. Vascular resistance is calculated on the basis of both direct and indirect measurements, all with intrinsic sources of error; therefore, of all the hemodynamic information obtained from the pulmonary artery catheter, vascular resistance values are the least accurate and the most sensitive to inaccuracies in data acquisition.

Clinical Use of Hemodynamic Measurements

Hemodynamic monitoring allows differentiation of shock states, determination of intravascular volume status and cardiac performance, and monitoring of interventions such as volume challenges, diuresis, and the infusion of vasoactive agents. Certain cardiopulmonary disorders are associated with characteristic hemodynamic profiles (**Table 6–6**).

A point of much debate has been the choice between the PA catheter and CVP monitoring in mechanically ventilated patients in the ICU.[29] Clinicians who advocate for the use of the PA catheter note that the ability to predict intravascular pressure by CVP correlates poorly with pulmonary artery wedge pressure. Others argue that no clear clinical benefit has been associated with the use of the PA catheter and that clinicians often misinterpret the information provided. A randomized controlled trial in patients with acute lung injury reported that PA catheter–guided therapy did not improve survival or organ function and was associated with more complications than CVP-guided therapy.[30] These results suggest that the PA catheter should not be routinely used, and its use has fallen out of favor in recent years. The PA catheter is no longer used commonly for fluid management. Its use is reserved for assessment of left heart failure, pulmonary hypertension, and when knowledge of cardiac output is needed.

A fluid resuscitation protocol known as *early goal-directed therapy* is commonly used in the management of sepsis.[31,32] This protocol (**Figure 6–14**) addresses CVP, arterial blood pressure, and $Scvo_2$ in a systematic manner. There are also guidelines for sepsis management available from the Surviving Sepsis Campaign, which condense management for severe sepsis into two bundles: an acute resuscitation bundle (within 6 hours) and an ongoing management bundle (within 24 hours). Early goal-directed therapy is one of the components of these care bundles.

KEY POINTS

- The heart rate can be measured by counting the peripheral pulse or by using bedside monitors.
- Arterial blood pressure can be measured noninvasively or invasively.
- Pulse pressure variation is an indicator of fluid responsiveness.
- Central venous pressure can guide fluid and blood volume replacement.
- The pulmonary artery catheter is used to measure the pulmonary artery pressure, wedge pressure, cardiac output, and mixed venous oxygen saturation.
- Techniques to measure cardiac output include thermodilution, the Fick method, and pulse contour analysis.

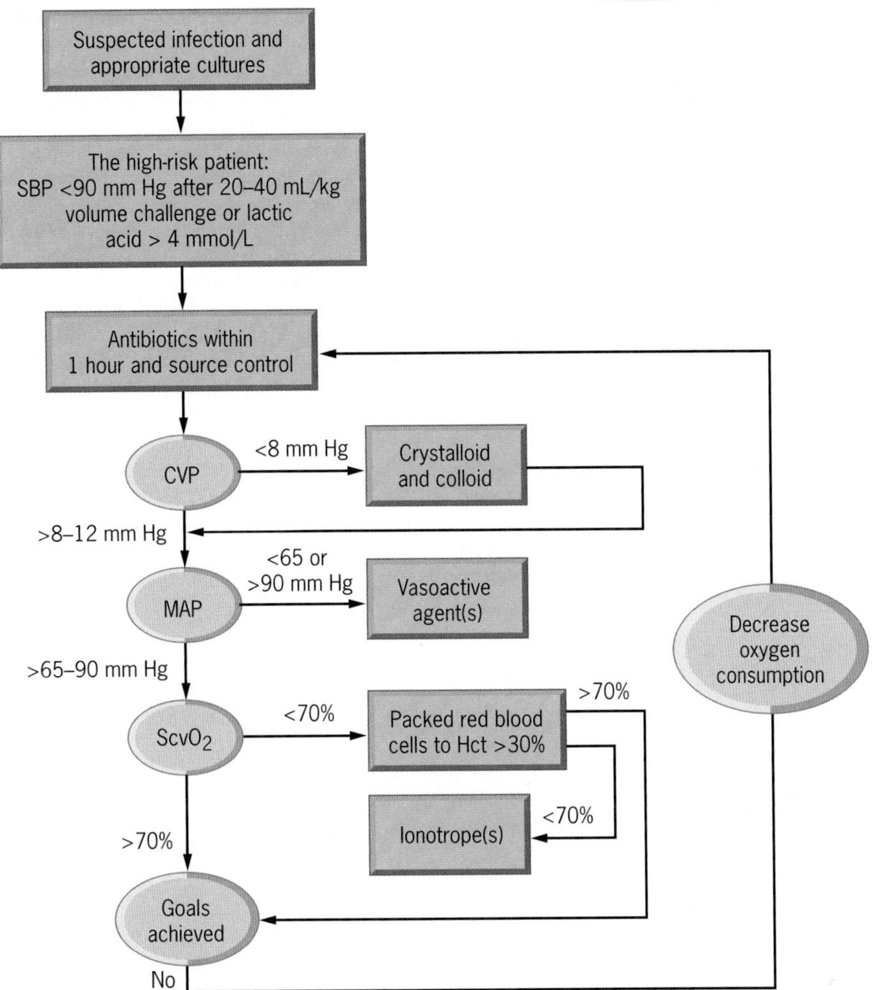

FIGURE 6–14 Algorithm for early management of the septic patient. Adapted from Rivers EP, et al. Early goal-directed therapy in severe sepsis and septic shock: a contemporary review of the literature. *Curr Opin Anesthesiol.* 2008;21:128–140.

REFERENCES

1. Perloff D, Grim C, Flack J, et al. Human blood pressure determination by sphygmomanometry. *Circulation.* 1993;88:2460–2467.
2. Reeves RA. Does this patient have hypertension? How to measure blood pressure. *JAMA.* 1995;273:1211–1218.
3. Clark VL, Kruse JA. Arterial catheterization. *Crit Care Clin.* 1992;8:687–697.
4. Dorman T, Breslow MJ, Lipsett PA, et al. Radial artery pressure monitoring underestimates central arterial pressure during vasopressor therapy in critically ill surgical patients. *Crit Care Med.* 1998;26:1646–1649.
5. Michard F, Teboul JL. Using heart-lung interactions to assess fluid responsiveness during mechanical ventilation. *Crit Care.* 2000;4:282–289.
6. Michard F. Changes in arterial pressure during mechanical ventilation. *Anesthesiology.* 2005;103:419–428.
7. Bendjelid K, Romand JA. Fluid responsiveness in mechanically ventilated patients: a review of indices used in intensive care. *Intensive Care Med.* 2003;29:352–360.
8. Huang CC, Fu JY, Hu HC, et al. Prediction of fluid responsiveness in acute respiratory distress syndrome patients ventilated with low tidal volume and high positive end-expiratory pressure. *Crit Care Med.* 2008;36:2810–2816.
9. Morgan P, Al-Subaie N, Rhodes A. Minimally invasive cardiac output monitoring. *Curr Opin Crit Care.* 2008;14:322–326.
10. de Waal EE, Wappler F, Buhre WF. Cardiac output monitoring. *Curr Opin Anaesthesiol.* 2009;22:71–77.
11. Agee KR, Balk RA. Central venous catheterization in the critically ill patient. *Crit Care Clin.* 1992;8:677–686.
12. Randolph AG, Cook DJ, Gonzales CA, et al. Ultrasound guidance for placement of central venous catheters: a meta-analysis of the literature. *Crit Care Med.* 1996;24:2053–2058.
13. Swan HJC, Ganz W, Forrester J, et al. Catheterization of the heart in man with the use of a flow-directed balloon-tipped catheter. *N Engl J Med.* 1970;283:447.
14. Summerhill EM, Baram M. Principles of pulmonary artery catheterization in the critically ill. *Lung.* 2005;183:209.
15. Weed HG. Pulmonary "capillary" wedge pressure not the pressure in the pulmonary capillaries. *Chest.* 1991;100:1138.
16. O'Quin R, Marini JJ. Pulmonary artery occlusion pressure: clinical physiology, measurement, and interpretation. *Am Rev Respir Dis.* 1983;128:319.

17. Putterman C. The Swan-Ganz catheter: a decade of hemodynamic monitoring. *J Crit Care.* 1989;4:127.
18. Sharkey SW. Beyond the wedge: clinical physiology and the Swan-Ganz catheter. *Am J Med.* 1987;83:111.
19. Raper R, Sibbald WJ. Misled by the wedge? The Swan-Ganz catheter and left ventricular preload. *Chest.* 1986;89:427.
20. Kleinman B, Powell S, Kumar P, Gardner RM. The fast flush test measures the dynamic response of the entire blood pressure monitoring system. *Anesthesiology.* 1992;77:1215.21.
21. Snyder RW, Glamann B, Lange RA, et al. Predictive value of prominent pulmonary arterial wedge v waves in assessing the presence and severity of mitral regurgitation. *Am J Cardiol.* 1994;73:568.
22. Pinsky MR. Pulmonary artery occlusion pressure. *Intensive Care Med.* 2003;29:19.
23. Pinsky MR. Clinical significance of pulmonary artery occlusion pressure. *Intensive Care Med.* 2003;29:175.
24. West JB, Dollery CT, Naimark A. Distribution of blood flow in isolated lung: relation to vascular and alveolar pressures. *J Appl Physiol.* 1964;19:713.
25. Teboul JL, Besbes M, Andrivet P, et al. A bedside index assessing the reliability of pulmonary artery occlusion pressure measurements during mechanical ventilation with positive end-expiratory pressure. *J Crit Care.* 1992;7:22.
26. Hess DR, Bigatello LM. The chest wall in acute lung injury/acute respiratory distress syndrome. *Curr Opin Crit Care.* 2008;14:94–102.
27. Yelderman ML, Ramsay MA, Quinn MD, et al. Continuous thermodilution cardiac output measurement in intensive care unit patients. *J Cardiothorac Vasc Anesth.* 1992;6:270.
28. Nelson LD. The new pulmonary arterial catheters: right ventricular ejection fraction and continuous cardiac output. *Crit Care Clin.* 1996;12:795–818.
29. Pulmonary Artery Catheter Consensus Conference. Consensus statement. *Crit Care Med.* 1997;25:910–925.
30. Wheeler AP, Bernard GR, Thompson BT, et al. Pulmonary-artery versus central venous catheter to guide treatment of acute lung injury. *N Engl J Med.* 2006;354:2213–2224.
31. Rivers E, Nguyen B, Havstad S, et al. Early goal-directed therapy in the treatment of severe sepsis and septic shock. *N Engl J Med.* 2001;345:1368–1377.
32. Rivers EP, Coba V, Whitmill M. Early goal-directed therapy in severe sepsis and septic shock: a contemporary review of the literature. *Curr Opin Anaesthesiol.* 2008;21:128–140.

CHAPTER 7

Cardiac Assessment

Jaspal Singh

OUTLINE

Evaluation of Ventricular Function
Valvular Function
Coronary Artery Disease
Cardiac Conduction System

OBJECTIVES

1. Compare the similarity of symptoms and the interaction between the respiratory and cardiovascular systems.
2. Compare systolic and diastolic dysfunction.
3. Describe tests of cardiac function, their use in clinical practice, and their advantages and disadvantages.
4. Describe tests used to assess left ventricular function and right ventricular function.
5. Describe tests used to evaluate valvular function.
6. Discuss tests to evaluate coronary circulation.
7. Interpret common arrhythmias.
8. Integrate cardiac evaluation into the assessment of the patient with cardiopulmonary disease.

KEY TERMS

afterload
angina
cardiac catheterization
cardiac output ($\dot{Q}c$)
cor pulmonale
diastolic dysfunction
echocardiography
ejection fraction (EF)
electrocardiography (ECG)
ischemia
myocardial perfusion imaging
pulmonary hypertension
radionuclide angiocardiography
stress test
stroke volume
systolic dysfunction
transesophageal echocardiography (TEE)
valvular heart disease
valvular regurgitation
valvular stenosis
ventriculography

INTRODUCTION

Diseases of the respiratory and cardiovascular systems interact in pathophysiology, symptoms, treatment, and prognosis. Although primary diseases of either organ system may not involve the other, a significant interaction is more common. This interaction between the respiratory and cardiovascular systems often confounds the diagnosis of the primary problem and complicates its management. Understanding the basics of cardiac evaluation is important for the respiratory therapist in numerous respects, some of which are described in this chapter.

Evaluation of Ventricular Function

Case 1. Congestive Heart Failure

A 50-year-old man comes to the emergency department with several days of worsening shortness of breath. He has a history of hypertension, diabetes, and high cholesterol. Vital signs show hypertension, hypoxia, and respiratory distress but no fever. On examination he is obese and has an elevated jugular venous pressure (JVP), S_3 gallop, crackles in his lung bases, and prominent bilateral leg swelling. His chest x-ray shows pulmonary edema, and his electrocardiogram (ECG) shows no signs of acute myocardial infarction (MI), although there are signs of chronic ischemic heart disease.

This patient may have dyspnea for several reasons, but the clinical clues in this case are derived from the history and physical, with supportive information from the chest x-ray and ECG. All these clues suggest that the patient has acute congestive heart failure (CHF). He has risk factors for heart disease (obese, diabetic, hypertensive, high cholesterol), and the examination demonstrates physical findings of left-sided heart failure (S_3 gallop, crackles in his lung bases) as well as right heart failure (leg edema). The absence of fever helps to exclude an active infectious process such as pneumonia, and additional supportive information is gleaned from the chest x-ray, ECG, and perhaps other laboratory tests. The ECG also points away from an active MI or other diagnosis complicating his picture. At this point, it would be very helpful to understand the patient's cardiac physiology (especially left ventricular function). A transthoracic echocardiogram would be an excellent way to evaluate this quickly and noninvasively and would provide the greatest amount of functional and prognostic information.

Left Ventricular Dysfunction

The primary symptom of patients with left ventricular dysfunction is dyspnea, but additional symptoms of CHF such as orthopnea or paroxysmal nocturnal dyspnea may suggest that the primary cause of dyspnea is ventricular dysfunction rather than a pulmonary disorder. The initial diagnostic step used to evaluate patients with symptoms of ventricular dysfunction is to determine whether **systolic dysfunction** (impaired contractility) or **diastolic dysfunction** (impaired filling) is the major pathophysiologic mechanism.

Symptoms of CHF (dyspnea on exertion, orthopnea, paroxysmal nocturnal dyspnea) can also occur with normal systolic function of the left ventricle. Diastolic dysfunction increasingly is recognized as a cause of the symptoms of CHF and may be present with or without systolic dysfunction. Although the history and physical examination are useful for differentiation of cardiac causes from respiratory causes of dyspnea, it may be more difficult to determine whether CHF is due to systolic or diastolic dysfunction without an imaging study of left ventricular function. Moreover, many patients have findings of both systolic and diastolic heart failure.

Echocardiography uses ultrasonography to examine the heart structures and function. Because of its portability and noninvasiveness (safety), echocardiography often is the primary test used in the assessment of ventricular function. Echocardiography provides information on the **ejection fraction (EF)**, which is the percentage of blood pumped from the ventricle during a single cardiac contraction. The normal left ventricular ejection fraction is more than 50%. Because the ejection fraction is easily obtained, fairly reproducible, and is an important prognostic factor in critical illness, it is an extremely useful measurement.[1]

Echocardiography also examines the wall motion of the heart. Wall motion abnormality may suggest the cause of left ventricular systolic dysfunction. A disease such as viral myocarditis may affect all segments of the myocardium equally (a global process), whereas an MI that occurred previously or ischemia in a specific coronary artery distribution results in a focal wall motion abnormality (a regional or localized process).[1] Moreover, different features of echocardiography (M-mode, Doppler modes) allow more sophisticated assessment of cardiac structure and function.

RESPIRATORY RECAP

Tests to Assess Left Ventricular Function

- » Electrocardiography
- » Radionuclide angiocardiography
- » Echocardiography: M-mode, two-dimensional
- » Left ventriculography by cardiac catheterization
- » Cardiac magnetic resonance imaging
- » Brain natriuretic peptide elevation

In summary, echocardiography is often useful in simultaneously confirming the presence of both systolic and diastolic heart dysfunction, excluding other potentially confounding diagnoses or other complicating factors, giving prognostic information, and formulating a treatment plan.

Other Tests to Assess Left Ventricular Function

In general, **electrocardiography (ECG)** is an insensitive and nonspecific test used to evaluate ventricular function and cannot reliably differentiate systolic dysfunction from diastolic dysfunction. However, it is a simple and specific test to detect hypertrophy of either ventricular chamber. ECG evidence of left ventricular hypertrophy (LVH) is commonly found in patients with both systolic and diastolic dysfunction.[2] ECG manifestations of LVH include an increase in voltage, a shift in the QRS axis, prolongation of depolarization, and repolarization abnormalities (characterized by changes in the ST segment and T waves in a direction opposite to the major

S wave amplitude in lead V1 or V2 + R in V5 ≥ 35 mm
S in V1 or V2 + R in V5 or V6 > 35 mm
Any R + S > 40 mm
S in V1 ≥ 24 mm
R in VL ≥ 11 mm
R in lead 1 > 15 mm

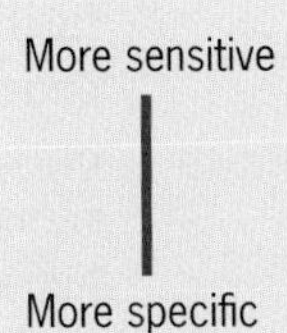

FIGURE 7–1 Commonly used electrocardiographic voltage criteria for the diagnosis of left ventricular hypertrophy.

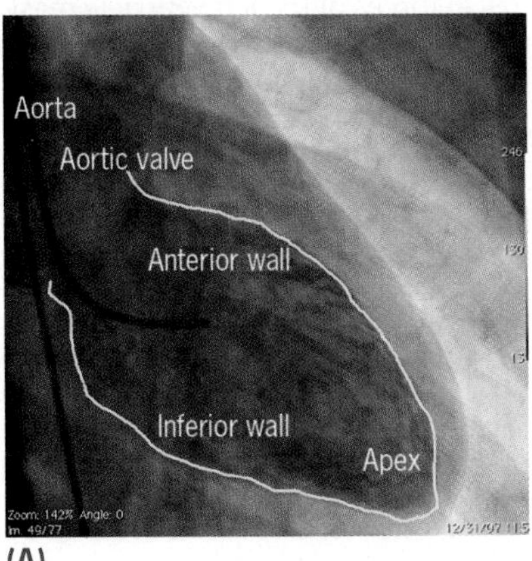

(A)

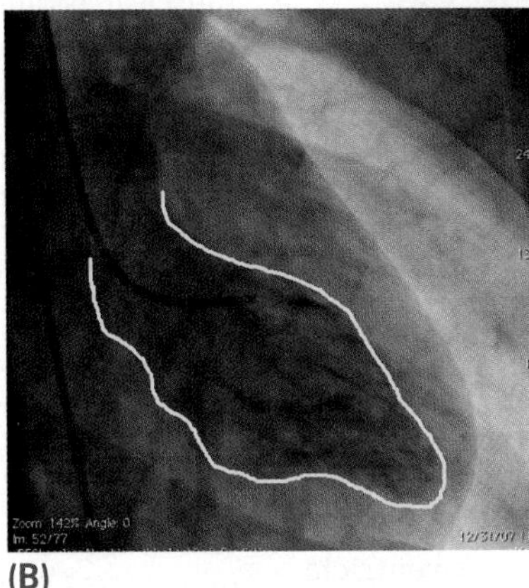

(B)

FIGURE 7–2 Left ventriculogram performed during cardiac catheterization, demonstrating (**A**) left ventricular cavity at end-diastole and (**B**) left ventricle at end-systole, with normal contractility of all regions of the myocardium.

QRS deflection). A number of QRS voltage criteria exist for the diagnosis of LVH (**Figure 7–1**).

Left **ventriculography** performed during **cardiac catheterization** is the gold standard of cardiac imaging modalities, although the risks of the procedure are higher than noninvasive methods. The left ventriculogram typically involves injection of a radiocontrast agent directly into the chamber through a catheter passed retrograde via a large artery (usually the femoral or radial artery) through the aorta and into the left ventricle. The radiographic absorbency of the contrast agent increases the radiographic density of the blood in the chamber so that the internal contours are visualized throughout cardiac contraction (**Figure 7–2**).

Cardiac catheterization techniques include other methods used to evaluate ventricular function. **Cardiac output ($\dot{Q}c$)** reflects forward blood flow from the heart into the peripheral vasculature and provides an overall assessment of cardiovascular function. Cardiac output can be calculated by a number of different techniques, including the Fick method, indicator dilution, and thermodilution. Numerous assumptions are involved in validating the calculation of $\dot{Q}c$ with such methods, which is why these may not be as reliable as other methods that are discussed in more detail in this chapter.

Other tests for evaluating left ventricular function include **radionuclide angiocardiography** and cardiac magnetic resonance imaging (cardiac MRI). Radionuclide tests involve intravenous injection of a radioisotope (most commonly technetium) and the use of a γ-ray scintillation camera to detect the isotope's signal in the left ventricle to allow a reflection of the ejection fraction. Cardiac MRI not only images the heart and assesses ventricular function, but it also can examine tissues surrounding the heart and may have more interesting applications in the future. Currently, due to technical limitations, expense, and lack of true standardization of its applications, the role of cardiac MRI is still evolving.

Elevated brain natriuretic peptide (BNP), or B-type natriuretic peptide, levels can be used as a diagnostic tool to evaluate for cardiac dysfunction as a cause of dyspnea and have also been shown to correlate with the presence and severity of cardiac diseases such as CHF. The diagnostic role of BNP values in such a setting is still evolving, with different institutions using different tests and different definitions of what constitutes abnormal levels in making diagnoses; measurement is confounded by factors such as obesity, tobacco use, and other diseases, such as chronic obstructive pulmonary disease (COPD).[3] Moreover, an elevated BNP level does not give more insight into overall cardiac systolic and diastolic dysfunction; knowing such information may affect treatment options. BNP testing is becoming more rapidly available and can help discern a cardiac cause of the patient's dyspnea, as opposed to other common pulmonary diseases.

Case 2. Right Ventricular Failure

A 53-year-old woman presents with worsening shortness of breath and leg swelling after a long plane ride. She has a history of COPD that was previously well controlled. Vital signs show moderate hypoxemia, tachycardia, and tachypnea. On examination she is obese, has a prominent right ventricular heave, diminished lung sounds throughout, and prominent bilateral leg swelling. Her chest x-ray is clear, and a subsequent ECG stress test is unremarkable but was stopped short due to her dyspnea. A computed tomography (CT) scan of the chest with IV contrast shows bilateral pulmonary emboli (**Figure 7–3**).

Her clinicians are trying to decide whether to administer lytic therapy, which is more likely to rapidly dissolve the clot than systemic heparin anticoagulation. However, lytic therapy is associated with a higher risk of bleeding complications. Therefore, it often is reserved for patients with cardiac dysfunction, generally those patients with either left or right ventricular compromise. At this time,

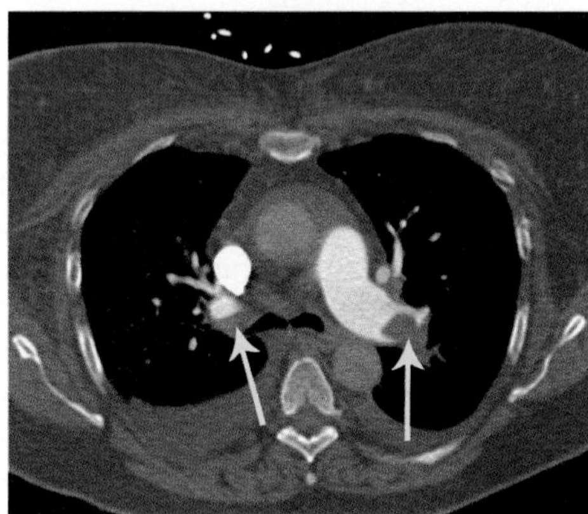

FIGURE 7–3 Bilateral pulmonary emboli.

an echocardiogram can be used to evaluate the patient's right ventricular function and size; if a pulmonary embolism is large, it may cause strain on the right heart that is visible by the echo.

An echocardiogram demonstrated elevated right ventricular systolic pressures and evidence of strain. The strain was impairing the function of the left ventricle as well. Based on this information, the patient received thrombolytic therapy and resolved the clot burden without further complications.

Right Ventricular Function

Evaluation of right ventricular function is important to determine the effects and severity of pulmonary disease. For example, in patients with severe COPD or severe obstructive sleep apnea, the pulmonary artery pressure may be elevated, resulting in hypertrophy and dilation of the right ventricle, a condition known as **cor pulmonale**. **Pulmonary hypertension** with chronic respiratory disease (such as COPD) is a poor prognostic finding.[4] Right ventricular dysfunction, or right-sided heart failure, may be suspected in patients with lung disease by the findings of peripheral edema, elevated JVP, hepatomegaly, and ascites.

> **RESPIRATORY RECAP**
>
> **Tests to Evaluate Right Ventricular Function**
> - » Echocardiography
> - » Electrocardiogram
> - » Right heart catheterization (i.e., Swan-Ganz)

The right ventricle is a thin-walled structure that ejects blood into the low resistance of the pulmonary vasculature. Because of its lower muscle mass, it is very sensitive to an acute increase in **afterload** (pulmonary artery pressure), and right ventricular systolic dysfunction may develop. If pulmonary hypertension develops more slowly, the right ventricle may adapt by the process of hypertrophy so that the right ventricular ejection fraction remains normal at rest but may decrease during exercise because of an increase in pulmonary artery pressure. A lack of increase in the cardiac output during exercise may result in the symptom of dyspnea. If the pulmonary artery pressure continues to increase over time, further elevation of the right ventricular systolic pressure, and subsequently diastolic pressure, occurs. The elevation in right ventricular diastolic filling pressure results in the signs of right-sided CHF, such as lower extremity edema, hepatomegaly, and ascites.

Analysis of right ventricular function is complicated and has not been standardized. The ECG is less sensitive for the diagnosis of right ventricular hypertrophy (RVH) than for LVH because in the normal ECG, the larger muscle mass and electrical forces of the left ventricle mask right ventricular forces. These right ventricular forces are most apparent in the right precordial leads (V_1 and V_2). Although ECG criteria for RVH are insensitive, the commonly used ECG criteria for the diagnosis of RVH are very specific: right axis deviation, 110 degrees or more; R/S ratio in lead V_1 more than 1; and R in V_1 of 7 mm or more.[5]

Characteristic ECG changes may occur with other pulmonary conditions, such as acute pulmonary embolism or obstructive lung disease. If an acute pulmonary embolus results in a significant increase in pulmonary arterial pressure, a number of electrocardiographic features suggestive of acute right ventricular strain may be present: (1) $S_1Q_3T_3$ (development of an S wave in lead I, and Q wave and T wave inversion in lead III); (2) rightward QRS axis shift; (3) transient right bundle branch block; and (4) T wave inversion in the right precordial leads (V_{1-2}).[5] However, these changes are relatively insensitive and transient (as resolution or thrombolysis of the pulmonary embolus occurs).

COPD also may cause characteristic electrocardiographic changes, which are thought to be due to hyperinflation of the lungs and a low position of the diaphragm. As a result, the heart becomes more vertical in the chest and rotates clockwise along its longitudinal axis. Other electrocardiographic abnormalities include right atrial abnormality, right axis deviation, low QRS voltage, T wave abnormalities in the right precordial leads (V_{1-2}), and leftward shift of the transitional zone.

Echocardiography provides valuable information about global right ventricular function. In addition to quantitative assessment of right ventricular function and qualitative assessment of right ventricular size and wall thickness, Doppler echocardiography can be used to estimate the pulmonary artery systolic pressure and suggest whether right ventricular dysfunction is caused by pressure overload or volume overload.

Right heart catheterization with the use of a pulmonary artery catheter (Swan-Ganz catheter) can be used to measure right heart dysfunction. Although this is a much more accurate means of measuring right ventricle and pulmonary artery pressures than echocardiogram,[4] it is an invasive test. As such, it not only exposes the patient to more risks, but also may be difficult to perform when the patient is having acute issues. Moreover, there is literature to suggest that right heart catheterization may actually worsen clinical outcomes.[6] Therefore, its use has somewhat fallen out of favor when less invasive means are available.

Valvular Function

Case 3. Valvular Disease

A 26-year-old man comes to the emergency department with 1 day of severe shortness of breath and high fever. He is in respiratory distress, hypoxemic, and unable to provide a history. On examination he is thin, hypotensive, and has a loud, harsh murmur near his left nipple. In addition, bilateral crackles are heard on examination. Further inspection shows poor dentition and needle track marks indicating prior intravenous drug use. His chest x-ray shows pulmonary edema, but no discrete infiltrate suggestive of pneumonia. ECG shows only sinus tachycardia. The patient is intubated and placed on mechanical ventilation. Labs show a markedly elevated white blood cell (WBC) count. Blood cultures are drawn, and the patient is started on intravenous antibiotics. He is seen by several specialists in the emergency department, who suspect the patient has developed mitral valve endocarditis (a potentially life-threatening infection of the mitral valve). At this time, a transthoracic or transesophageal echocardiogram would be most useful.

This patient may have several reasons to be dyspneic, but the clinical clues in this case are derived from the history and physical, with supportive information from the chest x-ray. These in summation lead one to suspect the patient has mitral valve endocarditis. The high fever and elevated WBC count are indicative of an acute infectious process. The ensuing hypotension, loud apical murmur, and pulmonary edema are the salient clues to the diagnosis of endocarditis. The chest x-ray and the murmur point away from community-acquired pneumonia as the etiology, whereas the ECG also points away from an active MI or other gross arrhythmia.

In this case, the valve has been infected and thereby damaged, creating an incomplete closure of the valve during each systolic contraction. Such mitral regurgitation results not only in the murmur auscultated but also in symptoms of left heart failure (dyspnea from pulmonary edema, and hypotension due to lack of forward flow). The optimal confirmatory test here is then an echocardiogram, which may be performed via a transthoracic approach (simpler, noninvasive, but lower resolution of the valve) or a transesophageal approach (more invasive but much more sensitive to valvular pathology).

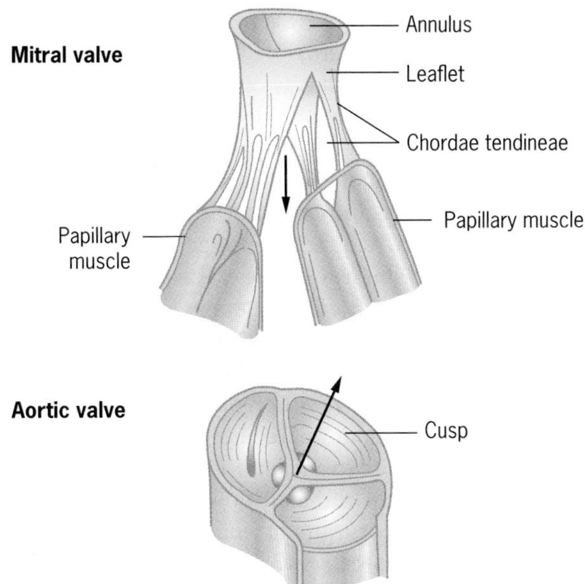

FIGURE 7–4 Normal cardiac valve anatomy. This article was published in *Textbook of Medical Physiology*. 8th ed. Guyton AC, Hall JE. Copyright Elsevier (WB Saunders) 1991.

Evaluation of Valvular Function

Acquired or congenital heart disease may affect valvular function. **Figure 7–4** shows the normal valvular anatomy. Hemodynamically, **valvular heart disease** can be differentiated into two types: stenotic lesions resulting from a decrease in the size of the valve orifice or impaired valve opening, or regurgitant lesions caused by impaired valve closure. The two types may be present concurrently. Valvular heart lesions may remain stable for years or may increase in severity because of the underlying disease or degenerative changes. Of note, the severity of the valvular lesion may not correlate with the symptoms or indicate the need for treatment, particularly if the valvular abnormality has progressed slowly and adaptive changes in cardiac function have occurred.

Normally, a valve opens when the pressure in the proximal chamber of the heart exceeds the pressure in the distal chamber. Although the pressure difference (gradient) is responsible for opening of the valve and blood flow across the valve, the normal valve gradient is minimal as blood flows between chambers of the heart. When disease causes narrowing of the valve orifice, a higher pressure difference develops between the chambers of the heart that are separated by the stenotic valve. Stenotic valvular lesions result in pressure overload of the proximal or upstream heart chamber, eventually resulting in abnormal diastolic function and the symptoms and signs of heart failure.

> **RESPIRATORY RECAP**
>
> **Types of Valvular Heart Disease**
>
> » Stenotic lesions
>
> » Regurgitant lesions

The severity of valvular stenosis is determined by measurement of either the pressure gradient across the valve or the valve area. The pressure gradient reflects not only the severity of stenosis but also on the rate of blood flow across the valve. In general, valve area measurements have been correlated with severity of disease for left-sided valvular lesions (mitral and aortic stenosis), but the clinical application of valve areas is less clear for the right-sided heart valves; therefore, pressure gradients are used to express the severity of stenosis. Using mean gradients alone, severe stenosis is defined as a measurement greater than 50 mm Hg across the aortic or pulmonic valve, greater than 10 mm Hg across the mitral valve, and greater than 5 mm Hg across the tricuspid valve.

Valvular regurgitation is caused by abnormal or impaired valve closure. Normally, when pressure in the downstream chamber exceeds pressure in the upstream chamber, the leaflets of the interceding valve close and coapt to prevent regurgitation of blood flow into the proximal chamber. Acquired or congenital valvular disease may result in abnormal valve closure. In such cases a proportion of the ventricular **stroke volume** flows backward rather than contributing to forward blood flow.

With mitral regurgitation, for instance, instead of the blood flowing forward, a portion of this flows backward, depending on the amount of regurgitation. The left ventricle therefore needs to increase its workload to meet the forward demands of blood flow as well as account for the additional regurgitant volume going back into the left atrium. This extra work due to chronic severe regurgitation results in volume overload and dilation of the ventricle, and symptoms may develop from resulting systolic dysfunction.

Electrocardiography

Electrocardiography may offer clues to the presence of a valvular lesion. Pressure overload caused by a stenotic valve may result in changes of hypertrophy (for example, LVH with aortic stenosis or right ventricular hypertrophy with pulmonic stenosis), and volume overload may result in changes of chamber enlargement (for example, left atrial enlargement with chronic mitral regurgitation). However, these ECG changes are insensitive and nonspecific for the diagnosis of the particular valvular lesion or its hemodynamic severity.

> **RESPIRATORY RECAP**
>
> **Tests to Assess Valvular Function**
>
> » Electrocardiography
> » Radionuclide angiography
> » Echocardiography
> » Cardiac catheterization

Echocardiography

Echocardiography is the most useful initial test to evaluate valvular function. Two-dimensional echocardiography allows visualization of valve leaflet anatomy and mobility. The appearance of thickened, calcified leaflets with poor mobility suggests **valvular stenosis** (**Figure 7–5**). In addition, with different angles of ultrasound transmission, the orifice of the valve can be visualized and measured. Echocardiography is also useful in evaluating the sequelae of valvular stenosis, such as LVH secondary to aortic stenosis or left atrial enlargement secondary to mitral stenosis.

Although no echocardiographic techniques can measure pressure gradients directly, Doppler echocardiography allows calculation of the pressure difference across a stenotic valve, helping to better delineate the severity of the stenosis. This can often be useful for planning interventions, such as the timing of surgery. Two-dimensional echocardiography is also useful in the assessment of secondary changes of valvular regurgitation, such as increased ventricular size and impaired systolic function, factors that are also used to decide when to intervene. Particularly relevant to the respiratory therapist is the ability of echocardiography to estimate right ventricular systolic pressure, which may reflect the presence of pulmonary hypertension as well as signs of right heart failure. Moreover, when evaluating patients for persistent hypoxemia, agitated saline may be used as a contrast agent (i.e., bubble echo). This method works on the principle that if there is a large shunt process, then bubbles from the venous side of the circulation should travel quickly from the right side of the heart to the left side. Normally, in the absence of any shunt, the pulmonary capillaries filter out the bubbles, so no bubbles appear in the left heart.

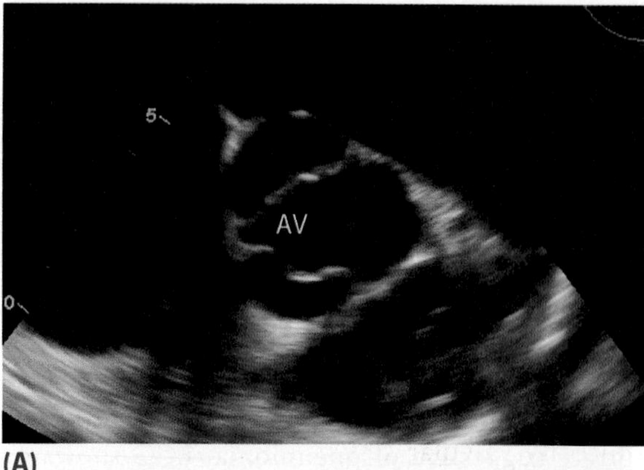

(A)

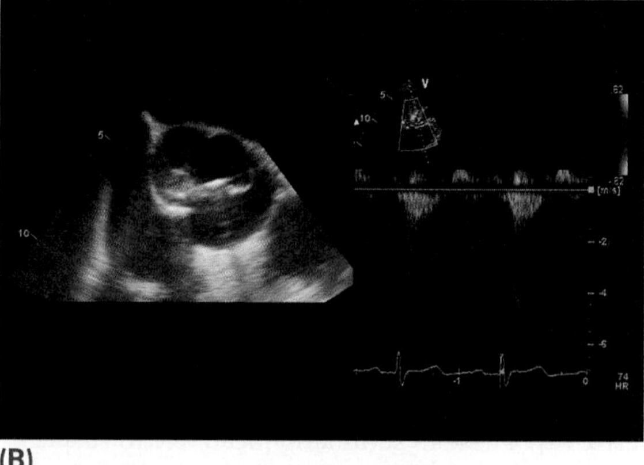

(B)

FIGURE 7–5 Two-dimensional echocardiography (short-axis view). (**A**) Normal aortic valve (AV) orifice. (**B**) Calcified, stenotic aortic valve. The continuous wave Doppler analysis across the aortic valve demonstrates a high-velocity jet (>4 meters per second), consistent with severe aortic stenosis.

Transesophageal echocardiography (TEE) is a more invasive procedure in which a smaller ultrasound transducer is passed posterior to the heart via the esophagus. This allows closer investigation of valvular heart disease because of the proximity of the transesophageal probe to the heart and the absence of intervening anatomic barriers such as the thoracic ribs. TEE includes all aspects of transthoracic imaging, including two-dimensional, Doppler, and color Doppler techniques, and is useful in assessments of valve morphology and function. It is particularly advantageous in evaluations of both the mitral valve, because of this valve's posterior position (**Figure 7–6**), and prosthetic valves, which may be difficult to visualize by transthoracic echocardiography because of shadowing of the ultrasound beam.

Cardiac Catheterization

Cardiac catheterization is an invasive, accurate means to quantify valvular stenosis and regurgitation. The pressure gradient can be directly assessed with the use of fluid-filled or micromanometer catheters to measure the pressure in the distal and proximal heart chambers across the stenotic valve. The pressure gradient across a stenotic valve is inversely related to the valve area (i.e., the smaller the valve area, the larger the pressure gradient). What is important for the clinician to understand is that the gradients across valves depend on mathematical concepts that are subject to some assumptions that may not be valid at any given moment. For instance, if a valve has regurgitation and stenosis, or the individual is in an unstable hemodynamic state, the gradient measurements will not take both factors into account accurately and therefore may be inaccurate.

Coronary Artery Disease

Case 4. Coronary Artery Disease

A 60-year-old woman comes to the emergency department with several hours of crushing substernal chest pain. Previously this occurred while she was exerting herself and would abate with rest. This time, however, it developed while standing at work. The pain is severe, radiates down her left arm and up to her left face, and is causing her to feel sweaty, nauseated, and lightheaded. Her medical history is notable for hypertension, high cholesterol, and a family history of heart disease. Her coworker calls for emergency help, and she is given sublingual nitroglycerin and oxygen, which lessen her pain. She is given aspirin therapy and thereafter transported to the local emergency department, where an ECG shows ST segment elevation (**Figure 7–7**). On examination, she is diaphoretic, tachycardic, in mild respiratory distress, and obviously still in pain. A chest-x-ray is clear. Cardiac troponin assay and creatine kinase MB fraction (CK-MB) levels are moderately elevated.

This patient has classic symptoms of **angina**, which is chest pain that is presumed to be due to coronary **ischemia** (lack of oxygen to the heart muscle tissues that are dependent on the blood flow from the blocked vessel). This usually affects the left ventricle, but occasionally may affect the right side of the heart. Before the presentation that brought her to the emergency department, the patient's symptoms would have been classified as stable angina (abates easily with rest), but now her symptoms would be deemed unstable, and in fact she likely has an occluded coronary artery that, if it persists, may result in more extensive cardiac damage. Her elevated cardiac troponin and CK-MB (cardiac proteins that are leaked into the bloodstream when there is heart damage such as ischemia) levels already indicate that there has been cardiac injury, so there is little time to waste in preventing more heart damage.

She therefore undergoes emergent left heart catheterization, not only because it would be diagnostic for occluded vessels but also because there is a chance that it may in fact be therapeutic if an occluded coronary vessel can be visualized and opened successfully (by means of angioplasty and possibly placing a stent to maintain the patency of the opened artery).

Evaluation of the Coronary Circulation

The most common cause of abnormal coronary circulation is coronary artery disease (CAD) caused by atherosclerosis. Significant CAD primarily affects the left

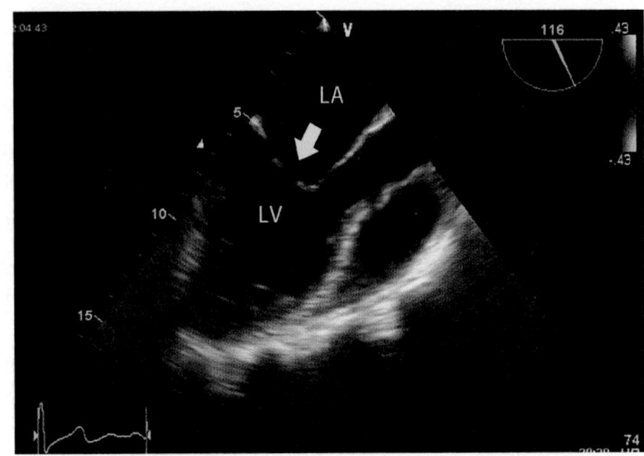

FIGURE 7–6 Transesophageal echocardiography demonstrating significant mitral stenosis. The left atrium (LA) and left ventricle (LV) are depicted, along with the stenotic mitral valve opening (arrow).

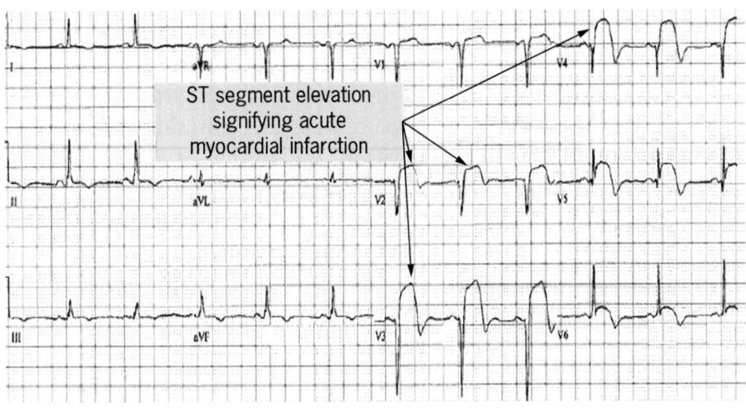

FIGURE 7–7 ECG with ST segment elevation characteristic of cardiac ischemia.

ventricle of the heart because of the relative mass of this chamber and the distribution of the coronary arteries. Therefore, left ventricular diastolic dysfunction, systolic dysfunction, or mitral valve dysfunction may occur as a result of limited blood supply to the coronary circulation (i.e., coronary ischemia). Resulting symptoms such as chest pain and dyspnea are common symptoms of CAD.

Longitudinal, epidemiologic studies have revealed that patients with certain clinical characteristics, or risk factors, have a greater likelihood of developing CAD. These risk factors include older age, tobacco use, hypertension, diabetes mellitus, hyperlipidemia, and a family history of premature CAD.[7] The presence of risk factors and the clinical history of the patient's symptoms may suggest CAD, and a test for the purpose of diagnosis should then be pursued.

Clinical tests used to evaluate the coronary circulation can be divided into two categories: anatomic or functional. Both types of tests provide diagnostic and prognostic information, and the rationale for the choice of one test over another is based on the information sought for treatment and the clinical scenario.

Anatomic Tests

Anatomic tests provide information on the presence, distribution, and severity of CAD. In some cases the anatomy of CAD provides important prognostic information. For instance, significant stenosis of the left main coronary artery or stenoses involving the proximal segments of all three coronary arteries are known to be associated with a decrease in long-term survival with medical therapy alone, indicating the need to consider revascularization either by percutaneous or surgical means.

In Case 4, the patient's history, physical, ECG, and laboratory tests all indicate that she is very likely having an acute coronary event. An anatomic test, such as cardiac catheterization, would better depict where the lesion or lesions might be in the acute event. However, what if she had presented earlier, before her acute event? In that situation, there might be an evolving role for cardiac CT scanning to anatomically visualize the coronary circulation.

Functional Tests

Functional tests assess for impaired blood flow with resultant ischemia or impaired cardiac function. With impaired coronary circulation, the supply of blood to the myocardial tissue may be unable to meet metabolic demands, and ischemia results. Major determinants of myocardial oxygen demand include the myocardial wall tension, contractility, and the heart rate. Furthermore, the response of the heart to ischemia is progressive (the ischemic cascade); therefore, as ischemia persists, additional abnormalities of cardiac function develop. **Figure 7–8** summarizes the ischemic response. When blood flow via a coronary artery is diminished significantly, diastolic dysfunction of the left ventricle is the first demonstrable abnormality of cardiac function. Continued ischemia leads to systolic dysfunction, electrocardiographic changes, and finally, the symptom of angina. Prolonged lack of blood flow results in an MI (myocardial cell death or necrosis).

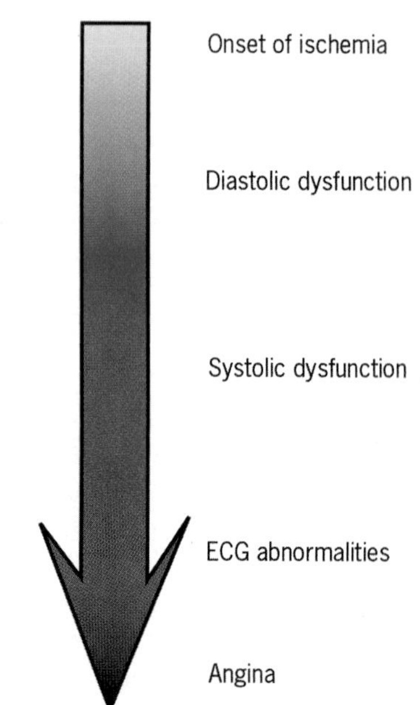

FIGURE 7–8 The ischemic cascade of cardiac dysfunction during coronary artery occlusion. Adapted from Nesto RW, Kowalchuck GJ. The ischemic cascade: temporal sequence of hemodynamic, electrocardiographic and symptomatic expressions of ischemia. *Am J Cardiol.* 1987;57:23C–27C.

In Case 4, a functional test might have been helpful in the preceding weeks to diagnose and target therapy for stable angina, but now, when the patient is having an acute coronary event, additional stress such as exercise can cause more damage. Therefore, functional tests at this time are not indicated.[8] That being said, functional tests can be quite helpful to elicit cardiac disease in an earlier stage as well as to identify potential areas of cardiac interest that might need more directed therapies.

Specific Tests to Assess Coronary Circulation

The ECG is a simple, readily available technique that should be the first test performed in the diagnosis of CAD. However, up to one-third of patients with CAD may have a normal ECG at rest. Therefore, this test is relatively insensitive for diagnostic purposes. Similar to the spectrum of clinical manifestations of CAD, a range of ECG changes may occur that may reflect ischemia, injury, or infarction, or all three.

Ischemia typically is manifested as changes in the T wave, which reflects abnormalities of repolarization of the myocardium. Displacement of the ST segment (depression or elevation) is an indicator of myocardial injury, as in Case 4. The diagnostic feature of MI, either acute or old, is the Q wave. Infarction signifies that the lack of oxygen, or ischemia, to the myocardium has been so profound that significant cardiac cell damage has occurred. The location of myocardial ischemia, injury, or infarction (i.e., anterior, inferior, or lateral) often is suggested by the specific leads in which the abnormalities occur. The ability to localize the region of affected myocardium is limited for T wave changes and ST segment depression but greater for findings of ST segment elevation or Q waves. Furthermore, all the ECG changes mentioned may be apparent in conditions other than CAD, such as metabolic abnormalities, LVH, or COPD. For these reasons, such ECG abnormalities must be interpreted in the context of the individual patient's symptoms, history, and physical examination results.

> **RESPIRATORY RECAP**
>
> **Tests to Assess Coronary Circulation**
>
> » Electrocardiogram: ST segment changes
> » Exercise stress testing
> » Radionuclide angiocardiography
> » Echocardiography
> » Myocardial perfusion imaging
> » Coronary arteriography
> » Cardiac CT scanning

Functional studies, specifically **stress tests**, of the coronary circulation use a stressor to induce an imbalance between the coronary blood supply and myocardial demand and a means to detect the ischemic response. The simplest and perhaps most informative stressor is exercise, because it provides additional evidence of the patient's functional status (exercise capacity). Typically, a target heart rate to be achieved during exercise is calculated based on the patient's age (85% to 90% of the predicted maximum heart rate), and attainment of the target heart rate is thought to represent an adequate stress.

Of course, some patients may be unable to exercise because of coexisting medical problems or may be unable to achieve an adequate heart rate response. In such cases a pharmacologic stressor, such as dobutamine, may be used to increase the myocardial oxygen demand. Dobutamine is a catecholamine with a β_1-adrenergic agonist effect, which stresses the heart in several ways (increases heart rate, increases systolic blood pressure, and increases cardiac contractility). Intravenous administration of dobutamine at increasing doses is used to increase the myocardial oxygen demand above the threshold of ischemia, similar to exercise.

Either exercise or dobutamine may be used as a stressor in combination with different methods used to detect ischemia, although if the patient is able to exercise, then this is preferred. Other pharmacologic agents include dipyridamole and adenosine, which result in vasodilation rather than a true ischemic response.

Markers of an ischemic response commonly used in clinical practice include ECG changes, systolic wall motion abnormalities, or myocardial perfusion changes. ECG is used in conjunction with exercise as a simple, readily available, and less expensive stress test. The most common ischemic response detected by ECG is a change in the ST segment. The standard criterion for an abnormal result is horizontal or down-sloping ST segment depression of 0.10 mV or more for 60 to 80 ms or longer after the end of the QRS complex, either during or after exercise (**Figure 7–9**).[9] Other factors related to the presence and severity of CAD include the amount, time of appearance, duration, and number of leads with ST segment depressions.[9] In patients with ST segment depression at baseline, an additional 0.10 mV or more of ST depression should be present to improve the specificity of the test result. It is important to remember that ST segment depression does not localize the region of myocardial ischemia or the coronary artery involved.

ST segment elevation is a less common finding during exercise stress testing, yet the site of ST segment

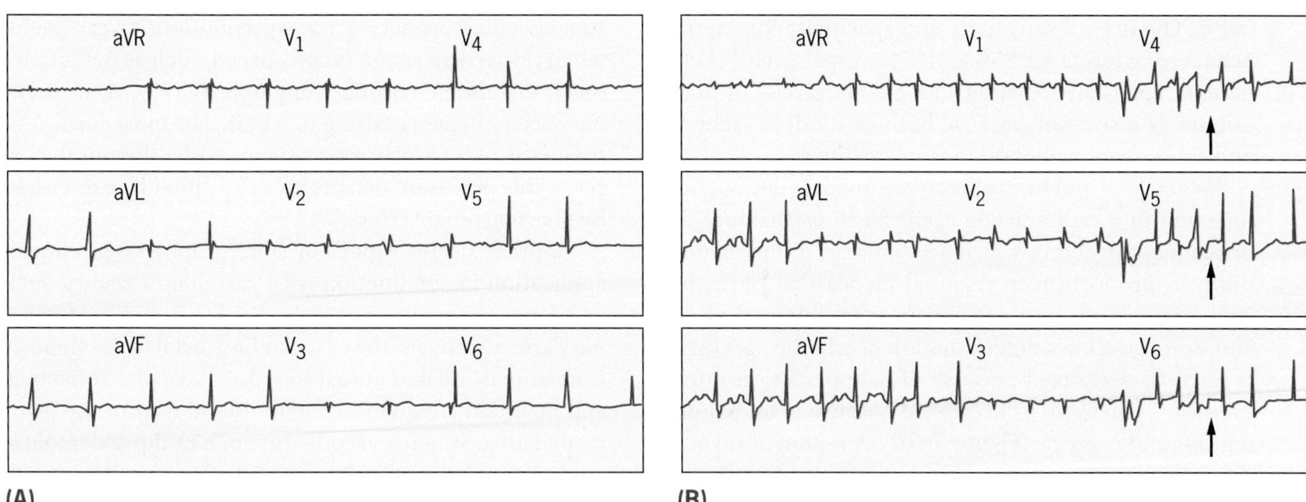

FIGURE 7–9 Electrocardiogram at (**A**) baseline and (**B**) during exercise treadmill test at peak heart rate, demonstrating ST segment depression in leads V_4 through V_6 (arrows) due to myocardial ischemia.

elevation is relatively specific for the coronary artery involved in patients who have not had a previous Q wave MI. ST segment elevation in ECG leads with evidence of previous Q wave infarction may reflect wall motion abnormality or a ventricular aneurysm. Exercise ECG may not be diagnostic for ischemia in other clinical conditions that affect the interpretation of ST segment changes, such as left bundle branch block, ventricular paced rhythms, LVH, or treatment with digitalis. In these settings, another marker of ischemic response, such as wall motion or myocardial perfusion, should be used instead of electrocardiography alone.

In most studies the sensitivity (percentage of patients with the disease who have an abnormal test result) of exercise stress testing for the diagnosis of CAD is approximately 70%. The specificity (percentage of patients without the disease who have a normal test result) of exercise stress testing is approximately 70% to 80%,[10] although certain factors, such as the number of vessels affected, may affect these numbers.

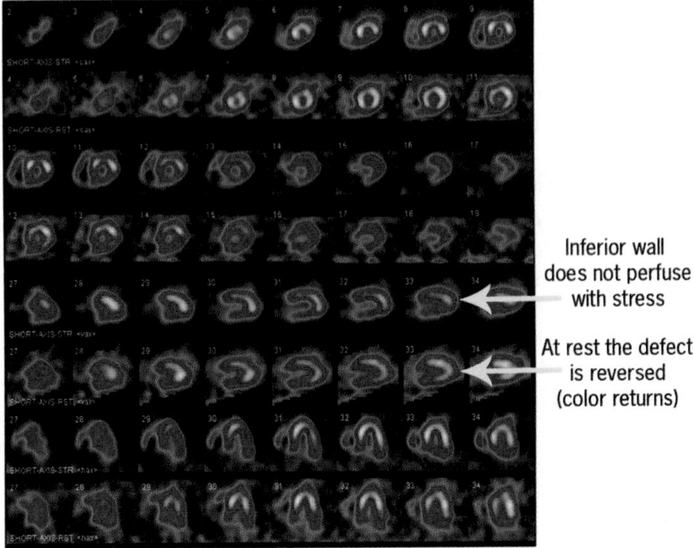
Inferior wall does not perfuse with stress
At rest the defect is reversed (color returns)

FIGURE 7–10 Nuclear cardiology perfusion imaging of the left ventricular myocardium during exercise and rest. The left ventricle is depicted in three different views during exercise and rest. The perfusion images demonstrate hypoperfusion (decreased blood flow) to the inferior wall during exercise (yellow arrows). After the patient rests, the blood flow returns, consistent with myocardial ischemia in that region.

Other functional tests for the diagnosis of CAD use different markers of ischemia, such as left ventricular systolic dysfunction or perfusion abnormalities, in conjunction with ECG changes. These tests, such as radionuclide angiocardiography, generally have the advantages of greater sensitivity with similar specificity as well as the ability to localize the region of ischemic myocardium. Similarly, stress echocardiography can also be used to detect wall motion abnormalities during exercise as a marker of ischemia. With a significant coronary artery lesion, the region of myocardium supplied by the artery may have normal contractile function at rest, but decreased function during exercise. Chronic ischemia, which may be difficult to detect clinically, may result in a wall motion abnormality or segmental hypocontractility at rest (known as hibernating myocardium), which, with exercise and more severe ischemia, becomes akinetic. The overall sensitivity and specificity for exercise echocardiography are 85% and 77%, respectively.[10] Echocardiography can be paired with either exercise or dobutamine as a stressor because both can induce ischemia and subsequent wall motion abnormalities.

Myocardial perfusion imaging involves intravenous injection of a radionuclide agent (such as thallium-201 or technetium-99m), which accumulates in the myocardium in proportion to regional myocardial perfusion. The comparison of perfusion images obtained at rest and exercise allows determination of whether perfusion is normal, decreased because of hypoperfusion during exercise (ischemia), or decreased because of an MI during rest and exercise (**Figure 7–10**). A region of myocardium that is hypoperfused during exercise but appears normal at rest is called a *reversible perfusion defect.* This abnormality is consistent with the presence of a significant lesion in the coronary artery that limits the increase in myocardial blood flow to that region normally seen during exercise; hopefully this can be treated. A region of myocardium that is hypoperfused both during exercise and at rest is called a *fixed perfusion defect* and is consistent with an MI (i.e., the cardiac tissue of the affected area has essentially been replaced by scar tissue, which does not carry the same type of blood flow as healthy cardiac tissue).

The sensitivity of perfusion imaging, or *scintigraphy,* is higher (approximately 85%), with comparable specificity, than electrocardiography alone.[10] The ability to predict accurately the number of diseased vessels and to identify specific ischemic regions is improved with tomographic imaging. This ability to localize ischemia to a specific coronary artery distribution is very useful when revascularization is considered, such as percutaneous transluminal coronary angioplasty (PTCA) or coronary artery bypass grafting (CABG). The most consistent predictor of a cardiac event seems to be the number of reversible perfusion defects induced either by exercise or by pharmacologic stress.[11]

Another useful aspect of scintigraphy is its clinical application in conjunction with vasodilator agents, such as adenosine or dipyridamole. With a significant coronary artery stenosis, the vascular bed distal to the stenosis is maximally dilated at rest to reduce vascular resistance and maintain adequate coronary blood flow to the myocardial area. When a vasodilator such as dipyridamole is administered, the vascular territory of a normal coronary artery dilates further, whereas the territory supplied by a diseased artery is nearly maximally dilated at rest. As a result, there is a relative decrease in perfusion to the region of the diseased artery compared with the normal artery, and this heterogeneous perfusion of the myocardium can be detected by scintigraphy. In actuality, this type of pharmacologic stress does not induce ischemia (as provoked by exercise or dobutamine), but rather is a test of coronary flow reserve. For this reason, vasodilator pharmacologic tests are not useful in tests with ischemic markers as endpoints, such as wall motion abnormalities during exercise echocardiography.

In addition to their role in the diagnosis of CAD, functional tests provide significant prognostic information. These tests can determine the effect of CAD on the patient's functional capacity, electrocardiogram, left ventricular function, or myocardial perfusion; therefore, they may be performed in patients known to have CAD. For instance, the evaluation of a patient who has experienced a recent MI often includes a functional test (such as an exercise perfusion study) to assess for ischemia and define the patient's risk of a recurrent infarction. In such cases the functional test result is used to *risk stratify* the patient as having a high risk (presence of a partly reversible perfusion defect, or residual ischemia) or low risk (fixed perfusion defect, or infarction only) of a cardiac event in the near future. Functional tests also are commonly used for risk stratification of patients known to have CAD who are scheduled for noncardiac surgery to assess their risk of a perioperative MI.

An abnormal functional test may suggest the presence of significant CAD and prompt further evaluation to confirm the condition and define the extent of disease. Coronary arteriography performed during cardiac catheterization is the gold-standard anatomic assessment of the coronary circulation. In this procedure, radiocontrast is injected directly into the coronary arteries via a catheter passed retrograde through the aorta. As with left ventriculography, the radiographic density of blood is increased by the radiologic contrast, allowing visualization of the internal contour of the epicardial coronary arteries (**Figure 7–11**), particularly focused on stenoses (narrowing of the arteries). In general, a 50% stenosis is considered significant.

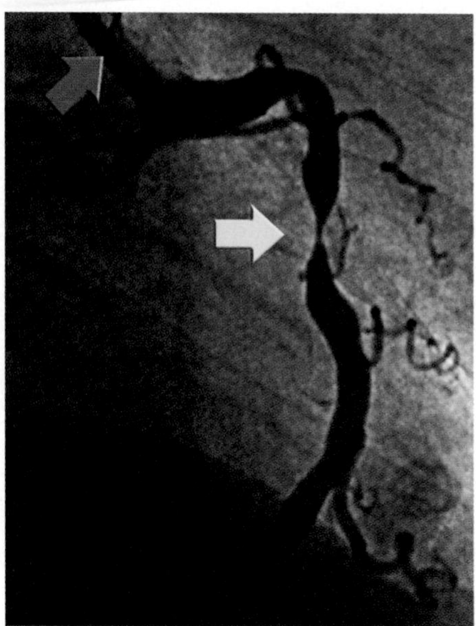

FIGURE 7–11 Right coronary angiogram of a patient with angina and abnormal exercise treadmill test result. The purple arrowhead demonstrates the catheter in the ostium of the right coronary artery. The yellow arrowhead demonstrates a 95% mid–right coronary artery stenosis.

However, despite demonstration of the anatomic presence of a coronary artery lesion by coronary arteriography, the functional significance of the lesion on coronary blood flow is less certain. A decrease in blood flow is not apparent during resting conditions until the artery is severely narrowed (90% of luminal diameter), but a less significant stenosis may limit blood flow during exercise. The effect of a stenosis on coronary blood flow depends not only on the severity of the stenosis but also on other factors, such as the extent of the lesion and its geometry, the presence of other lesions in series, the shape of the artery immediately proximal and distal to the narrowed segment, the blood flow velocity, and the presence of collateral circulation to the region of myocardium. Commonly, the degree of stenosis and its geometry are estimated visually in a qualitative manner. Because of the subjective nature of this assessment, interpretation may vary according to the observer and may be affected by factors such as the location of the stenotic lesion, the degree of stenosis, and the quality of the images.

One of the most interesting technologies of late is the application of CT to the coronary circulation (CT angiocardiography). The technology is based on the principle that diseased coronary arteries become calcified over time, and that the amount of calcium detected in the coronary arteries, by means of a low-radiation rapid CT scan, can assess the presence and degree of CAD, or atherosclerosis. Essentially, the amount of calcium detected by the scan results in a quantified calcium score; studies have shown that higher scores correlate with the greater risk of CAD in symptomatic patients, with sensitivities and specificities close to that of myocardial nuclear imaging.[12] Newer CT scans and CT software and further refinement of the technology can accurately image the coronary arteries without cardiac catheterization, thus saving the patient from a potentially unnecessary procedure with its associated risks.

The technology and its standards of interpretation are evolving, however, and there is still controversy as to what the calcium score signifies in asymptomatic patients.[13] Moreover, there is a radiation risk to CT scanning that may place the patient at higher risk for cancer during his or her lifetime.[14] In summary, CT scanning of the coronary arteries needs more standardization and refinement, but will likely evolve into a significant means of defining the coronary circulation noninvasively in the very near future.

Cardiac Conduction System

Case 5. Cardiac Arrhythmia

A 75-year-old woman with a history of CAD develops lightheadedness and diaphoresis, and almost has a syncopal episode. On examination, her pulse and blood pressure are low, and she is taken to the local emergency department. An electrocardiogram (**Figure 7–12**) reveals third-degree block. She is taken immediately for a pacemaker insertion and has a full recovery.

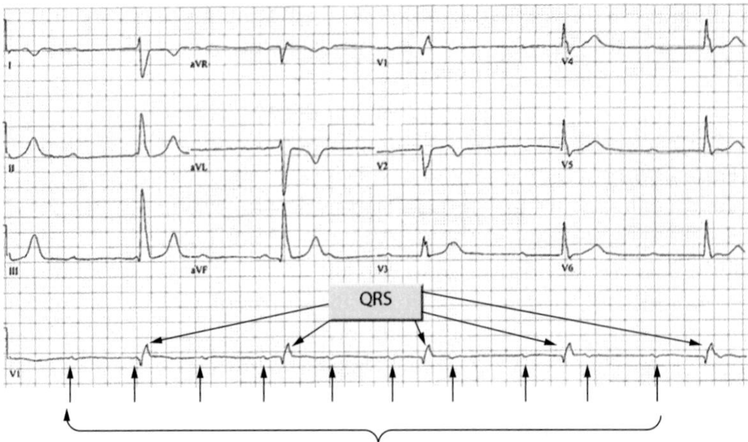

FIGURE 7–12 Complete heart block (third degree).

Evaluation of the Cardiac Conduction System

Cardiac arrhythmias are fairly common occurrences encountered by respiratory therapists. Arrhythmias can develop from many medical conditions, both cardiac and noncardiac, as well as from medications or other interventions. Therefore, a basic understanding of the cardiac conduction system is important. **Appendix 7–1** and **Table 7–1** provide a more complete discussion of the different types of cardiac arrhythmias and give some fundamental guidance on the major types of blocks and their severity.

Clinical severity is dependent on several important variables, including the type of arrhythmia, the patient's current physical state, and the patient's other comorbidities. **Figure 7–13** shows the cardiac conduction system. Typically, the heart conducts sequentially from the sinoatrial (SA) node in the right atrium (the heart's intrinsic pacemaker), to the atrioventricular (AV) node, and then to the Purkinje system and ventricular fibers. Interestingly, the AV node and the conduction fibers in the His/Purkinje system have their own backup rates of pacing the heart, so if there's a problem with, say, the SA node, the fibers just downstream from that can sometimes compensate adequately. Generally speaking, the farther down the circuit the problem lies, the more severe the problem becomes (refer to Table 7–1).

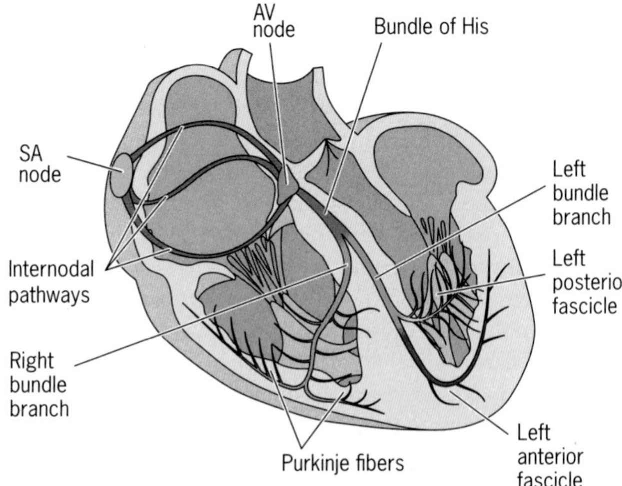

FIGURE 7–13 Electrical activity in the heart. The electrical signal normally starts at the sinus node, which causes the right and left atria to contract. The atrioventricular (AV) node is triggered next. The AV node sends a signal through the His/Purkinje system via the conduction pathways. The conduction pathways then signal the right and left ventricles to contract.

In Case 5, the patient has third-degree heart block, whereby the AV node is firing on its own, but the electrical stimulus is not getting through at all to the ventricle, which is necessary for the ventricle to contract in a normal fashion. Instead, the ventricle's pacing system is firing at its own slower pace, resulting in a much slower heart rate. This slow rate is not enough of a heart rate and cardiac output to meet the body's demands, and hence the patient is having severe symptoms that may worsen shortly. An artificial pacemaker is required to relieve her symptoms.

KEY POINTS

- Proper cardiac assessment is an important element in the care of patients with symptoms of pulmonary disease or documented pulmonary conditions because of the overlap of symptoms between cardiac and pulmonary disease.
- Clinical assessment involves integrating the history, physical examination, and laboratory studies with other diagnostic studies.
- Clinical tests such as blood tests, electrocardiography, nuclear cardiology, echocardiography, and cardiac catheterization have an important role in the diagnosis and prognosis of cardiac conditions, and each test may be used to assess various elements of cardiac function.
- Newer tests for coronary anatomy and functional status are being developed and validated to assist clinicians in cardiac assessments.
- A single test can provide information about several elements of cardiac function, and the

TABLE 7–1 Summary of Cardiac Rhythms

	Normal Sinus*	Paroxysmal Supraventricular Tachycardia	Atrial Flutter	Atrial Fibrillation	Ventricular Tachycardia	Ventricular Fibrillation	First- Degree AV Block	Second-Degree AV Block, Type I	Second-Degree AV Block, Type II	Complete AV Block (Type III)
Rate (beats per minute)	60–100	150–250	250–350 atrial; ventricular rate varies	Atrial rate >400; ventricular rate varies	100–250 ventricular	Difficult to discern	Normal	Atrial > ventricular; both usually normal	Atrial > ventricular; both usually normal	Atrial > ventricular; both usually normal
Rhythm	Regular	Regular	Atrial is regular; ventricular can be regular or irregular	Irregular	Regular ventricular	Rapid and chaotic	Regular	Atrial regular; ventricular pauses	Atrial regular; ventricular irregular with pauses	Regular
P waves	Uniform, upright, one before each QRS	May be hard to see	Sawtooth P waves	No P waves identifiable	Usually not discernible	Not discernible	Prolonged, constant PR interval	Progressive widening, then dropped	Some P waves not followed by QRS	No relationship between P and QRS
QRS†	Narrow	Narrow	Narrow	Narrow	Wide	Not discernible	Narrow	Narrow; sometimes dropped	Can be wide	Narrow or wide
Clinical severity‡	Normal	Mild to moderate	Usually mild to moderate	Mild to severe, depending on context	Severe to life threatening	Life threatening	Mild	Mild to moderate, depending on context	Severe to life threatening	Life threatening

*If rate is less than 60, it would be called sinus bradycardia. If rate is greater than 100, it would be sinus tachycardia.

†*Narrow* is defined as less than or equal to 0.12 second and *wide* as greater than 0.12 second.

‡This clinical severity is used as a general guide for clinicians in training, but the actual severity takes into account numerous factors of a patient's illness and the clinical context and thus should be interpreted accordingly.

advantages and disadvantages of the specific test must be considered in the clinical context of the individual patient.

- Tests of cardiac function may be used not only to help diagnose cardiac disease but also to evaluate the prognosis of patients with these conditions and to guide therapeutic interventions.

REFERENCES

1. Sheikh KH, de Bruijn NP, Rankin JS, et al. The utility of transesophageal echocardiography and Doppler color flow imaging in patients undergoing cardiac valve surgery. *J Am Coll Cardiol.* 1990;15:363–372.
2. Davie AP, Francis CM, Love MP, et al. Value of the electrocardiogram in identifying heart failure due to left ventricular systolic dysfunction. *BMJ.* 1996;312:222.
3. Felker GM, Petersen JW, Mark DB. Natriuretic peptides in the diagnosis and management of heart failure. *CMAJ.* 2006;175:611–617.
4. McLaughlin VV, Presberg KW, Doyle RL, et al. Prognosis of pulmonary arterial hypertension. *Chest.* 2004;126:78S–92S.
5. McGoon M, Gutterman D, Steen V, et al. Screening, early detection, and diagnosis of pulmonary arterial hypertension. *Chest.* 2004;126:14S–34S.
6. Shah MR, Hasselblad V, Stevenson LW, et al. Impact of the pulmonary artery catheter in critically ill patients: meta-analysis of randomized clinical trials. *JAMA.* 2005;294:1664–1670.
7. Wilson PWF, D'Agostino RB, Levy D, et al. Prediction of coronary heart disease using risk factor categories. *Circulation.* 1998;97:1837–1847.
8. Antman EM, Hand M, Armstrong PW, et al. 2007 focused update of the ACC/AHA 2004 guidelines for the management of patients with ST-elevation myocardial infarction. *J Am Coll Cardiol.* 2008;51:210–247.
9. Gibbons RJ, Balady GJ, Beasley JW, et al. ACC/AHA guidelines for exercise testing. Executive summary: a report of the American College of Cardiology/American Heart Association Task Force on Practice Guidelines (Committee on Exercise Testing). *Circulation.* 1997;96:345–354.
10. Greenland P, Smith SC Jr, Grundy SM. Improving coronary heart disease risk assessment in asymptomatic people: role of traditional risk factors and noninvasive cardiovascular tests. *Circulation.* 2001;104:1863–1867.
11. Gibbons RJ, Balady GJ, Timothy Bricker J, et al. ACC/AHA 2002 guideline update for exercise testing. Summary article: a report of the American College of Cardiology/American Heart Association Task Force on Practice Guidelines (Committee to Update the 1997 Exercise Testing Guidelines). *J Am Coll Cardiol.* 2002;40:1531–1540.
12. Budoff MJ, Achenbach S, Blumenthal RS, et al. Assessment of coronary artery disease by cardiac computed tomography: a scientific statement from the American Heart Association Committee on Cardiovascular Imaging and Intervention, Council on Cardiovascular Radiology and Intervention, and Committee on Cardiac Imaging, Council on Clinical Cardiology. *Circulation.* 2006;114:1761–1791.
13. Piers LH, Dikkers R, Willems TP, et al. Computed tomographic angiography or conventional coronary angiography in therapeutic decision-making. *Eur Heart J.* 2008;29:2902–2907.
14. Brenner DJ, Hall EJ. Computed tomography: an increasing source of radiation exposure. *N Engl J Med.* 2007;357:2277–2284.

APPENDIX 7–1

ECG Monitoring and Dysrhythmia Recognition

Locations for Chest Electrodes

Lead I

- Positive electrode placed just below the left clavicle
- Negative electrode placed just below the right clavicle
- Provides information about the left lateral wall of the heart

Lead II

- Positive electrode just below the left pectoral muscle
- Negative electrode just below the right clavicle
- Provides information about the inferior wall of the heart

FIGURE 7A–1 Location for chest electrodes: Lead I. G, ground. Adapted from Aehlert B. *ACLS Quick Review Study Guide.* Mosby; 1994.

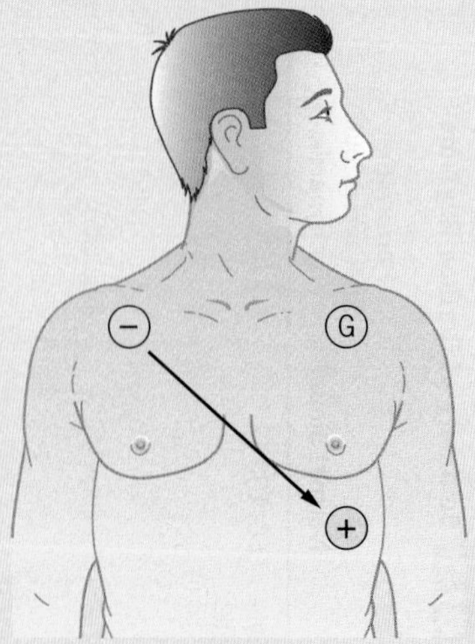

FIGURE 7A–2 Location for chest electrodes: Lead II. G, ground. Adapted from Aehlert B. *ACLS Quick Review Study Guide.* Mosby; 1994.

Appendix 7–1 *(continued)*

Lead III

- Positive electrode placed just below the left pectoral muscle
- Negative electrode placed just below the left clavicle
- Provides information about the inferior wall of the heart
- P waves seen in this lead usually are of lower amplitude than in leads I and II and are more likely to be biphasic (partly positive and partly negative)

Lead MCL_1 (Modified Chest Lead)

- Negative electrode placed just below the left clavicle
- Positive electrode placed to the right of the sternum at the fourth intercostal space
- Provides information about the anterior wall of the heart
- May prove useful in assessment of the width of the QRS complex to differentiate supraventricular tachycardia (SVT) from ventricular tachycardia (VT)

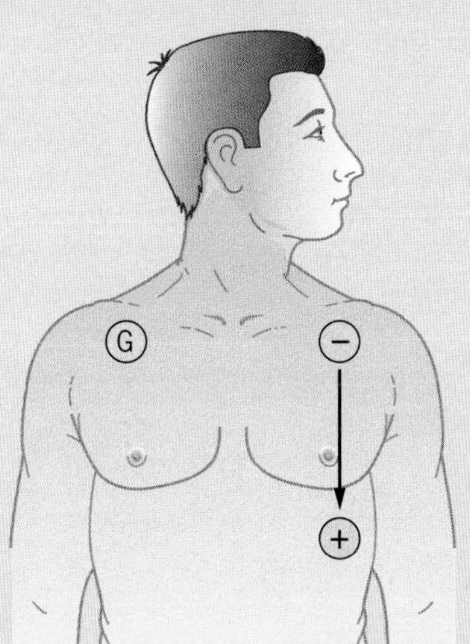

FIGURE 7A–3 Location for chest electrodes: Lead III. G, ground. Adapted from Aehlert B. *ACLS Quick Review Study Guide.* Mosby; 1994.

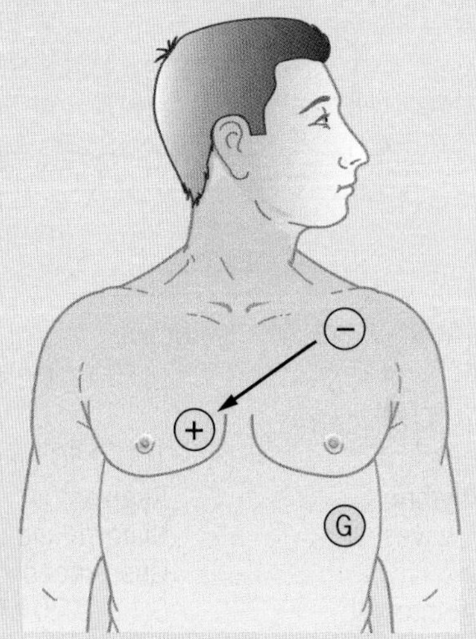

FIGURE 7A–4 Location for chest electrodes: Lead MCL_1. G, ground. Adapted from Aehlert B. *ACLS Quick Review Study Guide.* Mosby; 1994.

Because the speed of ECG paper is 25 mm/s, the distance between two vertical lines is 1 mm and represents 0.04 second. Thus, the time between two bold vertical lines (five small lines, or 5 mm) represents 0.2 second. The distance between two horizontal lines is also 1 mm. An upward deflection of 10 small lines (or two bold lines) represents 1 mV.

Dysrhythmia Recognition

Normal Sinus Rhythm (NSR)

Rate	60 to 100 beats/min
Rhythm	Regular
P waves	Uniform and upright in appearance One preceding each QRS complex
PR interval	0.12–0.20 s
QRS	<0.10 s

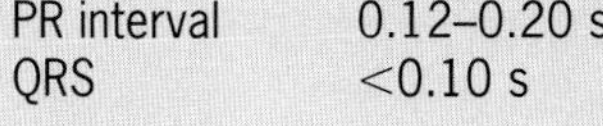

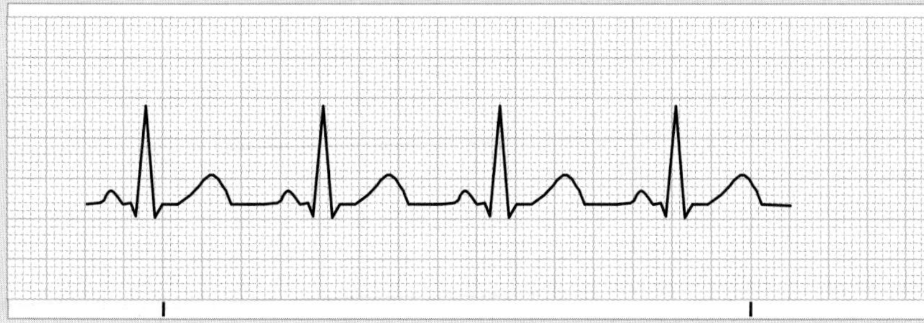

FIGURE 7A–5 Normal sinus rhythm.

(continues)

Appendix 7–1 *(continued)*

Sinus Bradycardia

Rate	<60 beats/min
Rhythm	Regular
P waves	Uniform and upright in appearance One preceding each QRS complex
PR interval	0.12–0.20 s
QRS	<0.10 s

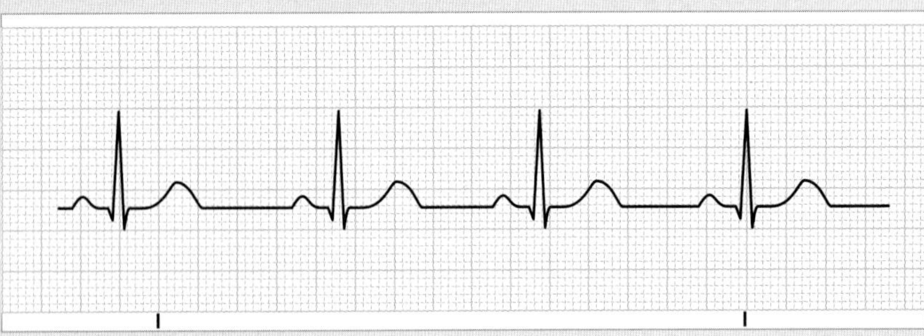

FIGURE 7A–6 Sinus bradycardia.

Sinus Tachycardia

Rate	100–160 beats/min
Rhythm	Regular
P waves	Uniform and upright in appearance One preceding each QRS complex
PR interval	0.12–0.20 s
QRS	<0.10 s

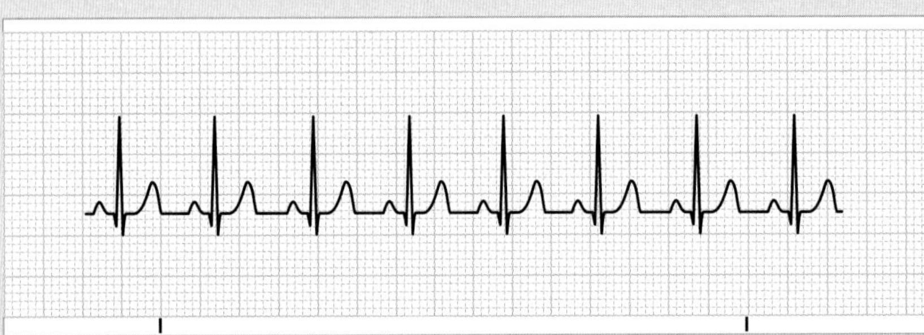

FIGURE 7A–7 Sinus tachycardia.

Sinus Arrhythmia

Rate	Usually 60–100 beats/min but may be faster or slower
Rhythm	Irregular
P waves	Uniform and upright in appearance One preceding each QRS complex
PR interval	0.12–0.20 seconds
QRS	<0.10 s

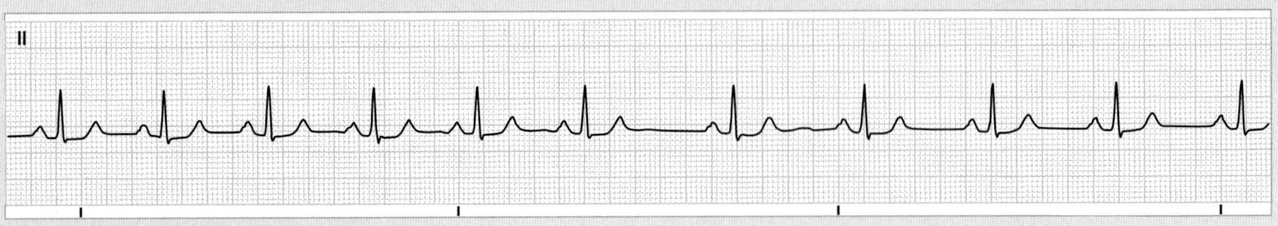

FIGURE 7A–8 Sinus arrhythmia.

Appendix 7–1 *(continued)*

Premature Atrial Complexes (PACs)

Rate	Usually normal, but depends on underlying rhythm
Rhythm	Irregular because of PACs
P waves	P wave of the early beat differs from sinus P waves Is premature May be flattened or notched May be lost in the preceding T wave
PR interval	Varies from 0.12–0.20 s when the pacemaker site is near the SA node to 0.12 s when the pacemaker site is nearer the AV node
QRS	Usually <0.10 s but may be prolonged

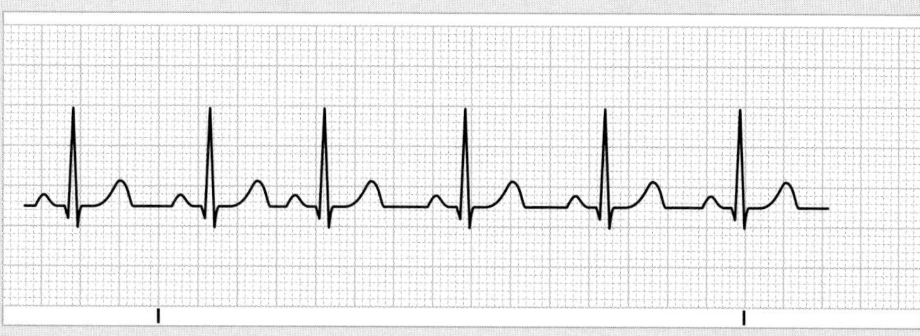

FIGURE 7A–9 Premature atrial complexes.

Supraventricular Tachycardia

Rate	150–250 beats/min
Rhythm	Regular
P waves	Atrial P waves different from sinus P waves P waves usually identifiable at the lower end of the rate range but seldom identifiable at rates >200 May be lost in preceding T wave
PR interval	Usually not measurable because the P wave is difficult to distinguish from the preceding T wave; if measurable, is 0.12–0.20 s
QRS	<0.10 s

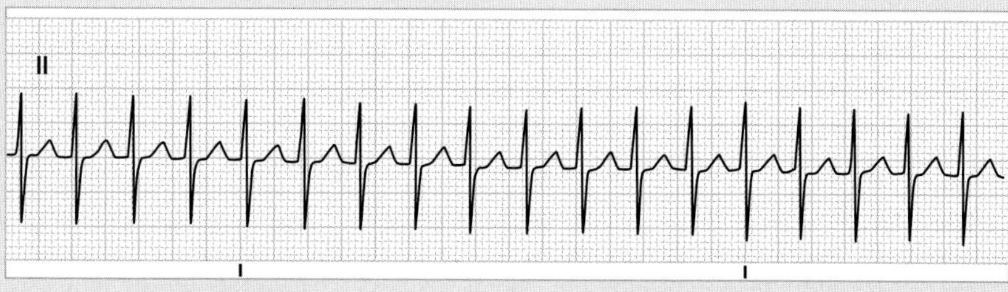

FIGURE 7A–10 Supraventricular tachycardia.

(continues)

Appendix 7–1 *(continued)*

Atrial Flutter

Rate	Atrial rate 250–350 beats/min Ventricular rate variable
Rhythm	Atrial rhythm regular Ventricular rhythm usually regular but may be irregular
P waves	Sawtooth flutter waves
PR interval	Not measurable
QRS	Usually <0.10 s but may be widened if flutter waves are buried in the QRS complex

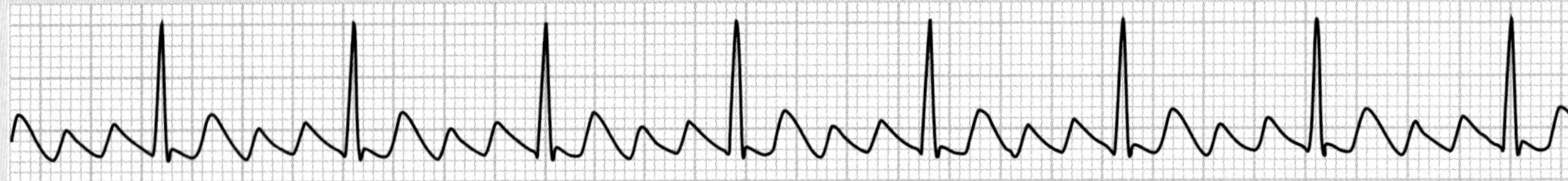

FIGURE 7A–11 Atrial flutter.

Atrial Fibrillation

Rate	Atrial rate usually >400 beats/min Ventricular rate variable
Rhythm	Atrial and ventricular very irregular (regular, bradycardic ventricular rhythm may occur as a result of digitalis toxicity)
P waves	No identifiable P waves Erratic, wavy baseline
PR interval	None
QRS	Usually <0.10 s

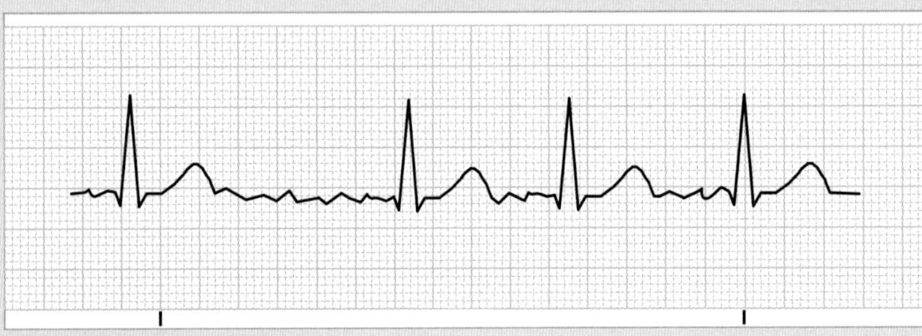

FIGURE 7A–12 Atrial fibrillation.

Premature Junctional Complexes (PJCs)

Rate	Atrial and ventricular rates depend on underlying rhythm
Rhythm	Irregular because of premature complex
P waves	May occur before, during, or after the QRS; if seen, will be inverted (retrograde)
PR interval	If the P wave occurs before the QRS, the PR interval will usually be ≤0.12 s
QRS	<0.10 s

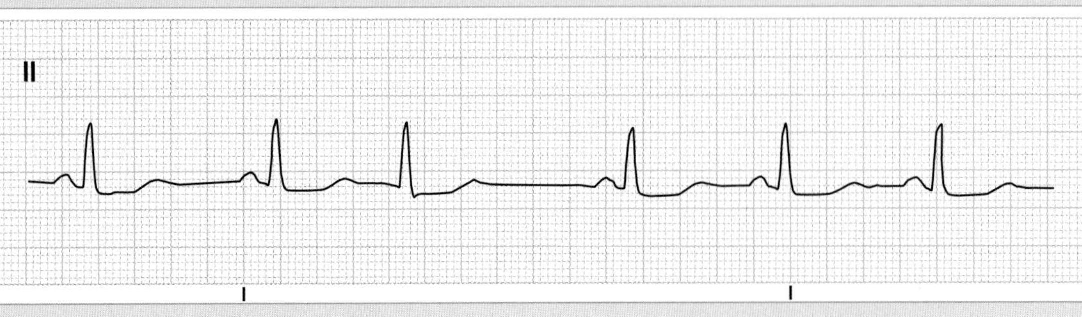

FIGURE 7A–13 Premature junctional complexes.

Appendix 7–1 *(continued)*

Accelerated Junctional Rhythm

Rate	60–100 beats/min
Rhythm	Atrial and ventricular very regular
P waves	May occur before, during, or after the QRS; if seen, will be inverted (retrograde)
PR interval	Not measurable unless the P wave precedes the QRS; when present, will usually be ≤0.12 s
QRS	<0.10 s

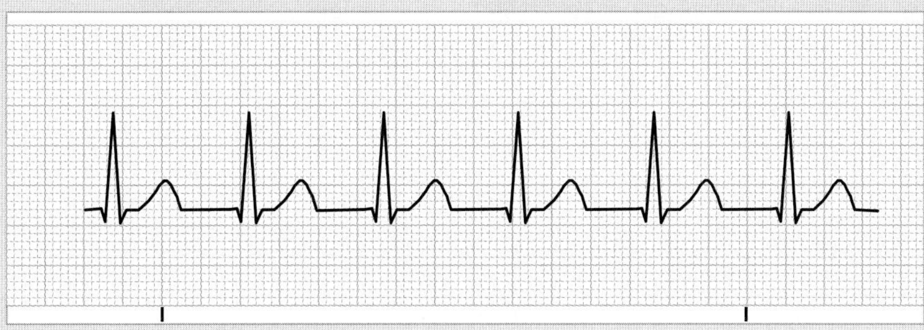

FIGURE 7A–14 Accelerated junctional rhythm.

Junctional Tachycardia

Rate	100–180 beats/min
Rhythm	Atrial and ventricular very regular
P waves	May occur before, during, or after the QRS; if seen, will be inverted (retrograde)
PR interval	Not measurable unless the P wave precedes the QRS; when present, will usually be ≤0.12 s
QRS	<0.10 s

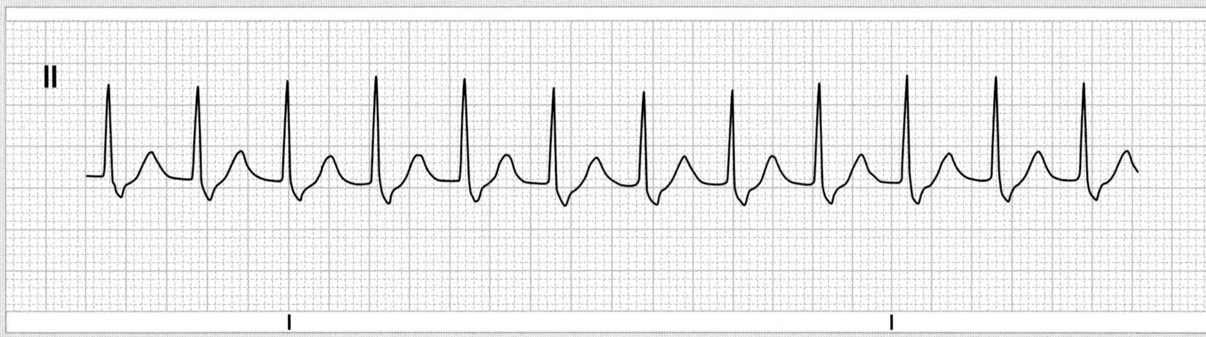

FIGURE 7A–15 Junctional tachycardia.

(continues)

Appendix 7–1 *(continued)*

Premature Ventricular Complexes (PVCs)

Rate	Atrial and ventricular rate depend on the underlying rhythm
Rhythm	Irregular because of PVC If the PVC is interpolated (sandwiched between two normal beats), the rhythm will be regular
P waves	No P wave is associated with the PVC
PR interval	None with the PVC because the ectopic originates in the ventricles
QRS	>0.12 s Wide and bizarre T wave frequently in opposite direction of the QRS complex

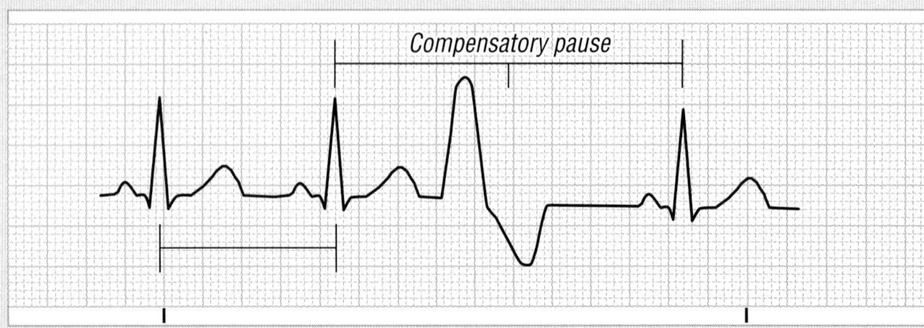

FIGURE 7A–16 Premature ventricular complexes.

Ventricular Escape Rhythm (Idioventricular Rhythm [IVR])

Rate	Atrial not discernible; ventricular 20–40 beats/min
Rhythm	Atrial not discernible; ventricular essentially regular
P waves	Absent
PR interval	None
QRS	>0.12 s

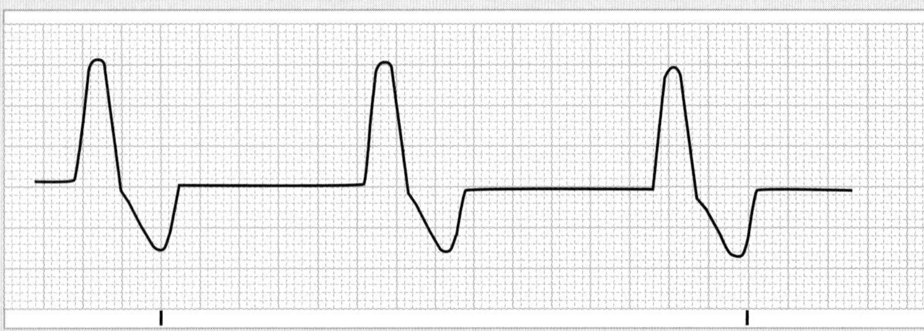

FIGURE 7A–17 Ventricular escape (idioventricular) rhythm.

Accelerated Idioventricular Rhythm (AIVR)

Rate	Atrial not discernible; ventricular 40–100 beats/min
Rhythm	Atrial not discernible; ventricular essentially regular
P waves	Absent
PR interval	None
QRS	>0.12 s

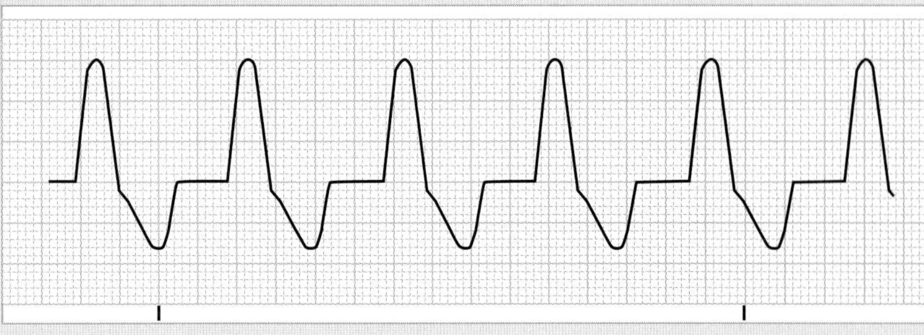

FIGURE 7A–18 Accelerated idioventricular rhythm.

Appendix 7–1 *(continued)*

Ventricular Tachycardia (Monomorphic VT)

Rate	Atrial not discernible; ventricular 100–250 beats/min
Rhythm	Atrial not discernible; ventricular essentially regular
P waves	May be present or absent; if present, they have no set relationship to the QRS complexes, appearing between the QRSs at a rate different from that of the VT
PR interval	None
QRS	>0.12 s Often difficult to differentiate between the QRS and the T wave

Note: Three or more PVCs occurring sequentially are referred to as a "run" of VT.

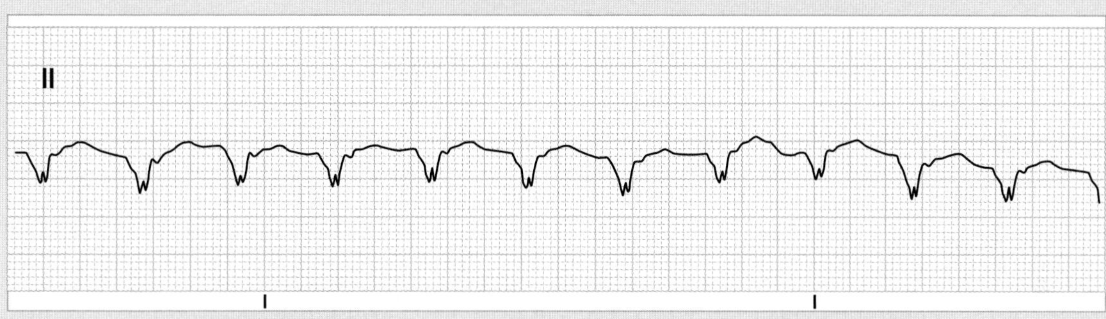

FIGURE 7A–19 Ventricular tachycardia.

Torsades de Pointes

Rate	Atrial not discernible; ventricular 150–250 beats/min
Rhythm	Atrial not discernible; ventricular may be regular or irregular
PR interval	None
QRS	>0.12 s Gradual alteration in the amplitude and direction of the QRS

Torsades de pointes (French for *twisting of the points*) is a type of polymorphic VT associated with a prolonged QT interval. Symptoms associated with torsades de pointes are related to the decrease in cardiac output, which occurs as a result of the fast ventricular rate. Patients may complain of palpitation or lightheadedness or experience seizures or a syncopal episode. Torsades de pointes is usually initiated by a premature ventricular contraction and may occasionally terminate spontaneously and recur after several seconds or minutes, or it may deteriorate into ventricular fibrillation.

The causes of long QT are many and include the following:

- Drug-induced
  - Cyclic antidepressants (doxepin, imipramine, amitriptyline)
  - Phenothiazines (haloperidol, chlorpromazine, thioridazine)
  - Type I antidysrhythmics (quinidine, procainamide, disopyramide, tocainide, mexiletine)
  - Organophosphate insecticides
- Eating disorders (bulimia, anorexia)
- Electrolyte abnormalities (hypomagnesemia, hypokalemia, hypocalcemia)

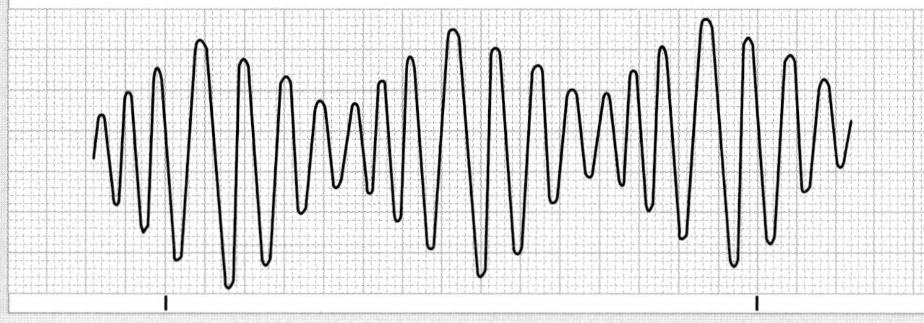

FIGURE 7A–20 Torsades de Pointes.

(continues)

Appendix 7–1 *(continued)*

Ventricular Fibrillation

Rate	Cannot be determined because waves or complexes are not discernible to measure
Rhythm	Rapid and chaotic with no pattern or regularity
P waves	Not discernible
PR interval	Not discernible
QRS	Not discernible

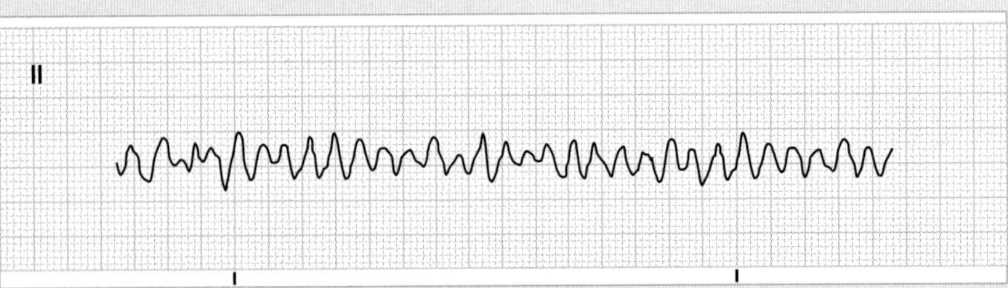

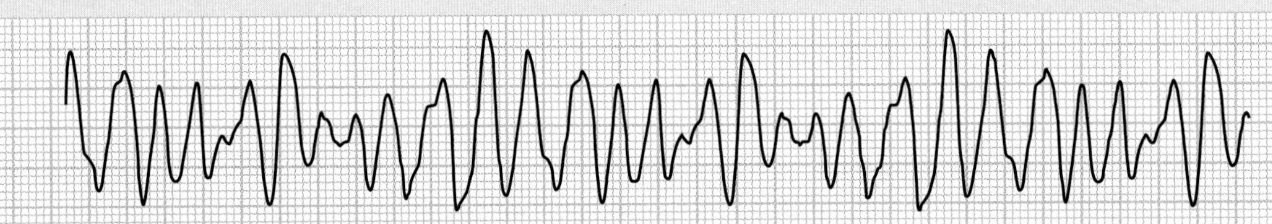

FIGURE 7A–21 Ventricular fibrillation.

Asystole (Ventricular Asystole, Ventricular Standstill)

Rate	Ventricular usually indiscernible, but may see some atrial activity
Rhythm	Atrial may be discernible; ventricular indiscernible
P waves	Usually not discernible
PR interval	Not measurable
QRS	Absent

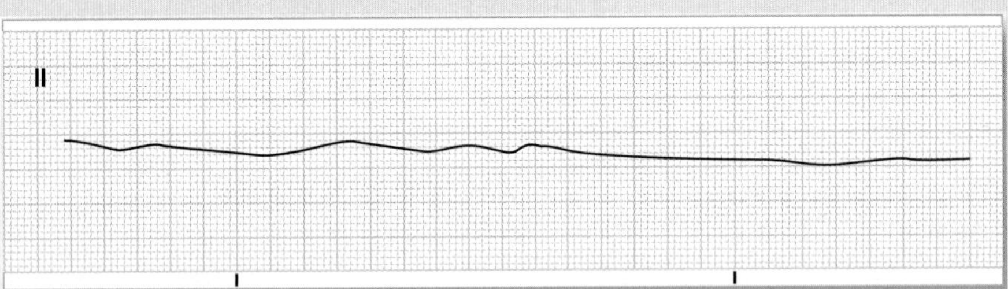

FIGURE 7A–22 Asystole.

Appendix 7–1 *(continued)*

First-Degree AV Block

Rate	Atrial and ventricular within normal limits and the same
Rhythm	Atrial and ventricular regular
P waves	Normal in size and configuration One P wave for each QRS
PR interval	Prolonged (>0.20 s) but constant
QRS	<0.10 s

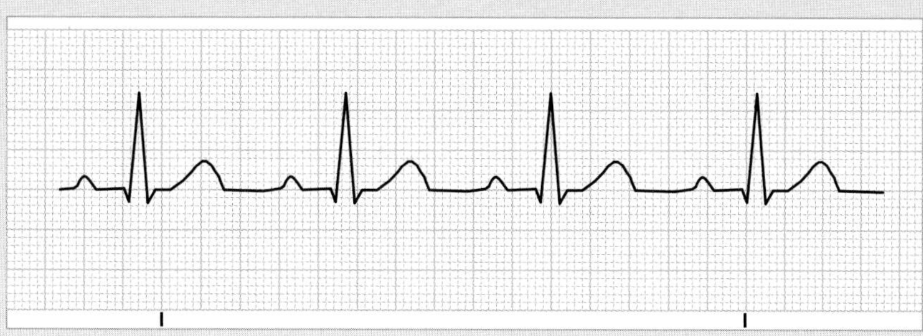

FIGURE 7A–23 Sinus rhythm with first-degree AV block.

Second-Degree AV Block, Type I (Wenckebach, Mobitz I)

Rate	Atrial rate > ventricular rate; both are usually within normal limits
Rhythm	Atrial regular (P waves plot through) Ventricular irregular
P waves	Normal in size and configuration Some P waves are not followed by a QRS (more P waves than QRS complexes)
PR interval	Lengthens with each cycle (although lengthening may be slight) until a P wave appears without a QRS
QRS	<0.10 s but is dropped periodically

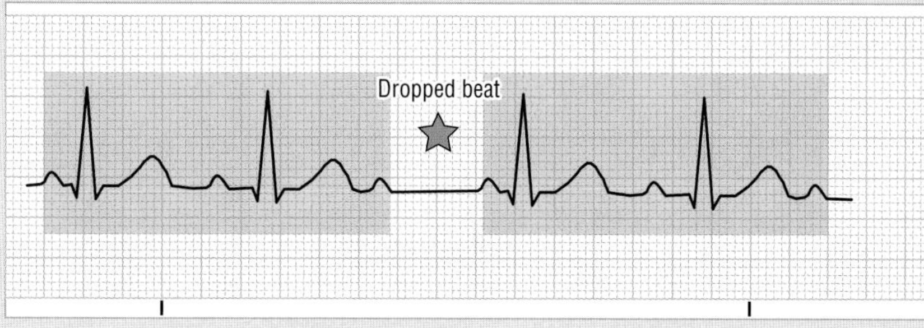

FIGURE 7A–24 Second-degree AV block, type I.

(continues)

Appendix 7–1 *(continued)*

Second-Degree AV Block, Type II (Mobitz II)

Rate	Atrial rate > ventricular rate
Rhythm	Atrial regular (P waves plot through) Ventricular irregular
P waves	Normal in size and configuration Some P waves are not followed by a QRS (more P waves than QRS complexes)
PR interval	May be within normal limits or prolonged but is constant for each conducted QRS
QRS	>0.10 s but is dropped periodically

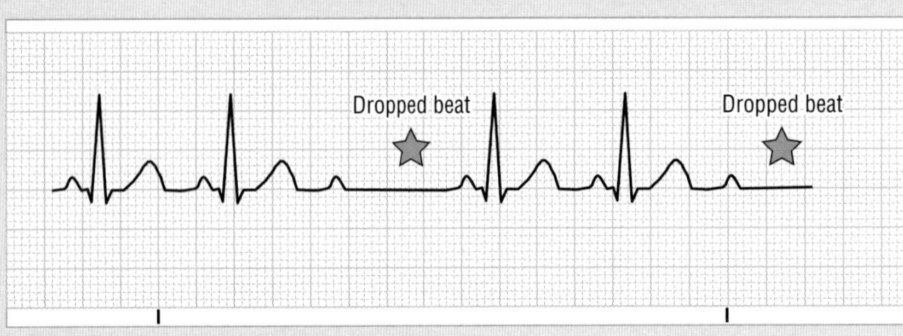

FIGURE 7A–25 Second-degree AV block, type II.

Second-Degree AV Block, 2:1 Conduction

Rate	Atrial rate > ventricular rate
Rhythm	Atrial regular (P waves plot through) Ventricular regular
P waves	Normal in size and configuration Every other P wave is followed by a QRS (more P waves than QRS complexes)
PR interval	Constant
QRS	Within normal limits if the block occurs above the bundle of His (probably type I) Wide if the block occurs at or below the bundle of His (probably type II) Absent after every other P wave

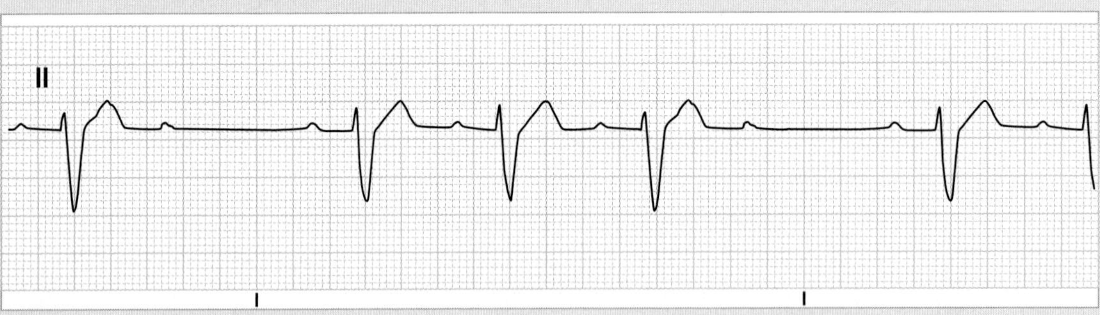

FIGURE 7A–26 Second-degree AV block, 2:1 conduction, probably type I.

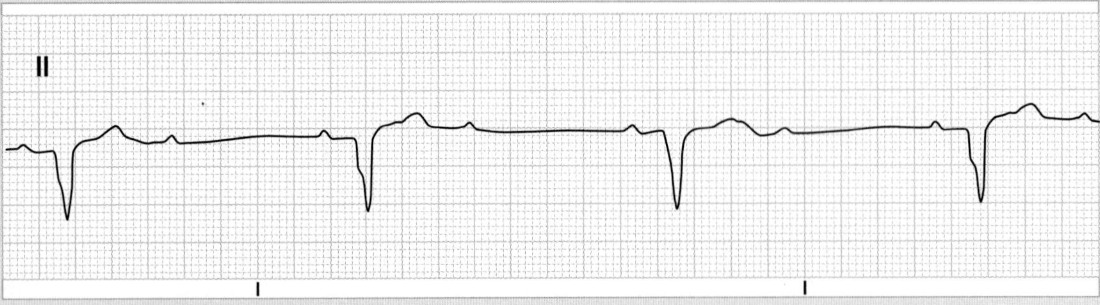

FIGURE 7A–27 Second-degree AV block, 2:1 conduction, probably type II.

Appendix 7–1 *(continued)*

Complete (Third-Degree) AV Block

Rate	Atrial rate > ventricular rate; ventricular rate determined by the origin of the escape rhythm
Rhythm	Atrial regular (P waves plot through) Ventricular regular
P waves	Normal in size and configuration Some P waves are not followed by a QRS (more P waves than QRS complexes)
PR interval	None—the atria and ventricles beat independently of each other; no relationship between the P waves and QRS complexes
QRS	Narrow or wide depending on the location of the escape pacemaker and the condition of the interventricular conduction system Narrow → junctional pacemaker Wide → ventricular pacemaker

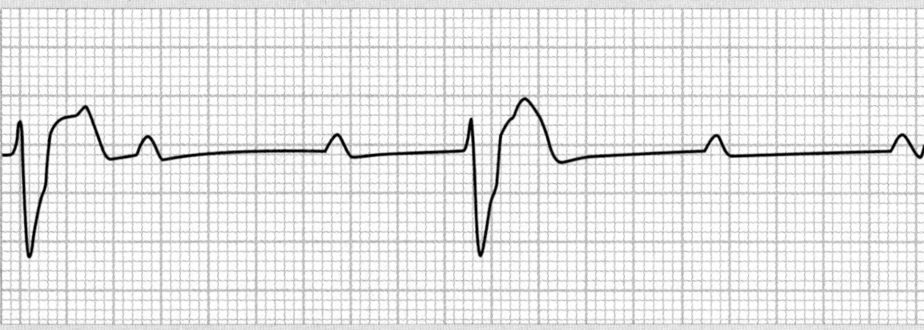

FIGURE 7A–28 Complete (third-degree) AV block.

Modified from Aehlert B. *ACLS Quick Review Study Guide.* St. Louis: Mosby; 1994.

CHAPTER 8

Blood Chemistries and Hematology

Rafat O. Mohammed
Rajesh Bhagat
Neil R. MacIntyre

OUTLINE

OBJECTIVES

1. Discuss the physiology of normal fluid and electrolyte balance.
2. List causes of abnormal electrolyte levels.
3. Discuss the effects of renal function on serum chemistry.
4. Discuss the role of serum enzymes in assessing liver and cardiac function.
5. Describe laboratory tests used to assess coagulation.
6. Discuss abnormalities of hemoglobin, platelets, and leukocytes.

KEY TERMS

activated partial thromboplastin time (aPTT)
anion gap
anions
bilirubinemia
blood urea nitrogen (BUN)
brain natriuretic peptide (BNP)
cardiac enzymes
cation
C-reactive protein (CRP)
creatinine
diabetic ketoacidosis
extracellular fluid
hematocrit
hemoglobin
hypercalcemia
hyperchloremia
hyperkalemia
hypermagnesemia
hypernatremia
hyperosmolar
hyperphosphatemia
hypocalcemia
hypochloremia
hypokalemia
hypomagnesemia
hyponatremia
hypophosphatemia
intracellular fluid
lactate
leukocytes
leukocytosis
leucopenia
oncotic pressure
platelets
procalcitonin
proteins
prothrombin time (PT)
troponin
serum electrolytes
unmeasured anions

INTRODUCTION

Circulating blood is composed of water, proteins, electrolytes, and cells. Fluid left after removing the cells from blood is the *plasma*. When both cells and coagulation proteins are removed from blood, the leftover fluid is the *serum*. The water component of blood moves across both tissue barriers and cell membranes, depending on hydrostatic and **oncotic pressures** (osmotic pressure exerted by colloids in a solution; for example, serum proteins in intravascular blood). On the other hand, protein and electrolyte movements into and from blood vessels often depend on complex tissue or cell membrane pumps. Blood cells generally remain within the blood vessels except under conditions of blood vessel injury or inflammation.

Measuring the chemical and cellular properties of blood can yield considerable information about disease states. These measurements are often expressions of concentrations of a substance. Some measurements, however, measure a functional property, such as coagulation activity or osmotic pressure. This chapter covers the common measurements performed on blood samples from patients. For each measurement the discussion includes a review of the physiologic (and pathophysiologic) importance of the blood substance or property, followed by a brief review of commonly used measurement techniques. Diagnoses that should be considered in the event of an abnormal value also are reviewed.

Serum Electrolytes

Body Water

In an average person, approximately 60% of total body weight is water. Two-thirds is in the intracellular compartment (i.e., within cells) and one-third is in the extracellular compartment (i.e., interstitium and blood, which make up 75% and 25%, respectively, of this compartment). The compartments are separated by cell membranes that set up active and passive forces regulating water, electrolyte, and solute movement, with resulting electrolyte concentration gradients and oncotic pressures. The most common **serum electrolytes** are the **cations** Na^+, K^+, Ca^{+2}, and Mg^{+2} and the **anions** HCO_3^-, PO_4^-, and SO_4^-.

> **RESPIRATORY RECAP**
>
> **Body Water**
>
> » Approximately 60% of total body weight is water.
>
> » Two-thirds of body water is in the intracellular space.
>
> » One-third of body water is in the extracellular space.

Extracellular fluid is characterized by higher amounts of Na^+, Cl^-, and HCO_3^-, whereas **intracellular fluid** has higher amounts of K^+, Mg^{+2}, PO_4^-, and SO_4^-. These cations and anions are regulated in the compartments over a narrow normal range. Mechanical, inflammatory, and other pathologic processes frequently affect the integrity of these compartments, with consequent movement of electrolytes, proteins, and water. A change in body or compartment level of one substance often sets off a sequence of compensatory events in the body to maintain fluid homeostasis.

Thus, initial assessment of the overall water volume status is critical in any evaluation of a patient's fluid and electrolyte status. No single test precisely quantifies total body water (TBW) easily in the clinical setting. Instead, clinicians rely on history taking and physical examination. The intent is to decide whether the patient is hypovolemic, euvolemic, or hypervolemic with respect to TBW (**Box 8–1**).

Sodium

The sodium cation (Na^+) is the most common electrolyte in extracellular fluid, and the normal serum values range from 135 to 145 mmol/L. Na^+ is important for a variety of cell membrane functions and in determinations of serum osmotic pressure. In the hypovolemic patient with normal total body Na^+ content, the relationship between Na^+ and TBW allows for calculation of the free water deficit, as follows:

$$\text{Free water deficit} = \text{TBW} \times \left(1 - \frac{140}{\text{Serum Na}^+}\right)$$

$$= 0.6 \times \text{Weight (kg)} \times \left(1 - \frac{140}{\text{Serum Na}^+}\right)$$

This formula is useful in calculations of the appropriate amount of free water to be administered in water-deficit states. The relationship between Na^+ and TBW also can be used to predict the change in serum Na^+ after administration of various intravenous fluids, as follows:

$$\text{Change in serum Na}^+ = \frac{(\text{Infusate Na}^+ + \text{Infusate K}^+) - \text{Serum Na}^+}{\text{TBW} + 1}$$

Both low-Na^+ (**hyponatremia**) and high-Na^+ (**hypernatremia**) conditions are evident in a number of disease states and produce important clinical manifestations.

The physiologic effects of Na^+ depend on its concentration in extracellular water. If the serum sample has significant amounts of substances that increase the

> **BOX 8–1**
>
> **Assessment Tools Used to Evaluate Total Body Water**
>
> Decreased total body water (hypovolemia) is associated with the following:
>
> - *Symptoms*: Thirst, decreased urine output, dizziness on standing up.
> - *Signs*: Thready rapid pulse, low blood pressure, orthostatic hypotension, low skin turgor, sunken eyes, depressed fontanelle in infants, dry coated tongue; also associated with muscle tremors, rigidity, and even seizures and rarely with hallucinations, delirium, and maniac behavior; development of tachypnea and respiratory arrest before death.
> - *Laboratory data*: Elevated hematocrit (if hypovolemia is not due to blood loss), sodium (hypernatremia), and protein levels. Urine is concentrated, and urine potassium loss (kaliuresis) is seen, associated with decreased serum potassium levels.
>
> Increased total body water (hypervolemia) is associated with the following:
>
> - *Symptoms*: Weight gain, loss of diurnal rhythm of diuresis, pedal edema, dyspnea.
> - *Signs*: Orthopnea, pedal edema, elevated jugular venous pressure, wheezing, ascites.
> - *Laboratory data*: Are not characteristic but may show serum hyponatremia (dilutional) and hypoproteinemia.

serum volume but not the water volume, the measured serum Na^+ will appear low even though its water concentration is normal (pseudohyponatremia). Substances that expand serum volume but not blood volume include the toxins methanol and ethylene glycol, as well as glucose, mannitol, proteins, and lipids. To assess this instance, osmolality can be measured directly and compared with an estimated value, as follows:

$$\text{Estimated osmolality} = 2Na^+ + \left(\frac{\text{BUN mg/dL}}{2.8}\right) + \left(\frac{\text{Glucose mg/dL}}{18}\right)$$

If the measured osmolality is within 20 of the estimated serum osmolality (that is, no osmolar gap), the Na^+ value reflects the true value and rules out the presence of unmeasured substances.

Decreased serum Na^+ levels are associated with water moving osmotically within cells and creating a significant shift in the relationship between intracellular and extracellular fluid compartments. This shift is associated with weakness, giddiness, lassitude, faintness, muscle cramps, anorexia, nausea, vomiting, confusion, delirium, stupor, and coma. On examination the skin turgor is low, blood pressure may be decreased, and orthostatic hypotension is usually present.

Because the relationship between Na^+ and fluid is so intertwined, a useful practice is to divide the causes of hyponatremia into hypovolemic, euvolemic, and hypervolemic categories, depending on the estimation of TBW by physical examination and the response of the kidney in moving Na^+ into the urine (**Box 8–2**).

Clinically increased Na^+ serum concentrations (hypernatremia) is of concern because it suggests dehydration. In contrast, increased total body sodium levels are seen in patients with hypervolemic hyponatremia; however, their serum sodium levels are diluted because of excess water. Hypernatremia is associated with an increased serum osmolality, and its clinical features are classically the same as those associated with water loss. **Box 8–3** lists the causes of hypernatremia.

Laboratory techniques used to estimate sodium concentration include flame atomic emission spectroscopy, ion selective electrode (ISE) potentiometry (direct and indirect), chromogenic ionophore technique, and enzymatic (or enzyme activation) methods. ISE (either direct or indirect) is the most commonly used method. The direct ISE method has the advantage that hyperproteinemic and hyperlipidemic states do not affect accuracy. A potential source of error is protein buildup on membrane surfaces of the measuring electrode.

Potassium

Approximately 90% of total body potassium (K^+) is intracellular. K^+ homeostasis is regulated by acid–base status, insulin, catecholamines, and aldosterone. Alkalosis and elevated insulin, catecholamine, and aldosterone levels lower serum K^+ through either renal excretion or intracellular potassium shifting. Acidosis and reduced insulin, catecholamine, and aldosterone levels raise serum potassium levels. K^+ is essential for maintenance of the electrical membrane potential; thus, changes in serum K^+ levels affect neuromuscular activity as well as cardiac electrical impulses. Normal serum range is from 3.5 to 5.5 mmol/L.

Serum K^+ levels below normal (**hypokalemia**; **Box 8–4**) affect neuromuscular function, causing muscular weakness, malaise, fatigue, and myalgias. Severe K^+ depletion has been associated with paralysis and rhabdomyolysis. Life-threatening cardiac arrhythmias with electrocardiogram (ECG) changes (U waves, QT prolongation, T wave changes) are commonly associated with severe hypokalemia. Paresthesias, abdominal cramps, and ileus also are

BOX 8–2

Classification of Hyponatremia

Hypovolemic Hyponatremia

- Total body sodium deficit higher than TBW deficit
  - *Renal loss (urine sodium >20 mmol/L)*
    - Diuresis: osmotic or diuretic excess
    - Mineralocorticoid deficiency
  - *Extrarenal loss (urine sodium <10 mmol/L)*
    - Vomiting
    - Diarrhea
    - Fluid movement into the third space*

Euvolemic Hyponatremia

- Increased TBW undetectable by clinical evaluation
- Syndrome of inappropriate ADH secretion: malignancy, drugs, CNS lesions
- Hypothyroidism
- Immediate postoperative period (first 24 hours)
- Glucocorticoid deficiency

Hypervolemic Hyponatremia

- Dilutional: TBW increase greater than total body sodium
- Congestive heart failure
- Nephrotic syndrome
- Cirrhosis
- Acute and chronic renal failure

*Extracellular space is sometimes grouped into three volumes. The first is plasma volume, the second is interstitial fluid volume, and the third refers to various actual or potential cavities, such as the pleural space, peritoneal space, and gut lumen.

TBW, total body water; ADH, antidiuretic hormone; CNS, central nervous system.

BOX 8–3

Causes of Hypernatremia

Water Loss More Than Sodium Loss

Osmotic and loop diuretics
Postobstructive nephropathy
Sweating
Diarrhea and fistulas

Pure Water Loss

Diabetes insipidus: central, peripheral, and combination
Excessive sweating: exercise, fever, and hot environment

Increase in Total Body Sodium

Primary hyperaldosteronism
Cushing syndrome
Hypertonic sodium bicarbonate administration in situations such as cardiac arrest

BOX 8–4

Causes of Hypokalemia

Increased loss of potassium
- *GI losses*: vomiting, especially with pyloric obstruction; villous adenoma of colon; diarrhea; non-β islet cell tumor of pancreas
- *Renal losses*: diuretics, such as thiazides and furosemide; renal tubular acidosis I and II; hyperaldosteronism; massive doses of penicillin G, ureteroenterostomy

Intracellular shift of potassium: insulin, testosterone, β_2 agonists, respiratory and metabolic alkalosis, hypokalemic periodic paralysis
Decreased intake: malnutrition, alcoholism, and anorexia nervosa
Miscellaneous: magnesium depletion, Bartter syndrome, Liddle syndrome, licorice abuse

common manifestations. Spuriously reduced potassium levels—pseudohypokalemia—may accompany markedly elevated white blood cell (WBC) counts, as in cases of leukemia. Prompt laboratory processing of the sample helps prevent such false-positive results. Hypokalemia may be associated with hypomagnesemia.

Serum K^+ levels above normal (**hyperkalemia**; **Box 8–5**) produce hyporeflexia and muscle weakness. Paralysis can occur in cases of severe hyperkalemia, but death due to cardiac arrhythmias usually takes place beforehand. On the ECG, peaked T waves, widened QRS, and eventually sine waves develop before the appearance of actual cardiac arrest. Falsely elevated K^+ levels may be seen when the blood sample is hemolyzed or the WBC or platelet count is unusually elevated. Elevated serum potassium levels are frequently encountered in patients with renal disease or failure.

Techniques used to estimate sodium and potassium levels include flame atomic emission spectroscopy, ISE (direct and indirect), chromogenic ionophore, and enzymatic (enzyme activation). ISE is the most frequently used technique.

Chloride

Chloride (Cl^-) is the most common anion in the extracellular space. Usually, changes in serum Cl^- follow changes in serum sodium levels. Exceptions are hyperchloremic (elevated serum Cl^-) acidoses and chloride-responsive, hypochloremic (reduced serum Cl^-) alkaloses. Although **hypochloremia** in experimental situations is associated with vasoconstriction and increased reactivity to norepinephrine (especially in cerebral vessels), clinically important isolated chloride changes are almost never seen. Normal Cl^- levels are 98 to 107 mmol/L in the serum and 110 to 250 mmol/L in the urine. Estimation of Cl^- is affected by other halides. Erroneously high values (**hyperchloremia**) may be found with bromide present

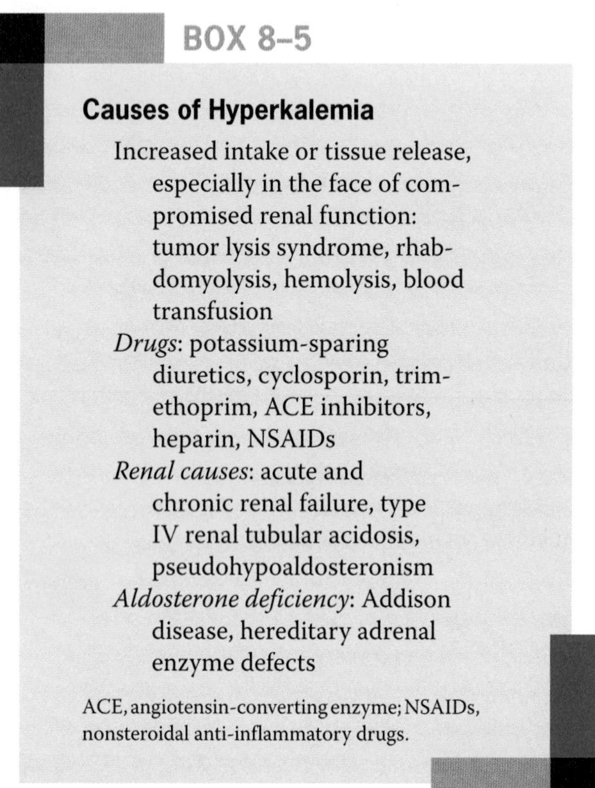

BOX 8–5

Causes of Hyperkalemia

Increased intake or tissue release, especially in the face of compromised renal function: tumor lysis syndrome, rhabdomyolysis, hemolysis, blood transfusion

Drugs: potassium-sparing diuretics, cyclosporin, trimethoprim, ACE inhibitors, heparin, NSAIDs

Renal causes: acute and chronic renal failure, type IV renal tubular acidosis, pseudohypoaldosteronism

Aldosterone deficiency: Addison disease, hereditary adrenal enzyme defects

ACE, angiotensin-converting enzyme; NSAIDs, nonsteroidal anti-inflammatory drugs.

in the sample. Four laboratory methods are used to estimate Cl^- levels: colorimetric method (mercuric/ferric thiocyanate), coulometric titration, ISE, and enzymatic method. ISE methods are the most commonly used.

Total Serum Carbon Dioxide

Serum contains carbon dioxide in the form of dissolved carbon dioxide (CO_2), carbon dioxide loosely bound to the amine group of plasma proteins, bicarbonate anion (HCO_3^-), carbonate anion (CO_3^{-2}), and carbonic acid. It acts as one of the major buffering systems to control the acid–base milieu of the body. The normal range is 22 to 32 mmol/L. The Henderson-Hasselbalch equation describes the relationship of dissolved CO_2, pH, and HCO_3^-.

Methods used to estimate total serum CO_2 include gas release, pH indicator, carbon dioxide electrodes, enzymatic methods, and calculation from the acid–base estimation. Commonly used methods include the ISE or colorimetric method. Accuracy requires anaerobic handling of the sample. Most autoanalyzers permit immediate analysis of the sample. However, if the sample is left uncapped, the total CO_2 levels can decrease by 6 mmol/L per hour.

RESPIRATORY RECAP

Serum Electrolytes

- » Sodium
- » Potassium
- » Chloride
- » Total carbon dioxide
- » Unmeasured anions
- » Calcium
- » Magnesium
- » Phosphorus
- » Lactate

BOX 8–6

Unmeasured Anions

Lactate (liver disease, tissue hypoxia)
Ketones (diabetic and alcoholic ketoacidosis)
Salicylates (toxic ingestion)
PO_4^- and SO_4^-
Uremic acidosis
Formate and lactate
Glycolate and oxalate
Ethylene glycol
Free fatty acids
Methyl malonate

Unmeasured Anions

Anionic proteins and other substances (**Box 8–6**) also can exist in serum. Generally these are not measured in routine serum electrolyte determinations. However, their presence can be suspected by calculation of the **anion gap**, as follows:

$$\text{Anion gap} = ([Na^+] + [K^+]) - ([CO_2] + [Cl^-])$$

If the anion gap exceeds 12 mmol/L, excessive **unmeasured anions** are likely present. Because its concentration is normally low, $[K^+]$ often is omitted from this calculation.

Calcium

Calcium (Ca^{+2}) performs multiple functions in the body. Besides being a major structural substance in bone, it plays an important role in maintaining cellular conduction in the neuromuscular system. Ca^{+2} is also an important participant or catalyst in several metabolic cascades (e.g., the coagulation pathways). Ca^{+2} is mainly absorbed in the bowel and excreted in the urine. Bones serve as a major calcium reservoir. The important Ca^{+2} regulators levels are vitamin D, calcitonin, phosphate, and parathyroid hormone. In general, vitamin D and parathyroid hormone increase Ca^{+2} levels, whereas calcitonin and phosphate reduce them.

In serum, most Ca^{+2} is bound to albumin. Measured Ca^{+2} levels are thus sensitive to all the factors regulating or affecting serum protein levels (especially albumin). Because unbound (i.e., ionized) calcium is what is metabolically important, measured total serum Ca^{+2} should be corrected for albumin concentration (i.e., a reduction in Ca^{+2} level of 0.8 mg/dL for every gram per deciliter of albumin below normal). Ionized calcium also can be measured directly. In adults, normal total serum Ca^{+2} levels are 8.6 to 10.0 mg/dL (2.15 to 2.50 mmol/L). Normal ionized Ca^{+2} levels are 4.6 to 5.3 mg/dL (1.16 to 1.32 mmol/L).

BOX 8–7

Causes of Hypercalcemia

Abnormal Protein Syndromes
Multiple myeloma and paraproteinemias

Increased Parathyroid Hormone or Related Peptides
Malignancy of lung or kidney

Increased Absorption
Usually vitamin D related (milk alkali syndrome), granulomatous diseases (such as tuberculosis and sarcoidosis), lymphoma

Excessive Renal Phosphate Excretion
Familial syndrome, sarcoidosis

Abnormal Bone Resorption or Formation
Prolonged bed rest, Paget disease

Miscellaneous
Bone metastases, especially from breast and prostate cancers, drugs such as thiazides (rarely)

A low ionized calcium level (**hypocalcemia**) is usually due to either decreased absorption or decreased mobilization of calcium from the bones. Causes include malnutrition, parathyroid hormone activity, vitamin D abnormalities, certain drugs, and renal dysfunction (which produces hyperphosphatemia). Pancreatitis, massive blood transfusions, and tumor lysis syndrome can precipitate Ca^{+2} and thus reduce serum levels. Low Ca^{+2} levels frequently coexist with low magnesium levels, especially in malnourished alcoholics. Alkalosis can disrupt calcium ion balance and cause the symptoms of hypocalcaemia. Clinical features of hypocalcemia consist of perioral numbness and tingling progressing to tetany. Physical examination evidence of protein-energy malnutrition, previous parathyroidectomy, pancreatitis, and tumor lysis syndrome should increase the suspicion for reduced Ca^{+2} levels.

Increases in Ca^{+2} levels (**hypercalcemia**) are caused by multiple factors (**Box 8–7**). The clinical features of hypercalcemia include anorexia, vomiting, polyuria, mental confusion, obtundation, and death. The ECG may show a shortened QT interval.

Laboratory tests used to measure serum Ca^{+2} include atomic absorption, cresolphthalein complex formation, arsenazo III dye, and ISE methods to estimate ionic calcium levels. Autoanalyzers frequently use ISE methods. Atomic absorption remains the gold standard, although it is not frequently used for clinical work.

Magnesium

Magnesium (Mg^{+2}) is the other major cation in the serum (besides Ca^{+2}) that helps maintain membrane potentials at the cellular level. Mg^{+2} also is important in maintaining potassium homeostasis through regulation of cell membrane potassium channels. Only 1% to 2% of total body Mg^{+2} is present in the serum, and one-third of this amount is bound to proteins. Mg^{+2} is mainly absorbed in the small bowel (mostly in the initial parts) and is excreted by the kidneys. In adults the normal serum Mg^{+2} range is 1.8 to 3.0 mg/mL (0.7 to 1.1 mmol/L).

Box 8–8 lists causes of low Mg^{+2} levels (**hypomagnesemia**). Low levels often are associated with hypokalemia. Indeed, concurrent hypomagnesemia and hypokalemia makes it difficult to correct the potassium levels until the Mg^{+2} levels are corrected. Hypomagnesemia also is associated with hyponatremia, hypocalcemia, and hypophosphatemia. Low Mg^{+2} levels result in tremulousness, hyperreflexia, ataxia, convulsions, and death in extreme cases.

Hypomagnesemia-induced cardiac dysrhythmias originating in the atria or the ventricles can be fatal. In patients with rapid polymorphic ventricular tachycardia (torsades de pointes), intravenous magnesium infusion can be life saving. Hypertension in hypomagnesemic patients can be difficult to control. Hypomagnesemic dysmotility in gastrointestinal muscles is clinically manifested as dysphagia.

High Mg^{+2} levels (**hypermagnesemia**) are uncommon but can be seen in patients suffering from renal failure, especially those undergoing inappropriate dialysis or alimentation regimens. Another cause of hypermagnesemia is abuse of magnesium-based laxatives. In addition, hypermagnesemia is sometimes induced to treat eclampsia. The condition's clinical manifestations include hyporeflexia, muscle weakness, hypotension, bradycardia, coma, and death.

BOX 8–8

Causes of Hypomagnesemia

Absorption Problems

Malnutrition per se or due to alcoholism, diarrhea, intravenous alimentation, intestinal bypass surgery

Psychological problems: bulimia, laxative abuse, or aggressive weight reduction

Others: short bowel syndrome or malignancies, especially in the bowel

Excessive Loss in Urine

Use and abuse of diuretics, postobstructive diuresis, acute tubular necrosis, hypercalcemia, and hereditary renal magnesium wasting

Miscellaneous

Association with hyperaldosteronism, diabetic ketoacidosis, and excessive lactation

Exchange transfusions

Acute intermittent porphyria

Laboratory methods used to estimate serum levels of Mg^{+2} include colorimetric methods using calmagite, methyl thymol, or chlorophosphonazo III; ISE methods; and atomic absorption, the latter of which remains the gold standard. However, ISE methods are increasingly being used to estimate serum Mg^{+2} levels.

Phosphorus

More than 80% of total body phosphorus is found in bones. Phosphate ion (PO_4^-) is a major intracellular anion participating primarily as a cofactor in intracellular metabolic processes. Extracellular phosphate salts function as buffers and play a role in calcium homeostasis. (That is, serum PO_4^- and Ca^{+2} exist in a reciprocal, balanced relationship.) PO_4^- is absorbed through the gastrointestinal tract (vitamin D dependent) and excreted through the kidneys (enhanced by parathyroid hormone). In adults, normal serum PO_4^- levels range between 2.7 and 4.5 mg/dL (0.87 to 1.45 mmol/L).

Low PO_4^- (**hypophosphatemia**) levels are primarily caused by decreased absorption, intracellular shifts, or increased excretion (**Box 8–9**). Severe stress causing glucagon and cortisol release may be responsible for the low serum PO_4^- levels seen in trauma patients. Clinical features of hypophosphatemia include decreased contractility of muscles, causing cardiomyopathy, hyporeflexia, and hypoventilation. If severe, this condition can lead to rhabdomyolysis. Hypophosphatemia also can produce confusion, seizures, and coma. Chronic deficiency can cause osteomalacia.

High PO_4^- levels (**hyperphosphatemia**) are unusual but can be seen in individuals with chronic renal failure, in which the hyperphosphatemia is often overshadowed by other metabolic and electrolyte abnormalities. Other conditions producing hyperphosphatemia include hypoparathyroidism (with low calcium levels also being seen), pseudohypoparathyroidism, and Paget disease of the juvenile, which is characterized by muscle weakness and high alkaline phosphatase levels.

BOX 8–9

Causes of Hypophosphatemia

Decreased Absorption

Malnutrition, alcohol abuse, vitamin D deficiency, laxative abuse, and antacid abuse

Intracellular Shift

High-energy states and parenteral nutrition with carbohydrate overload

Increased Excretion

Hyperparathyroidism, diuretics, hyperglycemia, and alcohol abuse

To estimate serum PO_4^- levels, ammonium phosphomolybdate complex levels are read directly by an ultraviolet monitor, or the complex is reduced to molybdenum and its levels estimated.

Lactate

An increase in **lactate** is caused by either increased production as a result of anaerobic metabolism or reduced degradation of lactate as a result of problems in the liver. Lactate is most commonly formed in ischemic cells as a consequence of anaerobic glycolysis and the use of pyruvate for generation of adenosine triphosphate (ATP). Thus, it is frequently used to indicate the severity of shock and provides a rough idea of tissue perfusion, oxygen delivery, and oxygen use. For individuals in shock, increased lactate is associated with increased mortality.

Increased lactate also is seen in patients with bowel ischemia. An elevated serum lactate level is an important cause of anion gap metabolic acidosis. Lactate has both D and L isomers. Humans normally produce L-lactic acidosis, which most laboratories easily estimate. Theoretically, D-lactate (normally produced by ruminants and bacteria) can be elevated in certain types of individuals (e.g., those with bowel abnormalities). Currently D-lactic acidosis is a research curiosity, with rare cases involving humans. Normal values for lactate in adults are less than 2 mmol/L.

Methods used to estimate lactate levels include chemical oxidation, enzyme reactions, and enzyme electrodes. Other methods use gas chromatography and photometry. Thus, enzyme electrodes have made estimation of serum lactate levels much simpler. Because lactate is unstable, samples should be processed immediately. Lactate increases by 0.4 mmol/L in whole blood kept at room temperature for 30 minutes (0.1 mmol/L on ice).

Serum Chemistries Associated with Renal Function

Good urine production (quantitative as well as qualitative) is a marker of end organ perfusion as well as renal function. The most important tests are the quantity of urine produced and the characteristics of that urine (i.e., pH, specific gravity, microscopic analysis, and culture). However, two other measurements are frequently used to assess renal function: the serum blood urea nitrogen (BUN) and creatinine levels.

Blood Urea Nitrogen

Serum **blood urea nitrogen (BUN)** levels indicate the body's ability to clear nitrogenous wastes in the form of urea in the urine. Urea (along with ammonia) is a breakdown product of amino acids. Thus, it can be increased by increases in gastrointestinal protein absorption from either dietary factors or heme in the bowels (i.e., gastrointestinal bleeding). Similarly, urea levels can be decreased with decreases in protein intake or liver impairment. Urea is readily filtered in the glomeruli, but approximately half of it is reabsorbed. It also is broken down into ammonia in the bowel. Levels of BUN thus reflect protein intake and metabolism, as well as glomerular and proximal tubule function in the kidney. In the adult, normal BUN values are between 7 and 21 mg/dL.

BUN is estimated from serum urea levels. Almost all the tests used—calorimetric methods, indicator dye, and ISE methods—directly or indirectly estimate the amount of ammonia present in the sample.

Creatinine

Serum **creatinine** levels are a function of skeletal muscle breakdown. Thus, the levels are directly related to the muscle mass of a person. Most creatinine is filtered in the glomeruli, with very little reabsorption. A small amount also is secreted by the tubules into the urine. Thus, if the individual's muscle mass is relatively stable, serum creatinine level is a good indicator of glomerular filtration and, hence, renal function. Increased creatinine levels, however, also can occur in conjunction with increased muscle breakdown (e.g., corticosteroids, rhabdomyolysis) or with decreased tubular excretion, such as that seen with use of trimethoprim. Decreased creatinine levels reflect decreased muscle mass, such as those in states of malnutrition or muscle atrophy. In the adult, normal values for creatinine are 0.7 to 1.4 mg/dL.

> **RESPIRATORY RECAP**
>
> **Laboratory Tests Associated with Renal Function**
>
> » Urine analysis
> » Blood urea nitrogen
> » Creatinine

Serum creatinine level is a relatively insensitive monitor of renal function and may not increase until more than 50% of renal function has deteriorated. With complete renal shutdown, creatinine levels rise approximately 1 mg/dL per day. Creatinine levels also can be used to describe creatinine clearance (the amount of blood per minute cleared of creatinine by the kidney), a more precise measurement of renal function, as follows:

$$\text{Creatinine clearance} = \frac{\text{Urine creatinine concentration} \times \text{24-hour urine volume}}{\text{Plasma creatinine concentration}}$$

A simpler method used to estimate creatinine clearance is as follows:

$$\text{Creatinine clearance} = (140 - \text{Age}) \times \frac{\text{Weight (kg)}}{72} \times \text{Serum creatinine}$$

Normal creatinine clearance is 97 to 137 mL/min (for men) and 88 to 128 mL/min (for women). Creatinine clearance decreases 6.5 mL/min per decade after 40 years of age.

Estimation of creatinine is done by spectrophotometric analysis of the Jaffe reaction, enzymatic hydrolysis of creatinine, and cation-exchange high-performance liquid chromatography.

Serum Enzyme Activity

Enzymes are chemical substances that facilitate chemical reactions. Most enzymatic reactions occur intracellularly. Nevertheless, a number of these enzymes appear in serum under physiologic conditions. In pathologic conditions, many enzymes appear in serum in increased concentrations because of either cell injury or metabolic abnormalities within the cell.

A number of serum enzymes reflect liver function but also may reflect dysfunction elsewhere. Alanine aminotransferase (ALT) is present in liver cells, and an increased serum level indicates liver cell injury. Aspartate aminotransferase (AST) is present in liver cells but

TABLE 8–1 Lactate Dehydrogenase Abnormalities

LDH Type	Normal (U/L)	Source	Significance of Elevations
HHHH	14–26	Cardiac, RBC, kidney	Myocardial infarct, renal infarct, hemolytic anemia, megaloblastic anemia
HHHM	29–39	Cardiac, RBC, kidney	Myocadial infarct, renal infarct, hemolytic anemia, megaloblastic anemia
HHMM	20–26	Lung, lymphocytes, pancreas, spleen, platelets	Pulmonary emboli, pneumonia, cancer
HMMM	8–16	Liver	Hepatic injury
MMMM	6–16	Skeletal muscle	Skeletal muscle injury

LDH, lactate dehydrogenase; RBC, red blood cell.

also is present in cardiac, skeletal, kidney, and brain tissue. Serum alkaline phosphatase (ALP) comes from either liver or bone. Elevation of liver ALP indicates intrahepatic or collecting system bile drainage abnormalities (cholestasis). Elevated γ-glutamyltransferase (GGT) serum levels also indicate cholestasis. An AST:ALT ratio greater than 2 suggests alcoholic liver injury.

Lactic dehydrogenase (LDH) enzymes are a family of enzymes in which elevations can reflect liver, bone, cardiac, red blood cell, or pancreatic abnormalities. LDH assays can be fractionated (isoenzymes) to indicate the organ involved (**Table 8–1**).

Amylase and lipase are two enzymes that appear elevated as a consequence of pancreatic injury. Both may be elevated in individuals with other gastrointestinal abnormalities as well. Pancreatic disease caused by biliary tract disease usually has accompanying liver-associated abnormalities in the serum.

Cardiac Enzymes and Proteins

Cardiac Enzymes

The term **cardiac enzymes** refers to a group of enzymes that are released from myocardial tissue and appear in the serum as a result of myocardial injury (usually ischemia). As the understanding of cardiac ischemia has changed, so has the use of various enzymes to estimate cardiac muscle damage. Nevertheless, cardiac enzyme abnormalities remain a standard used to diagnose cardiac ischemia, in conjunction with history and ECG changes. The initial panel of cardiac enzymes included serum lactate dehydrogenase (LDH), serum glutamic-oxaloacetic transaminase (SGOT), and creatine kinase (CK). The myocardial-specific creatine kinase MB isoform (CK-MB) was used for diagnosing myocardial injury, but recently serum troponin levels have become the standard of care. CK-MB levels begin rising within 4 to 8 hours of myocardial injury, with peak activity by 24 hours. CK-MB levels return to baseline within 2 to 3 days.

RESPIRATORY RECAP

Cardiac Injury Markers

- » Cardiac enzymes (CK-MB)
- » Troponins T and I
- » Brain natriuretic peptide

Troponins

Serum **troponins** are cardiac regulatory proteins that are involved in the calcium-mediated interaction of actin and myosin in the cardiac muscle. Many centers are now measuring cardiac troponin I or T isoform for diagnosing myocardial injury. Cardiac troponins begin to rise 2 to 3 hours following an acute myocardial injury, peak by about 14 to 20 hours, and return to baseline within 5 to 10 days. Unfortunately, nonuniformity in the measurement of troponins has made the comparison of values from various laboratories difficult. CK, CK-MB, troponin I, and troponin T are estimated by different methods. Rapid assays of these enzymes are very helpful in the quick triaging of patients with suspected acute coronary syndrome. In renal failure and rhabdomyolysis, reduced clearance from the serum or increased production, or both, makes interpretation of the increased serum levels of these proteins difficult. In the future other proteins and enzymes, such as fatty acid-binding protein (FABP) and glycogen phosphorylase isoenzyme (BB), may also prove useful for diagnosing myocardial injury.

Methods used to estimate CK include electrophoresis, ion exchange chromatography, immunoinhibitors, and mass assay (specific for CK-MB). Normal total serum CK is 15 to 130 U/L, and CK-MB is less than 6% of total CK. Potential sources of error are hemolysis, exposure of sample to daylight, and the muscle mass of the patient (either too large or too small). For troponin estimation, enzyme-linked immunosorbent assay (ELISA), immunoenzyme techniques, and rapid immunochromatographic assays are available. The normal range is less than 0.1 ng/mL to 3.1 ng/mL.

Brain Natriuretic Peptide

Brain natriuretic peptide (BNP), also know as B-type natriuretic peptide, is a natriuretic hormone similar to atrial natriuretic peptide (ANP). BNP's physiologic actions include an increase in natriuresis (discharge of sodium through urine) and decrease in systemic vascular resistance and central venous pressure. These actions lead to a decrease in cardiac output and in blood volume. In humans the cardiac ventricles are the major source of BNP.

The N-terminal part of the propeptide of BNP (NT-ProBNP) is an active metabolite of BNP. BNP has a shorter half-life than NT-ProBNP (15–20 min versus 90 min, respectively). Thus, BNP may more closely relate to rapid neurohormonal and hemodynamic changes after acute coronary syndrome. However, elevated NT-ProBNP has a higher circulating concentration, is more stable, and has less biological variability. Nevertheless, elevated serum BNP and NT-ProBNP levels both help to differentiate dyspnea due to heart failure from pulmonary disease. They are elevated in both systolic and diastolic heart failure.

BNP is also useful to guide therapy in and prognostication of heart failure, acute coronary syndrome, and stable angina. BNP levels tend to be higher in people with renal failure and in older people, and lower in obese people and in women. Elevated BNP levels in medical intensive care patients are seen in mild heart failure, values of 600 to 900 pg/mL are seen in moderate heart failure, and values greater than 900 pg/mL are seen in severe heart failure. Recombinant BNP (Nesiritide) is also used for the treatment of acute decompensated congestive heart failure.

BNP and NT-ProBNP are measured by ELISA and chemiluminescent immunometric assay, respectively. Kits are commercially available.

Miscellaneous Serum Chemistries

C-Reactive Protein

C-reactive protein (CRP) was first recognized by its ability to precipitate in the presence of the somatic C polysaccharide of *Pneumococcus*. CRP is a nonspecific marker of acute inflammation produced by the liver and adipocytes. CRP levels are elevated in infections and several long-term diseases, including cancer; rheumatologic diseases such as lupus, rheumatoid arthritis, and giant cell arteritis; inflammatory bowel disease; and osteomyelitis. Recent data suggest that elevation of CRP from baseline within the normal range as well as CRP levels above normal are predictive of risk for myocardial infarction, stroke, peripheral vascular disease, and sudden cardiac death. The availability of high-sensitivity CRP (hs-CRP) measurement techniques has helped to reduce variation and provide reproducible CRP measurements.

CRP values for early risk stratification should be checked in conjunction with serum troponins as soon as possible after a patient presents with acute coronary syndrome to limit the influence of the extent of necrosis. For assessment of long-term risk, CRP values should be assessed at least 4 to 6 weeks after a myocardial infarction to allow for resolution of the acute phase reaction. Several different ELISA-based assays are available for measuring CRP. All have their own reproducibility as well as characteristics. Ultrasensitive microchip-based systems to measure CRP in other body fluids are currently under investigation.

Bilirubin

Bilirubin is a breakdown product of hemoglobin that is metabolized in the liver. Total serum bilirubin concentration is less than 1.1 mg/dL. Approximately 80% of serum bilirubin is indirect or unconjugated. Elevation of indirect bilirubin levels suggests prehepatic **bilirubinemia** caused by increased bilirubin production (e.g., hemolysis) or decreased liver uptake, as seen in Gilbert syndrome. Parenchymal liver injury and bile collecting system abnormalities (i.e., posthepatic lesions) cause bile stasis (cholestasis) and lead to an increase of conjugated bilirubin levels.

Proteins

Serum **proteins** include albumin, globulins, and immunoglobulins. Serum albumin is exclusively synthesized in the liver. Its half-life is approximately 3 weeks, and it can be used as a marker of liver synthetic function. Serum albumin also is a useful marker of nutritional status. Ferritin is an iron-binding protein that also is taken as an index of nutritional status. Serum globulins are mediators of the humoral immune system. Elevations can be seen in individuals with tumors secreting these globulins (e.g., multiple myeloma) and other paraproteinemias. Low values are seen in individuals with various congenital immune deficiency states.

Glucose

Glucose metabolism is heavily influenced by a number of nutritional, liver, hormonal, and pancreatic factors. Glucagon and adrenal steroids increase glucose concentrations by promoting liver breakdown of stored glycogen. Insulin is produced by islet cells in the pancreas and is critical for the transfer of glucose into cells. Pancreatic injury or islet cell dysfunction (type 1 diabetes) impairs insulin production and results in serum hyperglycemia. If severe, this condition can produce **diabetic ketoacidosis**. Severe hyperglycemia also can cause a **hyperosmolar** state with coma. In addition, type 2 diabetes (cellular resistance to insulin) can produce hyperglycemia and deranged glucose metabolism. Insulin-secreting tumors or exogenous insulin overdoses produce hypoglycemia. Severe liver injury also can produce hypoglycemia because of a depletion or failure to metabolize liver glycogen; if severe, hypoglycemia can bring about coma and death.

Procalcitonin

Ongoing studies suggest that serum **procalcitonin** levels might be a more useful marker for distinguishing bacterial infections from aseptic inflammation than erythrocyte sedimentation rate (ESR) or CRP. Procalcitonin is a precursor protein of the hormone calcitonin and is produced in C cells of the thyroid gland. Procalcitonin is believed to be released during infections by microbial toxins or indirectly by humoral factors or the cell-mediated host response. This induction is not as significant in viral or other inflammatory conditions. Thus, serum procalcitonin levels help to distinguish inflammation caused secondary to bacterial or fungal infection from viral or other aseptic inflammatory conditions.

Early data suggest that serum procalcitonin levels may be used to guide the need as well as duration of antibiotic therapy. This has the potential to safely reduce the number of antibiotic prescriptions and the duration of antibiotic use in patients. Various studies have reported varying sensitivity and specificity for procalcitonin in diagnosing bacteremia. A meta-analysis reported a sensitivity of 76% and a specificity of 76%. Rapid semiquantitative strip-based and quantitative luminometric immunoassays are being developed to measure serum procalcitonin levels. Soluble triggering receptors expressed on myeloids cells–1 (sTREM-1) also are under investigation as a marker of infections.

Coagulation Tests

The coagulation system (**Figure 8–1**) can be assessed in a number of ways. A simple and direct way to evaluate overall coagulation status is the bedside bleeding time. However, this method is time consuming and difficult to standardize. More commonly used techniques are measurements of the prothrombin time, activated partial thromboplastin time, and platelet count.

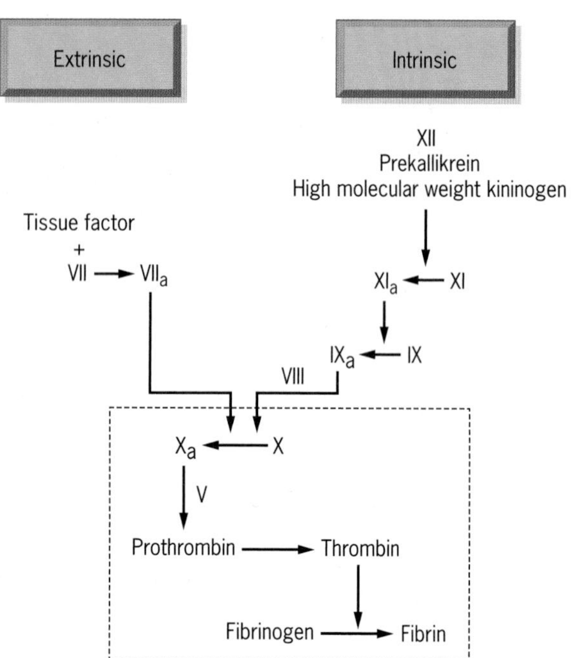

FIGURE 8–1 A simplified version of the role of various clotting factors in the coagulation cascade. This article was published in *Cecil Textbook of Medicine*. 21st ed. Goldman L, Bennett JC. Copyright Elsevier (WB Saunders) 2001.

> **RESPIRATORY RECAP**
>
> **Coagulation Studies**
>
> » Prothrombin time (PT)
>
> » Activated partial thromboplastin time (aPTT)
>
> » Thrombin time

Prothrombin Time

The **prothrombin time (PT)** is used to evaluate the extrinsic pathway, which involves tissue factor, factor VII, and coagulation factors in the common pathway (prothrombin, V, X, and fibrinogen) (refer to Figure 8–1). It often is used to monitor adequate anticoagulation in patients on Coumadin, which acts on these factors. The result is usually expressed as either a time or ratio of the values with respect to normal pooled sera. To standardize PT monitoring for oral anticoagulation therapy, PT is expressed as an international normalized ratio (INR). The goals of Coumadin therapy are to increase the INR to 2–3. However, in specific conditions, such as mechanical prosthetic heart valves, this ratio must be increased further.

PT can be prolonged in vitamin K deficiency; liver disease; deficiency or inhibition of factors VII, X, II, V, or fibrinogen; and in the presence of antiphospholipid antibodies and sometime heparin treatment, especially after bolus administration of heparin. In the presence of severe, acute liver injury, the PT may rapidly (i.e., within 24 hours) become abnormal. Vitamin K absorption also is impaired in the presence of hepatocellular disease and cholestasis, contributing to the abnormal PT.

Activated Partial Thromboplastin Time

The **activated partial thromboplastin time (aPTT)** is used to assess the intrinsic clotting pathway, especially the early stages involving factors XII, XI, IX, and VIII (refer to Figure 8–1). It often is used to monitor patients on heparin therapy. The goals of heparin therapy are to extend the aPTT to about twice the upper level of normal. In individuals not on anticoagulant therapy, abnormal PT or aPTT values indicate abnormalities in the coagulation system, possibly reflecting liver disorders, hematologic disorders, toxins or drugs, or disseminated intravascular coagulation (DIC) associated with a multiorgan failure syndrome. Further workup might include a number of specific clotting factor assays to identify the exact abnormality. Adding normal clotting factors to the test sample can help determine whether a coagulation abnormality is due to factor deficiency (coagulation normalizing with mix) or a circulating anticoagulant (coagulation not normalizing with mix).

In the clinical setting, prolonged aPTT is frequently seen in patients on intravenous heparin therapy. Heparin is an indirect thrombin inhibitor that complexes with antithrombin (AT) and converts it into a rapid inactivator of thrombin, factor Xa, and to a lesser extent factors XIIa, XIa and IXa. The goal of heparin therapy is to elevate the aPTT to 1.5 times the upper limit of normal range within 24 hours. The goal of maintenance therapy is to maintain the aPTT in the range of 1.5 to 2.5 times the patient's baseline aPTT value. Activated PTT can be prolonged due to a deficiency of, or an inhibitor to, any of the clotting factors except factor VII. Certain lupus anticoagulants can cause aPTT prolongation by interfering with in vitro assembly of the prothrombinase complex. This also causes paradoxical increased risk of venous and arterial thrombus.

Thrombin Time

The thrombin time measures the final step of the clotting pathway, which is the conversion of fibrinogen to fibrin. Thrombin time can be prolonged in the presence of heparin, a direct thrombin inhibitor such as hirudin or argatroban, fibrin degradation products, and hypofibrinogenemia.

Hematology

The complete blood count (CBC) is the most frequently ordered diagnostic test in the hospital. Under the heading of CBC is a long list of indices that vary among laboratories. Automated machines usually directly measure the hemoglobin, WBC count, RBC count, platelet count, differential leukocyte fractions, and RBC distribution list, as well as calculate the hematocrit, mean corpuscular volume, mean corpuscular hemoglobin, mean corpuscular hemoglobin concentration, and differential leukocyte count.

Hemoglobin and Hematocrit

Hemoglobin is an iron-containing globular protein consisting of two pairs of polypeptides. Its primary function is the transport of oxygen from the lungs to the tissues. Approximately 1 g of hemoglobin binds with 1.34 mL of oxygen. Normal values for hemoglobin in the adult are 13.5 to 15.5 g/dL (for men) and 12.5 to 14.5 g/dL (for women). The **hematocrit** is the proportion of whole blood that is composed of RBCs (the hemoglobin-carrying cell). Normal hematocrit values in the adult are 42% to 52% (for men) and 37% to 48% (for women). **Box 8–10** lists causes of abnormal hemoglobin and hematocrit levels. High hemoglobin levels are associated with chronic hypoxia and hematologic diseases, such as polycythemia vera. High hemoglobin or hematocrit values, or both, also may be seen in individuals with dehydration and hemoconcentration.

Estimation of hemoglobin levels and types of hemoglobin is done by electrophoresis (alkaline or acid), other tests used to estimate abnormal hemoglobin (e.g., solubility test for sickle cell disease), and autoanalyzers.

BOX 8–10

Causes of Low Hemoglobin and Hematocrit Values

Abnormal Hemoglobin

- Iron in the ferric form: methemoglobinemia
- Abnormalities in the polypeptide chain: hemoglobinopathies, such as thalassemias and sickle cell disease

Decreased Hemoglobin Production

- *Bone marrow problems*: aplastic anemia, myelosuppressive drugs, idiosyncratic reaction to drugs, infiltration of bone marrow by other cells
- *Deficiencies*: iron, vitamin B_{12} cofactors, erythropoietin
- *Miscellaneous*: malignancy, chronic diseases, hypothyroidism, hypopituitarism

Increased Loss or Breakdown of RBCs

- Fault in the RBCs: membrane defects, enzymatic deficiencies, hemoglobin disorders
- Acquired causes of hemolysis: drugs, toxins, infections
- Hypersplenism
- Bleeding

RBC, red blood cell.

Platelets

Platelets are blood cells critical to clot formation after vascular injury. They are produced in the bone marrow, with normal blood concentrations ranging from 150,000 to 400,000/μL. **Box 8–11** lists abnormalities in platelet function.

Total and Differential Leukocyte Count

The primary role of **leukocytes** (WBCs) is in fighting infections, and an elevated WBC count (**leukocytosis**) is often a sign of significant infection. Leukocytosis, however, also can be associated with elevated glucocorticoids (e.g., stress reaction, steroid administration) and can be seen in a number of cases of hematologic malignancies (**Box 8–12**). A marked elevation in white cell count, such as is seen in patients with leukemia, may interfere with the interpretation of arterial blood gas values. A low WBC count (**leukopenia**) is invariably

RESPIRATORY RECAP

Hematology

» Hemoglobin and hematocrit
» Platelets
» Leukocytes

BOX 8–11

Abnormalities in Platelet Function

Thrombasthenia

Abnormal platelet function with uremia
von Willebrand disease
Drugs

Thrombocytopenia (Decreased Platelet Count)

Bone marrow problems: malignancies, drugs, myelodysplasias
Increased breakdown: structural platelet defects, immune problems (heparin-induced thrombocytopenia)
Hypersplenism

Thrombocytosis (Increased Platelet Count)

Essential or idiopathic
After splenectomy
Acute blood loss
Pregnancy

BOX 8–12

Causes of Leukocytosis

Physiologic

Exercise
Pregnancy
Stress: pain, psychologic, cold exposure, anesthesia, anoxia
Trauma, hemorrhage
Menstruation, pregnancy, and labor
Seizure

Pathologic

Infections: bacterial, fungal, viral, and parasitic
Leukemoid reaction due to any of the previous causes
Leukemias: uncontrolled malignant proliferation of any of the WBCs in the bone marrow

WBC, white blood cell.

a bad sign in any disease process, especially in infections, in which it often indicates overwhelming infection (**Box 8–13**). The differential percentage of various WBCs in the peripheral smear helps identify the disease process. Once the percentage of different cells is known, the absolute numbers can be calculated from the total WBC

BOX 8–13

Causes of Leukopenia

Overwhelming infection, especially in the very young or very elderly
Drug actions and adverse events
Malignant involvement of the bone marrow
Collagen vascular diseases such as lupus (infrequent cause)
Idiopathic or not-well-understood disease processes, such as myelodysplastic syndromes

counts. Normal WBC counts in adults range from 4000 to 11,000/μL.

Leukocytes are classified into two groups: granulocytes and agranulocytes. The granulocytes (neutrophils, eosinophils, and basophils) have granules in their cell cytoplasm and a multilobed nucleus. They also are called polymorphonuclear leukocytes or polys. The agranuloctyes (lymphocytes and monocytes) do not have granules and have a nonlobular nuclei. When immature leukocytes are first released from the bone marrow into the peripheral blood, they are called bands or stabs. The normal differential for leukocyte count is:

- Bands or stabs: 3–5%
- Neutrophils: 50–70% relative value
- Eosinophils: 1–3% relative value
- Basophils: 0.4–1% relative value
- Lymphocytes: 25–35% relative value
- Moncytes: 4–6% relative value

The differential always adds up to 100%.

Earlier hematology laboratories used visual counting techniques to estimate WBC concentrations. Today, most laboratories have automated instruments that use either resistance changes or flow characteristics to estimate the cell count and size of the cells. To enhance accuracy, RBCs are usually destroyed by chemicals in the blood sample before the WBC counts are performed. Currently, flow-through techniques using electrical resistance (or flow) changes or cytometry alone or in combination with cytochemical techniques are used. The sophistication of the instrument depends on whether it provides a three-, five-, or six-part differential. Ideally, the false-negative rate varies from 2% to 4%, with a false-positive rate of 8% to 15%. Falsely elevated WBC counts may be seen in individuals with undestroyed nucleated RBCs or large or aggregated platelets. Falsely low numbers may be seen in individuals with leukoagglutination; abnormal cells, such as blasts; immature granulocytes; and atypical lymphocytes. Further limitations include an inability to separate mature polymorphonuclear cells from band forms.

Autoanalyzers for CBC using spectrophotometric methods, electric impedance technique, or light-scattering phenomenon can provide reliable numbers for all the parameters in the majority of samples. Results may be compromised in the presence of hyperlipidemia, cryoproteinemia, agglutination of various cells (e.g., RBC, WBC, platelets), and abnormally shaped and sized cells (e.g., schistocytes, sickled cells). Atypical features are usually flagged by the machine and must be assessed by a visual review of the smear.

Laboratory Standards and Quality Control

An enormous amount of clinical information can be derived from examination of blood chemistries and hematology. Indiscriminate or routine ordering of these tests, however, should be discouraged because such practices consume resources unnecessarily, cause potential harm from false-positive or false-negative results, and waste patient blood. Indeed, one of the most important causes of ICU anemia is blood drawing.

The clinical relevance and significance of results are a composite product of not only the appropriateness of the test request but also patient sample identification, criteria for sample acceptance, and running of the tests by appropriate standardized methods followed by communication and interpretation of results. Point-of-care testing has made the task even more difficult. All hematology and blood chemistry testing procedures must be standardized to ensure optimal accuracy and precision. To this end, the U.S. federal government in 1988 established published standards under the Clinical Laboratory Improvement Amendment (CLIA). Other organizations, such as the College of American Pathologists (CAP) and the Joint Commission (TJC), also have published certification standards for laboratories. All laboratories must adhere to these standards, not only to ensure quality care but also to ensure appropriate reimbursement.

As testing methodologies are made more portable, so-called point-of-care devices for measuring electrolytes, glucose, lactate, hemoglobin, and blood gases have become available. In addition to more rapid turnaround times, these devices offer the ability to use smaller samples of blood or even to return the blood to the patient after testing. However, the same quality standards mandated for central laboratories should also be applied to these devices.

Regardless of the device used, the limitations of various methods must be kept in mind. Interpretation of values requires knowledge of other medical conditions that may affect the numbers. Indeed, an appropriate first step in the assessment of an unexpected abnormality might be to simply repeat the test. Laboratory tests can provide significant information that drives clinical decision making. The clinician assessing the results should fully appreciate both the significance of the results and the potential errors that might exist.

KEY POINTS

- The most common serum electrolytes are sodium, potassium, calcium, magnesium, chloride, total carbon dioxide, and phosphorus.
- Two-thirds of body water is intracellular.
- Sodium is the most common electrolyte in extracellular fluid.
- Hyponatremia and hypernatremia are associated with a number of disease states.
- Potassium is found primarily in the intracellular space.
- Changes in serum potassium concentrations affect neuromuscular activity and cardiac electrical impulses.
- Changes in serum chloride concentrations usually follow changes in serum sodium concentrations.
- Unmeasured anions are estimated through calculation of the anion gap.
- Most calcium is bound to albumin, but only ionized calcium is metabolically important.
- Magnesium plays an important role in maintaining membrane potential.
- Phosphorus is a major intracellular anion that participates in many metabolic processes.
- Increased lactate concentrations are usually due to anaerobic metabolism.
- Blood urea nitrogen and serum creatinine levels are used to assess renal function.
- Serum enzyme levels are used to assess liver and cardiac function.
- Bilirubin is a breakdown product of hemoglobin that is metabolized in the liver.
- Serum albumin level is a useful marker of nutritional status.
- Hyperglycemia and hypoglycemia result from derangements in glucose metabolism.
- Brain natriuretic peptide levels are elevated in patients with congestive heart failure.
- Elevated serum C-reactive protein levels are a marker for nonspecific inflammation.
- High-sensitivity CRP is used to monitor patients with coronary artery disease.
- Serum procalcitonin levels are currently under evaluation to help distinguish inflammation caused by septic bacterial and fungal sources from viral infections and noninfectious conditions.
- Prolonged prothrombin time and activated partial thromboplastin time are indicative of problems in blood coagulation.
- Reduced hemoglobin and hematocrit values are seen in anemia.
- Reduced platelet counts are indicative of problems in clot formation, which can be a problem in patients undergoing bronchoscopic biopsy or arterial blood gas testing.
- Reduced leukocytes suggest an immunocompromised state. Moderate elevation of leukocyte

count is seen in infections or steroid treatment, and a marked elevation in leukemia and leukemoid reactions.

SUGGESTED READING

Adrogue HJ, Madias NE. Hypernatremia. *N Engl J Med.* 2000;342: 1493–1499.

Barth JH, Fiddy JB, Payne RB. Adjustment of serum total calcium for albumin concentration: effects of non-linearity and of regression differences between laboratories. *Ann Clin Biochem.* 1996;33:55–58.

Bartlett RH. Fluids and electrolytes. In: Bartlett RH, ed. *Critical Care Physiology.* Boston: Little Brown; 1996:155–175.

Bishop ML, Duben-Engelkirk JL, Fody EP. *Clinical Chemistry: Principles, Procedures, Correlations.* 4th ed. Philadelphia: Lippincott Williams & Wilkins; 2000.

Black S, Kushner I, Samols D. C-reactive protein. *J Biol Chem.* 2004;279:48487–48490.

Carrigan SD, Scott G, Tabrizian M. Toward resolving the challenges of sepsis diagnosis. *Clin Chem.* 2004;50:1301–1314.

Dirks JL. Diagnostic blood analysis using point-of-care technology. *AACN Clin Issues Crit Care Nurs.* 1996;7:249–259.

Eklund U, Forberg JL. New methods for improved evaluation of patients with suspected acute coronary syndrome in the emergency department. *Emerg Med J.* 2007;24:811–814.

Fulop M. Algorithms for diagnosing some electrolyte disorders. *Am J Emerg Med.* 1998;16:76–84.

Gailani D, Renne T. Intrinsic pathway of coagulation and arterial thrombosis. *Arterioscler Thromb Vasc Biol.* 2007;27:2507–2513.

George JN. Platelets. *Lancet.* 2000;355:1531–1539.

Gulati GL, Hyun BH. The automated CBC: a current perspective. *Hematol Oncol Clin North Am.* 1994;8:593–601.

Harvey MA. Point-of-care laboratory testing in critical care. *Am J Crit Care.* 1999;8:72–83.

Hood VL, Tannen RL. Mechanisms of disease: protection of acid-base balance by pH regulation of acid production. *N Engl J Med.* 1998;339:819–826.

James JH, Luchette FA, McCarter FD, et al. Lactate is an unreliable indicator of tissue hypoxia in injury or sepsis. *Lancet.* 1999;354:505–508.

Jospe N, Forbes G. Fluids and electrolytes: clinical aspects. *Pediatr Rev.* 1996;11:395–403.

Kamath PS. Clinical approach to the patient with abnormal liver test results. *Mayo Clin Proc.* 1996;71:1089–1095.

Kaplan LA, Pesce AJ, Kaznierzak SC. *Clinical Chemistry: Theory, Analysis and Correlation.* 3rd ed. St. Louis: Mosby; 1996.

Kellum JA. Metabolic acidosis in critically ill: lessons from physical chemistry. *Kidney Int.* 1998;53(suppl 66):S81–S86.

Kokko JP, Tannen RL. *Fluids and Electrolytes.* 3rd ed. Philadelphia: WB Saunders; 1996.

Krause JR. The automated white blood cell differential: a current perspective. *Hematol Oncol Clin North Am.* 1994;8:605–616.

Ledue TB, Rifai N. Preanalytic and analytic sources of variations in C-reactive protein: implications for cardiovascular disease risk assessment. *Clin Chem.* 2003;49:1258–1271.

Lum G. Evaluation of a laboratory critical limit (alert value) policy for hypercalcemia. *Arch Pathol Lab Med.* 1996;120:633–636.

Mackman N, Tilley RE, Key NS. Role of extrinsic pathway in blood coagulation in hemostasis and thrombosis. *Arterioscler Thromb Vasc Biol.* 2007;27:1687–1693.

Mandal AK. Renal disease: hypokalemia and hyperkalemia. *Med Clin North Am.* 1997;81:611–639.

McGee S, Abernethy WB, Simel DL. Is this patient hypovolemic? *JAMA.* 1999;281:1022–1028.

Reynolds RM, Padfield PL, Seckl JR. Disorders of sodium balance. *BMJ.* 2006;332:702–705.

Roberts R. Rapid MB CK subform assay and the early diagnosis of myocardial infarction. *Clin Lab Med.* 1997;17:669–683.

Schrier RW. Body water homeostasis: clinical disorders of urinary dilution and concentration. *J Am Soc Nephrol.* 2006;17:1820–1832.

Spital A. Diuretic induced hyponatremia. *Am J Nephrol.* 1999;19:447–452.

Toffaletti J. Elevations in blood lactate: overview of use in critical care. *Scand J Clin Lab Invest.* 1996;56(suppl 224):107–110.

Uribarri J, Oh MS, Carroll HJ. D-Lactic acidosis: a review of clinical presentation, biochemical features and pathophysiologic mechanisms. *Medicine.* 1998;77:73–82.

Whang R, Burns JA. Clinical disorders of magnesium metabolism. *Compr Ther.* 1997;23:168–173.

Workman ML. Magnesium and phosphorus: the neglected electrolytes. *AACN Clin Issues Crit Care Nurs.* 1992;3:655–663.

CHAPTER 9

Imaging the Thorax

Paolo Formenti
Vinko F. Tomicic
Dean R. Hess

OUTLINE

Density and Contrast
The Normal Chest Radiograph
Abnormalities Seen on Chest Radiographs
Cross-Sectional Imaging Techniques

OBJECTIVES

1. Describe the underlying principles of radiography, including densities and contrast.
2. Outline the features of a normal chest radiograph, including the different projections and a systematic inspection.
3. Describe the major abnormalities seen on chest radiographs.
4. Explain the use of a chest radiograph in locating and quantifying abnormal pockets of air of fluid within the chest.
5. Explain how the chest radiograph is used to verify the proper positioning of monitoring and therapeutic catheters, tubes, and devices.
6. Describe how computed tomography, compared with the chest radiograph, improves diagnostic imaging capabilities.
7. Describe the use of ultrasound, magnetic resonance imaging, and positron emission tomography in imaging studies.

KEY TERMS

air bronchogram
anteroposterior (AP) projection
apical lordotic
chest radiograph
computed tomography (CT)
deep sulcus sign
ground glass appearance
Hampton hump
honeycomb appearance
Hounsfield units (HU)
Kerley B lines
lateral decubitus
Macklin effect
magnetic resonance imaging (MRI)
mediastinal shift
nodular appearance
opacifications
positron emission tomography (PET)
posteroanterior (PA) projection
radiodensity
radiolucent
radiopaque
silhouette sign
voxels
Westermark sign

INTRODUCTION

Medical radiographs for diagnostic imaging have been used for over a century. Their application depends on the differential reduction of the radiograph beam when traveling through the human body. This reduction produces a superimposed gray- or white-on-black shadow of the internal anatomy of the patient. More recently, a three-dimensional representation of the anatomy has become available by acquiring multiple, angular projections synthesized into tomographic images using **computed tomography (CT)**.[1] CT has revolutionized the use of radiographs in diagnostic imaging even if the traditional radiograph remains the first step in the diagnostic assessment.

Radiographs are produced when electrons interact with matter and convert their kinetic energy into electromagnetic radiation.[1,2] A **chest radiograph** is produced by x-ray beams (energy) passing through the thorax and exposing a photographic plate or film. Radiographic imaging is based on the anatomy of the patient blocking x-ray transmission by varying degrees, which results in an image caused by the degree of exposure of the photographic plate. Before computers and digital imaging, a photographic plate sensitive to x-rays was used to produce radiographic images, and the images were produced directly on film.[3] Digital radiography is replacing film in medicine.[4] The major difference between the analog and digital detectors is the digitalization of the continuous output signal into discrete spatial sampling locations performed by an analog-digital converter.[3,4] The radiograph image can be a still photograph or video display.

Density and Contrast

The x-ray beam transmitted through the patient will vary in intensity and, when unblocked, completely expose the photographic film, converting it from white to black. *Blocking* is the reduction of an x-ray beam, which depends on the penetrating characteristics of the beam and the physical characteristics of the tissue.[3] The blocking of x-rays by intervening tissue is potentially harmful radiation exposure. Therefore, the range of energies used is chosen to optimize the diagnostic information and minimize the radiation absorbed by the patient.

> **RESPIRATORY RECAP**
>
> **Densities Seen on Chest Radiographs**
>
> » Gas
> » Fat
> » Soft tissue (water)
> » Bone (metal)

When there is minimal tissue density, such as air or air-filled structures, black areas are produced on the radiograph; these areas are referred to as **radiolucent**. Areas or body tissues that cannot be penetrated by x-rays are **radiopaque** and appear white on the radiograph. Each body tissue or structure has a different **radiodensity**. The four basic radiodensities are as follows:

- Gas, which appears black or radiolucent; an example is gas in the airways or stomach.
- Fat, which appears gray or less radiolucent than air; an example is lipid tissue around muscle.
- Soft tissue (water), which appears gray or less radiolucent than air; examples are heart, blood vessels, and muscles.
- Bone (or metal), which appears all white or completely radiopaque; examples are bones, calcium deposits, prostheses, and contrast media. Objects placed into the patient, such as endotracheal tubes and vascular catheters, are radiopaque.

Density is determined not only by the composition of an object but also by its thickness. Thus, two objects of different composition can appear to be the same density if they have different thicknesses. Contrast occurs when two objects of different densities are side by side. Radiodense materials are sometimes injected into the body to improve contrast between anatomic structures (e.g., arteriograms, bronchograms, barium swallows).

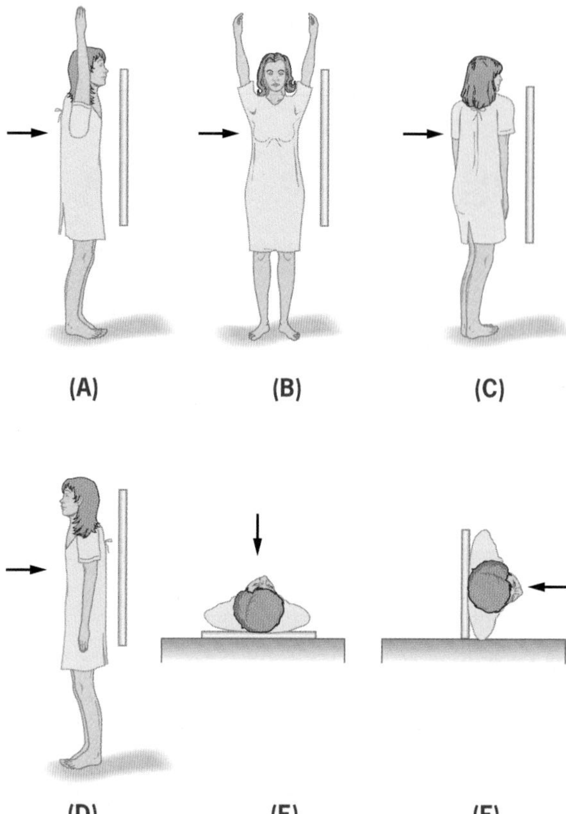

FIGURE 9–1 Various radiographic positions. (**A**) Posteroanterior. (**B**) Lateral. (**C**) Right anterior oblique. (**D**) Anteroposterior. (**E**) Anteroposterior supine. (**F**) Right lateral decubitus. Adapted from Goodman LR. *Principles of Chest Roentgenology: A Programmed Text.* 3rd ed. Saunders Elsevier; 2007.

The Normal Chest Radiograph

Technical Factors

Frontal views of the thorax are **posteroanterior (PA)** and **anteroposterior (AP) projections**. In ambulatory patients, PA and lateral projections are commonly obtained (**Figure 9–1**). Other projections, such as **lateral decubitus** and **apical lordotic**, are used to better visualize the pleural space and the lung apices, respectively (**Box 9–1**).[5,6] Frontal and lateral radiographs allow the chest to be viewed from two directions (thus, three dimensions) to more easily localize infiltrates and lesions. The lateral view is used to evaluate the mediastinum, the tracheal air column, the inferior vena cava, the retrosternal space, the posterior margin of the heart, the diaphragmatic contour, and the presence of pleural effusions.

For the PA projection, the x-ray beam passes through the chest from the back to the front. For the AP view, the beam passes through the chest from the front to the back. For patients in the intensive care unit (ICU), supine AP views are obtained with a portable x-ray machine. The supine AP view is typically of inferior technical quality. The diaphragm is elevated because of the supine position. Objects that are further away from the x-ray film are magnified. Thus, the heart appears larger on the AP film.

It is important to assess the technical quality of the chest radiograph. *Penetration* refers to the amount of x-ray exposure. An overpenetrated film will be too black, and an underpenetrated film will appear too white (**Figure 9–2**). With a properly penetrated film, the vertebral bodies should be just visible through the cardiac shadow. The patient should be oriented correctly and not rotated

BOX 9–1

Chest Radiograph Projections

Posteroanterior (PA)

The PA position is the most commonly used position.

X-ray energy passes posterior to anterior through the chest of the patient, with the radiograph film anterior to the patient's chest.

The radiograph is taken with the patient upright, with maximal inspiration, and the scapulae are rotated away from the lung fields.

Anteroposterior (AP)

The AP position is commonly used for portable radiographs in the critical care unit.

X-ray energy passes anterior to posterior through the chest of the patient.

The heart size is magnified.

The quality of the image is inferior to the PA projection.

Lateral

X-ray energy passes laterally through the chest of the patient. The lateral position allows visualization of the lung bases and lung parenchyma behind the heart.

Oblique

X-ray energy passes obliquely through the chest of the patient. The oblique position is used to project abnormalities away from overlying structures.

Lordotic

The lordotic position provides a better view of the lung apex, lingula, and right middle lobe.

Expiratory

The expiratory position is used to demonstrate a small pneumothorax or unilateral airway obstruction.

Lateral Decubitus

The radiograph is taken with the patient in a side-lying position.

The lateral decubitus position is used to identify the presence of free pleural fluid or to confirm the presence of an air–fluid level in the lung.

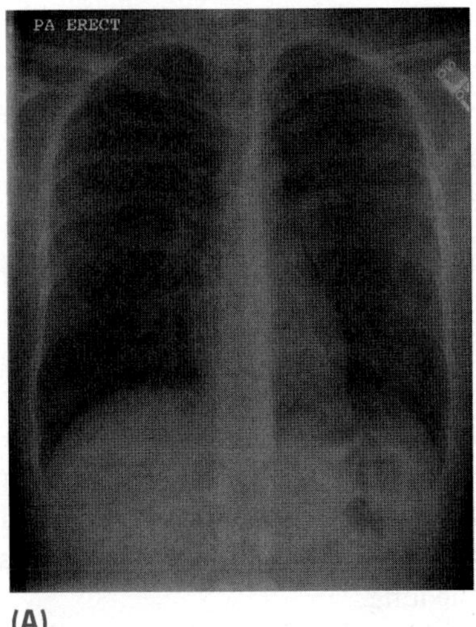

(A)

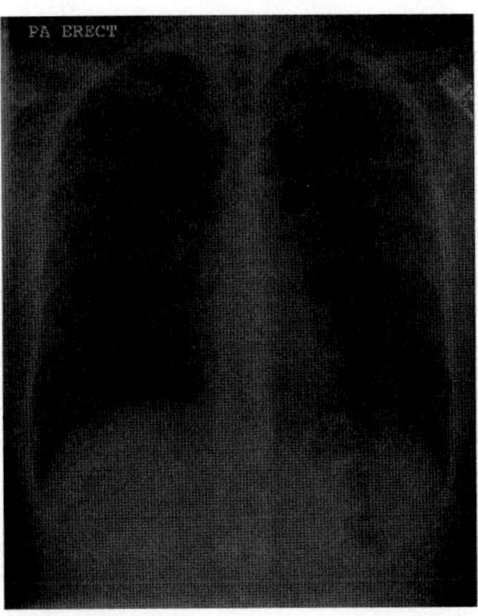

(B)

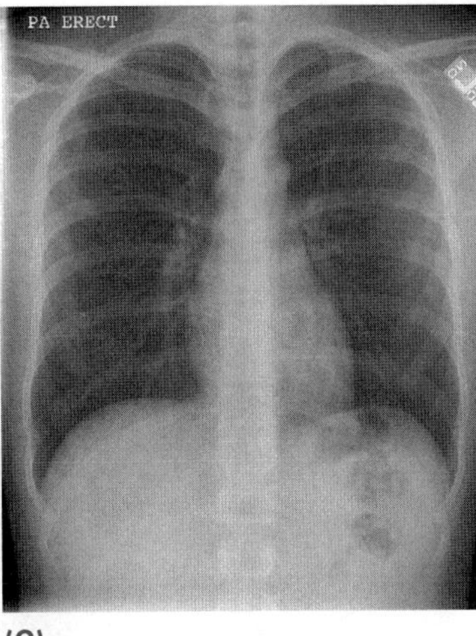

(C)

FIGURE 9–2 (**A**) Correctly penetrated chest radiograph. (**B**) Overpenetrated chest radiograph. (**C**) Underpenetrated chest radiograph.

to one side or the other. With proper position, the clavicles appear symmetric. The radiograph should be taken at full inspiration. A poor inspiration will make the heart look larger and produce appearance of basilar infiltrates (**Figure 9–3**). The scapulae should be rotated out of position on PA film, but will be present on an AP film. The heart should be oriented to the left unless the patient has dextrocardia or situs inversus.

Examination of the Chest Radiograph

Examination of the chest radiograph should include systematic inspection of the extrathoracic soft tissues, bony thorax, mediastinal contour, hilar region, pleural surfaces, vascular pattern, and lung fields. The frontal chest radiograph is viewed as though the patient were facing you; in other words, the patient's left is to your right. **Figure 9–4** and **Figure 9–5** show normal chest radiographs.

> **RESPIRATORY RECAP**
>
> **Normal Chest Radiograph**
>
> » Right hemidiaphragm higher than the left
> » Clear and sharp costophrenic angles
> » Left hilum higher than right
> » Air tracheogram midline under sternum
> » Aortic arch to left of spine
> » Heart toward left thorax
> » Gastric air bubble on left

The trachea appears as a vertically oriented radiolucent structure midway between the clavicles and over the spine.[7] The carina is normally positioned at the level of the sixth posterior rib or T4. Causes of tracheal deviation are chest rotation, tumor, **mediastinal shift**, pneumothorax, or major atelectasis.[8]

Twelve pairs of symmetric ribs should be seen. Each intercostal space is numbered according to the rib above it. Widened intercostal spaces occur in conditions such as chronic obstructive pulmonary disease (COPD), pneumothorax, and pleural effusion. Narrowed intercostal spaces are associated with decreased lung volume (e.g., atelectasis).[9]

The right hemidiaphragm is normally higher than the left because of the liver. The apex of the diaphragm lies at the level of the sixth anterior rib on the PA projection.[9] Flattening of the diaphragm is associated with hyperinflation of the lungs or thorax, as in COPD or pneumothorax.[10] The costal, diaphragmatic, and mediastinal pleura are not visible on plain radiographs.[11] The costophrenic angle should appear sharp. A gastric air bubble is often present under the left hemidiaphragm.

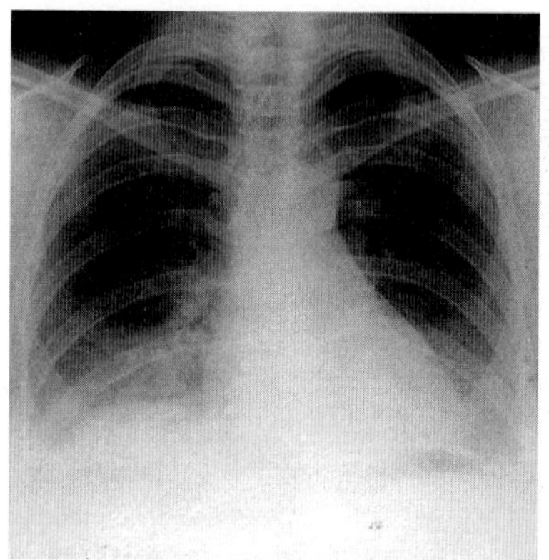

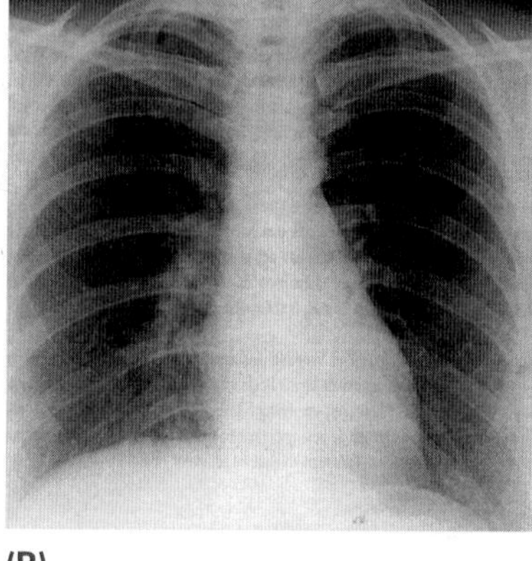

(A) (B)

FIGURE 9–3 (**A**) Expiratory film. (**B**) Inspiratory film.

The mediastinum is a narrow, vertically oriented structure between the medial parietal pleural layers of the lung that contains the central cardiovascular structures (heart and major vessels), tracheobronchial structures (trachea and main bronchi), esophagus, lymphatic chain, thoracic duct, and autonomic nerves.[5] The normal heart presents a homogeneous shadow on the chest film without any internal detail. The heart projects toward the left thorax unless the patient has dextrocardia or situs inversus. Detection and identification of heart disease depends mainly on changes in the size and shape of the cardiac silhouette and the great vessels. The cardiothoracic ratio is measured by the horizontal width of the heart divided by the widest width of the thorax and is normally 1:2 or less.[12,13] The aortic arch is normally to the left of the spine.

The left hilum is slightly higher than the right because the left pulmonary artery is higher than the right.[6,14] Bronchovascular markings branch out from the hila to the periphery of the lung fields. Hilar elevation is usually present in collapse of the upper lobes of the lung, and hilar depression occurs in collapse of the lower lobes of the lung.

The lung fields are radiolucent because they consist mainly of air and very little tissue or blood. The basis of visualization of a border of a structure depends on its contiguity with another structure of different density. It is possible to recognize a silhouette of the mediastinal structures and diaphragm

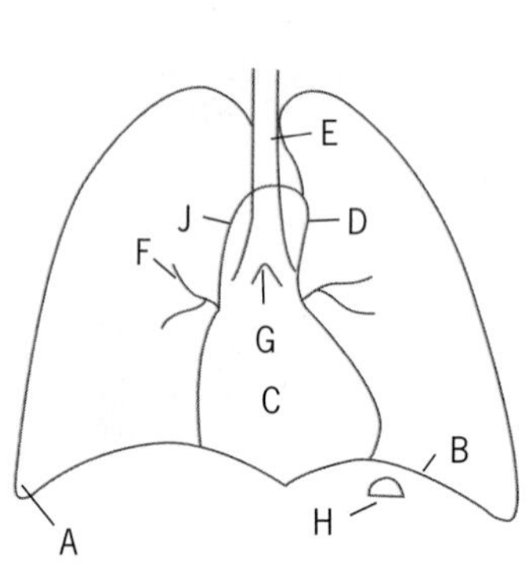

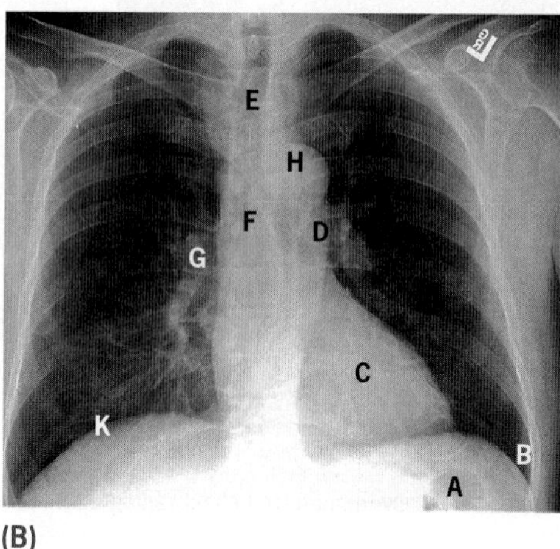

(A) (B)

FIGURE 9–4 (**A**) Landmarks on posteroanterior chest radiograph. A, costophrenic angle (sulcus); B, left hemidiaphragm; C, heart; D, aortic arch; E, trachea; F, hilum; G, carina; H, stomach bubble; J, ascending aorta. (**B**) Normal posteroanterior chest radiograph. A, stomach bubble; B, costophrenic angle (sulcus); C, heart; D, descending aorta; E, trachea; F, carina; G, hilum; H, aortic arch; K, right hemidiaphragm. (**A**) Adapted from Goodman LR. *Principles of Chest Roentgenology: A Programmed Text.* 3rd ed. Saunders Elsevier; 2007.

because they are outlined by adjacent air density of the lung. The minor fissure is located in the middle of the right lung fields, where it appears as a horizontal line on the frontal radiograph. The major or oblique fissures separate the upper lobes of the lung from the lower lobes. They cannot be seen on a frontal view but are visible on a lateral view.[5,6]

Abnormalities Seen on Chest Radiographs

Abnormalities of the lung fields on chest radiographs include signs and patterns. Two common and important signs are the air bronchogram sign and the silhouette sign. Normally, the airways cannot be visualized on a chest radiograph because there is no contrast between the airway and the surrounding alveoli. If the alveoli become filled with fluid or if they are consolidated or collapsed, an **air bronchogram** will appear; this indicates that the underlying opacity is of pulmonary rather than pleural or mediastinal origin. The **silhouette sign** indicates an obliteration of the borders of the heart, mediastinal structures, or diaphragm by an adjacent opacity of similar density. An intrathoracic lesion that is not anatomically contiguous with one of these structures will not obliterate its border.

> **RESPIRATORY RECAP**
>
> **Signs and Patterns on Chest X-Ray**
>
> » *Signs:* air bronchogram and silhouette
>
> » *Patterns:* honeycomb, nodular, and ground glass

Processes involving the medial segment of the right middle lobe obliterate the right heart border. If the lingual is involved, the left heart border is obliterated. Lower lobe processes involving the basilar segments result in obliteration of the border of the diaphragm.

The honeycomb pattern, the nodular pattern, and the ground glass pattern are common patterns seen on the chest radiograph. The **honeycomb appearance** is characterized by the presence of cystic air spaces with thick fibrous walls lined by bronchiolar epithelium. This pattern occurs with idiopathic pulmonary fibrosis, collagen vascular diseases, asbestosis, chronic hypersensitivity pneumonitis, and drug-related fibrosis. A **nodular appearance** refers to multiple round **opacifications** on the chest radiograph. This pattern occurs with sarcoidosis, pneumoconiosis, and metastasis. **Ground glass appearance** is a hazy increased attenuation of the lungs with preservation of bronchial and vascular margins. The ground glass pattern may be associated with air bronchograms. It occurs with pneumonia, pulmonary edema, pulmonary hemorrhage, and pulmonary alveolar proteinosis.

Chronic Obstructive Pulmonary Disease

There are several major chest radiograph findings that indicate the presence of COPD. The radiograph appears hyperlucent, and bullae may be present. The diaphragms are lowered and flattened. An increased retrosternal airspace is seen on the lateral projection. Two conditions cause the lungs to be more radiolucent: hyperinflation and interstitial destruction. Both of these are present in COPD.

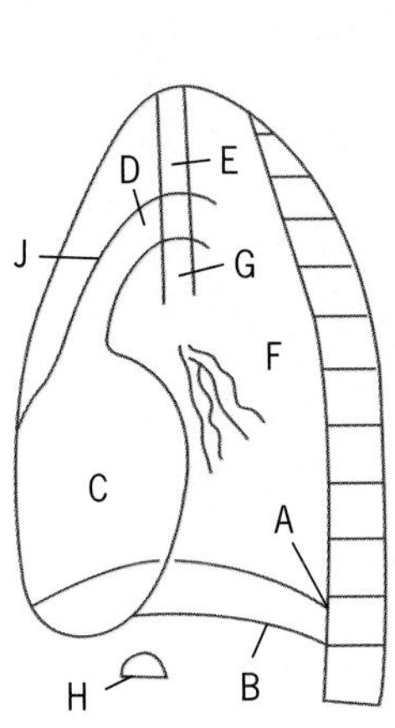

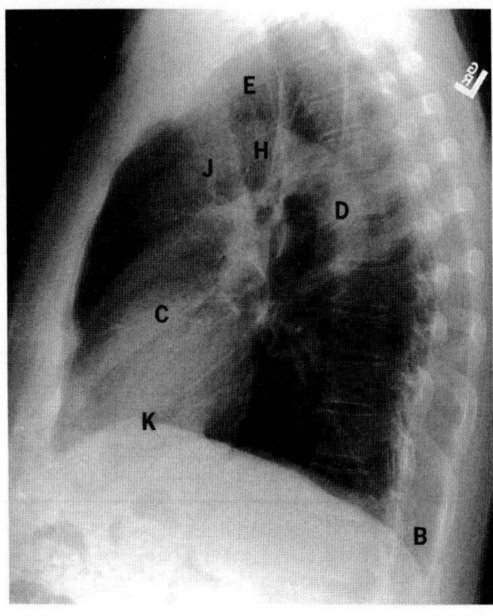

(A) (B)

FIGURE 9–5 **(A)** Landmarks on lateral chest radiograph. A, costophrenic angle (sulcus); B, left hemidiaphragm; C, heart; D, aortic arch; E, trachea; F, hilum; G, carina; H, stomach bubble; J, ascending aorta. **(B)** Normal lateral chest radiograph. B, costophrenic angle (sulcus); C, heart; D, descending aorta; E, trachea; H, aortic arch; J, ascending aorta; K, right hemidiaphragm. **(A)** Adapted from Goodman LR. *Principles of Chest Roentgenology: A Programmed Text.* 3rd ed. Saunders Elsevier; 2007.

Pneumonia

Pneumonia can cause a wide variety of abnormalities on the chest radiograph, resulting in segmental or lobar homogenous opacities or scattered nonsegmental opacities. There may be an extensive and diffuse airspace process. In pneumonia, as opposed to atelectasis, lung volume is preserved and findings persist for days to weeks. Air bronchograms may be present, and there may be associated pleural effusions. The silhouette sign can be used to identify the lobes and segments of the lungs that are involved.

Atelectasis

Direct signs of atelectasis on the chest radiograph include displacement of fissures toward the collapsed lung, increased radiopacity, and air bronchograms (**Figure 9–6** and

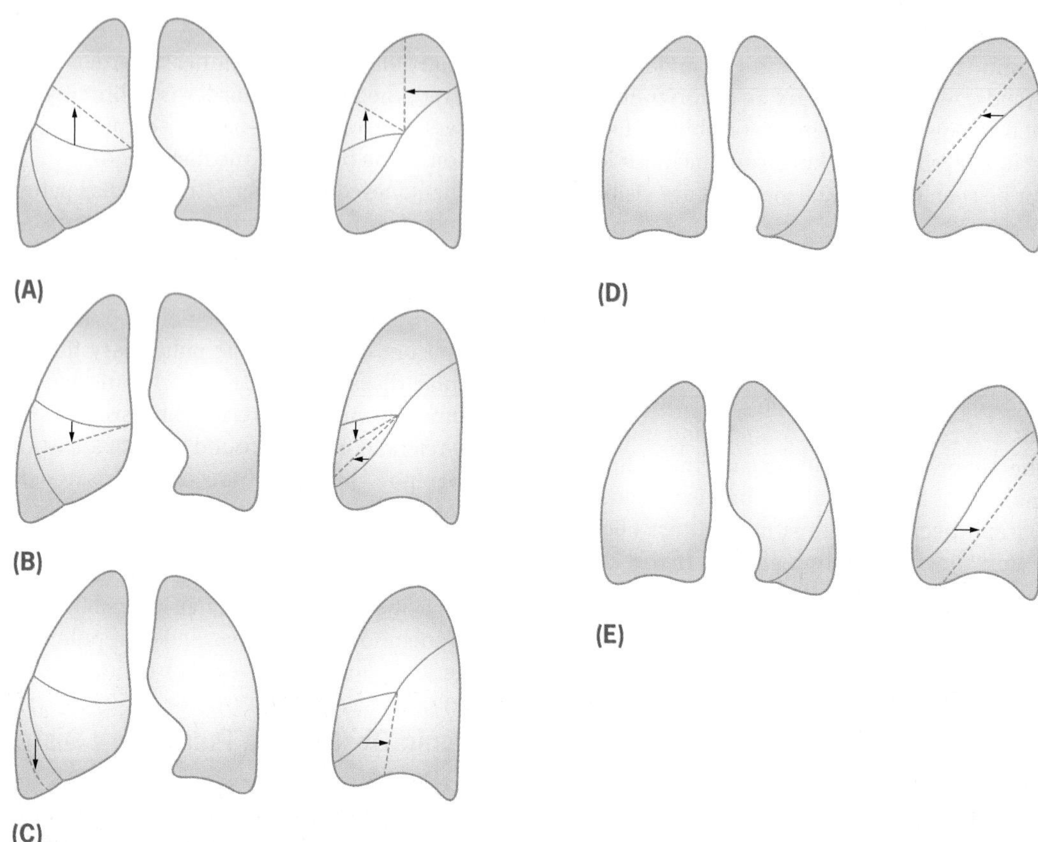

FIGURE 9–6 The best sign of lobar collapse is shift of a fissure. (**A**) Right upper lobe collapse. (**B**) Right middle lobe collapse. (**C**) Right lower lobe collapse. (**D**) Left upper lobe collapse. (**E**) Left lower lobe collapse. This article was published in *Felson's Principles of Chest Roentgenology: A Programmed Text*. 3rd ed. Goodman LR. Copyright Elsevier (Saunders) 2007.

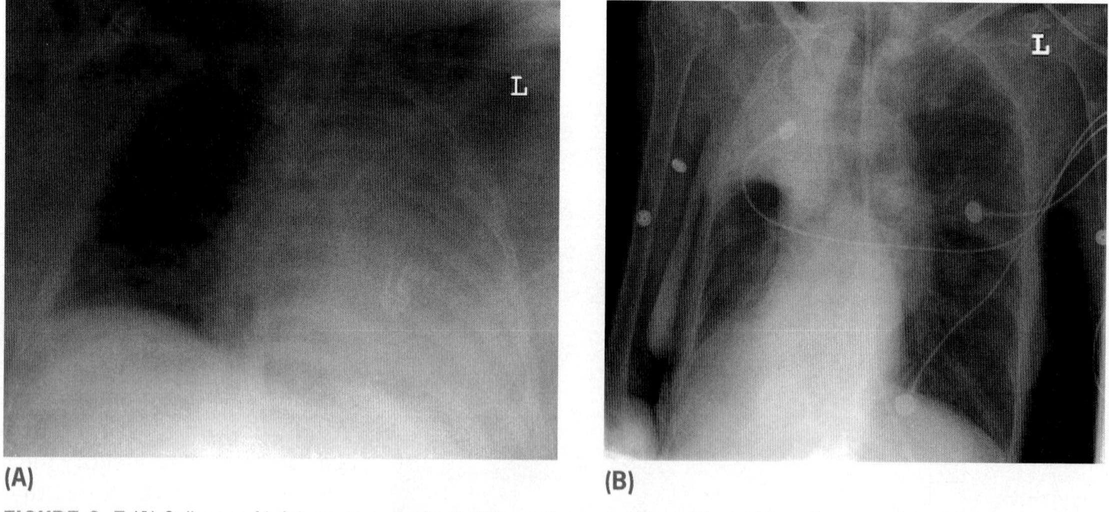

FIGURE 9–7 (**A**) Collapse of left lung. Note tracheal shift, mediastinal shift, and loss of the silhouette of the left hemidiaphragm. (**B**) Right upper lobe collapse. Note upward shift of horizontal fissure and right shift of trachea.

Figure 9–7). Indirect signs of atelectasis include hemidiaphragm elevation, displacement of the mediastinum or hilum, and compensatory overinflation of the remainder of the other lung.

Atelectasis can mimic pneumonia, particularly when other specific signs are absent. Distinguishing atelectasis from pneumonia may be difficult and at times impossible, often requiring corroborative clinical information and follow-up radiographs. If small airways are obstructed, subsegmental opacities result, which often are described as discoid or platelike in appearance. They appear as thin, linear, horizontally or obliquely oriented opacities and frequently are seen in postsurgical patients at the lung bases (**Figure 9–8**). Obstruction of a large airway may result in lobar atelectasis, most commonly involving the left lower lobe or the right lower lobe.[15] Involvement of the left lower lobe is particularly common after cardiac surgery.[16]

Left Heart Failure

With left heart failure (congestive heart failure), the cardiac silhouette is enlarged. With mild failure, interstitial edema develops, and the pulmonary vessel margins become less sharp and the peripheral interstitial markings become more prominent. With moderate failure, fluid thickens the interlobular septa, causing short lines to appear perpendicular to the pleural surface. These are called **Kerley B lines** and indicate interstitial edema. Severe failure causes alveolar edema, resulting in opacification (water density) of the lower lung zones. Pleural effusions can also occur with congestive heart failure.

Pneumothorax and Air Leaks

The pathophysiology of extra-alveolar air generally begins with the rupture of distal alveoli into the interstitial space and the subsequent dissection of air into the mediastinum, tissues, and pleural space.[17] Air dissects along bronchovascular bundles, producing the appearance of a pulmonary vessel surrounded by air. Air dissecting into the mediastinum creates vertical linear streaks, which is called the **Macklin effect**.[18] Subcutaneous emphysema results from air leak into the tissues (**Figure 9–9**).

The radiographic diagnosis of pneumothorax is established by identification of the visceral pleural line (**Figure 9–10**). Other radiographic features suggestive of pneumothorax include the absence of vascular markings and increased lucency in the hemithorax. Visualization of the visceral pleura can be enhanced by exposure of the film in expiration. With expiration, the volume of the pneumothorax remains constant, whereas the volume

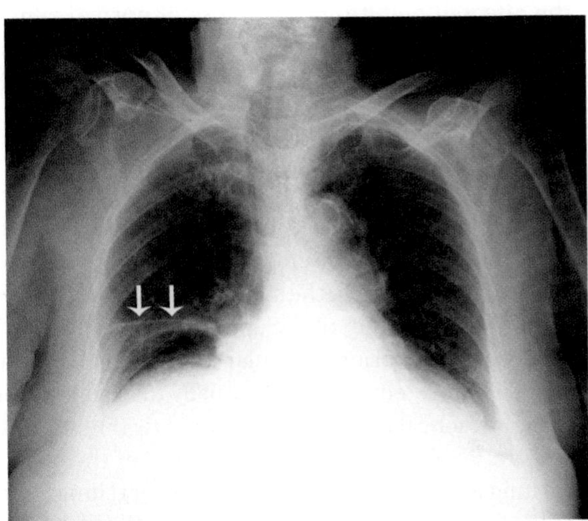

FIGURE 9–8 Platelike atelectasis (arrows).

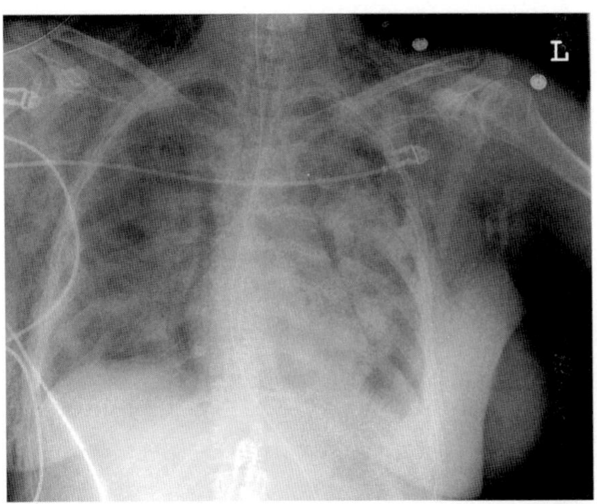

FIGURE 9–9 Pneumomediastinum and subcutaneous emphysema.

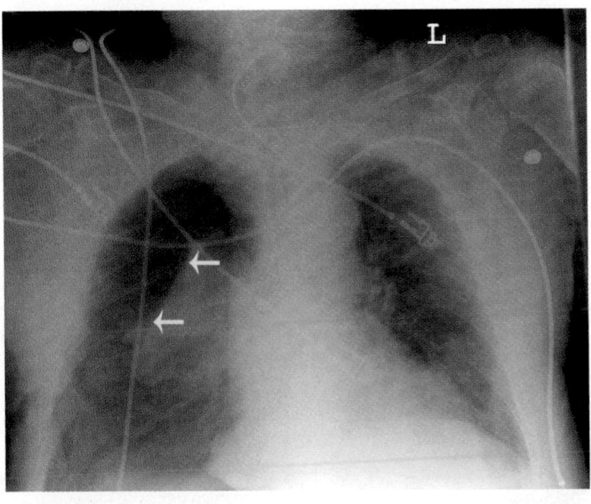

(A)

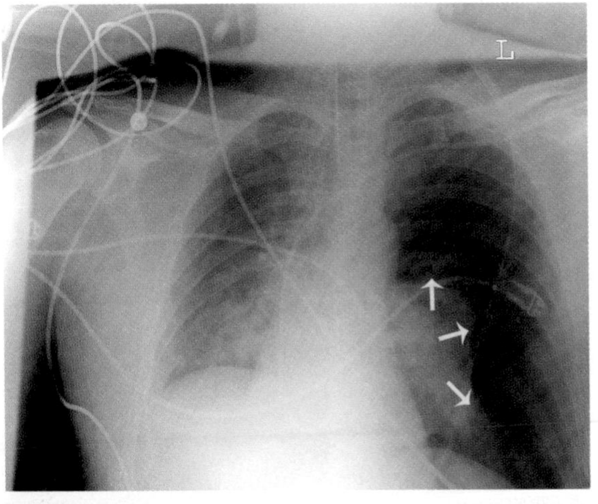

(B)

FIGURE 9–10 (**A**) Right-sided pneumothorax with visceral pleura line. (**B**) Left-sided tension pneumothorax. Note depression of left hemidiaphragm, widened intercostal spaces on left, shift of mediastinum to right, and collapsed left lung.

of the hemithorax in which it is contained is reduced. Pneumothorax is treated by insertion of a chest tube (**Figure 9–11**). A skin fold (**Figure 9–12**) may mimic the visceral pleural line, but whereas the visceral pleural line is a thin line with air on both sides, a skin fold is represented as an interface in which one edge is sharp but gradually fades away.[19]

In the upright position, free air in the pleural space generally collects over the apex of the lung. Most clinicians have been trained to look for air in this location when they suspect a pneumothorax. In patients in the supine position, the highest portion of the thorax is generally the anterior costophrenic sulcus. Free air within the pleural space rises to this position, projecting over the upper abdomen and diaphragm. This results in a distinctive radiographic appearance that is called the **deep sulcus sign** (**Figure 9–13**).[20] If the pneumothorax is on the left side, the apex of the heart and the pericardial fat pad often will be sharply outlined. In addition, the edge of the lung and the visceral pleural line may be identified.

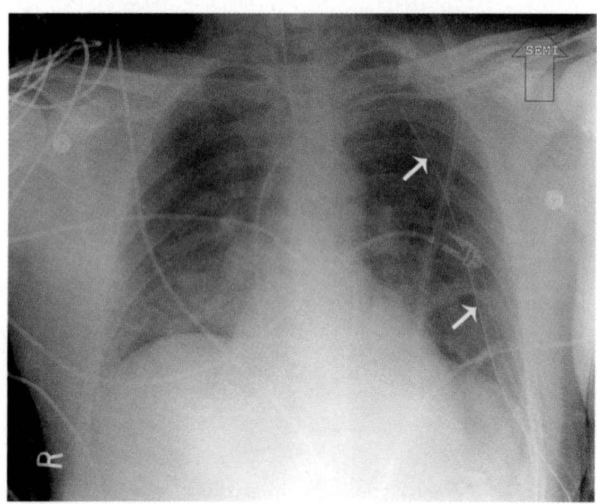

FIGURE 9–11 Note presence of left chest tube (arrows) and reexpansion of the lung after pneumothorax.

However, in the supine projection, recognition of the deep sulcus sign and increased lucency over the upper abdomen is critical because direct visualization of the visceral pleura in this projection is difficult.

Pleural Effusion

In the supine position, free fluid in the pleural space tends to layer posteriorly. Significant amounts of fluid create a generalized increased opacity over the affected hemithorax. The supine radiograph is relatively insensitive in the detection of pleural fluid and could underestimate its amount. The lateral radiograph is more sensitive than a frontal radiograph to identify a pleural effusion. Decubitus projection allows confirmation of the presence of free fluid in the pleural space (**Figure 9–14**). The presence of pleural effusion should be suspected with a blunted costophrenic angle, which normally appears sharp. Free fluid can track up the pleural space, forming a meniscus, called the *meniscus sign*. There can be an increased homogeneous density on the affected hemithorax and loss of normal silhouette of the hemidiaphragm. There can also be an apparent elevation of the hemidiaphragm, which is actually due to subpulmonic fluid.

Evaluation of Tubes and Catheters

The optimal position of the tip of the endotracheal tube is approximately 4 to 6 cm above the carina with the neck in the neutral position. In the supine position, the correct position of the distal tip of the endotracheal tube should be between the superior clavicular margin and T5. Intubation of a main stem bronchus, usually the right, occurs when endotracheal tube position is too low (**Figure 9–15** and **Figure 9–16**). This results in collapse of the contralateral lung and overinflation of the ipsilateral lung.[21] The tube diameter should be one-half to two-thirds that of the trachea lumen, and the inflated cuff should not cause bulging of the tracheal wall (**Figure 9–17**). Esophageal

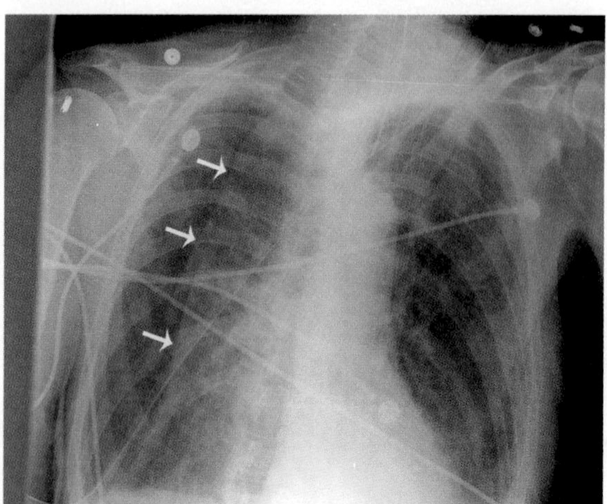

FIGURE 9–12 Skin fold (arrows), which can be confused with a visceral line and pneumothorax.

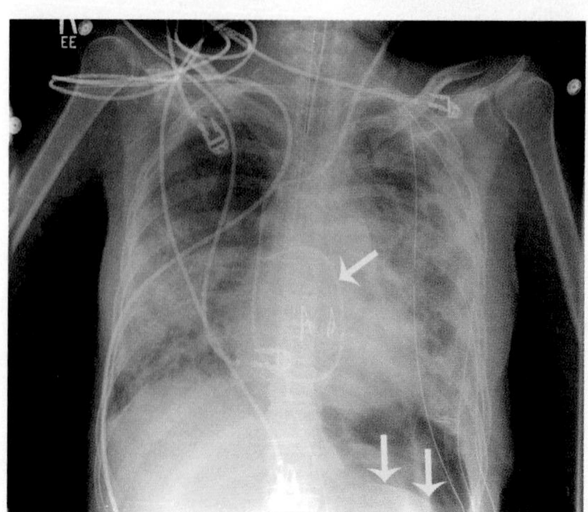

FIGURE 9–13 Deep sulcus sign on left (double arrows) and pulmonary artery catheter (arrow).

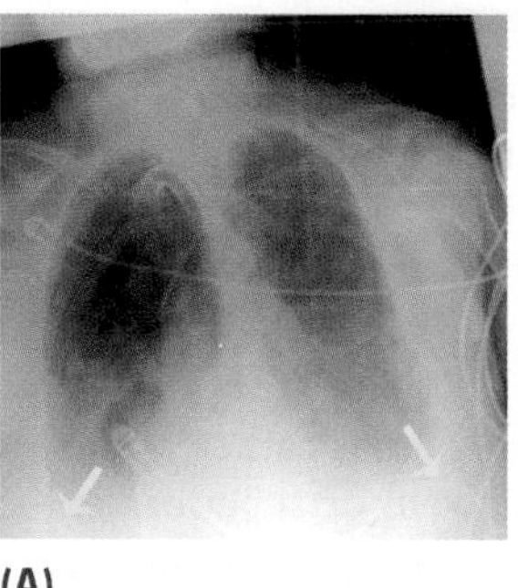
(A)

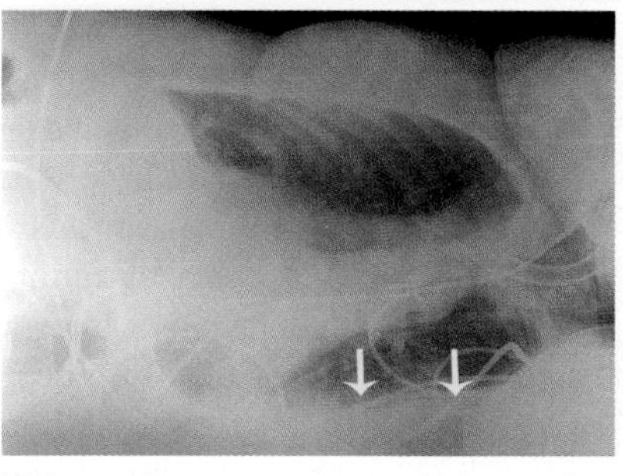
(B)

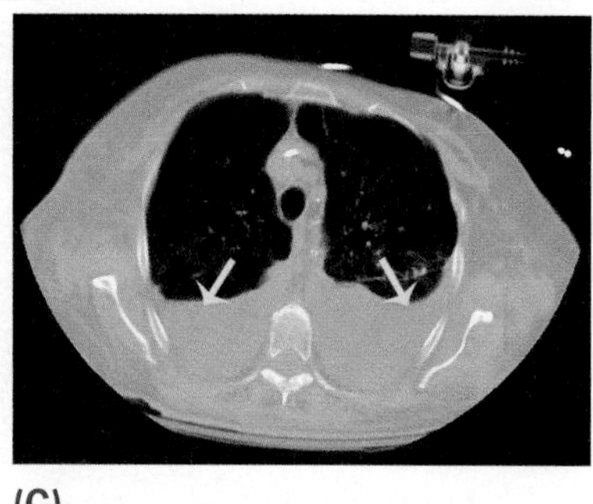
(C)

FIGURE 9–14 (**A**) Anteroposterior projection of patient with bilateral pleural effusions. Note blunted costophrenic angles. (**B**) Lateral decubitus projection. Note layering of the pleural effusion. (**C**) Computed tomographic scan showing large dependent pleural effusions. Lack of air bronchograms suggests this is in the pleural space and not in the lungs.

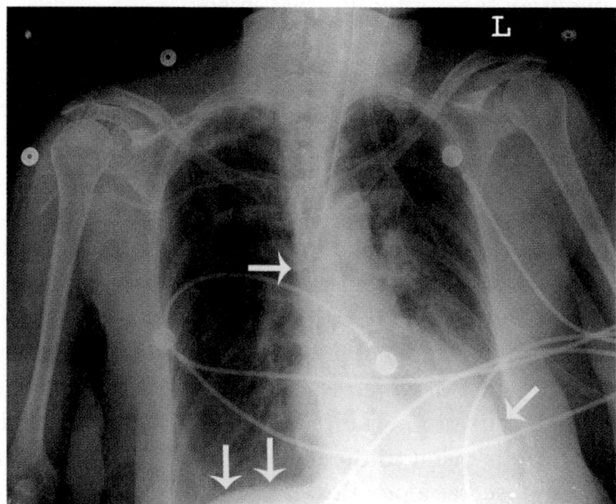

FIGURE 9–15 Right main stem intubation. Also note hyperinflation of right lung and atelectasis on left.

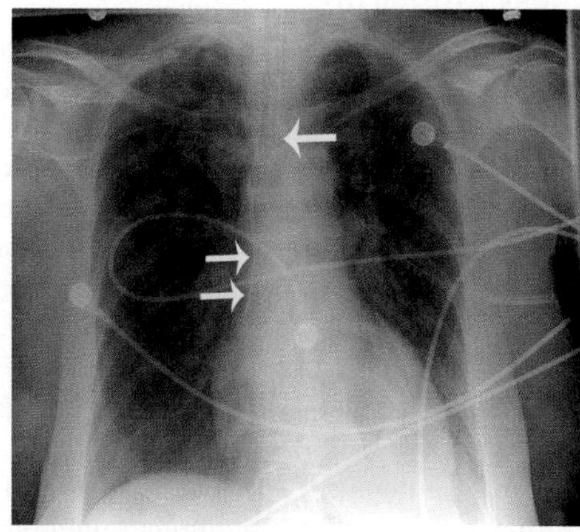

FIGURE 9–16 Endotracheal tube in good position (single arrow). Also note presence of central venous catheter (double arrows).

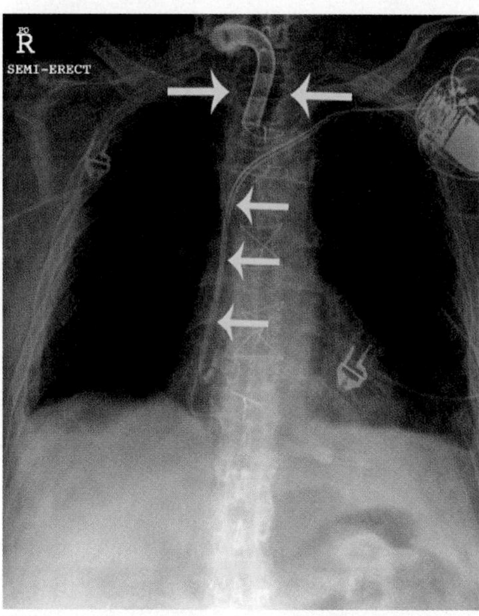

FIGURE 9–17 Tracheal dilation due to overinflation of the cuff of the tracheostomy tube. Also note the presence of a pacemaker. Lowered, flattened diaphragms suggest the presence of chronic obstructive pulmonary disease.

intubation occasionally occurs and should be considered when significant gastric distension is observed.

A tracheostomy tube should be midline, and optimal positioning of the tip is one-half to two-thirds of the distance between the stoma and the carina. After insertion of a tracheostomy tube, it is important to be certain that it is in the trachea and not inserted into a false track (**Figure 9–18**).

The tip and the side hole of a feeding tube should be beyond the gastroesophageal junction. Misplacement of the nasogastric tube into the airway may occur (**Figure 9–19**). Radiographic confirmation of feeding tube position is essential before use.[22]

Chest tubes have a radiopaque line that is interrupted by a side hole proximal to the tip, which should be seen medial to the inner margin of the ribs. The side hole should be within the pleural space to ensure proper drainage. Inadvertent insertion of the tube into the soft tissues may be suspected by silhouetting of the non-opaque wall of the tube within the adjacent soft tissue density. Normally, the nonopaque wall is rendered visible by surrounding lucent lung.[23] Optimal positioning of the

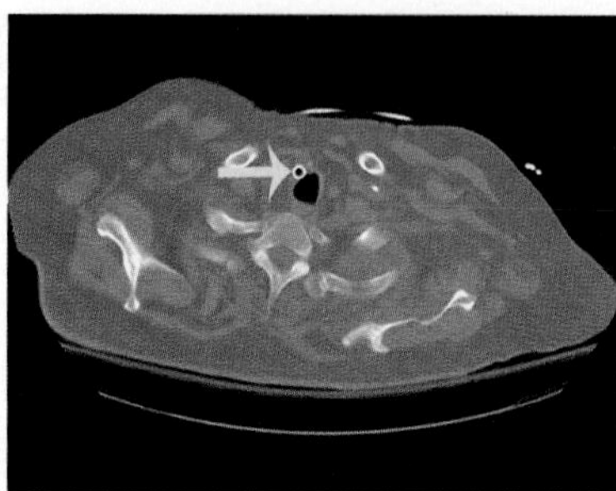

FIGURE 9–18 Computed tomographic scan showing tracheostomy tube in false track.

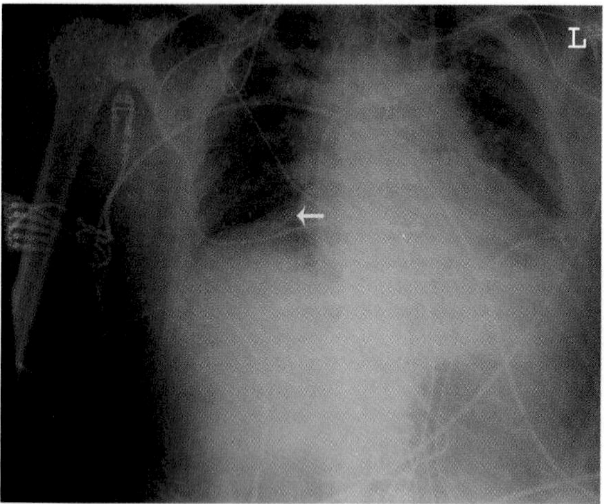

(A)

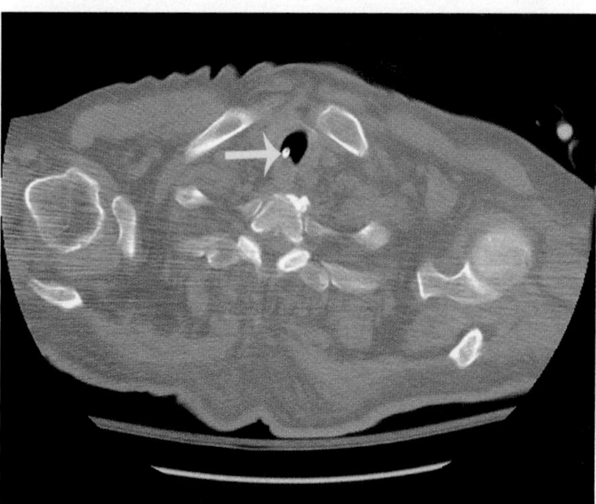

(B)

FIGURE 9–19 (A) Gastric tube in right lower lobe bronchus. (B) Computed tomographic scan showing gastric tube in trachea.

tube depends on whether the air or fluid collection is free or loculated within the pleural space. Intraparenchymal placement may be complicated by a bronchopleural fistula, pulmonary laceration, or hematoma. When a chest tube is inserted into the pulmonary parenchyma, a pulmonary contusion may be seen as an opacity near the chest tube. Placement into a fissure is associated with unsatisfactory drainage.[23,24]

Central venous catheters are inserted peripherally into upper extremity veins or, more commonly, into the subclavian or internal jugular vein. The optimal position of the distal tip of a central venous catheter is the junction of the brachiocephalic vein or superior vena cava, or just proximal to the right atrium in the superior vena cava. Common malpositions of central venous catheters include insertion into the internal mammary and azygous veins, or insertion into the internal jugular vein in the case of a subclavian catheter. A chest radiograph should be used to evaluate the possibility of hemothorax or pneumothorax after line placement.

The optimal position of a pulmonary artery catheter is the right or left pulmonary artery, approximately 5 cm distal to the bifurcation of the main pulmonary artery. Placement of the distal tip into the right ventricle predisposes to arrhythmias and myocardial perforation. Placement too distal in the pulmonary artery may result in pulmonary infarction, hemorrhage, or rupture of the pulmonary artery. The inflated cuff should never be seen on a radiographic study.

An intra-aortic balloon pump catheter is radiolucent, except for the tip, which is radiopaque to permit radiographic localization. The recommended position of the balloon tip is distal to the aortic knob.[25] The carina has been proposed as a practical landmark for positioning of the intra-aortic balloon pump.[26] If the balloon is too high, occlusion of the great vessels may result.

Pulmonary Embolism

Many patients with pulmonary embolism have abnormal chest radiographs. However, the findings are generally nonspecific and may be difficult to appreciate.[27] The most common findings are platelike or discoid atelectasis, peripheral airspace consolidation, and pleural effusion. Other less common abnormalities include enlargement of one or both pulmonary arteries secondary to large emboli, signs of right-sided heart failure, and hemidiaphragm elevation. Decreased vascularity in one lung causing a unilateral increase in radiographic lucency (**Westermark sign**) suggests the presence of a large pulmonary embolus.[28] A wedge-shaped peripheral infiltrate may be seen after a pulmonary embolus that occludes distal vessels in the pulmonary arterial tree (**Hampton hump**). Emboli in the ambulatory patient are more frequent in the lower lobes because of increased blood flow in this region.

Traditionally, the initial investigation of pulmonary embolism has relied on ventilation-perfusion scanning. However, contrast-enhanced spiral CT of the thorax is more sensitive and specific than radionuclide scanning for the detection of pulmonary embolism.[29] Resolution

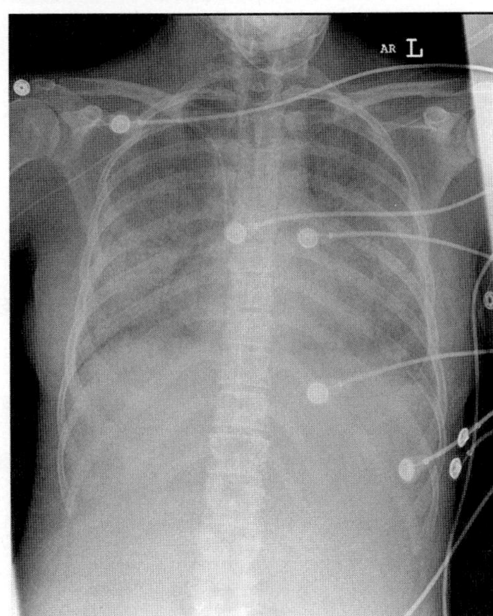

FIGURE 9–20 Anteroposterior projection of patient with severe acute respiratory distress syndrome.

occurs from the periphery, which has been described as the melting of an ice cube. Occasionally, cavitation from an ischemic necrosis or infection occurs during the course of resolution.

Acute Respiratory Distress Syndrome

The chest radiograph in acute respiratory distress syndrome (ARDS) has been traditionally characterized by bilateral diffuse infiltration of the lungs (**Figure 9–20**). The radiographic findings are often progressive, expanding from centrally located, poorly defined opacities to the periphery of the lung fields. The opacified areas often have a fluffy alveolar appearance that progresses to a patchy pattern. Eventually, a reticular pattern develops, and microabscesses with small cavities may become apparent. The CT reveals a gravity-dependent opacity with normal-appearing nondependent regions of the lungs.

Chest Trauma

Chest trauma may be associated with a number of abnormalities on the chest radiograph. These include broken ribs, chest contusion, pneumothorax, and hemothorax.

Cross-Sectional Imaging Techniques

Computed Tomography

The fundamental principle of computed tomography is to acquire multiple views of an object over a range of angular orientations.[1,7] By this means, additional dimensional data are obtained in comparison with conventional radiographs, in which there is only one view. The CT image is typically called a *slice*, which corresponds to a thickness of the object being scanned. Whereas a digital image is composed of pixels (picture elements), a CT slice image is composed of **voxels** (volume elements). The gray levels in a CT slice correspond to x-ray attenuation, which reflects the proportion of x-rays scattered or absorbed as they pass through each voxel.

> **RESPIRATORY RECAP**
>
> **Cross-Sectional Imaging Techniques**
> » Computed tomography
> » Ultrasonography
> » Magnetic resonance imaging
> » Positron emission tomography

A CT image is created by directing x-rays from multiple orientations and measuring their resultant decrease in intensity. A specialized algorithm is then used to reconstruct the distribution of x-ray densities in the slice plane. Medical systems generally use **Hounsfield units (HU)**, in which air is given a value of –1,000 and water is given a value of 0, causing most soft tissues to have values ranging from –100 to 100 and bone to range from 600 to over 2,000.[30] Conventional medical CT exams provide resolution on the order of 1 to 2 mm, whereas high-resolution instruments provide resolution on the order of 100 to 200 micrometers. Ultra-high-resolution instruments provide resolution on the order of a few tens of microns.

Cross-sectional CT images can be viewed in axial, sagittal, coronal, and oblique projections (**Figure 9–21**). New scanners have made it possible to scan the thorax in a single breath hold, thereby eliminating breathing artifact, with advances including high-resolution imaging for the evaluation of interstitial lung disease and a helical technique. Because CT provides exquisite anatomic detail of the thorax, it can be used for a number of different problems (**Figures 9–22 through 9–25**), including soft tissue or bony abnormalities, pleural abnormalities, lung parenchyma and interstitial disease, hilar or mediastinal pathology including the heart and great vessels, pulmonary embolism, and aortic dissection. CT is also useful to guide procedures such as drainage of pleural effusions or to assess the position of drainage catheters. Intravenous contrast, which can be useful for delineating vascular structures, is required in situations such as aortic dissection and the detection of pulmonary embolism. However, most CT studies of the thorax do not require IV contrast.

A portable chest radiograph may demonstrate a nonspecific area of consolidation. CT can reveal signs of volume loss not otherwise apparent, favoring the diagnosis of atelectasis over pneumonia. Pneumonia on CT is typically space-occupying, involving a lobe or part of a lobe and the presence of air bronchograms.[31] Air bronchograms are also seen with atelectasis, noninfectious lung inflammation, and in neoplastic etiologies, including bronchioloalveolar carcinoma and pulmonary lymphoma.

CT is the most accurate examination for detecting and characterizing pleural effusions. Pleural effusion can

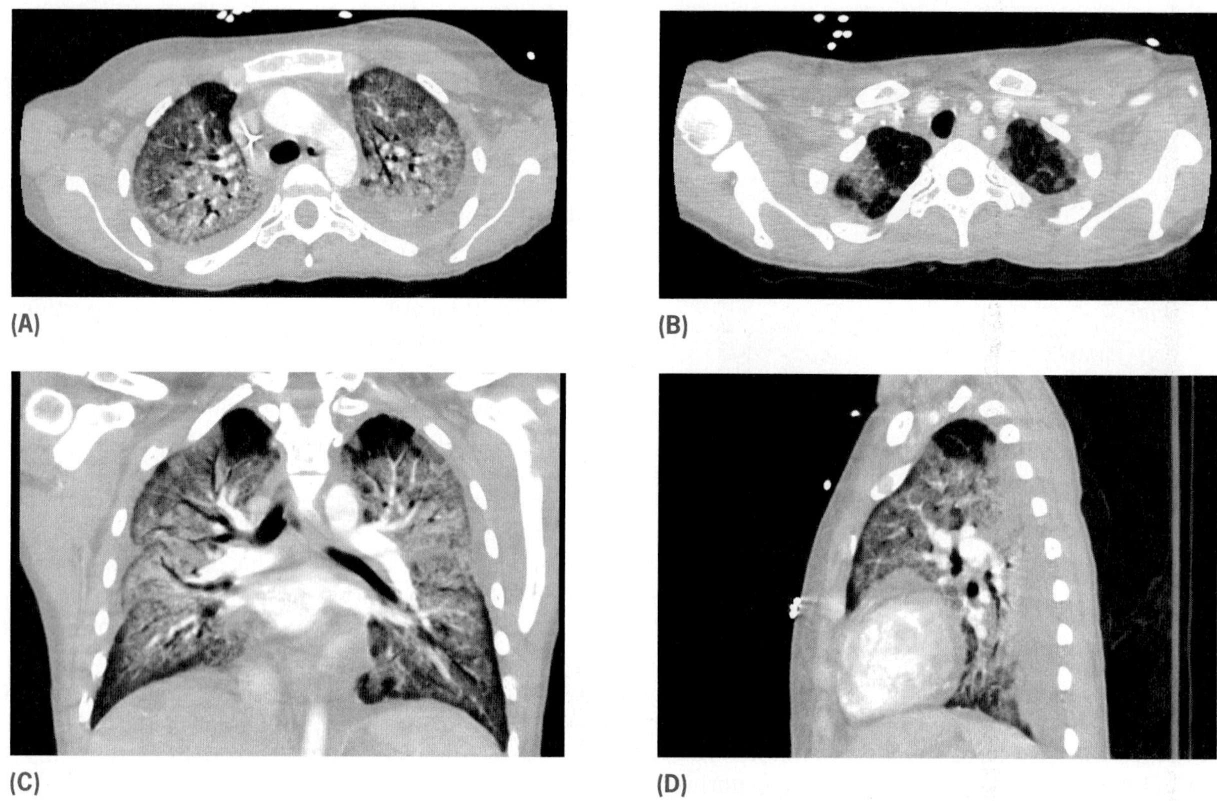

FIGURE 9–21 Computed tomographic scan of patient in Figure 9–20. (**A**) Axial image from mid-lung. (**B**) Axial image from apex. (**C**) Coronal reconstruction. (**D**) Sagittal reconstruction.

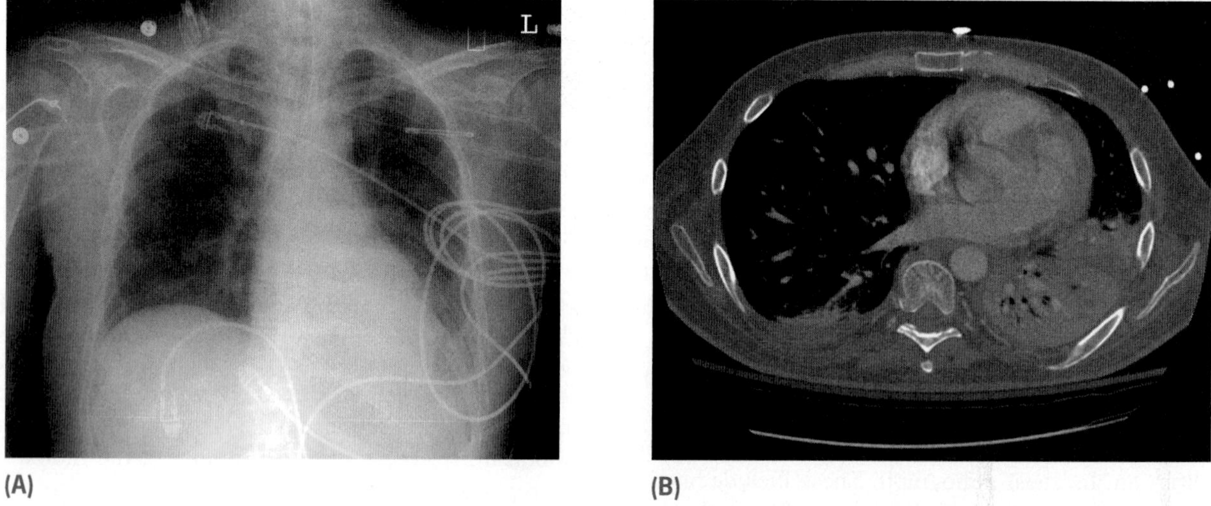

FIGURE 9–22 Left lower lobe pneumonia. (**A**) Note loss of diaphragm border on anteroposterior projection. (**B**) Computed tomography image. Note presence of air bronchograms, indicating that the abnormality is in the lung and not the pleural space.

be difficult to detect on a portable chest radiograph, and its appearance can mimic airspace consolidation. Thus, chest CT in many cases may be the only way to accurately assess the size of a pleural effusion. Small pleural effusions can be overlooked easily or be difficult to identify accurately on a supine portable chest radiograph. If an effusion is uncomplicated and free flowing, its appearance will differ with a change in patient position. Pneumothorax is missed frequently when interpreting the portable chest radiograph. CT may be helpful especially for evaluating loculated air collections and the proper location of chest tubes when a pneumothorax persists.

The older generation of CT scanners were very sensitive (85% to 90%) and specific (90%) in diagnosing central and subsegmental emboli,[32,33] but were less accurate in the detection of more peripheral clots. With newer multidetector CT scanners, however, small emboli to the subsegmental level can be diagnosed confidently.

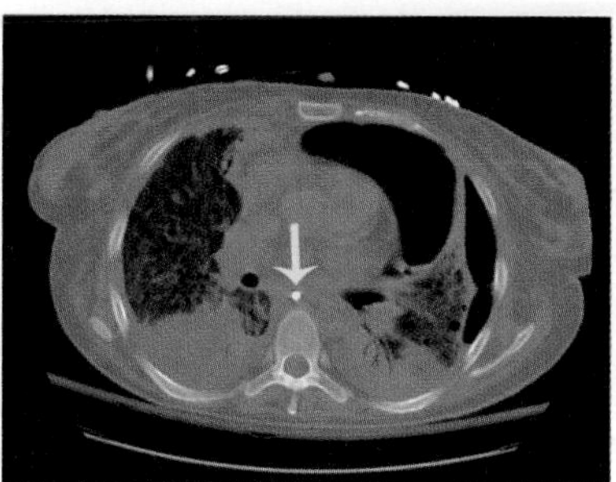

FIGURE 9–23 Computed tomography of the chest of a patient with right pleural effusion and left pneumothorax. Note that the pleural effusion is in the dependent thorax and the pneumothorax is in the nondependent thorax. Also note the air bronchograms in the left lower lobe and the gastric tube in the esophagus (arrow).

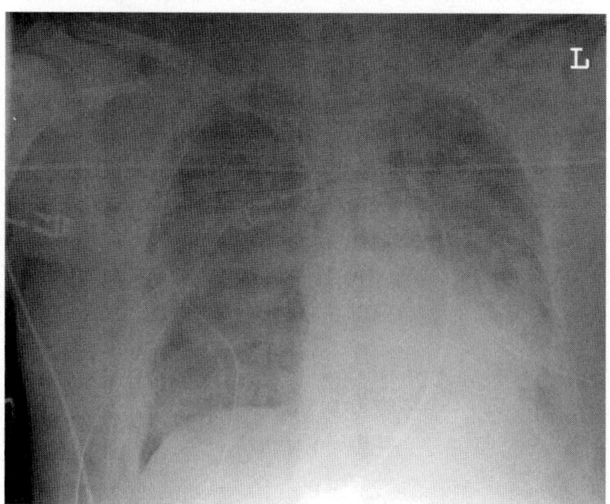

(A)

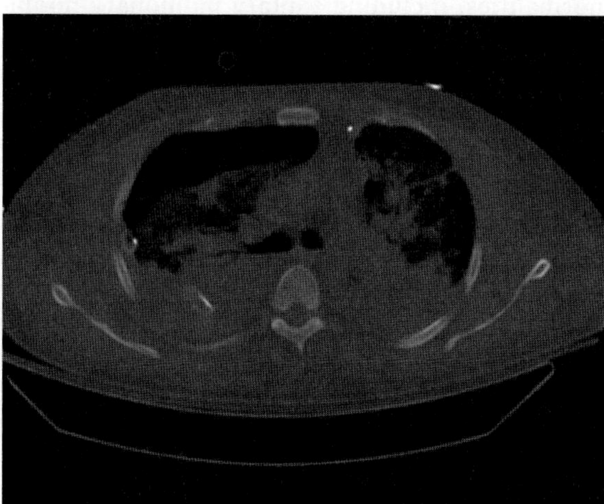

(B)

FIGURE 9–24 **(A)** Anteroposterior projection of patient with bilateral whiteout of the lung fields. **(B)** Computed tomography of the same patient showing large right-sided pneumothorax and dependent consolidation.

CT pulmonary angiography has reported sensitivities ranging from 53% to 100% and specificities of 83% to 100% when the examination is performed on the newer generation of CT scanners. The clinical validity of using a CT to rule out pulmonary embolism is similar to that reported for conventional pulmonary angiography.[33] A major advantage of CT compared with other diagnostic tests for pulmonary embolism is its ability to diagnose other potential causes of the patient's symptoms.

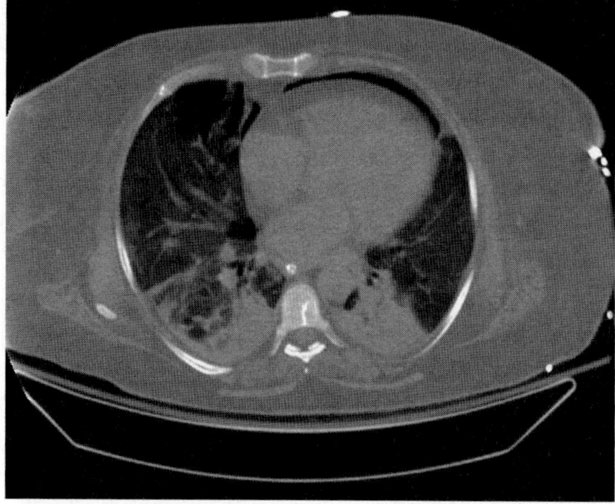

FIGURE 9–25 Computed tomographic scan showing dependent consolidation and pneumopericardium.

Ultrasonography

Ultrasonography is a diagnostic tool that provides a quick approach to assess the acutely ill patient and can be easily performed at bedside. This method has been introduced into the emergency department and subsequently into ICUs.[34] Pneumothorax, empyema, and pleural effusions are the most frequent processes studied.[35] Ultrasonography has expanded to include other less common pleural diseases as well as peripheral parenchymal lesions, mediastinal lesions, consolidation, and atelectasis.[36–41]

Ultrasound does not transmit through normal lung tissue due to characteristics of the pleura and an inability to penetrate air within the lungs. Instead, when the loss of aeration is massive, such as in lung consolidation or when a pleural effusion is present, ultrasound does adequately transmit. This characteristic makes it possible to visualize the magnitude of consolidation, estimate pleural effusion volume, and identify deep intrathoracic structures, such as cardiac fossa and great vessels.

The increasing availability of ultrasonography has improved the ability to diagnose, quantify, and safely drain pleural fluid accumulations at bedside.[37–39] The specificity and sensitivity of ultrasound for the diagnosis of pleural effusions are 93% and 97%, respectively.[37,40] If the pleural effusion is large enough to be compressive, the lung appears consolidated and floating on the pleural effusion. Ultrasonography can detect a pleural effusion as small as 100 mL in mechanically ventilated patients.[41] It can also be used to identify a pneumothorax.

Ultrasound guidance has been demonstrated to accommodate the insertion of central venous catheters, especially into the internal jugular vein. A systematic review showed a clear benefit from two-dimensional ultrasound guidance for central venous access compared with the landmark method.[42] This is manifest in a lower technical failure rate (overall and on first attempt), a reduction in complications, and faster access. Ultrasound has also been used for arterial cannulation (**Figure 9–26**).[43] The artery is distinguished from nearby veins due to the pulsating nature of the artery or by the use of color Doppler ultrasound. Ultrasound has been used to identify the radial, femoral, axillary, and dorsalis pedis arteries.

Magnetic Resonance Imaging

Magnetic resonance imaging (MRI) takes advantage of nuclear magnetic resonance, in which nuclei with odd numbers of protons and a magnetic moment become aligned when placed in a strong magnetic field. These protons then can be excited to a more energetic state with the addition of a radio-frequency pulse. Once allowed to relax, excited protons emit a resonance signal that reflects the number of protons and their nuclear environment. Different relaxation signals are generated depending on the pulse sequence, that is, the way in which the protons within the nuclei are excited. In the body, the greatest source of odd-number protons, that is, hydrogen nuclei, is used to create a resonance signal. Although some signals have features suggestive of a particular disease process, signal characteristics often are nonspecific.

Once a resonance signal has been generated, the information can be mathematically transformed to produce an image. MRI provides accurate anatomic detail of the thorax. Its current indications include soft tissue and bone marrow pathology, complicated pleural and diaphragmatic diseases, hilar and mediastinal abnormalities (including congenital heart disease, cardiac abnormalities, and vascular pathology), pulmonary embolism, and aortic dissection.

Although MRI often is complementary to CT, it has several advantages. Patients with renal dysfunction often are better served by MRI because intravenous contrast, which can be nephrotoxic, usually is not required. MRI has several other disadvantages, including limited patient monitoring capabilities and motion artifacts caused by cardiac and respiratory motion, which can obscure the images. MRI is contraindicated in patients with cardiac pacemakers. Despite these limitations, MRI offers information not available from other modalities. In addition, MRI, unlike CT, uses no ionizing radiation.

Positron Emission Tomography

The newest imaging modality, **positron emission tomography (PET)**, has become a recognized tool for the assessment of thoracic pathologic processes, particularly for tumor imaging. Previous PET investigations were performed almost exclusively on the brain, but now some of the same principles have been applied to thoracic abnormalities. Unlike CT and MRI, PET provides physiologic and metabolic information. This test, which focuses on the biochemical properties of cells, has the ability to analyze abnormalities quantitatively. Currently, the positron emitting agent most commonly used in the thorax is F18-fluorodeoxyglucose (FDG). Metabolically active cells take up and trap this D-glucose analogue. The activity then can be measured and mapped to a specific region within the thorax. Data from multiple studies demonstrate that more metabolically active tumor cells show increased FDG uptake compared with normal tissues or a benign process.

Indications for PET imaging of the thorax include distinguishing benign and malignant focal pulmonary abnormalities, including solitary pulmonary nodules, staging lung cancer, and differentiating fibrosis from tumor in patients treated for lung cancer. PET imaging has a sensitivity of approximately 95% for the detection of cancer in patients who have indeterminate lesions on CT. The specificity of 85% with PET in these lesions is less than the sensitivity because some inflammatory

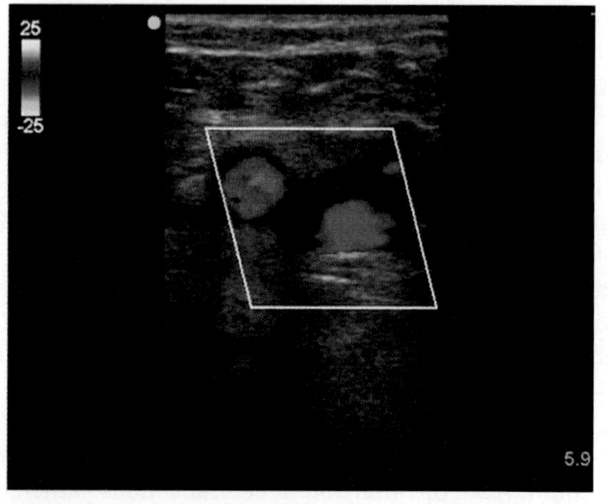

(A)

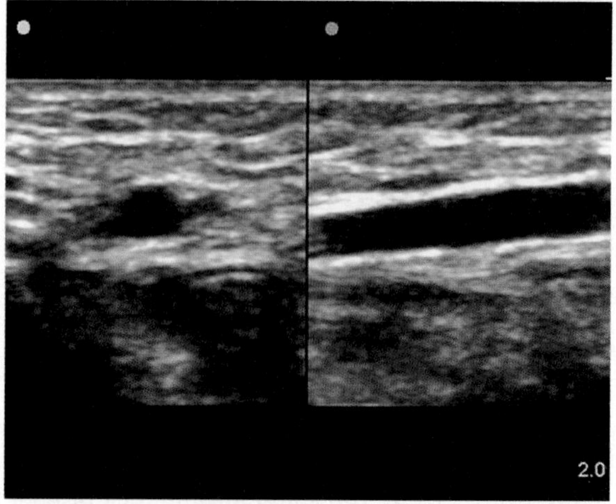

(B)

FIGURE 9–26 (**A**) Femoral artery and vein: color Doppler ultrasound. (**B**) Radial artery in transverse and longitudinal orientations.

processes, such as granulomatous infection, avidly accumulate FDG. PET is more accurate than CT in determination of the presence or absence of intrathoracic metastatic nodal disease. Intrathoracic and extrathoracic disease can be staged in a single examination with whole-body PET. This allows the detection of occult metastasis. PET is most useful in the management of cancer patients, and its role in critically ill patients is limited.

KEY POINTS

- Structures are seen on the chest radiograph due to density and contrast.
- Positions used for chest radiography include anteroposterior, posteroanterior, lateral decubitus, and apical lordotic.
- The chest radiograph displays anatomic and pathophysiologic features for determining the presence of disorders in the thorax.
- The location and size of abnormal air or fluid pockets within the chest can be evaluated by chest radiography.
- The proper positioning of tubes and catheters is determined by chest radiography.
- The multiple slices of computed tomography provide three-dimensional viewing of the thorax.
- Computed tomography improves the ability to discriminate pneumonia versus atelectasis as well as the location and extent of an effusion or pulmonary emboli.
- Ultrasonography has become useful in vascular cannulation, central venous catheter placements, and bedside assessment of pleural diseases including the presence of air or fluid.
- Magnetic resonance imaging is indicated for detection of soft tissue pathology that includes complicated pleural and diaphragmatic diseases as well as hilar and mediastinal abnormalities.
- Positron emission tomography is indicated for monitoring thoracic pathologic processes, particularly tumor imaging.

REFERENCES

1. Seibert A. X-ray imaging physics for nuclear medicine technologists. Part 1. Basic principles of x-ray production. *J Nucl Med Technol.* 2004;32:139–147.
2. McCollough C. The AAPM/RSNA physics tutorial for residents X-ray production. *Radiographics.* 1997;17:967–984.
3. Seibert A, Boone JM. X-ray imaging physics for nuclear medicine technologists. Part 2. X-ray interactions and image formation. *J Nucl Med Technol.* 2005;33:3–18.
4. McAdams HP, Samei E, Dobbins J III, et al. Recent advances in chest radiography. *Radiology.* 2008;241:663–683.
5. Brant WE, Helms CA. *Fundamentals of Diagnostic Radiology.* 2nd ed. Philadelphia: Lippincott Williams & Wilkins; 1999.
6. Siela D. Chest x-ray evaluation and interpretation. *AACN Adv Crit Care.* 2008;19:444–473.
7. Hill JR, Horner PE, Primack SL. ICU imaging. *Clin Chest Med.* 2008;29:59–76.
8. Dennie CJ, Coblentz CL. The trachea: normal features, imaging and causes of displacement. *Can Assoc Radiol J.* 1993;44:81–89.
9. Ellis H. The ribs and intercostal spaces. *Anaesthesia Intensive Care Med.* 2008;9:518–519.
10. Ottenheijm AC, Heunks L. Diaphragm muscle fiber dysfunction in chronic obstructive pulmonary disease: toward a pathophysiological concept. *Am J Respir Crit Care Med.* 2007;175:1233–1240.
11. Seow A, Kazerooni EA, Pernicano PG, Neary M. Comparison of upright inspiratory and expiratory chest radiographs for detecting pneumothoraces. *AJR Am J Roentgenol.* 1997;168:842–843.
12. Baron MJ. The cardiac silhouette. *J Thorac Imaging.* 2000;15:230–242.
13. Bruzzi JF, Rémy-Jardin M, Delhaye D, et al. When, why, and how to examine the heart during thoracic CT. Part 1, basic principles. *AJR Am J Roentgenol.* 2006;186:324–332.
14. Whitten CR, Khan S, Munneke GJ, Grubnic S. A diagnostic approach to mediastinal abnormalities. *Radiographics.* 2007;27:657–661.
15. Shevland JE, Hirleman MT, Hoang KA, et al. Lobar collapse in the surgical intensive care unit. *Br J Radiology.* 1983;56:531–534.
16. Tripp HF, Bolton JW. Phrenic nerve injury following cardiac surgery: a review. *J Card Surg.* 1998;13:218–223.
17. Unger JM, England DM, Bogust GA. Interstitial emphysema in adults: recognition and prognostic implications. *J Thorac Imaging.* 1989;4:86–94.
18. Carlton RR, Adler AM. *Principles of Radiographic Imaging: An Art and a Science.* 3rd ed. Albany, NY: Delmar Thomson Learning; 2000.
19. Spillane RM, Shepard JO, Deluca SA. Radiographic aspects of pneumothorax. *Am Fam Physician.* 1995;51:459–464.
20. Kong A. The deep sulcus sign. *Radiology.* 2003;228:415–416.
21. Ramez M, Salem MD. Verification of endotracheal tube position. *Anesthesiol Clin North Am.* 2001;19:813–839.
22. Lee J, Eve R, Bennett MJ. Evaluation of a technique for blind placement of post-pyloric feeding tubes in intensive care: application in patients with gastric ileus. *Intensive Care Med.* 2006;32:553–556.
23. Webb WR, Godwin JD. The obscured outer edge: a sign of improperly placed pleural drainage tubes. *Am J Roentgenol.* 1980;131:1062–1064.
24. Mauser JR, Friedman PJ, Wing VW. Thoracostomy tube in an interlobar fissure: radiologic recognition of a potential problem. *Am J Roentgenol.* 1982;139:1155–1161.
25. Attili A, Kazerooni E. Postoperative cardiopulmonary thoracic imaging. *Radiol Clin North Am.* 2004;42:543–564.
26. Kim JT, Lee JR, Kim JK, et al. The carina as a useful radiographic landmark for positioning the intraaortic balloon pump. *Anesth Analg.* 2007;105:735–738.
27. Bounameaux H, Righini M, Perrier A. Venous thromboembolism: contemporary diagnostic and therapeutic aspects. *Vasa.* 2008;37:211–226.
28. Westermark N. On the roentgen diagnosis of lung embolism. *Acta Radiol.* 1938;19:357.
29. Michiels JJ, Gadisseur A, Van Der Planken M, et al. A critical appraisal of non-invasive diagnosis and exclusion of deep vein thrombosis and pulmonary embolism in outpatients with suspected deep vein thrombosis or pulmonary embolism: how many tests do we need? *Int Angiol.* 2005;24:27–39.
30. Hounsfield GN. Nobel Award address. Computed medical imaging. *Med Phys.* 1980;7:283–390.
31. Goodman LR. *Felson's Principles of Chest Roentgenology: A Programmed Text.* 3rd ed. Philadelphia: Saunders Elsevier; 2007.
32. Roach PJ, Bailey DL, Harris BE. Enhancing lung scintigraphy with single-photon emission computed tomography. *Semin Nucl Med.* 2008;38:441–449.
33. Quiroz R, Kucher N, Zou KH, et al. Clinical validity of a negative computed tomography scan in patients with suspected pulmonary embolism: a systematic review. *JAMA.* 2005;293:2012–2017.

34. Bouhemad B, Zhang M, Lu Q, Rouby JJ. Clinical review: bedside lung ultrasound in critical care practice. *Crit Care.* 2007;11:205.
35. Overfors C, Hedgecock MW. Intensive care unit radiology: problems of interpretation. *Radiol Clin North Am.* 1978;16:407–409
36. Yang PC, Luh KT, Sheu JC, et al. Peripheral pulmonary lesions: ultrasonography and ultrasonically guided aspiration biopsy. *Radiology.* 1985;155:451–456.
37. Lichtenstein D, Goldstein I, Mourgeon E, et al. Comparative diagnostic performances of auscultation, chest radiography, and lung ultrasonography in acute respiratory distress syndrome. *Anesthesiology.* 2004;100:9–15.
38. Vignon P, Chastagner C, Berkane V, et al. Quantitative assessment of pleural effusion in critically ill patients by means of ultrasonography. *Crit Care Med.* 2005;33:1757–1763.
39. Mayo PH, Goltz HR, Tafreshi M, Doelken P. Safety of ultrasound-guided thoracentesis in patients receiving mechanical ventilation. *Chest.* 2004;125:1059–1062.
40. Lichtenstein D, Hulot JS, Rabiller A, et al. Feasibility and safety of ultrasound-aided thoracocentesis in mechanically ventilated patients. *Intensive Care Med.* 1999;25:955–958.
41. Eibenberger K, Dock W, Ammann M, et al. Quantifications of pleural effusions: sonography versus radiography. *Radiology.* 1994;191:681–684.
42. Hind D, Calvert N, McWilliams R, et al. Ultrasonic locating devices for central venous cannulation: meta-analysis. *BMJ.* 2003;327(7411):361.
43. Shiloh AL, Eisen LA. Ultrasound-guided arterial catheterization: a narrative review. *Intensive Care Med.* 2010;36:214–221.

SUGGESTED READING

Collins J, Stern EJ. *Chest Radiology: The Essentials.* 2nd ed. Philadelphia: Lippincott Williams & Wilkins; 2008.

CHAPTER 10

Pulmonary Function Testing

Ellen Cannefax
Paul Enright

OUTLINE

Goals of Pulmonary Function Testing
Spirometry
Lung Volumes and Capacities
Diffusing Capacity
Specialized Pulmonary Function Tests

OBJECTIVES

1. Describe the clinical use of pulmonary function tests.
2. Identify the features of normal and abnormal spirometry tracings.
3. Recognize the common errors seen in spirometry testing.
4. Specify the spirometry values seen in patients with normal lungs, obstructive disease, and restrictive disorders.
5. Explain the importance of spirometry testing before and after administering a bronchodilator.
6. Recognize upper airway obstruction.
7. State the purpose of complete pulmonary function testing.
8. Define lung volumes and capacities.
9. Compare methods used to measure functional residual capacity.
10. Discuss the American Thoracic Society's standards for pulmonary function testing.
11. Explain the importance of diffusing capacity.
12. List the goals of bronchial challenge testing, airways resistance, and tests of respiratory muscle strength.

KEY TERMS

airways resistance
body plethysmography
diffusing capacity
helium dilution
hyperinflation
lung volumes
maximum expiratory pressure
maximum inspiratory pressure
nitrogen washout
obstructive lung disease
pulmonary function tests (PFTs)
restrictive lung disease
spirometer
spirometry
total lung capacity
vital capacity

INTRODUCTION

Pulmonary function tests (PFTs) are a primary diagnostic tool for evaluating patients complaining of shortness of breath or intermittent wheezing and for management of such patients' diagnosed lung disease. The first lung function test, vital capacity, was invented in the 1840s to assess lung size (volume) in patients with consumption (tuberculosis, or TB). Patients with TB who had a low vital capacity lived for shorter periods of time compared to those with a higher vital capacity. Since 1950, the most common use of pulmonary function testing has been the assessment of obstructive lung diseases, such as asthma and chronic obstructive pulmonary disease (COPD). Cigarette smokers with lower lung function due to COPD have higher rates of morbidity and mortality. PFTs have a long, rich history, and the tests performed regularly are relatively well standardized. Spirometry is done in many settings, but tests that require expensive instruments are usually done in a hospital-based PFT laboratory. This chapter describes patient testing guidelines and the parameters commonly measured in a PFT laboratory.

Goals of Pulmonary Function Testing

Pulmonary function tests (PFTs) provide valuable information about the presence of ventilatory defects and their effect on gas exchange, the degree of lung impairment, and patients' responsiveness to therapy. Like most medical tests, the results of PFTs often change the pretest probability of a disease but do not make the diagnosis by themselves. Unlike most medical tests, in which the patient may remain passive, most PFTs require complex and sometimes athletic-like breathing maneuvers. Submaximal efforts often cause errors in the measurements, so respiratory therapists performing spirometry and other PFTs must have training and experience. The training of personnel conducting the tests should meet minimal criteria as recommended by the American Thoracic Society (ATS).

> **RESPIRATORY RECAP**
>
> **Goals of Pulmonary Function Testing**
>
> » Detecting airflow limitation
> » Detecting restriction
> » Detecting impaired gas transfer abnormalities
> » Respiratory muscle weakness

The primary goal of PFTs is the detection of restrictive and/or obstructive lung defects, the gas transfer abnormalities that accompany some restrictive and some obstructive lung diseases, and respiratory muscle weakness. **Restrictive lung disease** is detected by measurement of reduced lung volumes, whereas **obstructive lung disease** causes airflow limitation (a reduced flow of air out of the lungs due to narrow airways).

Spirometry

Spirometry is the most commonly performed PFT. The importance of spirometry has been emphasized by at least three major initiatives to diagnose and treat obstructive lung disease: the National Lung Health Education Program (NLHEP), the Global Initiative for Chronic Obstructive Lung Disease (GOLD), and the Global Initiative for Asthma (GINA). **Box 10–1** lists the most common clinical indications for spirometry.

Equipment

Spirometers can be categorized by their measurement method. In the 1950s, spirometers measured exhaled volume by accumulating exhaled air inside a cylindrical canister. Volume-sensing spirometers, such as water-sealed or dry-rolling seal models, maintain a high accuracy for many years, but are large, difficult to clean, and require leak checks, so they were largely replaced by flow-sensing spirometers in the 1990s. Flow can be measured by several methods, including a turbine, a laminar flow element (Fleisch pneumotachometer), a Pitot tube, a metal or fiber screen, heated wires, a vane that bends, or an ultrasonic flow sensor. Some models are relatively inaccurate at low and very high flows, and some become inaccurate when clogged by exhaled secretions or condensed moisture. Many use single-patient, disposable mouthpieces or filters. As is true with most other electronic devices, the size and cost of spirometers has declined while their ease of use and functionality has improved. **Figure 10–1** shows an example of a modern portable spirometer. Pocket spirometers, which cost less than $100, are now widely available for screening, although most spirometers used in a PFT lab remain connected to personal computers and cost more than $2000.

The ATS has established guidelines for equipment selection and maintenance (**Box 10–2**). Precision and

> **BOX 10–1**
>
> **Indications for a Spirometry Test**
>
> **Diagnostic**
> - Evaluate symptoms, signs, or abnormal laboratory tests
> - Measure effect of disease on pulmonary function
> - Screen individuals at risk of having pulmonary disease (e.g., smokers over 40)
> - Assess preoperative risk and/or health status prior to exercise program
>
> **Monitoring**
> - Assess the change in lung function over time or after administration of or change in therapy
> - Monitor for adverse reactions to drugs with known pulmonary toxicity
> - Assess the potential effects of environmental or occupational exposures
>
> **Disability**
> - Assess impairment or disability from lung disease
> - Assess risks as part of insurance evaluation
>
> **Public Health**
> - Epidemiologic surveys
> - Derivation of reference equations
> - Clinical research
>
> Adapted from Miller MR, Hankinson J, Brusasco V, et al. ATS/ERS Task Force: standardisation of spirometry. *Eur Respir J.* 2005;26:319–338. Reprinted with permission.

accuracy are key to obtaining reliable test data. In addition, equipment must have the capacity, linearity, and output for measuring lung parameters. **Table 10–1** summarizes the ATS quality control criteria. Once equipment selection has been made, a quality assurance program should be implemented to ensure that minimal ATS standards are met (**Box 10–3**). The respiratory therapist is responsible for maintaining a log of staff competency, equipment performance, policies and procedures, and reporting guidelines. Medical decisions are made on the basis of a PFT report, and it is the responsibility of the respiratory therapist to ensure reliable results.

Pretest Procedures

To determine predicted values, measure the patient's standing height and abdominal size (or weight). Also determine age, gender, and race or ethnicity. These are necessary because predicted reference values are determined according to the person's age, height, sex, and race. Height is the most important factor in determining lung size and is measured in stocking feet. For persons with spinal deformities (e.g., kyphoscoliosis), the arm span measurement from fingertip to fingertip is used to estimate height without the spinal deformity (**Figure 10–2**). Abdominal obesity (best measured by waist circumference) commonly causes a reduction in forced vital capacity. For a given height and age, healthy males have larger lung volumes than healthy females. Finally, lung function has been shown to differ among races.

> **RESPIRATORY RECAP**
>
> **Pretest Procedures**
>
> » Calculate reference values using age, height, gender, and race.
>
> » Ascertain the patient's pulmonary history and the number of hours since the patient inhaled a bronchodilator.

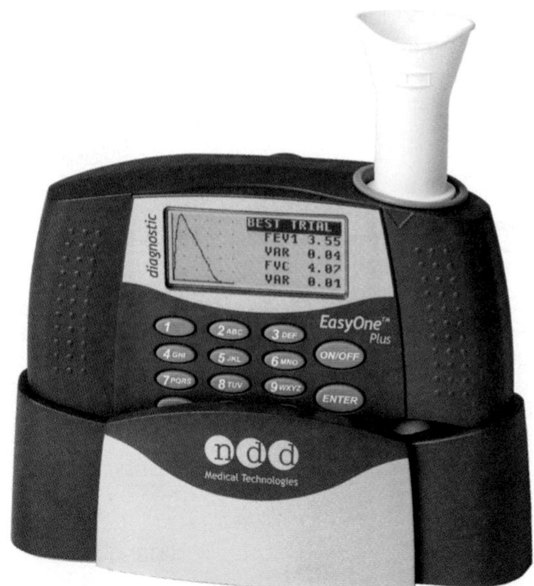

FIGURE 10–1 One of many modern models of portable spirometers that measure air flow. This model measures flow through the disposable white breathing tube using an ultrasonic Doppler technique. A microprocessor converts flow to FEV_1 and FVC.

TABLE 10–1 Quality Control for Spirometers

Test	Minimum Interval	Action
Volume	Daily	Calibration check with a 3-L syringe
Leak	Daily	3 cm H_2O (0.3 kPa) constant pressure for 1 minute
Volume linearity	Quarterly	1-L increments with a calibrating syringe
Flow linearity	Weekly	Test at least three different flow ranges
Time	Quarterly	Mechanical recorder check with stopwatch
Software	New versions	Log installation date and perform test using known subject

Note: The leak, volume linearity, and time checks only apply to volume-sensing spirometers. From Miller MR, Hankinson J, Brusasco V, et al. ATS/ERS Task Force: standardisation of spirometry. *Eur Respir J.* 2005;26:319–338, Table 3. Reprinted with permission.

BOX 10–2

Performance Standards for Spirometers

1. Volume accuracy must be within 3% (using a 3-L calibration syringe).
2. FEV_1 and FVC must be corrected to BTPS conditions.
3. A calibration check using a 3-L syringe is required daily.
4. Volumes up to 8 L and flows up to 14 L/s must be measured.
5. Both a volume–time and flow–volume curve must be printed on the report.
6. The highest FEV_1 and the highest FVC should be reported.

FEV_1, forced expiratory volume in 1 second; FVC, forced vital capacity; BTPS, body temperature and pressure saturated.

BOX 10–3

Quality Assurance of Spirometry

Volume verification (calibration): at least daily prior to testing, use a calibrated known-volume syringe with a volume of at least 3 L to ascertain that the spirometer reads a known volume accurately. The known volume should be injected and/or withdrawn at least three times, at flows that vary between 2 and 12 L/s (3-L injection times of approximately 1 second, 6 seconds, and somewhere between 1 and 6 seconds). The tolerance limits for an acceptable calibration are ±3.5% of the known volume. Thus, for a 3-L calibration syringe, the acceptable recovered range is 2.90 to 3.11 L. We encourage the practitioner to exceed this guideline whenever possible (i.e., reduce the tolerance limits to less than ±3.5%).

Leak test: volume-displacement spirometers must be evaluated for leaks daily.

Manual: a spirometry procedure manual should be maintained.

Log: a log that documents daily instrument calibration, problems encountered, corrective action required, and system hardware and/or software changes should be maintained.

Calculation verifications: computer software for measurement and computer calculations should be checked against manual calculations. In addition, biologic laboratory standards (i.e., healthy, nonsmoking individuals) can be tested periodically to ensure historic reproducibility, to verify software upgrades, and to evaluate new or replacement spirometers.

Syringe verification: the known-volume syringe should be checked for accuracy at least quarterly using a second known-volume syringe.

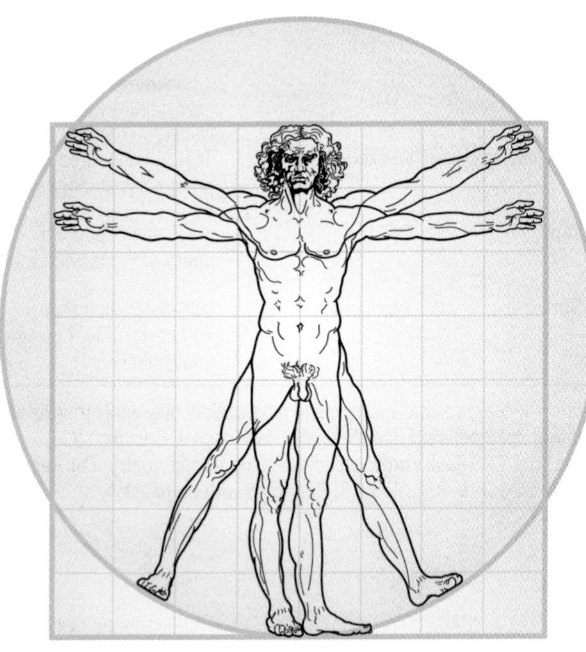

FIGURE 10–2 Height is approximately equal to arm span in healthy individuals.

The pulmonary history should include current medications, known respiratory disease, cough, allergies, chest surgeries, and occupational exposures. The number of hours since the patient inhaled a bronchodilator should be determined.

The ordering physician may ask the patient to withhold some respiratory medications before spirometry testing (**Table 10–2**). It is imperative for testing personnel to explain each test clearly and concisely and then to demonstrate the correct breathing maneuvers before the patient tries them.

TABLE 10–2 Withholding Medications Before Spirometry (Optional)

Medication	Time to Withhold
Albuterol	4 hours
Long-acting β-agonists	12 hours
Slow-release methylxanthines	24 hours
Ipratropium	4 hours
Tiotropium	24 hours
Inhaled steroids	Maintain dosage

Modified from Ruppel GL. *Manual of Pulmonary Function Testing*. 9th ed. St. Louis: Mosby; 2009: Table 2–2. Reprinted with permission.

Spirometry Tests

Most spirometers can perform four types of breathing tests. The most common is the forced vital capacity (FVC) test, for which the patient exhales rapidly into the spirometer. A forced inspiratory vital capacity (FIVC) can also be measured by many spirometers. When the FIVC is measured at the end of each FVC maneuver, a flow–volume loop is produced. The slow vital capacity (SVC) measures the vital capacity (VC) during a slow and deep inhalation. Less frequently, a maximal voluntary

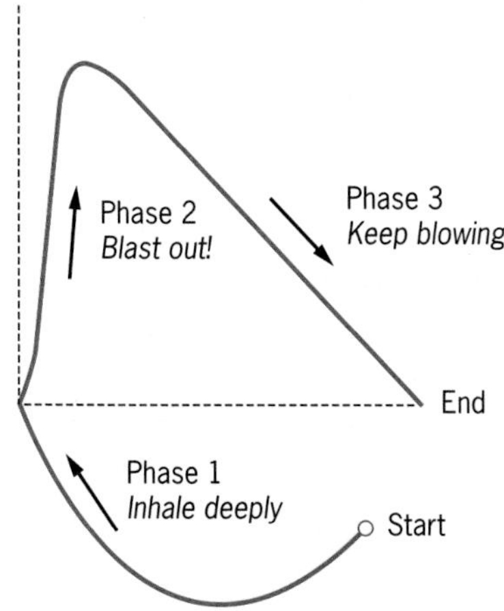

FIGURE 10–3 The forced vital capacity test consists of three breathing maneuvers performed in sequence.

ventilation (MVV) test can be performed with rapid breathing over 12 to 15 seconds using a flow-sensing spirometer.

FVC tests may be performed sitting or standing; however, sitting is recommended to avoid falling due to syncope. Three breathing maneuvers are performed during FVC tests, as shown in **Figure 10–3**. The first phase, a maximally deep inhalation, often is done before the patient inserts the disposable mouthpiece into his or her mouth. The second phase lasts for only one-tenth of a second as the respiratory therapist loudly coaches the patient to "blast out the air." The third phase is continued exhalation for several seconds.

FVC and FEV_1 are reported in liters at body temperature and pressure saturated (BTPS), which is the condition of the air in the lungs before it is exhaled and cools toward room temperature. The BTPS calculation is done automatically by multiplying the measurements by a temperature correction factor.

RESPIRATORY RECAP

Spirometry Technique

» The FVC maneuver is the most basic and commonly performed PFT.
» Skilled instruction, coaching, and feedback are needed to avoid errors.
» The FVC and FEV_1 must be from three acceptable and repeatable maneuvers.

The validity of numeric spirometry results depends largely on the cooperation and effort of the patient. For the results to be valid, the therapist must follow the ATS guidelines for acceptability and repeatability (**Figure 10–4** and **Box 10–4**). For a test to be *acceptable,* it must be performed at least three times in the appropriate manner and be free from artifact. To be *repeatable,* efforts obtained must be in close agreement with each other (within 0.15 L). Both the flow–volume and volume–time graphs for each maneuver should be reviewed for quality and repeatability (**Figure 10–5**). Because some patients may not be able to achieve acceptable end-of-test criteria, FVC and FEV_1

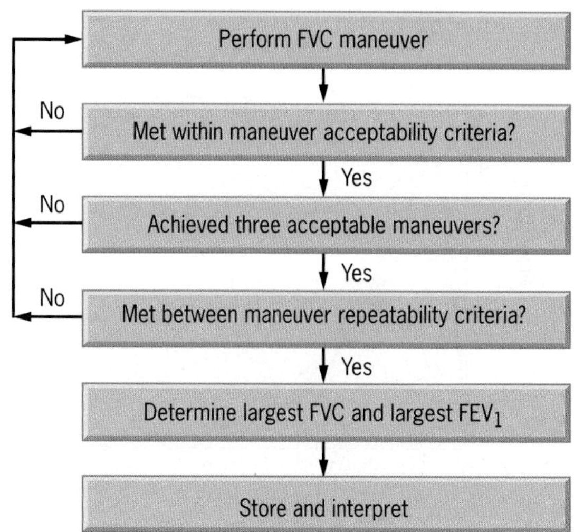

FIGURE 10–4 The American Thoracic Society's acceptability algorithm. FVC, forced vital capacity; FEV_1, forced expiratory volume in 1 second. From Miller MR, Hankinson J, Brusasco V, et al. ATS/ERS Task Force: standardisation of spirometry. *Eur Respir J.* 2005; 26: 319–338, Figure 3. Reprinted with permission.

BOX 10–4

American Thoracic Society Spirometry Quality Goals

Acceptability Criteria

Individual spirometry maneuvers are "acceptable" if they are free from all of the following conditions:

1. Slow start
2. A cough in the first second
3. Early termination*
4. A Valsalva maneuver (glottis closure)
5. A leak
6. An obstructed mouthpiece
7. Evidence of an extra breath

Repeatability Criteria

The difference between the largest and the next largest FVC is 0.150 L or less

The difference between the largest and the next largest FEV_1 is 0.150 L or less

No more than eight maneuvers should be attempted

Adapted from Miller MR, Hankinson J, Brusasco V, et al. ATS/ERS Task Force: standardisation of spirometry. *Eur Respir J.* 2005;26:319–338.

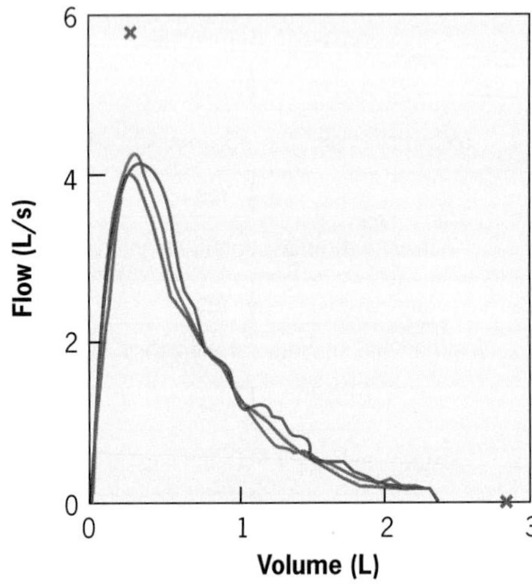

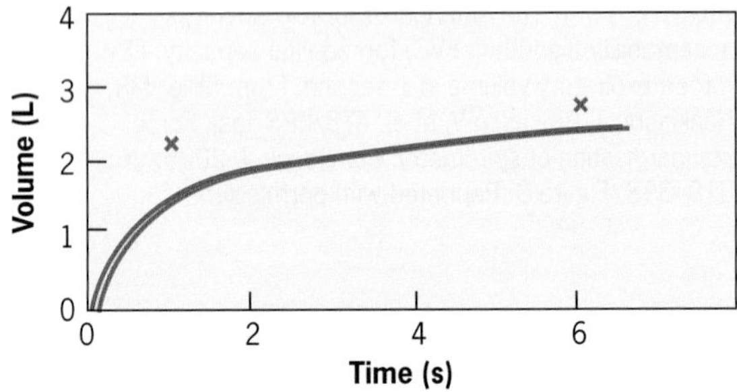

FIGURE 10–5 These two graphs were produced by the same forced vital capacity (FVC) maneuver. The top flow–volume curve enables easy recognition of poor efforts during the first second of the maneuver, and the patterns of obstruction. The blue Xs indicate predicted normal values. Multiple FVC maneuvers are usually superimposed on the same graph, in order to recognize the repeatability of the patterns. From the volume–time graph (spirogram), volumes at specific time intervals are easily identified, such as the important FEV_1 (at 1 second) and the FEV_6 (at 6 seconds). The volume–time curve also allows examination of the duration of the tracing and whether a plateau is achieved (indicating maximal exhalation).

may be measured from curves with an acceptable start of test and without cough or artifact in the first second. Curves obtained using these criteria are referred to as useable curves.

Vital capacity measured without a forced effort is called the slow vital capacity (SVC), or relaxed vital capacity. In many patients with airflow limitation, the SVC provides a larger, more accurate determination of the VC than the FVC. The difference between SVC and FVC is due to increased trapping of air in the lungs when the effort is forced. The FVC value in comparison with predicted values is most commonly examined in routine spirometry testing as an indicator of a restrictive process. FEV_6 has been introduced as an acceptable replacement for FVC that avoids prolonged expiratory efforts.

> **RESPIRATORY RECAP**
>
> **FEV_1/FVC Ratio**
>
> » A decreased ratio indicates airflow obstruction
>
> » A reduced FVC with a normal ratio suggests restriction.

FEV_1 is the volume of air exhaled in the first second of the FVC maneuver and is the most commonly measured (and most clinically important) PFT. The normal value for FEV_1 is predicted from the subject's height, age, gender, and race. A low FEV_1/FVC ratio detects airway obstruction, and a low FEV_1 measures the severity of the airway obstruction. In the normal adult, this ratio ranges from 0.75 to 0.85; after age 30 years, this ratio decreases with aging (**Figure 10–6**). The ratio is a sensitive and reliable indicator of airway obstruction and is valuable in identifying the cause of a low FEV_1.

Other Spirometry Numbers

The FEV_1, FVC, and their ratio are the most important spirometry results, but many spirometers also report other parameters, such as various forced expiratory flow (FEF) measures (e.g., $FEF_{25-75\%}$, FEF_{50}, FEF_{75}). These may help determine the quality of the expiratory effort, but do not provide clinically important information. (See **Figure 10–7**.)

PEF is the maximum flow rate attained during an FVC maneuver and usually is reported in liters per second. PEF can be easily measured with disposable, handheld devices. Although the PEF measurement is effort dependent, it can be an indicator of airway obstruction. For this reason it is useful in home monitoring of patients with asthma. Home monitoring of PEF or FEV_1 can evaluate the effectiveness of bronchodilator therapy and detect exacerbation of the disease.

The maximum voluntary ventilation (MVV) is the largest volume that a patient can move in and out of his or her lungs during a 12- to 15-second interval (but expressed in L-min). Patients are instructed to breathe as

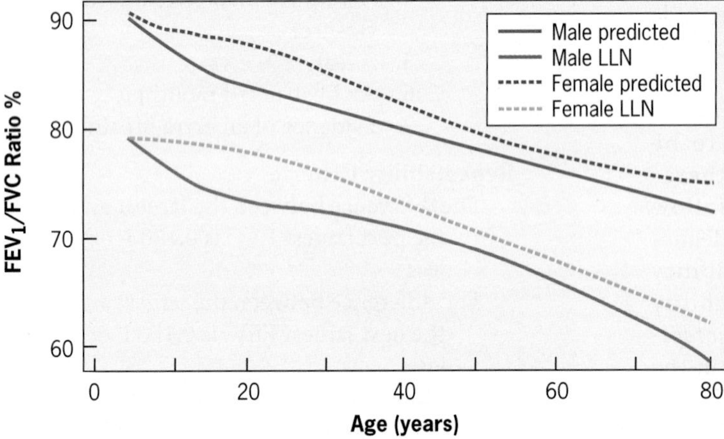

FIGURE 10–6 The lower limit of the normal range (LLN) for FEV_1/FVC declines with age; therefore, a fixed LLN should not be used to define airway obstruction. The predicted (mean) values are from healthy subjects in the NHANES III study. Adapted from Stanojevic S, et al. Reference range for spirometry across all ages: a new approach. *Am J Respir Crit Care Med.* 2008; 177(3):253–260. Courtesy of Sanja Stanojevic.

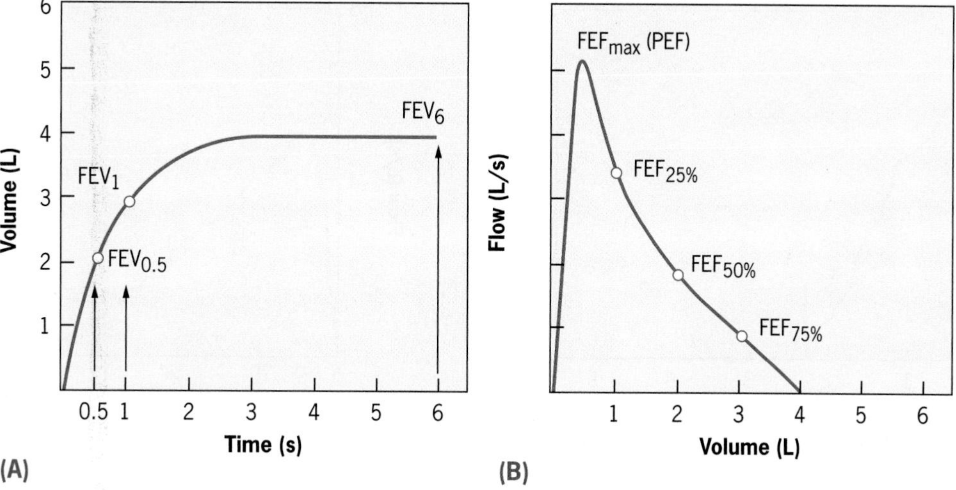

FIGURE 10–7 The volume–time curve (**A**) and the flow–volume curve (**B**). $FEF_{25\%}$, $FEF_{50\%}$, and $FEF_{75\%}$ are the forced expiratory flows after 25%, 50%, and 75% of the forced vital capacity have been exhaled.

rapidly and deeply as possible. It is now performed less frequently. A low MVV can occur in obstructive, restrictive, or neuromuscular disorders.

Quality Assurance

Respiratory therapists are responsible for providing good-quality test results. Physicians who order PFTs are usually unable to recognize poor quality, and thus may be misled by inaccurate PFT results. False-positive diagnoses or treatment decisions may be made based on poor-quality PFTs. The best method of recognizing poor-quality tests is to watch the body language of patients as they perform the maneuvers. After the tests are completed, a careful review of the graphs and numbers can also reveal poor-quality PFTs. Three acceptable efforts must be performed for the spirometry test to be valid. Types of unacceptable maneuvers (errors) include a delayed or slow start, a suboptimal "blast out" effort, and early termination. A slow or hesitant start leaks volume and alters the start-of-test time. If the volume leaked is more than 5% of the FVC or 0.150 L, that maneuver should be discarded and repeated. Newer computerized equipment automatically provides an error message so that the therapist can coach the patient appropriately.

> **RESPIRATORY RECAP**
>
> **Common Spirometry Errors**
>
> » Submaximal inhalation (before the forced exhalation)
> » Slow or hesitating start
> » Early termination (before 6 seconds in adults)

Several cases can be used to illustrate spirometry errors. Sammy is a 75-year-old car salesman with a chronic cough who has smoked a pack a day since age 18. His flow–volume curve (**Figure 10–8**) shows a slow start during phase 2 of the FVC maneuver. The peak flow is not sharp, and the BEV is about 400 mL. This caused the FEV_1 to be inaccurate. The respiratory therapist repeated a demonstration of the correct maneuver and coached the patient for a longer duration. His spirometry was then normal, ruling out COPD.

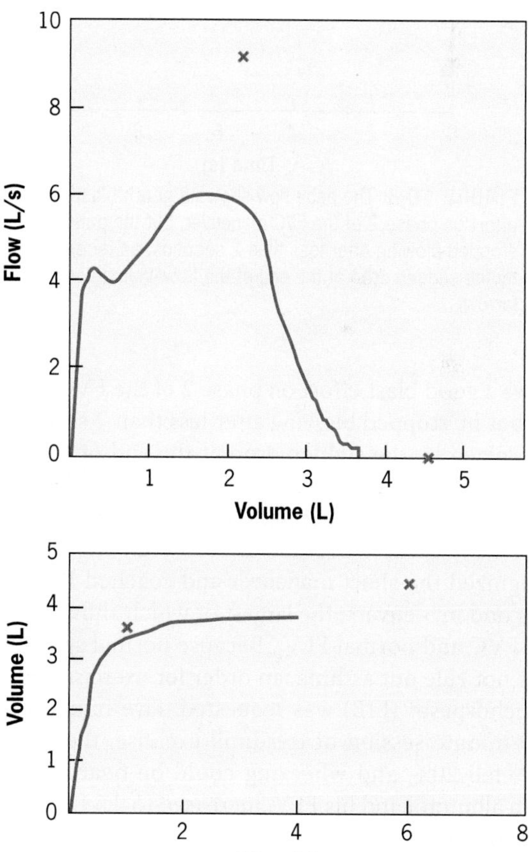

FIGURE 10–8 The flow–volume curve shows a slow start during phase 2 of the FVC maneuver. This causes a high back extrapolated volume.

A 12-year-old boy has a history of chest tightness and wheezing while playing soccer in relatively cold weather. His pediatrician ordered spirometry because she was worried that Reggie might have asthma. His peak flow

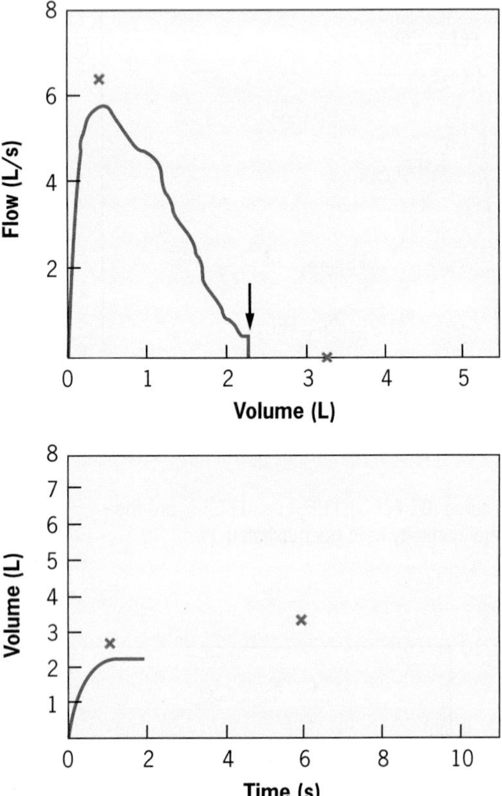

FIGURE 10–9 The peak flow shows a good "blast" effort on phase 2 of the FVC maneuver, but the patient stopped blowing after less than 2 seconds, as recognized by the sudden drop at the end of the flow–volume curve (arrow).

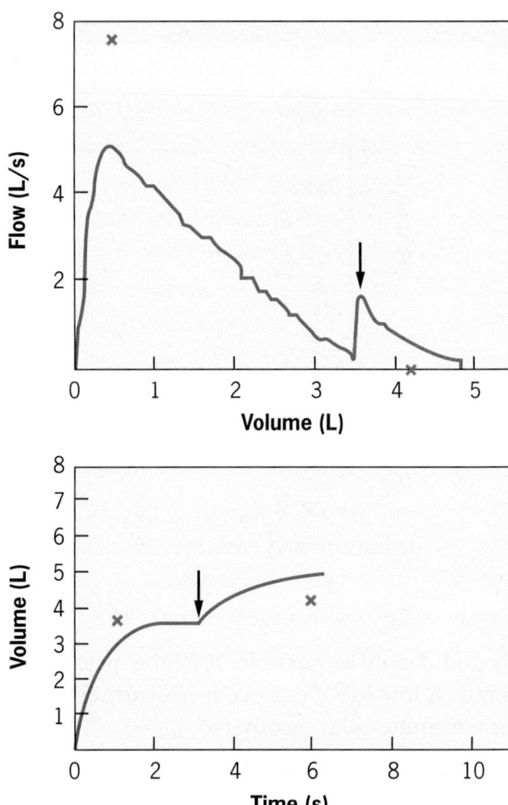

FIGURE 10–10 Note that the forced vital capacity is falsely increased due to an extra breath (arrows).

shows a good blast effort on phase 2 of the FVC maneuver, but he stopped blowing after less than 2 seconds, as recognized by the sudden drop at the end of the flow–volume curve after he exhaled 2.2 L (**Figure 10–9**). The spirometer interpretation was "mild restriction" because the FVC was 69% predicted. However, the therapist recognized the short maneuver and coached Reggie for 6-second maneuvers, the largest of which showed a normal FVC and normal FEV_1. Because normal spirometry does not rule out asthma, an order for exercise-induced bronchospasm (EIB) was requested. Five minutes after a 10-minute session of treadmill exercise, the patient's FEV_1 fell 20%, and wheezing could be heard. He was given albuterol and his FEV_1 increased to 2.5 L, confirming asthma.

A 70-year-old stockbroker has a 20-year history of smoking cigars. The interpretation from the spirometry interpretation was mild obstruction because the FEV_1/FVC was 0.60. However, the physician recognized that the FVC was falsely increased due to an extra breath (**Figure 10–10**). These are caused by cyclical breathing, in which a quick sniff of air is inhaled through the nose and then exhaled through the mouth. When nose clips were used for repeat spirometry testing, his true FVC of 4.0 L was measured, ruling out airway obstruction due to COPD, since his FEV_1/FVC was then 0.75.

Spirometry errors are correctable in 90% of patients, even preschool children and elderly patients, with good demonstrations, enthusiastic coaching, and patience. Most patients are extremely cooperative and provide excellent tests with the proper instruction and coaching. However, about 10% of patients do have difficulties with the maneuvers. Many modern spirometry systems include software that alerts therapists to maneuver errors, but respiratory therapists must also learn how to recognize these errors and correct them.

Infection Control

The goal of infection control is to prevent the transmission of infection from either direct or indirect contact. The guidelines in **Box 10–5** should be applied whenever PFTs are performed.

Spirometry Patterns

The flow–volume curve from a healthy person looks like a sail (**Figure 10–11**). Nonuniform emptying of airways is reflected by a concave upward configuration of the flow–volume curve, like a bowl, which is an obstructive pattern (**Figure 10–12**). The flow–volume curve in patients who cannot take a deep breath has a normal shape but a low FVC, which is a restrictive pattern (**Figure 10–13**).

The most common causes of airway obstruction are asthma (in patients of any age) and COPD in

BOX 10-5

Infection Control for Spirometry

Use universal precautions.

For patients with suspected infectious airborne diseases, wear an N-95 respirator.

Wear gloves when handling contaminated equipment.

Mouthpieces or flow sensors should be disposable or disinfected between patients.

The use of inline filters does not eliminate the need for regular cleaning and disinfection.

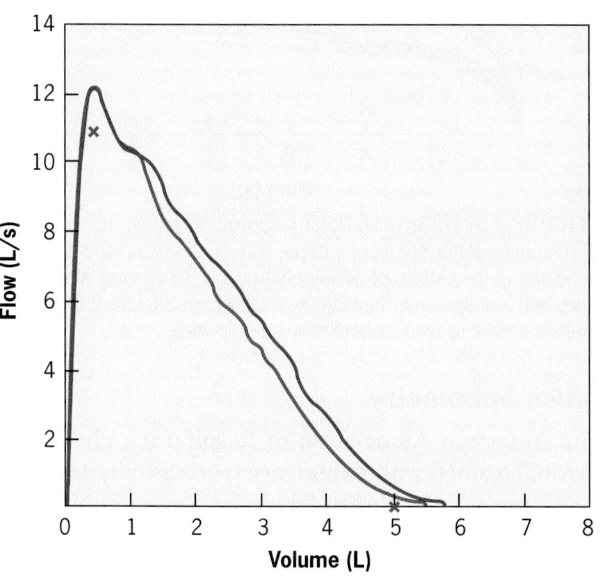

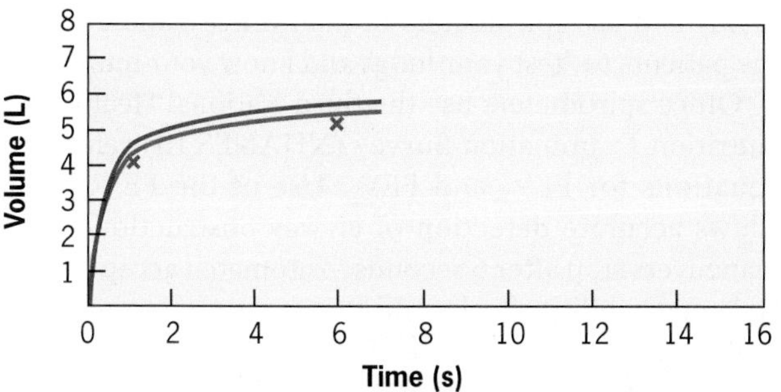

FIGURE 10–11 Normal spirometry. The patient performed two FVC maneuvers, which lasted 7 seconds each (note the duration of the volume–time graphs in the bottom frame). The shape of the flow–volume curve is normal (like the fully extended sail on a sailboat). The FEV_1 values are about 4.5 L and 4.6 L (matching closely), above the predicted value of 4.1 L (marked as a blue X on the volume–time graph). The FVC values are about 5.5 L and 5.8 L, also above the predicted FVC of 5.1 L. The FEV_1/FVC is 4.6/5.8 = 0.79, which is also normal.

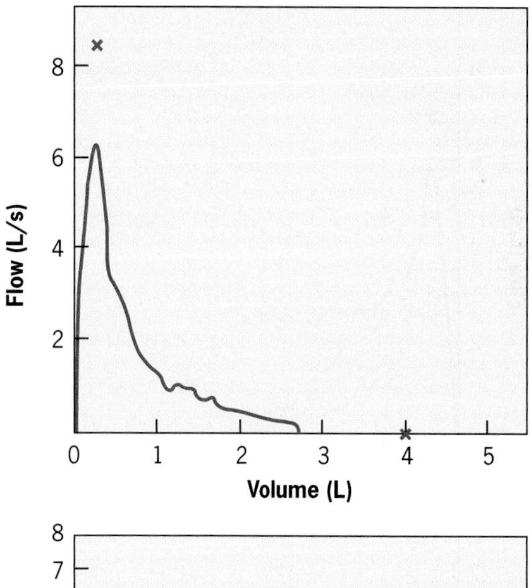

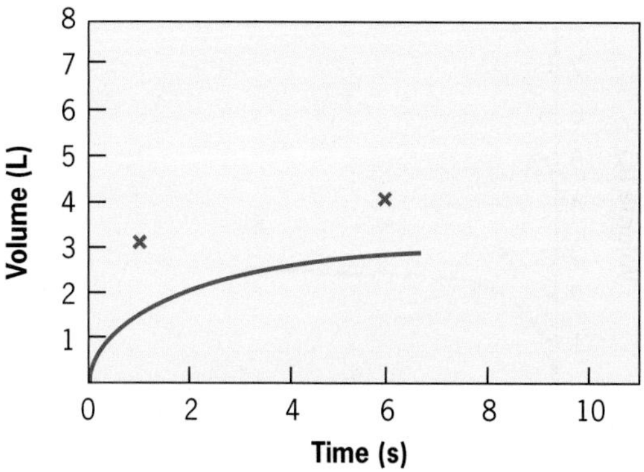

FIGURE 10–12 Spirometry graphs from a patient with a history of asthma. The flow–volume curve has the shape of airway obstruction (like a bowl). The airflow limitation is confirmed by the FEV_1/FVC of 0.52. The FEV_1 of 48% predicted suggests a moderate to severe impairment. The patient's FVC also is decreased, probably due to the hyperinflation that is associated with poorly controlled asthma.

smokers over age 40. If the patient has asthmalike symptoms and demonstrates airway obstruction on spirometry (prebronchodilator, or pre-BD), and the spirometry then becomes normal (or there is a very large improvement) after the patient is given an inhaled bronchodilator (post-BD), asthma is confirmed. Pre- and post-BD spirometry can thus be very helpful clinically to confirm asthma. However, because asthma is episodic, the patient who is currently not experiencing respiratory symptoms may have normal spirometry. The FEV_1 is commonly measured by respiratory therapists in the emergency department for patients seen with asthma exacerbations (attacks) after 30 to 60 minutes of bronchodilator treatment (post-BD). The results help determine whether to admit the patient to the hospital for prolonged asthma therapy.

> **RESPIRATORY RECAP**
>
> **Bronchodilator Response**
>
> » A 12% increase in FEV_1 or FVC is considered significant.

In adult patients with pre-BD airway obstruction, repeating spirometry post-BD may help clinicians to

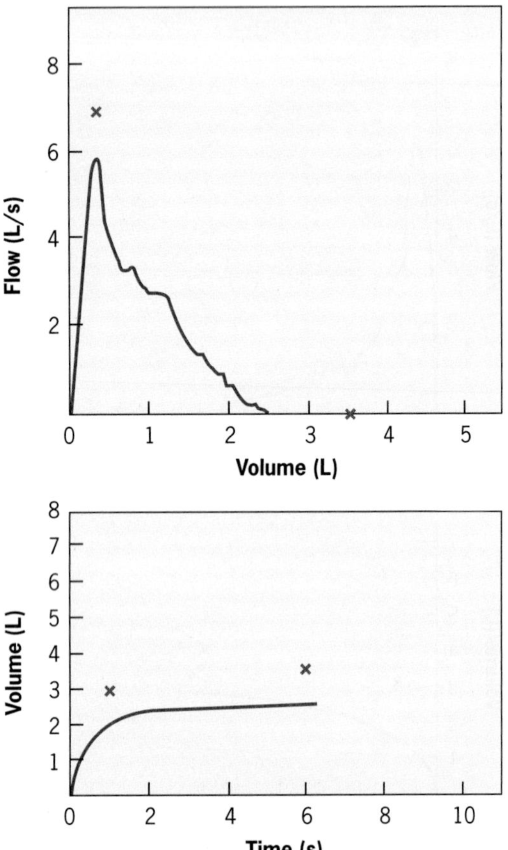

FIGURE 10–13 Spirogram of a patient with a restrictive pattern. The flow–volume curve has a normal shape, but the FVC is low (68% predicted). The FEV_1/FVC is normal (0.77).

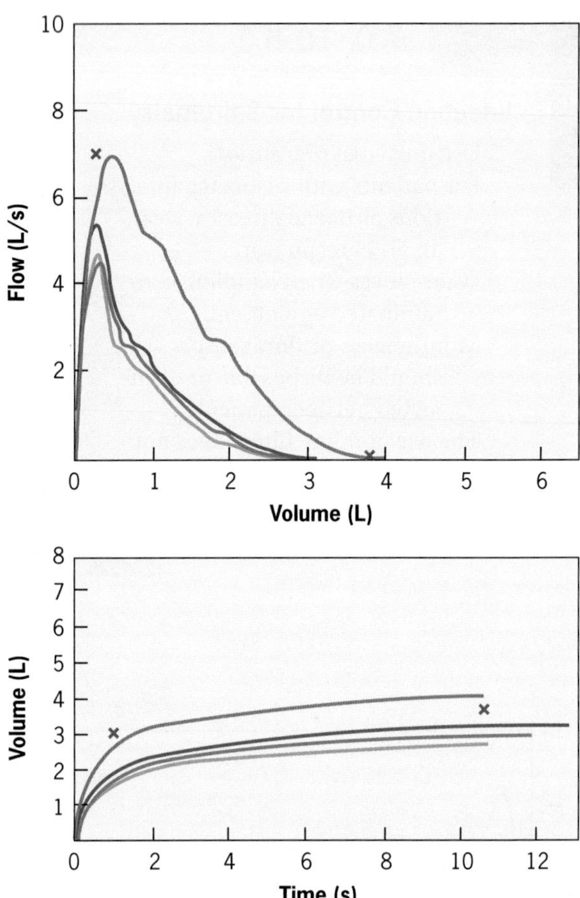

FIGURE 10–14 Bronchodilator response on spirogram. Prebronchodilator spirometry (three blue curves) was repeatable and shows the pattern of airway obstruction. 15 minutes after two puffs of albuterol, the FEV_1 increased from 2.0 L to 2.8 L, a 40% increase (postbronchodilator, green curve).

differentiate between asthma and COPD. If post-BD spirometry is normal, COPD is ruled out (**Figure 10–14**). If airway obstruction remains post-BD, the patient may have poorly controlled asthma (with considerable airway inflammation and mucus) or COPD (if the patient has more than a 20 pack year history of cigarette smoking). The amount of improvement in FEV_1 from pre-BD to post-BD spirometry is calculated by spirometers as bronchodilator responsiveness, and an increase of 12% or more is considered significant. However, patients with either asthma or COPD can have significant bronchodilator responsiveness.

When post-BD spirometry is ordered, good-quality pre-BD spirometry is obtained, and then the respiratory therapist administers two or four puffs of albuterol using a metered dose inhaler (MDI) with a spacer or holding chamber and waits 10 to 15 minutes before repeating spirometry (post-BD). In adults with a higher pretest probability of COPD, a combination of albuterol and a short-acting anticholinergic bronchodilator (ipratropium) may be administered by a nebulizer. When this is done, a wait of more than 30 minutes is necessary before repeating spirometry (to allow the ipratropium to become maximally effective). Some patients may develop temporary, but not serious, side effects from inhaled bronchodilators.

Office Spirometry

The American Association of Respiratory Therapists (AARC) teamed with pulmonary specialist physicians in the National Lung Health Education Program (NLHEP) to encourage spirometer manufacturers to make easy-to-use, simple spirometers; encourage primary care doctors to buy and use spirometers in their offices; and encourage patients to "test your lungs and know your numbers."

Office spirometers use the third National Health and Nutrition Examination Survey (NHANES III) reference equations for FEV_1 and FEV_6. Use of the FEV_1/FEV_6 allows accurate detection of airway obstruction when maneuvers stop after 6 seconds. Automated acceptability and repeatability checks and messages are required, as well as A through F test-session quality grades. A quality grade of B indicates that ATS quality goals were met. Automated interpretations are not provided when the quality grade is D (only one acceptable maneuver) or F (no acceptable maneuvers).

Upper Airway Obstruction

Most spirometers can also measure forced *inspiratory* flows and volumes in addition to the forced expiratory maneuvers needed to measure the FEV_1 and FVC.

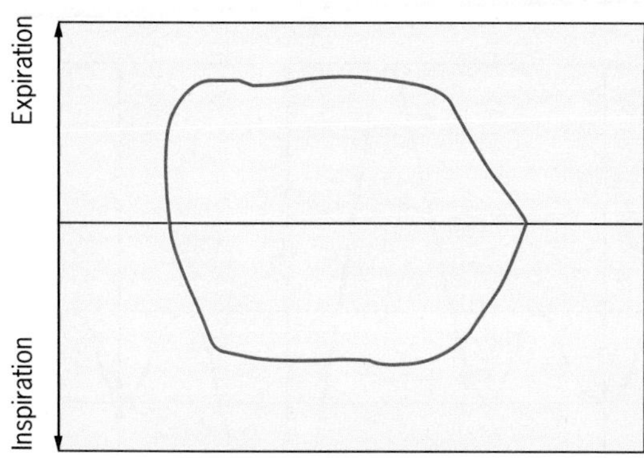

FIGURE 10–15 Flow–volume loop showing a fixed upper airway obstruction due to tracheal stenosis.

When a forced inspiratory maneuver follows the forced expiratory maneuver, the resulting graph is called a flow–volume *loop*. The inspiratory (bottom) half of the flow–volume loop can detect narrowing of the airway in the neck (also known as the extrathoracic or upper airway). Upper airway obstruction (UAO) is much less common than lower airway obstruction, which is often caused by asthma or COPD.

If the UAO decreases flow only during forced inhalation but not forced exhalation, as in vocal cord paralysis, it is categorized as a variable lesion. If the flow is decreased equally during inspiration and expiration, the lesion is considered fixed, as in tracheal stenosis. Narrowing of the upper airway causes relatively flat plateaus on flow–volume graphs (unlike the bowl-shaped flow–volume curves caused by asthma or COPD) (**Figure 10–15**).

Vocal cord paralysis and tracheal stenosis (due to prolonged intubation with an overinflated cuff) are two relatively common causes of UAO. The shape of the flow–volume loop can help to differentiate between them, although confirmation of the location of the UAO will almost always be done by direct visualization (fiberoptic endoscopy) or radiologic imaging.

Forced inspiratory flows (FIFs) depend greatly on inspiratory effort, which depends on enthusiastic coaching by the respiratory therapist. False-positive interpretations of UAO due to submaximal inspiratory efforts are unfortunately very common, so the therapist must strive to obtain maximal inspiratory efforts with repeatable forced inspiratory flows and volumes (FIVCs). The FEF_{50}/FIF_{50} is often calculated by the spirometer, is normally about 1.0, and increases with variable extrathoracic UAO (**Figure 10–16**). However, the upper limit of the normal range (ULN) for this ratio is poorly established, remains normal with fixed UAO, and is normal when both upper and lower airway obstruction exist, such as in patients with asthma who also have vocal cord paralysis. Therefore, the pattern of repeatable flat plateaus is the best method of reliably detecting UAO.

The following cases are illustrative of UAO. A 40-year-old minister complains of hoarseness after thyroid surgery. His physician observed inspiratory stridor over his neck and ordered flow–volume loops. The patient's forced expiratory flows were normal, but forced inspiratory flows were limited to about 2 L/s, causing a repeatable plateau during forced inhalations. This pattern was interpreted as variable extrathoracic UAO. He was referred to an otolaryngologist, who saw vocal cord paralysis during upper airway fiberoptic endoscopy.

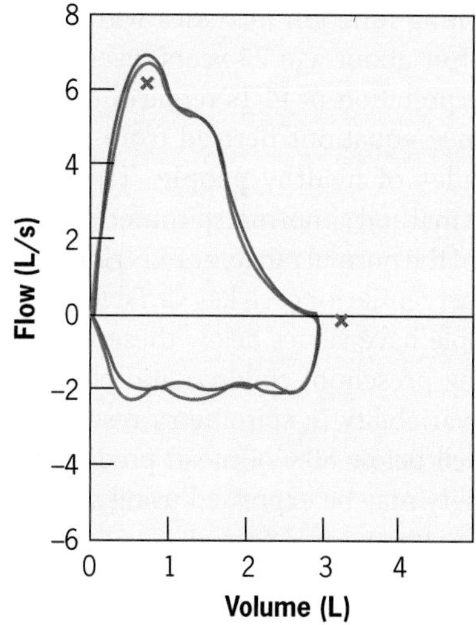

FIGURE 10–16 This pattern is interpreted as variable extrathoracic upper airway obstruction.

TABLE 10–3 Categorizing the Severity of Impairment Using the FEV_1

FEV_1	Severity
<LLN to 65% predicted	Mild
50% to 65% predicted	Moderate
35% to 50% predicted	Severe
<35% predicted	Very severe

FEV_1, forced expiratory volume in 1 second; LLN, lower limit of the normal range.

A 25-year-old real estate salesperson developed flu symptoms 1 month ago, rapidly progressing to respiratory failure that required mechanical ventilation for 1 week. Since hospital discharge, she has noted shortness of breath while climbing stairs. Her flow–volume loop shows a plateau during both forced exhalation and forced inhalation. This pattern was interpreted as a fixed UAO. A magnetic resonance image of her neck confirmed tracheal stenosis.

Spirometry Interpretation

The assessment and monitoring of restrictive and obstructive lung diseases always starts with spirometry results. A low FEV_1/FVC indicates airway obstruction. A low FVC with a normal FEV_1/FVC suggests spirometric restriction. The percent predicted FEV_1 is usually used to grade the severity of impairment, although the thresholds are arbitrary (**Table 10–3**). Regardless of the type of lung disease causing the impairment, and regardless of the patient's age, height, and sex, it is difficult for patients to survive with an FEV_1 below 0.5 L.

Because lung function increases with height and decreases after about age 25 years, even in healthy people, interpretation of PFTs requires comparisons with reference equations derived from population-based samples of healthy people. The threshold between normal and abnormal spirometry results (the lower limit of the normal range, or LLN) is determined by the fifth percentile for each key variable. Only 5% of healthy people have values below these fifth percentiles. Healthy preschool children and elderly adults have more variability in spirometry results, so their LLNs are well below 80% of mean predicted values. This variability may be expressed using standardized residuals (also known as Z scores).

Spirometry reference equations are incorporated into the software of modern spirometers, so there is no need to calculate normal values and LLN when spirometry is performed. For FEV_1/FVC and FEV_6/FVC, normal values are only dependent on age and ethnicity.

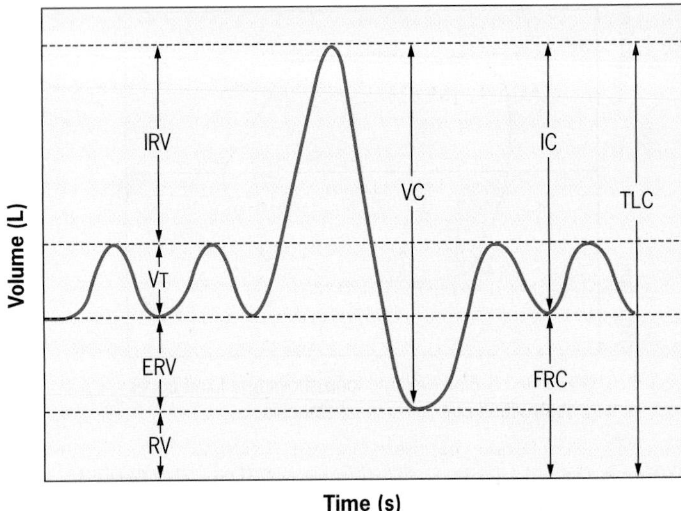

FIGURE 10–17 The volumes and capacities of the lungs. IRV, inspiratory reserve volume; VT, tidal volume; ERV, expiratory reserve volume; RV, residual volume; VC, vital capacity; IC, inspiratory capacity; FRC, functional residual capacity; TLC, total lung capacity.

Lung Volumes and Capacities

Spirometry provides screening information that identifies restrictive and obstructive impairments. Complete testing in a PFT laboratory can characterize the impairment by assessing the lung volumes, capacities, and diffusing capacity. Specialized tests can also determine airway responsiveness to a challenge and respiratory muscle strength.

A measure of lung size, the **vital capacity**, was first measured systematically by Hutchinson in 1846. When obstructive lung disease became more clearly defined in the 1960s, the emphasis of testing shifted to measurement of airflow limitation. Nevertheless, for more than 100 years, pulmonary function testing was primarily the measurement of static **lung volumes**. *Static* refers to volumes measured between the four resting or static positions: maximal inhalation, end inspiration, end expiration, and maximal exhalation.

> **RESPIRATORY RECAP**
>
> **Lung Volumes and Capacities**
>
> » *Lung volumes:* tidal volume, inspiratory reserve volume, expiratory reserve volume, residual volume
>
> » *Lung capacities:* vital capacity, inspiratory capacity, functional residual capacity, total lung capacity

A lung capacity is two or more lung volumes (**Figure 10–17**). Of the eight lung volume and capacity measurements, four provide the most useful information: vital capacity, **total lung capacity**, functional residual capacity, and residual volume. The patient is connected to the spirometer and instructed to perform maneuvers that measure the lung volumes and capacities. The four lung volumes are as follows:

- *Tidal volume* (VT) is the volume of gas inhaled or exhaled during normal breathing.
- *Inspiratory reserve volume* (IRV) is the maximum volume of gas that can be inspired from the end of a normal inspiration.
- *Expiratory reserve volume* (ERV) is the maximum volume of gas that can be expired from the end of a resting expiration.
- *Residual volume* (RV) is the volume of gas remaining in the lungs after a maximal expiration. By definition, this volume cannot be exhaled.

The four lung capacities are as follows:

- *Vital capacity* (VC) is the maximum volume of gas that can be exhaled from the lungs after a maximal inspiration (expiratory vital capacity) or inhaled from a point of maximal exhalation (inspiratory vital capacity). The VC includes the VT, IRV, and ERV.
- *Inspiratory capacity* (IC) is the maximum volume of gas that can be inspired from the normal end-expiratory position. The IC is the sum of VT and IRV.
- *Functional residual capacity* (FRC) is the volume of gas remaining in the lungs at the end of a resting expiration. The FRC is the sum of RV and ERV.
- *Total lung capacity* (TLC) is the volume of gas in the lungs at the end of a maximal inspiration and the total volume of air in the lungs seen on most chest radiographs and lung computed tomography (CT) scans.

Measurement of Lung Volumes

Although IC and ERV can be measured with a spirometer during a slow VC maneuver, FRC must be measured separately, using more expensive instruments, because the lungs cannot be emptied completely to zero lung volume. In PFT labs, FRC is measured using **nitrogen washout**, **helium dilution**, or **body plethysmography**. TLC can be estimated from posteroanterior (PA) and lateral chest radiographs and determined accurately from lung CT scans. **Box 10–6** lists clinical indications for lung volume tests.

In the nitrogen measurement method, the subject is switched from breathing room air (≈ 21% O_2) to inhaling

BOX 10-6

Indications for Lung Volume Measurements

In patients with airway obstruction and a low FVC, to determine whether a superimposed restrictive process exists (low TLC)

In patients with a low FVC, but without airway obstruction on spirometry, to determine whether the low FVC is due to a nonspecific abnormality (normal TLC) or a classic restriction of lung volumes (low TLC)

In patients with airway obstruction, to determine the presence and severity of hyperinflation (a high RV/TLC) or to measure the trapped air volume

To correct airway resistance measurements for the lung volume at which airway resistance was measured (usually FRC)

To measure FRC in infants and preschool children who cannot perform spirometry

FVC, forced vital capacity; TLC, total lung capacity; RV, residual volume; FRC, functional residual capacity.

from a reservoir of 100% oxygen and exhaling through a nitrogen analyzer and spirometer. This is called an *open-circuit method* because rebreathing does not occur. The 100% oxygen dilutes the residual nitrogen during each breath (initially ≈ 79% N_2) until almost all of the nitrogen in the lungs is washed out (**Equation 10–1**). The nitrogen concentration of the exhaled gas is measured continuously by a fast gas analyzer. The FRC then can be calculated from the dilution formula. In practice, the procedure is terminated after 7 minutes. This method can underestimate the FRC with airway obstruction because poorly communicating lung regions (also called slow spaces) are not allowed to wash out their nitrogen.

RESPIRATORY RECAP

Lung Volume Tests

» Nitrogen washout
» Helium dilution
» Body plethysmography

Helium, argon, or neon can be used to measure FRC by inert gas dilution, although helium (He) is usually used. The patient is connected to the circuit and switched to breathing from a spirometer with a known volume containing helium of a known concentration (**Figure 10–18** and **Equation 10–2**). This is called a *closed-circuit method* because rebreathing occurs. The procedure is stopped when the He concentration falls to a new plateau or steady value. The rate of fall in He concentration (time to equilibrium) is rapid in patients with

EQUATION 10-1

Nitrogen Washout Technique

FRC is calculated from the dilution formula as follows:

$$C_1 \times V_1 = C_2 \times V_2$$

where

C_1 = Nitrogen concentration in the lungs at the beginning of the procedure (≈ 79%)

C_2 = Nitrogen concentration in the pooled exhaled volume

V_2 = Total exhaled volume from the washout

FRC (V_1) then is calculated as follows:

$$V_1 = \frac{C_2 \times V_2}{C_1}$$

The nitrogen often is not completely removed from the lung by 7 minutes so a correction for this is made.

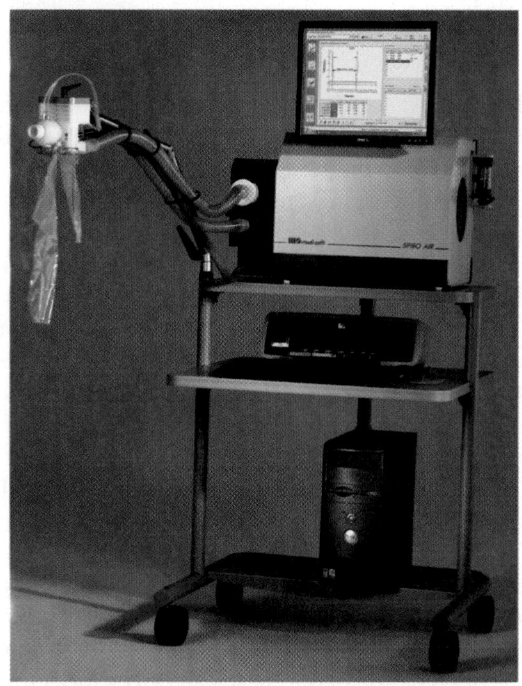

FIGURE 10–18 An instrument used to measure functional residual capacity using the helium dilution technique.

EQUATION 10–2

Helium Dilution Technique

FRC also measured by this method is determined by the standard dilution calculation as follows:

$$C_1 \times V_1 = C_2 \times V_2$$

where

C_1 = Initial helium concentration
V_1 = Spirometer volume
C_2 = Final helium concentration
$V_2 = V_1 + FRC$

Therefore,

$$V_2 = \frac{C_1 \times V_1}{C_2}$$

because

$$V_2 = V_1 + FRC$$

Therefore,

$$FRC = \frac{C_1 \times V_1}{C_2} - V_1$$

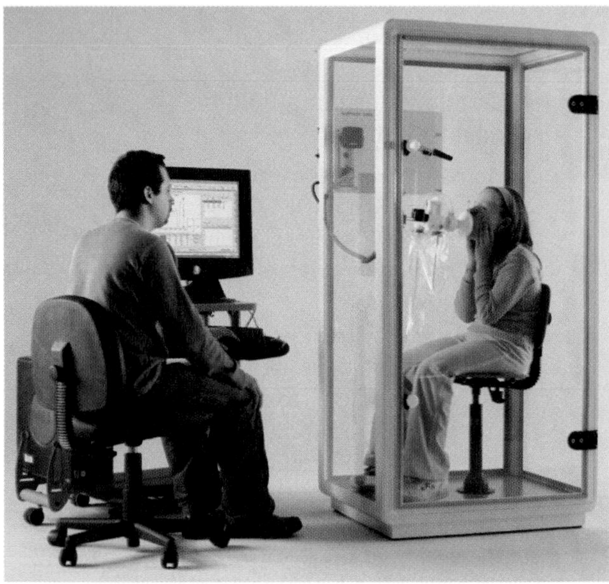

FIGURE 10–19 A body box used to measure static lung volumes and airway resistance. Patients sit on the chair and breathe quietly though the white mouthpiece. Mouth pressure is measured when a shutter in the mouthpiece assembly is closed.

healthy lungs, but slow in patients with substantial airway obstruction. The FRC measured by this method is determined by the standard dilution calculation. Any leaks occurring during the procedure will give a falsely high FRC.

The accuracy of the gas analyzers used by the nitrogen washout or inert gas dilution instruments should be verified at least daily, using a two-point calibration. The first point is zero concentration of the gas, and the second point is the concentration of the test gas near the middle or high end of the normal range (such as 5% to 10% for helium).

The measurement of FRC using a body box (plethysmograph) is based on Boyle's law ($P_1V_1 = P_2V_2$), wherein the product of one pressure and volume (P_1V_1) of a gas is equal to the product of another pressure and volume related to that gas (P_2V_2). In practice, the patient is placed inside a fixed-volume, air-sealed body box in which the effects of excursion of the chest wall can be measured by small pressure changes in the box and airway.

The patient sits in the box and breathes quietly through a mouthpiece with a shutter (**Figure 10–19**). The shutter is closed at the end of an exhalation (when the lungs contain the FRC volume to be measured). By occluding the airway and allowing the subject to decompress the chest by making an inspiratory effort, a new airway or lung pressure (P_1) and new body box pressure (P_2) are generated. The slope of change in airway and box pressures (P_1/P_2) is then used to calculate the missing volume (V_1 or FRC). The box volume (V_1) is known.

The advantage of the body box technique is its speed. About 30 minutes or longer usually is required to measure FRC by helium dilution or nitrogen washout. FRC can be determined multiple times in 10 minutes by body plethysmography. The gas dilution methods measure only communicating gas spaces, whereas body plethysmography measures all gas spaces, regardless of whether they are communicating (e.g., bullae). The difference in the FRC measured by these two techniques is the trapped air volume, which is abnormally high in patients with airway obstruction.

To ensure instrument accuracy, three signals must be checked daily: mouth pressure, using a red oil manometer; mouth flow and volume, using a 3-L calibration syringe; and change in box volume, using a small sine-wave pump. Weekly checks using an isothermal lung are also recommended.

Interpretation of Lung Volumes

Measured static lung volumes and capacities are evaluated in comparison with predicted values. Prediction equations calculated from height, age, and gender exist for all pulmonary function parameters. The TLC is considered abnormal when it falls below the LLN, consistent with a restriction of lung volumes. On the other hand, the RV and FRC are considered abnormal when they are too high (above the ULN), consistent with the air trapping or **hyperinflation** that usually accompanies lung diseases causing airway obstruction.

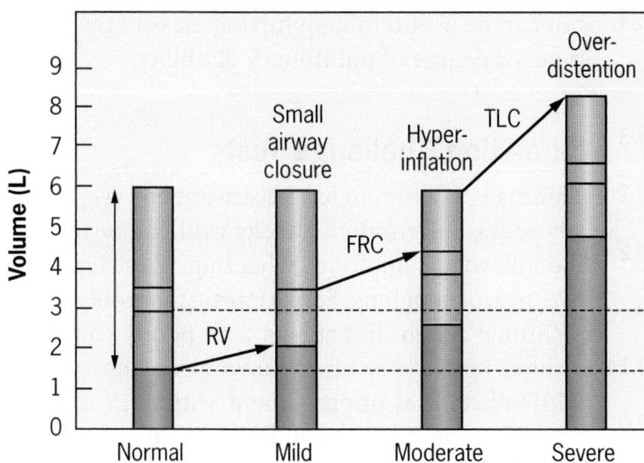

FIGURE 10–20 The effect of increasing airway obstruction on lung volumes. RV, residual volume; FRC, functional residual capacity; TLC, total lung capacity.

The size of the TLC is determined by the ability of the respiratory muscles to enlarge the chest wall to its maximum volume configuration (in other words, to fill completely). A lower-than-expected TLC could result from an increase in stiffness of the lung or chest wall, respiratory muscle weakness, or a less than maximal effort by the patient.

> **RESPIRATORY RECAP**
>
> **Abnormal Lung Volumes and Capacities**
>
> » Reduced lung volumes and capacities generally indicate restrictive disease.
>
> » Elevated residual volume or total lung capacity can indicate air trapping or hyperinflation.

FRC is another important lung volume measurement. In healthy individuals, the size of the FRC is determined by the balance between the elastic recoil of the lungs, which acts in an expiratory direction and tends to reduce the lung volume, and that of the chest wall, which acts in an inspiratory direction, tending to expand the chest. The RV is normally about 25% of the TLC in healthy individuals, and the FRC is normally 30% to 35% of TLC. Milder forms of airflow limitation have an elevated RV only, without a significant effect on TLC (**Figure 10–20**). Therefore, the ratio may be greater than 25% without an elevation in TLC. An elevated RV, FRC, RV/TLC, or FRC/TLC then can be interpreted as air trapping. An elevation in TLC is interpreted as overdistension. It is possible to have coexisting restrictive lung disease and air trapping, as seen in some cases of interstitial lung disease.

Diffusing Capacity

The **diffusing capacity** of the lung for carbon monoxide (DLCO) is the second most clinically valuable PFT, with many indications (**Box 10–7**). DLCO is an index of the uptake of oxygen from the alveoli into the blood. The uptake of oxygen itself is not measured because a mixed venous blood sample would be necessary (but highly invasive). A small concentration of carbon monoxide (CO) is inhaled during this test, since CO is normally not present in the blood but is quickly taken up by red blood cells. The major factors influencing DLCO are the area and thickness of the alveolocapillary membrane available for diffusion and the pulmonary capillary blood volume. Other factors that may alter DLCO but do not directly reflect the gas transfer properties of the lung include anemia, the inspired oxygen concentration, and a high carboxyhemoglobin level—usually caused by recent smoking, but sometimes caused by a leaky muffler or home heater. Patients should be instructed to avoid smoking for *at least* 1 hour before diffusing capacity tests.

> **BOX 10–7**
>
> **Indications for a DLCO Test**
>
> In a patient with a low FVC or TLC, to differentiate between a chest wall cause of restriction (normal DLCO) and an interstitial lung disease (low DLCO)
>
> In a patient with airway obstruction on spirometry, to differentiate between emphysema (low DLCO) versus asthma or simple chronic bronchitis (normal DLCO)
>
> In a patient with dyspnea but normal spirometry, to detect pulmonary vascular disease (low DLCO) or mild interstitial lung disease (low DLCO)
>
> To evaluate treatment effects (or disease progression) in patients with interstitial lung diseases
>
> To evaluate pulmonary involvement in systemic diseases, such as rheumatoid arthritis or systemic lupus erythematosus
>
> To detect pulmonary side effects from chemotherapy, radiation therapy, or drugs (e.g., amiodarone, bleomycin) known to induce pulmonary dysfunction
>
> To predict arterial desaturation during exercise in patients with moderate to severe lung disease (although a simple 6-minute walking test measures this directly)

DLCO is usually expressed in English units as mL CO/min/mm Hg (or SI units in some European countries). In this technique, the subject exhales to residual

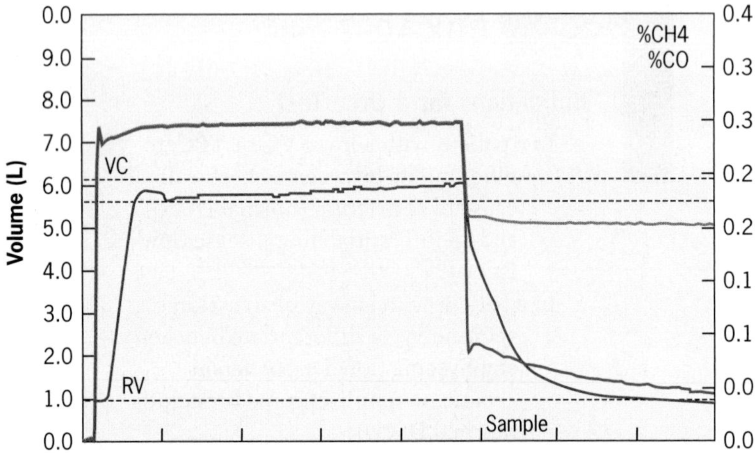

FIGURE 10–21 Graphs produced by a DLCO test. At the lower left corner, the patient begins to inhale the test gas. The red line shows the volume of inspired test gas (V_{in}) of about 6 L. The patient then holds his or her breath for about 10 seconds (the red line plateau), during which some of the carbon monoxide (CO) is absorbed by the red blood cells. The patient then exhales rapidly, and after the anatomic dead space air is discarded (about 1 L), a sample of air from the alveoli is obtained. The concentration of CO (blue line) and the tracer gas (green line) in the sample is measured by two gas analyzers or by gas chromatography.

volume, and then rapidly inhales a full breath of test gas (**Figure 10–21**). The test gas contains 0.3% CO, an inert gas such as 10% helium, nitrogen, and 21% to 25% oxygen. The patient is asked to hold his or her breath for 10 seconds and then exhale rapidly into a collection bag or chamber. Measurements include the volume of inspired test gas (Vin), the breath-hold time (BHT), and the inspired and expired alveolar gas concentrations for CO and the inert gas. The test is repeated at least once, until two tests of good quality match within 2 or 3 DLCO units.

> **RESPIRATORY RECAP**
>
> **Major Factors Influencing DLCO**
>
> » Area and thickness of the alveolocapillary membrane
>
> » Pulmonary capillary blood volume

Many technical and biologic variables affect the accuracy and reproducibility of the measured DLCO. The accuracy of the DLCO machine is ideally checked using a validation instrument; however, very few PFT labs currently own one. A two-point calibration of the gas analyzers is done automatically by the machine at the beginning of each test. The accuracy of the flow sensor should be checked every day using a 3-L syringe. The repeatability of DLCO for each machine should be checked at least weekly using a biologic control subject (usually a healthy therapist who works in the lab). The week-to-week coefficient of variation of DLCO should be less than 6%, and there should be no drift outside of 2 standard deviations of the mean value for each biologic control subject.

Specialized Pulmonary Function Tests

Several tests of specific aspects of lung function are performed in larger PFT laboratories. These tests are not considered in the context of routine outpatient testing but can be useful to help further classify the cause, type, or degree of pulmonary disability.

Inhalation Challenge Tests

Asthma is a common lung disease at any age. It usually causes intermittent attacks with one or more of the following symptoms: wheezing, chest tightness, dyspnea, or coughing. Sometimes asthma only causes a chronic cough. In patients with poorly controlled asthma, spirometry often shows airway obstruction with substantial improvement within 15 minutes after inhaling a bronchodilator (usually albuterol). However, most patients with mild asthma have normal spirometry results. In these patients, inhalation challenge tests often help to change the pretest probability of asthma. These tests are rarely done (except for research studies) when the diagnosis of asthma has previously been established.

The most frequently performed inhalation challenge test uses methacholine (Provocholine). Histamine is used in some countries, but more commonly causes uncomfortable systemic side effects, such as flushing or a headache, when compared with methacholine. The test is contraindicated in patients with moderate to severe airway obstruction, but is very safe in those with normal baseline spirometry. Methacholine acts directly on bronchial smooth muscle to cause bronchospasm, which lasts for up to an hour (without an intervention). The bronchoconstricting effect occurs only at relatively high concentrations of methacholine (more than 32 mg/mL) in people *without* asthma. Two methods of delivering the methacholine have been standardized by the ATS: 2-minute tidal breathing (from a nebulizer) and five-breath dosimeter-actuated nebulizer. The 2-minute tidal breathing method is more sensitive for detecting mild asthma and avoids the need for an expensive dosimeter.

The test starts at very low concentrations of methacholine, and if the FEV_1 remains above 80% of the baseline value, the concentration is doubled or quadrupled (**Figure 10–22**). Higher concentrations of methacholine are administered until the FEV_1 falls more than 20% or the highest concentration (32 mg/mL) has been given. The patient is then given albuterol to quickly reverse any bronchospasm caused by the methacholine. The results are summarized by the PC-20 (the provocative concentration of methacholine that caused a 20% fall in the FEV_1) (**Figure 10–23**).

> **RESPIRATORY RECAP**
>
> **Inhalation Challenge Tests**
>
> » The test is positive when there is a 20% decrease in the FEV_1.

Less commonly used inhalation challenge tests indirectly cause airway narrowing. These tests include cold and dry air challenges, ultrasonic nebulization of hypertonic saline, exercise (see the following section), and mannitol from a dry powder inhaler. Very rarely, specific

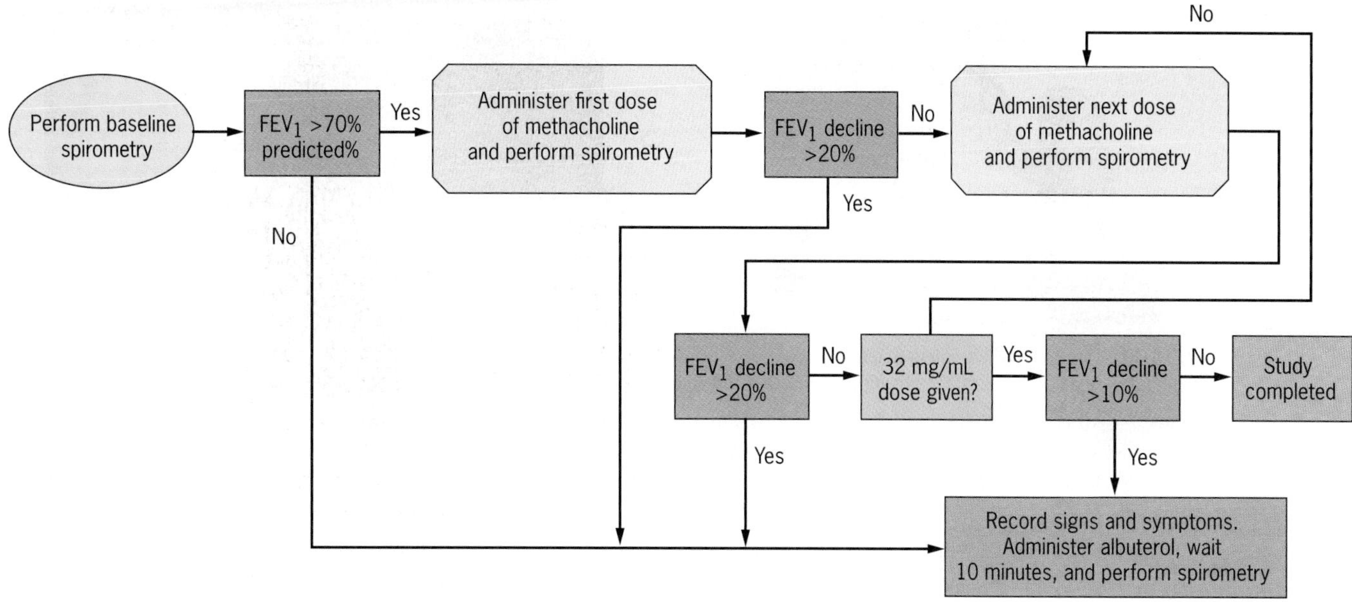

FIGURE 10–22 Algorithm for performance of methacholine challenge testing. Adapted from Crapo RO, et al. Guidelines for methacholine and exercise challenge testing—1999. *Am J Respir Crit Care Med.* 2000;161:309–329.

antigen challenges are done in specialized centers for research studies, or sometimes to confirm occupational asthma due to a single workplace pollutant. These patients are usually hospitalized for at least 24 hours because of the risk of a delayed response.

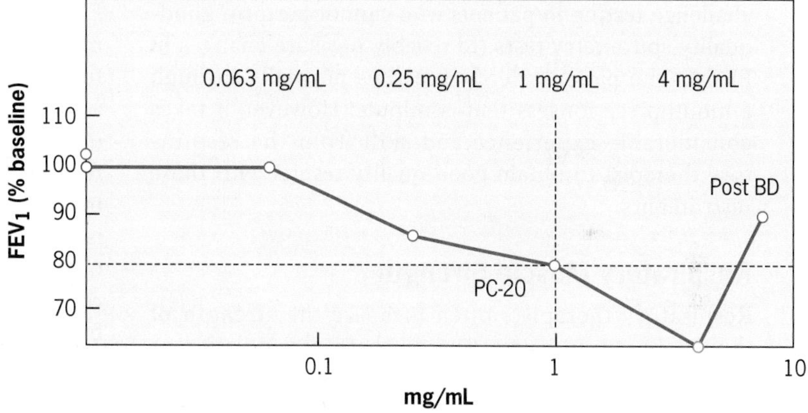

FIGURE 10–23 Methacholine challenge test from a patient with asthma-like symptoms. The PC-20 was 1 mg/mL. Courtesy of Pulmonary Function Laboratory, Saint Louis University Hospital.

Exercise-Induced Bronchospasm Test

Patients with asthma usually experience symptoms of exercise-induced bronchospasm (EIB) about 5 to 20 minutes after the end of a vigorous bout of exercise, especially in cold weather. These symptoms, like those of any asthma exacerbation, may include chest tightness, wheezing, coughing, or shortness of breath. EIB is due to drying of the lower airways, especially when the natural air conditioning of the nose is bypassed (during mouth breathing). EIB can often be reproduced in a PFT lab by exercising the patient using a bicycle ergometer or on a treadmill (while wearing nose clips to bypass the warming of inspired air by the nose) to achieve a heart rate above 80% of predicted maximal heart rate (220 – age) for 6 to 8 minutes. A positive test is suggested by a fall in FEV_1 of more than 10% from the preexercise baseline value. Maximum EIB occurs about 5 to 20 minutes after exercise is stopped. Albuterol is given to quickly reverse any symptoms of EIB.

Airways Resistance

A disadvantage of spirometry to measure airway obstruction is that athletic-like breathing maneuvers are necessary. Many preschool children and some elderly adults are unable to perform good-quality spirometry tests. Tests of **airways resistance** require very little cooperation since they are done during normal breathing or slow panting through a mouthpiece, while wearing nose clips and supporting the cheeks with hands (to minimize their motion).

The most common method of measuring airways resistance in a PFT lab is using a body box, done at the same time as the measurement of FRC. Airway resistance (Raw) is measured while the patient performs a slow panting maneuver with the mouth shutter open. Airway resistance changes according to the lung volume at which it is measured, so an advantage of measuring airway resistance in a body box (Raw) is the correction for FRC: specific airway conductance (sGaw) or the alternative, specific airway resistance (sRaw). Reference values for airway resistance are well established for children, but not for adults.

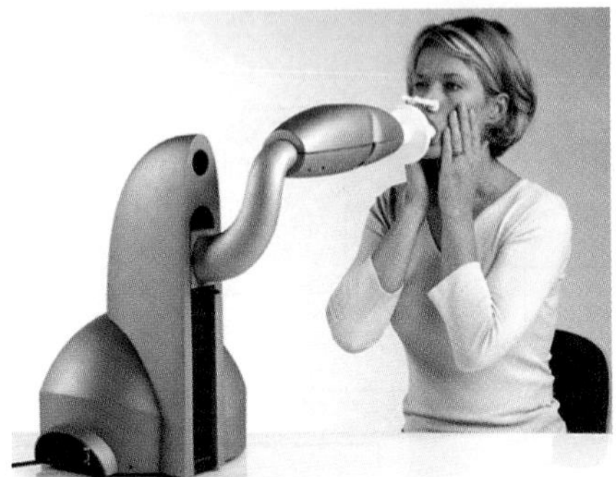

FIGURE 10–24 An instrument used to measure respiratory resistance using the forced oscillation technique (FOT).

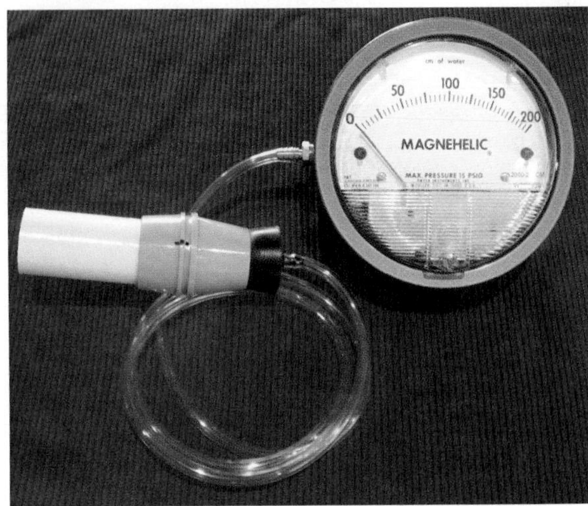

FIGURE 10–25 A pressure gauge used to measure maximum inspiratory pressure (PImax).

Airways resistance can also be measured using the forced oscillation technique (FOT) or interrupter technique (**Figure 10–24**). These instruments are much smaller and more portable than body boxes but are unable to measure lung volumes. However, they are clinically useful for measuring *changes* in airway resistance, such as bronchodilator responsiveness, or for inhalation challenge testing in patients who cannot perform good-quality spirometry tests (to reliably measure changes in FEV_1). The patient merely breathes normally through a mouthpiece for less than a minute. However, it takes considerable experience and skill from the respiratory therapist to obtain good-quality results with these instruments.

Respiratory Muscle Strength

Respiratory therapists often measure the strength of the diaphragm in patients on mechanical ventilation as an index of their ability to breathe independently again. For example, a **maximum inspiratory pressure** (MIP or PImax) of less than 20 cm H_2O suggests that the patient will be unable to take deep breaths due to inspiratory muscle weakness. On the other hand, the **maximum expiratory pressure** (MEP or PEmax) is a useful bedside measurement of the strength of the expiratory muscles to generate a forceful cough. Expiratory muscle weakness, as measured by a low MEP, is often caused by neuromuscular weakness and is clinically important because it increases the risk of aspiration pneumonia.

The maximum respiratory pressures, MIP and MEP, can also be measured for ambulatory patients in PFT labs (**Figure 10–25**). A simple mechanical pressure gauge can be used, much like at the bedside, or an electronic pressure gauge may be connected to the instrument used for other PFTs. In either case, a mouthpiece is usually connected by tubing to the pressure gauge. MIP can be measured using an inexpensive disposable cardboard mouthpiece. However, a firm rubber mouthpiece must be held firmly against the lips for accurate MEP measurements (because the MEP in healthy people often exceeds the strength of the lips to maintain a seal around mouthpieces placed into the mouth).

To measure MIP, the patient exhales slowly (from FRC toward RV), places the mouthpiece in his or her mouth, and then sucks from the mouthpiece as forcefully as possible (like sucking a thick milkshake through a narrow straw). The MIP is measured as the highest negative pressure maintained for about 1 second. Up to five MIP maneuvers are performed, with a goal of matching the highest value by less than 10%. The highest value is reported. MEP is measured similarly, but at maximal inhalation (near TLC). The lower limit of the normal range for MIP and MEP depends on age and gender, but not height or race. Other tests of respiratory muscle strength (such as sniff pressure) or endurance may also be measured in some PFT labs.

Ventilation Distribution

Ventilation distribution is sometimes measured using the single-breath nitrogen test. This test involves a maximal inspiration of 100% oxygen followed by a slow exhalation to RV. The slow, complete exhalation is directed by a one-way valve through a nitrogen meter and into a spirometer. The nitrogen meter continuously records the nitrogen concentration of the expired gas and simultaneously plots the expired nitrogen concentration against expired volume on an x–y plotter. The normal curve has four portions (**Figure 10–26**).

Phase III is an index of nonuniform ventilation. The onset of phase IV is considered an indication of the onset of airway closure in the dependent regions and often is called the *closing volume*. Relatively uniform gas distribution is identified by a flat phase III. With the onset of obstructive lung disease, closing volume and the slope of phase III are increased. If the distribution of ventilation becomes nonuniform, the slope of phase III

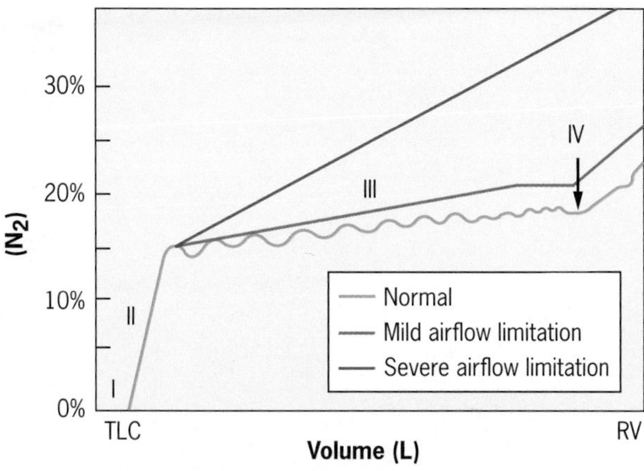

FIGURE 10–26 Single-breath nitrogen test for distribution of ventilation. Phase I is dead space gas, phase II is mixed gas (dead space and alveolar), phase III is alveolar gas, and phase IV is closing volume (arrow). TLC, total lung capacity; RV, residual volume.

becomes steeper. In advanced obstructive disease, phase IV becomes lost in the very steep slope of phase III. In obstructive lung disease, the distribution of ventilation worsens because regional differences in airway resistance and airspace compliance affect the rate at which airspace empties and fills.

KEY POINTS

- To avoid interpretation errors, spirometry requires attentive, vigorous coaching and careful scrutiny of the tracings.
- Spirometry detects airflow limitation due to lung disease, such as asthma or COPD.
- A low FEV_1/FVC indicates airway obstruction.
- A low FEV_1 and FVC with a normal FEV_1/FVC suggests restriction, which can be confirmed by a low TLC.
- Upper airway obstruction may be detected by a repeatable flat plateau on the inspiratory flow–volume curve.
- DLCO helps in the differential diagnosis when spirometry is abnormal.
- Decreases in lung volumes often indicate restrictive lung disease.
- Increases in residual volume and RV/TLC indicate air trapping, whereas an increase in TLC indicates overdistension.
- Specialized pulmonary function tests can be useful to help further classify the cause, type, or degree of respiratory impairment.

SUGGESTED READING

American Thoracic Society. Guidelines for methacholine and exercise challenge testing. *Am J Respir Crit Care Med.* 2000;161:309–329.

Anthonisen NR, Connett JE, Kiley JP, et al. Effects of smoking intervention and the use of an inhaled anticholinergic bronchodilator on the rate of decline in FEV_1: the Lung Health Study. *JAMA.* 1997;277:246–253.

ATS/ERS statement on respiratory muscle testing. *Am J Respir Crit Care Med.* 2002;166(4):518–624.

Cockcroft D, Davis B. Direct and indirect challenges in the clinical assessment of asthma. *Ann Allergy Asthma Immunol.* 2009;103:363–369.

Crapo RO, Casaburi R, Coates AL, et al. Guidelines for methacholine and exercise challenge testing—1999. *Am J Respir Crit Care Med.* 2000;161:309–329.

Enright PL, Kronmal RA, Manolio TA, et al. Respiratory muscle strength in the elderly: correlates and reference values. Cardiovascular Health Study research group. *Am J Respir Crit Care Med.* 1994;149(2 pt 1):430–438.

Evans JA, Whitelaw WA. The assessment of maximal respiratory mouth pressures in adults. *Respir Care.* 2009;54:1348–1359.

Ferguson GT, Enright PL, Buist AS, Higgins MW. Office spirometry for lung health assessment in adults: a consensus statement from the National Lung Health Education Program. *Respir Care.* 2000;45:513–530.

Hankinson JL, Odencranz JR, Fedan FB. Spirometric reference values from a sample of the general U.S. population [NHANES III]. *Am J Respir Crit Care Med.* 1999;159:179–187.

Hnizdo E, Glindmeyer HW, Petsonk EL, et al. Case definitions for chronic obstructive pulmonary disease. *COPD.* 2006;3(2):95–100.

Hyatt RE, Scanlon PD, Nakamura M. *Interpretation of Pulmonary Function Tests: A Practical Guide.* 2nd ed. Philadelphia: Lippincott-Raven; 2005.

MacIntyre N, Crapo RO, Viegi G, et al. for the ATS/ERS PFT Task Force. Standardisation of the single-breath determination of carbon monoxide uptake in the lung. *Eur Respir J.* 2005;26(4):720–735.

Miller MR, Hankinson J, Brusasco V, et al. ATS/ERS Task Force: standardisation of spirometry. *Eur Respir J.* 2005;26(2):319–338.

Pellegrino R, Viegi G, Brusasco V, et al. ATS/ERS Task Force: interpretative strategies for lung function tests. *Eur Respir J.* 2005;26(5):948–968.

Quanjer PH, Tammeling GJ, Cotes JE, et al. Lung volumes and ventilatory flows. *Eur Respir J.* 1993;6(suppl 16):5–40.

Ruppel GL. *Manual of Pulmonary Function Testing.* 9th ed. St. Louis: Mosby; 2009.

Stanojevic S, Wade A, Stocks J, et al. Reference ranges for spirometry across all ages: a new approach. *Am J Respir Crit Care Med.* 2008;177(3):253–260.

Stocks J, Quanjer PH. Reference values for residual volume, functional residual capacity and total lung capacity. *Eur Respir J.* 1995:8:492–506.

Swanney MP, Ruppel G, Enright PL, et al. Using the lower limit of normal for the FEV_1/FVC ratio reduces the misclassification of airway obstruction. *Thorax.* 2008;63(12):1046–1051.

Townsend MC, Hankinson JL, Lindesmith LA, et al. Is my lung function really that good? Flow-type spirometer problems that elevate test results. *Chest.* 2004;125(5):1902–1909.

Wanger J, Clausen JL, Coates A, et al. ATS/ERS Task Force: standardisation of the measurement of lung volumes. *Eur Respir J.* 2005;26(3):511–522.

CHAPTER 11

Interventional Pulmonary Procedures

Amy E. Treece
Momen M. Wahidi
Scott L. Shofer

OUTLINE

Diagnostic Bronchoscopy
Therapeutic Bronchoscopy
Airway Stenting
Pleural Disease
Future Directions

OBJECTIVES

1. Compare flexible fiberoptic bronchoscopy and rigid bronchoscopy.
2. Discuss appropriate patient selection for bronchoscopy.
3. List absolute and relative contraindications for bronchoscopy.
4. Discuss issues related to patient preparation for bronchoscopy.
5. Discuss issues related to sedation for bronchoscopy.
6. Describe the following techniques for flexible fiberoptic bronchoscopy: airway examination, bronchoalveolar lavage, bronchoscopic washing, bronchoscopic brushing, endobronchial biopsy, transbronchial biopsy, and transbronchial needle aspiration.
7. List complications of bronchoscopy.
8. List indications for bronchoscopy.
9. Describe the indications, equipment, and technique for rigid bronchoscopy.
10. Compare the types of stents used for airway stenting.
11. Describe the indications and procedure for thoracentesis.

KEY TERMS

airway stent
brachytherapy
bronchoalveolar lavage (BAL)
bronchoscopic brushing
bronchoscopic washing
bronchoscopy
conscious sedation
diagnostic bronchoscopy
endobronchial biopsy
exudative
flexible fiberoptic bronchoscope
hybrid stent
lung-volume reduction
metallic stent
nonprotected bronchial brush
pleural effusion
pleurodesis
protected bronchial brush
rigid bronchoscope
sclerosing agent
silicone stent
therapeutic bronchoscopy
thoracentesis
transbronchial biopsy (TBB)
transbronchial needle aspiration (TBNA)
transudative
videobronchoscope

INTRODUCTION

Interventional pulmonology is an evolving field within pulmonary medicine that focuses on procedural services provided to patients with airway disorders and pleural diseases. It encompasses three main areas in pulmonary medicine: malignant and nonmalignant airway disorders, pleural diseases, and artificial airways. The topics of **diagnostic bronchoscopy**, therapeutic bronchoscopy, and pleural interventions are covered in this chapter.

Diagnostic Bronchoscopy

Overview of Bronchoscopy

Bronchoscopy is the most commonly used invasive procedure in pulmonary medicine and can be used to perform both diagnostic and therapeutic procedures (**CPG 11–1**). In the United States alone, approximately 500,000 bronchoscopies are performed each year.[1]

Gustav Killian performed the first bronchoscopy in Germany in 1897 using a laryngoscope and a rigid esophagoscopy tube to remove a foreign body (a piece of pork bone) from the proximal right main stem bronchus. This led to the development of the rigid bronchoscope, consisting of a long, hollow, rigid tube with channels for light and other instruments. In the early 1900s, Chevalier Jackson of Philadelphia further refined the rigid bronchoscope and advocated for its use in clinical practice.

It was not until the late 1960s that the flexible fiberoptic bronchoscope was developed by Shigeto Ikeda in Tokyo, Japan.[2] The development of the flexible bronchoscope significantly simplified the procedure, and over time, it became widely used by pulmonary physicians, thoracic surgeons, and intensivists with the assistance of a respiratory therapist.

The Flexible Bronchoscope

The **flexible fiberoptic bronchoscope** (**Figure 11–1**) consists of a control unit (or head) and a soft, flexible shaft. The shaft has an external diameter of 3.5 to 6 mm and a tip that can rotate up to 210 degrees. The shaft contains a hollow internal operating channel for suctioning secretions and collecting specimens, and a working channel for administration of solutions (saline, lidocaine) and passage of instruments. The control unit is attached to a light source, and it can also be fitted with a camera for dynamic or still photography.

There are two types of flexible bronchoscopes: fiberoptic and video chip. The original flexible bronchoscopes were based on fiberoptic technology, with images being transmitted from the instrument's distal objective lens to the proximal eyepiece. The development of video chips led to the creation of the flexible **videobronchoscope**, which works by capturing digital images at the distal tip and transmitting these images via the bronchoscope to a remote television monitor.[3] The videobronchoscope has greatly enhanced the field of bronchoscopy, allowing images to be captured and saved with a camera and aiding in teaching and training purposes with its

CLINICAL PRACTICE GUIDELINE 11–1

Bronchoscopy Assisting

Indications

- The presence of lesions of unknown etiology on the chest radiograph film or the need to evaluate recurrent pneumonia, persistent atelectasis, or pulmonary infiltrates
- The need to assess patency or mechanical properties of the upper airway
- The need to investigate hemoptysis, persistent unexplained cough, dyspnea, localized wheeze, or stridor
- Suspicious or positive sputum cytology results
- The need to obtain lower respiratory tract secretions, cell washings, and biopsies for cytologic, histologic, and microbiologic evaluation
- The need to determine the location and extent of injury from toxic inhalation or aspiration
- The need to evaluate problems associated with endotracheal or tracheostomy tubes (tracheal damage, airway obstruction, or tube placement)
- The need for aid in performing difficult intubations or percutaneous tracheostomies
- The suspicion that secretions or mucous plugs are responsible for lobar or segmental atelectasis
- The need to remove abnormal endobronchial tissue or foreign material by forceps, basket, or laser
- The need to retrieve a foreign body (although under most circumstances, rigid bronchoscopy is preferred)
- Therapeutic management of endobronchial toilet in ventilator-associated pneumonia
- Achieving selective intubation of a main stem bronchus
- The need to place and/or assess airway stent function
- The need for airway balloon dilation in treatment of tracheobronchial stenosis

(continues)

Clinical Practice Guideline 11–1 *(continued)*

Contraindications

Absolute contraindications

- Absence of consent from the patient or his or her representative unless a medical emergency exists and the patient is not competent to give permission
- Absence of an experienced bronchoscopist to perform or closely and directly supervise the procedure
- Lack of adequate facilities and personnel to care for emergencies such as cardiopulmonary arrest, pneumothorax, or bleeding
- Inability to adequately oxygenate the patient during the procedure
- The danger of a serious complication from bronchoscopy is especially high in patients with the disorders listed, and these conditions are usually considered absolute contraindications unless the risk–benefit assessment warrants the procedure:
  - Coagulopathy or bleeding diathesis that cannot be corrected
  - Severe refractory hypoxemia
  - Unstable hemodynamic status, including dysrhythmias

Relative contraindications (or conditions involving increased risk), according to the American Thoracic Society guidelines for fiberoptic bronchoscopy in adults

- Lack of patient cooperation
- Recent (within 6 weeks) myocardial infarction or unstable angina
- Partial tracheal obstruction
- Moderate to severe hypoxemia or any degree of hypercarbia
- Uremia and pulmonary hypertension (possible serious hemorrhage after biopsy)
- Lung abscess (danger of flooding the airway with purulent material)
- Obstruction of the superior vena cava (possibility of bleeding and laryngeal edema)
- Debility and malnutrition
- Disorders requiring laser therapy, biopsy of lesions obstructing large airways, or multiple transbronchial lung biopsies
- Known or suspected pregnancy (safety concern of possible radiation exposure)
- Safety of bronchoscopic procedures in asthmatic patients is a concern, but presence of asthma does not preclude use of these procedures
- Recent head injury patients susceptible to increased intracranial pressures
- Inability to sedate (including time constraints of oral ingestion of solids or liquids)

Hazards and Complications

- Adverse effects of medication used before and during the bronchoscopic procedure
- Hypoxemia
- Hypercarbia
- Bronchospasm
- Hypotension
- Laryngospasm, bradycardia, or other vagally mediated phenomena
- Mechanical complications such as epistaxis, pneumothorax, and hemoptysis
- Increased airway resistance
- Death
- Infection hazard for healthcare workers or other patients
- Cross-contamination of specimens or bronchoscopes
- Nausea and/or vomiting
- Fever and chills
- Cardiac dysrhythmias

Modified from AARC clinical practice guideline: bronchoscopy assisting—2007 revision and update. *Respir Care*. 2007;52:74–80. Reprinted with permission.

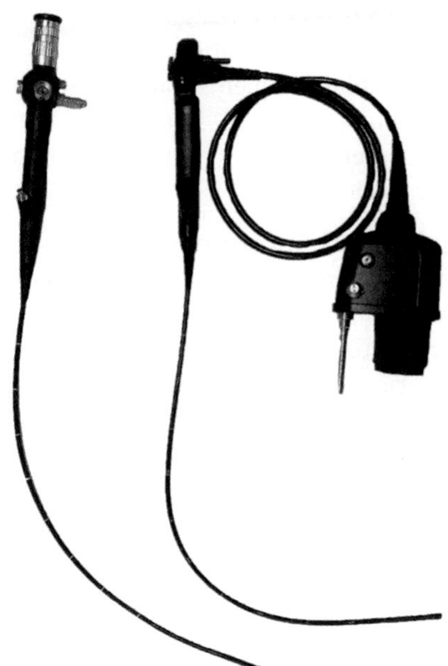

FIGURE 11–1 Flexible fiberoptic (on left) and video chip bronchoscope.

real-time display. The disadvantages of the flexible videobronchoscope include additional equipment and space requirements.[3]

Flexible Fiberoptic Bronchoscopy

Bronchoscopy is a safe and effective tool for diagnosing and treating a wide variety of pulmonary processes. However, this safety is dependent on several factors. The operator or bronchoscopist must master the technical skills of manipulating the bronchoscope safely through the airways and have a good understanding of respiratory anatomy. In addition, appropriate patient selection and preparation, careful use of sedatives, and a clear understanding of the indications and expected yields for the various bronchoscopic procedures are critical to making each bronchoscopy a success.

Patient Selection

The ideal patient for fiberoptic bronchoscopy is awake, able to understand and cooperate with the procedure, and free of other conditions that could elevate the risk of the procedure. In particular, major conditions to consider include ischemic or arrhythmic heart disease, bleeding diathesis (e.g., coagulopathy, thrombocytopenia, uremia), neurologic disease or head trauma, and respiratory insufficiency. Although bronchoscopy can be performed in patients who fall short of this ideal, the risk of the procedure increases accordingly, and options for more invasive manipulations (e.g., biopsies, lengthy procedures) can be limited. A careful history and physical should be targeted toward ascertaining the presence and severity of any risk factors or comorbidities, documenting previous anesthesia and associated complications, and defining ways in which the timing or nature of the procedure can be modified to minimize risk to the patient.

BOX 11–1

Contraindications to Fiberoptic Bronchoscopy and Transbronchial Biopsy

Absolute

- Inability to maintain adequate oxygenation
- Operator inexperience
- Inadequate facilities
- Lack of informed consent
- Status asthmaticus

Relative

- Active ischemic heart disease
- Active cardiac arrhythmia
- Refractory hypoxemia
- Bleeding diathesis
- Uncooperative patient
- Active or uncontrolled bronchospasm

Preoperative laboratory studies, including platelet count, coagulation studies, blood urea nitrogen level, and creatinine level, are often obtained to assess for bleeding tendencies. However, multiple studies examining the utility of preoperative lab work have determined that this is not universally necessary, but should be tailored to patients with medical histories suggesting an abnormality. In a retrospective study of 305 bronchoscopies with biopsy, Kozak and Brath identified five clinical risk factors that should prompt further preoperative evaluation: prior anticoagulant therapy, liver disease, family or personal history of bleeding tendencies, active bleeding or recent transfusion requirements, and presence of an unreliable historian.[4]

RESPIRATORY RECAP

Factors Necessary for Successful Bronchoscopy

- » Patient selection
- » Patient preparation
- » Appropriate sedation

Box 11–1 lists the absolute and relative contraindications for bronchoscopy and biopsy. Absolute contraindications to bronchoscopy are few and include inability to provide informed consent, status asthmaticus, severe hypoxemia, and unstable cardiovascular conditions. Some of the main factors to consider when selecting a patient for bronchoscopy are discussed next.

Asthma and Bronchospasm

Although bronchoscopy can be safely performed in asthmatic patients, it is associated with a significant drop in FEV_1 and PaO_2 after the procedure. This drop correlates inversely with the concentration of methacholine required to produce a 20% fall in FEV_1 at baseline but not with the usual measures of asthma severity, such as albuterol use, symptom scoring, and peak flow variation.[5] Therefore, bronchoscopy should be approached cautiously in the patient with asthma, and avoided entirely in the setting of status asthmaticus. In the case of elective bronchoscopy, the procedure should be deferred until bronchospasm is effectively controlled.

Cardiovascular Risk

Fiberoptic bronchoscopy can induce significant hemodynamic changes, including rise in heart rate by 43%, mean arterial pressure by 30%, and cardiac index by 28% when compared with prebronchoscopy controls.[6] Although these changes are well tolerated in a patient with normal cardiovascular function, they can cause significant stress in a patient with underlying heart disease. These hemodynamic changes in combination with episodic oxygen desaturation can lead to an imbalance between myocardial oxygen demand and delivery and precipitate myocardial ischemia, arrhythmias or both.[7] When possible, patients with active cardiac ischemia or recent myocardial infarction should have their bronchoscopy delayed until their cardiac status is stabilized. The British Thoracic Society's guidelines recommend deferring bronchoscopy a minimum of 6 weeks following myocardial infarction.[8]

Head Trauma and Elevated Intracranial Pressure

Increased intracranial pressure (ICP) has been anecdotally cited as a relative contraindication to bronchoscopy because of concerns that the rise in intrathoracic pressure induced by bronchoscopy-associated cough could abruptly raise ICP and precipitate herniation. A retrospective study found no increase in neurologic complications in patients with space-occupying central nervous system lesions undergoing bronchoscopy, although pretreatment with steroids was recommended to decrease cerebral edema.[9] More recently, a prospective study of 23 patients with intracranial drains in place revealed substantial, though transient, increases in ICP in patients undergoing bronchoscopy, despite adequate levels of sedation, analgesia, and paralysis.[10] No acute deterioration in the patients' clinical status was observed, but unfortunately, long-term complications or sequelae from these changes remain unknown.[10] Therefore, although fiberoptic bronchoscopy is often necessary in the care of patients after neurologic events, it should be used with caution in this patient population.

Hypoxemia and High Oxygen Requirement

Bronchoscopy carries a higher risk in patients who are hypoxemic at baseline, although determining the cause of hypoxemia is a common indication for bronchoscopy. Unfortunately, hypoxemia is also a complication of bronchoscopy, resulting from sedation-related hypoventilation and ventilation-perfusion mismatch secondary to partial airway occlusion (from the bronchoscope), atelectasis from frequent suctioning, airway bleeding, lavage fluid, and cough.[11] Although there is no absolute amount of supplemental oxygen that is a contraindication for bronchoscopy, caution should be used in patients with high oxygen requirements. Many pulmonologists advocate for elective intubation prior to bronchoscopy in patients with high supplemental oxygen requirements. Severe hypoxemia with $Pa{O_2}$ less than 65 to 70 mm Hg despite supplemental oxygen therapy is generally considered a contraindication.[12]

Anticoagulant and Antiplatelet Therapy

Use of anticoagulant and antiplatelet agents is common among patients referred for bronchoscopy. Therefore, it is important to carefully review all medications with the patient prior to bronchoscopy and make appropriate recommendations for continuing or holding medications prior to the procedure date.

- *Aspirin.* Aspirin was previously considered a contraindication to bronchoscopy due to its antiplatelet effects and prolongation of bleeding time. However, a large multicenter randomized trial found no difference in bleeding from transbronchial biopsies in the aspirin group compared with the no-aspirin group.[13] Therefore, it is generally accepted that patients can undergo bronchoscopy with transbronchial biopsy without holding aspirin therapy.
- *Clopidogrel.* In contrast to aspirin, clopidogrel significantly increases bleeding risks following transbronchial biopsy. When the effect of clopidogrel on the incidence of bleeding was studied during transbronchial biopsy, significant bleeding rates increased to 89% compared with 3.4% in the control group.[14] In a small number of patients receiving both aspirin and clopidogrel, the incidence of significant bleeding was 100% following transbronchial biopsy.[14] Given the relatively long half-life of clopidogrel, most practices require patients to discontinue clopidogrel a minimum of 5 days prior to undergoing bronchoscopy with transbronchial biopsy.
- *Warfarin and heparin.* No randomized trials exist regarding the use of warfarin in the setting of bronchoscopy. The British Thoracic Society recommends holding warfarin for 3 to 5 days prior to bronchoscopy and/or providing supplemental vitamin K prior to the procedure.[15,16] Laboratory studies should be obtained prior to the procedure to ensure appropriate clearance of anticoagulation effects. Guidelines from the American College of Chest Physicians suggest that an international normalized ratio (INR) of 1.5 is safe for most surgical procedures.[17] In patients who require bridging with therapeutic heparin, consensus statements recommend stopping unfractionated heparin a minimum of 4 to 6 hours prior to the procedure or holding low molecular weight heparin (such as enoxaparin) 24 hours in advance.[17] Heparin and/or warfarin can be resumed 12 to 24 hours after bronchoscopy in the absence of bleeding complications.

Thrombocytopenia

There are limited data available regarding what thresholds for platelets constitute safe levels for bronchoscopy. Transfusion guidelines and expert statements have recommended minimum platelet counts of 20,000 to 50,000/mm^3 for fiberoptic bronchoscopy and greater than 50,000/mm^3 for transbronchial biopsy.[18] When thrombocytopenia is present, an oral route for bronchoscope introduction is preferred to avoid unnecessary epistaxis.

Uremia and Renal Dysfunction

It is well established that uremia affects all aspects of platelet function, including secretion, adhesion, and aggregation.[19] No studies specifically examining the effect of uremia on bleeding complications in bronchoscopy currently exist. Some authors have suggested that the use of recombinant arginine vasopressin or desmopressin acetate (DDAVP) may decrease the bleeding time in uremic patients by increasing factor VIII levels and promoting platelet aggregation. The shortening of bleeding time with DDAVP is felt to occur within 1 hour of IV infusion with a dose of 0.3 μg/kg IV, and to last up to 6 to 8 hours.[20] However, the surgical literature reports mixed results in terms of benefit from vasopressin administration in the setting of renal insufficiency. Because of the substantial cost of vasopressin, and in the absence of a large randomized control trial showing clear benefit, its current use remains at the discretion of the physician and the bleeding risks of the individual patient.

Lung transplant recipients have been found to have higher bleeding risks from bronchoscopy independent of traditional risk factors such as coagulation parameters, aspirin use, and renal dysfunction.[21] Therefore, many centers are more aggressive about administering vasopressin in lung transplant recipients with coexistent renal insufficiency and have shown this to be beneficial in reducing bleeding complications.[22]

Patient Preparation

Informed Consent

Once the appropriate patient has been selected, informed consent can be obtained. All aspects of the procedure, from the initial application of topical anesthesia to the introduction of the bronchoscope through the nose or mouth, vocal cords, and distal airways, should be explained. The sensations that the patient can anticipate should be described, including the sensation of upper airway closure that is sometimes experienced as topical anesthesia takes effect, pressure in the nose as the bronchoscope is introduced, and the desire to cough as the bronchoscope is navigated through the airways. Reassurance should be provided about the steps taken to maximize patient comfort throughout the procedure, including the administration of topical anesthesia to alleviate cough and IV sedation as needed.

Procedure Risks and Complications

The risks of bronchoscopy and anesthesia should be specifically reviewed with the patient. The risk of major complications from bronchoscopy, including pneumothorax, pulmonary hemorrhage, infection, and respiratory failure, is 0.6%. When transbronchial biopsy is performed, the risk of serious complications is higher, at 1% to 6%.[23] Minor complications from bronchoscopy include fever, cough, bronchospasm, transient hypoxia, and hemoptysis. Additionally, cardiovascular complications can occur from the stress of the procedure itself, particularly in high-risk patients. Cardiac events can include vasovagal reactions, arrhythmias, myocardial ischemia, angina, and cardiac arrest.[7] The mortality rate from bronchoscopy is approximately 0.01% and has decreased in recent years as monitoring capabilities and technology have improved.[23]

Minimizing Complications

In an effort to minimize aspiration risk, the patient should be kept fasting after midnight prior to a morning procedure. If the procedure is planned for the afternoon, a light liquid breakfast is generally permitted.

Transient hypoxemia has been documented in up to 35% of patients undergoing fiberoptic bronchoscopy, but can often be alleviated with the use of supplemental oxygen therapy.[24] Therefore, oxygen supplementation of 2 to 3 L/min is recommended as a preventive measure for all patients undergoing bronchoscopy.[24]

Postprocedure Care and Education

Transient fever has been observed in up to 10% of patients after bronchoscopy, and typically resolves within 24 hours. For isolated postprocedure fever, no antibiotic therapy is needed.[25] Additionally, many patients experience a small amount of hemoptysis following bronchoscopy, which gradually subsides over the next 24 hours. Finally, patients receiving conscious sedation should be advised not to drive or operate heavy machinery for 24 hours following the procedure.

Patient Sedation

In one study examining patient perceptions of bronchoscopy, 62% of patients admitted to being anxious and fearful about potential pain, breathing difficulties, and discomfort from the procedure.[26] With careful explanation and reassurance, the physician, nurse, and respiratory therapist can help ease some of these fears. Additionally, use of intravenous sedation can be important in alleviating anxiety, improving patient comfort and cooperation, providing amnestic effects, and facilitating the bronchoscopic procedure.[27] Therefore, although bronchoscopy can be performed with topical anesthesia alone, many physicians and patients prefer the judicial use of adjunctive IV sedation.

Conscious sedation is generally used in the outpatient setting, which provides moderate levels of sedation and

TABLE 11-1 Common Pharmacologic Agents Used for Fiberoptic Bronchoscopy

Agent	Dose and Route	Onset	Duration	Effect	Side Effects
Anticholinergic					
Atropine	IM 0.4–1.0 mg	30–60 minutes	Variable	Reduce secretion, reduce vagal tone	Tachycardia, tachydysrhythmias, AV dissociation, urinary retention, dry mouth
Local Anesthetics					
Lidocaine	1–10%, topical or by inhalation Maximum dose 5–7 mg/kg	5–10 minutes	30–60 minutes	Cough suppression, local anesthesia	Early bronchospasm, dizziness, seizures in high doses; toxic reactions when plasma levels exceed 5 μg/mL
Sedation					
Midazolam	IV 2.5–10.0 mg (0.05–0.075 mg/kg)	1–3 minutes	2 hours	Amnesia, sedation	Respiratory depression
Diazepam	IV 2–7 mg (0.1 mg/kg) PO 5–10 mg	1–3 minutes 15–30 minutes	2–8 hours	Amnesia, sedation	Respiratory depression, thrombophlebitis, pain on injection
Narcotics					
Meperidine	IV/IM 20–75 mg (1 mg/kg)	IV 1–3 minutes IM 15–30 minutes	2–4 hours	Analgesia	Respiratory depression, nausea
Codeine	IM 20–120 mg	30 minutes	2–4 hours	Cough suppression	Urinary retention
Morphine	IV/IM 2–10 mg (0.1 mg/kg)	IV 5 minutes IM 15–30 minutes	2–6 hours	Analgesia	Respiratory depression, nausea, itching, bronchospasm, bradycardia, biliary spasm
Fentanyl	IV 50–100 μg (1 μg/kg)	2 minutes	30–60 minutes	Analgesia	Respiratory depression, nausea, chest wall rigidity, bradycardia
Alfentanil	IV 250–1000 μg (10 μg/kg)	1 minute	15–30 minutes	Analgesia	Respiratory depression, nausea, chest wall rigidity
Propofol	IV 50 μg/mg/kg (10–30 mg)	30 seconds	8–10 minutes	Sedation	Respiratory depression, hypotension
Antagonists					
Naloxone	IV 40 μg titrated to effect q 2–3 minutes	1 minute	Dose dependent, lasting 20–60 minutes	Reversal of opioid effect	Tachycardia, hypertension, dysrhythmias
Flumazenil	0.4–1 mg	2 minutes	1 hour	Reversal of benzodiazepine effect	CNS excitation, nausea, residual sedation

AV, atrioventricular; CNS, central nervous system.

From Matot I, Kramer MR. Sedation in outpatient bronchoscopy. *Respir Med.* 2000;94(12):1145–1153, Table 2. Reprinted with permission.

analgesia with short-acting agents while still maintaining adequate spontaneous ventilation and airway patency. Conscious sedation can only be performed in units where the medical team has had special training, and continuous monitoring and nursing capabilities must be available until the patient has recovered completely.[27]

Many possible sedation regimens are available for bronchoscopy. These regimens can include topical lidocaine for local anesthesia; anticholinergic drugs for reducing secretions and inhibiting vagal tone; codeine for antitussive effects; benzodiazepines for sedation, amnesia, and anxiolysis; and/or opioids for analgesia and cough suppression.[27] **Table 11-1** lists commonly used drugs for fiberoptic bronchoscopy as well as their typical doses, onset, duration of action, therapeutic roles, and side effects. Anticholinergic drugs, such as atropine, were previously considered standard premedications for bronchoscopy given their secretion-drying effects as well as their ability to prevent bradycardia and bronchoconstriction. However, more recent studies found no increase in bradycardia or excessive secretions when atropine was not used,[28] and many centers have abandoned these agents entirely.

Topical anesthesia is administered immediately prior to the start of the procedure, and can be given by a variety of routes. Many agents are available (e.g., tetracaine, benzocaine, cocaine), but lidocaine is the most commonly used because of its wide safety profile and short half-life.[27] An atomizer is often used to spray lidocaine onto the tongue, oropharynx, and pharynx. Lidocaine gel can also be used to lubricate the nose. Alternatively, nebulized lidocaine can be delivered through a face mask to anesthetize the entire airway, but takes approximately 20 minutes to administer. Whichever approach is used, careful attention must be given to the total dose of lidocaine delivered before and during the procedure because the serum concentration after topical administration can reach as high as 50% of what would be achieved by IV bolus.[27] The total lidocaine dose should not exceed 5 to 7 mg/kg. This dose should be adjusted downward in patients with significant hepatic or cardiac disease to avoid toxicity or adverse effects.

Entry into the nasopharynx can be facilitated by the application of topical vasoconstrictors such as 4% cocaine or 0.5% phenylephrine, both of which decrease local bleeding and mucosal edema. These can be applied directly into the nose with a cotton-tipped applicator, which can also be used to assess the patency of the nasopharynx and adequacy of topical anesthesia. Once the nasopharynx and/or oropharynx has been adequately anesthetized, additional aliquots (typically 2–3 mL each) of 1% to 2% lidocaine can be applied directly through the bronchoscope during the procedure to the visualized glottis, trachea, carina, and other airways as needed.

In addition to topical agents, IV medications are used both for premedication and sedative effects. Short-acting benzodiazepines, such as midazolam, are commonly used for their amnestic and anxiolytic properties. Although benzodiazepines have few cardiopulmonary effects alone, the risk of respiratory depression is potentiated when used in combination with opioids.[27] Similarly, short-acting opioids, such as fentanyl, can be used for their analgesic effects as well as to decrease the cough reflex and provide modest respiratory depressant effects. When these agents are used, their specific reversal agents (naloxone for narcotics and flumazenil for benzodiazepines) should be readily available.

Propofol is an alternative sedative-hypnotic agent for bronchoscopy given its rapid onset and short duration. It can be used for either conscious sedation or general anesthesia, depending on its dose-dependent sedative effects. Therefore, use of propofol often requires a trained anesthesia practitioner, should be reserved for use by experienced administrators, and is not yet approved for conscious sedation in many centers.

Patients should be monitored with telemetry, pulse oximetry, and noninvasive blood pressure measurements throughout the bronchoscopy procedure as well as the recovery period. Additionally, as noted earlier, supplemental oxygen at 2 to 3 L/min should be provided during the procedure to prevent transient hypoxia, and weaned appropriately at the conclusion of the procedure. Most bronchoscopies are performed on an outpatient basis, and patients are usually safe for discharge within 1 to 2 hours after the procedure. They should be advised not to drive or operate heavy machinery for 24 hours, given the potential for prolonged effects of sedative medications.

Flexible Fiberoptic Bronchoscopy Techniques

Airway Examination

The flexible bronchoscope can be introduced through the nose, mouth, endotracheal tube, or tracheostomy site. The most commonly used approach is transnasal, which is thought to provide more stability (and comfort) by anchoring the scope within the nose and preventing unnecessary fluctuation of the bronchoscope from side to side and interference from the patient's tongue. However, either a nasal or oral approach is acceptable, depending on operator preference and patient characteristics. In patients with unfavorable nasal anatomy, thrombocytopenia, or predilection for sinus infections (e.g., cystic fibrosis), the oral route often is preferred. Many interventional pulmonary procedures require larger bronchoscopes and more equipment, necessitating oral entry. With the oral route, a bite block is used to help anchor the scope and prevent trauma to the bronchoscope from biting. Bronchoscopy via tracheostomy requires a minimum trach size of 6 mm internal diameter or larger. Similarly, the endotracheal tube must be at least 1.5 mm larger than the bronchoscope (typically 8 mm internal diameter or larger).

The bronchoscope is lubricated with lidocaine gel and introduced under direct visualization into the preanesthetized nare, or alternatively, through a mouthpiece into the posterior hypopharynx. If introducing through a tracheostomy site or endotracheal tube, a medical-grade silicone spray is often necessary for additional lubrication. The nasal and, to a slightly lesser extent, oral approaches allow visualization of the anatomy of the posterior nasopharynx and larynx, including the eustachian tubes, base of the tongue, epiglottis, aryepiglottic folds, and vocal cords (**Figure 11–2**). All approaches allow examination of the trachea, carina, main stem bronchi, and, sequentially, the distal airways to the level of the fourth-order bronchi. A systematic approach to the airway exam is vital for complete evaluation of all upper and lower respiratory tract structures.

RESPIRATORY RECAP

Fiberoptic Bronchoscopy Techniques

- » Airway examination
- » Bronchoalveolar lavage
- » Bronchoscopic washing
- » Bronchial brushing
- » Endobronchial biopsy
- » Transbronchial lung biopsy
- » Transbronchial needle aspiration

The bronchoscopist should pay careful attention to the movement of the vocal cords (**Figure 11–3**) with respiration and phonation to screen for functional as well as structural abnormalities. Paralysis of the left true vocal cord is the most common abnormality seen, which manifests as inability to abduct the left cord. Patients with unilateral vocal cord paralysis are often symptomatic, with laryngospasm or recurrent aspiration.[3] Although sometimes no cause is identified, unilateral vocal cord paralysis, particularly on the left side, can be a sign of malignancy due to compression of the left recurrent

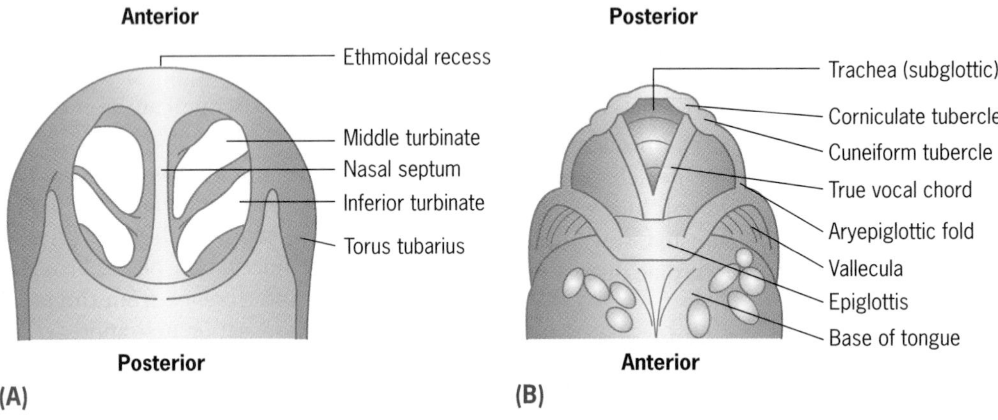

FIGURE 11–2 Normal nasopharyngeal (**A**) and laryngeal (**B**) structures as they appear to the bronchoscopist. This article was published in *Textbook of Respiratory Medicine*. 2nd ed. Murray JF, Nadel JA, eds. Copyright Elsevieer (WB Saunders) 1994.

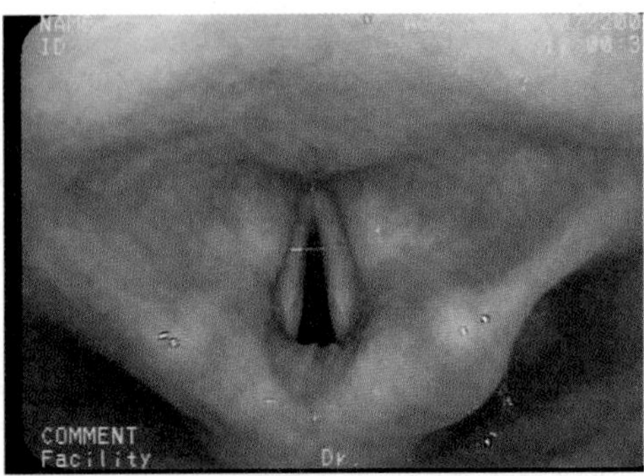

FIGURE 11–3 Normal vocal cord position and appearance.

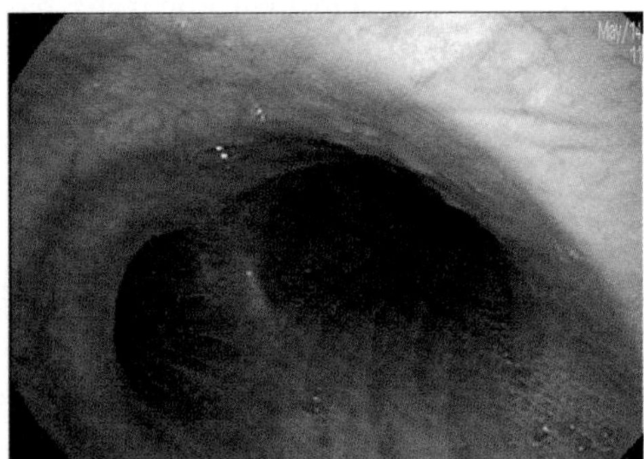

FIGURE 11–5 Normal-appearing main carina with sharply defined bifurcation.

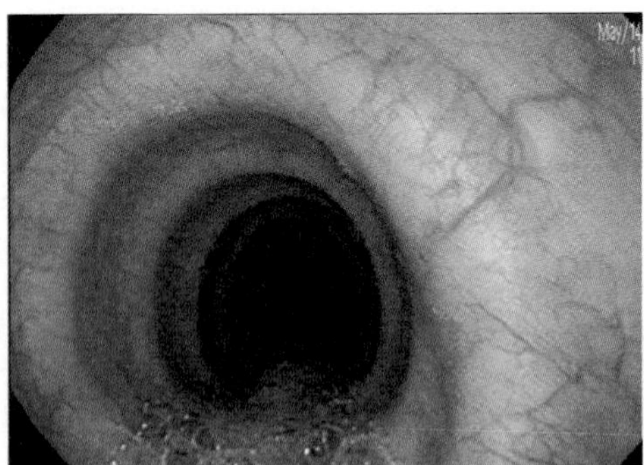

FIGURE 11–4 Normal tracheal anatomy with anterior cartilaginous wall and the posterior membranous wall.

laryngeal nerve by a cervical or mediastinal mass (or lymph node) and, in the setting of malignancy, could have important staging implications.[3]

The normal trachea (**Figure 11–4**) has well-defined cartilaginous C-shaped rings along the anterior wall, which serve to maintain airway patency during expiration and cough. The posterior wall consists of a highly organized series of connective tissue and smooth muscle fibers.[3] The shape of the trachea can provide valuable clinical information as well. The scabbard or sabre-sheath trachea, characterized by lateral narrowing and increased diameter of the posterior wall, can be seen in patients with obstructive lung disease such as emphysema and is felt to represent the chronic pressure on the trachea from forced exhalation. Tracheal stenosis can lead to areas of fixed narrowing, as opposed to the dynamic collapse observed with tracheomalacia. In the elderly, the trachea often appears elongated and buckled due to submucosal atrophy, making the tracheal cartilage appear more prominent.[29] Masses that occupy the anterior mediastinum may displace the anterior or lateral trachea, whereas esophageal tumors would displace or ulcerate into the posterior trachea.

The site where the trachea divides into the right and left main stem bronchi is termed the *carina*. The normal carina is a sharply angled structure with a smooth mucosal covering (**Figure 11–5**). When the lymph nodes in the subcarinal space become enlarged as a result of infection, inflammation, or malignancy, the carina may develop a splayed or deformed appearance (**Figure 11–6**).

The appearance of the respiratory mucosa can also provide diagnostic clues. For example, an inflamed hypopharynx may represent severe gastroesophageal reflux disease. A characteristic cobblestone appearance

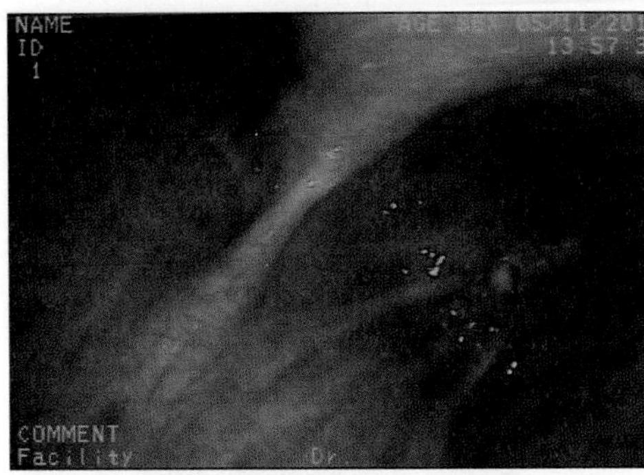

FIGURE 11–6 Tumor infiltrating the proximal right mainstem bronchus.

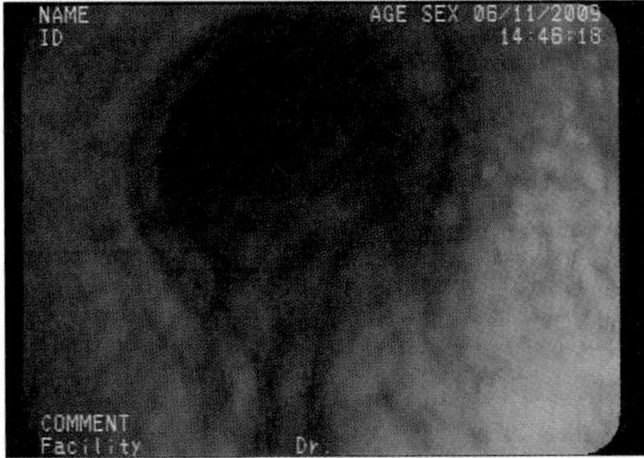

FIGURE 11–7 Cobblestone appearance of mucosa, a characteristic finding in sarcoidosis.

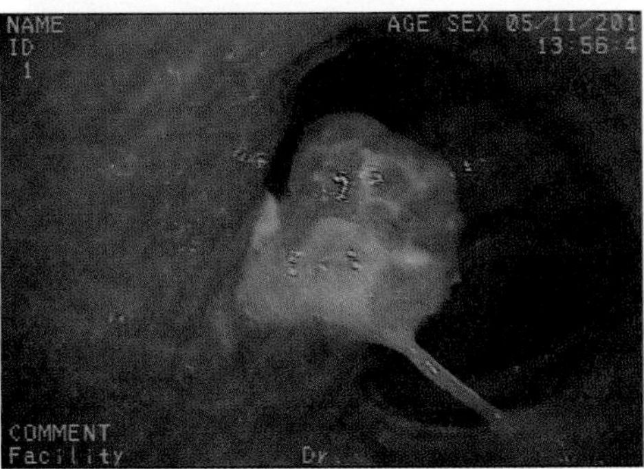

FIGURE 11–8 Endobronchial squamous cell carcinoma arising from the left upper lobe.

is often noted of endobronchial mucosa in sarcoidosis (**Figure 11–7**), and diffuse edema and inflammation is typically seen in chronic bronchitis. In contrast, a focal area of inflamed, friable, or irregular mucosa may represent the presence of submucosal tumor invasion (**Figure 11–8**).

After examination of the trachea and carina, the right and left bronchial trees are examined to the subsegmental level. Knowledge of normal endobronchial anatomy and nomenclature are essential for a complete and thorough exam. Each bronchial division is examined to the subsegmental level, with notation made of anatomic variant, mucosal abnormality, presence of endobronchial tumor or secretions, patency of bronchial lumens, and evidence of extrinsic compression. A complete airway exam should almost always precede any other diagnostic maneuvers.

Bronchoalveolar Lavage

Bronchoalveolar lavage (BAL) is the method traditionally used to sample the cellular and microbiologic components of the alveolar space. Although it has been used as a research tool to establish the cellular and biochemical features of several pulmonary diseases such as sarcoidosis, asthma, and interstitial lung disease, its primary use in daily clinical practice is for cytologic and microbiologic sampling. Additionally, BAL can be a tool for pulmonary toilet in rare diseases such as pulmonary alveolar proteinosis by helping to remove the abnormal surfactant material that accumulates with this disease.

Radiographic imaging is frequently used to determine the location for sample collection with the highest yield. The yield of bronchial lavage is generally better from nondependent areas such as anterior segments, the right middle lobe, or lingula. When a specific radiographic abnormality is present, the bronchoscope is directed to the closest correlating subsegmental bronchial lumen for lavage. However, in the presence of diffuse radiographic infiltrates, the right middle lobe or lingula is generally preferred due to the ease of intubation and occlusion so as to maximize return of lavage fluid.

When obtaining a BAL sample, the bronchoscope is advanced as far as possible into a third- or fourth-order bronchus to create a wedge or seal. Room-temperature sterile buffered saline is then introduced, allowed to wash out over the lung, and then retrieved by suction for analysis. The suction pressure is typically maintained below 120 cm H_2O to prevent premature collapse of the bronchus.[3] Some clinicians believe that having the patient hold a large breath also improves the volume of the BAL return.

Lavage amounts and techniques vary among bronchoscopists. The amount of normal saline used for diagnostic BAL should be limited to no more than 200 mL, even though most patients require less than 100 mL for adequate return. In most patients, approximately 60% of instilled fluid will be collected on lavage.[3] The most common lavage techniques include manual suction, gravity drainage, and mechanical suction at a moderate negative pressure. Additionally, multiple aliquots can be sequentially introduced before aspiration; alternatively, lavage fluid can be suctioned back after each 20- to 60-mL instillation. Some argue that serial lavage with manual suction produces a greater yield, although few data exist comparing the different bronchoscopic techniques.

If concern for diffuse alveolar hemorrhage (DAH) exists, serial lavage can be helpful for diagnosis because the return will become increasingly bloody as more alveolar fluid is sampled. This technique avoids false positives from scope trauma, in which fluid may initially appear hemorrhagic but will clear with additional aliquots of lavage fluid. Alternatively, DAH should be considered if BAL fluid exhibits more than 20% hemosiderin-laden macrophages on Prussian blue staining.[30]

Complications from bronchoalveolar lavage include hypoxemia and, rarely, bleeding. The incidence of bleeding from BAL in thrombocytopenic patients has been shown to be minimal.[31] Pneumothorax is an extremely rare complication of BAL and has been reported in the literature exclusively in intubated patients.

Bronchoscopic Washing

Bronchoscopic washing is similar to a lavage but is designed to sample the airway rather than the alveolar space. It is commonly used to obtain a cytologic specimen from an endobronchial mass, abnormal mucosa, or an obstructed orifice. When possible, bronchoscopic washing should be used in conjunction with other diagnostic methods such as bronchoscopic brushing or endobronchial biopsy. The timing of the wash, in respect to other procedures, is somewhat controversial. Some bronchoscopists advocate washing a lesion before any other manipulations to avoid contamination of the specimen with blood. Prior to biopsy, washing can also help to assess bleeding risk by evaluating how easily the lesion bleeds with suction alone. Others believe that the best yield for bronchoscopic washing is after biopsy or brushing, believing that more malignant cells may be recovered after the brush or biopsy disrupts the tumor surface. Additionally, bronchoscopic washings can be used when collection of fluid from BAL is inadequate or large amounts of secretions are present in the airway. However, in this setting, microbiology results can be difficult to interpret because of contamination from upper airway flora.

Similar to BAL, the suction apparatus is fitted with a collection trap reserved for the wash sample alone. The bronchoscope is then placed in close proximity to the lesion while 5- to 10-mL aliquots of sterile buffered saline are introduced and then suctioned back into the collection trap. The sample then is sent to cytology and/or microbiology for processing.

Bronchoscopic Brushing

Two types of brushes are available for **bronchoscopic brushing**. A standard **nonprotected bronchial brush** is used to collect cytologic samples of abnormalities in the proximal airways under direct visualization as well as peripheral lesions under fluoroscopic guidance. A catheter with a brush at its distal end (**Figure 11–9**) is introduced through the working channel of the bronchoscope. This brush may be open or enclosed within an open-ended sheath, which can be advanced and retracted by the assistant at the bronchoscopist's request. Because the sheath is open ended, the brush is not protected from upper airway contamination (within the bronchoscope) but is protected from losing samples when it is withdrawn from the bronchoscope at the conclusion of the procedure.

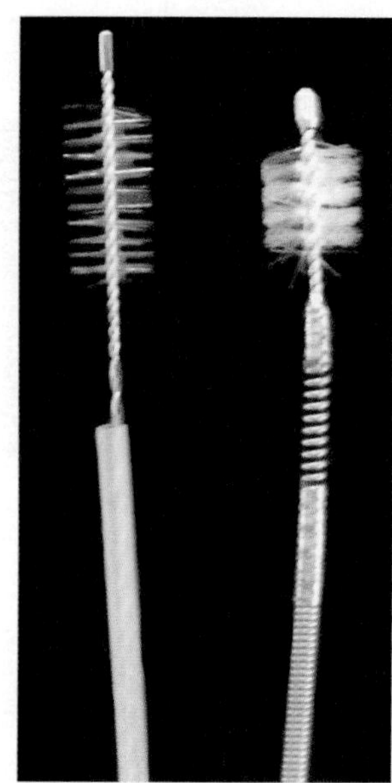

FIGURE 11–9 Brushes used for bronchoscopy.

Alternatively, a **protected bronchial brush** is available to collect microbiologic samples (for suspected infection) to ensure that the bacteria collected represent lower-tract pathogens and not upper airway contaminants. The protected specimen brush (PSB) is enclosed within two telescoping catheters, the outer of which is occluded at its tip by a biodegradable plug. This outer catheter protects the catheter tip from contamination as it is advanced through the bronchoscope and the proximal airways.[32] The protected brush is also designed with denser bristles and a more flexible head to maximize secretion recovery. When the area of interest is reached, the plug is dislodged, the inner catheter advanced, and the brush directed into the distal airway through the inner catheter. After the specimen is obtained, the brush is withdrawn into the inner catheter first, followed by the outer catheter, and then withdrawn from the bronchoscope. The outer catheter is cleaned with 70% alcohol and then cut off distal to the inner catheter in sterile fashion. The inner catheter is then advanced, cleaned with alcohol, and cut distal to the brush. Finally, the brush is advanced, cut off, and placed in sterile saline for processing.

With both brushes, the technique for sampling the airway itself is identical. For proximal lesions that are directly visualized, the brush is advanced through the tip of the bronchoscope, placed adjacent to the site of interest, and vigorously advanced back and forth in short strokes. This movement disrupts the mucosa and enables dislodged cells and tissue to become caught within the bristles. The brush is then withdrawn into its sheath and removed from the bronchoscope. For more peripheral lesions, the bronchoscope is advanced to the nearest

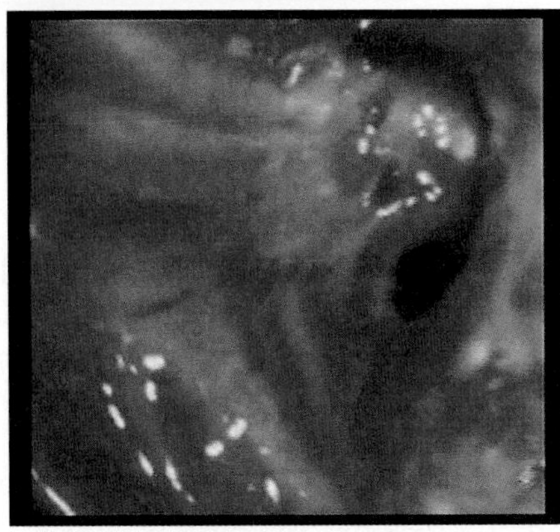

FIGURE 11–10 Endobronchial obstruction.

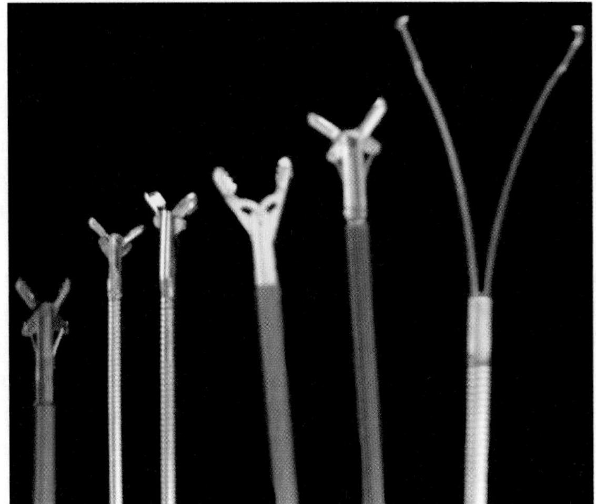

FIGURE 11–11 Biopsy forceps used for bronchoscopy.

segmental lumen and then the brush is advanced under fluoroscopic guidance to reach the lesion of interest.

The brush can be processed several ways, depending on the diagnostic goals. For cytologic analysis, including staining for special infections (such as acid-fast bacilli [AFB], fungi, *Pneumocystis carinii* pneumonia, or viral inclusions), the contents of the brush can be smeared directly onto glass slides that are then fixed by immediate immersion into 95% alcohol or application of a fixative spray. Alternatively, the entire brush can be placed in a sterile saline solution, vigorously agitated to dislodge its contents, and sent to a laboratory for culture.

Because of the vigorous brushing technique required to obtain samples, brushing does carry a slightly higher risk of bleeding than BAL or bronchial washing. This is particularly true if friable mucosa is being evaluated. In rare instances, pneumothorax can occur, particularly if very peripheral lesions are being sampled.

Endobronchial Biopsy

Endobronchial biopsy is the method used to sample abnormalities directly visualized within the airway, including visible tumors (**Figure 11–10**) or mucosal irregularities. A variety of tools are available, including cupped-tip forceps with a cutting edge, alligator forceps with a toothed jaw, and needle forceps with a sharp prong positioned between the jaws that can be used to help position the forceps over the area of interest.[2] Forceps with a central needle are particularly useful in obtaining biopsies from flat endobronchial lesions in the trachea or main stem bronchi, or when significant flexion of the bronchoscope is required.[2] However, in general, the choice of forceps depends on operator preference.

When the biopsy area has been identified, the forceps (**Figure 11–11**) are advanced through the working channel of the bronchoscope in the closed position. Once the forceps have been completely visualized within the airway lumen, the jaws can be opened and positioned directly over the lesion of interest. The bronchoscopist will then direct the assistant to close the jaws of the forceps, and the closed forceps and sample are removed together through the working channel of the bronchoscope. The sample is then dislodged from the forceps and placed in the appropriate medium for processing (formalin for histology, sterile saline for microbiologic culture). Multiple biopsy samples (three to six) should be obtained to maximize yield, particularly in the setting of an exophytic endobronchial mass, due to the common presence of surface necrosis and inflammation, which may otherwise preclude an actual pathologic diagnosis.[33] The major complication of endobronchial biopsy is bleeding.

Transbronchial Biopsy

Transbronchial biopsy (TBB) is used to collect small samples of lung tissue for histopathologic review. Careful study of a prebronchoscopy computed tomography (CT) scan is useful in determining the best pulmonary segment to access for biopsy. In diffuse pulmonary diseases, use of fluoroscopy is not necessary, although the risk of significant pneumothorax may be reduced. In focal disease that is visible on chest x-ray, use of fluoroscopy during the procedure may significantly increase the diagnostic yield of the study.

After a careful airway examination, the pulmonary segment of interest is intubated with the tip of the bronchoscope, and the pulmonary forceps are passed through the working channel of the bronchoscope. As the forceps are visualized entering the pulmonary subsegment, the fluoroscopy unit should be activated to visualize the forceps as they enter the distal segments of the lung. To take a biopsy of peripheral portions of the lung, the forceps should be gently advanced in the closed position until resistance is encountered. If fluoroscopy is used, the forceps may not appear to move very far within the lung if the direction of motion is within the plane of imaging due to the two-dimensional nature of fluoroscopic imaging. If the fluoroscopy unit is equipped with a C-arm, the camera head may be rotated out of plane from the forceps to detect movement in the anterior-posterior direction relative to the patient. Next, the forceps are withdrawn approximately 1 cm, and the command is given to open the forceps' jaws. The forceps are then advanced close to the area where resistance was encountered, and the forceps jaws are closed. With the fluoroscopy unit still activated, the forceps are retracted with firm, continuous pressure to allow the biopsy specimen to be removed from the surrounding lung parenchyma. The lung parenchyma should be watched on the fluoroscopy monitor for retraction during the collection of the biopsy sample. If there is excessive resistance or extensive retraction of the lung parenchyma during sampling, the forceps should be opened to release the lung tissue, and the biopsy procedure should be restarted. Once a sample is obtained, the forceps are removed from the working channel of the bronchoscope and the biopsy is placed in formalin.

Two schools of thought exist as to how best to manage the airway after a biopsy sample is collected. One school advocates use of the wedge technique, in which the tip of the bronchoscope is lodged firmly (wedge position) in the airway subsegment that was sampled to monitor for bleeding. It is thought that leaving the bronchoscope wedged permits control of potential bleeding by continuous suctioning to remove extravasated blood, thereby preventing soiling of the remainder of the lung. Continuous suctioning also allows the operator to assess the quantity of bleeding present, and collapsing the distal airways (with suction) produces a tamponade effect. When bleeding has slowed, the tip of the bronchoscope may be slowly withdrawn from the wedge position to allow observation of the bleeding segment and, if necessary, to facilitate repeating the wedge maneuver if the bleeding continues to be significant. The disadvantage of the wedge maneuver is that the bronchoscopist is not able either to visualize the airways due to blood obscuring the optics of the bronchoscope or to assess the effectiveness of the wedge in isolating the bleeding subsegment.

In the alternative strategy, the tip of the bronchoscope is withdrawn from the subsegment of interest so that the bronchoscopist can watch for welling up of blood from the distal lung. Blood is suctioned with a back-and-forth motion to clear the airway and maintain vision. This suctioning permits a more global assessment of the extent of bleeding and potential seepage of blood into the other portions of the lung. There are currently no data to support the superiority of either approach. Our practice is to have novice bronchoscopists maintain a wedge after each biopsy and use the observational technique after they have acquired more experience with the bronchoscope.

Several studies have examined how best to enhance biopsy yield in terms of number of samples to be collected and characteristics of the collected specimens. Most studies report a range of 4 to 10 pieces of tissue to optimize sampling sensitivity.[34–36] The British Thoracic Society's guidelines on flexible bronchoscopy recommend 4 to 6 samples in patients with diffuse lung disease and 7 to 8 in patients with focal lung disease.[8] Our practice is to obtain a minimum of 6 tissue pieces of a minimum size of 1 to 2 mm in the long axis for patients with either focal or diffuse lung disease.

Several studies have examined the optimal size of biopsy forceps for performing TBB. No clear difference has been established regarding size of tissue samples or diagnostic sensitivity between large and small forceps, although one study using large, alligator-type forceps showed lower yields compared with large or small forceps. The lower yield was attributed to difficulty in passing the larger forceps past the various subcarinae of the small airways.[37,38] A third study examined the size and quality of tissue samples obtained using a small round-cup, medium oval-cup, or large round-cup forceps. Tissue sample sizes were equal using the medium or large forceps, and larger in size than those obtained with the small forceps. However, the quality of samples was greater using the oval forceps, revealing less crush artifact and more intact basement membrane on pathologic analysis.[39]

An additional study examined the ability of physicians to predict the quality of TBB at the time of bronchoscopy. The authors found no significance of floating of the tissue sample in formalin (suggesting alveolated tissue), and no ability of the physicians to predict the quality of the sample at the time the specimen was obtained. The authors did find that alligator forceps obtained larger samples when compared with cup-type forceps of a similar size (3 mm), although the samples were graded for size using a technician's observation as the assessment tool (as opposed to the microscopic measurement used in the other studies described earlier).[40] Our practice is to use medium-sized oval-cup forceps for all of our TBBs because they do not entirely occlude the working channel of the bronchoscope while the forceps are extended, thereby permitting continued use of the working channel for suctioning. Larger forceps show no clear advantage in biopsy quality, but do preclude effective suctioning while they are deployed.

Following bronchoscopy with TBB, patients should be observed in a recovery unit, similar to other patients receiving conscious sedation. Given the increased risk of hemorrhage with TBB, outpatients should continue to hold their anticoagulant or antiplatelet agents until the morning after the procedure. Inpatients may resume anticoagulants such as heparin or enoxaparin 12 hours after the procedure.

Transbronchial Needle Aspiration

Transbronchial needle aspiration (TBNA) is a simple and safe procedure that can provide useful diagnostic information in benign and malignant conditions. It is used to evaluate mediastinal and hilar lymphadenopathy, exophytic endobronchial disease, and submucosal disease as well as extrinsic compression of the proximal airways.[41]

For endobronchial disease, the ability of TBNA to bypass surface necrosis and sample viable tumor from deeper within the mass can significantly increase bronchoscopic yield. The sensitivity of TBNA in exophytic mass lesions has been reported to be from 65% to 92% alone, and one study noted an increase in yield from 65% to 96% when TBNA was combined with other conventional methods.[33]

Successful TBNA in lymph node evaluation can provide important diagnostic as well as staging information. Until recently, surgical procedures, including mediastinoscopy, thoracotomy, and video-assisted thoracoscopy, have been the preferred methods for sampling hilar and mediastinal lymphadenopathy. In contrast to bronchoscopy, surgery is more invasive, carries higher risk, and requires general anesthesia. However, recent advances in TBNA techniques, including rapid on-site cytologic evaluation, the use of 19-gauge needles for performing core biopsies, and the availability of endobronchial ultrasound (EBUS) guidance, have significantly increased the diagnostic yield of this procedure.[42] Several studies have now documented reduced need for surgical procedures with the use of TBNA, both with and without EBUS guidance.[42,43]

The sensitivity of TBNA for mediastinal lymphadenopathy varies from 15% to 85% and depends largely on lymph node location, size, operator experience, needle type, and number of aspirates obtained.[44] TBNA has a higher yield in malignancy (compared with benign conditions), as well as in small cell lung cancer (SCLC) compared with non-small-cell lung cancer (NSCLC). Other predictors of positive aspirates include increased lymph node size, subcarinal or right tracheobronchial position, visible mucosal abnormalities, and exophytic endobronchial lesions.[45]

Herth et al. demonstrated an overall diagnostic yield of 80% using EBUS-guided TBNA, compared with 71% with conventional TBNA techniques. Although results were similar at the subcarinal location, the diagnostic yield significantly increased (from 58% to 84%) with EBUS guidance in all other stations.[46] Currently, the availability of EBUS guidance is limited to select centers because of its additional training requirements and equipment needs.

The diagnostic yield of TBNA can be enhanced by the on-site assessment of bronchoscopy specimens by cytopathologists. In one study, the diagnostic yield for malignancy was increased from 50% to 81% with the addition of rapid on-site cytologic evaluation (ROSE).[47] Additionally, ROSE can allow additional biopsy passes to be deferred without any loss in diagnostic yield, likely reducing procedural complications and overall costs.[48]

There is no clear consensus regarding the number of biopsy passes needed to establish a diagnosis. Diacon et al. documented diagnosis with the first, second, third, and fourth needle pass at 64%, 87%, 95%, and 98%, respectively, and ultimately concluded that three passes are adequate when only tissue diagnosis is needed or when TBNA is combined with other modalities.[45] However, for isolated lymph node aspiration in the setting of cancer staging, a minimum of four to five biopsies should be obtained.[45] Similarly, Chin et al. demonstrated a plateau effect in diagnostic yield by the seventh biopsy, with all positive results obtained in seven or fewer biopsies.[49]

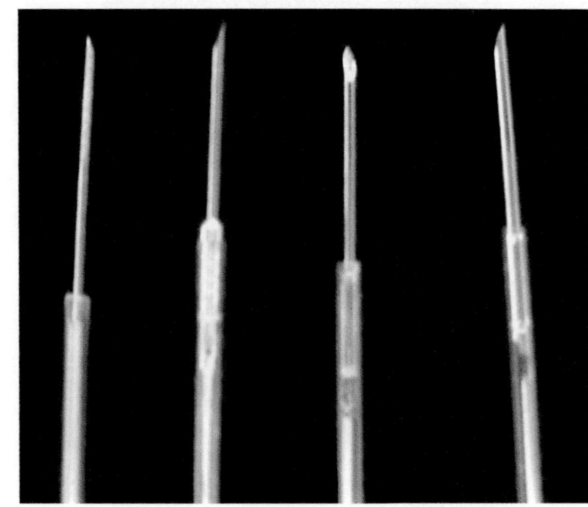

FIGURE 11–12 Needles used for bronchoscopy.

TBNA should be obtained before other procedures, such as endobronchial or transbronchial biopsies or brushings, to prevent contamination of the area causing false-positive results. The aspiration needle is available in 19-, 20-, 21-, and 22-gauge sizes, and is used to obtain cytologic specimens.[50] The apparatus (**Figure 11–12**) consists of a long, flexible plastic catheter or sheath with a needle retracted within the tubing and controlled by a metal spring.

When the site of interest is located, the sheathed needle can be passed through the working channel of the bronchoscope. Once the tip of the sheath is visualized within the bronchial lumen, the needle can be exposed and subsequently inserted into the intercartilaginous space adjacent to the lymph node targeted for aspiration.[3] Caution must be used to avoid deployment of the needle within the bronchoscope because this can cause significant damage to the bronchoscope itself. Once the needle has been completely inserted into the tissue (**Figure 11–13**), an assistant applies suction at the proximal end of the catheter. Typically, a 60-mL syringe filled with 2 mL of saline is attached to the proximal end of the bronchoscope, and the plunger is withdrawn to create negative suction.

If no resistance is felt when the syringe plunger is withdrawn, the needle is not adequately fixed in tissue and should be repositioned under direct visualization. Alternatively, aspiration of blood with negative pressure indicates inadvertent cannulation of a blood vessel and should

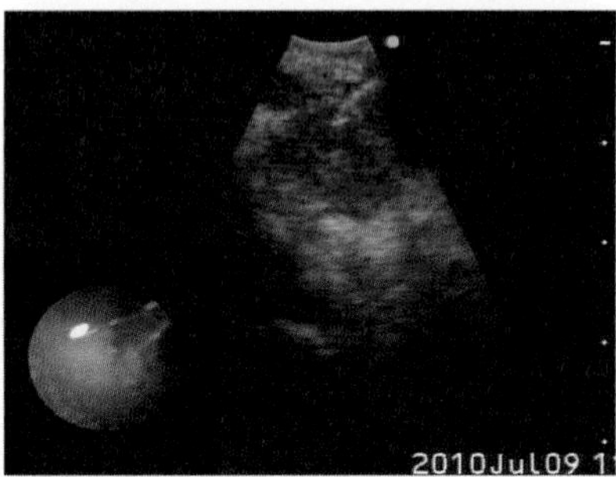

FIGURE 11–13 Ultrasonographic view of bronchoscopic needle aspiration of a right paratracheal lymph node. The visible light image of the needle catheter against the airway wall is shown on the inset.

result in removal of the needle, retraction of the needle in the sheath under direct endoscopic guidance, and observation of the site. Notably, vessel puncture during TBNA procedures rarely results in significant bleeding because of the small gauge of the needles used. If blood is obtained on aspiration, the catheter should be withdrawn from the bronchoscope and flushed before subsequent aspiration attempts because the presence of blood may obscure further cytologic diagnosis. If no blood is aspirated, then suction should be maintained for 1 to 2 minutes as the needle is gently advanced back and forth to maximize recovery of cells.[3] After the sample is obtained, the needle is removed from the aspiration site, retracted into the catheter under direct visualization, and then withdrawn from the bronchoscope. The sample is recovered by flushing the catheter/needle apparatus with saline.

Cytologic sampling by TBNA has inherent limitations. False-positive results can be obtained if malignant cells from the tracheobronchial tree contaminate the tip of the bronchoscope, particularly if the primary malignancy is close in proximity to the biopsy site or other maneuvers, including airway exam, are conducted prior to TBNA. Additionally, site contamination (and false positives) can occur from secretions that have migrated into the proximal airways with coughing. False-negative results can also occur as a result of the small sample size and the blind nature of the technique.

The bleeding at the site of needle puncture is usually negligible. Hemomediastinum, pneumothorax, pneumomediastinum, and bacteremia have been reported in sporadic cases.[3]

Complications of Bronchoscopy

Pneumothorax

Pneumothorax occurs in 1% to 6% of patients undergoing TBB.[23,51] Symptoms include chest pain, hemoptysis, and shortness of breath after the procedure. The need for chest radiography after TBB is controversial. In a single study examining the incidence of pneumothorax after TBB, pneumothorax was identified in 10 of 259 non-lung-transplant patients, 7 of whom developed symptoms suggestive of pneumothorax. The 3 patients who were asymptomatic had small pneumothoraces that did not require additional intervention, whereas 4 of 7 symptomatic patients had large pneumothoraces that required chest tube insertion. Severity of symptoms coincided with the size of the pneumothorax. The authors concluded that routine radiography is not necessary after TBB in patients who are able to describe symptoms after biopsy.[51] The use of fluoroscopy during TBB has not been shown to reduce risk of pneumothorax,[8] although a survey of 328 chest physicians in the United Kingdom showed a significantly lower incidence of reported pneumothorax requiring chest tube drainage in the past year for those who routinely used fluoroscopy.[52] No significant difference in the number of pneumothoraces was noted between the two groups (0.86% vs. 1.15%).

Bleeding Complications

Significant hemorrhage, defined as more than 50 mL of blood, is observed in 2% to 9% of patients undergoing TBB. No randomized studies have been published on the optimal management of hemorrhage related to TBB, although recognized experts have proposed several recommendations. Zavala first described the wedge technique in 1976, whereby the tip of the bronchoscope is placed within the subsegment that is being biopsied. The forceps used for the biopsy are passed through the working channel of the bronchoscope and extended into the subsegment, and the biopsy obtained. Afterward, the forceps are removed and the bronchoscope is left in position to isolate the subsegment and prevent the seepage of blood into the remainder of the bronchial tree. Blood is suctioned for a recommended period of 5 minutes to permit clotting, and the bronchoscope is cautiously withdrawn from the subsegment so that it can be observed for further bleeding.[12] As noted previously, no data exist to suggest that the wedge technique decreases significant bleeding or related complications.

Additional therapeutic modalities that have been suggested include the use of iced saline administered via the working channel of the bronchoscope placed in the wedge position. Our practice is to give a 20-mL bolus of iced saline and withhold suctioning for several minutes to allow the cold fluid to induce local vasoconstriction. If the first bolus is unsuccessful, the fluid is suctioned and a second bolus is administered, repeating the observation period for several minutes. If this process is unsuccessful in controlling bleeding, 20 mL of 1:20,000 epinephrine is administered, and the patient is placed with the hemorrhaging lung down to prevent soiling of the uninvolved lung.[8] Using these measures, the majority of hemorrhages related to TBB will be controlled. Occasionally, the bleeding may be severe enough to require placement of an endobronchial blocker.

Indications for Bronchoscopy

Acute Lung Collapse, Atelectasis, and Secretion Management

The use of bronchoscopy for acute atelectasis, lobar collapse, and clearance of retained secretions is common, particularly in the intensive care unit (ICU), although there has been very little research dedicated to the safety and utility of bronchoscopy in this clinical setting. Studies have reported success rates ranging from 19% to 89%.[53] When compared with bronchoscopy for subsegmental atelectasis or retained secretions alone, bronchoscopy for lobar collapse seems to be more beneficial, likely due to the presence of large central plugs that are easily accessible by the bronchoscope.[53] However, some studies indicate that the adjunctive use of bronchoalveolar lavage may be helpful in clearing more distal mucous plugs. Notably, the presence of an air bronchogram, suggesting a more distal obstruction, is considered a predictor of delayed resolution of the collapse, independent of the treatment interventions used.[54]

Practice opinions vary regarding when to use bronchoscopy instead of conservative therapy alone. In one study comparing bronchoscopy followed by chest physiotherapy with chest physiotherapy alone for acute atelectasis, Marini et al. observed no difference in improvement between the two groups.[54] There are many other new tools available for conservative management of secretions and atelectasis in addition to chest physiotherapy, including kinetic beds, mucolytic agents, percussion vests, and mechanical vibration therapy with handheld devices such as flutter valves.[53] The efficacy of most of these tools has not been formally compared with bronchoscopy. In general, conservative management should be tried first, particularly in patients with modest oxygen requirements who are able to cooperate with therapy. For selected patients in whom conservative management has failed, as well as those with rapidly progressive respiratory failure or distorted airway anatomy, bronchoscopy may have a role.

Hemoptysis

The role of bronchoscopy in the patient with hemoptysis remains controversial. Unfortunately, many of the studies designed to clarify bronchoscopy's role in this setting have been small cohort studies, with results that vary dramatically depending on geographic location, time of publication, and diagnostic studies available.[55] Therefore, it has been difficult to develop consensus recommendations for management of hemoptysis, and practice patterns vary widely.

Indications for bronchoscopy in hemoptysis include identifying the cause of bleeding, localizing the bleeding source, and evaluating for endobronchial malignancy. In massive or persistent hemoptysis, localizing the bleeding source can be helpful in planning surgical intervention or vascular embolization procedures. However, the most common reason for bronchoscopy in the setting of hemoptysis is for diagnosis of suspected malignancy.

The yield of bronchoscopy for diagnosing malignancy is highest when the chest radiograph is abnormal.[56] However, approximately 5% to 6% of patients presenting with hemoptysis and a normal chest radiograph are found to have an endobronchial malignancy.[57] Because hemoptysis can be the only clue to localized and potentially resectable disease, screening airway exams for hemoptysis are widely performed, particularly in patients with other risk factors for malignancy. The factors associated with the highest yield for lung cancer on bronchoscopy include significant smoking history (>40 pack years), male sex, and age greater than 40 years.[58] Other factors, including severity of bleeding, persistent hemoptysis for more than 1 week, and prior episodes of hemoptysis, have not been shown to correlate directly with risk of malignancy.[58]

> **RESPIRATORY RECAP**
>
> **Diagnostic Indications for Bronchoscopy**
> - » Lung collapse/atelectasis
> - » Hemoptysis
> - » Cough
> - » Suspected malignancy
> - » Infection
> - » Foreign body aspiration
> - » Interstitial lung disease
> - » Lung transplant
> - » Trauma

Bronchoscopy can also be useful in massive or life-threatening hemoptysis. In this setting, bronchoscopy is used primarily to assist efforts to maintain ventilation. Rigid bronchoscopy is often preferred because of its superior suctioning and ventilation capabilities.[59] However, rigid bronchoscopy does require general anesthesia and access to an operating room, which can limit its utility in emergency settings. Flexible bronchoscopy is more readily available, but limited in its ability to rapidly suction blood and prevent obstruction of visibility from blood. Therefore, when flexible bronchoscopy is used, endotracheal intubation should be performed first to secure the airway, facilitate selective intubation to protect the nonbleeding lung, and allow for repeated reintroduction of the bronchoscope should vision become obscured by blood. Bronchoscopy can then be used to direct endobronchial blockade maneuvers to isolate bleeding from other areas of the lung, as well as to guide the endotracheal tube into the main stem bronchus for protective ventilation strategies.[59]

Cough

Chronic cough is a common problem that can be very bothersome for patients. Asthma, postnasal drip/allergic rhinitis, and gastroesophageal reflux disease remain the most common etiologies for chronic cough. Diagnostic workup often includes pulmonary function testing, methacholine challenge, chest radiograph, empiric reflux treatment, 24-hour pH probe (to assess for silent reflux), allergy evaluation, and/or sinus CT, depending on patient history. Prior studies suggest that a diagnosis will be achieved in close to 100% of chronic cough patients when worked up systematically by a set algorithm or protocol screening for common conditions.[60] However, if cough persists despite aggressive workup and empiric treatment, bronchoscopy should be considered.

The largest study of bronchoscopy in refractory cough consisted of 82 patients referred from a dedicated specialty cough clinic. In this study, 11% of subjects received a diagnosis based on bronchoscopic findings. These diagnoses included tracheal or upper airway abnormalities and tracheal malformations such as tracheobronchopathia osteochondroplastica, stenosis, and broncholithiasis.[60] Ultimately, authors agreed that bronchoscopy does have a role in chronic cough evaluation but should be reserved for patients who elude diagnosis despite extensive workup.

Suspected Malignancy

Bronchoscopy has a variety of roles in the evaluation of suspected malignancy. An airway exam can be used to evaluate for the presence of endobronchial tumor, particularly when the possibility of obstruction is suggested on the radiograph by volume loss, hyperinflation, or recurrent or unresolving pneumonitis. Similarly, the presence of a localized wheeze, hemoptysis, or chronic cough can be due to endobronchial disease. In these settings, bronchoscopy is often used to evaluate for malignancy, even in the absence of a clear mass on chest radiograph. A careful airway exam will also include evaluation for oropharyngeal or nasopharyngeal lesions and vocal cord paralysis, which can be a sign of recurrent laryngeal nerve entrapment by bulky mediastinal disease.

Bronchoscopy is commonly used to evaluate specific lesions noted on chest radiograph or computed tomography. However, the diagnostic yield for suspected malignancy is highly dependent on the location of the tumor as well as the sampling technique used. The sensitivity of bronchoscopy for evaluating central lesions has been documented to be as high as 71%, compared with 49% for more peripheral lesions.[61] Adequate sampling of peripheral nodules is more difficult and relies on the ability to visualize the lesion fluoroscopically during the procedure as well as on accessibility from a nearby bronchus.[62] Overall, the diagnostic yield of bronchoscopy for detection of proven malignancy has been reported to be as high as 75%, and up to 92% in macroscopically visible endobronchial lesions.[63]

For endobronchial disease, the highest sensitivity is seen with endobronchial biopsy (74%), followed by brushing for cytology (59%), and washing (49%). When all modalities are combined, sensitivity can reach as high as 88%.[61] In contrast, for peripheral lesions, brushing demonstrated the highest sensitivity (52%), followed by transbronchial biopsy (46%) and BAL/washing (43%), with a combined sensitivity of 69% when all modalities were used.[61] The diagnostic yield was significantly less for peripheral lesions smaller than 2 cm in diameter (33%) compared with larger lesions (62%).[61]

Although less commonly used, transbronchial needle aspiration can also be helpful in evaluating endobronchial disease due to the prevalence of submucosal involvement. Even in visible endobronchial tumor, endobronchial biopsy results can be nondiagnostic due to the presence of surface necrosis and inflammation.[33] The ability of TBNA to bypass surface necrosis and sample viable tumor from deeper within the mass can increase the diagnostic yield of the bronchoscopy. The sensitivity of TBNA in exophytic mass lesions has been reported to be from 65% to 92% alone, and one study noted an increase in yield from 65% to 96% when added to other conventional methods.[33]

In addition to discreet masses, bronchoscopy can be helpful in evaluating mediastinal and hilar lymphadenopathy in both undiagnosed and known malignancy. Many lymph nodes, particularly in subcarinal and hilar regions, are easily accessible by bronchoscopy because of their location just beyond the tracheal or bronchial wall. The ability to sample lymph nodes has greatly enhanced the role of bronchoscopy in cancer staging, and it is now possible to provide patients with diagnosis and staging information from a single procedure.

Infection

Bronchoscopy is used in infection to help define the causative microbiological organism. It can also be helpful to rule out infection in the setting of other lung processes. Initially, bronchoscopy had little to offer as a diagnostic tool for pulmonary infection because of contamination of the instrument during passage through the upper airways. However, the development of protected catheters and quantitative cultures has significantly increased the utility of bronchoscopy in this setting.[64] Nonetheless, the yield of bronchoscopy in the diagnosis of pneumonia remains directly related to the immune status of the host, the index of suspicion for associated endobronchial disease based on radiographic findings, and the specific techniques used to obtain and process the sample. Although it has been shown to be very helpful in immunocompromised patients, its indication in the immunocompetent host is less clear.

The role of bronchoscopy in community-acquired pneumonia (CAP), particularly in the immunocompetent host, remains uncertain. According to most guidelines, testing for microbial diagnosis in outpatients with CAP is optional because these patients almost always respond to empiric antibiotics (such as a macrolide or fluoroquinolone), and isolation of an organism might not lead to changes in management. However, testing for microbial diagnosis is always recommended in patients who require hospitalization, have comorbid conditions, or have risk factors for more resistant pathogens.

In a study of 262 patients hospitalized with CAP, a microbial diagnosis was only achieved in 60% of cases, using routine measures such as blood and sputum cultures, urine serologic detection *Legionella* and pneumococcal antigens, and selective bronchoscopy.[65] Bronchoscopy was reserved for patients who did not expectorate sputum within 24 hours or patients with treatment failure 72 hours after antibiotic administration. In these cases, bronchoscopy provided microbial diagnosis in 49% of patients who did not expectorate sputum within 24 hours and 52% of patients presenting with treatment failure 72 hours after antibiotic administration. Bronchoscopy provided an additional diagnosis, not detected by other methods, in 25% of patients. These results were validated by Ortqvist et al., who reported obtaining a diagnosis with fiberoptic bronchoscopy in 54% of patients with antibiotic treatment failure.[64]

Therefore, although bronchoscopy should not be routinely used for microbial diagnosis in community-acquired pneumonia, it offers a reasonable adjunct to other forms of testing and can be helpful in hospitalized patients not responding to treatment, particularly those who are severely ill, immunocompromised, or require ICU care. Additionally, it is useful for patients who are unable to produce sputum samples and any patients with treatment failure, especially if suspicion of anatomic obstruction is considered. Interestingly, the presence of prior or ongoing antibiotic therapy did not appear to influence the bronchoscopic yield, since microbial diagnosis was obtained in 54% of patients with treatment failure.

Pulmonary infections account for significant morbidity and mortality in immunocompromised patients. Therefore, it is important to quickly identify the cause of lung infiltrates in these patients and institute specific treatment. Unfortunately, many infectious and noninfectious diseases can present with similar clinical and radiologic features in immunocompromised patients. The etiology of immunosuppression (e.g., HIV, malignancy, drug induced, rheumatologic) should also be considered when constructing a differential diagnosis. In general, common infections in immunocompromised patients include bacterial pneumonia, cytomegalovirus, *Legionella*, aspergillosis, *Pneumocystis carinii* (PCP), and tuberculosis. Other possibilities for pulmonary infiltrates in these patients can include diffuse alveolar hemorrhage, nonspecific interstitial pneumonitis (NSIP), drug-induced pneumonitis, radiation pneumonitis, congestive heart failure, and diffuse alveolar damage or adult respiratory distress syndrome (ARDS).[66] Flexible bronchoscopy was more likely to provide definitive diagnosis when infiltrate was due to infection (81%) than to a noninfectious etiology (56%).

In one study of 104 immunocompromised patients with pulmonary infiltrates, fiberoptic bronchoscopy was the primary source of diagnosis in 78% of patients; notably, all but one of these patients was receiving antibiotics at the time of bronchoscopy.[66] Additionally, similar to bronchoscopy for suspected malignancy, when multiple diagnostic modalities (BAL, brushing, biopsy, etc.) are used together, the overall diagnostic yield is enhanced. Notably, the yield of BAL for fungal infections, compared with bacterial infections, is reduced (47%), and multiple studies have advocated the importance of obtaining multiple sputum samples in addition to BAL to optimize the diagnostic yield for fungal infections.[30,67,68] In immunosuppressed patients, bronchoalveolar lavage samples should always be sent for cytologic evaluation (in addition to culture) because the diagnosis can often be made based on features such as viral inclusion bodies or fungal forms on special stains for various infectious organisms.[69] In addition, cytology may be available sooner than information from cultures, which can take days to weeks for growth and identification, depending on the organism in question.

Suspected Foreign Body Aspiration

Foreign body aspiration is a common (and serious) problem in children, but it can occur in any age group. Tracheobronchial foreign body aspiration can result in severe airway compromise and death, as well as more long-term complications such as bronchiectasis and/or recurrent or persistent pneumonia. Foreign body aspiration is often suspected by history alone, although the classic diagnostic triad includes the sudden onset of paroxysmal coughing, wheezing, and diminished breath sounds on one side.[70] The chest radiograph can also provide valuable information. In a study of 140 patients with foreign body aspiration, radiographic findings included visualization of a radiopaque foreign body (34%), hyperinflation (18%), atelectasis (12%), and lung infiltrate/consolidation (11%). Normal radiographs were seen in 34% of subjects.[71] Therefore, although suspected foreign body aspiration is a definite indication for bronchoscopy, it is also important to remember that the absence of appropriate history or lack of visualization of a radiopaque object on chest radiograph does not exclude this diagnosis, particularly because many aspirated objects, especially food, are radiolucent.

Successful foreign body extraction requires an experienced bronchoscopy team because unexpected complications often arise. When foreign body aspiration is suspected on clinical or radiographic grounds, either flexible or rigid bronchoscopy can be performed. Flexible bronchoscopy allows visualization of more distal airways and does not require general anesthesia. Objects can be extracted by forceps retrieval or use of a basket extraction device through the working channel of the scope. However, the bronchoscopist must be careful to avoid dislodging the object, which could lead to acute airway obstruction. In contrast, rigid bronchoscopy is sometimes preferred because of the wider range of extraction devices available, the ability to ventilate the patient throughout the procedure, better visualization (in the large airways), and the ability to provide rapid suctioning in the event of substantial bleeding. The rigid bronchoscope remains the instrument of choice for foreign body aspiration in the pediatric population.[70,72] More complicated cases may necessitate intubation or tracheotomy to maintain adequate ventilation and assist in extraction of large objects.

Although many opinions exist, most research suggests that early bronchoscopy is associated with a lower risk of complication. Delayed bronchoscopy can be complicated by the formation of granulation tissue around the foreign material, leading to less visibility and increased risk of bleeding with extraction.[71]

Interstitial Lung Disease

The diagnosis of interstitial lung disease often requires a tissue sample for pathology evaluation. Therefore, bronchoscopy with transbronchial biopsy is often considered. However, the yield of transbronchial lung biopsies in patients with interstitial lung disease depends heavily on the diagnosis in question. For example, a diagnosis of sarcoidosis may be easily obtained by transbronchial biopsy, in contrast to other forms of idiopathic interstitial lung disease, which require surgical biopsy for adequate diagnostic material.

Given the high rate of pulmonary involvement in patients with sarcoidosis, bronchoscopy is the diagnostic procedure of choice, with yields as high as 90% in some studies.[34] Transbronchial biopsy has a high yield in other interstitial lung diseases, such as Langerhans cell histiocytosis, pulmonary alveolar proteinosis, lipoid pneumonia, eosinophilic pneumonia, and drug-induced pneumonitis.[73] These diseases all have characteristic appearances under the microscope, and if the affected lung is adequately sampled, transbronchial biopsy can be reliable.[73] In contrast, the diagnosis of other lung diseases, such as various forms of interstitial fibrosis, requires that a larger surgical biopsy be obtained.

Lung Transplant

Lung transplantation is a well-recognized treatment for end-stage pulmonary disease. Flexible bronchoscopy with bronchoalveolar lavage and/or transbronchial biopsy has proven to be a valuable tool for evaluating lung allograft complications. These complications can include infection, rejection (acute or chronic), and airway compromise. Transbronchial biopsy remains the gold standard for determining the presence or absence of acute pulmonary allograft rejection in lung transplant patients.[74] The role of surveillance bronchoscopy, in the absence of clinical worsening, remains controversial and varies between institutions. Many transplant centers endorse routine surveillance bronchoscopy with the hope that early detection and treatment of clinically silent episodes of acute rejection or infection may lead to reduced rates of chronic rejection or bronchiolitis obliterans syndrome (BOS). However, the impact of surveillance bronchoscopy on overall survival remains unknown.[75]

In lung transplant patients, bronchoscopy also allows for visualization of the airway anastomosis and management of mechanical complications, such as airway stenosis, with interventional techniques such as stent placement, balloon dilatation, and laser therapy.[76]

Trauma

Blunt trauma to the chest can be associated with tracheal and bronchial injuries that are life threatening. Although tracheal rupture remains uncommon, its incidence has increased in recent years due to an increasing number of motor vehicle accidents as well as improved paramedic services, which enable patients with major chest trauma to survive transportation to a hospital.[77] Injuries to the tracheobronchial tree are found at autopsy in 3% to 11% of motor vehicle accident victims.[78] Tracheal injury can also occur as an iatrogenic complication of orotracheal intubation. Despite a lack of clear clinical symptoms, the need for early diagnosis and surgical repair is imperative.

Although most trauma patients do receive chest CT imaging, tracheal trauma is not always seen radiographically. In a retrospective analysis of 10 patients with tracheal rupture at a university trauma center, the diagnosis was only definitively made by CT in 1 case, with the remaining 9 diagnosed at bronchoscopy.[77] However, in many of these cases indirect clues were seen radiographically, including pneumomediastinum, pneumothorax, hemothorax, persistent atelectasis, and lung contusion. In addition to radiographic signs, the presence of mediastinal or cervical emphysema on clinical exam, unexplained hemoptysis, or continuous air leak through a chest tube following blunt trauma are also suggestive of tracheobronchial injury and should be considered urgent indications for bronchoscopy.[77] Bronchoscopy remains the gold standard for diagnosing tracheobronchial injuries following blunt trauma and should be obtained early in all patients with suspected tracheal injury to avoid the significant morbidity and mortality associated with untreated or unrecognized airway injuries.

Therapeutic Bronchoscopy

Therapeutic bronchoscopy is most commonly employed to treat patients with central airway obstruction due to benign or malignant etiology. Although the incidence of central airway obstruction is unknown, it is a commonly encountered clinical problem present in 20% to 30% of patients with primary lung cancer[79] and 7% to 18% of patients following lung transplantation.[80] Additional common causes of central airway obstruction include tracheal stenosis, either post-tracheostomy or idiopathic, tracheomalacia, and foreign body aspiration (**Box 11–2**).[79] Although many of the techniques

BOX 11–2

Causes of Central Airway Obstruction

Malignant Causes

- Primary endoluminal carcinoma
- Metastatic carcinoma to the airway
- Laryngeal carcinoma
- Esophageal carcinoma
- Mediastinal tumors
- Lymphoma

Nonmalignant Causes

- Sarcoidosis
- Infectious
  - Tuberculosis
  - Histoplasmosis
  - Human papilloma virus
- Vascular
- Relapsing polychondritis
- Granulation tissue formation
  - Wegener granulomatosis
  - Foreign bodies
  - Airway stents
  - Surgical anastomosis
- Amyloid
- Hamartomas
- Tracheomalacia

that are described in this section are amenable to use with the flexible bronchoscope, rigid bronchoscopy provides definitive control of the airway, permitting the use of general anesthesia to maximize patient comfort (**Box 11–3**).[81] In addition, the rigid bronchoscope becomes a conduit for use of a variety of tools and suction devices to perform minimally invasive airway surgery. The bronchoscope itself can become a therapeutic tool useful for dilation of airway stenoses and "coring out" of airway tumor, providing rapid relief of central airway obstruction.[81]

Rigid Bronchoscopy

The **rigid bronchoscope** was the only method of bronchoscopy available from the advent of bronchoscopy in 1897 by Gustav Killian until the introduction of the flexible fiberoptic scope in 1967 by Ikeda. After the introduction of flexible bronchoscopy, use of the rigid bronchoscope declined by pulmonologists in North America. However, its distinct advantages in controlling the airway while facilitating the passage of a wide variety of tools for minimally invasive airway surgery have been "rediscovered" by the pulmonary community resulting in an increased interest in training and application of the technique over the past 15 years.[82]

BOX 11–3

Indications for Rigid Bronchoscopy

- Massive hemoptysis
- Foreign body removal
- Dilation of airway stenosis
- Airway stent placement
- Resection of central airway tumor

Indications

Rigid bronchoscopy can be used for any bronchoscopic indication; however, the additional requirements of general anesthesia generally result in most centers limiting its use to therapeutic indications such as relief of central airway obstruction and foreign body removal, and for investigation of massive hemoptysis. Patient selection for rigid bronchoscopy is similar to that for flexible bronchoscopy. Patients should be able to tolerate general anesthesia, and not have an excessive oxygen requirement. Relative contraindications are similar to those described for diagnostic bronchoscopy, including uncontrolled coagulopathy and high O_2 requirement, with the addition of limitation in cervical neck extension due to the need to hyperextend the neck during bronchoscope insertion; an absolute contraindication is inability to provide informed consent.

Equipment

The rigid bronchoscope is essentially a stainless steel tube with a beveled tip at the distal end (**Figure 11–14**), while the proximal end usually contains a series of ports for ventilation, passage of suction catheters, grasping tools, a telescope, or a flexible bronchoscope. Fenestrated caps may be placed over the ports to permit closed ventilation during the procedure. Adult bronchoscopes are generally 9 to 13 mm in diameter and 40 cm long, whereas tracheoscopes are of similar diameter but are only 25 cm in length. Fenestrations are present in the side wall at the distal end of the bronchoscope to allow for continued ventilation of the opposite lung if the scope is passed down one of the main stem bronchi during the procedure.

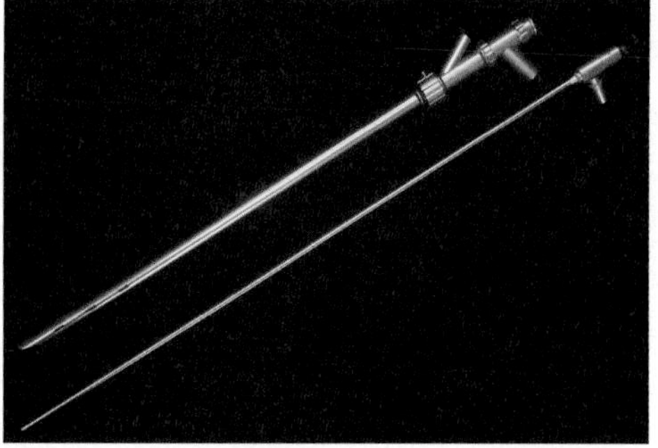

FIGURE 11–14 Rigid bronchoscope with articulated head and multiple ports for passage of a variety of tools or for connection to a closed ventilation system when the appropriate silicone caps are attached to the ports. Below is a telescope unit that may be used to visualize the airway directly or that may be fitted with a video camera for inspection of the airway using a video monitor.

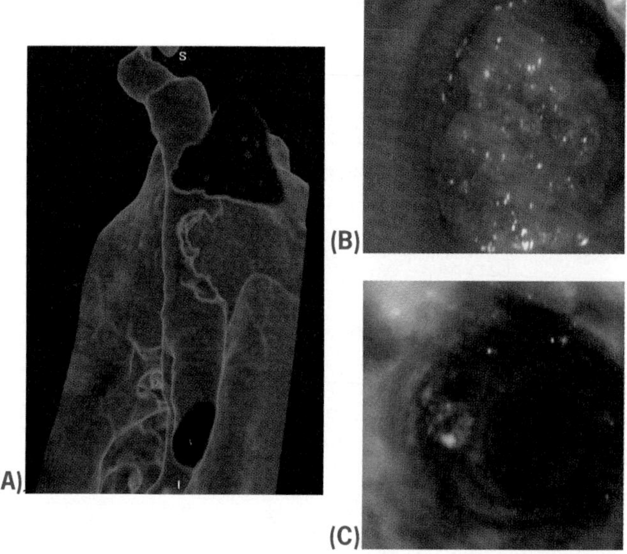

FIGURE 11–15 Intrinsic airway obstruction due to human papilloma virus (HPV) in a patient with HIV infection. (**A**) CT reconstruction of the trachea showing near complete obstruction by the mass of HPV-induced granulation tissue. (**B**) Bronchoscopic view of airway obstruction showing characteristic cluster-of-grapes appearance of HPV disease. (**C**) Trachea after removal of the mass using a combination of argon plasma coagulation and mechanical debridement. Note areas of superficial thermal injury on the tracheal mucosa due to argon plasma coagulation use.

Insertion

Prior to bronchoscope insertion, the patient must be adequately sedated with general anesthesia. Many centers choose to administer a muscle relaxant as well, although this is not absolutely required. The patient's neck is hyperextended, and with the fingers of the left hand, the upper lip and teeth are covered with the operator's thumb, the index finger is inserted into the patient's mouth to displace the tongue toward the left side of the patient's mouth, and the middle finger is used to cover the patient's lower lip and teeth to prevent injury to these structures. The bronchoscope is held in the right hand with the barrel of the scope resting between the thumb and first finger, with the bevel of the distal end of the scope facing down. The tip of the scope is inserted into the patient's mouth against the base of the tongue. The tongue is visualized via the telescope inserted through the bronchoscope, and the scope is advanced along the base of the tongue until the epiglottis is visualized. The bevel of the scope is advanced under the epiglottis, and the tip of the scope is rotated upward using the thumb located over the patient's upper mandible as a fulcrum to lift the epiglottis and bring the vocal cords into view. The scope is then rotated 90 degrees to allow the beveled tip to slide between the cords. Rotation is continued an additional 90 degrees as the bronchoscope enters the trachea to run the bevel against the posterior wall of the trachea to prevent injury to the membranous tracheal wall.[81]

Anesthesia and Ventilation

Because of the irritating nature of the rigid intubation, virtually all centers perform rigid bronchoscopy under general anesthesia. If the bronchoscope is capped appropriately, inhalational anesthesia may be used to maintain the patient's sedation; however, most centers in the United States use a total intravenous anesthetic approach in combination with either spontaneous assisted ventilation[83] or jet ventilation using a Sander's jet ventilator. Some centers provide jet ventilation via an automated system, which allows the anesthesiologist to be freed from managing the Sander's jet.[84,85] Limited data exist comparing outcomes between ventilation strategies; however, there is some evidence to suggest that spontaneous assisted ventilation may reduce rates of reintubation following rigid bronchoscopy.[83] This result may be partially explained by the need for use of muscle relaxants with jet ventilation.

Therapeutic Procedures

Central airway obstruction may result from benign or malignant conditions. Benign conditions include tracheal stenosis secondary to endotracheal intubation or following tracheostomy, tracheomalacia from disorders such as relapsing polychondritis, stenosis at anastomic sites following lung transplantation, and secondary to human papilloma virus infections of the airway. Virtually any type of malignancy can involve the airways, but the most common types are lung cancer, breast cancer, and renal cell carcinoma. Airway obstruction may take one of three forms: extrinsic compression, endobronchial obstruction (**Figure 11–15**), and mixed types.[86] Identification of the type of obstruction is important because it helps the physician determine the best course of treatment for relief of central airway obstruction and whether a procedure is likely to be effective.

A variety of therapeutic procedures are available to relieve airway obstruction due to malignancy or benign

TABLE 11-2 Currently Available Bronchoscopic Ablative Therapies

Modality	Mechanism	Effect	Advantages	Disadvantages
Nd:YAG	Thermal energy produced by laser light	Coagulation and vaporization of tissue	Excellent debulking	Expensive; cumbersome setup
Electrocautery	Thermal energy produced by an electrical current	Coagulation of tissue but more superficial than laser	Excellent safety profile; multiple instrument designs; inexpensive	Contact mode requiring frequent cleaning of probe
Argon plasma coagulation	Thermal energy produced by the interaction between argon gas and an electrical current	Superficial coagulation of tissue	No undesired deep tissue effects	Ineffective for in-depth tissue coagulation or debulking
Photodynamic therapy	Injection of a photosensitizer followed by the destruction of presensitized tumor cells through illumination with nonthermal laser	Delayed destruction of tissue (24–48 hours)	Relatively long-lasting effects	Expensive; need for multiple bronchoscopies; skin photosensitivity lasting up to 6 weeks
Brachytherapy	Direct delivery of radiation therapy into the airway	Delayed and in-depth destruction of tissue	Long-lasting effect; synergistic with external beam radiation	Higher incidence of complications, particularly hemorrhage
Cryotherapy	Destruction of tissue by alternating cycles of freezing to extreme cold temperatures and thawing	Delayed destruction of tissue (1–2 weeks)	Useful for retrieval of foreign objects and removal of large mucous plugs or clots	Not suitable for debulking in acute airway obstruction; need for multiple bronchoscopies

Adapted from Wahidi M, Herth F, Ernst A. State of the art interventional pulmonology. *Chest.* 2007;131:261–274, Table 2.

airway stenosis (**Table 11-2**). Rapid relief of airway obstruction may be obtained using heat therapy such as endobronchial laser or electrocautery. Laser (light amplification of stimulated emission of radiation) was first described for use in the airway in 1976,[87] and is used in many centers as the primary tool for rapid resection of central airway tumors. The most commonly used laser is the Nd:YAG device, which causes photocoagulation rather than vaporization of tumor tissue. This allows for devitalization of tumor tissue followed by removal with forceps to open the airway. When using heat therapy in the airway, care must be taken that the inspired FIO_2 is reduced to 40% or less to avoid ignition of flammable components in the airway. Using this technique, 70% of central airway obstructions are relieved.[86]

Similar effect can be obtained using a pulsed electrical field and an electrocautery probe extended through the rigid or flexible bronchoscope. In this case the tissue is devitalized using direct contact, permitting excellent control of tissue destruction. The electrocautery is fired in short bursts, with frequent observation of the underlying tissue injury to avoid unwanted extension of the coagulation effect. Similar to laser therapy, devitalized tissue may then be removed with the use of grasping forceps with a minimum of bleeding.[79,82] There have been no direct comparisons of laser therapy and electrocautery for the relief of central airway obstruction; however, reported efficacy has been similar with both techniques. Electrocautery has an advantage in that it requires less investment in equipment and does not require the use of special eye protection or the avoidance of reflective surfaces during its use.

An additional technique that uses heat therapy is argon plasma coagulation (APC). This technique employs argon gas to form a plasma that when exposed to high voltage conducts electricity to underlying tissue, resulting in a superficial coagulation effect. APC is a noncontact technique, in that the electrical energy is carried by the gas to the underlying tissue, and so this technique may be used to deliver energy around corners and in difficult-to-reach locations in the airway. The effect of APC is more superficial than either laser or electrocautery, causing coagulation to a depth of 2 to 3 mm within the airway.[88] This limited penetration provides the ability to spray the coagulating effect within the airway, making APC a useful tool for control of airway bleeding and devitalization of granulation tissue. The superficial coagulation effect also makes APC extremely safe, resulting in lower rates of complications such as airway perforation and massive hemorrhage,[89] although there are theoretical concerns about the development of gas embolism with higher flow rates and longer pulse duration with the use of APC.[90]

Treatment of airway stenosis following tracheostomy or lung transplantation may be performed using inflatable balloons or rigid dilators to disrupt the fibrous connective tissue that forms at the site of the prior airway injury.[91] Often, a combination of techniques, such as use of an electrocautery knife to cut the membranous region of a stenosis followed by dilation with an inflatable balloon and removal of granulation tissue with forceps, is required to achieve the desired result. Finally, the rigid bronchoscope itself can be used as a therapeutic instrument to core out central airway tumors after adequate dessication and coagulation have been performed using laser therapy or electrocautery.[86]

In addition to the rapidly acting procedures described earlier, there are several therapies that provide delayed effect in debulking airway malignancies. Cryotherapy is a safe and effective method that uses nitrous oxide gas to cool the tip of a metal probe placed through the working channel of the flexible bronchoscope. Once the gas flow is activated, the tip of the catheter rapidly cools to induce freezing of tissues at the point of contact and a small margin of surrounding tissue. The tissue thaws and the cycle may be repeated. The freeze-thawing of tissues results in delayed necrosis and sloughing of the treated area over the next several days.[92] This technique has been shown to be effective in debulking tumors and improving central airway obstruction. Cryotherapy is also useful for removal of foreign bodies.[93] The tip of the probe is placed on the foreign body, and the gas flow is activated, resulting in the foreign body being frozen to the catheter tip. The foreign body is then removed from the patient by removing the flexible bronchoscope with the catheter still in the working channel without turning off the gas flow.

Additional delayed-efficacy treatments include photodynamic therapy, which employs a systemically administered photosensitizing agent prior to the procedure that is preferentially concentrated by tumor cells. Photophrin is currently the only sensitizing agent licensed for use in the United States. When stimulated by light of 630 nm via an argon/dye or diode laser applied through a light guide, oxygen radicals are produced in tissues that have concentrated the previously administered medication, resulting in tissue necrosis.[94] Often necrosis is so exuberant that a repeat procedure is needed 24 to 48 hours after light administration to debride necrotic tumor that can cause airway obstruction. Efficacy is good in patients with central airway tumors, where up to 70% report improvement in symptoms of dyspnea.[92] Primary complications include severe sunburn due to the photosensitizing effect of the medication, which may last as long as 6 weeks, and bleeding due to the destruction of vascular tumors.[95]

Finally, **brachytherapy** is a palliative technique that employs locally delivered radionuclide for treatment of endobronchial tumor resulting in central airway obstruction. The advantages of this approach are the delivery of high-dose radiation directly to the tumor tissue with limited penetration to surrounding tissue due to the rapid drop-off of radiation dose with distance from the source, the ability to modify the area of treatment to conform to the shape of the tumor, and the ability to precisely target the tissue of interest.[95] The radionuclide most commonly used is iridium-192 delivered in an encapsulated form via a polyethylene catheter inserted via the working channel of the flexible bronchoscope. The catheter is placed adjacent to the area to be treated, and the bronchoscope is removed. The catheter is then secured at the nose or mouth, and the position is confirmed using fluoroscopy. The iridium source is then afterloaded into the catheter and dwells for a period of time until the desired dose is delivered, generally 7 Gy for high-dose applications; the catheter and source are then removed from the patient. Efficacy for symptom palliation ranges from 65% to 95%.[96–98] A Cochrane review compared the efficacy of external beam radiation therapy and high-dose endobronchial therapy and showed no difference between the two treatments.[99] Complications are rare, although fatal hemoptysis is reported in 2% to 11% of treated patients.[98]

Airway Stenting

Types of Stents

Modern airway stenting began as a modification of the Montgomery T-tube, with silicone stents popularized by Dumon in the late 1980s.[100] Shortly afterward, the self-expandable metal stent was developed and became widely used because of its ease of deployment without the need for rigid bronchoscopy as is required for silicone stent placement.[101] More recently, hybrid metal-silicone stents have been developed, which share some of the advantages and disadvantages of each type of **airway stent**.

> **RESPIRATORY RECAP**
>
> **Airway Stents**
>
> » Self-expandable metal stents, silicone stents, and hybrid metal-silicone stents are available.
>
> » Rigid bronchoscopy is required for silicone stent placement.
>
> » Stents are generally effective in improving airway patency.
>
> » Common complications include stent migration and occlusion by secretions.

Silicone Stents

Silicone stents are composed of silicone sleeves fitted with external studs to retard stent migration in the airway. The stent wall is relatively thick at 2 mm, and therefore significant portions of the airway lumen may be occupied in smaller (<10 mm outer diameter) stents. Stents are sized from 10 mm to 20 mm in outer diameter and come in lengths ranging from 2 to 8 cm. In addition, Y-shaped stents are available for placement at the main carina with limbs of the Y extending proximally into the trachea and distally into each of the main stem bronchi. The limbs of the Y are not symmetrically angled, but instead are more

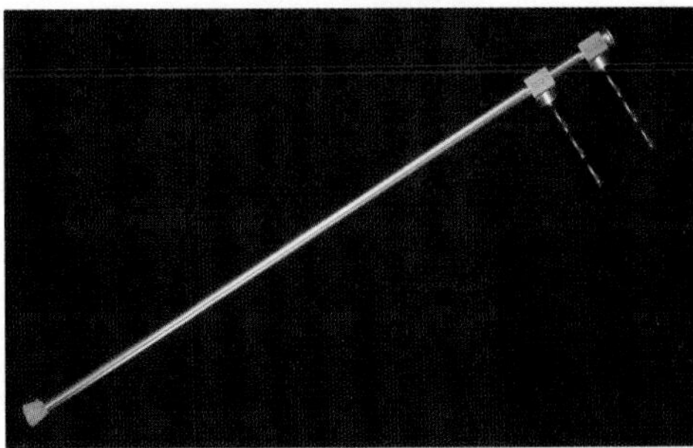

FIGURE 11–16 Silicone stent deployment system. A stent is pictured in partial deployment to illustrate the manner in which the stent is folded to be fitted into the deployment tube.

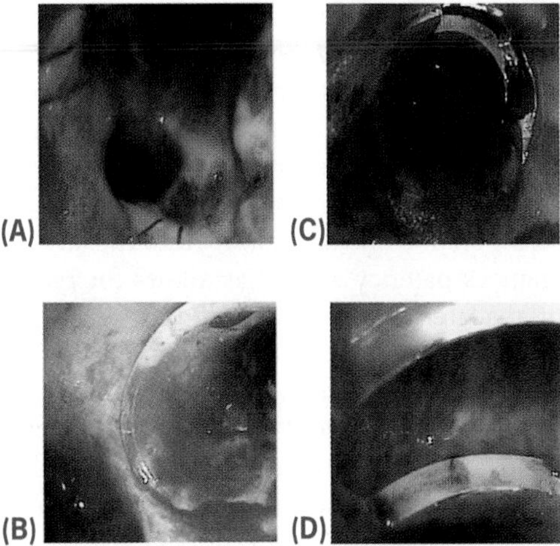

FIGURE 11–17 Lung transplant anastomosis dehiscence treated with a silicone stent. (**A**) Anastomosis dehiscence showing fistula in communication with the patient's mediastinum. (**B**) Proximal view of the silicone stent seen from the distal trachea. (**C**) Axial view of the stent that extends from the right main stem to the distal bronchus intermedius. Note complete occlusion of the underlying fistula, minimizing continued passage of secretions into the mediastinum. (**D**) View of window cut in the stent for ventilation of the right upper lobe.

acute for the left main stem bronchus take-off to accommodate the positioning of the two main stem bronchi.

Rigid bronchoscopy is required for silicone stent placement. During deployment, the stent is rolled along the long axis and placed into a steel delivery tube sized the same length as the rigid bronchoscope. The bronchoscope is advanced to the midpoint of the desired airway obstruction, and the deployment tube is inserted into the bronchoscope. The stent is then pushed forward using a pushrod placed down the deployment tube, followed by removal of both the pushrod and deployment tube (**Figure 11–16**). The rigid scope is then withdrawn while holding the incompletely expanded stent in place until the proximal end is free from the bronchoscope. Generally, the stent will fully expand, but occasionally may need to be opened using a dilation balloon. If the stent has been positioned distal to the area of narrowing, it may be dragged proximally using large forceps; however, stents that have been placed too proximally cannot be advanced, and must be removed and reinserted (**Figure 11–17**).

Self-Expanding Metal Stents

Self-expanding **metallic stents** were introduced in the mid-1990s as an alternative to silicone stents. The majority of these stents are constructed of nitinol, an alloy composed of nickel and titanium. This metal has the properties of being flexible while retaining excellent shape memory, and so the stent can be compressed onto a factory-packaged deployment rod and then will expand to its initial diameter after it is deployed. These stents are less likely to migrate than silicone stents[102] because they rapidly embed into the surrounding mucosa. They also are less likely to become occluded with secretions, because the open meshwork of the stent allows normal ciliary function of the underlying mucosa to move secretions into the upper airway. However, lumen occlusion with granulation tissue can be a significant problem with metallic stents. In addition, once metallic stents are placed, they are rapidly incorporated into the airway wall, making removal very difficult.[103] Over time, stress fractures often develop in the stents, resulting in loose wires, which may migrate through the airway wall and cause injury to the surrounding lung and mediastinal structures. Because of these complications, the American College of Chest Physicians and the Food and Drug Administration have issued warnings against the use of metallic airway stents for benign airway diseases.[104]

An advantage of metal stents over silicone stents is their ability to be placed without the need for rigid bronchoscopy, but rather using a flexible bronchoscope and fluoroscopic guidance. To achieve this, the patient is examined using conscious sedation with a flexible bronchoscope. The obstructed airway of interest is identified, the lesion is measured using the bronchoscope, and a guidewire is passed through the working channel of the bronchoscope across the area of stenosis. Next, the bronchoscope is positioned at the distal and proximal ends of the stenosis, and markers are placed on the patient's chest under fluoroscopy. The bronchoscope is removed with the guidewire left in place. The self-expandable metal stent is then passed over the guidewire, positioned in the airway using fluoroscopy and the previously placed surface markers, and deployed under fluoroscopy to ensure accurate positioning.

Hybrid Stents

Hybrid silicone and nitinol stents have been developed that share some of the characteristics of silicone and metallic stents. These **hybrid stents** are constructed of a polyurethane or silicone sleeve with supporting nitinol struts. They share many of the advantages of metal stents in that they are self-expanding and so may be deployed across a tight stenosis and act to open the lesion via the radial force exerted by the wire mesh. The silicone sleeve prevents tumor ingrowth through the stent, and also prevents the stent from granulating into the airway wall. This enhances patency as well as allows for removal of the stent at a later time if needed.

One disadvantage of these stents has recently been recognized related to the open nature of the nitinol struts. These struts may fold inward on themselves during vigorous coughing or breathing. Generally they will reexpand to their original dimensions, but occasionally they remain collapsed. Case reports exist describing severe shortness of breath associated with collapsed tracheal stents, requiring urgent removal.[105]

Efficacy and Complications of Stent Placement

Stents are generally effective in improving airway patency[106] and are associated with increases in FEV_1.[107] There are no randomized trials evaluating stent efficacy, survival benefit, or head-to-head comparisons of efficacy between types of stent. In addition, optimal placement of airway stents may be more complicated than previously perceived. Miyazawa et al. examined flow-limiting segments of malignant airway stenosis in 64 patients using ultrathin bronchoscopy, flow volume loops, and three-dimensional CT reconstruction before and after central airway stenting. They found that the flow-limiting segment migrated distally in 15% of patients after stent placement, requiring additional airway stent deployment to optimize respiratory function.[108] Significant complications are common and are as high as 50% in some series. Common complications include stent migration and occlusion by secretions, occasionally with significant airway obstruction requiring emergent procedures to clear the impacted secretions.

Choice of therapeutic approach is based on a variety of variables, including the patient's degree of dyspnea, the location of the tumor, whether the tumor is primarily endobronchial or the airway obstruction is secondary to extrinsic compression, available equipment, and the level of local experience with the various techniques. Generally speaking, the rapid effect of heat-based therapies may have a less durable effect in the absence of additional treatment such as airway stenting, palliative radiation, or chemotherapy. Treatments such as photodynamic therapy or brachytherapy may delay the recurrence of tumor, and thus may result in a longer-lasting tumor reduction. Currently, there are no data available comparing the efficacy of techniques. There is no demonstrated increase in life expectancy with use of any of the treatments described here; however, substantial data exist that suggest efficacy for providing symptomatic relief.[109–113]

Pleural Disease

Pleural effusions are a commonly encountered medical problem in both inpatient and outpatient medicine. Although no good data are available regarding the incidence of pleural effusions, it is estimated that over one million new effusions are diagnosed annually in the United States.[114] Pleural effusions may be caused by a variety of medical conditions (**Box 11–4**). However, the most common causes are related to congestive heart failure, malignancy, pneumonia, and pulmonary embolism.[114] The first step in determining the etiology of the newly recognized pleural effusion is to perform **thoracentesis**.

Thoracentesis

Indications

Thoracentesis is a safe procedure that may be performed at the bedside and is the first step in the diagnosis of a newly recognized pleural effusion. Indications include diagnosis of a new pleural effusion of unknown etiology and relief of dyspnea in a patient with a large pleural effusion resulting in significant loss of lung volume due to the occupation of the hemithorax with fluid.[115] Contraindications are few and include inability to provide informed consent, uncorrected coagulopathy, and operator inexperience.

Procedure

It is generally considered safe to perform a blind thoracentesis if the fluid layers to a depth of 1 cm on ipsilateral decubitus radiographs of the chest. Using percussion of the chest, the fluid level is identified by listening for loss

BOX 11–4

Causes of Pleural Effusions

Transudative
- Congestive heart failure
- Cirrhosis of the liver
- Renal failure
- Urinothorax

Exudative
- Malignancy
- Pneumonia
- Pulmonary embolism
- After thoracic surgery
- Tuberculosis
- Chyle
- Connective tissue diseases (e.g., rheumatoid arthritis, systemic lupus erythematosus)

of the resonant note as the examiner continues to firmly tap the chest wall of both hemithoraces moving from the cephalad to caudal position along the patient's back in the mid-scapular line. The first rib below the area where dullness is first encountered should be identified by palpation and a site marked at the superior aspect of the rib. To avoid injury to the neurovascular bundle that runs below each rib, the finder needle should be inserted at the middle of the rib body, below the marked site.

After the area is cleaned with an appropriate antiseptic such as chlorhexidine or Betadine, a fenestrated sterile drape is applied to the patient's back and a wheal of 1% lidocaine is raised using a 21- or 22-gauge needle and syringe at the needle insertion site. The tissues between the skin and rib are infiltrated with lidocaine until the rib body is contacted with the tip of the finder needle. The finder needle is then angled in the cephalad direction and "walked" over the top of the rib until it is able to pass into the intercostal space. While maintaining negative pressure on the syringe plunger, the needle is advanced into the pleural space. Often, the patient will flinch as the parietal pleura is contacted by the needle tip. Once the needle has passed through the pleural lining, fluid will be seen to fill the syringe. The needle should not be advanced at this point, but rather retracted 1 to 2 mm and lidocaine administered at this position to provide adequate analgesia to proceed with a sampling needle.

Once the fluid has been located, a clean 20-gauge needle and syringe should be inserted as just described to collect diagnostic pleural fluid samples. Approximately 100 mL should be collected to provide sufficient fluid for all necessary laboratory testing. If a large-volume therapeutic thoracentesis is to be performed, a 4-cm, 18-gauge angiocatheter may be inserted and connected to a three-way stopcock to withdraw fluid. Several convenient, commercially available kits for performing therapeutic thoracentesis have been produced that contain all of the necessary materials, including antiseptic, lidocaine, and long flexible catheters with one-way valves to prevent the entrainment of air into the thoracic cavity during drainage of pleural fluid.

Although no good data exist, it is generally thought that removal of 1500 mL of fluid at a time is safe to avoid the rare, but potentially fatal, complication of reexpansion pulmonary edema.[116,117] Fluid removal should be stopped if the patient develops intractable cough or sensation of chest discomfort during the procedure. To remove the catheter, the patient is asked to hum to produce positive intrathoracic pressure while the catheter is quickly removed. For an uncomplicated thoracentesis, it is not necessary to perform a postprocedure chest x-ray; although in any case in which air was aspirated, intractable cough was present, or chest pain occurred that persists after the procedure is completed an x-ray should be performed to evaluate for procedural complications.

In obese patients whose body habitus does not permit accurate physical exam, or in patients with small or loculated pleural effusions, thoracic ultrasonography may be useful in localizing pleural fluid for thoracentesis.[118] No randomized trials exist, but several studies suggest that ultrasound-guided thoracentesis is associated with lower complication rates than blind thoracentesis.[119–121] To perform ultrasound-guided thoracentesis, the patient should be placed in the seated position similar to the procedure for blind thoracentesis. The hemithorax of interest is examined, and the diaphragm with subdiaphragmatic structures (liver on the right and spleen on the left), visceral and parietal pleura, and pleural fluid are identified. A site is marked just superior to a rib where there is a clear path on ultrasound from the chest wall to underlying pleural fluid. Once the site is marked, the area is reexamined with the ultrasound probe to confirm the correct location, and the thoracentesis is performed as previously described. Ultrasound-guided thoracentesis should be performed in a single sitting. Use of ultrasound marking followed by performance of thoracentesis at a later time, such as when the patient returns to his or her room from the radiology suite, has not been shown to decrease procedural complications, because the patient is unlikely to be in the same position for both the imaging and thoracentesis.[122] Thoracic ultrasonographic images can be difficult for the novice operator to interpret, and thus ultrasound-guided thoracentesis should only be performed by an adequately trained operator.

RESPIRATORY RECAP

Thoracentesis

- » The most common causes of pleural effusions are related to congestive heart failure, malignancy, pneumonia, and pulmonary embolism.
- » Indications for thoracentesis include diagnosis of a new pleural effusion of unknown etiology and relief of dyspnea in a patient with a large pleural effusion.
- » Removal of 1500 mL of fluid at a time is safe.
- » Pleural fluid with pH < 7.20 and glucose < 60 mg/dL may indicate a complicated parapneumonic effusion.
- » Light's criteria are used to discriminate between exudative and transudative pleural fluid.
- » Pleurodesis is the traditional approach to recurrent pleural effusions.

Interpretation of Results

The primary purpose of performing diagnostic thoracentesis is to categorize pleural fluid as either **transudative**, suggesting benign, noninflammatory causes, or **exudative**, suggesting a malignant, infectious, or inflammatory etiology. Light's criteria were introduced in 1972 to discriminate between exudative and transudative pleural fluid and are composed of the measurement of pleural fluid and serum protein and lactate dehydrogenase (LDH).[123] A fluid is deemed exudative if the ratio of pleural fluid to serum protein is 0.5 or greater or if the ratio of pleural fluid to serum LDH is 0.6 or greater. Either criterion is adequate to classify the pleural fluid.

Alternatively, if the pleural fluid LDH is greater than two-thirds the upper limit of the normal local laboratory values, the fluid is considered to be an exudate.[124]

Additional studies may also be performed on the pleural fluid to establish particular diagnoses. Pleural fluid with pH less than 7.20 and glucose less than 60 mg/dL may indicate a complicated parapneumonic effusion, an indication for chest tube insertion to complete drainage of the pleural space.[125,126]

Pleural fluid cytology has a 70% sensitivity for diagnosis of a malignant pleural effusion,[127] whereas pleural fluid adenosine deaminase levels may be helpful when there is a high suspicion of a tuberculous effusion.[115] Should the cause of an exudative effusion not be determined after initial fluid analysis, medical pleuroscopy or surgical thoracoscopy may be indicated for direct visualization and biopsy of the pleura (**Figure 11–18**). Up to 15% of effusions may elude a definitive diagnosis.[115]

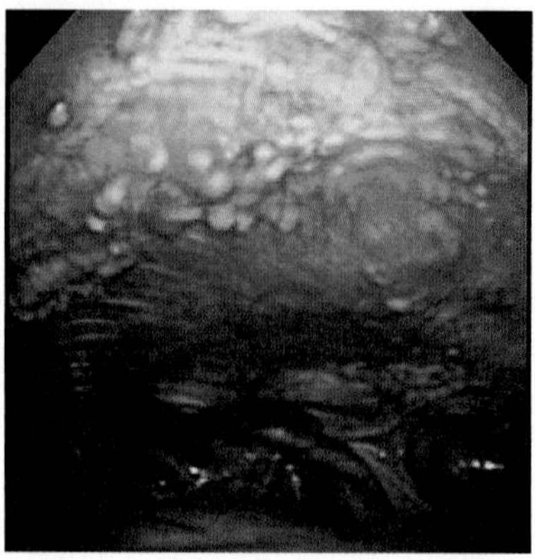

FIGURE 11–18 Thoracoscopic view of parietal pleura showing malignant nodules lining the interior aspect of the chest cavity. These were metastatic breast cancer.

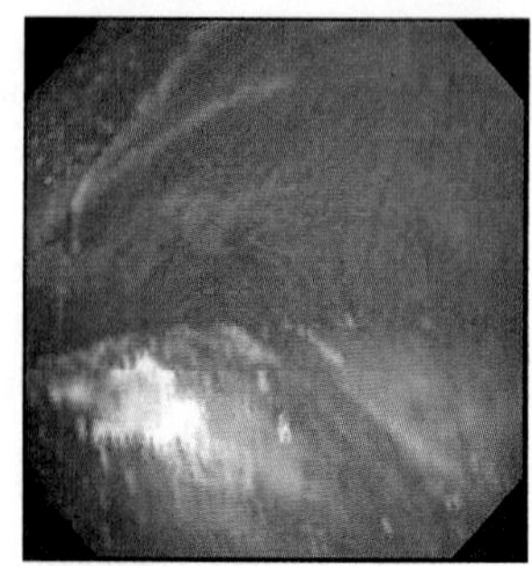

FIGURE 11–19 Thoracoscopic view of a talc poudrage pleurodesis. Note the characteristic "snowstorm" appearance of the insufflated talc sclerosant.

Management of Recurrent Pleural Effusions

Many pleural effusions are self-limited and resolve with treatment of the underlying etiology of the effusion; however, some effusions may be recurrent and result in significant dyspnea and limitation of functional status for the affected patient. Malignant effusions in particular result in substantial morbidity for the patient and often require palliative intervention to alleviate the dyspnea that results from the fluid.

The traditional approach to recurrent pleural effusions is to provide **pleurodesis**, either with mechanical abrasion during a thoracotomy or thorascopic surgery or by administering a **sclerosing agent** via tube thoracostomy. Many sclerosing agents have been evaluated, including tetracycline or doxycycline, bleomycin, and talc. Talc is currently considered to be the most efficacious agent available, with 30-day success rates of 80% for control of the recurrent effusion[128] as compared with a 60% success rate at 30 days for doxycycline[129] or bleomycin.[130] There is some controversy as to what is the best form in which to administer the talc, either as a slurry suspended in normal saline, or aerosolized as a talc poudrage during medical thoracoscopy or video-assisted thoracoscopy (**Figure 11–19**). The largest study available suggests a small increase in efficacy when talc is delivered as a poudrage in patients with effusions due to metastatic lung, renal, or breast cancer.[128] Although pleurodesis is generally effective, it requires an inpatient stay and usually several days of chest tube drainage following the administration of the sclerosing agent to allow for drainage of pleural fluid as the pleurodesis takes place.

An alternative to pleurodesis is the placement of a tunneled pleural catheter, which allows patients to manage their effusion in the outpatient setting. The catheter is a 15.5 Fr silicone tube fitted with a polyester cuff that is tunneled beneath the skin of the chest wall and into the pleural space (**Figure 11–20**). The catheter is fitted at the distal end with a one-way valve that is accessed using a specially designed catheter attached to a vacuum bottle for drainage at home. The tunneled catheter permits outpatient management of recurrent pleural effusions with simple insertion done in a radiology or endoscopy suite. Complications are primarily related to inability to adequately drain a loculated fluid collection, and infection rates are low, between 2% and 8%.[131,132] The catheter may be left in place as long as the effusion continues to recur. In one series, 42% of patients underwent spontaneous pleurodesis by repeated drainage of the effusion at 6 weeks, permitting removal of the catheter at that time.[132]

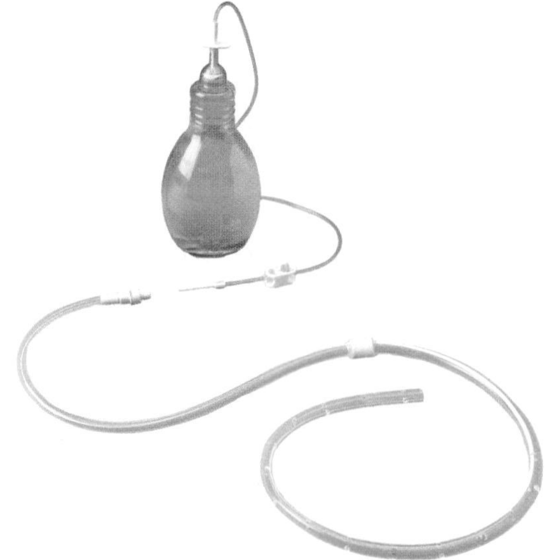

FIGURE 11–20 Pleurx tunneled pleural catheter system with attached drainage bottle. The catheter is tunneled below the skin and inserted into the chest cavity for repeated drainage of pleural fluid. The catheter has a polyester cuff that induces granulation tissue at the skin insertion site, reducing infectious risk with long-term use of the device.

Future Directions

Interventional pulmonology is a rapidly advancing, technologically driven field of medicine. One current area of intense interest is endoluminal **lung-volume reduction** for treatment of advanced emphysema using one-way endobronchial valves. The valves are inserted bronchoscopically into subsegmental airways with the goal of allowing air to escape via the one-way valve but not reenter the area of emphysema, producing an effective collapse of the abnormal area of lung. This is thought to permit the surrounding lung parenchyma to expand, resulting in improved ventilation-perfusion matching as well as permitting the diaphragm to assume a more normal position in the chest, improving muscle mechanics. Published studies to date show good safety and tolerance profiles, but significant changes in physiologic parameters are lacking.[133,134] Other techniques designed to alleviate hyperinflation due to emphysema that are currently under investigation include biologic lung-volume reduction that uses a fibrin gluelike substance to occlude target airways[135] and airway bypass that uses a small stainless steel stent across a central airway to provide a conduit for air escape from regions of emphysematous lung.[134]

Promising new diagnostic tools include an electromagnetic navigation system that allows use of a high-resolution CT scan of the chest to guide an endobronchial probe to a nodule of interest to permit histologic sampling. Preliminary data suggest yields of 67% for lesions smaller than 2 cm in diameter, far superior to yields with fluoroscopically guided techniques.[136] Addition of a radial endobronchial ultrasound probe in combination with the electromagnetic system enhances yield to 88%.[137] As promising as these new techniques are, further data are needed to establish their efficacy before they are widely accepted into general pulmonary practice.

In conclusion, diagnostic and therapeutic bronchoscopy are useful tools in appropriately trained hands for the management of patients with complex pulmonary disease. Although invasive, procedures may be safely performed when proper precautions are taken to prevent and avoid complications. Given the degree of interest in new technology associated with bronchoscopic techniques, we anticipate a growing role for the pulmonologist in patient care in the coming years.

KEY POINTS

- Bronchoscopy is the most commonly used invasive procedure in pulmonary medicine and can be used to perform both diagnostic and therapeutic procedures.
- The flexible fiberoptic bronchoscope consists of a control unit (or head) and a soft, flexible shaft.
- Bronchoscopy is a safe and effective tool for diagnosing and treating a wide variety of pulmonary processes.
- Factors necessary for a successful bronchoscopy include proper patient selection, patient preparation, and appropriate anesthesia.
- The ideal patient for fiberoptic bronchoscopy is awake, able to understand and cooperate with the procedure, and free of other conditions that could elevate the risk of the procedure.
- Although bronchoscopy can be performed with topical anesthesia alone, many physicians and patients prefer the judicial use of adjunctive IV sedation.
- Common bronchoscopy techniques include airway examination, bronchoalveolar lavage, bronchoscopic washing, bronchial brushing, endobronchial biopsy, transbronchial lung biopsy, and transbronchial needle aspiration.
- Indications for bronchoscopy include atelectasis, hemoptysis, cough, suspected malignancy, infection, foreign body aspiration, interstitial lung disease, lung transplant, and trauma.
- Rigid bronchoscopy can be used for any bronchoscopic indication; however, the additional requirements of general anesthesia generally result in most centers limiting its use to therapeutic indications such as relief of central airway obstruction and foreign body removal, and for investigation of massive hemoptysis.
- Modern airway stenting uses self-expandable metal stents, silicone stents, and hybrid metal-silicone stents.
- Pleural effusions may be caused by a variety of medical conditions.
- Indications for thoracentesis include diagnosis of a new pleural effusion of unknown etiology and relief of dyspnea in a patient with a large pleural effusion resulting in significant loss of lung volume due to the occupation of the hemithorax with fluid.
- Pleural fluid is deemed exudative if the ratio of pleural fluid to serum protein is 0.5 or greater or if the ratio of pleural fluid to serum LDH is 0.6 or greater.
- The traditional approach to recurrent pleural effusions is to provide pleurodesis, either with mechanical abrasion during a thoracotomy or thorascopic surgery or by administering a sclerosing agent via tube thoracostomy.

REFERENCES

1. Ernst A, Silvestri GA, Johnstone D. Interventional pulmonary procedures: guidelines from the American College of Chest Physicians. *Chest.* 2003;123(5):1693–1717.
2. Murray JF. *Textbook of Respiratory Medicine.* 3rd ed. Philadelphia: Saunders; 2000.
3. Murray JF, Nadel JA. *Murray and Nadel's Textbook of Respiratory Medicine.* 4th ed. Philadelphia: Elsevier Saunders; 2005.
4. Kozak EA, Brath LK. Do "screening" coagulation tests predict bleeding in patients undergoing fiberoptic bronchoscopy with biopsy? *Chest.* 1994;106(3):703–705.

5. Djukanovic R, Wilson JW, Lai CK, Holgate ST, Howarth PH. The safety aspects of fiberoptic bronchoscopy, bronchoalveolar lavage, and endobronchial biopsy in asthma. *Am Rev Respir Dis.* 1991;143(4 pt 1):772–777.
6. Lundgren R, Haggmark S, Reiz S. Hemodynamic effects of flexible fiberoptic bronchoscopy performed under topical anesthesia. *Chest.* 1982;82(3):295–299.
7. Matot I, Kramer MR, Glantz L, Drenger B, Cotev S. Myocardial ischemia in sedated patients undergoing fiberoptic bronchoscopy. *Chest.* 1997;112(6):1454–1458.
8. British Thoracic Society guidelines on diagnostic flexible bronchoscopy. *Thorax.* 2001;56(suppl 1):1–21.
9. Bajwa MK, Henein S, Kamholz SL. Fiberoptic bronchoscopy in the presence of space-occupying intracranial lesions. *Chest.* 1993;104(1):101–103.
10. Kerwin AJ, Croce MA, Timmons SD, et al. Effects of fiberoptic bronchoscopy on intracranial pressure in patients with brain injury: a prospective clinical study. *J Trauma.* 2000; 48(5):878–882; discussion 882–883.
11. Wahidi MM, Rocha AT, Hollingsworth JW, et al. Contraindications and safety of transbronchial lung biopsy via flexible bronchoscopy. A survey of pulmonologists and review of the literature. *Respiration.* 2005;72(3):285–295.
12. Zavala DC. Pulmonary hemorrhage in fiberoptic transbronchial biopsy. *Chest.* 1976;70(5):584–588.
13. Herth FJ, Becker HD, Ernst A. Aspirin does not increase bleeding complications after transbronchial biopsy. *Chest.* 2002;122(4):1461–1464.
14. Ernst A, Eberhardt R, Wahidi M, Becker HD, Herth FJ. Effect of routine clopidogrel use on bleeding complications after transbronchial biopsy in humans. *Chest.* 2006;129(3):734–737.
15. Guidelines on oral anticoagulation: third edition. *Br J Haematol.* 1998;101(2):374–387.
16. Baglin TP, Keeling DM, Watson HG. Guidelines on oral anticoagulation (warfarin): third edition—2005 update. *Br J Haematol.* 2006;132(3):277–285.
17. Douketis JD, Berger PB, Dunn AS, et al. The perioperative management of antithrombotic therapy: American College of Chest Physicians evidence-based clinical practice guidelines. 8th ed. *Chest.* 2008;133(6 suppl):299S–339S.
18. Rebulla P. Platelet transfusion trigger in difficult patients. *Transfus Clin Biol.* 2001;8(3):249–254.
19. Sohal AS, Gangji AS, Crowther MA, Treleaven D. Uremic bleeding: pathophysiology and clinical risk factors. *Thromb Res.* 2006;118(3):417–422.
20. Lohr JW, Schwab SJ. Minimizing hemorrhagic complications in dialysis patients. *J Am Soc Nephrol.* 1991;2(5):961–975.
21. Diette GB, Wiener CM, White P Jr. The higher risk of bleeding in lung transplant recipients from bronchoscopy is independent of traditional bleeding risks: results of a prospective cohort study. *Chest.* 1999;115(2):397–402.
22. Dransfield MT, Garver RI, Weill D. Standardized guidelines for surveillance bronchoscopy reduce complications in lung transplant recipients. *J Heart Lung Transplant.* 2004;23(1):110–114.
23. Pue CA, Pacht ER. Complications of fiberoptic bronchoscopy at a university hospital. *Chest.* 1995;107(2):430–432.
24. Milman N, Faurschou P, Grode G, Jorgensen A. Pulse oximetry during fibreoptic bronchoscopy in local anaesthesia: frequency of hypoxaemia and effect of oxygen supplementation. *Respiration.* 1994;61(6):342–347.
25. Witte MC, Opal SM, Gilbert JG, et al. Incidence of fever and bacteremia following transbronchial needle aspiration. *Chest.* 1986;89(1):85–87.
26. Poi PJ, Chuah SY, Srinivas P, Liam CK. Common fears of patients undergoing bronchoscopy. *Eur Respir J.* 1998;11(5):1147–1149.
27. Matot I, Kramer MR. Sedation in outpatient bronchoscopy. *Respir Med.* 2000;94(12):1145–1153.
28. Williams T, Brooks T, Ward C. The role of atropine premedication in fiberoptic bronchoscopy using intravenous midazolam sedation. *Chest.* 1998;113(5):1394–1398.
29. Adam A, Dixon AK, Grainger RG, Allison DJ. *Grainger and Allison's Diagnostic Radiology: A Textbook of Medical Imaging.* Philadelphia: Churchill Livingstone/Elsevier; 2008.
30. Peikert T, Rana S, Edell ES. Safety, diagnostic yield, and therapeutic implications of flexible bronchoscopy in patients with febrile neutropenia and pulmonary infiltrates. *Mayo Clin Proc.* 2005;80(11):1414–1420.
31. Weiss SM, Hert RC, Gianola FJ, Clark JG, Crawford SW. Complications of fiberoptic bronchoscopy in thrombocytopenic patients. *Chest.* 1993;104(4):1025–1028.
32. Baughman RP. Protected-specimen brush technique in the diagnosis of ventilator-associated pneumonia. *Chest.* 2000;117 (4 suppl 2):203S–206S.
33. Dasgupta A, Jain P, Minai OA, et al. Utility of transbronchial needle aspiration in the diagnosis of endobronchial lesions. *Chest.* 1999;115(5):1237–1241.
34. Gilman MJ, Wang KP. Transbronchial lung biopsy in sarcoidosis. An approach to determine the optimal number of biopsies. *Am Rev Respir Dis.* 1980;122(5):721–724.
35. Popovich J Jr, Kvale PA, Eichenhorn MS, et al. Diagnostic accuracy of multiple biopsies from flexible fiberoptic bronchoscopy. A comparison of central versus peripheral carcinoma. *Am Rev Respir Dis.* 1982;125(5):521–523.
36. Scott JP, Fradet G, Smyth RL, et al. Prospective study of transbronchial biopsies in the management of heart-lung and single lung transplant patients. *J Heart Lung Transplant.* 1991;10(5 pt 1): 626–636; discussion 636–637.
37. Loube DI, Johnson JE, Wiener D, et al. The effect of forceps size on the adequacy of specimens obtained by transbronchial biopsy. *Am Rev Respir Dis.* 1993;148(5):1411–1413.
38. Smith LS, Seaquist M, Schillaci RF. Comparison of forceps used for transbronchial lung biopsy. Bigger may not be better. *Chest.* 1985;87(5):574–576.
39. Aleva RM, Kraan J, Smith M, et al. Techniques in human airway inflammation: quantity and morphology of bronchial biopsy specimens taken by forceps of three sizes. *Chest.* 1998;113(1):182–185.
40. Curley FJ, Johal JS, Burke ME, Fraire AE. Transbronchial lung biopsy: can specimen quality be predicted at the time of biopsy? *Chest.* 1998;113(4):1037–1041.
41. Le Jeune I, Baldwin D. Measuring the success of transbronchial needle aspiration in everyday clinical practice. *Respir Med.* 2007;101(3):670–675.
42. Patel NM, Pohlman A, Husain A, et al. Conventional transbronchial needle aspiration decreases the rate of surgical sampling of intrathoracic lymphadenopathy. *Chest.* 2007;131(3):773–778.
43. Larsen SS, Vilmann P, Krasnik M, et al. Endoscopic ultrasound guided biopsy performed routinely in lung cancer staging spares futile thoracotomies: preliminary results from a randomised clinical trial. *Lung Cancer.* 2005;49(3):377–385.
44. Kennedy MP, Jimenez CA, Bruzzi JF, et al. Endobronchial ultrasound-guided transbronchial needle aspiration in the diagnosis of lymphoma. *Thorax.* 2008;63(4):360–365.
45. Diacon AH, Schuurmans MM, Theron J, et al. Transbronchial needle aspirates: how many passes per target site? *Eur Respir J.* 2007;29(1):112–116.
46. Herth F, Becker HD, Ernst A. Conventional vs endobronchial ultrasound-guided transbronchial needle aspiration: a randomized trial. *Chest.* 2004;125(1):322–325.
47. Diette GB, White P Jr, Terry P, et al. Utility of on-site cytopathology assessment for bronchoscopic evaluation of lung masses and adenopathy. *Chest.* 2000;117(4):1186–1190.
48. Baram D, Garcia RB, Richman PS. Impact of rapid on-site cytologic evaluation during transbronchial needle aspiration. *Chest.* 2005;128(2):869–875.
49. Chin R Jr, McCain TW, Lucia MA, et al. Transbronchial needle aspiration in diagnosing and staging lung cancer: how many aspirates are needed? *Am J Respir Crit Care Med.* 2002;166(3):377–381.

50. Prakash UB. Advances in bronchoscopic procedures. *Chest.* 1999;116(5):1403–1408.
51. Izbicki G, Shitrit D, Yarmolovsky A, et al. Is routine chest radiography after transbronchial biopsy necessary? A prospective study of 350 cases. *Chest.* 2006;129(6):1561–1564.
52. Smyth CM, Stead RJ. Survey of flexible fibreoptic bronchoscopy in the United Kingdom. *Eur Respir J.* 2002;19(3):458–463.
53. Kreider ME, Lipson DA. Bronchoscopy for atelectasis in the ICU: a case report and review of the literature. *Chest.* 2003;124(1):344–350.
54. Marini JJ, Pierson DJ, Hudson LD. Acute lobar atelectasis: a prospective comparison of fiberoptic bronchoscopy and respiratory therapy. *Am Rev Respir Dis.* 1979;119(6):971–978.
55. Hirshberg B, Biran I, Glazer M, Kramer MR. Hemoptysis: etiology, evaluation, and outcome in a tertiary referral hospital. *Chest.* 1997;112(2):440–444.
56. Weaver LJ, Solliday N, Cugell DW. Selection of patients with hemoptysis for fiberoptic bronchoscopy. *Chest.* 1979;76(1):7–10.
57. Colice GL. Detecting lung cancer as a cause of hemoptysis in patients with a normal chest radiograph: bronchoscopy vs CT. *Chest.* 1997;111(4):877–884.
58. Poe RH, Israel RH, Marin MG, et al. Utility of fiberoptic bronchoscopy in patients with hemoptysis and a nonlocalizing chest roentgenogram. *Chest.* 1988;93(1):70–75.
59. Karmy-Jones R, Cuschieri J, Vallieres E. Role of bronchoscopy in massive hemoptysis. *Chest Surg Clin N Am.* 2001;11(4):873–906.
60. Decalmer S, Woodcock A, Greaves M, Howe M, Smith J. Airway abnormalities at flexible bronchoscopy in patients with chronic cough. *Eur Respir J.* 2007;30(6):1138–1142.
61. Schreiber G, McCrory DC. Performance characteristics of different modalities for diagnosis of suspected lung cancer: summary of published evidence. *Chest.* 2003;123 (1 suppl):115S–128S.
62. Tan BB, Flaherty KR, Kazerooni EA, Iannettoni MD. The solitary pulmonary nodule. *Chest.* 2003;123(1 suppl):89S–96S.
63. Joos L, Patuto N, Chhajed PN, Tamm M. Diagnostic yield of flexible bronchoscopy in current clinical practice. *Swiss Med Wkly.* 2006;136(9–10):155–159.
64. Ortqvist A, Kalin M, Lejdeborn L, Lundberg B. Diagnostic fiberoptic bronchoscopy and protected brush culture in patients with community-acquired pneumonia. *Chest.* 1990;97(3):576–582.
65. van der Eerden MM, Vlaspolder F, de Graaff CS, et al. Value of intensive diagnostic microbiological investigation in low- and high-risk patients with community-acquired pneumonia. *Eur J Clin Microbiol Infect Dis.* 2005;24(4):241–249.
66. Jain P, Sandur S, Meli Y, et al. Role of flexible bronchoscopy in immunocompromised patients with lung infiltrates. *Chest.* 2004;125(2):712–722.
67. Horvath JA, Dummer S. The use of respiratory-tract cultures in the diagnosis of invasive pulmonary aspergillosis. *Am J Med.* 1996;100(2):171–178.
68. Yu VL, Muder RR, Poorsattar A. Significance of isolation of *Aspergillus* from the respiratory tract in diagnosis of invasive pulmonary aspergillosis. Results from a three-year prospective study. *Am J Med.* 1986;81(2):249–254.
69. Woods GL, Walker DH. Detection of infection or infectious agents by use of cytologic and histologic stains. *Clin Microbiol Rev.* 1996;9(3):382–404.
70. Eren S, Balci AE, Dikici B, Doblan M, Eren MN. Foreign body aspiration in children: experience of 1160 cases. *Ann Trop Paediatr.* 2003;23(1):31–37.
71. Soysal O, Kuzucu A, Ulutas H. Tracheobronchial foreign body aspiration: a continuing challenge. *Otolaryngol Head Neck Surg.* 2006;135(2):223–226.
72. Daines CL, Wood RE, Boesch RP. Foreign body aspiration: an important etiology of respiratory symptoms in children. *J Allergy Clin Immunol.* 2008;121(5):1297–1298.
73. Leslie KO, Gruden JF, Parish JM, Scholand MB. Transbronchial biopsy interpretation in the patient with diffuse parenchymal lung disease. *Arch Pathol Lab Med.* 2007;131(3):407–423.
74. Glanville AR. The role of bronchoscopic surveillance monitoring in the care of lung transplant recipients. *Semin Respir Crit Care Med.* 2006;27(5):480–491.
75. McWilliams TJ, Williams TJ, Whitford HM, Snell GI. Surveillance bronchoscopy in lung transplant recipients: risk versus benefit. *J Heart Lung Transplant.* 2008;27(11):1203–1209.
76. Chhajed PN, Tamm M, Glanville AR. Role of flexible bronchoscopy in lung transplantation. *Semin Respir Crit Care Med.* 2004;25(4):413–423.
77. Kunisch-Hoppe M, Hoppe M, Rauber K, Popella C, Rau WS. Tracheal rupture caused by blunt chest trauma: radiological and clinical features. *Eur Radiol.* 2000;10(3):480–483.
78. Dennie CJ, Coblentz CL. The trachea: pathologic conditions and trauma. *Can Assoc Radiol J.* 1993;44(3):157–167.
79. Ernst A, Feller-Kopman D, Becker H, Mehta A. Central airway obstruction. *Am J Respir Crit Care.* 2004;169:1278–1297.
80. Santacruz J, Mehta A. Airway complications and management after lung transplantation. *Proc Am Thorac Soc.* 2009;6:79–93.
81. Beamis J. Modern use of rigid bronchoscopy. In: Bollinger CT, Mathur PN, eds. *Interventional Bronchoscopy*. Basel, Switzerland: S. Karger; 2000.
82. Wahidi M, Herth F, Ernst A. State of the art: interventional pulmonology. *Chest.* 2007;131:261–274.
83. Perrin G, Colt HG, Martin C, et al. Safety of interventional rigid bronchoscopy using intravenous anesthesia and spontaneous assisted ventilation. A prospective study. *Chest.* 1992;102:1526–1530.
84. Conacher ID. Anaesthesia and tracheobronchial stenting for central airway obstruction in adults. *Br J Anaesthesia.* 2003;90:367–374.
85. Godden DJ, Willey RF, Fergusson RJ, et al. Rigid bronchoscopy under intravenous general anesthesia with oxygen venturi ventilation. *Thorax.* 1987;37:532–534.
86. Bollinger CT, Sutedja TG, Strausz J, Freitag L. Therapeutic bronchoscopy with immediate effect: laser, electrocautery, argon plasma coagulation and stents. *Eur Respir J.* 2006;27:1258–1271.
87. Laforet EG, Berger RL, Vaughan CW. Carcinoma obstructing the trachea. Treatment by laser resection. *N Engl J Med.* 1976;294:941.
88. Keller CA, Hinerman R, Singh A, Alvarez F. The use of endoscopic argon plasma coagulation in airway complications after solid organ transplantation. *Chest.* 2001;119:1968–1975.
89. Morice R, Ece T, Ece F, Keus L. Endobronchial argon plasma coagulation for treatment of hemoptysis and neoplastic airway obstruction. *Chest.* 2001;119:781–787.
90. Feller-Kopman D, Lukanich JM, Shapira G, et al. Gas flow during bronchoscopic ablation therapy causes gas emboli to the heart: a comparative animal study. *Chest.* 2008;33:892–896.
91. Vergnon J, Huber R, Moghissi K. Place of cryotherapy, brachytherapy and photodynamic therapy in therapeutic bronchoscopy of lung cancers. *Eur Respir J.* 2006;28:200–218.
92. Ferretti G, Jouvan FB, Thony F, Pison C, Coulomb M. Benign noninflammatory bronchial stenosis: treatment with balloon dilation. *Radiology.* 1995;196:831–834.
93. Reddy A, Govert J, Sporn T, Wahidi M. Broncholith removal using cryotherapy during flexible bronchoscopy. *Chest.* 2007;132:1661–1663.
94. Mang T. Lasers and light sources for PDT: past, present, and future. *Photodiag Photodyn Ther.* 2004;1:43–48.
95. Lee P, Kupeli E, Mehta A. Therapeutic bronchoscopy in lung cancer. *Clin Chest Med.* 2002;23:241–256.
96. Spratling L, Speiser BL. Endoscopic brachytherapy. *Chest Surg Clin N Am.* 1996;6:293–304.
97. Huber RM, Fischer R, Hautmann H, et al. Palliative endobronchial brachytherapy for central lung tumors: a prospective randomized comparison of two fractionation schedules. *Chest.* 1995;107:463–470.
98. Ozkok S, Karakoyun-Celik O, Goksel T, et al. High dose rate endobronchial brachytherapy in the management of lung cancer:

response and toxicity evaluation in 158 patients. *Lung Cancer.* 2008;62:326–333.
99. Cardona Zorrilla AF, Reveiz L, Ospina EG, Yepes A. Palliative endobronchial brachytherapy for non-small cell lung cancer. *Cochrane Database System Rev* 2008;2:CD004284.
100. Dumon JF. A dedicated tracheobronchial stent. *Chest.* 1990;97:328–332.
101. Freitag L. Tracheobronchial stents. In: Bollinger CT, Mathur PN, eds. *Interventional Bronchoscopy.* Basel, Switzerland: Karger; 2000:171–186.
102. Chan A, Juarez MM, Allen RP, Albertson TE. Do airway metallic stents for benign lesions confer too costly a benefit? *BMC Pulm Med.* 2008;8:7–15.
103. Lunn W, Feller-Kopman D, Wahidi M, et al. Endoscopic removal of metallic airway stents. *Chest.* 2005;127:2106–2112.
104. Lund W, Force S. Airway stenting for patients with benign airway disease and the Food and Drug Administration advisory: a call for restraint. *Chest.* 2007;132:1107–1108.
105. Trisolini R, Paioli D, Fornario V, et al. Collapse of a new type of self-expanding metallic tracheal stent. *Monaldi Arch Chest Dis.* 2006;65:56–58.
106. Dumon JF, Cavaliere S, Diaz-Jimenez JP, et al. Seven-year experience with the Dumon prosthesis. *J Bronchol.* 1996;2:6–10.
107. Vergnon JM, Costes F, Bayon MC, Emonot A. Efficacy of tracheal and bronchial stent placement on respiratory functional tests. *Chest.* 1995;107:741–746.
108. Miyazawa T, Miyazu Y, Iwamoto Y, et al. Stenting at the flow-limiting segment in tracheobronchial stenosis due to lung cancer. *Am J Respir Crit Care Med.* 2004;169:1096–1102.
109. Wood DE, Liu YH, Vallieres E, Karmy-Jones R, Mulligan MS. Airway stenting for malignant and benign tracheobronchial stenosis. *Ann Thorac Surg.* 2003;76:167–172.
110. Saad CP, Murthy S, Krizmanich G, Mehta AC. Self-expandable metallic airway stents and flexible bronchoscopy: long-term outcomes analysis. *Chest.* 2003;124:1993–1999.
111. Dasgupta A, Dolmatch BL, Abi-Saleh WJ, Mathur PN, Mehta AC. Self-expandable metallic airway stent insertion employing flexible bronchoscopy: preliminary results. *Chest.* 1998;114:106–109.
112. Bollinger CT, Probst R, Tschopp K, Soler M, Perruchoud AP. Silicone stents in the management of inoperable tracheobronchial stenosis: indications and limitations. *Chest.* 1993;104:1653–1659.
113. Lemaire A, Burfeind WR, Toloza E, et al. Outcomes of tracheobronchial stents in patients with malignant airway disease. *Ann Thorac Surg.* 2005;80:434–438.
114. Light RW. *Pleural Diseases.* 4th ed. Philadelphia: Lippincott Williams & Wilkins; 2001.
115. Light RW. Pleural effusion. *N Engl J Med.* 2002 346:1971–1977.
116. Feller-Kopman D, Walkey A, Berkowitz D, Ernst A. The relationship of pleural pressure to symptom development during therapeutic thoracentesis. *Chest.* 2006;129:1556–1560.
117. Feller-Kopman D, Parker MJ, Schwartzstein RM. Assessment of pleural pressure in the evaluation of pleural effusions. *Chest.* 2009;135:201–209.
118. Feller-Kopman D. Ultrasound-guided thoracentesis. *Chest.* 2006;129:1709–1714.
119. Seneff MG, Corwin RW, Gold LH, Irwin RS. Complications associated with thoracentesis. *Chest.* 1986;90:97–100.
120. Mayo PH, Goltz HR, Tafreshi M, Doelken P. Safety of ultrasound-guided thoracentesis in patients receiving mechanical ventilation. *Chest.* 2004;125:1059–1062.
121. Jones PW, Moyers JP, Rogers JT, et al. Ultrasound-guided thoracentesis: is it a safer method? *Chest.* 2003;123:418–423.
122. Raptopoulos V, Davis LM, Lee G, et al. Factors affecting the development of pneumothorax associated with thoracentesis. *Am J Roentgenol.* 1991;156:917–920.
123. Light RW, Macgregor MI, Luchsinger PC, Ball WC Jr. Pleural effusions: the diagnostic separation of transudates and exudates. *Ann Intern Med.* 1972;77:507–513.
124. Burgess LJ, Maritz FJ, Taljaard JJF. Comparative analysis of the biochemical parameters used to distinguish between pleural transudates and exudates. *Chest.* 1995;107:1604–1609.
125. Colice GL, Curtis A, Deslauriers J, et al. Medical and surgical treatment of parapneumonic effusions. *Chest.* 2000;118:1158–1171.
126. Maskell NA, Butland RJA. BTS guidelines for the investigation of a unilateral pleural effusion in adults. *Thorax.* 2003;58:ii8–ii17.
127. Prakash UBS, Reiman HM. Comparison of needle biopsy with cytologic analysis for the evaluation of pleural effusion: analysis of 414 cases. *Mayo Clin Proc.* 1985;60:158–164.
128. Dresler CM, Olak J, Herndon JE, et al. Phase III intergroup study of talc poudrage vs talc slurry sclerosis for malignant pleural effusion. *Chest.* 2005;127;909–915.
129. Diacon AH, Wyser C, Bolliger CT, et al. Prospective randomized comparison of thoracoscopic talc poudrage under local anesthesia versus bleomycin instillation for pleurodesis in malignant pleural effusions. *Am J Respir Crit Care Med.* 2000;162:1445–1449.
130. Seaton KG, Patz EF, Goodman PC. Palliative treatment of malignant pleural effusions: value of small-bore catheter thoracostomy and doxycycline sclerotherapy. *AJR.* 1995;164:589–591.
131. Putnam JB, Light RW, Rodriquez RM, et al. A randomized comparison of indwelling pleural catheter and doxycycline pleurodesis in the management of malignant pleural effusions. *Cancer.* 1999;86:1992–1999.
132. Tremblay A, Michaud G. Single-center experience with 250 tunnelled pleural catheter insertions for malignant pleural effusion. *Chest.* 2006;129:362–368.
133. Wood ED, McKenna RJ, Yusen RD, et al. A multicenter trial of an intrabronchial valve for treatment of severe emphysema. *J Thorac Cardiovasc Surg.* 2007;133:65–73.
134. Ingenito EP, Wood DE, Utz JP. Bronchoscopic lung volume reduction in severe emphysema. *Proc Am Thorac Soc.* 2008;5:454–460.
135. Criner GJ, Pinto-Plata V, Strange C, et al. Biologic lung volume reduction in advanced upper lobe emphysema. *Am J Respir Crit Care Med.* 2009;179:791–798.
136. Eberhardt R, Anantham D, Herth F, Feller-Kopman D, Ernst A. Electromagnetic navigation diagnostic bronchoscopy in peripheral lung lesions. *Chest.* 2007;131:1800–1805.
137. Eberhardt R, Anantham D, Ernst A, Feller-Kopman D, Herth F. Multimodality bronchoscopic diagnosis of peripheral lung lesions. *Am J Respir Crit Care Med.* 2007;176:36–41.

CHAPTER 12

Polysomnography

Bashir A. Chaudhary
Susan Whiddon
Shelley C. Mishoe

OUTLINE

Normal Sleep and Sleep Stages
Polysomnography Components
Scoring Criteria
Polysomnography Report

OBJECTIVES

1. Discuss the 10-20 system of electrode placement for electroencephalography (EEG).
2. Describe how amplifiers, gain, and sensitivity are applied in polysomnography.
3. Describe low-cut, high-cut, and notch filters.
4. Explain the basics of electrooculography and electromyography.
5. Identify common EEG rhythms.
6. Explain the scoring of sleep stages.
7. Apply the rules of disordered breathing.
8. Explain the scoring of leg movements.
9. Discuss the concepts and identification of arousals during sleep.
10. Describe the preparation of a polysomnography report.

KEY TERMS

amplifiers
apnea
arousals
arousal index
delta wave
EEG rhythms
electroencephalogram (EEG)
electromyogram (EMG)
electrooculogram (EOG)
hypopnea
international 10-20 system
K complexes
nonrapid eye movement (NREM) sleep
oximetry
periodic limb movements (PLMs) of sleep
polysomnogram
rapid eye movement (REM) sleep
respiratory effort–related arousal
sleep efficiency
sleep latency
sleep spindles
sleep stages

INTRODUCTION

We spend about one-third of our life sleeping. Although there is considerable variation, most young adults sleep about 7.5 hours during the weeknights and 8.5 hours during the weekends. During sleep, major changes to the organ systems of the body occur. The most important are the neurologic and respiratory systems. Sleep decreases the direct neurologic control of ventilation and ventilatory muscle tone. There are also changes to neurochemical reflexes that maintain respiration. These changes result in a reduced drive to breathe and increased airway resistance during normal sleep. Acute and chronic diseases can compound these normal changes, leading to apnea, hypopnea, and sleep-disordered breathing. This chapter focuses on the study of sleep.

Normal Sleep and Sleep Stages

Normal sleep consists of two states: **nonrapid eye movement (NREM) sleep** and **rapid eye movement (REM) sleep**. These sleep states alternate during the night. A combination of NREM and REM sleep makes one sleep cycle. Typically, there are three to five sleep cycles during one night of sleep. The average duration of a sleep cycle is about 100 ± 10 minutes (mean ± standard deviation). The first sleep cycle is usually the shortest (85 ± 15 minutes). Each sleep cycle starts with NREM sleep. After about 90 minutes, NREM sleep is followed by REM sleep. NREM sleep has been subdivided into three **sleep stages**: stages N1, N2, and N3 (**Table 12–1**). Stages N1 and N2 represent superficial sleep, whereas stage N3 sleep represents deep sleep.

> **RESPIRATORY RECAP**
>
> **Physiologic Changes During Sleep**
>
> » Alterations in neurochemical reflexes
> » Increased airway resistance
> » Reductions in airway space, drive to breathe, upper airway muscle tone, ventilatory muscle tone, ventilation (rate and depth of breathing)

The first sleep cycle starts with sleep stage N1, which lasts only 1 to 7 minutes. During this stage of sleep, the person wakes up easily and may not even realize that he or she was asleep. Stage N2 sleep lasts for 10 to 30 minutes, followed by 25 to 45 minutes of stage N3 sleep. Usually the stage N3 sleep changes back to stage N2 sleep for 5 to 10 minutes before the start of stage R (REM) sleep. The duration of stage R sleep in the first sleep cycle is usually less than 5 minutes. During the subsequent sleep cycles stage N3 sleep decreases in duration, and it is usually absent in the last sleep cycle. On the other hand, stage R increases in duration in the subsequent sleep cycles. The change to and from stage R sleep is through stage N2 sleep. The distribution of sleep stages in a given night can be affected by many factors, including age, the amount of sleep during the previous nights, medications, and the presence of sleep-related medical disorders.[1]

During the first year of life, the onset of sleep frequently is with stage R sleep instead of NREM sleep, and the sleep cycles are about 60 minutes long. The amount of stage N3 sleep is at maximum during the first decade of life and decreases significantly (by about 40%) in the second decade (**Figure 12–1**). The duration of stage N3 sleep decreases progressively with aging and is frequently absent after age 60, particularly in men. The percentage of REM sleep usually does not change much with age.

> **AGE-SPECIFIC ANGLE**
>
> During the first year of life, the onset of sleep frequently is with stage R sleep cycles that are about 60 minutes long. The duration of stage N3 sleep decreases progressively with aging and is frequently absent after age 60. The percentage of REM sleep usually does not change much with age.

TABLE 12-1 Sleep Stages in Young Adults

Sleep Stage	Time Spent
NREM Sleep	*75–80%*
Stage N1	2–5%
Stage N2	45–55%
Stage N3	15–20%
REM Sleep	*20–25%*

Sleep stage pattern changes significantly after sleep deprivation. Stage N3 sleep and stage R sleep are increased in duration, as if the body were trying to recover these components of sleep lost during the earlier nights. Stage N3 sleep is usually recovered the first night, and stage R sleep during the subsequent nights. Chronic sleep deprivation or disturbance of sleep and irregular sleep schedule can cause earlier onset of stage R sleep. Most antidepressants, particularly tricyclics, suppress stage R sleep. Benzodiazepines prolong the duration of sleep, but the amount of stage N3 sleep is actually decreased. Withdrawal of the medications suppressing stage N3 or R sleep results in rebound of these stages.

> **RESPIRATORY RECAP**
>
> **Sleep Stages**
>
> » Stage W (wakefulness)
> » Stage N1 (old NREM 1)
> » Stage N2 (old NREM 2)
> » Stage N3 (old NREM 3 and 4)
> » Stage R (old REM)

Any medical illness that disturbs sleep, causing arousal, can reduce the amount of stage N3 and stage R sleep. In severe sleep apnea these two stages are frequently reduced. Continuous positive airway pressure (CPAP) therapy is associated with rebound. Narcolepsy is characterized by early onset of stage R sleep.

Polysomnography Components

A typical **polysomnogram** (Current Procedural Terminology code 95810) includes recording of **electroencephalogram (EEG)**, **electrooculogram (EOG)**, **electromyogram (EMG)** of chin muscles, oronasal airflow, chest and abdominal movements, leg movements, snoring, and **oximetry**.[2]

Rechtschaffen and Kales (R&K) developed a manual in 1968 that had been used since that time as the standardized system for sleep stages.[3] In 2007, the American Academy of Sleep Medicine (AASM), previously called the American Sleep Disorders Association, published a

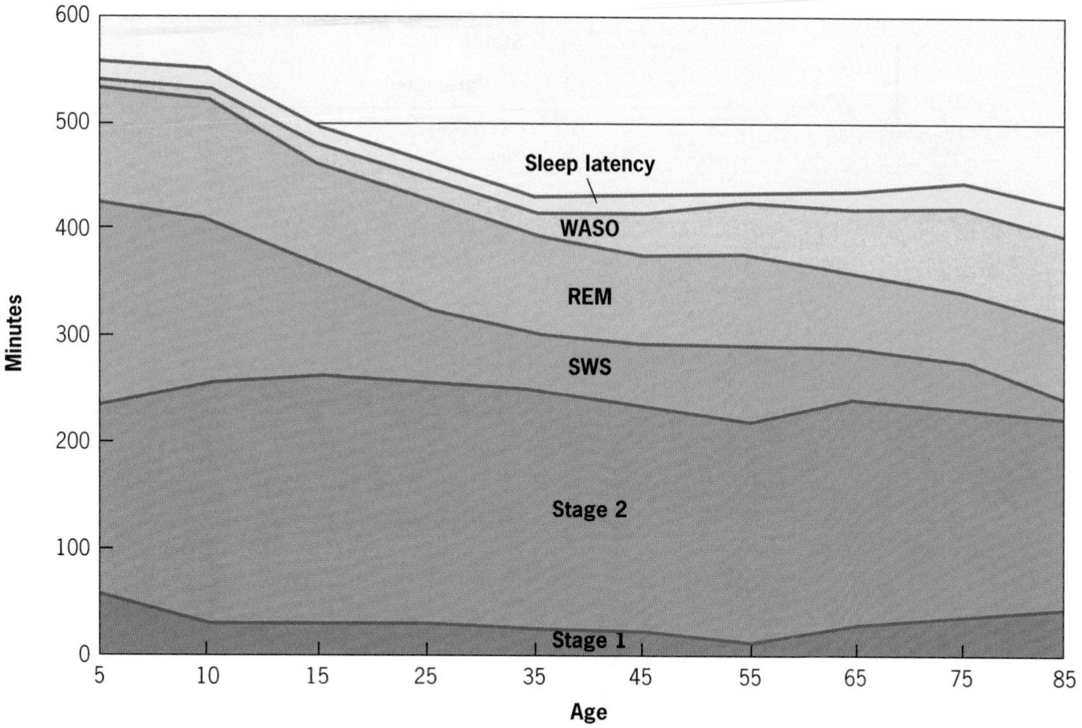

FIGURE 12–1 Age-related sleep stage changes. Reproduced from Ohayon MM, et al. Metaanalysis of quantitative sleep parameters from childhood to old age in healthy individuals: developing normative sleep values across the human lifespan. *Sleep*. 2004;27:1255–1273. Reprinted with permission.

> **RESPIRATORY RECAP**
>
> **Components of Polysomnography**
>
> » Electroencephalogram (EEG)
> » Electrooculogram (EOG)
> » Electromyogram (EMG) of chin muscles
> » Oronasal airflow
> » Chest and abdominal movements
> » Leg movements
> » Snoring
> » Oximetry

new manual. This new manual has made significant changes in sleep stages.[4] This manual also added rules about arousals, cardiac rhythm, muscle movements, and sleep-related breathing problems. The AASM rules became the new standard for performing and interpretation of polysomnograms in 2008. Following is a discussion of some of the basic aspects of polysomnography.

Electroencephalography

Brain electrical activity is recorded through surface electrodes placed on the skull in accordance with an internationally accepted method. These electrical signals pass from the electrodes and through amplifiers, where they are modified before being recorded on paper (analog) or digital recorders.

International 10-20 System

The **international 10-20 system** was developed in 1958 to standardize the placement of electrodes for EEG recording.[5] The system is termed *10-20* because electrodes are placed either at 10% or 20% of the total distance between two skull landmarks (**Figure 12–2**). The use of percentages instead of absolute distances allows for variation in head sizes. Based on specific anatomic correlates, this system of electrode placement allows for comparison of electrical activity from different areas of the brain and serial comparison of follow-up EEGs in a single patient. Also, it is consistent from one patient to another.

The four landmarks used are the nasion (the indentation between the forehead and the nose), the inion (the ridge at the back of the skull), and two preauricular points (indentations just in front of the tragus cartilage). The nomenclature gives each electrode a site pertaining to a certain area of the brain (F, frontal; P, parietal; T, temporal; C, central; O, occipital; A, auricular), with the exception of the "z" electrode, which refers to the midline or zero line. Appended numbers refer to the right (even numbers) and the left (odd numbers) side of the brain. The numbers also define the electrode location in relation to the midline. The smaller the number, the closer the electrode position is to the midline.

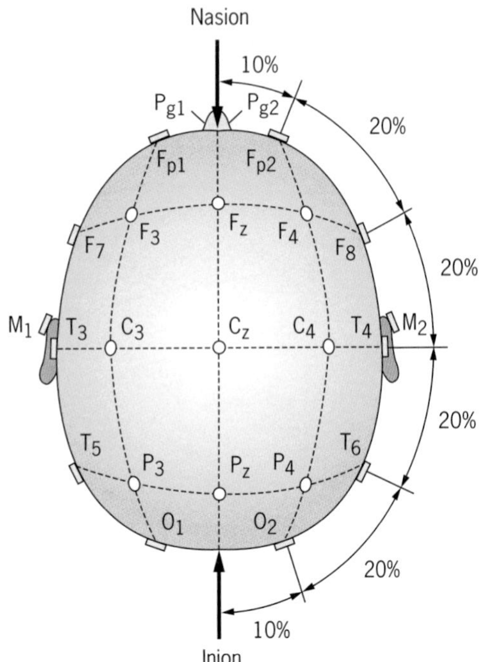

FIGURE 12–2 Electrode placement in the international 10-20 system.

Generally, the three measurements made to locate the electrode sites are the nasion to inion, right and left preauricular points, and the circumference of the head at the level of Fpz (which is at 10% of the distance from the nasion) and Oz (which is at 10% of the distance from inion). Frontal (F3 and F4) electrodes are located on the sides of Fz, which is at 30% of the distance from the nasion. Cz is located at the top of the head, at the crossing of the nasion-to-inion line and the line between the two preauricular points. The C3 and C4 electrodes are located on the line between the two auricular points at 20% of the distance from the Cz point or at 30% of the distance from the preauricular points. The O1 and O2 electrodes are separated by 10% of the circumference measurement. These electrodes are at the sides of the Oz electrode at 5% of the circumference measurement.

EEG is recorded using either referential or bipolar deviations. A referential deviation is used when the exploring electrode is compared with a relatively inactive reference site such as the mastoid. A bipolar derivation is used when the two exploring electrodes are compared with each other.

According to Rechtschaffen and Kales, the standard scoring channel for sleep stages was the central channel (C3/A2 or C4/A1).[3] Usually both of these channels were used to minimize the possibility of electrode displacement during the recording. Sleep spindles, K complexes, vertex waves, and delta waves are clearly recorded from these channels. Slow waves and K complexes are maximally expressed in the frontal region, spindles in the central region, and alpha rhythm in the occipital region. Occipital channels are helpful in defining sleep onset.

TABLE 12–2 Standard Montage for Monitoring of Sleep States

Parameter	Derivation
EEG	F4-M1 C4-M1 02-M1
EOG	E1-M2 E2-M2
EMG	One electrode above the inferior edge of mandible Two electrodes below the inferior edge of mandible

The AASM has recommended that EEG derivations be increased to three (**Table 12–2**). The major change is the addition of frontal electrodes (F) to better diagnose K complexes and delta waves. With three backup EEG derivations, the total number becomes six. The location of EEG electrodes has been modified, and the recommended derivations are F4-M1, C4-M1, and O2-M1. The back-up derivations are F3-M, C3-M2 and O2-M2. The alternative derivations are Fz-Cz, Cz-Oz, and C4-M1, with backup derivations of FPZ-C3, C3-O1, and C3-M2.

Amplifiers

The amplitudes (voltage) of the EEG signals recorded at the scalp are too small. Therefore, **amplifiers** are needed to increase the signal to make them suitable for interpretation. Modern amplifiers also have calibration devices and filters to reduce unwanted EEG frequencies. Amplifiers are able to receive large inputs (volts). Sometimes, amplifiers are arbitrarily referred to as *preamplifiers* if they receive small inputs (microvolts [μV] and millivolts [mV]).

An amplifier multiplies an input signal with a constant, which is usually in the range of 2 to 1000. This amplification factor is referred to as *gain*. The gain can also be expressed as V_{out}/V_{in}. Differential alternating-current (AC) amplifiers used for EEG monitoring receive voltage input from two sources (grid 1 and grid 2, or G1 and G2); the difference between the two voltages is passed through. For example, if the input at G1 is –70 μV and the input at G2 is –10 μV, the difference (i.e., 60 μV) will be amplified and passed further. Signals common to both inputs—for example, the noise from a 60-Hz line current—are called *in phase* or *common mode* and are not passed further. The ability of an amplifier to enlarge the difference in voltage and to reject the voltage common to both inputs is expressed as the *common-mode rejection ratio*.

The ability of a recording system to respond (i.e., pen deflection) to a given input signal is a function of its sensitivity. *Sensitivity* describes the amount of voltage needed to produce a fixed amount of pen deflection and is usually expressed in microvolts per centimeter. The usual sensitivity setting for sleep stages in adults is

50 μV/cm. That is, in order to have a pen deflection of 1 cm, an input of 50 μV is needed. If the amount of pen deflection needs to be increased, then the number of microvolts needed to produce 1 cm of pen deflection has to be decreased. This will give a lower numeric value for sensitivity (e.g., 25 μV/cm). Similarly, if the amplitude of the EEG waves is too high, as is often the case in children, this amplitude may have to be decreased by increasing the number of microvolts needed to produce 1 cm of pen deflection. This change (e.g., 75 μV/cm) will give a higher number for sensitivity even though the amplitude for pen deflection is being decreased. Because the electrocardiographic (ECG) signal is very strong compared with the EEG signal, the sensitivity of the ECG signal has to be very high. The typical sensitivity setting for the ECG signal is 1 to 10 millivolts per centimeter (mV/cm). The mV/cm value is 1000 times more than the μV/cm value.

The relationship of sensitivity, voltage, and pen deflection is similar to the relationship of voltage, current, and resistance in Ohm's law (voltage = current × resistance). In the EEG, sensitivity represents resistance, and pen deflection represents current. If the resistance (sensitivity) goes up, then the current (pen deflection) will decrease, provided there is no change in voltage.

Amplifiers not only increase the size of the input signal but also are able to filter out undesirable signals. The three main types of filters used are high-frequency filters, low-frequency filters, and notch filters. High-frequency filters (HFFs) are used to attenuate frequencies higher than the desired frequency (e.g., muscle activity–related artifacts). These filters are also called *low-pass filters.* Most frequencies of interest in EEG range from 0.16 to 100 Hz. The HFF for EEG is set at 35 Hz. Higher EEG frequencies are seen in patients with seizures. The upper frequency of spike discharge (with a 20-ms base) is 50 Hz. Spikes by definition have a base of 20 to 70 ms, with a frequency of 14 to 50 Hz. In such cases the HFF may be set at a higher frequency (e.g., at 70 Hz). A filter does not have a static or single level of attenuation. The HFF usually attenuates the designated frequency by 80%, and this percentage increases progressively for frequencies higher than the designated frequency of the HFF.

Low-frequency filters (LFFs) are used to attenuate undesirable frequencies in the lower frequency range. These filters are also called *high-pass filters.* These filters attenuate the signal at the designated frequency by 20%. For example, a standard LFF set at 0.3 Hz will attenuate a 0.3-Hz signal of 100 μV to 80 μV. EEG frequencies lower than the designated frequency of the LFF are progressively attenuated more. The *time constant* is another form of expressing filtration of low frequencies. The time constant is defined as the time it takes for a square wave signal to drop to 37% of the original baseline. Frequently, time constant and LFF are used interchangeably, although the numeric values are not the same. A time constant of 1 s represents an LFF of 0.1, and a time constant of 0.3 s represents an LFF of 0.5.

Notch filters are designed to sharply attenuate a narrow-frequency bandwidth within the range of 50 or 60 Hz. Notch filters are also known as 60-Hz filters. These filters are used to eliminate the noise from electric power lines. Routine use of notch filters is not appropriate because they can mask frequencies that may be of interest in seizure monitoring. This filter can also hide high electrode impedance and poor signal transmission. In EMG channels, the notch filter may excessively attenuate the muscle tone, leading to misinterpretation of the sleep stage.

Electrical interference can be minimized if the power cords are kept away from the circuit. Low impedance of the electrodes also helps in minimizing the electric line noise. By convention, EEG signals using differential amplifiers are displayed such that negative waveforms cause an upward deflection and positive waveforms cause a downward deflection.

Electrooculography

Using the R&K manual system, eye movements were recorded from electrodes placed near the outer canthus of each eye.[3] The right outer canthus electrode (ROC) was attached about 1 cm above and out from the outer canthus of the right eye. The left outer canthus electrode (LOC) was attached about 1 cm below and out from the outer canthus of the left eye. These electrodes were usually referred to the same auricular electrode (e.g., ROC/A1 and LOC/A1).

The AASM manual modified the placement of EOG electrodes. Because the highest amplitude of EOG signals is obtained when the electrodes are placed above and below the eyes at the level of the outer canthi, the lateral part of the electrodes' placement has been eliminated. The nomenclature has changed: E1 and E2 represent the left and right eye electrodes, and M1 and M2 represent the left and the right mastoid electrodes. The recommended EOG derivations are E1-M2 and E2-M2. The location of eye electrodes has also changed. E1 is placed 1 cm below the left outer canthus. The E2 electrode is placed 1 cm above the right outer canthus. This new arrangement provides higher-amplitude signals for the eye movements.

Eye movements occur in all directions. Generally only about 10% of eye movements are horizontal, whereas 30% are vertical and 60% are oblique. If it is important to evaluate the direction of eye movements, then an alternative derivation may be helpful. The alternative EOG electrodes are E1-Fpz and E2-Fpz. The alternative E1 electrode is placed 1 cm below and 1 cm lateral to the outer canthus of the left eye. Similarly, the alternative E2 electrode is placed 1 cm below and 1 cm lateral to the outer canthus of the right eye.

Placement of electrodes just above one eye and just below the opposite eye produces out-of-phase deflections for conjugate eye movements. This is helpful in distinguishing artifacts coming to the ROC and LOC from other channels. Delta waves are frequently seen in these channels, but can be distinguished by being in the same direction (i.e., in phase).

The small electropotential difference that normally exists between the front and the back of the eye is responsible for the eye movements recorded during polysomnography. The eyeball is like a dipole in which the cornea is positive and the retina is negative. When the eyes move to one side, the electrode placed on the same side as the eye movement will record a positive deflection (downward), while the other electrode will record a negative deflection (upward) because the other eye is going away from that electrode.

Eye movements can be divided into slow eye movements (SEMs) and rapid eye movements (REMs). There are no well-defined criteria to distinguish SEMs from REMs. The frequency of SEMs is usually less than 0.5 Hz (i.e., more than 2 s in duration) and the duration of the entire waveform of REMs is less than 1 s. The main feature that helps in distinguishing these two types of eye movements is that the duration of initial deflection of REMs is less than 500 ms, whereas the initial deflection of SEMs is greater than 500 ms.

The main reason for recording eye movements is to establish the presence of REM sleep. REM sleep cannot be diagnosed without the presence of REMs. The frequency of REMs per hour of REM sleep is designated as *REM density* and is a reflection of REM sleep intensity. The presence of SEMs usually means that sleep stage 1 either has begun or is about to begin. Hence it is helpful in defining the onset of sleep.

Electromyography

In routine polysomnography, EMG is recorded from chin muscles and anterior tibialis muscles. The AASM manual has recommended placing three electrodes for recording chin EMG. One electrode should be placed 1 cm above the inferior edge of the mandible. The second electrode should be placed 2 cm below the inferior edge of the mandible and 2 cm to the right of the midline. The third electrode should be placed 2 cm below the inferior edge of the mandible and 2 cm to the left of the midline. The EMG is recorded bipolarly, and a combination of any two electrodes can be used. The third electrode serves as the backup electrode and is particularly helpful for studies extending to the daytime, when there is a greater likelihood of electrodes coming off during eating and talking.

The limb electrodes are attached about 2 to 4 cm apart over the anterior tibialis muscle on both legs. Additional electrodes are attached in certain situations. EMG from the masseter muscle is helpful in the evaluation of bruxism. In patients suspected of having **periodic limb movements (PLMs) of sleep**, electrodes also may be attached to the upper limbs because PLMs of sleep occur in all four limbs.

Chin-muscle EMG is recorded mainly to distinguish REM sleep from NREM sleep. Reduction of muscle tone is one of the requirements for diagnosing REM sleep. PLMs of sleep are diagnosed from limb EMG channels. Because intercostal muscle activity ceases during REM sleep, sometimes an intercostal EMG is used to determine respiratory effort. The normal EMG frequency is between 20 and 200 Hz and generally is greater than 40 Hz. The use of a 60-Hz filter can substantially reduce the amplitude of the EMG signal. Conversely, reduction in muscle tone may be difficult to detect in the presence of significant 60-Hz artifact.

Respiratory Measurement

Respiratory effort can be measured in many ways, including esophageal pressure monitoring, flow monitoring by pneumotachometer, flow monitoring by thermistor and thermocouple, nasal pressure monitoring, intercostal EMG monitoring, and inductive plethysmography. As yet there is no consensus as to which method of monitoring is the best method for polysomnography.

Thermistors and thermocouples detect airflow indirectly and semiquantitatively by sensing the temperature change during breathing. The sensors sense the temperature difference between the cooler inspiration and warmer expiration. The change in temperature of the sensor is associated with a change in resistance. A thermistor measures this as a change in resistance, and a thermocouple as a change in electromotive force. These sensors are well tolerated by patients. The correlation between the temperature change and the flow is relatively poor. Although apneas are detected reliably, hypopneas are usually underestimated.

Pneumotachometers, placed in tightly fitted masks, measure total oronasal airflow by detecting changes in pressure between inspiration and expiration. In central sleep apnea, respiratory effort, and hence pressure change, is absent. Monitoring of airflow by this method requires a tightly fitting mask, which can cause discomfort and disruption of sleep. Because of these problems, mask pneumotachometry has not become popular for clinical studies.

Nasal pressure can be measured through nasal cannulas placed inside the nares and connected to pressure transducers. Airflow is estimated by measuring nasal airway pressure, which decreases during inspiration and increases during expiration. The flattened contour of inspiratory flow is suggestive of upper airway resistance. Nasal pressure monitoring is more sensitive but less specific than thermistors. This technique underestimates the degree of airflow reduction in patients with nasal obstruction and is not recommended in patients who are mouth breathers. Newer cannulas have been introduced that can detect both nasal and oral airflow. One advantage of nasal cannulas is the detection of inspiratory flow limitation, which was missed by thermistors.

Respiratory inductive plethysmography measures the volume changes in the chest and abdomen during a breathing cycle. The sum of these measurements provides an estimate of tidal volume. Asynchronous breathing can be detected with this method. Asynchronous breathing is paradoxical chest wall and abdominal movements associated with disordered breathing. This means that the chest and abdomen move in opposite directions, rather than together. This method does not allow for accurate distinction between apneas and hypopneas in the absence of an airflow measurement. This technique has been suggested for identification of upper airway resistance syndrome by looking at the ratio of the peak inspiratory flow to mean flow. The loops generated by this technique may also be useful for titration of continuous positive airway pressure.

The AASM manual[4] has made recommendations for the detection of sleep-related breathing events. The sensor to detect absence of airflow for identification of an apnea is an oronasal thermal sensor. The sensor for detection of airflow for identification of hypopneas is a nasal air pressure transducer. The sensor for detection of respiratory effort is either esophageal manometry or inductive plethysmography. Flattening of the nasal air pressure waveform leading to an arousal from sleep can also be used for detection of respiratory effort–related arousal.

TABLE 12-3 EEG Rhythms

Rhythm	Frequency (cycles/second)
Beta	≥14
Alpha	8 to 13
Theta	4 to 7
Delta	<4

Scoring Criteria

The main categories of scoring during polysomnography include sleep stages, respiratory events, leg movements, and arousals. Many other parameters, such as oximetry, ECG, snoring, continuous positive airway pressure titration, and effect of posture, also are evaluated.

Sleep Stages

Depending on the frequency (i.e., cycles per second), EEG waves are divided into **EEG rhythms** such as beta, alpha, theta, and delta rhythms (**Table 12-3**).

The sleep state is divided into NREM sleep and REM sleep. NREM sleep was once further subdivided into four stages, with stage 1 being the most superficial and stage 4 the deepest. The AASM manual has recommended that NREM stages be named stages N1, N2, N3, the latter of which represents the combined stages 3 and 4 of the R&K manual.[4,6] Sleep stages are scored in 30-s segments (epochs) based on EEG, EOG, and EMG.

Stage W (wakefulness) is characterized by low-amplitude, mixed-frequency EEG (**Figure 12-3**). When the eyes are closed, the alpha rhythm becomes prominent and then diminishes at sleep onset (**Figure 12-4**). Eye movements are present and muscle tone is high. Stage W is scored when more than 50% of the epochs have an alpha rhythm over the occipital region. In those subjects who do not have a discernible alpha rhythm, stage W can be scored if any of the following three items are present: eye blinks with a frequency of 0.5 to 2 Hz, reading eye movements, or irregular conjugate eye movements associated with normal or high chin muscle tone.

Stage N1 sleep is characterized by a change from alpha activity to theta activity (**Figure 12-5**). SEMs are usually present at sleep onset. Muscle tone usually diminishes at sleep onset compared with stage W. Ten percent to 20% of the

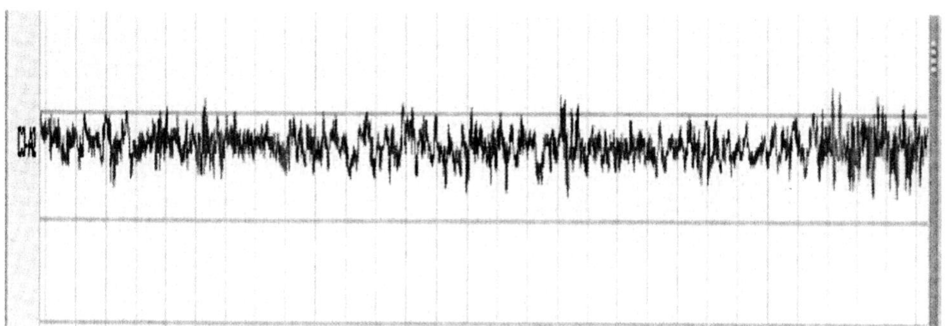

FIGURE 12-3 A thirty-second epoch of mixed-frequency EEG of stage W.

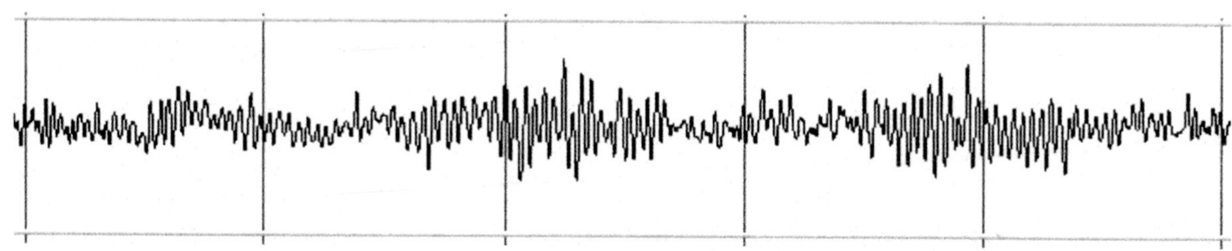

FIGURE 12-4 Ten-second epoch of stage W with eyes closed showing alpha frequency of EEG.

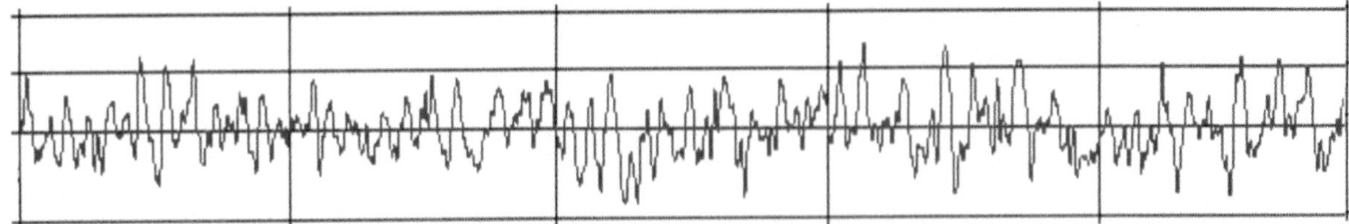

FIGURE 12–5 Ten-second epoch of stage N1 sleep showing predominantly theta frequency EEG.

population do not have a discernible alpha rhythm. In these subjects, N1 sleep can be scored by the presence of any of the following three items: theta activity with slowing of background frequencies greater than 1 Hz from those of stage W, vertex sharp waves, or slow eye movements.

Sleep onset was previously defined by the presence of sleep for at least three consecutive epochs of stage 1 sleep. The AASM manual has recommended that sleep onset be defined from the start of the first epoch scored as any stage other than stage W.

Stage N2 sleep is characterized by the continuation of the same low-amplitude, mixed-frequency EEG of stage 1 sleep and the appearance of two markers: sleep spindles and K complexes (**Figure 12–6**). **Sleep spindles** have a frequency of 12 to 14 cps (11–16 Hz) and duration of 0.5 to 1.5 s. Incipient (mini, baby) spindles are less than 0.5 s in duration and are seen in stage 1 sleep that precedes stage 2 sleep. Sleep spindles occur with a frequency of 3 to 8 spindles per minute in normal adults. **K complexes** have a sharp upward (negative) deflection followed by a downward (positive) component and are at least 0.5 s in duration. Amplitude is not a criterion for defining a K complex. The usual frequency of K complexes during stage 2 sleep is about 1 to 3 per minute. K complexes occur either spontaneously or are associated with arousals (K arousals). According to the AASM manual, only K complexes unassociated with arousal signal the presence of stage N2 sleep. The presence of K complexes associated with arousal signals the change from stage N2 sleep to stage N1 sleep. The muscle tone is lower than in stage W, and eye movements are uncommon.

Stage N2 continues to be scored as long as there is low-amplitude, mixed-frequency EEG activity even without K complexes or sleep spindles. The end of stage N2 sleep is determined by one of the following five events: (1) transition to stage W, (2) transition to stage N1 because of an arousal, (3) transition to stage N1 because of major body movement followed by slow eye movements, (4) transition to stage N3, or (5) transition to stage R.

Sleep stages 3 and 4 have been called delta sleep and are characterized by the presence of high-voltage ($\geq$75 μV) waves with slow frequency ($\leq$2 cps or slower) (**Figure 12–7**). A **delta wave** should be at least 0.5 s in duration. Stage 3 sleep is defined by the presence of delta waves that occupy at least 20% of an epoch. Stage 4 sleep was scored if delta waves covered at least 50% of an epoch. In the AASM manual system, stages 3 and 4 have been combined into stage N3. Stage N3 is scored when 20% or more of an epoch consists of slow wave activity. Occasional sleep spindles may be present in stage N3 sleep. K complexes may be present, but are difficult to distinguish from delta waves. Muscle tone is usually still high, but it can be low enough that it

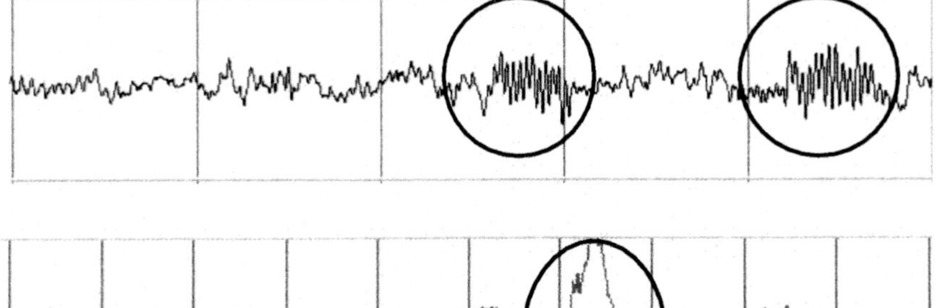

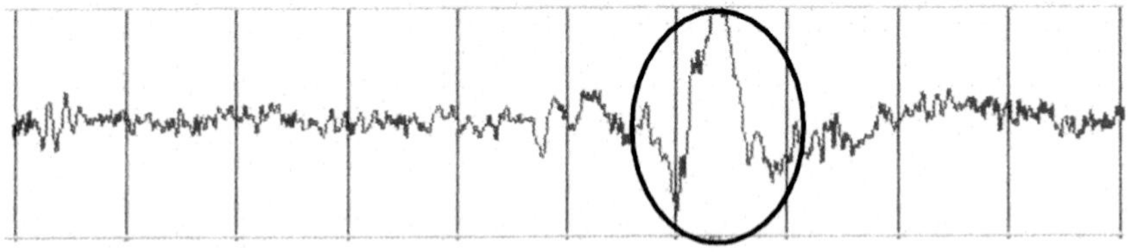

FIGURE 12–6 Ten-second epochs of stage N2 sleep showing sleep spindles in the upper tracing and a K complex in the lower tracing.

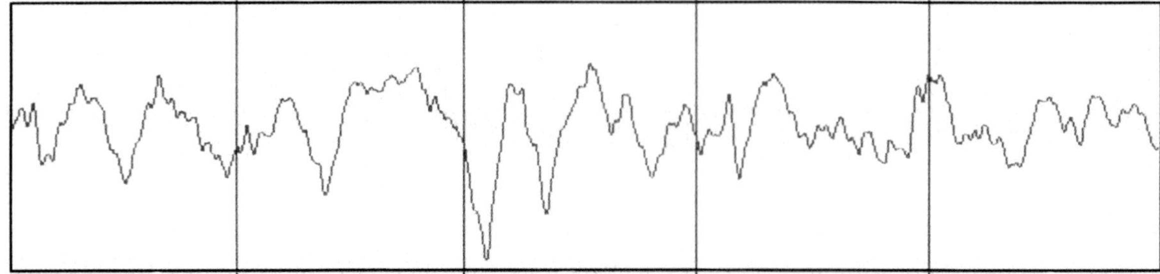

FIGURE 12–7 Ten-second epoch of stage N3 sleep showing high-amplitude, low-frequency delta waves.

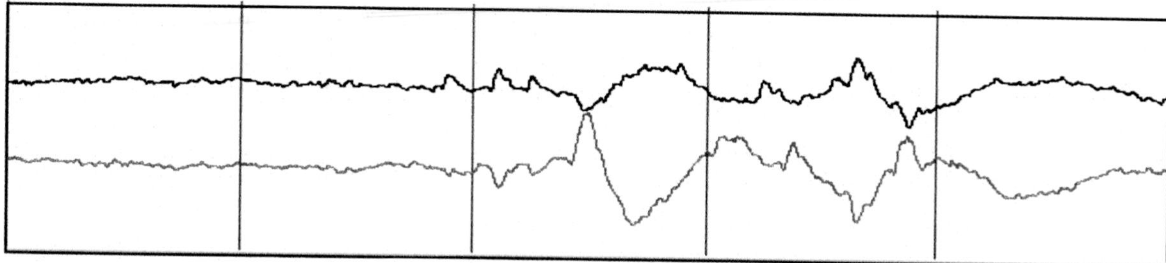

FIGURE 12–8 Ten-second epoch stage R sleep showing eye movements in EOG channels.

resembles the muscle tone of REM sleep. Eye movements are usually absent, but delta waves are frequently seen in eye channels because of the high voltage of delta waves.

REM sleep (stage R) has three cardinal features: low-amplitude, mixed-frequency EEG; bursts of REMs; and loss of muscle tone (**Figure 12–8**). The background EEG is similar to that seen in stage N1 or stage N2 sleep. During this stage, a notched morphology EEG pattern, referred to as *sawtooth waves,* can occur. The presence of this pattern alone does not define REM sleep. The frequency of sawtooth waves is in the theta range. Alpha rhythm is commonly present in REM sleep, and its frequency is 1 to 2 cps lower than in stage W. The EOG shows bursts of REMs. The EMG shows loss of muscle tone. There are occasional muscle twitches. REM sleep is divided into phasic and tonic components based on the presence or absence of eye movements and muscle twitches.

Once stage R sleep has been established, the stage is extended both forward and backward, even in the absence of REMs, until there is evidence of another stage of sleep, as long as there is no change in EMG and EEG. Because stage R can be extended in both directions, we often describe this "REM rule" as "REM rules."

The end of stage R sleep is determined by any of the following: (1) transition to stage W, (2) transition to stage N1 because of increase in muscle tone, (3) transition to stage N1 because of arousal followed by slow eye movements, (4) transition to stage N1 because of major body movement followed by slow eye movements, (5) transition to stage N2, or (6) transition to stage N3 sleep.

Major Body Movements

Movements occur frequently during sleep and obscure EEG and EOG recordings. It becomes difficult to ascertain whether the patient is awake or asleep. If movement occurred for 15 seconds or more, the epoch was scored as "Movement Time" according to the R&K manual.[3] The AASM manual has recommended the term *major body movements* for such artifacts.[4] If alpha rhythm is present for part of the epoch (even less than 15 s in duration), it should be scored as stage W. If stage W either precedes or follows the epoch with major body movement, then it should also be scored as stage W. In other cases the epoch should be scored as the epoch that follows it.

Sleep-Disordered Breathing

Sleep-disordered breathing includes apneas, hypopneas, and respiratory effort–related arousals.[7,8] There has been great deal of controversy about the definition of these events. The most recent recommendations for detection and scoring have come from the AASM manual.[4,9] **Apnea** is defined as cessation of airflow for more than 10 s. The reduction in airflow should be 90% or more of baseline. At least 90% of the event's duration should meet the amplitude reduction criteria for apnea. Baseline is defined as the mean amplitude of stable breathing and oxygenation in the preceding 2 minutes or the mean amplitude of the three largest breaths in the preceding 2 minutes.

Apnea is classified as *obstructive* if it is associated with continued or increased inspiratory effort throughout the entire period of absent airflow; it is classified as *central* if it is associated with absent inspiratory effort throughout the entire period of absent airflow. Apnea is classified as *mixed* if it is associated with absent inspiratory effort in the initial portion of the event, followed by resumption of inspiratory effort in the second portion of the event.

> **RESPIRATORY RECAP**
>
> **Sleep Disordered Breathing**
>
> » *Apnea*: Reduction of airflow by ≥ 90% of baseline for ≥ 10 seconds
> » *Obstructive apnea*: Apnea with continued respiratory effort
> » *Central apnea*: Apnea with absent respiratory effort
> » *Mixed apnea*: Apnea with initial absence and then resumption of respiratory effort
> » *Hypopnea*: Reduction of airflow by ≥ 30% for ≥ 10 seconds and O_2 desaturation by ≥ 4%

Hypopnea is defined as a 30% or more decrease (compared with baseline) in airflow or thoracoabdominal movements lasting at least 10 s associated with 4% or more oxygen desaturation. At least 90% of the event's duration should meet the amplitude reduction criteria for hypopneas. Hypopnea can also be scored by an alternative method that requires airflow reduction by 50% and associated oxygen desaturation of 3%.

A **respiratory effort–related arousal** event is defined as a sequence of breaths lasting 10 s characterized by increasing respiratory effort or flattening of the nasal pressure waveform leading to an arousal from sleep when the sequence of breaths does not meet the criteria for an

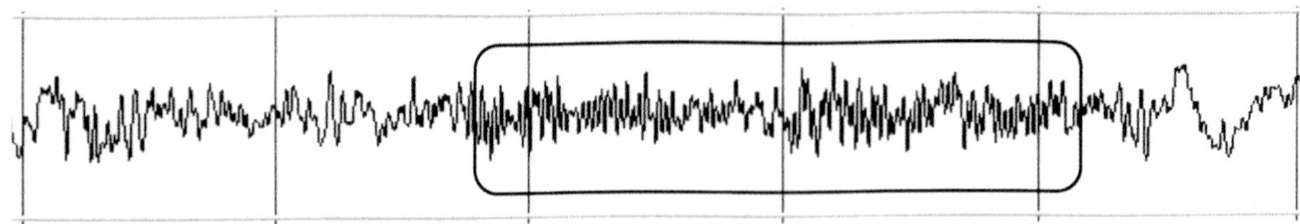

FIGURE 12–9 Ten-second epoch showing an EEG arousal in stage N1 sleep.

apnea or hypopnea. Esophageal pressure measurement is the preferred method of assessing change in respiratory effort, although nasal pressure and inductive plethysmography can be used.

Arousals

Cortical **arousals** (i.e., those seen on EEG) indicate sleep disruption and are important in defining upper airway resistance syndrome and in determining the clinical impact of nocturnal myoclonic episodes. Arousals were a part of the criteria used to define hypopneas; however, the recent recommendations of the Centers of Medicare and Medicaid Services did not include arousals as part of the definition of hypopneas.

Arousal is defined as an abrupt shift in EEG frequency that may include theta waves, alpha waves, or frequencies higher than 16 Hz, but not spindles (**Figure 12–9**).[10] Because this change in EEG activity lasts less than 15 s, it does not change the sleep stage. The epoch is scored as awake stage if the change in EEG activity lasts 15 s or more.

The AASM suggests the following rules for scoring of arousals:[4]

1. There should be at least 10 s of continuous sleep prior to an arousal.
2. There should be 10 s of continuous sleep prior to a second arousal.
3. An arousal should be at least 3 s long.
4. Arousal in NREM sleep can be scored without EMG elevation.
5. Arousals in REM sleep must have concurrent elevation of chin EMG.
6. Arousals should not be scored based on submental EMG alone.
7. Artifacts, K complexes, and delta waves are not arousals unless there is a change in EEG.
8. Pen-deflection artifacts are not arousals unless there is a change in EEG.
9. Nonconcurrent, but contiguous, EEG and EMG changes that last less than 3 s individually but more than 3 s together are not arousals.
10. Alpha sleep is not arousal.
11. Transition from one sleep stage to another sleep stage is not arousal.

Some authors use different duration criterion (e.g., 1.5 s) for defining an arousal. Arousals are also seen during normal sleep, and there is no consensus at the present time about the normal frequency of arousals. An **arousal index** (number of arousals per hour of sleep) of less than 10 is generally considered within the normal range. Arousal indices of more than 20 (or 25) may be abnormal.

Cardiac Rules

The AASM manual recommends the following rules for scoring of cardiac events:[4,11]

1. Sinus tachycardia is scored if the heart rate is greater than 90 beats/min.
2. Bradycardia is scored if the heart rate is less than 40 beats/min.
3. Asystole is scored if the cardiac pause is greater than 3 seconds.
4. Wide complex tachycardia is scored if the rhythm lasts for a minimum of three consecutive beats at a rate of greater than 100 beats/min and QRS duration of 120 ms or more.
5. Narrow complex tachycardia is scored for a rhythm lasting for a minimum of three consecutive beats at a rate of greater than 100 beats/min and QRS duration of less than 120 ms.
6. Atrial fibrillation is scored if there is an irregularly irregular ventricular rhythm associated with replacement of consistent P waves by rapid oscillations that vary in size, shape, and timing.

Periodic Limb Movements of Sleep

Limb movements are recorded from one or both anterior tibialis muscles. Sometimes the recordings are also made from upper extremities. A limb movement is a burst of muscle activity with a mean duration of 1.5 to 2.5 s (**Figure 12–10**).

The AASM manual has recommended the following rules for a significant leg movement (LM) event:[4,12]

1. The minimum duration of an LM is 0.5 s.
2. The maximum duration of an LM event is 10 s.
3. The minimum amplitude of an LM is an 8-μV increase in EMG voltage above resting EMG.

Limb movements are called *periodic* when they occur in a stereotypic manner at intervals of 20 to 40 s. Random aperiodic limb movements are not counted. The AASM has recommended the following rules for defining a periodic limb movement (PLM) series:

1. The minimum number of consecutive LM events needed is four.
2. The minimum period length between LMs is 5 s.

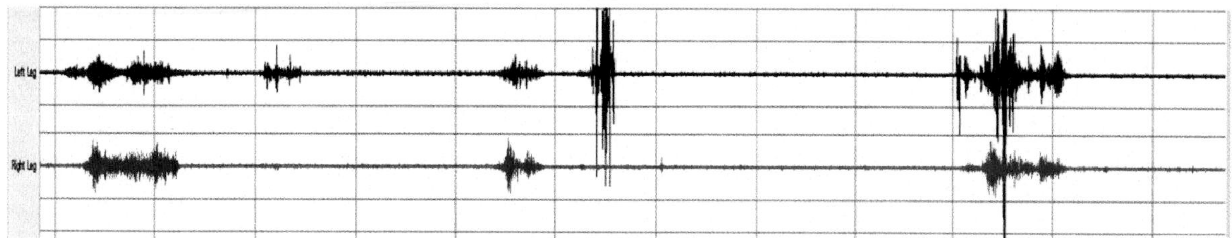

FIGURE 12–10 Two-minute epoch showing leg movements in two EMG channels.

3. The maximum period length between LMs is 90 s.
4. Leg movements on two different legs separated by less than 5 seconds between movement onsets are counted as a single leg movement.

The total number of limb movements divided by the number of hours of sleep is called the *PLM index*. Limb movements with arousals are counted separately, and the PLM with arousal index is calculated.

Leg movements occurring within 0.5 s of beginning or termination of apneas or hypopneas are not considered a part of periodic limb movements of sleep. On the other hand, leg movements associated with arousals may be a marker of upper airway resistance syndrome. Leg movements without arousals are very common in patients taking antidepressants.

Muscle twitches with duration shorter than 150 ms are called *fragmentary myoclonus*. Excessive fragmentary myoclonus (EFM) is diagnosed if at least 5 potentials per minute are present.

Polysomnography Report

The AASM manual[4] has recommended that the following be included in a polysomnography report:

A. *Parameters*. Nine parameters for a polysomnography report are EEG, EOG, chin EMG, leg EMG, airflow, respiratory effort, oxygen saturation, EKG and body position. Most sleep labs also include the monitoring of snoring.
B. *Sleep scoring data*. Ten respiratory events of data for sleep scoring are light-out time, light-on time, total sleep time, total recording time, **sleep latency**, stage R latency, wake after sleep onset (WASO), percent **sleep efficiency**, time in each sleep stage in minutes, and percentage of total sleep time in each stage.
C. *Arousal events*. Total number of arousals and the arousal index (i.e., arousals per hour of sleep).
D. *Respiratory events*. Eleven recommended respiratory events are number of obstructive apneas, mixed apneas, central apneas, hypopneas, total apneas and hypopneas, apnea index, hypopnea index, apnea-hypopnea index, mean oxygen saturation, minimum oxygen saturation, and the presence or absence of Cheyne-Stokes breathing. In addition, five optional respiratory events are total respiratory effort–related arousals, respiratory effort–related arousal index, total number of oxygen desaturation episodes (3% or 4%), oxygen desaturation index, and the occurrence or absence of hypoventilation.
E. *Cardiac events*. Three respiratory events are the average heart rate during sleep, highest heart rates during sleep, and total recording. In addition the presence or absence of bradycardia, tachycardia, asystole, narrow complex tachycardia, wide complex tachycardia, atrial fibrillation, or any other arrhythmia should be noted.
F. *Movement events*. Four recommended respiratory events are number of periodic limb movements of sleep, number of periodic limb movements with arousals, PLM index, and PLM arousal index.
G. *Summary statements*. Four respiratory events are the findings related to sleep diagnoses, EEG abnormalities, ECG abnormalities, and behavioral observations. Inclusion of sleep hypnogram is an option.

KEY POINTS

- Normal sleep consists of two states: nonrapid eye movement (NREM) sleep and rapid eye movement (REM) sleep.
- NREM and REM sleep states alternate during the night.
- The amount and type of sleep is affected by many variables, such as age, posture, circadian cycle, diseases, alcohol, and medications.
- Polysomnography is used to determine sleep stages and various sleep disorders.
- A typical polysomnogram includes recordings of electroencephalogram (EEG), electrooculogram (EOG), electromyogram (EMG) of chin muscles, oronasal airflow, chest and abdominal movements, leg movements, snoring, and oximetry.
- The main categories of scoring during polysomnography include sleep stages, respiratory events, leg movements, and arousals.
- Many other parameters, such as oximetry, ECG, snoring, continuous positive airway pressure titration, and the effects of posture, are also evaluated.

- The American Academy of Sleep Medicine (AASM) rules became the new standard for the performance and interpretation of polysomnograms in 2008.
- Knowing the basics of polysomnography is important for comprehension of sleep-disordered breathing and common sleep disorders.

REFERENCES

1. Ohayon MM, Carskadon MA, Guilleminault C, Vitiello MV. Metaanalysis of quantitative sleep parameters from childhood to old age in healthy individuals: developing normative sleep values across the human lifespan. *Sleep*. 2004;27:1255–1273.
2. Carskadon MA, Rechtschaffen A. Monitoring and staging of human sleep. In: Kryger M, Roth T, Dement W, eds. *Principles and Practice of Sleep Medicine*. 4th ed. Philadelphia: WB Saunders; 2005:1359–1377.
3. Rechtschaffen A, Kales A, eds. *A Manual of Standardized Terminology: Techniques and Scoring System for Sleep Stages of Human Subjects*. Los Angeles: UCLA Brain Information Service/Brain Research Institute; 1968.
4. Iber C, Ancoili-Israel S, Chesson A, Quan SF for the American Academy of Sleep Medicine. *The AASM Manual for the Scoring of Sleep and Associated Events: Rules, Terminology and Technical Specifications*. Westchester, IL: American Academy of Sleep Medicine; 2007.
5. Jasper H. The ten-twenty electrode system of the International Federation. *EEG Clin Neurophysiol*. 1958;10:371–375.
6. Silber MH, Ancoli-Israel S, Bonnet MH et al. The visual scoring of sleep in adults. *J Clin Sleep Med*. 2007;3:121–131.
7. Meoli AL, Casey KR, Clark RW, et al. Hypopnea in sleep-disordered breathing in adults. *Sleep*. 2001;24:469–470.
8. Sleep-related breathing disorders in adults: recommendations for syndrome definition and measurement techniques in clinical research. The report of an American Academy of Sleep Medicine Task Force. *Sleep*. 1999;22:667–689.
9. Redline S, Bhudiraja R, Kapur V, et al. Reliability and validity of respiratory event measurement and scoring. *J Clin Sleep Med*. 2007;3:169–200.
10. EEG arousals: scoring rules and examples. A preliminary report from the Sleep Disorders Atlas Task Force of the American Sleep Disorders Association. *Sleep*. 1992;15:173–184.
11. Caples SM, Rosen CL, Shen WK, et al. The scoring of cardiac events during sleep. *J Clin Sleep Med*. 2007;3:147–154.
12. Walters AS, Lavigne G, Hening W, et al. The scoring of movements in sleep. *J Clin Sleep Med*. 2007;3:155–167.

CHAPTER 13

Nutrition Assessment and Support

Charles D. McArthur

OUTLINE

Effects of Nutrition on Respiratory Function
Nutrition Assessment
Calculation of Energy Requirements
Nutritional Support Guidelines

OBJECTIVES

1. Discuss the effects of nutritional status on the respiratory system.
2. Explain the principles of nutrition assessment.
3. Compare methods used to estimate nutrient needs and provide nutritional support for patients with acute and chronic lung disease.
4. Discuss the role of indirect calorimetry in nutrition assessment.
5. Describe nutrition therapies for acute and chronic lung disease.

KEY TERMS

anthropometry
basal metabolic rate (BMR)
cell-mediated immunity
diet-induced thermogenesis
enteral nutrition
indirect calorimetry
metabolic cart
nitrogen balance
parenteral nutrition
protein-calorie malnutrition (PCM)
respiratory quotient
resting energy expenditure (REE)

INTRODUCTION

Nutrition is defined as a series of processes by which an organism uses food for energy, growth, and replacing tissues. Assessment of nutritional status is an important part of the overall assessment of a patient. The human body requires an adequate supply of energy, protein, vitamins, and minerals to maintain an optimal state of health and normal physiology. Without these life-sustaining nutrients, organ system functions become compromised. The respiratory system is no exception. During periods of prolonged semistarvation and hypercatabolism, the diaphragm and other respiratory muscle groups are not spared, but rather may be broken down for use as a fuel source. Caloric overfeeding, on the other hand, may also adversely affect lung function by increasing ventilatory demand and carbon dioxide production, which may result in hypercarbia and present problems for mechanically ventilated patients. A careful assessment of the nutritional status of individuals with pulmonary disease is essential.

Effects of Nutrition on Respiratory Function

Minute Ventilation

The waste products of metabolism are carbon dioxide and nonvolatile acids. The kidney removes approximately 2% of the waste products that are in the form of nonvolatile acids. The lungs remove 98% of the waste products in the form of carbon dioxide. Metabolic rate determines the amount of carbon dioxide produced and excreted by the process of ventilation. The amount of carbon dioxide produced by metabolizing nutrients is specific to the amount and type of nutrient being metabolized. **Diet-induced thermogenesis** is an increase in metabolic rate of 10% to 15% that occurs after eating as a result of the energy cost of digesting and storing nutrients. Starvation reduces the metabolic rate and results in the use of endogenous fat stores for energy. The reduction in metabolic rate and the metabolism of fat both reduce carbon dioxide production, resulting in lower ventilatory needs. Overfeeding of carbohydrates will result in the production of stored fats (lipogenesis); this process produces an excessive amount of carbon dioxide, resulting in higher ventilatory needs. Amino acids in proteins may increase respiratory drive, which in turn will also increase ventilatory needs. In a subject with limited ventilator reserves, overfeeding may lead to respiratory failure or prolonged mechanical ventilation.

Muscle Compromise

When the body is faced with an energy deficit, it turns to its own reserves of glycogen, fat, and protein for the release of fuel. Initially protein is spared, because the body mobilizes and oxidizes fat to serve as the principal fuel source in starvation. However, if the deficit continues and undernutrition is prolonged, catabolism of muscle tissue occurs. In a stressed, critically ill patient, this muscle breakdown occurs within days as a result of the body's hypermetabolic response to injury. This circumstance has important implications for an individual with respiratory disease, because the diaphragm, intercostal muscles, and other accessory muscles make up part of the body's skeletal muscle pool and are preyed on in time of need. Patients whose body weight is approximately 70% below their ideal weight for height have 43% to 60% less diaphragmatic muscle tissue than individuals at healthier weights.

It also appears that, although **protein-calorie malnutrition (PCM)** affects all types of muscle fibers, it impairs fast twitch fibers most profoundly, resulting in diminished contractile strength. This effect is seen clinically as a decline in maximum inspiratory and expiratory pressures, vital capacity, and voluntary ventilation. Malnutrition also contributes to muscle weakness by depleting the body of phosphorus, which is essential for the production of adenosine triphosphate and 2,3-diphosphoglycerate, without which oxygen release to tissues is limited. This results in impairment of the expiratory muscles' contractility and endurance. Magnesium deficiency also has been associated with muscle weakness and may hinder attempts at weaning from mechanical ventilation. Malnutrition, however, is not the only precipitating factor. Hypophosphatemia and hypomagnesemia may be caused by gastrointestinal losses, the use of antacids and diuretics, and severe malabsorption conditions. With aggressive repletion of these minerals, diaphragmatic strength and contractility improve.

Immune Function

The primary component of the immune system adversely affected by PCM is **cell-mediated immunity**. However, secretory immunoglobulin A (IgA) antibody response, neutrophilic bactericidal capacity, and the complement system also are adversely affected. Protein deficiency triggers a reduction in T4 helper cells and T8 cytotoxic cells and through these T cells impairs B cell activity as well. With the reduction in IgA secretion, the lungs may be more susceptible to bacterial colonization and infection.

RESPIRATORY RECAP

Effects of Poor Nutrition on Respiratory Function

- Muscle compromise
- Impaired immune function
- Impaired surfactant production
- Hypoalbuminemia
- Overnutrition and obesity

Surfactant Production

Severe starvation causes loss of pulmonary surfactant, which is essential for maintaining alveolar stability and reducing the work of breathing. The size, number, and internal surface area of the alveoli are reduced. Lung lipid content also declines because of multiple factors associated with malnutrition, including alterations in elastin metabolism and a decrease in lipogenesis. PCM has also been shown to reduce the number and size of the lamellar bodies of the granular alveolar pneumocytes, which are the storage sites for surfactant.

Hypoalbuminemia

In a critically ill or malnourished patient, the serum albumin level is likely to be low. In critical illness this is a consequence of the body's metabolic response to injury, inflammatory damage, or sepsis because the synthesis of albumin is deferred to allow for the manufacture of other acute-phase proteins such as fibrinogen, haptoglobin, and ceruloplasmin. Albumin is essential for the maintenance of plasma colloid oncotic pressure, which controls the movement of fluid from the interstitial space into the capillaries or intracellular space. When the serum albumin concentration is low, interstitial lung fluid increases, which may compromise lung function by increasing the risk of pulmonary edema.

Obesity

Mass loading of the chest wall in obesity causes restriction of lung volumes. The most common finding is a decreased expiratory reserve volume, but in extreme obesity vital capacity may also be reduced. The decrease of functional residual capacity may create ventilation-perfusion mismatch, which could cause hypoxemia. The work of breathing may be increased, which increases metabolic rate and carbon dioxide production and may lead to carbon dioxide retention. Weight loss in obese patients can improve lung function, presumably by reducing the work of breathing. Obesity also contributes to problems such as obstructive sleep apnea. Persons with morbid obesity are also prone to obesity hypoventilation syndrome (also known as Pickwickian syndrome).

TABLE 13–1 Objective Parameters of Malnutrition

Parameter	Malnutrition		
	Mild	*Moderate*	*Severe*
Ideal body weight	80–90%	70–79%	<70%
Usual weight	80–95%	80–89%	<80%
Triceps skinfold thickness	40th–50th percentile	30th–39th percentile	<30th percentile
Serum albumin	2.8–3.4 g/dL	2.1–2.7 g/dL	<2.1 g/dL
Serum transferrin	150–200 mg/dL	100–149 mg/dL	<100 mg/dL
Serum prealbumin	12–17 mg/dL	7–11 mg/dL	<7 mg/dL

Nutrition Assessment

The components of a nutrition evaluation are the patient history, a physical examination, anthropometric measurements, biochemical tests, and indicators of immune system function. Information from the patient's history should help determine the individual's baseline nutritional state and should reveal signs of nutrition compromise such as weight loss, anorexia, dysphagia, early satiety, nausea, or vomiting.

Anthropometry is the study of human body measurements and components. It includes measurement of height, weight, body mass index, midarm muscle circumference, skinfold thicknesses, and skeletal breadths. Determination of an individual's weight as a percentage of usual weight and calculation of the percentage of weight loss over time are particularly important indices of nutritional risk and the extent of illness. A weight loss of 10% or more of the usual body weight over a 6-month period or a body weight below 80% of ideal is considered a sign of significant nutritional risk and indicates a need for aggressive nutritional intervention.

Biochemical assessment of nutritional status should accompany the physical and historical assessments. Along with other objective tests (**Table 13–1**), laboratory measurements help reflect the status of a subject's protein stores and therefore the degree of nutritional risk. The serum albumin, transferrin, and transthyretin (prealbumin) levels, along with the retinol-binding protein level, are commonly used to assess the visceral protein stores (**Table 13–2**). Studies of **nitrogen balance**, which involve a 24-hour urine collection and calculation of the difference between nitrogen intake and excretion, can help determine protein requirements and assess changes in visceral protein stores over time. However, interpretation of these values as indicators of nutritional status is difficult because serum concentrations of proteins are affected by many factors, such as acute illness, infection, inflammation, stress, sepsis, hepatic disease, renal disease, malignancy, and hydration status.

TABLE 13–2 Biochemical Measurements of Nutritional Status

Marker	Normal Range
Albumin	3.5–5 g/dL
Transferrin	200–400 mg/dL
Prealbumin	18–50 mg/dL
Retinol-binding protein	30–80 mg/L

The ideal protein for use as a marker of nutritional status has a short half-life, a relatively small body pool, and a rapid rate of synthesis and remains unaffected by a disease or its severity. Albumin, transferrin, and transthyretin all have been used in attempts to fit this role.

> **RESPIRATORY RECAP**
>
> **Components of Nutrition Assessment**
>
> » Anthropometric measurements
>
> » Biochemical assessments

Albumin, a protein synthesized by the liver, is required for the transport of molecules, maintenance of the vascular system, and prevention of edema. Its body pool is large, and most of this protein (60%) is present in the extravascular space. The 40% found in the intravascular compartment functions primarily to maintain the plasma colloid oncotic pressure. Because of its abundance in the body and its long half-life (18 to 21 days), albumin does not respond quickly to acute changes in nutritional status. It more often reflects the severity of disease and the metabolic response to injury or infection and therefore can be used as an important prognostic indicator; low albumin levels have been associated with morbidity and mortality and with longer hospitalization.

Transferrin is a β-globulin synthesized by the liver, which functions as a transport protein for iron. Its

EQUATION 13–1

Equations Used to Estimate Energy Expenditure

Harris-Benedict Equation

$$\text{BMR (men)} = 66 + (13.7 \times W) + (5.0 \times H) - (6.8 \times A)$$

$$\text{BMR (women)} = 655 + (9.6 \times W) + (1.7 \times H) - (4.7 \times A)$$

where:

BMR = Basal metabolic rate
W = Weight (kg)
H = Height (cm)
A = Age (years)

Ireton-Jones Formula

$$\text{EEE (obese person)} = [(606 \times G) + (9 \times W) - (12 \times A)] + (400 \times V) + 1444$$

where:

EEE = Estimated energy expenditure
G = Gender (male = 1; female = 0)
W = Actual body weight (kg)
A = Age (years)
V = Ventilator (present = 1; absent = 0)

$$\text{EEE (ventilated person)} = 1925 - (10 \times A) + (5 \times W) + (281 \times G) + (292 \times T) + (851 \times B)$$

where:

EEE = Estimated energy expenditure
A = Age (years)
G = Gender (male = 1; female = 0)
T = Trauma (present = 1; absent = 2)
B = Burn (present = 1; absent = 0)
W = Weight (kg)

biologic half-life is 8 to 10 days, and its body pool is small. It therefore may be a more sensitive indicator of protein status than the serum albumin level, although its levels also may be affected by disease and should be interpreted with caution. Transferrin levels may be low with liver disease, after surgery or trauma, or with infection, even in patients with good nutritional status. Its serum levels may be elevated in individuals with iron deficiency anemia, acute hepatitis, dehydration, or acute blood loss.

Transthyretin (thyroxine-binding prealbumin) is a carrier protein that aids in the transport of thyroxine and retinol-binding protein. It has a small body pool and a short half-life of 2 to 3 days. Transthyretin is not affected by iron deficiency, but decreased levels may be seen with zinc deficiency and with inflammation, hepatitis, or cirrhosis. Increased levels are seen in patients with renal disease, presumably because of a decrease in protein breakdown by the kidneys. Even so, changes and trends in the serum level of this protein can be monitored and used to assess acute changes in protein status and response to nutritional support.

Immune function measurements also can be used as objective markers of nutritional status. The measurements most commonly evaluate cell-mediated immunity, the immune system component most affected by malnutrition. A reduced total lymphocyte count, lack of delayed cutaneous hypersensitivity to antigens, and abnormal lymphocyte stimulation assay results all may reveal poor immune function. At least one study has shown that nutrition therapy for malnourished individuals with chronic obstructive pulmonary disease (COPD) resulted in improvements in these markers.

Calculation of Energy Requirements

Equations Versus Measurements

Inadequate energy and protein nutrition may compromise the ability to heal and thrive. Overfeeding of calories may impair bodily functions and lead to respiratory compromise in subjects with limited ventilatory reserve. Energy requirements may be estimated by prediction equations or measured by calorimetry. The use of prediction equations is the most common method to estimate **resting energy expenditure (REE)**. The equations (**Equation 13–1**) work well to predict REE in healthy nonobese subjects, but they work less well in obese or critically ill patients.

The original work of Harris and Benedict (see Equation 13–1) in 1919 first described the amount of energy required to maintain the most basic bodily functions. This amount of energy, expressed as kilocalories (kcal) per day, is known as the **basal metabolic rate (BMR)**. The BMR has a fixed relationship with gender, weight in kilograms, height in centimeters, and age in years. The BMR does not take into account stress factors due to illness. For this reason the term *resting energy expenditure* is used in the clinical setting. Critically ill patients may not be at their BMR due to the stress of the disease process. This makes predictions based on BMR invalid for some critically ill patients. In obese subjects, adipose tissue does not contribute to the BMR. For this reason, an ideal body weight or adjusted body weight is usually substituted for actual weight in the equation, which diminishes the ability to predict energy expenditure. The Ireton-Jones formula (refer to Equation 13–1) is a commonly used equation and adjusts for obesity and mechanical ventilation. Energy needs also may be estimated with calories per kilogram of body weight (usually 25 to 35 kcal/kg) if other data are unavailable. Prediction equations may fail to predict REE in a significant number of obese subjects or critically ill patients.

Calorimetry

In direct measurement of energy expenditure (direct calorimetry), an individual is placed in a sealed, thermally insulated chamber. The heat liberated from the individual is determined by measurement of the temperature change in water circulated through the walls of the chamber. The energy produced during metabolism is equal to the heat generated when the organism is at rest. Direct calorimetry is impractical in the clinical setting and is rarely performed even in research studies. For clinical purposes, the most common technique to measure energy requirements is **indirect calorimetry**, which is based on the measurement of inspired and expired gases. The amount of oxygen consumed ($\dot{V}O_2$) and carbon dioxide produced ($\dot{V}CO_2$) is equal to the energy produced and at rest equals the metabolic rate.

Open-circuit calorimetry measures $\dot{V}O_2$ and $\dot{V}CO_2$. The simplest example of this approach is the Douglas bag technique. In this configuration oxygen and carbon dioxide concentrations are measured in samples of inspired and expired gases. These concentrations can be precisely determined by mass spectrometry or, more routinely, by infrared carbon dioxide and paramagnetic or zirconium oxide oxygen analyzers. Accurate measurement of exhaled or inhaled minute volume is also required, usually by a precision volume pneumotachometer.

Indirect calorimetry can be performed in mechanically ventilated and spontaneously breathing patients (**CPG 13–1; Figure 13–1, Figure 13–2,** and **Figure 13–3**). Devices designed for spontaneous breathing use various methods, including a ventilated canopy, masks, and mouthpieces with nose clips. The devices are commonly

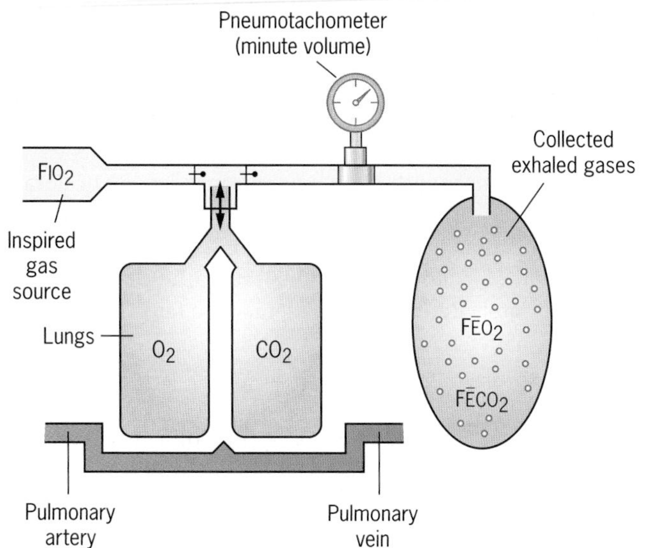

FIGURE 13–1 Diagram illustrating measurement of $\dot{V}O_2$ and $\dot{V}CO_2$ by indirect calorimetry. This article was published in *Comprehensive Respiratory Care*. Dantzker DR, MacIntyre NR, Bakow ED, eds. Copyright Elsevier (WB Saunders) 1995.

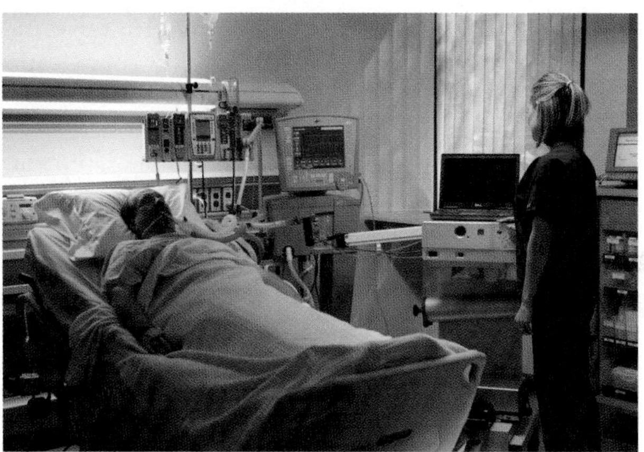

FIGURE 13–2 Use of a metabolic cart (indirect calorimetry) in a mechanically ventilated patient.

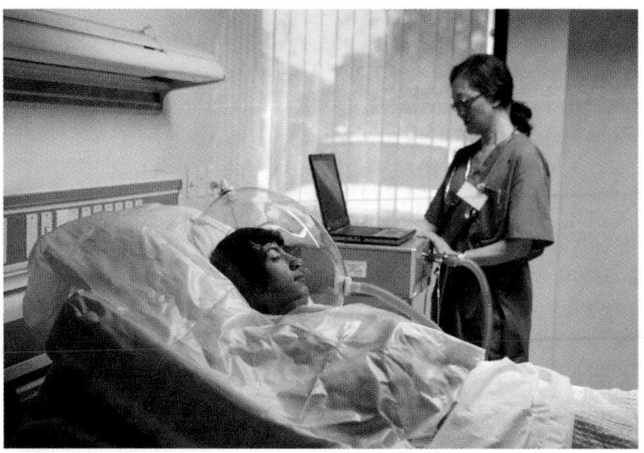

FIGURE 13–3 Use of a metabolic cart (indirect calorimetry) in a spontaneously breathing patient using a hood.

CLINICAL PRACTICE GUIDELINE 13–1

Metabolic Measurement with Indirect Calorimetry During Mechanical Ventilation

Indications

- Patients with known nutritional deficits or derangements. A number of nutritional risk and stress factors may considerably skew prediction by the Harris-Benedict equation, including neurologic trauma; paralysis; chronic obstructive pulmonary disease; acute pancreatitis; cancer with residual tumor burden; multiple trauma; amputation; patients whose height and weight cannot be accurately determined; patients who fail to respond adequately to estimated nutritional needs; new patients receiving home total parenteral nutrition; patients unable to eat who require mechanical ventilation for longer than 5 days; transplant patients; morbidly obese patients; and severely hypermetabolic or hypometabolic patients.
- To measure the O_2 cost of breathing in mechanically ventilated patients.
- To assess ($\dot{V}O_2$) in mechanically ventilated patients to evaluate hemodynamic support.
- To measure cardiac output ($\dot{Q}C$) by the Fick method.
- To determine the cause(s) of increased ventilator requirements.

Contraindications

- When a specific indication is present, no contraindications exist to the performance of metabolic measurement with indirect calorimetry unless short-term disconnection of ventilatory support to allow connection of measurement lines results in hypoxemia, bradycardia, or other adverse effects.

Hazards and Complications

- Obtaining metabolic measurements with an indirect calorimeter is a safe, noninvasive procedure with few hazards or complications. However, under certain circumstances and with particular equipment, the following hazards or complications may be seen:
  - Short-term disconnection of ventilatory support to allow connection of the indirect calorimetry apparatus may result in hypoxemia, bradycardia, or discomfort for the patient.
  - Inappropriate calibration or system setup may produce erroneous values, resulting in incorrect patient management.
  - Isolation valves may increase circuit resistance and cause increased work of breathing or dynamic hyperinflation, or both.
  - Inspiratory reservoirs may cause a reduction in alveolar ventilation due to increased compressible volume of the breathing circuit.
  - Manipulation of the ventilator circuit may cause leaks that may lower alveolar ventilation.

Modified from AARC clinical practice guideline: metabolic measurement using indirect calorimetry during mechanical ventilation—2004 revision and update. *Respir Care.* 2004;49:1073–1079. Reprinted with permission.

called **metabolic carts**. $\dot{V}O_2$ is determined by subtraction of the volume of expired oxygen from the volume of inspired oxygen. Mixed exhaled gas analysis is a simple, accurate method of indirect calorimetry in relatively healthy individuals breathing room air. However, the accuracy of this technique requires precise knowledge of the inspired oxygen content (FIO_2). With mechanical ventilation, the FIO_2 may vary during the breath or between breaths. Commercial devices currently measure the peak FIO_2 to determine FIO_2. This is not a problem with interbreath variation, but these devices cannot measure intrabreath variation. Small errors in the measurement of FIO_2 cause large errors in $\dot{V}O_2$, and this error is magnified as the FIO_2 rises. For these reasons, this method of indirect calorimetry generally is limited to patients who are spontaneously breathing in room air and to those who are mechanically ventilated with an FIO_2 below 60%.

When gas exchange measurements are performed for nutritional assessment, every effort must be made to ensure that the measurement conditions are at steady state. Generally, the patient should be resting and recumbent during the measurement period. If the patient is mechanically ventilated, appropriate adjustments should be made to duplicate the patient's usual FIO_2, minute ventilation, and airway pressure. If the patient is breathing spontaneously, measurements should be taken only after the patient has adjusted to breathing through the interface. After steady-state conditions have been confirmed, gas exchange measurements should be averaged over a period of at least 15 minutes. The patient's body

TABLE 13-3 Energy and Respiratory Values of Energy Substrates

Energy Substrate	Caloric Value (kcal/g)	Caloric Equivalent (kcal/L O_2)	Respiratory Quotient
Carbohydrate	4.1	5.05	1.0
Protein	4.1	4.46	0.82
Fat	9.3	4.74	0.71
Alcohol	7.1	4.86	0.6

temperature and other vital signs should be noted at the time of measurement as a reference for future studies.

After a measurement has been completed, a quality assessment should be performed. The **respiratory quotient** (RQ = $\dot{V}CO_2/\dot{V}O_2$) should be in the physiologic range (0.67–1.3) and be consistent with the patient's condition and nutritional status. The collection time should be sufficient to ensure at least a 5-minute period with the variability of the $\dot{V}CO_2$ and $\dot{V}O_2$ measurements less than 5%. If these conditions have not been met, technical errors such as calibration mistakes, non-steady-state conditions, or tubing leaks may have occurred during the measurement period. After these factors have been corrected, the gas exchange measurement should be repeated. After the results of a gas exchange measurement have been confirmed, the corresponding energy expenditure can be calculated.

A caloric equivalent has been derived for each class of foodstuffs (substrates). The caloric equivalent of a given energy substrate is the amount of heat (in kilocalories) liberated when the substrate is burned in 1 L of oxygen. Similarly, each class of foodstuffs has a unique respiratory quotient (**Table 13–3**). Through measurement of $\dot{V}O_2$, $\dot{V}CO_2$, and urinary nitrogen excretion (in grams), the de Weir equation can be used to determine the REE:

$$\text{REE (kcal)} = [(3.581 \times \dot{V}O_2) + (1.448 \times \dot{V}CO_2)] \times 1440 - (1.773 \times \text{Nu})$$

where $\dot{V}O_2$ is oxygen consumption (L/min), $\dot{V}CO_2$ is carbon dioxide production (L/min), and Nu is daily urinary nitrogen excretion. Determination of the REE without the measurement of Nu is acceptable because it results in an error of 2% or less.

Fick Method

If $\dot{V}CO_2$ is unavailable, the REE can be determined from $\dot{V}O_2$ alone with the use of an estimated respiratory quotient of 0.8 (to generate a value for $\dot{V}CO_2$). The Fick equation also may be used to determine $\dot{V}O_2$ and the corresponding energy expenditure (**Equation 13–2**). This technique requires the presence of a pulmonary artery catheter. The range of error for this calculation is significant when the individual errors of thermodilution, cardiac output, blood gas determinations, hemoglobin measurement, and estimation of the oxygen-carrying capacity of hemoglobin are added. For these reasons, the Fick method to calculate $\dot{V}O_2$ and energy expenditure should be regarded as only an approximation of the metabolic rate. This method does not allow for determination of $\dot{V}CO_2$ and the respiratory quotient.

Protein Requirements

In both acute and chronic disease, focusing nutritional support efforts on the maintenance of protein stores is important. With prolonged inadequate nutrient intake, endogenous protein catabolism occurs, with most of the loss from muscle tissue. As mentioned previously, this includes the respiratory muscles, and weakness and fatigue are likely to result, causing increased difficulty breathing. Therefore, providing patients with an adequate supply of nutrients for nitrogen building and endogenous protein sparing is important. It generally is suggested that 25 to 35 nonprotein calories per kilogram of body weight be provided to allow for metabolic utilization of 1 g of protein. For most patients, in the absence of renal or liver disease, 1.2 to 1.5 g of dietary protein per kilogram of body weight is recommended. Visceral protein stores are difficult to monitor, but attempts should be made to evaluate the adequacy of a feeding regimen, the response to nutrition therapy, and changes in protein status. Common tools include measurement of transferrin and transthyretin and 24-hour urine collections to calculate urinary urea nitrogen (UUN).

The UUN, or calculation of nitrogen balance, requires an accurate 24-hour urine collection and can be helpful in the assessment of a patient's response to nutrition therapy. The goal of nutritional support is to achieve positive nitrogen balance, which occurs when protein in the diet provides nitrogen in excess of its loss. Nitrogen balance is calculated as follows:

$$\text{Nitrogen balance (g)} = \left[\frac{\text{24-hour protein intake (g)}}{6.25}\right] - [\text{24-hour urinary urea nitrogen (g)} + 4\text{g}]$$

The 4 g added to the UUN value is an estimate of insensible nitrogen loss (e.g., from the feces, skin, and hair). A negative nitrogen balance indicates protein catabolism, whereas a positive nitrogen balance reflects an anabolic state. The clinician should aim for a positive nitrogen balance of approximately 1 to 4 g a day. In certain

EQUATION 13–2

Calculation of Oxygen Consumption with the Fick Equation

$$\dot{V}O_2 = \dot{Q}c \times C(a - \bar{v})O_2$$

where:

$\dot{V}O_2$ = Oxygen consumption
$\dot{Q}c$ = Cardiac output
$C(a - \bar{v})O_2$ = Difference between arterial and mixed venous oxygen content

To perform this calculation, an indwelling pulmonary artery catheter is required to determine the $\dot{Q}c$ (by thermodilution) and obtain a mixed venous blood sample (which must be obtained from the distal port of the catheter positioned in the pulmonary artery). An arterial blood sample also must be obtained. Blood gas analysis is performed on both samples, and the $C(a - \bar{v})O_2$ is then calculated, as follows:

$$C(a - \bar{v})O_2 = [(SaO_2 - S\bar{v}O_2) \times Hb \times 1.34] + [0.003 \times (PaO_2 - P\bar{v}O_2)]$$

where:

$C(a - \bar{v})O_2$ = Difference between arterial and mixed venous oxygen content
SaO_2 = Oxygen saturation of arterial blood
$S\bar{v}O_2$ = Oxygen saturation of venous blood
Hb = Hemoglobin
PaO_2 = Partial pressure of arterial oxygen
$P\bar{v}O_2$ = Partial pressure of oxygen in mixed venous blood

diseases and conditions, however, this measurement may be misleading. In patients with renal disease, gastrointestinal fistulas, severe diarrhea, or other conditions that may involve excessive nitrogen loss, calculation of nitrogen balance is most likely to present the clinician with unreliable results and may not accurately reflect the patient's nutritional state. It also should be kept in mind that in critically ill patients with infection, sepsis, or inflammatory disease and in those receiving steroid therapy, a positive nitrogen balance may not be achieved even with aggressive nutritional support. In these cases, only when the inflammatory process subsides and the patient's condition becomes less critical are improvements in protein stores reflected by serum protein levels and UUN studies.

Nutritional Support Guidelines

The primary goal of nutrition therapy in patients with respiratory disease is to improve respiratory function through the prevention or minimization of the loss of muscle mass. Other goals are to prevent infection, enhance the immune system, increase exercise tolerance, and improve the patient's quality of life.

Nutrition Delivery

The preferred and most convenient method of nutrient delivery is the oral route. However, it may be difficult for many individuals with severe respiratory disease to consume enough to maintain their weight and meet their increased nutrient needs. This may occur for several reasons, such as dyspnea on food preparation and consumption, early satiety, gastroesophageal reflux, bloating caused by air swallowing, nausea, and vomiting. Much of the gastrointestinal discomfort can be caused or exacerbated by medications commonly prescribed to treat respiratory symptoms and infection, including bronchodilators, anticholinergics, corticosteroids, antibiotics, and mucolytics. The reflux many patients experience may also be attributed to the effects of lung hyperinflation on the position of the stomach or an increase in abdominal pressure associated with coughing.

If oral intake is inadequate to meet daily energy needs despite the use of high-calorie, high-protein supplements and snacks, enteral delivery of nutrients by means of a feeding tube should be considered. This should also be the method of choice to feed patients requiring ventilatory support.

Enteral nutrition should always be considered when a patient has a functioning gastrointestinal (GI) tract. The benefits of enteral nutrient delivery are well documented. Nutrients absorbed via the portal system with delivery to the liver may allow for better absorption and result in enhanced immune competence. The presence of nutrients in the gut prevents intestinal atrophy and maintains the absorptive capacity of the GI mucosa by directly nourishing the enterocytes, supporting epithelial cell repair and replication. Enteral nutrition also helps preserve normal gut flora and gastric pH, which may guard against bacterial overgrowth in the small intestine. Finally, nutrients, especially fats and proteins, stimulate feeding-dependent neuroendocrine activity, which results in the secretion of immunoglobulins. These substances, particularly secretory IgA, are important in the prevention of bacterial translocation and gut sepsis. Although enteral nutrition is not entirely devoid of risk, if administered carefully and sensibly, it is safer than parenteral nutrition and considerably less expensive.

The route of delivery varies and may depend on the ease and availability of enteral access; the patient's risk of aspiration, tolerance to feedings, and clinical condition; and the length of time feeding is likely to be needed. Nasogastric or orogastric tubes often are used because they are easy to place at the bedside and are also needed for medication administration. They are considered short-term feeding tubes (less than 3 to 4 weeks) and may be contraindicated in patients who have severe reflux or delayed gastric emptying or gastroparesis, or who are otherwise at high risk of aspiration. In these latter cases a feeding tube placed past the stomach (postpyloric) into the small intestine should be considered. These tubes are also indicated for short-term tube feeding and allow for uninterrupted duodenal or jejunal feeding in patients with gastric dysmotility and large gastric residual volumes, which would otherwise prevent the administration of adequate nutrition support. In this case, the feeding would be infused via the small-bowel (enteric) tube, and a larger gastric tube could be used to decompress the stomach and allow for the drainage of gastric secretions. Presumably the more distal to the stomach the feeding is delivered, the less likely aspiration related to the feeding is to occur. Thus, the optimal postpyloric tube placement is past the ligament of Treitz, or in the fourth portion of the duodenum.

RESPIRATORY RECAP

Routes of Nutrition Delivery

» Oral
» Enteral
» Parenteral

A Dobhoff tube is a small-bore, flexible, nasogastric feeding tube that typically has an inside diameter of 4 mm. It is smaller and more flexible than other NG tubes, and, therefore, is usually more comfortable for the patient. The tube is inserted by use of a guide wire (stylet), which is removed after the tube's correct placement has been confirmed. A Dobhoff tube typically has a weighted end that helps guide it through the digestive system. Peristalsis helps to move the weight through the esophagus into the stomach or beyond.

If long-term feeding is anticipated, tubes can be placed through the skin into the stomach or small intestine by surgical, endoscopic, radiologic, or laparoscopic techniques. The percutaneous endoscopic gastrostomy (PEG) tube is placed endoscopically. The patient is sedated, and an endoscope is passed through the mouth and esophagus into the stomach. The position of the endoscope can be visualized on the outside of the patient's abdomen because it contains a powerful light source. A needle is inserted through the abdomen and visualized within the stomach by the endoscope, and a suture passed through the needle is grasped by the endoscope and pulled up through the esophagus. The suture is then tied to the end of the PEG tube and pulled back down through the esophagus and stomach and out through the abdominal wall. The insertion takes about 20 minutes. The tube is kept within the stomach either by a balloon or by a retention dome. Gastric tubes are suitable for long-term use and can be replaced without an additional endoscopic procedure. The PEG tube is useful when there is difficulty with swallowing because of neurologic or anatomic disorders and to avoid the risk of aspiration pneumonia. These tubes generally are more comfortable than the nasogastric, orogastric, or enteric tubes.

Many enteral formulas are available (**Table 13–4**), and selection of the most cost-effective, beneficial product presents a great challenge to the clinical nutrition specialist. General-purpose formulas are quite cost effective, palatable, and well tolerated by most patients, except those individuals with malabsorption syndromes or other special conditions. These formulas generally provide 1 calorie (cal) per milliliter and are approximately 50% carbohydrate, 30% fat, and 15% to 20% protein.

Many specialized enteral nutrition formulas have been developed for patients with specific conditions, such as diabetes mellitus, hepatic disease, renal disease, and pulmonary

TABLE 13–4 Composition of Select Enteral Formulas

Formula	Kcal/mL	Carbohydrate (g/mL)	Protein (g/mL)	Fat (g/mL)
Ensure Plus*	1.5	200	55	53
Boost High Protein†	1.06	140	61	23
Boost Plus	1.5	190	61	57
Isocal†	1.06	138	34	44
Isocal HN†	1.06	123	44	46
TraumaCal†	1.5	162	82	68
Deliver 2.0†	2.0	200	75	102
TwoCal HN†	2.0	217	84	91
Pulmocare*	1.5	106	63	93
Oxepa*	1.5	106	63	93
Respalor†	1.5	148	76	71

*Ross Products Division, Abbott Laboratories, Columbus, Ohio; †Mead-Johnson Nutritionals, Evansville, Indiana.

disease. The composition of these formulas is different from that of more general formulas, and they tend to be higher in price. The formula designed for patients with pulmonary disease is based on the theory that through the provision of fewer calories from carbohydrate and more from fat, total carbon dioxide production will be decreased, reducing carbon dioxide retention. These formulas contain a higher percentage of calories from fat, or 40% to 55% of total calories. The carbohydrate sources typically contribute less than 40% of total calories. The caloric density typically is 1.5 cal/mL, which reduces the amount of overall volume necessary to provide full nutritional support. This may be beneficial for patients at risk for the development of fluid overload and pulmonary edema. Studies that have shown positive outcomes with these specialty formulas have been criticized for their small sample sizes, and frequently reports of carbohydrate overfeeding have been based on studies with patients receiving excessive calorie loads (approximately 50 kcal/kg) via parenteral nutrition. If overall calories are not excessive, carbon dioxide production is more affected by total calories than by the percentage of carbohydrate calories. Use of higher-priced specialized formulas for pulmonary patients therefore is controversial.

Intravenous delivery of substrate may be necessary when the GI tract is not functioning or if stimulation of the gastrointestinal or pancreatic systems would worsen the patient's condition. **Parenteral nutrition**, which bypasses the GI system, may be indicated for nutritional support in patients with severe pancreatitis, gastrointestinal fistulas, short bowel syndrome, prolonged ileus, and some cancers. It should not be initiated if the expected duration of support is less than 7 days. Placement of a central or peripheral venous catheter is required for the infusion of nutrients into the bloodstream; central venous access usually is preferred. Complications involved in the placement of a central venous catheter include pneumothorax, arterial puncture, catheter malposition, catheter embolization, site infection, air embolus, thoracic duct injury, mediastinal injury, and cardiac injury. The most common complication of percutaneously placed subclavian catheters is pneumothorax, with an incidence rate of 1% to 4%. Pericardial tamponade, a lethal complication, has a mortality rate of 65% to 90%. Furthermore, the infusion of nutrients into the central circulation leaves the GI tract unstimulated, which can lead to gut atrophy, mucosal compromise, and a weakening of the gut barrier, which may increase the risk of bacterial contamination.

Nutritional Support in Mechanically Ventilated Patients

The importance of nutrition in the hospital setting cannot be overstated. This is particularly important in critical illness, which is associated with a catabolic stress state in which patients commonly demonstrate a systemic inflammatory response. Nutritional support in critically ill patients has three objectives: to preserve lean body mass, to maintain immune function, and to avert metabolic complications. Important aspects of nutritional support in critically ill patients include early enteral nutrition, appropriate macronutrient and micronutrient delivery, and meticulous glycemic control. Early nutritional support using the enteral route is a proactive therapeutic strategy that may reduce disease severity, diminish complications, decrease length of stay in the intensive care unit, and favorably affect patient outcome.

A nutritional product rich in antioxidants and supplemented with omega-3 fatty acids such as eicosapentenoic acid and gamma-linoleic acid can modulate proinflammatory properties in patients with acute respiratory distress syndrome (ARDS) and septic shock, resulting in improved oxygenation. However, recent results of a study performed by the ARDS Network did not find that omega-3 and antioxidant supplementation had any benefit in terms of important patient outcomes. Glycemic control is important in critically ill patients, and some have advocated for intensive insulin therapy to maintain blood glucose levels at or below 110 mg/dL. However, current evidence does not support tight glucose control in terms of improved patient outcomes and is associated with a higher risk of hypoglycemia.

> **RESPIRATORY RECAP**
>
> **Nutritional Support in Critically Ill Patients**
> » Early enteral nutrition
> » Macronutrient and micronutrient delivery
> » Glycemic control

The following recommendations are adapted from guidelines of the Society of Critical Care Medicine.

- Enteral feeding should be started within the first 24 to 48 hours following admission.
- Enteral feeding is the preferred route of feeding over parenteral nutrition for critically ill patients.
- In critically ill patients, neither the presence nor the absence of bowel sounds or evidence of passage of flatus and stool is required for the initiation of enteral feeding.
- Either gastric or small bowel feeding is acceptable. Critically ill patients should be fed via an enteral access tube placed in the small bowel if at high risk for aspiration or after showing intolerance to gastric feeding. Withholding of enteral feeding for repeated high gastric residual volumes may be a sufficient reason for small bowel feeding.
- If unable to meet energy requirements after 7 to 10 days by the enteral route alone, consider initiating supplemental parenteral nutrition. Initiating supplemental parenteral nutrition before this time in the patient receiving enteral nutrition does not improve outcome and may be detrimental.
- In the critically ill obese patient, permissive underfeeding or hypocaloric feeding with enteral nutrition is recommended.
- The following measures have been shown to reduce risk of aspiration: elevation of the head of the bed

BOX 13–1

Nutritional Guidelines for Patients with Chronic Respiratory Disease

Choose high-calorie, nutrient-dense foods.
Plan for small frequent meals or snacks rather than fewer large ones.
Drink liquids between meals, not with them.
Add fats to foods to increase calories, and add dry milk powder to boost the protein content.
Set alarm clocks as reminders to eat, and keep your favorite foods visible.
Avoid gas-forming foods (e.g., cabbage, onions, beans) that may cause bloating and indigestion.
Use home-delivered meal services, frozen foods, and convenience foods to decrease food preparation time.
Supplement your food intake with medical nutritional products (e.g., Ensure, Boost) if you are unable to consume an adequate diet.
Review your medications and consult your physician about adjusting the dosage or type, if possible, of those that have an adverse effect on your food intake.

30 to 45 degrees; continuous infusion of enteral feeding; use of agents to promote motility; and postpyloric tube placement.

- Blue food coloring and glucose oxidase strips as surrogate markers for aspiration should not be used in the critical care setting.
- Specialty high-lipid, low-carbohydrate formulations designed to manipulate the respiratory quotient and reduce $\dot{V}CO_2$ are not recommended for routine use.
- Fluid-restricted calorically dense formulations should be considered for patients with acute respiratory failure.

Nutritional Support in Chronic Respiratory Disease

The goals of nutrition therapy in acute respiratory disease are the same as for patients suffering from chronic disease. Maintaining nutritional status with an adequate energy, protein, vitamin, and mineral intake is essential. For individuals participating in pulmonary rehabilitation programs, poor nutrition may adversely affect their state of health and well-being in several ways. It decreases exercise tolerance, hinders the body's ability to regenerate healthy muscle tissue, increases susceptibility to infection, and ultimately may prevent successful progression through the program. These individuals need practical, simple guidelines to optimize their nutrient intake, such as those listed in **Box 13–1**.

KEY POINTS

- Respiratory function is affected by nutritional status, which also can affect muscle function, immunity, fluid balance, and surfactant production, in addition to other systems.
- Caloric overfeeding should be avoided in patients requiring mechanical ventilation because it may result in increased hypercarbia and a prolonged ventilatory period.
- Indirect calorimetry is the most accurate method to determine energy expenditure in hospitalized patients.
- Enteral delivery of nutrients is preferred to parenteral nutrition because it carries fewer risks of infection, may have a protective effect on the gastrointestinal mucosa, and is less costly.
- The objectives of nutritional support in critically ill patients are to preserve lean body mass, to maintain immune function, and to avert metabolic complications.
- A complete nutrition assessment and subsequent support should be included in the plan of care for patients with acute or chronic lung disease.

SUGGESTED READING

Afifi S. Glycemic control in critical care: current benefits and future needs. *Int Anesthesiol Clin.* 2009;47:139–151.

Aliprandi G, Bissolotti L, Turla D, Vallet M, Scarazzato M, Fredi M. The use of REE determination in a clinical setting applied to respiratory disease. *Acta Diabetol.* 2001;38:27–30.

Baudouin SV, Evans TW. Nutritional support in critical care. *Clin Chest Med.* 2003;24:633–644.

Compher C, Frankenfield D, Keim N, Roth-Yousey L. Best practice methods to apply to measurement of resting metabolic rate in adults: a systematic review. *J Am Diet Assoc.* 2006;106:881–903.

Cresci G, Cue JI. Nutrition support for the long-term ventilator-dependent patient. *Respir Care Clin North Am.* 2006;12:567–591.

da Rocha EE, Alves VG, da Fonseca RB. Indirect calorimetry: methodology, instruments and clinical application. *Curr Opin Clin Nutr Metab Care.* 2006;9:247–256.

da Rocha EE, Alves VG, Silva MH, Chiesa CA, da Fonseca RB. Can measured resting energy expenditure be estimated by formulae in daily clinical nutrition practice? *Curr Opin Clin Nutr Metab Care.* 2005;8:319–328.

de Aguilar-Nascimento JE, Kudsk KA. Early nutritional therapy: the role of enteral and parenteral routes. *Curr Opin Clin Nutr Metab Care.* 2008;11:255–260.

Dominguez-Cherit G, Borunda D, Rivero-Sigarroa E. Total parenteral nutrition. *Curr Opin Crit Care.* 2002;8:285–289.

Elamin EM. Nutritional care of the obese intensive care unit patient. *Curr Opin Crit Care.* 2005;11:300–303.

Elamin EM, Camporesi E. Evidence-based nutritional support in the intensive care unit. *Int Anesthesiol Clin.* 2009;47:121–138.

Eslami S, de Keizer NF, de Jonge E, et al. A systematic review on quality indicators for tight glycaemic control in critically ill patients: need for an unambiguous indicator reference subset. *Crit Care.* 2008;12:R139.

Fahy BG, Sheehy AM, Coursin DB. Glucose control in the intensive care unit. *Crit Care Med.* 2009;37:1769–1776.

Griffiths RD, Bongers T. Nutrition support for patients in the intensive care unit. *Postgrad Med J.* 2005;81:629–636.

Haugen HA, Chan LN, Li F. Indirect calorimetry: a practical guide for clinicians. *Nutr Clin Pract.* 2007;22:377–388.

Iapichino G, Radrizzani D, Destrebecq A, Vincenzi M, Zanello M. Metabolic support of the critically ill: 2008 update. *Minerva Anesthesiol.* 2008;74:709–713.

Jeejeebhoy KN. Enteral feeding. *Curr Opin Clin Nutr Metab Care.* 2002;5:695–698.

King DA, Cordova F, Scharf SM. Nutritional aspects of chronic obstructive pulmonary disease. *Proc Am Thorac Soc.* 2008;5:519–523.

Koretz RL. Enteral nutrition: a hard look at some soft evidence. *Nutr Clin Pract.* 2009;24:316–324.

Levine JA. Measurement of energy expenditure. *Public Health Nutr.* 2005;8:1123–1132.

Martindale RG, McClave SA, Vanek VW, et al. Guidelines for the provision and assessment of nutrition support therapy in the adult critically ill patient: Society of Critical Care Medicine and American Society for Parenteral and Enteral Nutrition: executive summary. *Crit Care Med.* 2009;37:1757–1761.

McClave SA. Indirect calorimetry: relevance to patient outcome. *Respir Care Clin North Am.* 2006;12:635–650.

McClave SA, Heyland DK. The physiologic response and associated clinical benefits from provision of early enteral nutrition. *Nutr Clin Pract.* 2009;24:305–315.

McClave SA, Kleber MJ, Lowen CC. Indirect calorimetry: can this technology impact patient outcome? *Curr Opin Clin Nutr Metab Care.* 1999;2:61–67.

Miles JM. Energy expenditure in hospitalized patients: implications for nutritional support. *Mayo Clin Proc.* 2006;81:809–816.

Oltermann MH. Nutrition support in the acutely ventilated patient. *Respir Care Clin North Am.* 2006;12:533–545.

Rinaldi S, Landucci F, De Gaudio AR. Antioxidant therapy in critically septic patients. *Curr Drug Targets.* 2009;10:872–880.

Scurlock C, Mechanick JI. Early nutrition support in the intensive care unit: a US perspective. *Curr Opin Clin Nutr Metab Care.* 2008;11:152–155.

Singer P, Shapiro H, Theilla M, et al. Anti-inflammatory properties of omega-3 fatty acids in critical illness: novel mechanisms and an integrative perspective. *Intensive Care Med.* 2008;34:1580–1592.

Stapleton RD, Jones N, Heyland DK. Feeding critically ill patients: what is the optimal amount of energy? *Crit Care Med.* 2007;35(9 suppl):S535–540.

Vanhorebeek I, Langouche L, Van den Berghe G. Tight blood glucose control: what is the evidence? *Crit Care Med.* 2007;35(9 suppl):S496–502.

Walker RN, Heuberger RA. Predictive equations for energy needs for the critically ill. *Respir Care.* 2009;54:509–521.

Wooley JA. Indirect calorimetry: applications in practice. *Respir Care Clin North Am.* 2006;12:619–633.

CHAPTER 14

Cardiopulmonary Exercise Assessment

Neil R. MacIntyre

OUTLINE

OBJECTIVES

1. Describe the normal physiologic responses of the respiratory, cardiac, skeletal muscle, and peripheral and pulmonary vascular systems to exercise.
2. Describe the various approaches to exercise assessment and the primary measurements obtained during exercise testing.
3. Describe interpretation strategies for exercise testing.
4. Discuss the indications for exercise testing.
5. Discuss safety issues related to exercise testing.
6. Compare cardiopulmonary exercise testing and timed walk tests.

KEY TERMS

carbon dioxide production ($\dot{V}CO_2$)
cardiopulmonary exercise testing (CPET)
lactate
lactate threshold
metabolic equivalent (MET)
oxygen consumption ($\dot{V}O_2$)
oxygen delivery (DO_2)
oxygen extraction
oxygen pulse
respiratory exchange ratio
timed walk test
ventilatory equivalent
work rate

INTRODUCTION

Exercise testing can help document impairment and distinguish abnormal cardiopulmonary physiologic responses from inorganic causes associated with anxiety or malingering. In this chapter, the normal cardiopulmonary response to exercise will be described. Approaches to cardiopulmonary exercise testing and timed walk tests are discussed as well as interpretation strategies for exercise testing.

Normal Cardiopulmonary Response to Exercise

With increasing muscle activity (e.g., exercise), cellular metabolism increases and the cardiopulmonary system must provide the necessary oxygen and nutrients to fuel this activity. The system must also help clear the byproducts of metabolism, including carbon dioxide and other substances (e.g., lactate). To accomplish this, both the lungs and the heart have the capability to increase ventilation and cardiac output, respectively, severalfold over resting values.

Oxygen Consumption and Carbon Dioxide Production

Exercise is often quantified by measuring **oxygen consumption ($\dot{V}O_2$)**. $\dot{V}O_2$ at rest is approximately 3.5 mL/kg/min. With slow walking, $\dot{V}O_2$ is 8 to 10 mL/kg/min, which is the minimal requirement to perform simple daily activity. At maximal exertion, $\dot{V}O_2$ increases to 30 mL/kg/min in a sedentary 70-year-old and to more than 80 mL/kg/min in a young, elite athlete.[1–4] The maximum $\dot{V}O_2$ ($\dot{V}O_2$max) depends on genetics, level of conditioning, and presence of disease.[3] At low to moderate levels of exercise, cellular metabolism is largely aerobic (i.e., O_2 reacts with nutrients to produce energy, H_2O, and CO_2). Under these conditions, increases in $\dot{V}O_2$ and **carbon dioxide production ($\dot{V}CO_2$)** parallel each other as a function of the **respiratory exchange ratio** or respiratory quotient (RQ). RQ values depend on the relative contributions of fat versus carbohydrate as the mitochondrial nutrient.

At higher levels of exercise when oxygen delivery to the tissues begins to plateau, cellular metabolism converts to nonaerobic mechanisms that produce metabolic acids (e.g., **lactate**). This point in exercise has often been called the *anaerobic threshold*, but a better term is the **lactate threshold**, reflecting the fact that lactate buildup is multifactorial and includes hormonal and regional blood flow effects as well as anaerobic metabolism.[1–4] Lactate is buffered by bicarbonate ion, which then results in $\dot{V}CO_2$ rising faster than $\dot{V}O_2$. This change is RQ is a commonly used indicator for the lactate threshold. Ultimately, bicarbonate buffering capacity may be exceeded at higher levels of exertion. The resulting acidemic stimulus to the medullary receptor and carotid bodies produces levels of exercise ventilation disproportionate to the level of $\dot{V}CO_2$. This relative hyperventilation results in decreased $PaCO_2$ at higher levels of exertion.

Ventilatory Responses

As oxygen demand and $\dot{V}CO_2$ increase, the lungs will increase minute ventilation ($\dot{V}E$) to meet these demands. However, the ultimate alveolar ventilation requirement is driven by two variables—$\dot{V}CO_2$ and the $PaCO_2$:

$$\dot{V}A = (0.86 \times \dot{V}CO_2)/PaCO_2$$

where $\dot{V}A$ is alveolar ventilation (i.e., minute ventilation minus dead space ventilation), $\dot{V}CO_2$ is carbon dioxide production, and $PaCO_2$ is the partial pressure of arterial carbon dioxide.

$\dot{V}E$ increases initially as an increase in tidal volume, up to 55% of the vital capacity with a relatively stable end-expiratory lung volume.[1–4] Thereafter, $\dot{V}E$ increases are largely driven by breathing frequency increases. Measurements of $\dot{V}E$ often are referenced to the maximal ventilatory capacity of the subject, a value commonly represented by the maximum voluntary ventilation (MVV), in L/min, from a maximal effort over 12 to 15 seconds. In referencing $\dot{V}E$ to this maximal capacity ($\dot{V}E$/MVV%), a ventilatory reserve can be defined. The normal range for this ratio at maximal exercise is 70% to 80%, indicating that 20% to 30% of the maximal ventilatory capacity remains unused at this level of exercise. This reserve reflects the fact that in normal subjects, cardiovascular factors reach limits at maximal exercise before ventilatory factors do. It is important to recognize that this notion of ventilatory reserve assumes that the MVV is indeed reflective of the maximal ventilatory capacity during exercise, an assumption that may not be valid if respiratory system mechanics change with exercise (e.g., bronchospasm, air trapping, edema formation, muscle fatigue).

The ratio of dead space to tidal volume (V_D/V_T) represents the proportion of each breath that is not involved in gas exchange. This ratio represents both the anatomic dead space (upper airway and bronchi) and physiologic dead space (high $\dot{V}/\dot{Q}$). Although absolute dead space rises normally during exercise, it is generally less than the rise in V_T, and thus the V_D/V_T ratio should fall with exercise. V_D/V_T should be less than 0.35 at rest and less than 0.25 at maximal exertion.

Gas Exchange Responses to Exercise

Despite severalfold increases in ventilation and cardiac output ($\dot{Q}C$) with exercise, the ventilation-perfusion ratio ($\dot{V}/\dot{Q}$) is remarkably stable.[3,4] As a consequence, the alveolar–arterial oxygen gradient increases only slightly with exercise and thus the PaO_2 is maintained in the normal range throughout exercise in normal subjects. Interestingly, at extremely high $\dot{Q}C$ in elite athletes, the exposure time of red blood cells to alveolar gas in the pulmonary capillaries (transit time) can become so brief that alveolocapillary O_2 transfer can be cut short and mild hypoxemia can develop.

Cardiovascular Responses to Exercise

The cardiac response to exercise is an increase in $\dot{Q}C$.[1–4] In normal subjects, up to a fivefold increase in $\dot{Q}C$ can occur, and trained athletes can increase this further. Importantly, it is the limit on $\dot{Q}C$ that ultimately limits exercise capabilities in normal subjects. The increase in

$\dot{Q}C$ involves an increase in stroke volume during the initial phase of exercise. However, at higher levels of exercise, the entire increase in $\dot{Q}C$ is related to increases in heart rate. Of note is that the heart rate is higher for any given power output with exercise that uses smaller muscle mass. Therefore, heart rate during arm exercise is greater than during bicycle exercise, which is greater than during treadmill exercise for any given power output.

Oxygen Delivery

The integrated effect of increases in the output of the cardiopulmonary system is often expressed as **oxygen delivery (Do_2)**, which is determined by $\dot{Q}C$ and arterial oxygen content (Cao_2). At rest in normal subjects, Cao_2 is 200 mL/L of blood and $\dot{Q}C$ is approximately 5 L/min. Thus, Do_2 is roughly 1000 mL/min at rest; this can increase severalfold with exercise. Cao_2 is not only determined by alveolocapillary gas transport properties but also by the ability of the blood to carry oxygen. This is heavily dependent on the hemoglobin concentration and its oxygen-binding properties (expressed as the oxyhemoglobin dissociation curve). In the lungs, the higher pH and lower temperature of the alveolar spaces shift this oxyhemoglobin dissociation curve to the left to increase oxygen loading. The lower pH and increased temperature of exercising muscle result in shifts of the oxyhemoglobin dissociation curve to the right to facilitate the unloading of oxygen into the contracting muscle.

Oxygen Extraction

Similar to $\dot{V}/\dot{Q}$ matching in the lungs, the peripheral circulation responds to exercise with an increase in blood flow to active skeletal muscle to ensure that oxygen delivery is matched to oxygen demand.[3,4] Peripheral vascular resistance decreases with exercise, but blood pressure rises because of disproportionate increases in $\dot{Q}C$. The oxygen delivered to the tissues (muscles) must be extracted (i.e., delivered to muscle mitochondria) to provide energy for muscle contraction. **Oxygen extraction** is quantified by the extraction ratio:

$$\text{Extraction ratio} = \dot{V}o_2/Do_2 = (Cao_2 - C\bar{v}o_2)/Cao_2$$

In normal subjects at rest, the extraction ratio is 25%, but this can increase to over 50% at maximal exercise. Oxygen extraction can be further increased with endurance training through increases in muscle mitochondrial density, capillary density, and metabolic enzymes. Oxygen extraction can be decreased in a variety of pathologic states that impair cellular metabolism and oxygen utilization (e.g., congenital mitochondrial disorders).

Incremental Exercise Testing

Exercise stresses the cardiopulmonary system, and thus assessing physiologic responses can give valuable information on cardiopulmonary function. The most comprehensive way to assess this is **cardiopulmonary exercise testing (CPET)** using incremental or ramped exercise to a symptom-limited maximum. Both bicycles and treadmills have been used for this purpose, with the increment or ramped increases designed to get 8 to 12 minutes of data before symptoms terminate the test.[3,4] A practical approach uses bicycle exercise ramped at 12.5-watt increases per minute for poorly conditioned subjects and at 25-watt increases per minute for better conditioned subjects. The optimal duration, however, may be disease specific. For example, in patients with chronic obstructive pulmonary disease (COPD), a 5- to 9-minute duration may produce a higher maximal workload.[5]

Symptom-Limited Work Rate

A useful way to quantify exercise capacity is to measure the maximal work performed (watts). The relationship between $\dot{V}o_2$ and **work rate** ($\Delta\ \dot{V}o_2/\Delta$watts) reflects the change in the internal metabolic demand of exercise for a given change in external load and thus remains relatively constant under most circumstances (approximately 10 mL/min/watt during bicycle exercise). Values less than 8.8 mL/min/watt may be associated with significant impairments in oxygen delivery or use, such as severe cardiac disease or myopathy. Sudden drops in this value during an exercise study may indicate cardiac ischemia. If this value is consistently less than 10 in all patients tested in a given laboratory, the calibration of the ergometer should be questioned.

Symptoms at Maximal Exercise

Subjects stop exercising because they achieve intolerable symptoms. Thus the sense of effort at maximal exercise is a useful parameter to collect. The Borg ratings for dyspnea and leg effort (**Figure 14–1**) offer a validated technique to assess symptoms during exertion.[6,7]

Oxygen Consumption and Carbon Dioxide Production

$\dot{V}o_2$ is calculated either breath-to-breath or averaged over short periods of time. When inspired gas is room air, it is a straightforward calculation using the measured mixed exhaled O_2 concentration ($F\bar{E}o_2$) and the minute ventilation:

$$\dot{V}o_2 = (0.21 - F\bar{E}o_2) \times \dot{V}E$$

Analysis of inhaled O_2 concentration must be included if the patient requires supplemental O_2. A simple way to express $\dot{V}o_2$ is a **metabolic equivalent (MET)**. One MET approximates the resting $\dot{V}o_2$ (3.5 mL/kg), and exercise increases in $\dot{V}o_2$ can be reported in METs.

$\dot{V}o_2$ is usually the single most important parameter used to quantify exercise tolerance, and many other variables derived during exercise testing are often plotted

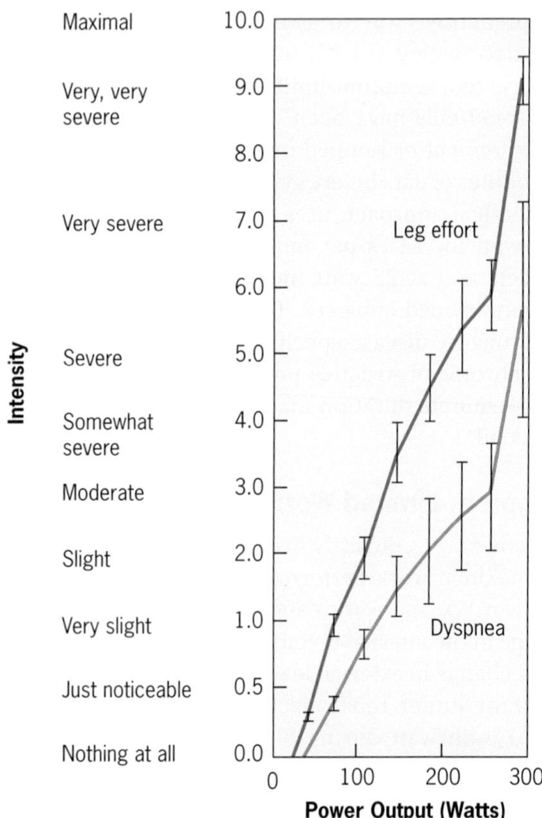

FIGURE 14–1 Exertion scale for perceived effort and sense of dyspnea during incremental exercise testing in normal subjects. From Kearon MC, et al. Effort and dyspnea during work of varying intensity and duration. *Eur Respir J.* 1991;4:917–925. Reprinted with permission.

TABLE 14–1 Predictive Equations for Maximum Oxygen Consumption

Author	Equation
Hansen	Men: mL/min = (50.75 − 0.372A) × W
	Women: mL/min = (22.78 − 0.17A) × (W + 43)
Jones	Men: L/min = 0.046H − 0.021A − 4.31
	Women: L/min = 0.046H − 0.021A − 4.93
Blackie	Men: L/min = 0.0142H − 0.0494A + 0.00257W + 3.015
	Women: L/min = 0.0142H − 0.0115A + 0.00974W + 0.651
Fairbarn	Men: L/min = 0.023H − 0.031 A + 0.0117W − 0.322
	Women: L/min = 0.0158H − 0.027A + 0.00899W + 0.207

A, age (years); W, weight (kg); H, height (cm).

as a function of $\dot{V}O_2$ to measure the appropriateness of their responses throughout exertion. At maximal exertion, this function is called $\dot{V}O_2$max and represents an individual's cardiopulmonary fitness and level of conditioning. $\dot{V}O_2$max is reported as a percentage of predicted normal values (**Table 14–1**) or is adjusted for weight as mL/kg/min.[3] Normal $\dot{V}O_2$max percentage is often taken as greater than 80%. Differences in exercise protocol may result in differences in $\dot{V}O_2$max. Treadmill exercise results in values approximately 10% higher than those achieved with cycle ergometry. Protocol durations that are too short or too long may decrease maximal achieved values.

$\dot{V}CO_2$ can also be measured breath-to-breath or over short time intervals. It is a straightforward calculation that requires an analysis of exhaled CO_2 ($F\bar{E}CO_2$) and minute ventilation:

$$\dot{V}CO_2 = F\bar{E}CO_2 \times \dot{V}E$$

$\dot{V}CO_2$ changes with $\dot{V}O_2$ at low to moderate levels of exercise, with the ratio expressed as the RQ. At higher levels of exercise, when oxygen delivery is reaching maximums and lactate generation is occurring, the buffering by bicarbonate causes $\dot{V}CO_2$ to increase faster than $\dot{V}O_2$. This change in slope can be plotted, and that level of exercise is often taken as an estimate of the lactate threshold (V slope method).[3] Normal lactate threshold occurs at 50% to 60% of $\dot{V}O_2$max, but the confidence limits extend as low as 40% in groups of individuals without known disease. Lactate threshold can be protocol dependent and varies with rate of incremental work increases and type of exercise, with cycle ergometry resulting in values approximately 10% lower than those seen with treadmill exercise.

The **ventilatory equivalents** for both CO_2 and O_2 are commonly reported during exercise ($\dot{V}E/\dot{V}CO_2$ and $\dot{V}E/\dot{V}O_2$, respectively). $\dot{V}E/\dot{V}CO_2$ has been used as an indirect estimate of dead space in the absence of arterial blood gas measurements to calculate VD/VT. Normal values for $\dot{V}E/\dot{V}CO_2$ and $\dot{V}E/\dot{V}O_2$ at the lactate threshold are less than 34 and 31, respectively. Increases in the $\dot{V}E/\dot{V}CO_2$ and $\dot{V}E/\dot{V}O_2$ can be associated with psychogenic hyperventilation, malingering, metabolic acidosis, or other causes of increased ventilatory drive.

Plots of $\dot{V}E/\dot{V}CO_2$ and $\dot{V}E/\dot{V}O_2$ as a function of $\dot{V}O_2$ are alternative approaches commonly used in the detection of the lactate threshold. Both values initially fall and then plateau up to moderate levels of exertion. In cases of early lactic acidosis, during which time bicarbonate buffering results in increasing $\dot{V}CO_2$ but not in acidemia (the isocapnic buffering period), the $\dot{V}E/\dot{V}O_2$ rises while the $\dot{V}E/\dot{V}CO_2$ remains constant. With increasing acidemia, $\dot{V}E/\dot{V}CO_2$ increases. In respiratory conditions such as COPD, increased tissue stores of CO_2 associated with hypoventilation may make the noninvasive determination of lactate threshold impossible.[3]

Exercise Ventilation

Exercise ventilation is largely driven by pH and PCO_2 (and thus $\dot{V}CO_2$). $\dot{V}E$ can be measured breath-to-breath or over discrete intervals. In normal subjects, the maximal ventilatory capacity of the lung is generally much larger than the ventilation requirements at maximal exercise. There thus exists a substantial ventilatory reserve in normal subjects at maximal exercise (i.e., $\dot{V}E/MVV$ is less than 70% to 80% at maximal exercise).

An additional ventilation assessment is the end-expiratory lung volume (EELV). EELV should remain relatively stable during increases in exercise ventilation. Increases suggest that air trapping is developing. Changes in EELV can be estimated by changes in the inspiratory capacity (IC). Multiple IC maneuvers can be performed throughout exertion, and EELV then is calculated as the difference between total lung capacity and IC.

Arterial Blood Gas Measurements

Arterial blood gas values can be analyzed at different levels of exercise either from an indwelling arterial catheter or intermittent sampling. Because ventilation-perfusion matching is well maintained even at exercise with maximal $\dot{Q}c$, Pao_2 does not change significantly during exercise in healthy individuals. However, the gradient between alveolar and arterial Po_2 [$P(A - a)o_2$] increases with exertion. Both resting and exercise $P(A - a)o_2$ increase with aging.[8] $Paco_2$ and pH are generally well maintained through low and moderate exercise by appropriate increases in the minute ventilation. Above the lactate threshold, however, accelerated increases in ventilation will lower $Paco_2$ in order to preserve the pH. Because ventilatory capacity is not the limiting step to exercise in normal subjects, this ability to protect the pH is well maintained until the very highest levels of exercise.

Ratio of Dead Space to Tidal Volume

In addition to calculating $\dot{V}co_2$, exhaled CO_2 can be used either alone or with a measurement of $Paco_2$ to calculate VD/VT. One weakness with the use of VD/VT to represent parenchymal disease is that it is influenced by the ventilatory pattern. Because of the 150 to 200 mL of anatomic dead space, respiratory patterns with shallow VT have a greater proportion of dead space independent of parenchymal gas exchange characteristics. Importantly, in the computation of the dead space and the VD/VT, subtraction of the dead space of the measuring device used to perform the gas analysis is necessary.

In healthy individuals, the end-tidal Pco_2 ($PETCO_2$) can be used to estimate $Paco_2$. Both the $Paco_2$ and the $PETCO_2$ remain unchanged at moderate levels of exertion. However, they both drop during the hyperventilation associated with the lactate threshold. Even with healthy lungs, small differences exist between the $Paco_2$ and the $PETCO_2$. In diseased lungs with significant increases in physiologic dead space, the $PETCO_2$ may differ considerably from the $Paco_2$.

Cardiovascular Assessment

$\dot{Q}c$ increases with exercise are initially stroke volume increases followed by heart rate increases until maximal exercise. Because of this, heart rate approaches the predicted maximum of 220 minus age as maximal exercise is approached in normal subjects. A maximal heart rate less than 80% to 90% of predicted should raise the suspicion of noncardiovascular limitations to exertion (e.g., ventilatory/gas exchange limitation, submaximal effort). On the other hand, identification of significant metabolic acidosis in the presence of a large heart rate reserve may indicate chronotropic insufficiency (as with β-blocker, calcium-channel blocker, or conduction system abnormalities or heart transplantation). However, it also may reflect large-extremity ischemia if associated with symptoms of claudication.

Cardiac assessment during CPET in most pulmonary laboratories usually consists of heart rate, blood pressure, and cardiac rhythm. Heart rate is often plotted as a function of $\dot{V}o_2$ to assess the appropriateness of its response. Elevations in the heart-rate-versus-$\dot{V}o_2$ slope are associated with abnormal stroke volume because heart rate must increase to maintain $\dot{Q}c$ for a given $\dot{V}o_2$. Hemoglobin, Sao_2, and peripheral muscle function independently affect the body's ability to increase $\dot{V}o_2$ and may result in increases in the heart-rate-versus-$\dot{V}o_2$ slope independent of stroke volume. The **oxygen pulse** ($\dot{V}o_2$/heart rate) is another way to represent this concept:

$$O_2pulse_{max} = \frac{\dot{V}o_2\,max}{fc_{max}} = \text{Stroke volume}_{max} \times Cao_2 \times \text{Muscle extraction rate}_{max}$$

where $\dot{V}o_2max$ is maximum $\dot{V}o_2$, Cao_2 is oxygen content of arterial blood, and fc_{max} = maximum heart rate. Although maximal O_2 pulse has been considered the noninvasive surrogate to stroke volume, influences of pathologic processes exist in the blood and muscle as well. Normal values for O_2 pulse are determined by the ratio of predicted $\dot{V}o_2$ to predicted heart rate. Normal values are greater than 80% predicted.

In some laboratories, measurements of $\dot{Q}c$ can be made.[9] The gold standard for $\dot{Q}c$ assessment is the direct Fick method, which requires invasive placement of a pulmonary artery catheter. A mixed venous gas is sampled from the pulmonary artery catheter, arterial blood is sampled, and $\dot{V}o_2$ measurements are made from expired gas. $\dot{Q}c$ is then calculated from the Fick equation. This technique is reliable during submaximal steady-state exercise, but its use is limited because of its invasive nature and inaccuracy in non-steady-state exercise.

Acetylene and other inert soluble gas rebreathing or single-breath methods can also be used to assess $\dot{Q}c$ based on the assumption that the rate of disappearance of such gases is directly proportional to the flow of blood through the lungs.[10] The technique is accurate and simple to perform at maximal exercise in healthy individuals but is inaccurate in persons with gas exchange abnormalities caused by lung disease. Doppler echocardiography has shown promise as a noninvasive accurate technique to measure beat-by-beat changes in $\dot{Q}c$. The downside of this technique is its expense and the requirement of trained personnel, although recent advances may improve access to this technology.

Interpreting the Results of Incremental Cardiopulmonary Exercise Testing

A common approach to interpreting the results of symptom-limited CPET first describes the level of impairment, often using maximal $\dot{V}O_2$ as a percent of predicted (refer to Table 14–1). The exercise-limiting factors can then be defined as ventilatory limitations, gas exchange limitations, or cardiovascular limitations.[3,4,11,12]

The first question that then should be answered is whether an individual has a normal exercise capacity. A $\dot{V}O_2max$ of greater than 80% of predicted indicates a normal physiologic capacity to perform metabolic work. In obese or otherwise inefficient individuals, significant discrepancies may exist between their physiologic capacity to perform work ($\dot{V}O_2max$) and the actual work performed on their environment, or power output, which may be abnormally decreased. Furthermore, in obese individuals $\dot{V}O_2max$ adjusted for weight (mL/min/kg) may be decreased into the mild (<25 mL/min/kg) or even severe (<15 mL/min/kg) disability range in the setting of normal $\dot{V}O_2max$% predicted, which is calculated based on height or lean body mass.

Cardiovascular limitation to exercise occurs when the cardiac and peripheral vascular components of the Fick equation are maximized. Thus, further increases in $\dot{V}O_2$ cannot occur, resulting in unbearable symptoms that lead to exercise termination. The most common indicator is a heart rate greater than 80% to 90% of predicted maximum. In addition, a decrease in base excess or a lactate increase of more than 3 mmol/L can indicate cardiovascular limitation. Healthy individuals exhibit a cardiovascular limitation at normal maximal exercise; thus, reaching this limit at a normal maximal $\dot{V}O_2$ does not imply abnormalities in the cardiovascular system. The differential diagnosis for isolated abnormalities in the cardiovascular response includes any condition that affects the delivery or use of oxygen, including severe deconditioning, left or right heart systolic or diastolic dysfunction, anemia, hemoglobinopathy, carboxyhemoglobin, myopathy, or peripheral shunt.

Ventilatory limitation occurs when an individual approaches the mechanical limits of the respiratory system, resulting in intolerable dyspnea that leads to exercise termination. Thus, $\dot{V}O_2$ cannot increase further despite significant reserves in the cardiovascular system. Indicators of ventilatory limitation include a $\dot{V}Emax$/MVV ratio of greater than 0.70 to 0.80, a rising $PaCO_2$, or a developing respiratory acidosis.

Individuals demonstrating ventilatory limitation nearly all have abnormalities in ventilatory mechanics and thus MVV. Exceptions include the elite athlete, who has trained the cardiovascular system to challenge the limits of the capacity for the ventilatory system, and the individual with increased ventilatory drive, as may occur in cases of severe acute or chronic metabolic acidosis. Importantly, because MVV is conventionally measured at rest, acute reductions in MVV because of bronchospasm or because of development of air trapping may be unappreciated as a cause of ventilatory limitations. Thus, intraexercise measurements of inspiratory capacity and postexercise spirometry should be performed in these subjects.[13,14]

Gas exchange limitations (i.e., hypoxemia) leading to intolerable dyspnea are commonly considered a separate category of exercise limitation. Parameters indicating an abnormal gas exchange response include increased V_D/V_T, abnormally widened $P(A-a)O_2$, a decrease in PaO_2 or SpO_2, elevated $\dot{V}E/\dot{V}O_2$ at the lactate threshold, and increased $P(a-ET)CO_2$. Common criteria defining a gas exchange limit to exercise are a PaO_2 less than 55 to 60 mm Hg or an SpO_2 less than 88% to 89%. The finding of abnormalities in gas exchange supports the presence of, and quantifies the magnitude of, overt or occult parenchymal lung disease or airways disease. Note that the impairment in oxygen delivery associated with hypoxemia and the elevation in $\dot{V}E$ associated with dead space abnormalities may contribute to premature cardiovascular and ventilatory limitations.

> **RESPIRATORY RECAP**
>
> **Interpretative Strategies for CPET**
>
> » Is the subject's maximal exercise capacity abnormal?
> » What is the major limiting factor to maximal exertion: cardiac, ventilatory, gas exchange, or combined?
> » Are non-exercise-limiting abnormalities present in the cardiovascular and ventilatory gas exchange response?

Combined limitation occurs when cardiovascular, gas exchange, and/or ventilatory parameters approach physiologic limits together. In such cases, symptoms from each process likely contribute to exercise termination.[3] Combined abnormalities involving cardiovascular, gas exchange, and ventilatory parameters may be characteristic of disease processes, such as primary pulmonary vascular disease. In other cases the response pattern helps subcategorize disease. For example, although COPD is primarily associated with significant deficits in gas exchange, abnormalities in the cardiovascular parameters may indicate the presence of secondary pulmonary hypertension, myopathy, deconditioning, or left ventricular comorbidity. Whereas subjects with idiopathic pulmonary fibrosis have qualitatively similar findings, that disease process is characterized by more profound arterial desaturation and rapid respiratory rates, which often exceed 60 breaths/min at maximal exertion. More subtle abnormalities in gas exchange can be observed in subjects with cardiomyopathy, in whom abnormalities in cardiovascular response are prominent.

TABLE 14–2 A General Scheme for Interpretation of CPET Responses

Parameter	Exercise-Limiting Criteria	Abnormal Response, Not Exercise Limiting
Ventilatory Factors		
$\dot{V}E/MVV$	> 0.80	0.70–0.80
$PaCO_2$	Increases more than 5 mm Hg	
VD/VT	Increases with exercise	Elevated at rest, decreases with exercise
Exercise-induced bronchospasm	Present	
Gas Exchange Factors		
PaO_2	< 60 mm Hg	60–75 mm Hg
SpO_2	< 88%	88%–92%, drop of > 4%
O_2 supplementation		Needed to keep SpO_2 > 90%
Cardiovascular Factors		
Heart rate	> 80% predicted (220 – age)	
$\dot{V}O_2$/heart rate (O_2 pulse)		< 80% predicted
ECG rhythm	Heart block, sustained tachycardia or bradycardia	Increasing extrasystoles
Blood pressure	Diastolic > 120 mm Hg or systolic fall > 20 mm Hg	

CPET, cardiopulmonary exercise testing; $\dot{V}E$, minute ventilation; MVV, maximum voluntary ventilation; ECG, electrocardiogram.

A submaximal response occurs when exercise is symptom terminated but cardiovascular, gas exchange, and ventilatory system parameters have not approached their physiologic limits. This finding may be a valid measure of exercise capacity if symptoms arise from peripheral muscle weakness or musculoskeletal pain, but the values are less meaningful if exercise is terminated due to a lack of effort, dry mouth, or sore buttocks.

Importantly, abnormalities in the various cardiovascular and ventilatory/gas exchange parameters can occur without these abnormalities actually limiting maximal exercise. For example, a low MVV may still be more than enough to provide $\dot{V}E$ for an exercise test limited by cardiovascular factors. Similarly, a PaO_2 reduction of 87 to 69 mm Hg with exercise is an abnormal response but would not be the exercise-limiting factor in a subject with other limitations. **Table 14–2** provides suggested criteria for defining abnormalities as being exercise limiting.

Timed Walk Tests

Timed walk tests focus primarily on functional performance.[15] They are generally easy to perform, and patients usually prefer them to other forms of exercise testing because the exercise is familiar to them and the tests allow patients to set their own pace (including rests) and adaptive maneuvers (e.g., pursed-lip breathing). A timed walk test generally involves a request for the patient to walk over a measured course for a set duration of time (e.g., 6 or 12 minutes). Patients are encouraged to go as far as they can, and supplemental oxygen is provided as necessary. A practice walk may result in a very slight (7%) increase in the subsequent walk test.[16] **Box 14–1** gives the protocol used for the National Emphysema Treatment Trial,[17] and **Equation 14–1** lists predicted normal values.[18] A less commonly used timed walk test is the shuttle walk, which involves a metronome to pace the subject's walk.

Walk test distance has a fair correlation with maximal exercise tolerance but a very strong correlation with an individual's ability to perform activities of daily living and quality of life. Indeed, this latter correlation makes the timed walk test attractive in the evaluation of novel therapies such as vasodilator response or lung volume reduction surgery. In a study of individuals who had experienced heart failure, a 20- to 40-meter change correlated with clinically important improvements in quality of life.[19] In COPD patients, 54-meter changes correlated with clinically important functional improvement.[20] Walk tests do not determine maximal exercise capabilities, nor do they routinely record ventilatory or cardiovascular responses. However, blood pressure, heart rate, FEV_1, and pulse oximetry (or arterial blood gas values) can be determined at the end of the walk test to further define the exercise response.

Indications for Cardiopulmonary Exercise Testing

When routine history, physical, and basic pulmonary function and blood tests fail to determine the cause of dyspnea, CPET can help document impairment and distinguish abnormal cardiopulmonary physiologic responses from inorganic causes associated with anxiety or even malingering.[11,12,21] A normal study can serve to reassure the individual and avoid expensive and invasive testing. An abnormal study may direct the workup toward more invasive testing, such as right or left heart catheterization, pulmonary angiography, lung biopsy, or muscle biopsy or may indicate specific therapy, such

BOX 14–1

Six-Minute Walk Test Procedures

Walk Course

Course should be unobstructed, flat, and indoors.
If testing site is moved, configuration should remain constant.

Patient Preparation

Prewalk bronchodilator should be administered at least 15 minutes in advance.
Oxygen supplementation should be provided as necessary.
The test should take place 2 hours after the last meal.
The patient should sit at rest at least 10 minutes before the test.
The patient should wear comfortable clothes and shoes.

Procedure

Instruct the patient to cover as much ground as possible.
Allow the patient to slow down or rest as needed (included in the 6 minutes).
Ask the patient not to talk or carry oxygen.
Provide the patient with encouragement and the time remaining at each 1-minute mark.
At the end of 6 minutes, ask the patient to stop. Then perform the following:

- Record the distance traveled.
- Record dyspnea (Borg scale).
- Record the patient's heart rate, blood pressure, and Sp_{O_2} (optional).

Data from the National Emphysema Treatment Trial Research Group. A randomized trial comparing lung-volume-reduction surgery with medical therapy for severe emphysema. *N Engl J Med.* 2003;348:2059–2073.

EQUATION 14–1

Prediction Equations for Healthy Subjects for Six-Minute Walk (in Meters)

Men: $(7.57 \times H) - (5.02 \times A) - (1.76 \times W) - 309$

Women: $(2.11 \times H) - (2.29 \times W) - (5.78 \times A) + 667$

H, height in centimeters; A, age in years; W, weight in kilograms. For the lower limit of normal, subtract 153 for men and 139 for women.

Data from Enright PL, Sherrill DL. Reference equations for the 6-minute walk in healthy adults. *Am J Respir Crit Care Med.* 1998;158:1384–1387.

as exercise training or specific medication use. Because of the wide variation of normal values, serial tests in the case of persistent or progressive symptoms may be necessary to document progression of an abnormal physiologic response. CPET can help determine the relative contributions of cardiovascular and ventilatory abnormalities to exercise impairment in individuals with known disease. Such determinations can direct therapy toward the appropriate organ system.

CPET has shown promise for research and clinical use in the assessment of physiologic and functional change associated with an intervention. For example, CPET has been used to document the effects of immunosuppressive therapy in those with idiopathic pulmonary fibrosis,[22] lung transplantation in those with COPD,[23] and prostacyclin therapy in individuals with primary pulmonary hypertension[24] as well as the effects of lung volume reduction surgery.[25,26]

Measurements of $\dot{V}O_2max$ are predictive of survival in individuals with cystic fibrosis and congestive heart failure.[27,28] In COPD, exercise tolerance and exercise hypoxemia have also been shown to predict mortality. For example, in COPD patients a $\dot{V}O_2max$ below 10 mL/min/kg was associated with a 5-year mortality of 62%, and a $Pa_{O_2}/\dot{V}O_2$ slope of less than −80 mm Hg/L was associated with a 5-year mortality of 80%.[29] Moreover, incorporating 6-minute walk distance into an integrated index including dyspnea, body mass index, and FEV_1 (the

BODE index) is an easy technique that allows for accurate mortality predictions in COPD.[30]

$\dot{V}O_2$ measurements have been used to assess preoperative risk before thoracotomy in individuals with cardiopulmonary disease.[31] The rationale for its use is that CPET mimics the hypermetabolism and tachycardia of the perioperative state and represents an objective evolution of the stair-climbing techniques traditionally used by surgeons. Other investigators have demonstrated low morbidity rates in patients with a good response to CPET who were otherwise considered high risks for thoracotomy by use of traditional criteria.[32,33] **Table 14–3** presents risk stratification based on the $\dot{V}O_2$ and extent of the operation. In elderly patients undergoing abdominal surgery, cutoff values for $\dot{V}O_2$ of 11 mL/kg/min have been shown to accurately identify patients with significantly higher mortality rates.[34]

TABLE 14–3 Risk Stratification Based on Type of Procedure and Maximum Oxygen Consumption

Procedure	$\dot{V}O_2$max (mL/kg/min) <10	10 to 15	15 to 20	>20
Pneumonectomy	High risk	High risk	Moderate risk	Low risk
Lobectomy	High risk	Moderate risk	Low risk	Low risk
VATS/wedge	Moderate risk	Low risk	Low risk	Low risk

High risk: avoid surgery; moderate risk: consider alternatives; low risk: proceed with surgery. $\dot{V}O_2$max, maximum oxygen consumption; VATS/wedge, video-assisted thoracic surgery/wedge resection.

In a large, randomized, controlled trial of lung volume reduction surgery (LVRS) in severe emphysema, low exercise tolerance was a key marker of patients likely to benefit from the surgery (i.e., less than 25 watts for females and 40 watts for males).[17] On the other hand, very low exercise tolerance (as reflected in 6-minute walk distances of less than 200 meters) predicted high postoperative mortality from LVRS.[27]

RESPIRATORY RECAP

Indications for CPET

- Unexplained or disproportionate dyspnea
- Assessment of the impact of an intervention
- Determination of prognosis
- Disability assessment
- Determination of a pulmonary rehabilitation prescription

Resting pulmonary function measurements clearly do not adequately predict functional status in disability assessments.[35] One standard commonly used to determine disability is to compare $\dot{V}O_2$ measurements in the laboratory to published energy requirements for different jobs.[36,37] The average energy requirement on the job should not exceed 40% to 50% of an individual's maximal work capacity.

CPET before pulmonary rehabilitation is recommended to define safety and determine exercise prescription.[37,38] CPET permits supervised observation of cases of potential ischemia, arrhythmia, hypotension, and hemoglobin oxygen desaturation. Although optimum exercise intensity is not well defined in respiratory patients, individuals who do not reach the lactate threshold are known to be able to train at a higher percentage of maximal exercise tolerance than those who reach the lactate threshold.[39] Although some argue that beneficial effects of pulmonary rehabilitation can be gained with lower-intensity work, evidence suggests that higher-work-intensity training results in greater reductions in lactic acidosis and ventilation requirements.[40]

Assessment for exercise-induced asthma can be performed as an add-on to CPET or as a separate diagnostic maneuver. If performed as an add-on to routine CPET, spirometry measurements are made before and then every 5 minutes for 30 minutes after a maximal exercise maneuver.[41,42] A decrease in FEV_1 of greater than 15% to 20% is considered diagnostic. If the testing is performed as a stand-alone procedure, the work rate is incremented until the subject achieves an exercise heart rate of 80% of the maximum predicted value and continues at this pace for 6 to 10 minutes. Spirometry is again performed.

The European Respiratory Society published an evidence-based report on the use of exercise testing in clinical practice.[43] **Figure 14–2** summarizes the relationship of various specific CPET measurements and outcomes found in the report. **Table 14–4** and **Table 14–5** summarize the society's recommendations and evidence grades for cardiopulmonary exercise testing and timed walk tests, respectively.

	COPD	ILD	PVD	CF	CHF
$\dot{V}O_2$, peak	+	+	+	+	+
Lactate threshold					+
$\dot{V}E$–$\dot{V}CO_2$ slope and $\dot{V}E$–$\dot{V}CO_2$ at lactate threshold		+			++
Arterial desaturation		++	+	+	
6-minute walking test distance	+		+		+

+, sensitive; ++, more sensitive.

COPD, chronic obstructive pulmonary disease; ILD, interstitial lung disease; PVD, pulmonary vascular disorders; CF, cystic fibrosis; CHF, chronic heart failure; $\dot{V}O_2$, peak, peak oxygen uptake; $\dot{V}E$–$\dot{V}CO_2$, ventilatory equivalent for carbon dioxide.

FIGURE 14–2 Exercise indices that have been shown to predict the prognosis of patients with chronic cardiopulmonary diseases. From Palange P, et al. Recommendations on the use of exercise testing in clinical practice. *Eur Respir J.* 2007;29:185–209. Reprinted with permission.

TABLE 14–4 Indications for CPET in Clinical Practice, with Strength of Evidence Supporting the Recommendation

Indication	Recommendation Grade
Detection of exercise-induced bronchoconstriction	A
Detection of exercise-induced arterial oxygen desaturation	B
Functional evaluation of subjects with unexplained dyspnea and/or exercise intolerance and normal resting lung and heart function	D
To recognize specific disease exercise response patterns that may help in the differential diagnosis of ventilatory versus circulatory causes of exercise limitation	C
Functional and prognostic evaluation of patients with COPD	B, C
Functional and prognostic evaluation of patients with ILD	B, B
Functional and prognostic evaluation of patients with CF	C, C
Functional and prognostic evaluation of patients with PPH	B, B
Functional and prognostic evaluation of patients with CHF	B, B
Evaluation of interventions:	
Maximal incremental test	C
High-intensity constant-work-rate "endurance" tests	B
Prescription of exercise training	B

With the use of this grading system, A is relatively rare and B is usually considered the best achievable grade. COPD, chronic obstructive pulmonary disease; ILD, interstitial lung disease; CF, cystic fibrosis; PPH, primary pulmonary hypertension; CHF, chronic heart failure.

From Palange P, Ward SA, Carlsen KH, et al. Recommendations on the use of exercise testing in clinical practice. *Eur Respir J.* 2007;29: 185–209. Reprinted with permission.

TABLE 14–5 Indications for Six-Minute Walk Test in Clinical Practice, with Strength of Evidence Supporting the Recommendation (A through C)

Indication	Recommendation Grade
Diagnosis of exercise-induced arterial desaturation	B
Functional evaluation of patients with COPD, ILD, PPH, and CHF	B
Prognostic evaluation of patients with CF	B
Functional evaluation of patients with CF	C
Prognostic evaluation of patients with COPD or CHF prior to surgery (LVRS, transplantation)	C
Evaluation of the benefits of therapeutic interventions (oxygen supplementation, rehabilitation, surgery)	B

With the use of this grading system, A is relatively rare and B is usually considered the best achievable grade. COPD, chronic obstructive pulmonary disease; ILD, interstitial lung disease; PPH, primary pulmonary hypertension; CHF, chronic heart failure; CF, cystic fibrosis; LVRS, lung volume reduction surgery.

From Palange P, Ward SA, Carlsen KH, et al. Recommendations on the use of exercise testing in clinical practice. *Eur Respir J.* 2007;29: 185–209. Reprinted with permission.

Safety Issues

CPET is generally a very safe procedure if patients are carefully screened for unstable medical conditions (especially cardiac, orthopedic, and neuromuscular issues).[1–4] Appropriate resuscitation equipment and personnel trained in its use are critical to have immediately available, however. After a maximal exercise maneuver, the patient must continue to pedal with unloaded or low resistance on the bicycle to maintain venous return. This action is especially important for patients with primary or secondary pulmonary hypertension who have a poorly compliant right ventricle and are particularly prone to postexercise hypotension and syncope. **Box 14–2** lists criteria for exercise termination.[3]

BOX 14–2

Criteria for Exercise Test Termination

Chest pain suggestive of angina
Evolving mental confusion or lack of coordination
Evolving lightheadedness
ECG evidence of ischemia or serious arrhythmia or conduction system abnormality (evolving complex ventricular ectopy, sustained SVT, new LBBB, second- or third-degree heart block)
Blood pressure: systolic > 250 mm Hg; diastolic > 120 mm Hg
Fall in systolic blood pressure > 20 mm Hg
Chronotropic insufficiency in absence of β-blockers
Spo_2 < 80%
Inability to sustain cadence above 40 rpm
Subject's request to stop despite encouragement because of symptoms of dyspnea, leg or global fatigue, or otherwise

ECG, electrocardiogram; SVT, supraventricular tachycardia; LBBB, left bundle branch block; Spo_2, oxygen saturation measured by pulse oximetry.

KEY POINTS

- The normal physiologic response to exercise includes increases in cardiac output and ventilation along with alterations in peripheral circulation, hemoglobin oxygen affinity, and cellular metabolism.
- CPET stresses the cardiopulmonary system and allows better assessment of the limits of this system.
- Important indications for exercise testing include diagnosis of unexplained dyspnea, determination of prognosis and risk, and evaluation of responses that follow interventions such as pulmonary rehabilitation.
- A global interpretive strategy involves definition of the physiologic systems responsible for exercise limitation and subsequent determination of the abnormal responses within these systems.
- Timed walk tests focus primarily on functional performance.

REFERENCES

1. Johnson BD, Badr MS, Dempsey JA. Impact of the aging pulmonary system on the response to exercise. *Clin Chest Med.* 1994;15:229–246.
2. Johnson B, Saupe K, Dempsey J. Mechanical constraints on exercise hyperpnea in endurance athletes. *J Appl Physiol.* 1992;73;874–886.
3. Sciurba FC, Patel SA. Exercise assessment. In: Hess DR, et al., eds. *Respiratory Care: Principles and Practice.* Philadelphia: WB Saunders; 2002.
4. Wasserman K, Hansen J, Sue D, et al. Principles of exercise testing and interpretation. Philadelphia: Lea & Febiger; 1994.
5. Benzo RP, Paramesh S, Patel SA, et al. Optimal protocol selection for cardiopulmonary exercise testing in severe COPD. *Chest.* 2007;132:1500–1505.
6. Jones N, Killian, KJ. Mechanisms of disease; exercise limitation in health and disease. *N Engl J Med.* 2000;343:632–641.
7. Kearon MC, Summers E, Jones NL, et al. Effort and dyspnea during work of varying intensity and duration. *Eur Respir J.* 1991;4:917–925.
8. Hansen J, Sue D, Wasserman K. Predicted values for clinical exercise testing. *Am Rev Respir Dis.* 1984;129(suppl):S49–S55.
9. Warburton DER, Haykowsky MJF, Quinney HA, et al. Reliability and validity of measures of cardiac output during incremental to maximal aerobic exercise. Part 1. Conventional techniques. *Sports Med.* 1999;1:23–41.
10. Huang YC, Helms MJ, MacIntyre NR. Normal values for single exhalation diffusing capacity and pulmonary capillary blood flow in sitting, supine positions and during mild exercise. *Chest.* 1994;105:501–508.
11. Weisman I, Zeballos R. An integrated approach to the interpretation of cardiopulmonary exercise testing. *Clin Chest Med.* 1994;15:421–445.
12. Wasserman K. Diagnosing cardiovascular and lung pathophysiology from exercise gas exchange. *Chest.* 1997;112:1091–1101.
13. Babb T, Viggiano R, Hurley B, et al. Effect of mild-to-moderate airflow limitation on exercise capacity. *J Appl Physiol.* 1991;70:223–230.
14. O'Donnell DE, Webb KA. Exertional breathlessness in patients with chronic airflow limitation; the role of lung hyperinflation. *Am Rev Respir Dis.* 1993;148:1351–1357.
15. Guyatt GW, Sullivan MJ, Thompson PJ, et al. The 6 minute walk: a new measure of exercise capacity in patients with chronic heart failure. *CMAJ.* 1985;132:919–923.
16. Sciurba F, Criner G, Lee SM, et al. Six minute walk distance in COPD. *Am J Respir Crit Care Med.* 2003;167:1522–1527.
17. National Emphysema Treatment Trial Research Group. A randomized trial comparing lung-volume-reduction surgery with medical therapy for severe emphysema. *N Engl J Med.* 2003;348:2059–2073.
18. Enright PL, Sherrill DL. Reference equations for the 6 minute walk in healthy adults. *Am J Respir Crit Care Med.* 1998;158:1384–1387.
19. O'Keefe ST, Lye M, Donnellan C, et al. Reproducibility and responsiveness of quality of life assessment and six minute walk test in elderly heart failure patients. *Heart.* 1998;80:377–382.

20. Solway S, Brooks D, Lacasse Y, Thomas S. A qualitative systematic overview of the measurement properties of functional walk tests used in the cardiorespiratory domain. *Chest.* 2001;119:256–270.
21. Martinez F, Stanopoulos I, Acero R, et al. Graded, comprehensive, cardiopulmonary exercise testing in the evaluation of dyspnea unexplained by routine evaluation. *Chest.* 1994;105:168–174.
22. Watters L, Schwarz M, Cherniack R, et al. Idiopathic pulmonary fibrosis: pretreatment bronchoalveolar lavage cellular constituents and their relationships with lung histopathology and clinical response to therapy. *Am Rev Respir Dis.* 1987;135:696–704.
23. Kawut SM, O'Shea MK, Bartels MN, Wilt JS, Sonett JR, Arcasoy SM. Exercise testing determines survival in patients with diffuse parenchymal lung disease evaluated for lung transplantation. *Respir Med.* 2005;99:1431–1439.
24. Oudiz RJ. The role of exercise testing in the management of pulmonary arterial hypertension. *Semin Respir Crit Care Med.* 2005;26:379–384.
25. Sciurba FC. Early and long-term functional outcomes following lung volume reduction surgery. *Clin Chest Med.* 1997;18:259–276.
26. Szekely S, Oldberg DA, Wright C, et al. Preoperative predictors of operative morbidity and mortality in COPD patients undergoing bilateral LVRS. *Chest.* 1997;111:550–558.
27. Nixon P, Orenstein D, Kelsey S, et al. The prognostic value of exercise testing in patients with cystic fibrosis. *N Engl J Med.* 1992;327:1785–1788.
28. Mancini D, Eisen H, Kussmaul W, et al. Value of peak exercise oxygen consumption for optimal timing of cardiac transplantation in ambulatory patients with heart failure. *Circulation.* 1991;83:778–786.
29. Hiraga T, Maekuar R, Okuda Y, et al. Prognostic predictors for survival in patients with COPD using cardiopulmonary exercise testing. *Clin Physiol Funct Imaging.* 2003;23:324–331.
30. Martinez FJ, Han MK, Adin-Cristian A, et al. Longitudinal change in the BODE index predicts mortality in severe emphysema. *Am J Respir Crit Care Med.* 2008;178:491–499.
31. Benzo R, Kelley GA, Recchi L. Complications of lung resection and exercise capacity: a meta analysis. *Respir Med.* 2007;101:1790–1797.
32. Morice RC, Peters EJ, Ryan MB, et al. Exercise testing in the evaluation of patients at high risk for complications from lung resection. *Chest.* 1992;101:356–361.
33. Bolliger C, Jordan P, Soler M, et al. Exercise capacity as a predictor of postoperative complication in lung resection candidates. *Am J Respir Crit Care Med.* 1995;151:1472–1480.
34. Older P, Smith R, Courtney P, et al. Preoperative evaluation of cardiac failure and ischemia in elderly patients by cardiopulmonary exercise testing. *Chest.* 1993;104:663–664.
35. Roca J, Whipp BJ, Agusti AGN, et al. Clinical exercise testing with reference to lung diseases; indications, standardization and interpretation strategies. *Eur Respir J.* 1997;10:2662–2689.
36. Cotes J, Zejda J, King B. Lung function impairment as a guide to exercise limitation in work-related lung disorders. *Am Rev Respir Dis.* 1988;137:1089–1093.
37. Passmore R, Durnin JY. Human energy expenditure. *Physiol Rev.* 1955;35:801–840.
38. Ries AL, Bauldoff GS, Carlin BW, et al. Pulmonary rehabilitation: joint ACCP/AACVPR evidence-based clinical practice guidelines. *Chest.* 2007;131(5 suppl):4S–42S.
39. Punzal PA, Ries AL, Kaplan RM, et al. Maximum intensity exercise training in patients with chronic obstructive pulmonary disease. *Chest.* 1991;100:618–623.
40. Casaburi R, Patessio A, Ioli F, et al. Reductions in exercise lactic acidosis and ventilation as a result of exercise training in patients with obstructive lung disease. *Am Rev Respir Dis.* 1991;143:9–18.
41. Cypcar D, Lemanske RF. Asthma and exercise. *Clin Chest Med.* 1994;15:351–368.
42. American Thoracic Society. Guidelines for methacholine and exercise challenge testing—1999. *Am J Respir Crit Care Med.* 2000;161:309–329.
43. Palange P, Ward SA, Carlsen KH, et al. Recommendations on the use of exercise testing in clinical practice. *Eur Respir J.* 2007;29:185–209.

SECTION II

Respiratory Therapeutics

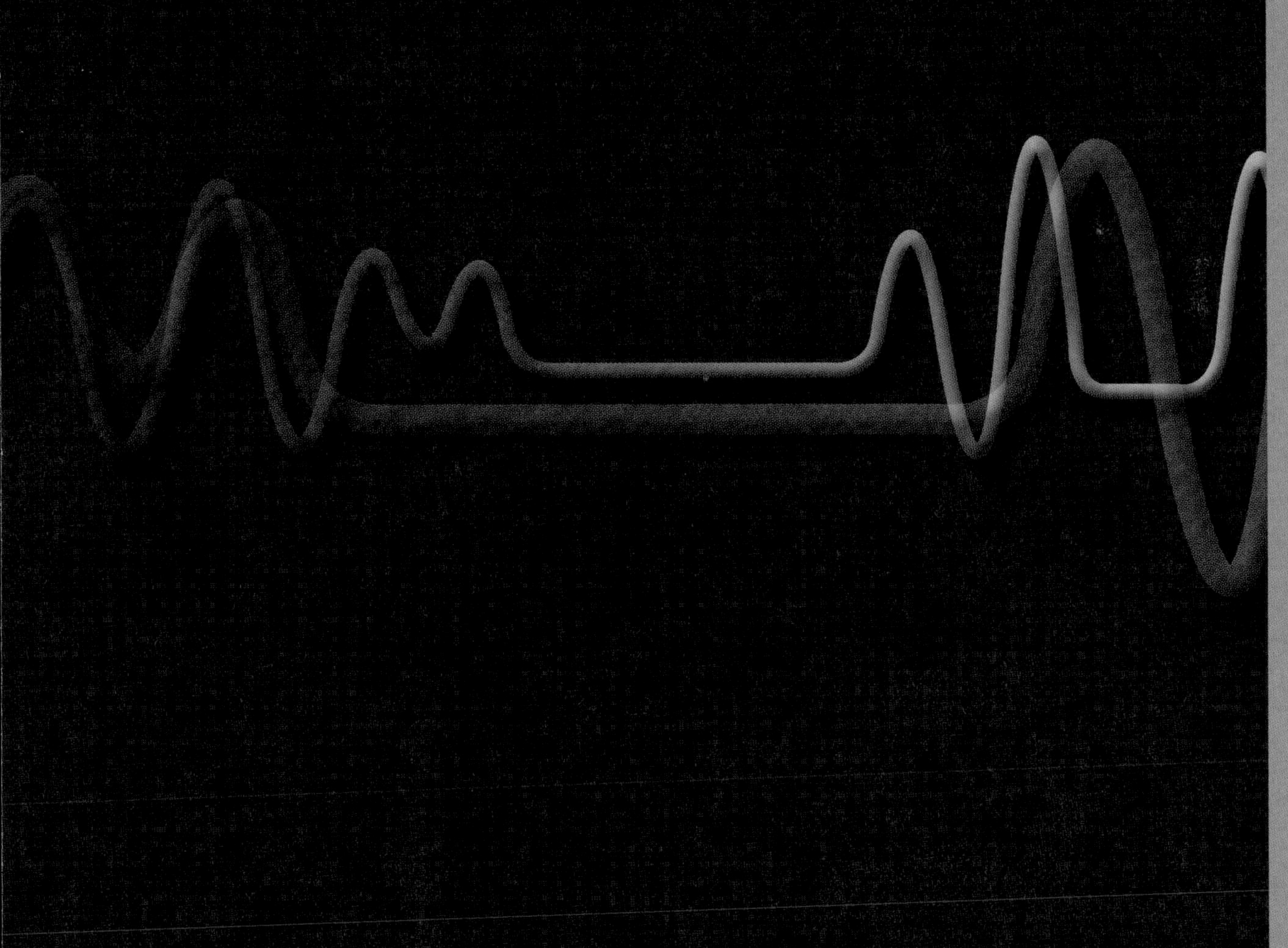

CHAPTER 15

Therapeutic Gases: Manufacture, Storage, and Delivery

John Boatright
Jeffrey J. Ward

OUTLINE

OBJECTIVES

1. Describe the manufacture, storage, distribution, and regulation (to working outlet pressure/flows) of medical therapeutic gases.
2. Describe the physical properties, chemical symbols, and uses of air, oxygen, carbon dioxide, helium, nitric oxide, and nitrogen.
3. Describe the processes for production of various medical gases.
4. Compare and contrast gaseous and liquid storage methods.
5. Describe the production, safety features, types, and uses of medical gas cylinders.
6. Discuss the established safety systems for the various equipment connections to ensure delivery of a specific gas, such as oxygen.
7. Calculate the duration of flow from a gas cylinder.
8. Describe the design, use, and troubleshooting of various bulk gas supply systems.

KEY TERMS

American Standard Safety System (ASSS)
carbogen
carbon dioxide
Compressed Gas Association (CGA)
Department of Transportation (DOT)
Diameter Index Safety System (DISS)
Food and Drug Administration (FDA)
fractional distillation of liquefied air
heliox
helium
hydrostatic testing
medical gas cylinders
nitric oxide
nitrogen
Pin Index Safety System (PISS)

INTRODUCTION

Because many therapeutic and diagnostic procedures routinely used in respiratory therapy involve the use of one or more medical gases, the respiratory therapist must have a thorough understanding of their properties, safe handling, and use. In addition, the therapist must know when and how to troubleshoot equipment malfunction to ensure the delivery of medical gases as needed by patients. This chapter provides descriptions of the physical and chemical characteristics of commonly used therapeutic gases, followed by information about their manufacture, storage, and distribution and the regulation of these gases typically used in acute care hospitals. This chapter does not specifically address the application of therapeutic gases in the home care setting, although the home care therapist will find much of the information generalizable to those settings.

Chemical and Physical Properties of Therapeutic Gases

Table 15–1 summarizes the physical properties of the therapeutic gases discussed in this chapter, as well as of nitrogen, which is provided for comparison. The following sections describe these various properties in more detail.

Flammability

All medical gases can be classified either as nonflammable or as flammable or inflammable (terms that are used interchangeably). Nonflammable gases do not burn; examples include nitrogen, oxygen, helium, air, and carbon dioxide. In fact, some nonflammable gases (such as nitrogen and carbon dioxide) are actually used to extinguish fire because they displace the oxygen that is necessary for combustion to occur. In contrast, a flammable or inflammable gas is one that can ignite, burn, and potentially explode. Cyclopropane and natural gas, not currently used for medical purposes, are examples of flammable gases. Oxygen, although not explosive or combustible, must be present for combustion to occur, and thus oxygen and air support combustion, meaning that their presence aids and accelerates combustion.

RESPIRATORY RECAP

Gas Flammability

- » Nonflammable gases do not burn, but some support combustion.
- » The terms *flammable* and *inflammable* are used interchangeably.
- » Inflammable gases burn and are rarely used for medical purposes.
- » Oxygen is a nonflammable gas; it does not burn and will not explode.
- » Oxygen supports combustion, making burning brighter, hotter, and faster.

Life Support

Oxygen and air are life supportive because the presence of appropriate quantities of these gases supports the metabolic production of energy in the carbon-based organisms found on earth. Gases that do not support life do not contain substances that are essential for the production of energy, but are also included in this discussion because they have physiologic effects and therapeutic potential for humans.

Atmospheric Concentration (by Volume)

Atmospheric concentrations are given in percentage values (%), which represent the relative quantities of gases as they are present in the earth's atmosphere. Most clinical discussions of gas quantities use this unit of measure.

Atmospheric Partial Pressure

The partial pressure of gas in the earth's atmosphere is an expression of absolute quantity rather than a relative value as in concentration amounts. Atmospheric partial pressure (ATPD) is an abbreviation that means that

TABLE 15–1 Physical Properties of Commonly Used Therapeutic Gases

Gas	Symbol	Molecular Weight	Atmospheric Concentration (% by volume)	Atmospheric Partial Pressure (mm Hg)	Viscosity (× 10^{-6} Pa-s)	Density (kg/m³)	Relative Density	Boiling Point (° C)
Air	Air	28.975	—	—	182.7	1.2	—	−194.3
Nitrogen	N_2	28.013	78.084	593.44	—	1.153	0.967	−195.9
Oxygen	O_2	31.99	20.946	158	201.8	1.326	1.105	−182.9
Carbon dioxide	CO_2	44.01	0.0335	0.25	148.0	1.833	1.522	−29.0
Helium	He	4.003	0.00052	—	194.1	0.166	0.138	−268.9
Nitric oxide	NO	30.006	0	—	—	1.245	1.040	−151.8

the physical conditions for a given gas are at ambient temperature and 760 mm Hg pressure without any humidity (dry gas). (STPD, standard temperature and pressure of dry gas, is a related abbreviation designating that the physical conditions for a gas are a temperature of 0° C at a pressure of 760 mm Hg [dry].) *Ambient* refers to the actual atmospheric temperature and pressure conditions experienced around an observer, such as you would find in your classroom or hospital. The term *dry* describes a condition that would rarely be experienced on earth—that is, an atmospheric condition without any humidity—because even the most dry, cold earth environments have some amount of gaseous water present in the ambient atmosphere (also known as PIH_2O, water vapor, or humidity). In situations where no specific ATPD is specified, the default total ambient pressure is assumed to be the ambient pressure at sea level (760 mm Hg). The Atmospheric Partial Pressure column in Table 15–1 represent the partial pressure of each gas in mm Hg under ATPS conditions with the total atmospheric pressure of 760 mm Hg. Respiratory therapists use partial pressures of gases for more precise clinical quantification of pulmonary function (e.g., $P(A - a)O_2$).

Viscosity

The viscosity, density, and specific gravity of gases have relevance under special clinical or environmental conditions, such as treatment of patients with extreme airflow obstruction or under highly hyperbaric conditions. In fluid mechanics, which apply to the behavior of liquids and gases, viscosity is best described as the thickness of a substance. Viscosity affects the resistance or friction of a substance to flow. For example, the viscosity of water is thin, whereas the viscosity of oil or honey is thick. The SI unit used for viscosity in Table 15–1 is the pascal-second (Pa-s).

Density

Density can be described as a measure of how close the molecules of a substance are to each other. Density is most easily defined as the mass per unit of volume, and the formula used to determine it is mass/volume (m/V). With regard to gases, mass is the molecular weight (grams) compared with the standard molar volume at ATPD 22.4 L. The unit of measure for density in Table 15–1 is kilograms per cubic meter (kg/m^3).

Relative Density

Sometimes, relative density is used to quantify the density of a gas. The relative density (specific gravity) of a liquid is a relative measurement that compares the density of a fluid with the density of water (at 4° C, 760 mm Hg). For the relative density of a gas, the density of gases at 4° C, 760 mm Hg are compared with the density of air. For example, a relative density of 1.00 indicates that the density of the gas in question is identical to the density of air (for a gas).

TABLE 15–1 (Continued)

Critical Temperature (° C)	Critical Pressure (psia)	Triple Point	Solubility in H_2O	Color	Odor	Taste	Life Support	Flammability	Physical State in Cylinder
−140.7	547	—	0.292	Colorless	Odorless	Tasteless	Supports life	Nonflammable/ supports combustion	Gas
−146.9	493	−210° C @ 1.81 psia	0.023	Colorless	Odorless	Tasteless	Does not support life	Nonflammable	Liquid or gas
−18.6	731.4	−218.8° C @ 60.4 psia	0.049	Colorless	Odorless	Tasteless	Supports life	Nonflammable/ supports combustion	Gas
31.1	1076.6	−56.6° C @ 60.4 psia	0.900	Colorless	Odorless/ pungent	Tasteless/ slightly acidic	Does not support life	Nonflammable	Liquid and gas
−297.9	33	—	0.009	Colorless	Odorless	Tasteless	Does not support life	Nonflammable	Gas
−92.9	949.4	—	0.073	Colorless	Slightly metallic	Tasteless	Does not support life	Nonflammable	Gas

All values are at ATPD (21.1° C, 760 mm Hg, and dry) unless otherwise noted.

Adapted from Langenderfer R, Branson R. Compressed gases: manufacture, storage, and piping systems. In: Branson R, Hess D, Chatburn R. *Respiratory Care Equipment*. 2nd ed. Philadelphia: Lippincott Williams & Wilkins; 1999.

Boiling Point

Boiling point, critical temperature, critical pressure, and triple point are relevant to the respiratory therapist in understanding the mechanism of humidification and in the use of gas and liquid storage systems. The boiling point of a substance is the temperature at which a substance changes its state from a liquid to a gas (at 760 mm Hg). The change of state between a liquid and a gas is known as evaporation or vaporization.

Critical Temperature

Critical temperature (T_C) is the temperature at which a substance no longer can be characterized as either a liquid or a gas, nor can it be forced into a liquid state by applying pressure, although with enough pressure it can be changed into a solid. Gases can be more easily converted to liquids at certain temperatures, because as a gas's temperature increases, it becomes more difficult to get it to change from a gas to a liquid. For example, oxygen's T_C is –118.6° C. Above this temperature, oxygen cannot become a liquid no matter how much pressure is applied.

Critical Pressure

The critical pressure (P_C) is the pressure (1 = one earth atmosphere) required at a critical temperature to change a gas to a liquid. For example, oxygen will become a liquid if 49.7 atmospheres of pressure is applied to –118.6° C gas. It should be noted that H_2O is considered an anomalous substance because water's critical temperature and pressure do not correspond to the typical change of state model. In a solid state, water is a crystalline form (ice), which is in fact less dense than the liquid form of water (which is why ice floats in a glass of water).

Triple Point

The triple point of a substance is the pressure and temperature at which the substance can exist in the three phases of matter in equilibrium. That is, the substance could just as easily exist in a liquid, gas, or solid, especially with a small shift in pressure or temperature in any direction. For example, when the temperature is –219° C and the pressure is 0.220 psia (pounds per square inch, absolute), oxygen can exist as a liquid, gas, or solid. Note that at this very cold temperature, the pressure condition is nearly a total vacuum (0 psia).

Solubility in Water

Solubility is the physical property of a substance to dissolve in a solvent—in this case, water. Water solubility is relevant to the respiratory therapist in understanding gas transport physiology. For example, the solubility of oxygen is much less than the solubility of carbon dioxide, which affects differences in the rate of solution and dissolution in plasma, and the migration of the two gases through the alveolocapillary membrane and the cell wall.

Physical State in Cylinder

The physical state of some gases, as contained in a cylinder, may be as a liquid or as a gas. This occurs because some gases assume a liquid state at the pressures required to store them in a cylinder. For example, the degree of compression that is required to store carbon dioxide in a cylinder causes it to change states and become a liquid. When the cylinder valve is opened and the pressure in the cylinder drops a little (below critical pressure), the liquid at the surface evaporates and returns to the gaseous state. When the liquid in the cylinder has completely evaporated, the cylinder pressure will begin to drop and will reach zero when the cylinder is empty.

Therapeutic Gases in Respiratory Care

Air

At normal atmospheric conditions, air is an odorless, colorless, transparent, tasteless mixture of gases and water vapor that is nonflammable and supports combustion. Air is composed of about 78% nitrogen and 21% oxygen by volume. The remaining 1% consists of extremely small amounts of chemically inert trace and rare gases, such as argon, neon, helium, krypton, and xenon (**Figure 15–1**). The largest component of air is nitrogen, which is not directly involved in metabolic reactions and is thus considered inert. Nonetheless, nitrogen gas is important in maintaining the inflation of gas-filled body cavities such as alveoli, sinus cavities, and the middle ear.

Compressed air may also be referred to in medical settings as *room air* or *ambient air*. **Table 15–2** shows the relative quantities of the various gases that compose our atmosphere (in both volume percent concentration and fractional concentration). The composition of the major components in dry air is relatively constant. For clinical purposes, gas quantities are commonly referred to as percentages (of concentrations by volume). For the respiratory therapist, fractional concentrations (F_IX) are commonly required in certain physiologic calculations.

Therapeutic Uses

Compressed air has two primary uses in respiratory therapy: (1) to dilute 100% O_2 to provide 22% to 99% mixtures, and (2) as a driving gas for breathing devices when used on patients who do not require O_2 supplementation.

Manufacture

Compressed air can be manufactured by a precise mixing of nitrogen and oxygen. More commonly, however, atmospheric air is filtered, compressed, and stored in cylinders or directly delivered through a central piping system. The **Compressed Gas Association (CGA)** specifies grades of gaseous air. Medical-grade compressed air (CGA grade J) contains 19.5% to 23.5% oxygen, no water

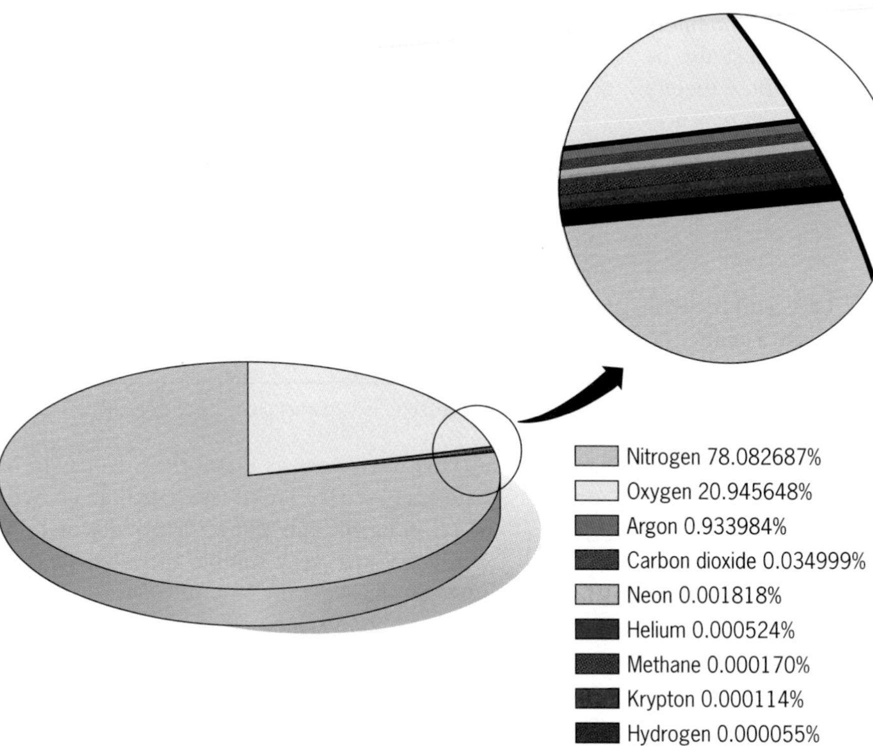

FIGURE 15-1 Constituents of the atmosphere. Values represent percent concentration in the earth's atmosphere. Data from the Encyclopedia of Earth. Atmospheric composition. Available at: http://www.eoearth.org/article/atmospheric_composition.

TABLE 15-2 Composition of Room Air

Gas	Concentration by Volume (%)	Fractional Concentration
Nitrogen	78.083	0.78084
Oxygen	20.946	0.20946
Argon	0.934	0.00934
Carbon dioxide	0.033	0.00033
Neon	0.001818	—
Helium	0.000524	—
Methane	0.00016	—
Krypton	0.000114	—
Hydrogen	0.00005	—
Nitrous oxide	0.00003	—

Modified from Compressed Gas Association. *Handbook of Compressed Gases*. 4th ed. Boston: Kluwer Academic; 1999. Reprinted with kind permission from Springer Science and Business Media.

vapor, and minimal amounts of hydrocarbons and other impurities. Aside from its medical applications, compressed air is the breathing gas that is supplied in many self-contained breathing devices used in industry, scuba diving, aerospace technology, and firefighting.

Distribution

Cylinders

Compressed air is supplied in cylinders that are color-coded yellow. Compressed air cylinders are similar in composition and size to oxygen cylinders. Regulators (for both compressed air and O_2 cylinders) reduce the high cylinder pressure (greater than 200 pounds per square inch, gauge [psig]) to working pressure (50 psig [345 kPa]), the pressure needed to adequately operate clinical equipment such as flow meters and other respiratory therapy equipment. The size and shape of the regulator cylinder connections are specifically designed to prevent the inadvertent application of an oxygen regulator on a helium cylinder. The design for these connections is designated the **American Standard Safety System (ASSS)** and has been established by agreement among the various manufacturers of gas cylinders. Further reductions of working pressure for more refined control of flow or pressure are standardized specifically for compressed air via the Diameter Index Safety System (DISS) of connections or brand-specific quick-connects.

Piped Air Systems

Piped compressed air is commonly provided in hospital medical gas systems for use in areas such as the operating room and intensive care units. Many mechanical ventilators and oxygen–air blenders require separate sources of both medical air and oxygen. The supply of compressed air for these piped distribution systems is provided by large compressors. Various designs of these large compressors are available, but the piston type appears to be the industrial standard. A pressure-sensitive switch senses changes in the line pressure and turns the compressor on and off to maintain line pressures of 50 psig (345 kPa). Normally a holding reservoir is added to the system to provide a ready supply and prevent the compressor from running all the time. In large institutions, it is common to have two compressors that alternate operation, prolonging compressor life.

Portable Compressors

Smaller, portable air compressors are available for hospital or home use. Because the air source of these systems is the hospital's ambient air, high humidity and dust may foul the mechanism of these compressors and contaminate the delivered air. It is therefore important that portable compressed air systems incorporate condensers and filters to remove water and dust. Water trap drains must also be maintained to prevent wet air from fouling flow meters and ventilators. Inline desiccant dryers or filters may also be needed, especially during humid months.

Oxygen

Physical Characteristics

The specific individual who should be credited with the scientific discovery of oxygen has been a matter of dispute. For many years, English theologian-scientist and politician Joseph Priestley was credited with first publishing findings on "dephlogisticated air" in 1774. Yet Swedish apothecary Carl Scheele, who copublished Priestley's findings, appears to have been the first to have chemically generated what he termed "fire air." Neither scientist, however, developed a clear, complete comprehension of oxygen; that distinction belongs to France's Antoine Lavoisier, who named the gas *oxygen*, meaning "acid generator."

RESPIRATORY RECAP

Properties of Oxygen

- » Oxygen is a colorless, transparent, odorless, tasteless, nonflammable gas, only slightly heavier than air at STP.
- » Only 3.3 mL of oxygen dissolves in 100 mL of water at STP.
- » Gaseous oxygen can be liquefied when its temperature is lowered to −297.3° F (−182.9° C).
- » Liquid oxygen has a pale-blue color and is 1.1 times heavier than water.
- » Oxygen stays in the liquid oxygen state as long as its temperature remains below the boiling point.
- » O_2 forms when two oxygen atoms combine by sharing two electrons in their outer orbital shell.
- » F_{IO_2} in air is 0.2095 and remains constant with changes in altitude.
- » P_{O_2} varies depending on the P_B.

The atomic weight of oxygen (O) is 16 g/mole, and its gram molecular weight (O_2) is 32 g/mole. There is some difference in the proportion of atomic and molecular oxygen with changes in altitude. At about 20 km, photodissociation produces atomic oxygen, which is accompanied by an increase in ozone (O_3); these reach their maximum concentrations at 30 km (0.003%) and 90 km (7%), respectively. Radiation strips off an electron from atomic oxygen, producing the ionized species O^+ and O^{++}. The ionic forms are quite reactive, however, occurring only at high altitudes, and oxygen most commonly exists in molecular form.

The element oxygen exists in molecular form in the atmosphere, and in combination with other elements is present in a large number of compounds. Molecular oxygen (O_2) is formed when two oxygen atoms combine by sharing two electrons in their outer orbital shell. This unique molecular bonding characteristic gives oxygen a paramagnetic property—that of being attracted to a magnet—that can be used to determine oxygen concentration in a gas mixture. At standard temperature and pressure (STP), oxygen is a colorless, transparent, odorless, tasteless gas, only slightly heavier than air, with a density of 1.326 kg/m^3 and a specific gravity of 1.051 at STPD. Oxygen is not very soluble in water. At STP, 3.3 mL of oxygen dissolves in 100 mL of water, which nonetheless is enough to sustain all aquatic life.

TABLE 15–3 Effects of Altitude on Barometric Pressure and Partial Pressure of Inspiratory Oxygen

Altitude (Feet)	Atmospheres (atm)	P_B (mm Hg)	P_{IO_2} (mm Hg)
Sea level	1.0	760	159
5000	0.83	630	132
10,000	0.69	523	109
20,000	0.46	349	73
30,000	0.30	226	47

P_B, barometric pressure; P_{IO_2}, partial pressure of oxygen.

About half of the earth's crust by weight is oxygen, and gaseous O_2 makes up 20.95%, or 0.2095 fractional concentration (F_{IO_2}) by volume, of the atmosphere. Although the F_{IO_2} does not normally change, the partial pressure of oxygen inspiratory gas (P_{IO_2}) will vary considerably. Oxygen's fractional concentration in air normally remains constant at 0.2095 to an altitude of 60 miles (96.5 km) above sea level. The P_{IO_2}, however, varies with changes in barometric pressure (P_B), which decreases at higher or lower altitudes compared with sea level. At 1 atmosphere (P_B = 760 mm Hg), the P_{IO_2} is 159 mm Hg. The P_{IO_2} for any P_B can be calculated with the following formula:

$$P_{IO_2} = P_B \times F_{IO_2}$$

where P_{IO_2} is the partial pressure of oxygen in inspiratory gas, P_B is the barometric pressure, and F_{IO_2} is the fractional concentration of oxygen in the inspiratory gas.

The above equation is a demonstration of an application of Dalton's law, which quantifies oxygen's portion of the total atmospheric gas pressure, that is, its partial pressure (P_{IO_2}). For example, on Mount Everest the P_B is about 220 mm Hg (29.26 kPa), whereas the P_{IO_2} is only 47 mm Hg (6.25 kPa), which is the sea level equivalent of 6% O_2 (F_{IO_2} is 0.062 under normobaric conditions). These changes in P_{IO_2} account for the need for some mountain climbers to use supplemental O_2 and for pressurizing aircraft during high-altitude flights. This also relates to and explains in part why scuba divers need to stage their return to the surface in order to normalize their bodies to the normobaric P_B. **Table 15–3** illustrates several examples of the effect of altitude on P_{IO_2}.

Below sea level, 1 atm (760 mm Hg) is added for each 33 ft (10 m) of seawater. (*Note*: In freshwater, which has a slightly lower density than saltwater, the pressure increases 1 atm in each 34 feet of depth.) Because the density of water is so much greater than that of atmospheric air, the pressure increases experienced by a diver

TABLE 15–4 Effects of Depth on Barometric Pressure and Partial Pressure of Inspiratory Oxygen

Depth (Feet of Seawater)	Atmospheres (atm)	PB (mm Hg)	P_{IO_2} (mm Hg)
Sea level (0)	1	760	159
33	2	1520	318
66	3	2280	478
99	4	3040	637
132	5	3800	796

are dramatically more rapid than the pressure decreases experienced by the climber at altitude. Therefore, for a diver 66 ft below sea level (or for a patient in a hyperbaric chamber at 3 atm), the total gas pressure is 2280 mm Hg (303.24 kPa), the P_{IO_2} is 478 mm Hg (64 kPa), and the equivalent F_{IO_2} is 0.63 (**Table 15–4**).

Support of Combustion

Oxygen is a nonflammable gas; that is, it is not capable of being ignited. However, oxygen vigorously accelerates and supports combustion. The higher the partial pressure of O_2, the hotter, faster, and brighter is the burning. Burning (combustion) commonly occurs in air at 21% oxygen. A burning match exposed to a 42% oxygen atmosphere (which contains twice the quantity of O_2 as room air) will burn twice as hot, bright, and fast as with 21% oxygen. In concentrations greater than 21%, therefore, oxygen not only supports combustion but also accelerates the burning process. In the presence of high concentrations of oxygen, certain combustible items, especially petroleum-based products (e.g., oil, grease, petroleum jelly, clothing), can easily and violently ignite with great force from a spark, friction, pressure, or impact.

Manufacture

Photosynthesis

Oxygen is produced naturally by all green land and aquatic plants through photosynthesis, a process in which chlorophyll-containing plants, in the presence of sunlight, convert carbon dioxide and water into glucose and release oxygen as a by-product into the atmosphere. This process of biologic photosynthesis is the main source and regulator of oxygen levels in the atmosphere. Chlorophyll is the chemical agent necessary for this transformation. A normal human must consume 2 to 5 lb of oxygen a day (4.5 to 11.2 kg) to convert carbohydrates, fats, and proteins into heat, energy, and CO_2. As a result of photosynthesis by green land and aquatic plants, the CO_2 produced by animals and the burning of fossil fuels is converted to O_2. The formula for photosynthesis is as follows:

RESPIRATORY RECAP

Ways to Produce Oxygen

- » Photosynthesis
- » Electrolysis of water
- » Fractional distillation of air
- » Molecular filtration

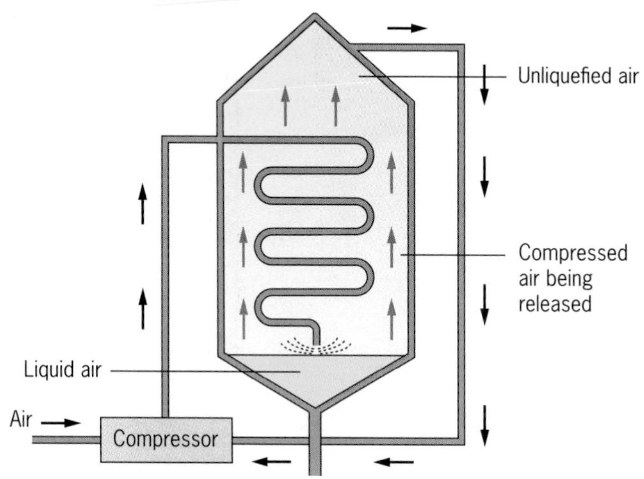

FIGURE 15–2 The process of fractional distillation. Because the boiling points of N_2 and O_2 are different, the two gases can be separated on the basis of the temperature of the distillation chamber.

$$6\ CO_2 + 6\ H_2O + \text{Sunlight} + \text{Chlorophyll} \rightarrow C_6H_{12}O_6 + 6\ O_2$$

Isolating Metallic Oxides

The laboratory or commercial manufacture of oxygen can be accomplished using one of the four following methods: (1) heating and isolating metallic oxides, (2) electrolysis, (3) fractional distillation of liquefied air, and (4) filtration by membrane or molecular sieve. Scheele and Priestley, the scientists who first discovered and described O_2, generated oxygen by heating metallic oxides of mercury, silver, or barium. This method is not commonly used to mass manufacture O_2.

Electrolysis of Water

An electric current passed through water causes the water to separate into its component parts—hydrogen and oxygen—with hydrogen bubbling off at the cathode in a 2:1 ratio to the oxygen at the anode. This process, the electrolysis of water, is impractical for the commercial production of oxygen.

Fractional Distillation of Liquefied Air

The two major components of air—oxygen and nitrogen—can be produced in bulk, commercial quantities by a process first described in 1907 by Karl von Linde. This process, the **fractional distillation of liquefied air**, relies on the Joule-Kelvin principle, which states that when gases under pressure are released into a vacuum, the gas molecules tend to lose their kinetic energy. In a vacuum, the reduction in kinetic energy causes a decrease in temperature and a reduction in the cohesive forces between the molecules, leading to liquefaction.

Air liquefaction plants are large, complex industrial sites that somewhat resemble a small oil refinery. The actual fractional distillation process consists of multiple stages and steps (**Figure 15–2**). The process begins with

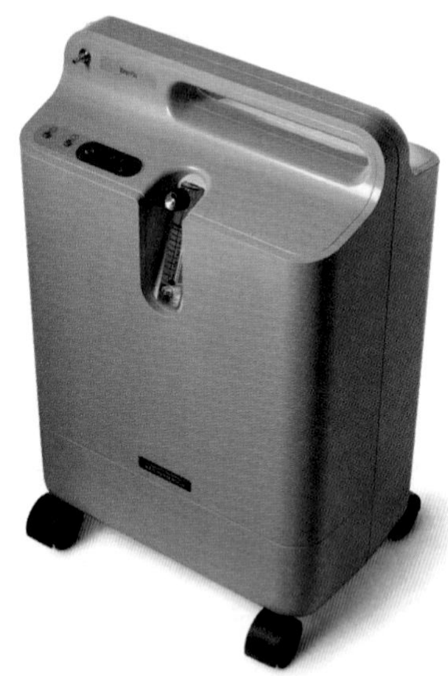

FIGURE 15–3 Molecular sieve. Oxygen concentrators concentrate oxygen from ambient air by filtering out nitrogen.

atmospheric air being drawn through filters and scrubbers to remove airborne contaminants, then compressed and cooled in several stages to 2000 psig and −50° F. Along the way, water vapor in the air freezes and is removed. The air then is cooled further to −265° F at a pressure of 200 psig, then allowed to expand to 90 psig in a separator, where partial liquefaction takes place. The liquefied air from the separator is pumped to the top of the fractional distillation column. As it flows down the column, the nitrogen boils off and can be captured and stored in a gaseous or liquid state. Oxygen collects at the bottom of the column in liquid form. This liquid oxygen still contains a number of trace gas contaminants, primarily argon and krypton, and is further distilled to recover the argon. Distillation continues with careful control of temperature and pressure until the remaining liquid exceeds 99.0% oxygen, the standard of purity required by the United States Pharmacopoeia/National Formulary (USP/NF) for medical-grade oxygen.

Molecular Filtration

Another method used to produce oxygen is molecular filtration. This process is used widely in respiratory home care with oxygen concentrator devices. *Molecular filtration* is a generic term that refers to the filtering out of gas molecules other than oxygen through various methods. A common method for O_2 production by molecular filtration is the molecular sieve or pressure swing absorbent method (**Figure 15–3**). In this method, a vacuum draws room air into cylinders packed with crystallized zeolite, a silicate with ion exchange properties. The air is compressed (to 100 to 300 psig [690 to 2069 kPa]), and environmental nitrogen is filtered out, that is, temporarily absorbed by the zeolite. The process is reversed by switching to a depressurization phase, which causes the crystals to release the nitrogen as exhaust. The final concentration of oxygen, as well as the flow setting exiting the sieve, varies among manufacturers. Most concentrators deliver oxygen in the 1 to 5 L/min range at between 0.95 and 0.98 but fall to 0.92 to 0.95 when run at higher flows. This decrease in oxygen concentration is caused by the increasing concentration of argon gas.

An alternative type of commercial device for O_2 production is the membrane oxygen concentrator. Membrane O_2 concentrators use a set of plastic polymer membranes through which room air is filtered. A pump provides the pressure gradient across the membrane cells, and oxygen and water vapor, which are more permeable than nitrogen, move through the membranes to be collected. These concentrators are less commercially popular because they produce only 30% to 40% oxygen and are not currently being manufactured.

All O_2 concentrators require routine mechanical maintenance and should be periodically checked (with an O_2 analyzer and calibrated flow-measuring device) to verify proper flow setting and oxygen concentration.

Distribution

Oxygen's normal physical state is as a gas. As a gas, oxygen can be stored in cylinders and may easily be distributed by flexible and rigid piping systems. Because liquid O_2 can be stored in much larger volumes more efficiently, most hospitals and many patients have liquid O_2 (LOX) storage systems designed to contain O_2 in the liquid state. These systems are designed to maintain the storage tanks at the pressure and temperature required to maintain oxygen in the liquid state: 716 psig (4937 kPa) and −118° C. The process of returning the liquid oxygen to gaseous O_2 (which is more easily distributed and therapeutically usable) involves heating the liquid oxygen and subsequent evaporation. To accomplish this heat gain, large liquid oxygen storage and distribution systems use evaporator coils in which external ambient heat is absorbed to raise the temperature of the liquid oxygen above its boiling point (which is still very cold). The heat absorption from the atmosphere needed to accomplish liquid oxygen's evaporation and its conversion to a gas results in ice formation on the evaporative coils of the storage system.

Carbon Dioxide

Physical Characteristics

Carbon dioxide (CO_2) is a colorless, transparent, odorless to pungent, and tasteless or slightly acid-tasting gas with a specific gravity of 1.522, making it heavier than air. CO_2 is nonflammable and does not support combustion or animal life. Carbonic acid (H_2CO_3), which forms when carbon dioxide dissolves in water, is corrosive to metals. Under normal atmospheric conditions, the atmospheric concentration of carbon dioxide gas is very low, 0.03% (F_{CO_2} of 0.0003). Carbon dioxide in an unrefined form is released by the combustion of wood, coal, coke, natural gas, or oil, and by lime kilns, the fermentation process, volcanoes, and natural springs. Animals exhale CO_2 as a by-product of metabolism:

$$O_2 + \text{Glucose} \rightarrow \text{ATP} + H_2O + CO_2$$

Humans exhale 5% CO_2 ($F\bar{E}CO_2 = 0.05$), which, along with exhaled H_2O, constitutes the vast majority of the hydrocarbon by-product resulting from energy production by the mitochondria. Adenosine triphosphate (ATP) is the energy molecule produced by the mitochondria.

Because CO_2 is a by-product of animal metabolism and the burning of carbonaceous fuels, the atmospheric concentration of CO_2 is increasing. The increase of atmospheric CO_2 (along with increases in methane gas concentrations) has resulted in an abnormal retention of planetary heat (the greenhouse effect) and is implicated in global warming.

Therapeutic Uses

Pure, or 100%, CO_2 is not used therapeutically. Small amounts of 100% CO_2 gas have also been added to breathing gas for control-ventilated patients to increase $PaCO_2$ and correct respiratory alkalosis. This application has served as an alternative to the addition of mechanical dead space to ventilator breathing circuits. Because CO_2 does not support life, CO_2 must be mixed with O_2 to create **carbogen** if it is to be administered via inhalation. The usual available carbogen mixtures are 90% O_2 to 10% CO_2 or 95% O_2 to 5% CO_2. There are significant differences in the density, specific gravity, and viscosity of carbon dioxide when compared with oxygen or air (refer to Table 15–2). Accurate metering of gas through tubes and orifices must accommodate this factor.

Carbogen has historically been used to treat hiccups (singultus), atelectasis, retinal revascularization after reattachment, anxiety-related hyperventilation, and cerebrovascular conditions. In fact, breathing elevated CO_2 by inspiring and expiring into a paper bag is still a common treatment for anxiety-related hyperventilation. The theorized mechanism of action in this treatment is that increasing the CO_2 concentration of inspiratory gas through rebreathing the patient's own exhaled CO_2 will correct the hypocarbia (low $PaCO_2$) that accompanies hyperventilation. Although this technique can no doubt be an effective distraction from the events that induced the patient's anxiety-related hyperventilation, whether the suggested mechanism of action is at all related to increasing the CO_2 in breathing gas—that is, whether the inspiratory CO_2 level is in fact increased by the technique—requires further study. When carbogen is used therapeutically, it is used for short treatment intervals of about 10 minutes, during which the patient must be carefully monitored. The current Occupational Safety and Health Act (OSHA) standard for the maximal allowable concentration is 0.5% for 8 hours of continuous exposure, or 3% carbon dioxide over a 10-minute period. Today, CO_2 mixtures are used primarily in medicine for the calibration of capnographs, blood gas analyzers, and other laboratory and diagnostic equipment.

Nonmedical uses of CO_2 include carbonated beverage bottling, food preservation, refrigeration, and fire extinguishing. Solid carbon dioxide (dry ice) exists at temperatures below its triple point of 69° F (21° C) and at a pressure above 60 psig (416 kPa). At temperatures below its triple point, 70° F (56° C) and 1 atm pressure, dry ice will sublimate into a gas without passing through a liquid phase. Carbon dioxide also has a low thermal conductivity, which allows dry ice to remain relatively stable.

Manufacture and Distribution

The manufacture of CO_2 for medical purposes involves refining atmospheric CO_2. This refinement process removes carbon monoxide, hydrogen sulfide, nitric acid, water, and other pollutants and impurities. For medical purposes, the purity of CO_2 gas must be at least 99.5%. Three forms of carbon dioxide are available: cylinders at ambient temperatures, liquid at subambient temperatures, and solid carbon dioxide (dry ice). Cylinders of CO_2 commonly contain both liquid and gas if the temperature is below 31° C with pressures above 60 psig (414 kPa). This possibility requires that cylinders be weighed to determine the quantity of liquid CO_2 in the cylinder. This phenomenon does not occur with medical mixtures of 95%-to-5% and 90%-to-10% oxygen–carbon dioxide. **Figure 15–4** illustrates a cylinder containing both liquid and gas CO_2.

Helium

Physical Characteristics

Helium (He) is a rare gas naturally occurring in the atmosphere in extremely small amounts (0.000524% by volume). It is colorless, transparent, odorless, tasteless, and nonflammable; it does not support combustion or life. Helium is the second-lightest element (hydrogen being lighter), with an extremely low density (0.165 kg/m^3) and specific gravity (0.138), slightly more than one-eighth that of air. It is a rare gas in the sense that it is not generally present in the atmosphere (less than 5 parts per million [ppm]) and is chemically and physiologically nonreactive (inert).

Therapeutic Uses

Because helium is an inert, non-life-supporting gas, it must be mixed with at least 20% O_2. Helium and oxygen mixtures are often referred to as **heliox**. In higher concentrations (>50%), it is used medically for its low-density and low-viscosity properties in palliative treatment of large airway obstructions (such as encountered in asthma, chronic obstructive pulmonary disease, croup, and bronchiolar cancer), because it decreases the work of breathing. Clinical applications may be via mask or via mechanical ventilation.

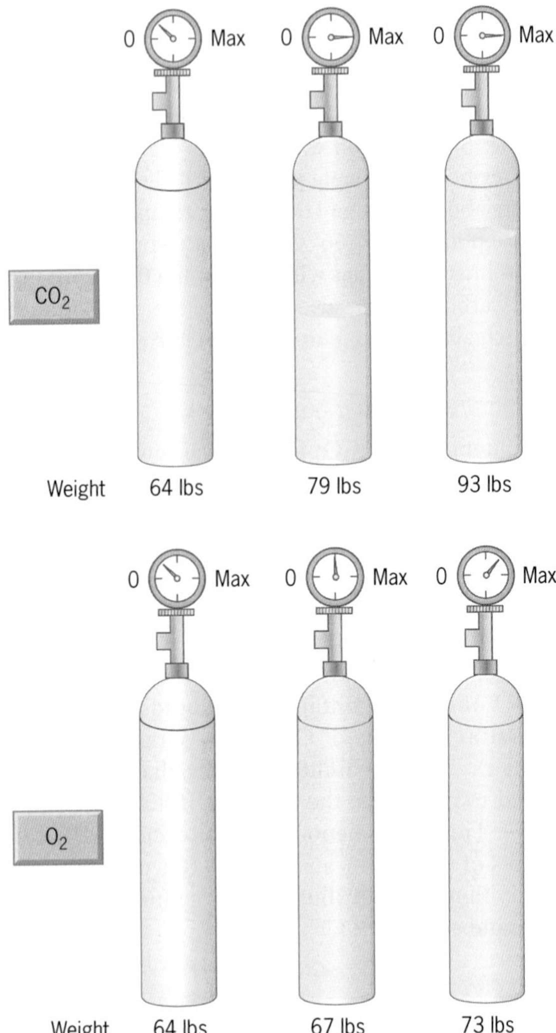

FIGURE 15–4 A cylinder containing liquid and gas carbon dioxide (top) compared to a cylinder containing oxygen (bottom). In gases that assume the liquid state under typical cylinder pressure conditions, gas quantity and flow duration evaluation will require accounting for the amount of liquefied gas that remains in the cylinder. Modified from Dorsch JA, Dorsch SE. *Understanding Anesthesia Equipment.* 4th ed. Lippincott Williams & Wilkins; 1994. Reprinted with permission.

Heliox is also used in place of normal compressed nitrogen and oxygen mixtures (N_2/O_2) for extreme hyperbaric conditions, such as in commercial and scientific deep-water operations. The use of heliox rather than N_2/O_2 decreases the risk of nitrogen narcosis. Low concentrations ($<5\%$) of helium are also used in pulmonary function laboratories as a test gas in lung volume and diffusing testing. Commercially, helium is also used as a nuclear reactor coolant, in cryogenic research, as a shield in arc welding, in silicon and germanium crystal-growing atmospheres, in lighter-than-air aircraft, and for breathing mixtures in deep-water diving.

Manufacture and Distribution

Helium is not manufactured. On earth, natural gas containing up to 2% helium is found only in wells in the southern United States, Canada, and the Black Sea. Helium also is produced by fusion reaction from hydrogen in nuclear weapons and in stars. In medical settings, helium gas is supplied in compressed gas cylinders containing 100% helium or various concentrations blended with at least 20% oxygen.

Nitric Oxide

Physical Characteristics

Nitric oxide (NO) is a colorless, tasteless gas with a slight metallic odor. This nonflammable and non-life-supporting gas supports combustion, is toxic, and is found in the atmosphere in extremely small amounts (10 to 100 parts per billion) as an air pollutant by-product of combustion. Nitric oxide, also known as nitrogen monoxide, is an unstable free radical that was originally regarded as an environmental pollutant (e.g., in smog and cigarette smoke) and an impurity of nitrous oxide manufacture. The NO molecule is highly diffusible and lipid soluble. The half-life of NO ranges from 3 to 50 seconds because its conversion to nitrates, nitrites, and higher oxides of nitrogen increases the rate of conversion with higher oxygen tensions.

Therapeutic Uses

In 1987 NO was found to normally biosynthesize in vascular endothelial cells. It is an important signaling messenger molecule, a mediator of physiologic functions including vasodilation, neurotransmission, long-term memory, and immunologic defense. Nitric oxide plays an important role in vascular smooth muscle relaxation, inhibition of platelet aggregation, neurotransmission, and immune regulation. Abnormally low NO levels in humans have been implicated in atherosclerosis, hypertension, diabetes, erectile dysfunction, and immune deficiency diseases. Exhaled NO (eNO) is a marker of airway inflammation associated with asthma and is gaining importance as a diagnostic adjunct in its care.

The inhalation administration of nitric oxide (iNO) in very low concentrations (5 to 80 ppm) causes selective pulmonary vascular dilation, which has led to the use of nitric oxide to treat persistent pulmonary hypertension of the newborn (PPHN), meconium aspiration, bronchopulmonary dysplasia, refractory hypoxemia, and hypertension-associated congenital heart disease in infants. In conjunction with ventilatory support and other appropriate agents, iNO is indicated for the treatment of term and near-term neonates with hypoxic respiratory failure associated with clinical or echocardiographic evidence of pulmonary hypertension, where it improves oxygenation and reduces the need for extracorporeal membrane oxygenation. This gas has also been used for treatment of acute respiratory distress syndrome in adult patients, primarily as a method to improve oxygenation. At the present time, however, the use of iNO as a therapeutic practice in patients other than term neonates with hypoxic respiratory failure remains controversial. Research regarding the prevention of adverse long-term outcomes for iNO-treated patients remains inconclusive.

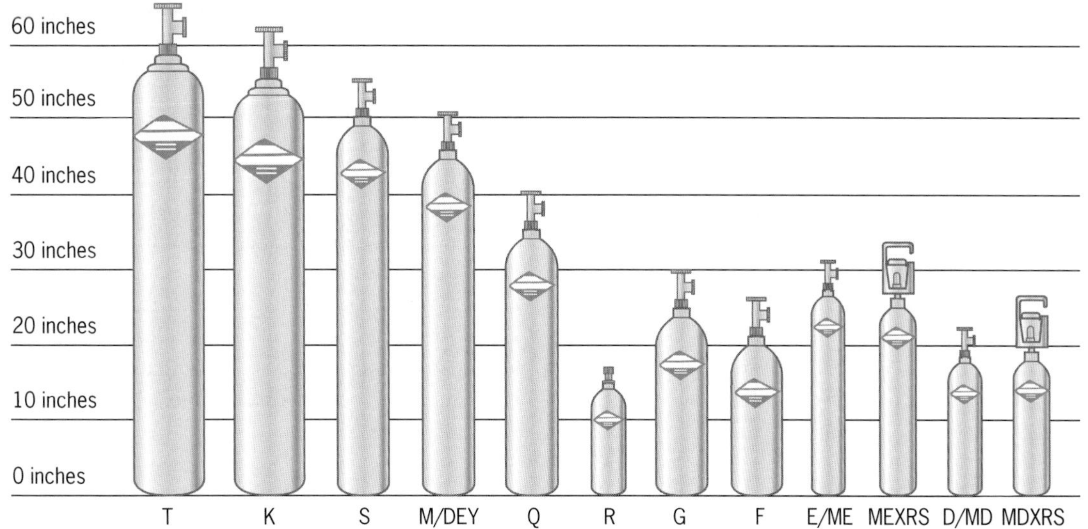

FIGURE 15–5 Cylinder sizes. Cylinders are available in many sizes for a variety of applications (not all sizes are pictured here).

Manufacture and Distribution

Nitric oxide is produced in the reaction of sulfur dioxide with nitric acid and through the oxidation of ammonia at temperatures above 500° C in the presence of platinum as a catalyst. Nitric oxide is also produced as a by-product of the anesthetic gas nitrous oxide (N_2O). Medical NO is supplied in concentrations of 100 to 2200 ppm diluted by nitrogen (N_2) for a purity of 99.0%. The usual concentration is 800 ppm, which is further reduced before delivery to the patient. Nitric oxide is supplied in specially cleaned, high-pressure aluminum cylinders. In a cylinder, NO will remain in stable form and not convert to nitrogen dioxide for approximately 18 months.

Nitrogen

Physical Characteristics

Nitrogen (N_2) is the major component of the atmosphere, 78% by volume. Nitrogen gas is responsible for the blue color of the sky on earth.

Therapeutic Uses

100% nitrogen gas is used in surgery to inflate the abdomen for some minimally invasive procedures and, because N_2 does not support combustion, is also used to power pneumatic instruments in the operating room. N_2 also is used to provide the zero-point reference in some oxygen analyzers, as a diagnostic gas in pulmonary function testing, and is applied in a subatmospheric pressure dressing (SPD) to treat aerobic wound infections such as are sometimes encountered with burns, frostbite, or diabetes. There are also reports of the use of inhaled administration of subatmospheric or subambient oxygen concentrations (created by adding N_2 to gaseous air or oxygen) to temporarily increase pulmonary vascular resistance and thus reduce pulmonary blood flow in congenital heart defects such as hypoplastic left heart syndrome.

Manufacture and Distribution

Nitrogen gas is produced in large quantities (along with O_2) during fractional distillation of liquefied air. In medical settings, it is usually supplied as compressed gas in cylinders.

Storage and Distribution of Medical Gases

Since as early as the 1890s, steel cylinders have been used to store compressed oxygen and other gases. They continue to be frequently used in medical care today despite the widespread use of piped gas supply systems. Properly handled, they are quite safe, and small cylinders offer portability for patient transport or ambulation. Medical gases can be stored and transported in the gaseous state or as liquefied gas in various-sized cylinders and cryogenic bulk containers. Available high-pressure **medical gas cylinders** range from small, lightweight units containing a few cubic feet of gas to large cylinders of several hundred cubic feet (**Figure 15–5**).

Medical Gas Cylinders

Federal regulation of the construction of cylinders used to transport compressed gas began in 1948 under the jurisdiction of the U.S. Interstate Commerce Commission (ICC) and in 1968 was transferred to the U.S. **Department of Transportation (DOT)**. (In Canada, cylinder standards have been set by Transport Canada [TC] since 1980.) DOT regulations specify that high-pressure medical

> **RESPIRATORY RECAP**
>
> **Safe Use of Cylinders**
>
> » Cylinder markings
> » Color-coding
> » Labeling
> » Standardized testing
> » Standardized valves
> » Connection indexing systems
> » Regulation and standardization of filling and refilling of cylinders

gas cylinders be made with seamless construction from high-quality steel, chromium-molybdenum alloy, or aluminum. Today, numerous federal, state, and local statutes as well as industry standards and guidelines regulate the storage, transport, distribution, and use of medical gases. **Table 15–5** summarizes these government agencies and private organizations and their areas of responsibilities and expertise.

Steel cylinders are produced by one of two methods. One involves the pressing of soft steel into a tubular form and using heat to shape and seal the bottom and form the shoulder and neck at the outlet end. Hot steel also can be spun to form a seamless cylinder. Aluminum cylinders are produced by extrusion with an alloy often containing a blend of magnesium and silicon. Aluminum cylinders are as much as 40% lighter than those constructed of steel. Another type of construction available for cylinders, the composite cylinder, is up to 70% lighter than steel. Composite cylinders are manufactured by overwrapping a thin-walled aluminum cylinder with multiple layers of carbon, fiberglass, or Kevlar fibers in an epoxy resin wrap. Steel and aluminum cylinders have flat bottoms, whereas composite cylinder bottoms are rounded. Composite cylinders are available only in small sizes, up to 22 cubic feet of gas (623 liters), whereas steel and aluminum cylinders are available in a wide range of sizes, as described in **Table 15–6**.

TABLE 15–5 Regulatory and Standards Organizations in the Manufacture, Storage, and Distribution of Medical Gases

ANSI—American National Standards Institute: a private, not-for profit organization that coordinates U.S. private-sector voluntary standards development

ASME—American Society of Mechanical Engineers: an organization that issues design, mechanical, and structural standards for items such as components of central piping systems

ASTM—American Society for Testing and Materials: a not-for-profit organization that aids in the development and publication of voluntary consensus standards for medical devices and many consumer products

CGA—Compressed Gas Association: an industry technical trade organization that has developed numerous safety standards involving cylinders, fittings, and connections

CSA—Canadian Standards Association: an independent Canadian organization that recommends standards for the safety, quality, and performance of equipment

DOT—(U.S.) Department of Transportation: the federal body that regulates cylinder manufacture and testing and the transport of hazardous materials, including compressed gases and cryogenic liquids

EPA—(U.S.) Environmental Protection Agency: the government agency that establishes standards and administers regulations concerning potential and actual environmental hazards

FDA—(U.S.) Food and Drug Administration: an agency of the Department of Health and Human Services (HHS) that enforces regulations and standards concerning the purity of medical gases and their manufacture, packaging, and labeling

HHS—(U.S.) Department of Health and Human Services: the principal government agency dealing with health and social services, with the following subsets: FDA, Centers for Disease Control and Prevention (CDC), National Institutes of Health (NIH), and Centers for Medicare and Medicaid Services (CMS)

ICC—(U.S.) Interstate Commerce Commission: a government bureau that before 1967 set and administered the regulations currently the domain of the DOT

ISO—International Standards Organization: a worldwide agency that coordinates and establishes technologic standards in manufacturing and safety

NFPA—(U.S.) National Fire Protection Association: a private independent agency that recommends standards related to fire and safety, which are routinely adopted as regulations by state and local government building and safety codes

NIOSH—(U.S.) National Institute for Occupational Safety and Health: a part of the CDC responsible for conducting research and making recommendations for the prevention of work-related disease and injury

OSHA—(U.S.) Occupational Safety and Health Administration: an agency of the Department of Labor that establishes and enforces standards of safety in the workplace

TC—Transport Canada: Canadian government agency that administers regulations concerning the manufacture and testing of compressed gas cylinders and their distribution

USP/NF—United States Pharmacopoeia/National Formulary: a not-for-profit private organization founded to develop officially recognized quality standards for drugs, including medical gases

Z-79: a committee of ANSI that establishes standards for oxygen and respiratory and anesthesia equipment and devices

TABLE 15–6 Physical Characteristics of Common-Sized Aluminum and Steel Cylinders

	Aluminum					
	B or M6	*ML6*	*C or M9*	*D*	*E*	*N or M60*
Service pressure (psig)	2216.0	2015.0	2015.0	2015.0	2015.0	2216.0
Height without valve (inches)	11.6	7.7	10.9	16.5	25.6	23.0
Diameter (inches)	3.2	4.4	4.4	4.4	4.4	7.25
Weight empty (without valve, pounds)	2.2	2.9	3.7	5.3	7.9	21.7
Capacity (oxygen, cubic feet)	6.0	6.0	9.0	15.0	24.0	61.4
Capacity (oxygen, liters)	170.0	170.0	255.0	425.0	680.0	1738.0

Cylinder Markings

Figure 15–6 shows the typical DOT-required markings found permanently struck into the shoulder of all cylinders. (In Canada, the mark "TC" would replace "DOT.") The DOT specifications to which cylinders are manufactured are DOT 3A, seamless carbon-steel; DOT 3AA, seamless heat-treated, tempered alloy-steel; or DOT 3AL, seamless cylinders made from specified aluminum alloys. The service pressure in psig immediately follows the DOT specification marking and is 2015 for most medical gas cylinders. Cylinders may be filled to 10% more than the service pressure, most being filled to 2200 psig. Also struck into the cylinder are the name or mark of the manufacturer, the serial number of the cylinder, and the original hydrostatic test date followed by the date(s) of subsequent tests.

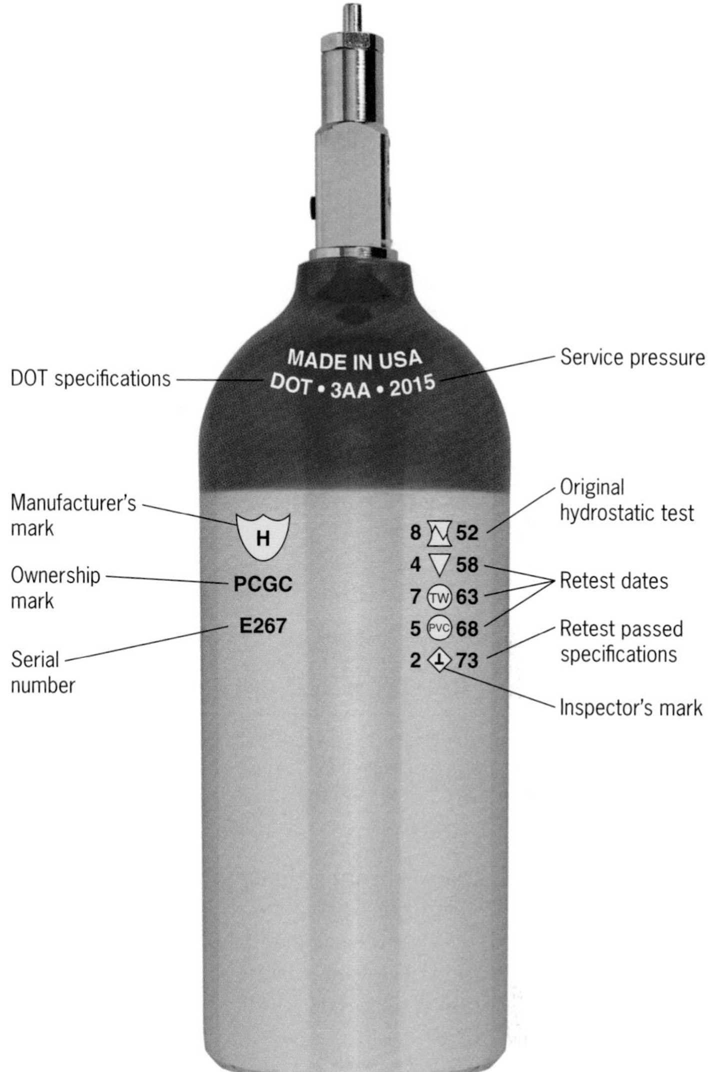

FIGURE 15–6 Typical cylinder markings.

Cylinder Testing

The DOT and TC require that cylinders be tested at regular intervals to ensure that they remain safe for filling to their specified pressures. Steel medical cylinders (3A, 3AA) must be tested at least once every 10 years, and aluminum cylinders (3AL) every 5 years. The cylinder exterior is inspected for signs of damage from rust, corrosion, dents, or deep scarring. After the valve is removed, the interior is inspected for signs of rust, corrosion, and scaling and then hydrostatically tested to a pressure at least five-thirds its normal working pressure. For most cylinders, that would be a test pressure of 3358 psi (2015 × 5⁄3).

The hydrostatic challenge procedure used to periodically test the integrity of cylinders involves measuring the expansion behavior of the cylinder when it is exposed to internal pressures two-thirds greater than normal. This process is done through suspending the entire cylinder in a tank of water and pumping water into the cylinder. The increased pressure causes the cylinder to expand. The amount of this expansion is measured by the water displaced. The amount of elastic expansion is directly related to the thickness of the cylinder wall. As the wall thickness diminishes over time due to normal wear, the cylinder expands more during **hydrostatic testing**, eventually failing the test and being removed from service before becoming unsafe. This challenge process ensures that cylinders can accommodate the typical pressure increases that may occur when cylinders are used in warm environments.

TABLE 15–6 (Continued)

Steel					
M or MM	*D*	*E*	*M*	*H or K*	*T*
2216.0	2015.0	2015.0	2015.0	2265.0	2400.0
35.75	16.75	25.75	43.0	51.0	55.0
8.0	4.2	4.2	7.0	9.0	9.25
38.6	7.9	11.3	58.0	117.0	139.0
122.0	15.0	24.0	110.0	250.0	300.0
3455.0	425.0	680.0	33,113.0	7075.0	8490.0

Cylinder Color-Coding and Labeling

To decrease the possibility of inadvertent administration of the wrong therapeutic gas, a safety system using color-coding, labels, and connection devices is used. A standard color-coding system for medical gas cylinders was suggested by the CGA and adopted by the U.S. Department of Commerce on the recommendation of the Bureau of Standards. **Table 15–7** shows this system and a slightly different color-coding scheme used internationally. In addition to the color code, each medical gas cylinder

TABLE 15–7 Color Codes and Purity of Medical Gases

Gas	Chemical		Color Code	
	Symbol	*Purity* (%)*	*U.S.*	*International*
Oxygen	O_2	99.0	Green	White
Air	—	99.0	Yellow	Black and white
Nitrogen	N_2	99.0	Black	Black
Nitrogen/oxygen†	N_2/O_2	99.0	Black and green	Pink
Carbon dioxide	CO_2	99.0	Gray	Gray
Carbon dioxide/oxygen (carbogen)†	CO_2/O_2	99.0	Gray and green	Gray and white
Helium	He	99.0	Brown	Brown
Helium/oxygen (heliox)†	He/O_2	99.0	Brown and green	Brown and white
Nitrous oxide	N_2O	97.0	Blue	Blue
Nitric oxide/nitrogen†	NO/N_2	99.0	Teal and black	Teal and black
Cyclopropane‡	C_3H_6	99.0	Orange	Orange
Ethylene‡	C_2H_4	99.0	Red	Red

*U.S. Pharmacopoeia/National Formulary standards.
†Labels should always be checked for the percentage of each gas.
‡Flammable anesthetic gas (rarely used).

must feature a label meeting the specifications of the U.S. **Food and Drug Administration (FDA)** that indicates the gas contained, that the gas meets U.S. Pharmacopeia (USP) specifications, relevant warnings and dangers, and that a prescription is necessary for dispensing.

Cylinder Valves

Many of the safety systems involved in gas storage systems involve the manufacturer's use of the cylinder valve. Most high-pressure medical gas cylinders use a direct-acting valve, shown in **Figure 15–7**, in which turning the handle moves the stem up or down, thereby raising or lowering the seat and allowing gas to flow from the cylinder or stopping the gas flow. Small cylinders (sizes A through E) use a four-sided rectangular post valve, whereas larger cylinders feature a faucet-like valve with a threaded outlet.

Because the pressure in a closed cylinder is directly related to the temperature (Gay-Lussac's law), all cylinder valves have pressure-relief safety devices that allow for the controlled release of excessive pressure from the cylinder if it is exposed to high temperatures, thus preventing an explosive rupture. If a cylinder is exposed to fire or heat that raises its internal pressure to 1.5 times its normal filled pressure, a safety valve opens and vents the gas. This response prevents the cylinder wall from exploding. Some valves use a frangible (breakable) disk or fusible (meltable) metal plug or a combination. Wood's metal, an alloy of bismuth, lead, cadmium, and tin, is commonly used for the fusible plug material and will yield when the temperature reaches 208° F (97.8° C) to 220° F (104° C). Copper is used as a frangible disk material. **Figure 15–8** illustrates examples of cylinder valve pressure-relief safety devices.

Safe Storage and Handling of Cylinders

Most medical gas cylinders of any size are filled to the same high pressure—2200 to 2500 psig. This pressure involves a formidable force of more than a ton pushing against every square inch of the inside of the cylinder. Because cylinders are shaped awkwardly and steel cylinders are quite heavy, they may fall or be dropped. Therefore, respiratory therapists should practice pressure awareness and lifting precautions whenever handling gas cylinders. Cylinder rupture may result in metal shrapnel or a spinning or rapidly moving cylinder. Additionally, many therapeutic gases accelerate combustion or are themselves flammable; the use of these gases therefore requires fire safety vigilance by the respiratory therapist. Respiratory therapists should be alert for potential sources of ignition, such as smoking, static, or electrical arcs, as well as the presence of flammable fuels (such as plastics, petroleum-based oils or jelly, or synthetic clothing and bed linens). **Table 15–8** summarizes the CGA's recommendations for safe practices in the handling and storing of medical gas cylinders.

Gas-powered respiratory therapy equipment in the United States is designed and calibrated to operate with an inlet gas pressure of 50 psig, which is referred to as the *working pressure*. Central piping systems incorporate

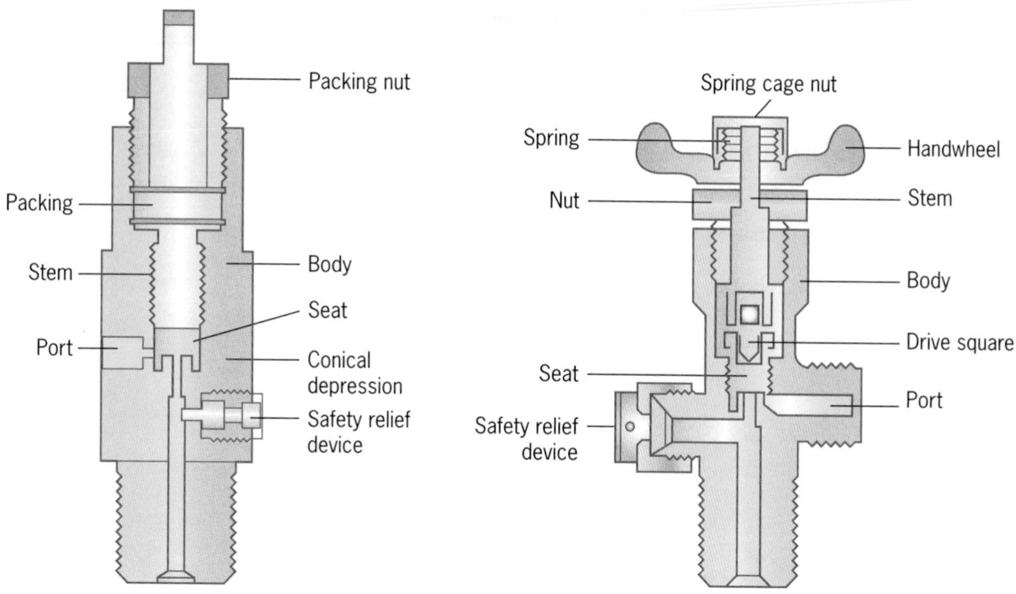

FIGURE 15–7 Direct-acting cylinder valve. When closed, the stem and seat are screwed together by the handwheel. To open the valve, the stem is screwed away from the seat using the handwheel.

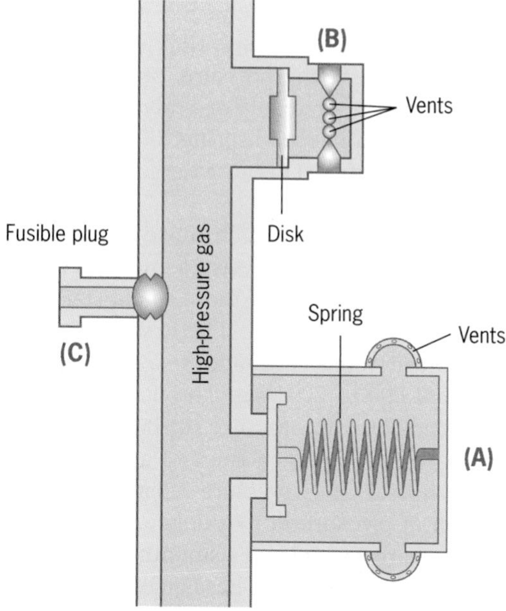

FIGURE 15–8 Cylinder pressure-relief systems. (**A**) Spring loaded device. When gas pressure exceeds the spring tension, the spring is compressed to the top, allowing gas to escape through the vents. When gas pressure is reduced to normal, the spring tension re-seats the valve. (**B**) Frangible disk. When gas pressure exceeds safe limits, the disk ruptures, allowing all of the contents of the cylinder to escape into the atmosphere through the vents. (**C**) Fusible plug. If the temperature inside or outside the cylinder exceeds safe limits, the plug melts, allowing all of the gas in the cylinder to safely escape. Adapted from Branson RD, Hess DR, Chatburn RL. *Respiratory Care Equipment*. 2nd ed. Lippincott Williams & Wilkins; 1999.

pressure-reducing valves that regulate and maintain the pressure at the station (room) outlets at 50 psig. Ventilators, blenders, and flow meters can be connected directly to the station outlets without further need for pressure control.

When cylinders of gas are used, the pressure in a full cylinder may be 2200 to 2500 psig and must be reduced to the standard and safe working pressure of 50 psig through attachment of a high-pressure-reducing valve called a *regulator* to the cylinder outlet. High-pressure regulators can be direct acting or indirect acting; configured in single or multiple stages; and preset or adjustable.

For most respiratory therapy applications, the single-stage regulator is adequate. **Figure 15–9** illustrates the basic components and operating functions of a direct-acting, single-stage, preset high-pressure-reducing regulator. The regulator is connected to the cylinder by a pin-indexed or ASSS fitting. The high-pressure source of gas enters at the inlet, usually passing through a fine-sintered brass filter to remove any debris. A pressure gauge is positioned at the inlet to indicate the pressure in the cylinder, which is directly related to the volume of gas in the cylinder. The body of the regulator is divided by a flexible diaphragm into two chambers: a high-pressure chamber and a chamber open to ambient pressure. A spring is attached to the ambient-pressure side of the diaphragm. A valve stem is attached to the high-pressure side of the diaphragm, and its end is positioned in the high-pressure inlet. In the regulator, the very high pressure from the cylinder is exerted on a very small area of the valve stem, which is balanced by the much larger area of the diaphragm. The tension of the spring exerts a preset pressure on the diaphragm and moves the valve stem to hold the high-pressure inlet open. When the gas outlet is open, the high-pressure inlet remains open and

TABLE 15-8 Guidelines for Safe Cylinder Storage and Handling

Storage
Cylinder storage must be in compliance with NFPA standards and all local, state, and federal regulations.
Cylinders must be stored in a cool, dry, fire-resistant enclosure that has good ventilation to prevent accumulation of gas if leaks occur.
Cylinder storage areas must be protected from the elements to prevent exposure to rain, snow, ice, and temperatures above 125° F.
Cylinder storage areas must be locked and secured from access and tampering by all unauthorized persons and should not be located near flammable or combustible substances.
Segregated locations for full and empty cylinders within the cylinder storage area must be clearly labeled to prevent their commingling.
Flammable gases must not be stored with gases that support combustion.
Large cylinders must be stored upright, with their protective caps screwed on tightly, and secured by a chain or other restraint mechanism to prevent their falling over.
Small cylinders may be stored upright or horizontally. In either position, they must be secured in racks, holders, or carts.
Cylinder storage areas must be clearly posted with signs inside and out indicating no smoking, open flames, combustible materials, oil or grease, etc.
Transport and Handling
Cylinders must be transported on an appropriate cart secured with a restraining chain or strap. They must never be dragged, rolled, or slid.
Large cylinders must be transported with their protective caps screwed on tightly.
A cylinder should never be lifted by its protective cap. Cylinders should be transported and handled only by properly trained personnel.
Cylinders must never be handled with oily or greasy hands, gloves, or clothing.
Petroleum-based products and lubricants must never be used on cylinder valves, regulators, fittings, or connections. Oxygen and petroleum-based products coming into contact under pressure may cause an explosive oxidation reaction.
Cylinders and cylinder valves should always be treated with care and respect.

Derived with permission from NFPA 99, *Health Care Facilities*. Copyright © 1999 National Fire Protection Association, Quincy, MA. This reprinted material is not the official position of the NFPA on the referenced subject, which is represented only by the standard in its entirety.

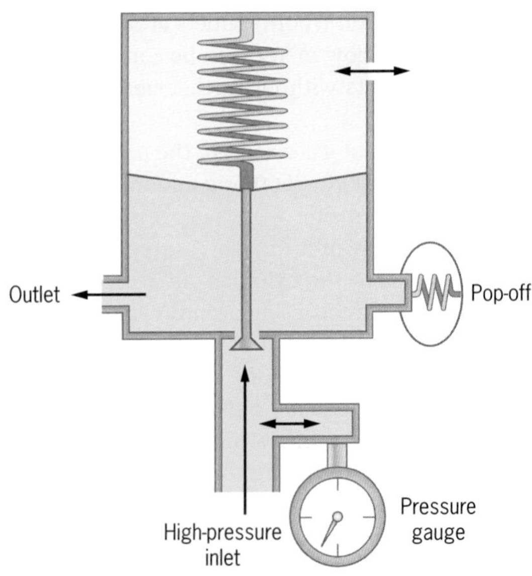

FIGURE 15-9 Single-stage regulator. These regulators are commonly used in clinical settings to regulate gas pressures. This article was published in *Egan's Fundamentals of Respiratory Care*. 7th ed. Scanlan CL, Wilkins RL, Stoller JK. Copyright Elsevier (Mosby) 1999.

a balance is maintained between the flow through the outlet and the pressure at the high-pressure inlet. This balance between the force of the spring upward on the diaphragm and the gas pressure above the diaphragm maintains a near-constant outlet pressure, usually preset at 50 psig. When the outlet is closed, pressure increases in the chamber above the diaphragm until it exceeds that of the spring, causing the diaphragm to move downward, pulling the valve stem down and closing the high-pressure inlet. A pressure relief (pop-off) valve is part of the high-pressure chamber. If a malfunction occurs, allowing excessive pressure to develop, this safety valve will open and vent the pressure, preventing a rupture of the diaphragm or regulator body. Modern regulator design has added a second spring, allowing regulators to become more compact because the size of the diaphragm can be reduced.

For applications in which more precise control of pressure and flow are necessary, a multistage regulator is used by connecting two or more single-stage regulators in a series (**Figure 15-10**). The first stage reduces the high pressure from the cylinder to a preset intermediate pressure of 500 to 700 psig. The next stage (or stages) further reduces the pressure until the 50-psig outlet pressure is reached. Each stage of a multistage regulator must have a safety pressure-relief valve. The gradual reduction of pressure in two or more stages allows for better pressure control and a smoother flow than can be attained in a single stage. These qualities may be important when precise instrumentation is being used, such as in research and diagnostic applications. Multistage regulators are larger, heavier, and more expensive than the more common single-stage units.

Safety-Indexed Connection Systems

The outlets of cylinder valves are manufactured so that only the regulator or connector specific for that gas or mixture can be attached. Three indexed safety systems are available for medical gases: the American Standard Compressed Gas Cylinder Outlet and Inlet Connections, usually referred to as the American Standard Safety System (ASSS); the Pin Index Safety System (PISS); and the Diameter Index Safety System (DISS). **Figure 15-11** compares these three safety systems.

American Standard Safety System

The threaded outlets of the faucet-like valves found on large cylinders (larger than E) conform to the American Standard Safety System. This system uses a combination of the following factors specific for each gas or gas combination:

- Diameter of the outlet (in thousandths of an inch)
- Number of threads per inch
- Right-handed or left-handed threads
- External or internal threads
- The shape of the mating nipple on the corresponding regulator

The large high-pressure oxygen cylinder (G, H, or K) has an outlet that meets the specification of 0.903-14-RH-Ext; that is, its outlet diameter is 0.903 inch with 14 threads to the inch, the connections will screw on with a turn to the right, and the threads are external. This configuration is referred to as CGA 540 by the CGA. **Figure 15–12** illustrates selected ASSS valve outlets and connections.

> **RESPIRATORY RECAP**
>
> **Indexed Safety Systems**
>
> » American Standard Safety System for large-capacity cylinders (above 200 psig)
>
> » Pin Index Safety System for small cylinders (above 200 psig)
>
> » Diameter Index Safety System for low-pressure connections (below 200 psig)

Pin Index Safety System

High-pressure medical gas cylinders, size E and smaller, use another indexing system known as the **Pin Index Safety System (PISS)**. This system uses a

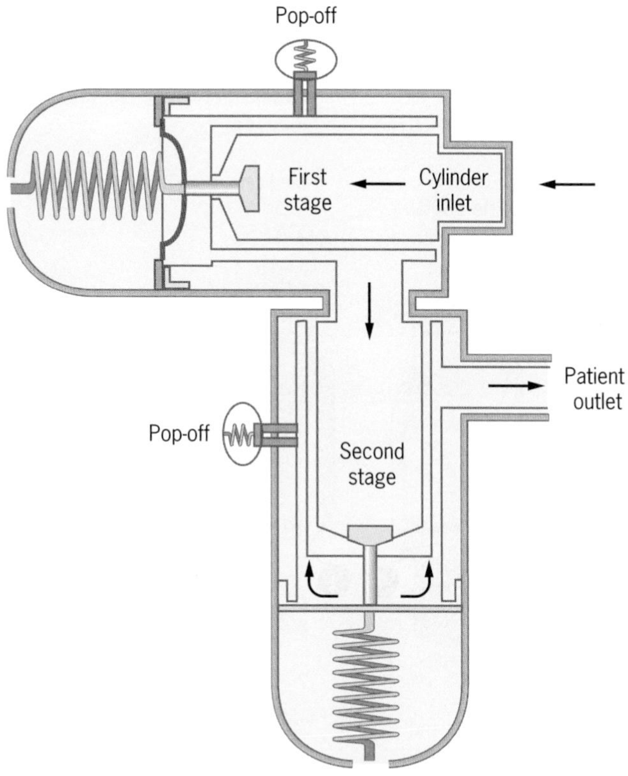

FIGURE 15–10 Multiple-stage regulator. These regulators are more complex than single-stage regulators and are thus more expensive. Multiple-stage regulators may be needed for situations in which very consistent gas pressures are necessary. Modified from Cairo JM, Pilbeam SP. *Mosby's Respiratory Care Equipment*. 6th ed. Mosby; 1999. Reprinted with permission.

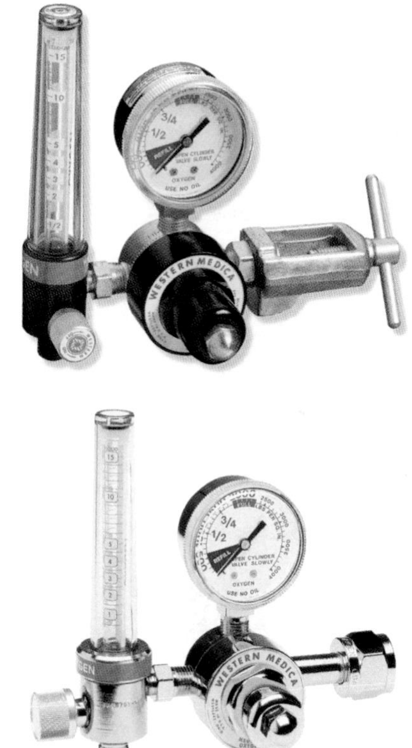

FIGURE 15–11 ASSS, PISS, and DISS connections. These safety systems prevent the inadvertent application of regulators or flow meters designed and calibrated for one gas to a different gas.

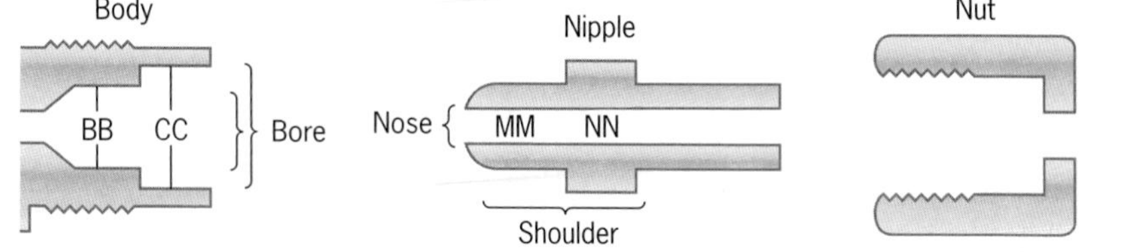

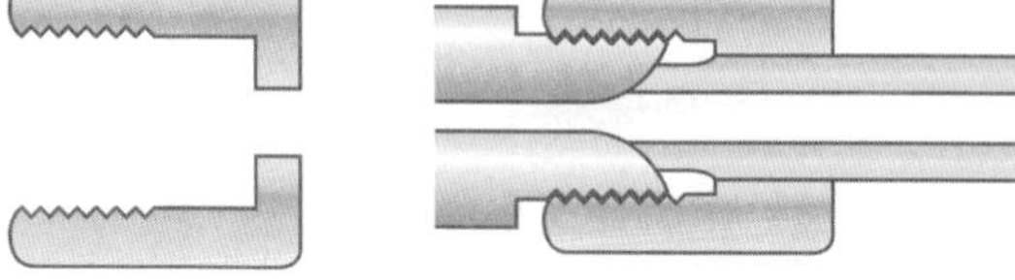

FIGURE 15–12 ASSS valve outlets. Modified from Dorsch JA, Dorsch SE. *Understanding Anesthesia Equipment*. 3rd ed. Lippincott Williams & Wilkins; 1994.

specific combination of two holes in the post valve just below the gas outlet for each gas or gas mixture. Any regulator or device intended to connect to the valve has pins that correspond to those holes, allowing for a proper connection. The pin index for oxygen is 2–5, which also is referred to as CGA 870. **Figure 15–13** shows the connection of a pin-indexed regulator to the post valve. **Figure 15–14** illustrates the pin-indexed positions for some common therapeutic gases.

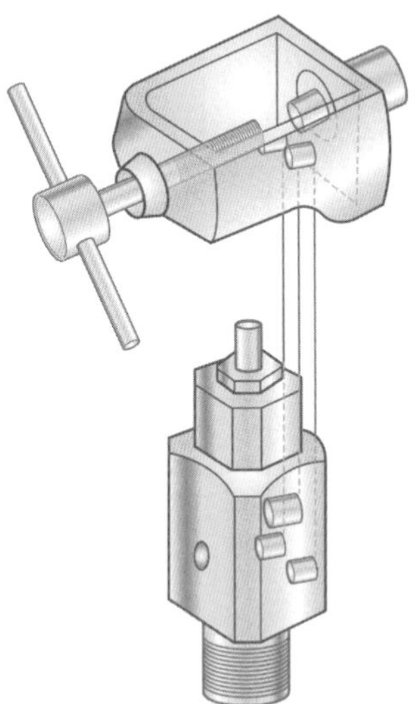

FIGURE 15–13 PISS valve outlet. Modified from Barnes TA, ed. *Core Textbook of Respiratory Care Practice*. 2nd ed. Mosby; 1994.

Diameter Index Safety System

The PISS and ASSS systems are designed for use on high-pressure cylinders. In contrast, the **Diameter Index Safety System (DISS)** was designed by the CGA for low-pressure (0–200 psig) connections and fittings. The DISS utilizes specific diameter-threaded male outlets that mate with a corresponding female nut and nipple. Different diameters, thread pitch, and nipple configurations are assigned to various gases and gas mixtures. The common oxygen DISS connection (CGA 1240) has a diameter of 9/16 of an inch and 18 threads to the inch,

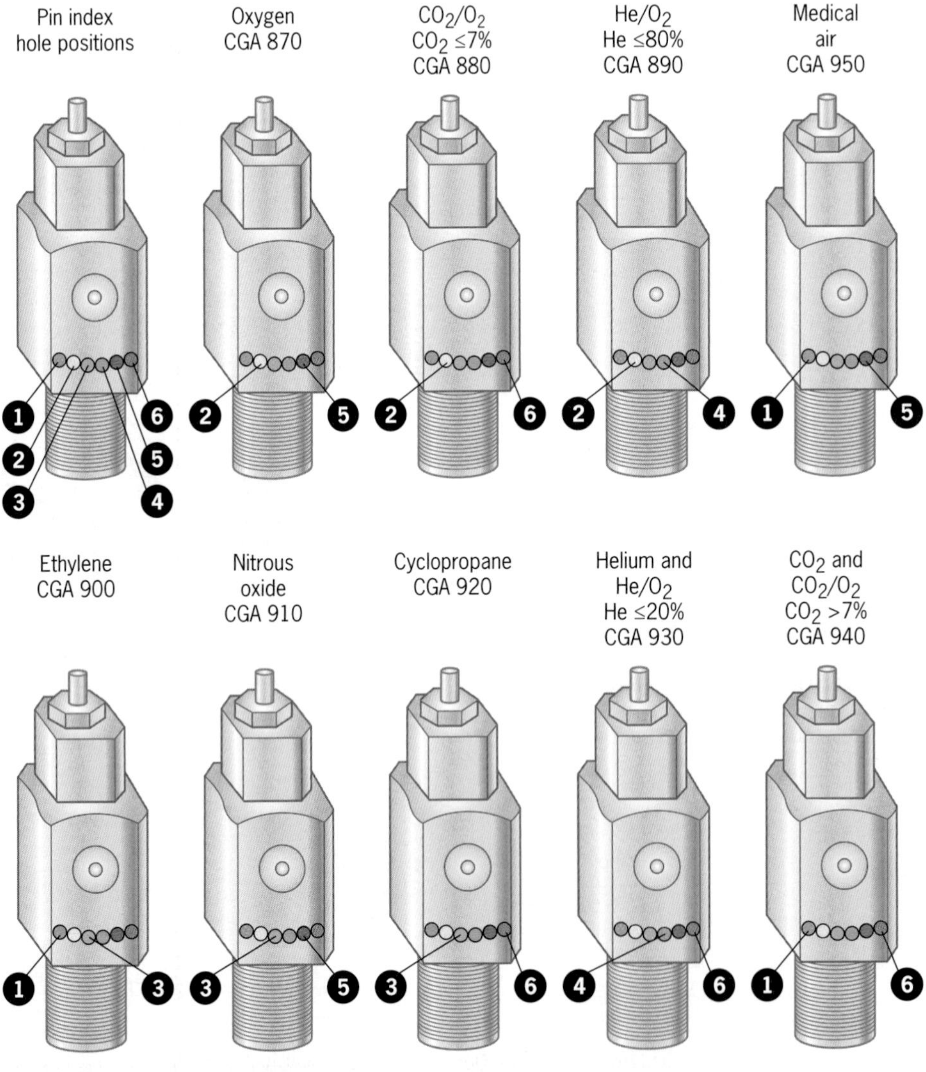

FIGURE 15–14 PISS pin positions.

often indicated as 9/16 − 18. This number will be found at the outlet of an oxygen flow meter, the inlet to a bubble humidifier, and the threaded connection at the end of an oxygen hose. It is important that the respiratory therapist recognize that this means that the relatively low gas flows that emerge from a flow meter and the threaded 50-psig working gas pressure connections have the same DISS connection. **Figure 15–15** illustrates the DISS safety systems for both flow meter outlets and 50-psig working-pressure outlets.

One factor that reduces the incidence of inadvertent connection of respiratory therapy equipment requiring relatively low flows (such as a nasal cannula) directly to working-pressure outlets in modern clinical settings is the common use of quick-connect connectors rather than threaded DISS connections.

Calculating Duration of Flow from a Gas Cylinder

Providers of gas therapy cannot expect that a bulk gas distribution system will always be available, and cylinders must be used in transport, during bulk system repair or failure, and whenever wall outlets are inaccessible. In such cases, it is important to calculate how long the contents of any size cylinder will last at a specified flow.

Calculating the remaining volumes of cylinder gas or duration at a specific flow requires data in both English and metric units, because cylinders are commonly sized by cubic foot (ft^3), whereas gas is administered in liters per minute (L/min). This simple calculation requires knowledge of how many liters of gas are in the cylinder and the prescribed L/min utilization rate. Dividing the contents of the cylinder (in liters) by the rate of flow (in L/min) provides the time (in minutes) available.

To make this calculation easier, conversion factors are commonly used. The conversion factor can be determined for any cylinder via multiplication of the cubic feet of gas in the full cylinder by 28.3 and division of that product by 2200 psig (the pressure in a full cylinder). As an example, the following equation illustrates the calculation of the conversion factor for an E cylinder:

$$\frac{22 \text{ Cubic feet of gas} \times 28.3 \text{ L/ft}^3}{2200 \text{ psig}} = 0.28 \text{ L/psig}$$

Table 15–9 presents the conversion factors for a number of cylinder sizes. The duration of flow can be accurately calculated by multiplying the actual pressure in the cylinder (psig) by the conversion factor for that size cylinder and dividing that product by the prescribed flow rate (L/min). **Equation 15–1** provides an example of the duration calculation.

> **RESPIRATORY RECAP**
>
> **Determining Duration of Flow**
>
> » Such calculations are necessary to determine how long an oxygen supply will last when a patient is transported.
>
> » For compressed gas cylinders, duration of flow is calculated by use of the actual pressure in the cylinder, the conversion factor for the size of the cylinder, and the oxygen flow rate.
>
> » For cylinders containing liquefied gas, the weight of the cylinder is used to infer the amount remaining because the gauge shows a constant pressure.

It also is important to realize the serious consequences of allowing a cylinder to run completely out when in clinical use. For this reason, most respiratory therapists consider cylinders with 500 psig to be effectively empty. A modified formula that takes this into account is the following:

$$\frac{(1600 - 500 \text{ psig}) \times 0.28}{4 \text{ L/min}} = 77 \text{ minutes}$$

By using the conversion described in Equation 15–1, 77 minutes is equivalent to 1 hour and 17 minutes. In this example, the cylinder needs to be changed in 1 hour and 17 minutes (at which time the cylinder will contain 500 psig, which is effectively empty).

It also is important to note that cylinders of pure carbon dioxide and nitrous oxide contain a mixture of liquid and gas and that the cylinder pressures will remain constant until the last bit of liquid has evaporated. A pressure gauge on a cylinder containing liquefied gas shows a constant pressure—the vapor pressure of that

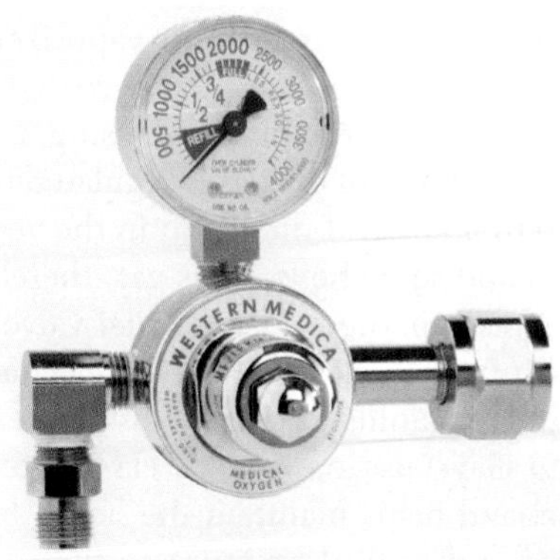

FIGURE 15–15 DISS safety systems: flow meter and 50-psig outlet.

TABLE 15–9 Cylinder Conversion Factors

	Conversion Factors		
Cylinder Size	O_2, Air, O_2/N_2	O_2/CO_2	He/O_2
D	0.16	0.20	0.14
E	0.28	0.35	0.23
G	2.41	2.94	1.93
H or K	3.14	3.84	2.50
T	3.54		

O_2, oxygen; N_2, nitrogen; CO_2, carbon dioxide; He, helium.

EQUATION 15–1

Calculation of Duration of Flow

When an E cylinder with 1600 psig of oxygen is used at a flow rate of 4 L/min, the duration of flow is calculated as follows:

$$\frac{1600 \text{ psig} \times 0.28 \text{ L/psig}}{4 \text{ L/min}} = 112 \text{ minutes}$$

This can be converted to hours by dividing the number of minutes by 60:

$$\frac{112 \text{ minutes}}{60} = 1 \text{ hour and } 52 \text{ minutes}$$

Respiratory therapists must be careful to recognize that decimal fractions of hours do not indicate minutes; 0.5 hour equals 30 minutes, for instance.

gas. This pressure bears no relationship to the contents until all the liquid gas has been vaporized, when the pressure will begin to drop. Therefore, cylinders containing these gases must be weighed to determine their remaining contents. The contents are directly related to the weight of the contents minus the weight of the cylinder. For example, if the weight of the liquid in the full cylinder is 30 pounds, it follows that when the weight decreases by 15 pounds, half of the contents would have been used.

Central Medical Gas Distribution

Today medical gases are available to medical consumers in portable high-pressure gas cylinders, bulk (liquid) cylinders, and fixed liquid systems that feed pipelines for gas supply. Containers of liquefied gases such as oxygen are portable, containing a few liters or gallons to several hundred gallons in a delivery vehicle or several thousand gallons in a tanker truck or railway car. Bulk liquid oxygen storage vessels, such as those found at most hospitals, contain from 500 to 10,000 gallons. Oxygen and other medical gases from bulk storage containers are distributed where needed through a piping system throughout the hospital.

Most hospitals and many other healthcare facilities, such as skilled nursing homes, rehabilitation centers, and outpatient surgical or diagnostic clinics, commonly feature piped medical gas distribution systems for oxygen, air, and vacuum. Depending on usage, systems for nitrous oxide and occasionally for nitrogen and other gases may also be centrally distributed from a bulk source. Central oxygen, air, and vacuum piping systems have made these commodities as common as water faucets and available at every bedside and other locations throughout most healthcare facilities.

Because of the potential hazards medical gases pose to the general public during transportation and to handlers and patients in healthcare settings, a fairly complex array of regulatory and recommending agencies have become involved, each providing extremely detailed information, specifications, regulations, and safety procedures that are beyond the scope of this text.

Systems for Gas Storage and Distribution

Acute care facilities use an enormous amount of oxygen daily. As an example, 50 patients using oxygen at 2 L/min require a total of 144,000 liters of oxygen gas in 24 hours, the equivalent of 21 H cylinders a day, or 625 a month. A large, active facility may require many times more. To satisfy this demand, a bulk liquid oxygen storage system is generally used.

Containers for the bulk supply of liquid oxygen are referred to as *stand tanks, vessels,* or *dewars* (named for Scottish chemist and physicist Sir James Dewar, its inventor). These containers are available in sizes ranging from as small as 500 gallons to 6000 gallons or more. Because 1 gallon of liquid oxygen is equal to 3.785 liters of liquid oxygen, and 1 liter of liquid converts to 861 liters of gaseous oxygen, a 500-gallon stand tank can deliver 1.6 million liters of gas, and a 6000-gallon vessel can deliver 19.5 million liters. Refilling a liquid bulk supply tank is much more cost effective than physically handling and exchanging the equivalent amount of gas stored in cylinders. (For example, a full H or K cylinder only contains 7075 L of O_2.)

Because the boiling point of liquid oxygen is –297.3° F, liquid oxygen must be stored in a container resembling a thermos bottle to keep heat transfer to a minimum and maintain the liquid state. All liquid storage containers, from small portable units for individual patient use to the largest stand tanks, are similarly designed and constructed, as shown in **Figure 15–16**. The liquid oxygen is held in an inner stainless steel vessel surrounded by an outer exterior shell. Between the inner vessel and the outer shell is an insulation-filled space in which a vacuum is drawn. The inner reservoir contains oxygen both as a liquid and as a gas.

As oxygen is needed in the facility, liquid oxygen flows from the reservoir and is quickly converted to gas through exposure to the ambient temperature as it passes through the vaporizing coils. So much heat is necessary for this vaporization process that the vaporizer plates are kept extremely cold and are frequently coated with ice as a result of moisture in the air condensing and freezing on them. The pressure of the gas is regulated to enter the facility at 50 to 55 psig. If the liquid in the vessel warms up too much and some boils off as gas, thereby increasing the gas pressure, the pressure-relief valve will open, allowing a controlled release of pressure. This release of gas causes the remaining gas in the vessel to expand and, according to Gay-Lussac's law, lowers the temperature in the vessel and helps maintain the liquid between its boiling point and critical pressure so that most of the contents remain in the liquid state.

The National Fire Protection Association (NFPA) issues standards concerning the placement, construction, and maintenance of bulk vessels and piping systems that have been widely adopted by local and state regulatory authorities.

Liquid oxygen is transported to the facility by tanker truck or rail and filled on location, as shown in Figure 15–16. The liquid reservoirs are similar to cold/hot beverage thermos bottles in which a vacuum between inner and outer walls provides the insulation. As the liquid oxygen (No. 1) continuously warms and decompresses, it evaporates into the head of the stand tank (No. 2.). It flows out through pressure regulation (No. 3) and vaporizer systems (No. 4) to the hospital. A pressure-relief valve will vent off pressure if it becomes excessive.

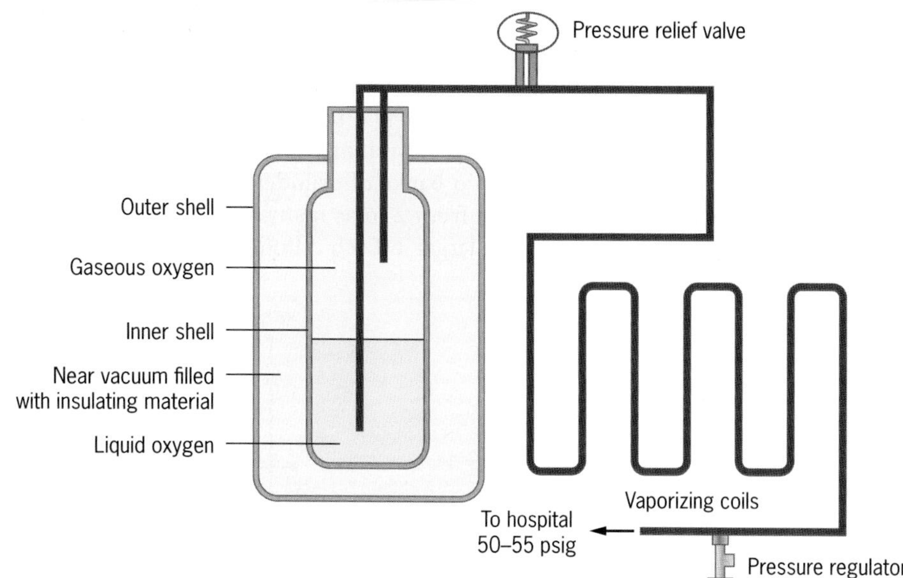

FIGURE 15–16 Bulk O_2 storage. Adapted from Branson RD, Hess DR, Chatburn RL. *Respiratory Care Equipment*. 2nd ed. Lippincott Williams & Wilkins; 1999.

Incidents involving bulk oxygen systems are not rare. A lack of preventive maintenance or miscommunication between respiratory care and facilities management departments can lead the oxygen system to abruptly stop, which is a major emergency. Oxygen loss in the operating room or critical care unit must be quickly corrected with easily available backup cylinder gas. Without predetermined emergency protocols in place, the response will usually be slow and disorganized. Analysis of catastrophic loss of the oxygen supply in hospitals has implicated the following causes:

- False alarms caused by calibration drift of pressure sensors
- Excessive depletion of the reserve supply because of pressure imbalance between the main and reserve supply
- Failure of the vacuum seal on the reserve supply
- Inappropriate manipulation of supply valves
- Leakage around valves and ruptured piping
- Failure of monitoring personnel to notify appropriate service personnel
- Occlusion of pressure sensors with foreign substance

Other potentially serious problems include the following:

- Filling bulk cylinders with the wrong gas
- Misconnection of pipelines following remodeling
- Damage from high winds, tornadoes, earthquakes, and fires

Because of the potential for catastrophic failure of oxygen supply systems and the serious injury that would occur under such circumstances, hospitals and clinics should have procedures in place for response to such a failure. Procedures should minimally include standards for maintaining adequate numbers of backup cylinders as well as a rapid distribution plan for operating rooms and critical care areas. It has also been suggested that institutions should regularly provide practice opportunities for such a possibility. For extreme catastrophic failures of the bulk storage facility, an emergency connection to the distribution system is also provided so that a liquid oxygen delivery truck can be directly connected into the distribution system to provide a temporary gas supply.

The NFPA requires that the reserve supply be equal to a 1-day average supply. A reserve supply in a second liquid bulk reservoir may be used. Besides acting as a backup, this second reservoir also continuously adds a small amount of gas as normal vaporization occurs. Check valves (one-way valves) prevent any leaks in either system from inadvertently draining the other. Facilities with less volume demand may need only a reserve bank of large gas cylinders (as discussed in the following section concerning alternating supply systems). Alarms that alert personnel to problems in a bulk system traditionally signal the following:

- Low liquid level in either primary or reserve systems
- Reserve in use following a switchover when the main supply falls to approximately 85 psig (586 kPa)
- Main supply line pressure variations exceeding ±20%

Oxygen piping systems may be supplied from the central source of liquid oxygen or combination of liquid and gas or from cylinders of gaseous oxygen. The volume of gas used and the costs of supply dictate the choice of the supply source. Three central bulk supply systems are used: alternating supply systems with or without a reserve emergency supply, and continuous supply systems.

Alternating Supply Systems

Alternating supply systems are used in smaller facilities to supply oxygen or specialty gases such as nitrous oxide and nitrogen (**Figure 15–17**). Figure 15–17A shows the arrangement of an alternating supply system without a reserve supply. It consists of two banks of cylinders, each of which contains anywhere from 2 to as many as 20 cylinders, usually size H or the larger T. Each cylinder is connected by a flexible pigtail pipe containing a one-way check valve that allows flow from the cylinder only to a high-pressure header and a pressure regulator. The combination of the header with its pigtails, valves, and regulator is often referred to as a *manifold*.

Gas flows from one bank of cylinders, the supply bank, through its manifold valve and regulator, where the pressure is reduced to 100 to 200 psig, and then to the

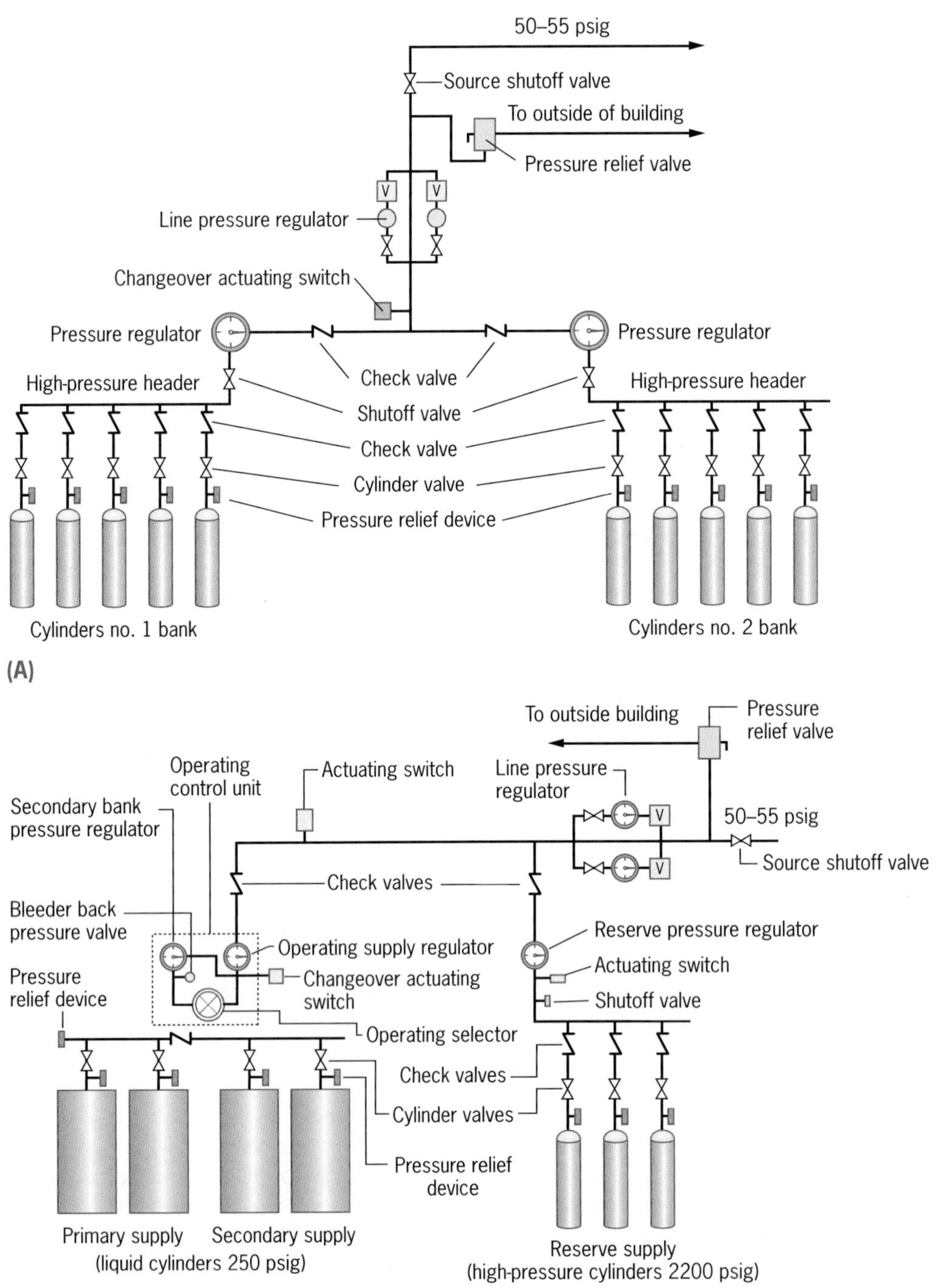

FIGURE 15–17 (**A**) Alternating supply system without a reserve supply (used to back up a bulk storage system). (**B**) Alternating supply system with an emergency reserve supply (used as a primary supply system). Reprinted with permission from NFPA 99, *Health Care Facilities*. Copyright © 1999, National Fire Protection Association, Quincy, MA. This reprinted material is not the official position of the NFPA on the referenced subject, which is represented only by the standard in its entirety.

main-line pressure regulator, where it is further reduced to 50 to 55 psig and proceeds through the main shut-off valve and into the piping system. Flow continues until the pressure in the supply bank approaches 100 to 200 psig, which activates the changeover switch, automatically opening the valve from the second bank of cylinders, which now becomes the supply bank, and closing the valve from the first bank. The switch-over process also activates an alarm, usually located in a manned location, such as the security, maintenance, or central telephone operator area, to alert the responsible party that one bank is empty and needs to be refilled or replaced.

Figure 15–17B shows an alternating supply system with an emergency reserve supply. This system is similar to that in the previous description but adds a third gas supply as an emergency reserve in case either the primary or the secondary supply or both fail. The system depicted shows liquid vessels being used as the primary and secondary sources of the oxygen supply. Banks of cylinders of gaseous oxygen also can be used.

Gas Piping Systems

Gases stored in bulk quantities are distributed throughout the facility via a system of pipes, valves, and outlets, as shown in **Figure 15–18**. The entire system must meet the standards of the NFPA for construction, installation, testing, and maintenance. The pipe must be type K or L seamless copper tubing specially cleaned to remove all traces of oxidizable material. Engineering studies determine the size (diameter) of pipe required to maintain 50 psig and maximum flows throughout the system. In most cases the pipe decreases in diameter size the further it is from the main supply. Each pipe must be clearly labeled at regular intervals to indicate the gas contained. All joints and fittings are sweat-soldered with silver solder.

Before any outlets are attached or added to the piping system, the system is blown clean with oil-free dry air or nitrogen to dislodge and eliminate debris such as solder, flux, and metallic filings. When construction is completed, the entire system is pressurized to a minimum of 150 psig with oil-free dry air or nitrogen. Every fitting, connection, valve, and outlet is individually inspected for leaks, and the system then must hold that pressure for at least 24 hours. This cleaning and testing procedure is conducted on each of the piping systems, including those for oxygen, air, nitrous oxide, and any others. Before any piping system can be put into use, the test gas must be

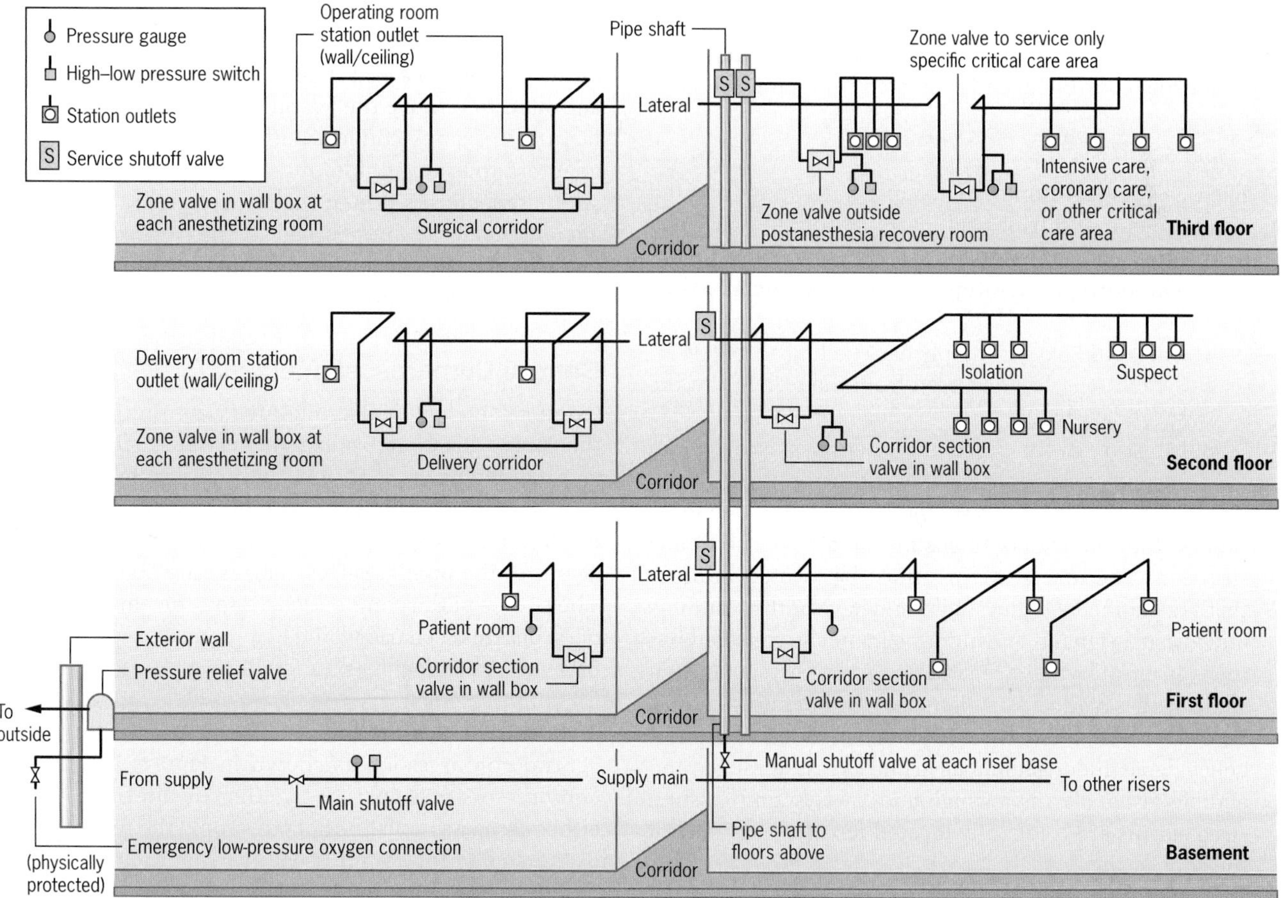

FIGURE 15–18 Gas distribution system in an acute care facility. Reprinted with permission from NFPA 99, *Heath Care Facilities*. Copyright © 1999, National Fire Protection Association, Quincy, MA. This reprinted material is not the official position of the NFPA on the referenced subject, which is represented only by the standard in its entirety.

purged and the gas supply for that system attached. Every outlet must then be tested to ensure that it functions properly, that flow and pressure meet specifications, and that the correct gas is present.

Valves

A primary supply shut-off valve must exist at the point at which the main distribution pipe leaves the bulk supply and, when the bulk supply is located outside the building, at the point at which the main supply pipe enters the facility. From the main line, pipes extend laterally and usually further branch into zones serving groups of patient rooms or other service areas. Risers proceed vertically from the main line to service upper floors.

A shut-off valve must be located at the beginning of each lateral branch and at the base of each riser. Additionally, zone valves are placed in strategic locations so as to isolate specific areas in case of fire or during maintenance or construction. Zone valves are frequently grouped so that several gases may be controlled from the same box, as shown in Figure 15-18. In addition to groups of patient rooms, zone valves would be located to control gas flow to nurseries, each intensive care unit, the emergency department, recovery rooms, and other necessary areas. Each anesthetizing location (operating rooms or special procedures rooms, for example) must have its own dedicated shut-off valve. All shut-off valves must be easily accessible, clearly marked to indicate the area being controlled, and protected from tampering.

Gauges and Alarms

Each gas distribution system must have an automated continuous-monitoring and alarm system to alert personnel to such changes in the system as the following:

- The normal operating pressure has increased or decreased.
- The liquid oxygen supply has reached a low level.
- Switch-over has occurred from the primary to the secondary bank.
- Moisture in the piped air system has exceeded an acceptable level.

A master set of alarms should be located in two locations within the facility to ensure rapid response to any situation. The master alarms must be located in areas that are manned 24 hours a day and have both an audible and a visual signal that cannot be manually canceled but turns itself off when the situation is corrected. Certain critical areas of the hospital, such as the operating rooms, recovery room, intensive care units, nurseries, and emergency department, should have line-pressure gauges and audible/visual alarms for high and low system pressure. Area alarms are frequently located next to or as part of the zone valves.

Zone Valves

For safety, a system of partitioning off branches of the system is required. Zone valves are strategically installed to allow isolation of outlets in a certain area or zone (**Figure 15–19**). Valves are required immediately adjacent to anesthetizing areas, life-support rooms, or intensive care units to shut flow down in case of a leak, repair, or fire. Practitioners must secure alternative gas sources for patients before closing a zone valve.

Station Outlets

The station outlet is the working end of the gas distribution piping system. It is where the gas can be accessed and used by delivery devices such as flow meters and ventilators. Outlets, like cylinders, must be color-coded and labeled for the gas they deliver and have indexed fittings that allow connection only to compatible delivery devices. Two safety systems are in common use: the DISS and the quick-connect system.

A DISS-type station outlet is shown in Figure 15–19. As the female nut and nipple is manually tightened onto the outlet, it makes contact with the plunger, which moves it forward until it seats on the stem, allowing gas to flow from the piping system. Representative examples of quick-connect adapters are shown in **Figure 15–20**. The internal mechanism of both types of outlet systems is similar, but in quick-connect adapters, instead of tightening a screw fitting to engage the plunger, a male adapter is inserted into the outlet to push the plunger against the seat and allow air flow. Once inserted, the adapter is locked in place and a release mechanism, such as the pressing of a button or twisting of a collar, must be activated to remove the adapter from the outlet. Manufacturers of quick-connect outlet stations have designed adapters that are usable only in their brand of outlet. All manufacturers design their adapters so that only an adapter made for oxygen can fit into an oxygen outlet and would be physically incompatible with an air, nitrous oxide, or vacuum outlet.

Central Compressed Medical Air Distribution

Compressed medical-grade air is commonly used as the source gas to aerosolize medications, activate large-volume nebulizers, and mix with oxygen in ventilators and blenders to provide a specific FIO_2. The central air distribution system is similar to the oxygen system in the layout of the piping, valves, alarms, and station outlets. The source of the compressed air may be banks of cylinders, but this scenario would be practical only in the case of a very small facility or a facility with a minimal need for compressed air.

In most cases the bulk of the air comes from dual central compressors, as shown in **Figure 15–21**. The compressors can operate together or alternate, but in either case each must be able to supply the full demands of the facility for compressed air when the other needs maintenance. For medical use, the compressors must deliver oil-free air. The compressors used for central systems are usually of the piston or centrifugal/rotary type. Piston compressors use carbon or Teflon rings to create

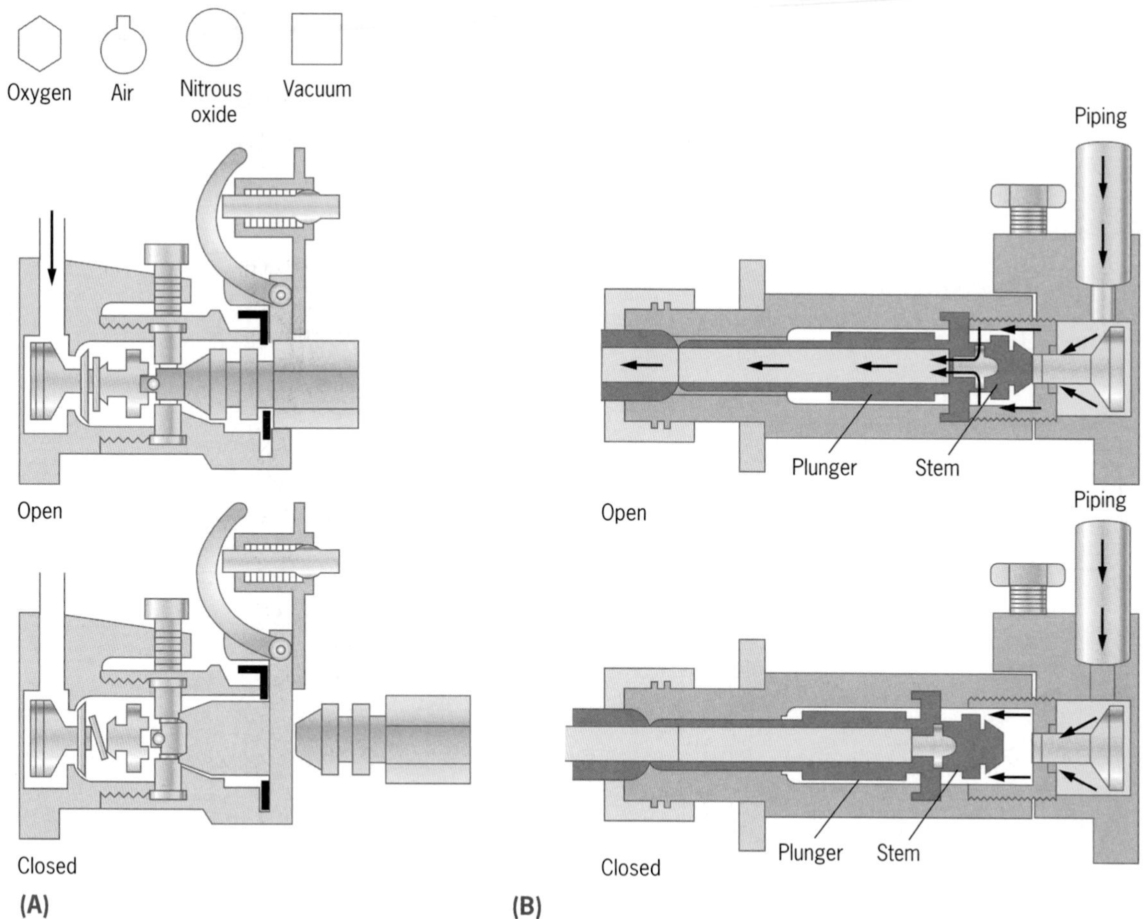

FIGURE 15–19 (**A**) Quick-connect station outlets and (**B**) DISS. Modified from Cairo JM, Pilbeam SP. *Mosby's Respiratory Care Equipment*. 6th ed. Mosby; 1999. Reprinted with permission.

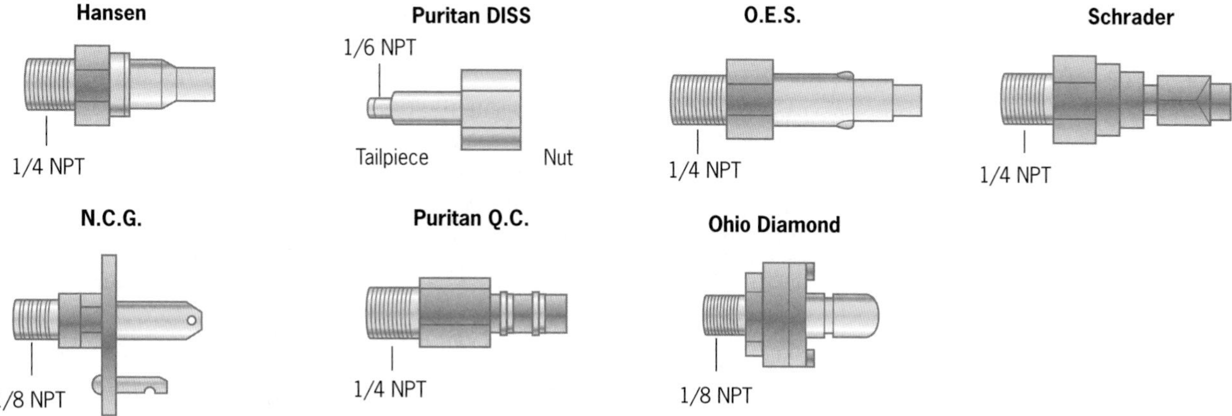

FIGURE 15–20 Quick-connects. Wall outlets only open when a quick-connect is fully locked in place. Modified from Cairo JM, Pilbeam SP. *Mosby's Respiratory Care Equipment*. 6th ed. Mosby; 1999. Reprinted with permission.

the seal against the cylinder wall and eliminate the need for an oil lubricant. High-pressure rotary compressors use a liquid sealant, usually water, between the impeller blades and the housing, again eliminating the need for oil lubrication.

To meet NFPA standards, the air being drawn into the compressor must come from an intake located outside the building, above the roof, and in a location where the air is free from particulates, odors, engine exhaust, and vacuum system discharges. The air is

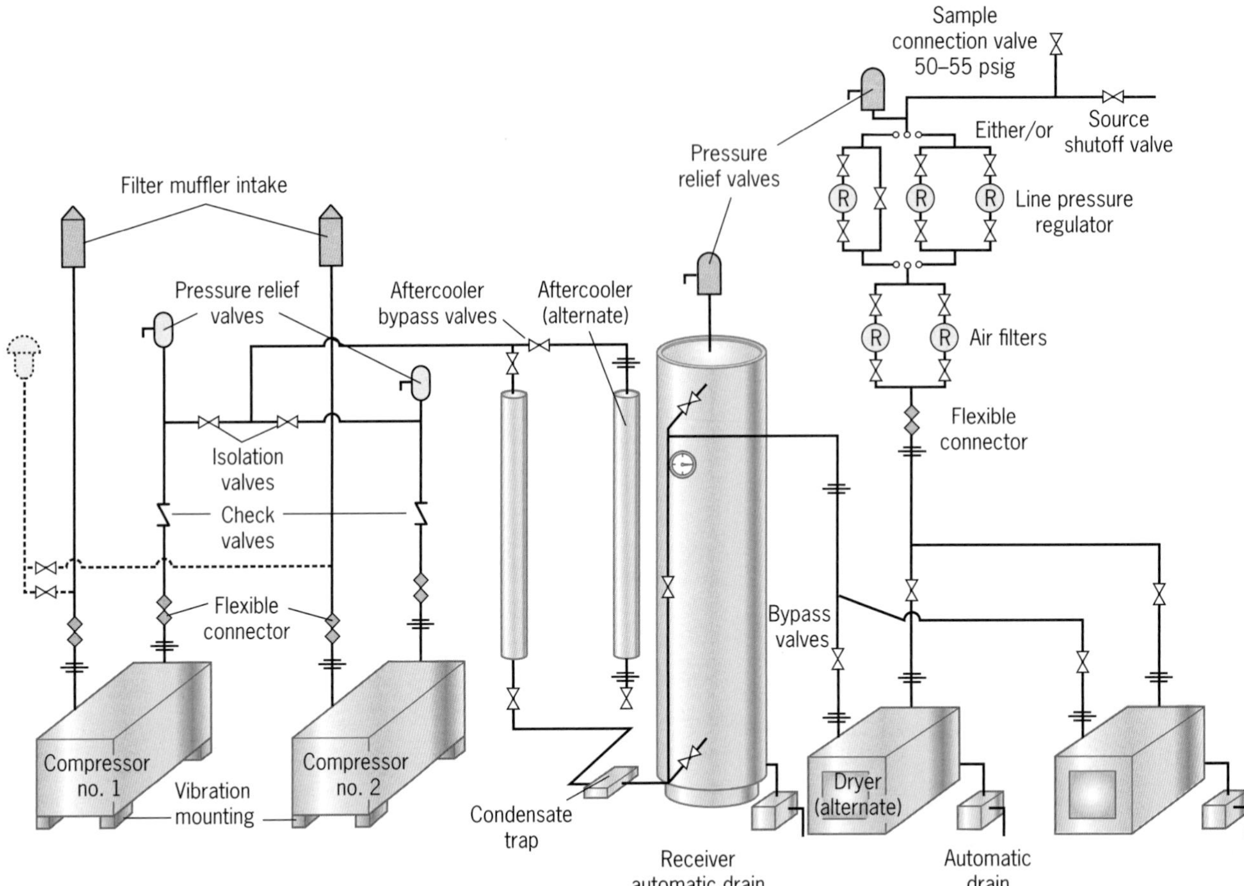

FIGURE 15–21 Bulk air supply compressor system. Dual compressors ensure that the supply of compressed air will be maintained. Note the engineering required to manage the considerable amount of water produced in compressing ambient air. Modified from Cairo JM, Pilbeam SP. *Mosby's Respiratory Care Equipment*. 6th ed. Mosby; 1999. Reprinted with permission.

filtered, compressed, and passed through an after-cooler, where cooling causes water vapor to condense and be removed. The air then is stored in a large tank called a reservoir or receiver. Air is stored in the receiver tank at a pressure higher than the 50 to 55 psig required in the facility's piping system, allowing the air to flow in a steady stream from the line pressure regulator. In addition, the compressor turns off when a sufficient supply of air is stored in the reservoir, thus minimizing wear, and additional water vapor condenses in the tank and is eliminated.

After leaving the reservoir, the air passes through a dryer to remove any remaining water vapor. Removal of water vapor, water droplets, and humidity from the compressed air supply is important to prevent microbial growth (e.g., bacteria, fungi, molds) within the piping system. Water in the air supply causes serious damage to ventilators, blenders, and other devices. Alarm systems to monitor dew point (humidity) and carbon monoxide in the main air supply are required by NFPA standards. Although the compressed air delivered to the station outlets is dry, oil free, and clean, it is not sterile, and thus appropriate filters should be used between the air supply and delivery devices.

SUGGESTED READING

Cairo JM, Pilbeam SP. *Mosby's Respiratory Care Equipment.* 8th ed. St. Louis: Mosby; 2009.

Compressed Gas Association. *Handbook of Compressed Gases.* 4th ed. Boston: Kluwer Academic; 1999.

Kacmarek R, Dimas S. *Essentials of Respiratory Care.* 4th ed. St. Louis: Mosby; 2005.

National Fire Protection Association. *NFPA 99: Standard for Health Care Facilities.* Quincy, MA: NFPA; 2005.

West JB. *Respiratory Physiology: The Essentials.* 8th ed. Philadelphia: Lippincott Williams & Wilkins; 2008.

Wilkins RL, Dexter JR, Heuer A. *Clinical Assessment in Respiratory Care.* 6th ed. St. Louis: Mosby; 2009.

CHAPTER 16

Therapeutic Gases: Management and Administration

John Boatright
Jeffrey J. Ward

OUTLINE

OBJECTIVES

1. Discuss the scientific basis for oxygen therapy.
2. Compare flow control devices.
3. Discuss the effect of downstream resistance on the accuracy of flow control devices.
4. Compare low-flow and high-flow oxygen delivery systems.
5. Calculate the F_{IO_2} delivered by a nasal oxygen cannula.
6. Describe the principles of oxygen analysis.
7. Describe the therapeutic application of medical gases, including equipment selection, dosage regulation, patient interface, and therapy outcome monitoring.
8. Discuss the application of heliox, carbogen, and nitric oxide.

KEY TERMS

air-entrainment mask
air–oxygen blenders
air-to-oxygen mix ratios
Bourdon gauge flow meter
carbogen
carboxyhemoglobin
diffusion defect
flow restrictor
heliox
high-flow nasal cannula
high-flow/fixed-performance devices
hyperbaric oxygen therapy
hypercarbia
hypoxemia
hypoxemic drive
hypoxia
low-flow/variable-performance devices
nasal oxygen cannula
nasal oxygen catheter
nitric oxide (NO)
nitrogen washout atelectasis
nonrebreathing mask
oxygen analyzers
oxygen hoods
oxygen-induced hypoventilation
oxygen tents
oxygen toxicity
partial rebreathing mask
retinopathy of prematurity (ROP)
shunt
simple oxygen mask
Thorpe tube flow meter
ventilation-perfusion ($\dot{V}/\dot{Q}$) mismatch

INTRODUCTION

This chapter presents information relevant to the therapeutic application of gases typically used in respiratory care. Not discussed are anesthetic gases, gases used for diagnostic purposes, or invasive oxygenation using extracorporeal membrane (ECMO) techniques. The primary focus of the chapter is the use of oxygen (O_2) to treat hypoxemia, but other gases are also discussed, including helium–oxygen mixtures (heliox), inhaled nitric oxide (iNO), and carbon dioxide–oxygen mixtures (carbogen).

The Rationale for Supplemental Oxygen

Supplemental oxygen is indicated when **hypoxemia** is suspected by history or physical examination or is documented by laboratory data (**CPG 16–1**). The short-term application of high concentrations of oxygen is relatively free of complications, and withholding oxygen can have grave consequences. Tachycardia, cardiac dysrhythmias, dyspnea, tachypnea, use of accessory muscles, increased difficulty breathing, mental confusion, and disorientation may indicate the need for oxygen therapy. In adults, children, and infants (older than 1 month) at rest breathing room air, a Pa_{O_2} below 60 mm Hg or Sp_{O_2} below 90% indicates the need for O_2 therapy. In neonates, a Pa_{O_2} below 50 mm Hg, Sp_{O_2} below 88%, or capillary P_{O_2} below 40 mm Hg indicates the need for O_2 therapy. In the non–critically ill patient, the medical history and previous laboratory findings are key data.

Hypoxemia can be caused by low ambient O_2, hypoventilation, **ventilation-perfusion ($\dot{V}/\dot{Q}$) mismatch**, **shunt**, or **diffusion defect**. Hypoxemia caused by $\dot{V}/\dot{Q}$ mismatching or diffusion defects is accompanied by an increased $P(A-a)_{O_2}$. Only with hypoxemia due to rarified atmosphere (e.g., altitude) or hypoventilation is the $P(A-a)_{O_2}$ normal. Further differentiation requires either testing after 100% oxygen breathing or carbon monoxide diffusion lung testing.

The physiologic mechanism by which increased inspiratory O_2 concentration (expressed either as a percentage of O_2 in the total atmosphere or as a fractional concentration [F_{IO_2}]) increases the Pa_{O_2} is by an increase in the partial pressure of oxygen in inspiratory air (P_{IO_2}), resulting in the increased partial pressure of oxygen in alveolar units that are ventilated (P_{AO_2}). The increased P_{AO_2} results in an increase in Pa_{O_2} and oxygen saturation of hemoglobin.

O_2 therapy is only a stopgap measure and does not address the underlying pulmonary pathology that resulted in hypoxemia. The ultimate cause of the hypoxemia must be addressed. For example, if the clinical problem is atelectasis (alveolar collapse), recruitment of collapsed alveoli is the definitive care, even if O_2 therapy is temporarily needed to prevent vital organ injury related to the hypoxemia and the resultant tissue **hypoxia** caused by the maldistribution of ventilation.

CLINICAL PRACTICE GUIDELINE 16–1

Oxygen Therapy in the Acute Care Hospital

Indications

- Documented hypoxemia, defined as a decreased Pa_{O_2} in the blood below normal range (Pa_{O_2} of less than 60 mm Hg or Sp_{O_2} below 90% in subjects breathing room air or with Pa_{O_2} and/or Sp_{O_2} below the desirable range for the specific clinical situation)
- An acute care situation in which hypoxemia is suspected; substantiation of hypoxemia is required within an appropriate period of time following initiation of therapy
- Severe trauma
- Acute myocardial infarction
- Short-term therapy or surgical intervention (e.g., postanesthesia recovery, hip surgery)

Contraindications

- No specific contraindications to oxygen therapy exist when indications are judged to be present.

Precautions and Possible Complications

- With $Pa_{O_2} \geq 60$ mm Hg, ventilatory depression may occur in spontaneously breathing patients with elevated Pa_{CO_2}.
- With $F_{IO_2} \geq 0.5$, absorption atelectasis, oxygen toxicity, and/or depression of ciliary and/or leukocytic function may occur.
- Supplemental oxygen should be administered with caution to patients suffering from paraquat poisoning and to patients receiving bleomycin.
- During laser bronchoscopy, minimal levels of supplemental oxygen should be used to avoid intratracheal ignition.
- Fire hazard is increased in the presence of increased oxygen concentrations.
- Bacterial contamination associated with certain nebulization and humidification systems is a possible hazard.

Modified from AARC clinical practice guideline: oxygen therapy for adults in the acute care facility—2002 revision and update. *Respir Care*. 1991;36:1470–1413. Reprinted with permission.

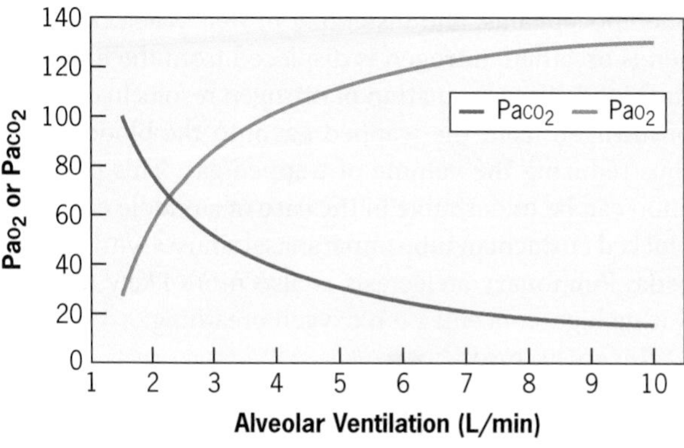

FIGURE 16–1 Relationship between alveolar ventilation, PaO_2, and $PaCO_2$. Note that a reduction in alveolar ventilation causes $PaCO_2$ to increase and PaO_2 to decrease.

RESPIRATORY RECAP

Oxygen Therapy

- » O_2 therapy should be considered for hypoxemic conditions.
- » Short-term use of high O_2 concentrations is relatively free of serious complications.
- » Hypoxemia can be caused by low ambient O_2, hypoventilation, $\dot{V}/\dot{Q}$ mismatch, shunt, or diffusion defect.
- » O_2 therapy increases the PaO_2.
- » The cause of hypoxemia must be corrected; O_2 therapy is a stopgap measure.
- » Shunt cannot be corrected with O_2 therapy.

The net improvement in Pao_2 with supplemental oxygen is variable. Previously normal subjects with carboxyhemoglobinemia who are given 100% O_2 can achieve a Pao_2 of more than 500 mm Hg very rapidly. At the opposite extreme, patients with a very high shunt will have only a small increase in Pao_2 breathing 100% O_2. With hypoventilation, an increase in F_{IO_2} increases Pao_2 sufficiently to compensate for the effect of the increased $Paco_2$ on Pao_2 until the primary hypoventilation can be corrected. Under normal barometric conditions, patients cannot tolerate the arterial hypoxemia that will result from $Paco_2$ levels of over 90 mm Hg without oxygen-enriched atmospheres due to the level of displaced Pao_2 (**Figure 16–1**).

Patient Conditions Commonly Warranting Oxygen Therapy

Patients with hypoxemia due to $\dot{V}/\dot{Q}$ mismatch or diffusion defect require O_2 therapy until more definitive therapies take effect. With chronic obstructive pulmonary disease (COPD), hypoxemia is caused by $\dot{V}/\dot{Q}$ mismatch with or without hypercapnia. Continuous long-term oxygen therapy in COPD has been shown to be life prolonging. Its usefulness during exercise or for sleep-related hypoxemia has not been as well established. Patients with interstitial pulmonary fibrosis may also require supplemental oxygen if a diffusion defect becomes significant.

TABLE 16-1 Summary of Conditions Commonly Requiring Treatment with Oxygen

Condition Causing Hypoxemia	General Approach
Perioperative	Treat with O_2 to maintain adequate SpO_2 or PaO_2.
Chronic obstructive pulmonary disease	Use care to identify patients with chronic hypercarbia because CO_2 retention may occur with O_2 administration. Patients who are chronically hypoxemic may tolerate a lower PaO_2.
Adult respiratory distress syndrome	Treat with O_2 and PEEP to maintain adequate PaO_2.
Cardiopulmonary resuscitation	Use of 100% O_2 is standard practice with bag-valve ventilation.
Myocardial infarction	Use of low-flow nasal cannula is standard practice for myocardial infarction patients.
Cardiogenic pulmonary edema	Treat with O_2 to maintain adequate SpO_2 or PaO_2.
Cor pulmonale	Treat with O_2 to maintain adequate SpO_2 or PaO_2.
Carbon monoxide poisoning	Treat with high-concentration O_2. SpO_2 or PaO_2 may not be reflective of the degree of disruption in O_2 transport caused by carboxyhemoglobin. Consider hyperbaric oxygen treatment.
Absorption of air in body cavities	Unusual indication for O_2 therapy, such as pneumocephalus, subcutaneous emphysema, or small pneumothorax.

PEEP, positive end-expiratory pressure.

The perioperative state predisposes patients to the need for supplemental oxygen (**Table 16–1**). General anesthesia commonly causes a decrease in Pao_2 secondary to increased $\dot{V}/\dot{Q}$ mismatch and decreased functional residual capacity. The effects are greatest with thoracic and abdominal surgery, elderly or obese patients, and preexisting pulmonary disease. Hypoxemia usually responds to intraoperative or postoperative supplemental oxygen. General anesthetics can also reduce the normal respiratory center's responsiveness to hypoxemia. Postoperative oxygen administration has been used to decrease the risk of surgical site infection, but the effectiveness of this is controversial.

Acute respiratory distress syndrome (ARDS) is a nonspecific pulmonary response to a range of pulmonary and nonpulmonary insults. ARDS is characterized by interstitial infiltrates, alveolar hemorrhage, diffuse atelectasis, and reduced functional residual capacity. Intrapulmonary shunting results in hypoxemia that is difficult to correct with supplemental oxygen. Patients often require a high F_{IO_2} and mechanical ventilation with positive end-expiratory pressure (PEEP). Although based on a different etiology, respiratory distress syndrome of the newborn also results in pulmonary atelectasis, causing increased work of breathing and hypoxemia. Supplemental oxygen is used to improve PaO_2 in the setting of pulmonary (and/or intracardiac) right-to-left shunting and $\dot{V}/\dot{Q}$ mismatch; adjuncts of continuous positive airway pressure (CPAP) or PEEP with mechanical ventilation are added as indicated.

During cardiopulmonary resuscitative (CPR) efforts in adults, as much O_2 as possible should be provided. Typically, manual bag-mask ventilators are equipped to deliver 100% O_2 when connected to an adequate O_2 supply. Respiratory therapists on code teams should ensure that adequate O_2 flows are provided to such equipment as soon as practicable. To minimize the possibility of retinopathy of prematurity, it is advisable that premature infants requiring frequent or repeated resuscitative efforts be ventilated using concentrations of O_2 that have been previously determined to meet the patient's oxygenation needs.

Although there is a lack of data to suggest that it alters mortality in uncomplicated care of patients after a myocardial infarction (MI), it is rational to use supplemental oxygen to avoid hypoxemia and decrease the incidence of dysrhythmias. Tissue hypoxia and lactic acidemia often occur after MI as the result of reduced cardiac output rather than hypoxemia. Cardiogenic pulmonary edema commonly requires the use of high-concentration oxygen therapy to sustain the patient while diuretics and vasoactive drugs reduce the effects of the left ventricular failure. If present, tissue hypoxia is commonly the result of reduced cardiac output and hypoxemia from $\dot{V}/\dot{Q}$ mismatching, shunting, and diffusion defect in the lung. Oxygen therapy is indicated in such cases. It can be administered in conjunction with CPAP or noninvasive ventilation.

Cor pulmonale is a common manifestation of chronic hypoxemia. Chronically low P_{AO_2} induces hypoxic pulmonary vasoconstriction. Oxygen administration can reverse the arteriolar constriction unless the vascular changes have become fixed or destructive vascular disease has occurred. One of the goals of long-term oxygen therapy is to reverse or prevent cor pulmonale.

In carbon monoxide poisoning, **carboxyhemoglobin** reduces the oxygen saturation. The treatment of choice for carbon monoxide poisoning is 100% O_2, sometimes in conjunction with hyperbaric conditions, to achieve the highest PaO_2 possible. The use of 100% oxygen is considered an essential therapy in the treatment of carbon monoxide poisoning. In addition to maximizing the quantity of O_2 dissolved in serum, the high PaO_2 resulting from breathing 100% O_2 causes a rapid dissociation of carbon monoxide from hemoglobin. High oxygen concentrations are also a valuable stopgap measure in severe acquired methemoglobinemia until treatment with methylene blue.

High concentrations of oxygen have been used to treat patients who have collection of air in body cavities or tissues. Such conditions include pneumothorax, pneumomediastinum, subcutaneous emphysema, pneumocephalus, and distended bowel. When pure oxygen is breathed, nitrogen is displaced from the lungs and the blood. The elimination of nitrogen results in diffusion of nitrogen from the trapped gas into the bloodstream, thus reducing the volume of trapped gas. This phenomenon can be undesirable in the case of a middle ear with a blocked eustachian tube or paranasal sinuses with blocked ostia. Pulmonary atelectasis is also more likely to occur during high-concentration oxygen breathing.

Recently, brain tissue Po_2 (Pbo_2) monitoring has been introduced in clinical practice to guide management of patients with severe traumatic brain injury. Brain tissue oxygenation is measured by an electrode that is inserted through the same bur hole as an intracranial pressure monitor. The target Pbo_2 is above 15 mm Hg. One of the strategies that is used to increase Pbo_2 is an increase in PaO_2 by increasing FIO_2. Whether this results in improved patient outcomes is currently controversial.

RESPIRATORY RECAP

Oxygen Therapy

» O_2 therapy is used for perioperative conditions, COPD, ARDS, CPR, MI, pulmonary edema, carbon monoxide poisoning, and traumatic brain injury.
» O_2 may be of limited usefulness for anemia, low cardiac output, or high shunt.
» Nitrogen washout with high O_2 concentrations may accelerate air absorption.

Limitations of Supplemental Oxygen

Supplemental oxygen should not be used as a substitute for ventilation when ventilation is indicated; in this case, O_2 therapy should be used in conjunction with ventilation. Patients with hypoxic conditions produced by acute anemia (Hb $<$ 10 g/dL) can be temporarily supported by high-concentration supplemental oxygen, but only a small portion of resting oxygen needs can be met with supplemental O_2. Patients with hypoxia produced by low cardiac output or low tissue perfusion may also be placed on O_2 therapy, but again only a small portion of resting oxygen needs can be met with supplemental O_2. The goal of oxygen therapy in these situations is to maximize the blood's oxygen content. However, once hemoglobin is 100% saturated, further increases in PaO_2 have a marginal effect on oxygen content and oxygen delivery. Patients with large cardiac or pulmonary right-to-left shunts will have a disappointing response to oxygen therapy because increasing the P_{AO_2} in the areas of good $\dot{V}/\dot{Q}$ matching cannot supersaturate hemoglobin to overcompensate for poorly saturated blood from areas with shunting.

Complications and Hazards of Oxygen Therapy

Supplemental oxygen is a relatively benign drug. Far more patients die from hypoxia than suffer complications from oxygen therapy. However, respiratory

TABLE 16–2 Summary of Complications and Hazards of Oxygen Therapy

Complication or Hazard	Patients Affected	Etiology	Prevention
O_2 toxicity	All ages, patients on 50% or higher O_2	Additional free radicals of O_2 in increased O_2 atmospheres	Use minimal O_2 to maintain normal SpO_2 and/or PaO_2.
Nitrogen washout atelectasis	All ages, patients receiving 90% to 100% O_2	Sedentary breathing, obstruction, absorption of PaO_2 by hemoglobin	Alveolar recruitment; deep breathing; ambulate patient as soon as possible; avoid use of 90% to 100% O_2.
Oxygen-induced hypoventilation	Patients with chronic hypercarbia	Haldane effect, $\dot{V}/\dot{Q}$ change, or ventilatory drive suppression	Limit O_2 to minimum necessary to correct hypoxemia (SpO_2 88% to 92%).
Retinopathy of prematurity	Premature infants	Retinal vasoconstriction in the presence of $PaO_2 > 80$ mm Hg	Maintain PaO_2 of premature infants between 50 and 80 mm Hg.
Closure of the ductus arteriosis	Infants with congenital heart defects that require ductal blood flow	High PaO_2 triggers closure of the ductus	Maintain modest PaO_2.
Support of combustion	All patients	O_2 accelerates combustion	Maintain fire-safe environment: no sparks, open flames, or smoking. Use no oil or other petroleum products with O_2 therapy. Avoid the use of flammable clothing and plastics.

therapists must take precautions to minimize untoward effects of O_2 therapy. **Table 16–2** summarizes possible complications caused by supplemental oxygen and how to prevent them.

Oxygen Toxicity

Pulmonary **oxygen toxicity** refers to cellular injury of lung parenchyma and airway epithelium. When intracellular Po_2 is elevated, cytotoxic free radicals are generated in excessive amounts. The free radicals include superoxide anions (O_2^-), singlet oxygen molecules, hydroxyl radicals (OH), and partially reduced oxygen metabolites such as hydrogen peroxide (H_2O_2). Some free radical production occurs as a normal aspect of cellular metabolism; intracellular enzymes such as superoxide dismutase and catalase eliminate most toxic products. Nonenzymatic antioxidants include vitamin A, ascorbate, cysteine carotene, tocopherol, and hemoglobin.

Toxic effects depend on the concentration, length of exposure to oxygen, and underlying lung condition. Because cellular levels cannot be directly measured, dosage relationships can only be presumed. To date, no exact threshold concentration has been established at which toxicity occurs. Onset and severity are more severe in hyperbaric oxygen therapy and may include neuropathologic effects such as vertigo and nausea followed by altered behavior, clumsiness, and finally convulsions.

Clinical manifestations of high-concentration oxygen breathing include symptoms of mild to severe substernal pain, dyspnea, fatigue, and paresthesias. There is tracheobronchitis, and ciliated airway cells have depressed activity within 6 hours of 100% oxygen exposure. Clinical signs of gas exchange abnormalities can occur within 24 to 48 hours at an FIO_2 of 1.0. They include hypoxemia caused by right-to-left shunting from atelectasis, decreased lung compliance, and infiltrates on chest radiograph that reflect the cellular pathology. Inflammatory changes, edema, and fibrosis occur with exposure longer than 72 to 96 hours.

Multiple factors affect tolerance, including hormones, catecholamine levels, vitamin E levels, and drugs such as paraquat. It has been suggested that bleomycin therapy may accelerate the onset of O_2 toxicity, but this claim remains controversial because of the difficulty of human research.

In clinical practice, high-concentration oxygen should not be withheld from critically ill patients or for transport. Breathing concentrations of up to 0.5 for 2 to 7 days does not result in clinically significant lung impairment. Extended exposure to an FIO_2 above 0.6 should be avoided when possible. A goal of respiratory therapists is to use the minimum concentration required to achieve adequate tissue oxygenation. Mechanical ventilation with PEEP should be considered when a high FIO_2 is required.

Nitrogen Washout Atelectasis

Absorption atelectasis can occur with high-concentration oxygen breathing, secondary to washout of nitrogen from the lungs (**nitrogen washout atelectasis**). During room air breathing, the partial pressure of nitrogen in the lungs is approximately 570 mm Hg. When FIO_2 is increased, nitrogen molecules are replaced with O_2 in the alveoli. Any airway obstruction or reduction in ventilation may result in oxygen being removed by pulmonary blood. Alveolar collapse is more likely in the absence of nitrogen, and hypoxemia from increased physiologic shunting will result.

Oxygen-Induced Hypoventilation

To understand **oxygen-induced hypoventilation**, it is necessary to understand the neurologic control of ventilation. Under normoxic conditions, the minute-to-minute control of ventilation is managed by the CO_2 drive (carbic ventilatory drive). Chemoreceptors in the central nervous system respond to the hydrogen ion concentration ($[H^+]$) of the cerebral spinal fluid (CSF). The $[H^+]$ in the CSF is determined primarily by the $Paco_2$. That is, when the $Paco_2$ increases, so does the $[H^+]$ of the CSF. Receptors on the surface of the brain stem sense changes in $[H^+]$ of the CSF and respond by changing the level of ventilation to maintain a normal $Paco_2$. These central chemoreceptors are very sensitive to small changes in H^+ and will maintain the $Paco_2$ very closely.

A second, more primitive chemoventilatory drive is the **hypoxemic drive** (also called the *hypoxic drive*). The peripheral chemoreceptors, which are located in the chest and neck (in the aortic arch and the carotid bodies), respond when the Pao_2 falls below about 60 mm Hg. Whenever the Pao_2 decreases below the hypoxemic threshold of about 60 mm Hg, increased ventilation will be stimulated. For example, when a person climbing a mountain reaches an altitude where Pio_2 causes a Pao_2 of less than 60 mm Hg, the climber will experience an increased ventilatory rate and tidal volume. Although the hypoxemic drive will always override the CO_2 drive, the two chemical drives act independently of each other.

Oxygen-induced hypoventilation may occur in patients who have adapted to long-term **hypercarbia** (elevated baseline $Paco_2$). Examples of diagnoses associated with chronic hypercarbia are chronic bronchitis, cystic fibrosis, and obesity hypoventilation syndrome. In these patients, the carbic drive is no longer appropriately responsive to $Paco_2$ levels, and the hypoxemic drive becomes the primary ventilatory drive. These patients require hypoxemia to stimulate their ventilation ($Pao_2 <$ 60 mm Hg). Administration of supplemental oxygen to return the Pao_2 to normal levels may suppress the hypoxemic ventilatory drive, and ventilation may diminish. As a result of the oxygen-induced hypoventilation, the $Paco_2$ increases and the patient becomes more hypoxemic.

Recently, the role of hypoxemic drive suppression to explain oxygen-induced hypoventilation has been challenged. Studies have shown that the hypoxemic drive is only marginally affected when oxygen is administered. Oxygen-induced hypercarbia has been attributed to changes in ventilation-perfusion relationships resulting in an increased dead space and/or the influence of O_2 on the ability of hemoglobin to bind CO_2 (the Haldane effect). Regardless of the mechanism, clinicians must be alert to the possibility of an increase in $Paco_2$ with supplemental O_2 in patients with chronic hypercapnia. Oxygen should be titrated to produce a Pao_2 of 50 to 60 mm Hg with an Spo_2 in the 88% to 92% level. Oxygen must never be withdrawn in the face of high or rising $Paco_2$. If oxygen-induced hypercapnia results in a severely elevated $Paco_2$, mechanical ventilation is indicated.

Retinopathy of Prematurity

Retinopathy of prematurity (ROP) is an insult to the developing retinal vasculature from an elevated Pao_2. It was first described in 1942 and termed *retrolental fibroplasia* (RLF). In ROP, oxygen radicals attack the incompletely developed retinal tissue, resulting in vasoconstriction, which can progress to complete obliteration and retinal detachment. It was initially thought that supplemental oxygen was the iatrogenic culprit in ROP. However, elevated Pao_2 in retinal vessel walls is only one of several predisposing factors that can result in visual defects, which can progress to total blindness. Low birth weight, sepsis, gestational age, apnea, acidemia/hypercarbia, oxygen levels, and length of exposure all interact as multiple causes. ROP is also seen in low-birth-weight babies who did not receive supplemental oxygen. Occurrence of blindness varies from 1% to 3% in all live births and from 40% to 70% in infants weighing less than 1 kg. The incidence is inversely proportional to birth weight and highest in neonates weighing less than 1 kg.

In the 1940s and 1950s, the incidence of ROP reached epidemic proportions because oxygen was used without monitoring. Arbitrary guidelines limiting oxygen concentration to 0.4 resulted in increased infant mortality and cerebral palsy, complications reduced by the development of blood gas monitoring and pulse oximetry. Dietary supplementation with vitamin E can also ameliorate the effect and reduce the incidence of ROP through its antioxidant action. The Fio_2 of critically ill infants should be analyzed, and Pao_2 and Spo_2 monitored both by periodic blood gases and continuous pulse oximetry. Supplemental oxygen should be given to keep the Pao_2 above 50 mm Hg. Although the safe upper level is unknown, guidelines recommend less than 80 to 90 mm Hg. The duration of oxygen use as well as the Pao_2 is critical in developing ROP.

RESPIRATORY RECAP

Complications of Oxygen Therapy

- Oxygen toxicity is damage to lung tissue caused by breathing high concentrations of O_2.
- A patient's need for O_2 must override concerns about O_2 toxicity.
- Nitrogen washout atelectasis can occur with high concentrations of O_2.
- Oxygen-induced hypoventilation may occur in patients who rely on their hypoxemic drive.
- ROP only occurs in infants.
- Some infants with congenital heart defects need a low PaO_2 to maintain an open ductus.
- Oxygen is not explosive, but it increases the combustibility of other flammable materials.

Closure of the Ductus Arteriosis

Neonates with congenital heart lesions depend on patency of the ductus arteriosus for either pulmonary or systemic blood flow. Those with pulmonary atresia form the majority of cases, but cases also include those with coarctation of the aorta, tricuspid atresia, and aortic arch interruption. Many newborns will have profound hypoxia or circulatory collapse as the ductus closes spontaneously. Prostaglandin E_1 has been an important drug for management. Increasing PO_2 is the chief trigger of ductal smooth muscle contraction, and thus a modest PaO_2 is also indicated as a palliative measure or until corrective surgery is performed.

Support of Combustion

Fire hazard is a concern when dealing with normobaric oxygen and a major hazard in hyperbaric applications. Oxygen-enriched atmospheres in patient enclosures are a risk during laser bronchoscopy and head and neck surgery. Ignition can result in a flash flame via fine surface fibers of fabric or body hair. Combustible materials (e.g., cigarettes), sparking friction toys, and electric razors should be avoided in enclosures or close to open sources of oxygen.

Dosage Regulation and Administration Devices

Once the gas pressure has been reduced to the safe working pressure of 50 psig (by a cylinder/pressure regulator system or as supplied by a bedside gas distribution station connector), a device to provide more refined control of flow is usually needed. For example, when oxygen or gas mixtures are administered directly to the patient via mask, aerosol, or nasal cannula, a method for metering the flow is necessary. On the other hand, some equipment (such as blenders and ventilators) meter flow internally and do not need an external flow metering device. The respiratory therapist must understand this difference. Flow control devices can be categorized as follows:

- *Flow restrictor:* A preset, fixed flow controller.
- *Bourdon gauge flow meter:* An adjustable flow controller, with adjustable inlet pressure from a fixed outlet orifice.
- *Thorpe tube flow meter:* An adjustable flow controller, with preset inlet pressure from an adjustable outlet orifice.

Flow Restrictor

The most basic flow meter is commercially known as a **flow restrictor**. It is a carefully machined orifice attached to a 50-psig gas source. There are no adjustments and no gauges. A flow restrictor (**Figure 16–2**) has a specific-size orifice that allows a specific flow of gas to pass, provided the inlet pressure is a constant 50 psig. Flow restrictors are uncomplicated, require no maintenance (because they have no moving parts), can be used in any position, and do not allow accidental changes in flow. When a flow change is necessary, however, the single-flow flow restrictor must be removed and replaced by another with an orifice delivering the appropriate flow.

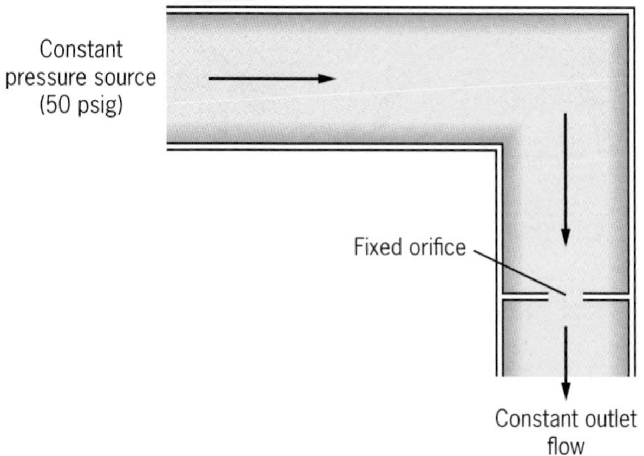

FIGURE 16–2 Fixed orifice flow restrictor. This article was published in *Egan's Fundamentals of Respiratory Care, Seventh Edition.* Scanlan CL, Wilkins RL, Stoller JK. Copyright Elsevier (Mosby) 1999.

This need can be met by the use of an adjustable flow restrictor that allows the selection of one of a number of orifices, depending on the flow required. Adjustable multiorifice flow meters in combination with an indirect single-stage, preset regulator are commonly used on small cylinders in home care or patient transport because of their compact and lightweight configuration. Other applications include emergency resuscitation packs, in which compact, lightweight devices require relatively high flows to a bag-valve-mask device. Because there is no way to indicate the actual flow, flow restrictors should be periodically checked with a calibration flow meter.

The outlet flow on a flow restrictor can be calculated using the following equation:

$$\dot{V} = (P_1 - P_2)/R$$

where $\dot{V}$ is the flow per unit of time (L/min), P_1 is the inlet pressure (50 psig), P_2 is the outlet pressure (atmospheric), and R is the resistance to gas flow through the orifice. Any change to the $P_1 - P_2$ relationship alters the accuracy of the output flow, which occurs if the inlet pressure varies from 50 psig or if increased resistance is present downstream from the orifice outlet, creating back pressure.

Bourdon Gauge Flow Meters

Like the flow restrictor just described, the **Bourdon gauge flow meter** has a fixed outlet orifice, but the pressure regulator is adjustable, which facilitates the adjustment of flow output by varying the pressure supply. The change in pressure is displayed on the Bourdon gauge face, which has been calibrated (labeled) in L/min, corresponding to the predictable flows at the variable inlet pressures. The Bourdon gauge is positioned between the pressure source and the fixed orifice. The gas pressure is transmitted to the gauge through a hollow tube. As the pressure increases, the closed distal end of the

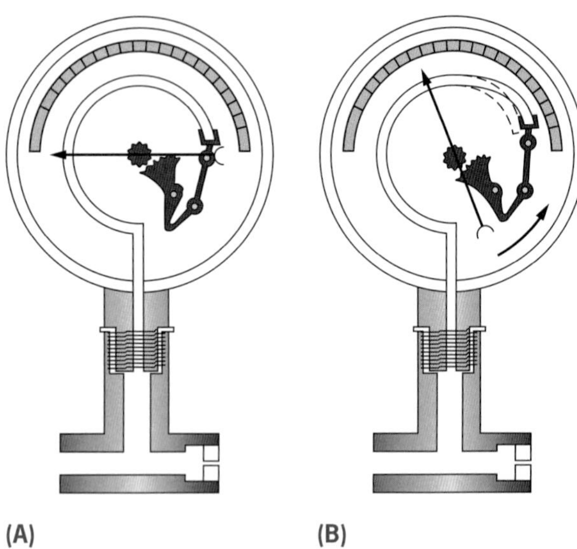

FIGURE 16–3 Bourdon flow gauge, showing the hollow pressure tube and gearing mechanism in an unpressurized state (**A**) and pressurized state (**B**). An increase in pressure causes straightening of the tube and movement of the indicator needle. Modified from Ward JJ. Equipment for mixed gas and oxygen therapy. In: Barnes TA, ed. *Core Textbook of Respiratory Care Practice*. 2nd ed. Mosby; 1994.

curved hollow tube is straightened (**Figure 16–3**). It is linked to a gear system and an indicator needle pointing to the calculated output flow for that pressure. Clinical devices frequently have two gauges: one that indicates cylinder pressure, and one that indicates the flow output (**Figure 16–4**). The gauge closest to the cylinder indicates the pressure contents of the cylinder.

With Bourdon gauge flow meters, the flow meter will deliver accurate flow rates if the outlet flow is unrestricted. However, when resistance is added downstream of the fixed outlet orifice, such as the addition of a long length of tubing and respiratory equipment, the outlet pressure (P_2) rises and the actual outlet flow is decreased (**Figure 16–5**). In fact, if the Bourdon gauge outlet were completely obstructed, the gauge would continue to show flow when in fact none would be present. Because pneumatic nebulizers present a large downstream resistance to the flow meter, they should not be used with a Bourdon gauge if accurate indication of flow rate is necessary.

Bourdon gauges are commonly used on medical gas cylinders for transport and when a mask or nasal cannula is used. These compact flow meters are handy because flow can be changed (in contrast to flow restrictors) and they can be read correctly without being held in a vertical (gravity-dependent position).

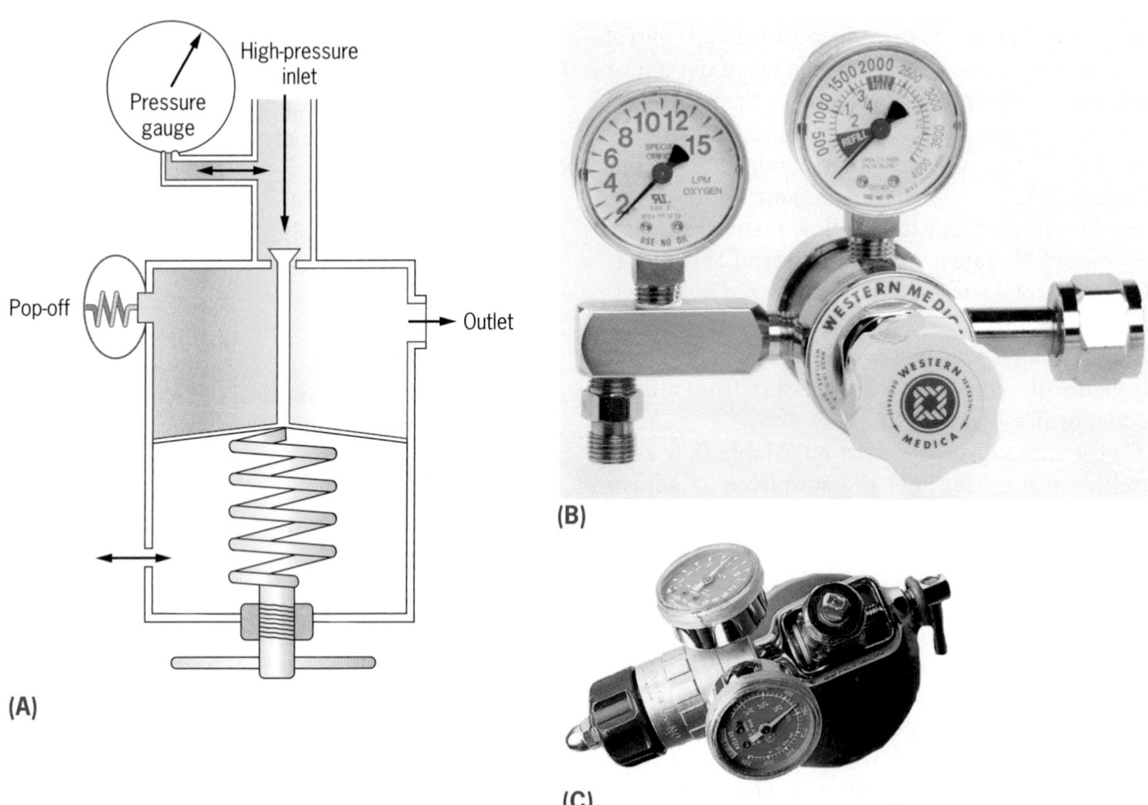

FIGURE 16–4 (**A**) Adjustable, direct-acting, single-stage, high-pressure-reducing regulator. (**B**) A single-stage, adjustable regulator with two Bourdon gauges. The gauge to the right, closest to the connection to the gas source, is calibrated in pounds per square inch (psi), indicating the contents of the cylinder. The Bourdon gauge closest to the outlet is calibrated in liters per minute (L/min). Flow is set by turning the knob, increasing or decreasing the regulator pressure and thus the outlet flow through the fixed orifice. (**C**) Bourdon gauge flow meter on an oxygen cylinder. (**A**) This article was published in *Egan's Fundamentals of Respiratory Care, Seventh Edition*. Scanlan CL, Wilkins RL, Stoller JK. Copyright Elsevier (Mosby) 1999.

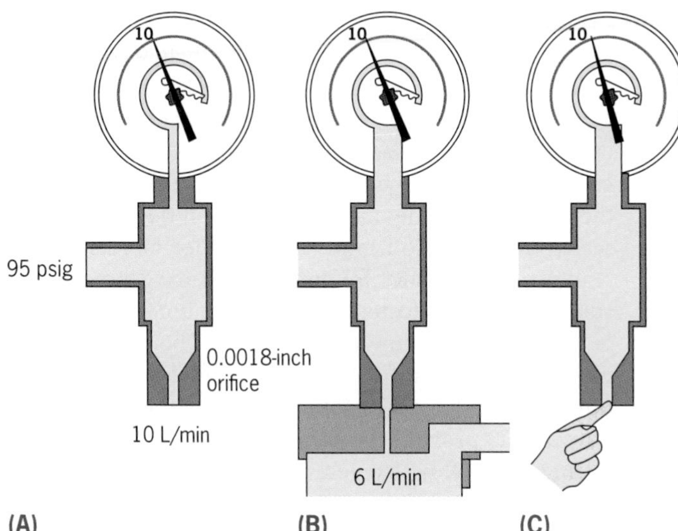

FIGURE 16–5 Bourdon gauge illustrating (**A**) that with a constant inlet pressure and a known fixed outlet orifice size, a predictable outlet flow is achieved and is indicated on the gauge face. Adding resistance downstream of the fixed outlet orifice (**B**) causes flow to be diminished, yet the gauge reading remains unchanged because it measures the pressure prior to the resistance. If the outlet orifice is completely obstructed (**C**), allowing no flow, the gauge continues to read a flow even though there is none because it continues to read preobstruction pressure.

Thorpe Tube Flow Meters

The most common type of medical gas flow meter has a needle valve for adjustment of flow and a hollow tube with an indicator float device. These are called pressure-compensated **Thorpe tube flow meters** or rotameters—or, more commonly, simply flow meters. The name *rotameter* implies use of a rotating bobbin or float instead of a spherical-type indicator. Rotameters are often used to administer anesthetic gases, which require greater accuracy in flow indication.

Unlike flow resistors and Bourdon gauges, a pressure-compensated Thorpe tube flow meter displays the actual outlet flow regardless of downstream resistance. As long as the inlet pressure remains constant, the pressure-compensated Thorpe tube flow meter displays correct readings of outlet flow. For this reason, these flow control and flow measurement devices are the most common type of dosage regulation device used in hospitals for direct, quick-connect application to piped outlet stations.

A Thorpe tube flow meter consists of a clear, tapered glass tube with a diameter that is larger at the top than at the bottom. The tube has graduated markings calibrated to indicate flow (usually liters or milliliters per minute). The gas flow is indicated by a float in the glass tube, and a needle valve controls the flow. When the needle valve is opened, gas flows from the pressure source. Gas entering the bottom of the Thorpe tube creates a pressure differential significant enough to lift the float. As the float rises in the tapered tube, the diameter of the tube increases (equivalent to an increase in the outlet orifice size) and more gas is able to flow around the float. Eventually the float stabilizes when the upward force of the pressure differential across the float equals the downward force of gravity.

The location of the needle valve in the Thorpe tube flow meter is important. It can be located distal or proximal to the Thorpe tube (**Figure 16–6**). Placing the needle valve distal to the Thorpe tube creates a pressure-compensated flow meter. With increasing back pressure applied to the outlet of the flow meter, the float drops, reflecting the decrease in outlet flow. The pressure-compensated Thorpe tube flow meter is preferred for clinical applications because it provides an accurate display of flow in the face of downstream resistance, provided it is in a vertical position and the inlet pressure is constant. **Figure 16–7** shows the effects of back pressure on pressure-compensated Thorpe tube flow meters, non-pressure-compensated flow meters, and Bourdon gauge flow meters.

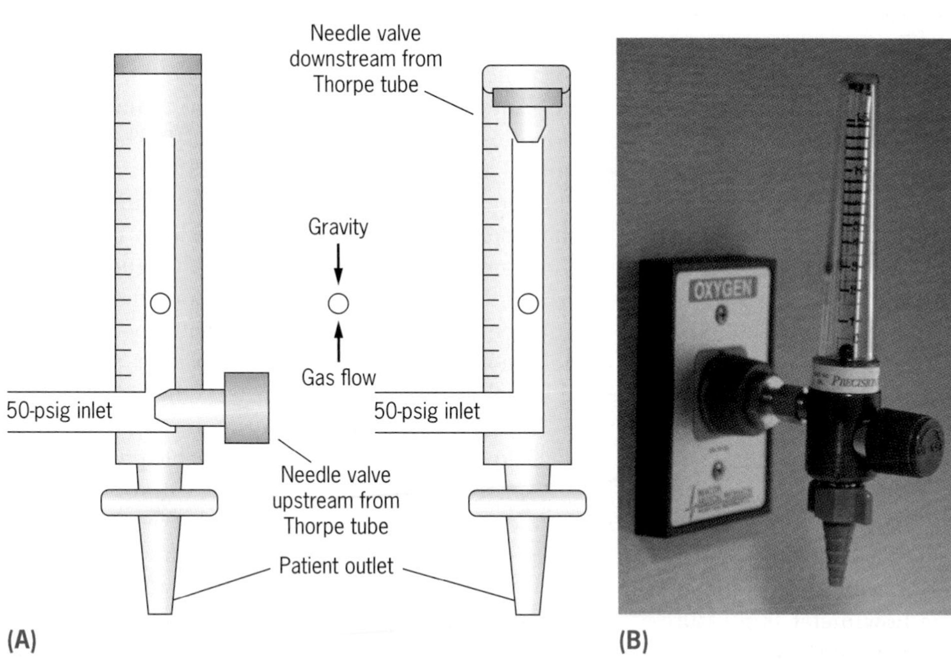

FIGURE 16–6 Thorpe tube flow meters. (**A**) Non-pressure compensated design with needle valve prior to indicator ball (left) and pressure-compensated with needle valve after indicator ball (right). (**B**) Commercially available Thorpe tube flow meter. (**A**) Modified from Cairo JM, Pilbeam SP. *Mosby's Respiratory Care Equipment.* 6th ed. Mosby; 1999.

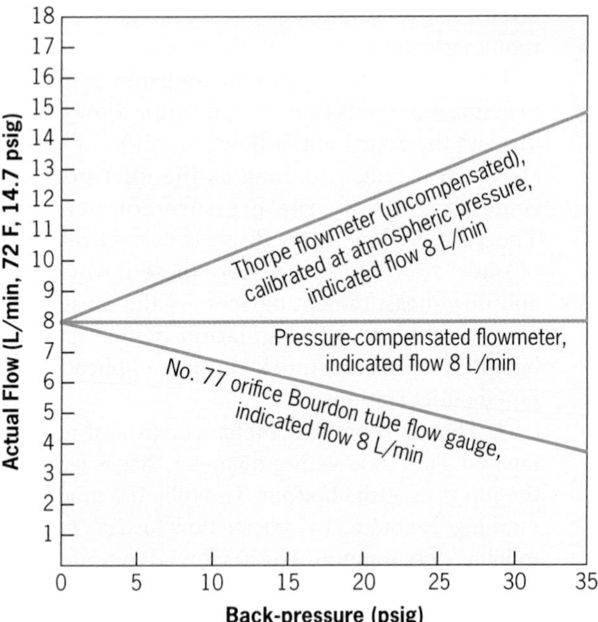

FIGURE 16–7 Comparison of the accuracy of pressure-compensated and non-compensated Thorpe tube flow meters and a Bourdon gauge when faced with increasing levels of downstream back pressure. The pressure-compensated Thorpe tube's indicated flow is the actual flow regardless of back pressure. With a non-compensated Thorpe tube, actual flow is higher then the indicated flow at increasing downstream pressure. With the Bourdon gauge, indicated flow is progressively higher than actual flow as back pressure increases. Modified from McPherson SP, Spearman CB. *Respiratory Therapy Equipment.* 5th ed. Mosby; 1995.

In the past, non-pressure-compensated flow meters were commonly used for medical applications. They are still used for laboratory or industrial applications. The non-pressure-compensated version of the Thorpe tube flow meter has the needle valve located proximal to the Thorpe tube. When a flow-restricting device is attached to a non-pressure-compensated Thorpe tube flow meter, increasing the downstream resistance, the pressure is increased within the Thorpe tube, which forces the float downward and provides a reading lower than the actual flow.

Determining whether a Thorpe tube flow meter is pressure compensated can be done when the needle valve is closed and the flow meter subsequently pressurized as the cylinder valve is opened or is connected to a station outlet. If the Thorpe tube flow meter is pressure compensated, the float will jump to the top of the tube and then fall back as gas rushes in and fills the tube to the needle valve.

RESPIRATORY RECAP

Flow Meters

» Flow restrictors are preset, fixed flow meters.
» Pressure-compensated Thorpe flow meters indicate actual flow unless the source gas pressure varies from 50 psig or the float tube is not set in the vertical position.
» Bourdon gauges, although less accurate, are used whenever a patient application requires that the regulator not be vertical.

Most Thorpe tube flow meters commonly used in respiratory therapy use a ball as the float, although the float may assume various shapes and configurations. Sighting the float at eye level is important to avoid inaccuracy due to parallax. A ball float is read through the center of the ball, whereas rotameter floats are read at the top surface. The majority of clinical flow meters are scaled from 0 to 16 L/min. The need for more accurate reading of low flows for infants and oxygen-sensitive adult patients has fostered development of 0- to 1-L/min or 0- to 5-L/min flow meters. Most Thorpe-type flow meters also have a flush setting beyond the calibrated range. Although there is no industry standard, most flow meters provide greater than 60 L/min on the flush setting. High-flow oxygen delivery systems (requiring calibrated flow measurements) have prompted manufacturers to develop 0- to 75-L/min Thorpe tubes.

Oxygen Administration Devices

O_2 therapy systems generally are categorized as either **low-flow/variable-performance** or **high-flow/fixed-performance** devices. Variable-performance devices (commonly referred to as low-flow devices) provide variable and approximate F_{IO_2}, whereas fixed-performance devices (commonly referred to as high-flow devices) are designed to provide a fixed and known F_{IO_2}.

The descriptive names most commonly employed (low flow and high flow) can be confusing to the respiratory therapy student because the distinguishing characteristic of the two devices is actually whether the device in question provides a premixed, precise, and known F_{IO_2} (fixed performance) or whether the F_{IO_2} received by the patient will be a function of the patient's breathing pattern and volume in combination with supplemental 1.0 F_{IO_2} gas administered by the device (variable performance).

For example, a patient using a nasal cannula (which is a low-flow device) receives a flow of 100% O_2 at 0 to 6 L/min. The flow of gas coming from the nasal cannula is continuous across both inspiration and expiration, but during inspiration the patient will inhale an inspiratory volume composed of some of the 100% O_2 and some air present in the room (0.21 F_{IO_2}). Therefore, the final F_{IO_2} mix that enters the trachea and is eventually conducted to the alveolus varies from patient to patient, and in fact from breath to breath, depending on the tidal volume and respiratory rate and pattern.

Thus, low-flow devices provide variable performance in the sense that the delivered F_{IO_2} cannot be accurately known. On the other hand, high-flow devices are designed to produce flow outputs that meet or exceed the patient's full inspiratory flow demand and thus maintain a fixed F_{IO_2}. High-flow devices accomplish this by presenting the patient with a very high flow of premixed F_{IO_2} gas in quantities that meet or exceed the patient's inspiratory demands.

Again, as with low-flow devices, high-flow devices provide gas continuously (throughout inspiration and expiration) but at the desired O_2 dosage (FIO_2). The major difference between high-flow and low-flow devices is that the high-flow device provides such a high flow of premixed gas that the patient is not required to inhale any room air. Examples of high-flow devices include air-entrainment devices such as masks and large-volume nebulizers.

Low-Flow (Variable-Performance) Devices

As previously stated, the primary distinguishing feature of low-flow O_2 administration devices is that the patient experiences a variable FIO_2 as changed through variations in minute ventilation (especially changes in tidal volume, inspiratory flow, and respiratory rate). This is because the device delivers 100% O_2 to the patient's upper airway, which is mixed during inspiration with variable amounts of inhaled room air to produce the final delivered FIO_2.

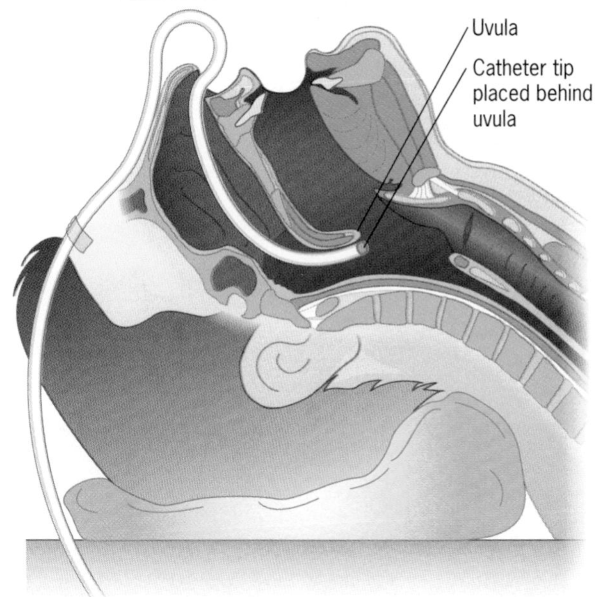

FIGURE 16–8 Nasal catheter for oxygen administration. Adapted from Scanlan CL, et al. *Egan's Fundamentals of Respiratory Care.* 7th ed. Mosby; 1999.

Nasal Catheter

The nasal catheter was widely used as the standard low-flow oxygen delivery system of choice until the late 1960s. The nasal cannula and other less invasive oxygen appliances have since replaced the catheter because of the frequency of complications with the latter's use. The **nasal oxygen catheter** is a soft, pliable plastic tube about 12 inches long with a series of small holes at the distal end and a fitting at the other end to connect it to the oxygen supply tubing. Nasal oxygen catheters for adults are 12 or 14 Fr (3.96 mm and 4.72 mm outside diameter [OD]), whereas those for pediatric use are 8 and 10 Fr (Fr = French size). At flow rates of 1 to 5 L/min, the delivered FIO_2 ranges from 0.22 to 0.35.

The nasal catheter is usually inserted blindly, and the appropriate distance for insertion estimated by measuring the length from the nose to the external ear. Inserting the catheter for that distance should place it in the approximate location. The catheter is inserted into either external naris and along the floor of the nasal cavity. After the catheter is advanced into the nose, the conscious patient should be asked to open his or her mouth; with the tongue depressed, the catheter should be visualized with a light as it emerges from behind the uvula. The catheter is correctly placed when it is moved to a position in which it just disappears behind the uvula (**Figure 16–8**).

This procedure produces some discomfort in all patients. Insertion can be complicated if there is a nasal pathologic condition or the catheter is inserted upward, injuring the nasal turbinates. A defect in the blood clotting mechanism is a contraindication for the use of the nasal catheter because insertion or removal may cause nasal bleeding. A deviated septum, severe mucosal congestion, and nasal polyps may prevent passage of the catheter. Because the catheter is held in place by taping it externally to the nose, external trauma to the nose can make securing the device problematic; the alternative naris or (more likely) a different appliance should be selected. The catheter is usually changed periodically (e.g., every 8 hours) to prevent secretions from encasing the catheter, which causes bleeding and pain problems on withdrawal.

Nasal Cannula

The **nasal oxygen cannula** (**Figure 16–9**) is the most widely used device for administering low-flow oxygen to infants, children, and adults in the hospital and the home. The nasal cannula is easily applied and well tolerated by most patients when used with flow rates of 6 L/min or less and held in place with an elastic band around the head or, more commonly, by looping the delivery tubing over the ears and holding it in place with an adjustable slide placed

> **RESPIRATORY RECAP**
>
> **Oxygen Delivery Devices**
>
> » FIO_2 is the actual dose of O_2 administered.
> » In low-flow devices, *flow* refers to the amount of 100% O_2 gas administered.
> » Low-flow devices have variable performance in terms of delivered O_2 concentration.
> » Low-flow devices are titrated to achieve acceptable PaO_2 or SpO_2.
> » The nasal catheter, while historically interesting, is no longer used.
> » The nasal cannula consists of nasal prongs delivering 1 to 6 L/min (0.24–0.40 FIO_2).
> » The transtracheal O_2 catheter is a surgically placed O_2 catheter that lowers O_2 utilization for long-term O_2 administration.
> » With a high-flow nasal cannula, nasal prongs are fitted to nearly fill the naris, and warmed, humidified O_2 is delivered at flows typically exceeding those of the traditional nasal cannula.
> » The partial rebreathing mask is a high-concentration reservoir mask (0.60–0.80 FIO_2).
> » The nonrebreathing mask is a high-concentration reservoir mask (0.60–1.0 FIO_2).

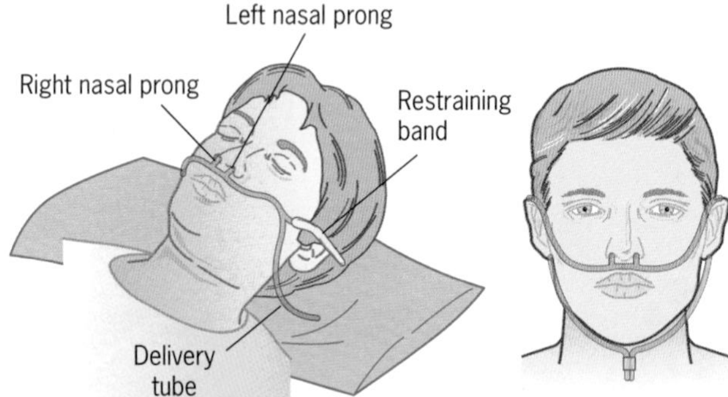

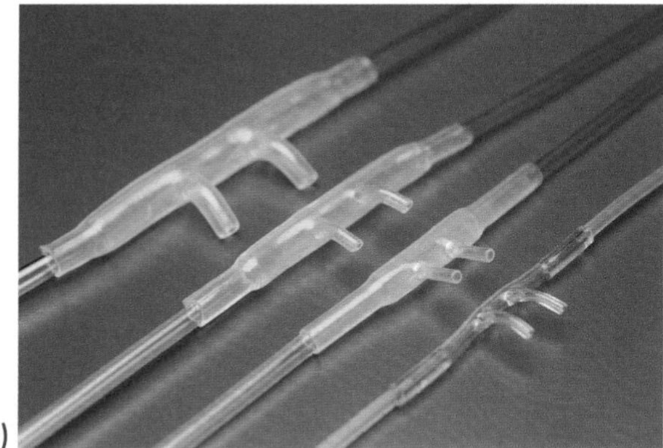

FIGURE 16–9 **(A)** Elastic strap (left) and over-the-ear (right) nasal cannula styles. **(B)** Various styles of nasal prongs. **(A)** Adapted from Scanlan CL, et al. *Egan's Fundamentals of Respiratory Care*. 7th ed. St. Louis: Mosby; 1999.

under the chin. The nasal cannula consists of a delivery tube that ends in two short prongs, each about one-half inch long and made of soft, pliable plastic. Cannula prongs are available curved or straight, tapered to a flair or nontapered.

When oxygen is delivered by nasal cannula to an adult, the expected delivery may be an F_{IO_2} of 0.24 at 1 L/min and up to about 0.40 at 5 to 6 L/min. Actual F_{IO_2} levels achieved with a nasal cannula at specific oxygen flows have been debated for many years. Investigators using human subjects and bench tests have reported a wide range of F_{IO_2} levels delivered to the trachea because of the variability of this device. The nasal cannula is usually used at flows of 1 to 6 L/min. Flows of 10 and 15 L/min can achieve tracheal concentrations of 0.35 to 0.45, although that level of flow is uncomfortable and should be considered only for short-term use.

Although not clinically practical, calculating the theoretical F_{IO_2} delivered by the nasal oxygen cannula is a useful learning tool. Assumptions include the O_2 flow, tidal volume, respiratory frequency, inspiration-to-expiration (I:E) ratio, and anatomic reservoir, as illustrated in **Equation 16–1**. The rule of fours is a useful clinical guideline commonly used as a memory tool to provide an estimated F_{IO_2} for any of the acceptable nasal cannula flow rates (1 to 6 L/min). According to this rule, each liter of O_2 delivered by the nasal cannula will provide approximately four additional percentages of O_2, starting at 24%. For example, 1 L/min will provide 24%; 2 L/min, 28%; and 3 L/min, 32%. Remember, however, that this is just an estimate. Because liter flow settings with any low-flow O_2 device are ultimately guided by patient conditions, oximetry, and blood gas values, the most practical application of estimated F_{IO_2} is to determine the approximate F_{IO_2} needs for patients whose pulmonary conditions have worsened in order to establish a starting point for the application of high-flow O_2 therapy.

An issue of controversy is the effect of an open mouth on F_{IO_2} with a nasal cannula. Some studies have reported no effect of an open mouth, others have reported a decrease in F_{IO_2}, and others have reported an increase in F_{IO_2}. Thus, one cannot be dogmatic about the effect

EQUATION 16–1

Estimation of F_{IO_2} from a Nasal Cannula

Cannula flow	2 L/min (33 mL/s)
Tidal volume	500 mL
Anatomic reservoir	50 mL (nasal passages and nasopharynx)
Inspiratory time	1 s

Volume of O_2 inspired:

50 mL	(anatomic reservoir)
33 mL	(O_2 flow)
84 mL	(amount of O_2 in the inspired air; 420 mL × 0.21)

Volume O_2 inspired = 167 mL

F_{IO_2} = 167 mL (O_2)/500 mL (tidal volume) = 0.33

For a flow of 6 L/min, volume of O_2 inspired:

50 mL	(anatomic reservoir)
100 mL	(O_2 flow)
150 mL	(amount of O_2 in the inspired air; 350 mL × 0.21)

Volume O_2 inspired = 220 mL

F_{IO_2} = 220 mL (O_2)/500 mL (tidal volume) = 0.44

If tidal volume is decreased to 250 mL, the F_{IO_2} increases to 0.64. If tidal volume is increased to 1000 mL, the F_{IO_2} decreases to 0.32.

Similar calculations can be used to calculate the effects of changes in O_2 flow or inspiratory time.

of an open mouth on F_{IO_2} with oxygen administration by nasal cannula. Although not commonly appreciated clinically, nasal obstruction will decrease F_{IO_2} when a nasal cannula is used.

The nasal cannula flow rate should be titrated using vital signs, pulse oximetry, and arterial blood gas (Pa_{O_2}) measurements. At a minimum, respiratory therapists should monitor the patient by recording the oxygen flow and respiratory rate. Devices other than the nasal cannula should be used if blood oxygen levels are critical and the patient requires a higher F_{IO_2}. Some clinicians combine a cannula with an oxygen mask in an attempt to provide a higher F_{IO_2}. Clinicians should confirm actual flow from the distal prongs by feeling for gas flow. Absent or low flows should prompt the operator to check for flow meter accuracy, a twisted cannula or connecting tubing, or a leaky humidifier bottle seal (if a humidifier is used).

A frequent patient complaint while using a nasal cannula is drying of the nasal mucosa. This problem has been addressed by use of disposable bubble humidifiers. These devices are relatively inefficient, and most hospitals do not routinely use them. Patients may also experience discomfort where the tubing or elastic is in contact with the face or ears. Foam or gauze padding can be added to protect pressure points on the ears or over the cheekbones.

Nasal cannulas are available in sizes appropriate for infants, toddlers, and children. Because of these patients' small tidal volumes and rapid respiratory frequencies, the oxygen flow to infants and children should be precisely controlled by use of flow meters with an appropriate scale (0 to 2 L/min in increments of 0.25 or 0.0625 L/min). A flow of 0.25 L/min by nasal cannula to an infant can achieve an F_{IO_2} of 0.35, and more than 0.60 at 1 L/min is possible. The maximum flow to a nasal cannula for an infant is 2 L/min.

Simple Mask

The **simple oxygen mask** is used when a higher F_{IO_2} is needed than can be attained with a nasal cannula or when a cannula is not appropriate because of nasal obstruction, such as in emergency situations and during and after minor surgical procedures. The simple oxygen mask is a disposable plastic product, available in infant, child, and adult sizes, with a length of small-diameter oxygen supply tubing connected to the base of the mask. The masks fit over the bridge of the nose and often are held in place with a malleable aluminum strip, which helps minimize leakage toward the eyes. They cover the nose and mouth down to below the lower lip or to under the chin and are held in place by an elastic band around the head (**Figure 16–10**).

The simple O_2 mask increases the inspired oxygen concentration by acting as an oxygen reservoir, adding a volume in an adult mask of 100 to 200 mL, which is inhaled at the beginning of inspiration. The patient also inhales room air through a series of small holes in the mask. The amount of oxygen enrichment of the inspired air depends on mask volume, pattern of ventilation, and the oxygen flow to the mask. It is difficult to predict the delivered F_{IO_2} at specific flows. During normal breathing, it is reasonable to expect a range from 0.3 to 0.6 with flows of 5 to 10 L/min, respectively. Oxygen levels can be higher with small tidal volumes or slow breathing rates. With higher flows and ideal conditions, F_{IO_2} may approach 0.7 to 0.8.

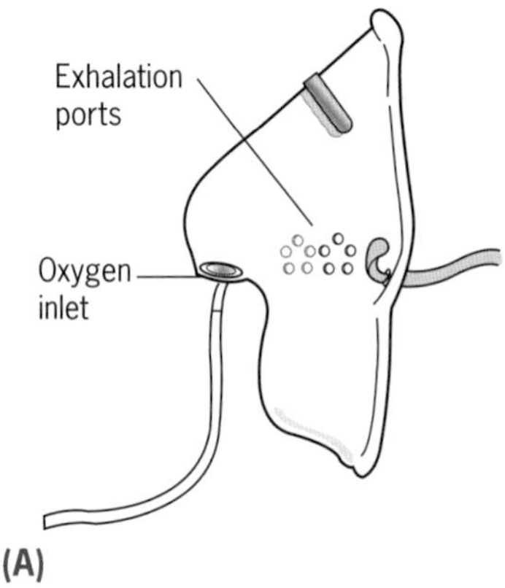

(A)

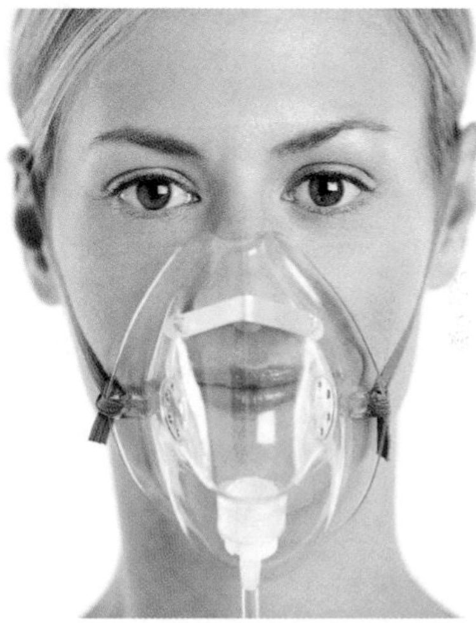

(B)

FIGURE 16–10 Simple O_2 mask. (**A**) Modified from Scanlan CL, et al. *Egan's Fundamentals of Respiratory Care*. 7th ed. Mosby; 1999.

Because the mask accumulates CO_2 during exhalation, the oxygen flow rate must be sufficient to wash out the mask and prevent rebreathing. A general recommendation is that a minimum flow of 5 L/min should be used to avoid accumulation of exhaled CO_2. The simple mask is a low-flow, variable-performance oxygen delivery system capable of providing an F_{IO_2} of from 0.3 to 0.6 at flows of 5 to 10 L/min, depending on the size of the mask and the patient's respiratory pattern.

All oronasal masks present the same problems, which include claustrophobic feelings for some patients, speech muffling, and difficulty with eating and drinking. Additionally, any mask administration device increases the possibility of aspirating regurgitated stomach contents.

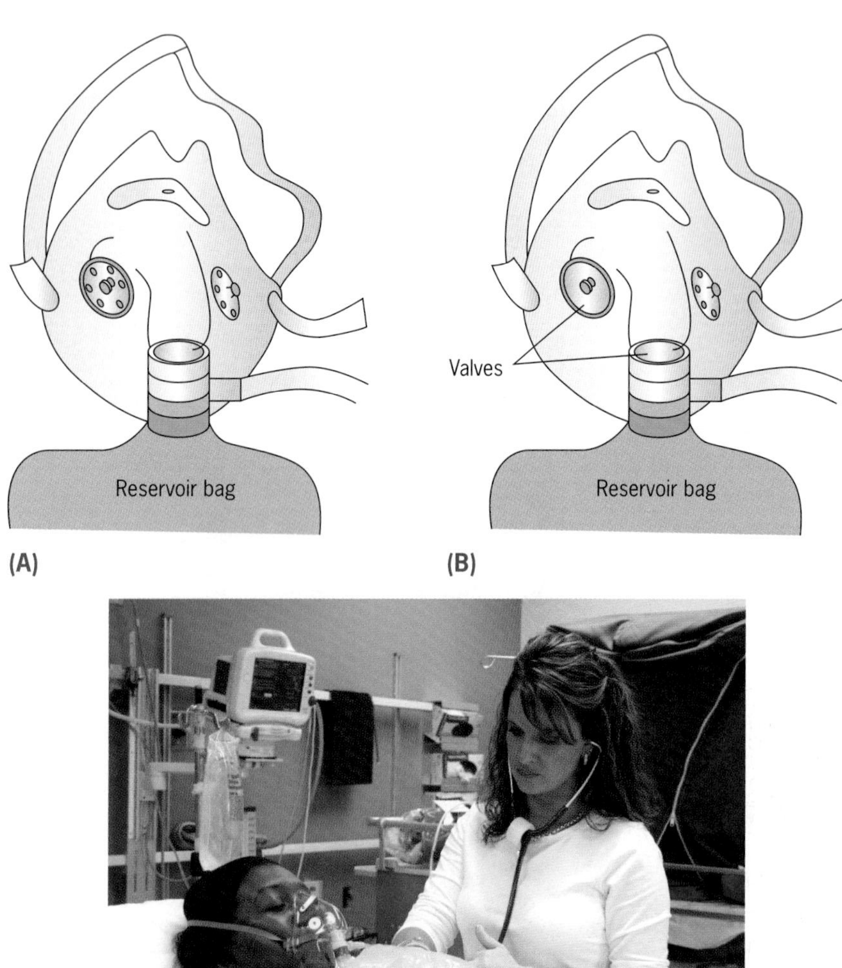

FIGURE 16–11 (**A**) Partial rebreathing mask. (**B**) Nonrebreathing mask. (**C**) Commercially available nonrebreathing mask. (**A** and **B**) Modified from Scanlan CL, et al. *Egan's Fundamentals of Respiratory Care*. 7th ed. Mosby; 1999.

Partial Rebreathing Mask

The **partial rebreathing mask** (**Figure 16–11**) is a simple mask with the addition of a 300- to 600-mL reservoir bag. The partial rebreathing mask is somewhat misnamed because although there is some insignificant rebreathing of exhaled gas, the mask's actual indication is primarily for administering relatively high O_2 concentrations to severely hypoxemic patients. The oxygen supply tube is positioned between the mask and the reservoir bag. The oxygen flow is set at a rate sufficient to keep the bag at least partially inflated throughout inspiration. This flow varies depending on the patient's respiratory pattern, but is usually between 8 and 15 L/min, which produces an F_{IO_2} in the range of 0.4 to 0.7, depending on the patient's respiratory pattern.

During inspiration, the patient inhales 100% O_2 from the reservoir bag, partially deflating it, and draws in an additional volume of air through the mask ports. When the patient exhales, the first part of the exhaled gas (usually about a third of the exhaled tidal volume) enters the reservoir bag; because of the pressure in the partially full reservoir, the remaining two-thirds exit the mask through the mask ports. When the patient then takes the next breath, the inspiratory gas will be composed of a mixture of the captured exhaled gas, the 100% O_2 that fills the remaining volume in the reservoir bag, and some room air inhaled from the mask ports. However, because the exhaled gas that entered the reservoir bag comes from the uppermost parts of the airway, it will be high in oxygen and low in carbon dioxide. If the O_2 flow is set correctly (so that the reservoir bag remains half or more full), the rebreathed gas will contain little CO_2.

To increase O_2 delivery from a partial rebreathing mask, a modification called the Tusk mask has been described. The Tusk mask consisted of a partial rebreathing mask with corrugated ventilator tubing (15 cm long; 2.5 cm in diameter) placed into the holes made by cutting out the exhalation ports of the mask.

Nonrebreathing Mask

The **nonrebreathing mask** uses the same basic system as the partial rebreathing mask but incorporates valves between the bag and mask and on at least one of the exhalation ports. Oxygen is directed into the mask and into the reservoir bag by small-bore tubing. A valve prevents exhaled gas from entering the reservoir; the entire exhaled volume exits the mask through the mask ports. While the patient is exhaling, the reservoir bag fills with O_2. At the beginning of inspiration, the mask exhalation port valves close, minimizing room air from being drawn in, and the reservoir valve opens, allowing the patient to inhale 300 to 500 mL of O_2 from the reservoir in addition to the oxygen flow. If the system were perfect, delivery of 100% oxygen would be possible. However, these inexpensive disposable masks cannot provide an airtight fit on the face, and their valves are simple rubber or vinyl disks that do not provide a perfect seal. However, at flows of 10 to 15 L/min, an F_{IO_2} of 0.6 to 0.8 is achievable. As with the partial rebreathing mask, the O_2 flow must be set at a rate high enough to prevent the bag from emptying more than half. A nonrebreathing mask is indicated for patients who require a high F_{IO_2}. Such patients may include victims of trauma, MI, or carbon monoxide exposure.

Because there is a risk of suffocation if the mask valves stick or the O_2 supply fails, some system must be provided to allow room air to enter. Some manufacturers provide spring-loaded antisuffocation valves at the neck of the reservoir bag. The spring-loaded antisuffocation valve opens if the pressure in the mask becomes subatmospheric, as happens when the O_2 supply fails. Other manufacturers provide the nonrebreathing mask with a valve on only one side of the mask.

High-Flow (Fixed-Performance) Devices

Precise delivery of FIO_2 is required to supply therapeutic levels of O_2 and avoid complications. Several methods exist for control of FIO_2 and delivery of adequate flow to meet inspiratory demands. High-flow O_2 administration devices blend 100% O_2 and room air (21% O_2) to produce a gas with the desired FIO_2, and provide a flow of the gas high enough to prevent the patient from diluting the FIO_2 with room air. High-flow O_2 delivery devices accomplish this by exceeding any tidal volume, respiratory frequency, or inspiratory flow that the patient might produce.

RESPIRATORY RECAP

High-Flow Oxygen Delivery Devices

- » High-flow, fixed-performance O_2 administration devices deliver a predictable FIO_2.
- » Mix ratios can be calculated or memorized.
- » FIO_2 and flow are important to delivered FIO_2.
- » FIO_2 is reduced if patient inspiratory flow exceeds the device flow output.
- » Flow minimum may be established by tripling or quadrupling the minute ventilation.
- » Minimum flow for infants is 4 to 6 L/min, and for adults it is 40 L/min.
- » Large-volume nebulizers use an air-entrainment mechanism for FIO_2 mixing.
- » Air-entrainment masks deliver a precise low FIO_2.
- » High-flow generators are engineered to deliver a higher FIO_2 and flow.
- » Dual flow meters can be used to mix O_2 and air.
- » Air–oxygen blenders require 50-psig sources of both air and O_2.

Although high-flow O_2 administration devices potentially offer a constant FIO_2, this may not occur in all clinical situations; thus, the respiratory therapist must understand the performance characteristics, design, and engineering constraints of each device. For example, if the patient's inspiratory flow exceeds the flow from the device, the patient will dilute the FIO_2 by breathing in additional room air. If this is not recognized, clinicians might be misled into falsely thinking that the patient is receiving a specific concentration of oxygen.

Proportioning 100% O_2 and 21% O_2 (room air) to produce a specific FIO_2 is actually very much like making any solution, except that the solvent and the solute each contain some amount of O_2. For example, if the respiratory therapist wishes to provide a 40% mixture of O_2, each liter of 100% O_2 must be diluted with approximately 3 liters of 21% room air. Because of quality differences between devices and discrepancies in the calibration of flow meters, it is clinically important to verify any O_2 concentration from any high-flow O_2 administration device with an oxygen analyzer.

TABLE 16–3 **Air-to-Oxygen Mix Ratios for Various FIO_2 Levels**

FIO_2	Mix Ratio ($Air:O_2$ Ratio)
0.24	25:1
0.28	10:1
0.30	8:1
0.35	5:1
0.40	3:1
0.50	1.7:1
0.60	1:1
0.70	0.6:1
0.80	0.3:1

Air-to-oxygen mix ratios are highly predictable and can be mathematically modeled using relatively simple processes. One strategy used by some respiratory therapists is to simply memorize key mix ratios for common FIO_2 levels (**Table 16–3**). Another common strategy is to use a variant of the volume-concentration formula:

$$V_1 \times C_1 = V_2 \times C_2$$

For example, if one wishes to find the mix ratio for a 0.40 FIO_2 high-flow O_2 administration device, the calculation will look like this:

$$\text{Air-to-oxygen} = (100 - O_2\%)/(O_2\% - 21){:}1$$

$$\text{Air-to-oxygen} = (100 - 40)/(40 - 21){:}1$$

$$\text{Air-to-oxygen} = (60/19){:}1$$

$$\text{Air-to-oxygen} = 3{:}1$$

Most likely, in clinical use this mix ratio would be rounded to 3:1, because the output would be verified by an O_2 analyzer. Another approach to find a mix ratio is to use an ancient mathematical shortcut, which is known as the *alligation alternate* (sometimes referred to as the magic box). **Figure 16–12** illustrates this approach.

Once the mix ratio is determined, the total gas flow must be taken into account. A total flow of 40 L/min is sufficient to meet or exceed almost all adult patients' inspiratory demands. To obtain the desired FIO_2 in sufficient quantities, one can simply plug in various increasing 100% O_2 flows, proportionally increasing the air flow to maintain the desired FIO_2, noting the increasing sum as the increases are made, as is demonstrated in **Table 16–4**. Note that in order to reach an acceptable total flow of 40 L/min, the O_2 flow will need to be set at at least 10 L/min for an FIO_2 of 0.40.

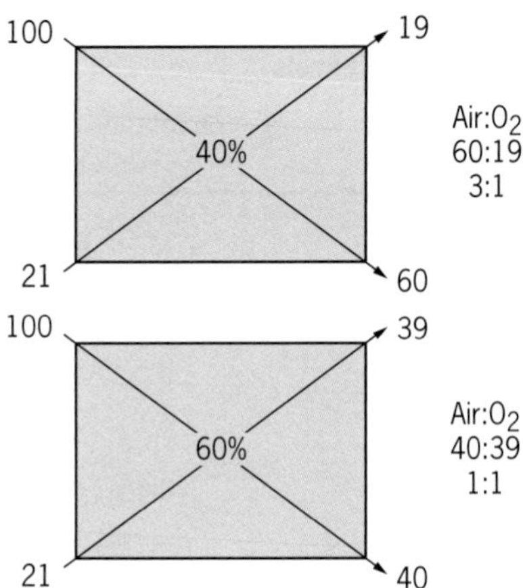

FIGURE 16–12 Magic box to determine air-to-oxygen ratio when mixing O_2 and air. Examples are shown for 40% and 60% O_2.

TABLE 16–4 Flows of Oxygen, Air, and Total Flow for a 40% O_2 Mixing Device

L/min of Oxygen	L/min of Air	Total Flow in L/min
1	3	4
2	6	8
3	9	12
4	12	16
10	30	40

It is important to note that the 40-L/min minimum flow rate guideline is based on the assumption that the patient's minute ventilation will not exceed 10 L/min and that the I:E ratio will on average be 1:3. The therapist should realize that some patients have a higher minute ventilation and may therefore require more total gas flow to be certain that the F_{IO_2} delivery is as desired. A general rule is that more gas flow is better, from an F_{IO_2} delivery standpoint; however, higher gas flows produce more noise, can be annoying, and may deplete the gas source.

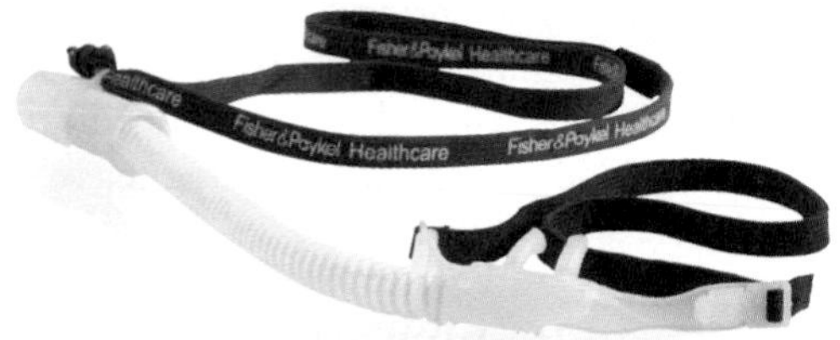

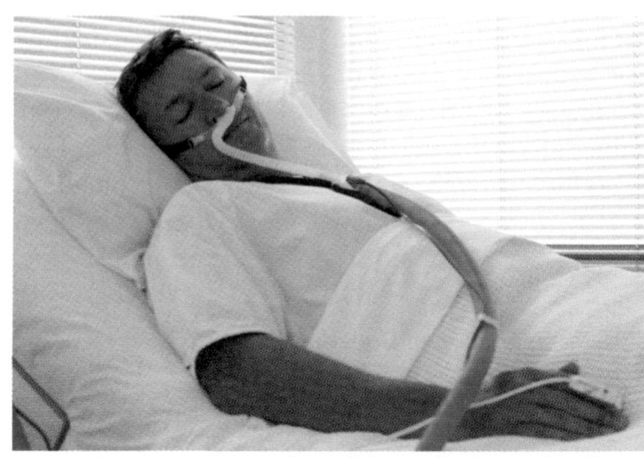

FIGURE 16–13 High-flow nasal cannula.

High-Flow Nasal Cannula

The **high-flow nasal cannula** (HFNC) has gained favor as a more comfortable alternative to mask-delivered O_2 therapy and nasal CPAP (**Figure 16–13**). HFNC devices are designed to administer higher O_2 flows than the standard nasal cannula. They utilize larger delivery prongs intended to entirely fill each naris. Flows of up to 50 L/min are used for adults, with lower flows (1–8 L/min) for neonates. Humidification via high-efficiency heated humidifiers is also used for this therapy to ameliorate the mucosal drying effects of such high gas flow. These flows are also likely to result in variable amounts of increased upper airway positive pressure, and thus some of the therapeutic effects of the HFNC relate to the CPAP effect that occurs. The degree of CPAP effect varies according to many factors but is especially affected by the flow.

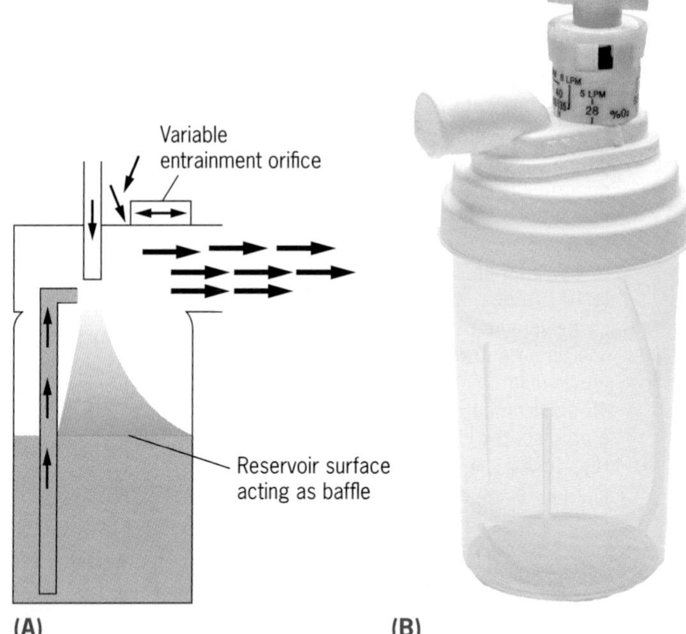

FIGURE 16–14 Large-volume nebulizers. (**A**) Modified from Cohen N, Fink J. Humidity and aerosols. In: Eubanks DH, Bone RC, eds. *Principles and Applications of Cardiorespiratory Care Equipment*. Mosby; 1994.

Large-Volume Air-Entrainment Nebulizers

Large-volume, high-output, all-purpose nebulizers with either cool or heated aerosols have been used in respiratory therapy for many years to provide bland mist therapy with some control of the F_{IO_2} (**Figure 16–14**). They are the most commonly applied O_2 administration devices

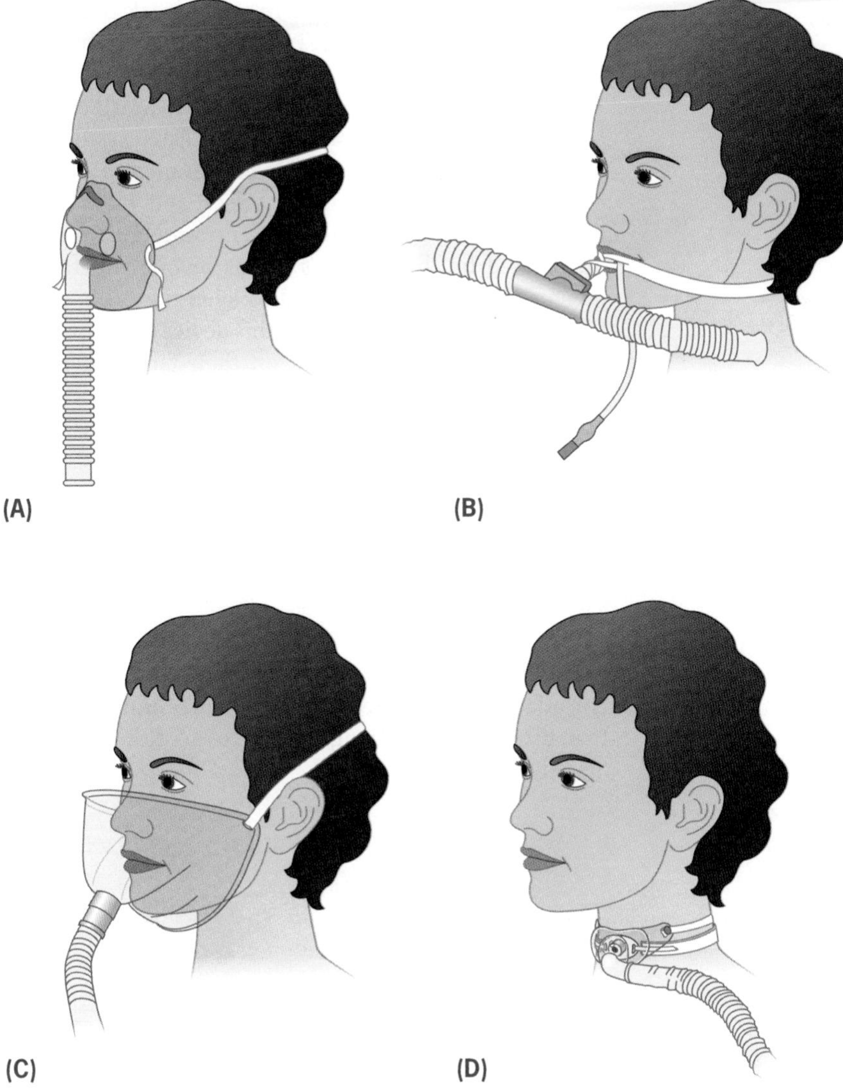

FIGURE 16–15 Aerosol mask (**A**), Briggs T-piece (**B**), face tent (**C**), and tracheostomy collar (**D**). Adapted from Fink JR, Hunt GE. *Clinical Practice of Respiratory Care*. Lippincott Williams & Wilkins; 1999.

after the nasal cannula. They use an adjustable dilution setting collar to vary F_{IO_2} from approximately 0.3 to 1.0. In the typical device, as the F_{IO_2} is increased, less room air is entrained and total flow output decreases. Nebulizer systems can be applied to the patient through many different devices. The aerosol mask, tracheostomy collar, face tent, and T piece or Briggs adapter (**Figure 16–15**) are attached to the large-volume nebulizer by corrugated, large-bore tubing. All of these attachments provide an open system that freely vents inspiratory and expiratory gases around the patient's face or out a distal port of a Briggs adapter.

Most commercial units have an inlet orifice diameter that will allow only 12 to 15 L/min (at 50 psig). When the O_2 input flow is 15 L/min, the total flows at 0.6, 0.7, and 1.0 are 30, 24.5, and 15 L/min, respectively. The problem with air-entrainment systems is that the most tachypneic and hypoxemic patients need the highest F_{IO_2} setting, but this results in the lowest total flow, and thus the F_{IO_2} is limited due to air entrainment. Without special modifications, such inexpensive large-volume nebulizers are acceptable for use in patients who require no more than 50% O_2. Another clinical concern is that excess water in the tubing can collect and obstruct gas flow completely or offer increased flow resistance.

Respiratory therapists should be alert to patients who, as a result of clinican deterioration, increase their minute ventilation when on an aerosol system. In such circumstances, a system should be substituted that ensures the required F_{IO_2} with an adequate flow. One approach is to use two nebulizers in tandem, which doubles the flow delivery to the patient (**Figure 16–16**). Another approach is to use a gas injector nebulizer, in which an additional flow is added downstream from the nebulizer output (**Figure 16–17**).

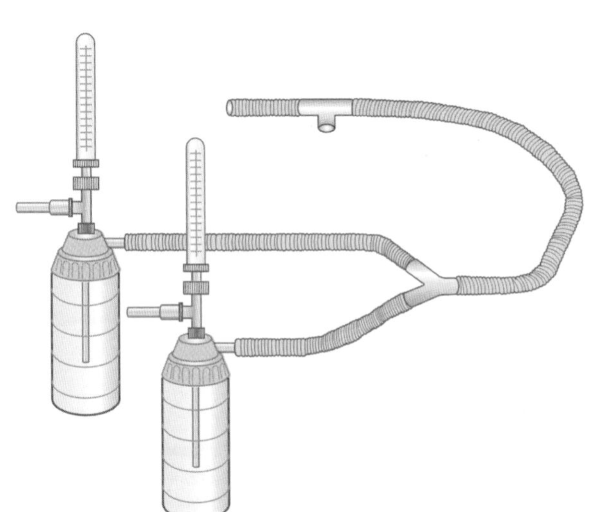

FIGURE 16–16 Flow can be increased by attaching two nebulizers in tandem.

Air-Entrainment Masks

An **air-entrainment mask** consists of a single-patient-use, disposable mask, a jet nozzle, and entrainment ports. 100% O_2 is delivered through the jet nozzle, which increases its velocity. This gas at high velocity entrains

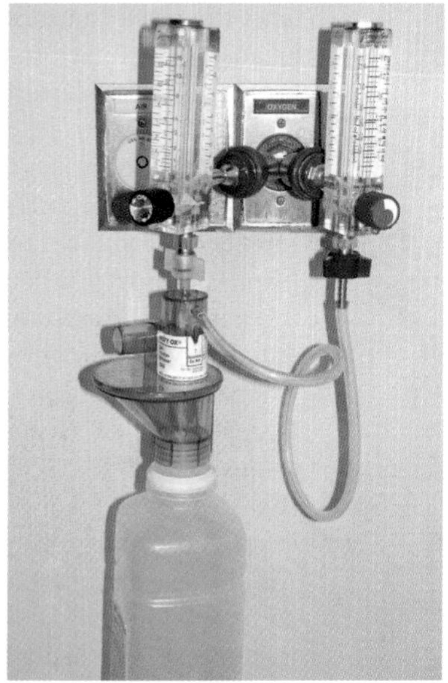

FIGURE 16–17 Injection nebulizer, in which additional flow is injected at the outlet of the nebulizer.

(or slipstreams) ambient air into the mask because of the viscous shearing forces between the gas traveling through the nozzle and the stagnant ambient air. The FIO_2 depends on the nozzle size and the size of the entrainment ports. Commercially available systems use interchangeable jets, adjustable entrainment ports, or a combination of these (**Figure 16–18** and **Table 16–5**). FIO_2 levels will increase if the entrainment ports are obstructed by the patient's hands or bed sheets. The patient should be encouraged to keep the mask on the face constantly. A limitation of this device is that patients often do not keep the mask on their face, potentially resulting in hypoxemia unless an alternative device such as a nasal cannula is used. Air-entrainment masks are a reasonable choice for patients whose hypoxemia cannot be controlled on lower-FIO_2 devices such as the cannula (because of changes in breathing pattern). Patients who hypoventilate with a moderate FIO_2 are candidates for the air-entrainment mask.

Downs Flow Generator

An adaptation of the classic air-entrainment device that provides gas mixing is the Downs flow generator

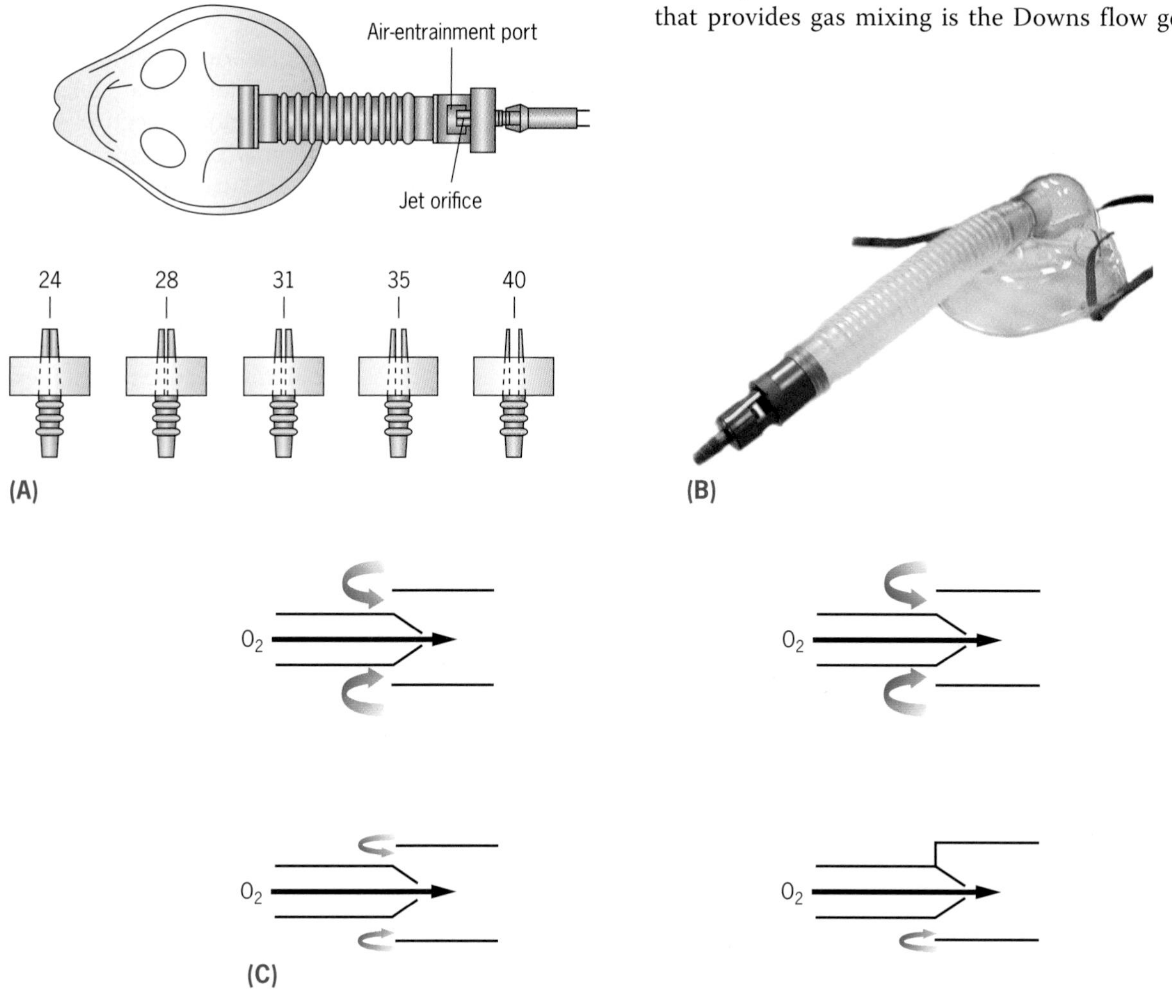

Air-entrainment port

Jet orifice

24 28 31 35 40

(A)

(B)

O_2

O_2

O_2

O_2

(C)

FIGURE 16–18 (**A**) Air-entrainment mask. (**B**) Commercially available air-entrainment mask. (**C**) Changes in air entrainment by changing jet size or changing size of the entrainment port. (**A**) Modified from Kacmarek RM. Methods of oxygen delivery in the hospital. *Prob Respir Care.* 1990;3:536–574.

TABLE 16–5 FIO_2, **Minimum Flow Requirements, Outputs, and Entrainment Ratios for an Air-Entrainment Mask**

FIO_2 Setting	Minimum O_2 Flow (L/min)	Entrainment Ratio (Air:O_2)	Total Flow (L/min)
0.24	4	25:1	104
0.28	4	10:1	44
0.31	6	7:1	48
0.35	8	5:1	48
0.40	8	3:1	32
0.50	12	1.7:1	32
0.60	12	1:1	24
0.70	12	0.6:1	19

Data from Branson RD. The nuts and bolts of increasing arterial oxygenation: devices and techniques. *Respir Care.* 1993;38:672–686.

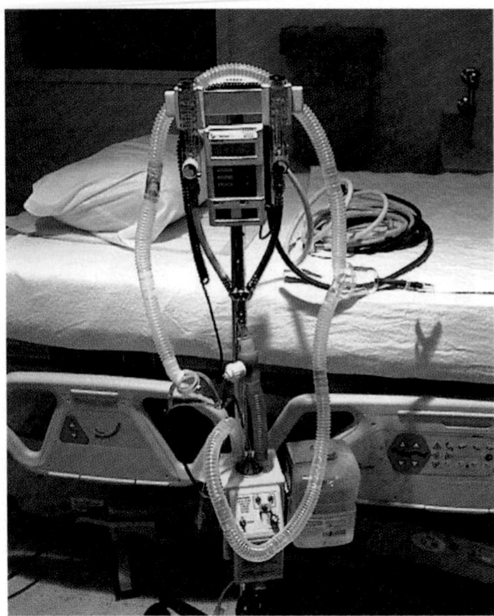

FIGURE 16–20 High-flow oxygen delivery system using two flow meters.

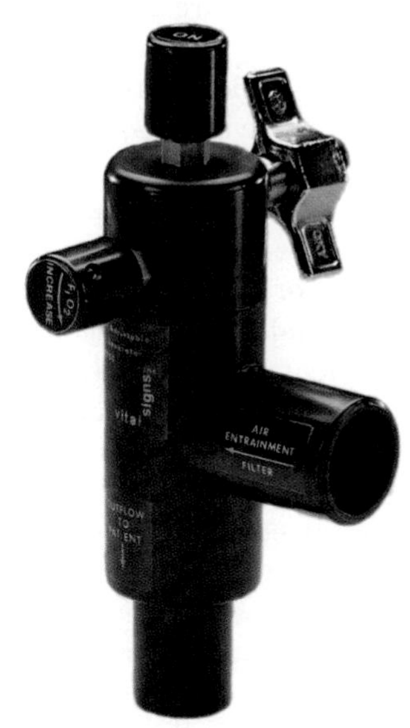

FIGURE 16–19 Downs flow generator.

(**Figure 16–19**). This device is designed to provide high gas flows in situations in which downstream resistance occurs, such as a CPAP system. In contrast to the air-entrainment nebulizer systems discussed earlier (which can be used only in low-FIO_2 situations), the Downs flow generator has the advantages that it can provide both a consistent FIO_2 and the high gas flows required to meet or exceed patient inspiratory needs (up to 100 L/min) and that it provides an FIO_2 of 0.3 to 1.0.

The mechanism by which the flow generator increases the FIO_2 is by redirecting the O_2 inlet flow in increasing amounts away from the jet. As greater proportions of the 100% O_2 are shifted away from the jet, less room air is entrained and the FIO_2 increases. The higher flow of O_2 (which directly enters the device's output gas flow) compensates for lesser amounts of entrained room air; thus, the FIO_2 increases and total device output flow is maintained. The needle valve at the top of the tube controls the total amount of source oxygen into the system and is adjusted to supply the appropriate total flow of mixed gas. Disadvantages of the Downs high-flow generator include high gas consumption and noise levels. A bacterial filter can be fitted over the air inlet port to reduce noise.

Air–Oxygen Blending Using Dual Flow Meters

Dual flow meters are the simplest and most economical method of delivering a specific FIO_2 and total flow. Two flow meters, one for air and one for O_2, can be used to mix and deliver precise oxygen concentrations (**Figure 16–20**). The gas flow delivered to the patient through large-bore corrugated tubing is simply the sum of the flows from the two flow meters. The mixed gas will be very dry and should be humidified before it is delivered to the patient. The patient interface can be the standard aerosol mask, tent, tracheostomy mask, or Briggs adapter with reservoir.

Air–Oxygen Blenders (Proportioners)

Air–oxygen blenders, sometimes referred to as *mixers* or *proportioners* (**Figure 16–21**), provide a convenient, compact device for dialing in a specific FIO_2; however, they are expensive in comparison with dual flow meter manual techniques. The principal component of the

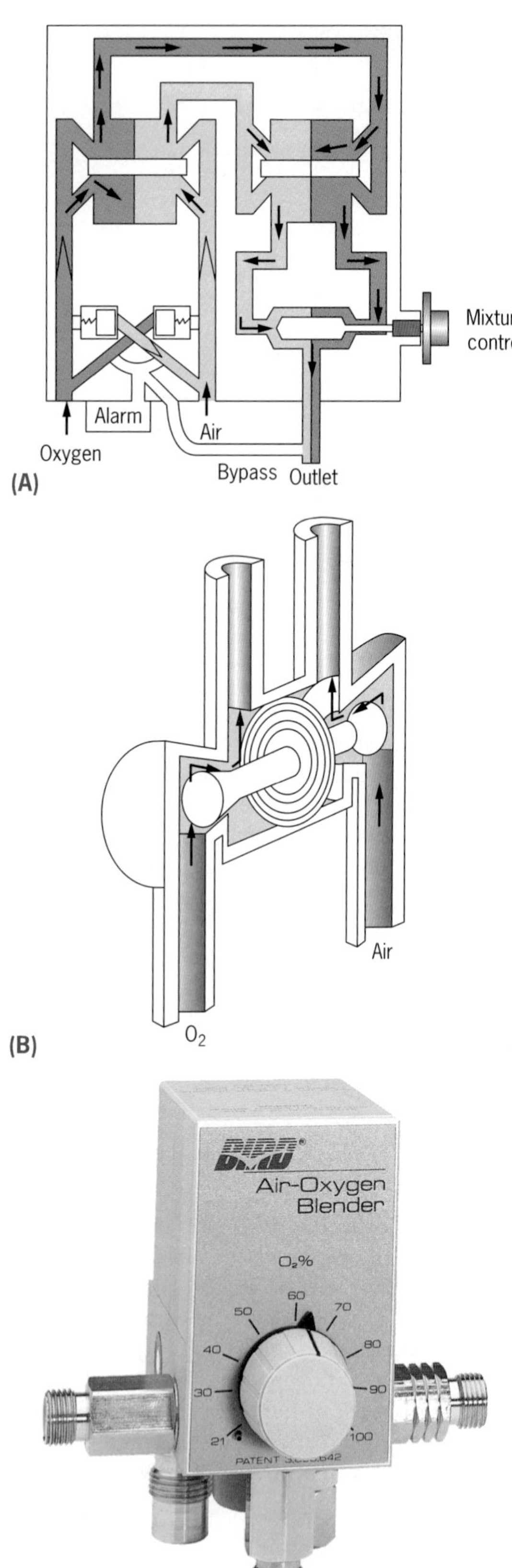

FIGURE 16–21 (**A**) Air–oxygen blender or proportioner. (**B**) Proportioning valve in an air-oxygen blender. (**C**) Commercially available air–oxygen blender. (**A** and **B**) Modified from Ward JJ. Equipment for mixed gas and oxygen therapy. In: Barnes TA, ed. *Core Textbook of Respiratory Care Practice*. 2nd ed. Mosby; 1994.

blender is a proportioning module, in which a 50-psig source of air and O_2 is proportioned to produce the required F_{IO_2}. The blender outlet usually produces 50 psig of the mixed gas, which can then be directly attached to devices by using a flow meter.

Air–oxygen proportioners receive each gas separately from a pipeline or compressed gas cylinder. Ideally, the supply pressures of both gases are nearly equal, usually 50 psig. In clinical practice, this does not always occur, so blenders have internal pressure-regulating systems. Once the pressures for air and oxygen are sufficiently similar, a dual-orifice needle valve controls the amount of each gas flowing out of the orifices. For higher concentrations, the valve would simultaneously open for more O_2 flow as it decreases the air flow. Blender manufacturers provide built-in alarm systems and sometimes pressure gauges that allow the respiratory therapist to confirm the proper inlet pressures.

Aside from imbalances in the inlet gas pressure supply lines, another common problem is contamination of one gas supply by another because of retrograde flow. This problem has been reported when blenders are connected to gas inlets but are not running to patient systems. The higher-pressure gas (usually oxygen) can flow into the medical air gas lines if inlet check valves are defective. When blenders are not in use, the path of least resistance for the higher-pressure oxygen is the piped air system. Contaminates from gas lines can prevent these pressure valves from sealing properly. Corrosion due to moisture and particulate matter can build up and restrict flow or prevent sealing of check valves. Routine inspection and cleaning twice a year are recommended. Replacement of inlet sintered metal filters and use of water trap filters should reduce this problem. In more serious cases, more complex filter systems may be required.

It is difficult for manufacturers to build blenders with the desired accuracy over the complete range of flows needed clinically. Low-flow blenders are most accurate at low-flow applications requiring less than about 20 L/min. High-flow blenders must be accurate in providing controlled F_{IO_2} levels at flows in the 80 to 100 L/min range. High-flow blenders tend to be more inaccurate at low flow rates, and low-flow blenders at high flows. Evaluations of commercially available medical air–oxygen blenders have found that all blenders were quite accurate when both inlet pressures were 50 psig.

Given the above technical challenges to the accuracy of air–oxygen blenders, it is important that all blenders be calibrated initially and verified periodically by O_2 analyzers. Although the devices are relatively reliable and the air–oxygen mixing equations are valid, inaccurately calibrated equipment and calculation errors may affect the delivered F_{IO_2}. To avoid potentially lethal medical mistakes, all fixed-performance devices and air–oxygen blender systems should always have the F_{IO_2} confirmed by direct oxygen analysis.

Oxygen Enclosures

Placing the patient into an oxygen-enriched environment was one of the earliest methods of O_2 administration. Adult **oxygen tents**, infant incubators, and pediatric croup tents were all introduced between the mid-1920s and the 1940s. The adult tent was widely used for both oxygen administration and high-humidity therapy through the 1960s. Today enclosures are used primarily in infant and pediatric applications and include hoods, incubators, and croup tents. Oxygen and aerosol tents, even for children, have been virtually abandoned.

> **RESPIRATORY RECAP**
>
> **Oxygen Enclosures**
>
> » O_2 enclosures include O_2 tents and hoods.
>
> » HBO therapy is currently indicated for treatment of carbon monoxide poisoning, wounds (especially those infected by anaerobic bacteria), air embolism, and decompression sickness.

Infant **oxygen hoods** are used, but infant nasal cannulas are being used increasingly as an alternative. The hood covers only the head, allowing access to the infant's lower body while still permitting use of a standard incubator or radiant warmer. The oxygen hood (**Figure 16–22**) is a round or rectangular, bottomless, clear rigid plastic device with a half-moon cutout that allows it to be placed over an infant's neck to enclose the entire head. O_2 is delivered to the hood through either a blender with a heated humidifier or a heated air-entrainment nebulizer. Providing a minimum flow of 6 to 8 L/min is necessary to prevent the accumulation of CO_2. Frequent or continuous monitoring of the O_2 concentration and internal hood temperature is necessary.

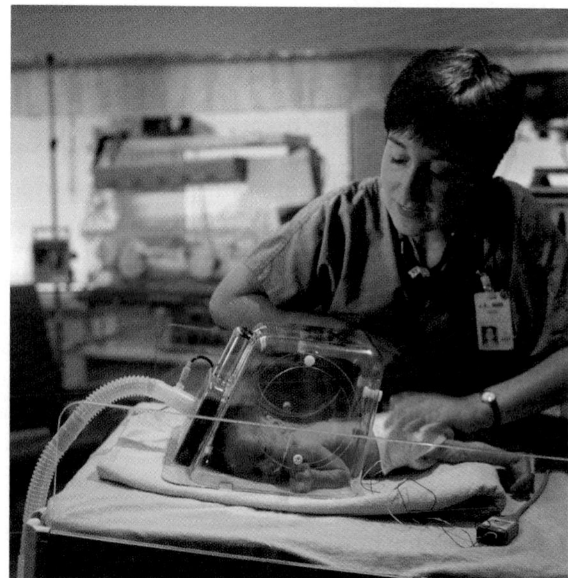

FIGURE 16–22 Oxygen hood.

Hyperbaric Oxygen Therapy

Hyperbaric oxygen (HBO) therapy involves administration of gas at an increased atmospheric pressure; its use in medicine has varied over the years. HBO patients are placed inside an airtight chamber that can be pressurized to several times the normal atmospheric pressure of 760 mm Hg. The goal of HBO is to dissolve more gas (particularly O_2) into the blood and body tissues of the patient. The increased O_2 dissolved in blood and body tissues facilitates metabolism in the absence of O_2Hb (when used for CO poisoning) and exposes anaerobic bacteria to a fatal level of O_2 (for treatment of wounds with *Clostridium* infections, such as gas gangrene).

Hyperbaric chambers can contain several patients and caretakers or can be designed to contain only one patient, with the care personnel remaining outside. Smaller HBO apparatuses designed to enclose individual affected limbs are also in use. There are many significant differences between conventional O_2 therapy and HBO therapy, and thus specialized training of respiratory therapy personnel involved with HBO is required. For example, gas volumes differ in relation to the chamber pressure, and O_2 toxicity occurs in both a pulmonary and cerebral form that occur much more rapidly under HBO conditions.

Since hyperbaric treatment is indicated for clinical situations arising from recreational or occupational diving accidents, many of the available HBO chambers are found in coastal areas or on rescue ships. Divers are trained to incrementally gas-off by ascending slowly or in stages, but when divers surface too rapidly, they may develop decompression sickness and air embolisms. In these cases, the affected divers are returned to their lowest depth pressure and decompressed more slowly in the chamber. Because of the frequent use of HBO equipment in diving accidents, gauges are calibrated in feet of sea water (fsw) (33 fsw is the equivalent of 1 atmosphere). Treatment of recreational or occupational decompression sickness does not necessarily involve use of supplemental oxygen.

HBO treatment is indicated for carbon monoxide poisoning (from attempted suicide or furnace venting accidents), *Clostridium* myonecrosis (gas gangrene), air embolism (the bends), decompression sickness (N_2 narcosis, rapture of the deep), and accelerating healing of selected wounds, grafts, burns, or infections. Because of the biochemical complexity of CO poisoning, the advantages of HBO therapy in comparison to normobaric, ambient 100% oxygen therapy continue to be debated. HBO treatment for the bends (nitrogen coming out of solution in the joints of the body) has never been questioned.

Monitoring the Physiologic Effects of Oxygen

O_2 therapy is often initiated in response to patient complaints of shortness of breath. The actual symptoms of hypoxia, however, are cognitive impairment, cardiac rhythm and conduction dysfunction, and renal dysfunction. The signs of hypoxia may include high respiratory frequency, cyanosis, chest pain, low PaO_2, and low SaO_2. Effective oxygen treatment of these conditions requires careful monitoring.

Blood Gases and Oximetry

Monitoring the clinical signs and the results of arterial blood gas analysis is standard for documenting oxygenation, ventilation, and acid–base balance. The blood gas measurement of PaO_2 and SaO_2 and the measurement of Hb and cardiac output are excellent methods for assessing the presence and common causes of hypoxia. However, these measurements are sometimes not easily obtained or are intermittent, meaning that the measurements may have once been accurate but have since changed. In an attempt to overcome the periodic nature of oxygen analysis, more continuous technologies have evolved.

Pulse oximetry has become the most common form of continuously monitoring oxygen saturation (SpO_2) and is the standard of care in the operating or recovery room, pulmonary function or sleep laboratory, intensive care unit, emergency room, and other clinical areas throughout the hospital. Clinicians can use oximetry to detect episodes of desaturation during patient transport, cardiac catheterization, bronchoscopy, or airway suctioning. Its noninvasive approach, ease of use, and real-time feedback have led to its widespread acceptance in titrating oxygen levels to ventilated and spontaneously breathing patients. It may be used to spot check or continuously measure patients' condition. Clinicians can select among such features as portability, recording methods, amount of memory for trend analysis, alarms, electrocardiogram synchronization, and probe styles, depending on their application and budget. Some units allow clinicians to adjust the average time between signals to allow for closer real-time correlation with the patient's data.

Oxygen Analysis

When an accurate analysis of oxygen concentrations can be performed, it should be part of a safe therapy protocol. **Oxygen analyzers** are used to measure the concentration of oxygen (O_2%) administered to patients (**Figure 16–23**). Analysis is routinely performed in infant oxygen hoods, incubators, mechanical ventilators, anesthetic circuits, and some fixed-performance oxygen administration devices (e.g., an aerosol-entrainment T piece). Clinicians should check dual air–oxygen flow meters and blenders to confirm the desired oxygen concentrations. Monitoring can consist of spot samples, periodic checks, or continuous monitoring with high-low limit alarms.

> **RESPIRATORY RECAP**
>
> **Evaluation of Oxygen Therapy**
>
> » Arterial blood gas measurements are the best way of evaluating hypoxemia.
>
> » Pulse oximetry provides a real-time, noninvasive estimate of oxygenation.
>
> » O_2 analyzers are used to measure the O_2 concentration of a gas mixture.

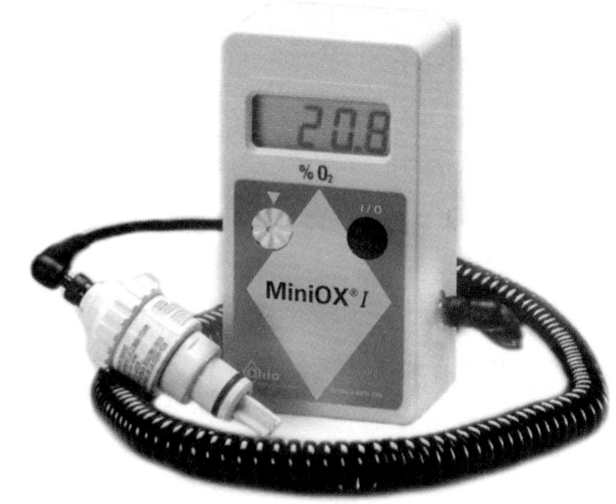

FIGURE 16–23 Oxygen analyzer.

Polarographic analyzers use a Clark electrode to measure oxygen. Galvanic cell analyzers, like polarographic analyzers, use an electrochemical principle. Although both analyzers actually measure PIO_2, they display O_2%. Therefore, analyzers used at high altitudes require recalibration. Calibration is usually accomplished by exposing the electrode to room air (21% oxygen) and then to 100% oxygen. The O_2 analyzer is then adjusted to read the two calibrating gas concentrations correctly. An inability to calibrate the analyzer usually means that the electrolyte in the electrode needs to be changed. O_2 analyzers should be checked relatively frequently for calibration and should be repaired if they are unable to read within ±2%.

Clinical Application of Oxygen Therapy

Respiratory therapists are frequently asked to integrate patient information and recommend a medical gas therapy. This process begins with patient assessment and is usually based on clinical circumstances or specific signs or symptoms that suggest hypoxemia or hypoxia. Sometimes laboratory data (e.g., blood gases) reveal an unnoticed problem. After determining that the patient has a problem that oxygen or other gas therapy may treat, the decision process is made complex by the many factors related to oxygen transport. For instance, there may be problems with ventilation, oxygen content of arterial blood, or perfusion. **Figure 16–24** shows all of the factors to be considered in the decision-making process for clinical application of O_2 therapy.

A complete history and laboratory profile are commonly absent when a patient has acute problems

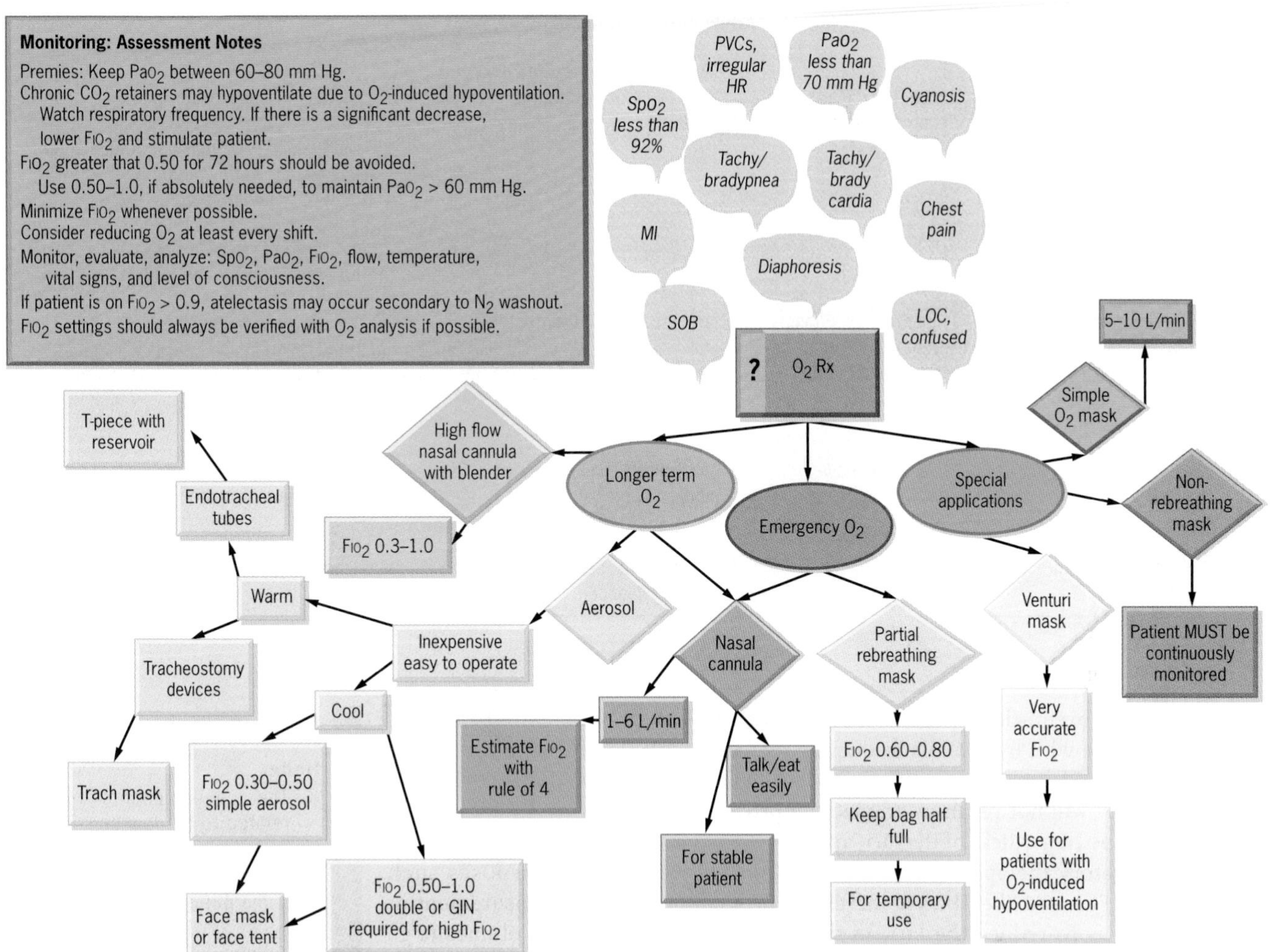

FIGURE 16–24 Oxygen administration guide.

indicating medical gas therapy, and thus clinical signs and symptoms may be the clinician's only guides. As a general guideline, it is usually safer to provide liberal flows and concentrations than to restrict oxygen. There are always exceptions, but side effects of O_2 therapy are usually less significant than the profound brain damage secondary to hypoxia. In the past there has been too much emphasis on withholding oxygen because of a relatively small number of COPD patients with chronic hypercarbia who may hypoventilate when O_2 is administered.

The initial assessment may also provide information about the cause of the dyspnea or hypoxemia. In the case of partial upper airway obstruction caused by severe acute asthma, heliox may allow time to further evaluate the pathology, prepare a definitive therapy, or await effects of pharmacologic therapy. Following initial assessment, clinicians should determine whether the patient requires hyperbaric O_2 therapy or traditional ambient medical gas therapy. Severe carbon monoxide poisoning can be treated with hyperbaric therapy if there is immediate access to a chamber.

The next decision is the initial concentration of oxygen and appropriate O_2 therapy device (**Table 16–6**). Respiratory therapists often apply oxygen based on bedside assessment and clinical judgment. An O_2 mask is often more uncomfortable than a nasal cannula, but a mask may be more appropriate if the O_2 requirement is high. A room air blood gas analysis is quite valuable if it can be obtained without significant delay to assist with diagnosis and guide selection of the level of oxygen concentration needed. An O_2 therapy system should be selected based on the FIO_2 and inspiratory flow requirement. High-flow devices allow more consistent levels for patients who have rapid respiratory rates and those who require a high FIO_2. Inspired O_2 is then titrated to achieve a PaO_2 above 60 mm Hg or an SpO_2 above 90%. Pulse oximetry can useful for the initial O_2 titration. It should also be kept in mind that O_2 therapy alone may not

TABLE 16–6 Oxygen Delivery Devices for Adult Applications

Device	Usual Flow Range	Approximate Inspired Oxygen Concentration	Comments
Nasal cannula	1 to 6 L/min	24% to 40%	F_{IO_2} is reduced with nasal obstruction; can be less effective with mouth breathing; F_{IO_2} varies with breathing pattern.
Simple mask	5 to 10 L/min	30% to 60%	Flows <5 L/min result in rebreathing; F_{IO_2} varies with breathing pattern.
Nonrebreathing mask	Flow must be high enough to prevent full collapse of reservoir bag during inhalation; ≥12 L/min often is required	Theoretically, a nonrebreathing mask will deliver close to 100% O_2. In reality, it delivers 60% to 80% because the mask does not fit tightly over the face.	If Sp_{O_2} remains low despite use of a nonrebreathing mask, consider using a high-flow O_2 delivery device.
Air entrainment mask	Use at least the flow stamped on the colored adapter	O_2 concentration is stamped on the colored adapter.	When mask is removed, administer O_2 by nasal cannula to provide target Sp_{O_2}.
High-flow oxygen system	>30 L/min	24% to 100%, set by air and O_2 flow meters or blender.	Gas should be humidified with high-flow system.

correct hypoxemia in all patients. Patients with profound hypercapnia with hypoxemia frequently require ventilatory support. For patients with a large right-to-left shunt, O_2 therapy will not result in dramatic improvements in Pa_{O_2} or Sp_{O_2} regardless of the F_{IO_2} applied.

Respiratory therapists should be conservative when reducing F_{IO_2} and liberal when increasing it. A common guideline is to reduce the F_{IO_2} in decrements of 0.05, monitoring Pa_{O_2} or Sp_{O_2} as the F_{IO_2} is decreased and allowing at least 20 minutes to reflect the actual physiologic response to any F_{IO_2}. For increases in F_{IO_2}, it is always wise to overshoot or exceed the predicted Pa_{O_2} or Sp_{O_2} and then titrate down.

Therapist-driven protocols and clinical pathways (**Figure 16–25**) allow clinicians to apply oxygen therapy within a predetermined decision-making algorithm. Each patient must be considered as a special case, however, and clinicians should not be bound by guidelines if the clinical situation dictates an alternative approach.

Helium–Oxygen Therapy

Since Barach established the value of low-density gas therapy in 1934, helium–oxygen mixtures have had a notable, if limited, role in respiratory care. Beyond their use in industry and deep sea diving, there are a number of medical reasons for patients to breathe these mixtures, generally referred to as **heliox**. Heliox is used clinically because of its low density. The only gas with a density less than helium is hydrogen. Unlike hydrogen, helium is an inert gas and is thus nonreactive. Helium is relatively insoluble in body fluids. Because helium does not support life, for clinical applications it must always be delivered in a gas mixture containing at least 20% oxygen. In addition to its use for diagnostic purposes such as measurement of lung volumes (e.g., functional residual capacity), it may be of therapeutic use in patients with obstructive lung diseases.

> **RESPIRATORY RECAP**
>
> **Heliox**
>
> » Therapeutic benefits are related to the low density of heliox.
>
> » Use of heliox is beneficial in some patients with partial upper airway obstruction or asthma.
>
> » Heliox adversely affects the function of equipment such as flow meters, nebulizers, and ventilators.

The physical properties of helium are different from those of air or oxygen (**Table 16–7**). These physical properties of helium affect its flow through airways of the lungs (**Equation 16–2**). Because turbulent flow is density dependent, whereas laminar flow is density independent, use of heliox is expected to have a greater effect on turbulent flow. Because of its lower density and higher viscosity, heliox produces a lower Reynolds number and a greater tendency for laminar flow. Laminar flow is desirable because it is more energy efficient than turbulent flow. According to the Reynolds number, gas flow tends to be laminar in small peripheral airways of the lungs and turbulent in larger central airways. Therefore, heliox may have limited benefit for diseases affecting small airways (e.g., emphysema, asthma), whereas it may be useful for diseases affecting larger airways (e.g., postextubation stridor, croup). For gas flow through an orifice (i.e., axial acceleration), flow through the orifice (e.g., constricted airway) will increase if the density of the gas decreases (e.g., heliox). Because of the Bernoulli

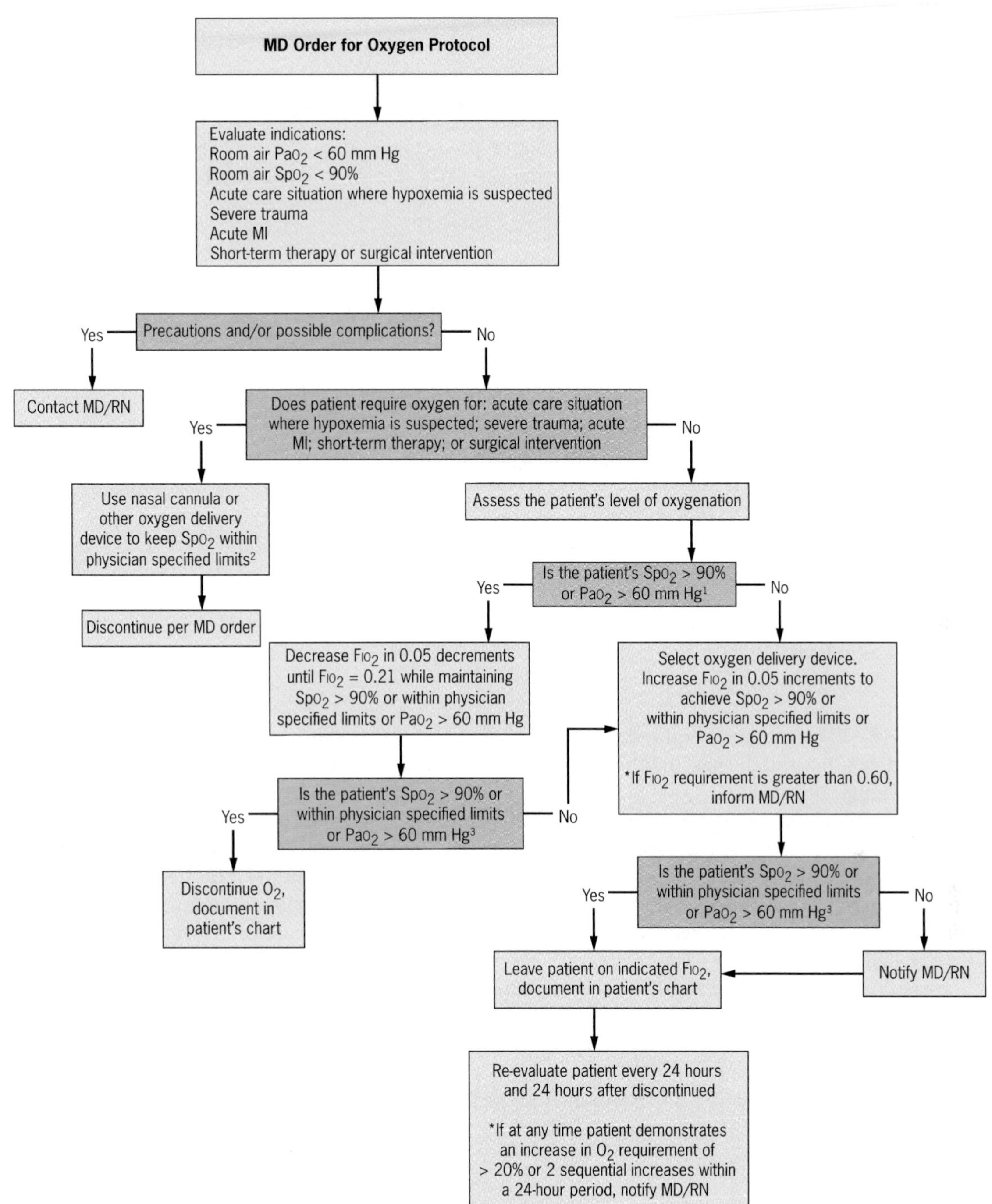

FIGURE 16–25 Protocol for oxygen administration.

TABLE 16–7 Physical Properties of Oxygen, Air, and Helium

Gas	Density (g/L)	Viscosity (μpoise)	Thermoconductivity (μcal × cm × 5 × °K)
Air	1.293	170.8	58.0
Oxygen	1.429	192.6	58.5
Helium	0.179	188.7	352.0

principle, less pressure is required to produce flow with heliox than with air or oxygen. According to Graham's law, heliox (80% helium/20% oxygen) diffuses at a rate 1.8 times greater than oxygen.

Helium is available premixed with oxygen in several standard mixtures in large compressed gas cylinders. The most popular mixtures are 80%/20% and 70%/30% helium–oxygen. The densities are 1.805 and 1.586 less dense, respectively, than pure oxygen. In any heliox

EQUATION 16–2

Physical Principles That Explain the Benefits of Heliox Therapy

For turbulent flow, the Hagen-Poiseuille equation predicts that flow is affected by the radius of the conducting tube, the pressure gradient, the density of the gas (ρ), and the length of the conducting tube (l) as follows:

$$\dot{V} = (4\pi r^5 \Delta P)/(\rho l)$$

where $\dot{V}$ is flow and ΔP is the pressure gradient.

Whether flow is laminar or turbulent is determined by the Reynolds number (Re), as follows:

$$\text{Re} = \text{Inertial forces/Viscous forces} = (vr\rho)/\eta$$

where v is the velocity of gas movement, r is the radius, and η is viscosity. A low Reynolds number causes flow to be laminar.

For gas flow through an orifice (e.g., axial acceleration), flow has only a weak dependence on the Reynolds number and is affected by density as follows:

$$\dot{V}^2 = (\Delta P)/\rho$$

In other words, flow through an orifice (e.g., constricted airway) will increase if the density of the gas decreases (e.g., heliox).

The Bernoulli principle states that the pressure required to produce flow is affected by the mass of the gas as follows:

$$(P_1 - P_2) = \tfrac{1}{2} \times m \times (v_2^2 - v_1^2)$$

where $(P_1 - P_2)$ = pressure required to produce flow, $(v_2^2 - v_1^2)$ = difference in velocity between P_1 and P_2, and m = mass of the gas. In other words, less pressure is required to produce flow with heliox than with air or oxygen.

Graham's law states that the rate of diffusion is inversely related to the square root of gas density. Thus, heliox (80% He/20% O_2) will diffuse at a rate 1.8 times faster than oxygen, which explains why the flow of heliox through an oxygen flow meter is 1.8 times faster than the indicated flow.

According to wave speed theory, flow through an airway cannot be greater than the flow at which gas velocity equals wave speed. Wave speed is the speed at which a small disturbance travels in a compliant tube filled with a fluid. The wave speed (c) in an airway depends on the cross-sectional area of the airway (A), the density of the fluid, and the slope of the pressure–area curve of the airway (dP/dA), as follows:

$$c^2 = A/\rho \times dP/dA$$

Note that maximal flow ($\dot{V}_{max}$) is the product of the fluid velocity at wave speed and the airway area (cA). If $\dot{V}_{max} = cA$, then the following occurs:

$$\dot{V}_{max} = (A/\rho \times dP/dA)^{1/2}$$

According to wave speed theory, $\dot{V}_{max}$ increases as gas density decreases. However, wave speed theory is useful only when gas flow is density dependent. In small airways, and particularly at low lung volumes, gas flow is density independent, and viscous flow limitation becomes more important than wave speed.

breathing system, a tightly sealed, closed system is required because helium will easily leak through small holes. To avoid administration of a hypoxic gas mixture, 20% O_2/80% He should be mixed with oxygen to provide the desired helium concentration and F_{IO_2}. The F_{IO_2} requirement limits the helium concentration that can be administered. If an F_{IO_2} greater than 0.40 is required, the limited concentration of helium is unlikely to produce clinical benefit. However, the F_{IO_2} requirement may decrease if heliox therapy is effective.

Although a consensus on the clinical indications for the use of heliox has not yet formed, it has been used

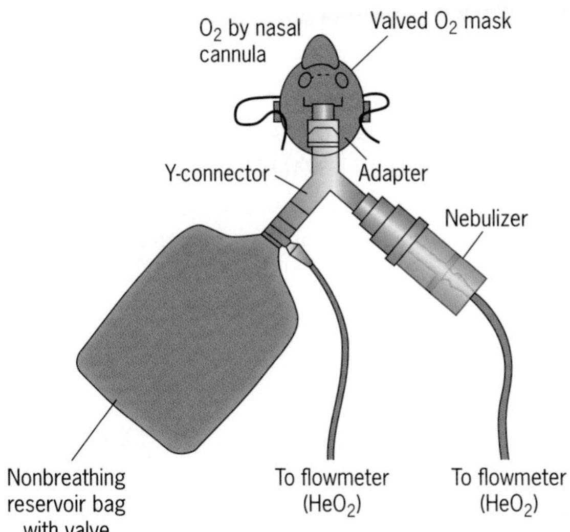

FIGURE 16–26 Equipment for heliox administration to spontaneously breathing patients.

to treat two types of cases: as a temporary measure for patients with stridor and for those with airway obstruction, such as in patients with life-threatening asthma. The benefit of heliox for postextubation stridor is anecdotal. Although it may improve the symptoms related to stridor, aggressive treatment of the underlying problem must occur concurrently. In spontaneously breathing patients with asthma, heliox has been reported to decrease $Paco_2$, increase peak flow, and decrease pulsus paradoxus. The reduction in pulsus paradoxus may be particularly important because it reflects a reduction in inspiratory muscle work. Heliox has also been used with intubated and mechanically ventilated asthmatic patients, in whom it reportedly produces a reduction in $Paco_2$ with a lower peak airway pressure and an improvement in oxygenation. The role of heliox in the treatment of COPD is unclear. COPD is a disease of the small airways, a region of the lungs in which flow is density independent.

Nonintubated patients may receive therapy via a well-fitting simple mask or a mask with a reservoir bag (**Figure 16–26**). A Y piece attached to the mask allows concurrent delivery of aerosolized medications. Sufficient flow is required to keep the reservoir bag inflated. This is often 12 to 15 L/min and requires three to six H-size cylinders per day. Using an oxygen-calibrated flow meter for heliox therapy causes the flow of heliox (80% helium/20% oxygen) to be 1.8 times greater than the indicated flow. Accurate flows are not required in administering helium–oxygen mixtures. The objective when using a reservoir bag and mask is to keep the reservoir bag nearly full at all times. Nasal cannulas have been found to be ineffective in such treatment.

Heliox administration during mechanical ventilation can be problematic. Ventilators are designed to deliver a mixture of air and oxygen. The density, viscosity, and thermal conductivity of helium can affect the delivered tidal volume and the measurement of exhaled tidal volume. With some ventilators, no reliable tidal volume is delivered with heliox. Use of other ventilators may result in a much higher delivered tidal volume than desired. A number of ventilators are currently approved for heliox delivery.

Several studies reported improved aerosol penetration and deposition in the lungs with the nebulizer powered with heliox rather than air, but studies reported no benefit with the use of heliox-driven nebulizer therapy. Heliox can affect nebulizer function, resulting in a smaller particle size, reduced output, and longer nebulization time. When heliox (rather than air or oxygen) is used to power the nebulizer, the flow should be increased by 50% to 100% to ensure adequate output from the nebulizer. Heliox has been shown also to improve aerosol delivery during mechanical ventilation.

Some clinicians are interested in combining the beneficial effects of noninvasive ventilation and heliox. In COPD patients, several studies have reported that heliox reduced $Paco_2$, dyspnea, and work of breathing to a greater extent than oxygen alone without heliox. However, outcome studies to date have not been able to show an improvement in patient outcomes when using a combination of noninvasive ventilation and heliox.

Carbon Dioxide Therapy

In the past, CO_2 therapy was commonly used for its pharmacologic effects. Today, however, such therapeutic applications are quite limited or controversial. Carbon dioxide therapy has several dangerous side effects, and its efficacy remains unproved in many of the following applications.

Historically, it was thought that increasing inspired CO_2 levels could treat hysterical hyperventilation (anxiety attacks) by lessening syncopal attacks due to hypocarbia. Five percent carbon dioxide in oxygen (**carbogen**) or rebreathing into a paper bag or tubing reservoir was used. Anxiety attacks may still be relieved by breathing into a paper bag, but current treatment standards recommend treating most cases with anxiolytic medications such as diazepam (Valium) or lorazepam (Ativan).

Carbogen historically was also used to stimulate spontaneous breathing in postoperative patients to hasten the removal of volatile anesthetics and to prevent atelectasis. This use of carbogen was an indirect means of encouraging patients to take deep breaths. Currently, mechanical or nonmechanical methods to cause sustained inspiration (such as incentive spirometry or CPAP therapy) are used to prevent or treat postoperative pulmonary complications.

Treatment of hiccoughs (singultus) with carbogen or by rebreathing exhaled CO_2 is occasionally successful, but the mechanisms by which such treatment works are unknown. Carbogen has also been used to terminate seizures (petit mal) by the mechanism of decreasing brain excitability. CO_2 was also used in the past to improve regional blood flow by dilating vessels in the brain for the treatment of strokes. More recently, carbogen has been used to encourage ophthalmic artery blood flow.

Because expired air normally contains approximately 5% CO_2 (normal F_{ECO_2} is approximately 0.05), rebreathing that gas can provide CO_2 gas therapy. The paper bag is the simplest device. The Adler rebreather and Dale-Schwartz tube are commercial adaptations. Administration of specific mixtures of carbon dioxide can be provided by premixed high-pressure gas cylinders. Regulators that attach to the cylinder valves must be specific for the concentration used. Most common are mixtures of 5% CO_2 and 95% O_2 and of 7% CO_2 and 93% O_2, although no more than 5% CO_2 is normally used. Although CO_2 concentrations greater than 10% are available, their use is not recommended because of the risk of rapidly developing side effects.

Administration devices for CO_2/O_2 gas therapy include the disposable nonrebreathing mask with reservoir and the well-fitted mask with reservoir. As with any mask therapy, patients must be observed for vomiting and aspiration. Administration times are normally limited to fairly short periods of 5 to 15 minutes. Patients on carbogen therapy must be carefully monitored for pulse, respiratory rate, blood pressure, and mental state. Pulse rate, minute ventilation, and blood pressure usually increase somewhat when carbogen treatments are administered, but significant changes in any of these should prompt the discontinuance of the therapy. Carbogen therapy may also depress the patient's mental state and can result in convulsions, coma, and ultimately death.

Nitric Oxide Therapy

In 1987, it was found that **nitric oxide (NO)** is normally biosynthesized in vascular endothelial cells and is an important mediator of physiologic function, including vasodilation, neurotransmission, long-term memory, and immunologic defense. The NO molecule is highly diffusible and lipid soluble. Its half-life ranges from 3 to 50 seconds as it converts to nitrates, nitrites, and higher oxides of nitrogen. Nitric oxide is a ubiquitous, highly reactive, gaseous, diatomic radical that is important physiologically at low concentrations (**Box 16–1**). Atmospheric concentrations of NO usually range from 10 to 100 ppb.

RESPIRATORY RECAP

Inhaled Nitric Oxide

- » Inhaled nitric oxide is a selective pulmonary vasodilator.
- » Inhaled nitric oxide is an FDA-approved treatment of hypoxic respiratory failure of the newborn.
- » Toxicity is low at usual clinical doses.
- » Inhaled NO is administered via a specially designed delivery system.

BOX 16–1

Typical Expression of Concentration of Nitric Oxide and Nitrogen Dioxide

Concentrations are usually expressed in concentrations of parts per million (ppm) or parts per billion (ppb).

% = 1:100
ppm = 1:1,000,000
10,000 ppm = 1%
1000 ppb = 1 ppm

L-Arginine is the substrate for NO synthesis in biologic systems. NO is produced in the presence of nitric oxide synthase (NOS). NO is lipophilic and readily diffuses across cell membranes to adjacent cells, thus serving as a local messenger molecule. It typically diffuses from its cell of origin to a neighboring cell, where it binds with guanylate cyclase. Activation of guanylate cyclase results in the production of cyclic guanosine 3′,5′-monophosphate (cGMP) from guanosine triphosphate (GTP), which produces a biologic effect within the cell (e.g., smooth muscle relaxation).

The term *selective pulmonary vasodilation* is used to indicate two physiologic phenomena (**Figure 16–27**). First, selective pulmonary vasodilators reduce pulmonary vascular resistance without affecting systemic vascular resistance. Second, a selective pulmonary vasodilator affects vascular resistance only near ventilated alveoli. Inspired vasodilators are delivered to those lung units that are ventilated. NO is not a selective pulmonary vasodilator but becomes one when inhaled. Inhaled NO selectively improves blood flow to ventilated alveoli and produces a reduction in intrapulmonary shunt and improved arterial oxygenation. The selective pulmonary vasodilation demonstrated by inhaled NO is due to the high affinity of hemoglobin for NO, which is about 10^6 times as great as the affinity of hemoglobin for O_2. In contrast to inhaled NO, intravenous vasodilators (e.g., sodium nitroprusside, nitroglycerin, prostacyclin) are not selective. Although intravenous vasodilators lower pulmonary artery pressure, they also lower systemic blood pressure. These agents increase blood flow to both ventilated and unventilated lung units, resulting in an increased intrapulmonary shunt and a lower Pa_{O_2}.

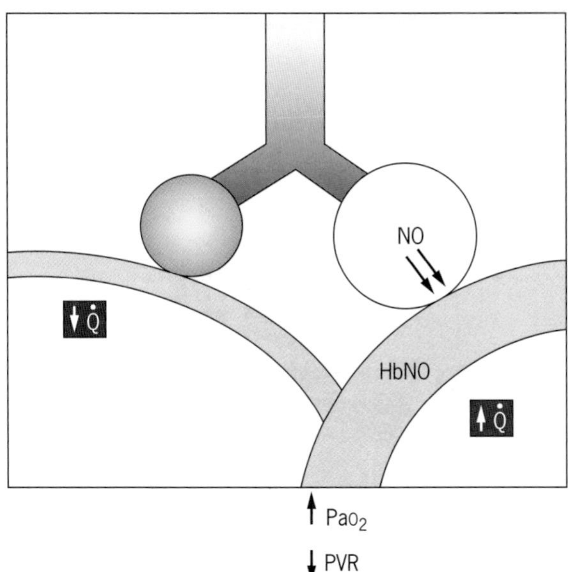

FIGURE 16–27 Inhaled nitric oxide is a selective pulmonary vasodilator because vasodilation occurs primarily in parts of the lungs that are ventilated, and because systemic vasodilation does not occur.

Multicenter, randomized, double-blind, placebo-controlled studies of inhaled NO for persistent pulmonary hypertension of the newborn (PPHN) have reported improvements in Pa_{O_2} and a reduction in the requirement for extracorporeal life support with the use of inhaled NO. These studies established a role for inhaled NO in term infants with PPHN and led to approval by the FDA in 1999 for use of inhaled NO, as noted by DailyMed:

> INO_{max}, in conjunction with ventilatory support and other appropriate agents, is indicated for the treatment of term and near-term (>34 weeks) neonates with hypoxic respiratory failure associated with clinical or echocardiographic evidence of pulmonary hypertension, where it improves oxygenation and reduces the need for extracorporeal membrane oxygenation.

This is the only FDA-approved indication for inhaled NO, and all other uses are off-label. Nitric oxide should not be used for hypoxemic newborns with congenital cardiac defects who are dependent upon right-to-left shunt. The usual starting dose of inhaled NO is 20 ppm. This dose is then weaned to the lowest effective dose (e.g., 5 ppm) and continued until the condition of the baby is improved. Inhaled NO produces an initial improvement in Pa_{O_2} for patients with ARDS, but this effect is lost after several days. Randomized multicenter trials failed to report improvements in important patient outcomes such as mortality with the use of inhaled NO.

AGE-SPECIFIC ANGLE

The only FDA-approved indication for inhaled nitric oxide is hypoxic respiratory failure of the newborn.

The toxicity of inhaled NO appears to be low when administered by clinicians familiar with its use. Nitrogen dioxide (NO_2) is produced spontaneously from NO and O_2. The conversion rate of NO to NO_2 is determined by the O_2 concentration, NO concentration, and the residence time of NO with O_2. The Occupational Safety and Health Administration (OSHA) has set safety limits for NO_2 at 5 ppm, but airway reactivity and parenchymal lung injury have been reported with inhalation of 2 ppm NO_2 or less. Methemoglobin production after NO exposure is uncommon at the NO doses used for therapeutic inhalation (20 ppm or less). Inhibition of platelet adhesion, aggregation, and agglutination has been reported with inhaled NO. At high doses (40 to 80 ppm), inhaled NO reportedly decreases pulmonary vascular resistance and increases pulmonary capillary wedge pressure in some patients with severe left ventricular dysfunction.

Withdrawal of inhaled NO is problematic for some patients. In some cases, the degree of hypoxemia and pulmonary hypertension is greater after discontinuation of NO than at baseline, leading to hemodynamic instability. Reinstitution of NO inhalation promptly corrects the hemodynamic instability, and NO withdrawal is postponed until the patient is less severely ill. The reasons for rebound are not known but may relate to feedback inhibition of NOS activity. The following guidelines may prevent the deleterious effects of rebound during withdrawal of inhaled NO:

1. Use the lowest effective NO dose (5 ppm or less).
2. Do not withdraw inhaled NO until the patient's clinical status has improved sufficiently.
3. Set the NO dose at 1 ppm for a short time (30 minutes to 1 hour) before discontinuing NO.
4. Increase the F_{IO_2} before withdrawal of inhaled NO and prepare to support the patient's hemodynamics if necessary.

The INOvent, NOmax DS, and INOblender (**Figure 16–28**) allow for operator-determined concentrations of inhaled NO without excessive inhaled NO_2. These devices can be used with neonatal ventilators, adult ventilators, and anesthesia machines, and with spontaneously breathing patients. The system is configured for 0 to 80 ppm with an 800-ppm NO source cylinder. These cylinders are either D size or size 88 (1963 L at 2000 psig), are constructed of aluminum alloy, and have threaded connections specific for NO (CGA 626). NO is stored as nitrogen gas. The injection module of the INOvent is inserted into the inspiratory circuit at the outlet of the ventilator. The injection module consists of a hot-film flow sensor and a gas injection tube. Flow in the ventilator circuit is precisely measured, and NO is injected proportional to that flow to provide the desired NO dose. The delivery system includes gas monitoring of O_2, NO, and NO_2 downstream from the point of injection.

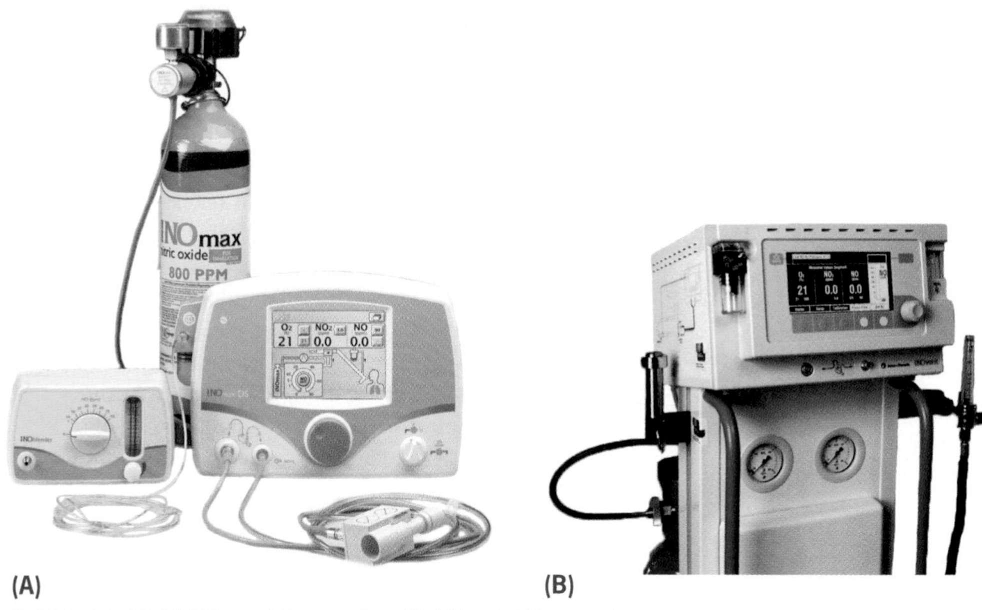

(A) (B)

FIGURE 16–28 (**A**) INOmax delivery system. (**B**) INOvent delivery system.

KEY POINTS

- Supplemental oxygen is indicated to treat hypoxemia.
- O_2 therapy is used for perioperative conditions, COPD, ARDS, CPR, MI, pulmonary edema, CO poisoning, and traumatic brain injury.
- O_2 is not explosive, but increases the combustibility of other flammable materials.
- Complications of O_2 therapy include oxygen toxicity, nitrogen washout atelectasis, oxygen-induced hypoventilation, retinopathy of prematurity, and failure of ductus closure in infants with congenital heart disease.
- O_2 may be of limited usefulness for anemia, low cardiac output, or high shunt.
- Flow control devices include flow restrictors, Bourdon gauges, and Thorpe tubes.
- Back-pressure-compensated Thorpe tubes are accurate regardless of downstream resistance.
- Nasal catheters, nasal cannulas, simple masks, partial rebreathing masks, and nonrebreathing masks are low-flow oxygen delivery devices.
- The F_{IO_2} from a low-flow oxygen delivery device is determined by the oxygen flow, reservoir volume, and inspiratory flow of the patient.
- High-flow oxygen delivery systems meet the entire inspiratory needs of the patient.
- Hoods, incubators, and tents are oxygen enclosure devices.
- Hyperbaric oxygen therapy is currently indicated for treatment of carbon monoxide poisoning, wounds (especially those infected by anaerobic bacteria), air embolism, and decompression sickness.
- Oxygen analyzers use polarography or galvanic cells to measure oxygen concentration.
- Heliox is used clinically because of its low density.
- Therapeutic applications of CO_2 therapy are limited or controversial.
- Inhaled nitric oxide is a selective pulmonary vasodilator.

SUGGESTED READING

Adhikari NK, Burns KE, Friedrich JO, et al. Effect of nitric oxide on oxygenation and mortality in acute lung injury: systematic review and meta-analysis. *BMJ*. 2007;334:779.

Annane D, Troche G, Delisle F, et al. Effects of mechanical ventilation with normobaric oxygen therapy on the rate of air removal from cerebral arteries. *Crit Care Med*. 1994;22:851–857.

Arul N, Konduri GG. Inhaled nitric oxide for preterm neonates. *Clin Perinatol*. 2009;36:43–61.

Aubier M, Murciano D, Milic-Emili J, et al. Effects of the administration of O_2 on ventilation and blood gases in patients with chronic obstructive pulmonary disease during acute respiratory failure. *Am Rev Respir Dis*. 1980;122:747–754.

Barnes TA. Equipment for mixed gas and oxygen therapy. *Respir Care Clin North Am*. 2000;6:545–595.

Bazuaye EA, Stone TN, Corris PA, Gibson GJ. Variability of inspired oxygen concentration with nasal cannulas. *Thorax*. 1992;47(8):609–611.

Boumphrey SM, Morris EA, Kinsella SM. 100% inspired oxygen from a Hudson mask—a realistic goal? *Resuscitation*. 2003;57:69–72.

Branson RD. The nuts and bolts of increasing arterial oxygenation: devices and techniques. *Respir Care*. 1993;38:672–686.

Campbell DJ, Fairfield MC. The delivery of oxygen by a venturi T piece. *Anaesthesia*. 1996;51:558–560.

Campbell EJ, Baker MD, Crites-Silver P. Subjective effects of humidification of oxygen for delivery by nasal cannula. A prospective study. *Chest*. 1988;93(2):289–293.

Carvalho CR, Schettino GP, Maranhao B, Bethlem EP. Hyperoxia and lung disease. *Curr Opin Pulm Med*. 1998;4:300–304.

Chevrolet JC. Helium oxygen mixtures in the intensive care unit. *Crit Care*. 2001;5:179–181.

Chien JW, Ciufo R, Novak R, et al. Uncontrolled oxygen administration and respiratory failure in acute asthma. *Chest.* 2000;117:728–733.

Christopher KL. Transtracheal oxygen catheters. *Clin Chest Med.* 2003;24:489–510.

Colebourn CL, Barber V, Young JD. Use of helium-oxygen mixture in adult patients presenting with exacerbations of asthma and chronic obstructive pulmonary disease: a systematic review. *Anaesthesia.* 2007;62:34–42.

Creagh-Brown BC, Griffiths MJ, Evans TW. Bench-to-bedside review: inhaled nitric oxide therapy in adults. *Crit Care.* 2009;13:221.

Crossley DJ, McGuire GP, Barrow PM, Houston PL. Influence of inspired oxygen concentration on deadspace, respiratory drive, and $PaCO_2$ in intubated patients with chronic obstructive pulmonary disease. *Crit Care Med.* 1997;25:1522–1526.

DailyMed. INOmax (nitric oxide) for inhalation (Initial U.S. approval in 1999.) Available at: http://dailymed.nlm.nih.gov/dailymed/getFile.cfm?id=11080&type=pdf&name=762b51be-1893-4cd1-9511-e645fc420d3a.

Dexter F, Reasoner DK. Theoretical assessment of normobaric oxygen therapy to treat pneumocephalus. *Anesthesiology.* 1996;84:442–447.

Dick CR, Liu Z, Sassoon CS, et al. O_2-induced change in ventilation and ventilatory drive in COPD. *Am J Respir Crit Care Med.* 1997;155:609–614.

Dunlevy CL, Tyl SE. The effect of oral versus nasal breathing on oxygen concentrations received from nasal cannulas. *Respir Care.* 1992;37:357–360.

Dunn WF, Nelson SB, Hubmayr RD. Oxygen-induced hypercarbia in obstructive pulmonary disease. *Am Rev Respir Dis.* 1991;144:526–530.

Estey W. Subjective effects of dry versus humidified low flow oxygen. *Respir Care.* 1980;25:1143–1144.

Fairfield JE, Goroszeniuk T, Tully AM, Adams AP. Oxygen delivery systems—a comparison of two devices. *Anaesthesia.* 1991;46:135–138.

Fink JB. Opportunities and risks of using heliox in your clinical practice. *Respir Care.* 2006;51:651–660.

Foust GN, Potter WA, Wilons MD, Golden EB. Shortcomings of using two jet nebulizers in tandem with an aerosol face mask for optimal oxygen therapy. *Chest.* 1991;99:1346–1351.

Gentile MA. The role of inhaled nitric oxide and heliox in the management of acute respiratory failure. *Respir Care Clin North Am.* 2006;12:489–500.

Gibson RL, Comer PB, Beckham RW, McGraw CP. Actual tracheal oxygen concentrations with commonly used oxygen equipment. *Anesthesiology.* 1976;44:71–73.

Gomersall CD, Joynt GM, Freebairn RC, et al. Oxygen therapy for hypercapnic patients with chronic obstructive pulmonary disease and acute respiratory failure: a randomized, controlled pilot study. *Crit Care Med.* 2002;30:113–116.

Griffiths MJ, Evans TW. Inhaled nitric oxide therapy in adults. *N Engl J Med.* 2005;353:2683–2695.

Hanson CW, Marshall BE, Frasch HF, Marshall C. Causes of hypercarbia with oxygen therapy in patients with chronic obstructive pulmonary disease. *Crit Care Med.* 1996;24:23–28.

Hedenstierna G, Rothen HU. Atelectasis formation during anesthesia: causes and measures to prevent it. *J Clin Monit.* 2000;16:329–335.

Hess DR. Heliox and noninvasive positive-pressure ventilation: a role for heliox in exacerbations of chronic obstructive pulmonary disease? *Respir Care.* 2006;51:640–650.

Hess D, D'Agostino D, Magrosky S, et al. Effect of nasal cannula displacement on arterial PO_2. *Respir Care.* 1984;29:21–24.

Hess D, Figaszewski E, Henry D, et al. Subjective effects of dry versus humidified low flow oxygen on the upper respiratory tract. *Respir Ther.* 1982;12:71–75.

Hess DR, Fink JB, Venkataraman ST, et al. The history and physics of heliox. *Respir Care.* 2006;51:608–612.

Hill SL, Barnes PK, Hollway T, Tennant R. Fixed performance oxygen masks: an evaluation. *Br Med J (Clin Res Ed).* 1984;288:1261–1263.

Hoffman LA. Novel strategies for delivering oxygen: reservoir cannula, demand flow, and transtracheal oxygen administration. *Respir Care.* 1994;39:363–379.

Hunter J, Olson LG. Performance of the Hudson Multi-Vent oxygen mask. *Med J Aust.* 1988;148:444–447.

Ingrassia TS, Ryu JH, Trastek VF, Rosenow EC. Oxygen-exacerbated bleomycin pulmonary toxicity. *Mayo Clin Proc.* 1991;66:173–178.

Jensen AG, Johnson A, Sandstedt S. Rebreathing during oxygen treatment with face mask. The effect of oxygen flow rates on ventilation. *Acta Anaesthesiol Scand.* 1991;35:289–292.

Jobe AH, Bancalari E. Bronchopulmonary dysplasia. *Am J Respir Crit Care Med.* 2001;163:1723–1729.

Koh Y, Hurford WE. Inhaled nitric oxide in acute respiratory distress syndrome: from bench to bedside. *Int Anesthesiol Clin.* 2003;41:91–102.

Lorch SA, Cnaan A, Barnhart K. Cost-effectiveness of inhaled nitric oxide for the management of persistent pulmonary hypertension of the newborn. *Pediatrics.* 2004;114:417–426.

Martini RP, Deem S, Yanez ND, et al. Management guided by brain tissue oxygen monitoring and outcome following severe traumatic brain injury. *J Neurosurg.* 2009;111:644–649.

McBrien ME, Sellers WF. A comparison of three variable performance devices for postoperative oxygen therapy. *Anaesthesia.* 1995;50:136–138.

McGarvey JM, Pollack CV. Heliox in airway management. *Emerg Med Clin North Am.* 2008;26:905–920.

Milross J, Young IH, Donnelly P. The oxygen delivery characteristics of the Hudson Oxy-one face mask. *Anaesth Intensive Care.* 1989;17:180–184.

Moloney ED, Kiely JL, McNicholas WT. Controlled oxygen therapy and carbon dioxide retention during exacerbations of chronic obstructive pulmonary disease. *Lancet.* 2001;357:526–528.

Myers TR. Use of heliox in children. *Respir Care.* 2006;51:619–631.

Nolan KM, Winyard JA, Goldhill DR. Comparison of nasal cannulae with face mask for oxygen administration to postoperative patients. *Br J Anaesth.* 1993;70:440–442.

Nortje J, Gupta AK. The role of tissue oxygen monitoring in patients with acute brain injury. *Br J Anaesth.* 2006;97:95–106.

Ooi R, Joshi P, Soni N. An evaluation of oxygen delivery using nasal prongs. *Anaesthesia.* 1992;47:591–593.

Poulton TJ, Comer PB, Gibson RL. Tracheal oxygen concentrations with a nasal cannula during oral and nasal breathing. *Respir Care.* 1980;25:739–741.

Redding JS, McAfee DD, Gross CW. Oxygen concentrations received from commonly used delivery systems. *South Med J.* 1978;71:169–172.

Robinson BR, Athota KP, Branson RD. Inhalational therapies for the ICU. *Curr Opin Crit Care.* 2009;15:1–9.

Robinson TD, Freiberg DB, Regnis JA, Young IH. The role of hypoventilation and ventilation-perfusion redistribution in oxygen-induced hypercapnia during acute exacerbations of chronic obstructive pulmonary disease. *Am J Respir Crit Care Med.* 2000;161:1524–1529.

Schacter EN, Littner MR, Luddy P, Beck GJ. Monitoring of oxygen delivery systems in clinical practice. *Crit Care Med.* 1980;8:405–409.

Sheridan RL, Hess D. Inhaled nitric oxide in inhalation injury. *J Burn Care Res.* 2009;30:162–164.

Sim MAB, Dean P, Kinsella J, et al. Performance of oxygen delivery devices when the breathing pattern of respiratory failure is simulated. *Anaesthesia.* 2008;63:938–940.

Sokol J, Jacobs SE, Bohn D. Inhaled nitric oxide for acute hypoxic respiratory failure in children and adults: a meta-analysis. *Anesth Analg.* 2003;97:989–898.

Soll RF. Inhaled nitric oxide in the neonate. *J Perinatol.* 2009;29(suppl 2):S63–S67.

Statement on the care of the child with chronic lung disease of infancy and childhood. *Am J Respir Crit Care Med.* 2003;168:356–396.

Stausholm K, Rosenberg-Adamsen S, Skriver M, et al. Comparison of three devices for oxygen administration in the late postoperative period. *Br J Anaesth.* 1995;74:607–609.

Valli G, Paoletti P, Savi D, et al. Clinical use of heliox in asthma and COPD. *Monaldi Arch Chest Dis.* 2007;67:159–164.

Wagstaff TAJ, Soni N. Performance of six types of oxygen delivery devices at varying respiratory rates. *Anaesthesia.* 2007;62:492–503.

Waldau T, Larsen VH, Bonde J. Evaluation of five oxygen delivery devices in spontaneously breathing subjects by oxygraphy. *Anaesthesia.* 1998;53:256–263.

Ward JJ, Gracey DR. Arterial oxygen values achieved by COPD patients breathing oxygen alternately via nasal mask and nasal cannula. *Respir Care.* 1985;30:250–255.

Weaver LK, Hopkins RO, Chan KJ, et al. Hyperbaric oxygen for acute carbon monoxide poisoning. *N Engl J Med.* 2002;347:1057–1067.

Wettstein RB, Shelledy DC, Peters JI. Delivered oxygen concentrations using low-flow and high-flow nasal cannulas. *Respir Care.* 2005;50:604–609.

White AC. The evaluation and management of hypoxemia in the chronic critically ill patient. *Clin Chest Med.* 2001;22:123–134.

Williams AB, Jones PL, Mapleson WW. A comparison of oxygen therapy devices used in the postoperative recovery period. *Anaesthesia.* 1988;43:131–135.

CHAPTER 17

Humidity and Aerosol Therapy

Dean R. Hess

OUTLINE

OBJECTIVES

1. Describe the normal gas warming and humidification functions of the upper airway.
2. List the goals of aerosol and humidity therapy.
3. Compare active and passive humidifiers.
4. Compare heated and unheated humidifiers.
5. Compare jet nebulizers, ultrasonic nebulizers, pressurized metered dose inhalers, and dry powder inhalers for aerosol drug administration.
6. Distinguish between spacers and valved holding chambers.
7. Discuss issues involved in the selection of a device for aerosol delivery.
8. Discuss issues pertinent to aerosol drug delivery during mechanical ventilation.

KEY TERMS

active humidifier
aerosol
artificial nose
bland aerosol therapy
bubble humidifier
dry powder inhaler (DPI)
geometric standard deviation (GSD)
gravitational sedimentation
humidity therapy
isothermic saturation boundary (ISB)
jet nebulizer
large-volume nebulizer
mass median aerodynamic diameter (MMAD)
mesh nebulizer
nebulizer
passive humidifier
passover humidifier
pressurized metered dose inhaler (pMDI)
spacer
ultrasonic nebulizer
valved holding chamber

INTRODUCTION

Administration of humidity and aerosol therapy is a common task for the respiratory therapist. Humidification of inspired gas is particularly important in the care of mechanically ventilated patients, and many respiratory drugs are administered as aerosols. The selection of appropriate devices for humidity and aerosol production may have an important impact on the outcome of the patient's condition.

Humidity

The interface between the atmosphere and the lungs is mediated through the fluid lining of the airways. Water in inspired gas is essential to a healthy respiratory tract. Administration of dry, cold gas bypassing the upper airway can change the balance of the fluid lining the airways and may result in either short-term or irreversible structural damage of the airway.[1–9] Exposure of the airways to cold, dry air from the ambient environment increases mucus production and thickening of secretions, reduces the motility of the cilia, and increases airway irritability. Administration of dry gases via an endotracheal tube can damage the tracheal epithelium.[3] **Humidity therapy** is the addition of water to the gas delivered to the airways.

The nose is an efficient humidifier, which adds heat and humidity to the inspired gas. The respiratory mucosa lining the sinuses, trachea, and bronchi assists in heating and humidifying inspired gas.[2] The respiratory mucosa is covered by secretions produced by mucous glands, goblet cells, and transudation of fluid through cell walls (**Figure 17–1**). Heat is transferred from capillary beds close to the surface of the mucosa. The nasal mucosa is particularly well suited for this function, having the highest concentration of mucous glands in the airway and a rich vascular bed close to the surface that provides heat and water. The turbinates and conchae provide a convoluted path for gas to travel, creating turbulent flow and a large surface area for contact with respiratory gases. This large surface area gives up heat and moisture to inspired gas and efficiently recovers heat and water on exhalation.

> **RESPIRATORY RECAP**
>
> **Normal Heat and Moisture Exchange**
>
> » The upper airway is an effective humidifier.
> » The isothermic saturation boundary (ISB) is the point at which inspired gas reaches body temperature and humidity.
> » Breathing dry gas moves the ISB deeper into the respiratory tract.

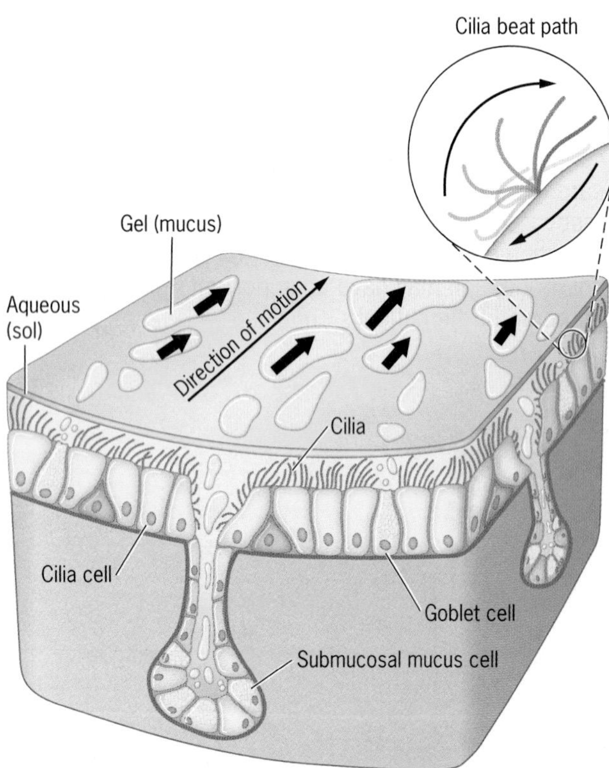

FIGURE 17–1 The cellular, aqueous, and mucous components of the airway mucosa. Adapted from Williams R, et al. Relationship between humidity and temperature of inspired gas and the function of the airway mucosa. *Crit Care Med.* 1996;24:1920–1929.

Normal Heat and Moisture Exchange

By the time inspired gas reaches the lung parenchyma, it is fully saturated with water vapor at body temperature (44 mg/L at 37° C [98.6° F]). See **Figure 17–2**. The point at which this occurs is known as the **isothermic saturation boundary (ISB)**, which is approximately 5 cm below the carina at the level of the third-generation airways.[1] Above the ISB, temperature and humidity fall during inspiration and rise during exhalation. Below the ISB, temperature and relative humidity do not fluctuate. A drop in environmental temperature and humidity, mouth breathing, an increase in tidal volume, or endotracheal intubation (which bypasses the upper airway) moves the ISB deeper into the lungs, although it never reaches the level of the respiratory bronchioles or alveoli.

At the end of inspiration, the temperature of the nasal mucosa is 31° C (87.8° F) or lower because of heat loss caused by turbulent convection and loss of the latent heat of vaporization. As inspired gas warms, water vapor is transferred by evaporation from the mucosal lining through the latent heat of vaporization. Warming and humidification continue until the inspired gas is fully saturated at body temperature. Although the latent heat of vaporization remains as water vapor and does not contribute to warming of gases, the loss of latent heat of vaporization does cause the mucosa to cool. During exhalation, heat is transferred from exhaled gas to the cooler tracheal and nasal mucosa by convection. As these gases cool, their capacity to hold water vapor diminishes, and condensation occurs. Water accumulates on the tracheal surfaces, where it is reabsorbed by the mucus. Heat

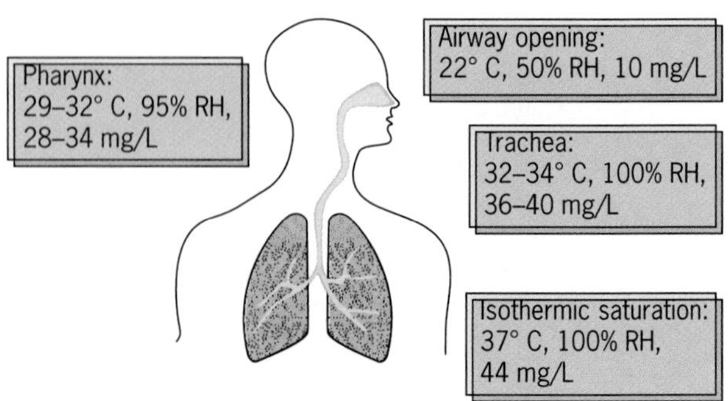

FIGURE 17–2 Normal temperature and humidity of gas at various points along the respiratory tract.

is transferred back to the mucosa, resulting in warming and rehydration. Latent heat and water are held until the next inspiration. With mouth breathing, the flow is more laminar, requiring heat transfer by radiation. Because air is a poor conductor of heat, the mouth is less efficient than the nose at heating inspired air.

The measured temperature and water vapor at the oropharynx during oral and nasal breathing of room air is about 22° C (71.6° F), with a relative humidity (RH) of 15% to 39%.[6] At the pharynx, the temperature difference between inspired and expired gas is 4° C (39.2° F) during nose breathing and 7° C (44.6° F) during mouth breathing. The inspired gas temperature increases 5° C (41° F) during mouth breathing and 9° C (48.2° F) during nose breathing. During inspiration with nose breathing, the RH is 95% at the oropharynx; this measurement is 75% during mouth breathing. On exhalation, the RH is nearly 95% at the pharynx and 90% at the airway opening. This suggests that the normal airway can condition inspired gas to add humidity with either nose or mouth breathing. However, more heat and moisture are lost with exhalation in mouth breathing than with exhalation in nose breathing. Even with mouth breathing, the ISB is not typically lower than the third generation of the bronchi.

Heat and moisture normally are lost from the mucosa above the ISB, from a surface area of approximately 300 cm^2 that is covered by 240 μL of airway lining fluid 8 μm deep. With normal tidal volume for an adult male, 22 μL of water and 61 J of heat are required to condition each breath from normal ambient conditions to 100% RH at body temperature. The water and heat losses per breath are 15 μL and 42 J, respectively. Over a 24-hour period, these losses total 250 mL of water and 726 kJ.[5]

When dry, cold gases are inhaled, the ISB is shifted deeper into the respiratory tract, and ciliary function and mucus production are compromised. Bypassing the upper airway eliminates the normal efficient mechanisms used to retain heat and humidity in the lungs.[10] Recruitment of airways that are less efficient for humidification changes their mucosal characteristics. The lower gas temperature farther down the airways reduces ciliary activity within 10 minutes. Once compromised, ciliary function can take several weeks to recover. Respiratory secretions become thicker, contributing to mucous plugging and inability to maintain normal bronchopulmonary hygiene. When absolute humidity drops below 24 mg/L in the inhaled gas, the beat frequency of the cilia is reduced.

Goals of Humidity Therapy

The primary goal of humidity therapy is to maintain normal physiologic conditions by providing adequate heat and humidity to inspired gas to approximate normal inspiratory conditions. Administration of heat and humidity is also advocated, with less supporting data, for the treatment of hypothermia, reactive airway response to cold air, and thickened secretions.

Medical gases are processed to remove all water vapor. When this gas is delivered to the nose and mouth, ideally it should be heated and humidified to normal ambient room air conditions (22° C [71.6° F] at 50% RH or an absolute humidity of 10 mg/L). For gas delivered to the trachea through an endotracheal or tracheotomy tube, heat and humidity should be at least 32° to 35° C (89.6° to 95° F) at 100% RH (absolute humidity of 36 to 40 mg/L).[10]

For premature and newborn infants, a neutral thermal environment should be maintained, with adequate warmth and humidity to minimize insensible heat and water loss. Low-birth-weight infants provided adequate heat and humidity showed a reduced morbidity rate compared with infants breathing colder and dryer inspired gas.[11] The body loses considerable heat through normal ventilation. For hypothermic patients, rewarming and reduction of further heat loss can be facilitated by heating the inspired gases.[12] However, this technique is less useful than other warming treatments (e.g., wrapping the patient in blankets and warming intravenous solutions). Individuals with reactive airways develop increased airway resistance when they breathe cold air.[13] This response can be diminished by warming of the inspired gases and provision of gas humidified with at least 20 mg/L of water at 23° C (73.4° F).

> **RESPIRATORY RECAP**
>
> **Goals of Humidity Therapy**
>
> » To provide adequate heat and humidity
> » To treat hypothermia
> » To prevent airway response to cold air
> » To aid removal of thick secretions

Heated humidity has been used in the treatment of patients with thick, tenacious secretions. However, no studies have reported a benefit from the use of external humidifiers to try to improve the character and mobilization of thick secretions. Most patients with an artificial airway require humidification of inspired gas to prevent the formation of thick, tenacious secretions. However, evidence is lacking to support the use of humidity therapy (i.e., cool mist or heated aerosol) for patients with an intact upper airway. Cool (colder than room temperature) humidified gases and aerosols commonly are used in the treatment of upper airway inflammation caused by croup, epiglottitis, and swelling resulting from extubation.[14] The cold gas promotes localized vasoconstriction, thereby reducing swelling and relieving the discomfort associated with upper airway inflammation.

Excessive humidity is defined as a level greater than 100% RH at body temperature. The water volume of a vapor stream is 20 to 50 μL of water per liter of air and is unlikely to cause overhumidification. To exceed that water volume, gas temperatures would have to be grossly in excess of body temperature. Humidification of inspired gas reduces insensible water loss from the airway but is unlikely to add significant water to the body. Inspired gas warmer than 45° C (113° F) may cause thermal injury to the airway.[5]

Devices Used for Humidification

A humidifier adds molecular water to gas (**CPG 17–1**).[15–20] An **active humidifier** adds water or heat or both to the inspired gas. A **nebulizer** produces an **aerosol**, or suspension of particles in gas. A **passive humidifier** uses exhaled heat and moisture to humidify inspired gas; heat and moisture exchangers are passive humidifiers. The American National Standards Institute (ANSI) recommends that heated humidifiers have a water output level of at least 30 mg/L (100% RH at 30° C [86° F]).[21–23] This is considered the minimum level of humidity to avoid mucosal damage and inspissation of secretions

CLINICAL PRACTICE GUIDELINE 17–1

Humidification During Mechanical Ventilation

Indication

- Humidification of inspired gas during mechanical ventilation is mandatory when an endotracheal or tracheostomy tube is present.

Contraindications

- There are no contraindications to the provision of physiologic conditioning of inspired gas during mechanical ventilation.
- A heat and moisture exchanger (HME) is contraindicated under some circumstances:
  - Use of an HME is contraindicated for patients with thick, copious, or bloody secretions.
  - Use of an HME is contraindicated for patients with an expired tidal volume less than 70% of the delivered tidal volume (e.g., those with large bronchopleurocutaneous fistulas or incompetent or absent endotracheal tube cuffs).
  - Use of an HME is contraindicated for patients with a body temperature below 32° C (90° F).
  - Use of an HME may be contraindicated for patients with high spontaneous minute volumes (over 10 L/min).
  - An HME must be removed from the patient circuit during aerosol treatments when the nebulizer is placed in the circuit.

Hazards and Complications

- Hazards and complications associated with the use of humidification devices include the potential for electrical shock (heated humidifier); hypothermia (HME or heated humidifier); hyperthermia (heated humidifier); thermal injury to the airway from heated humidifiers; burns to the patient and tubing meltdown if heated-wire circuits are covered or circuits and humidifiers are incompatible; underhydration and impaction of mucous secretions (HME or heated humidifier); hypoventilation or alveolar gas trapping (or both) caused by mucous plugging of airways (HME or heated humidifier); possible increased resistive work of breathing caused by mucous plugging of airways (HME or heated humidifier); possible increased resistive work of breathing through the humidifier (HME or heated humidifier); possible hypoventilation caused by increased dead space (HME); inadvertent overfilling, resulting in unintentional tracheal lavage (heated reservoir humidifier); potential for burns to caregivers from hot metal (heated humidifier); inadvertent tracheal lavage from pooled condensate in patient circuit (heated humidifier); elevated airway pressures caused by pooled condensation (heated humidifier); patient–ventilator dyssynchrony and improper ventilator performance as a result of pooled condensation in the circuit (heated humidifier); and ineffective low-pressure alarm during disconnection as a result of resistance through an HME.
- When disconnected from the patient, some ventilators generate a high flow through the patient circuit that may aerosolize contaminated condensate, putting both the patient and clinician at risk for nosocomial infection (heated humidifiers).

Limitations

- Insufficient heat and humidification can occur with heated humidifiers and result in complications if improper temperature settings are selected or the water level in the humidifier falls below the manufacturer's suggested level.
- The HME selected should be appropriate to the patient's size and tidal volume.

Modified from AARC clinical practice guideline: humidification during mechanical ventilation. *Respir Care*. 1992;37:887–890. Reprinted with permission.

for patients who have a bypassed upper airway (i.e., an endotracheal or tracheostomy tube). The Emergency Care Research Institute (ECRI) recommends that active humidifiers have an output of 37 mg of water per liter of inspired gas (85% RH at body temperature or 100% RH at 34° C [93.2° F]).[24] Active heated water humidifiers are the devices of choice for intubation, tracheostomy, and long-term mechanical ventilation. The ANSI recommends a water output of 10 mg/L for unheated humidifiers; this provides approximately 50% RH at 22° C (71.6° F) ambient conditions, which enhances the dissipation of static electricity to prevent fires. This humidity level is thought to be the lowest acceptable level to minimize mucosal damage to the upper airway in a variety of environments.

Active Humidifiers

A **passover humidifier** (**Figure 17–3**) directs gas over the surface of a body of water (Figure 17-3A and Figure 17-3B). The passover wick humidifier incorporates a wick of absorbent paper or cloth that draws water from the reservoir and becomes saturated; the wick comes in contact with the gas stream. A passover/barrier humidifier uses a hydrophobic barrier that allows water molecules but not droplets to cross from the water reservoir into the gas stream.

In a **bubble humidifier**, dry gas is directed toward the bottom of a water-filled reservoir, where the stream of gas is broken up (diffused) into bubbles, which gain humidity as they rise through the water (Figure 17-3C). This commonly is accomplished with a tube that directs gas beneath the surface of the water; with a tube that has small holes along its length; or with a tube that is attached to a diffuser made of plastic foam, sintered metal, or mesh that breaks the stream of gas into small bubbles. Bubble humidifiers typically are not heated and are used with simple oxygen delivery devices. The higher the flow through a bubble humidifier, the lower the water vapor content and temperature of the gas leaving the device. Commercially available bubble humidifiers are capable of humidifying dry medical gas to an absolute humidity of 10 to 20 mg/L at flows of 2 to 10 L/min. Bubble humidifiers are most efficient at flows of 5 L/min or less.[25] When flows greater than 10 L/min are required, other humidifying options should be considered. At flows under 10 L/min, bubble humidifiers are safe for extended single-patient use without risk of infection.[26] Heating the reservoir improves the efficiency of these humidifiers; however, the small-bore tubing used to connect the humidifier to the administration appliance is easily obstructed by condensate as the humidified gas cools en route to the patient. Low-flow, unheated bubble humidifiers typically have a gravity or spring-loaded pressure-relief valve to protect against obstructed or kinked tubing and an alarm that sounds when a pressure of 2 psi or higher develops in the humidifier.

The addition of humidity to low-flow medical gas is not an evidence-based practice, and eliminating the use of humidifiers for low-flow oxygen reduces the cost of routine oxygen administration.[27] Humidification of the inspired gas should be considered for patients who complain of discomfort associated with nasal dryness or irritation. However, this is accomplished better by devices that are more efficient than simple bubble humidifiers. Topical application of water-based lubricants to the nostrils may be a reasonable response to complaints of dryness.

Heated bubble humidifiers (Figure 17-3D) can be used with intubated patients. These humidifiers can accommodate flows of 10 to 120 L/min and use tubing with a 22-mm inside diameter (ID). These devices are used corrugated 22-mm ID tubing between the humidifier and the patient. At high flows bubble humidifiers produce aerosols that may transmit bacteria from the humidifier's reservoir to the patient. Heated passover humidifiers are used most commonly during mechanical ventilation (**Figure 17–4**).

A **jet nebulizer** (**Figure 17–5**) uses a jet of compressed gas that passes through a restricted orifice, creating a low-pressure area near the tip of a narrow tube. Fluid is drawn from a reservoir and sheared or shattered into droplets by the airstream. Jet nebulizers incorporate baffles to minimize aerosol exiting particle size and use the aerosol in the device to maximize surface contact with the gas. Because jet nebulizers pose a risk of infection from bacteria that might colonize the reservoir, they should always

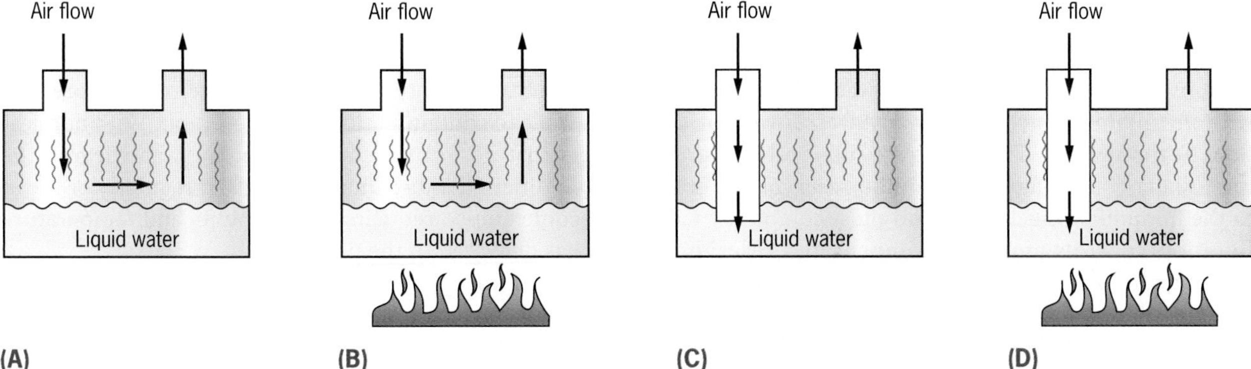

FIGURE 17–3 (**A**) Passover humidifier. (**B**) Heated passover humidifier. (**C**) Bubble humidifier. (**D**) Heated bubble humidifier. Adapted from Peterson BD. Heated humidifiers. *Respir Care Clin North Am.* 1998;4:243–260.

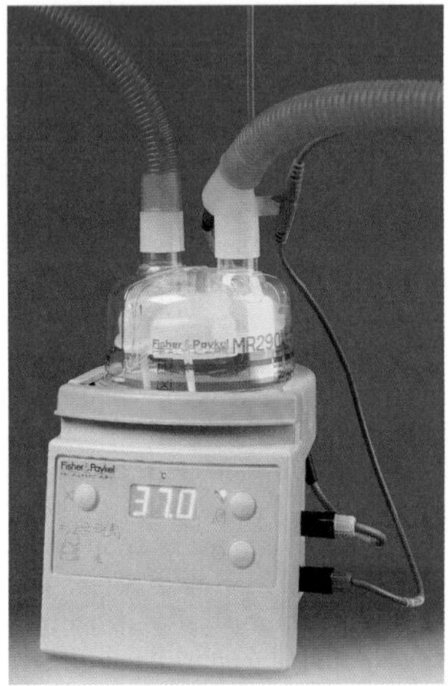
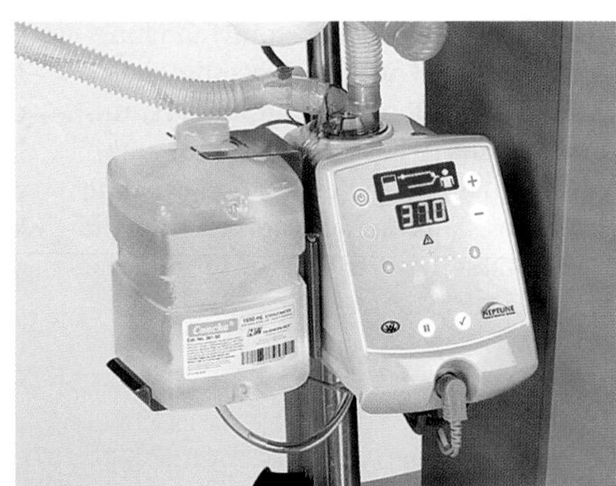

FIGURE 17–4 Commercially available heated humidifiers used during mechanical ventilation.

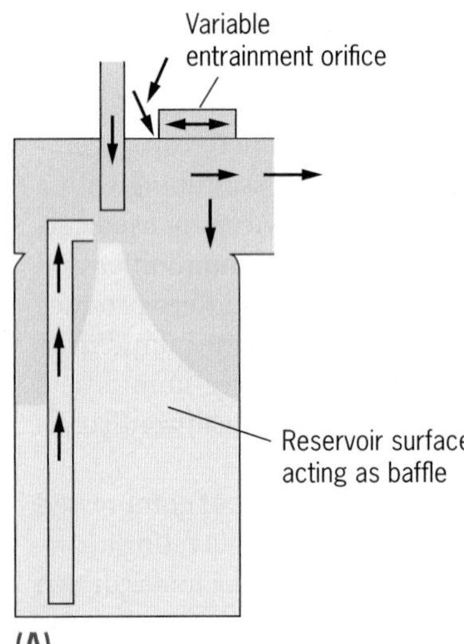

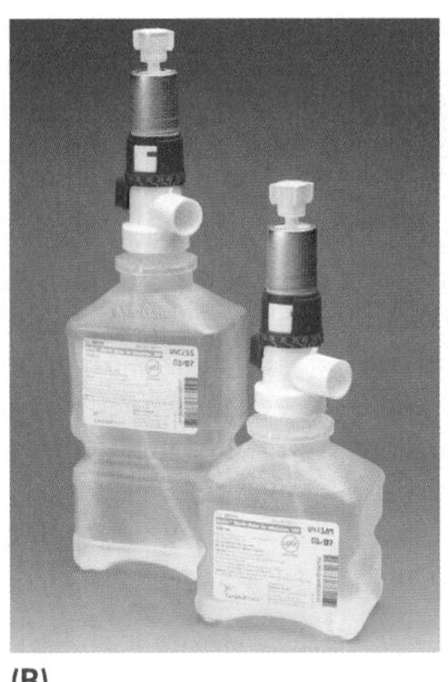
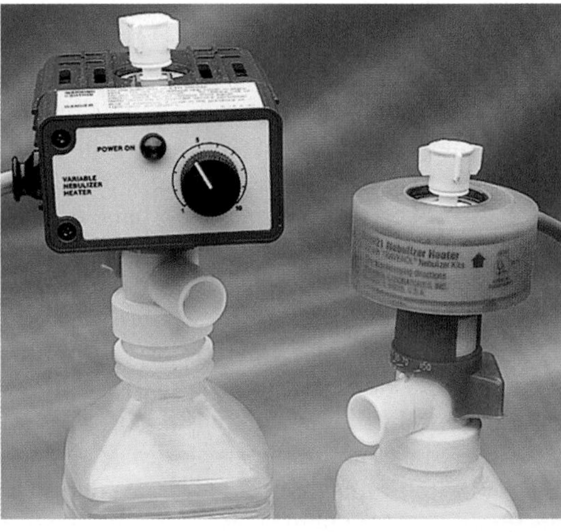

FIGURE 17–5 (**A**) Schematic drawing of large-volume jet nebulizer. (**B**) Commercially available large-volume nebulizers. (**A**) Modified from Cohen N, Fink J. Humidity and aerosols. In: Eubanks DH, Bone RC, eds. *Principles and Applications of Cardiorespiratory Care Equipment.* Mosby; 1994.

be filled with sterile fluids and changed daily, and residual fluids should be discarded before refilling.

Systems used to replace the water in the humidifier should ensure continuity of therapy and minimize disruption of gas flow to the patient. Continuous-feed systems are desirable because the water is replenished without operator intervention or interruption of gas flow to the patient. These systems often rely on gravity, usually consisting of a mounted reservoir external to the humidifier mechanism and most commonly with flotation controls and level-compensated reservoirs. Continuous feed systems typically maintain a constant compressible volume, which is important when they are used in the neonatal or pediatric ventilator circuit.

Intermittent-feed systems have disadvantages compared with continuous-feed systems. Changing the water level in a fixed-volume container changes the compressible volume in both the humidifier and the ventilator, resulting in fluctuations in the delivered tidal volume. This problem is of greatest concern for mechanically ventilated newborns and pediatric patients. Open intermittent-feed systems are more susceptible to contamination of the reservoir. With humidifiers that do not have alarms for low water levels, the humidifier chamber must be checked regularly or it can become empty, reducing the humidity and temperature of gas delivered to the patient.

Humidifier heaters most commonly use controllers to regulate electrical power to the heater element. The most basic units do not monitor the temperature of the heater, providing power to the heating element based on the setting of the temperature control knob rather than

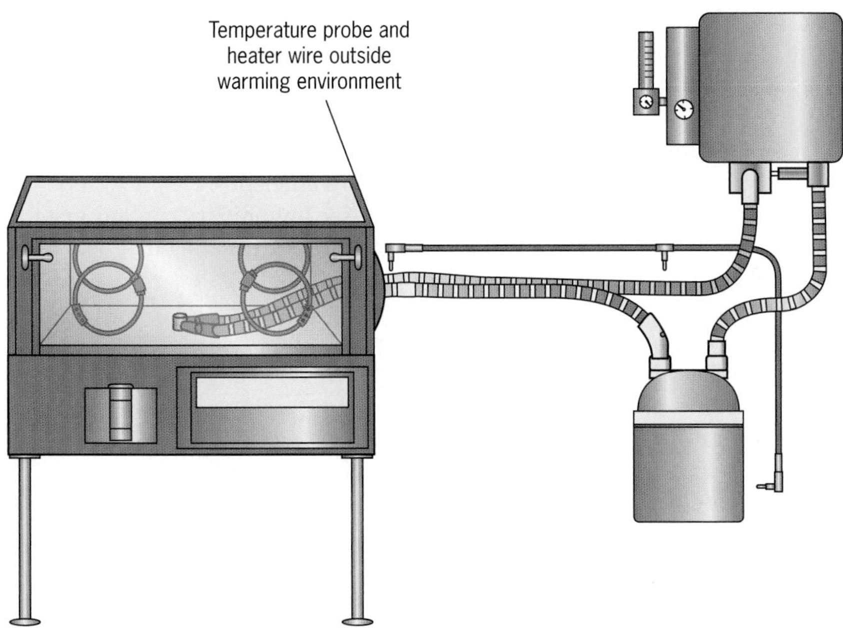

FIGURE 17–6 Position of temperature probe outside of incubator when using heated humidification system. Adapted from Peterson BD. Heated humidifiers. *Respir Care Clin North Am.* 1998;4:243–260.

the patient's airway temperature. Active humidifiers use one of several types of heating elements: a heating plate located under the reservoir, a curved element wrapped around the humidifier chamber, a yoke or collar between the water reservoir and the active mechanism of the nebulizer, a plate or rod immersed in the water reservoir, or a set of wires or elements that heat an absorbent wick or tubes containing water.

Servo-controlled humidifiers monitor the temperature of gas delivered to the patient, adjusting the power to the heating elements according to the temperature monitored by a thermistor probe placed downstream from the humidifier, near the patient's airway connection. When the temperature at the patient's airway is lower than desired, the controller supplies more power to the heater. As this distal temperature nears or exceeds the set temperature, power to the heating system is reduced. Thermistor probes are best placed in the inspiratory limb of the ventilator circuit, far enough from the patient that the temperature of the exhaled gas is not detected. The sensor probe in the inspiratory limb must be located outside the heated environment to allow the heated-wire controller to maintain the desired temperature and water content of inspired gases (**Figure 17–6**).

> **AGE-SPECIFIC ANGLE**
>
> The temperature probe of a humidifier should not be placed inside an incubator or under a radiant heater because the surrounding air temperature affects humidifier function.

As heated and humidified gas cools, its ability to hold water vapor declines, and condensation (rain out) occurs. The amount of condensate is affected by the ambient temperature, gas flow, and the patient's airway temperature and by the length, diameter, and thermal mass of the tubing between the humidifier and the patient. In a traditional ventilator circuit, the humidifier is heated to 50° C (122° F) or higher and saturated gas contains more than 80 mg of water per liter. As the gas cools to 35° C (95° F) en route to the patient, it can hold only 40 mg of water per liter; therefore, any amount over that condenses in the tubing. The circuit must be drained frequently to prevent pooling condensate from obstructing the gas flow or inadvertently pouring into the patient's airway.

Often the ventilator circuit, and subsequently condensate, becomes contaminated with bacteria from the patient within the first hour that the patient is attached to the ventilator. The tubing should be positioned such that drainage is away from the patient's airway to avoid accidental lavage of the airway. Condensate presents a risk to the staff and should always be treated and disposed of as contaminated waste. Water traps placed in dependent positions in both the inspiratory and expiratory limbs drain condensate from the ventilator circuit, reducing the obstruction to gas flow. Water traps should minimize changes in circuit compliance and allow emptying without disrupting ventilation of the patient.

Techniques used to reduce the formation of condensate include an increase in the thermal mass of the circuit, use of a coaxial circuit with the inspiratory limb surrounded by the expiratory limb, or addition of heated wires to the circuit.[12] Increasing the passive thermal mass of the circuit with thick tubing or wrapping the tubing with insulating material insulates the gas inside the tubing from ambient air. Surrounding the inspiratory limb of the circuit with the expiratory limb in a coaxial manner uses the patient's exhaled gas as a heated air bath surrounding the inspiratory limb.

Placing heated wires in the inspiratory and expiratory tubing of the ventilator circuit heats the gas in the circuit, reducing the temperature differential between humidifier and patient. The humidifier operates at a lower temperature with heated-wire circuits than it does with conventional circuits. The humidifier's RH control regulates the temperature differential between the humidifier and the circuit temperature. When the humidifier is cooler than the gas in the inspiratory limb, the absolute humidity remains the same although the relative humidity is decreased, and the circuit has no condensate (**Figure 17–7**). An increase in inlet chamber temperature induced by high ambient temperature reduces the performance of heated-wire humidifiers, leading to a risk of endotracheal tube occlusion (**Figure 17–8**).[27–29] When inlet chamber temperature is high, the humidifier heater plate stops heating. The water contained in the chamber remains too cold for evaporation to occur, leading to low levels of humidity. Inlet chamber temperature is influenced by both ambient temperature and ventilator output temperature. High ambient temperature prevents the gas from cooling in the circuit between the ventilator output and the humidification chamber. Ventilator output gas temperature is also influenced by minute ventilation. To avoid overhumidification, the temperature of gas delivered under conditions of induced hypoventilation should be set to the patient's core body temperature.[30]

When no condensate is visible in the inspiratory limb of the ventilator circuit, it is impossible to know whether the gas is being humidified without direct humidity measurements. To ensure humidification of the inspired gas, the temperature differential should be adjusted to the point at which condensation forms near the patient's airway; this is the most reliable indicator that gas is fully saturated. If no condensate is visible, the relative humidity could be anything from zero to 99%, and the clinician has no way of knowing what it is without using a hygrometer. If the humidity control is set incorrectly, dry gas can be delivered to the patient's airway, resulting in mucous obstruction of the airway (refer to Figure 17–7).

RESPIRATORY RECAP

Assessment of Adequate Humidity Delivery

» The delivered relative humidity is 100% if condensate is seen in the delivery tubing near the patient's airway.

Passive Humidifiers

A heat and moisture exchanger (HME), or **artificial nose**, is a passive humidifier. The HME captures exhaled heat and moisture and transfers part of that heat and humidity to the next inspired breath (**Figure 17–9**). The ideal HME should add minimal dead space, weight, and resistance to the airway, should incorporate standard connections, and should operate at 70% efficiency or higher. Efficiency is defined as the ratio of the humidity of exhaled gas to the humidity returned to the patient by the HME.

HMEs include condensers, hygroscopic condensers, and hygrophobic condensers. Condenser humidifiers are constructed of metallic gauze, corrugated metal, or parallel metal tubes that provide high thermal conductivity. The condenser cools to room temperature during inspiration. During exhalation, saturated gas cools as it contacts the condenser, water condenses and collects on the elements of the condenser, and the temperature of the condenser core rises. On the next inspiration, air is warmed and humidified by the condenser through evaporation of water from the surface. Condenser humidifiers usually are only about 50% efficient.

Hygroscopic condenser humidifiers contain materials of low thermal conductivity (meaning that heat from

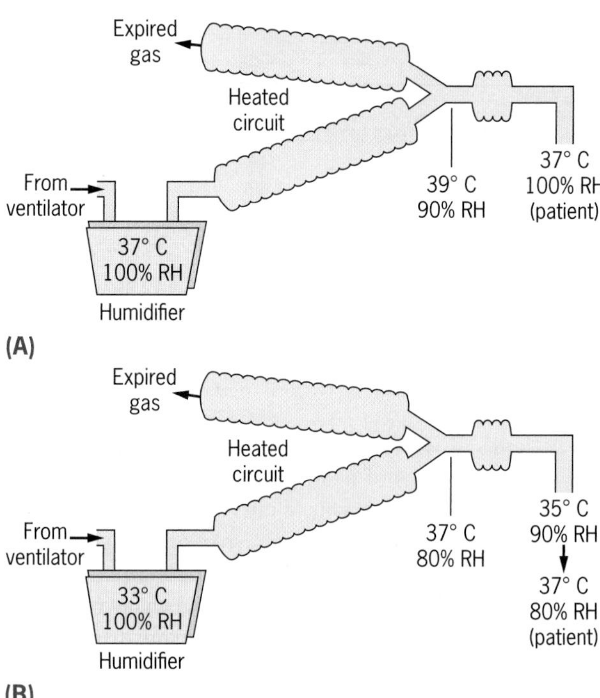

FIGURE 17–7 (**A**) Appropriate settings for a heated-wire circuit, such that gas delivered to the patient is 100% body humidity. (**B**) Settings too low for a heated-wire circuit, such that gas delivered to the patient is too dry.

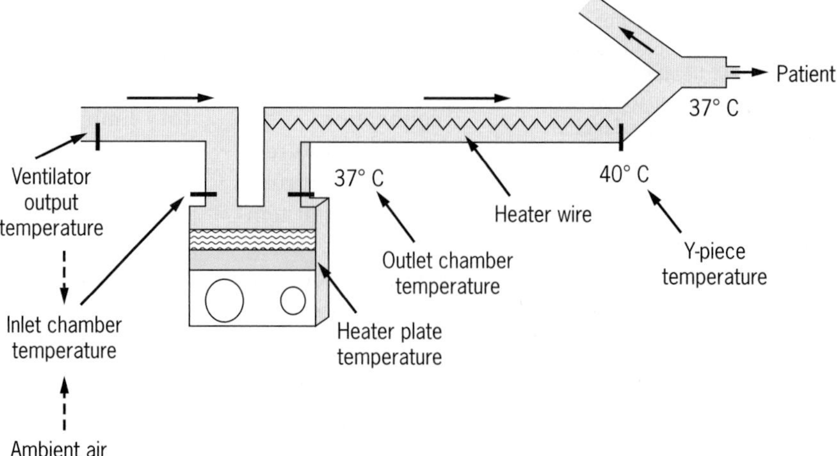

FIGURE 17–8 The heated humidifier outlet temperature is regulated through the heater plate. When the inlet temperature is low, the heater plate heats the water and evaporation occurs, ensuring sufficient humidification. When the inlet temperature is high, the water may not be warmed, and consequently the gas may remain dry. From Lellouche F, et al. Influence of ambient and ventilator output temperatures on performance of heated-wire humidifiers. *Am J Respir Crit Care Med.* 2004;170:1073–1079.

conduction and the latent heat of condensation are not dissipated), such as paper, wool, or foam, that are impregnated with a hygroscopic chemical such as calcium chloride or lithium chloride. During exhalation, warm saturated gas precipitates water on the cool condenser element while water molecules bind to the salt without transition from vapor to liquid state. During inspiration, the lower water vapor pressure in the inspired gas liberates water molecules from the hygroscopic compound without a fall in temperature from vaporization. The efficiency of these devices can be as high as 70%.

Hydrophobic condenser humidifiers use a water-repellent element with a large surface area and low thermal conductivity. During exhalation, the condenser temperature rises to about 25° C (77° F). On inspiration, cool gas and evaporation cool the condenser to about 10° C (50° F). This large temperature shift results in more water condensation in the humidifier on exhalation, and this water is used to humidify the next inspiration. These devices are about 70% efficient. Hydrophobic humidifiers can also serve as efficient microbiologic filters.

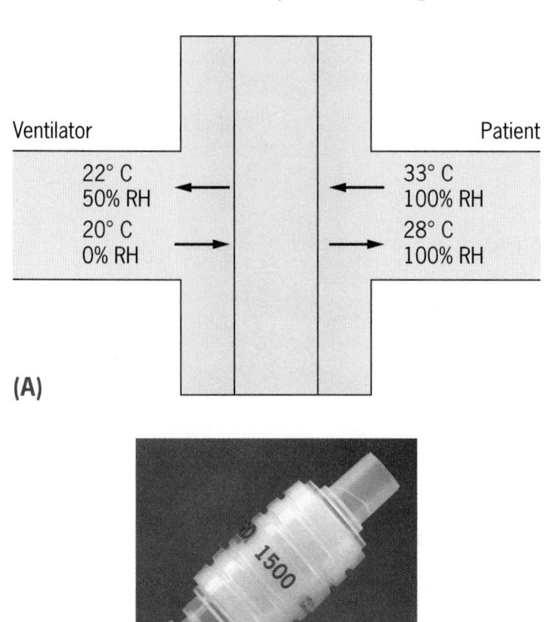

FIGURE 17–9 **(A)** Function of heat and moisture exchanger. **(B)** Commercially available heat and moisture exchanger.

The efficiency of HMEs declines as the tidal volume, inspiratory flow, or fractional inspired oxygen concentration (F_{IO_2}) increases. Resistance through the HME increases as the water load of the device increases. When the HME is dry, resistance across the device is minimal, but after several hours of use, resistance may increase as water is absorbed onto a hygroscopic HME. The increased work of breathing imposed by HMEs may not be well tolerated by patients.[31,32] HMEs also increase mechanical dead space. Although HMEs increase the minute ventilation requirement and work of breathing, these drawbacks can be overcome by use of a low level of pressure support ventilation.

> **RESPIRATORY RECAP**
>
> **Heat and Moisture Exchangers**
>
> » Efficiency declines as the tidal volume, inspiratory flow, and fractional inspired oxygen concentration (F_{IO_2}) increase.
>
> » HMEs increase dead space and resistive work of breathing.
>
> » HMEs do not need to be changed more often than every 48 hours.

The HME forms a barrier between the patient and the ventilator circuit.[33] However, the value of the HME as a filter, in terms of patient outcomes and the safety of the healthcare provider, is unclear. HMEs are an inexpensive alternative to humidifiers.[34,35] A clinical algorithm can be used to guide the use of HMEs (**Figure 17–10**). Although manufacturers recommend that these devices be changed daily, current evidence suggests that they can be safely used for at least 48 hours.[36,37]

The choice of an HME should be based on efficiency, dead space, weight, and cost. In a study of 48 HMEs,[38] it was reported that the humidity efficiency of the devices ranged from 37.8% to 91.1%. In this study, several HMEs performed poorly and should not be used. The resistance of these devices ranges from a maximum of 3.9 cm H_2O/L/s to a minimum of 0.4 cm H_2O/L/s. The dead space of the HMEs ranged from 22 mL to 95 mL. The most important result of this study was the heterogeneity of the humidification performance of HMEs.

Contraindications for HME use include the presence of thick, copious, or bloody secretions; a large leak

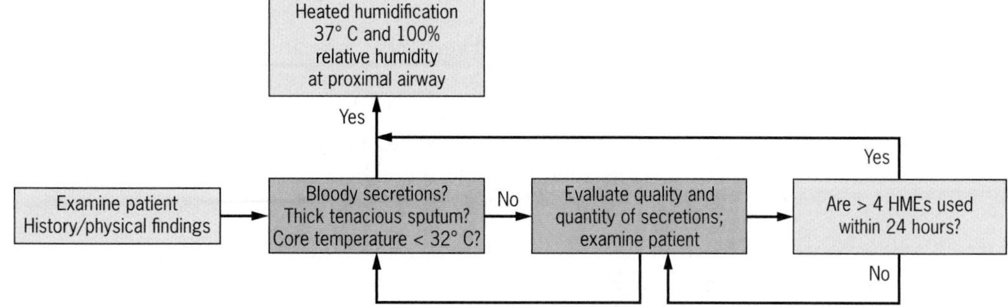

FIGURE 17–10 Clinical algorithm for use of heat and moisture exchanger. Adapted from Branson RD, Campbell RS. Humidification in the intensive care unit. *Respir Care Clin North Am.* 1998;4:305–320.

around an endotracheal tube, such as might occur with a large bronchopleural fistula or leaking endotracheal tube cuff; a body temperature below 32° C (89.6° F); and a minute ventilation greater than 10 L/min. Hazards associated with the use of HMEs include underhydration, impaction of pulmonary secretions, increased resistive work of breathing, mucous plugging of the airways, increased dead space, and hypothermia. During aerosol administration, HMEs must be removed, bypassed, or placed between the HME and the patient.

With use of an HME, the circuit remains dry, and some HMEs are effective filters. This has led some to recommend that an HME can be used as part of a ventilator-associated pneumonia (VAP) prevention program. However, recent studies have not found that HME use is effective in prevention of VAP compared with active humidification.[39–41] Of concern is the fact that the dead space of the HME can result in an increase in $Paco_2$ or ventilatory requirement, or both, particularly in the patient with a low tidal volume as part of a lung-protective ventilation strategy.[42–45]

Bland Aerosol Therapy

Bland aerosol therapy provides humidification with solutions such as saline for therapeutic and diagnostic purposes (**CPG 17–2**). Large-volume pneumatic nebulizers and ultrasonic nebulizers are commonly used for

CLINICAL PRACTICE GUIDELINE 17–2

Bland Aerosol Administration

Indications

- The presence of upper airway edema (cool bland aerosol)
- Laryngotracheobronchitis (LTB)
- Subglottic edema
- Postextubation edema
- Postoperative management of the upper airway
- The presence of a bypassed upper airway
- The need for sputum specimens or mobilization of secretions

Contraindications

- Bronchoconstriction
- History of airway hyperresponsiveness

Hazards and Complications

- Wheezing or bronchospasm
- Bronchoconstriction when artificial airway is employed
- Infection
- Overhydration
- Patient discomfort
- Caregiver exposure to droplet nuclei of *Mycobacterium tuberculosis* or other airborne contagious microorganisms produced as a consequence of coughing, particularly during sputum induction
- Edema of the airway wall
- Edema associated with decreased compliance and gas exchange and with increased airway resistance
- Sputum induction by hypertonic saline inhalation can cause bronchoconstriction with patients who have chronic obstructive pulmonary disease, asthma, cystic fibrosis, or other pulmonary diseases

Limitations

- The efficacy of intermittent or continuous use of bland aerosol as a means of reducing mucus has not been established. Bland aerosol is not a substitute for systemic hydration.
- The physical properties of mucus are only minimally affected by the addition of water aerosol.
- Bland aerosol for humidification when the upper airway has been bypassed is not as efficient or effective as are heated water humidifiers or adequately designed heat and moisture exchangers (HMEs) because of the difficulties in maintaining temperature at patient airway, possible irritation to the airway, and infection risk.

Modified from AARC clinical practice guideline: bland aerosol administration—2003 revision and update. *Respir Care.* 2003;48(5):529–533. Reprinted with permission.

these purposes. Large-volume pneumatic nebulizers, which have reservoir volumes greater than 100 mL, are commonly used to aerosolize solutions such as normal saline (0.9% NaCl), half normal saline (0.45% NaCl), and distilled water for prolonged periods. They are primarily indicated to provide humidification of medical gases for patients with bypassed upper airways, as treatment of upper airway inflammation with cold mist for local vasoconstriction, to prevent occlusion of airway stents, and to induce sputum production for diagnostic purposes. There is little evidence to support the use of bland aerosols to hydrate a dehydrated patient. For delivery of humidified inspired gases, a large-volume nebulizer offers little advantage over alternative methods such as heated wick humidifiers.

Device Selection for Humidity Therapy

Selection of an appropriate humidification device should include consideration of the following questions:

- What source, temperature, and humidity of gas is the patient breathing?
- What is the point of entry of gas into the airway?
- What is the rate of inspiratory flow or minute volume?
- Does the patient have an intact or a bypassed upper airway?
- Does the patient have normal or diseased lungs?
- Is there evidence of increased, thick secretions or a humidity deficit?
- Are special needs imposed by dead space or the patient's size, age, ability to tolerate administration, or sensitivity to changes in the work of breathing?

Table 17–1 compares the relative attributes of common humidification systems.

Aerosol Drug Administration

Aerosol drug therapy has a number of advantages: a smaller dose can be targeted to the site of action, the onset of action occurs more quickly, and the therapeutic effect is achieved with fewer systemic side effects.[46,47] When aerosolized drugs are delivered directly to the airways, systemic absorption is limited, systemic side effects are minimized, and a high therapeutic index is achieved compared with systemic administration. In contrast, a variety of medications, including peptides and other macromolecules, can be targeted to the lung parenchyma for systemic administration across the alveolocapillary membrane into the pulmonary vascular bed. Aerosol devices can deliver a wide variety of medications, from bronchodilators to insulin, and many types of devices are used, including nebulizers, pressurized metered dose inhalers, and dry powder inhalers.[47–49] For medical use, aerosol generators produce respirable particles with a mass median aerodynamic diameter of 1 to 5 μm.[31]

RESPIRATORY RECAP

Primary Factors Affecting Aerosol Delivery

» Deposition
» Inertia
» Gravity
» Diffusion

Basic Concepts of Aerosol Therapy

An aerosol is composed of particles suspended in air. The time that particles can remain suspended depends on their low terminal settling velocity (v_t), or the velocity at which the aerosol particles fall in air because of gravity, a

TABLE 17–1 Comparison of Common Humidification Systems

Parameter	Bubble Humidifiers*	Passover Humidifiers†	Unheated Nebulizers	Heated Nebulizers	Heat and Moisture Exchangers
Output (mg/L)	15–20	30–50	15–30	20–40	13–32
Temperature (°C)	10–20	30–40	10–20	22–28	22–30
Flow limitation	Yes	No	Yes	Yes	Yes
Retains body temperature	No	Yes	No	Yes	Yes
Infection risk	Yes	No	Yes	Yes	No
Potential for overheating	No	Yes	No	Yes	No
Potential for overhydration	No	No	Yes	Yes	No
Potential for underhydration	Yes	No	Yes	No	Yes
Increases work of breathing	Yes	No	Yes	Yes	Yes
Possible electrical hazard	No	Yes	No	Yes	No

*Unheated.

†Heated.

value related to the size and density of the particle. The geometric size of the particles is commonly expressed as the **mass median aerodynamic diameter (MMAD)**. The deposition of inhaled aerosols onto airway surfaces varies with the size of the particles. For example, the v_t of a 5-μm water droplet is 0.074 cm/s, almost 22 times greater than a 1-μm water droplet but one-fourth that of a 10-μm water droplet. Half the mass of particles in an aerosol is less than the MMAD, and the other half is greater. Relatively few particles larger than the median particle diameter comprise the mass above the MMAD, with a much greater number of particles less than the median particle diameter required to reach comparable mass. **Geometric standard deviation (GSD)** is a measure of the magnitude of variation of particle size distribution. A monodisperse aerosol, in which all particles are basically the same size, has a GSD under 1.2, whereas a heterodisperse aerosol, with a wider range of particle sizes, has a GSD of more than 1.2. Most therapeutic aerosols are heterodisperse.

RESPIRATORY RECAP

Characterization of Aerosols

» Mass median aerodynamic diameter (MMAD)
» Geometric standard deviation (GSD)

Inertia is the tendency of an object with mass, once it is in motion, to travel in a straight line. The greater the mass and velocity of a particle, the greater is the inertia that keeps it in motion. Inertial impaction is the primary mechanism of deposition of aerosol particles 5 μm or larger and an important mechanism for particles as small as 2 μm. As aerosol is inhaled and the stream of gas is diverted in the airway, particles tend to continue along their initial trajectory, impacting and depositing on the airway. The higher the inspiratory flow, the greater the velocity and inertia of the particles, increasing the tendency of smaller particles to impact and deposit in airways. Turbulent flow, complex passageways, bifurcation of the airways, and inspiratory flows greater than 30 L/min increase the impaction of particles larger than 2 μm in the larger airways.

Gravitational sedimentation occurs when aerosol particles settle out of suspension because of gravity. The greater the mass of the particle, the faster it settles. Very small particles (those less than 0.5 μm in diameter) do not settle at all. Holding the breath for 4 to 10 seconds after inhalation of an aerosol lengthens the residence time for particles in the lungs, increasing the time for deposition through gravitational sedimentation, especially in the last six generations of the airway. Breath holding increases deposition of aerosol by as much as 10%, with up to a fourfold increase in peripheral distribution. This marginal increase in deposition may explain why breath holding has not been demonstrated to significantly improve the clinical response to aerosolized medications conducted to targeted airways.

Diffusion, or Brownian movement, is the primary mechanism of deposition of particles less than 3 μm in the airway. As gas reaches the distal regions of the lungs, gas flow stops. Aerosol particles bouncing against air molecules and each other deposit on contact with the airway surfaces. Preferential deposition for particles 0.5 to 3 μm is divided between the central and peripheral airways. Coalescence, the attraction of particles to each other, occurs when particles come within a distance 25 times or less their diameter.

Aerosol droplets in the respirable range (1 to 5 μm MMAD) are more likely to deposit in the lower respiratory tract than are larger or smaller particles. For particles larger than 0.5 μm, the depth of penetration into the lungs is inversely proportional to the particle size. Particles between 0.1 and 1 μm are so small that a significant proportion of those that enter the lungs may be exhaled. Particles larger than 5 μm impact in the upper airway before reaching the lower respiratory tract.

Aerosol Deposition, Targeting, and Translocation

Once an aerosol deposits on the airway, it must translocate across the mucous barrier and retain bioactivity to be effective as a therapeutic agent. The optimum site of action depends on the agent administered. Bronchodilators and steroids must reach the epithelium to be effective. Aerosolized antibiotics and mucokinetic agents are most effective when dispersed in infected airway secretions at sites of maximum airway obstruction. Gene transfer therapy must not only access the epithelium through the mucous barrier but also must then gain access to the submucous glands or basal (progenitor) cells of the epithelium.

Particle charge, solubility, and size and the biophysical properties of secretions all affect the ability of an aerosol to penetrate the mucous barrier. Turbulent flow and airway obstruction affect the airway deposition pattern. Other factors that limit efficacy, especially of macromolecules, include binding to constituents of mucus, including mucin and deoxyribonucleic acid (DNA), and the breakdown of bioactive molecules by proteases and other enzymes. Molecular weight and particle diffusion through mucus are inversely related. The antibiotic diffusion barrier represented by mucin may be significant in vitro, particularly for aerosol antibiotics. Translocation of macromolecules can be further compromised by the hypersecretion that accompanies inflammation and chronic pulmonary disease. These secretions can act as a barrier to the penetration of any aerosol.

Factors that promote translocation of medicated aerosols to the airway include an effective surfactant layer and increased particle retention time. Mucus discontinuity in the airway may assist deposition and translocation. The translocation of particles through the mucous layer depends partly on the presence of bronchial surfactant. Pulmonary surfactant promotes the displacement of some particles from air to the aqueous phase. The extent of particle immersion depends on the surface tension of the surface active film. For particles smaller than 100 μm, the surface tension force is several orders of magnitude greater than forces related to gravity.

Factors Affecting Drug Dose Distribution

Dosing of aerosolized medication is imprecise. It is unclear how much drug is delivered to targeted areas of the lung with progressive disease states and during acute exacerbations. These factors reduce aerosol deposition in the respiratory tract to as little as 1% of the medication dose placed in a nebulizer, regardless of whether the patient is breathing spontaneously or is mechanically ventilated. There is no established correlation between tidal volume and aerosol effectiveness. Theoretically, larger breaths capture more aerosol, but this relationship has not been shown clinically. This may be the result of partitioning of the tidal volume, which is regulated both by the delivered volume and by the airway dimensions. High inspiratory flow increases aerosol impaction in larger airways, whereas low inspiratory flow may result in a reduced amount of medication being available for inhalation from a dry powder inhaler.

Humidity also influences the delivery of aerosol medications. This has been well demonstrated with ventilator circuits, in which humidity can result in a 40% or greater reduction in aerosol delivered to the lungs. Droplets of solution evaporate or grow, depending on the water content and temperature of the gas, and powder can clump or aggregate in high humidity.

Drug formulations dictate, in part, which aerosol options are available for delivery of a specific medication. Most solutions can be nebulized if the medication is soluble (corticosteroids are an exception), but the physical characteristics of the solution (or suspension) can affect particle size and nebulizer output. Furthermore, some macromolecules may not enter suspension well and can be shattered into nonbioactive forms by the force of air required to generate an aerosol.

Aerosol Generators

Jet Nebulizers

Pneumatic jet nebulizers use the Bernoulli principle to drive a high-pressure gas through a restricted orifice across the top of a capillary tube, with the bottom of the tube immersed in the solution (**Figure 17–11**).[50,51] An aerosol is formed when the jet stream shears fluid from the capillary tube and drives the particles against a solid or liquid surface that acts as a baffle. Impaction against a baffle removes larger particles from suspension and allows them to return to the reservoir, whereas smaller particles remain suspended in the gas and travel from the nebulizer. A number of factors affect the delivery of aerosols by nebulizer (**Box 17–1**). **Box 17–2** describes the technique for the use of a medication nebulizer.

An effective small-volume pneumatic nebulizer should deliver more than 50% of its total dose as aerosol in the respirable range (1 to 5 μm MMAD) in 10 minutes or less of nebulization time. Nebulizer performance varies with fill volume, flow, gas density, and nebulizer model.[52] The amount of drug nebulized increases as the fill volume increases. The residual volume of solution (dead volume) that remains in commercial small-volume nebulizers varies from 0.5 to 1.5 mL, depending on the

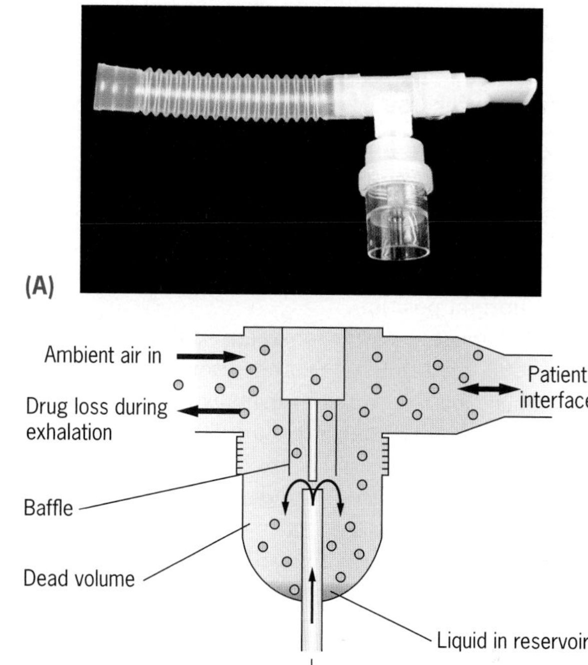

FIGURE 17–11 (**A**) Small-volume jet nebulizer for drug delivery. (**B**) Schematic drawing of small-volume jet nebulizer.

BOX 17–1

Factors That Affect Aerosol Delivery by Nebulizer

Technical Factors
- Manufacturer flow
- Fill volume
- Solution characteristics
- Characteristics of driving gas
- Designs to enhance output
- Continuous versus intermittent delivery

Patient Factors
- Breathing pattern
- Nose versus mouth breathing
- Characteristics of gas
- Airway obstruction
- Positive pressure delivery
- Artificial airway and mechanical ventilation

BOX 17-2

Technique for Use of a Jet Nebulizer

1. Assemble tubing, nebulizer cup, and mouthpiece (or mask).
2. Place medicine into the nebulizer cup; use fill volume of 4 to 5 mL.
3. The patient should be seated in an upright position.
4. Connect to power source; use a flow of 6 to 8 L/min or a compressor.
5. Have patient breathe normally with occasional deep breaths until sputter or no more aerosol is produced.
6. Keep nebulizer vertical during treatment.
7. Rinse nebulizer with sterile or distilled water and allow to air dry.

specific device. Therefore, increasing the fill volume allows a greater proportion of the medication to be nebulized. For example, with a 1-mL residual volume, a fill of 2 mL provides only 50% of the nebulizer charge available for nebulization. However, a fill of 4 mL makes 3 mL, or 75%, of the medication available for nebulization. Droplet size and nebulization time vary inversely with flow. Within the design limits of the nebulizer, the higher the flow to the nebulizer, the smaller the particle size generated and the shorter the time required to nebulize the full dose.

Gas density affects both aerosol generation and delivery of aerosol to the lungs. This is most evident with low-density helium–oxygen mixtures.[53,54] A carrier gas of lower density produces less turbulent flow, reducing aerosol impaction losses during inspiration and improving delivery of aerosol to the lungs. However, when helium–oxygen is used to drive a jet nebulizer, aerosol output is reduced, requiring a twofold increase in flow to produce a comparable respirable aerosol output per minute. Consequently, helium–oxygen mixtures may increase the percentage of aerosol available to the lungs but impair the production of the aerosol by the nebulizer. Humidity and temperature affect the particle size and concentration of drug remaining in the nebulizer. Evaporation of water and adiabatic expansion of gas reduce the temperature of the aerosol more than 5° C (41° F) below the ambient temperature. Aerosol particles entrained into a warm and water-saturated gas stream may increase in size. These larger particles tend to coalesce, increasing the MMAD.

Clinicians and patients commonly tap a nebulizer periodically to shake droplets of medication from the walls of the nebulizer into the reservoir. However, in

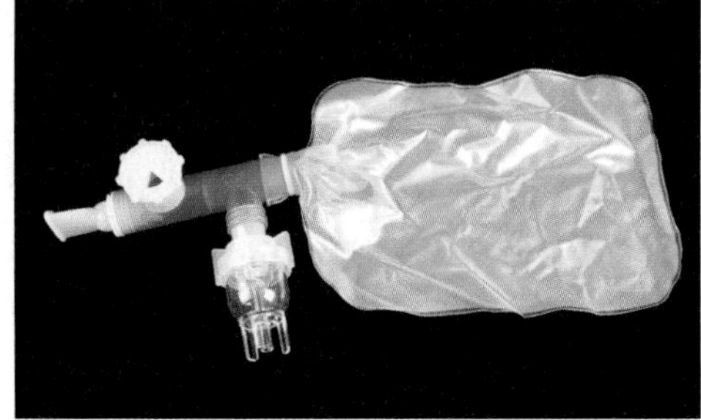

FIGURE 17–12 Nebulizer with reservoir bag to capture aerosol during the expiratory phase.

one study, albuterol delivery from the nebulizer stopped with the onset of inconsistent nebulization (sputtering).[55] Continuation past the point of initial jet nebulizer sputter is ineffective and should indicate an end of the treatment. Because the nebulizer selected affects aerosol delivery, a nebulizer should be chosen that reliably delivers specific medications. When a compressor is used to power the nebulizer, the performance of the compressor also is important.

Nebulizers commonly are operated continuously—that is, throughout the patient's respiratory cycle. This wastes the aerosol produced during the expiratory phase. A typical inspiration-to-expiration ratio of 1:3 results in 75% of the aerosol emitted from the nebulizer being lost to the atmosphere. This is a major factor in the poor efficiency associated with pneumatic nebulizers. If 50% of the nominal dose is emitted, 50% in the respirable range, and 25% of that is inhaled by the patient, then 12.5% of the nominal dose is inhaled by the patient and 20% of that is exhaled. This results in the 10% deposition observed with in vivo measurements.

A reservoir on the expiratory limb of the nebulizer conserves drugs by collecting some of the nebulizer output that otherwise would be wasted to the atmosphere. A reservoir can be created through placement of 15 cm of aerosol tubing on the expiratory side of the nebulizer. As an alternative, commercial devices such as simple bag reservoirs (**Figure 17–12**) provide a greater volume reservoir in which the smaller aerosol particles remain in suspension for inhalation and larger particles rain out.

Vented breath-enhanced nebulizer systems (**Figure 17–13**) allow the patient to inhale additional air through the nebulizer, increasing drug delivery on inspiration. The inlet vent closes on exhalation, and aerosol exits via a one-way valve in the mouthpiece. This design reduces aerosol waste and increases the inhaled dose by as much as 50% without increasing the treatment time.

Breath-actuated nebulization synchronizes aerosol generation with inspiration, increasing the amount of drug available for inspiration by up to fourfold. The inhaled aerosol per breath is similar, but the amount of drug inhaled and the treatment time increase by a factor of four. Inspiratory phase nebulization can be accomplished with a thumb control port that allows the patient to manually direct gas to the nebulizer only on

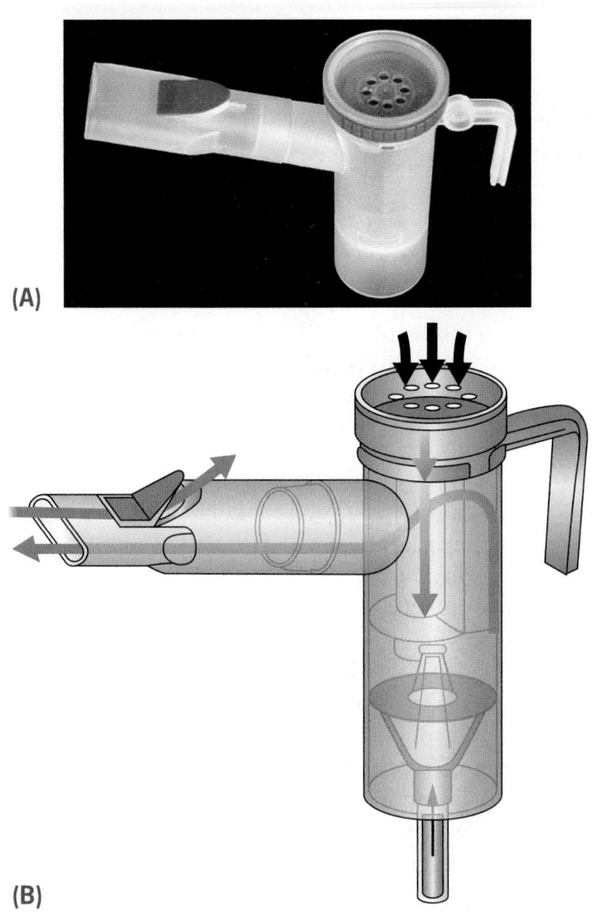

FIGURE 17–13 (**A**) Vented breath-enhanced nebulizer. (**B**) Schematic drawing of a vented breath-enhanced nebulizer.

inspiration. This improves the efficiency of the nebulizer if the patient has good hand–breath coordination. More effective systems do not require hand–breath coordination and operate by the synchronizing of aerosol production to the patient's inspiratory phase.

The I-Neb system uses a microprocessor and pneumotachometer to regulate nebulization during the first half of inspiration, monitoring the inspiratory time of the first threew breaths and creating a template for nebulization during inspiration of subsequent breaths (**Figure 17–14**). This is called adaptive aerosol delivery (AAD). The Monaghan AeroEclipse (**Figure 17–15**) is a pneumatic breath-actuated nebulizer that responds to the patient's inspiratory flow, producing aerosol during inspiration and ending nebulization when the inspiratory flow drops below a threshold.

Some nebulizers are valved and have expiratory filters (**Figure 17–16**); these are designed specifically for the delivery of pentamidine. The filter minimizes ambient contamination with the aerosol and the patient's exhaled gases. These nebulizers also produce very small particles to enhance parenchymal deposition.

Plastic nebulizers may show degradation of performance after many uses. A study of disposable nebulizers reported that repeated use did not alter performance as long as proper cleaning was performed.[56] Nebulizers should be cleaned and disinfected or rinsed with sterile water between uses and air dried. Contamination of nebulizer solutions is related to storage of multiple-dose solutions at room temperature and reuse of syringes to

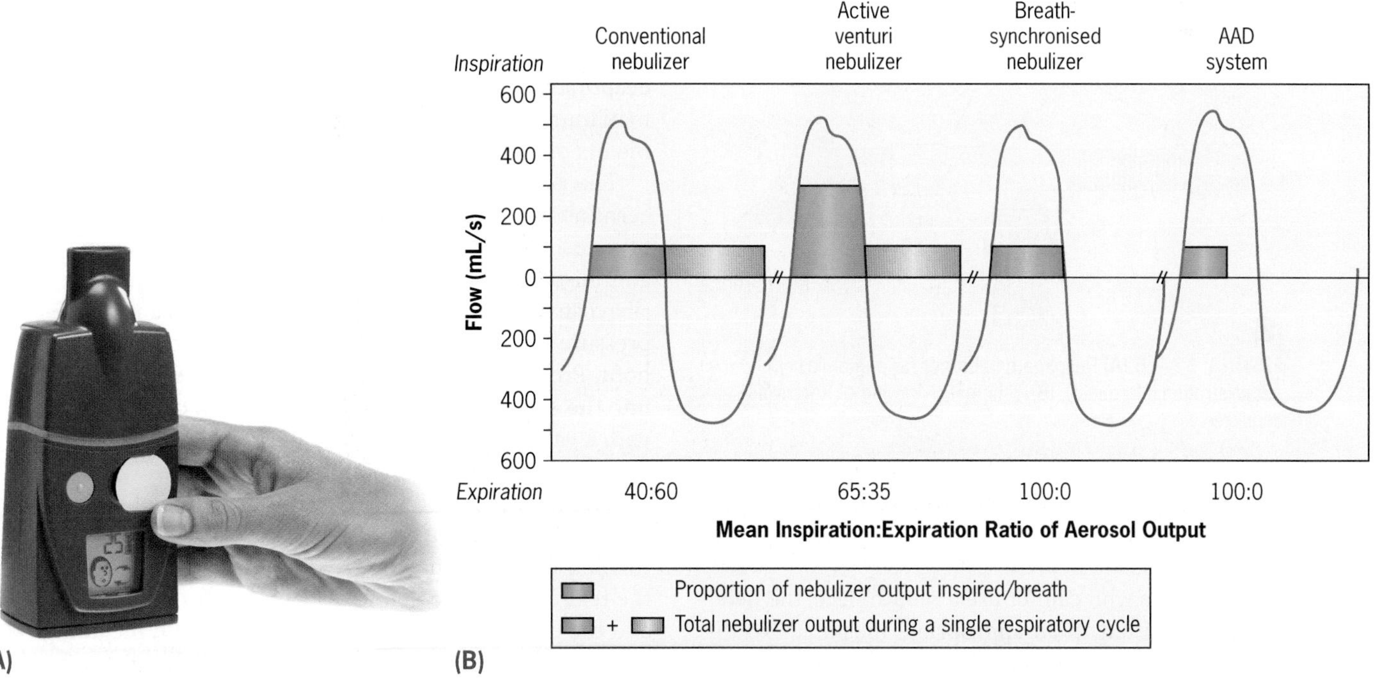

FIGURE 17–14 (**A**) Adaptive aerosol delivery system. (**B**) Schematic of the flow and inspiration-to-expiration ratios of aerosol output with four types of jet nebulizer. The drug available for inhalation is indicated by the darker shaded areas. The lighter shaded areas indicate the aerosol loss to the ambient air. These two areas are used to calculate the mean inspiration-to-expiration ratios for the aerosol output of the various types of nebulizers. AAD, adaptive aerosol delivery system. (**B**) Reproduced from Denyer J, et al. *Expert Opin Drug Deliv.* 2004:165–176. Reprinted by permission of the publishers (Taylor & Francis Group, www.informaworld.com).

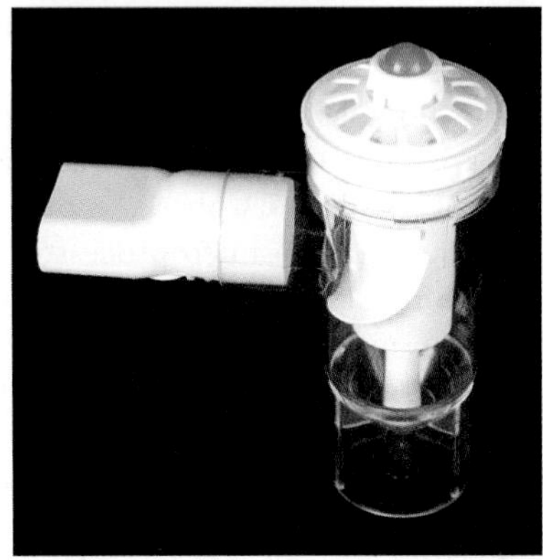

FIGURE 17–15 Breath-actuated nebulizer.

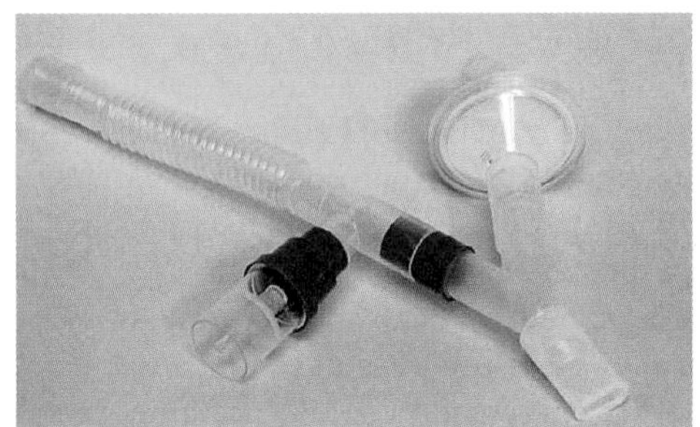

(A)

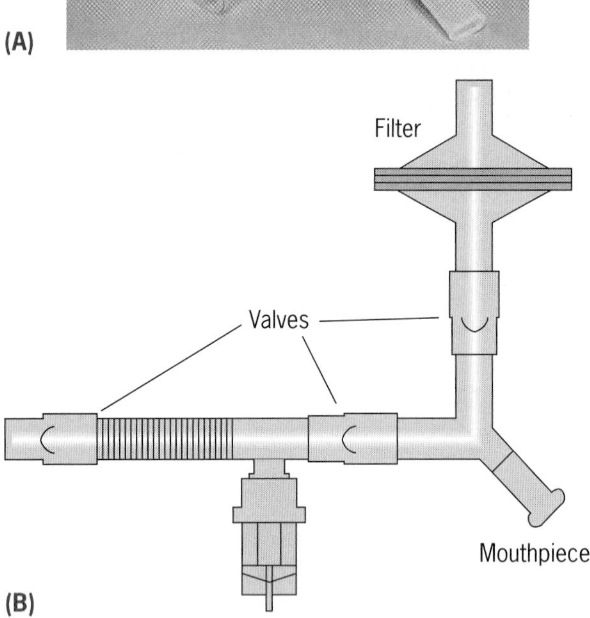

(B)

FIGURE 17–16 (**A**) Respirgard nebulizer for pentamidine administration (Marquest). (**B**) Schematic drawing of Respirgard nebulizer.

measure the solution. Refrigerating solutions and disposing of syringes every 24 hours eliminates bacterial contamination.

For patients who cannot use a mouthpiece, the nebulizer can be fitted to an appropriate mask.[57,58] No difference in clinical response has been found between mouthpiece and close-fitting mask treatment; therefore, patient compliance and preference should guide selection of the device.[59] If a mask is used, care should be taken to avoid aerosol delivery in the eyes (**Figure 17–17**).[60–65] However, a mouthpiece enhances medication delivery

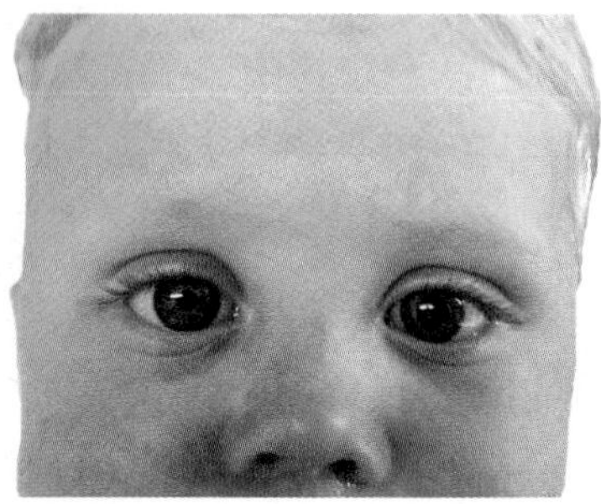

FIGURE 17–17 Unilateral left dilated pupil, which did not react to light, caused by the inadvertent aerosolization of ipratropium bromide into the eye.

to the airways in adults. Crying is a long exhalation preceded by a very short and rapid inhalation; this completely prevents lower airway deposition of an aerosol. Thus, aerosols should not be administered to a crying child. It is more efficient to deliver medication by close-fitting mask when the child is asleep. Blow-by, in which the clinician directs the aerosol from the nebulizer toward the patient's nose and mouth, is not supported by evidence; aerosol deposition studies suggest that virtually no drug enters the airway.[66,67]

The small particle aerosol generator (SPAG) is a jet-type aerosol generator used to administer ribavirin (**Figure 17–18**). It uses a secondary drying chamber that reduces the MMAD to 1.2 μm with a GSD of 1.4. The SPAG reduces the 50 psi of line-pressure medical gas to 26 psi, connected to two flow meters that control flow to the nebulizer and the drying chamber. The aerosol generated in the medication reservoir enters the long cylindric drying chamber, where additional flow of dry gas reduces the size of the aerosol particles through evaporation. The flow to the nebulizer is adjusted to a maximum of 7 L/min, with a total flow from both flow meters of 15 L/min.

The administration of ribavirin has highlighted concerns about secondhand exposure of healthcare workers to aerosol, resulting in recommendations that open-air administration be avoided.[68] To protect staff members, ribavirin administration should be limited to a negative-pressure, single-patient room with six air exchanges per hour. Procedures used to reduce the release of ribavirin into the environment include containment of the aerosol with a canopy over the delivery device (**Figure 17–19**),[69] use of a scavenging system, and filtering of the expiratory limb of the circuit of a mechanically ventilated patient. Practices that reduce caregiver exposure include the turning off of the nebulizer 5 minutes before opening the tent or 1 minute before disconnecting the ventilator and the use of personal protective equipment, including goggles, a respirator, gown, and gloves. Administrative policies should prevent pregnant or lactating women and staff members who have had reactions to the drug from coming into contact with ribavirin. Caution must be used when ribavirin is administered during mechanical ventilation because of the drug's tendency to occlude

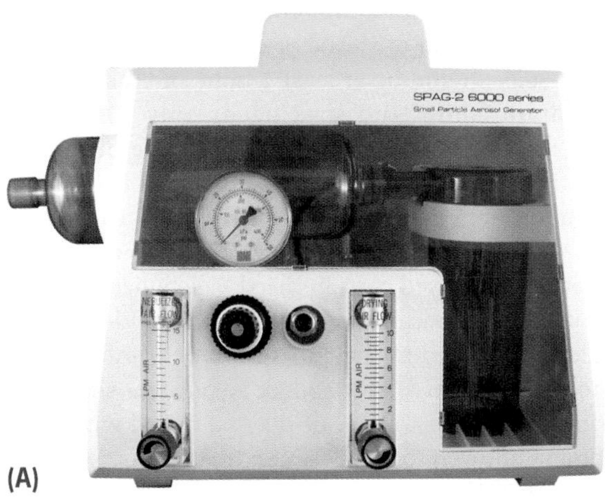

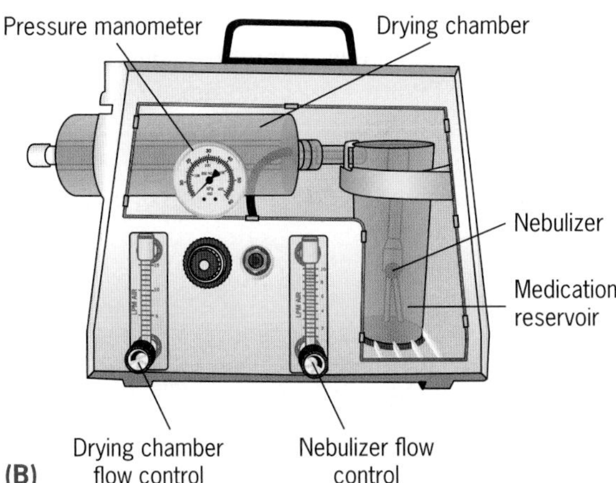

FIGURE 17–18 (**A**) Small particle aerosol generator (SPAG) for ribavirin administration. (**B**) Schematic drawing of SPAG. (**B**) Adapted from Scanlan CL, et al. *Egan's Fundamentals of Respiratory Care*. 7th ed. Mosby; 1999.

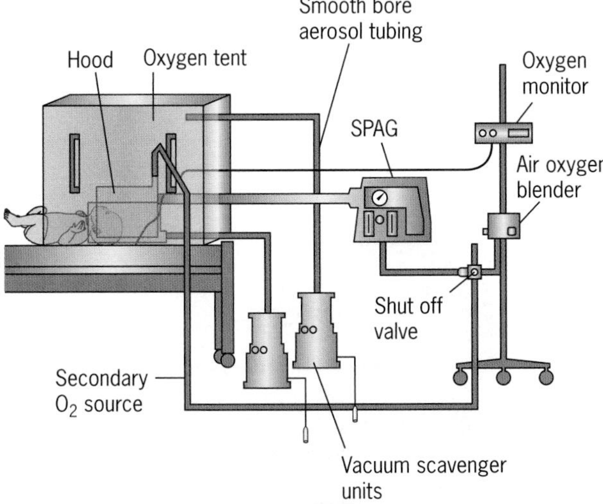

FIGURE 17–19 Scavenging system for ribavirin administration. Modified from Kacmarek RM, Kratohvil J. Evaluation of a double-enclosure double-vacuum unit scavenging system for ribavirin administration. *Respir Care*. 1992;37:37–45. Reprinted with permission.

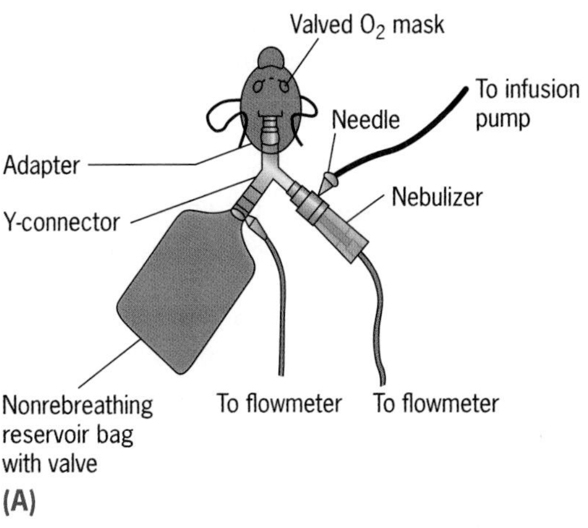

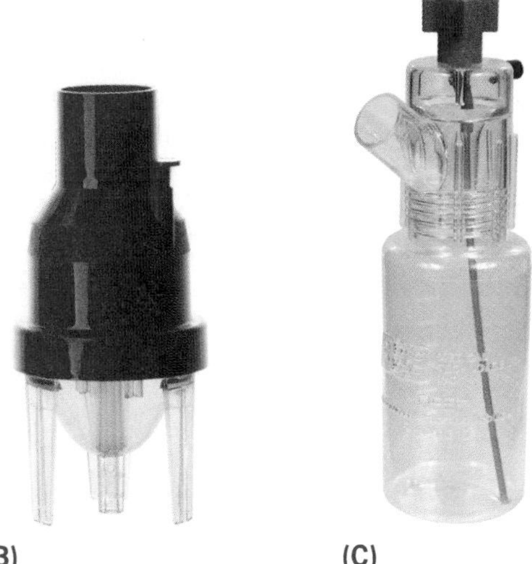

FIGURE 17–20 (**A**) Delivery systems for continuous aerosolized bronchodilator by continuous infusion of medications into a standard small-volume nebulizer. (**B**) Commercially available nebulizer for continuous aerosol administration. (**C**) Commercially available nebulizer for continuous aerosol administration. (**A**) Modified from Moler FW, et al. Continuous versus intermittent nebulized terbutaline: plasma levels and effects. *Am J Respir Crit Care Med*. 1995;151:602–606. (**C**) Courtesy of B&B Medical Technologies.

filters, valves, and endotracheal tubes. Tandem filters placed in series in the expiratory limb of the ventilator reduce expiratory valve occlusion but require frequent changing. Aerosol from the SPAG is entrained into the ventilator circuit distal to the output of the humidifier through a one-way valve.[70] A high-pressure alarm in the circuit alerts the clinician to an excessive baseline pressure should expiratory occlusion occur.

If the symptoms of a patient with acute exacerbation of asthma are not relieved with standard bronchodilator dosing, continuous aerosol can be provided at a controlled rate of medication delivery.[71,72] Doses of albuterol between 7.5 and 15 mg/h have proved effective in treating acute exacerbations of asthma. One strategy is to use an intravenous infusion pump to deliver a premixed bronchodilator solution into a jet nebulizer (**Figure 17–20**). Another strategy is to use a **large-volume nebulizer** that delivers a consistent output of medication at a specific flow. Albuterol solution and saline are mixed in the reservoir, and the nebulizer is operated at a flow recommended by the manufacturer to deliver the desired dose. The aerosol can be delivered with a mask or in-line with a ventilator circuit. For patients with moderately severe asthma, continuous or intermittent therapy has a similar effect with either low- or high-dose β-agonists.

> **RESPIRATORY RECAP**
>
> **Aerosol Medication Delivery Devices**
>
> » Jet nebulizer
> » Mesh nebulizer
> » Soft mist inhaler
> » Ultrasonic nebulizer (USN)
> » Pressurized metered dose inhaler (pMDI)
> » Metered dose inhaler with spacer or holding chamber
> » Dry powder inhaler (DPI)

Patients should be taught how to disinfect their nebulizers used in the home. After each treatment, the patient should shake the remaining solution from the nebulizer cup. The nebulizer cup should be rinsed with either sterile or distilled water and left to air dry on an absorbent towel. Once or twice a week, the nebulizer should be disassembled, washed in soapy tap water, and disinfected with either a 1.25% acetic acid (white vinegar) mixture or a quaternary ammonium compound at a dilution of 1 ounce to 1 gallon of sterile or distilled water. The acetic acid soak should be at least 1 hour, but a quaternary ammonium compound soak needs only 10 minutes. Acetic acid should not be reused, but the quaternary ammonium solution can be reused for up to 1 week.[73] Pneumatic nebulizers have been reported to function correctly in repeated uses provided that they are cleaned after each use, rinsed, and air dried.[56] Nebulizers for hospital use are disposable, single-patient-use devices and should be changed at the conclusion of the dose, every 24 hours, or when visibly soiled. Nebulizers should not be rinsed with tap water, but may be rinsed with sterile water and allowed to dry between treatments.

Mesh Nebulizers

Several manufacturers have developed aerosol devices that use a mesh or plate with multiple apertures to produce an aerosol (**Figure 17–21** and **Box 17–3**).[74–76] **Mesh nebulizers** use a vibrating mesh or a vibrating horn. For the vibrating mesh (e.g., Aerogen Aeroneb, Pari eFlow Technology), contraction and expansion of a vibrational

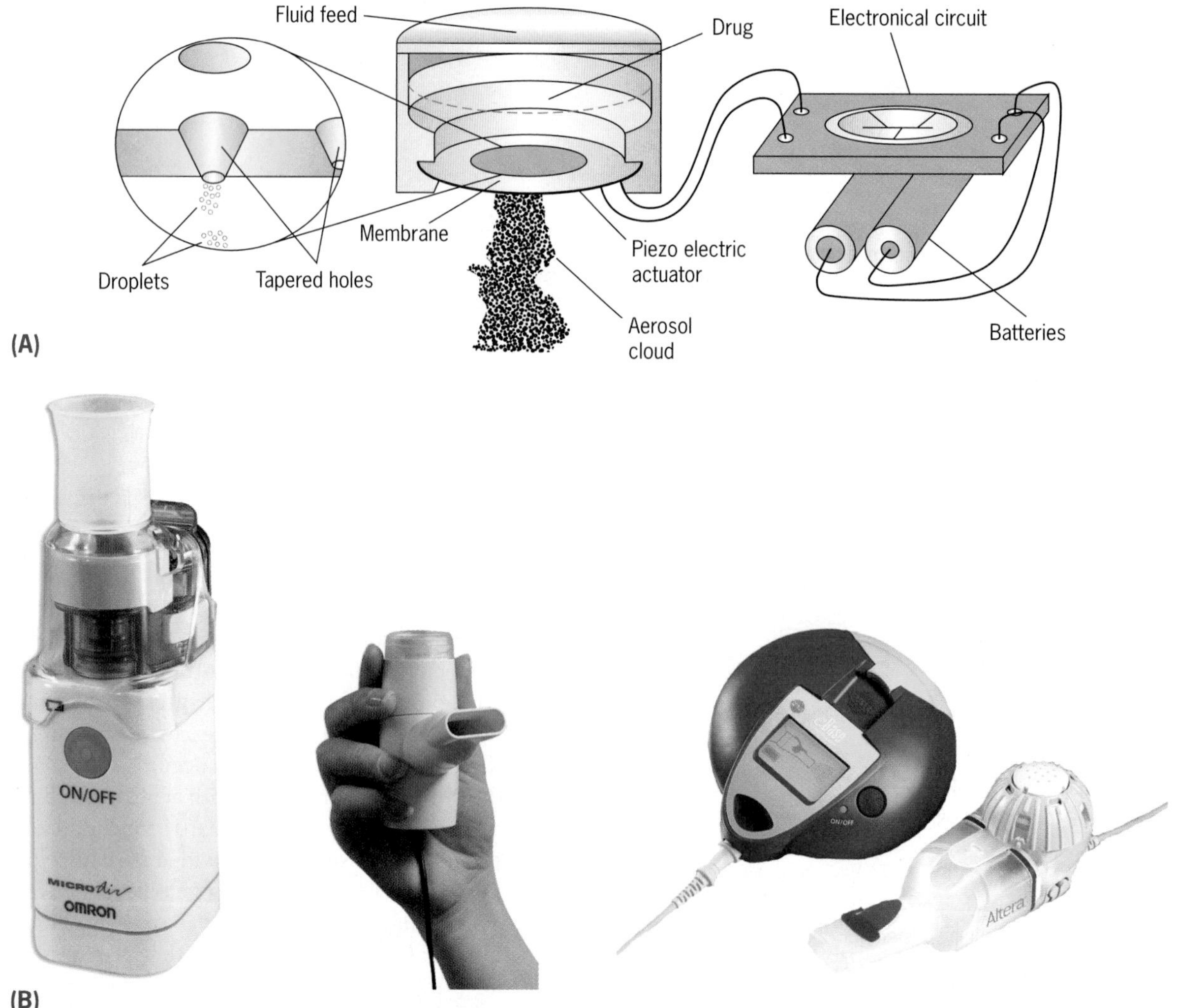

FIGURE 17–21 Mesh nebulizers. (**A**) Principle of operation. (**B**) Representative commercially available mesh nebulizers. (**A**) Adapted from Hess DR. Aerosol delivery devices in the treatment of asthma. *Respir Care*. 2008;53:699–725.

element produces an upward and downward movement of a domed aperture plate. The aperture plate contains up to 4000 tapered holes. The holes have a tapered shape with a larger cross section on the liquid side and a smaller cross section on the side the droplets emerge. The medication is placed in a reservoir above the domed aperture plate. Sound pressure is built up in the vicinity of the membrane, creating a pumping action that extrudes solution through the holes in the plate to produce an aerosol. The aerosol particle size and flow are determined by the exit diameter of the aperture holes. The size of the holes in the plate can be modified for specific clinical applications. eFlow Technology combines a vibrating mesh with an aerosol mixing chamber; eFlow Technology devices are drug-specific and are linked to one drug.

In the vibrating horn system (e.g., Omron) a piezoelectric crystal vibrates at a high frequency when electrical current is applied, and the vibration is transmitted to a transducer horn that is in contact with the solution. Vibration of the transducer horn forces the liquid passes through the apertures in the plate and forms an aerosol.

Nebulization with a mesh nebulizer is dependent on fluid characteristics.[77,78] These nebulizers may be unsuitable for viscous fluids, which suggests that matching the formulation to the device may be important for these aerosol generators. Mesh technology can be coupled with adaptive aerosol delivery, as in the I-neb.

BOX 17–3

Technique for Use of a Mesh Nebulizer

1. Correctly assemble the equipment.
2. Follow the manufacturer's instructions to perform a functionality test prior to the first use of a new device and after each disinfection to verify proper operation.
3. Pour the solution into the medication reservoir. Do not exceed the volume recommended by the manufacturer.
4. Turn on the power.
5. Hold the nebulizer in the position recommended by the manufacturer.
6. Breathe normally with occasional deep breaths.
7. If the treatment must be interrupted, turn off the unit to avoid waste.
8. At the completion of the treatment, disassemble and clean as recommended by the manufacturer.
9. Be careful not to touch the mesh during cleaning, as this will damage the unit.
10. Once or twice a week, disinfect the nebulizer following the manufacturer's instructions.

Soft Mist Inhaler

The Respimat Soft Mist Inhaler delivers a metered dose of medication as a fine mist (**Figure 17–22**).[79–81] Medication delivered by the Respimat is stored in a collapsible bag in a sealed plastic container inside the cartridge. With each actuation, the correct dosage is drawn from the inner reservoir, and the flexible bag contracts accordingly. A twist of the inhaler's base compresses a spring. A tube slides into a canal in the cartridge, and the dose is drawn through the tube into a micro-pump. When the dose-release button is pressed, the energy released from the spring forces the solution through the uniblock, and a slow-moving aerosol is released.

The fine nozzle system of the uniblock is the core element of the Respimat. When the medication solution is forced through the nozzle system, two jets of liquid emerge and converge at an optimized angle, and the impact of these converging jets generates the aerosol. The aerosol produced by the Respimat moves much slower and has a more prolonged duration than an aerosol cloud from a **pressurized metered dose inhaler (pMDI)**.[82] A dose indicator shows how many doses are left. Compared with a pMDI with fenoterol plus ipratropium bromide, the Respimat provides equivalent bronchodilation at half the cumulative dose in asthmatic patients.[83] Compared with a pMDI, lung deposition is doubled and oropharyngeal deposition reduced.[84–86] Low deposition on the face, and especially in the eyes, occurs when the Respimat is fired accidentally outside the body or is fired at the same time as the patient exhales.[87] It has been reported that a majority of patients preferred the Respimat to a pMDI.[88]

Ultrasonic Nebulizers

The **ultrasonic nebulizer** (USN) uses a piezoelectric crystal that vibrates at a high frequency to convert electricity to sound waves, creating standing waves in the liquid immediately above the transducer and disrupting the liquid's surface, forming a geyser of droplets (**Figure 17–23**). Because electronics are not readily sterilized, disposable medication cups with a flexible diaphragm are commonly used, with the sound waves communicated through a layer of water acting as a couplant. USNs are capable of greater aerosol output (0.4 to 5 mL/min) with greater aerosol density than conventional jet nebulizers.

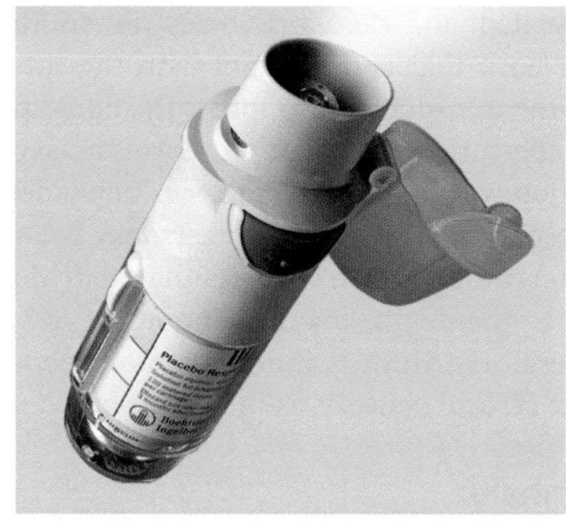

(A)

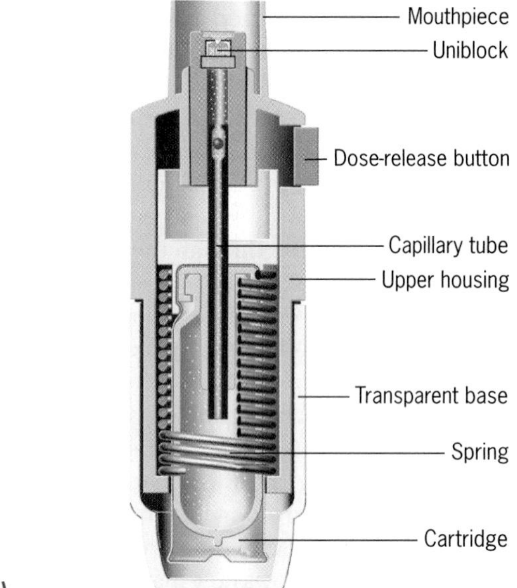

(B)

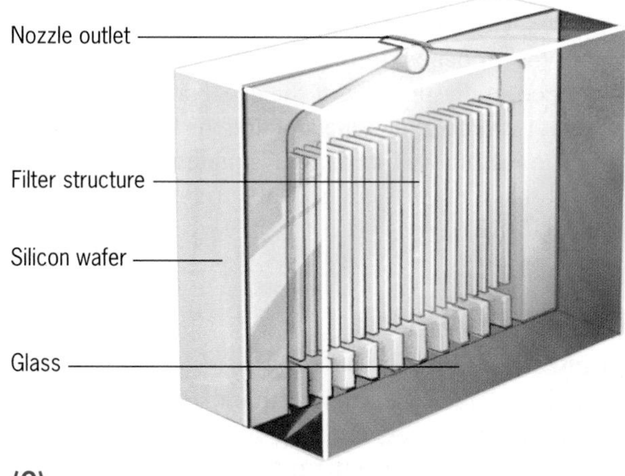

(C)

FIGURE 17–22 (**A**) Respimat Soft Mist Inhaler. (**B**) Components of the Respimat. (**C**) The uniblock, which is the core element of the Respimat.

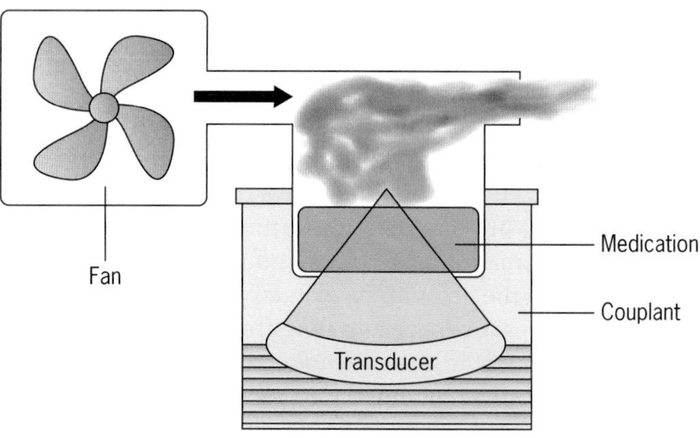

FIGURE 17–23 Schematic drawing of ultrasonic nebulizer. Adapted from Cohen N, Fink J. Humidity and aerosols. In: Eubanks DH, Borne RC, eds. *Principles and Applications of Cardiorespiratory Care Equipment.* Mosby; 1994.

Particle size is determined by frequency, and output by the amplitude of the signal. Within limits, the particle size is inversely proportional to the frequency and is not user adjustable. Two USNs from the same manufacturer can operate at different frequencies (1.24 to 2.25 MHz), producing a range of MMADs (2.5 to 6 μm).

Large-volume USNs, which are used primarily for bland aerosol therapy or sputum induction, incorporate air blowers to carry the mist to the patient. An inverse relationship exists between the aerosol density emitted by the USN and the flow of gas through the nebulizer. Because of the energy required, the temperature of the solution in a USN increases by as much as 15° C (59° F) over 15 minutes. As the temperature rises, the drug concentration also rises, increasing the likelihood of undesirable side effects such as denaturing proteins.

Small-volume ultrasonic nebulizers are available for aerosol drug delivery.[89] These systems may or may not use a water-filled couplant compartment, with the medication placed in a cup or directly onto the transducer connected to a battery-powered power source. The patient's inspiratory flow draws aerosol from the nebulizer into the lungs. As the USN operates, the aerosol remains in the medication cup or chamber until a flow of gas pushes or pulls the aerosol from the nebulizer. If a USN creates aerosol continuously, the patient draws aerosol from the nebulizer during inspiration and clears aerosol from the chamber during exhalation, with aerosol collecting in the chamber between end expiration and through inspiration. If exhalation is diverted away from the medication chamber, there is minimal waste to atmosphere and more drug available for inhalation.

Small-volume USNs may have less dead volume than small-volume nebulizers. The contained portable power source provides convenience and mobility. However, the advantages of ultrasonic nebulizers may be offset by their high cost relative to standard jet nebulizers. USNs have been promoted for administration of a wide variety of formulations ranging from bronchodilators to anti-inflammatory agents and antibiotics, but they generally have proved less effective than other delivery devices, especially with suspensions.[90]

The Optineb (**Figure 17–24**) uses an ultrasonic nebulizer to deliver treprostinil inhalation solution for the treatment of pulmonary arterial hypertension. It incorporates filters to minimize ambient contamination with the drug. The device prompts the patient to use correct inhalation technique. The recommended prescribed dose of treprostinil is up to 9 breaths (54 micrograms) per treatment session and up to 4 treatment sessions per day.

Overhydration has been associated with prolonged bland aerosol treatment by use of a USN in children and patients with renal insufficiency. The high-density aerosol from USNs may precipitate bronchospasm. An acoustic power output above 50 watts/cm^2 has been associated with disruption of the structure of some molecules. USNs recently have drawn attention for the administration of aerosols during mechanical ventilation because they do not require the addition of a driving gas flow to the circuit.[91] Disadvantages of the USN in the ventilator circuit include weight, position dependency, a tendency to heat medications, and the need for water couplants.

Pressurized Metered Dose Inhalers

The pressurized metered dose inhaler (**Figure 17–25**) is the most commonly prescribed method of aerosol delivery.[92] Pressurized MDIs are used to administer bronchodilators, anticholinergics, anti-inflammatory agents, and steroids. In the United States, more formulations are available by pMDI than by other aerosol delivery systems. When properly used, pMDIs are at least as effective for drug delivery as other nebulizers. For this reason, pMDIs often are the preferred method used to deliver bronchodilators to both spontaneously breathing and mechanically ventilated patients.

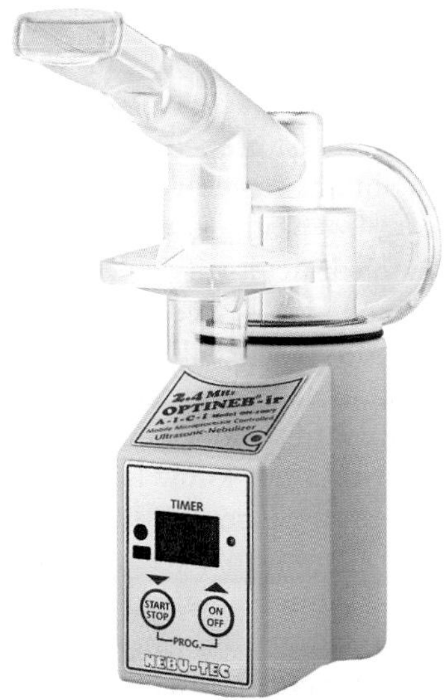

FIGURE 17–24 The TYVASO inhalation system.

A pMDI consists of a pressurized canister containing a drug in the form of a micronized powder or solution that is suspended with a mixture of propellants, surfactant, preservatives, flavoring agents, and dispersing agents. The concentrations of the dispersing agents are equal to or greater than that of the medication, and dispersing agents may be associated with coughing and wheezing. The active drug accounts for about 1% of the contents of the pMDI. As much as 80% by weight of the spray from the pMDI is composed of a propellant, which in the past was a chlorofluorocarbon (CFC) such as Freon. Because

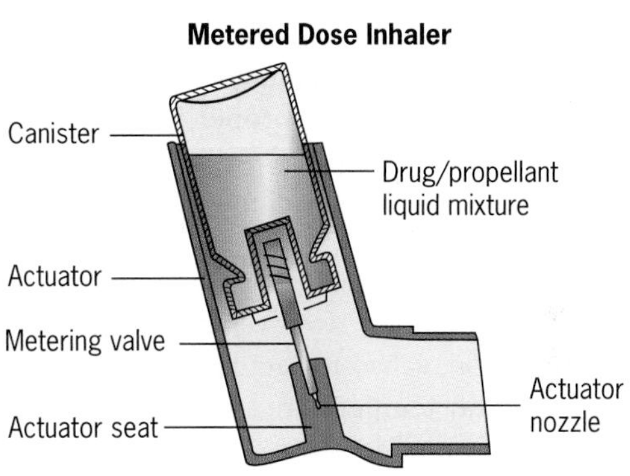

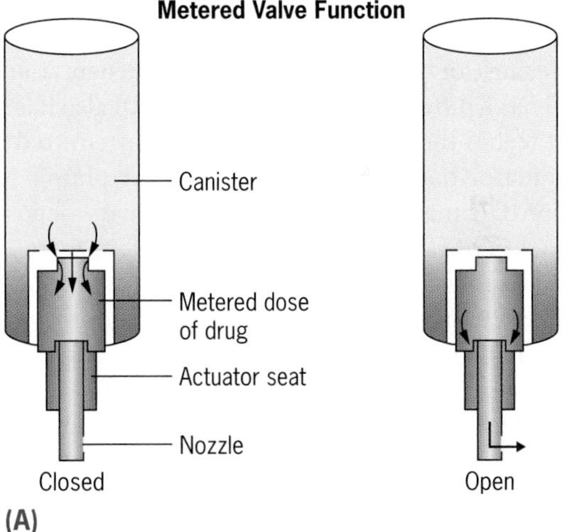

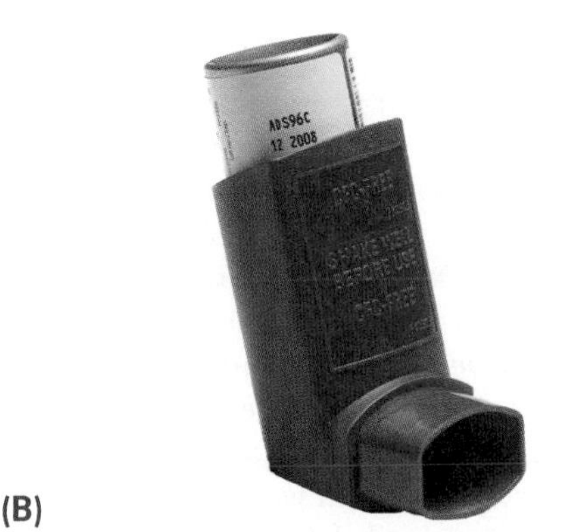

FIGURE 17–25 (**A**) Schematic drawing of metered dose inhaler. (**B**) Commercially available metered dose inhaler. (**A**) Adapted from Rau JL Jr. *Respiratory Care Pharmacology*. 5th ed. Mosby; 1998.

of international agreements to ban CFCs, most pMDIs now use hydrofluoroalkanes (HFAs), such as HFA133a, as the propellant.[93] By December 31, 2013, all pMDI using CFC will be removed from the U.S. market.

In a pMDI, the mixture is released from the canister through a metering valve and stem that fit into an actuator boot, and the device is designed and tested by the manufacturer to work with a specific medication formulation. Small changes in the actuator's design can change the characteristics and output of the aerosol. The metering valve volume varies from 30 to 100 μL and contains 20 μg to 5 mg of drug. The volume emitted by the pMDI is 15 to 20 mL after volatilization of the propellant.[94] Lung deposition ranges from 10% to 25% of the nominal dose in adults, with intersubject variability largely technique dependent. When proper technique and an effective accessory device are used, the pMDI delivers substantially more of the dose of medication to the lungs than a jet nebulizer.

HFA pMDI albuterol formulations are as effective as their CFC counterparts.[95] However, because of the redesigned formulation, valve, and actuator, the HFA version has a warmer spray temperature and less impact force at the back of the throat. Moreover, Proventil HFA does not suffer a loss of dose when the inhaler is stored inverted, nor is it subject to loss of dose in a cold climate, and there is less dose variability at the end of the canister's life. Because of the differences in the propellant, the HFA pMDI has a different taste. The HFA pMDI also has a different feel in the mouth because the spray emitted from the actuator has less force and a smaller plume. Some HFA pMDIs may provide greater pulmonary deposition than CFC pMDIs.[96] HFA steroid inhalers were engineered to generate aerosol particles with an average size of 1.2 μm, to more effectively reach the lower respiratory tract and have less oropharyngeal deposition, which may improve clinical outcomes. Each puff of Proventil HFA releases 4 μL of ethanol, which may be of concern for patients who abstain from alcohol. A breath alcohol level of up to 35 μg per 100 mL may be detected for up to 5 minutes after two puffs of Proventil HFA.[97] ProAir HFA and Xopenex HFA also contain ethanol. HFA propellant may cause false-positive readings in gas-monitoring systems, because the infrared spectra of HFAs overlap with common anesthetic gases.[98] Ventolin HFA contains no excipients other than the propellant but has a greater affinity for moisture than other HFA inhalers and is therefore packaged in a moisture-resistant protective pouch that contains a desiccant and has a limited shelf life once it is removed from the pouch. Clogging of HFA pMDI albuterol actuators has been reported.[99] They should be cleaned at least once a week by removing the metal canister, running warm water through the plastic actuator for 30 seconds, shaking the actuator to remove water, and then allowing it to air dry. The actuator should be cleaned more frequently if a reduction in the force of emitted spray is noted.

The nominal dose of medication with the pMDI is much smaller than that with a nebulizer. The amount of albuterol exiting the actuator nozzle of a pMDI is 100 μg with each actuation, or 90 μg from the opening of the actuator boot; this is how pMDI aerosol actuations are characterized in the United States. Thus, a dose of two to four actuations (200 to 400 μg nominal dose) usually is used. In ambulatory patients, 10% deposition may deliver a dose of 20 to 40 μg for an effective bronchodilation response.

Effective use of the pMDI is technique dependent. As many as two-thirds of patients who use pMDIs and health professionals who teach pMDI use do not perform the procedure properly.[100] **Box 17–4** lists the steps for administering a bronchodilator with a pMDI. Good patient instruction can take 10 to 30 minutes and should include demonstration, practice, and confirmation of the patient's performance (demonstration placebo units are available for this purpose). Repeated instruction improves performance.[101] Infants, young children, the elderly, and patients in acute distress may not be able to use a pMDI effectively. A cold Freon effect can occur when the aerosol plume reaches the back of the mouth and the patient stops inhaling. The pMDI can be used as often as every 30 seconds without affecting its performance. A new pMDI or one that has not been used recently should be actuated several times before use to prime the metering chamber properly. The pMDI should always be stored with the cap on, both to prevent foreign objects from entering the boot and to reduce humidity and microbial contamination.

AGE-SPECIFIC ANGLE

Infants, young children, the elderly, and patients in acute distress may not be able to use a pMDI effectively.

Pressurized MDIs should always be discarded when empty to avoid administration of propellant without medication. Although many pMDIs contain more than the labeled number of doses, drug delivery per actuation may be very inconsistent and unpredictable after the labeled number of actuations. Beyond the labeled number of actuations, propellant can release an aerosol plume that contains little or no drug, a phenomenon called tail-off.[102] A practical problem for patients who use pMDIs is the difficulty of determining the number of doses remaining in the device. Ideally the patient knows the number of doses in a full pMDI and keeps track of how many actuations have been used. However, many patients are unaware of the number of doses in a full pMDI, and most do not know how to determine when their pMDI is empty. Floating the canister in water has been suggested as a way to determine when it is depleted, but this method is unreliable and should not be used.[103–105] The Food and Drug Administration now recommends that manufacturers integrate a dose-counting device into new pMDIs, and several pMDIs have integrated dose counters (e.g., Ventolin HFA, Flovent HFA). Add-on

BOX 17-4

Technique for Use of a Pressurized Metered Dose Inhaler

1. Hold the pressurized metered dose inhaler (pMDI) in your hand to warm it.
2. Remove the mouthpiece cover.
3. Inspect the mouthpiece for foreign objects.
4. Hold the pMDI in a vertical position.
5. Shake the pMDI.
6. If the pMDI is new or has not been used recently, prime it by shaking and pressing the canister to deliver a dose into the room. Repeat several times.
7. Breathe out normally.
8. Open your mouth and keep your tongue from obstructing the mouthpiece.
9. Hold the pMDI in a vertical position, with the mouthpiece aimed at your mouth.
10. Place the mouthpiece between your lips or position it two finger widths from your mouth.
11. Breathe in slowly and press the pMDI canister down once at the beginning of inhalation.
12. Continue to inhale until your lungs are full.
13. Move the mouthpiece away from your mouth and hold your breath for 10 seconds (or as long as you comfortably can).
14. Wait at least 30 seconds between doses.
15. Repeat for the prescribed number of doses.
16. Recap the mouthpiece.
17. Rinse your mouth if using inhaled steroids.
18. Keep a diary of the number of uses so that you know when the canister is empty.
19. Clean the pMDI once a week and as needed.

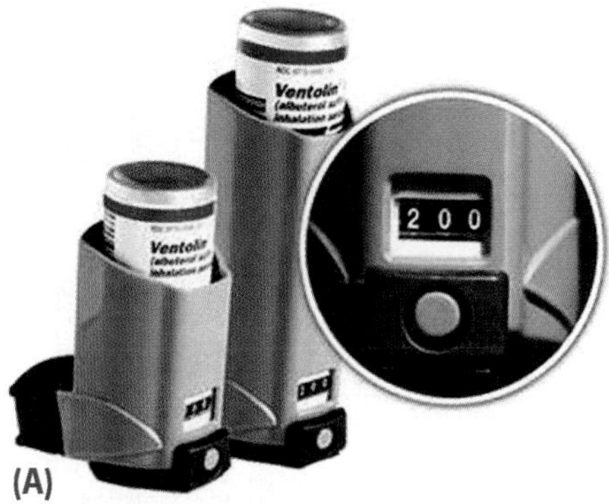

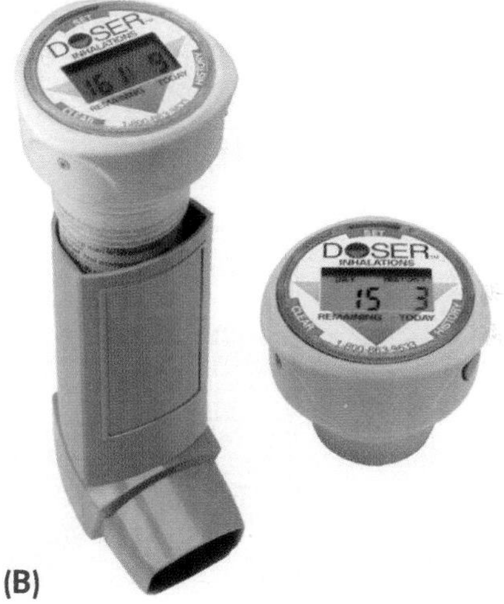

FIGURE 17–26 (**A**) Dose counter on a hydrofluoroalkane (HFA) pressurized metered dose inhaler (Ventolin HFA). (**B**) Doser.

devices can also be used that count down the number of puffs released from a pMDI (**Figure 17–26**).

The Autohaler is a flow-triggered pMDI designed to reduce the need for hand–breath coordination by firing in response to the patient's inspiratory effort (**Figure 17–27**). To use the Autohaler, the patient cocks a lever on top of the unit that spring loads the canister against a vane mechanism. When the patient's inspiratory flow exceeds 30 L/min, the vane moves, allowing the canister to be pressed into the actuator, firing the pMDI. In the United States this device is available only with the β-agonist pirbuterol. The flow required to actuate the device may be too great for some small children to generate, especially during acute exacerbations of disease.

Spacers and Valved Holding Chambers

Spacers and valved holding chambers (**Figure 17–28**) are accessory devices that reduce oropharyngeal deposition of drugs, ameliorate the bad taste of some medications, eliminate the cold Freon effect, and, in the case of valved holding chambers, reduce the need for hand–breath coordination. These devices reduce the pharyngeal dose of aerosol from the pMDI 10-fold to 15-fold. This

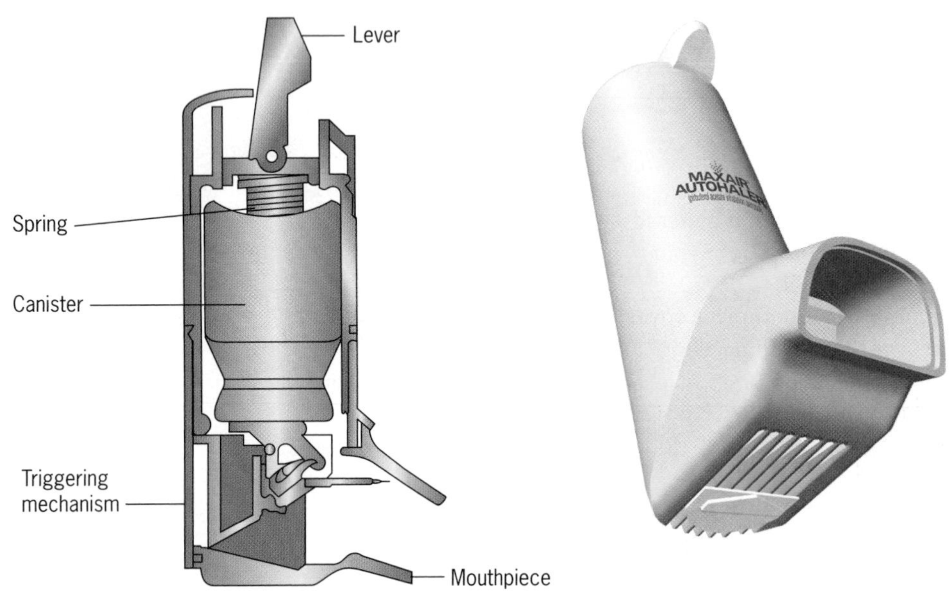

FIGURE 17–27 Breath-actuated metered dose inhaler.

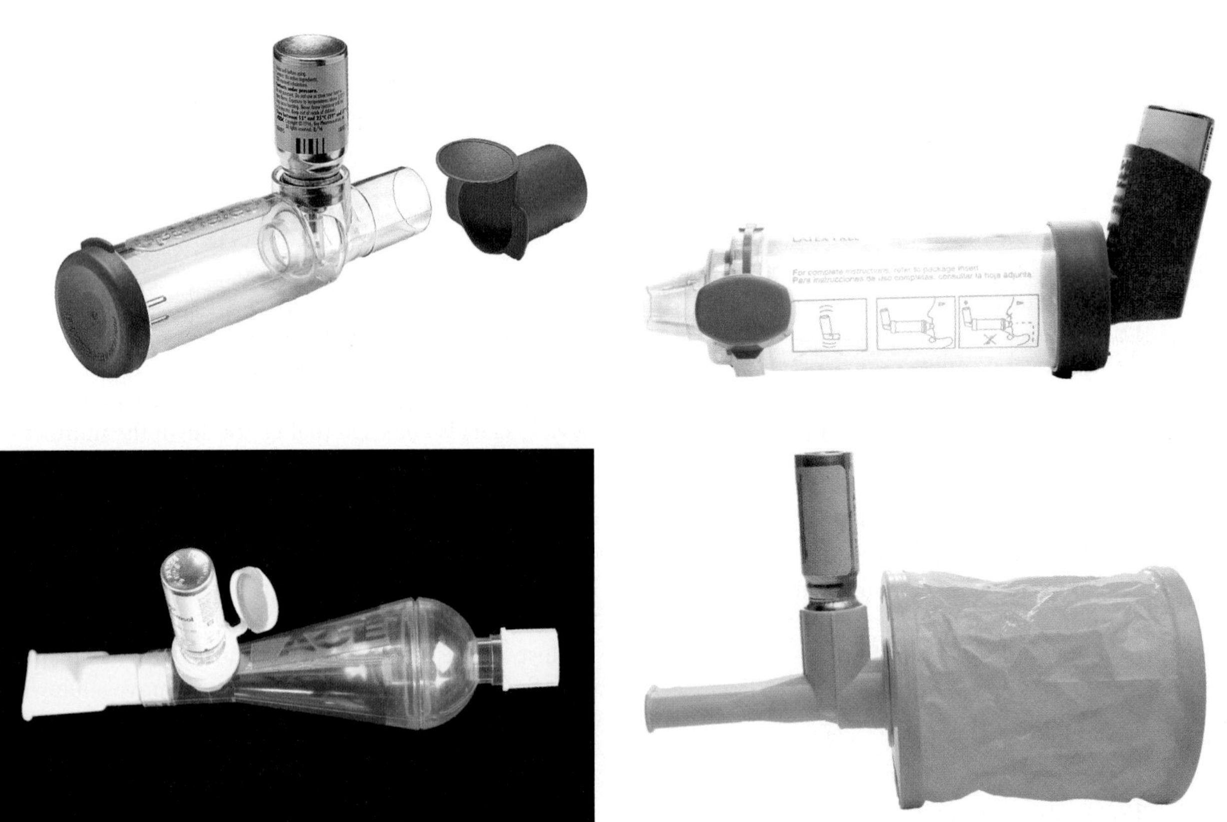

FIGURE 17–28 Spacers and valved holding chambers.

reduces the total body dose from swallowed medications, which is an important consideration with steroid administration. For the very young, the very old, or others unable to use the device with a mouthpiece, a face mask can be used (**Figure 17–29**).

A **spacer** is a simple open-ended tube or bag that, with sufficiently large device volume, provides space for the pMDI plume to expand by allowing the propellant to evaporate. To perform this function, a spacer must have an internal volume of more than 100 mL and provide a distance of 10 to 13 cm between the pMDI nozzle and the first wall or baffle. Smaller, inefficient spacers can reduce the respiratory dose by 60% and offer no protection against poor coordination of actuation and breathing

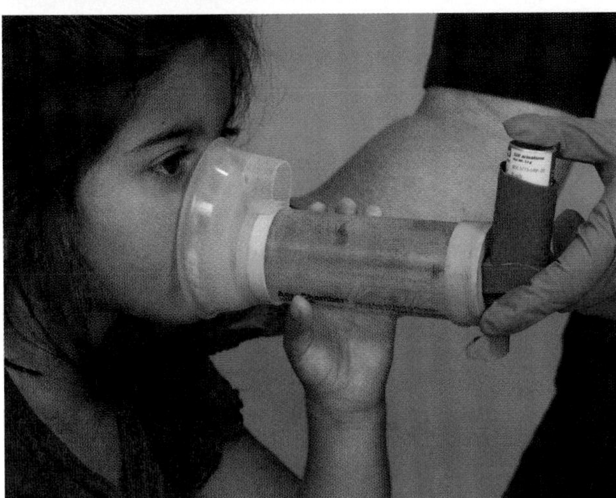

FIGURE 17–29 Valved holding chamber with face mask.

pattern. Spacers with internal volumes greater than 100 mL generally provide some protection against early firing of the pMDI, although exhalation immediately after the actuation clears most of the aerosol from the device, wasting the dose.

A **valved holding chamber** (usually 140 to 750 mL in volume) allows the plume from the pMDI to expand and incorporates a one-way valve that permits the aerosol to be drawn from the chamber during inhalation only, diverting the exhaled gas to the atmosphere and not disturbing remaining aerosol suspended in the chamber. Patients with small tidal volumes may empty the aerosol from the chamber with five to six breaths except when there is an exceptionally large dead space. A valved holding chamber (VHC) can also incorporate a mask for use with an infant, a child, or a patient unable to use a mouthpiece because of size, age, coordination, or mental status. With infants these masks must have minimal dead space and must be comfortable on the child's face, and the chamber must have a valve that opens or closes with the low inspiratory flow generated by the patient. **Box 17–5** describes the optimal technique for use of a valved holding chamber. The high oropharyngeal drug deposition with steroid pMDIs can increase the risk of oral yeast infections (thrush). Rinsing the mouth after steroid use can reduce this problem, but most pMDI steroid aerosol impaction occurs deeper in the pharynx, which is not easily rinsed. For this reason, steroid pMDIs should always be used in combination with a valved holding chamber.

Electrostatic charge acquired by the aerosol when generated, or present on the surface of the inhaler or add-on device, decreases aerosol delivery from VHCs.[106–122] Electrostatic charge may be particularly important with a delay in aerosol inhalation after actuation. VHCs made from conducting materials, such as stainless steel or aluminum, avoid this problem. Priming by firing 20 doses

BOX 17–5

Technique for Use of a Pressurized Metered Dose Inhaler with a Spacer or Valved Holding Chamber

1. Hold the pressurized metered dose inhaler (pMDI) in your hand to warm it.
2. Assemble the apparatus and check for foreign objects.
3. Remove the mouthpiece cover.
4. Shake the pMDI.
5. If the pMDI is new or has not been used recently, prime the device by shaking it and pressing the canister to deliver a dose into the room.
6. Repeat several times.
7. Hold the canister in a vertical position.
8. Breathe out normally.
9. Open your mouth and keep your tongue from obstructing the mouthpiece.
10. Place the mouthpiece into your mouth (or place the mask completely over your nose and mouth).
11. Breathe in slowly through your mouth and press the pMDI canister once at the beginning of inspiration.
12. If the device produces a "whistle," your inspiration is too rapid.
13. Allow 15 seconds between puffs.
14. Move the mouthpiece away from your mouth and hold your breath for 10 seconds (or as long as you comfortably can).
15. The technique is slightly different for a device with a collapsible bag:
    a. Open the bag to its full size.
    b. Remove the canister from the pMDI mouthpiece and insert it into the mouthpiece attached to the collapsible bag.
    c. Press the pMDI canister immediately before inhalation and inhale until the bag is completely collapsed (if you have difficulty emptying the bag, you can breathe in and out of the bag several times to evacuate the medication).
16. Rinse your mouth if using inhaled steroids.
17. Clean the holding chamber every two weeks and as needed.

into a new spacer coats the inner surface with surfactant and minimizes static charge, but this is not practical because it uses more than 10% of the doses in a new pMDI canister. Washing a nonconducting VHC with detergent is a commonly used method to reduce surface electrostatic charge, and detergent washing is now incorporated in most manufacturer instructions. Detergent washing greatly improves drug delivery and is easy for the patient to perform. After washing, the VHC should not be towel dried, which could impart electrostatic charge; instead, the device should be allowed to drip dry in ambient air. The Food and Drug Administration requires manufacturers of add-on devices to recommend that patients rinse them in clean water after washing in detergent, to avoid patient contact with detergent-coated surfaces, which could result in contact dermatitis. VHCs manufactured from transparent, charge-dissipative polymers, as an alternative to opaque conducting materials such as stainless steel or aluminum, have become available in recent years.

Accessory devices either use the manufacturer-designed boot that comes with the pMDI or incorporate a universal canister adapter to fire the pMDI canister. Different formulations of pMDI drugs operate at different pressures and have different-sized orifices in the boot designed by the manufacturer for use exclusively with that pMDI. The output characteristics of a pMDI change if an adapter with a different-sized orifice is used. For this reason, spacers or holding chambers with universal canister adapters should be avoided, and only those with a universal boot adapter should be used.

Particularly in young children, use of a VHC requires a face mask. When using a face mask, an adequate seal is necessary, and five to six breaths are taken through the chamber to deliver the full dose. Drug delivery is also influenced by mask dead space, VHC dead space, and the opening pressure of the inspiratory and expiratory valves. Drug delivery decreases when dead space increases, and drug delivery increases with smaller VHC volume and lower tidal volume.[123]

Dry Powder Inhalers

Dry powder inhalers (DPIs) create aerosols by drawing air through a dose of powdered medication. The powder contains micronized drug particles (less than 5 μm MMAD) with larger lactose or glucose particles (over 30 μm in diameter) or micronized drug particles bound into loose aggregates.[124] Micronized particles adhere strongly to each other and to most surfaces. Adding the larger particles of the carrier diminishes cohesive forces in the micronized drug powder so that separation into individual respirable particles (deaggregation) occurs more readily. Thus, the carrier particles aid the flow of the drug powder from the device. Carriers also act as fillers by adding bulk to the powder when the unit dose of a drug is very small. The drug particles usually are loosely bound to the carrier and are stripped from the carrier by the energy provided by the patient's inhalation (**Figure 17–30**). The release of respirable particles of the drug requires inspiration at relatively high flow (30 to 120 L/min).[125,126] A high inspiratory flow results in pharyngeal impaction of the larger carrier particles that make up the bulk of the aerosol. The oropharyngeal impaction of carrier particles gives the patient the sensation of having inhaled a dose.

Commercially available DPIs are either unit dose (the patient loads a single-dose capsule prior to each use) or multidose (the device contains a month's prescription) (**Figure 17–31**).[127] With unit-dose devices, it is important to instruct the patient that the capsules are not to be ingested; they should be administered only via inhalation, with the appropriate delivery device. Moreover, the capsules should be used only in the intended device and should not be administered in another device. For example, formoterol capsules should not be administered in the HandiHaler, and the powder should never be dumped from the capsule into a nebulizer for administration. Currently available DPIs are all passive systems, meaning that the patient must provide the energy to disperse the powder from the device. A primary advantage of DPIs is coordination of actuation with inspiration, because they are breath actuated. A primary disadvantage of unit-dose DPIs is the time needed to load a dose for each use. Another disadvantage of DPIs is that each operates differently from the others in loading and priming.[128]

The internal geometry of the DPI device influences the resistance offered to inspiration and the inspiratory flow required to deaggregate and aerosolize the medication. Devices with higher resistance require a higher inspiratory flow to produce a dose. Inhalation through high-resistance DPIs may improve drug delivery to the lower respiratory tract compared with pMDIs, provided the patient can reliably generate the required flow rate.[129] High-resistance devices have not been shown to improve either deposition or bronchodilation compared with low-resistance DPIs. DPIs with several components require correct assembly of the apparatus and priming of the device to ensure aerosolization of the dry powder. Some DPIs require periodic brushing to remove any residual powder that has accumulated in the device.

DPIs produce aerosols in which most of the drug particles are in the respirable range, with the distribution of particle sizes differing significantly among various DPIs. High ambient humidity causes the dry powder to clump, creating larger particles that are not as effectively aerosolized.[130] Air with a high moisture content is less efficient at deaggregating particles of dry powder than dry air, such that high ambient humidity increases the size of drug particles in the aerosol and may reduce drug delivery to the lungs. High ambient humidity also can result from exhalation into a DPI; from bringing a DPI into a warm indoor environment from the cold outdoors or a cold car, causing condensation to form inside the device; or from being using a DPI in a warm, humid environment. Newer DPIs contain individual doses that are better protected from humidity. Humidity also can accumulate if the DPI is stored with the cap off.

Because the energy from the patient's inspiratory flow disperses the drug powder, the magnitude and duration of the patient's inspiratory effort influences aerosol generation from a DPI.[131] Failure to perform inhalation at a sufficiently fast inspiratory flow reduces the dose of the drug emitted by the DPI and increases the distribution of particle sizes within the aerosol. Research on active DPI delivery devices is under way. These devices use either a small motor and impeller or compressed gas propulsion to disperse the powder. With active DPIs, aerosol production and airway deposition are less influenced by the patient's inspiratory flow than with DPIs that rely solely on patient effort for aerosol production.

Breath coordination is also important during use of a DPI. Exhalation into a DPI blows out the powder from the device and reduces drug delivery. Moreover, the humidity in the exhaled air reduces subsequent aerosol generation. For these reasons, patients must be instructed not to exhale into a DPI. Because DPIs are breath actuated, they reduce the problem of coordinating inspiration with actuation. Using a DPI (**Box 17–6**) differs in important respects from the technique used to inhale drugs from a pMDI. Although DPIs are easier to use than pMDIs, as many as 25% of patients may use DPIs improperly.[132] DPIs are critically dependent on inspiratory airflow to generate the aerosol; therefore, they should be used with caution, if at all, in very young or ill children, the weak, the elderly, and those with altered mental status. Patients may need repeated instruction before they can master the use of a DPI, and periodic assessment is necessary to ensure that patients continue to use optimum technique.

Aerosol Delivery During Mechanical Ventilation

Aerosolized drugs are often administered to mechanically ventilated patients (**CPG 17–3**).[133–143] The ventilator circuit is a closed system that is pressurized during operation, requiring the nebulizer or pMDI to be attached with connectors that maintain the integrity of the circuit during operation. DPI cannot be used in intubated mechanically ventilated patients. With mechanical ventilation the inspiratory flow pattern and respiratory rate are often different from those of spontaneous breathing,

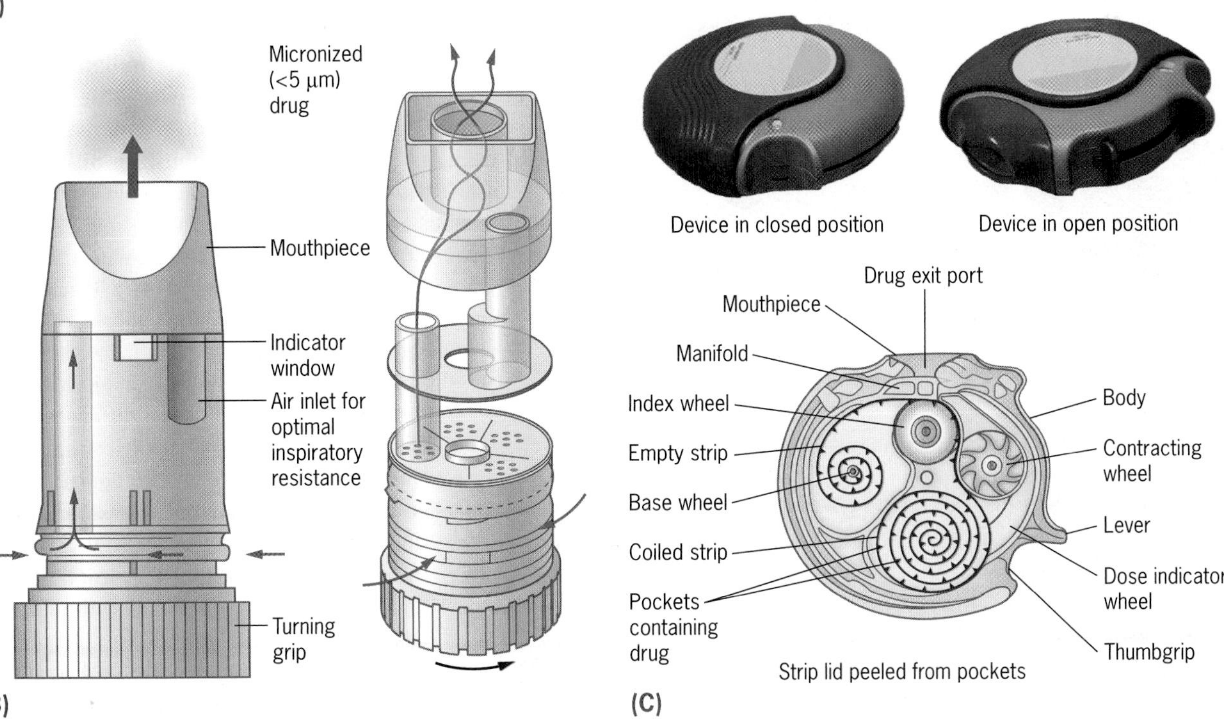

FIGURE 17–30 **(A)** Aerosolization of dry powder. **(B)** Component parts of Flexhaler. **(C)** Component parts of Diskus. **(A)** Modified from Dhand R, Fink JB. Dry powder inhalers. *Respir Care.* 1999;44:940–951. Reprinted with permission. **(B)** Modified from Crompton GK. Delivery Systems. In Kay AB. editor. *Allergy and Allergic Diseases.* London: Blackwell Science; 1997:1440–1450.

and this may influence aerosol delivery to the lower respiratory tract. **Box 17–7** and **Box 17–8** present the techniques used to deliver aerosolized bronchodilators during mechanical ventilation by nebulizer and pMDI, respectively. A number of factors affect aerosol delivery during mechanical ventilation (**Figure 17–32**).

(A) (B)

(C)

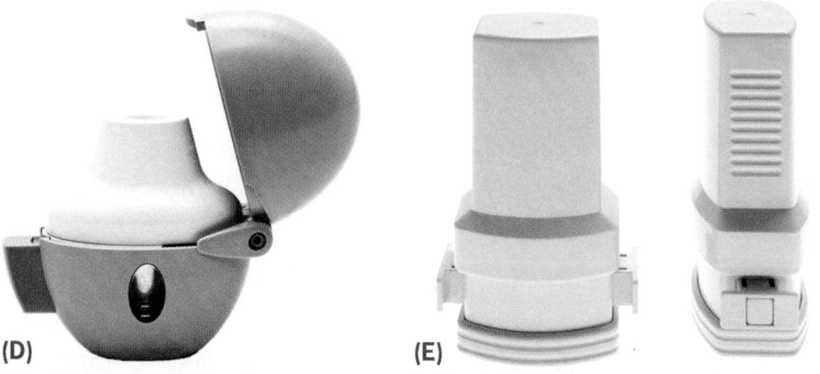

FIGURE 17–31 Multiple-dose dry powder inhalers: (**A**) Diskus, (**B**) Flexhaler, and (**C**) Diskhaler. Single-dose dry powder inhalers: (**D**) Handihaler and (**E**) Aerolizer.

Abrupt angles in the ventilator circuit, such as the 90-degree connector, often are used to connect the ventilator circuit Y piece to the endotracheal tube. This results in points of impaction and turbulence not found in the normal airway. Although the endotracheal tube is narrower than the trachea, its smooth interior surface may create a more laminar flow path than the structures of the glottis and larynx and may be less of a barrier to aerosol delivery than the ventilator circuit. Aerosol impaction in the endotracheal tube can reduce the efficiency of aerosol delivery in children, but the efficiency of aerosol delivery beyond the endotracheal tube does not vary among tube sizes that have internal diameters of 7 to 9 mm.

Ventilator circuits are designed to heat and humidify the inspired gas. Humidity can increase particle size and reduce deposition during mechanical ventilation. Humidification of inhaled gas reduces aerosol deposition by approximately 40%, probably because of an increase in particle loss in the ventilator circuit. Some experts have proposed bypassing the humidifier during aerosol administration. However, some nebulizers require as long as 30 minutes to complete aerosolization, and inhalation of dry gas for this length of time can damage the airway. In addition, disconnection of the ventilator circuit, which is required to bypass the humidifier, interrupts ventilation, and may increase the risk of ventilator-associated pneumonia.

Placement of a jet nebulizer 30 cm from the endotracheal tube is more efficient than placement between the inspiratory limb and the patient Y piece because the inspiratory ventilator tubing acts as a spacer for the aerosol to accumulate between breaths. Addition of a spacer between the nebulizer and the endotracheal tube modestly increases aerosol delivery. Operating the nebulizer only during inspiration is more efficient for aerosol delivery than continuous aerosol generation.

Because the pMDI cannot be used with the actuator designed by the manufacturer, a third-party actuator is required (**Figure 17–33**). The size, shape, and design of these actuators affect the amount of respirable drug available to the patient and may vary with different pMDI formulations. A pMDI with a spacer in the inspiratory limb of the ventilator circuit produces a fourfold to sixfold greater delivery of aerosol than pMDI actuation into a connector attached directly to the endotracheal tube or into an inline device that lacks a chamber. When an elbow adapter connected to the endotracheal tube is used, actuation of the pMDI out of synchrony with inspiratory airflow delivers very little aerosol to the lower respiratory tract. Unlike nebulizer use, dose

BOX 17-6

Technique for Use of Dry Powder Inhalers

Diskus

1. Open the device.
2. Slide the lever.
3. Breathe out normally; do not exhale into the device.
4. Place the mouthpiece into your mouth and close your lips tightly around the mouthpiece.
5. Keep device level while inhaling dose with a rapid and steady flow.
6. Remove the mouthpiece from your mouth and hold your breath for 10 seconds (or as long as you comfortably can).
7. When you exhale, be sure that you are not exhaling into the device.
8. Store the device in a cool, dry place.
9. Observe the counter for the number of doses remaining, and replace when appropriate.

Flexhaler

1. Twist and remove cap.
2. Hold inhaler upright (mouthpiece up).
3. In order to load the correct dose, the Flexhaler must be held in the upright position (mouthpiece up) whenever a dose of medication is being loaded. Do not hold the mouthpiece when you load the inhaler.
4. Twist the brown grip fully in one direction as far as it will go. Twist it fully back again in the other direction as far as it will go (it does not matter which way you turn it first). You will hear a click during one of the twisting movements.
5. Breathe out normally—do not exhale into the device. If you accidentally blow into your inhaler after loading a dose, simply follow the instructions for loading a new dose.
6. Place the mouthpiece into your mouth and close your lips tightly around the mouthpiece. Do not bite or chew on the mouthpiece.
7. Inhale dose with a rapid and forceful flow.
8. Remove the mouthpiece from your mouth and hold your breath for 10 seconds (or as long as you comfortably can).
9. When you exhale, be sure that you do not exhale into the device.
10. Replace the cover and twist to close. Store the device in a cool, dry place.
11. The dose indicator shows how many doses remain in the inhaler. Look at the middle of the window to find out how many doses are left in the inhaler. The dose indicator starts with either the number 60 or 120 when full, depending upon the strength of the product. The indicator is marked in intervals of 10 doses, alternating numbers and dashes. The dose indicator counts down each time a dose is loaded, not when a dose is inhaled. The grip will still twist and click even when the inhaler is empty, and you may still hear a sound if you shake it.

Aerolizer

1. Remove the mouthpiece cover.
2. Hold the base of the inhaler and twist the mouthpiece counterclockwise.
3. Remove capsule from foil blister immediately before use; do not store the capsule in the Aerolizer.
4. Place the capsule in the chamber in the base of the inhaler.
5. Hold the base of the inhaler and turn it clockwise to close.
6. Simultaneously press both buttons; this pierces the capsule.
7. Keep your head in an upright position.
8. Breathe out normally; do not exhale into the device.
9. Hold the device horizontal, with the buttons on the left and right.
10. Place the mouthpiece into your mouth and close your lips tightly around the mouthpiece.
11. Breathe in rapidly and as deeply as possible.
12. Remove the mouthpiece from your mouth and hold your breath for 10 seconds (or as long as you comfortably can).
13. When you exhale, be sure that you are not exhaling into the device.
14. Open the chamber and examine the capsule; if there is powder remaining, repeat the inhalation process.
15. After use, remove and discard the capsule.
16. Close the mouthpiece and replace the cover.
17. Store the device in a cool, dry place.

(continues)

Box 17–6 *(continued)*

HandiHaler

1. Immediately before using the HandiHaler, peel back the aluminum foil and remove a capsule; do not store capsules in the HandiHaler.
2. Open the dust cap by pulling it upward.
3. Open the mouthpiece.
4. Place the capsule in the center chamber; it does not matter which end is placed in the chamber.
5. Close the mouthpiece firmly until you hear a click; leave the dust cap open.
6. Hold the HandiHaler with the mouthpiece up.
7. Press the piercing button once and release; this makes holes in the capsule and allows the medication to be released when you breathe in.
8. Exhale normally; do not exhale into the device.
9. Place the mouthpiece into your mouth and close your lips tightly around the mouthpiece.
10. Keep your head in an upright position.
11. Breathe in slowly, at a rate sufficient to hear the capsule vibrate, until your lungs are full.
12. Remove the mouthpiece from your mouth and hold your breath for 10 seconds (or as long as you comfortably can).
13. When you exhale, be sure that you are not exhaling into the device.
14. To ensure you get the full dose, repeat the inhalation from the HandiHaler.
15. Open the mouthpiece, tip out the used capsule, and dispose of it.
16. Close the mouthpiece and dust cap for storage of the HandiHaler.

Diskhaler

1. Remove the mouthpiece cover.
2. Pull the tray out from the device.
3. Place the disk on the wheel (numbers up).
4. Rotate the disk by sliding the tray out and in.
5. Lift the back of the lid until fully upright so that the needle pierces both sides of the blister.
6. Breathe out normally; do not exhale into the device.
7. Place the mouthpiece into your mouth and close your lips tightly around the mouthpiece.
8. Keep the device level while inhaling the dose with a rapid and steady flow.
9. Remove the mouthpiece from your mouth and hold your breath for 10 seconds (or as long as you comfortably can).
10. When you exhale, be sure that you are not exhaling into the device.
11. Store the device in a cool, dry place.
12. Replace the disk when all of the blisters have been punctured.
13. Once every week, brush off any powder remaining within the device.

Do *not* clean DPIs.

delivery from a pMDI is relatively constant regardless of ventilator settings.[144]

Aerosol can be delivered during patient-triggered ventilation provided the patient is breathing in synchrony with the ventilator. Albuterol deposition has been reported to be more than 20% higher during simulated spontaneous breaths than with controlled breaths of equivalent tidal volume. For efficient aerosol delivery to the lower respiratory tract, the tidal volume of the ventilator-delivered breath must be larger than the volume of the ventilator tubing and endotracheal tube. Tidal volumes of 500 mL or greater in adults are associated with adequate aerosol delivery, but the larger tidal volumes can be detrimental to the lungs. During mechanical ventilation, delivery of a large tidal volume, use of an end-inspiratory pause, and use of a slow inspiratory flow have little effect on aerosol delivery and deposition.[145–147] Aerosol delivery by nebulizer is directly correlated with higher inspiratory time, because longer inspiratory times allow a higher proportion of the aerosol generated by the nebulizer to be inhaled with each breath. Because nebulizers generate aerosol over several minutes, longer inspiratory times have a cumulative effect in improving aerosol delivery. However, pMDIs produce aerosol only over a portion of a single inspiration, and the mechanism by which longer inspiratory times increase aerosol delivery is unclear. Aerosol particles that deposit in the ventilator tubing may be swept off the walls and entrained by longer periods of inspiratory flow. Helium–oxygen mixtures also affect aerosol deposition, and in vitro modeling has reported a 50% increase in deposition of albuterol from a pMDI.[148]

Nebulizers placed in-line in the ventilator circuit can become contaminated with bacteria, which are then carried as microaerosols directly to the lower respiratory tract. Such contamination has been reported even after a single use of a nebulizer.[149] The risk of VAP may be greater with a nebulizer than with a pMDI. The Centers

CLINICAL PRACTICE GUIDELINE 17–3

Selection of a Device for Administration of a Bronchodilator and Evaluation of the Response to Therapy in Mechanically Ventilated Patients

Indication

- Aerosol administration of a bronchodilator and evaluation of the response are indicated whenever bronchoconstriction or increased airway resistance is documented or suspected in mechanically ventilated patients.

Contraindications

- Some assessment maneuvers may be contraindicated for patients in extremis (e.g., a prolonged inspiratory pause for patients with high auto-PEEP).
- Certain medications may be contraindicated in some patients; the package insert should be consulted for these product-specific contraindications.

Hazards and Complications

- Specific assessment procedures may have inherent hazards or complications (e.g., inspiratory pause or expiratory pause).
- Inappropriate selection of a device or inappropriate use of a device and/or technique variables may result in underdosing.
- Device malfunction may result in reduced drug delivery and may compromise the integrity of the ventilator circuit.
- Complications may arise from specific pharmacologic agents. Higher doses of β-agonists delivered by a metered dose inhaler (MDI) or nebulizer may cause adverse effects secondary to systemic absorption of the drug or propellants. The potential for hypokalemia and atrial and ventricular dysrhythmias may exist with high doses in critically ill patients.
- Aerosol medications, propellants, or cold, dry gas that bypasses the natural upper respiratory tract may cause bronchospasm or irritation of the airway. Although the efficiency of aerosol delivery from an MDI can be increased by actuating the canister into a narrow-gauge catheter with the catheter positioned at the end of the endotracheal tube, a study in rabbits has shown that this technique produces necrotizing inflammation and mucosal ulceration, probably caused by the topical effect of the oleic acid used for its surfactant property and the chlorofluorocarbons (CFCs); therefore, such administration is not recommended. Further study of the practice is needed.
- The aerosol device or adapter used and the technique of operation may affect ventilator performance characteristics or alter the sensitivity of the alarm systems.
- Addition of gas to the ventilator circuit from a nebulizer may increase volumes, flows, and peak airway pressures, thereby altering the intended pattern of ventilation. Ventilator setting adjustments made to accommodate the additional gas flow during nebulization must be reset at the end of the treatment.
- Addition of gas from a nebulizer into the ventilator circuit may result in the patient becoming unable to trigger the ventilator during nebulization, leading to hypoventilation.

Modified from AARC clinical practice guideline: selection of a device for administration of a bronchodilator and evaluation of the response to therapy in mechanically ventilated patients. *Respir Care.* 1999;44:105–113. Reprinted with permission.

for Disease Control and Prevention (CDC) recommends that nebulizers be sterile at the start of nebulization, and that they be removed from the ventilator circuit after each use, disassembled, cleaned with sterile water, rinsed, and air dried. Care should be taken to store the nebulizer aseptically between uses. When the collapsible chamber spacer remains in the ventilator circuit between treatments, condensate collects inside it.[150,151] Care must be taken to prevent the condensate in the spacer from being washed into the patient's respiratory tract when the spacer is pulled open during use. When a noncollapsible spacer chamber is used to actuate a pMDI, it should be removed from the ventilator circuit between treatments. No studies have demonstrated contamination problems with administration of aerosol from a pMDI during mechanical ventilation.

Leaving a pMDI noncollapsible chamber device inline is not practical because of the increased compressible volume it adds to the circuit. Depending on the F_{IO_2} and the propellant gas volume, an inline pMDI actuation theoretically may result in a hypoxic gas mixture to an infant receiving a tidal volume less than 100 mL. It is

BOX 17–7

Technique for Aerosol Delivery by Nebulizer During Mechanical Ventilation

1. Fill the nebulizer with the drug solution to the optimum fill volume.
2. Place the nebulizer in the inspiratory line at least 30 cm from the patient's Y piece.
3. Ensure that the flow through the nebulizer is 6 to 8 L/min. Continuous gas flow from an external source also can be used to power the nebulizer.
4. The nebulizer may be operated continuously or only during inhalation. Some ventilators provide inspiratory gas flow to the nebulizer.
5. Adjust tidal volume as necessary.
6. Turn off the bias flow on the ventilator if possible and remove (or bypass) the heat and moisture exchanger if present.
7. Check the nebulizer for adequate aerosol generation throughout its use.
8. Disconnect the nebulizer when all the medication has been nebulized or when no more aerosol is being produced. Store the nebulizer under aseptic conditions.
9. Reconnect the ventilator circuit and reinstate the original ventilator settings.

BOX 17–8

Technique for Use of a Pressurized Metered Dose Inhaler During Mechanical Ventilation

1. Place a spacer situated in the inspiratory limb of the ventilator circuit. It is preferable to use a spacer that remains in the ventilator circuit so that the circuit need not be disconnected for each bronchodilator treatment.
2. Shake the pressurized metered dose inhaler (pMDI) canister vigorously.
3. Actuate the pMDI to synchronize with the precise onset of inspiration by the ventilator. Actuate the pMDI once only.
4. Repeat actuations at 30-second intervals until the total dose has been delivered.

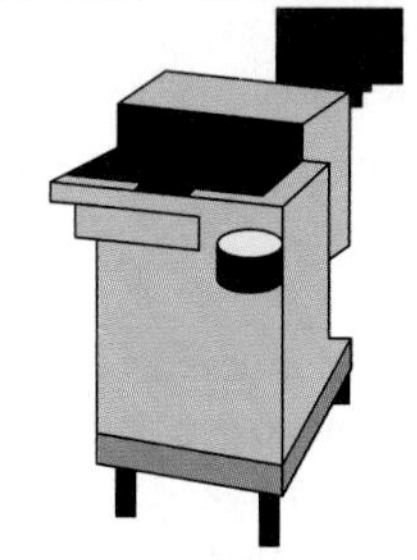
Ventilator Related
• Mode of ventilation
• Tidal volume
• Respiratory rate
• Duty cycle
• Inspiratory waveform
• Breath-triggering mechanism
Circuit Related
• Endotracheal tube
• Inhaled gas humidity
• Inhaled gas density

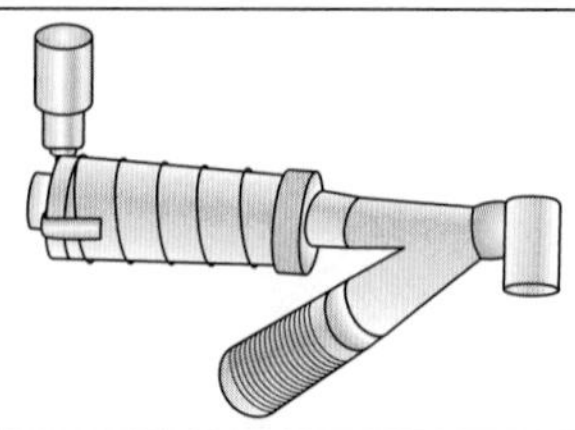

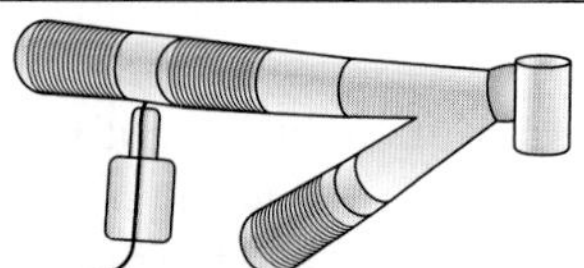

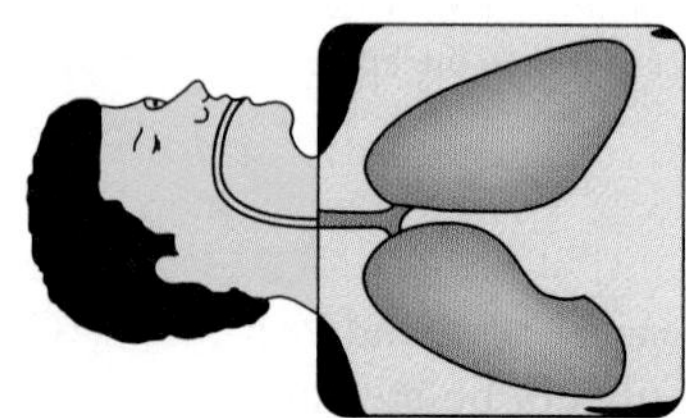

FIGURE 17–32 Summary of factors affecting delivery of aerosols during mechanical ventilation. Adapted from Dhand R, et al. Bronchodilator delivery by metered-dose inhaler in ventilator supported patients. *Eur Respir J.* 1996;9:585–595.

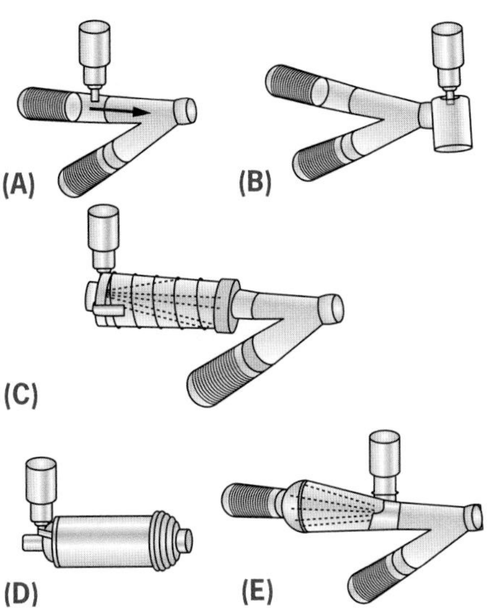

FIGURE 17–33 Devices to adapt a metered dose inhaler to a ventilator circuit. (**A**) Inline device. (**B**) Elbow device. (**C**) Collapsible chamber device. (**D**) Chamber device. (**E**) Chamber device in which aerosol is directed retrograde into the ventilator circuit. Modified from Dhand R, et al. Bronchodilator delivery by metered-dose inhaler in ventilator supported patients. *Eur Respir J.* 1996;9:585–595.

possible to deliver a pMDI aerosol medication to an intubated neonate, especially those medications available only in pMDI preparations. If a chamber adapter is used, the infant must be removed from the circuit, the chamber placed in-line, and the infant reattached to the circuit before the pMDI medication is administered. The large dead space volume created through placement of a spacer or chamber at the end of the endotracheal tube must also be considered during administration of pMDI medications to an infant.

> **RESPIRATORY RECAP**
>
> **Aerosol Delivery During Mechanical Ventilation**
>
> » Either a pMDI or nebulizer can be used.
>
> » Careful attention to technique is important.

Studies that have examined the dose response to bronchodilators in mechanically ventilated patients found effects with administration of 2.5 mg of albuterol via a standard nebulizer even under less than optimum conditions or with four actuations (400 μg) with a pMDI.[152–154] Although the efficiency is greater with a pMDI and spacer, the dose delivered with the nebulizer is greater because of the higher nominal dose placed into the nebulizer. In the routine clinical setting, higher doses of bronchodilators may be needed for patients with severe airway obstruction or if the technique of administration is not optimal. When the technique of administration is carefully executed, most mechanically ventilated patients in stable condition who have chronic obstructive pulmonary disease (COPD) achieve near-maximum bronchodilation after administration of four puffs of albuterol with a pMDI or 2.5 mg with a nebulizer. Dosing requirements for infants and small children during mechanical ventilation have not yet been established.

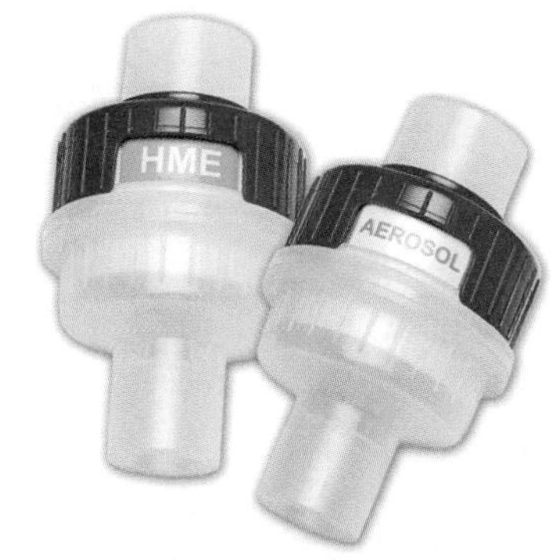

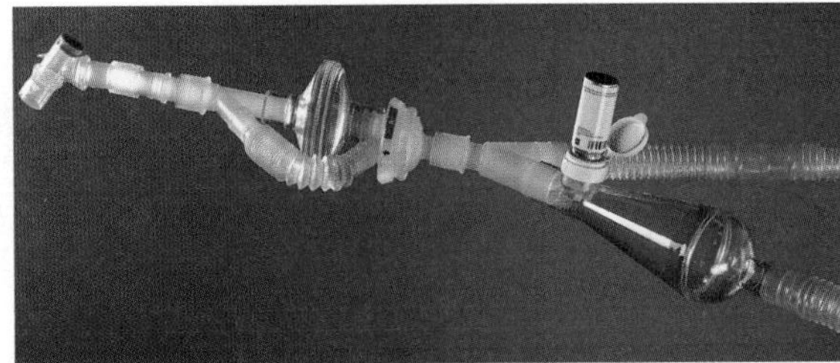

FIGURE 17–34 Devices that allow a heat and moisture exchanger to be bypassed during aerosol delivery.

With proper technique, nebulizers and pMDIs produce similar therapeutic effects in mechanically ventilated patients.[154] The use of pMDIs for routine bronchodilator therapy in ventilator-supported patients is preferred because of several problems associated with the use of nebulizers. The rate of aerosol production by nebulizers varies considerably, not only in nebulizers from different manufacturers but also in different batches of the same brand. The gas flow driving the nebulizer produces additional airflow in the ventilator circuit, requiring adjustment of tidal volume and inspiratory flow when the nebulizer is in use. When patients are unable to trigger the ventilator during assisted modes of mechanical ventilation (because of the additional nebulizer gas flow), hypoventilation can result.[155] Aerosol delivery by pMDI is easy to administer, involves less personnel time, provides a reliable dose of the drug, and is free of the risk of bacterial contamination. When pMDIs are used with a collapsible cylindric spacer, the ventilator circuit need not be disconnected with each treatment, thus reducing the risk of ventilator-associated pneumonia. If an HME is in-line, it must either be removed or a specially designed HME used that allows the HME to be bypassed during aerosol therapy (**Figure 17–34**).

Aerosol Delivery by Tracheostomy

Inhaled albuterol is occasionally used in spontaneously breathing patients with a tracheostomy tube.[156] A measurable amount of albuterol aerosol can be delivered through the tracheostomy tube during spontaneous

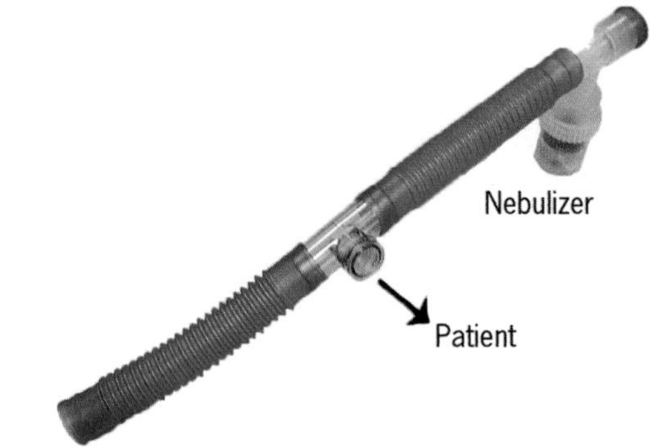

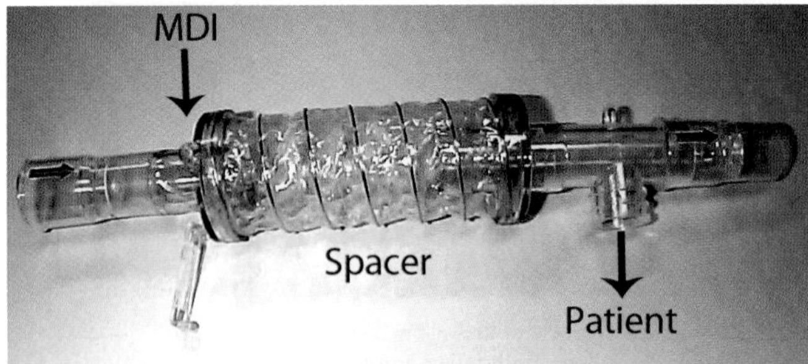

FIGURE 17–35 Equipment for aerosol delivery to tracheostomy.

breathing, whether a nebulizer or a pMDI with spacer is used. Delivery of albuterol aerosol into a high gas flow is inefficient for the nebulizer, and use of a T piece for albuterol delivery is more effective than use of a tracheostomy mask. The efficiency is greater for a pMDI with valved holding chamber than for a nebulizer, and the pMDI is most efficient when a valved T piece is used and the valve is placed proximal rather than distal to the spacer. **Figure 17–35** shows the proper equipment for aerosol delivery by nebulizer and pMDI for spontaneously breathing patients with a tracheostomy.

Selection of an Aerosol Delivery Device

Each type of aerosol delivery device has advantages and disadvantages (**Table 17–2**). The choice of device often is determined by patient preference or clinician bias. In some cases the choice of device is dictated by the drug to be delivered (e.g., antibiotics are available only for nebulizer delivery).[154] Whenever possible, patients should use only one type of aerosol delivery device. The technique for the use of each device is different, and repeated instruction is necessary to ensure that the patient uses the device appropriately. Using different devices can be confusing for patients and may reduce their compliance with therapy.

Each of the aerosol delivery devices can work equally well provided that patients can use them correctly. When selecting an aerosol delivery device, the following questions should be considered:[154]

- In what devices is the desired drug available?
- What device is the patient likely to be able to use properly, given the patient's age and the clinical setting?
- For which device and drug combination is reimbursement available?
- Which devices are the least costly?
- Can all types of inhaled asthma/COPD drugs that are prescribed for the patient be delivered with the same type of device? Using the same type of device for all inhaled drugs may facilitate patient teaching and decrease the chance of confusion among devices that require different inhalation techniques.
- Which devices are the most convenient for the patient, family (outpatient use), or medical staff (acute care setting) to use, given the time required for drug administration and device cleaning and the portability of the device?
- How durable is the device?
- Does the patient or clinician have any specific device preferences?

Proper patient education is critical. Respiratory therapists, physicians, and nurses caring for patients with respiratory diseases should be familiar with issues related to performance and with the correct use of aerosol delivery devices. If the selected delivery device should fail to provide satisfactory treatment, another option should be considered.

To improve compliance, aerosol therapy should be administered with some easily remembered activity of daily living. For twice-daily administration, medications can be kept with the toothbrush and inhaled just before teeth brushing. This also reduces aerosol corticosteroid deposition in the oropharynx. It is always best to avoid regular use of medication at school, because the inconvenience can significantly reduce compliance and may be an embarrassment to some children. However, rescue medication must be available at school or day care or the caretaker's home. It helps to prepare written guidelines for use of the medication, and the guidelines must be distributed to all places where the child stays, such as home, school, or the residences of both parents in cases of divorce or separation.

Lack of response to inhaled asthma medication can be related to a number of factors, including incorrect inhalation technique, inhalation from an empty canister, failure to take preventive medications as prescribed, a change in the patient's environment, or perhaps misdiagnosis. For example, children who have aspirated a foreign body or who have gastroesophageal reflux disease or psychogenic wheeze have a poor response to asthma therapy, and infants with tracheomalacia or bronchopulmonary dysplasia may even worsen after inhaling a bronchodilator aerosol because of increased dynamic airway collapse.

TABLE 17-2 Advantages and Disadvantages of Various Aerosol Delivery Devices

Device	Advantages	Disadvantages
Jet nebulizer	Patient coordination is not required Effective with tidal breathing High doses can be given Dose modification is possible Can be used with supplemental O_2 Can deliver combination therapies if drugs are compatible Some are breath actuated	Expense Device is not portable Pressurized gas source is required Lengthy treatment time Contamination is possible Device preparation required Not all medications are in solution form Performance variability
Mesh nebulizer	Patient coordination is not required Effective with tidal breathing High doses can be given Dose modification is possible Some are breath actuated Small dead volume Quiet Faster delivery than jet nebulizer Less drug is lost during exhalation Battery operated Portable and compact Dose reproducibility is high	Expense Contamination is possible Device preparation is required Not all medications are in solution form
Ultrasonic nebulizer	Patient coordination is not required High doses are possible Small dead volume Quiet Faster delivery than jet nebulizer Less drug is lost during exhalation Some are breath actuated	Expense Need for electrical power Contamination is possible Prone to malfunction Possible drug degradation Does not nebulize suspensions well Device preparation is required Potential for airway irritation exists
Pressurized metered dose inhaler (pMDI)	Portable and compact No drug preparation is required Dose reproducibility is high Device is difficult to contaminate Treatment time is short Some are breath actuated Some have a dose counter	Patient coordination is essential Patient actuation is required Large pharyngeal deposition occurs High doses are difficult to deliver Not all medications can be used with this device Many of these devices use CFC propellants
Metered dose inhaler with holding chamber	Less patient coordination is required Less pharyngeal deposition occurs	More complex for some patients More expensive than an pMDI alone Device is less portable than an pMDI
Dry powder inhaler	Less patient coordination is required Propellant is not required Breath activated Small and portable Short treatment time	Requires moderate to high inspiratory flow Some units are single dose High pharyngeal deposition is possible Not all medications are available High doses are difficult to deliver

CFC, chlorofluorocarbon.

Adapted from AARC consensus statement: aerosols and delivery devices. *Respir Care.* 2000;45:589–595; and Dolovich MB, Ahrens RC, Hess DR, et al. Device selection and outcomes of aerosol therapy: evidence-based guidelines. *Chest.* 2005;127:335–371.

KEY POINTS

- The upper airway is an efficient humidifier.
- The primary goal of humidity therapy is to maintain normal physiologic conditions by providing heat and humidity in the inspired gas.
- Humidifiers can provide active or passive humidification.
- Active humidifiers may be heated or unheated.
- Heated circuits can be used to maintain heat and humidity in gas delivery.
- The humidity delivery device should be assessed for condensate near the patient.
- Use of HMEs is limited by their effectiveness and their dead space.
- Bland aerosol therapy is used for therapeutic and diagnostic purposes.

- The MMAD of aerosols for medical purposes should be 1 to 5 μm.
- Devices used to deliver therapeutic aerosols include jet nebulizers, ultrasonic nebulizers, metered dose inhalers, metered dose inhalers with a spacer or holding chamber, and dry powder inhalers.
- Nebulizers and pMDIs can be used effectively in patients receiving mechanical ventilation and in spontaneously breathing patients with a tracheostomy.
- Either a nebulizer, pMDI, pMDI with a spacer or valved holding chamber, or DPI can be used effectively if the patient uses good technique.

REFERENCES

1. Shelley MP, Lloyd GM, Park GR. A review of the mechanisms and the methods of humidification of inspired gas. *Intensive Care Med.* 1988;14:1–9.
2. Irlbeck D. Normal mechanisms of heat and moisture exchange in the respiratory tract. *Respir Care Clin North Am.* 1998;4: 189–198.
3. Branson RD. The effects of inadequate humidity. *Respir Care Clin North Am.* 1998;4:199–214.
4. Rankin N. What is optimum humidity? *Respir Care Clin North Am.* 1998;4:321–328.
5. Williams RD. Effects of excessive humidity. *Respir Care Clin North Am.* 1998;4:215–228.
6. Primiano FP Jr, Montague FW Jr, Saidel GM. Measurement system for water vapor and temperature dynamics. *J Appl Physiol.* 1984;56:1679–1685.
7. Shelly MP. The humidification and filtration functions of the airways. *Respir Care Clin North Am.* 2006;12:139–148.
8. Rathgeber J. Devices used to humidify respired gases. *Respir Care Clin North Am.* 2006;12:165–182.
9. Sottiaux TM. Consequences of under- and over-humidification. *Respir Care Clin North Am.* 2006;12:233–252.
10. Chatburn RL, Primiano FP. A rational basis for humidity therapy. *Respir Care.* 1987;32:249–253.
11. Tarnow-Mordi WO, Reid R, Griffiths P, et al. Low inspired gas humidity and respiratory complications in very low birth weight infants. *J Pediatr.* 1988;114:438.
12. Anderson S, Herbring BG, Widman B. Accidental profound hypothermia. *Br J Anaesth.* 1970;42:653.
13. Greenspan JS, Wolfson MR, Shaffer TH. Airway responsiveness to low inspired gas temperature in preterm neonates. *J Pediatr.* 1991;118:443–445.
14. Hill TV, Sorbello JG. Humidity outputs of large reservoir nebulizers. *Respir Care.* 1987;32:225–260.
15. Peterson BD. Heated humidifiers. *Respir Care Clin North Am.* 1998;4:243–260.
16. Miyao H, Hirokawa T, Miyasaka K, et al. Relative humidity, not absolute humidity, is of great importance when using a humidifier with a heating wire. *Crit Care Med.* 1992;20:674–679.
17. Miyao H, Miyasaka K, Hirokawa T, et al. Consideration of the international standard for airway humidification using simulated secretions in an artificial airway. *Respir Care.* 1996;41:43–49.
18. Wilkes AR. Heat and moisture exchangers: structure and function. *Respir Care Clin North Am.* 1998;4:261–279.
19. Ploysongsang Y, Branson D, Rashkin MC, et al. Effect of flow rate and duration of use on the pressure drop across six artificial noses. *Respir Care.* 1989;343:902–907.
20. Züchner K. Humidification: measurement and requirements. *Respir Care Clin North Am.* 2006;12:149–163.
21. American National Standards Institute. *American National Standards for Nebulizers and Humidifiers.* Washington, DC: American National Standards Institute; 1979.
22. Emergency Care Research Institute. Heated humidifiers. *Health Devices.* 1987;16:223–250.
23. Darin J, Broadwell J, MacDonnell R. An evaluation of water vapor output from four brands of unheated prefilled humidifiers. *Respir Care.* 1981;27:41.
24. Seigel D, Romo B. Extended use of prefilled humidifier reservoirs and the likelihood of contamination. *Respir Care.* 1990; 35:806–810.
25. Lellouche F, Taillé S, Maggiore SM, et al. Influence of ambient and ventilator output temperatures on performance of heated-wire humidifiers. *Am J Respir Crit Care Med.* 2004;170: 1073–1079.
26. Carter BG, Whittington N, Hochmann M, Osborne A. The effect of inlet gas temperatures on heated humidifier performance. *J Aerosol Med.* 2002;15:7–13.
27. Nishida T, Nishimura M, Fujino Y, Mashimo T. Performance of heated humidifiers with a heated wire according to ventilatory settings. *J Aerosol Med.* 2001;14(1):43–51.
28. Lellouche F, Qader S, Taille S, et al. Under-humidification and over-humidification during moderate induced hypothermia with usual devices. *Intensive Care Med.* 2006;32:1014–1021.
29. Iotti GA, Olivei MC, Palo A, et al. Unfavorable mechanical effects of heat and moisture exchangers in ventilated patients. *Intensive Care Med.* 1997;23:399–405.
30. LeBourdelles G, Mier L, Fiquet B, et al. Comparison of the effects of heat and moisture exchangers and heated humidifiers on ventilation and gas exchange during weaning trials from mechanical ventilation. *Chest.* 1996;110:1294–1298.
31. Hedley RM, Alt-Graham J. A comparison of the filtration properties of heat and moisture exchangers. *Anaesthesia.* 1992; 47:414–420.
32. Branson RD, Davis K. Evaluation of 21 passive humidifiers according to the ISO 9360 standard: moisture output, dead space, and flow resistance. *Respir Care.* 1996;41:736–743.
33. Branson RD, Davis K Jr, Brown R, et al. Comparison of three humidification techniques during mechanical ventilation: patient selection, cost, and infection considerations. *Respir Care.* 1996;41:809–816.
34. Hess D. Prolonged use of heat and moisture exchangers: why do we keep changing things? *Crit Care Med.* 2000;28:1667–1668.
35. Hess DR, Kallstrom TJ, Mottram CD, et al. Care of the ventilator circuit and its relation to ventilator-associated pneumonia. *Respir Care.* 2003;48:869–879.
36. Lellouche F, Taillé S, Lefrançois F, et al. Humidification performance of 48 passive airway humidifiers: comparison with manufacturer data. *Chest.* 2009;135:276–286.
37. Lacherade JC, Auburtin M, Cerf C, et al. Impact of humidification systems on ventilator-associated pneumonia: a randomized multicenter trial. *Am J Respir Crit Care Med.* 2005;172: 1276–1282.
38. Ricard JD, Boyer A, Dreyfuss D. The effect of humidification on the incidence of ventilator-associated pneumonia. *Respir Care Clin North Am.* 2006;12:263–273.
39. Siempos II, Vardakas KZ, Kopterides P, Falagas ME. Impact of passive humidification on clinical outcomes of mechanically ventilated patients: a meta-analysis of randomized controlled trials. *Crit Care Med.* 2007;35:2843–2851.
40. Prin S, Chergui K, Augarde R, et al. Ability and safety of a heated humidifier to control hypercapnic acidosis in severe ARDS. *Intensive Care Med.* 2002;28:1756–1760.
41. Hinkson CR, Benson MS, Stephens LM, Deem S. The effects of apparatus dead space on $PaCO_2$ in patients receiving lung-protective ventilation. *Respir Care.* 2006;51:1140–1144.
42. Campbell RS, Davis K Jr, Johannigman JA, Branson RD. The effects of passive humidifier dead space on respiratory variables

in paralyzed and spontaneously breathing patients. *Respir Care.* 2000;45:306–312.

43. Pelosi P, Solca M, Ravagnan I, et al. Effects of heat and moisture exchangers on minute ventilation, ventilatory drive, and work of breathing during pressure-support ventilation in acute ventilatory failure. *Crit Care Med.* 1996;24:1184–1188.
44. Rau JL. The inhalation of drugs: advantages and problems. *Respir Care.* 2005;50:367–382.
45. AARC consensus statement: aerosols and delivery devices. *Respir Care.* 2000;45:589–596.
46. Hess DR. Aerosol delivery devices in the treatment of asthma. *Respir Care.* 2008;53:699–725.
47. Hess DR. Metered-dose inhalers and dry powder inhalers in aerosol therapy. *Respir Care.* 2005;50:1376–1383.
48. Rau JL. Design principles of liquid nebulization devices currently in use. *Respir Care.* 2002;47:1257–1278.
49. Hess DR. Nebulizers: principles and performance. *Respir Care.* 2000;45:609–622.
50. Hess D, Fisher D, Williams P, et al. Medication nebulizer performance: effects of diluent volume, nebulizer flow, and nebulizer brand. *Chest.* 1996;110:498–505.
51. Kim IK, Saville AL, Sikes KL, Corcoran TE. Heliox-driven albuterol nebulization for asthma exacerbations: an overview. *Respir Care.* 2006;51:613–618.
52. Hess DR, Acosta FL, Ritz RH, et al. The effect of heliox on nebulizer function using a beta-agonist bronchodilator. *Chest.* 1999;115:184–189.
53. Malone RA, Hollie MC, Glynn-Barnhart A, et al. Optimal duration of nebulized albuterol therapy. *Chest.* 1993;104:1114–1118.
54. Standaert TA, Morlin GL, Williams-Warren J, et al. Effects of repetitive use and cleaning techniques of disposable jet nebulizers on aerosol generation. *Chest.* 1998;114:577–586.
55. Harris KW, Smaldone GC. Facial and ocular deposition of nebulized budesonide: effects of face mask design. *Chest.* 2008;133:482–488.
56. Smaldone GC, Sangwan S, Shah A. Facemask design, facial deposition, and delivered dose of nebulized aerosols. *J Aerosol Med.* 2007;20(suppl 1):S66–S75.
57. Lowenthal D, Kanan M. Face masks versus mouthpieces for aerosol treatment of asthmatic children. *Pediatr Pulmonol.* 1992;14:192–196.
58. Bisquerra RA, Botz GH, Nates JL. Ipratropium-bromide-induced acute anisocoria in the intensive care setting due to ill-fitting face masks. *Respir Care.* 2005;50:1662–1664.
59. Brodie T, Adalat S. Unilateral fixed dilated pupil in a well child. *Arch Dis Child.* 2006;91:961.
60. Mulpeter KM, Walsh JB, O'Connor M, et al. Ocular hazards of nebulized bronchodilators. *Postgrad Med J.* 1992;68:132–133.
61. Reuser T, Flanagan DW, Borland C, Bannerjee DK. Acute angle closure glaucoma occurring after nebulized bronchodilator treatment with ipratropium bromide and salbutamol. *J R Soc Med.* 1992;85:499–500.
62. Rho DS. Acute angle-closure glaucoma after albuterol nebulizer treatment. *Am J Ophthalmol.* 2000;130:123–124.
63. Singh J, O'Brien C, Wright M. Nebulized bronchodilator therapy causes acute angle closure glaucoma in predisposed individuals. *Respir Med.* 1993;87:559–561.
64. Rubin BK. Bye-bye, blow-by. *Respir Care.* 2007;52:981.
65. Lin HL, Restrepo RD, Gardenhire DS, Rau JL. Effect of face mask design on inhaled mass of nebulized albuterol, using a pediatric breathing model. *Respir Care.* 2007;52:1021–1026.
66. Harrison R. Reproductive risk assessment with occupational exposure to ribavirin aerosol. *Pediatr Infect Dis J.* 1990;9(suppl):S102–S105.
67. Kacmarek RM, Kratohvil J. Evaluation of a double-enclosure double-vacuum unit scavenging system for ribavirin administration. *Respir Care.* 1992;37:37–45.
68. Adderly RJ. Safety of ribavirin with mechanical ventilation. *Pediatr Infect Dis J.* 1990;9(suppl):S112–S114.
69. Peters SG. Continuous bronchodilator therapy. *Chest.* 2007;131:286–289.
70. Camargo CA Jr, Spooner CH, Rowe BH. Continuous versus intermittent beta-agonists in the treatment of acute asthma. *Cochrane Database Syst Rev.* 2003;CD001115.
71. Chatburn RL, Kallstrom TJ, Bajaksouzian S. A comparison of acetic acid with a quaternary ammonium compound for disinfection of hand-held nebulizers. *Respir Care.* 1988;88:179–187.
72. Dhand R. Nebulizers that use a vibrating mesh or plate with multiple apertures to generate aerosol. *Respir Care.* 2002;47:1406–1416.
73. Lass JS, Sant A, Knoch M. New advances in aerosolised drug delivery: vibrating membrane nebuliser technology. *Expert Opin Drug Deliv.* 2006;3:693–702.
74. Knoch M, Keller M. The customised electronic nebuliser: a new category of liquid aerosol drug delivery systems. *Expert Opin Drug Deliv.* 2005;2:377–390.
75. Ghazanfari T, Elhissi AM, Ding Z, Taylor KM. The influence of fluid physicochemical properties on vibrating-mesh nebulization. *Int J Pharmacol.* 2007;339:103–111.
76. Zhang G, David A, Wiedmann TS. Performance of the vibrating membrane aerosol generation device: Aeroneb Micropump Nebulizer. *J Aerosol Med.* 2007;20:408–416.
77. Kassner F, Hodder R, Bateman ED. A review of ipratropium bromide/fenoterol hydrobromide (Berodual) delivered via Respimat Soft Mist Inhaler in patients with asthma and chronic obstructive pulmonary disease. *Drugs.* 2004;64:1671–1682.
78. Geller DE. New liquid aerosol generation devices: systems that force pressurized liquids through nozzles. *Respir Care.* 2002;47:1392–1404.
79. Dalby R, Spallek M, Voshaar T. A review of the development of Respimat Soft Mist Inhaler. *Int J Pharmacol.* 2004;283:1–9.
80. Hochrainer D, Holz H, Kreher C, et al. Comparison of the aerosol velocity and spray duration of Respimat Soft Mist inhaler and pressurized metered dose inhalers. *J Aerosol Med.* 2005;18:273–282.
81. Kunkel G, Magnussen H, Bergmann K, et al. Respimat (a new soft mist inhaler) delivering fenoterol plus ipratropium bromide provides equivalent bronchodilation at half the cumulative dose compared with a conventional metered dose inhaler in asthmatic patients. *Respiration.* 2000;67:306–314.
82. Newman SP. Use of gamma scintigraphy to evaluate the performance of new inhalers. *J Aerosol Med.* 1999;12(suppl 1):S25–S31.
83. Newman SP, Brown J, Steed KP, et al. Lung deposition of fenoterol and flunisolide delivered using a novel device for inhaled medicines: comparison of Respimat with conventional metered-dose inhalers with and without spacer devices. *Chest.* 1998;113:957–963.
84. Newman SP, Steed KP, Reader SJ, et al. Efficient delivery to the lungs of flunisolide aerosol from a new portable hand-held multidose nebulizer. *J Pharm Sci.* 1996;85:960–964.
85. Newman SP, Steed KP, Reader SJ, et al. An in vitro study to assess facial and ocular deposition from Respimat Soft Mist inhaler. *J Aerosol Med.* 2007;20:7–12.
86. Schurmann W, Schmidtmann S, Moroni P, et al. Respimat Soft Mist inhaler versus hydrofluoroalkane metered dose inhaler: patient preference and satisfaction. *Treat Respir Med.* 2005;4:53–61.
87. Phillips GD, Millard FJL. The therapeutic use of ultrasonic nebulizers in acute asthma. *Respir Med.* 1994;88:387–389.
88. Nakanishi AK, Lamb BM, Foster C, et al. Ultrasonic nebulization of albuterol is no more effective than jet nebulization for the treatment of acute asthma in children. *Chest.* 1997;97:1505–1508.
89. Thomas SH, O'Doherty MJ, Page CJ, et al. Delivery of ultrasonic nebulized aerosols to a lung model during mechanical ventilation. *Am Rev Respir Dis.* 1993;148:872–877.

90. Fink JB. Metered dose inhalers, dry powder inhalers, and transitions. *Respir Care.* 2000;45:623–625.
91. Leach CL. The CFC to HFA transition and its impact on pulmonary drug development. *Respir Care.* 2005;50:1201–1208.
92. Hess D, Daugherty A, Simmons M. The volume of gas emitted from five metered dose inhalers at three levels of fullness. *Respir Care.* 1992;37:444–447.
93. Hendeles L, Colice GL, Meyer RJ. Withdrawal of albuterol inhalers containing chlorofluorocarbon propellants. *N Engl J Med.* 2007;356:1344–1351.
94. Cheng YS, Fu CS, Yazzie D, Zhou Y. Respiratory deposition patterns of salbutamol pMDI with CFC and HFA-134a formulations in a human airway replica. *J Aerosol Med.* 2001;14:255–266.
95. Barry PW, O'Callaghan C. New formulation metered dose inhaler increases breath alcohol levels. *Respir Med.* 1999;93:167–168.
96. Levin PD, Levin D, Avidan A. Medical aerosol propellant interference with infrared anaesthetic gas monitors. *Br J Anaesth.* 2004;92:865–869.
97. Bamber MG. Difficulties with CFC-free salbutamol inhaler. *Lancet.* 1996;348:1737.
98. Guidry GG, Brown WD, Stogner SW, et al. Incorrect use of metered dose inhalers by medical personnel. *Chest.* 1992;1010:31–33.
99. Johnson DH, Robart P. Inhaler technique of outpatients in the home. *Respir Care.* 2000;45:1182–1187.
100. Schultz RK. Drug delivery characteristics of metered-dose inhalers. *J Allergy Clin Immunol.* 1995;96:284–287.
101. Cain WT, Oppenheimer JJ. The misconception of using floating patterns as an accurate means of measuring the contents of metered dose inhaler devices. *Ann Allergy Asthma Immunol.* 2001;87:417–419.
102. Wolf BL, Cochran KR. Floating patterns of metered dose inhalers. *J Asthma.* 1997;34:433–436.
103. Brock TP, Wessell AM, Williams DM, Donohue JF. Accuracy of float testing for metered-dose inhaler canisters. *J Am Pharm Assoc (Wash).* 2002;42:582–586.
104. Wildhaber JH, Devadason SG, Eber E, et al. Effect of electrostatic charge, flow, delay and multiple actuations on the in vitro delivery of salbutamol from different small volume spacers for infants. *Thorax.* 1996;51:985–988.
105. O'Callaghan C, Lynch J, Cant M, Robertson C. Improvement in sodium cromoglycate delivery from a spacer device by use of an antistatic lining, immediate inhalation, and avoiding multiple actuations of drug. *Thorax.* 1993;48:603–606.
106. Barry PW, O'Callaghan C. The effect of delay, multiple actuations and spacer static charge on the in vitro delivery of budesonide from the Nebuhaler. *Br J Clin Pharmacol.* 1995;40:76–78.
107. Clark DJ, Lipworth BJ. Effect of multiple actuations, delayed inhalation and antistatic treatment on the lung bioavailability of salbutamol via a spacer device. *Thorax.* 1996;51:981–984.
108. Barry PW, Robertson CF, O'Callaghan C. Optimum use of a spacer device. *Arch Dis Child.* 1993;69:693–694.
109. Mitchell JP, Coppolo DP, Nagel MW. Electrostatics and inhaled medications: influence on delivery via pressurized metered-dose inhalers and add-on devices. *Respir Care.* 2007;52:283–300.
110. Wildhaber JH, Devadason SG, Hayden MJ, et al. Electrostatic charge on a plastic spacer device influences the delivery of salbutamol. *Eur Respir J.* 1996;9:1943–1946.
111. Wildhaber JH, Waterer GW, Hall GL, Summers QA. Reducing electrostatic charge on spacer devices and bronchodilator response. *Br J Clin Pharmacol.* 2000;50:277–280.
112. Pierart F, Wildhaber JH, Vrancken I, et al. Washing plastic spacers in household detergent reduces electrostatic charge and greatly improves delivery. *Eur Respir J.* 1999; 13:673–678.
113. Dubus JC, Guillot C, Badier M. Electrostatic charge on spacer devices and salbutamol response in young children. *Int J Pharm.* 2003;261:159–164.
114. Chuffart AA, Sennhauser FH, Wildhaber JH. Factors affecting the efficiency of aerosol therapy with pressurised metered-dose inhalers through plastic spacers. *Swiss Med Wkly.* 2001;131:14–18.
115. Bisgaard H, Anhoj J, Klug B, Berg E. A non-electrostatic spacer for aerosol delivery. *Arch Dis Child.* 1995;73:226–230.
116. Bisgaard H. A metal aerosol holding chamber devised for young children with asthma. *Eur Respir J.* 1995;8:856–860.
117. Kenyon CJ, Thorsson L, Borgstrom L, Newman SP. The effects of static charge in spacer devices on glucocorticosteroid aerosol deposition in asthmatic patients. *Eur Respir J.* 1998;11:606–610.
118. Janssens HM, Devadason SG, Hop WC, et al. Variability of aerosol delivery via spacer devices in young asthmatic children in daily life. *Eur Respir J.* 1999;13:787–791.
119. Rau JL, Coppolo DP, Nagel MW, et al. The importance of nonelectrostatic materials in holding chambers for delivery of hydrofluoroalkane albuterol. *Respir Care.* 2006;51:503–510.
120. Coppolo DP, Mitchell JP, Nagel MW. Levalbuterol aerosol delivery with a nonelectrostatic versus a nonconducting valved holding chamber. *Respir Care.* 2006;51:511–514.
121. Everard ML, Clark AR, Milner AD. Drug delivery from holding chambers with attached face mask. *Arch Dis Child.* 1992;67:580–585.
122. Dhand R, Fink JB. Dry powder inhalers. *Respir Care.* 1999;44:940–951.
123. Engel T, Heinig JH, Madsen F, et al. Peak inspiratory flow rate and inspiratory vital capacity of patients with asthma measured with and without a new dry powder inhaler device (Turbuhaler). *Eur Respir J.* 1990;3:1037–1041.
124. Pederson S, Hansen OR, Fuglsang G. Influence of inspiratory flow rate upon the effect of a Turbuhaler. *Arch Dis Child.* 1990;65:308–310.
125. Atkins PJ. Dry powder inhalers: an overview. *Respir Care.* 2005;50:1304–1312.
126. Rau JL. Practical problems with aerosol therapy in COPD. *Respir Care.* 2006;51:158–172.
127. Svartengren K, Lindestad PA, Svartengren M, et al. Added external resistance reduces oropharyngeal deposition and increases lung deposition of aerosol particles in asthmatics. *Am J Respir Crit Care Med.* 1995;152:32–37.
128. Rajkumari NJ, Byron PR, Dalby RN. Testing of dry powder aerosol formulations in different environmental conditions. *Int J Pharmacol.* 1995;113:123–130.
129. Timsina MP, Martin GP, Van der Kolk H, et al. The effect of inhalation flow on the performance of a dry powder inhalation system. *Int J Pharmacol.* 1992;81:199–203.
130. Kesten S, Elias M, Cartier A, et al. Patient handling of a multidose dry powder inhalation device for albuterol. *Chest.* 1994;105:1077–1081.
131. Dhand R. Aerosol delivery during mechanical ventilation: from basic techniques to new devices. *J Aerosol Med Pulm Drug Deliv.* 2008;21:45–60.
132. Dhand R, Guntur VP. How best to deliver aerosol medications to mechanically ventilated patients. *Clin Chest Med.* 2008;29:277–296.
133. Dhand R. Inhalation therapy in invasive and noninvasive mechanical ventilation. *Curr Opin Crit Care.* 2007;13:27–38.
134. Dhand R, Mercier E. Effective inhaled drug administration to mechanically ventilated patients. *Expert Opin Drug Deliv.* 2007;4:47–61.
135. Dhand R. Inhalation therapy with metered-dose inhalers and dry powder inhalers in mechanically ventilated patients. *Respir Care.* 2005;50:1331–1335.
136. Dhand R. New frontiers in aerosol delivery during mechanical ventilation. *Respir Care.* 2004;49:666–677.
137. Dhand R. Basic techniques for aerosol delivery during mechanical ventilation. *Respir Care.* 2004;49:611–622.

138. Fink JB, Dhand R. Bronchodilator therapy in mechanically ventilated patients. *Respir Care*. 1999;44:53–69.
139. Dhand R, Tobin MJ. Bronchodilator delivery with metered dose inhalers in mechanically ventilated patients. *Eur Respir J*. 1996; 9:585–595.
140. Dhand R, Juran A, Tobin MJ. Bronchodilator delivery by metered dose inhaler in ventilator-supported patients. *Am J Respir Crit Care Med*. 1995;151:1827–1833.
141. Dhand R. Special problems in aerosol delivery: artificial airways. *Respir Care*. 2000;45:636–645.
142. Hess DR, Dillman C, Kacmarek RM. In vitro evaluation of aerosol bronchodilator delivery during mechanical ventilation: pressure-control vs. volume control ventilation. *Intensive Care Med*. 2003;29:1145–1150.
143. Mouloudi E, Katsanoulas K, Anastasaki M, et al. Bronchodilator delivery by metered dose inhaler in mechanically ventilated COPD patients: influence of tidal volume. *Intensive Care Med*. 1999;25:1215–1221.
144. Mouloudi E, Katsanoulas K, Anastasaki M, et al. Bronchodilator delivery by metered dose inhaler in mechanically ventilated COPD patients: influence of end-inspiratory pause. *Eur Respir J*. 1998;12:165–169.
145. Mouloudi E, Prinianakis G, Kondili E, et al. Effect of inspiratory flow rate on β-agonist-induced bronchodilation in mechanically ventilated COPD patients. *Intensive Care Med*. 2001;27:42–46.
146. Good M, Fink JB, Dhand R, et al. Improvement in aerosol delivery with helium-oxygen mixtures during mechanical ventilation. *Am J Respir Crit Care Med*. 2001;163:109–114.
147. Craven DE, Lichtenberg DA, Goularte TA, et al. Contaminated medication nebulizers in mechanical ventilator circuits: a source of bacterial aerosols. *Am J Med*. 1984;77:834–838.
148. Waugh JB, Waugh JB. Water accumulation in metered dose inhaler spacers under normal mechanical ventilation conditions. *Heart Lung*. 2000;29:424–428.
149. Lin HL, Fink JB, Zhou Y, Cheng YS. Influence of moisture accumulation in inline spacer on delivery of aerosol using metered-dose inhaler during mechanical ventilation. *Respir Care*. 2009;54: 1336–1341.
150. Thomas SHL, O'Doherty MJ, Fidler HM, et al. Pulmonary deposition of a nebulized aerosol during mechanical ventilation. *Thorax*. 1993;48:154–159.
151. Dhand R, Duarte AG, Jubran A, et al. Dose response to bronchodilator delivered by metered dose inhaler in ventilator-supported patients. *Am J Respir Crit Care Med*. 1996;154:388–393.
152. Dolovich MB, Ahrens RC, Hess DR, et al. Device selection and outcomes of aerosol therapy: evidence-based guidelines. *Chest*. 2005;127:335–371.
153. Beaty CD, Ritz RH, Benson MS. Continuous in-line nebulizers complicate pressure support ventilation. *Chest*. 1989;96: 1360–1363.
154. Piccuito CM, Hess DR. Albuterol delivery via tracheostomy tube. *Respir Care*. 2005;50:1071–1076.

CHAPTER 18

Sputum Collection, Airway Clearance, and Lung Expansion Therapy

Dean R. Hess

OUTLINE

Normal Mechanisms of Mucociliary Transport
Sputum Collection
Airway Clearance
Lung Expansion Therapy

OBJECTIVES

1. Describe the mechanism of normal mucus transport in the lungs.
2. Compare the following methods of sputum collection: cough, induced sputum, tracheal aspiration, bronchoscopy, mini-bronchoalveolar lavage, transtracheal aspiration.
3. Demonstrate the techniques of nasotracheal suctioning, mechanical insufflation–exsufflation, postural drainage, manually assisted coughing, active cycle of breathing, autogenic drainage, incentive spirometry, intermittent positive pressure breathing, positive expiratory pressure, oscillatory positive expiratory pressure, and high-frequency techniques.
4. List indications, contraindications, hazards, and precautions for nasotracheal suctioning, mechanical insufflation–exsufflation, postural drainage, manually assisted coughing, active cycle of breathing, autogenic drainage, incentive spirometry, intermittent positive pressure breathing, positive expiratory pressure, oscillatory positive expiratory pressure, and high-frequency techniques.
5. Compare the advantages and disadvantages of various secretion clearance techniques.
6. Compare techniques of lung inflation therapy.

KEY TERMS

active cycle of breathing
autogenic drainage
chest physiotherapy (CPT)
forced expiratory technique (FET)
high-frequency chest wall compression (HFCWC)
high-frequency chest wall oscillation (HFCWO)
huff coughing
incentive spirometry (IS)
intermittent positive pressure breathing (IPPB)
intrapulmonary percussive ventilation (IPV)
mechanical insufflation–exsufflation
mini-bronchoalveolar lavage (mini-BAL)
nasotracheal suctioning
percussion therapy
positive expiratory pressure (PEP)
postural drainage (PD)
sputum induction
vibration therapy

INTRODUCTION

Many acute and chronic respiratory diseases are associated with retained airway secretions due to increased mucus production, impaired mucociliary transport, or a weak cough. In normal lungs, mucociliary activity, breathing, and coughing are the primary mechanisms used to remove secretions. With disease, changes in volume and character of secretions, dyskinesia of the cilia, and instability of the airway reduce the ability to clear secretions from the airway. Difficulty with secretion clearance commonly occurs at the end of life.[1] A variety of breathing maneuvers and mechanical devices have been used to assist patients in mobilizing secretions from the lower respiratory tract. This chapter describes these maneuvers and devices.

Normal Mechanisms of Mucociliary Transport

Secretions from the submucosal glands and surface secretory cells cover the ciliated epithelium of the airway (**Figure 18–1**). The relatively thin and watery sol layer, through which the cilia normally beat, arises from serous cell secretions. The thicker, superficial gel layer is formed from the more viscous secretions contributed by mucous cells and surface goblet cells, possibly enriched by components from the sol layer as water evaporates. This gel layer traps and holds dust, pollens, contaminants, and microorganisms. In the central airways, the majority of the secretory capacity is attributed to submucosal glands rather than surface secretory cells.

The cilia beat in a coordinated wavelike motion through the sol layer, with the tips of the cilia extending to the gel layer, propelling it toward the pharynx during the forward power stroke. This action is followed by a return recovery stroke in which the cilia return to their starting position, closer to the cell surface and at a slower speed.[1–3] The normal respiratory tract produces about 100 mL of mucus per day, some of which is absorbed as the secretions converge on the trachea, the remainder being expelled from the respiratory tract and swallowed. This serves as a first-line defense and is protective of the lower respiratory tract. With airway mucus hypersecretion, the amount of mucus produced is abnormal, which is pathologic and no longer protective. In the case of mucus hypersecretion, there is submucosal gland hypertrophy, goblet cell hyperplasia, and increased mucin synthesis. There also is plasma exudation, decreased mucociliary transport, mucostasis, and mucous plugs (**Figure 18–2**).

Mucociliary transport is dependent on the rheologic properties of mucus.[3,4] The interaction of mucus and airflow can alter these properties. Mucous gel properties are primarily dependent on the concentration and molecular characteristics of the mucous glycoproteins (mucins). Deoxyribonucleic acid (DNA) and actin fibers resulting from infection and inflammation can contribute additional cross-linking to the mucous gel. The

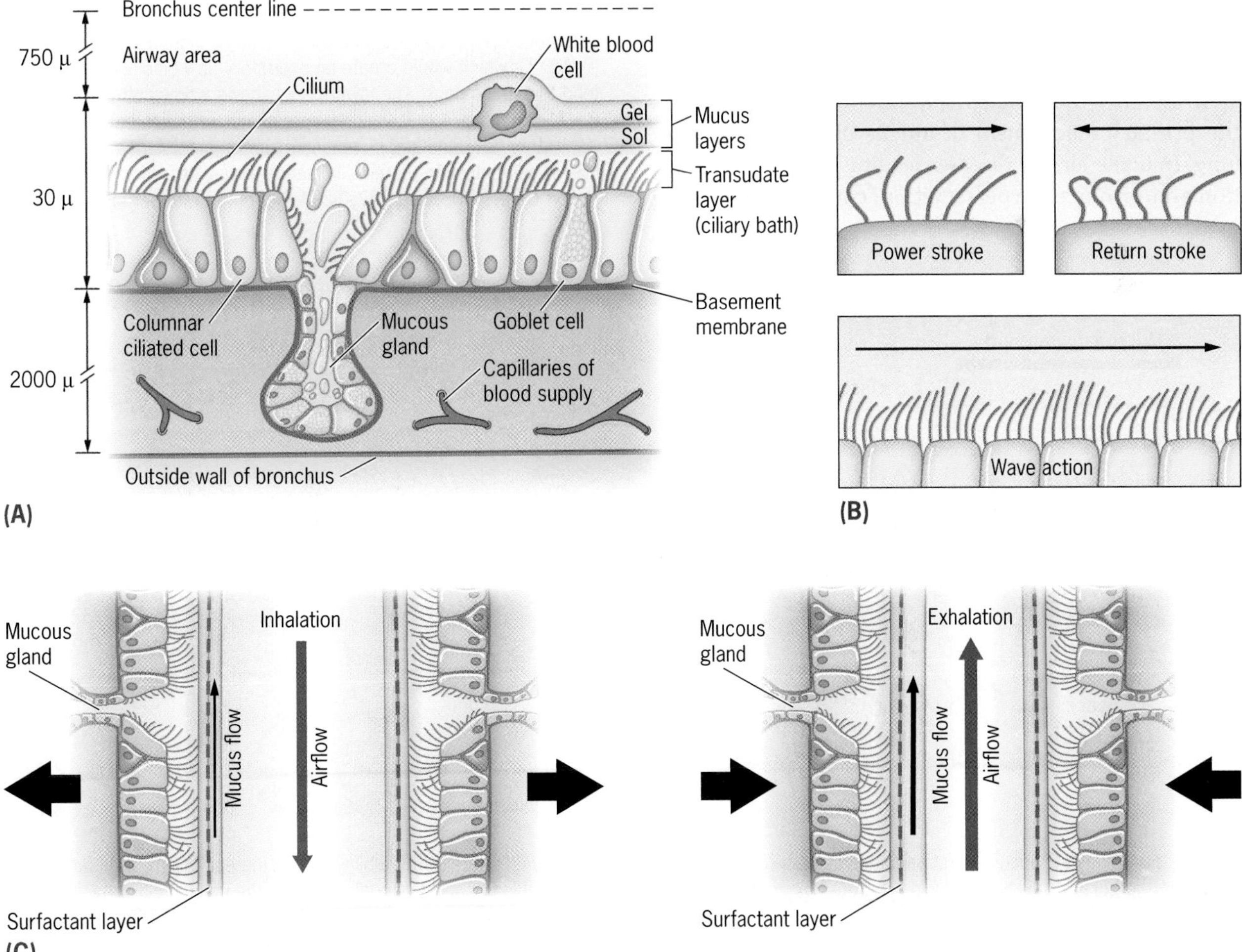

FIGURE 18–1 (**A**) Drawing of the surface of a typical ciliated epithelium. (**B**) Drawing of cilia at each phase of beat cycle. (**C**) Cephalad airflow bias. With normal mucociliary function, greater energy is applied to the mucous layer during expiration than during inspiration because of airway narrowing during expiration. (**C**) From Fink JB. Forced expiratory technique, directed cough, and autogenic drainage. *Respir Care.* 2007;52:1210–1223. Reprinted with permission.

purulent sputum from adult patients with cystic fibrosis (CF) has higher elasticity and viscosity than nonpurulent sputum from normal subjects.[5]

Cough and other high-airflow maneuvers reduce the cross-linking of mucus when airflow linear velocities are high enough (3 L/s in the trachea) to cause wave formation in the mucous layer.[6] Reduced mucus viscosity during the cough maneuver may improve sputum clearance. Mucus acts as a low-viscosity fluid during the short time of the rapidly changing, turbulent airflow associated with effective cough but resumes its high-viscosity character after cessation of the cough and does not flow backward under the influence of gravity. Airflows associated with tidal breathing have no effect on mucus viscoelasticity.

Cephalad airflow bias is responsible for the movement of mucus in airways during normal ventilation.[7,8] Airway diameters normally increase on inspiration and narrow on expiration. The narrowing of airways on exhalation increases the velocity and shearing forces in the airway, creating a cephalad airflow bias with tidal breathing. This bias is amplified during coughing, when increased transmural pressure causes the airways to fold and constrict, increasing airflow velocity even further. During mechanical ventilation, a peak expiratory flow greater than peak inspiratory flow favors mucus transport toward the airway opening (**Figure 18–3**).[8]

In healthy individuals the mucociliary escalator is the primary mechanism of mucus clearance from the lung. In acute airway diseases leading to ciliary dysfunction and/or mucus hypersecretion, cough is the primary mechanism for mucus clearance from the central airways, and cephalad airflow contributes increasingly to peripheral airway clearance. In chronic airway diseases involving mucus hypersecretion, these latter mechanisms become the major mechanisms responsible for keeping the airways patent. Gravity is not a primary mechanism for normal mucociliary transport because the viscosity of

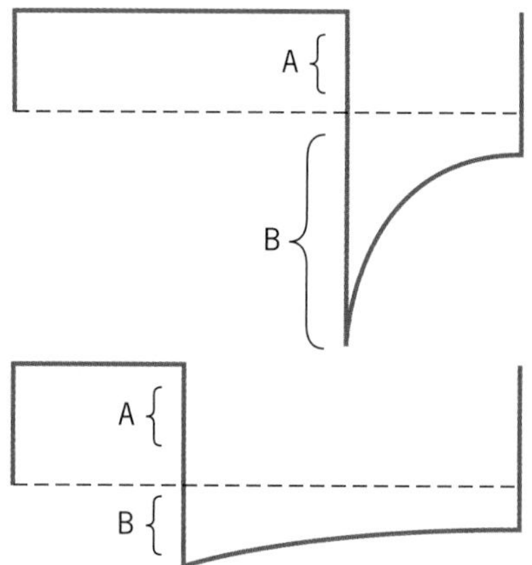

FIGURE 18–3 The upper panel displays an example of a flow pattern that gives a positive value for the expiratory–inspiratory flow difference (i.e., B – A > 0) and the expiratory–inspiratory flow ratio (B/A > 1), which would create an expiratory flow bias and therefore tend to expel mucus. The lower panel shows a flow pattern in which B – A < 0 and B/A < 1, which favors mucus retention because of inspiratory flow bias and increased expiratory resistance. From Volpe MS, et al. Ventilation patterns influence airway secretion movement. *Respir Care.* 2008;53:1287–1294. Reprinted with permission.

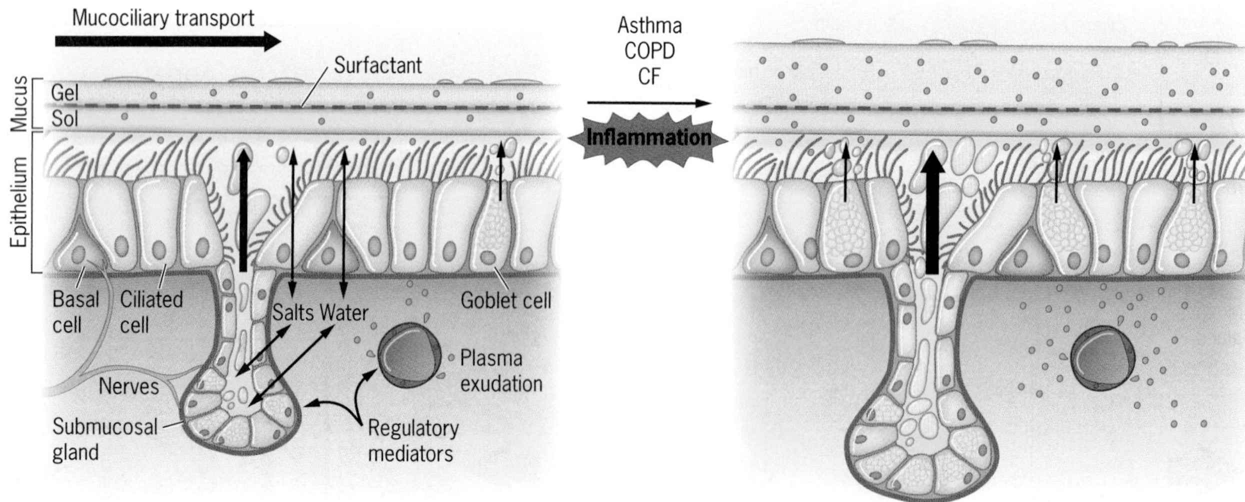

FIGURE 18–2 Airway mucus secretion and hypersecretion. (**Left**) In healthy airways, mucus forms a bilayer over the epithelium, with surfactant separating the gel and sol layers. Mucins secreted by goblet cells and submucosal glands confer viscoelasticity on the mucus, which facilitates mucociliary clearance of inhaled particles and irritants. Mucus hydration is regulated by salt (and hence water) flux across the epithelium. The glands also secrete water. Plasma proteins exuded from the tracheobronchial microvasculature bathe the submucosa and contribute to the formation of mucus. These processes are under the control of nerves and regulatory mediators. (**Right**) Airway inflammation (in asthma, chronic obstructive pulmonary disease [COPD], and possibly cystic fibrosis [CF]) induces changes associated with a mucus hypersecretory phenotype, including increased plasma exudation (more predominant in asthma than COPD or CF), goblet cell hyperplasia via differentiation from basal cells and associated increased mucus synthesis and secretion, and submucosal gland hypertrophy (with associated increased mucus production), leading to increased luminal mucus (and airway obstruction). Adapted from Rogers DF. Physiology of airway mucus secretion and pathophysiology of hypersecretion. *Respir Care.* 2007;52(9):1134–1149.

the normal mucous blanket is sufficient to resist flow of mucus into gravity-dependent terminal bronchioles.

Cough is one of the most common respiratory symptoms for which patients seek medical attention.[9] During a normal cough, the expiratory airflow rises to a maximum along with narrowing of the intrathoracic airways. The narrowing of the airways is a product of high airflows and pressure differentials across the lung. Airflow velocity varies inversely with the cross-sectional area of the airways, creating high linear velocities, increased turbulence, high shearing forces within the airway, and high kinetic energy. These forces shear secretions and debris from the airway walls, propelling them toward the central and upper airway, where they are expectorated or swallowed. A rapid series of coughs improves airway clearance. A number of complications are associated with excessive cough (**Table 18–1**).[10] In chronic obstructive pulmonary disease (COPD), narrowing airways may close prematurely, trapping gas, reducing expiratory flow rates, and limiting the effectiveness of the cough. There is an important balance between compression and collapse of airways; with collapse of the airway, clearance is obviously inhibited.

Sputum Collection

A sputum sample can be used as a diagnostic test for pulmonary infection or cancer. A sputum culture is a test to detect and identify bacteria or fungi that are infecting the lungs. A sputum sample is placed into a sterile container and then sent to the microbiology laboratory for Gram stain, culture, and sensitivity. If there is no growth of bacteria or fungi, the culture is negative. If pathogenic organisms grow, the culture is positive and the type of bacteria or fungus is identified. Additional tests are done to determine which antibiotics are most effective in treating the infection. This is called *susceptibility* or *sensitivity testing.* Bacteria usually need 2 to 3 days to grow, fungus often takes a week or longer to grow, and tuberculosis may take 6 weeks to grow. Any bacteria or fungi that grow will be identified under a microscope or by chemical tests. Sensitivity testing to determine the best antibiotic to use against the organism often takes 1 to 2 additional days.

> **RESPIRATORY RECAP**
>
> **Collection of Sputum for Diagnosis**
>
> » Cough
> » Induced sputum
> » Tracheal aspiration
> » Bronchoscopy
> » Mini-bronchoalveolar lavage
> » Transtracheal aspiration

The sputum sample is usually collected by coughing, most often first thing in the morning. The patient should not use mouthwash before collecting a sputum sample because it may contain antibacterial agents. Other factors that can affect the results of sputum culture include recent use of antibiotics, contamination of the sputum sample, an inadequate sputum sample, and waiting too long to deliver the sample to the laboratory.

Sputum cytology can be done when lung cancer is suspected or to detect certain noncancerous lung conditions. However, it is not used as a screening test for people at risk for developing lung cancer, such as smokers.

Induced Sputum

Aerosols of bland solutions, such as hypertonic saline, are used to stimulate cough and sputum production. Such therapy has been used for diagnostic **sputum induction.**[11] Hypertonic saline (e.g., 3% sodium chloride) is commonly used to induce sputum. Hypertonic saline on the mucosa moves water via osmosis from the airway into the secretions. This action causes a bronchorrhea, diluting the secretions and increasing their bulk to ease expectoration. The delivery of hypertonic saline by ultrasonic nebulizer is used to induce sputum for the diagnoses of *Pneumocystis carinii*, tuberculosis (acid-fast bacilli), *Legionella* species, and Mycobacteria atypical infections. The procedure involves the patient breathing hypertonic saline until about 5 mL of sputum is produced. It is important to instruct the patient to expectorate sputum from the lower respiratory tract; expectoration of saliva is not helpful. It is important for the respiratory therapist to observe appropriate infection control procedures during the procedure. Sputum induction is often repeated over 3 days. Induced sputum contains a higher proportion of viable cells than spontaneously produced sputum.[11] Sputum induction is safe and well tolerated for patients with asthma and COPD.[12]

Tracheal Aspirate

When secretions in the airway cannot be effectively expelled with a cough, mechanical aspiration may be required. Tracheal aspiration for sputum collection uses a Lukens trap. This is a plastic collection unit designed for specimens collected from the lungs during suction (**Figure 18–4**). Patients with artificial airways almost

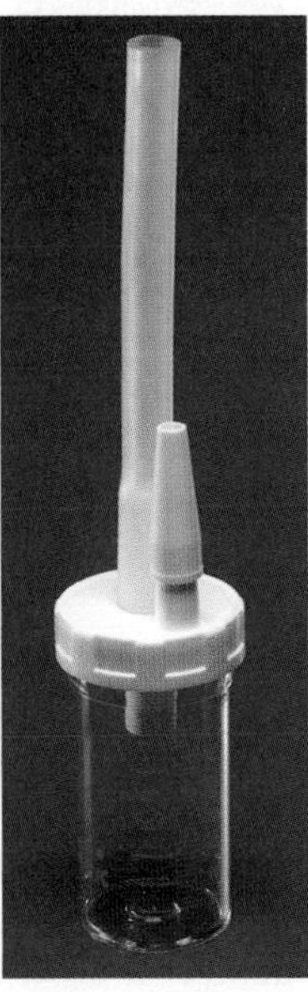

FIGURE 18–4 Lukens trap for sputum collection during tracheal suctioning.

TABLE 18–1 Complications of Excessive Cough

Cardiovascular	Arterial hypotension Bradyarrhythmias and tachyarrhythmias Dislodgement/malfunctioning of intravascular catheters Loss of consciousness Rupture of subconjunctival, nasal, and anal veins, and massive intraocular suprachoroidal hemorrhage during pars plana vitrectomy
Constitutional symptoms	Excessive sweating, anorexia, exhaustion
Gastrointestinal	Gastroesophageal reflux events Gastric hemorrhage following percutaneous endoscopic gastrostomy Hepatic cyst rupture Herniations (e.g., inguinal, through abdominal wall, small bowel through laparoscopic trocar site) Malfunction of gastrostomy button Mallory-Weiss tear Splenic rupture
Genitourinary	Inversion of bladder through urethra Urinary incontinence
Musculoskeletal	From asymptomatic elevations of serum creatine phosphokinase to rupture of rectus abdominus muscles Diaphragmatic rupture Rib fractures Sternal wound dehiscence
Neurologic	Acute cervical radiculopathy Cerebral air embolism Cerebral spinal fluid rhinorrhea Cervical epidural hematoma associated with oral anticoagulation Cough syncope Dizziness Headache Malfunctioning ventriculoatrial shunts Seizures Stroke due to vertebral artery dissection
Ophthalmologic	Spontaneous compressive orbital emphysema of rhinogenic origin
Psychosocial	Fear of serious disease Lifestyle changes Self-consciousness
Quality of life	Decreased
Respiratory	Exacerbation of asthma Herniations of the lung (e.g., intercostal, supraclavicular) Hydrothorax in peritoneal dialysis Laryngeal trauma (e.g., laryngeal edema, hoarseness) Pulmonary interstitial emphysema, with potential risk of pneumatosis intestinalis, pneumomediastinum, pneumoperitoneum, pneumoretroperitoneum, pneumothorax, and subcutaneous emphysema Tracheobronchial trauma (e.g., bronchitis, bronchial rupture)
Skin	Petechiae and purpura Disruption of surgical wounds

From Irwin RS. Complications of cough: ACCP evidence-based clinical practice guidelines. *Chest.* 2006;129(1 suppl):54S–58S. Reprinted with permission.

always require suctioning of airway secretions. Some patients without artificial airways may need suctioning of bronchial secretions. To remove secretions from the upper airway, oropharyngeal suction may be performed with a Yankauer tip or suction catheter. To remove secretions from the lower respiratory tract, **nasotracheal suctioning** is performed (**CPG 18–1**). **Box 18–1** outlines the nasotracheal suctioning procedure; **Box 18–2** lists possible complications. Patients who require frequent nasotracheal suctioning may benefit from placement of a nasopharyngeal airway to reduce the trauma of repeated catheter insertion. Many patients respond to nasopharyngeal insertion of the catheter with a cough, which effectively removes secretions.

BOX 18–1

Procedure for Nasotracheal Suctioning

1. Assess patient and preoxygenate.
2. Assemble equipment and select appropriate suction pressure.
3. Determine which nasal passage is most patent.
4. Lubricate suction catheter.
5. Gently insert catheter through the nose to the level of the glottis; if obstruction is encountered, use other nostril.
6. During inspiration, pass the catheter into the trachea.
7. Assess for signs that the catheter is in the trachea: airflow through the catheter (listening over thumb port), patient coughing.
8. If catheter is not in the trachea, withdraw to the level of the pharynx, assess patient, and re-advance catheter.
9. Insert catheter until resistance is met, then withdraw by 1 to 2 cm, apply suction for 1 to 2 seconds, release suction, withdraw catheter several centimeters, and repeat until catheter is withdrawn from the airway; do not exceed 15 seconds.
10. Assess patient and need to repeat procedure.

CLINICAL PRACTICE GUIDELINE 18–1

Nasotracheal Suctioning

Indications

- The need to maintain a patent airway and remove saliva, pulmonary secretions, blood, vomitus, or foreign material from the trachea in the presence of:
  - Inability to clear secretions when audible or visible evidence of secretions in the large/central airways persist in spite of patient's best cough effort (evidenced by one or more of the following: visible secretions in the airway; chest auscultation of coarse, gurgling breath sounds, rhonchi; or diminished breath sounds)
  - Feeling of secretions in the chest (increased tactile fremitus)
  - Suspected aspiration of gastric or upper airway secretions
  - Clinically apparent increased work of breathing
  - Deterioration of arterial blood gas values suggesting hypoxemia or hypercarbia
  - Chest radiographic evidence of retained secretions resulting in atelectasis or consolidation
- To stimulate cough or for unrelieved coughing
- To obtain a sputum sample for microbiologic or cytologic analysis

Contraindications

- Occluded nasal passages
- Nasal bleeding
- Epiglottitis or croup (absolute)
- Acute head, facial, or neck injury
- Coagulopathy or bleeding disorder
- Laryngospasm
- Irritable airway
- Upper respiratory tract infection
- Tracheal surgery
- Gastric surgery with high anastomosis
- Myocardial infarction
- Bronchospasm

(continues)

Clinical Practice Guideline 18–1 *(continued)*

Hazards and Complications

- Mechanical trauma (mucosal hemorrhage, tracheitis, epistaxis from laceration of nasal turbinates, and perforation of the pharynx)
    - Laceration of nasal turbinates
    - Perforation of the pharynx
    - Nasal irritation/bleeding
    - Tracheitis
    - Mucosal hemorrhage
    - Uvular edema
- Hypoxia/hypoxemia
- Cardiac dysrhythmias/arrest
- Bradycardia
- Increase in blood pressure
- Hypotension
- Respiratory arrest
- Uncontrolled coughing
- Gagging/vomiting
- Laryngospasm
- Bronchoconstriction/bronchospasm
- Discomfort and pain
- Nosocomial infection
- Atelectasis
- Misdirection of catheter
- Increased intracranial pressure, intraventricular hemorrhage, exacerbation of cerebral edema
- Pneumothorax

Modified from AARC clinical practice guideline: nasotracheal suctioning—2004 revision and update. *Respir Care*. 2004;49:1080–1084. Reprinted with permission.

BOX 18–2

Complications of Nasotracheal Suctioning

Trauma to upper airway and pain
Hypoxemia
Cardiac dysrhythmia, bradycardia, cardiac arrest
Hypertension or hypotension
Respiratory arrest
Uncontrolled coughing
Gagging/vomiting
Laryngospasm or bronchospasm
Nosocomial infection
Misdirection of catheter
Increased intracranial pressure

Bronchoscopy

Diagnostic bronchoscopy is used with bronchoalveolar lavage (BAL) or protected specimen brush to obtain respiratory secretions for diagnostic purposes. This is commonly performed in the setting of suspected ventilator-associated pneumonia (VAP). Therapeutic bronchoscopy is used for removal of retained secretions, such as in hospitalized patients with new atelectasis or collapse of a lung segment, when less invasive procedures have failed.[13,14]

Mini-Bronchoalveolar Lavage

Mini-bronchoalveolar lavage (mini-BAL) is a nonbronchoscopic bedside method of performing a small-volume BAL for quantitative culture results to guide antibiotic therapy prescribed for patients suspected of VAP. These catheters are smaller in diameter than a bronchoscope, so the risk of complications is minimized. The procedure typically only requires the sampling catheter to be in the airway for 1 to 2 minutes. Moreover, lavage volumes are significantly smaller than those used in bronchoscopy, so there is less residual fluid in the lung, resulting in faster postprocedure patient recovery time.

Some mini-BAL catheters are directional, meaning that they can be theoretically directed into one lung or the other. However, the procedure is blind, so the user

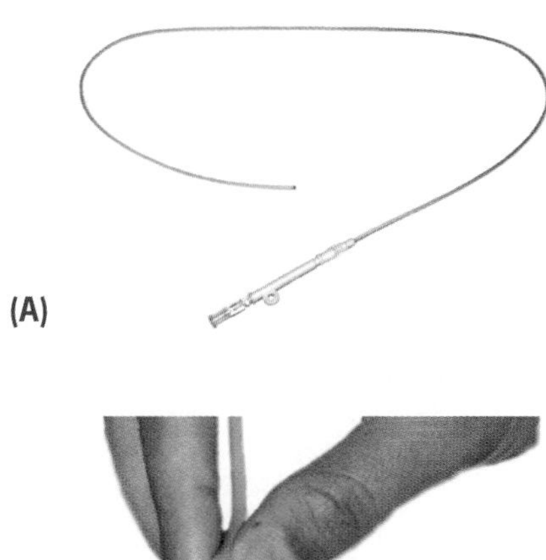

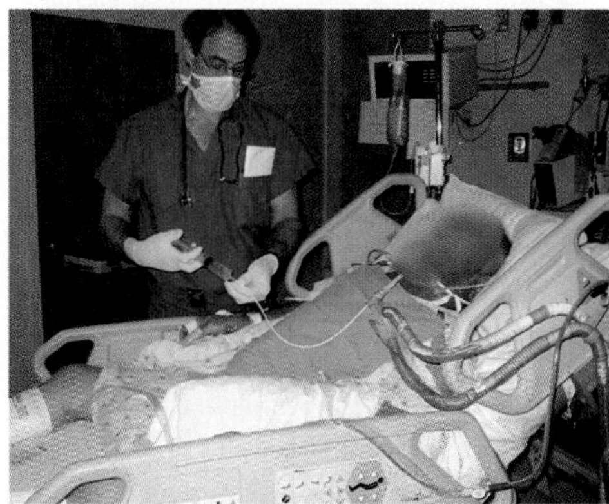

FIGURE 18–5 (**A**) Protected catheter for mini-bronchoalveolar lavage (mini-BAL). (**B**) Catheter tip. The red plug is removed to allow the inner protected catheter to exit. (**C**) Respiratory therapist performing mini-BAL procedure.

has no means of confirming the actual catheter location. It also has been shown that a blindly inserted protected catheter yields similar results as a bronchoscopically directed catheter. Some mini-BAL catheters have a plugged tip to avoid upper airway contamination. In this design, there is a polyethylene-glycol tip that protects the inner sampling catheter from contamination (**Figure 18–5**). The mini-BAL procedure typically uses a small lavage volume of 20 to 60 mL in one to three aliquots. Mini-BAL performed by respiratory therapists has results comparable to bronchoscopy and is less costly (**Box 18–3**).[15–19]

Transtracheal Aspiration

Transtracheal aspiration, or transtracheal wash, is a technique in which a needle is inserted through the skin overlying the trachea and through the cricothyroid ligament. A catheter is introduced into the trachea and passed to the level of the tracheal bifurcation. Saline is then injected, withdrawn, and sent to the laboratory for histologic and microbiologic examination.

Airway Clearance

Deep Breathing and Coughing

The normal mechanism for lung expansion and bronchial hygiene is spontaneous deep breathing (including yawn and sigh maneuvers) and an effective cough. Instructing and encouraging the patient to take sustained deep breaths is among the safest, most effective, and least expensive strategies to keep the lungs expanded and secretions moving.[20,21] The negative intrathoracic pressure generated during spontaneous deep breathing tends to better inflate the less compliant, gravity-dependent areas of the lung than mechanical methods relying on lung inflation by application of positive airway pressure. A deep breath is a key component of a normal effective cough.

An effective cough is the most important component of bronchial hygiene therapy (**CPG 18–2** and **Box 18–4**). The normal cough involves the taking of a deep breath, closure of the glottis, and compression of abdominal and thoracic muscles generating pressures in excess of 80 mm Hg, followed by an explosive release of gas as the glottis opens (**Figure 18–6**). In addition to mobilizing and expelling secretions, the high inspiratory volume generated during a cough may be an important factor in reexpanding lung tissue. Coughing can be painful for the patient, especially after upper abdominal surgery, and it has been reported to dislodge central venous catheters (refer to Table 18–1).[22] Paroxysms of uncontrolled coughing have been associated with neurologic symptoms[23] and gastroesophageal reflux.[24] In the patient with unstable airways, high pleural pressures cause dynamic compression of airways, trapping gas and secretions and rendering the cough ineffective. A variety of breathing techniques enhance cephalad airflow bias.

RESPIRATORY RECAP

Coughing

- » Forced expiratory technique
- » Manually assisted coughing
- » Active cycle of breathing
- » Autogenic drainage
- » Mechanical insufflation–exsufflation

Forced Expiratory Technique

For patients unable to generate an effective cough, sharp forced exhalations without glottis closure (**huff coughing**) may be the maneuver of choice.[25–34] Huff coughing is a **forced expiratory technique (FET)** that is performed through sharp exhalation from high to mid lung volumes through an open glottis.[20] The individual takes in a slow, deep breath, followed by a 1- to 3-second breath hold, and then performs short, quick forced exhalation with the glottis open. Toddlers can also be taught blowing games (e.g., pinwheel, bubbles) to encourage prolonged exhalation maneuvers.[35]

BOX 18–3

Procedure for Mini-Bronchoalveolar Lavage

1. Place the patient on 100% oxygen.
2. Assess for sedation level; if patient is agitated, obtain order for sedation.
3. Place the bronchoscopy adapter on the end of the endotracheal tube.
4. Suction if there are a lot of tracheal secretions.
5. Place the bed in the flat position. This makes it easier and keeps the instilled saline from moving away from the catheter tip.
6. Open the catheter using aseptic technique, but do not remove from packaging.
7. Open the sterile field.
8. Open three syringes onto the sterile field.
9. Open the bottle of saline solution and pour it into a sterile bowl. Don the sterile gloves.
10. Pick up one of the syringes and fill it with 20 mL sterile saline and a 10 mL air bolus. Repeat with the other two syringes.
11. Insert the blunt end of the catheter (the end with the red plug) into the endotracheal tube via the bronchoscopy adapter. As you advance the catheter, remove the polyethylene sheath covering the white outer catheter, taking care not to dislodge the spacer for the inner cannula.
12. Slowly advance the catheter into the lungs until you feel a resistance. The CombiCath should usually be advanced past the 40-cm mark to pass the carina.
13. Pull the catheter back about 3 cm.
14. Remove the spacer at the distal end of the catheter by sliding it off from the side channel.
15. Gently push the newly exposed inner cannula into the white portion of the catheter up to the hub of the Luer connector.
16. Connect the saline-filled syringe to the catheter.
17. Instill all 20 mL of the saline along with the 5 mL air bolus to ensure that all of the saline is pushed through the catheter.
18. Draw back on the syringe and retrieve the aspirate sample. *Note:* The size of the sample will be approximately 3 to 5 mL. A high-quality sample will have stable bubbles at the top of the meniscus, representing the presence of surfactant.
19. Assess the patient's vital signs.
20. Repeat with syringes 2 and 3. The procedure should be stopped if the patient is decompensating or the first or second instillation provided a good-quality sample.
21. Gently withdraw the entire catheter and syringe, taking care not to lose the sample.
22. Decant the samples into a sterile sputum trap. Send to laboratory for appropriate analysis.
23. Suction the patient if necessary. Return the bed to its original position. Return the ventilator to the original settings.
24. Document procedure.

Manually Assisted Coughing

Manually assisted coughing involves thrusts with hands and arms positioned on the patient's abdomen, coordinated with expiration (**Figure 18–7**). Compression of the lateral aspect of the chest also can be effective. Often this technique is augmented with manual hyperinflation for patients with a low vital capacity. This technique requires a cooperative patient, good coordination between patient and clinician, and a clinician with sufficient physical strength to reliably perform the maneuver. Efficacy is limited for patients with significant scoliosis and osteoporosis of the rib cage. This technique is used most commonly in patients with neuromuscular disease or quadriplegia and is sometimes called *quad coughing.*

Active Cycle of Breathing

Active cycle of breathing techniques are a combination of breathing control, thoracic expansion control, and forced expiration technique (**Box 18–5** and

CLINICAL PRACTICE GUIDELINE 18–2

Directed Cough

Indications

- The need to aid in the removal of retained secretions from central airways (with the suggestion that forced expiratory technique at lower lung volumes may be effective in preferentially mobilizing secretions in peripheral airways whereas larger volumes facilitate movement in the central airways lacking validation)
- The presence of atelectasis
- As prophylaxis against postoperative pulmonary complications
- As a routine part of bronchial hygiene in patients with cystic fibrosis, bronchiectasis, chronic bronchitis, necrotizing pulmonary infection, or spinal cord injury
- As an integral part of other bronchial hygiene therapies such as postural drainage therapy, positive expiratory pressure therapy, and incentive spirometry
- The need to obtain sputum specimens for diagnostic analysis

Contraindications

- Directed cough is rarely contraindicated. The contraindications listed must be weighted against potential benefit in deciding to eliminate cough from the care of the patient. The following listed contraindications are relative:
  - Inability to control possible transmission of infection from patients suspected or known to have pathogens transmittable by droplet nuclei (e.g., *Mycobacterium tuberculosis*)
  - Presence of an elevated intracranial pressure or known intracranial aneurysm
  - Presence of reduced coronary artery perfusion, such as in acute myocardial infarction
  - Acute unstable head, neck, or spine injury
  - Possibly manually assisted directed cough with pressure to the epigastrium in presence of increased potential for regurgitation/aspiration (e.g., unconscious patient with unprotected airway), acute abdominal pathologic process (abdominal aortic aneurysm, hiatal hernia, or pregnancy), a bleeding diathesis, untreated pneumothorax
  - Possibly manually assisted directed cough with pressure to the thoracic cage in presence of osteoporosis, or flail chest

Hazards and Complications

- Reduced coronary artery perfusion
- Reduced cerebral perfusion
- Incontinence
- Fatigue
- Headache
- Paresthesia
- Bronchospasm
- Muscular discomfort
- Barotraumas
- Cough paroxysms
- Chest pain
- Rib or costochondral junction fracture
- Incisional pain or evisceration
- Anorexia or vomiting and retching
- Visual disturbances including retinal hemorrhage, central line displacement, and gastroesophageal reflux

Modified from AARC clinical practice guideline: directed cough. *Respir Care.* 1993;38:495–499. Reprinted with permission.

BOX 18–4

Procedure for Directed Cough

1. Explain to the patient that deep breathing and coughing will help to keep the lungs expanded and clear of secretions.
2. Assist the patient to a sitting position, or to a semi-Fowler position if sitting position is not possible.
3. Directed cough procedure (see below for modifications):
   a. Instruct patient to take a deep breath, then hold the breath, using abdominal muscles to force air against a closed glottis, then cough with a single exhalation.
   b. Have the patient take several relaxed breaths before the next cough effort.
   c. Document teaching accomplished, procedures performed, and patient response in the patient record.
4. Huff cough procedure (forced expiratory technique):
   a. Instruct patient to take three to five slow, deep breaths, inhaling through the nose, exhaling through pursed lips, using diaphragmatic breathing. Have the patient take a deep breath and hold it for 1 to 3 seconds.
   b. Instruct patient to exhale from mid-to-low lung volume (to clear secretions from peripheral airways). Have the patient take a normal breath in and then squeeze it out by contracting the abdominal and chest wall muscles, with the mouth (and glottis) open during exhalation. Repeat several times.
   c. As secretions enter the larger airways, have the patient exhale from high-to-mid lung volume to clear secretions from more proximal airways. Repeat maneuver two to three times.
   d. Instruct patient to take several relaxed diaphragmatic breaths before the next cough effort.
   e. Document teaching accomplished, procedures performed, and patient response in the patient record.
5. Modified directed cough procedures:
   a. Patients who have had abdominal or thoracic surgery: Instruct patient to place hand or a pillow over the incision site and apply gentle pressure while coughing. Caregiver may assist with incision support during coughing. Support chest tubes as necessary.
   b. Quadriplegic patients: Clinician places palms on the patient's abdomen, below the diaphragm, and instructs the patient to take three deep breaths. On exhalation of the third breath, clinician pushes forcefully inward and upward as the patient coughs (similar to abdominal thrust maneuver performed on an unconscious patient with an obstructed airway).

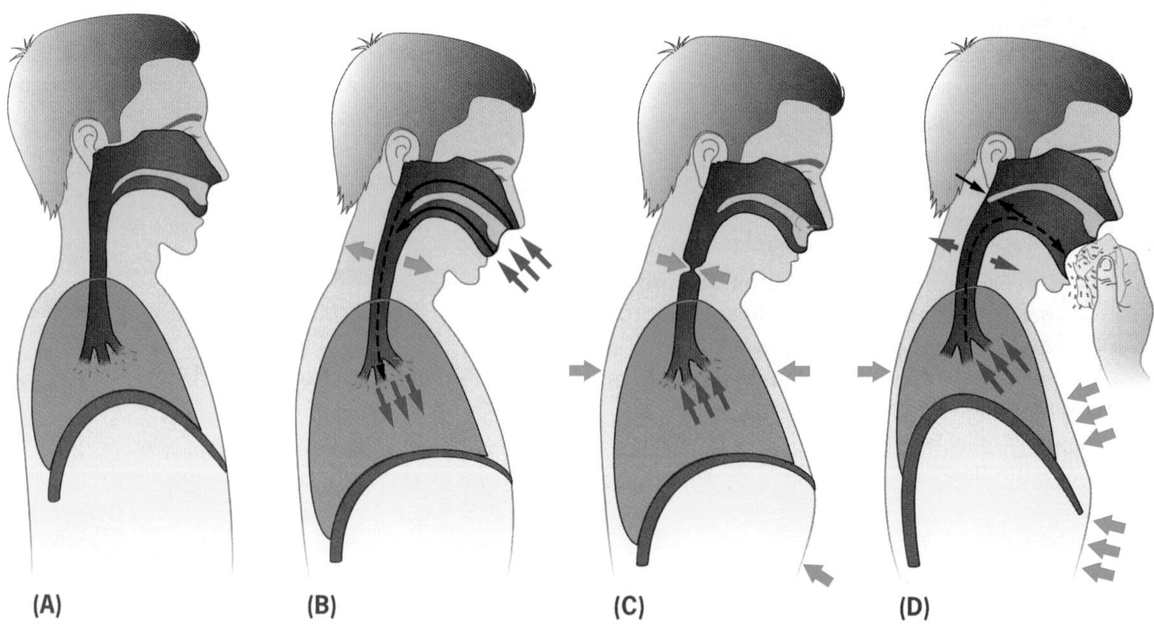

FIGURE 18–6 The cough reflex. (**A**) Irritation. (**B**) Inspiration. (**C**) Compression. (**D**) Expulsion.

BOX 18–5

Procedure for Active Cycle of Breathing

1. Patient should be in a relaxed, sitting, or reclined position.
2. Have the patient do several minutes of relaxed diaphragmatic breathing (breathing control).
3. Instruct the patient to take three to four active deep inspirations with passive relaxed exhalation (thoracic expansion exercises).
4. Have the patient do relaxed diaphragmatic breathing (breathing control).
5. As the patient feels secretions entering the larger central airway, instruct him or her to do two to three huffs (forced expiratory technique) starting at low volume, followed by two to three huffs at higher volume, followed by relaxed breathing control.
6. Repeat the cycle two to four times, as tolerated.

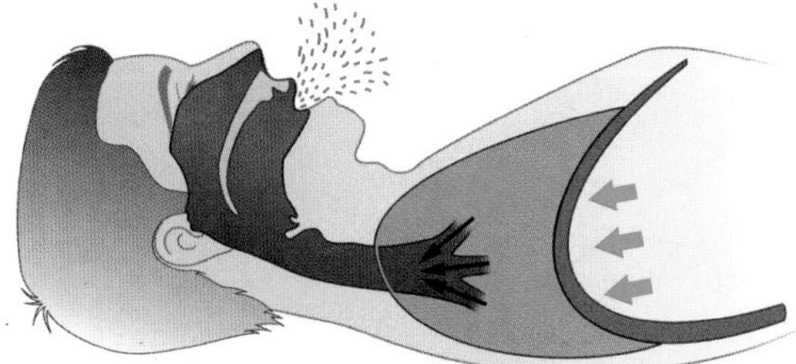

FIGURE 18–7 To produce manually assisted (quad) coughing, external abdominal pressure is applied under the diaphragm during exhalation following maximal inspiration, resulting in an increased expiratory flow and secretion clearance.

Figure 18–8).[20] Breathing control is described as gentle breathing with the lower chest. With the upper chest and shoulders relaxed, the patient breathes at normal tidal volume and rate. The patient should feel a swelling around the waist on inspiration, which subsides while breathing out. Breathing control is the default maneuver between the more active techniques. Thoracic expansion exercises are simply large breaths with active inspiration (involving both diaphragm and rib cage musculature) and relaxed expiration. Increasing lung volume increases flow through small airways and collateral ventilation channels, increasing the volume of gas available to help mobilize secretions on expiration. This is limited to three or four deep breaths to avoid fatigue and hyperventilation. The FET consists of one or two forced expirations or huffs, combined with a period of controlled breathing.[20,36,37] A normal breath is taken in, and then the air is squeezed out by contraction of the chest wall and abdominal muscles. The mouth and glottis are kept open. The huff should not be a violent or explosive exhalation.

Autogenic Drainage

Autogenic drainage aims to achieve the highest possible airflow in the different generations of bronchi to move secretions without forced expirations (**Figure 18–9**).[38,39] This technique depends on staged breathing at different lung volumes, starting with small tidal breaths from expiratory reserve volume (ERV), repeated until secretions are felt gathering in the central airways. At that point the cough is suppressed, and a larger tidal volume is taken for a series of 10 to 20 breaths, followed by a series of larger (approaching vital capacity) breaths, followed by several huff coughs. Although this technique is effective, it requires a great deal of patient cooperation.[20]

Mechanical Insufflation–Exsufflation

The mechanical insufflation–exsufflator (MIE), also called the Cough Assist, is a device (**Figure 18–10**) that inflates the lungs with positive pressure followed by a negative pressure to simulate a cough.[40–42] Treatment consists of five cycles of **mechanical insufflation–exsufflation** followed by 20 to 30 seconds of normal breathing, with repetitions until secretions are cleared. For each cycle the inspiratory pressure is 25 to 35 cm H_2O for 1 to 2 seconds, followed by an expiratory pressure of –30 to –40 cm H_2O for 1 to 2 seconds. The MIE can be used with an oronasal mask, with a mouthpiece, or attached to an artificial airway. Combining manual abdominal thrusts with expiration can help to increase expiratory flow expulsion of secretions. This procedure has been shown to be effective in patients with neuromuscular disease. In patients with bulbar disease, use of the MIE can be limited by upper airway closure during the active negative pressure expiratory phase.[42]

Aerosol Therapy

Aerosolized antibiotics and mucolytics are effective when dispersed in infected airway secretions at sites of maximal airway obstruction. Mucus is a nonhomogeneous, adhesive, viscoelastic gel consisting of high-molecular-weight, cross-linked glycoproteins mixed with serum, cellular proteins, lipids, and water. The antibiotic diffusion barrier represented by mucin may be significant in vitro, particularly for nebulized antibiotics.

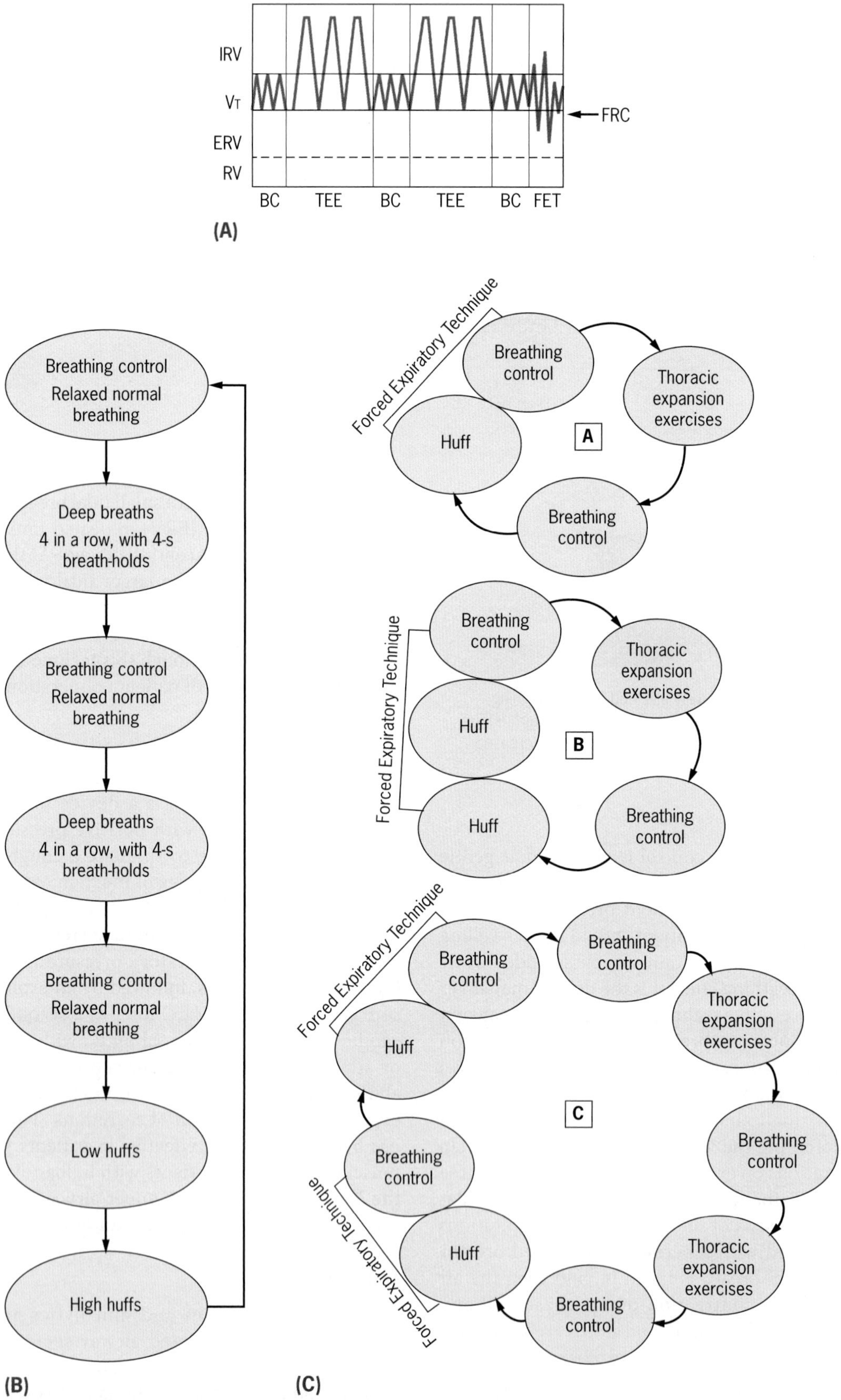

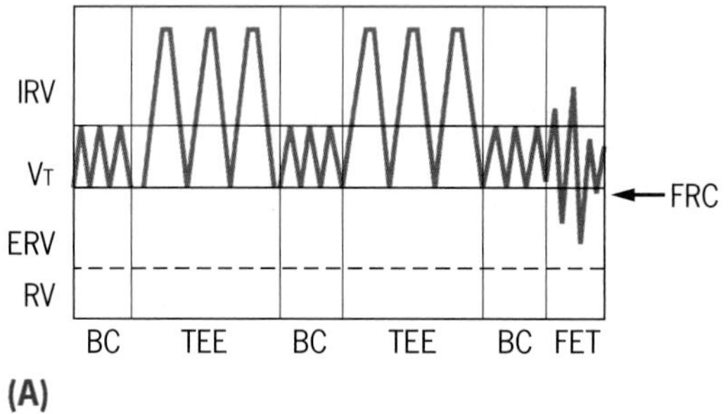

FIGURE 18–8 (**A**) Lung volumes during active cycle of breathing technique. (**B**) Active cycle of breathing technique. (**C**) Three active cycle of breathing routines. IRV, inspiratory reserve volume; VT, tidal volume; ERV, expiratory reserve volume; RV, reserve volume; BC, breathing control; TEE, thoracic expansion exercise; FRC, functional residual capacity; FET, forced expiratory technique. From Fink JB. Forced expiratory technique, directed cough, and autogenic drainage. *Respir Care.* 2007;52:1210–1223. Reprinted with permission.

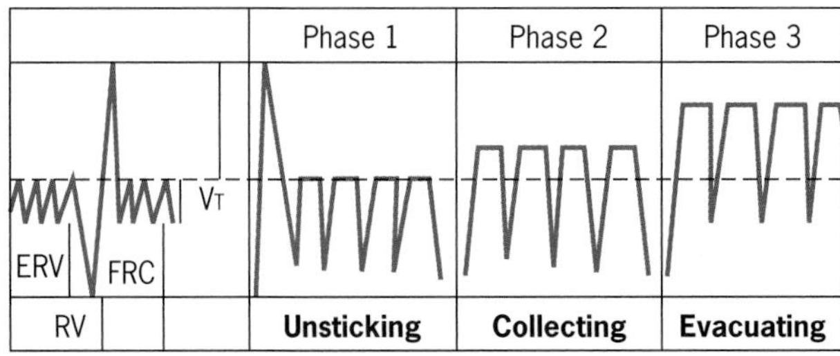

FIGURE 18–9 The three phases of autogenic drainage. ERV, expiratory reserve volume; RV, reserve volume; FRC, functional residual capacity; IRV, inspiratory reserve volume; VT, tidal volume. From Fink JB. Forced expiratory technique, directed cough, and autogenic drainage. *Respir Care.* 2007;52:1210–1223. Reprinted with permission.

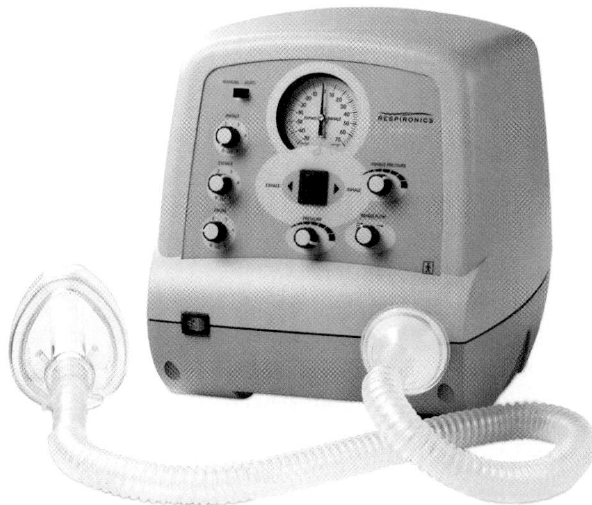

FIGURE 18–10 Cough Assist mechanical insufflation–exsufflation device.

Translocation of macromolecules can be further compromised by the hypersecretion that accompanies inflammation and chronic pulmonary disease. These secretions can be a barrier to the penetration of any aerosol.

Sputum is expectorated mucus mixed with inflammatory cells, cellular debris, polymers of DNA and F-actin, and bacteria. Recombinant human deoxyribonuclease (dornase alfa) was the first approved mucoactive agent for the treatment of CF. The efficacy of dornase alfa has not been demonstrated in treatment of other chronic airway diseases. Acetylcysteine (*N*-acetyl-L-cysteine sodium; Mucomyst) has been administered by aerosol or direct instillation based on its in vitro ability to break disulfide bonds of mucoprotein. However, little data support its in vivo efficacy. Mucomyst is an irritant to the airway that is capable of inducing bronchospasm, and it has a nauseating smell and taste. Hypertonic saline (7%) has been shown to improve outcomes in patients with CF,[43] but might not be useful for COPD.[44] Aerosolized isotonic saline from a small volume nebulizer is not an effective airway clearance therapy. Most guidelines for management of COPD do not advocate treatment with inhaled mucolytics.[45]

The involvement of the cholinergic and adrenergic neural pathways in the pathophysiology of mucus hypersecretion suggests the potential therapeutic role of bronchodilators as mucoactive agents. Although anticholinergics and adrenergic agonist bronchodilators have been used to enhance mucociliary clearance in patients with obstructive lung disease, the existing evidence does not consistently show clinical effectiveness.[46] Although short-acting beta-adrenergics have mucociliary-enhancing effects in healthy individuals, their effect in subjects with depressed airway clearance is minimal. There has historically been concern that inhaled anticholinergic agents used to treat airway disease could dry respiratory tract secretions. However, this is not clinically important for the anticholinergics commonly used to treat airway disease. Atropine or glycopyrrolate injection and scopolamine patch are used to reduce cholinergic symptoms such as sialorrhea, bronchorrhea, and excessive pharyngeal secretions. However, aerosolized anticholinergics are minimally effective in drying respiratory tract secretions.

Conventional Chest Physiotherapy

Conventional **chest physiotherapy (CPT)** consists of a combination of forced exhalation (directed cough or huff), postural drainage, percussion, and/or shaking.[47] Conventional CPT has become the standard to which all other bronchial hygiene techniques are compared. Patient satisfaction with conventional CPT is less than with other bronchial hygiene techniques.[48] Given the potential for hazard, the time required for therapy, and the paucity of evidence to support its use,[49] prudence is necessary regarding use of CPT.

Postural drainage (PD) results in greater expectoration than no treatment in patients with CF.[50] PD is used in the treatment of acute and stable conditions characterized by excessive sputum production that the patient has difficulty clearing or expectorating (**CPG 18–3**).[51–55] It consists of positioning so that secretions drain from specific segments and lobes of the lung toward gravity-dependent central airways, where they can be more readily removed with cough or mechanical aspiration. This action is accomplished by positioning of the patient so that the affected lung segments are superior to the carina, with each position maintained for 5 to 10 minutes (**Figure 18–11**). Typically, 11 to 12 positions are identified to drain all areas of the lungs, requiring at least 1 hour for a complete session. Because of this time commitment, therapy may be concentrated in those positions that drain the most affected segments. This time commitment is a major obstacle to prescription adherence by the patient.

PD has no benefit in conditions presenting with scant secretions (e.g., viral pneumonia, postoperative coronary artery bypass). The indications for PD are largely limited to patients diagnosed with CF or bronchiectasis, and specifically those who produce more than 30 mL of

CLINICAL PRACTICE GUIDELINE 18–3

Postural Drainage Therapy

Indications

- *Turning:* Inability or reluctance of patient to change body position (e.g., mechanical ventilation, neuromuscular disease, drug-induced paralysis), poor oxygenation associated with position (e.g., unilateral lung disease), potential for or presence of atelectasis, presence of artificial airway
- *Postural drainage (PD):* Evidence or suggestion of difficulty with secretion clearance; difficulty clearing secretions with expectorated sputum production greater than 25 to 30 mL/day (adult); evidence or suggestion of retained secretions in the presence of an artificial airway; presence of atelectasis caused by or suspected of being caused by mucous plugging; diagnosis of diseases such as cystic fibrosis, bronchiectasis, or cavitating lung disease; presence of foreign body in airway
- *External manipulation of the thorax:* Sputum volume or consistency suggesting a need for additional manipulation (e.g., percussion and/or vibration) to assist movement of secretions by gravity in a patient receiving PD

Contraindications

- The decision to use PD therapy requires assessment of potential benefits versus potential risks. Therapy should be provided for no longer than necessary to obtain the desired therapeutic results.
- All positions are contraindicated for intracranial pressure (ICP) greater than 20 mm Hg; head and neck injury until stabilized (absolute); active hemorrhage with hemodynamic instability (absolute); recent spinal surgery (e.g., laminectomy) or acute spinal injury; active hemoptysis; empyema; bronchopleural fistula; pulmonary edema associated with congestive heart failure; large pleural effusions, pulmonary embolism; aged, confused, or anxious patients who do not tolerate position changes; rib fracture, with or without flail chest; and surgical wound or healing tissue.
- The Trendelenburg position is contraindicated for ICP greater than 20 mm Hg; patients in whom increased ICP is to be prevented (e.g., because of neurosurgery, aneurysms, eye surgery); uncontrolled hypertension; distended abdomen; esophageal surgery; recent gross hemoptysis related to recent lung carcinoma treated surgically or with radiation therapy; and uncontrolled airway at risk for aspiration (tube feeding or recent meal). Reverse Trendelenburg is contraindicated in the presence of hypotension or vasoactive medication.
- External manipulation of the thorax is contraindicated with subcutaneous emphysema; recent epidural spinal infusion or spinal anesthesia; recent skin grafts, or flaps, on the thorax; burns, open wounds, and skin infections of the thorax; recently placed transvenous pacemaker or subcutaneous pacemaker (particularly if mechanical devices are to be used); suspected pulmonary tuberculosis; lung contusion; bronchospasm; osteomyelitis of the ribs; osteoporosis; coagulopathy; complaint of chest wall pain.

Hazards and Complications

- Hypoxemia
- Increased intracranial pressure
- Acute hypotension
- Pulmonary hemorrhage
- Pain or injury to chest wall
- Vomiting and aspiration
- Bronchospasm
- Dysrhythmias

Modified from AARC clinical practice guideline: postural drainage therapy. *Respir Care.* 1991;36:1418–1426. Reprinted with permission.

Upper and Middle Lobes

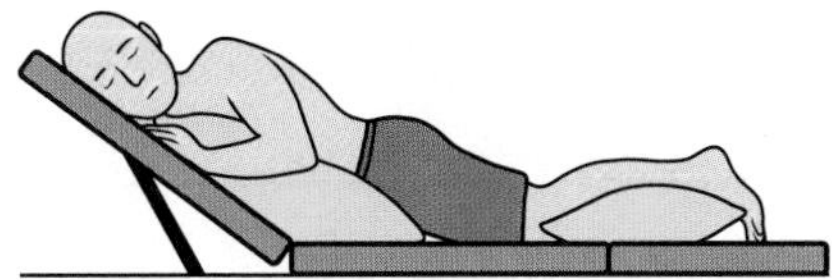

Apical posterior segment, left upper lobe

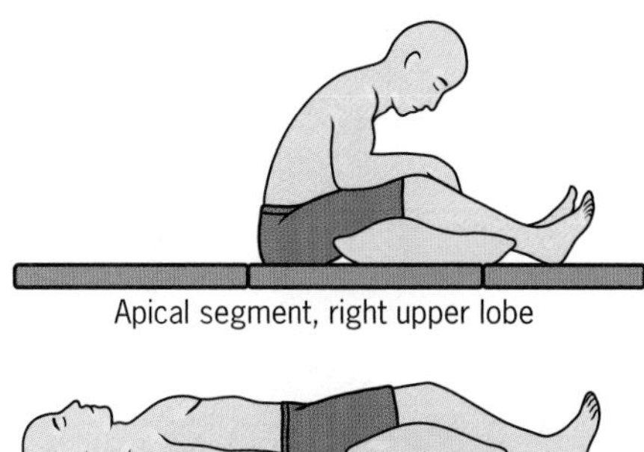

Apical segment, right upper lobe

Anterior segments, upper lobes

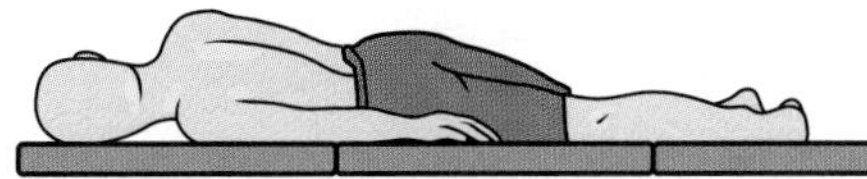

Posterior segment, right upper lobe

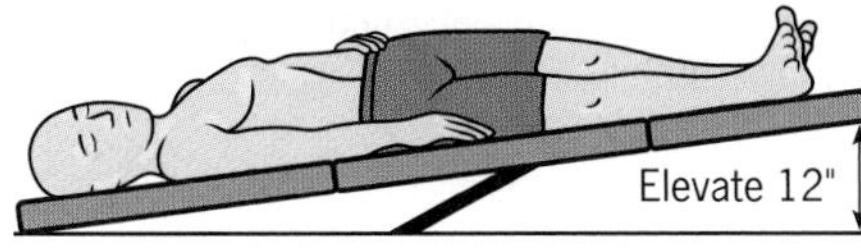

Left upper lobe, lingula

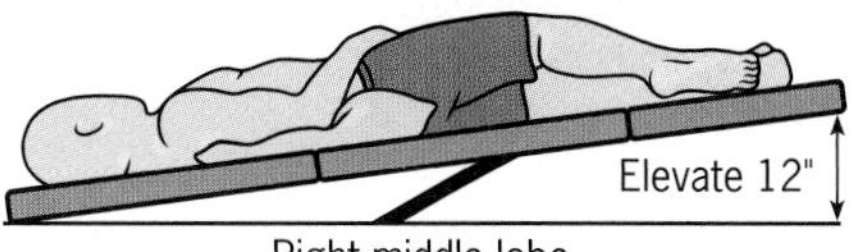

Right middle lobe

Lower Lobes

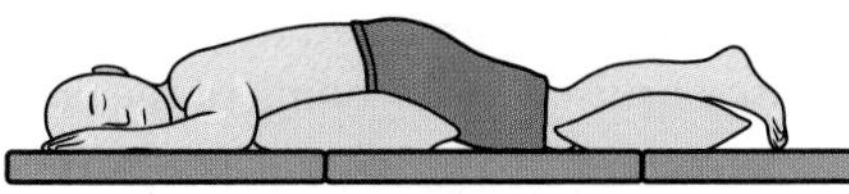

Superior segments, lower lobes

Elevate 18"

Posterior basal segments, lower lobes

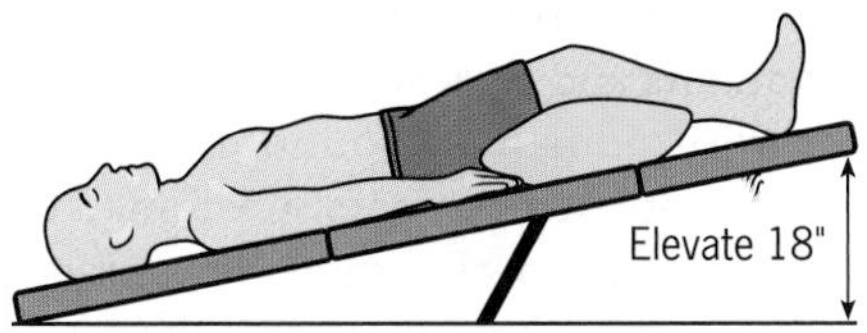

Right anterior basal and left anterior medial basal segments, lower lobes

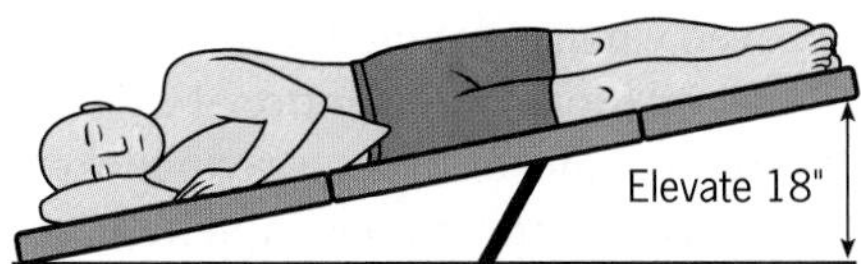

Lateral basal segment, left lower lobe

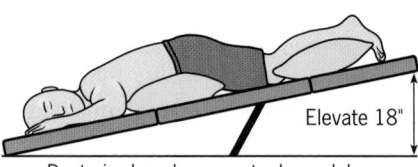

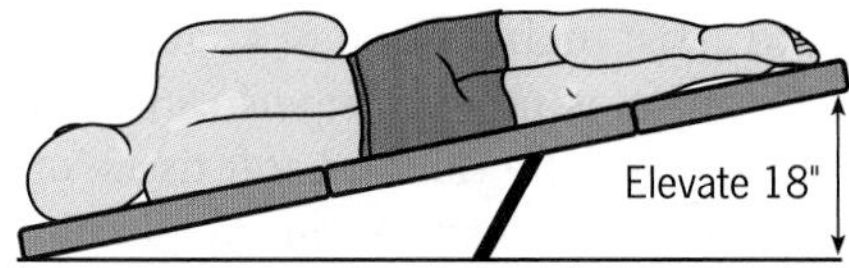

Lateral basal segment, right lower lobe

FIGURE 18–11 Positions for postural drainage.

sputum per day and have difficulty clearing that. Sputum production of less than 25 mL/day is insufficient to justify the application of PD therapy. Some patients have productive coughs with sputum production from 15 to 30 mL/day (occasionally as high as 70 or 100 mL/day) without need for PD. If PD does not increase sputum production in a patient who produces more than 30 mL/day of sputum without PD, the continued use of PD is not indicated.

Placing the patient in a head-down or Trendelenburg position affects both hemodynamics and interaction of physical forces between the thorax and the abdomen. With the head down, there is increased blood flow to the head. Therefore, the Trendelenburg position should be avoided in patients with head injury, uncontrolled hypertension, or gross hemoptysis.[56] Shifting of abdominal and thoracic contents with gravity in the Trendelenburg position may be deleterious in patients at risk for aspiration, with distended abdomens, or after recent esophageal surgery. Reverse Trendelenburg position may be hazardous for patients with hypotension or those receiving vasoactive medication.

RESPIRATORY RECAP

Conventional Chest Physiotherapy

- Postural drainage
- May be combined with percussion and vibration

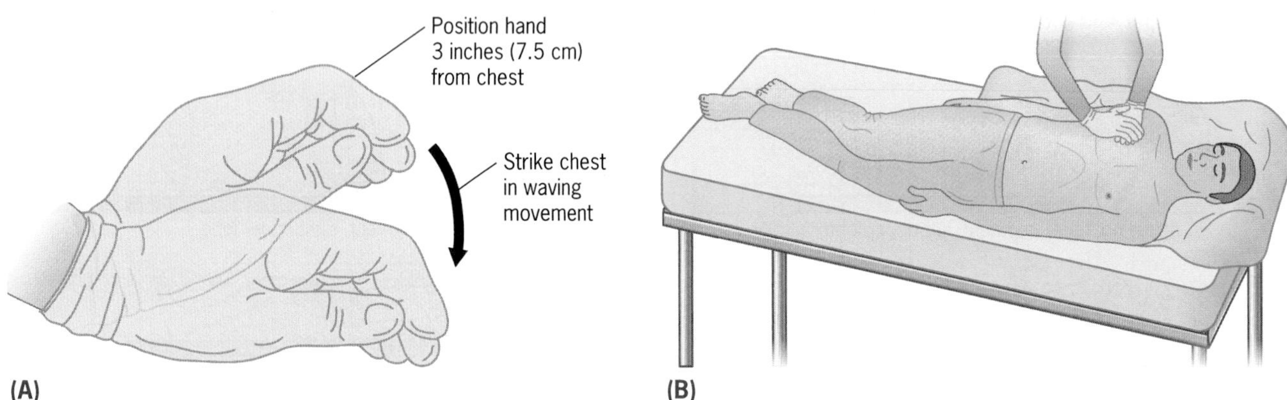

FIGURE 18–12 (**A**) Movement of cupped hand at wrist to percuss chest. (**B**) Chest vibration. This article was published in *Egan's Fundamentals of Respiratory Care, Seventh Edition.* Scanlan CL, Wilkins RL, Stoller JK. Copyright Elsevier (Mosby) 1999.

During PD therapy, care should be taken to identify hypoxemia, bronchospasm, acute hypotension, increased intracranial pressure, hemoptysis, pain or injury to the tissue, and vomiting with risk of aspiration. To minimize risk of vomiting and aspiration, therapy should be performed before meals or more than 1 hour after meals. For patients receiving tube feedings, feedings should cease 1 hour before and during therapy. For patients with a history of bronchospasm, bronchodilators are commonly administered before PD therapy.

Percussion therapy is a technique involving rapid clapping, cupping, or striking of the external thorax directly over the lung segment being drained, with either cupped hands or a mechanical device (**Figure 18–12**).[57,58] Percussion has been advocated to assist secretion mobilization by shaking loose secretions, similar to the shaking of ketchup from a bottle. Vibrating the chest wall over the draining area with a fine tremulous action also has been used to assist mobilization of secretion during PD. **Vibration therapy** is manually performed by pressing in the direction that the ribs and soft tissue of the chest normally move during exhalation. Mechanical devices can be used to perform chest percussion and vibration. These devices may be more convenient for the caregiver, but data are lacking that these devices improve airway clearance.

Percussion and vibration appear to be relatively ineffective and do not add to the effectiveness of the combination of coughing, breathing exercises, and PD.[59–63] Little evidence exists that percussion alone, without positioning of the patient, is of any value. Although the clinical efficacy of percussion and vibration is questionable, the techniques are associated with a number of potential hazards and complications. A variety of conditions may be exacerbated by performance of percussion or vibration to the thorax, such as irregularities of the skin (e.g., burns, open wounds, skin infections, recent skin grafts), subcutaneous emphysema, recently placed transvenous pacemaker or subcutaneous pacemaker, or recent epidural spinal infusion of anesthetic of the spinal type. Percussion and vibration are difficult for patients to apply without assistance. Potential damage to the thorax from percussion makes osteoporosis and osteomyelitis of the ribs, as well as complaints of chest pain, relative contraindications to this therapy. Lung contusion and coagulopathies may be aggravated by percussion, resulting in increased bruising or bleeding of the chest wall or in the lungs.

Conventional CPT has been suggested as the most stimulating and disturbing procedure in mechanically ventilated patients and thus should not be administered to patients with poor cardiopulmonary reserve.[64] In mechanically ventilated patients, CPT may be accompanied with manual hyperinflation. This practice is discouraged, however, because it may result in dangerously high airway pressures and tidal volumes in patients with acute lung injury.[65] In patients with CF, tolerance for CPT may be improved when combined with noninvasive pressure support ventilation.[66] Conventional CPT is overused in many hospitals, and efforts to reduce its unnecessary use have been successfully implemented without adversely affecting patient outcomes.[67]

A technique used to perform a complete PD session with minimal movement of the patient is the clockwise rotation of the patient, with each rotation draining a different segment of the lung. Each position should be maintained for 5 to 10 minutes as tolerated, with the patient being encouraged to deep breathe and cough during and between positions. This technique starts with the patient flat on his or her back and proceeds through eight partial turns in a clockwise direction (**Table 18–2**). **Box 18–6** describes the general procedure for CPT.

Positive Expiratory Pressure

Positive expiratory pressure (PEP) therapy is performed with the patient seated comfortably and with elbows resting on a table (**Box 18–7** and **CPG 18–4**).[68] Equipment

TABLE 18–2 **Clockwise Rotation for Complete Postural Drainage**

Procedure	Area Drained
Start with bed flat.	
Position patient supine, pillow under knees for comfort.	Anterior segments of both upper lobes
Roll patient prone. Use pillow to raise right chest.	Posterior segment, right upper lobe
Raise foot of bed to 12", as tolerated.	
Place patient supine on right side, pillow behind back and shoulder.	Lingula, left upper lobe
Raise foot of bed to 18", as tolerated.	
Place supine.	Right anterior basal and left anterior medial basal segments of the lower lobes
Position patient with right side down.	Lateral basal segment, left lower lobe
Lower foot of bed to flat position.	
Position patient prone, pillow under hips, bed flat.	Superior segments of both lower lobes
Raise foot of bed to 18", as tolerated.	
Position patient prone, pillow under hips.	Posterior basal segments of both lower lobes
Position patient with left side down.	Lateral basal segment, right lower lobe
Lower foot of bed to 12".	
Place patient supine on left side, pillow behind back and shoulders.	Right middle lobe
Place bed in semi-Fowler position.	
Roll patient to prone position, pillow beneath head and chest, pillows between knees for comfort.	Apical posterior segment, left upper lobe
Patient sits up, dangling legs over side of bed, and leans forward over pillows on a bedside table.	Apical segment, right upper lobe

BOX 18–6

Procedure for Chest Physiotherapy

1. Assess patient and need for chest physiotherapy.
2. Gather appropriate equipment: bed or table that can assume range of positions, pillows to support patient, light towel to cover chest percussion area, tissues or basin for secretions.
3. Explain therapy to patient and instruct patient in proper cough techniques.
4. Assist patient to each position and maintain for 5 to 10 minutes.
5. Assess patient response in each position; modify position if necessary.
6. Perform chest percussion and vibration over the affected area if necessary.
7. Encourage patient to take slow, deep breaths and cough between positions; note character of cough and secretions.
8. Document procedure and response to therapy in the medical record; communicate adverse effects to physician.

consists of a soft transparent mask or mouthpiece, T assembly with a one-way valve, a variety of fixed orifice resistors (or an adjustable expiratory resistor), and a manometer (**Figure 18–13**). The subject is instructed to relax while performing diaphragmatic breathing, inspiring a volume of air larger than normal tidal volume but not to the level of total lung capacity, through the one-way valve. Exhalation to functional residual capacity (FRC) is active but not forced, through the resistor chosen to achieve a peak airway pressure of 10 to 20 cm H_2O during exhalation. A series of 10 to 20 breaths are performed with the mask or mouthpiece in place. The mask (or mouthpiece) is then removed, and the patient performs several coughs to raise secretions. This sequence of 10 to 20 breaths, followed by huff coughing, is repeated four to six times per PEP therapy session. Each session requires 10 to 20 minutes and may be performed one to four times per day as needed. For lung

BOX 18–7

Procedure for Positive Expiratory Pressure Therapy

1. The patient should sit comfortably upright while holding the mask firmly over the nose and mouth or the mouthpiece tightly between the lips (a nose clip may be necessary).
2. Adjust the expiratory resistor dial to the prescribed setting.
3. Have the patient breathe from the diaphragm, taking in a larger than normal tidal breath, but not to total lung capacity.
4. Have the patient gently exhale, maintaining a prescribed pressure of 5 to 20 cm H_2O.
5. Exhalation time should last approximately three times longer than inhalation.
6. Patient should perform 10 to 20 positive expiratory pressure breaths, then perform two to three forced exhalation maneuvers or huffs.
7. Repeat steps 3 to 6 until secretions are cleared or until the predetermined treatment period has elapsed.

From Myers TR. Positive expiratory pressure and oscillatory positive expiratory pressure therapies. *Respir Care.* 2007;52:1308–1327. Reprinted with permission.

CLINICAL PRACTICE GUIDELINE 18–4

Use of Positive Airway Pressure Adjuncts to Bronchial Hygiene Therapy

Indications

- To reduce air trapping in asthma and chronic obstructive pulmonary disease
- To aid in mobilization of retained secretions (in cystic fibrosis and chronic bronchitis)
- To prevent or reverse atelectasis
- To optimize delivery of bronchodilators in patients receiving bronchial hygiene therapy

Contraindications

- Patients unable to tolerate the increased work of breathing
- Intracranial pressure greater than 20 mm Hg
- Hemodynamic instability
- Recent surgery to face or mouth or skull
- Acute sinusitis
- Epistaxis
- Esophageal surgery
- Active hemoptysis
- Nausea
- Known or suspected tympanic membrane rupture or other middle ear pathologic process
- Untreated pneumothorax

Hazards and Complications

- Increased work of breathing that may lead to hypoventilation and hypercarbia
- Increased intracranial pressure
- Cardiovascular compromise
- Air swallowing with increased likelihood of vomiting and aspiration
- Claustrophobia
- Skin breakdown and discomfort from mask
- Pulmonary barotrauma

Modified from AARC clinical practice guideline: use of positive airway pressure adjuncts to bronchial hygiene therapy. *Respir Care.* 1993;38:516–521. Reprinted with permission.

expansion, patients should be encouraged to take 10 to 20 breaths every hour while awake.

Selection of a resistor with an appropriate orifice size is critical to proper technique. The therapeutic goal is to achieve a PEP of 10 to 20 cm H_2O, with an inspiration-to-expiration (I:E) ratio of 1:3 to 1:4. When a fixed orifice is used, most adults achieve this pressure range with an orifice of 2.5 to 4.0 mm in diameter. A manometer is placed in-line to measure the expiratory pressure while the appropriate-sized orifice is selected. Once the proper resistor orifice has been determined, the manometer may be removed from the system. Selection of a resistor with too large an orifice produces a short exhalation, with failure to achieve the proper expiratory pressure. Too small an orifice prolongs the expiratory phase, elevates the pressure above 20 cm H_2O, and increases the work of breathing. Performing a PEP session for more than 20 minutes may lead to fatigue. During periods of exacerbation, individuals are encouraged to increase the frequency with which PEP is performed, rather than extending the length of individual sessions.

Although no absolute contraindications to the use of PEP therapy have been reported, common sense dictates that patients with acute sinusitis, ear infection, epistaxis, or recent facial, oral, or skull injury or surgery should be carefully evaluated before a decision is made to initiate PEP mask therapy. Patients experiencing active hemoptysis or those with unresolved pneumothorax should avoid using PEP therapy until these acute pulmonary problems have resolved.

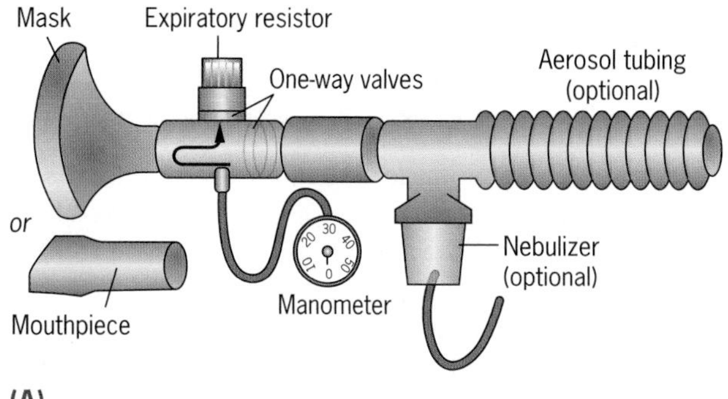

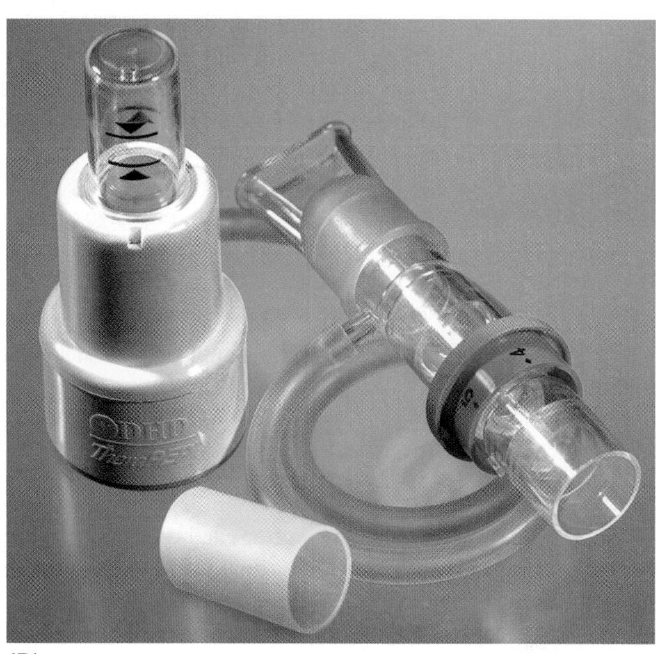

FIGURE 18–13 (**A**) Equipment for positive expiratory pressure (PEP) therapy. (**B**) Commercially available PEP device. (**A**) Adapted from Malmeister MJ, et al. Positive expiratory pressure mask therapy: theoretical and practical considerations and a review of the literature. *Respir Care.* 1991;36:1218–1229.

Oscillatory (or Vibratory) Positive Expiratory Pressure

Oscillatory, or vibratory, PEP combines the purported benefits of PEP with airway vibrations or oscillations.[68] Oscillations may decrease the viscoelastic properties of mucus, which makes it easier to mobilize mucus up the airways, and may create short bursts of increased expiratory airflow that assist in mobilizing secretions up the airways. Secretion removal is then facilitated by the patient forcing deep exhalations through the device or with subsequent coughing and/or huffing techniques.

The Flutter device is a pipe-shaped device with a steel ball in a bowl loosely covered by a perforated cap (**Figure 18–14**). The weight of the ball serves as a PEP device (approximately 10 cm H_2O), whereas the internal shape of the bowl allows the ball to flutter, generating oscillations of about 15 Hz (2 to 32 Hz), varying with the position of the device. **Box 18–8** describes the procedure for Flutter therapy. The Flutter can be used with the patient sitting upright or lying on either side. The Flutter bowl must be pointed upward for maximum efficacy

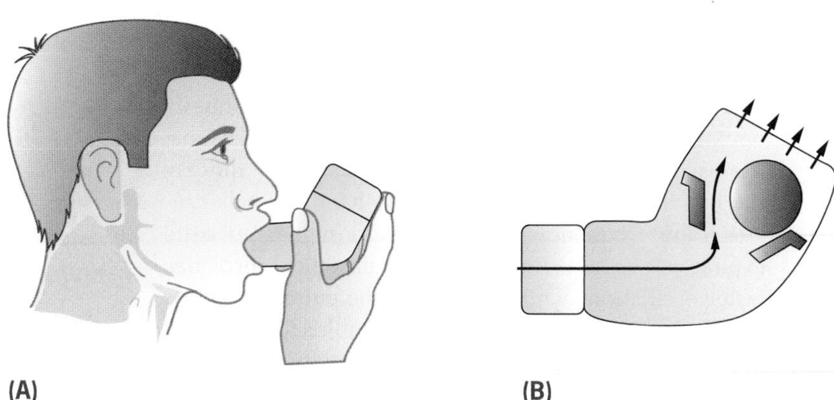

FIGURE 18–14 (**A**) Position of Flutter valve in patient's mouth. (**B**) During exhalation, the position of the steel ball is the result of an equilibrium between the pressure of the exhaled gas, the force of gravity on the ball, and the angle of the cone where the contact with the ball occurs. As the steel ball rolls and bounces up and down, it creates oscillations in the airway.

BOX 18–8

Procedure for Oscillatory Positive Expiratory Pressure with Flutter Device

1. Position the patient so that he or she is sitting upright with back straight and slightly extended, head upward, with relaxed breathing control technique.
2. Have the patient inhale at two to three times greater than a normal breath and breath-hold for 2 to 3 seconds.
3. Place the Flutter device mouthpiece in the mouth and have the patient exhale at twice the flow of a normal exhalation. Continue the exhalation until lungs reach functional residual capacity.
4. Discourage unproductive coughing episodes during the initial secretion-loosening breaths.
5. During exhalation through the Flutter device, advise the patient to adjust the horizontal tilt of the Flutter to the angle that best gives the sensation of vibration within the lungs.
6. Following multiple loosening breaths, instruct the patient to take a very deep breath, hold it for 2 to 3 seconds, and then forcefully exhale through the device until lungs reach functional residual capacity.
7. After one or two high-volume, high-expiratory-flow mucus-clearance breaths, have the patient do a huff or other effective expiratory maneuver.
8. Additional therapy sequences, identical to the above described procedure, should be performed during the therapy session, until lungs are clear or until the predetermined treatment period has elapsed.

From Myers TR. Positive expiratory pressure and oscillatory positive expiratory pressure therapies. *Respir Care.* 2007;52:1308–1327. Reprinted with permission.

and proper operation. The Flutter can be tilted (referred to as tuning) slightly upward or downward to change the vibration frequency.

The Acapella (**Figure 18–15**) uses a counterweighted plug and magnet to create airflow oscillations during expiratory flow.[68] It comes in three models: the green model, for patients with expiratory flow above 15 L/min; the blue model, for patients with expiratory flows below 15 L/min; and the Choice model, which can be disassembled and can withstand autoclaving, boiling, or dishwashing. A bench study comparison of the Acapella and Flutter devices concluded that both have similar operating performance characteristics.[69] The Acapella's performance is not gravity dependent, and the device may be easier to use for some patients.

The Quake device (**Figure 18–16**) has a manually operated rotating handle that creates the oscillations; the oscillation frequency is controlled by how quickly the handle is rotated.[68] Rotating the handle slowly creates a low-frequency oscillation and a higher pulsatile expiratory pressure. Rotating the handle quickly provides faster oscillations while decreasing the pulsatile expiratory pressure. The Quake can be dissembled for cleaning, and its operation and function are not gravity dependent.

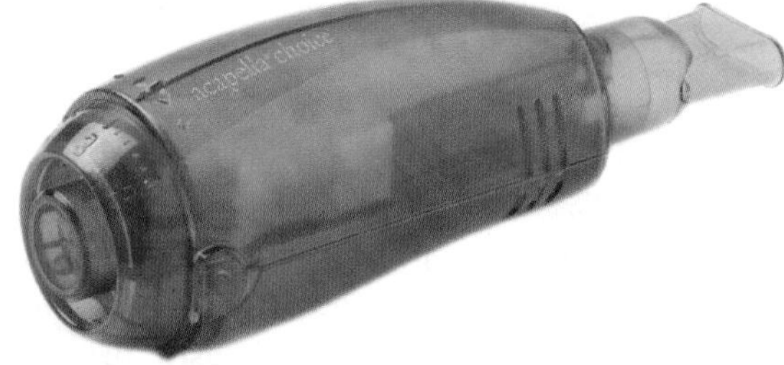

FIGURE 18–15 Acapella device.

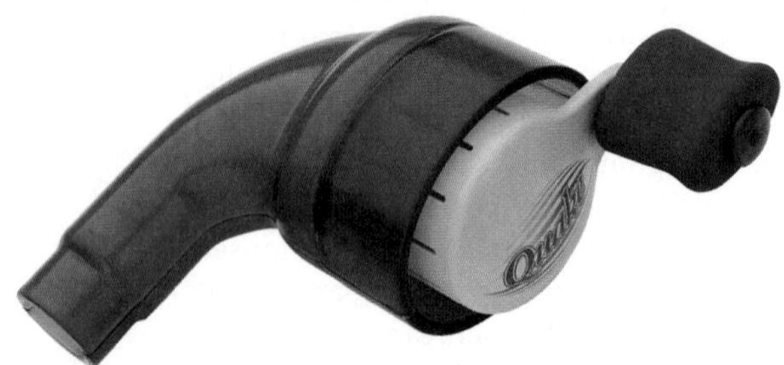

FIGURE 18–16 Quake device.

High-Frequency Chest Wall Compression

High-frequency chest wall compression (HFCWC) generates negative changes in transrespiratory pressure difference by compressing the chest externally (i.e., body surface pressure goes positive relative to the pressure at the airway opening, which remains at atmospheric pressure) to cause short, rapid expiratory flow pulses, and relies on chest wall elastic recoil to return the lungs to functional residual capacity. HFCWC is accomplished by encasing the chest in an inflatable vest.[70] A high-output compressor rapidly inflates and deflates the vest. On inflation, pressure is exerted on the body surface (range 5–20 cm H_2O), which forces the chest wall to compress and generates a short burst of expiratory flow. Pressure pulses are superimposed on a small (about 12 cm H_2O) positive pressure baseline. On deflation, the chest wall recoils to its resting position, causing inspiratory flow.

The Vest Airway Clearance System operates at 2 to 25 Hz and generates esophageal pressure and airflow oscillations as shown in **Figure 18–17**. HFCWC can generate volume changes of 17 to 57 mL and flows up to 1.6 L/s. This produces mini-coughs to mobilize secretions. HFCWC causes a decrease in end-expiratory lung volume, but the consequences of that decrease are debatable.[71] Other commercially available HFCWC devices include the InCourage system and the SmartVest (**Figure 18–18**). **Box 18–9** describes the procedure for use of HFCWC.

Intrapulmonary Percussive Ventilation

Intrapulmonary percussive ventilation (IPV) creates positive changes in transrespiratory difference by injecting short, rapid inspiratory flow pulses into the airway opening and relies on chest wall elastic recoil for passive exhalation.[70] It delivers high-flow mini-bursts of air, along with an aerosolized medication to the lungs, at a rate of 300 to 400 per minute. The Percussionator (**Figure 18–19**) operates at 1.7 to 5 Hz. Treatments last about 15 to 20 minutes. It can be used with a mouthpiece or mask. Similar devices include the Breas IMP2, which operates at about 1 to 6 Hz and can also deliver aerosol medication, and the single-patient-use PercussiveNeb. The PercussiveNeb operates at frequencies of 11 to 30 Hz and can also deliver an aerosolized medication. It cannot be used with a ventilator. All three devices produce roughly comparable pressure waveforms (**Figure 18–20**). These devices produce higher pressure amplitudes

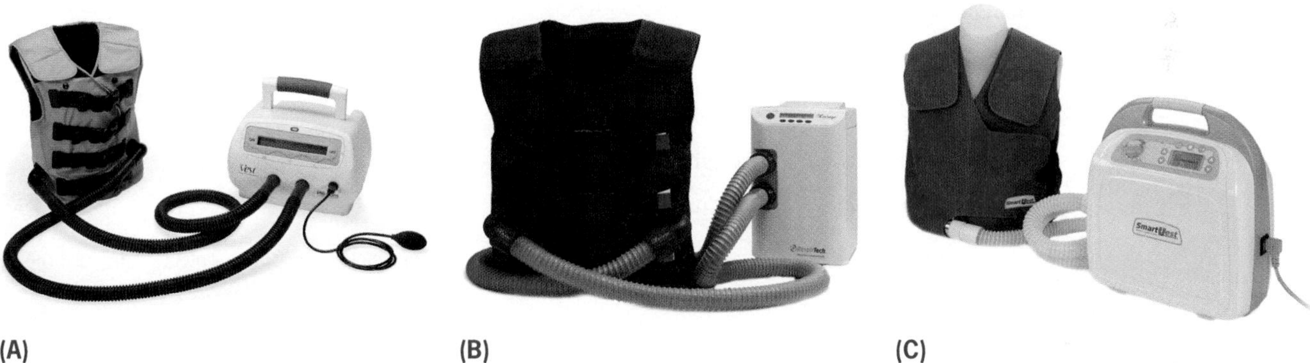

FIGURE 18–17 (**A**) Vest® Airway Clearance System. (**B**) InCourage device for high-frequency chest wall compression (HFCWC). (**C**) SmartVest device for HFCWC. (**A**) © 2010 Hill-Rom Services, Inc. Reprinted with permission—all rights reserved.

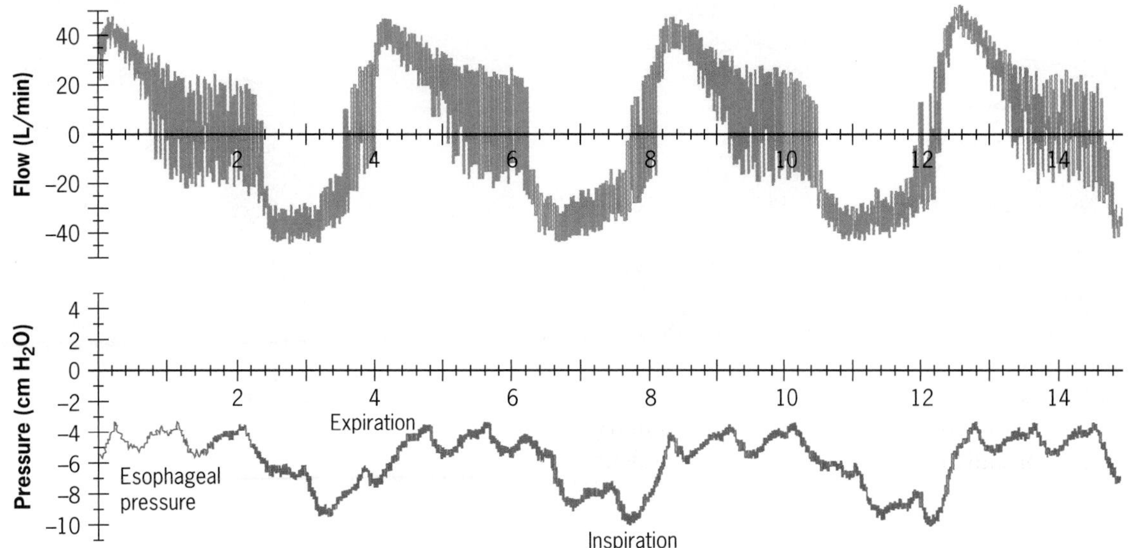

FIGURE 18–18 Flow, airway pressure, and esophageal pressure waveforms while breathing with the Vest Airway Clearance System. From Fink JB, Mahlmeister MJ. High-frequency oscillation of the airway and chest wall. *Respir Care.* 2002;47(7):797–807. Reprinted with permission.

BOX 18–9

Procedure for High-Frequency Chest Wall Compression

Ramping Session Using Hill-Rom Vest

Frequency	Pressure	Time
6, 8, 10 Hz	10	5 minutes at each frequency Pause machine and cough three times Resume session
16, 18, 20 Hz	6	5 minutes at each frequency Pause machine and cough three times Resume session

Therapy Session with InCourage

1. Push Quick Start button to initiate preprogrammed 30-minute automatic ramping session.
2. Pause button may be pushed at any time to allow for coughing.
3. Push Run button to resume therapy.
4. Pressure can be increased or decreased during therapy session.

Standard Protocol for SmartVest

Frequency	Duration
10 Hz	10 minutes, then huff cough
12 Hz	10 minutes, then huff cough
14 Hz	10 minutes, then huff cough

From Lester MK, Flume PA. Airway-clearance therapy guidelines and implementation. *Respir Care.* 2009;54:733–753. Reprinted with permission.

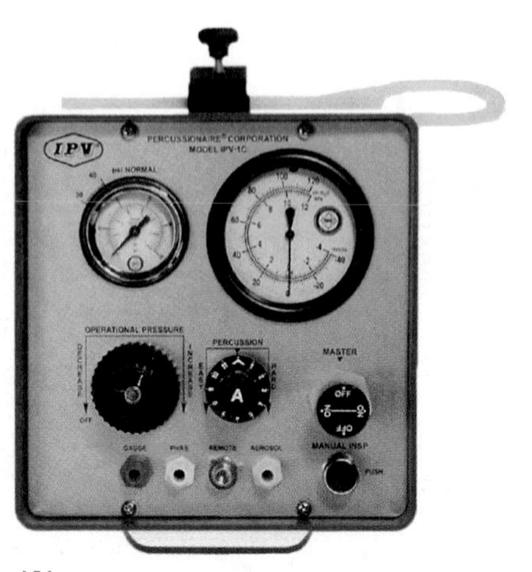

(A)

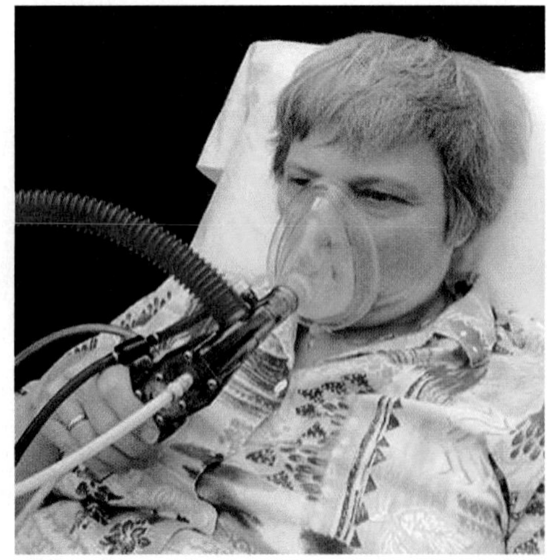

(B)

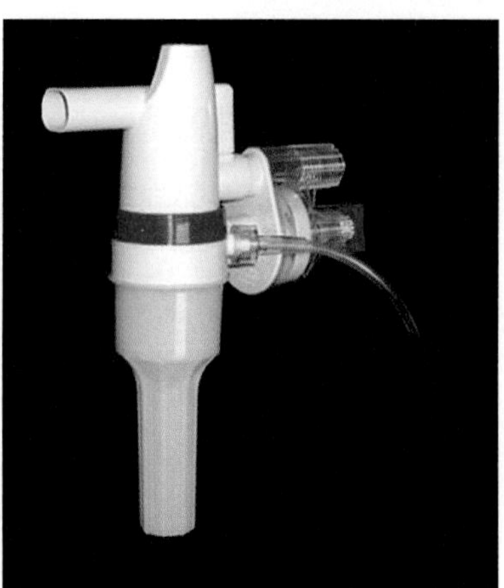

(C)

FIGURE 18–19 (**A**) Percussionaire Percussionator. (**B**) Patient using Percussionator. (**C**) VORTRAN® PercussiveNeb.

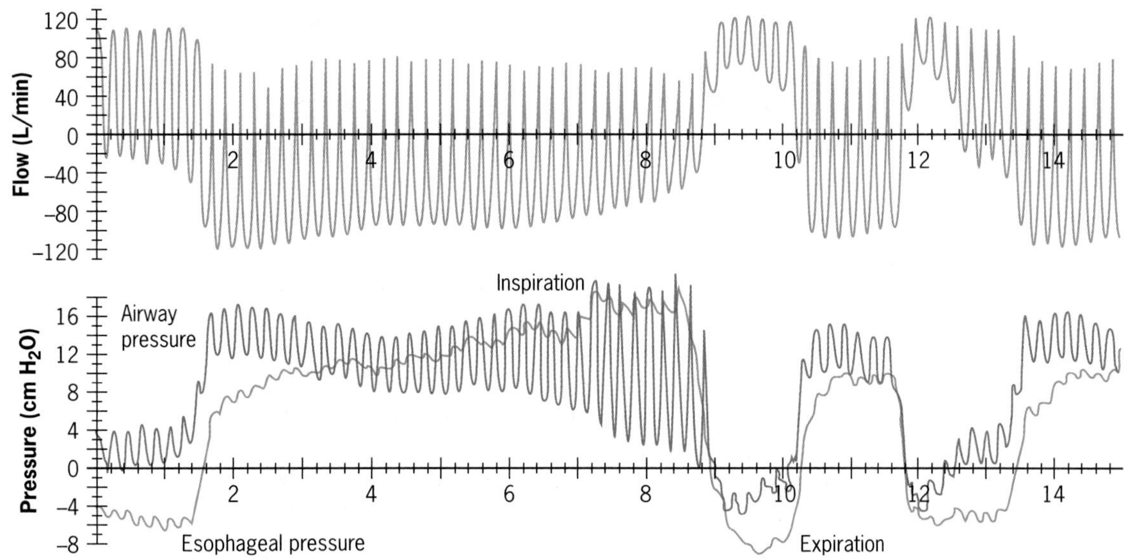

FIGURE 18–20 Flow, airway pressure, and esophageal pressure waveforms while breathing with an intrapulmonary percussive ventilator. From Fink JB, Mahlmeister MJ. High-frequency oscillation of the airway and chest wall. *Respir Care.* 2002;47(7): 797–807. Reprinted with permission.

than unassisted high-frequency airway clearance devices such as the Flutter and Acapella.[72] Each device delivers flow oscillations with normal spontaneous breathing.

High-Frequency Chest Wall Oscillation

High-frequency chest wall oscillation (HFCWO) uses a chest cuirass to generate biphasic changes in transrespiratory pressure difference.[70] The Hayek oscillator is an electrically powered, microprocessor-controlled, noninvasive oscillator ventilator that uses an external flexible chest enclosure (cuirass) to apply negative and positive pressure to the chest wall to deliver noninvasive oscillation to the lungs (**Figure 18–21**). The negative pressure generated in the cuirass causes the chest wall to expand for inspiration, whereas positive pressure compresses the chest to produce a forced expiration. Both inspiratory and expiratory phases may be active and not reliant on passive recoil of the chest. Expiratory pressure can be positive, atmospheric, or negative, allowing ventilation to occur above, at, or below the patient's normal FRC. Success has been reported with this device as a method of ventilatory support.[73] Four adjustable parameters with the Hayek include frequency range (to 999 oscillations per minute), I:E ratio (6:1 to 1:6), inspiratory pressure, and expiratory pressure (–70 to +70 cm H_2O).

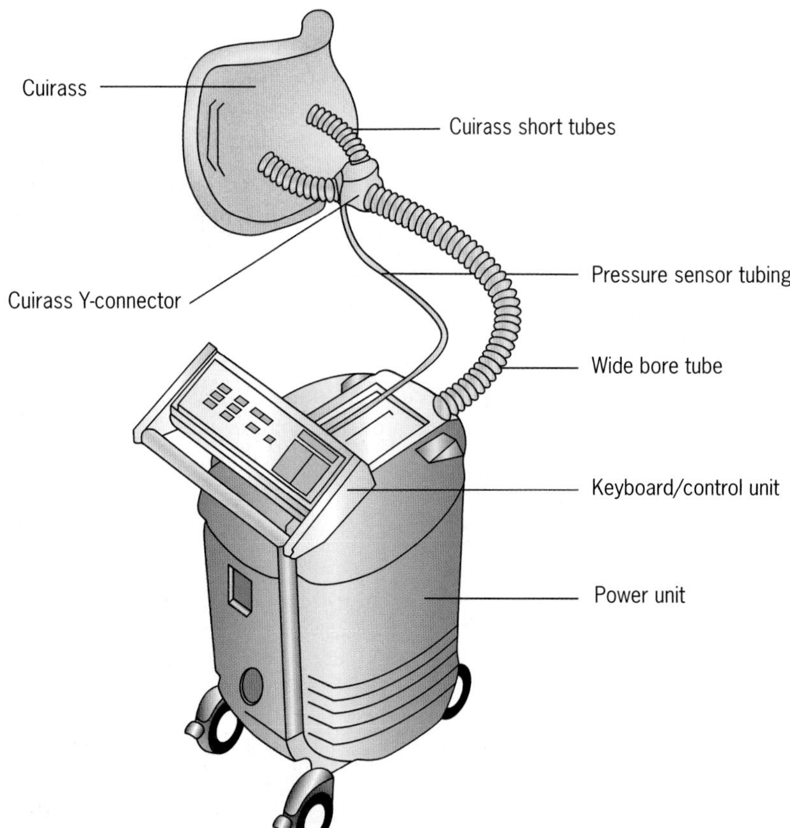

FIGURE 18–21 Schematic drawing of the Hayek oscillator. Adapted from materials courtesy of Breasy Medical Equipment, Stamford, Conn.

Clinicians' anecdotal observations of spontaneous expulsion of secretions during high-frequency ventilation have led to the development of several discrete secretion management program recommendations in which the chest is oscillated through two sets of cycles: several minutes at a high frequency of up to 999 per minute (usually 600 to 720 per minute) at an I:E ratio of 1:1, followed by 60 or 90 cycles per minute at an I:E ratio of 5:1. The setting can be changed according to the patient's need. Reports of efficacy of this or similar protocols for secretion management with the Hayek oscillator have yet to be published. It has been reported that high-frequency oscillation applied via the airway or via the chest wall and CPT have comparable augmenting effects on expectorated sputum.[73]

Exercise

Exercise causes increased sputum production compared with rest.[74,75] Exercise appears to augment bronchial hygiene and should be encouraged as tolerated; however, it should not substitute for other bronchial hygiene regimens.

Selection of Airway Clearance Technique

Several Cochrane reviews have evaluated airway clearance techniques for patients with cystic fibrosis. In a review that compared chest physiotherapy with no chest physiotherapy for cystic fibrosis, it was shown that airway clearance techniques have short-term effects in terms of increasing mucus transport; no evidence was found on which to draw conclusions concerning the long-term effects.[50] A review that compared conventional CPT with other airway clearance techniques for cystic fibrosis was unable to demonstrate any advantage of conventional CPT over other airway clearance techniques in terms of respiratory function, but there was a trend for participants to prefer self-administered airway clearance techniques.[76] Another review concluded that there was no clear evidence that PEP was a more or less effective intervention overall than other forms of physiotherapy, but there was limited evidence that PEP was preferred by participants compared with other techniques.[76] Similarly, there was no clear evidence that oscillation was a more or less effective intervention overall than other forms of physiotherapy.[77]

Guidelines of the Cystic Fibrosis Foundation recommend that airway clearance be performed on a regular basis in all patients with cystic fibrosis.[78] However, there is no airway clearance therapy that has been demonstrated to be superior to others. For the individual, one form of airway clearance therapy may be superior to the others. Thus, the prescription of airway clearance therapy should be individualized based on factors such as age, patient preference, and adverse events, among others. Aerobic exercise is recommended for patients with cystic fibrosis as an adjunctive therapy for airway clearance and its additional benefits to overall health. One of the important considerations in selection of an airway clearance technique is the age of the patient (**Figure 18–22**), because some therapies are not appropriate for all age groups.

Guidelines of the British Thoracic Society (BTS) and the Association of Chartered Physiotherapists in Respiratory Care (ACPRC) recommend the following regarding airway clearance.[79] For COPD:

- Consider the active cycle of breathing techniques (which include the forced expiratory technique), autogenic drainage, and plain or oscillating positive expiratory pressure for patients with stable COPD who need an airway clearance technique to assist in the removal of secretions.
- Incorporate postural drainage only if it further aids clearance and has no detrimental effects.

For cystic fibrosis:

- Teach patients with cystic fibrosis an airway clearance technique to increase mucus transport in the short term.
- Self-administered techniques should be the first-line airway clearance techniques offered in order to improve adherence to treatment.
- Patient preference for techniques should be considered in order to improve adherence to treatment.
- Individually assess the effect and acceptability of gravity-assisted positioning in patients with cystic fibrosis.
- Individually assess the effect and acceptability of modified gravity-assisted positioning in individual patients with cystic fibrosis.

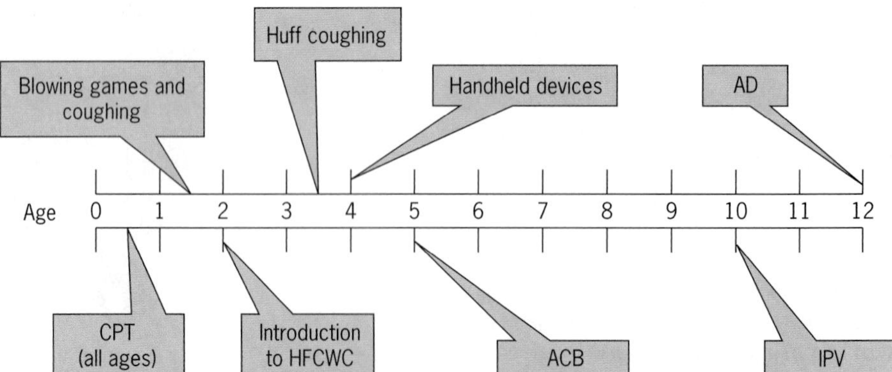

FIGURE 18–22 Various airway clearance techniques based on the patient's age and ability to perform the therapy. AD, autogenic drainage; CPT, conventional chest physiotherapy; HFCWC, high-frequency chest wall compression; ACB, active cycle breathing technique; IPV, intrapulmonary percussive ventilation. From Lester MK, Flume PA. Airway-clearance therapy guidelines and implementation. *Respir Care.* 2009;54:733–753. Reprinted with permission.

- If patients using independent techniques are unable to clear secretions effectively, chest wall vibration should be considered.
- Consider the active cycle of breathing techniques when recommending an airway clearance technique for adults with cystic fibrosis.
- Consider autogenic drainage when recommending an airway clearance technique for adults with cystic fibrosis.
- Consider positive expiratory pressure when recommending an airway clearance technique for adults with cystic fibrosis.
- Consider oscillating positive expiratory pressure devices when recommending an airway clearance technique for adults with cystic fibrosis.
- Exercise in isolation should not be used as an airway clearance technique for patients with cystic fibrosis unless adherence to other techniques is problematic.
- The addition of exercise to an appropriate physiotherapy regimen should be considered to increase airway clearance further.
- Consider high-frequency chest wall compression or oscillation when recommending an airway clearance technique for adults with cystic fibrosis.
- High-frequency chest wall oscillation is not recommended during an infective exacerbation.
- Consider mechanical vibration when recommending an airway clearance technique for adults with cystic fibrosis.
- Consider intrapulmonary percussive ventilation when recommending an airway clearance technique for adults with mild to moderate cystic fibrosis.
- Consider the addition of hypertonic saline when enhancing the effectiveness of an airway clearance technique.
- A predose bronchodilator should be used to minimize bronchospasm with inhalation of hypertonic saline.
- A bronchoconstriction trial should be carried out at the initial dose of hypertonic saline to ensure safety and suitability for the patient.
- Recombinant human deoxyribonuclease (dornase alfa) should be prescribed as per national and local guidelines.
- Consider the use of inhaled dornase alfa for enhancing airway clearance effectiveness.
- Consider inhalation therapy with dornase alfa for increasing exercise capacity.

For neuromuscular disease:

- Peak cough flow should be measured regularly in patients with neuromuscular disease.
- Measure peak cough flow additionally at the time of an acute respiratory tract infection.
- When peak cough flow is equal to or less than 270 L/min in a medically stable patient, introduce strategies for assisted airway clearance to raise it above 270 L/min.
- When peak cough flow is equal to or less than 160 L/min, additional strategies to assist secretion clearance must be used.
- If peak cough flow remains equal to or less than 160 L/min despite additional strategies, contact medical colleagues to discuss ventilation and/or airway management needs.
- When oxygen saturation falls below 95%, the use of noninvasive ventilation and/or strategies to aid airway clearance should be considered.
- Use some form of maximal insufflation strategy to improve effective cough generation when vital capacity falls below 1500 mL or 50% predicted.
- Use single maximal insufflation techniques for patients with bulbar dysfunction who are unable to breath stack.
- Teach patients without bulbar muscle involvement unaided breath stacking to improve cough effectiveness independently where possible.
- Regular breath stacking (10–15 times three times per day) to maximal insufflation capacity should be performed by patients with vital capacity of less than 2000 mL or 50% predicted.
- Consider teaching glossopharyngeal breathing to patients with reduced vital capacity to maintain range of chest wall movement and pulmonary compliance.
- Consider teaching glossopharyngeal breathing as one of the means of achieving maximal insufflation capacity in patients who have difficulty in clearing secretions.
- Consider teaching glossopharyngeal breathing to ventilator-dependent patients to allow some ventilator-free breathing time.
- Consider teaching glossopharyngeal breathing to patients with decreased voice strength.
- Manually assisted coughing should be used to increase peak cough flow in patients with neuromuscular disease.
- Combine manually assisted coughing with a maximal insufflation capacity strategy.
- Abdominal thrusts should be performed standing in front of the patient when possible to assist communication.
- Consider mechanical insufflation–exsufflation as a treatment option in patients with bulbar muscle involvement who are unable to breath stack.
- Consider mechanical insufflation–exsufflation for any patient who remains unable to increase peak cough flow to effective levels with other strategies.

- Where cough effectiveness remains inadequate with mechanical insufflation–exsufflation alone, combine it with manually assisted coughing.
- Intrapulmonary percussive ventilation may be considered for patients with neuromuscular disease to aid loosening of secretions prior to removal where there is evidence of sputum retention and other techniques have failed.
- In patients with ineffective cough, assisted cough strategies must be used additionally to increase cough effectiveness.
- Patients using intrapulmonary percussive ventilation must be monitored closely during and after treatment for any adverse response.

For patients in the intensive care unit, recommendations for airway clearance have been made by the European Respiratory Society and the European Society of Intensive Care Medicine Task Force on Physiotherapy for Critically Ill Patients.[80] Following are their recommendations for the nonintubated patient:

- Interventions for increasing inspiratory volume should be used if reduced inspiratory volume is contributing to ineffective forced expiration.
- Interventions for increasing expiratory flow should be used to assist airway clearance if reduced expiratory force is contributing to ineffective forced expiration.
- Manually assisted cough techniques and/or insufflation–exsufflation should be applied in the management of nonintubated patients with retained secretions secondary to respiratory muscle weakness.
- Oronasal suctioning should be used only when other methods fail to clear secretions.
- Nasal suctioning should be used with extreme caution in patients with anticoagulation, bony or soft tissue injuries, or after recent surgery of the upper airways.

Their recommendations for the intubated patient are as follows:

- Body positioning and mobilization can be used to enhance airway secretion clearance.
- Manual or ventilator hyperinflation and suctioning are indicated for airway secretion clearance.
- Manual hyperinflation should be used judiciously in patients at risk of barotrauma and volutrauma or who are hemodynamically unstable.
- Care must be taken to ensure that overventilation or underventilation does not occur with manual hyperinflation.
- Airway pressures must be maintained within safe limits (e.g., by incorporating a pressure manometer into the manual hyperinflation circuit).
- Reassurance, sedation, and preoxygenation should be used to minimize detrimental effects of airway suctioning.
- Neither suctioning nor instillation of normal saline should be performed routinely.

It has been suggested that the following hierarchy of questions might be asked when considering secretion clearance therapy for a patient.[81–83]

1. Is there a pathophysiologic rationale for use of the therapy? Is the patient experiencing difficulty clearing secretions? Are retained secretions affecting lung function in an important way, such as gas exchange or lung mechanics? Note that the production of large amounts of sputum does not necessarily mean that the patient is experiencing difficulty clearing sputum.
2. What is the potential for adverse effects from the therapy? Which therapy is likely to provide the greatest benefit with the least harm?
3. What is the cost of the equipment for this therapy? The cost of the device may not be covered by third-party insurers, resulting in considerable out-of-pocket expense for the patient or the hospital.
4. What are the preferences of the patient? Lacking evidence that any technique is superior to another, patient preference is an important consideration.

When a clinical decision is made to try a secretion clearance technique, a simple clinical trial can be conducted (*n*-of-1 trial).[81–83] Imagine that a decision is made to try PEP therapy for a patient with chronic obstructive pulmonary disease. The clinician and patient agree that a clinically useful outcome measure is fewer symptoms related to chest congestion and coughing up phlegm. A randomized controlled trial is designed. PEP is used for 2 weeks, a sham device is used for 2 weeks, and this process is repeated three times. The patient, who is naive to the therapy, does not know which device is potentially therapeutic. The order of treatments is randomized (the patient flips a coin), and the sequence is repeated four times. Each day, the sputum produced during the therapy session is weighed. A diary also is kept, in which events such as chest infections and other symptoms are logged. At the end of 12 weeks, the results are analyzed (which may include statistical analysis), reviewed together by the clinician and patient, and a collaborative decision is made regarding the benefit of the therapy. In this manner, an objective decision is made regarding the benefits of this therapy for this individual patient.

Lung Expansion Therapy

Incentive Spirometry

Incentive spirometry (IS) is a technique designed to mimic natural sighing or yawning maneuvers, also referred to as *sustained maximal inspiration* (**CPG 18–5**).[84] Because postoperative patients often adopt a pattern of rapid, shallow breathing, they should be encouraged to take 5 to 10 deep breaths every hour. Incisional pain

CLINICAL PRACTICE GUIDELINE 18–5

Incentive Spirometry

Indications

- Presence of conditions predisposing to the development of pulmonary atelectasis, such as upper abdominal surgery, thoracic surgery, surgery in patients with chronic obstructive pulmonary disease
- Presence of pulmonary atelectasis
- Presence of a restrictive lung defect associated with quadriplegia and/or dysfunctional diaphragm

Contraindications

- Patient cannot be instructed or supervised to ensure appropriate use of the device.
- Patient cooperation is absent, or patient is unable to understand or demonstrate use of the device.
- Incentive spirometry is contraindicated in patients unable to deep breathe effectively (e.g., with vital capacity less than about 10 mL/kg or inspiratory capacity less than about one-third of predicted).
- The presence of an open tracheal stoma is not a contraindication but requires adaptation of the spirometer.

Hazards and Complications

- Ineffective unless closely supervised or performed as ordered
- Inappropriate as sole treatment for major lung collapse or consolidation
- Hyperventilation
- Barotraumas
- Discomfort secondary to inadequate pain control
- Hypoxia secondary to interruption of prescribed oxygen therapy
- Exacerbation of bronchospasm
- Fatigue

Modified from AARC clinical practice guideline: incentive spirometry. *Respir Care.* 1991;36:1402–1405. Reprinted with permission.

RESPIRATORY RECAP

Inflation Therapy

» Incentive spirometry
» Intermittent positive pressure breathing

and splinting may make those breaths painful after upper abdominal surgery, so IS provides patients with sensory feedback to quantify the depth of the breath. IS should provide patients with an objective comparison to the volumes (of flows) they were generating preoperatively, with the goal of attaining or returning to that preoperative volume in spite of the pain experienced. In addition, the IS device instruction should include recording how long breaths are to be held, how many times the breaths were attempted, and how many times the patient succeeded in meeting his or her volume goals (**Box 18–10**).

Objectives of IS are to increase transpulmonary pressure and inspiratory volumes to near-preoperative vital capacity, improve inspiratory muscle performance, and reestablish the normal pattern of periodic deep breathing. It should not be used as the sole treatment for major lung collapse or consolidation, but rather as a part of a more comprehensive program of lung reexpansion. Because IS requires patient cooperation, as well as the ability to understand and demonstrate proper use of the device, IS is not a viable therapeutic option for the obtunded, confused, or uncooperative patient.

Evidence suggests that deep breathing alone, without mechanical aids, may be as beneficial as IS in preventing or reversing pulmonary complications, and controversy exists concerning overuse of IS. If the patient can take deep breaths without IS, he or she should be encouraged to do so at regular intervals. Deep breathing, coughing, and IS work best as shared tasks among all clinicians in the surgical units, with each clinician providing frequent reminders to the patient.

BOX 18–10

Procedure for Incentive Spirometry

1. Explain to the patient the importance of deep breathing and coughing.
2. Establish the volume goal for incentive spirometry.
3. Assist the patient to a sitting or semi-Fowler position.
4. Instruct or assist the patient to splint incision when appropriate.
5. Instruct patient to do the following:
   a. Place the spirometer on a flat surface or hold in an upright position.
   b. Place lips firmly around the mouthpiece.
   c. After a normal exhalation, inhale slowly through the mouthpiece, raising the flow/volume indicator while taking as deep a breath as possible.
   d. Hold breath for 3 to 5 seconds.
   e. Remove mouthpiece and exhale normally.
   f. Relax and breathe normally for several breaths.
   g. Repeat the maneuver for 10 breaths each session.
6. Have patient repeat series of breaths once each hour while awake.
7. Visit patient periodically to reinforce instruction.
8. Document procedure and patient response in the medical record.

The need for IS should focus on factors such as surgical procedures involving the upper abdomen or thorax, conditions predisposing to development of atelectasis (e.g., immobility, poor pain control, abdominal binders), and the presence of neuromuscular disease involving the respiratory muscles. Outcome assessment should include improvement of atelectasis (e.g., decreased respiratory rate, improved breath sounds, normal chest x-ray films, improved Pa_{O_2}), increased vital capacity to preoperative values (in absence of lung resection), and improved inspiratory muscle performance.

Most IS devices direct the patient's inspiratory flow through a tube to lift one or more light balls (or disks). The higher the patient's inspiratory flow, the higher the ball is raised or the greater the number of balls that are raised (**Figure 18–23**). The longer the flow is maintained, the larger the volume, so the patient is encouraged to take slow, deep breaths. Unfortunately, high flows can be generated (with low volumes) to raise the flow indicator to target levels without the patient meeting therapeutic volume or breath-holding objectives. Although flow-oriented IS devices impose an additional work of breathing,[84] it is unclear whether this additional workload is deleterious or a beneficial part of the therapy.

Successful use of IS devices depends on patient education and compliance. Although there are no clinically important differences among IS devices, a reduced frequency of use decreases their efficacy.[85] IS is comparable in therapeutic effect to deep breathing exercises, coughing, early mobilization, and intermittent positive pressure breathing in the postoperative patient. IS is comparable to CPT after abdominal surgery,[86] whereas mounting evidence suggests that IS may not have a viable role in treatment of patients who have had thoracic surgery and have healthy lungs.[87]

Intermittent Positive Pressure Breathing

Intermittent positive pressure breathing (IPPB) is short-term or episodic mechanical ventilation for the primary purpose of assisting ventilation and providing short-duration hyperinflation therapy (**CPG 18–6**). IPPB is usually administered with pneumatically driven, pressure-triggered, and pressure-cycled ventilators (**Figure 18–24** and **Box 18–11**). IPPB was first described in 1947. In the 1950s, it gained popularity as a method to treat and prevent postoperative atelectasis. In the 1960s, IPPB became a popular therapy for patients with pulmonary disease. In the 1970s, IPPB came under scrutiny both scientifically and by healthcare payers. Although IPPB has been used as a method for administration of aerosolized medication, it has no advantage over nebulizers or metered dose inhalers. In fact, it has been demonstrated that aerosols administered with IPPB deposit 32% less of the drug in the lungs than a handheld nebulizer.[88] All of the mechanical effects of IPPB are short lived, lasting an hour or less after the treatment. Efficacy of IPPB for ventilation and aerosol delivery is technique dependent (e.g., coordination, breathing pattern, selection of appropriate inspiratory flow, peak pressure, inspiratory hold). Efficacy is dependent on the design of the device (e.g., flow,

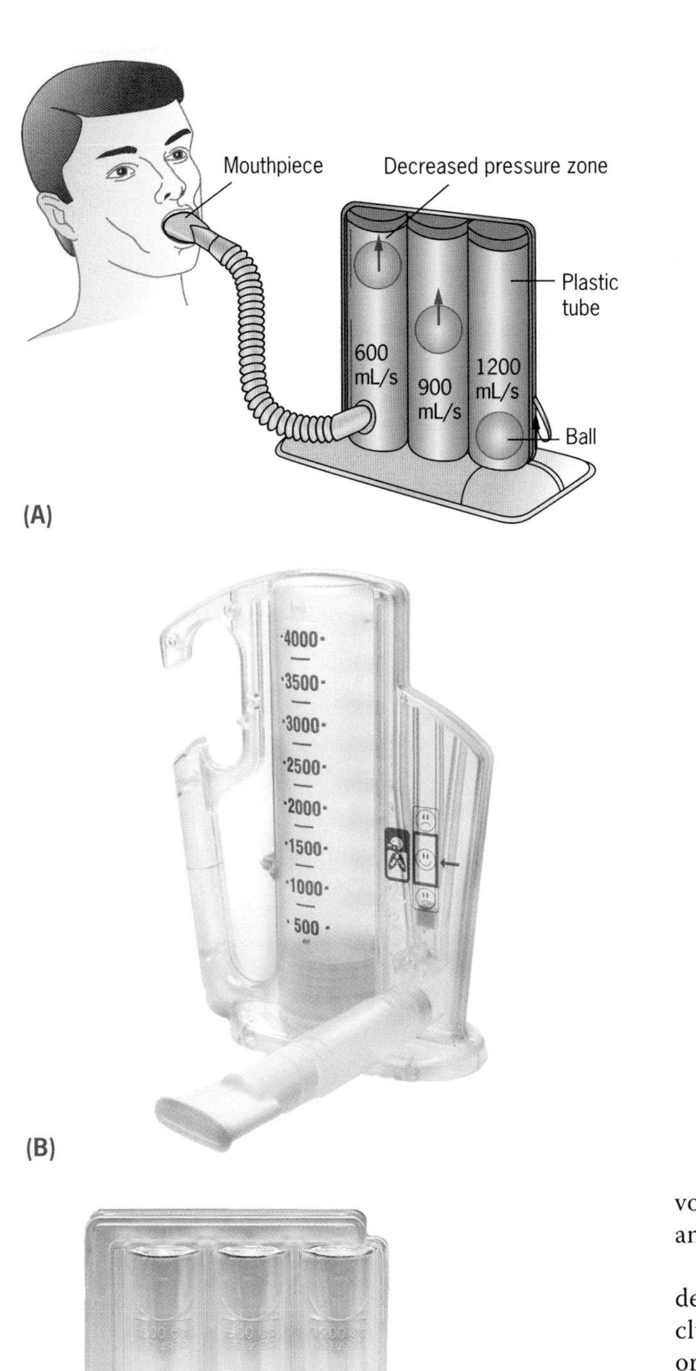

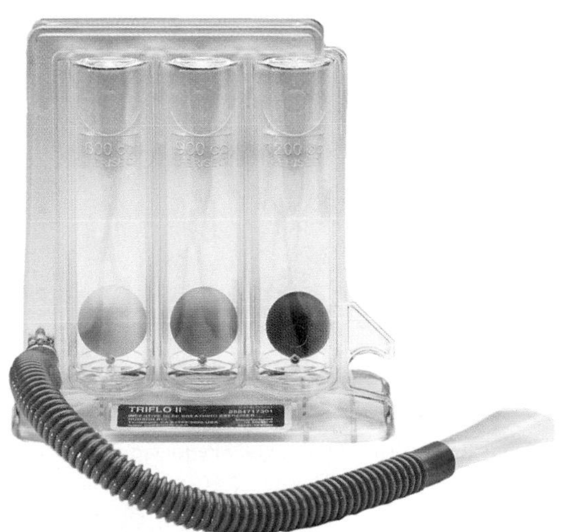

FIGURE 18–23 (**A**) Flow-oriented incentive spirometer. (**B**) Commercially available incentive spirometers. (**A**) Adapted from Eubanks DH, Bone RC. *Comprehensive Respiratory Care.* Mosby; 1985.

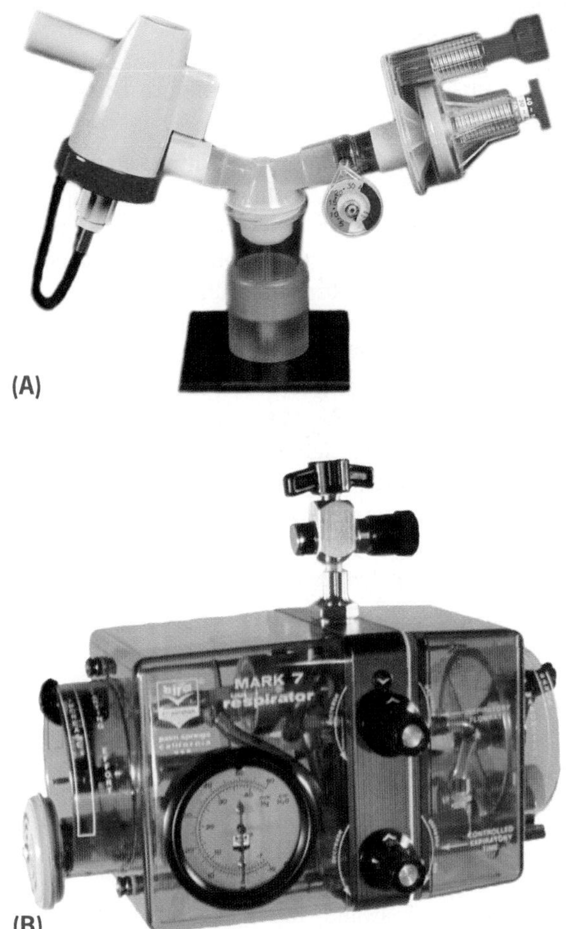

FIGURE 18–24 (**A**) VORTRAN® intermittent positive pressure breathing (IPPB) device. (**B**) Bird Mark 7 from IPPB therapy.

volume, pressure capability) and on the aerosol output and particle size.

Assessment of the need for IPPB should include evidence of atelectasis, reduced pulmonary function precluding an effective cough, neuromuscular disorders, or kyphoscoliosis with decreased lung volumes. IPPB may be applicable in situations of fatigue or muscle weakness with impending respiratory failure, in the presence of acute severe bronchospasm, and in COPD exacerbation that fails to respond to other therapy. IPPB should be volume oriented, with tidal volume during IPPB adjusted to deliver breaths that are at least 25% larger than the patient's tidal volume. The effects of IPPB can be assessed by improved secretion clearance, breath sounds, chest x-ray film, and dyspnea. IPPB has not been shown to have any benefit greater than other lung expansion techniques in spontaneously breathing patients.[89–91] Its use for lung expansion should be considered only after other alternatives have been exhausted.

CLINICAL PRACTICE GUIDELINE 18–6

Intermittent Positive Pressure Breathing

Indications

- The need to improve lung expansion; the presence of clinically important pulmonary atelectasis when other forms of therapy have been unsuccessful (e.g., incentive spirometry, chest physiotherapy, deep breathing exercises, positive airway pressure) or the patient cannot cooperate; inability to clear secretions adequately because of pathologic process that severely limits the ability to ventilate or cough effectively; and failure to respond to other modes of treatment.
- The need for short-term ventilatory support for patients who are hypoventilated as an alternative to tracheal intubation and continuous ventilatory support.
- The need to deliver aerosol medication. Intermittent positive pressure breathing (IPPB) may be used to deliver aerosol medications to patients with fatigue as a result of ventilatory muscle weakness (e.g., failure to wean from mechanical ventilation, neuromuscular disease, kyphoscoliosis) or chronic conditions in which intermittent ventilatory support is indicated (e.g., ventilatory support for home care patients and the more recent use of nasal intermittent positive pressure ventilation for respiratory insufficiency).

Contraindications

- Pneumothorax
- Intracranial pressure >15 mm Hg
- Hemodynamic instability
- Recent surgery to face or mouth or skull
- Tracheoesophageal fistula
- Recent esophageal surgery
- Active hemoptysis
- Nausea
- Air swallowing
- Active untreated tuberculosis
- Radiographic evidence of bleb
- Singultations (hiccups)

Hazards and Complications

- Increased airway resistance
- Barotrauma
- Nosocomial infection
- Hypocarbia
- Hemoptysis
- Hyperoxia when oxygen is the gas source
- Gastric distention
- Impaction of secretions associated with inadequately humidified gas mixture
- Psychologic dependence
- Impedance of venous return
- Exacerbation of hypoxemia
- Hypoventilation
- Increased mismatch of ventilation and perfusion
- Air trapping

Modified from AARC clinical practice guideline: incentive spirometry. *Respir Care.* 1993;38:1189–1195. Reprinted with permission.

BOX 18-11

Procedure for Intermittent Positive Pressure Breathing (IPPB) Therapy

1. Assess the need for IPPB and determine whether another therapy might be equally efficacious or superior.
2. Assemble necessary equipment.
3. Explain therapy to patient.
4. Determine appropriate interface: mouthpiece with lip seal, or mask.
5. Instruct patient to do the following:
   a. Sit comfortably.
   b. If using a mask, apply it tightly but comfortably over the nose and mouth; if mouthpiece is used, place lips firmly around it and breathe through mouth.
   c. Begin breathing to trigger the IPPB machine.
   d. Allow the machine to passively inflate the lungs to a volume that is larger than normal.
6. Make appropriate adjustments on the IPPB machine:
   a. Flow for I:E ratio of approximately 1:3
   b. Pressure to deliver an appropriate volume
7. Monitor inspiratory time and observe patient to prevent hyperventilation.
8. Encourage the patient to rest and cough as needed; do not exceed 20 minutes of treatment.
9. Rinse mouthpiece or mask, nebulizer, and manifold assembly with sterile water.
10. Document settings used, volume achieved, and patient response.

KEY POINTS

- Mucociliary transport is responsible for normal clearance of secretions from the lower respiratory tract.
- Cough is responsible for secretion clearance in acute and chronic respiratory disease.
- Techniques for sputum collection include cough, induced sputum, tracheal aspiration, bronchoscopy, mini-bronchoalveolar lavage, and transtracheal aspiration.
- Airway suctioning, nasotracheal suctioning, and bronchoscopy are used to mechanically clear secretions from the lower respiratory tract.
- Conventional chest physiotherapy consists of postural drainage, percussion, and vibration.
- Active cycle of breathing techniques consist of breathing control, thoracic expansion control, and forced expiratory technique.
- Autogenic drainage aims to achieve the highest possible airflow in different generations of bronchi to move secretions.
- Positive expiratory pressure, oscillating positive expiratory pressure, intrapulmonary percussive ventilation, and external chest wall compression are techniques that can be used for airway clearance.
- Incentive spirometry is used to facilitate deep breathing in postoperative patients.
- Intermittent positive pressure breathing is used for short-term hyperinflation therapy.

REFERENCES

1. Rogers DF. Physiology of airway mucus secretion and pathophysiology of hypersecretion. *Respir Care*. 2007;52(9):1134–1149.
2. Van der Schans CP. Bronchial mucus transport. *Respir Care*. 2007;52:1150–1158.
3. King M. Viscoelastic properties of airway mucus. *Fed Proc*. 1980; 39:3080–3085.
4. King M. Rheological requirements for optimal clearance of secretions: ciliary transport versus cough. *Eur J Respir Dis*. 1980; 110(suppl):39–45.
5. King M. Is cystic fibrosis mucus abnormal? *Pediatr Res*. 1981; 15:120–122.
6. King M, Kelly S, Cosio M. Alteration of airway reactivity by mucus. *Respir Physiol*. 1985;62:47–59.
7. Warwick WJ. Mechanisms of mucus transport. *Eur J Resp Dis*. 1983;127(suppl 64):162–167.
8. Volpe MS, Adams AB, Amato MB, Marini JJ. Ventilation patterns influence airway secretion movement. *Respir Care*. 2008; 53:1287–1294.
9. Irwin RS, Madison JM. The diagnosis and treatment of cough. *N Engl J Med*. 2000;343:1715–1721.
10. Irwin RS. Complications of cough: ACCP evidence-based clinical practice guidelines. *Chest*. 2006;129(1 suppl):54S–58S.
11. Pizzichni MM, Popov TA, Efthimiadis A, et al. Spontaneous and induced sputum to measure indices of airway inflammation in asthma. *Am J Respir Crit Care Med*. 1996;154:866–869.
12. Bhowmik A, Seemungal TA, Sapsford RJ, et al. Comparison of spontaneous and induced sputum for investigation of airway inflammation in chronic obstructive pulmonary disease. *Thorax*. 1998;53:953–956.
13. Jaworski A, Goldberg SK, Walkenstein MD, et al. Utility of immediate postlobectomy fiber-optic bronchoscopy in preventing atelectasis. *Chest*. 1988;94:38–43.
14. Marini JJ, Pierson DJ, Hudson LD. Acute lobar atelectasis: a prospective comparison of fiber-optic bronchoscopy and respiratory therapy. *Am Rev Respir Dis*. 1979;19:971–978.

15. Kollef MH, Bock KR, Richards RD, et al. The safety and diagnostic accuracy of minibronchoalveolar lavage in patients with suspected ventilator-associated pneumonia. *Ann Intern Med.* 1995;122:743–748.
16. Campbell GD Jr. Blinded invasive diagnostic procedures in ventilator-associated pneumonia. *Chest.* 2000117(4 suppl 2): 207S–211S.
17. Fujitani S, Cohen-Melamed MH, Tuttle RP, et al. Comparison of semi-quantitative endotracheal aspirates to quantitative non-bronchoscopic bronchoalveolar lavage in diagnosing ventilator-associated pneumonia. *Respir Care.* 2009;54:1453–1461.
18. Tuttle RP, Cohen MH, Augustine AJ, et al. Utilizing simulation technology for competency skills assessment and a comparison of traditional methods of training to simulation-based training. *Respir Care.* 2007;52:263–270.
19. Boots RJ, Phillips GE, George N, Faoagali JL. Surveillance culture utility and safety using low-volume blind bronchoalveolar lavage in the diagnosis of ventilator-associated pneumonia. *Respirology.* 2008;13:87–96.
20. Fink JB. Forced expiratory technique, directed cough, and autogenic drainage. *Respir Care.* 2007;52:1210–1223.
21. Partridge C, Pryor J, Webber B. Characteristics of the forced expiratory technique. *Physiotherapy.* 1989;75:193–194.
22. Jacobs WR, Zaroukian MH. Coughing and central venous catheter dislodgement. *JPEN.* 1991;15:491–493.
23. Stern RC, Horwitz SJ, Doerslock CF. Neurologic symptoms during coughing paroxysms in cystic fibrosis. *J Pediatr.* 1988; 112:909–912.
24. Ing AJ, Ngu MC, Breslin AB. Chronic persistent cough and gastroesophageal reflux. *Thorax.* 1991;46:479–483.
25. Pryor JA, Webber BA. An evaluation of the forced expiration technique as an adjunct to postural drainage. *Physiotherapy.* 1979;65:304–307.
26. Pryor JA, Webber BA, Hodson ME, et al. Evaluation of the forced expiration technique as an adjunct to postural drainage in the treatment of cystic fibrosis. *Br Med J.* 1979;2:417–418.
27. Bateman JRM, Newman SP, Daunt KM, et al. Is cough as effective as chest physiotherapy in the removal of excessive secretions? *Thorax.* 1981;36:683–687.
28. De Boeck C, Zinman R. Cough versus chest physiotherapy: a comparison of the acute effects on pulmonary function in patients with cystic fibrosis. *Am Rev Respir Dis.* 1984;129:182–185.
29. Webber BA, Hofmeyer JL, Morgan MOL, et al. Effects of postural drainage, incorporating the forced expiration technique, on pulmonary function in cystic fibrosis. *Br J Dis Chest.* 1986; 80:353–359.
30. Bain J, Bishop J, Olinsky A. Evaluation of directed coughing in cystic fibrosis. *Br J Dis Chest.* 1988;82:138–148.
31. Hie T, Pas BG, Roth RD, et al. Huff coughing and airway patency. *Respir Care.* 1979;24:710–713.
32. Sutton PP, Parker RA, Webber BA, et al. Assessment of the forced expiration technique, postural drainage, and directed coughing in chest physiotherapy. *Eur J Respir Dis.* 1983;64:62–68.
33. Hardy KA. A review of airway clearance: new techniques, indications, and recommendations. *Respir Care.* 1994;39:440–452.
34. Pryor JA, Webber BA, Hodson ME, et al. Evaluation of the forced expiration technique as an adjunct to postural drainage in the treatment of cystic fibrosis. *Br Med J.* 1979;2:417–418.
35. Lester MK, Flume PA. Airway-clearance therapy guidelines and implementation. *Respir Care.* 2009;54:733–753.
36. Hasani A, Pavia D, Agnew JE, et al. Regional lung clearance during cough and forced expiration technique (FET): effects of flow and viscoelasticity. *Thorax.* 1994;49:557–561.
37. Hasani A, Pavia D, Agnew JE, et al. Regional mucus transport following unproductive cough and forced expiration technique in patients with airways obstruction. *Chest.* 1994;105:1420–1425.
38. Schom MH. Autogenic drainage: a modern approach to physiotherapy in cystic fibrosis. *J R Soc Med.* 1989:82(suppl 16):32–37.
39. Miller S, Hall DO, Clayton CB, et al. Chest physiotherapy in cystic fibrosis. A comparative study of autogenic drainage and the active cycle of breathing techniques with postural drainage. *Thorax.* 1995;50:165–169.
40. Bach JR. Update and perspective on noninvasive respiratory muscle aids. Part 2. The expiratory aids. *Chest.* 1994;105:1538–1544.
41. Homnick DN. Mechanical insufflation-exsufflation for airway mucus clearance. *Respir Care.* 2007;52(10):1296–1305; discussion 1306–1307.
42. Sancho J, Servera E, Díaz J, Marín J. Efficacy of mechanical insufflation-exsufflation in medically stable patients with amyotrophic lateral sclerosis. *Chest.* 2004;125:1400–1405.
43. Elkins MR, Robinson M, Rose BR, et al. A controlled trial of long-term inhaled hypertonic saline in patients with cystic fibrosis. *N Engl J Med.* 2006;354:229–240.
44. Valderramas SR, Atallah AN. Effectiveness and safety of hypertonic saline inhalation combined with exercise training in patients with chronic obstructive pulmonary disease: a randomized trial. *Respir Care.* 2009;54:327–333.
45. Rogers DF. Mucoactive agents for airway mucus hypersecretory diseases. *Respir Care.* 2007;52:1193–1197.
46. Restrepo RD. Inhaled adrenergics and anticholinergics in obstructive lung disease: do they enhance mucociliary clearance? *Respir Care.* 2007;52:1159–1173.
47. van der Schans CP. Conventional chest physical therapy for obstructive lung disease. *Respir Care.* 2007;52:1198–1209.
48. Oermann CM, Swank PR, Sockrider MM. Validation of an instrument measuring patient satisfaction with chest physiotherapy techniques in cystic fibrosis. *Chest.* 2000;118:92–97.
49. Wallis C, Prasad A. Who needs chest physiotherapy? Moving from anecdote to evidence. *Arch Dis Child.* 1999;80:393–397.
50. Thomas J, Cook DJ, Brooks D. Chest physical therapy management of patients with cystic fibrosis. *Am J Respir Crit Care Med.* 1995;151:846–850.
51. Oberwaldner B. Physiotherapy for airway clearance in paediatrics. *Eur Respir J.* 2000;15:196–204.
52. van der Schans C, Prasad A, Main E. Chest physiotherapy compared to no chest physiotherapy for cystic fibrosis. *Cochrane Database Syst Rev.* 2000;2:CD001401.
53. Jones AP, Rowe H. Bronchopulmonary hygiene physical therapy for chronic obstructive pulmonary disease. *Cochrane Database Syst Rev.* 2000;2:CD000045.
54. van der Schans C, Prasad A, Main E. Conventional chest physiotherapy compared to any form of chest physiotherapy for cystic fibrosis. *Cochrane Database Syst Rev.* 2000;2.
55. Flenady VJ, Gray PH. Chest physiotherapy for preventing morbidity in babies being extubated from mechanical ventilation. *Cochrane Database Syst Rev.* 2000;2:CD000283.
56. Tyler ML. Complications of positioning and chest physiotherapy. *Respir Care.* 1982;27:458–466.
57. Murphy MB, Concannon D, Fitzgerald MX. Chest percussion: help or hindrance to postural drainage? *Irish Med J.* 1983;76:189–190.
58. Sutton PP, Lopez-Vidriero MT, Pavia D, et al. Assessment of percussion, vibratory shaking and breathing exercises in chest physiotherapy. *Eur J Respir Dis.* 1985;66:147–152.
59. Maxwell M, Redmond A. Comparative trial of manual and mechanical percussion technique with gravity-assisted bronchial drainage in patients with cystic fibrosis. *Arch Dis Child.* 1979;54:542–544.
60. Holody B, Goldberg HS. The effect of mechanical vibration physiotherapy in arterial oxygenation in acutely ill patients with atelectasis or pneumonia. *Am Rev Respir Dis.* 1981;124:372–375.
61. Wollmer P, Ursing K, Midgren B, et al. Inefficiency of chest percussion in the physical therapy of chronic bronchitis. *Eur J Respir Dis.* 1985;66:233–239.

62. van der Schans CP, Peris DA, Postma DS. Effect of manual percussion on tracheobronchial clearance in patients with chronic airflow obstruction and excessive tracheobronchial secretion. *Thorax.* 1986;41:448–452.
63. Radford R, Barutt J, Billingsley JG, et al. A rational basis for percussion-augmented mucociliary clearance. *Respir Care.* 1982;27:556–563.
64. Krause MF, Hoehn T. Chest physiotherapy in mechanically ventilated children: a review. *Crit Care Med.* 2000;28:1648–1651.
65. Clarke RCN, Kelly BE, Convery PN, et al. Ventilatory characteristics in mechanically ventilated patients during manual hyperventilation for chest physiotherapy. *Anaesthesia.* 1999;54:936–940.
66. Fauroux B, Boule M, Lofaso F, et al. Chest physiotherapy in cystic fibrosis: improved tolerance with nasal pressure support ventilation. *Pediatrics.* 1999;103:658–659.
67. Alexander E, Weingarten S, Mohsenifar Z. Clinical strategies to reduce utilization of chest physiotherapy without compromising patient care. *Chest.* 1996;110:430–432.
68. Myers TR. Positive expiratory pressure and oscillatory positive expiratory pressure therapies. *Respir Care.* 2007;52:1308–1327.
69. Volsko TA, DiFiore JM, Chatburn RL. Performance comparison of two oscillating positive expiratory pressure devices: Acapella versus Flutter. *Respir Care.* 2003;48:124–130.
70. Chatburn RL. High-frequency assisted airway clearance. *Respir Care.* 2007;52:1224–1237.
71. Dosman CF, Jones RL. High-frequency chest compression: a summary of the literature. *Can Respir J.* 2005;12:37–41.
72. Spitzer SA, Fink G, Mittelman M. External high-frequency ventilation in severe chronic obstructive pulmonary disease. *Chest.* 1993;104:1698–1701.
73. Scherer TA, Barandun J, Martinez E, et al. Effect of high-frequency oral airway and chest wall oscillation and conventional chest physical therapy on expectoration in patients with stable cystic fibrosis. *Chest.* 1998;113:1019–1027.
74. Zach MS, Purrer B, Oberwaldner B. Effect of swimming on forced expiration and sputum clearance in cystic fibrosis. *Lancet.* 1981;ii:1201–1203.
75. Bilton D, Dodd M, Webb AK. Evaluation of exercise as an adjunct to physiotherapy in the treatment of cystic fibrosis in the treatment of cystic fibrosis. *Thorax.* 1989;44:859.
76. Elkins MR, Jones A, van der Schans C. Positive expiratory pressure physiotherapy for airway clearance in people with cystic fibrosis. *Cochrane Database Syst Rev.* 2006;19(2):CD003147.
77. Morrison L, Agnew J. Oscillating devices for airway clearance in people with cystic fibrosis. *Cochrane Database Syst Rev.* 2009;1:CD006842.
78. Flume PA, Robinson KA, O'Sullivan BP, et al. Cystic fibrosis pulmonary guidelines: airway clearance therapies. *Respir Care.* 2009;54:522–537.
79. Bott J, Blumenthal S, Buxton M, et al. Guidelines for the physiotherapy management of the adult, medical, spontaneously breathing patient. *Thorax.* 2009;64(suppl 1):1–51.
80. Gosselink R, Bott J, Johnson M, et al. Physiotherapy for adult patients with critical illness: recommendations of the European Respiratory Society and European Society of Intensive Care Medicine Task Force on Physiotherapy for Critically Ill Patients. *Intensive Care Med.* 2008;34:1188–1199.
81. Hess DR. The evidence for secretion clearance techniques. *Respir Care.* 2001;46:1276–1293.
82. Hess DR. Secretion clearance techniques: absence of proof or proof of absence? *Respir Care.* 2002;47:757-758.
83. Hess DR. Airway clearance: physiology, pharmacology, techniques, and practice. *Respir Care.* 2007;52:1392–1396.
84. Mang H, Obermayer A. Imposed work of breathing during sustained maximal inspiration: comparison of six incentive spirometers. *Respir Care.* 1989;34:1122–1128.
85. Celli BR, Rodriguez KS, Snider GL. A controlled trial of intermittent positive pressure breathing, incentive spirometry, and deep breathing exercises in preventing pulmonary complication after abdominal surgery. *Am Rev Respir Dis.* 1984;130:12–15.
86. Hall JC, Tarala R, Harris J, et al. Incentive spirometry versus routine chest physiotherapy for prevention of pulmonary complications after abdominal surgery. *Lancet.* 1991;337:953–956.
87. Gooselink R, Schever K, Cops P, et al. Incentive spirometry does not enhance recovery after thoracic surgery. *Crit Care Med.* 2000;28:679–683.
88. Dolovich MB, Killian D, Wolff RK, et al. Pulmonary aerosol deposition in chronic bronchitis: intermittent positive pressure breathing versus quiet breathing. *Am Rev Respir Dis.* 1977;115:397–402.
89. The IPPB Trial Group. Intermittent positive pressure breathing therapy of chronic obstructive pulmonary disease: a clinical trial. *Ann Intern Med.* 1983;99:612–620.
90. Paul WL, Downs JB. Postoperative atelectasis: intermittent positive pressure breathing, incentive spirometry, and facemask positive end-expiratory pressure. *Arch Surg.* 1981;116:861–863.
91. Ricksten SE, Bengtsson A, Soderberg C, et al. Effects of periodic positive airway pressure by mask on postoperative pulmonary function. *Chest.* 1986;89:774–781.

CHAPTER 19

Airway Management

John D. Davies
Robert A. May
Pamela L. Bortner

OUTLINE

OBJECTIVES

1. Compare oropharyngeal and nasopharyngeal airways.
2. Demonstrate the techniques for inserting oropharyngeal and nasopharyngeal airways.
3. Describe the construction of an endotracheal tube.
4. Describe the technique for orotracheal and nasotracheal intubation.
5. Demonstrate the technique used to secure an endotracheal tube.
6. Demonstrate the technique used to measure cuff pressure.
7. Compare conventional and percutaneous dilational tracheostomy.
8. Compare various designs of tracheostomy tubes.
9. Compare conventional and closed suction catheters.
10. Describe techniques used to prevent complications from suctioning.
11. Discuss the important points of extubation and decannulation.

KEY TERMS

airway cuff
bite block
cricothyrotomy
decannulation
endotracheal intubation
endotracheal tube
extubation
gum elastic bougie
laryngeal mask airway (LMA)
laryngoscope
nasopharyngeal airway
nasotracheal intubation
oropharyngeal airway
orotracheal intubation
speaking valve
suction catheter
tracheostomy tube
tube exchanger

INTRODUCTION

Airway management is an important aspect of respiratory care (**CPG 19–1**). It involves the insertion of oropharyngeal airways, nasopharyngeal airways, endotracheal tubes, and tracheostomy tubes, as well as all aspects of the care of patients with artificial airways. The use of artificial airways is the topic of this chapter.

CLINICAL PRACTICE GUIDELINE 19–1

Management of Airway Emergencies

Indications

- Conditions requiring management of the airway, in general, are impending or actual airway compromise, respiratory failure, and the need to protect the airway. Specific conditions include, but are not limited to, airway emergency before endotracheal intubation, obstruction of the artificial airway, apnea, acute traumatic coma, penetrating neck trauma, cardiopulmonary arrest and unstable dysrhythmias, severe bronchospasm, severe allergic reactions with cardiopulmonary compromise, pulmonary edema, sedative or narcotic drug effect, foreign body airway obstruction, choanal atresia in neonates, aspiration, risk of aspiration, severe laryngospasm, and self-extubation.
- Conditions requiring emergency tracheal intubation include, but are not limited to, persistent apnea, traumatic upper airway obstruction (partial or complete), accidental extubation of a patient unable to maintain adequate spontaneous ventilation, obstructive angioedema (edema involving the deeper layers of the skin, subcutaneous tissue, and mucosa), massive uncontrolled upper airway bleeding, coma with potential for increased intracranial pressure, infection-related upper airway obstruction (partial or complete, such as epiglottitis in children or adults, acute uvular edema, tonsillopharyngitis or retropharyngeal abscess, or suppurative parotitis), laryngeal and upper airway edema, neonatal- or pediatric-specific conditions (perinatal asphyxia, severe adenotonsillar hypertrophy, severe laryngomalacia, bacterial tracheitis, neonatal epignathus, obstruction from abnormal laryngeal closure caused by arytenoid masses, mediastinal tumors, congenital diaphragmatic hernia, thick and/or particulate meconium in amniotic fluid), and absence of airway protective reflexes, such as cardiopulmonary arrest or massive hemoptysis.
- When airway control is not possible by other methods, surgical placement of an airway (needle or surgical cricothyrotomy) may be required.
- Conditions in which endotracheal intubation may not be possible and in which alternative techniques may be used include, but are not limited to, restriction of endotracheal intubation by policy or statute; situations in which endotracheal intubation is not immediately possible; and failed intubation in the presence of risk factors associated with difficult tracheal intubations, such as a short or bull neck, protruding maxillary incisors, receding mandible, reduced mobility of the atlantooccipital joint, temporomandibular ankylosis, congenital oropharyngeal wall stenosis, anterior osteophytes of the cervical vertebrae associated with diffuse idiopathic skeletal hyperostosis, large substernal and/or cancerous goiters, Treacher Collins syndrome, Brailsford Morquio syndrome, or endolaryngeal tumors.

Contraindications

- Aggressive airway management (intubation or establishment of a surgical airway) may be contraindicated if the patient's desire not to be resuscitated has been clearly expressed and documented in the patient's medical record or other valid legal document.

Hazards and Complications

- Failure to establish a patent airway
- Failure to intubate the trachea
- Failure to recognize intubation of the esophagus
- Upper airway trauma; laryngeal and esophageal damage
- Aspiration
- Cervical spine trauma
- Unrecognized bronchial intubation
- Eye injury
- Vocal cord paralysis
- Problems with endotracheal tubes (cuff perforation, cuff herniation, pilot tube valve incompetence, tube kinking during biting, inadvertent extubation, tube occlusion)
- Bronchospasm
- Laryngospasm
- Dental accidents
- Dysrhythmias

(continues)

Clinical Practice Guideline 19–1 *(continued)*

- Hypotension and bradycardia caused by vagal stimulation
- Hypertension and tachycardia
- Inappropriate tube size
- Bleeding
- Mouth ulceration
- Specific problems arising from nasal intubation (nasal damage, including epistaxis; tube kinking in the pharynx; sinusitis; and otitis media)
- Tongue ulceration
- Tracheal damage (tracheoesophageal fistula, tracheal innominate fistula, tracheal stenosis, and tracheomalacia)
- Pneumonia
- Laryngeal damage with consequent laryngeal stenosis, laryngeal ulcer, granuloma, polyps, or synechiae
- Specific problems arising from surgical cricothyrotomy or tracheostomy (stomal stenosis, innominate erosion)
- Specific problems arising from needle cricothyrotomy (bleeding at the insertion site with hematoma formation, subcutaneous and mediastinal emphysema, esophageal perforation)

Modified from AARC clinical practice guideline: management of airway emergencies. *Respir Care.* 1995;40:749–760. Reprinted with permission.

Oropharyngeal Airways

The **oropharyngeal airway** is a useful tool to promote airway patency in patients without a gag reflex. It is designed to be inserted into the mouth between the lips and teeth and extends from the lips to the pharynx, following the natural curvature of the tongue and palate, without entering the larynx or esophagus (**Figure 19–1**). Oropharyngeal airways are usually made of hard plastic and are relatively rigid. They generally consist of a flange, a bite portion (body), and an air channel. The flange at the mouth opening prevents the airway from falling back into the mouth and becoming an obstruction. It also provides a means to stabilize the airway in place against the lips or teeth. The bite portion, which fits between the teeth or gums, is straight and firm enough to prevent the patient from closing the air channel by biting down. The air channel, or curved portion, extends upward and backward along the curve of the tongue, pulling it and the epiglottis away from the posterior pharyngeal wall to provide a patent air passage.

RESPIRATORY RECAP

Oropharyngeal Airways

» Prevent upper airway obstruction
» May be used as a bite block
» May make bag-valve-mask ventilation more effective
» Should not be used in semicomatose or alert patients

Oropharyngeal airways are designed to prevent the patient's tongue from falling backward into the hypopharynx and partly or completely obstructing the upper airway. Use of an oropharyngeal airway may be indicated during spontaneous, manual, or mouth-to-tube ventilation. Oropharyngeal airways allow ready access to the mouth and pharynx for suctioning, and they may be inserted instead of a **bite block** to prevent a patient from biting an oral endotracheal tube. These airways also may help in facilitating airway patency to optimize bag-valve-mask ventilation, for example, in a patient who is edentulous or who has facial trauma that causes the cheeks to collapse, making an airtight mask seal impossible. It is important to note that because of its position in the pharynx, an oropharyngeal airway may gag a semicomatose or an alert patient, which could induce vomiting and increase the risk of aspiration.

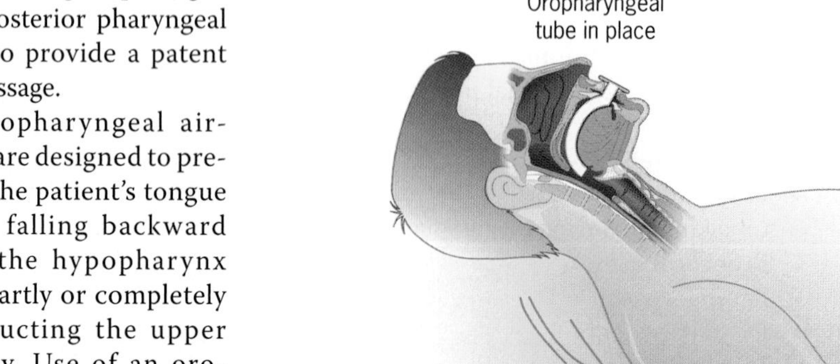

FIGURE 19–1 Oropharyngeal airway in place.

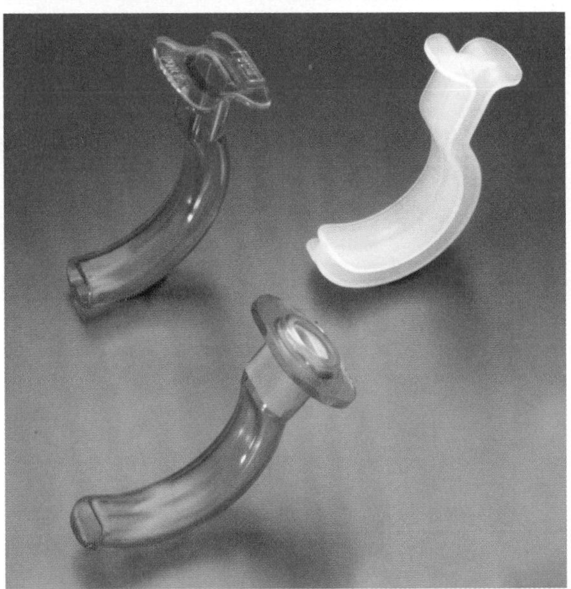

FIGURE 19–2 Guedel (left) and Berman airways (right).

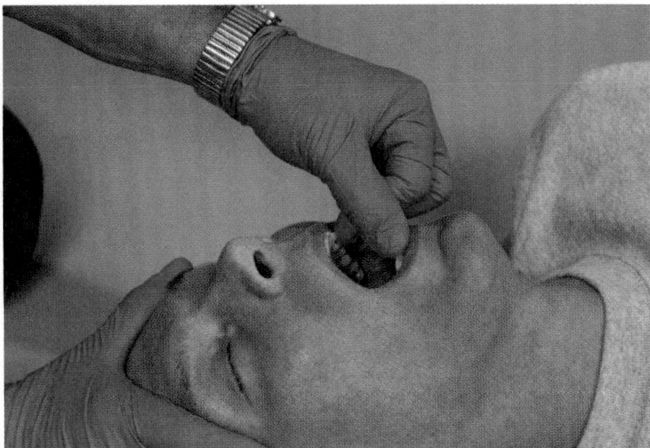

FIGURE 19–3 Cross-finger technique to open the mouth.

Types

The Berman airway (Figure 19–2) has a flange at the oral end, a rigid support beam through the center, and open sides.[1] The open sides allow suctioning and serve as air channels. The center may have openings for suctioning should the airway become lodged sideways in the mouth. The advantages of the Berman airway are ease of cleaning and the fact that the dual side air channels are less likely to be obstructed by mucus or foreign bodies. Because the Berman airway is uniformly rigid over its full length, it has an advantage over the Guedel airway in resistance to occlusion by the patient's bite.[2]

The Guedel airway (refer to Figure 19–2) has a large flange at the oral end and a supportive bite, and the curved portion that follows the curve of the tongue is made of a semirigid material. The Guedel airway differs from the Berman airway in that it is reinforced only in the bite region. This may pose a problem if the patient should bite down on the Guedel airway before it is completely inserted, causing an unreinforced portion to occlude the airway and preventing complete insertion. The Guedel airway also differs from the Berman airway in that it has an enclosed tubular channel to facilitate air exchange and suctioning.

Insertion

Before inserting an oropharyngeal airway, there should be an assessment for proper sizing. To get the right size, the device itself can be used to measure. When you place it on the patient's cheek with the flange parallel to his or her front teeth, the tip of the oropharyngeal airway should reach no further than the angle of the jaw. If the oropharyngeal airway selected is too large, its tip may press the epiglottis against the posterior pharyngeal wall or the larynx, obstructing both the device and the patient's physiologic airway. If the airway is inserted improperly or is too small, the tongue may be pushed against the posterior pharynx, causing obstruction. Oropharyngeal airways come in a variety of different sizes to accommodate adults, children, and infants.

To insert an oropharyngeal airway, stand at the patient's head, hyperextend the head and neck, and use the cross-finger technique to open the mouth (Figure 19–3). One method of insertion is to turn the airway 180 degrees from its resting position as it is passed over the tongue to avoid pushing the tongue back into the pharynx. When the tip of the airway reaches the uvula, the airway is rotated 180 degrees so that the tip is positioned behind the tongue and facing the larynx. In the second method the airway can be inserted from the lateral aspect of the mouth and rotated 90 degrees to the position in which it will rest (Figure 19–4). Once it is in place, the airway should be assessed for proper size and position through determination of whether it allows unobstructed breathing.

Complications

Regurgitation and aspiration are the major risks when an oral airway is employed. Laryngospasm and coughing can be induced in a patient who is awake or by insertion of an oropharyngeal airway that is too long and consequently comes into contact with the epiglottis or vocal cords. Another problem with oral airways is dental damage. Teeth can be broken or torn forcibly from the mouth as the patient bites down on the oral airway. Oral airways should be used judiciously if the patient has disease or decay of the teeth or caps, crowns, or other dental appliances. In such cases, use of a nasopharyngeal airway or bite block may be indicated.[3] When the oral airway is in place, the lip may be damaged if it is pinched between the teeth and the airway, or continuous chewing motions by a comatose patient may damage the tongue. Pressure necrosis of the tongue can occur if the airway is left in place for a prolonged period.

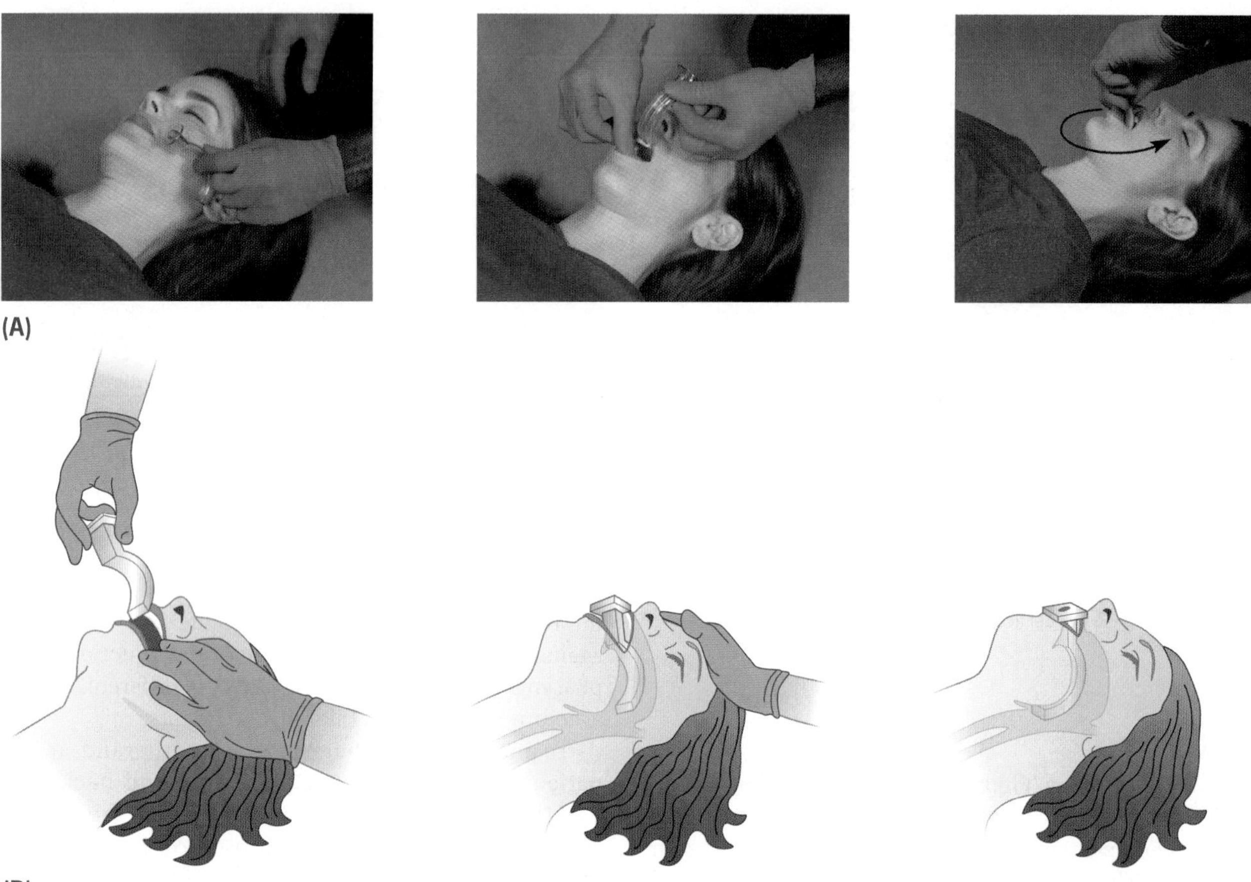

FIGURE 19–4 (**A**) Anti-anatomic insertion of an oral airway. (**B**) Insertion of an oral airway from the side of the mouth. (**B**) Adapted from Cairo JM, Pilbeam SP. *Mosby's Respiratory Care Equipment*. 7th ed. Mosby; 2004.

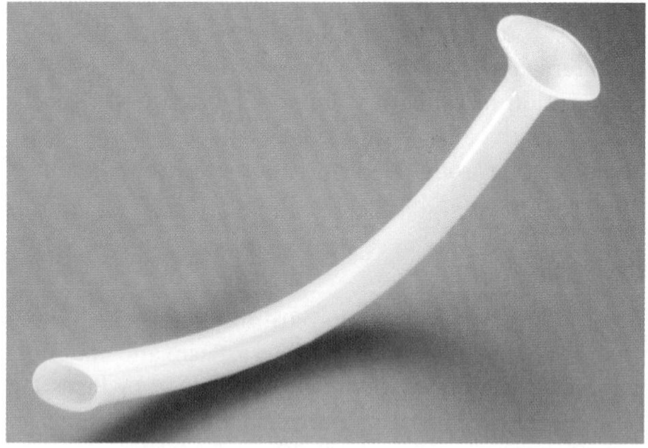

FIGURE 19–5 Nasopharyngeal airway.

Nasopharyngeal Airways

The **nasopharyngeal airway** (**Figure 19–5**) is an alternative to the oropharyngeal airway. Nasopharyngeal airways are inserted into the nose and directed along the floor of the nose parallel to the hard palate. They are curved to follow the anatomy of the nasopharynx so that the tip rests behind the tongue, just above the epiglottis. These airways are made of plastic or rubber and resemble a shortened endotracheal tube. All types have some degree of flange at the nasal end to facilitate insertion and prevent accidental aspiration of the tube. The proper length of airway can be determined by measurement of the distance from the tip of the nose to the meatus of the ear or from the tip of the nose to the tragus of the ear plus 2 cm.

> **RESPIRATORY RECAP**
>
> **Nasopharyngeal Airways**
> - May be used to bypass an upper airway obstruction
> - Aid passage of a bronchoscope
> - Reduce trauma caused by repeated nasotracheal suctioning

The nasopharyngeal airway can be an alternative to the oropharyngeal airway to provide a patent airway. In some situations the mouth cannot be opened, an active gag reflex minimizes the efficiency of an oral airway (and actually can lead to vomiting and aspiration), or an oral airway does not relieve the obstruction. In these cases a nasopharyngeal airway is better tolerated and more comfortable in a semiawake patient than an oral airway. A nasopharyngeal airway also eliminates the risk of trauma of the tongue and teeth seen with oral airways. Nasopharyngeal airways are used as conduits to perform fiberoptic bronchoscopy, provide easy access to the trachea for nasotracheal suctioning, and protect the nasopharyngeal mucosa from the traumatic effects of repeated nasotracheal suctioning.[4]

Insertion

After proper measurement, the nasopharyngeal airway first should be lubricated with a water-soluble gel. It is then introduced into the naris, and the end is pointed parallel to the hard palate. It is advanced gently to prevent trauma and bleeding (**Figure 19–6**). If resistance is met, the airway should be redirected. If excessive resistance is met, the attempt is made through the other nostril, or a smaller airway is chosen. Incorrect sizing of a nasopharyngeal airway, like its oral counterpart, carries risks. If the nasopharyngeal airway is too long, laryngospasm may occur. If it is too short, complete airway patency will not be achieved. As is the case with oropharyngeal airways, nasopharyngeal airways come in a variety of sizes.

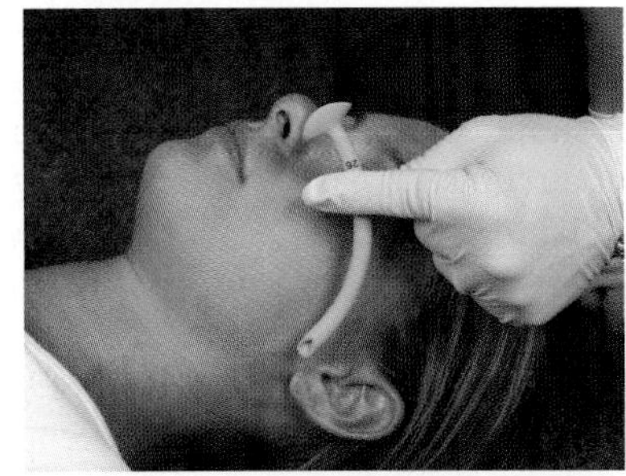

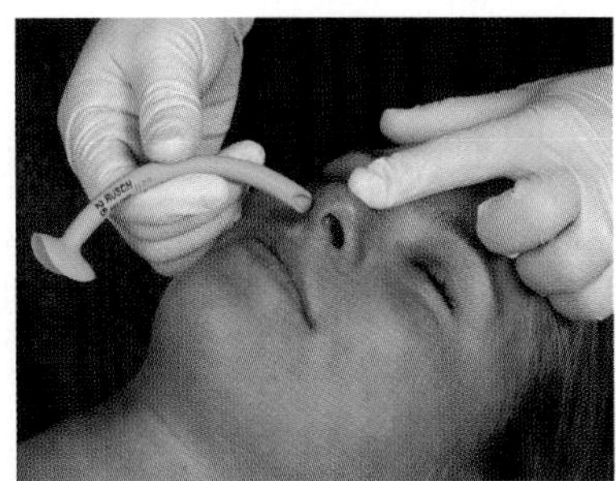

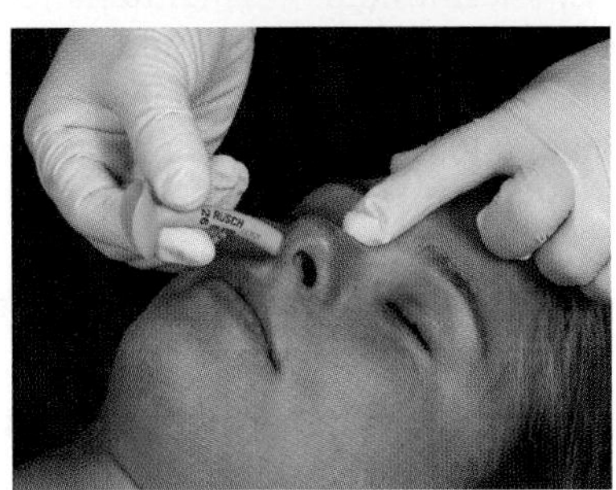

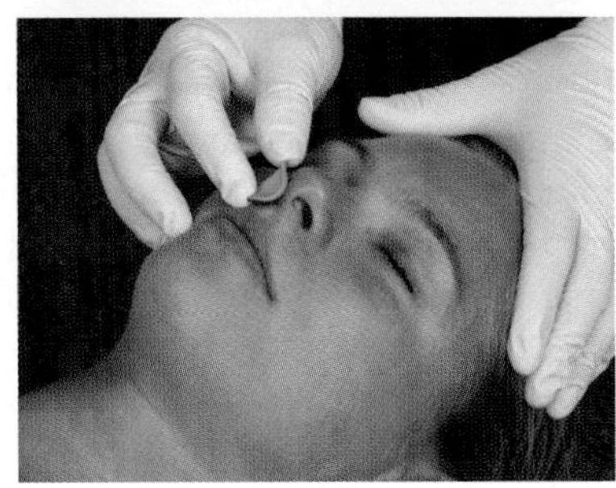

FIGURE 19–6 Insertion of a nasopharyngeal airway.

Complications

Laryngospasm and coughing can be induced by insertion of a nasopharyngeal airway that is too long and comes into contact with the epiglottis or vocal cords. Nosebleeds can occur from insertion of a nasopharyngeal airway, particularly if it is too large. These airways should be used with caution in patients with low platelet counts or undergoing anticoagulation therapy because excessive bleeding can occur. Improper insertion of nasopharyngeal airways may damage the turbinate, and insertion of a nasopharyngeal airway into a patient who is draining blood or cerebrospinal fluid may cause infection. Prolonged use of this airway may result in sinus infections. In patients with severe facial or head trauma, insertion of a nasopharyngeal airway may result, in rare cases, in cranial vault intubation, the risk being greatest in patients with basilar skull fractures.

History of Intubation

The use of tracheotomy to relieve upper airway obstruction dates to Asclepiad's first surgical tracheostomy in approximately 100 BC. Even several hundred years earlier, crude attempts to open airways had been made with swords or other instruments.[5,6] In the mid-1600s, Robert Hooke performed an experiment in which he kept animals alive by blowing air into their lungs with a bellows by use of a tracheotomy.[7] In the early 1700s, Trendelenburg fitted an inflatable cuff to a tracheostomy tube, creating the prototype for current airway devices.[5,6] In the 1880s, MacEwen,[8] O'Dwyer,[9] and Fell[10] all described the use of endotracheal intubation for delivery of positive pressure ventilation. The fundamental design of current endotracheal tubes was established in 1941 by Murphy.[11] In 1971, Grillo et al.[12] showed that low-pressure, high-compliance cuffs caused less frequent and less severe tracheal injury than the standard high-pressure tubes.

Selection and Training of Personnel

Understanding the concepts of airway management and becoming proficient in the techniques used to establish and maintain a patent airway are paramount in the practice of respiratory care. The airway should never be taken for granted. At times, a simple maneuver to reestablish a patent airway may prove to be life-saving. The major objectives of airway education are (1) recognizing the need for airway management, (2) properly identifying airway anatomy, (3) developing skills using bag-valve-mask ventilation, laryngoscopy, and intubation, (4) developing strategies for the difficult airway, and (5) maintaining airway management skills on an ongoing basis. The airway is the first concern in life support protocols.[13]

It is of vital importance that a logical sequence be followed in the evaluation and establishment of an airway. The respiratory therapist must be able to determine the adequacy of an airway and, when appropriate, implement corrective action to establish patency of an airway. As mentioned earlier, a simple maneuver may be all that is required to restore airway patency. However, when this is not sufficient, more intensive steps may have to be taken to resume adequate patient ventilation. It is imperative that airway patency be reevaluated properly after any interventional technique to determine whether the corrective action has indeed improved the situation. These techniques need also to be performed in a timely manner so as not to risk hypoxic- or hypercarbic-related decompensation.

Because of the significant impact airway management can have on the patient's outcome, guidelines should be established that address which personnel should perform endotracheal intubation and under what circumstances, and how appropriate training of these individuals should be accomplished. The literature offers very little guidance in the medicolegal aspects of who should manage the airway, and regional practices vary from locale to locale. The standard of care usually prevails but may be poorly defined. In the surgical areas, anesthesiologists and certified registered nurse anesthetists manage the airway. In the nonhospital setting, most regions are comfortable with paramedics performing endotracheal intubation. Because most hospitals have code teams, and respiratory therapists are part of the team, it is reasonable that respiratory therapists should manage the airway in the absence of more highly trained personnel.

The National Board for Respiratory Care (NBRC) includes endotracheal intubation in its examination outline for registered respiratory therapists. Most respiratory therapy training programs instruct their students in the technique of endotracheal intubation.[14] Anesthesia personnel have the highest skill level, but in the hospital setting, the practitioner with the highest level of experience and training outside the operating room probably is the respiratory therapist. Opportunities to practice live intubations are limited in the clinical setting, and perhaps the best-controlled setting in which to learn is in the operating room. The anesthesiologist and the operating room provide a logical means to implement a program that uses the skills of respiratory therapists in acute airway management.[15,16] Initial training is given by an anesthesiologist, followed by 10 to 15 supervised intubations in the operating room. After the operating room experience, a set number of supervised intubations should be performed before airway management competency can be achieved. How many that is will depend on the experience level of the clinician and skills of the supervisors. It might take as many as 57 training intubations before competency is achieved.[17]

RESPIRATORY RECAP

Healthcare Workers Who Perform Endotracheal Intubation

» Anesthesia personnel (anesthesiologists and nurse anesthetists)
» Critical care and emergency physicians
» Paramedics
» Respiratory therapists

A standard manikin model can help augment intubation technique but should not be used as the sole training method. Using only manikins for laryngoscopic training is inadequate.[18] Innovative methods are emerging that may help bridge the gap between standard manikin training and the live scenario. Manikins with difficult airway features and airway simulators can help add a wider range of situations. Video imaging during an intubation can be the next best thing to the clinician actually performing the procedure. Although an observer may not be actually manipulating the laryngoscope, imaging allows for identification of the various airway structures.

Skill decay is a concern in many institutions where intubations may not be a commonplace procedure. Not performing intubations on a regular basis has the potential of leading to time-related competency erosion. Therefore, it is very important to have a periodic skill maintenance program. Trained respiratory therapists should perform 10 intubations a year to be requalified or should undergo a repeat training course in the operating room. If the requirement for intubation outside the operating room is infrequent, training may need to be limited to supervisors or designated members of the code team to achieve continued competence.

Indications for Endotracheal Intubation

The indications for endotracheal intubation are numerous, with many involving emergency intubation, whereas others allow for a more structured, relaxed approach. **Box 19–1** lists specific conditions that require emergency endotracheal intubation. Generally accepted indications include establishment and maintenance of a patent airway, protection of the airway from aspiration, establishment of a conduit for mechanical ventilation, facilitation of clearance of secretions, and delivery of high oxygen concentrations.[19,20]

Establishment of a patent airway is the most basic intervention in all of health care and probably the most important. Without an adequate airway, meaningful survival is impossible. Establishment of an airway has retained its position as the first step in cardiopulmonary resuscitation for decades because all other treatment is futile unless a patent airway exists. However, because of the development of new techniques and equipment, endotracheal intubation may not necessarily be the first step to establish the airway; use of supraglottic devices may precede or replace it. Nevertheless, endotracheal intubation remains the gold standard used to establish an airway.

Aspiration of foreign objects into the airway can result in significant morbidity and mortality. Although not 100% effective, placement of an endotracheal tube in the trachea minimizes the risk of aspiration. Aspiration also can occur during insertion or removal of the endotracheal tube, and strong evidence suggests that aspiration of pharyngeal secretions occurs with high-volume, low-pressure endotracheal tube cuffs, resulting in ventilator-associated pneumonia.[1,21,22] Unquestionably, in a patient with compromised upper airway reflexes and function, the risk of aspiration is lower with an endotracheal tube in place.

BOX 19–1

Indications for Emergency Intubation

Persistent apnea
Traumatic upper airway obstruction
Accidental extubation of a patient unable to maintain adequate spontaneous ventilation
Obstructive angioedema
Massive uncontrolled upper airway bleeding
Coma with potential for increased intracranial pressure
Infection-related upper airway obstruction (e.g., epiglottitis, acute uvular edema, tonsillopharyngitis or retropharyngeal abscess, supportive parotitis)
Laryngeal and upper airway edema
Absence of airway protective reflexes
Cardiopulmonary arrest
Massive hemoptysis
Neonatal or pediatric disorders (e.g., perinatal asphyxia, severe tonsillar hypertrophy, severe laryngomalacia, bacterial tracheitis, neonatal epignathus, obstruction from abnormal laryngeal closure caused by arytenoid masses, mediastinal tumors, congenital diaphragmatic hernia, thick and/or particulate meconium in the amniotic fluid)

From Hess DR. Indications for translaryngeal intubation. *Respir Care.* 1999;44:604–609. Reprinted with permission.

Ever since the development of positive pressure ventilation, the endotracheal tube has been the mainstay for delivery of this type of ventilation. However, the use of noninvasive ventilation (NIV) and continuous positive airway pressure (CPAP) has increased over the last decade; for some indications, these techniques can be used to effectively ventilate patients without the use of an endotracheal tube.[23–27] The need for endotracheal intubation to deliver positive pressure ventilation will always exist, although practitioners certainly can be more selective and avoid intubation in some cases. Facilitation of the evacuation of pulmonary secretions by suctioning through an endotracheal tube is a common indication for endotracheal intubation.

RESPIRATORY RECAP

Indications for Endotracheal Intubation

- Bypass an upper airway obstruction
- Protect the airway from aspiration
- Apply positive pressure ventilation
- Aid clearance of secretions
- Correct hypoxemia and/or respiratory acidosis

When high oxygen concentrations are required to correct hypoxemia, placement of an endotracheal tube may be necessary. Most oxygen delivery devices fall well short of a 100% oxygen concentration because of air entrainment caused by poorly fitting devices or inadequate flow delivery.[28] Tight-fitting masks work well for high oxygen delivery if the inspiratory flows are high enough, but patients find these devices uncomfortable and often remove them, dropping the inspired oxygen concentration (F_{IO_2}) to dangerous levels. When high oxygen concentrations are needed, administration is required for several hours; therefore, positive pressure may be used to reduce the levels of inspired oxygen.

The Difficult Airway: Assessment and Strategy

Intubation will remain the mainstay to secure a patent airway and increasingly will be performed by nonanesthesia healthcare workers as outlined in emergency protocols. Of significant concern is the difficult airway. Healthcare workers who do not intubate regularly may not have the experience to recognize, evaluate, or manage a patient with a difficult airway. The American Society of Anesthesiologists (ASA) Task Force on Management of the Difficult Airway has described a difficult airway as a "clinical situation in which a conventionally trained anesthesiologist experiences difficulty with face mask ventilation of the upper airway, difficulty with tracheal intubation, or both."[29] Conventionally trained individuals have average skills for their specialty, which implies that the person is not a regional expert but has performed hundreds of tracheal intubations for operative anesthesia care. In emergency situations an individual with much less experience than a conventionally trained anesthesiologist may have to perform endotracheal intubation and may encounter a difficult airway.

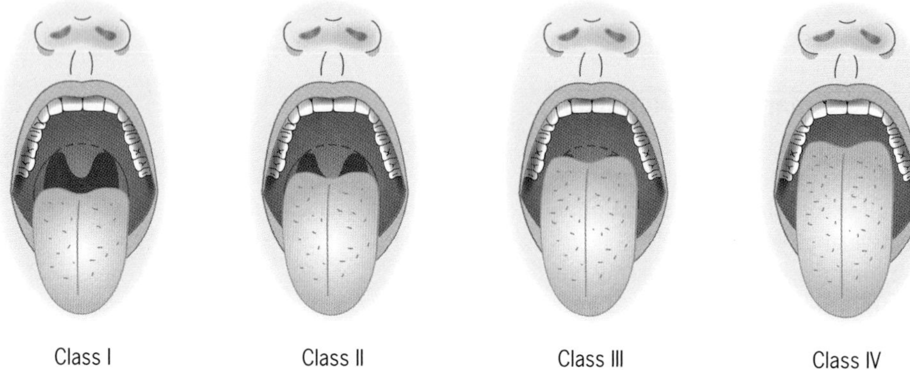

FIGURE 19–7 Mallampati classification. Adapted from Mallampati SR, et al. A clinical sign to predict difficult tracheal intubation: a prospective study. *Can Anaesth Soc J.* 1985;32:429–434; and Samsoon GLT, Young JRB. Difficult tracheal intubation: a retrospective study. *Anesthesiology.* 1987;42:487–490.

For this reason, training in the recognition and management of a difficult airway must occur concomitantly with training in basic intubation.

The incidence of difficult direct laryngoscopy and intubation is reported to be 1.5% to 15%, and impossible intubation during anesthesia has been reported in less than 1% of patients.[30–32] **Figure 19–7** and **Table 19–1** present a difficulty-class scale based on visualization of airway structures during direct laryngoscopy. **Table 19–2** presents a difficulty-class scale based on structures visualized during an oropharyngeal examination. Any laryngoscopy is complicated by tissue trauma, failed attempts, esophageal intubation, cardiovascular and respiratory instability, and aspiration of gastric or esophageal contents. Prediction of the ability to perform direct laryngoscopy and intubation is also associated with structural and anatomic factors (**Table 19–3**). It must be noted that although many of these factors seem obvious, some are subtle and often are not appreciated in an emergency situation. The ASA task force has recommended preintubation assessment as a guide to plan intubation; use of awake techniques if direct laryngoscopy is likely to be difficult; selection of alternative airways and techniques in a methodical fashion when direct laryngoscopy is unexpectedly difficult; and use of an airway management algorithm (**Figure 19–8**) to improve the outcome.[29]

Endotracheal Intubation

Endotracheal intubation is the establishment of an artificial airway by placement of a tube through the mouth or nose, through the glottis, and into the trachea.[33] This procedure can be performed electively under preplanned conditions or on an emergency basis if respiratory failure occurs. The type of endotracheal tube and the placement technique are determined by the factors dictating its use. Instrumentation of the airway stimulates intense reflexive responses in all individuals except severely obtunded patients. For this reason,

TABLE 19–1 Difficulty Class Based on Structures Visible on Direct Laryngoscopy

Class	Visible Structures
I	Supraglottic structures Laryngeal inlet Vocal cords
II	Epiglottis Laryngeal inlet Posterior aryepiglottic folds
III	Epiglottis only
IV	Epiglottis not visible

From Watson CB. Prediction of difficult intubation: methods for successful intubation. *Respir Care.* 1999;44:777–796. Reprinted with permission.

TABLE 19–2 Difficulty Class Based on Structures Visible During the Oropharyngeal Examination

Class	Visible Structures
I	Tongue Hard palate Soft palate Uvula Posterior pharynx
II	Tongue Hard palate Soft palate Part of the uvula and the posterior pharynx
III	Tongue Hard palate Soft palate Posterior pharynx not visible
IV	Anterior tongue Hard palate

From Watson CB. Prediction of difficult intubation: methods for successful intubation. *Respir Care.* 1999;44:777–796. Reprinted with permission.

TABLE 19–3 Complicating Anatomic Factors in Intubation

Factor	Common Condition	Primary Problem
Disproportionate soft tissues	Lingual hypertrophy Down syndrome Lingual tonsillar hypertrophy Marked obesity Supraglottic inflammation Previous neck dissection Expanding neck hematoma	Oversized tongue Mass effect Redundant soft tissue Swelling Torsion Deviation Obstructive edema
Distorted anatomy	Peritonsillar abscess Pharyngeal mass and brachial cleft cyst Thyroid tumor or goiter Developmental craniofacial anomalies Spinal subluxation or osteophytes Maxillofacial trauma	Lateral compression and risk of rupture Deviated larynx or trachea Bony incongruity and disproportionate anatomy Extrinsic mass effect Displacement or bleeding or both
Inadequate jaw mobility	Temporomandibular joint dysfunction Short mandibular ramus Trauma Malignant hyperthermia Myotonic crisis Neuroleptic-malignant syndrome Drug intoxication Infections	Fixed or limited motion Inadequate hinge length Trismus or locked jaw or both Masseter tetanus and generalized rigidity Rigidity, trismus, tetanus
Inadequate neck mobility	Degenerative cervical arthritis Morbid obesity Facial or neck burn scarring Dwarfism Hydrocephalus Cranial dysplasia Cervical meningomyelocele Cervical trauma Fractures Thoracic kyphosis	Fused or irregular intervertebral joints Tissue limits movement Fusion and contractures Short, thick neck Limited neck extension Inadequate space External fixation Fractures Hematoma Limited cervical extension

From Watson CB. Prediction of difficult intubation: methods for successful intubation. *Respir Care.* 1999;44:777–796. Reprinted with permission.

preplanning is imperative whenever possible, including a combination of topical application of local anesthetics, establishment of an intravenous line, intravenous sedation, general anesthesia, electrocardiographic monitoring, oximetry, suction capability, and availability of various types of equipment to meet unforeseen circumstances. In a true emergency, establishing an airway precludes many of these procedures. If ventilation can be performed with a bag-valve-mask system while some of this equipment is gathered, the chances of successful intubation increase.

Anatomy of the Upper Airway

An understanding of the basic anatomy of the airway is paramount to airway management, regardless of the technique used. The airway consists of five regions: the nose and nasopharynx, oral cavity and oropharynx, hypopharynx, larynx, and tracheobronchial tree (**Figure 19–9**).

The nose and nasopharynx region consist of the nasal cavity, turbinates, nasal septum, and adenoids. Warming, humidification, and filtering of inspired air are the primary functions of the nasopharyngeal structures, which are well suited to these tasks because of the region's large mucosal surface area and rich blood supply. If the nose is bypassed with an endotracheal tube, these important functions are lost and must be substituted artificially. The vascular supply to the area is received from the ethmoid artery and the maxillary artery. Sensory innervation is supplied by the trigeminal nerve through the pterygopalatine branches of the maxillary division. Openings to the paranasal sinuses also are present in the nasal cavity, and drainage of these sinuses may be interrupted if they are occluded by an endotracheal tube or nasogastric tube (this may result in sinusitis). Endotracheal intubation also interferes with the sense of olfaction.

The oral cavity and oropharynx consist of the teeth, tongue, buccal mucosa, faucial pillars, hard palate, soft

1. Assess the likelihood and clinical impact of basic management problems:
   A. Difficult Ventilation
   B. Difficult Intubation
   C. Difficulty with Patient Cooperation or Consent
   D. Difficult Tracheostomy

2. Actively pursue opportunities to deliver supplemental oxygen throughout the process of difficult airway management

3. Consider the relative merits and feasibility of basic management choices:

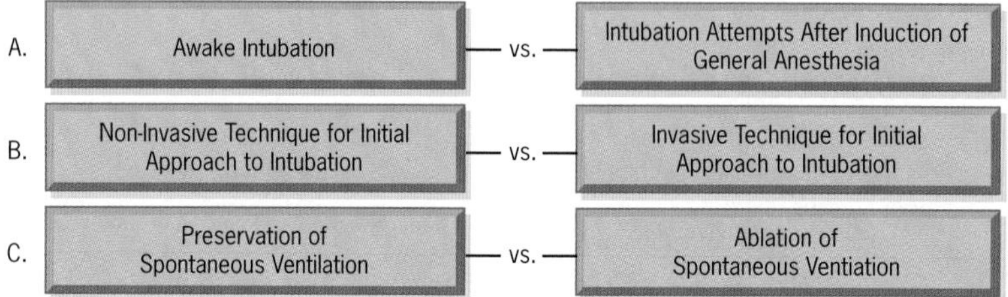

4. Develop primary and alternative strategies:

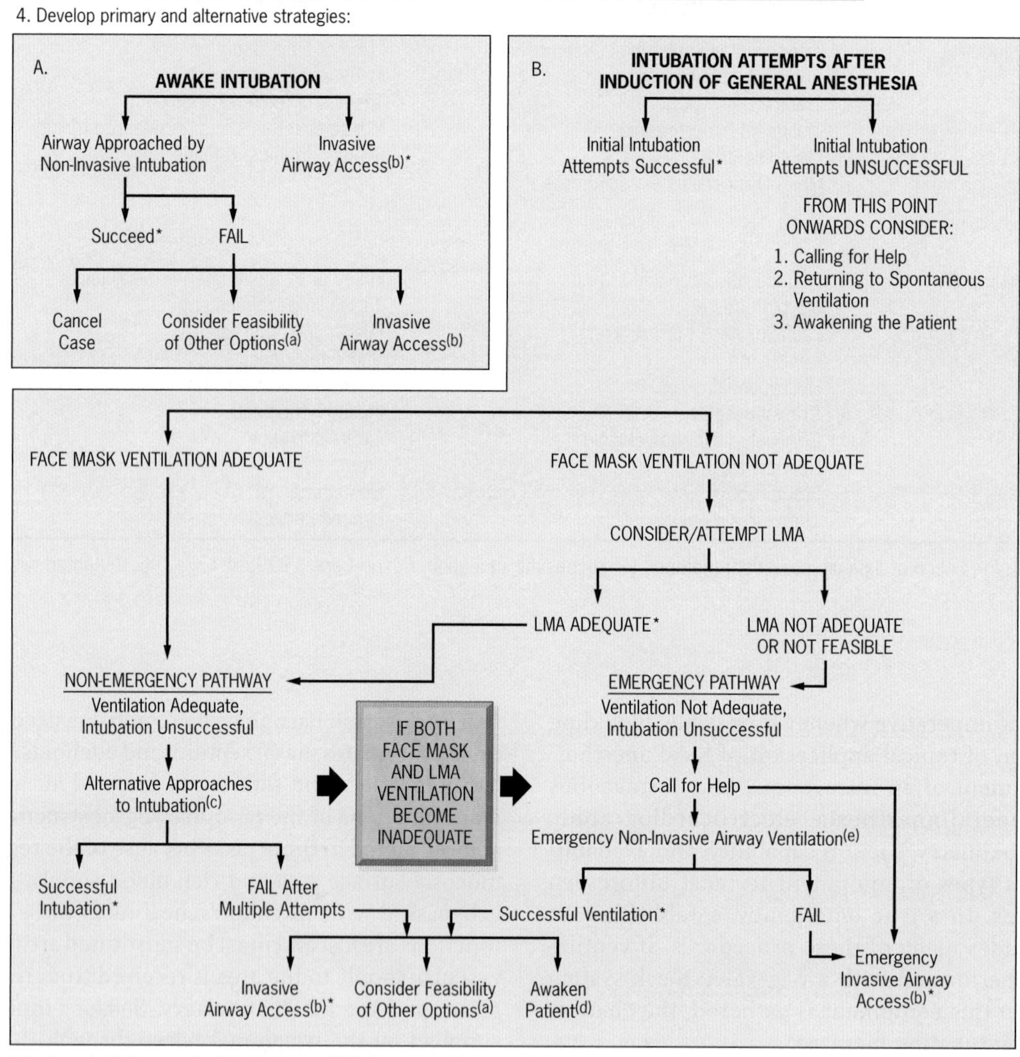

***Confirm ventilation, tracheal intubation, or LMA placement with exhaled CO_2**

a. Other options include (but are not limited to): surgery utilizing face mask or LMA anesthesia, local anesthesia infiltration, or regional nerve blockade. Pursuit of these options usually implies that mask ventilation will not be problematic. Therefore, these options may be of limited valve if this step in the algorithm has been reached via the Emergency Pathway.
b. Invasive airway access includes surgical or percutaneous tracheostomy or cricothyrotomy.
c. Alternative non-invasive approaches to difficult intubation include (but are not limited to): use of different laryngoscope blades, LMA as an intubation conduit (with or without fiberoptic guidance), fiberoptic intubation, intubating stylet or tube changer, light wand, retrograde intubation, and blind oral or nasal intubation.
d. Consider repreparation of the patient for awake intubation or canceling surgery.
e. Options for emergency noninvasive airway ventilation include (but are not limited to): rigid bronchoscope, esphageal-tracheal combitube ventilation, or transtracheal jet ventilation.

FIGURE 19–8 Algorithm for a difficult airway. From American Society of Anesthesiologists. Practice Guidelines for management of the difficult airway. *Anesthesiology.* 2003;98:1269–1277. http://www.asahq.org/publicationsAndServices/Difficult%20Airway.pdf. Reproduced with permission.

palate, uvula, tonsils, and posterior pharyngeal wall. Functionally these structures are important for mastication, taste, phonation, and humidification and warming of inspired gas. As swallowing occurs, the soft palate closes the entrance to the nasopharynx. This area has a rich mucosal blood supply, and innervation is complex, involving mandibular branches of the trigeminal nerve, the facial nerve, and the glossopharyngeal nerve. The mandible houses the tongue, and the temporomandibular joint (TMJ) determines the ability to mobilize these structures. Reduced mobility of the TMJ may make direct laryngoscopy difficult or impossible. Teeth may also form obstructions to direct laryngoscopy, depending on their position and shape. Dental appliances should be removed prior to intubation attempts to prevent damage and possible migration of the device into the trachea.

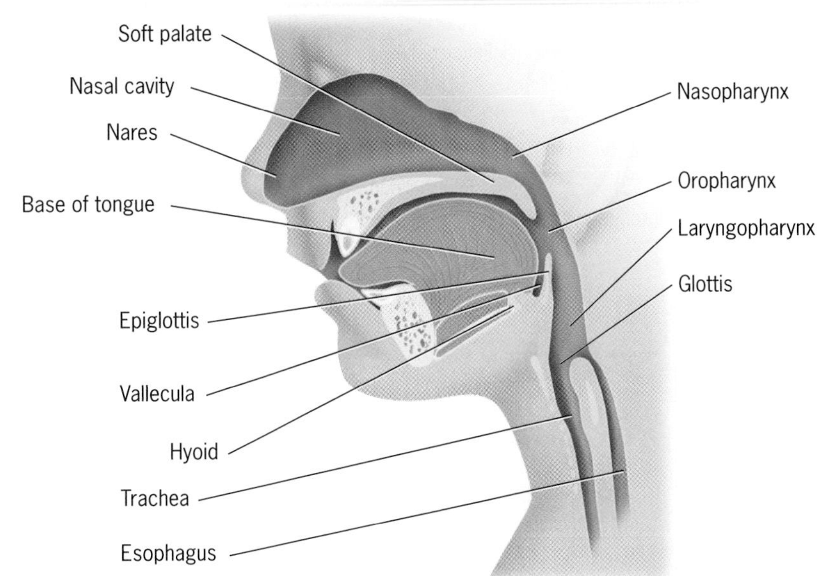

FIGURE 19–9 Anatomy of the upper airway.

Below the oropharynx and above the larynx is the hypopharynx. This area contains the epiglottis and the opening to the esophagus. It is an extension of the oropharynx and the position where a laryngeal mask airway seats. The larynx is a complex structure composed of nine cartilages, seven muscles, and the vocal ligaments (**Figure 19–10**). The space between the vocal cords is the glottis; in adults this is the narrowest part of the upper airway, whereas in children the narrowest point is the cricoid ring. The vocal cords protect the lower airway from aspiration of foreign objects and produce phonation. The cartilaginous structures and complex muscle groups of the larynx are responsible for the intricate vocal abilities of human beings. With nerve or muscle damage, the vocal cords may not open, causing airway obstruction, or may be unable to close, which leaves the lower airway unprotected.

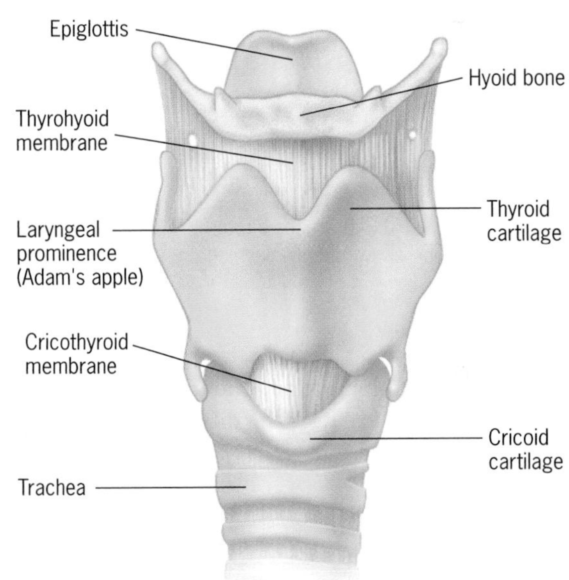

FIGURE 19–10 Anatomy of the larynx.

The trachea is inferior to the larynx, starting just below the cricoid ring. C-shaped cartilaginous rings connected by fibromuscular tissue extend approximately 10 to 12 cm to where the trachea bifurcates into the left and right main stem bronchi at the carina. The carina usually is located at the level of the fourth thoracic vertebra. Posteriorly the tracheal cartilages are open, and the wall is formed by a longitudinal fibromuscular band that allows expansion into the trachea as food traverses the esophagus en route to the stomach.

> **AGE-SPECIFIC ANGLE**
>
> In adults the glottis is the narrowest point of the upper airway, whereas in children the cricoid ring is the narrowest point.

Endotracheal Tubes

The construction of **endotracheal tubes** is dictated by the standards of the American Society for Testing and Materials (ASTM) (**Figure 19–11**).[34,35] The tubes usually are made of polyvinyl chloride (PVC). PVC is rigid, to facilitate insertion of the tube, but becomes softer at body temperature. The material used in endotracheal tubes is implant tested (i.e., it does not react with tissue), and it is smooth, to facilitate passage of a suction catheter. The distal end of the tube is beveled and rounded to

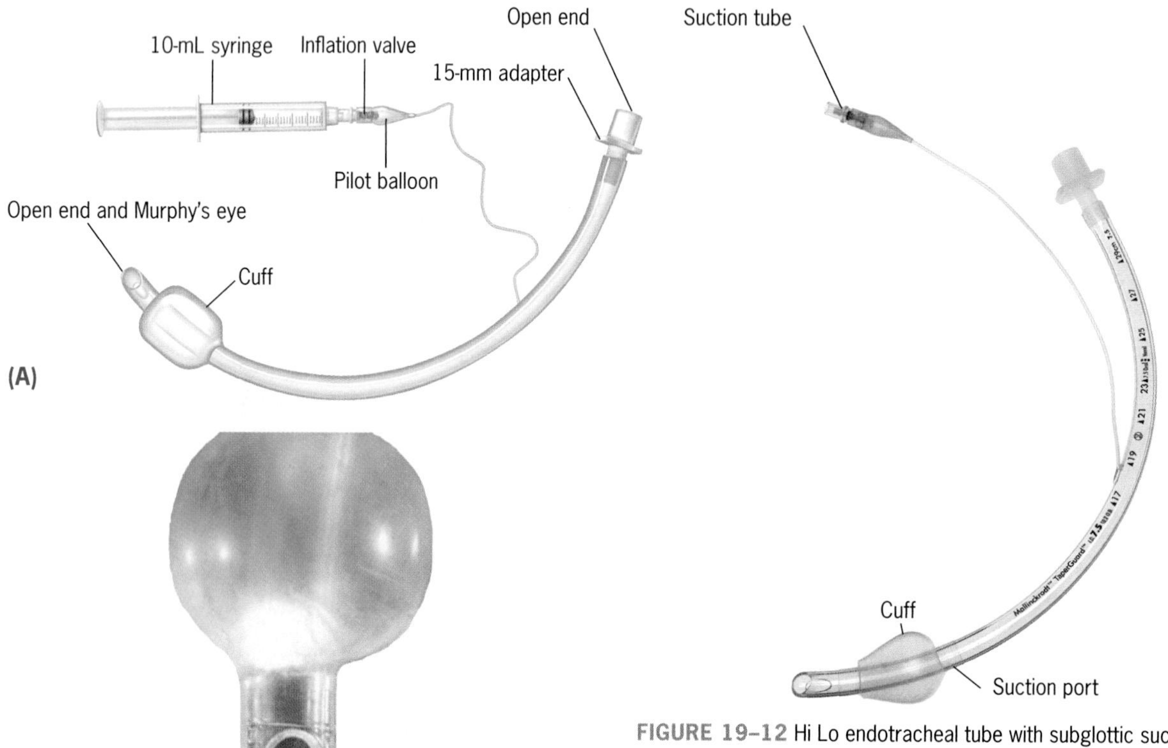

FIGURE 19–11 (**A**) Endotracheal tube. (**B**) Distal end of endotracheal tube showing cuff, beveled end, and Murphy eye.

FIGURE 19–12 Hi Lo endotracheal tube with subglottic suction.

minimize trauma on insertion. Endotracheal tubes usually have a Murphy eye near the distal tip, which allows the passage of gas if the end of the tube becomes occluded by secretions or the wall of the patient's airway. Near its distal end the tube has a cuff, which can be inflated by a pilot tube that extends past the proximal end of the tube and terminates with a pilot balloon and spring-loaded valve. A radiopaque line is molded into the tube to allow visualization of the tube on radiography.

> **RESPIRATORY RECAP**
>
> **Components of a Typical Endotracheal Tube**
>
> » Cuff
> » Pilot balloon
> » Radiopaque line
> » Proximal 15-mm connector

The tube's inner diameter (ID) and outer diameter (OD) measurements (in millimeters) are marked on it, as are the distance from the distal tip (in centimeters), the manufacturer's name, whether the tube is for oral or nasal use (an oral tube has a 45-degree angle at the tip; a nasal or oronasal tube has a 60-degree angle), and an indication that the tube material has been implant tested (IT). The proximal end of the tube is fitted with a standard 15-mm OD connection for respiratory and anesthesia equipment. By convention, the size of the endotracheal tube is given by its ID measurement.

Many variations in the design of the endotracheal tube can be seen. Given the recognized importance of preventing ventilator-associated pneumonia (VAP), several design modifications have emerged that show promising results. The Hi Lo Evac tube (**Figure 19–12**) allows continuous aspiration of subglottic secretions above the endotracheal tube cuff and has been shown to reduce the incidence of VAP.[36–39] An endotracheal tube with a polyurethane cuff has been introduced with an ultrathin cuff membrane, which may create a better seal by minimizing channel openings within folds formed when the cuff is inflated, thus preventing fluid and air leakage.[40,41] This design might decrease microaspiration of upper airway secretions, thus reducing the risk of VAP. In a prospective, single-blinded, randomized study, polyurethane cuffed endotracheal tubes reduced the frequency of early postoperative pneumonia in cardiac surgical patients. Unfortunately, the final diagnosis of pneumonia in this study was based on clinical criteria.[42] Further studies are needed to determine whether the benefit of these types of endotracheal tubes justify their additional expense.

Endotracheal tubes lined with a silver coating are thought to produce an enhanced antimicrobial activity by blocking bacterial adhesion to the tube itself.[43,44] The anode tube has a steel reinforcing wire that is wound spirally within the wall of the tube. This allows the tube to

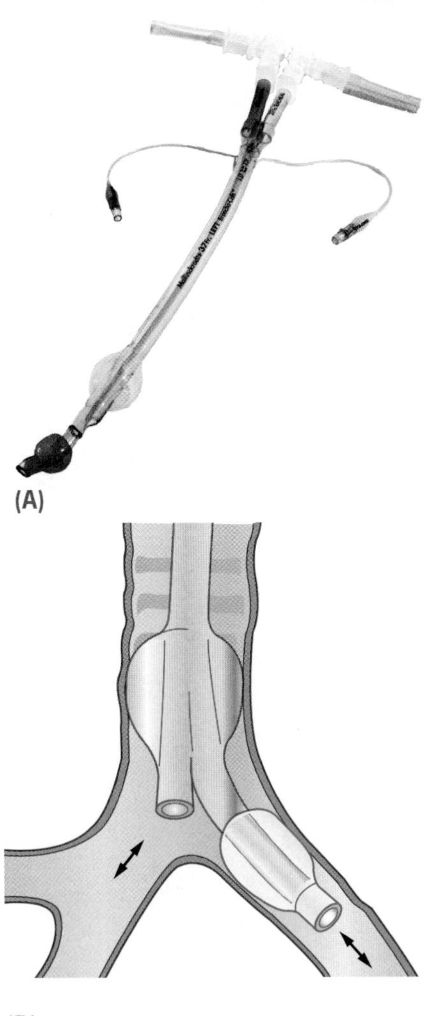

FIGURE 19–13 (**A**) Double-lumen tube. (**B**) Position of the left-sided endobronchial tube, showing the inflated cuffs and direction of gas flow.

be made of a softer material, yet prevents kinking when the tube must be bent at an angle to clear the surgical field or for bronchospirometry. The Endotrol allows the practitioner to control the direction of the distal tip of the endotracheal tube during intubation by pulling a loop near the tube's proximal end. A flexible, spiral stainless steel tube called the Laser-Flex can be used for laser surgery. Tubes for selective endobronchial intubation (**Figure 19–13**) are used during thoracic surgery (such as pneumonectomy), independent lung ventilation, or bronchospirometry.

Technique for Orotracheal Intubation

Once it has been determined that endotracheal intubation is required, proper preparation must follow. Each institution should have an emergency airway kit designed by the healthcare workers most likely to use it. This kit should be checked on a regular basis to assure proper function in an emergency situation. A difficult airway may be encountered unexpectedly, or a marginal airway may deteriorate rapidly, leaving little time to obtain an item from elsewhere.

It is imperative that the process of intubation be approached calmly. Frantic and rushed attempts often result in failure and worsening of the situation. Some method of oxygenation must be provided while the following preparatory steps are taken.

1. Obtaining a brief history is important, and the few seconds this requires may prevent surprises during the process. This is especially important when there have been prior intubations. A previously difficult airway or visualization could be uncovered, and the clinician can take the appropriate steps to be prepared for the scenario.
2. Positioning is a key aspect of preparation. The patient should be positioned as optimally as possible within the limits of the environment. Some positioning tips include moving the bed away from the wall and raising its height, bringing the patient as close to the head of the bed as possible to limit the amount of reaching, adjusting the patient into an even supine position, and placing a folded blanket or towels under the head to achieve the sniffing position (**Figure 19–14**), which aligns the oral, pharyngeal, and laryngeal axes for optimum visualization of the larynx. In essence, this is flexion of the lower cervical spine and extension of the upper cervical spine. However, this position is contraindicated in a patient with a confirmed or suspected neck injury. In such cases an assistant should maintain the head and neck in a neutral position as intubation is attempted.
3. Suction must be ready, preferably with a tonsil-tip suction apparatus, and a functioning intravenous line must be in place before any attempts at intubation are made.
4. Sedation or neuromuscular blocking agents may be necessary in a responsive patient to facilitate the intubation process. However, abolishing spontaneous ventilation shortens the available intubation time, eliminates airway reflexes, and further compromises airway patency.

When all preparations are complete, the procedure can be started. **Orotracheal intubation** is most commonly performed with a **laryngoscope**. The laryngoscope is composed of a handle and a blade. The handle may be made of metal or plastic, may be disposable or nondisposable, and may have a detachable or permanently affixed blade (**Figure 19–15**). Batteries in the body of the handle provide power to a lighting device in the blade or the handle. When the lighting mechanism is in the handle, a fiberoptic bundle in the blade transmits light to the distal end of the blade. The fiberoptic laryngoscope has several advantages over the traditional type. Because the light bulbs are in the handle in fiberoptic laryngoscopes, they do not contact the patient and cannot be dislodged in the airway. Also, fewer bulbs are needed because a laryngoscopy set with a handle and several blades requires only one light bulb, whereas the older system requires a bulb in each blade. The proper function of the handle and its light bulb and batteries must be determined before use.

Laryngoscope blades vary in construction and are available in several shapes and sizes. The three standard blades are the curved (MacIntosh) blade, the straight (Wisconsin) blade, and the straight with a slightly curved tip (Miller) blade. Many specialty blades also are available, all designed for the occasional unusual circumstance that requires a minor variation of these standard blades. The operator's preference, training, and experience determine which blade is used. Most clinicians choose the blade they have used most often, but an experienced intubator is comfortable with all three types, so that when one does not work, an alternative is available. Nearly all blades come in sizes 0 through 4, a range that accommodates neonates up through large adults.

The laryngoscope is introduced into the mouth from the right side, displacing the tongue to the left. This maneuver is used with either a curved or straight blade to prevent the tongue from reducing visualization of the glottis. As the posterior pharyngeal wall comes into view, the person performing the intubation looks for the epiglottis (**Figure 19–16**). When the epiglottis can be seen, and a curved blade is used, the laryngoscope is gently readjusted to place the tip of the blade into the vallecula (the junction of the base of the tongue and the epiglottis) (**Figure 19–17**). If a straight blade is used, the laryngoscope is readjusted to lift the tip of the epiglottis (**Figure 19–18**). The proper motor action of readjustment of the laryngoscope is to direct a force on a vector caudal and anterior without a prying action. Using the laryngoscope in a prying action increases the likelihood of dental damage during the procedure. The above maneuvers usually bring the glottis into view, with the opening into the lower airway between the vocal cords. With spontaneous ventilation, the appropriately sized endotracheal tube is introduced gently between the vocal cords during inspiration. If difficulty is encountered with passing the tube into the trachea, a stylet can be used to change the tube's curvature.

RESPIRATORY RECAP

Equipment Required for Endotracheal Intubation

- » Correct size endotracheal tube
- » Lubricant
- » Suction
- » Syringe
- » Laryngoscope
- » Stylet
- » Carbon dioxide detector
- » Bag-valve-mask device
- » Oxygen
- » Sedative and paralytic agents
- » Tape to secure tube

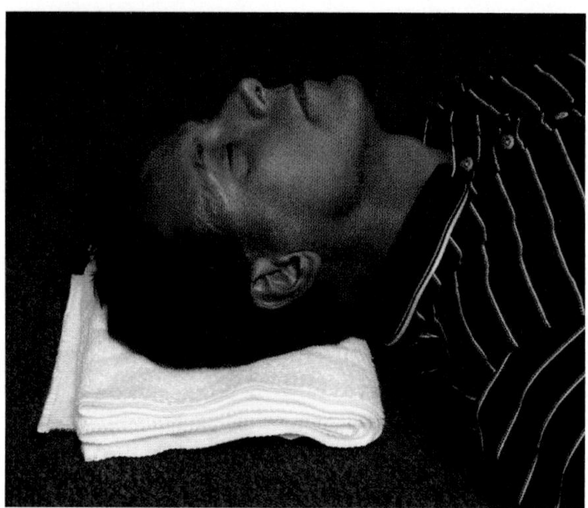

FIGURE 19–14 Sniffing position.

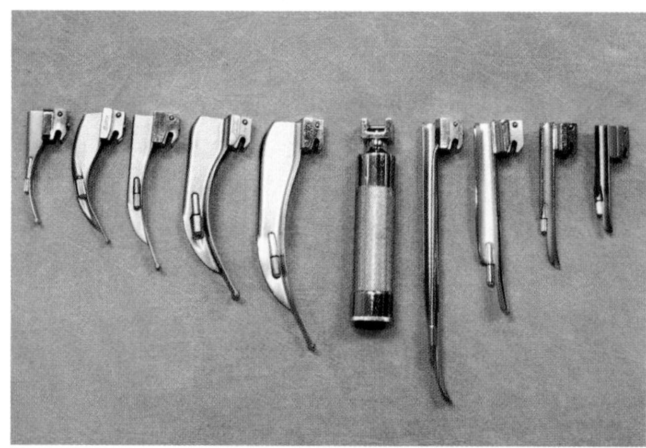

FIGURE 19–15 Laryngoscope handle (center), curved (Macintosh) blades (left), and straight (Miller) blades (right).

A stylet is generally used to help guide the endotracheal tube though the vocal cords and can be shaped to aid in the passage to the trachea. This may be of particular importance in the case of anterior airway presentation.

In adults, a 7- to 7.5-mm ID endotracheal tube is used for women and an 8- to 8.5-mm ID tube is used for men. The tube is advanced 2 to 4 cm below the level of the vocal cords into the trachea, and bilateral breath sounds are then verified by auscultation. Correct placement is then checked by other means, such as measurement of expired carbon dioxide, negative auscultation of air movement over the epigastrium, and chest radiograph. As a general rule, the tube should be secured at the 21-cm mark (at the teeth) in women and at the 23-cm mark in men.[45] The tube is secured to the upper lip and maxilla, and another check is made for bilateral breath sounds. An appropriate oxygen delivery and ventilation system is then connected.

As described previously with difficult airways, direct visualization of the laryngeal structures sometimes is inadequate or even impossible. Repeated attempts at intubation can cause trauma, can make subsequent attempts even more difficult, and also can interfere with ventilation. A disciplined approach must be used, including the abandonment of attempts that could make a bad situation worse. The difficult airway algorithm (refer to Figure 19–8) presents a problem-based approach to proceeding in this situation.

A **gum elastic bougie** can be an effective adjunct for difficult intubation. This is a blunt-ended, malleable rod that is passed through the poorly or nonvisualized larynx by putting a J-shaped bend at the tip and passing it blindly in the midline upward beyond the base of the epiglottis. The endotracheal tube is passed over the bougie and the bougie is withdrawn. A similar device is the endotracheal **tube exchanger**. This device facilitates quick, efficient endotracheal tube exchange or replacement without using a laryngoscope. It is constructed of flexible material and usually has depth marks to aid precise placement. Some tube exchangers have an internal lumen that allows for spontaneous breathing during the tube exchange.

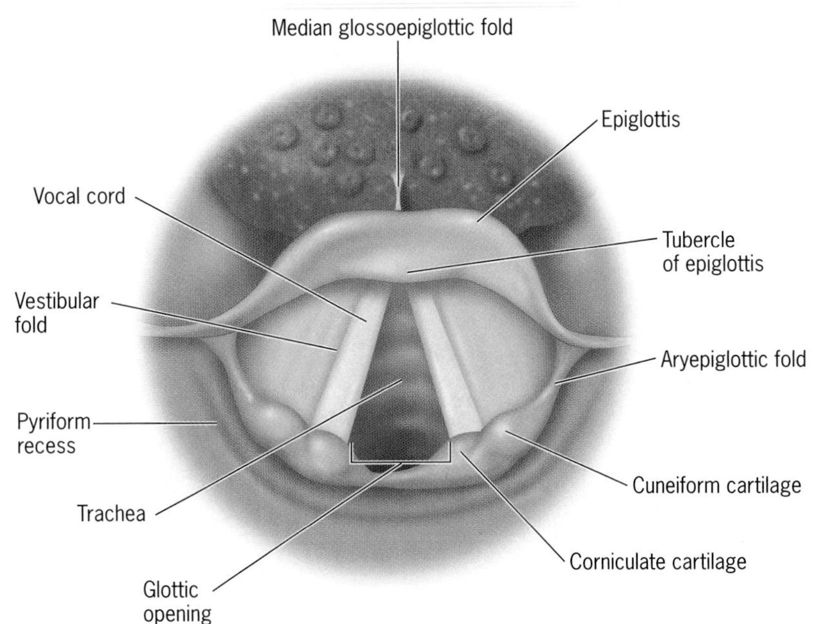

FIGURE 19–16 View of the glottis.

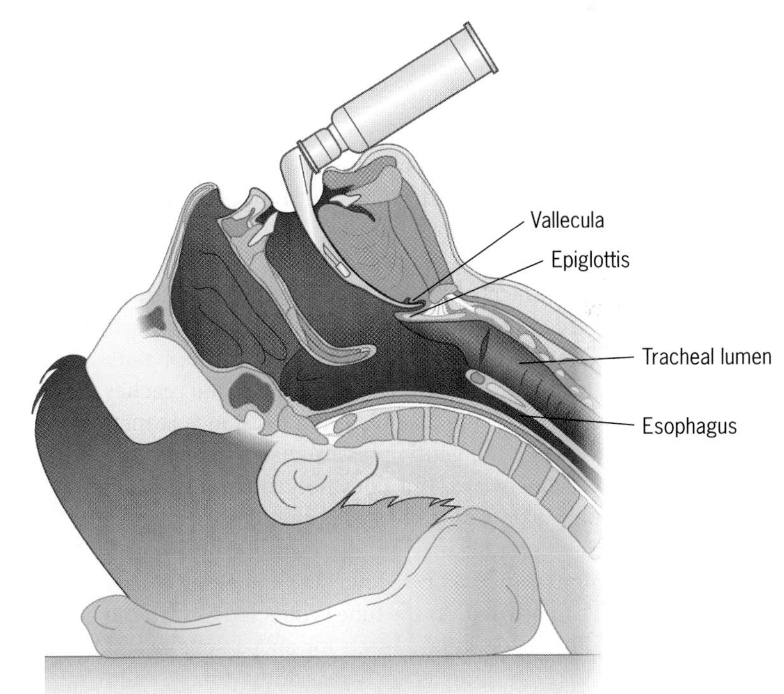

FIGURE 19–17 Use of curved blade.

Technique for Nasotracheal Intubation

Nasotracheal intubation generally is used for specific indications and has some special characteristics compared with orotracheal intubation.[46] Nasotracheal intubation is useful when access to the mouth is unavailable, as in oral surgery or oral trauma, or when the mouth cannot be opened adequately, as in trauma, TMJ dysfunction, or mandibular fixation. Some experts feel that a nasotracheal tube is more easily tolerated once inserted. Because the lips are not distorted, communication with the patient and oral care are easier. In addition, uncooperative patients often bite on an orotracheal tube, causing occlusion of the tube and difficulty with mechanical ventilation. However, the development of sinusitis often is associated with nasotracheal intubation. Although the nasotracheal tube may be easier to secure, it is more difficult to suction secretions through this tube. A nasotracheal tube is more stable because of the immobility of the nose and maxilla in contrast to mandibular movement, which can affect an orotracheal tube. Because movement of the endotracheal tube in the trachea is one of the determining factors in airway trauma from intubation, nasotracheal intubation may be less likely to cause tracheal injury.

For nasotracheal intubation, as with orotracheal intubation, equipment for oxygen delivery, manual ventilation, and suction is required. A Magill forceps and a fiberoptic laryngoscope also are useful. When access to the mouth is difficult, spontaneous breathing should not be suppressed, but light sedation is beneficial. A topical anesthetic spray or jelly and a vasoconstricting spray are applied to the

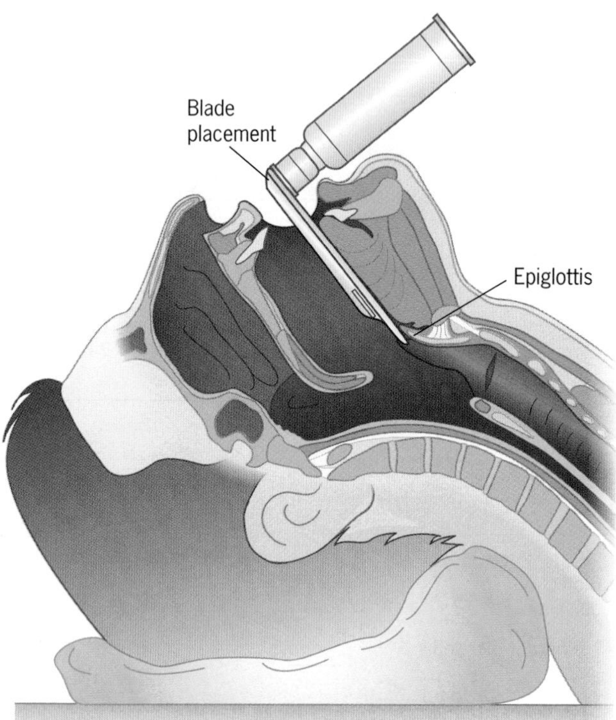

FIGURE 19–18 Use of straight blade.

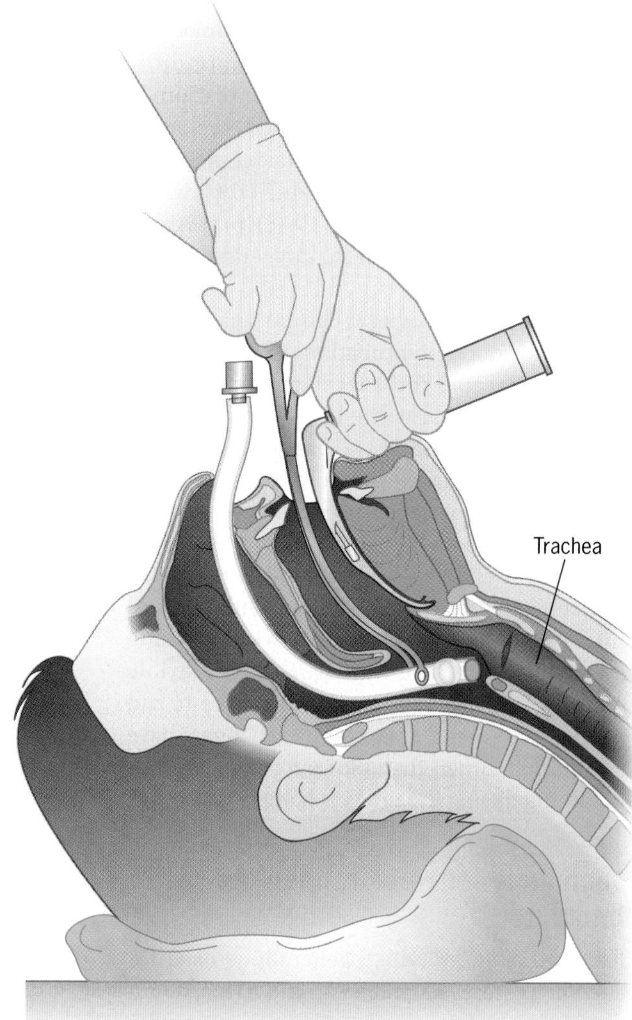

FIGURE 19–19 Use of Magill forceps.

nares and nasopharynx to minimize sensation, trauma, and bleeding. The nasal passage can be gently dilated with lubricated, soft nasopharyngeal airways to facilitate introduction of the firmer and larger endotracheal tube. The endotracheal tube should be inserted with an initial upward motion until it just passes into the naris and then continued on a course parallel to the palate with firm, gentle pressure. As the tip of the tube reaches the posterior wall of the nasopharynx, resistance is met. Slightly increasing the gentle pressure usually causes the tip to deflect downward. If it does not, rotating the tube slightly usually works. It is important not to use excessive force, or a false passage may be created in the pharyngeal wall, causing trauma and bleeding. As an alternative, the other naris can be tried. As the tube is directed toward the glottis, the intubator should listen for air passing in and out of the tube. As long as air is heard, the tube should be superior to the larynx. The tube is inserted into the glottis during inspiration (when the vocal cords are the widest apart), and as it passes the cords, a cough usually is produced. If the tube does not blindly pass into the glottis, it can be directed fiberoptically or directly with a Magill forceps and laryngoscope if the mouth can be opened (**Figure 19–19**). When the tube has been inserted to the appropriate depth, verification of breath sounds, carbon dioxide measurement, and verification of placement by chest radiograph should be performed.

Nasotracheal intubation may be contraindicated in some cases. Alternate techniques should be seriously considered for cases involving a suspected basilar skull fracture, nasal fracture, nasal polyps, epistaxis, coagulopathy, or planned thrombolysis.[47] Nasotracheal intubation with a basilar skull fracture is very controversial, although there is an increase in the complication rate with this condition.[47] Epistaxis is the most common complication of nasotracheal intubation and usually can be easily managed in patients with normal coagulation processes. Because the tube causes mucosal trauma and edema, the opening to the maxillary sinuses may become occluded, with subsequent development of sinusitis.[48]

Drugs to Facilitate Intubation

Rapid sequence intubation is used in patients who have a gag reflex who would otherwise be difficult to intubate. In these patients, intubation is accomplished by use of sedation and paralysis. The three phases of medication administration are pretreatment, induction, and paralysis. The patient is preoxygenated for 3 to 5 minutes. Pretreatment agents are used to lessen the physiologic response to laryngoscopy and include lidocaine, opioid analgesic (fentanyl, sufentanil alfentanil), atropine, and defasciculating agents. Induction agents provide a rapid loss of consciousness that facilitates ease of intubation. Various agents can be used for induction, including etomidate, propofol, midazolam, sodium thiopental, and ketamine. The most common induction agent is etomidate, which has a rapid onset and short duration, is cerebroprotective, is not associated with a significant drop in blood pressure, and is hemodynamically neutral compared with other agents, such as sodium thiopental. Paralyzing agents provide neuromuscular blockade and depolarizing agents such as succinylcholine or nondepolarizing agents such as rocuronium.

Video Laryngoscopy Devices

In recent years, technological advances have been made to improve the success of intubation both in controlled and emergency situations. Perhaps the most significant impact involves use of video laryngoscopes. These devices generally provide a digitally produced real-time view of the larynx without having to directly view through the patient's open mouth. The image is visualized on a screen attached to the scope or on a separate monitor and is particularly useful when mouth opening or neck positioning may be compromised to some degree. It is also useful in difficult airways or in situations characterized as failed intubation.

Several manufacturers have developed video laryngoscopes, and some are in common use today. The Airtraq by King Systems is a single-use device that is battery powered and portable. It has an L-shaped design and two channels, one for the optics and one a delivery channel for introduction of the endotracheal tube (**Figure 19–20**). The Airtraq is introduced above the epiglottis similar to a MacIntosh laryngoscope blade, and the endotracheal tube is advanced into the glottis under visualization and then moved out of the channel as the Airtraq is removed. Comparative studies with the MacIntosh laryngoscope have shown superior viewing with the Airtraq.[49–51]

Two multiple-use devices with single-use blade covers are the GlideScope (**Figure 19–21**) and McGrath video laryngoscopes (**Figure 19–22**). The McGrath is more portable because its small LCD screen is mounted directly on the handle, but the small size of the screen limits the view clarity at times. The view obtained with the McGrath is slightly better than the view obtained with the Airtraq, and the LCD screen is also adjustable to some degree. The GlideScope has a larger monitor attached by a video cable, which improves the quality and size of the image but limits its portability. A more portable version is the GlideScope Ranger (**Figure 19–23**), which has a handheld monitor that can be placed on the patient's chest during intubation for easier viewing. Several other manufacturers have developed variations of the three mentioned devices, and most are functional and improve visualization over the classic direct laryngoscopy, particularly in difficult visualization situations.

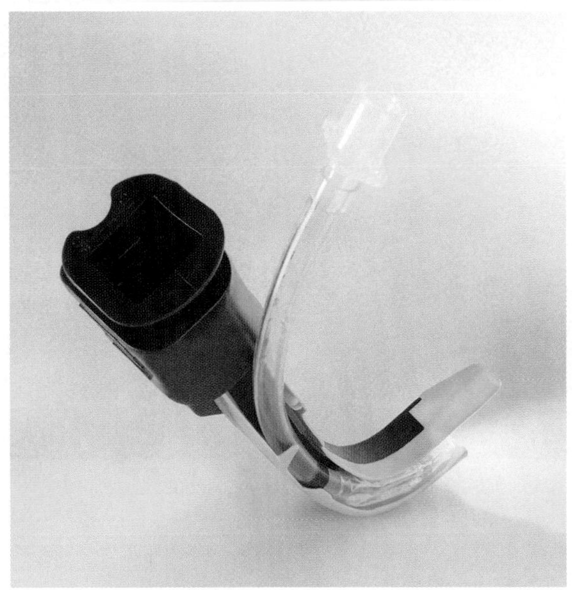

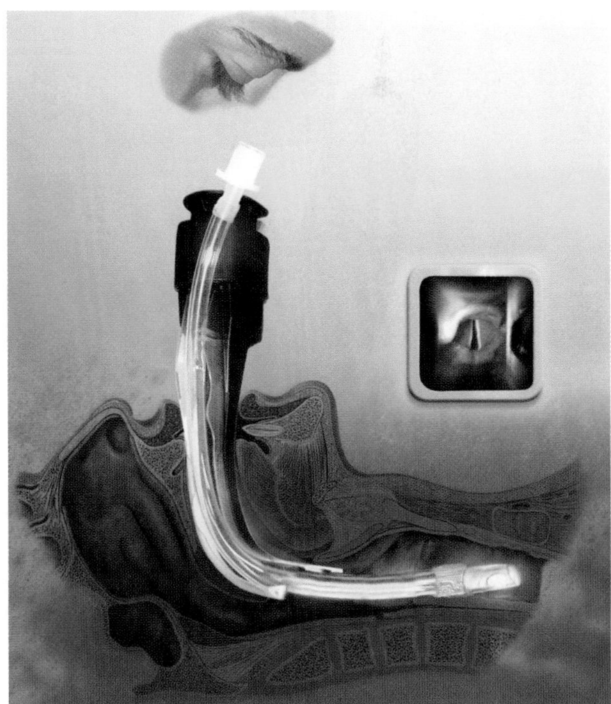

FIGURE 19–20 Airtraq laryngoscope with a tracheal tube in place in the side channel.

Supraglottic Ventilatory Devices

The **laryngeal mask airway (LMA)** (**Figure 19–24**) has evolved over a relatively short time and is currently in wide use both for routine management of the airway during general anesthesia and as an emergency airway adjunct for difficult airways. Brain began developing the LMA in 1981, modifying more than 100 prototypes to achieve the current LMA.[52] This device provides access to the upper airway with minimal potential for involving the upper gastrointestinal tract. The LMA allows more direct ventilation than bag-mask ventilation by isolating

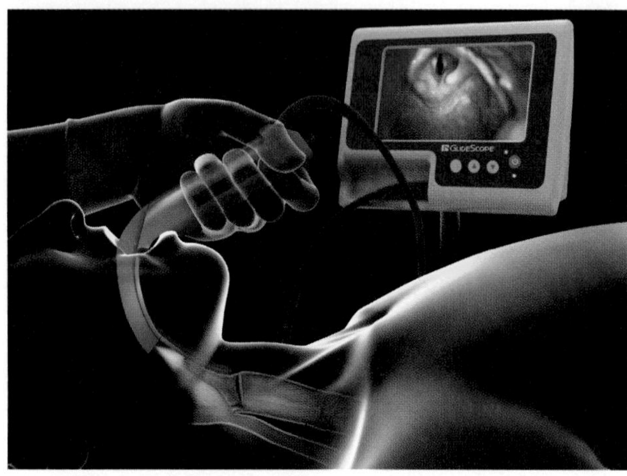

FIGURE 19–21 GlideScope video laryngoscope.

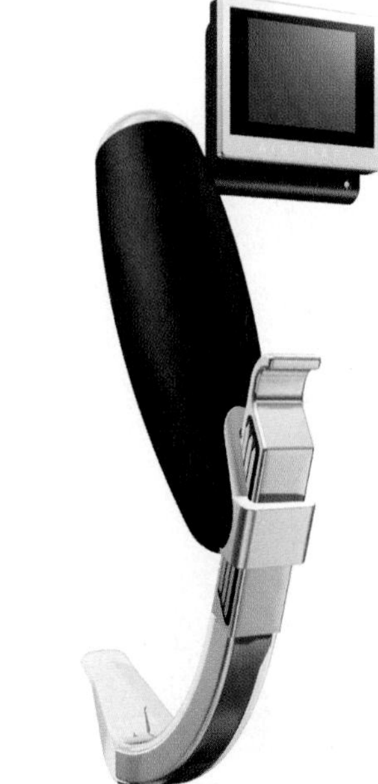

FIGURE 19–22 McGrath video laryngoscope.

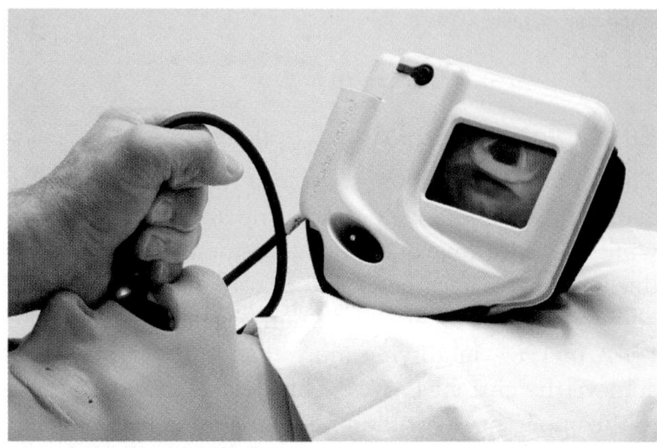

FIGURE 19–23 GlideScope Ranger.

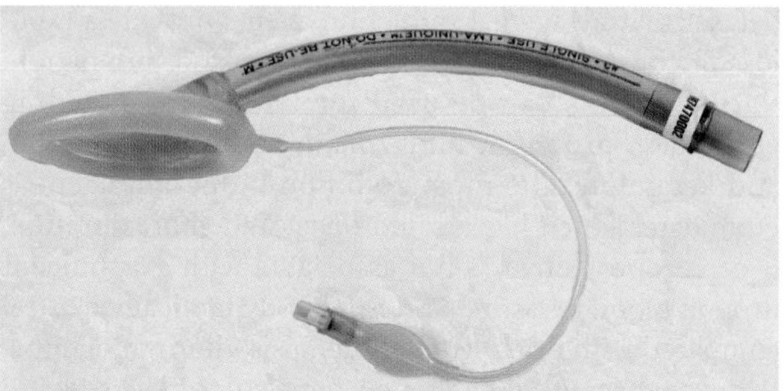

FIGURE 19–24 Laryngeal mask airway.

the laryngeal structures from the esophageal structures in most cases. Ventilation provided by an LMA generally is superior to bag-mask ventilation. The LMA does not, however, provide the same level of airway protection and security as an endotracheal tube. On the other hand, it does not require instrumentation of the laryngeal or tracheal structures and is relatively easy to place. Training for correct LMA placement only requires a few hours, and it is usually associated with a high rate of success.

The LMA is available in a range of sizes, from neonate to large adult. A No. 5 LMA is used for large adults, and sizes 3 and 4 are most often appropriate for small to average-sized adults. The LMA is a large-bore tube with a small inflatable mask at its distal end. A locking valve inflation port and tube allow inflation of the mask after it has been inserted and placed. The proximal end has the standard 15-mm adapter for connection to a ventilating or gas delivery device. The shape and design of this device, which has been refined over the past two decades and many prototypes, allows it to form a seal around the glottic opening while excluding the esophageal opening from the airway. This facilitates optimum ventilation with little risk of gastric insufflation or regurgitation. The risk of aspiration is not eliminated, but there is little evidence that this complication occurs with significant incidence. The technique for insertion of an LMA is shown in **Figure 19–25**.

The LMA has made a significant contribution to the management of the difficult airway. When attempts at intubation fail, an LMA can be inserted and often rescues a potentially disastrous situation. Introduction of a fiberoptic bronchoscope down the lumen of an appropriately placed LMA nearly always reveals the glottic opening in plain view. Threading a small endotracheal tube over the bronchoscope through the LMA lumen accomplishes intubation in this otherwise difficult circumstance. The widespread use of this technique and its inclusion in the difficult airway algorithm prompted the development of a special intubating LMA that has found its way onto most difficult-airway carts. Its rigid, preformed, and larger lumen makes passage of an endotracheal tube through it much easier. It also has special endotracheal tubes and pushers that allow removal of the LMA after successful endotracheal intubation. In contrast, removal

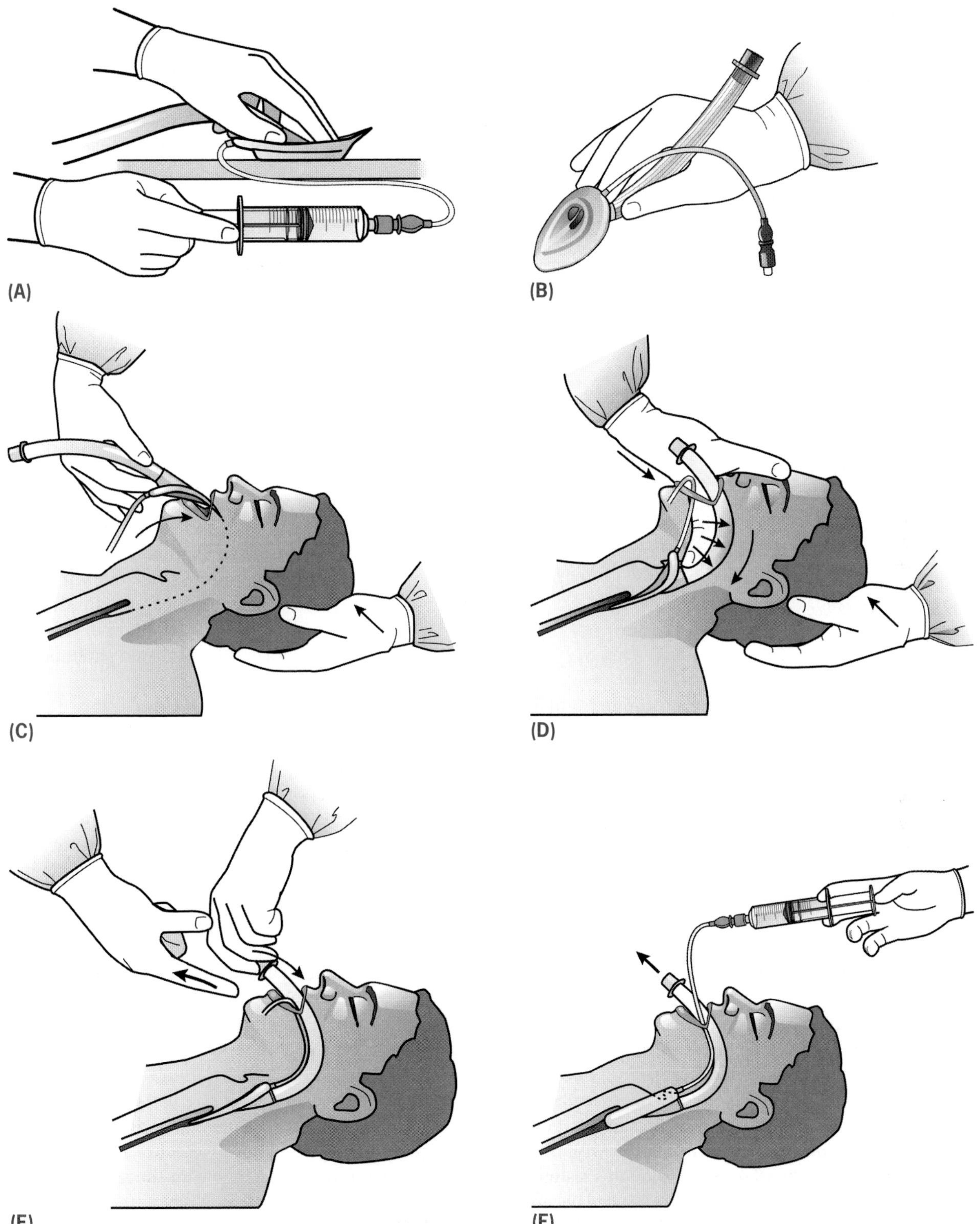

FIGURE 19–25 Insertion technique for laryngeal mask airway. Courtesy of LMA North America, Inc.

of the standard LMA after placement of an endotracheal tube can be cumbersome and is not without risk.

Other supraglottic devices have been developed to improve on the basic LMA for specific indications and to introduce disposability of the device. Specific modifications were made to (1) enable easier endotracheal intubation through the LMA, (2) provide portals for evacuation of gastric contents while the device is in place (**Figure 19–26**),[53,54] (3) provide for temperature monitoring, and (4) enhance the anatomic shape of the device. Conditions limiting the use of supraglottic devices include morbid obesity, known gastric contents,

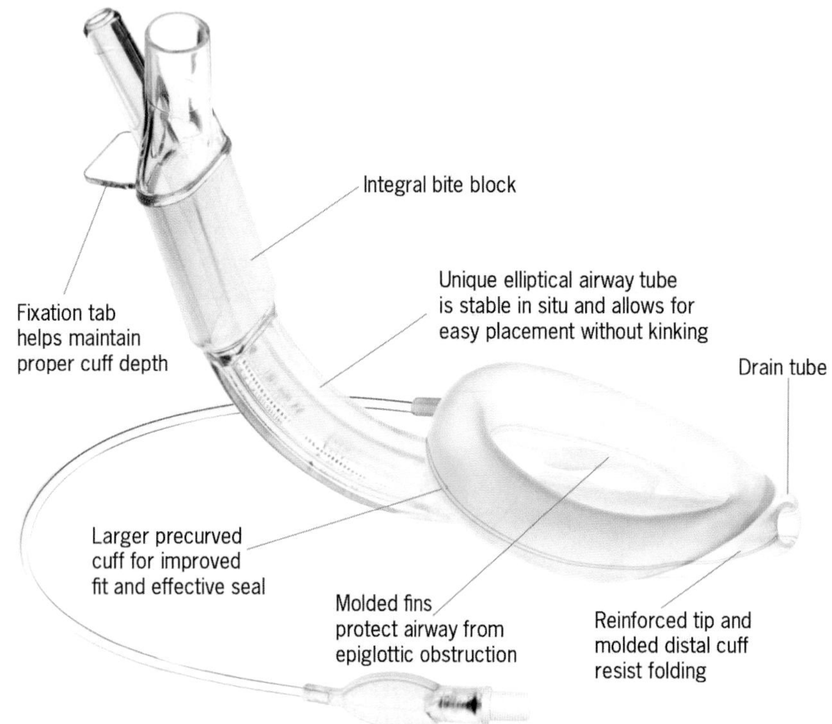

FIGURE 19–26 LMA Supreme.

or guidewire is then passed from the larynx back up to the oral cavity. An endotracheal tube is passed over the guidewire to the larynx and trachea.[56] This technique is also rarely used because of its invasiveness and complexity.

Complications of Endotracheal Intubation

A number of complications have been associated with endotracheal intubation (**Box 19–2**).[57,58] These have been classified temporally as complications that occur during the intubation procedure, those that occur while the endotracheal tube is in place, those that occur during and immediately after extubation, and those that occur late after extubation. The risk of complications associated with endotracheal intubation is reduced by meticulous attention to care of the airway in intubated patients.

oropharyngeal swelling, airway trauma, tumors, and distorted facial anatomy.

Cricothyrotomy

Creating an airway through the cricothyroid membrane is called a **cricothyrotomy**. Emergent cricothyrotomy is a valuable weapon in the airway arsenal when conventional airway access cannot be obtained. Access can be gained using a needle (needle cricothyrotomy) or surgically with a scalpel. In a needle cricothyrotomy a 12- to 16-gauge over-the-needle catheter is passed through the cricothyroid membrane. Once access to the trachea is gained, the needle is removed and the catheter can then be attached to an oxygen/ventilation source. The surgical cricothyrotomy is done in four steps: (1) palpation of the cricothyroid membrane, (2) making of a vertical or horizontal incision (3–4 cm), (3) insertion of a dilator, and (4) intubation with a tracheostomy tube (**Figure 19–27**).[55] Although a valuable airway technique, cricothyrotomy is rarely used because of its invasive nature; therefore, clinicians may lack the appropriate experience level. This technique should be used only when glottis visualization is impeded (e.g., due to trauma, vomitus, secretions, bleeding) and intubation cannot be done either orally or nasally through standard techniques.

Another airway technique that is used on rare occasions is retrograde intubation. In a retrograde intubation, the cricothyroid membrane again is accessed with a through-the-needle catheter or a guidewire. The catheter

Securing the Endotracheal Tube

Securing the endotracheal tube is an extremely important aspect of airway management. Although not well established, the reported rates of unplanned extubation (accidental extubation or self-extubation) are anywhere from 2% to 13%.[59–71] Although reintubation is not necessary in every case of unplanned extubation, it is more likely than with planned extubation and may occur under more dire circumstances due to patient instability. Unplanned extubation may result in serious complications and even death. Factors associated with unplanned extubation include chronic respiratory failure, orotracheal intubation, lack of intravenous sedation, and securing of the endotracheal tube with only thin adhesive tape.

The American Heart Association's advanced life support guidelines recommend the use of either tape or commercial devices to secure the endotracheal tube.[13] The traditional method used to secure an endotracheal tube has been to apply benzoin to the skin and secure the tube with adhesive tape (Lillehei technique) (**Figure 19–28**).[72] Tape 2.5 cm wide is cut long enough to go around the circumference of the patient's head one and one-half to two times. A second piece of tape is cut long enough to fit over the midportion of the first piece, thus preventing the tape from sticking to the patient's neck. The tape is then placed around the patient's neck. The skin surface is dried, and tincture of benzoin is placed on both of the patient's cheeks where the tape will come into contact with the skin. The tape is pulled snug against the patient's neck and applied on the patient's cheeks to

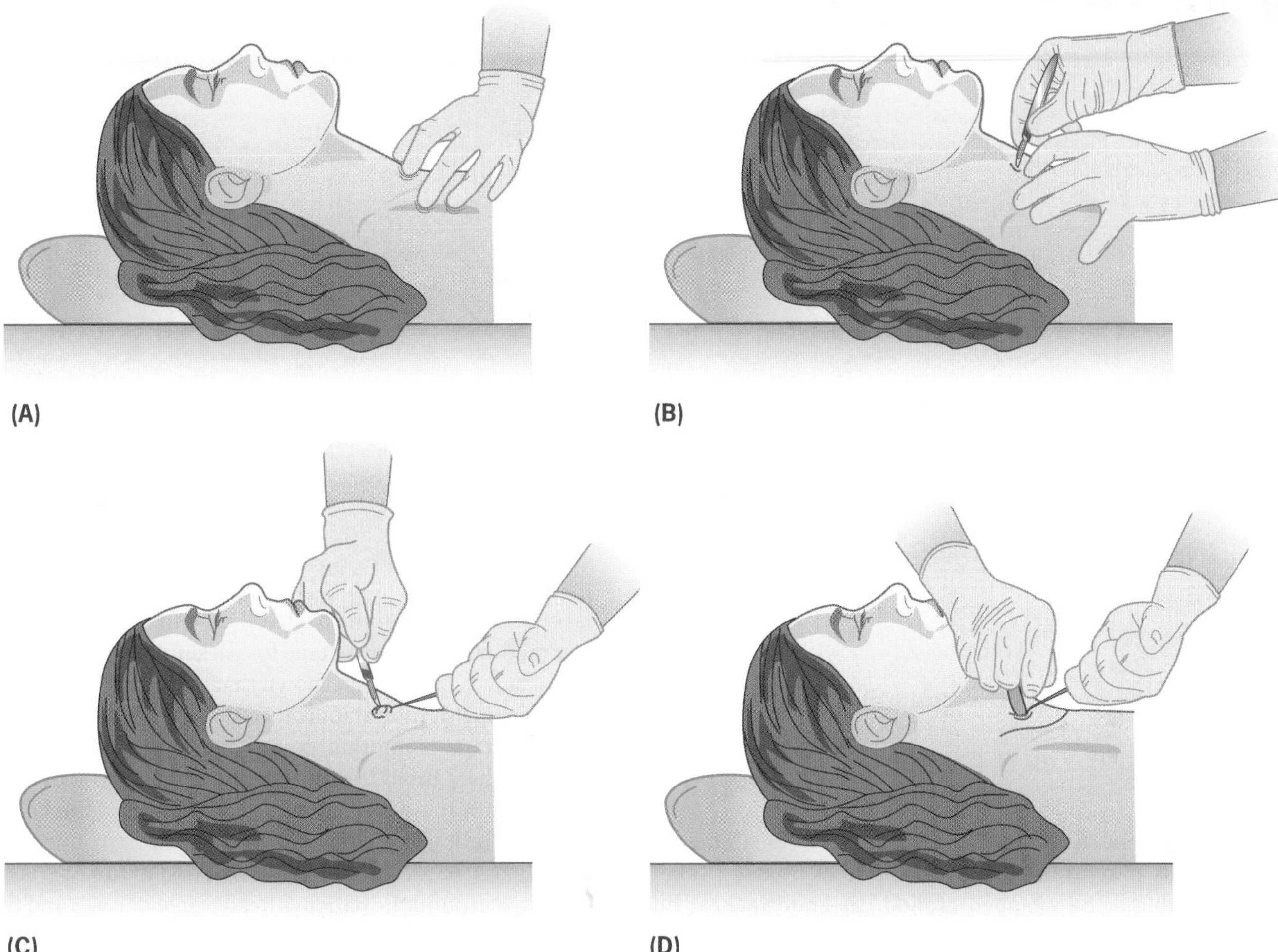

FIGURE 19–27 Approach to cricothyrotomy. (**A**) Step 1. The operator palpates the cricoid membrane. (**B**) Step 2. A horizontal stab incision is made into the inferior aspect of the cricothyroid membrane. (**C**) Step 3. The tracheal hook is placed flush against the caudal surface of the scalpel blade and pushed into the trachea. The scalpel is removed, and traction is maintained. (**D**) Step 4. A cuffed tracheostomy or endotracheal tube is inserted into the incision. Adapted from Brofeldt T, et al. An easy crichothyrotomy approach: the rapid four-step technique. *Acad Emerg Med.* 1996;3:1060–1063.

BOX 19–2

Complications of Intubation

During the Intubation Procedure
- Cardiac arrest
- Nasal and oral trauma
- Pharyngeal and hypopharyngeal trauma
- Laryngeal and tracheal trauma
- Main bronchus intubation
- Pulmonary aspiration
- Esophageal intubation

While the Endotracheal Tube Is in Place
- Nasal and oral ulceration (oral cellulitis)
- Sinus effusions and sinusitis
- Otitis
- Laryngeal injury
- Tracheal injury
- Pulmonary complication
- Self-extubation
- Mechanical problems with the tube or cuff
- Patient discomfort

During and Immediately After Extubation
- Sore throat
- Stridor
- Hoarseness
- Odynophagia
- True vocal cord immobility
- Pulmonary aspiration
- Cough

Late Complications After Extubation
- Laryngeal injury
  - Stenosis
  - Granuloma formation
- Tracheal injury
  - Stenosis

From Stauffer JL, Silvester RC. Complications of endotracheal intubation, tracheostomy, and artificial airways. *Respir Care.* 1982;27:417–434. Reprinted with permission.

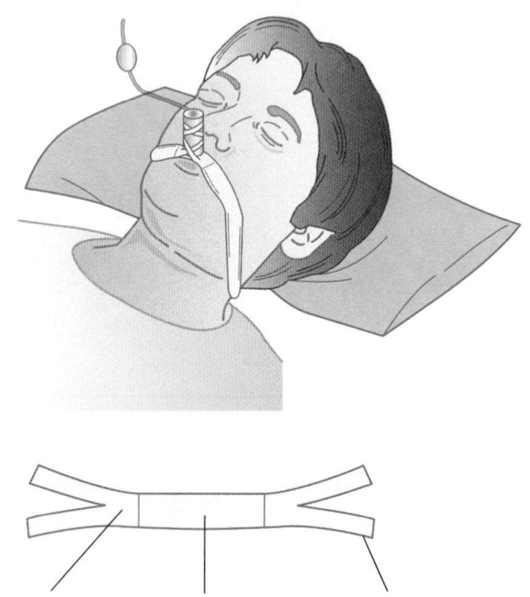

FIGURE 19–28 Securing the endotracheal tube (Lillehei technique).

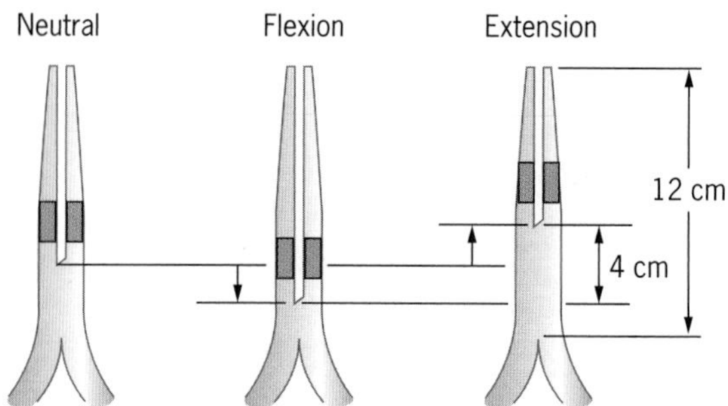

FIGURE 19–29 Movement of the distal endotracheal tube tip with flexion and extension of the head. Reproduced from Conrardy PA, Goodman LR, Lainge F, et al. Alteration of endotracheal tube position: flexion and extension of the neck. *Crit Care Med.* 1976;4(1):8–12. Reprinted with permission from Wolters Kluwer Health.

the edge of the endotracheal tube. The remaining tape is split longitudinally so that at least 5 cm of tape is available to be wrapped around the endotracheal tube at the lips. Later removal of the tape can be facilitated if the end of the tape is folded back on itself to form a tab. Some clinicians wrap both ends of the split tape around the tube, whereas others wrap one piece around the tube and pass the other piece over the lip and fasten it to the contralateral cheek. The tape is applied snugly but not so tight as to cause breakdown of the facial skin. The advantage of this method is that tape passes completely around the neck, which is preferable to techniques in which one or two pieces of tape are used to tape the tube to the patient's cheeks. A similar method can be used for nasally placed tubes. The endotracheal tube, gastric tube, and oral airway (if present) should be taped separately. In this way, one device can be repositioned or removed without affecting the other. The tube should not be taped to the mandible, because this increases the likelihood of tube movement if the jaw is moved.

> **RESPIRATORY RECAP**
>
> **Means of Securing Endotracheal Tubes**
>
> » Adhesive tape
> » Twill tape
> » Commercially available devices

Adhesive tape can pose some problems. Mouth care is difficult when too much tape is used. When an oral airway is added for stabilization and to prevent the patient from biting the tube, airway care becomes even more difficult. The patient's oral cavity and lips and the skin around the mouth must be carefully observed for signs of complications. The skin around the mouth of debilitated or immunosuppressed patients may become excoriated by tape on the face. In addition, the tape has been shown to promote bacterial growth. Although there are methods of securing tape for patients with beards and moustaches, it has been shown that these methods create problems with tube stabilization.[73]

Twill tape is another common means to secure the endotracheal tube.[72] With this method, a 1-m length of twill tape is folded in half and looped around the endotracheal tube. The ends are brought through this loop and tightened around the tube. One end of the twill tape is passed around the patient's head below one ear, and the other end is passed above the other ear. The two ends are tied in a bow on the cheek. This technique sometimes is repeated with a second piece of twill tape so that two ties are used to secure the endotracheal tube.

Tube movement is considered a major cause of airway trauma. Movement of the tube against the tracheal mucosa causes a raking motion along the soft tissues of the airway. The contact is greatest at the pressure points of the lips, posterior pharynx, and posterior of the glottis and at the site of the cuff.[73–80] In adults, the tip of the endotracheal tube should be positioned 3 to 7 cm above the carina when the neck is in a neutral position.[72] Flexion of the neck causes the distal tip to move toward the carina, and extension of the neck causes the tube to move toward the glottis (**Figure 19–29**). If the tube advances too far distally, it may enter a main stem bronchus (usually the right).[76] If the tube moves proximally with the cuff inflated, laryngeal damage may occur. Displacement into the esophagus or pharynx may result in gastric insufflation and inadequate lung ventilation.

There are now a number of non-tape devices available for securing endotracheal tubes. One study looked at the minimum force required for extubation with newer endotracheal tube holders compared with the conventional taping method.[80] Only the Thomas tube holder (**Figure 19–30**) required more force to extubate than conventional taping. No one retention device has been universally accepted. Many nontape devices tend to be on the large side, which could hinder mouth care. The ideal method would allow minimal tube migration, would be comfortable for the patient, would allow oral

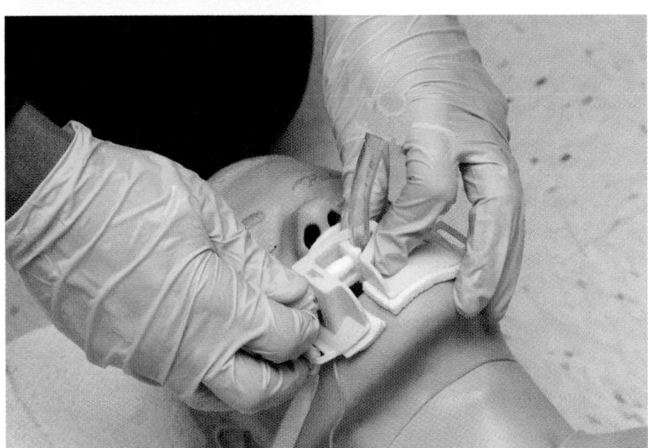

FIGURE 19–30 Thomas tube holder.

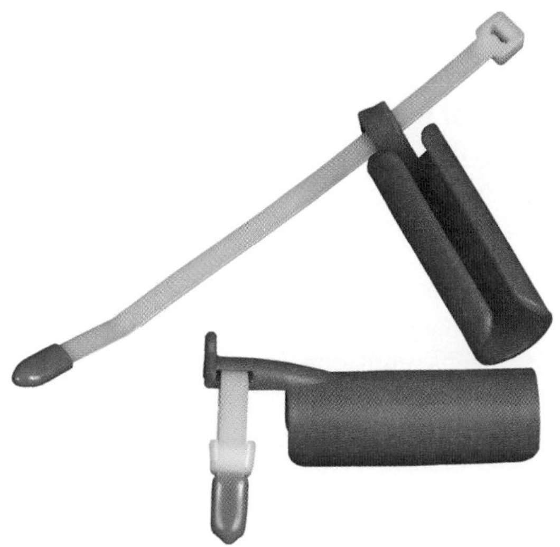

FIGURE 19–31 Universal bite block. Courtesy of B&B Medical Technologies.

hygiene, and would preserve skin integrity; it also would be easy to apply and would require minimal maintenance time from nurses or respiratory therapists.

The endotracheal tube should be repositioned in the mouth periodically to allow provision of mouth care and to prevent pressure sores of the lips, gums, and mouth.[72] Two people should be present when the endotracheal tube is unsecured for this care. One person is responsible for maintaining the tube's position, and the other person is responsible for providing mouth care and resecuring the tube. In some units it is also common practice to trim the excess endotracheal tube length. This may reduce the risk of tube malposition or kinking. However, it is important to ensure that the tube is properly positioned before it is trimmed. A swivel connector should be used between the endotracheal tube and the breathing circuit, and the breathing circuit should be supported so that it does not promote tube movement.

A bite block can be placed between the teeth to prevent the patient from biting an orotracheal airway or from biting the tongue or lips, causing bleeding and trauma to the mouth. The material should be tough but not rigid and may have channels for air passage. A variety of materials and adaptations of other airways have been used as bite blocks. Oropharyngeal airways are sometimes used but may damage the teeth. Also, the complications of oropharyngeal airways when endotracheal tubes are in place for prolonged periods are problematic. Oral airways have been modified for this purpose by removal of the pharyngeal portion. An airway gag was developed for patients receiving electroconvulsive therapy. The device, a wedge-shaped piece of surgical rubber, consists of a body with air channels, a flange, and a tongue depressor and retractor that hold the tongue in place but do not extend into the pharynx deep enough to induce a gag reflex.

In patients with an endotracheal tube, bite blocks may be used to prevent occlusion due to either active biting or large teeth. Oropharyngeal tubes also can be used to serve this purpose. However, they tend to be somewhat large and have the potential to cause dental or mucosal damage. Another option is a device that surrounds a portion of the endotracheal tube to prevent occlusive biting but has minimal impact on surrounding tissue (**Figure 19–31**). Once placed around the appropriate portion of the endotracheal tube, it can be secured to minimize slippage. Devices such as these have the advantages of being smaller and of posing less risk of migrating away from the tube as well as of causing unwanted gag stimulation.

Extubation

Because endotracheal tubes are considered a temporary measure, clinicians must determine the appropriate time to remove them from patients. Some patients require a permanent artificial airway, but these should receive a tracheostomy. **Extubation** is defined as the removal of an endotracheal tube (**CPG 19–2**).[81] A patient is generally ready to be extubated when the initial reason for intubation has been corrected. However, several criteria must also be met. These criteria include the ability to protect the lower airway from aspiration, the ability to clear secretions (cough strength), the nature of secretions (quantity and character), and the ability to prevent obstruction of the upper airway (level of consciousness). Quantity of secretions is assessed by suction frequency, and strength of cough can be assessed by peak cough flow using a peak flow meter attached to the endotracheal tube. It has been shown that patients with a cough peak flow of 60 L/min or less were nearly five times as likely to fail extubation.[82] Patients with secretions of more than 2.5 mL/h were three times as likely to fail. Patients who were unable to complete four simple tasks (i.e., open eyes, follow with eyes, grasp hand, stick out tongue) were more than four times as likely to fail as those who completed the four commands. The failure rate was 100% for patients with all three risk factors (cough, secretions,

CLINICAL PRACTICE GUIDELINE 19–2

Removal of the Endotracheal Tube

Indications

- When the airway control afforded by the endotracheal tube is deemed to be no longer necessary for the continued care of the patient, the tube should be removed. Subjective or objective determination of improvement of the underlying condition impairing pulmonary function and/or gas exchange capacity is made prior to extubation. To maximize the likelihood for successful extubation, the patient should be capable of maintaining a patent airway and generating adequate spontaneous ventilation. In general, this requires the patient to possess adequate central inspiratory drive, respiratory muscle strength, cough strength to clear secretions, laryngeal function, nutritional status, and clearance of sedative and neuromuscular blocking effects.
- Occasionally, acute airway obstruction of the artificial airway due to mucus or mechanical deformation mandates immediate removal of the artificial airway. Reintubation or other appropriate techniques for reestablishing the airway (i.e., surgical airway management) must be used to maintain effective gas exchange.
- Patients in whom an explicit declaration of the futility of further medical care is documented may have the endotracheal tube removed despite failure to meet the above indications.

Contraindications

- There are no absolute contraindications to extubation; however, to maintain acceptable gas exchange after extubation, some patients may require one or more of the following: noninvasive ventilation, continuous positive airway pressure, high inspired oxygen fraction, or reintubation. Airway protective reflexes may be depressed immediately following and for some time after extubation. Therefore, measures to prevent aspiration should be considered.

Assessment of Extubation Readiness

- The endotracheal tube should be removed as soon as the patient no longer requires an artificial airway. Patients should demonstrate some evidence for the reversal of the underlying cause of respiratory failure and should be capable of maintaining adequate spontaneous ventilation and gas exchange. The determination of extubation readiness may be individualized using the following guidelines.
- Patients with an artificial airway to facilitate treatment of respiratory failure should be considered for extubation when they have met established extubation readiness criteria.
- Resolution of the need for airway protection may be assessed by, but is not limited to, appropriate level of consciousness, adequate airway protective reflexes, and easily managed secretions.
- Issues that should be considered in all patients prior to extubation are no immediate need for reintubation anticipated; known risk factors for extubation failure; presence of upper airway obstruction or laryngeal edema as detected by diminished gas leak around the endotracheal tube with positive pressure breaths; evidence of stable, adequate hemodynamic function; evidence of stable nonrespiratory functions; electrolyte values within normal range; and evidence of malnutrition decreasing respiratory muscle function and ventilatory drive. Anesthesia literature indicates the patient must have no intake of food or liquid by mouth for a period of time prior to airway manipulation. The continuation of transpyloric feedings during an extubation procedure remains controversial.
- Prophylactic medication prior to extubation to avoid or reduce the severity of postextubation complications (e.g., steroids).

Hazards and Complications

- Hypoxemia after extubation may result from, but is not limited to, failure to deliver adequate inspired oxygen fraction through the natural upper airway, acute upper airway obstruction secondary to laryngospasm, postobstruction pulmonary edema, bronchospasm, atelectasis, pulmonary aspiration, and hypoventilation.
- Hypercapnia after extubation may be caused by, but is not limited to, upper airway obstruction resulting from edema of the trachea, vocal cords, or larynx; respiratory muscle weakness; excessive work of breathing; and bronchospasm.
- Death may occur when medical futility is the reason for removing the endotracheal tube.

Modified from AARC clinical practice guideline: removal of the endotracheal tube—2007 revision and update. *Respir Care.* 2007;52:81–93. Reprinted with permission.

noncompletion of four simple tasks), compared with 3% for those with no risk factors.

In some cases the upper airway may be at risk for swelling and inflammation during the period of intubation. Before extubation can be performed in these patients, the absence of these conditions is often assessed as the amount of leakage around the endotracheal tube during positive pressure ventilation with the cuff deflated.[83,84] Qualitatively, the leak test can be done by deflating the cuff and assessing for the presence of leak through the upper airway. Quantitatively, the leak can be assessed as the volume of the leak or the percentage of the tidal volume that leaks. The value of the leak test is controversial because false positives and false negatives are common.[85,86] When upper airway edema is suspected, prophylactic administration of corticosteroids decreases the risk of postextubation stridor and reintubation.[87,88]

RESPIRATORY RECAP

Extubation

- » Extubation is the removal of an endotracheal tube.
- » Adequacy of airway clearance and ability to protect the airway must be assessed before extubation.
- » Prophylactic corticosteroids decrease the risk of postextubation stridor and reintubation.

Two methods have been described for extubation, each intended to reduce the risk of aspiration of subglottic secretions. For the trailing suction catheter method, a suction catheter is placed through the endotracheal tube, the cuff is deflated, and suction is applied as the tube is removed. The other method uses a subglottic purge maneuver. A positive pressure hyperinflation is provided, the cuff is deflated, and secretions in the subglottic space are propelled upward into the oral pharynx and cleared.

Extubation failure, or the need to reintubate, occurs in 5% to 15% of cases for a variety of reasons.[89–91] Most commonly, the patient cannot sustain adequate spontaneous ventilation. Reintubation is not benign and has been associated with increased morbidity and mortality. However, prolonged intubation when successful extubation is possible also is associated with increased morbidity and mortality. Some patient populations may be at a higher risk of extubation failure; therefore, equipment and preparations for a timely reintubation should be present. Because some risk of extubation failure exists in all patients, it is important that a clinician who can perform reintubation be present at the time of extubation.

Tracheostomy

Advantages and Disadvantages of Tracheostomy

Tracheostomy is defined as the surgical introduction of a tube into the trachea. A tracheostomy is unusually done for three main reasons: to bypass an upper airway obstruction, to aid in removal of secretions from the airway, and to provide long-term mechanical ventilation. Although tracheostomy is the preferred method for these indications, there is much controversy over when it should be performed.[92] A tracheostomy should be performed only after the clinical benefits and risks for the individual patient have been considered, not because a certain number of days of intubation have elapsed.

Compared with endotracheal intubation, a tracheostomy has the advantages of lowering airway resistance, causing less tube movement in the trachea, affording greater patient comfort, and allowing the patient to swallow secretions and nourishment. The patient can communicate by moving the lips and can even talk with the aid of special **tracheostomy tubes** and devices. If accidental decannulation occurs, the tube can be reinserted into the mature stoma more easily than reintubation with an endotracheal tube can be accomplished after accidental extubation. Because the tracheostomy tube is shorter than an endotracheal tube, more of the airway below the cuff may be suctioned with greater efficiency. Tracheostomy also avoids the oral, nasal, pharyngeal, and laryngeal complications of translaryngeal intubation.

A tracheostomy does have disadvantages. It is a surgical procedure and has greater morbidity and mortality risks than endotracheal intubation. Additional risks include incisional hemorrhage, subcutaneous emphysema, pneumothorax, and pneumomediastinum. Tracheal stenosis is common, and a permanent scar is unavoidable. As with endotracheal intubation, the tracheostomy tube bypasses normal defense mechanisms and impedes an effective cough because the glottis is bypassed. Many of the complications experienced during conventional tracheostomy may be avoided if the surgery is performed by a skilled surgeon as an elective procedure under optimum conditions when the patient's airway has already been stabilized, rather than at the bedside as an emergency effort.

Timing of Tracheostomy

Tracheostomy is among the most commonly conducted procedures in critically ill patients. The timing of tracheostomy in patients receiving prolonged mechanical ventilation is controversial.[92] On one hand, earlier tracheostomy avoids complications of prolonged endotracheal intubation, improves patients' ability to communicate, and makes nursing care easier. However, the procedure is not without risk. Evidence to guide practice is limited. In 1989 the National Association of Medical Directors of Respiratory Care recommended that translaryngeal (endotracheal) intubation be used only for patients requiring fewer than 10 days of artificial ventilation and that a tracheostomy tube should be placed in patients who still require artificial ventilation 21 days after admission.[20] Although these recommendations are based only on expert opinion, modern practice broadly seems to follow them. A systematic review by Maziak et al.[93] concluded that there was insufficient evidence to support the view that the timing of tracheostomy alters the duration of mechanical ventilation or extent of airway injury in critically ill patients. Another meta-analysis concluded that in adult patients who require prolonged mechanical ventilation, performing a tracheostomy at an earlier stage than is currently practiced may shorten the duration of artificial ventilation and length of stay in intensive care.[94] In recent years, there has been a move toward earlier tracheostomy in these patients.

Open Tracheostomy

An open tracheostomy can be done in the intensive care unit at the bedside, under local anesthesia, or under general anesthesia in the operating room. The patient's head is hyperextended over a shoulder roll (unless there is a contraindication). The endotracheal tube is positioned so that the cuff is midway at the vocal cord level. A vertical or horizontal surgical incision is made, usually between the second and third tracheal ring, and the tube is inserted into the trachea. A mature tract does not form for 10 to 14 days, and attempted reinsertion of the tracheostomy tube before maturation can lead to bleeding, tracheal injury, and death. If accidental decannulation occurs, the patient should be reintubated orally to control the airway.

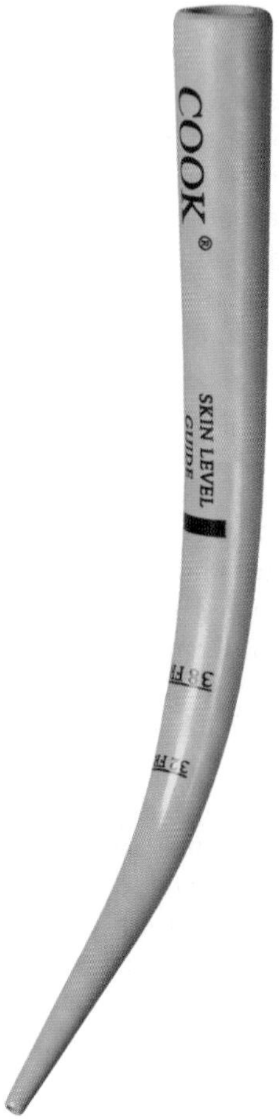

FIGURE 19–32 Dilator to form stoma for placement of percutaneous dilatation.

Percutaneous Dilational Tracheostomy

Another common technique is the percutaneous dilational tracheostomy (PDT). PDT is a comparatively new procedure that is less traumatic than the conventional surgical method.[95] It can be performed safely and expeditiously at the bedside without the risk and cost of transportation to the operating room.[96–103] The patient is positioned with the neck extended, and the skin in the area of puncture and incision is infiltrated with a local anesthetic with epinephrine. A small incision is made midway between the cricoid cartilage and the sternal notch, and a 14-gauge cannula is inserted into the trachea between the first and second tracheal rings. A guidewire is introduced into the trachea under direct bronchoscopic observation, and the stoma is dilated with increasing sizes of specially designed plastic dilators by use of the Seldinger catheter-over-wire technique (**Figure 19–32**). Once the dilation is complete, an appropriately sized tracheostomy tube is inserted over a small dilator and placed in position in the trachea.

The advantages of PDT are that it can be performed at the bedside in the intensive care unit, eliminating the risks involved in moving a high-risk patient to the operating room, and that it greatly reduces the potential for hemorrhage. The dilation creates an opening that fits tightly around the tracheostomy tube for several days, rather than the large, secured opening created during a conventional tracheostomy. If accidental decannulation occurs within the first several days following PDT, the patient should be reintubated orally. Once the airway is secure, the tract can be explored, the guidewire and dilators replaced, and the tracheostomy tube reinserted. The tracheostomy tube can usually be safely changed or downsized 5 days after PDT. Long-term problems with PDT, such as tracheal stenosis, have not yet been seen. In fact, the quality of the stoma is often better following PDT than with open tracheostomy. PDT, when done properly, has proved to be a safe, cost-effective procedure. Compared with surgical tracheostomy procedures, PDT has a lower incidence of pneumothorax, bleeding complications, and stenosis. With bronchoscopic guidance, PDT can be considered for patients with a difficult anatomy due to morbid obesity or abnormalities of the neck.

Tracheostomy Tubes

Metal Tracheostomy Tubes

Metal tracheostomy tubes of various types were used throughout the 19th century to relieve upper airway obstruction. In the early 1930s, Chevalier Jackson developed a systematic approach to the management of airway obstruction that became universally accepted. This approach made tracheostomy with double-lumen silver tubes the standard for treatment of airway obstruction.

Silver has long been used in the manufacture of tracheostomy tubes because the metal walls can be kept very thin, which is an advantage when the inner cannula is used. Silver was selected for construction of the tracheostomy tube because it is nonreactive when in contact with human tissue. The disadvantages of silver for tracheostomy tubes are that it is expensive and rigid. The curved shape does not conform well to the trachea, which can lead to compression damage along the tracheal wall and even erosion of major vessel walls.

The Jackson tracheostomy tube is constructed completely of silver. It has a rigid outer cannula with an attached fixed neck plate and a rigid inner cannula. These metal tracheostomy tubes are cuffless, but a rubber, reusable, high-pressure cuff can be added to prevent leaks during mechanical ventilation. The size of the metal tubes is identified by the Jackson system,[104] which uses the outer tube diameter. Disadvantages of metal tracheostomy tubes are their narrow IDs, the rigid structure of the neck plate, and the lack of a 15-mm adapter for connection to most ventilatory devices. Problems associated with the reusable high-pressure cuffs are nonuniform expansion along the tracheal wall, lack of cuff strength, and the danger of the cuff slipping over the end of tracheostomy tube, causing airway occlusion. Metal tracheostomy tubes are available in pediatric and adult sizes. However, because of improvements in material design, clinical use of metal tracheostomy tubes is almost nonexistent.

Current Construction

Tracheostomy tubes may be made of metal, rubber, silicone, Teflon, polyethylene, and PVC materials.[105] Like endotracheal tubes, tracheostomy tubes must satisfy ASTM requirements. Because the tubes are in direct contact with body tissue, the ideal material is nontoxic and determined by implant testing. Modern plastic tracheostomy tubes (**Figure 19–33**) are available in sizes 2.5 to 11.5 mm according to their ID. On most tracheostomy tubes, the manufacturer should mark both the ID and the OD as a guide for the user. Besides materials, standard requirements cover surface characteristics, dimensions, tolerances, cuff characteristics, and labeling of tubes and packages.

The shape of the tracheostomy tube should conform as closely as possible to the anatomy of the airway. Two main types of tracheostomy tubes are available—those that are curved, and those that are angled to fit the trachea at one end and the area between the skin and the trachea at the other end. Curved tracheostomy tubes usually have an inner cannula that can be removed for cleaning while the outer cannula remains in place. The outer cannula may have a window, or fenestration, to allow for speech when the inner cannula is removed. Because the trachea is mostly straight, the curved tracheostomy tube often does not conform to the shape of the trachea, which may allow compression of the membranous part of the trachea, and the tip may traumatize the anterior portion. These tubes may also damage the area of the stoma.

Extended-length tracheostomy tubes (**Figure 19–34**) are angled and provide extra length in the proximal or distal portions of the tube for a more customized fit. Extra length in the proximal portion accommodates

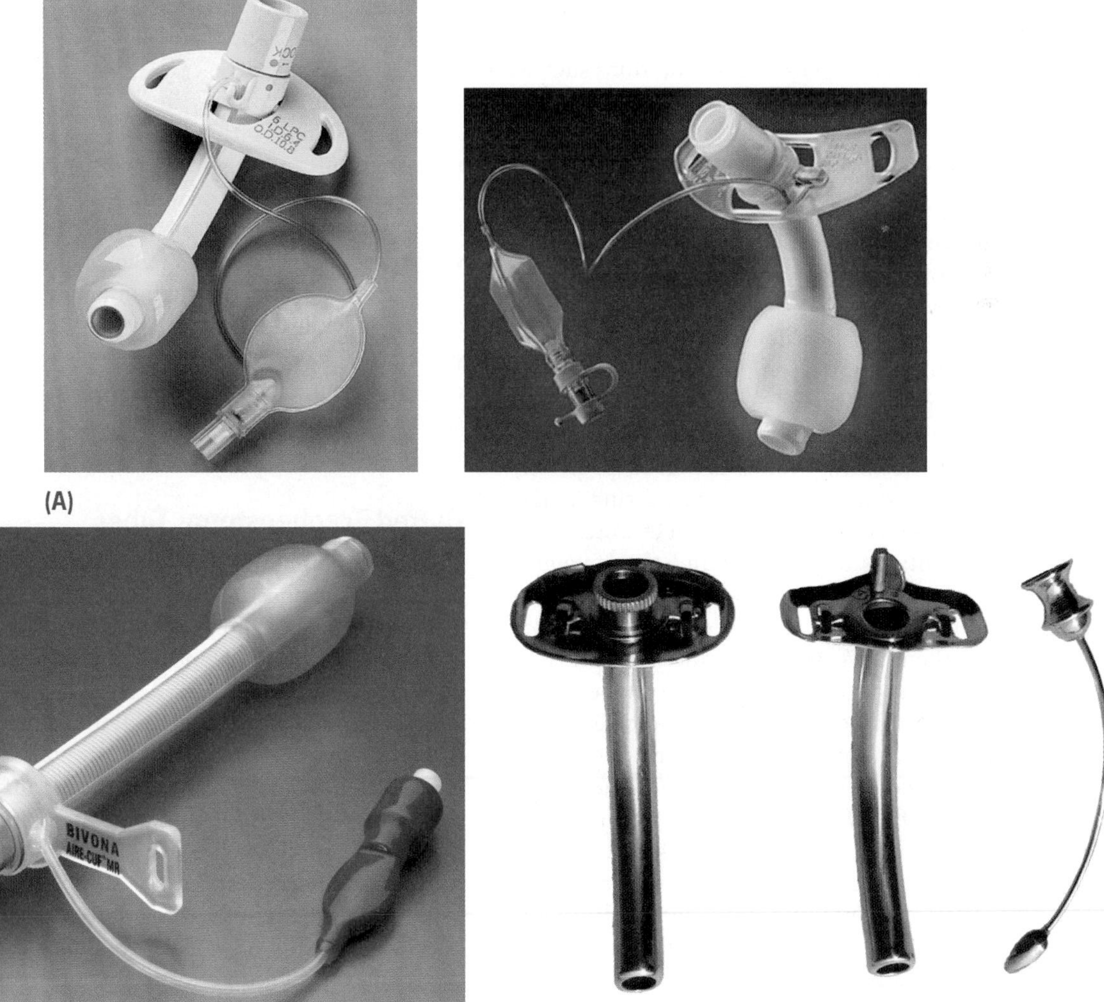

FIGURE 19–33 (**A**) Standard cuffed tracheostomy tubes. (**B**) Flexible tracheostomy tube. (**C**) Metal tracheostomy tube.

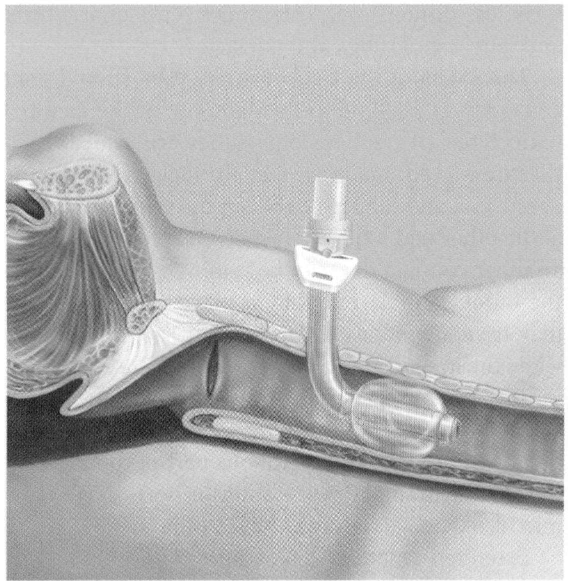

(A)

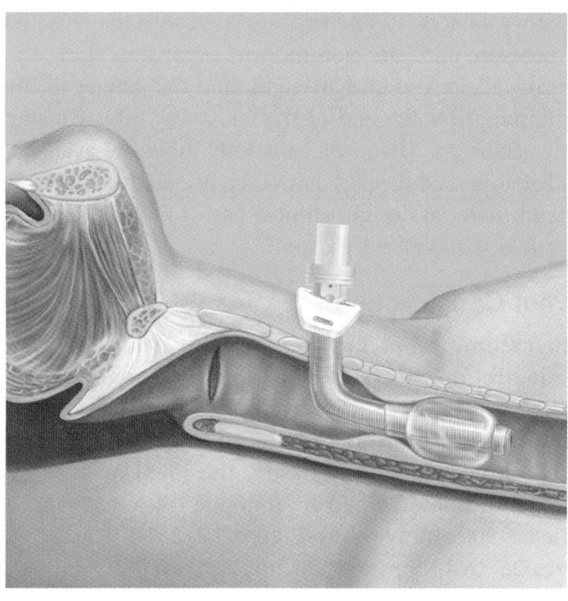

(B)

FIGURE 19–34 Examples of extra length angled tracheostomy tubes. (**A**) Increased proximal length. (**B**) Increased distal length. Images used by permission from Nellcor Puritan Bennett LLC, Boulder, Colorado, part of Covidien.

patients with thick necks who have increased skin-to-tracheal-wall distances. Extra length in the distal portion of the tube is used to compensate for conditions such as tracheal stenosis or malacia.

Uncuffed Tracheostomy Tubes

Standard uncuffed tracheostomy tubes have the same basic design as those described previously. On the flange attachment of some uncuffed adult tracheostomy tubes, UNCUFFED designates that the tube is uncuffed, and *FEN* indicates that the tube is fenestrated. If the tracheostomy tube chosen uses a removable inner cannula, the package of the inner cannula should list the size and make of the tube into which it is intended to fit.

Uncuffed tracheostomy tubes are used primarily in pediatric patients, in whom the cricoid ring is narrower than the glottis. Because the tissues anterior to the trachea in infants are thinner and the laryngeal and tracheal cartilages are softer, use of cuffed tracheostomy tubes in infants and children up to 6 years of age makes them susceptible to tracheal deformation. In children, especially infants, the shape of the neck plate of the tracheostomy tube is important. The usual straight neck plate does not fit well because of anatomic differences between infants and adults. The newer, flexible, soft, swivel-neck flange on most current tracheostomy tubes solves this problem. Uncuffed tracheostomy tubes are intended to allow a small leak during ventilation. Unfortunately, some clinicians tend to use a tube that fits rather snugly to reduce this leak. The large stomal opening required to accommodate the tube increases the chances of stomal stenosis. Silastic tubes with a single lumen that do not require an inner cannula are available for pediatric patients.

AGE-SPECIFIC ANGLE

Uncuffed tracheostomy tubes are used primarily for pediatric patients.

In adults, uncuffed tracheostomy tubes are used primarily after laryngectomy and in patients with neuromuscular disease who need frequent suctioning but not mechanical ventilation. Uncuffed tubes have also been used as a method of weaning from the tracheostomy tube. Progressively smaller diameters of uncuffed tubes are used to allow suctioning and maintenance of the stoma while allowing the patient to adapt to the normal airway. The absence of a cuff on a tracheostomy tube does not help prevent aspiration, and this type of tube should not be used in unconscious patients or in those in whom airway defenses have been lost.

Cuffed Tracheostomy Tubes

Like the uncuffed standard tracheostomy tubes, the typical cuffed tracheostomy tube is composed of outer and inner cannulas. The outer cannula forms the primary structure of the tube and also has the cuff assembly attached to its distal end. A standard 15-mm adapter is present on the proximal end of the tube. Also at the proximal end are the inflation tube and pilot balloon with spring-loaded valve assembly for cuff inflation and deflation. An obturator with a rounded tip is placed into the outer cannula before insertion of the tracheostomy tube. The rounded obturator tip extends beyond the distal end of the tube far enough to round the otherwise blunted end; this minimizes trauma to the mucosa of the tracheal wall during insertion of the tube. The tubes have a radiopaque marker on the distal tip to provide confirmation of the tube's position on radiographs. Tracheostomy tubes are constructed primarily of PVC or other synthetic materials and are tissue compatible as determined by acceptable implant test methods. Modern tracheostomy tubes are disposable and offer the practitioner a variety of models ranging from a standard system similar to the silver tracheostomy tube to one with single and double fenestrations and pressure-limiting automatic relief valves.

A controversy in the selection of the proper tracheostomy tube involves the choice of a single-lumen tube or a tube with an inner cannula. With a dual-cannula tracheostomy tube, the inner cannula can be removed for cleaning. In some cases, the ventilator connection is to the inner cannula. It is important to appreciate that an inner cannula (dual-cannula design) results in a decrease in the inner diameter of the tube or an increase in the outer diameter of the tube. An inner cannula is necessary to block the opening in a fenestrated tracheostomy tube.

Foam Cuff Tracheostomy Tubes

The Bivona foam cuff consists of a large-diameter, high-residual-volume cuff composed of polyurethane foam covered by a silicone sheath. This cuff was designed to address the problem of high lateral tracheal wall pressures that lead to complications such as tracheal necrosis and stenosis. Before insertion, air in the cuff is evacuated by a syringe attached to the pilot port, which makes the foam contract (**Figure 19–35**). This allows insertion of the tracheostomy tube. Once the tube is in place, the syringe is removed to allow the cuff to reexpand until it reaches the tracheal wall. The pilot tube remains open to the atmosphere so that the intracuff pressure is at ambient levels. The open pilot port also permits compression and expansion of the cuff during the ventilatory cycle, which allows intermittent perfusion of the tracheal tissue in contact with the tube without loss of volume during ventilation. The degree of foam expansion is a determining factor in the amount of pressure exerted on the tracheal wall. As the foam expands further, lateral tracheal wall pressure increases. However, when the device is used properly, this pressure rarely exceeds 20 mm Hg.

When a foam cuff tracheostomy tube is selected, the proper size is important to maintain a seal and still benefit from the pressure-limiting advantages of the foam-filled cuff. If the tube is too small, the foam will inflate to its unrestricted size and the cuff may leak, causing loss of ventilation and loss of protection against aspiration. If the tube is too large, the foam is unable to expand properly to provide the desired cushion, with resultant increased pressure against the tracheal wall. If air is injected into the cuff to increase the lateral wall pressure and provide a seal, the purpose and pressure-limiting benefits of the foam cuff are defeated and the cuff may leak, which can result in a loss of ventilator volume during inspiration. The manufacturer recommends periodic cuff deflation to assess the integrity of the cuff and prevent the silicone sheath from adhering to the tracheal mucosa.

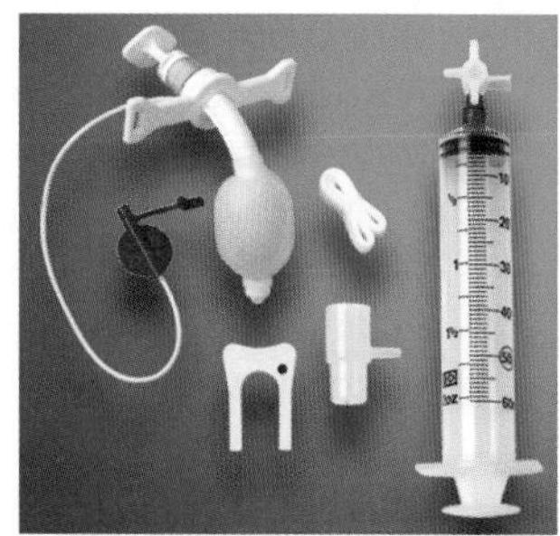

FIGURE 19–35 Foam cuff trach tube kit.

Tight-to-Shaft Cuff Tracheostomy Tubes

The tight-to-shaft tracheostomy tube is used for patients requiring short-term cuff inflation, such as avoidance of aspiration during feeding or nocturnal-only ventilation. When the silicone cuff is totally deflated, it adds no distinguishable dimension to the outer diameter of the tube's shaft. This cuff is unique because it is inflated with water rather than air.

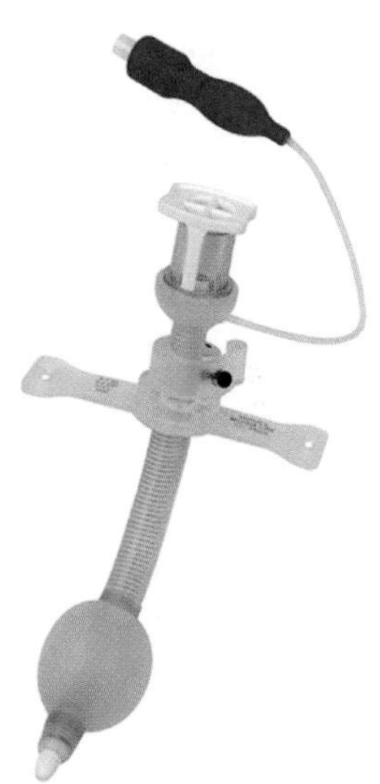

FIGURE 19–36 Adjustable flange tracheostomy tube.

Sleep Apnea Tracheostomy Tubes

These tubes are uncuffed tubes designed for use in patients with obstructive sleep apnea who do not tolerate continuous positive airway pressure (CPAP) therapy. They have a flexible all-silicone construction that improves patient comfort and minimizes skin irritation, encrustation, and mucus occlusion. These tubes have a low-profile design and are easily capped and concealed during waking hours. They also are used when airway access for pulmonary hygiene and suctioning is required. These tubes cannot be used in patients who require invasive ventilator assistance.

Adjustable Flange Tracheostomy Tubes

Adjustable neck flange tracheostomy tubes (**Figure 19–36**) can be adjusted for horizontal and vertical shaft drop to accommodate unusual anatomy or pathology. They are used for patients with thick necks and can also be used to position the cuff to avoid tracheal pathology. Adjustable neck flange tracheostomy tubes are intended for temporary use until the proper length fixed neck flange tube can be obtained. They should only be used in a clinically supervised setting. They are not for home care use.

Fenestrated Tracheostomy Tubes

A fenestrated tracheostomy tube can be useful in the assessment of a patient's readiness to be decannulated, and it allows the patient to talk when the tube is occluded and the cuff deflated. The fenestrated tracheostomy tube is similar in construction to a regular tracheostomy tube, with the addition of an opening in the posterior portion of the tube above the cuff (**Figure 19–37**). Fenestrated tubes are composed of a tracheostomy tube with a fenestration, a removable inner cannula, and a plastic plug. When the inner cannula is removed, the cuff deflated, and normal air passage occluded with the plug, the patient can inhale and exhale through the fenestration and around the tube. This allows for assessment of the patient's ability to breathe through the normal oral/nasal route (preparing the patient for decannulation) and permits air to pass by the vocal cords, creating phonation.

Healthcare workers must be properly trained in the use of fenestrated tracheostomy tubes. If the patient has been receiving humidified, oxygen-enriched air via the tube, an alternate source must be provided, such as a nasal cannula. Also, before the proximal end is blocked, the cuff must be completely deflated by evacuating all of the air. The tracheal cap is then put in place to allow the patient to breathe through the fenestrations and around the tube. If the cuff is left inflated during the capping procedure, airway resistance will be excessive, and the patient will experience respiratory distress. The patient must be observed carefully for aspiration of secretions or oral fluids while the cuff is deflated. This type of tube should be considered only for patients with normal upper airway reflexes.

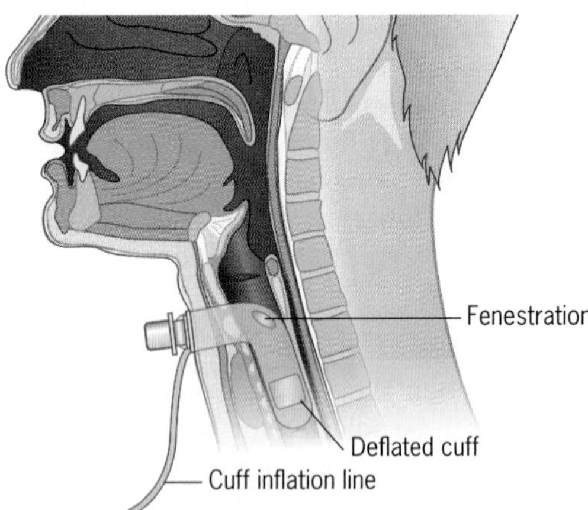

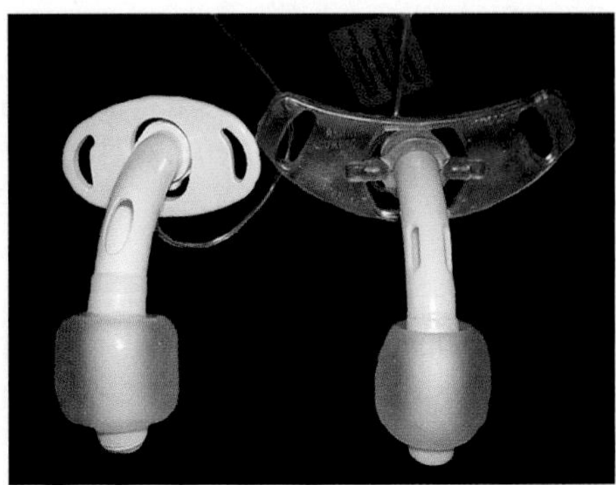

FIGURE 19–37 Fenestrated tracheostomy tubes.

Talking Tracheostomy Tubes

Specialized tracheostomy tubes allow communication for ventilator-dependent patients. The talking tracheostomy tube (**Figure 19–38**) operates using an external gas flow (4–6 L/min) that is routed through the larynx via a separate flow line with a thumb port. When the thumb port is occluded, gas passes though the larynx and can be used for phonation. The cuff stays inflated, separating speech from ventilation. A couple of drawbacks to this system are that a specialized tube has to be placed (perhaps replacing the existing tube) and that someone must be available to occlude the thumb port (e.g., the caregiver or, in some instances, the patients themselves).

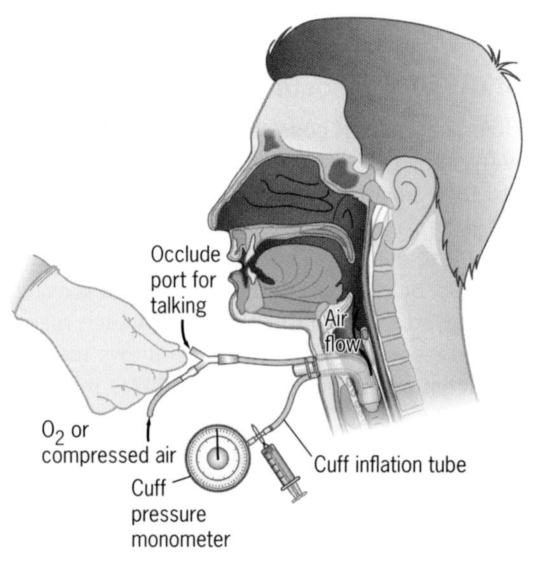

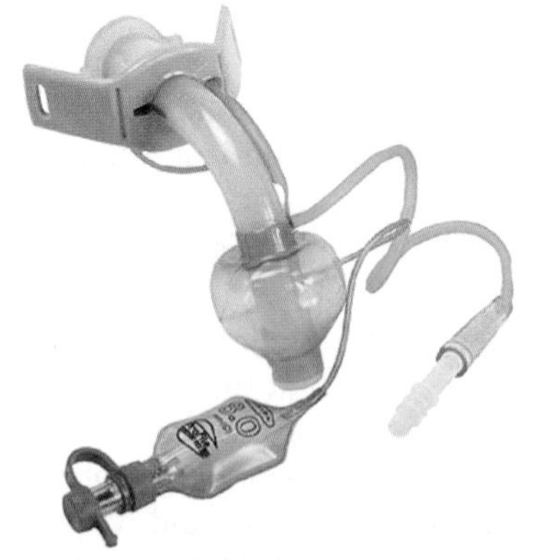

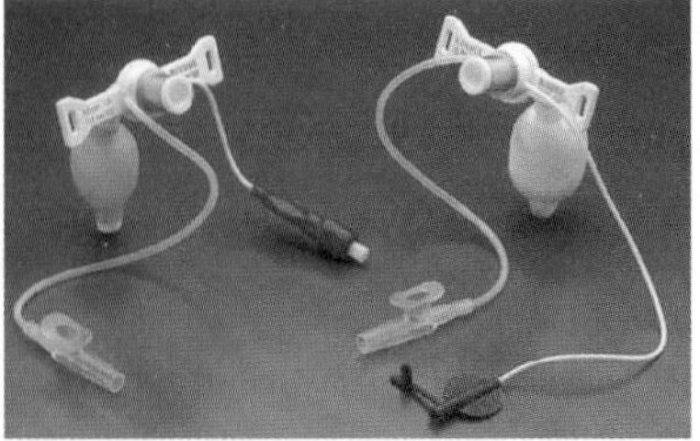

FIGURE 19–38 Talking tracheostomy tubes.

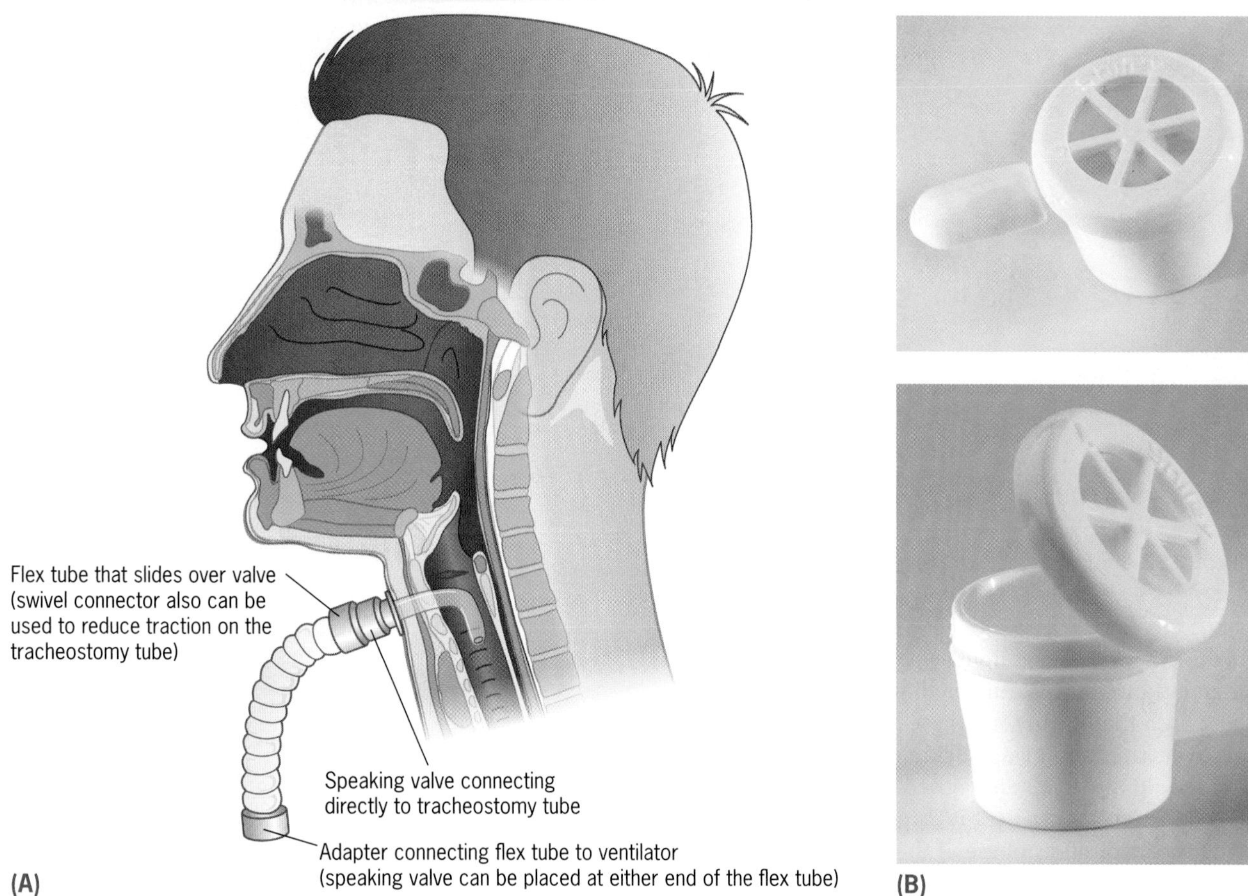

FIGURE 19–39 (**A**) Speaking valve in-line during mechanical ventilation. (**B**) Speaking valves.

Speaking Valves

The tracheostomy **speaking valve** (**Figure 19–39**) is designed to eliminate the need for finger occlusion to communicate by speaking.[106] The valve attaches to the 15-mm universal adapter of all tracheostomy tubes and can be used in adult and pediatric patients. The valve opens on inspiration, with air passing through to the lungs, and closes on expiration, with the air directed into the trachea and up past the vocal cords to permit speech. This device can be used in either spontaneously breathing or ventilator-dependent patients. Some patients may immediately adjust to breathing with the valve in place. Others may need to gradually increase the time the valve is worn. Breathing out with the valve in place is harder work than breathing through the tracheostomy tube, and some patients may need to build up strength and ability to use the valve. The speaking valve should be used with caution in patients at risk of aspiration because the cuff of the tracheostomy tube must be deflated to use this device. Increases in ventilator-delivered tidal volume may be needed to compensate for leakage around the tracheostomy tube during mechanical ventilation. After the speaking valve is removed and the tracheostomy cuff is reinflated, overventilation of the patient must be avoided. The speaking valve may also be used to wean patients from the tracheostomy tube as a means to reorient them to use of the upper airway for breathing.

Contraindications to the use of a speaking valve include an unconscious or comatose patient, situations in which the cuff cannot be deflated, use with a foam cuffed tube, copious secretions, and severe upper airway obstruction. Humidity and oxygen can both be delivered with the valve in place. The valve must be removed during the administration of aerosolized medications, because these may cause the valve to stick or not work well. It is important to consider the input of the speech-language pathologist to assess the patient's ability to produce voice in different situations that may include using a speaking valve. Also important is assessment of upper airway resistance when the cuff is deflated and the speaking valve is in place. This can be conducted by measuring the tracheal pressure with the speaking valve in place (**Figure 19–40**).[107] If the expiratory tracheal pressure is greater than 10 cm H_2O, the speaking valve should be removed and causes of increased upper airway resistance should be explored. In most cases, this can be addressed by downsizing the tracheostomy tube.

Speaking in Ventilator-Dependent Patients with a Tracheostomy Tube

In mechanically ventilated patients, speech can be provided by the use of a talking tracheostomy tube, using a cuff-down technique with a speaking valve, and using a

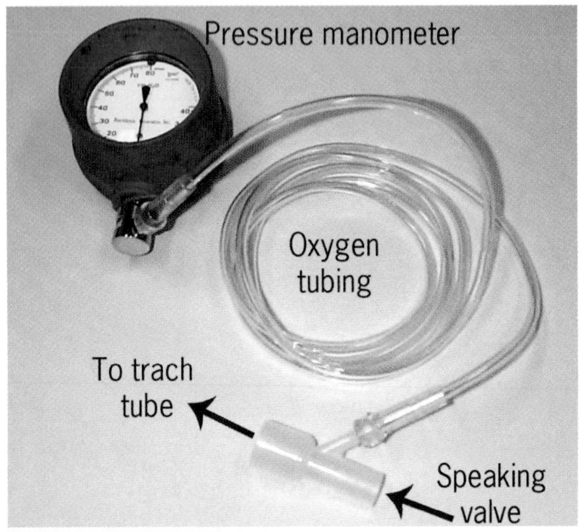

FIGURE 19–40 Equipment used to measure tracheal pressure with a speaking valve in place.

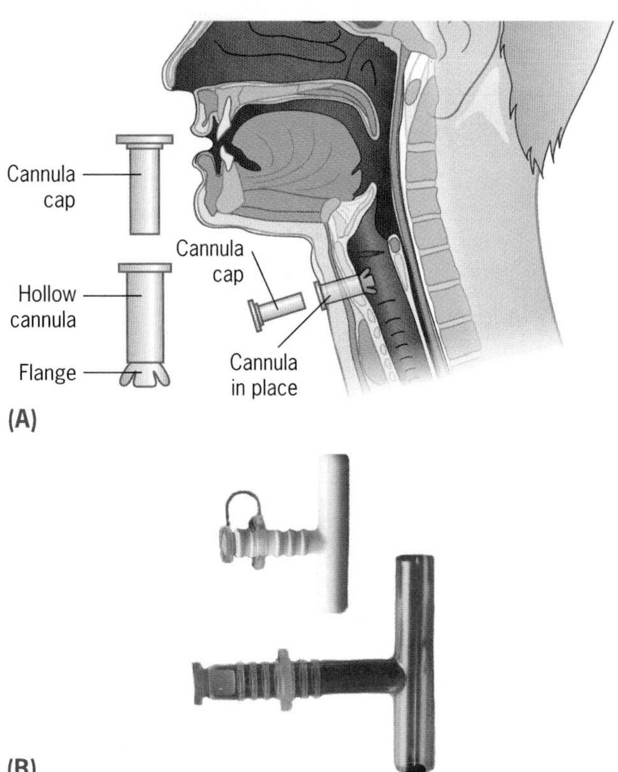

FIGURE 19–41 **(A)** Tracheostomy button. **(B)** Montgomery Standard Safe-T-Tube.

cuff-down technique without a speaking valve.[108] Simple manipulations of the ventilator allow the patient to speak during both the inspiratory phase and expiratory phase. Moreover, the lack of a speaking valve may increase safety should the upper airway become obstructed. If the cuff is deflated, gas can escape through the upper airway during the inspiratory phase. If the leak is excessive, the cuff can be partially inflated. This leak results in the ability to speak during the inspiratory phase. Increasing the inspiratory time setting on the ventilator increases the leak. If the positive end-expiratory pressure (PEEP) setting on the ventilator is zero, most of the exhaled gas exits through the ventilator circuit rather than the upper airway. In this situation, there is little ability to speak during the expiratory phase. If PEEP is set on the ventilator, then expiratory flow is more likely to occur through the upper airway, which increases speaking rate. Longer inspiratory time and higher PEEP are additive in their ability to improve speaking rate. Tracheal pressure (important for speech) is similar with the use of PEEP and the use of a speaking valve. By prolonging the inspiratory time and using PEEP, mechanically ventilated patients with a tracheostomy may be able to use 60% to 80% of the breathing cycle for speaking. Such patients may be able to speak throughout the entire ventilatory cycle without any pauses for breathing. This is unlike normal subjects without tracheostomy tubes, who speak only during the expiratory phase. The ventilator is normally flow cycled during pressure-support ventilation. In the presence of a leak through the upper airway, the ventilator may fail to cycle appropriately and thus result in a prolonged inspiratory phase. Although this would usually be considered undesirable, it might facilitate speech.

Eating with a Tracheostomy

Having a tracheostomy usually does not affect the patient's eating or swallowing patterns. Sometimes there are changes in swallowing dynamics that require adjusting to, but it is rare not to be able to overcome such issues in a short period of time. If swallowing problems do occur, they are usually due to limited elevation of the larynx or to poor closure of the epiglottis and vocal cords, which allows food or liquids in to the trachea. A speech pathologist can be consulted for an evaluation, which may include a videofluoroscopic swallowing study or other procedures to make sure the patient is swallowing safely. If the patient eats by mouth, it is recommended that the tracheostomy tube be suctioned prior to eating. This often prevents the need for suctioning during or after meals, which may stimulate excessive coughing and could result in vomiting. Always observe the patient while eating to be sure food does not get into the trachea.

Trach and Stoma Buttons

Trach buttons and stoma buttons (**Figure 19–41**) are used to maintain the tracheostomy stoma. They are temporary appliances generally made of Teflon or silicone. Some consist of a hollow outer cannula and an inner solid cannula. The device fits from the skin to just inside the anterior wall of the trachea. They should be used when the tracheostomy stoma must be maintained, either for later replacement of a tracheostomy tube or for suctioning. A button does not have a cuff. Therefore, it is of limited value in cases involving a risk of aspiration or during positive pressure ventilation.

The Montgomery Safe-T-Tube is a silicone T-shaped tube with internal and external limbs. Its primary indication is to maintain a patent airway in instances of tracheal stenosis, after laryngeal injuries such as crushing or laryngeal fractures, and after tracheal reconstruction and reanastamosis. It ranges in size from 6 to 16. The most common adult sizes are 11 to 13. The external limb can be gently tilted to allow the suction catheter to pass beyond the 45-degree angle of the tube. Ring washers assist in preventing posterior displacement. Several versions are available for specific patient needs. It is important to provide constant humidification to avoid obstruction of the tube by secretions. Capping the tube allows for normal humidification and phonation to occur.

Securing Tracheostomy Tubes

A major complication of tracheostomy is accidental decannulation. It is important to secure the tube appropriately while maintaining patient comfort by minimizing friction and pressure on the neck. It is also important to ensure that the tracheostomy tube is properly aligned in the trachea. A 10% rate of tracheostomy tube malposition has been reported,[109] suggesting that proper position should be regularly assessed.

Twill tape may be used to secure the tracheostomy tube. It must be tied securely, yet with enough give to enable the caregiver to slip two fingers under the tape. One technique is to use one long piece of twill tape and thread half the length through one side of the faceplate. Then bring one end around the back of the neck and through the other side of the faceplate and tie the two ends in a triple knot at the back of the neck. A second technique using twill tape recommends cutting two lengths of twill, each long enough to fold in half and still reach around the neck. Thread the folded end of one of the ties through one of the holes on the tracheostomy tube until it forms a loop, pulling it tightly. Repeat on the other side of the tracheostomy tube. Bring the loose ends of both ties around to the back of the neck and tie them together in a knot.

Specialized tracheostomy tube holders, such as the Dale tracheostomy holder, are available. This holder has a wider diameter neck band that distributes pressure and prevents skin irritation. Velcro-type hook fasteners are used to secure the tube, making it easier and faster to apply. The holder has elastic in the back, promoting tube security and allowing patient movement. Regardless of the type of tracheostomy tube holder that is used, the device must be changed whenever wet or soiled.

Decannulation

Decannulation is the removal of the tracheostomy tube once the patient no longer needs it. The patient should be alert and responsive to commands, no longer dependent on a ventilator for assisted breathing, and no longer requiring frequent suctioning for removal of tracheal secretions. Weaning from the tracheostomy tube typically is done through placement of a smaller tracheostomy tube, perhaps one that is fenestrated or cuffless; patients should not have breathing difficulty in the presence of this tube. The smaller tracheostomy tube can then have either a speaking valve or cap placed on it for several hours to assess the patient's ability to talk and clear his or her own secretions with no evidence of breathing difficulty. It has been reported that physicians and respiratory therapists based their decision to recommend decannulation on patients' level of consciousness, cough effectiveness, secretions, and oxygenation.[110] Most clinicians defined decannulation failure as the need to reinsert an artificial airway within 48 to 96 hours of planned tracheostomy removal. Once this process is tolerated, the patient is placed supine in bed, the tube is removed, and the opening in the neck is covered with sterile gauze and tape placed over the gauze. Decannulation should be done in the hospital where there is emergency support should it be needed.

Airway Cuff Concerns

An **airway cuff** is classified as a high-volume, low-pressure cuff or a low-volume, high-pressure cuff (**Figure 19–42**). Because high tracheal wall pressures exerted by an inflated cuff can injure the tracheal mucosa, most cuffs used today are high-volume, low-pressure. The tracheal capillary perfusion pressure normally is 25 to 35 mm Hg. Because the pressure transmitted from the cuff to the tracheal wall usually is less than the pressure in the cuff, it is generally agreed that 30 cm H_2O is the maximum acceptable intracuff pressure. If the cuff pressure is too low (<20 cm H_2O), micro-aspiration is more likely.[111,112] Therefore, it is reasonable to maintain cuff

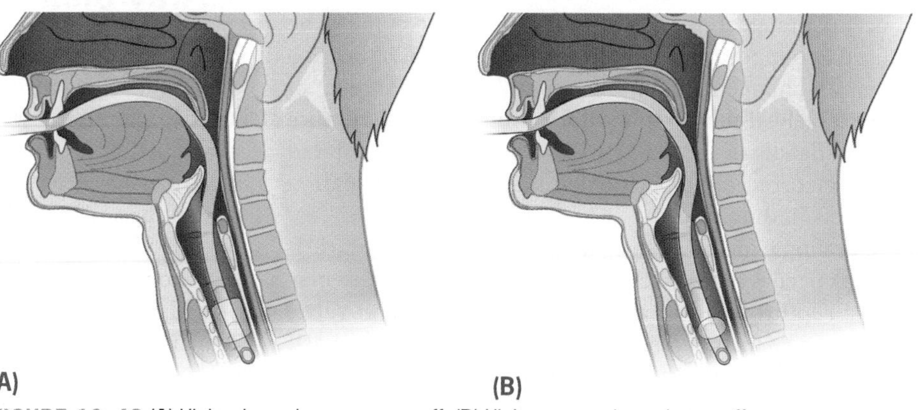

FIGURE 19–42 **(A)** High-volume, low-pressure cuff. **(B)** High-pressure, low-volume cuff.

pressures at 20 to 30 cm H_2O to minimize the risks of tracheal wall injury and aspiration.

The cuff typically is inflated with a minimum occlusion pressure or minimum leak technique. With the minimum occlusion pressure method, the cuff is inflated to a volume that just eliminates an end-inspiratory leak during positive pressure ventilation. With the minimum leak technique, the cuff is inflated to a volume that allows a small leak to occur at end-inspiration. With either method, leakage around the cuff is assessed by auscultation over the suprasternal notch or the lateral neck.

Monitoring of the cuff pressure is standard respiratory care practice. The intracuff pressure should be monitored and recorded at least once per shift and more often if the tube position is changed, if the volume of air in the cuff is changed, or if a leak occurs. Cuff pressure is measured with a syringe, stopcock, and manometer (**Figure 19–43**). With this method, the cuff pressure can be measured simultaneously with adjustment of the cuff volume. Methods in which the manometer is attached directly to the pilot balloon are discouraged, because they cause air to escape from the cuff to pressurize the manometer. Commercially available systems can also be used to measure cuff pressure.

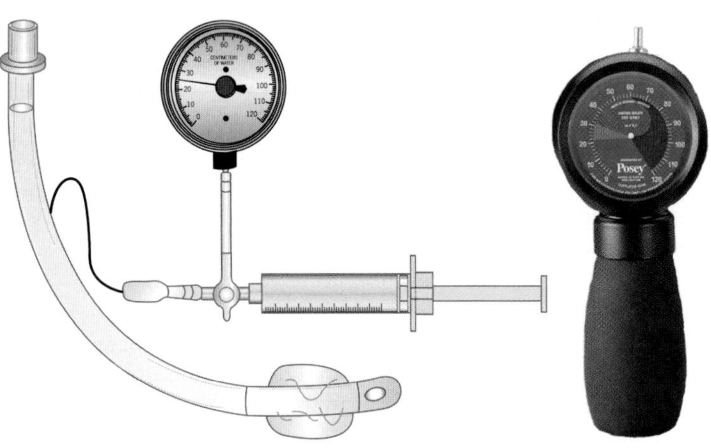

FIGURE 19–43 Equipment to measure cuff pressure.

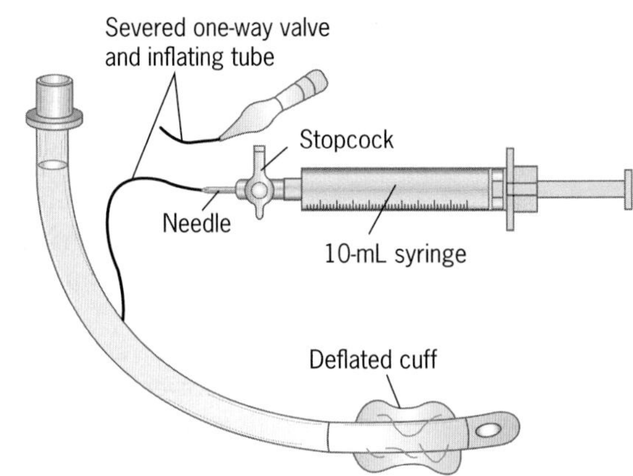

FIGURE 19–44 Technique to inflate cuff with severed inflating tube. Adapted from Sills J. An emergency cuff inflation technique. *Respir Care*. 1986; 31:199–201.

A common cause of high cuff pressure is a tube that is too small, which results in overfilling of the cuff to achieve a seal in the trachea. If the volume of air in the cuff required to achieve a seal exceeds the cuff's nominal volume, the tube is too small. The nominal cuff volume is the volume below which the cuff pressure is less than 20 cm H_2O ex vivo. Another common cause of high cuff pressure is incorrect positioning of the endotracheal tube, particularly a cephalad position in which the cuff is inflated in the larynx and pharynx. Other causes of high cuff pressure are overfilling of the cuff, tracheal dilation, and use of a low-volume, high-pressure cuff.

Occasionally the pilot tube may become severed. To correct this problem, a short, blunt needle can be passed into the pilot tube and a stopcock attached to the needle hub to add and maintain air in the cuff until the tube can be replaced (**Figure 19–44**).[113] Cuff leaks also can occur, and a continuous flow of gas into the cuff can be used to temporarily maintain cuff inflation until the tube can be changed.[114,115] Interestingly, a large number of endotracheal tubes removed for presumed cuff rupture were flawless, and some researchers have speculated that incorrect tube positioning may be the explanation for this finding.[116]

A simple method can be used to assess cuff rupture. If a leak occurs during a cuff inflation maneuver, there may be a ruptured cuff or an ineffective pilot balloon valve. This can be further assessed by clamping the pilot tube. If a leak occurs without the clamp, but not with the clamp, the pilot balloon or valve is incompetent. **Figure 19–45** presents an algorithm for cuff management. Occasionally an endotracheal tube must be changed, such as when the cuff has ruptured. A tube changer can be used to facilitate this procedure. The tube changer is passed through the endotracheal tube into the trachea, and the endotracheal tube is withdrawn while the tube changer is kept in place. The new endotracheal tube then is passed over the tube changer into the trachea.

Airway Clearance

Open Suction

Suctioning is a procedure that uses negative pressure to remove secretions from the trachea, pharynx, nose, or mouth either through the natural orifice (nose or mouth) or artificial airways such as endotracheal tubes, tracheostomy tubes, or nasal or oral airways. Suctioning should be considered whenever physical examination reveals secretions in the airway or whenever secretions are suspected and may be hindering oxygenation and ventilation or increasing the work of breathing. Suspected secretions can be identified through direct auscultation or from visual clues on the expiratory flow graphic display on the

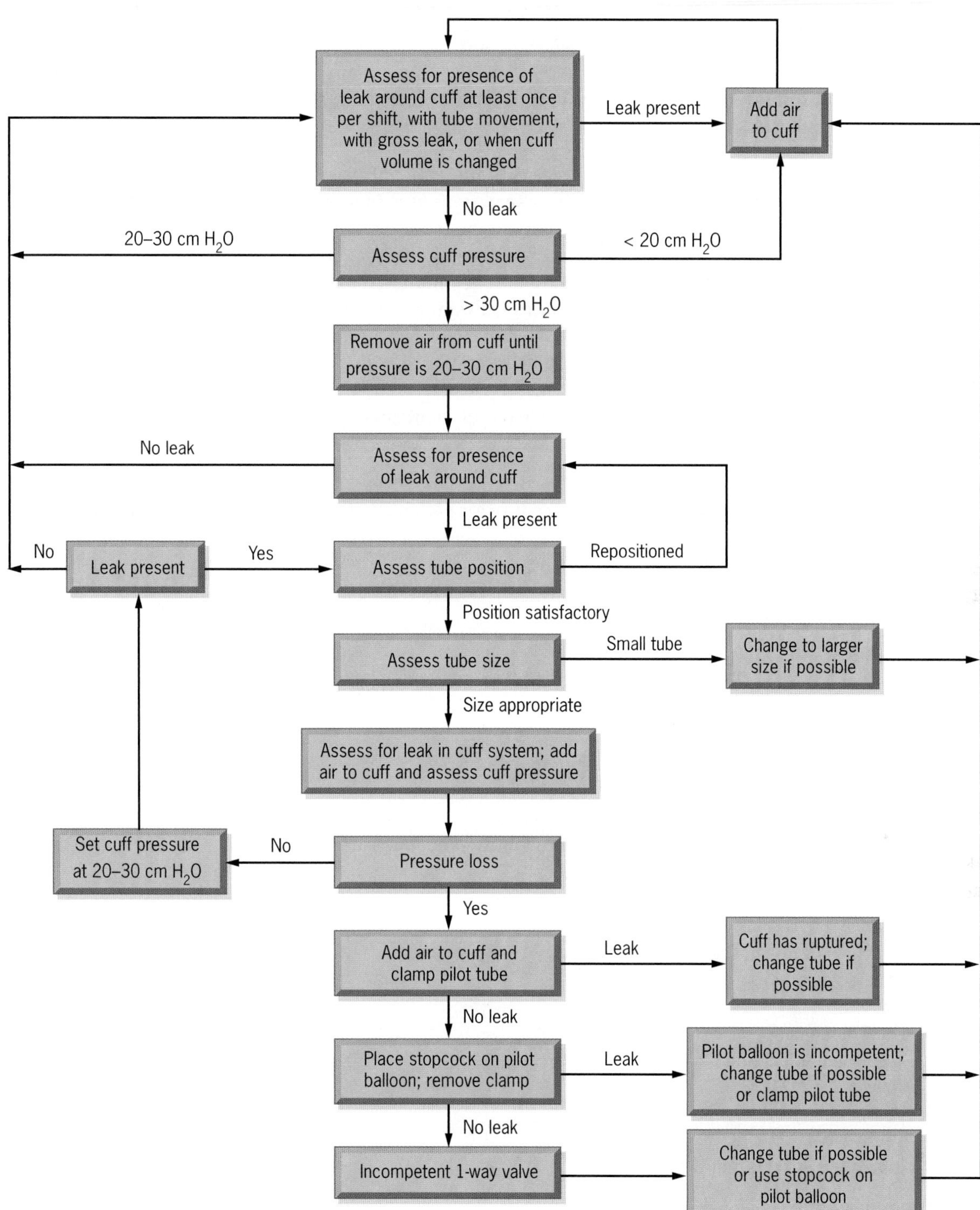

FIGURE 19–45 Algorithm to address issues with an artificial airway cuff leak. From Hess DR. Managing the artificial airway. *Respir Care*. 1999; 44:759–772. Reprinted with permission.

ventilator (sawtooth pattern). Because tracheal suctioning is uncomfortable for the patient and carries some risk, it should be performed only when indicated and not at fixed intervals. The presence of the catheter in the trachea can induce coughing and may stimulate bronchospasm in patients with reactive airways. In the absence of an artificial airway, nasotracheal suctioning can be performed if secretions need to be removed. In this scenario a **suction catheter** can be passed through a naris and into the trachea. This can be even more uncomfortable due to the added irritation of the nasal passage. This procedure is used on patients who have a decreased or absent cough reflex. **CPG 19–3** lists indications and contraindications for endotracheal suctioning.

The upper airway should be suctioned periodically to remove oral secretions. **Figure 19–46** depicts mouth/

CLINICAL PRACTICE GUIDELINE 19–3

Endotracheal Suctioning of Mechanically Ventilated Patients with Artificial Airways

Indications

- The need to maintain the patency and integrity of the artificial airway
- The need to remove accumulated pulmonary secretions as evidenced by one of the following: (1) sawtooth pattern on the flow–volume loop on the monitor screen of the ventilator and/or the presence of coarse crackles over the trachea are strong indicators of retained pulmonary secretions; (2) increased peak inspiratory pressure during volume-controlled mechanical ventilation or decreased tidal volume during pressure-controlled ventilation; (3) deterioration of oxygen saturation and/or arterial blood gas values; (4) visible secretions in the airway; or (5) patient's inability to generate an effective spontaneous cough, acute respiratory distress, or suspected aspiration of gastric or upper airway secretions
- The need to obtain a sputum specimen to rule out or identify pneumonia or other pulmonary infection or for sputum cytology

Contraindications

- Endotracheal suctioning is a necessary procedure for patients with artificial airways. Most contraindications are relative to the patient's risk of developing adverse reactions or worsening clinical condition as result of the procedure. When indicated, there is no absolute contraindication to endotracheal suctioning because the decision to withhold suctioning in order to avoid a possible adverse reaction may, in fact, be lethal.

Hazards and Complications

- Decrease in dynamic lung compliance and functional residual capacity
- Atelectasis
- Hypoxia/hypoxemia
- Tissue trauma to the tracheal and/or bronchial mucosa
- Bronchoconstriction/bronchospasm
- Increased microbial colonization of lower airway
- Changes in cerebral blood flow and increased intracranial pressure
- Hypertension
- Hypotension
- Cardiac dysrhythmias
- Routine use of normal saline instillation may be associated with the following adverse events:
    - Excessive coughing
    - Decreased oxygen saturation
    - Bronchospasm
    - Dislodgement of the bacterial biofilm that colonizes the endotracheal tube into the lower airway
    - Pain, anxiety, and dyspnea
    - Tachycardia
    - Increased intracranial pressure

Recommendations

The following recommendations are made following the Grading of Recommendations Assessment, Development, and Evaluation (GRADE) criteria.

- It is recommended that endotracheal suctioning should be performed only when secretions are present and not routinely (1C).
- It is suggested that pre-oxygenation be considered if the patient has a clinically important reduction in oxygen saturation with suctioning (2B).
- Performing suctioning without disconnecting the patient from the ventilator is suggested (2B).
- Use of shallow suction is suggested instead of deep suction, based on evidence from infant and pediatric studies (2B).
- It is suggested that routine use of normal saline instillation prior to endotracheal suction should *not* be performed (2C).

(continues)

Clinical Practice Guideline 19–3 *(continued)*

- The use of closed suction is suggested for adults with high F_{IO_2} or PEEP or who are at risk for lung derecruitment (2B) and neonates (2C).
- Endotracheal suctioning without disconnection (closed system) is suggested in neonates (2B).
- Avoidance of disconnection and use of lung-recruitment maneuvers are suggested if suctioning-induced lung derecruitment occurs in patients with acute lung injuries (2B).
- It is suggested that a suction catheter is used that occludes less than 50% of the lumen of the ETT in children and adults, and less than 70% in infants (2C).
- It is suggested that the duration of the suctioning event be limited to less than 15 seconds (2C).

Modified from AARC clinical practice guideline: endotracheal suctioning of mechanically ventilated patients with artificial airways. *Respir Care.* 2010;55(6):758–764. Reprinted with permission.

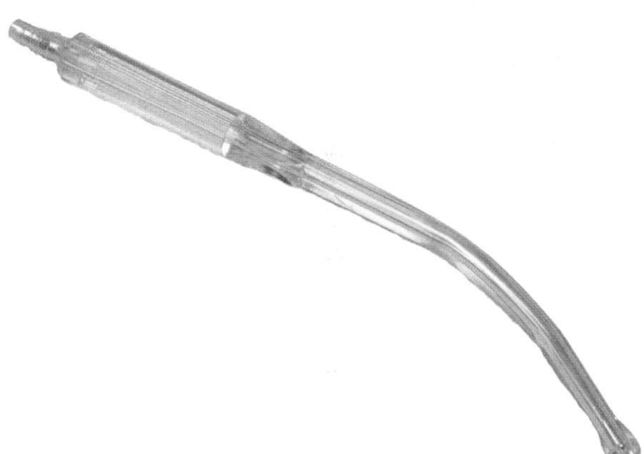

FIGURE 19–46 Yankauer mouth/pharyngeal suction.

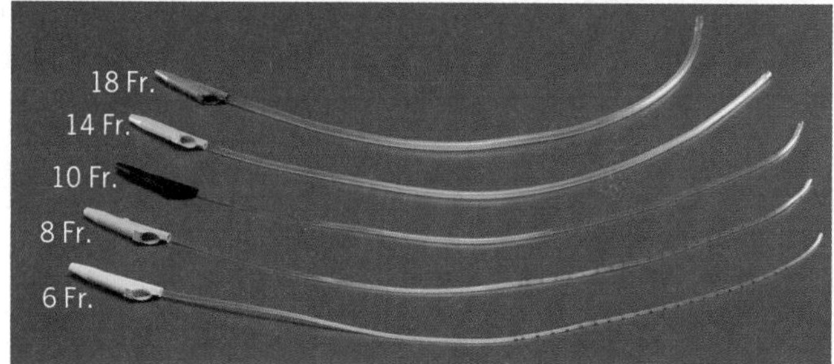

FIGURE 19–47 Suction catheter.

pharyngeal suctioning. This is generally used when secretions are visible in the oral cavity or prior to extubation. For suctioning through artificial airways, a suction catheter is used (**Figure 19–47**). A suction catheter must be long enough to enter the main stem bronchi. A thumb port at the proximal end controls suction to the catheter. The catheter must be rigid enough to allow passage through an artificial airway but flexible enough to prevent damage to the airway mucosa. Also to prevent damage to the airway mucosa, the catheter should have smooth, molded ends, one or more side holes near the catheter tip, and minimum frictional resistance when passed through the airway. The catheter should be transparent so that the aspirated secretions can be assessed.

The suction pressure should be no greater than that required to remove secretions adequately. It should not exceed 100 mm Hg in infants, 125 mm Hg in children, and 150 mm Hg in adults. Suction catheters are available in a variety of sizes. The catheter size is determined by its OD in French (Fr) units, which refers to the circumference of the tube. Because circumference equals 3.14 (π) $\times$ diameter, the French size is estimated by multiplication of the diameter by 3. The OD of the suction catheter should not exceed one-half to two-thirds the ID of the artificial airway. A 14 Fr catheter usually is acceptable for adults. CPG 19–3 lists indications and contraindications for artificial airway suctioning.

Although viewed as a beneficial therapeutic procedure, suctioning is not without risks to the patient. Potential complications associated with suctioning include hypoxemia, atelectasis, hyperinflation (if a manual resuscitator is used), airway trauma, contamination of the lower respiratory tract, arrhythmias, and increased intracranial pressure.

A number of factors contribute to suction-related hypoxemia, including interruption of mechanical ventilation during the suctioning procedure (i.e., loss of ventilation, inspired oxygen, and PEEP), aspiration of gas from the respiratory tract during the application of suction, entrainment of room air into the lungs, the duration of suctioning, and suction-related atelectasis. To prevent suction-related hypoxemia, the patient should be hyperoxygenated prior to the procedure. This most commonly is accomplished by an increase in the F_{IO_2} to 1.

Atelectasis can occur during suctioning as the result of evacuation of gases from the lower respiratory tract. This is more likely to occur when excessive suction pressures are used and when the size of the suction catheter is large in relation to the size of the endotracheal or tracheostomy tube. Derecruitment of lung units will then lead to some hypoxemia. The duration of suctioning also affects the degree of hypoxemia. A suctioning attempt should be as brief as possible to achieve the desired effect, which is removal of secretions, but should last no longer than 15 seconds.

Hyperinflation or hyperventilation (or both) to prevent suction-related hypoxemia should be used cautiously because of the hazards of overdistension lung injury. In some critical care units a manual ventilator (resuscitator) is used for hyperinflation and hyperoxygenation during suctioning procedures. The use of a manual resuscitator (especially without a pressure gauge) poses a significant threat of lung hyperinflation, which increases the potential risks of barotrauma.

Airway edema, hyperemia, mucosal ulceration, hemorrhage, and diminished mucociliary transport can occur with suctioning. These effects are related to operator technique and the amount of suction pressure used. Intermittent, rather than continuous, suctioning may be less traumatic to airway mucosa, but little evidence is available regarding this issue. The catheter tip should be smooth, molded, and atraumatic, and side holes near the tip of the catheter can minimize trauma to the airway mucosa. Pneumothorax that occurs secondary to bronchial perforation by a suction catheter has been reported in infants.[117–119] In infants, the suction catheter should not be inserted more than 1 cm beyond the tip of the endotracheal tube. A similar practice should be used for patients who have had a recent tracheal reconstructive surgery or pneumonectomy.

RESPIRATORY RECAP

Complications of Suctioning

- » Hypoxemia
- » Atelectasis
- » Hyperinflation
- » Airway trauma
- » Contamination of the lower respiratory tract
- » Arrhythmias
- » Increased intracranial pressure
- » Preferential suctioning of the right bronchus

AGE-SPECIFIC ANGLE

Pneumothorax that occurred secondary to bronchial perforation by a suction catheter has been reported in infants.

Contamination of the lower respiratory tract can occur during tracheal suctioning. This complication can be avoided with the use of sterile technique during the procedure. Care must be taken during suctioning to avoid contamination of the suction catheter, the ventilator circuit or the valve of the manual ventilator, and the clinician performing the procedure. Bedside manual ventilators can also be a source of contamination of the lower respiratory tract, which may increase the chance of pulmonary infection. Arrhythmias may occur during tracheal suctioning as a result of hypoxemia or vagal stimulation. This complication often can be avoided by hyperoxygenation of the patient during suctioning.

Because the left main stem bronchus has a smaller diameter than the right bronchus and leaves the trachea at a more acute angle, the suction catheter is more likely to enter the right main stem bronchus. Secretions therefore are more likely to be suctioned from the right lung than the left. Several techniques can be used for selective endobronchial suctioning, particularly of the left bronchus, including use of curved-tip catheters, turning the patient's head to the side (e.g., turning of the head to the right to facilitate suctioning of the left bronchus), and lateral positioning (turning of the patient onto the left side to facilitate passage of the catheter into the left main stem bronchus). Use of a curved-tip catheter (**Figure 19–48**) has proved to be the best means to accomplish endobronchial suctioning. When a curved-tip catheter with a guide mark is used for this purpose, successful endobronchial placement may occur in as many as 90% of cases. Factors that affect the success of the selective introduction of a catheter into a main stem bronchus include the anatomy of the carinal bifurcation, the patient's head and body positions, the route of tracheal tube placement (endotracheal or tracheostomy), the shape and direction of the endotracheal tube's bevel, the configuration and rigidity of the suction catheter, and the location of the tip of the endotracheal tube. Curved-tip catheters may be more effective with tracheostomy tubes than with endotracheal tubes.

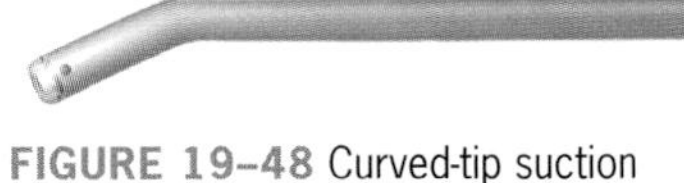

FIGURE 19–48 Curved-tip suction catheter.

An increase in intracranial pressure (ICP) can occur during tracheal suctioning, which may be clinically important in patients with a closed head injury. If a patient's ICP is being monitored, it should be watched closely during suctioning. Preoxygenation, hyperventilation, and pharmacologic support may be necessary for suctioning patients with an elevated ICP.

Closed Suction

With the closed suction system (**Figure 19–49**), the catheter becomes part of the ventilator circuit.[120–137] Closed suction and conventional suction catheters are equally effective at secretion clearance. However, the closed

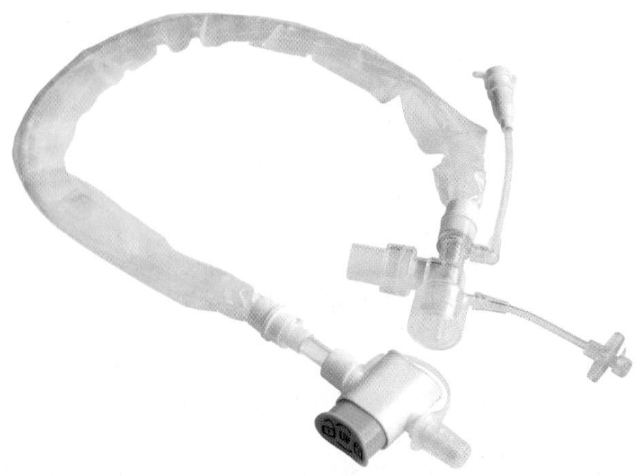

FIGURE 19–49 Closed suction catheter.

system may cause significantly fewer physiologic disturbances, such as dysrhythmias and desaturation, and environmental contamination is lower with the closed system. Perhaps the main advantage of a closed system is the minimization of circuit breaks, thus maintaining end-expiratory lung volume. A potential problem with closed suction catheters involves the catheter remaining in the airway after suctioning or migrating into the airway between suctioning procedures. This may be of particular concern during pressure ventilation, because the patient's tidal volume may be considerably compromised. Care must also be taken to avoid accidental patient lavage (which may wash some pathogens to the lower respiratory tract) when the catheter is rinsed with saline. Prolonged use of closed suction catheters does not affect the rate of ventilator-associated pneumonia,[136] and they do not need to be changed at regular intervals.[137]

Saline Instillation

Although saline may be instilled into the airway as part of the suctioning procedure to facilitate the removal of secretions, this practice is controversial.[138–145] Typically, more saline is instilled than is retrieved by the suctioning, which may result in an increase in the volume of secretions and worsening of airway obstruction. Saline instillation during suctioning may have an adverse effect on arterial oxygen saturation and may dislodge large numbers of bacteria from the lumen of the endotracheal tube, which may increase the likelihood of organisms being washed from the endotracheal tube into the lower respiratory tract. In a very few patients, saline instillation may be useful to loosen and remove thick secretions. However, this practice should be used judiciously and should *not* be a routine procedure each time a patient is suctioned.

KEY POINTS

- Oropharyngeal airways extend from the lips to the pharynx, following the natural curvature of the tongue, without entering the larynx or esophagus.
- Nasopharyngeal airways follow the anatomy of the nasopharynx so that the tip rests behind the tongue just above the epiglottis.
- Anesthesia personnel have the highest level of intubation skills, but in the hospital setting, the clinician with the highest level of experience and training outside the operating room may be the respiratory therapist.
- Indications for endotracheal intubation include bypassing of an upper airway obstruction, protection of the airway from aspiration, application of positive pressure ventilation, facilitation of secretion clearance, and delivery of high oxygen concentrations.
- Endotracheal intubation is the establishment of an artificial airway by use of a tube passed through the mouth or nose, then through the glottis, and into the trachea.
- The airway consists of five regions: the nose and nasopharynx, oral cavity and oropharynx, hypopharynx, larynx, and tracheobronchial tree.
- Endotracheal intubation should be approached calmly; frantic and rushed attempts at intubation often result in failure and worsening of the situation.
- Nasotracheal intubation generally is used for specific indications.
- The shape and design of the laryngeal mask airway allows it to form a seal around the glottic opening that excludes the esophageal opening from the airway.
- The risk of complications associated with endotracheal intubation is reduced by meticulous attention to care of the airway in intubated patients.
- The traditional method used to secure an endotracheal tube is to apply benzoin to the skin and secure the tube with adhesive tape, but commercial holding systems also are available.
- A bite block is placed between the teeth to prevent the patient from biting an orotracheal airway.
- The primary reason to perform a tracheostomy is to maintain a secure airway in patients who require long-term intubation.
- Percutaneous dilational tracheostomy is a comparatively new procedure that is less traumatic than the conventional tracheostomy.
- The fenestrated tracheostomy tube can be useful for assessment of a patient's readiness for decannulation.
- The primary goal of a talking tracheostomy tube is to allow cognitively intact, ventilator-dependent patients to communicate by speaking.
- Speaking valves are designed to eliminate the need for finger occlusion for oral communication.
- Tracheal buttons are used to maintain tracheostomy stomas.
- Cuff pressure should be kept at 20 to 30 cm H_2O to minimize the risks of tracheal wall injury and aspiration.
- Intubated patients should be suctioned whenever a physical examination reveals secretions in the airway.
- Numerous complications are possible with airway suctioning.
- With the closed suction system, the catheter becomes part of the ventilator circuit.
- Saline instillation during suctioning should be used judiciously and should not be performed each time a patient is suctioned.
- The most frequent cause of extubation failure is inability of the patient to sustain adequate spontaneous ventilation.

REFERENCES

1. Berman RA, Lilienfeld SM. The Berman airway. *Anesthesiology.* 1950;11:136–137.
2. Kupp PJ, Crewe TC. An airway for the edentulous adult. *Anesthesia.* 1974;29:601–602.
3. Pollard BJ, O'Leary J. Guedel airway and tooth damage. *Anesth Intensive Care.* 1981;9:395.
4. Wanner A, Zighelboim A, Sacker MA. Nasopharyngeal airway: a facilitated access to the trachea for nasotracheal suction, bedside bronchofiberoscopy, and selective bronchoscopy. *Ann Intern Med.* 1975;75:593–595.
5. Colice GL. Historical perspective on the development of mechanical ventilation. In: Tobin MJ, ed. *Principles and Practice of Mechanical Ventilation.* New York: McGraw-Hill; 1994.
6. Stoller JK. The history of intubation, tracheotomy, and airway appliances. *Respir Care.* 1999;44:595–601.
7. Hooke R. [title unknown.] *Phil Trans Roy Soc.* 1667;2:539.
8. MacEwen W. Clinical observations on the introduction of tracheal tubes by the mouth instead of performing tracheostomy or laryngotomy. *Br Med J.* 1880;2:122–124, 163–165.
9. O'Dwyer J. Intubation of the larynx. *N Y Med J.* 1885;4:145.
10. Fell GE. Forced respiration in opium poisoning: its possibilities and the apparatus best adapted to produce it. *Buffalo Med Surg J.* 1887;28:145.
11. Murphy FJ. Two improved intratracheal catheters. *Anesth Analg.* 1941;27:102–105.
12. Grillo HC, Cooper JD, Geffin B, et al. A low-pressure cuff for tracheostomy tubes to minimize tracheal injury: a comparative clinical trial. *J Thorac Cardiovasc Surg.* 1971;62:898–907.
13. 2005 American Heart Association guidelines for cardiopulmonary resuscitation and emergency cardiovascular care. *Circulation.* 2005;112:IV-19–IV-34.
14. Kacmarek RM. The role of the respiratory therapist in emergency care. *Respir Care.* 1992;37:523–530.
15. Bishop MJ. Who should perform intubation? *Respir Care.* 1999;44:750–758.
16. Bishop MJ, Michalowski P, Hussey JD, et al. Recertification of respiratory therapists' intubation skills one year after initial training: analysis of skill retention and retraining. *Respir Care.* 2001;46:234–237.
17. Konrad C, Schupfer G, Wietlisbach M, et al. Learning manual skills in anesthesiology: is there a recommended number of cases for anesthetic procedures? *Anesth Analg.* 1998;86:635–639.
18. Mulcaster JT, Mills J, Hung OR, et al. Laryngoscopic intubation: learning and performance. *Anesthesiology.* 2003;98:23–27.
19. Hess DR. Indications for translaryngeal intubation. *Respir Care.* 1999;44:604–609.
20. Plummer AL, Gracey DR. Consensus conference on artificial airways in patients receiving mechanical ventilation. *Chest.* 1989;96:178–180.
21. Kollef MH. What is ventilator-associated pneumonia and why is it important? *Respir Care.* 2005;50:714–772.
22. Coffin SE, Klompas M, Classen D, et al. Strategies to prevent ventilator-associated pneumonia in acute care hospitals. *Infect Control Hosp Epidemiol.* 2008;19:S31–S40.
23. Vital FM, Saconato H, Ladeira MT, et al. Non-invasive positive pressure ventilation (CPAP or bilevel NPPV) for cardiogenic pulmonary edema. *Cochrane Database Syst Rev.* 2008;3:CD005351.
24. Ram FSF, Picot J, Lightowler J, Wedzicha JA. Non-invasive positive pressure ventilation for treatment of respiratory failure due to exacerbations of chronic obstructive pulmonary disease. *Cochrane Database Syst Rev.* 2004;3:CD004104.
25. Nava S, Hill N. Noninvasive ventilation in acute respiratory failure. *Lancet.* 2009;374(9685):250–259.
26. Hess DR. The evidence for noninvasive positive-pressure ventilation in the care of patients in acute respiratory failure: a systematic review of the literature. *Respir Care.* 2004; 49:810–829.
27. Keenan SP, Mehta S. Noninvasive ventilation for patients presenting with acute respiratory failure: the randomized controlled trials. *Resp Care.* 2009;54:116–124.
28. Branson RD. The nuts and bolts of increasing arterial oxygenation: devices and techniques. *Respir Care.* 1993;38:686.
29. American Society of Anesthesiologists, Task Force on Management of the Difficult Airway. Practice guidelines for management of the difficult airway. *Anesthesiology.* 2003;98:1269–1277.
30. Williamson JA, Webb RK, Szekely S, et al. The Australian Incident Monitoring Study: difficult intubation: an analysis of 2000 incident reports. *Anesth Intensive Care.* 1993;78:597–602.
31. Wilson ME, Spiegelhalter D, Robertson JA, et al. Predicting difficult intubation. *Br J Anaesth.* 1988;61:211–216.
32. Nath G, Sekar M. Predicting difficult intubation: a comprehensive scoring system. *Anesth Intensive Care.* 1997;25:482–486.
33. Hurford WE. Techniques of endotracheal intubation. *Int Anesth Clin.* 2000;38:1–28.
34. Dunn PF, Goulet RL. Endotracheal tubes and airway appliances. *Int Anesth Clin.* 2000;38:65–94.
35. Jaeger JM, Durbin CG. Special-purpose endotracheal tubes. *Respir Care.* 1999;44:661–683.
36. Rello J, Sonora R, Jubert P, et al. Pneumonia in intubated patients: role of respiratory airway care. *Am J Respir Crit Care Med.* 1996;154:111–115.
37. Valles J, Artigas A, Rello J, et al. Continuous aspiration of subglottic secretions in preventing ventilator-associated pneumonia. *Ann Intern Med.* 1995;122:179–186.
38. Kollef MH, Skubas NJ, Sundt TM. A randomized clinical trial of continuous aspiration of subglottic secretions in cardiac surgery patients. *Chest.* 1999;116:1339–1346.
39. Smulders K, van der Hoeven H, Weers-Pothoff I, et al. A randomized clinical trial of intermittent subglottic secretion drainage in patients receiving mechanical ventilation. *Chest.* 2002;121:858–862.
40. Dezfulian C, Shojania K, Collard HR, Kim HM, et al. Subglottic secretion drainage for preventing ventilator-associated pneumonia: a meta-analysis. *Am J Med.* 2005;118:11–18.
41. Dullenkopf A, Gerber A, Weiss M. Fluid leakage past tracheal tube cuffs: evaluation of the new Microcuff endotracheal tube. *Intensive Care Med.* 2003;29:1849–1853.
42. Poelaert J, Depuydt P, De Wolf A, Van de Velde S, Herck Blot S. Polyurethane cuffed endotracheal tubes to prevent early postoperative pneumonia after cardiac surgery: a pilot study. *J Thorac Cardiovasc Surg.* 2008;135:771–776.
43. Olson ME, Harmon BG, Kollef MH. Silver-coated endotracheal tubes associated with reduced bacterial burden in the lungs of mechanically ventilated dogs. *Chest.* 2002;121:863–870.
44. Kollef MH, Afessa B, Anzueto A, et al. Silver-coated endotracheal tubes and incidence of ventilator-associated pneumonia: the NASCENT randomized trial. *JAMA.* 2008;300:805–813.
45. Owen RL, Cheney FW. Endobronchial intubation: a preventable complication. *Anesthesiology.* 1987;67:255–257.
46. Hurford WE. Nasotracheal intubation. *Respir Care.* 1999;44:643–647.
47. Rosen CL, Wolfe RE, Chew SE, et al. Blind nasotracheal intubation in the presence of facial trauma. *J Emerg Med.* 1997;15:141–145.
48. Rouby JJ, Laurent P, Gosnach M, et al. Risk factors and clinical relevance of nosocomial maxillary sinusitis in critically ill patients. *Am J Respir Crit Care Med.* 1994;150:776–783.
49. Maharaj CH, O'Croinin D, Curley G, Harte BH, Laffey JG. A comparison of tracheal intubation using the Airtraq or the MacIntosh laryngoscope in routine airway management: a randomized, controlled clinical trial. *Anaesthesia.* 2006;61(11):1093–1099.
50. Maharaj CH, Buckley E, Harte BH, Laffey JG. Endotracheal intubation in patients with cervical spine immobilization: a comparison of Macintosh and Airtraq laryngoscopes. *Anesthesiology.* 2007;107(1):53–59.

51. Maharaj CH, Costello JF, McDonnell JG, Harte BH, Laffey JG. The Airtraq as a rescue device following failed direct laryngoscopy: a case series. *Anaesthesia.* 2007;62(6):598–601.
52. Asai T, Morris S. The laryngeal mask airway: its features, effects, and roles. *Can J Anaesth.* 1994;41:930–960.
53. Verghese C, Ramaswamy B. LMA-Supreme—a new single-use LMA with gastric access: a report on its clinical efficiency. *Br J Anaesth.* 2008;101:405–410.
54. Theiler LG, Kleine-Brueggeney M, Kaiser D, et al. Crossover comparison of the Laryngeal Mask Supreme and the i-gel in simulated difficult airway scenario in anesthesized patients. *Anesthesiology.* 2009;111:55–62.
55. Brofeldt T, Panacek E, Richards JR. An easy crichothyrotomy approach: the rapid four-step technique. *Acad Emerg Med.* 1996;3:1060–1063.
56. Blanda M, Gallo UE. Emergency airway management. *Emerg Med Clin North Am.* 2003;21:1–26.
57. Stauffer JL, Silvester RC. Complications of endotracheal intubation, tracheostomy, and artificial airways. *Respir Care.* 1982;27:417–434.
58. Stauffer JL, Olson DE, Petty TL. Complications and consequences of endotracheal intubation and tracheostomy: a prospective study of 150 critical ill adult patients. *Am J Med.* 1981;70:65–76.
59. Tominga GT, Rudzwick H, Scannell G, et al. Decreasing unplanned extubations in the surgical intensive care unit. *Am J Surg.* 1995;170:586–590.
60. Boulain T. Unplanned extubations in the adult intensive care unit: a prospective multicenter study. *Am J Respir Crit Care Med.* 1998;157:1131–1137.
61. Listello D, Sessler CN. Unplanned extubation: clinical predictors for reintubation. *Chest.* 1994;105:1496–1503.
62. Scott PH, Eigen H, Moye LA, et al. Predictability and consequences of spontaneous extubation in a pediatric ICU. *Crit Care Med.* 1985;13:228–232.
63. Christie JM, Dethlefsen M, Cane RD. Unplanned endotracheal extubation in the intensive care unit. *J Clin Anesth.* 1996;8:289–293.
64. Vassal T, Anh NG, Gabillet JM, et al. Prospective evaluation of self-extubations in a medical intensive care unit. *Intensive Care Med.* 1993;19:340–342.
65. Whelan J, Simpson SQ, Levy H. Unplanned extubation: predictors of successful termination of mechanical ventilatory support. *Chest.* 1995;105:1808–1812.
66. Atkins PM, Mion LC, Mendelson W, et al. Characteristics and outcomes of patients who self-extubate from ventilatory support: a case-control study. *Chest.* 1997;112:1317–1323.
67. Betbese A, Perez M, Rialp G, et al. A prospective study of unplanned endotracheal extubation in intensive care unit patients. *Crit Care Med.* 1998;26:1180–1186.
68. Chiang AA, Lee KC, Lee JC, et al. Effectiveness of a continuous quality improvement program aiming to reduce unplanned extubation: a prospective study. *Intensive Care Med.* 1996;22:1269–1271.
69. Sessler CN. Unplanned extubations: making progress using CQI. *Intensive Care Med.* 1997;23:143–145.
70. Kapadia FN, Bajan KB, Raje KY. Airway accidents in intubated intensive care unit patients: an epidemiological study. *Crit Care Med.* 2000;28:659–664.
71. Carrion MI, Ayuso D, Marcos M, et al. Accidental removal of endotracheal and nasotracheal tubes and intravascular catheters. *Crit Care Med.* 2000;28:63–66.
72. Hess DR. Managing the artificial airway. *Respir Care.* 1999;44:759–772.
73. Tasota FJ, Hoffman LA, Zullo TG, et al. Evaluation of two methods used to stabilize oral endotracheal tubes. *Heart Lung.* 1987;16:140–146.
74. Levy H, Griego L. A comparative study of oral endotracheal tube securing methods. *Chest.* 1993;104:1537–1540.
75. Kaplow R, Bookbinder M. A comparison of four endotracheal tube holders. *Heart Lung.* 1994;23:59–66.
76. Conrardy PA, Goodman LR, Lainge F, et al. Alteration of endotracheal tube position: flexion and extension of the neck. *Crit Care Med.* 1976;4:8–12.
77. Carlson J, Mayrose J, Krause R, et al. Extubation force: tape versus endotracheal tube holders. *Ann Emerg Med.* 2007;50:686–691.
78. Barnson S, Graham J, Wild C, et al. Comparison of two endotracheal tube securement techniques on unplanned extubation, oral mucosa, and facial skin integrity. *Heart Lung.* 1998;27:409–417.
79. Patel N, Smith C, Pinchak A, et al. Taping methods and tape types for securing oral endotracheal tubes. *Can J Anaesth.* 1997;44:330–336.
80. Carlson J, Mayrose J, Krause R, et al. Extubation force: tape versus endotracheal tube holders. *Ann Emerg Med.* 2007;50:686–691.
81. Campbell RS. Extubation and the consequences of reintubation. *Respir Care.* 1999;44:799–806.
82. Salam A, Tilluckdharry L, Amoateng-Adjepong Y, Manthous CA. Neurologic status, cough, secretions, and extubation outcomes. *Intensive Care Med.* 2004;30:1334–1339.
83. Miller RL, Cole RP. Association between reduced cuff leak volume and postextubation stridor. *Chest.* 1996;110:1035–1040.
84. Fisher MM, Raper RF. The "cuff leak" test for extubation. *Anaesthesia.* 1992;47:10–12.
85. Kriner EJ, Shafazand S, Colice GL. The endotracheal tube cuff leak test as a predictor for post-extubation stridor. *Respir Care.* 2005;50:1632–1638.
86. Shin SH, Heath K, Reed S, Collins J, Weireter LJ, Britt LD. The cuff leak test is not predictive of successful extubation. *Am Surg.* 2008;74:1182–1185.
87. Jaber S, Jung B, Chanques G, Bonnet F, Marret E. Effects of steroids on reintubation and post-extubation stridor in adults: meta-analysis of randomized controlled trials. *Crit Care.* 2009;13(2):R49.
88. Fan T, Wang G, Mao B, et al. Prophylactic administration of parenteral steroids for preventing airway complications after extubation in adults: meta-analysis of randomized controlled trials. *BMJ.* 2008;337:a1841.
89. Esteban A, Alia I, Gordo F, et al. Extubation outcome after spontaneous breathing trials with T-tube or pressure support ventilation. *Am J Respir Crit Care Med.* 1997;156:459–465.
90. Epstein SK, Ciubotaru RL. Independent effects of etiology of failure and time to reintubation on outcome for patients failing extubation. *Am J Respir Crit Care Med.* 1998;158:489–493.
91. Torres A, Gatell JM, Aznar E, et al. Reintubation increases the risk of nosocomial pneumonia in patients needing mechanical ventilation. *Am J Respir Crit Care Med.* 1995;152:137–141.
92. Heffner JE. Tracheostomy: indications and timing. *Respir Care.* 1999;44:807–815.
93. Maziak DE, Meade MO, Todd TR. The timing of tracheotomy: a systematic review. *Chest.* 1998;114:605–609.
94. Griffiths J, Barber VS, Morgan L, Young JD. Systematic review and meta-analysis of studies of the timing of tracheostomy in adult patients undergoing artificial ventilation. *BMJ.* 2005; 330:1243–1248.
95. Reibel JE. Tracheotomy/tracheostomy. *Respir Care.* 1999;44:820–823.
96. Hill BB, Zweng TN, Maley RH, et al. Percutaneous dilational tracheostomy: report of 356 cases. *J Trauma.* 1996;41:238–243.
97. Cobean R, Beals M, Moss C, et al. Percutaneous dilatational tracheostomy: a safe, cost-effective bedside procedure. *Arch Surg.* 1996;131:265–271.
98. Fernandez L, Norwood S, Roettger R, et al. Bedside percutaneous tracheostomy with bronchoscopic guidance in critically ill patients. *Arch Surg.* 1996;131:129–132.
99. Nates JL, Cooper J, Myles PS, et al. Percutaneous tracheostomy in critically ill patients: a prospective randomized comparison of techniques. *Crit Care Med.* 2000;28:3734–3739.

100. Freeman BD, Isabella K, Lin N, et al. A meta-analysis of prospective trials comparing percutaneous and surgical tracheostomy in critically ill patients. *Chest.* 2000;118:1412–1418.
101. Higgins KM, Punthakee X. Meta-analysis comparison of open versus percutaneous tracheostomy. *Laryngoscope.* 2007;117:447–454.
102. Walz MK, Peitgen K, Thurauf N, et al. Percutaneous dilatational tracheostomy: early results and long-term outcome of 326 critically ill patients. *Intensive Care Med.* 1998;24:685–690.
103. Beltrame F, Zussino M, Martinez B, et al. Percutaneous versus surgical bedside tracheostomy in the intensive care unit: a cohort study. *BMC Bioinformatics.* 2007;8(suppl 1):S18.
104. Downes JJ, Schreiner MS. Tracheostomy tubes and attachments in infants and children. *Int Anesth Clin.* 1985;23:37–60.
105. Hess DR. Tracheostomy tubes and related appliances. *Resp Care.* 2005;50:497–510.
106. Hess DR. Facilitating speech in the patient with a tracheostomy. *Respir Care.* 2005;50:519–525.
107. Johnson DC, Campbell SL, Rabkin JD. Tracheostomy tube manometry: evaluation of speaking valves, capping and need for downsizing. *Clin Respir J.* 2008;3:8–14.
108. Hoit JD, Banzett RB, Lohmeier HL, Hixon TJ, Brown R. Clinical ventilator adjustments that improve speech. *Chest.* 2003;124:1512–1521.
109. Schmidt U, Hess D, Kwo J, et al. Tracheostomy tube malposition in patients admitted to a respiratory acute care unit following prolonged ventilation. *Chest.* 2008;134:288–294.
110. Stelfox HT, Crimi C, Berra L, et al. Determinants of tracheostomy decannulation: an international study. *Crit Care.* 2008;12(1):R26.
111. Pavlin EG, Van Mimwegan D, Hornbein TE. Failure of a high-compliance low-pressure cuff to prevent aspiration. *Anesthesiology.* 1975;42:216–219.
112. Bernhard WN, Cottrell JE, Sivakumaran C, et al. Adjustment of intracuff pressure to prevent aspiration. *Anesthesiology.* 1979;50:363–366.
113. Sills J. An emergency cuff inflation technique. *Respir Care.* 1986;31:199–201.
114. Ho AM, Contrardi LH. What to do when an endotracheal tube cuff leaks. *J Trauma.* 1990;40:486–487.
115. Tinkoff G, Bakow ED, Smith RW. A continuous flow apparatus for temporary inflation of damaged endotracheal tube cuffs. *Respir Care.* 1990;35:423–426.
116. Kearl RA, Hooper RG. Massive airway leaks: an analysis of the role of endotracheal tubes. *Crit Care Med.* 1993;21:518–521.
117. Vaughan RS, Menke JA, Giacoia GP. Pneumothorax: a complication of endotracheal tube suctioning. *J Pediatr.* 1978;92:633–634.
118. Grosfeld JL, Lemons JL, Ballantine TVN, et al. Emergency thoracotomy for acquired bronchopleural fistula in the premature infant with respiratory distress. *J Pediatr Surg.* 1980;15:416–421.
119. Anderson KD, Chandra R. Pneumothorax secondary to perforation of sequential bronchi by suction catheters. *J Pediatr Surg.* 1976;11:687–693.
120. Witmer MT, Hess D, Simmons M. An evaluation of the effectiveness of secretion removal with the Ballard closed-circuit suction catheter. *Respir Care.* 1991;36:844–848.
121. Craig KC, Benson MS, Pierson DJ. Prevention of arterial oxygen desaturation during closed airway endotracheal suction: effect of ventilator mode. *Respir Care.* 1984;29:1013–1018.
122. Carlon GC, Fox SJ, Ackerman NJ. Evaluation of a closed tracheal suction system. *Crit Care Med.* 1987;15:522–525.
123. Johnson KL, Kearnery PA, Johnson SB, et al. Closed versus open endotracheal suctioning: costs and physiologic consequences. *Crit Care Med.* 1994;22:654–666.
124. Hrashbarger SA, Hoffman LA, Zullo TG, et al. Effects of a closed tracheal suction system on ventilatory and cardiovascular parameters. *Am J Respir Crit Care Med.* 1992;3:57–61.
125. Deppe SA, Kelly JW, Thoi LL, et al. Incidence of colonization, nosocomial pneumonia, and mortality in critically ill patients using a Trach Care closed suction system versus an open suction system: prospective, randomized study. *Crit Care Med.* 1990;18:1389–1393.
126. Cobley M, Arkins M, Jones PL. Environmental contamination during tracheal suction. *Anaesthesia.* 1991;46:957–961.
127. Ombes P, Fauvage B, Oleyer C. Nosocomial pneumonia in mechanically ventilated patients: a prospective randomized evaluation of the Stericath closed suctioning system. *Intensive Care Med.* 2000;26:878–882.
128. Ritz R, Scott LR, Coyle MB, et al. Contamination of a multiple-use suction catheter in a closed circuit system compared to contamination of a disposable, single-use suction catheter. *Respir Care.* 1986;31:1086–1091.
129. Blackwood B, Webb CH. Closed tracheal suctioning systems and infection control in the intensive care unit. *J Hosp Infect.* 1998,39:315–321.
130. Hamori CA, O'Connell JM. Improperly positioned closed system suction catheter causes elevated peak inspiratory airway pressures. *Respir Care.* 1991;36:1441–1442.
131. DePew CL, Moseley MJ, Clark EG, et al. Open versus closed system endotracheal suctioning: a cost comparison. *Crit Care Nurse.* 1994;14:94–100.
132. Combes P, Fauvage B, Oleyer C. Nosocomial pneumonia in mechanically ventilated patients: a prospective randomized evaluation of the Stericath closed suctioning system. *Intensive Care Med.* 2000;26:878–882.
133. Rabitsch W, Kostler WJ, Fiebiger W, et al. Closed suctioning system reduces cross-contamination between system and gastric juices. *Anesth Analg.* 2004;99:886–892.
134. Maggiore SM, Lellouche F, Pigeot J, et al. Prevention of endotracheal suctioning-induced alveolar derecruitment in acute lung injury. *Am J Respir Crit Care Med.* 2003;167:1215–1224.
135. Cereda M, Villa F, Colombo E, et al. Closed system endotracheal suctioning maintains lung volume-controlled mechanical ventilation. *Intensive Care Med.* 2001;27:648–654.
136. Vonberg RP, Eckmanns T, Welte T, Gastmeier P. Impact of the suctioning system (open vs. closed) on the incidence of ventilation-associated pneumonia: meta-analysis of randomized controlled trials. *Intensive Care Med.* 2006;32:1329–1335.
137. Kollef MH, Prentice D, Shapiro SD, et al. Mechanical ventilation with or without daily changes of in-line suction catheters. *Am J Respir Crit Care Med.* 1997;156(2 pt 1):466–472.
138. Gray JE, MacIntyre NR, Kronenberger WG. The effects of bolus normal saline instillation in conjunction with endotracheal suctioning. *Respir Care.* 1990;35:785–790.
139. Ackerman MH, Ecklund MM, Abu-Jumah M. A review of normal saline instillation: implications for practice. *Dimensions Crit Care Nurs.* 1996;15:31–38.
140. Ackerman MH. The effect of saline lavage prior to suctioning. *Am J Crit Care.* 1993;2:326–330.
141. Hagler DA, Traver GA. Endotracheal saline and suction catheters: sources of lower airway contamination. *Am J Crit Care.* 1994;3:444–447.
142. Kinlock D. Instillation of normal saline during endotracheal suctioning: effects on mixed venous oxygen saturation. *Am J Crit Care.* 1999;8:231–242.
143. Ji YR, Kim HS, Park JH. Instillation of normal saline before suctioning in patients with pneumonia. *Yonsei Med J.* 2002;43:607–612.
144. Ackermann MH, Mick DJ. Instillation of normal saline before suctioning in patients with pulmonary infections: a prospective randomized controlled trial. *Am J Crit Care.* 1998;7:261–266.
145. Caruso P, Denari S, Ruiz SA, Demarzo SE, Deheinzelin D. Saline instillation before tracheal suctioning decreases the incidence of ventilator-associated pneumonia. *Crit Care Med.* 2009;37:32–38.

CHAPTER 20

Cardiopulmonary Resuscitation

Rhonda Bevis
Christine J. Moore

OUTLINE

Cardiopulmonary Resuscitation
Basic Life Support
Advanced Cardiovascular Life Support
Ethical Concerns

OBJECTIVES

1. Compare basic life support and advanced cardiovascular life support.
2. Discuss the rationale for rapid response resuscitation teams.
3. Describe the CABD survey.
4. Describe the techniques of external chest compression, airway opening, and emergency ventilation for a cardiac-arrested patient.
5. Compare one-rescuer and two-rescuer cardiopulmonary resuscitation.
6. Describe the emergency management of foreign body airway obstruction.
7. Compare the techniques of adult, pediatric, and neonatal resuscitation.
8. Describe the treatment of bradycardia and tachycardia during advanced cardiovascular life support.

KEY TERMS

advanced cardiovascular life support (ACLS)
automated external defibrillator (AED)
basic life support (BLS)
CABD survey
cardiopulmonary resuscitation (CPR)
chest compressions
defibrillation
face shield
foreign body obstruction (FBO)
impedance threshold valve (ITV)
manual resuscitator
rapid response team

INTRODUCTION

Resuscitation of patients in cardiopulmonary arrest requires assessment of the problem, training, and an organized response. Code teams and rapid response teams have a respiratory therapist on the team. This chapter addresses the administration of **cardiopulmonary resuscitation (CPR)**, namely the concepts of **basic life support (BLS)**; the use of automated external defibrillation (AED), CPR in adults, children and infants; the principles of advanced life support (ALS); and the ethical issues encountered.

BLS includes all aspects of care required to treat life-threatening events (sudden cardiac arrest, acute myocardial infarction, stroke, and foreign body airway obstruction), CPR, and **defibrillation** with an automated external defibrillator.[1] Respiratory therapists, nurses, and physicians work together as members of rapid response teams providing rapid assessment and quick intervention or as code teams providing BLS and **advanced cardiovascular life support (ACLS)** in healthcare settings. A **rapid response team**, known by some as a *medical emergency team*, is a team of clinicians who bring critical care expertise to the patient's side wherever it is needed. In many situations, rapid response teams can prevent the patient's deterioration to the point where BLS or ACLS is not needed to resuscitate the patient.

Cardiopulmonary Resuscitation

Recommendations and guidelines for resuscitation procedures are provided by the American Heart Association (AHA) and are based on recommendations from the Emergency Cardiovascular Care (ECC) committee. In 2005[2] and again in 2010,[3] the ECC evaluated the sequences, priorities, and steps of BLS and ACLS to determine which factors were most likely to have the greatest positive effect on the successful resuscitation of individuals who suffered a cardiopulmonary arrest. It emphasized the need for high-quality compressions and a minimization of interruptions to chest compressions to facilitate better perfusion to the patient's vital organs.

Over the last 25 years the AHA has made several changes in the recommended ratio of ventilations to compressions for CPR. Its 2005 guidelines were based on research indicating that during the first few minutes of a cardiac arrest with ventricular fibrillation, management of the airway, oxygenation, and ventilation are probably not as important as chest compressions. This is because the total amount of oxygen delivered to the vital organs is limited more by the amount of arterial blood flow to the organs than by the oxygen content of the arterial blood itself. During resuscitation, chest compressions are responsible for restoring blood flow to vital organs, and any interruption results in a lower perfusion pressure for the coronary and cerebral arteries and a higher rate of deaths for patients following a cardiac arrest.[3–5] In fact, current guidelines emphasize chest compressions rather than ventilation during CPR. Healthcare providers commonly provide excessive ventilation and chest compressions that are inadequate and frequently interrupted during the resuscitation. Laypersons commonly provide ventilations ineffectively, and therefore compression-only CPR is taught to laypersons.

The worldwide survival rate of people who suffer an out-of-hospital cardiac arrest averages only about 6% or less.[6–9] With properly trained caregivers, the survival rates for a witnessed ventricular fibrillation (VF) increase to 49% to 74%.[10] Proper training includes rapid recognition of the cardiopulmonary arrest, rapid response, CPR, and early defibrillation (within 5 minutes).[10] Factors affecting resuscitation outcomes include the initial cardiac rhythm, time to initiate CPR, time to defibrillate, duration of CPR, and whether the arrest was witnessed. Because a longer duration of VF leads to greater myocardial deterioration, late defibrillation is less likely to provide conversion to a spontaneous rhythm. The chain of survival illustrates the sequence of actions that improves the rate of survival after cardiac arrest (**Figure 20–1**): early access, early CPR, early defibrillation, and early advanced life support. The highest hospital discharge rate has been achieved in patients for whom CPR was initiated within 4 minutes of arrest and advanced life support was initiated within 8 minutes.

> **RESPIRATORY RECAP**
>
> **Chain of Survival**
>
> » Early access
> » Early CPR
> » Early defibrillation
> » Early ACLS

Each hospital defines the respiratory therapist's involvement on rapid response teams and code teams. Therapists utilize their skills and expertise in patient assessment, airway management, oxygen therapy and mechanical ventilation, electrocardiographic (ECG) recognition, chest compressions, defibrillation, hemodynamic monitoring, and administration of ACLS drugs. This chapter summarizes the BLS and ACLS responsibilities of respiratory therapists who work in these capacities. The clinical practice guidelines of the American Association for Respiratory Care (AARC) describe the role of respiratory therapists in providing patient support (**CPG 20–1**). Healthcare workers and respiratory therapists should modify their sequence of actions based on their location, whether or not immediate help is available, and their hospital or department protocol.[11]

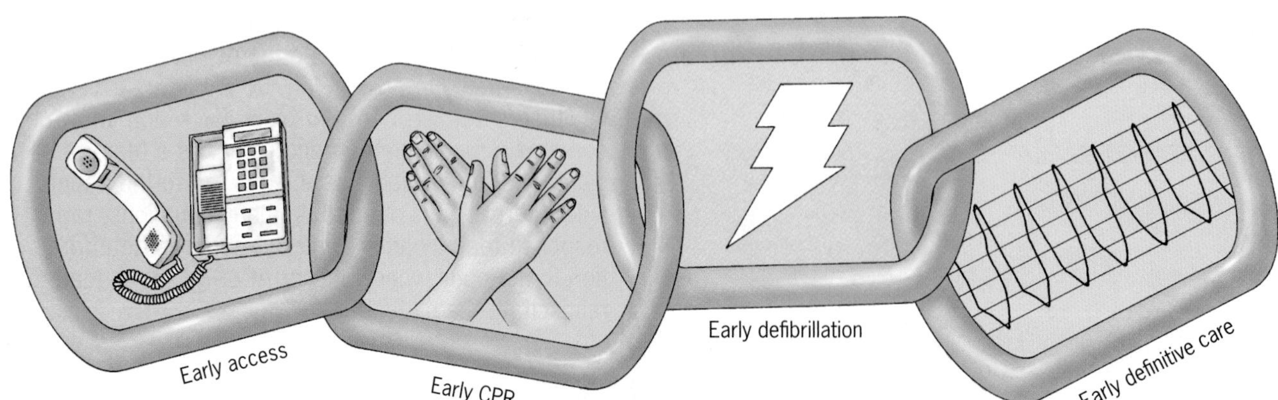

FIGURE 20–1 The emergency cardiac care system's concept displayed schematically as the chain of survival. Source: American Heart Association.

CLINICAL PRACTICE GUIDELINE 20–1

Resuscitation and Defibrillation in the Healthcare Setting

Specialty resuscitation teams trained to meet the needs of different hospital populations are desirable (e.g., trauma, stroke). Team members should be notified simultaneously. All hospital workers must know how to activate the hospital's emergency response system.

Level I

- *Training:* All Level I personnel should be trained, evaluated by performance, and retrained as necessary in basic life support (BLS) and the use of automated external defibrillators (AEDs) at frequent intervals that do not exceed 2 years.
- *Responsibilities:* First responders must be able to recognize that the patient is unresponsive, apneic, and pulseless. They should be able to attach automated defibrillator electrodes and operate AEDs. Level I personnel also assist the primary (Level II) members of the resuscitation team by (l) assessing patients for respiratory and/or cardiac arrest, (2) activating the resuscitation team, (3) administering BLS, (4) providing mouth-to-mask ventilation, (5) attaching electrocardiogram (ECG) and automatic defibrillator electrodes, (6) assisting with tracheal intubation, (7) defibrillating with automatic electronic defibrillators, (8) attaching pulse oximeter and capnograph, (9) preparing a written record of resuscitation effort, and (10) collecting arterial blood for analysis.

Level II

- *Training:* Level II personnel should be trained, evaluated by performance, and retrained as necessary in emergency cardiac care (ECC) and advanced cardiac life support (ACLS) as appropriate at intervals that should not exceed 2 years.
- *Responsibilities:* Level II health professionals should be capable of serving as primary members of the resuscitation team and as team leader when they are the best-qualified respondents. They are skilled in the use of all adjunctive equipment and special techniques for ECC/ACLS. They have the skills of Level I personnel and the following capabilities: (1) advanced ECG monitoring and dysrhythmia recognition, (2) tracheal intubation, (3) capability to deliver shocks with defibrillators, (4) use of mechanical ventilators, (5) preparation and administration of cardiac drugs, (6) stabilization of patients in the postarrest period, (7) provision of access for rapid administration of intravenous fluids, (8) managing ventilation via transtracheal catheter and cricothyrotomy, (9) emergency treatment of tension pneumothorax or hemothorax with large-bore needle, (10) interpretation of hemodynamic data, and (11) evaluating oxygenation, ventilation, and acid–base balance from blood gas reports.

Adapted from AARC clinical practice guideline: resuscitation and defibrillation in the health care setting—2004 revision and update. *Respir Care*. 2004;49:1085–1099. Reprinted with permission.

Sudden death related to coronary heart disease (CHD) is the most prominent medical emergency in the United States. **Box 20–1** lists risk factors for CHD. A prudent heart lifestyle is a lifestyle that includes weight control, physical fitness, smart eating habits, and avoidance of stress and cigarette smoking. The most important risk factor is cigarette smoking. The CHD death rate is 70% greater for smokers than nonsmokers, and the risk from smoking increases when combined with other factors (most notably elevated cholesterol and hypertension).

Indications for CPR are cardiac arrest or respiratory arrest or both. Cardiac arrest is usually secondary to ventricular fibrillation but may be the result of other arrhythmias (i.e., supraventricular tachycardia, ventricular tachycardia). Recognition of VF is particularly important because prompt defibrillation improves the success of CPR. Respiratory problems causing respiratory arrest include an obstructed airway (partial or complete), interference with the respiratory drive mechanism (spinal cord or head injury), and disorders of pulmonary gas transport (pulmonary edema or pulmonary embolus).

Basic Life Support

The Initial Steps

The initial step of cardiopulmonary resuscitation is a quick assessment of whether or not the patient truly needs to be resuscitated (**Algorithm 20–1**). Check for responsiveness by tapping the patient and asking in a loud voice "Are you all right?" If there is no response, activate the emergency response system according to the guidelines of the institution. Place the patient in a supine

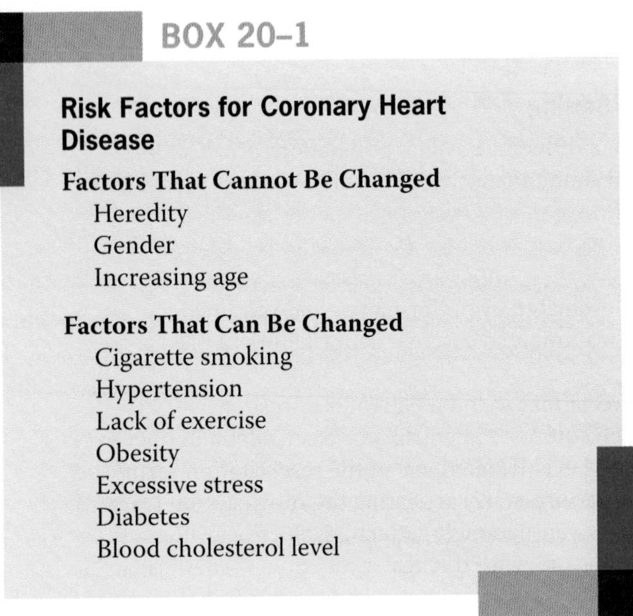

BOX 20-1

Risk Factors for Coronary Heart Disease

Factors That Cannot Be Changed
- Heredity
- Gender
- Increasing age

Factors That Can Be Changed
- Cigarette smoking
- Hypertension
- Lack of exercise
- Obesity
- Excessive stress
- Diabetes
- Blood cholesterol level

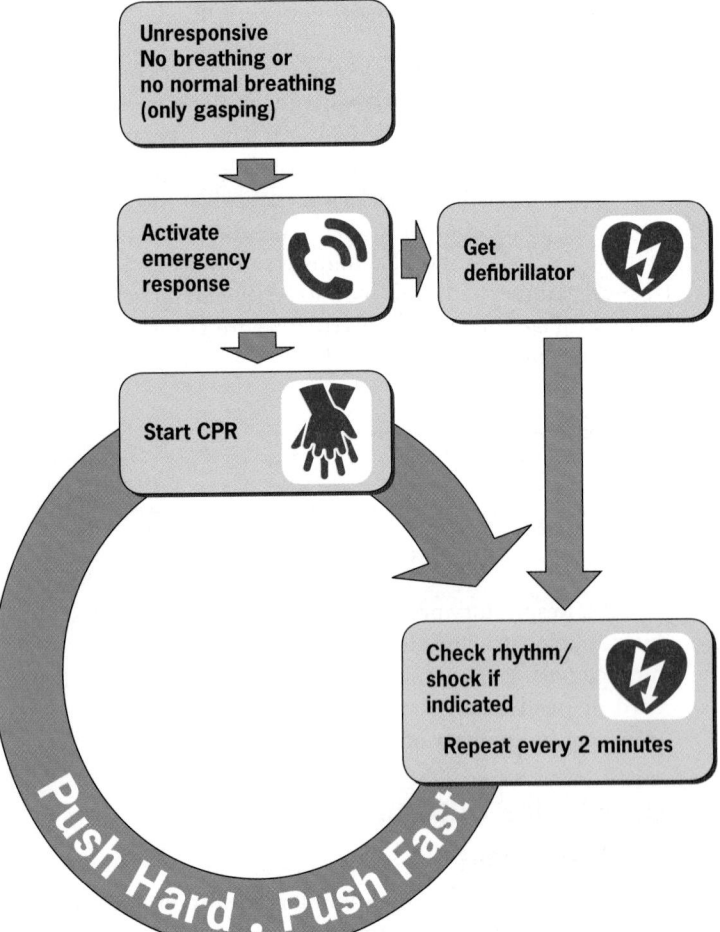

Unresponsive
No breathing or
no normal breathing
(only gasping)
Activate
emergency
response
Get
defibrillator
Start CPR
Check rhythm/
shock if
indicated
Repeat every 2 minutes
Push Hard . Push Fast

ALGORITHM 20-1 Simplified Basic Life Support Algorithm. Reprinted with permission. 2010 American Heart Association Guidelines for Cardiopulmonary Resuscitation and Emergency Cardiovascular Care. Part 5: Adult Basic Life Support. *Circulation.* 2010;122:S685–S705. © 2010 American Heart Association, Inc.

position on a hard surface and position yourself where you can do CPR by standing or kneeling at the level of the patient's upper chest.

A respiratory arrest is considered to be present when the patient's respirations are completely absent or when there is evidence that they are clearly inadequate to maintain adequate ventilation or oxygenation, or both. The agonal gasps that may occur in the first few minutes after a cardiac arrest are not interpreted as adequate breathing.[12] A cardiac arrest is considered to be present when the pulse is absent or when it is not sufficient to support perfusion. Either of these situations requires quick action by the rescuers.

Primary CABD Survey

Airway

Traditionally, opening the airway was the first step in providing CPR. However, in 2010 this changed from ABCD (airway, breathing, circulation, and defibrillation) to CABD (circulation, airway, breathing, and defibrillation). The AHA Guidelines indicate that chest compressions are the foundation for CPR, and the AHA recommends that chest compressions are done before opening the airway and providing ventilation by following the **CABD survey**. The rationale for initiation of CPR with chest compressions ensures that the victim receives this critical intervention early. Additionally, the 2010 Guidelines recognize the varying levels of rescuer proficiency by stressing the need for the untrained rescuer to provide hands-ony (compressions-only) CPR whereas health care providers incorporate rescue breathing and teamwork (**Box 20–2**).

Opening the airway can be done using one of two methods—the head tilt–chin lift maneuver or the jaw-thrust maneuver—depending on whether there is a possibility of a cervical spine injury. It is estimated that approximately 2% of all victims of blunt trauma have a spinal cord injury; this risk increases threefold if the patient has a craniofacial injury.[13]

The head tilt–chin lift method is performed by standing to the side of the patient and placing the palm of one hand on the patient's forehead and the fingers of the other hand under the bony part of the lower jaw near the chin. The head is then tilted backward using the palm of one hand while the chin is lifted forward using the finger of the other hand (**Figure 20–2**).

The jaw-thrust maneuver is accomplished by positioning yourself behind the top of the patient's head, placing the fingers of both hands under the angles of both jaws, and moving the mandible forward and upward. If there is a possibility of cervical spine injury, the jaw-thrust maneuver should

BOX 20–2

CABD Survey

Primary CABD Survey

(Begin basic life support algorithm.)
Activate emergency response system.
Call for defibrillator.

- **C** CPR: check pulse; if no pulse, proceed to the following step.
- **C** Start chest compressions.
- **A** Airway: open airway.
- **B** Breathing: give two slow breaths.
- **D** Defibrillator: attach automated external defibrillator (AED) when available.

Secondary CABD Survey

- **C** Initiate oxygen, IV, monitor, and fluids.
  - Rhythm-appropriate medications.
- **C** Check vital signs: temperature, blood pressure, heart rate, respirations.
- **A** Intubate as soon as possible.
- **B** Confirm tube placement; use two methods to confirm.
  - Primary physical examination criteria *plus* secondary confirmation device (qualitative and quantitative measures of end-tidal CO_2).
- **B** Secure tracheal tube.
  - Prevent dislodgment; purpose-made tracheal tube holders are recommended over tie-and-tape approaches.
  - If the patient is at risk for transport movement, cervical collar and backboard are recommended.
- **B** Confirm initial oxygenation and ventilation.
  - End-tidal CO_2 monitor.
  - Oxygen saturation monitor.
- **D** Perform differential diagnosis.

Adapted from Adult basic life support. *Circulation*. 2000;102:1–22; and 2010 American Heart Association Guidelines for Cardiopulmonary Resuscitation and Emergency Cardiovascular Care. Part 5: Adult Basic Life Support. *Circulation*. 2010;122:S685–S705.

be used to avoid the possibility of further injuries (**Figure 20–3**).[14] If the airway remains obstructed after the jaw-thrust maneuver is performed, the head should be tilted gently backward until the airway opens to provide an open airway and ventilation.[14]

Posterior displacement of the tongue is the most common cause of airway obstruction in the unconscious person (**Figure 20–4**). Loss of control of the submandibular muscles allows the tongue to drop and obstruct the oropharynx. Because the tongue is attached to the lower jaw, movement of the jaw forward using either maneuver moves the tongue up and away from the posterior pharynx, which opens the airway. Because positioning of the head can block the airway and prevent adequate breathing, in some patients opening the airway may allow the patient to resume sufficient breathing without the rescuer having to take further actions. Once

RESPIRATORY RECAP

Primary Airway Management During CPR

- » Posterior displacement of tongue obstructs airway.
- » Use head tilt–chin lift maneuver to open airway.
- » Use jaw-thrust maneuver with spinal injury.
- » Clean foreign objects from airway.

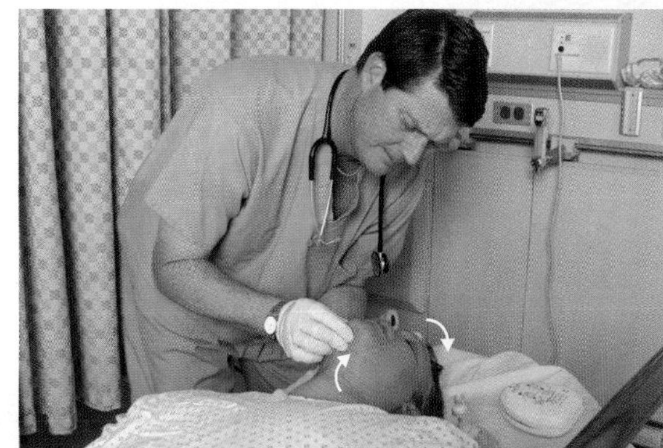

FIGURE 20–2 Opening the airway using the head tilt-chin method.

the mouth is open, the upper airway can be inspected for foreign objects, vomit, or blood. If foreign objects are seen they should be removed using a finger sweep or by suctioning, being careful not to push the object further into the airway.

Breathing

Once the airway has been opened, it has been traditionally taught to employ the "look, listen, and feel" technique: assess whether the patient is breathing by placing your ear over the patient's mouth and nose, listening for air movement, and looking for chest wall movement (**Figure 20–5**). However, a major change has been made to the 2010 CPR Guidelines in which the "look, listen, and feel" technique is removed from the algorithm. If the patient is breathing, place the patient in the recovery position and monitor (**Figure 20–6**).

After 30 chest compressions and opening the airway, emergency ventilation should be performed for patients with agonal breathing or apnea. Provide two breaths lasting no more than 1 second each using either the mouth-to-mouth, mouth-to-mask, mouth-to-stoma, or bag-to-mask method to deliver enough air to cause a rise of the patient's chest (**Figure 20–7** and **Figure 20–8**). If the first breath does not achieve chest rise, reposition the airway and attempt to deliver a second breath. Usually tidal volumes of 6 to 7 mL/kg are sufficient for normal oxygenation and ventilation during CPR.[15] Because cardiac output is reduced to about 25% to 33% of normal, there is a reduced uptake of oxygen from the lungs and reduced delivery of carbon dioxide to the lungs.[13] The emphasis of the 2005 AHA guidelines is that the volume delivered during a breath should be

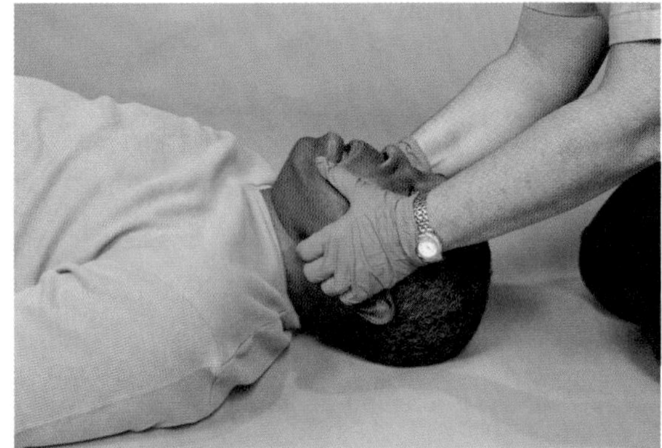

FIGURE 20–3 Jaw-thrust maneuver.

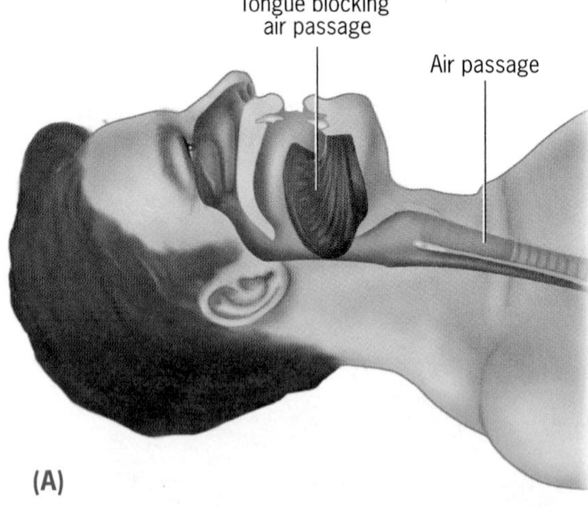

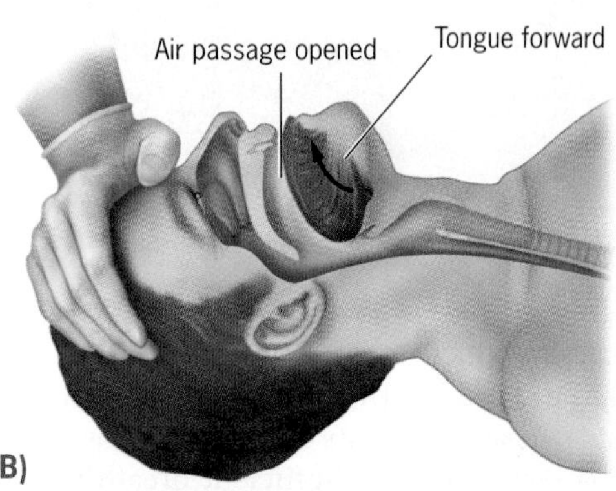

FIGURE 20–4 (**A**) Obstruction of upper airway by the tongue in an unconscious patient. (**B**) Opening the airway by tilting the head backward.

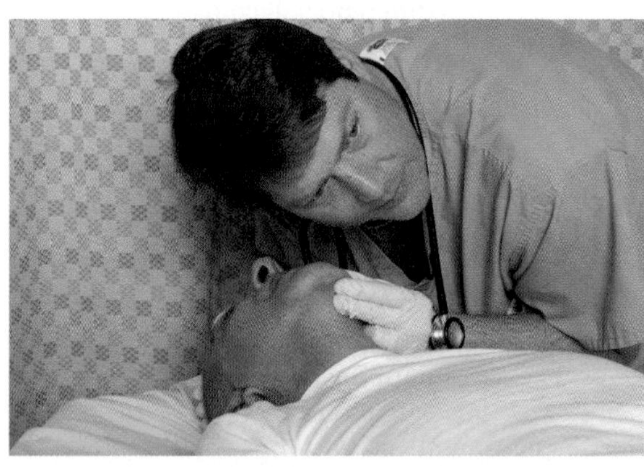

FIGURE 20–5 Opening the airway and checking for apnea.

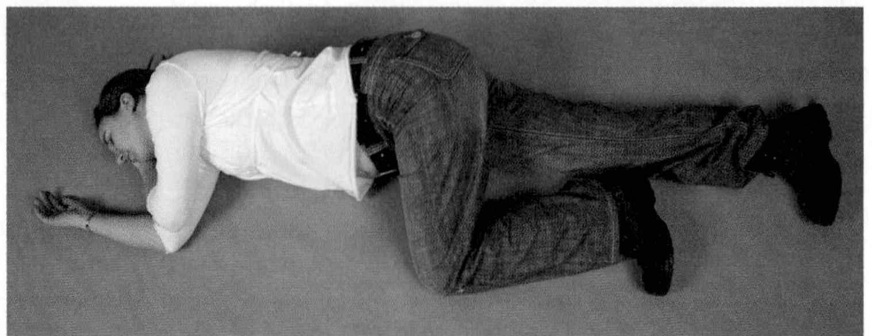

FIGURE 20–6 Recovery position.

just enough to produce visible rise and fall of the chest. The 2010 AHA guidelines emphasize chest compressions rather than ventilation. The 2010 guidelines not only recommend avoiding excessive ventilation but also beginning CPR with 30 chest compressions followed by 2 ventilations.

With delivery of the breaths too quickly or with too much force, it is likely that air will enter the stomach rather than the lungs and cause gastric inflation to occur.[16] Gastric inflation is the result of a breath that is too large, resulting in an airway pressure that exceeds the esophageal opening pressure and allowing air to enter the stomach.[17] This can result in serious complications such as vomiting, aspiration, and the later development of pneumonia.

Mouth-to-mouth breathing is done by the rescuer holding the patient's mouth open with one hand, pinching the nose with the other hand, taking in a breath, placing his or her mouth over the patient's mouth to make a seal, and blowing air directly into the patient's mouth to cause a chest rise.[18] When necessary, the rescuer can modify the delivery of breaths by doing mouth-to-nose or mouth-to-stoma breaths. Mouth-to-nose ventilation is necessary when it becomes impossible to ventilate through the patient's mouth in situations in which the mouth cannot be sealed or opened or the mouth is injured. To perform mouth-to-nose ventilation, the mouth is closed with the hand that normally maintains the jaw thrust; then the rescuer makes a seal with his or her mouth over the patient's nose and blows air into the nose while watching for a chest rise. In patients with a tracheal stoma, mouth-to-stoma ventilation is provided using a seal made over the stoma to inflate the lungs. With mouth-to-mouth, mouth-to-nose, or mouth-to-stoma ventilation, after the delivery of a breath, the rescuer quickly removes his or her mouth from the patient's airway to allow the patient to exhale and the rescuer to inhale another breath. The most common cause of difficulty providing ventilation for an apneic patient is an improperly opened or an occluded airway.[19]

> **RESPIRATORY RECAP**
>
> **Primary Breathing Management During CPR**
> - Mouth to mouth, mouth to nose, mouth to stoma
> - Face shield
> - Mouth to mask
> - Bag-valve-mask ventilation
> - Tidal volume 6 to 7 mL/kg
> - Slow inflation

The risk of infection from CPR is very low, but the Occupational Safety and Health Administration (OSHA) requires that all healthcare workers use standard precautions in the workplace anytime there is

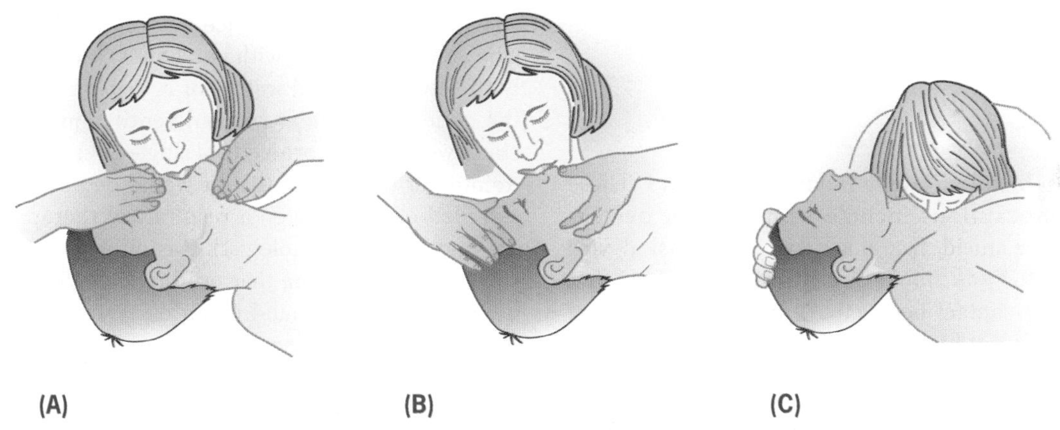

FIGURE 20–7 **(A)** Mouth-to-mouth ventilation. **(B)** Mouth-to-nose ventilation. **(C)** Mouth-to-stoma ventilation.

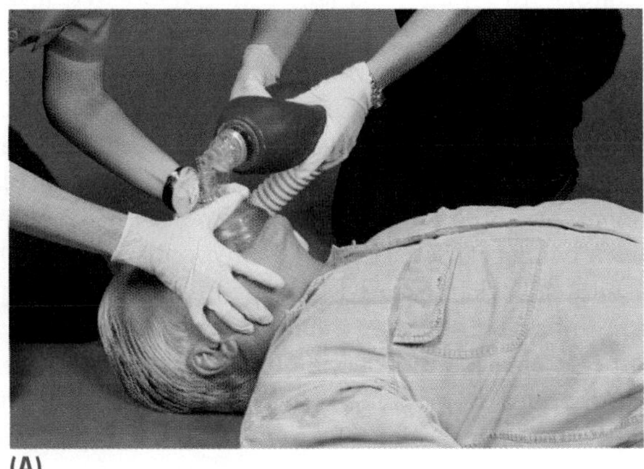

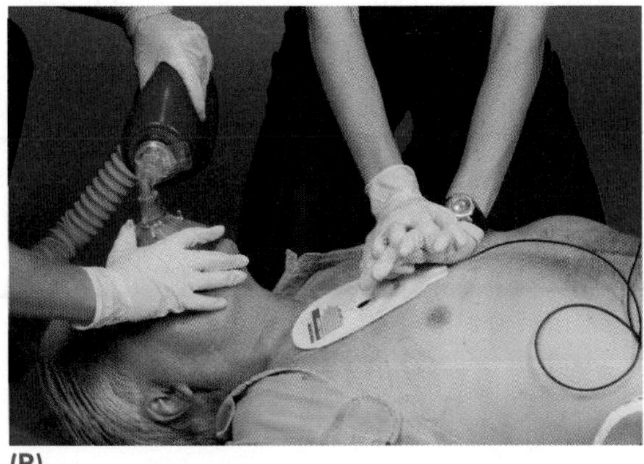

FIGURE 20–8 **(A)** Two-person bag-mask ventilation. **(B)** One-person bag-mask ventilation.

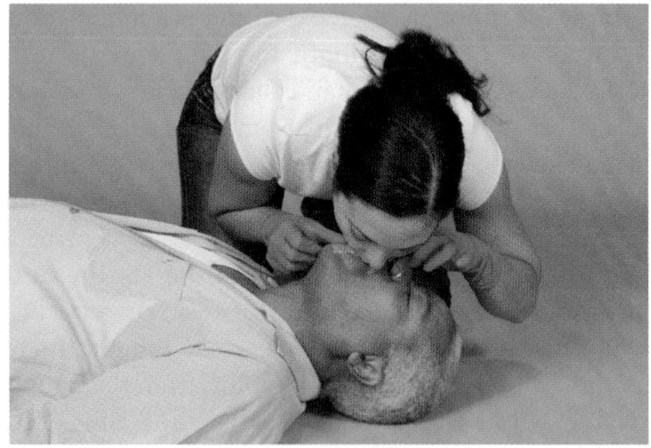

(A)

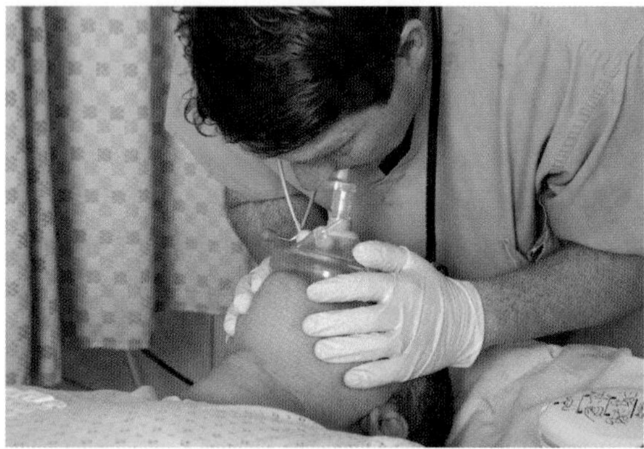

(B)

FIGURE 20–9 Barrier devices. (**A**) Face shield with duckbill valve. (**B**) Mouth-to-mask ventilation device.

exposure to blood or bodily fluids (e.g., saliva).[20] These standard precautions include using barrier devices such as a face shield, face mask, or a bag-mask device (**Figure 20-9**). **Face shields** are clear plastic sheets that reduce direct contact between the patient and the rescuer.[18] They do not prevent contamination of the rescuer if used incorrectly and may increase the resistance to air flow.[21–23] The rescuer should use a face mask or bag-mask ventilation as soon as possible.[24]

Mouth-to-mask devices are very effective for delivering adequate ventilation. These masks have a one-way valve that diverts the patient's exhaled air away from the rescuer's face. Some of these masks have an oxygen inlet that allows the use of supplemental oxygen. To use the mask, the rescuer is positioned at the patient's head and to the side, the airway is opened, and the mask is placed over the patient's nose and mouth using the bridge of the patient's nose as a guide. The mask is held in place using the thumbs and first fingers of each hand on top of the mask pressing firmly around the outside of the mask against the patient's face to create a seal, while the remaining fingers lift the jaw up and into the mask as the head is tilted back. The exhaled gas of the individual doing rescue breathing contains approximately 17% oxygen and 4% carbon dioxide. Mouth-to-mask or mouth-to-mouth breathing is a quick and effective way to provide sufficient oxygen to the patient for a short time until a manual resuscitator and mask can be provided.[18]

Manual resuscitators (bag-mask devices) consist of a self-inflating bag, a nonjamming air intake valve, a nonrebreathing valve, an oxygen inlet nipple, and an oxygen reservoir (**Figure 20–10**). A variety of manufacturers produce disposable manual resuscitator bags capable of ventilating patients during CPR. They are designed so that one end of the nonrebreathing valve connects to the self-inflating bag and the other end is connected to the face mask.[24] The masks should be made of a transparent material to allow the rescuer to detect whether the patient regurgitates into the mask. When the bag is compressed, the nonrebreathing valve directs gas from the bag through the mask and to the patient. When the bag is released, the exhaled gas is directed through the exhalation port, and at the same time the bag reinflates. During a cardiac arrest, it is important to administer the highest oxygen concentration possible. When supplemental oxygen is available, the devices provide a minimum oxygen flow rate of 10 to 12 L/min.

One rescuer providing manual ventilation by bag-valve-mask device may not provide adequate tidal volumes. This is improved when ventilation is performed by two persons simultaneously: one who opens the airway and holds the mask in place with two hands and one who squeezes the bag with two hands (see Figure 20–8). Both rescuers should watch for a visible rise and fall of the patient's chest.[25,26] Manual ventilation may be less effective when performed by a single operator with little training or experience than it would be in the hands of a skilled clinician (e.g., a respiratory therapist, nurse anesthetist, anesthesiologist). It is difficult to deliver an adequate tidal volume that produces a sufficient rise of the chest with one hand compressing the bag and the other hand holding the airway open and creating a seal with the mask.

The use of a bag-valve device to provide oxygen for a spontaneously breathing patient is discouraged because of the increased effort required to breathe through the nonrebreathing valve of a self-inflating manual resuscitator.[27] In an adult patient with a depressed level of consciousness (i.e., with no cough or gag reflex), a Sellick maneuver should be performed during ventilation with a manual resuscitator bag if gastric inflation is suspected (**Figure 20–11**).[28] To perform the Sellick maneuver, a second person applies pressure to the cricoid cartilage to compress the esophagus and prevent gastric contents from being regurgitated into the hypopharynx and then aspirated back into the trachea. Because cricord pressure can impede ventilation, the routine use of cricord pressure is not recommended in the 2010 AHA guidelines.

Opening the patient's airway and delivering the two initial breaths should take between 5 and 10 seconds.

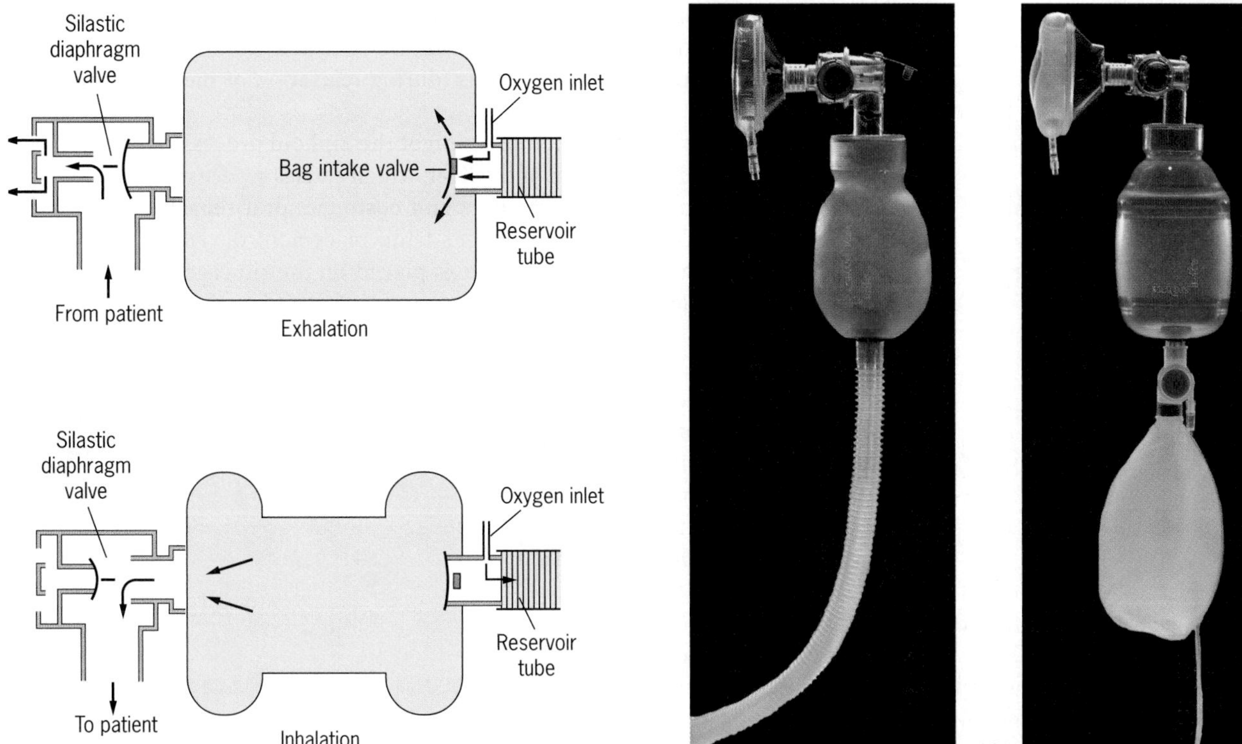

FIGURE 20–10 (**A**) Manual resuscitator with gas intake located at the bottom of the bag. (**B**) Manual resuscitator with tube reservoir. (**C**) Manual resuscitator with bag reservoir. (**A**) This article was published in *Respiratory Therapy Equipment, Fourth Edition*. McPherson SP. Copyright Elsevier (Mosby) 1990.

According to the 2005 AHA guidelines, when adequate ventilation and chest rise can be accomplished using mouth-to-mask or bag-mask ventilation, early placement of an endotracheal tube is not as important as providing compressions for circulation when necessary.[16]

Circulation

The presence of a heartbeat is determined by palpation of the carotid artery on the side of the neck nearest to the rescuer (**Figure 20–12**). The rescuer should take no more than 10 seconds to do this. If a pulse is not present, or if it is uncertain, immediately administer 30 chest compressions.[29] According to the AHA, providing unnecessary compressions is less harmful than not performing them when a patient truly needs them.[2] If the patient is on a soft surface, a firm surface should be placed under the patient. However, compressions should not be withheld while waiting for a firm surface. Move a sitting patient to a flat surface as safely and quickly as possible before beginning compressions.

Chest compressions are the rhythmic application of pressure on the lower half of the sternum to facilitate blood flow by compressing the heart. When performed properly they produce a low arterial blood flow, which delivers critically needed oxygen to the brain and myocardium.[30] Several studies have reported that healthcare

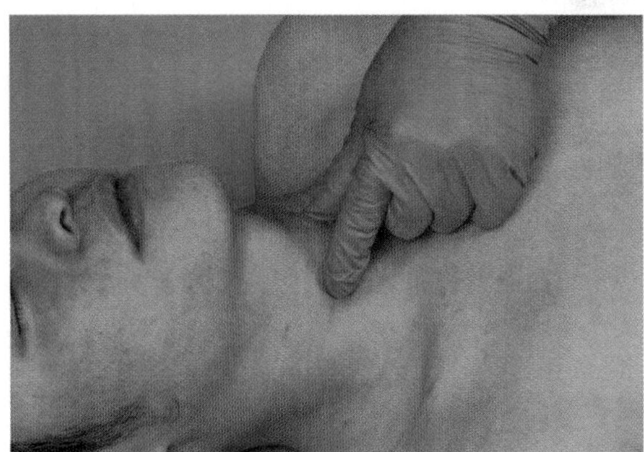

FIGURE 20–11 Sellick maneuver.

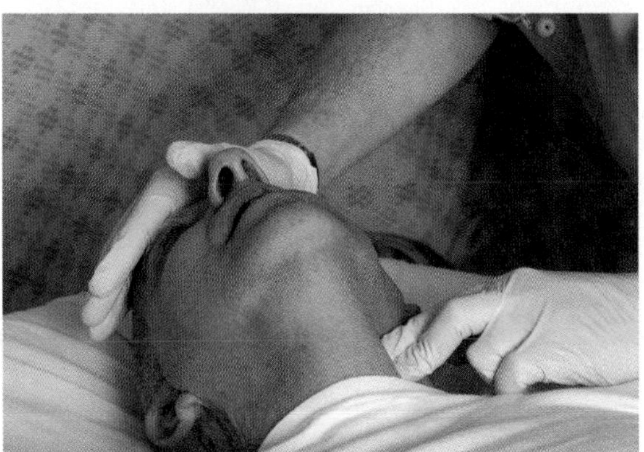

FIGURE 20–12 Carotid pulse check.

providers did not provide an adequate number or depth of compressions. The same studies reported that ventilation was excessive after the patient's airway was secured. The combination of inadequate compressions, interruptions in compressions for ventilation, and excessive ventilation rates resulted in lower than expected blood flow to vital organs.[31–33] Due to the importance of chest compressions, lay rescuers are encouraged to perform compressions-only CPR.

RESPIRATORY RECAP

Primary Circulation Management During CPR

- » Press hard and fast.
- » Compress over the lower half of the sternum.
- » Do not interrupt chest compression.
- » Use a compression-to-ventilation ratio of 30:2.
- » Defibrillate as soon as possible if indicated.

The 2005 and 2010 Consensus Conferences promulgated the following guidelines regarding chest compressions.[2,3] External chest compressions are performed on the lower half of the adult sternum, above the notch where the ribs meet the lower sternum or between the nipples (**Figure 20–13**). The heel of the first hand is placed on the lower half of the sternum, with the second hand on top of the hand on the sternum. The fingers are extended or interlaced to keep them up and off the chest. The rescuer's arms are kept straight, with the elbows locked and the shoulders of the rescuer directly over the patient's sternum. Pressure is exerted downward to depress the sternum at least 2 inches (5 cm) at a rate of at least 100 per minute (**Figure 20–14**). The rescuer's hands should not be removed from the chest between compressions (during relaxation of the heart and recoil of the chest).

Compression of the xiphoid process can cause laceration of the liver, which causes severe internal bleeding. Rib fractures and costochondral separation can occur if the rescuer's hand placement deviates from midline or if pressure is placed on the rib cage with the fingers during compressions. The broken ends of a rib can in

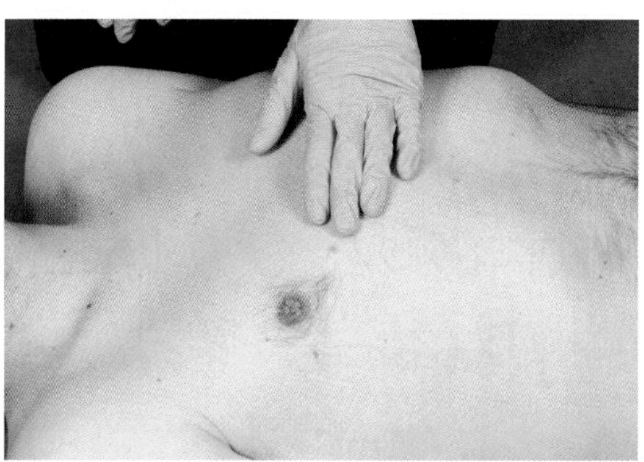

FIGURE 20–13 Identifying proper hand position for chest compressions. Chest compressions are performed on the lower half of the sternum, above the notch where the ribs meet the lower sternum or between the nipples.

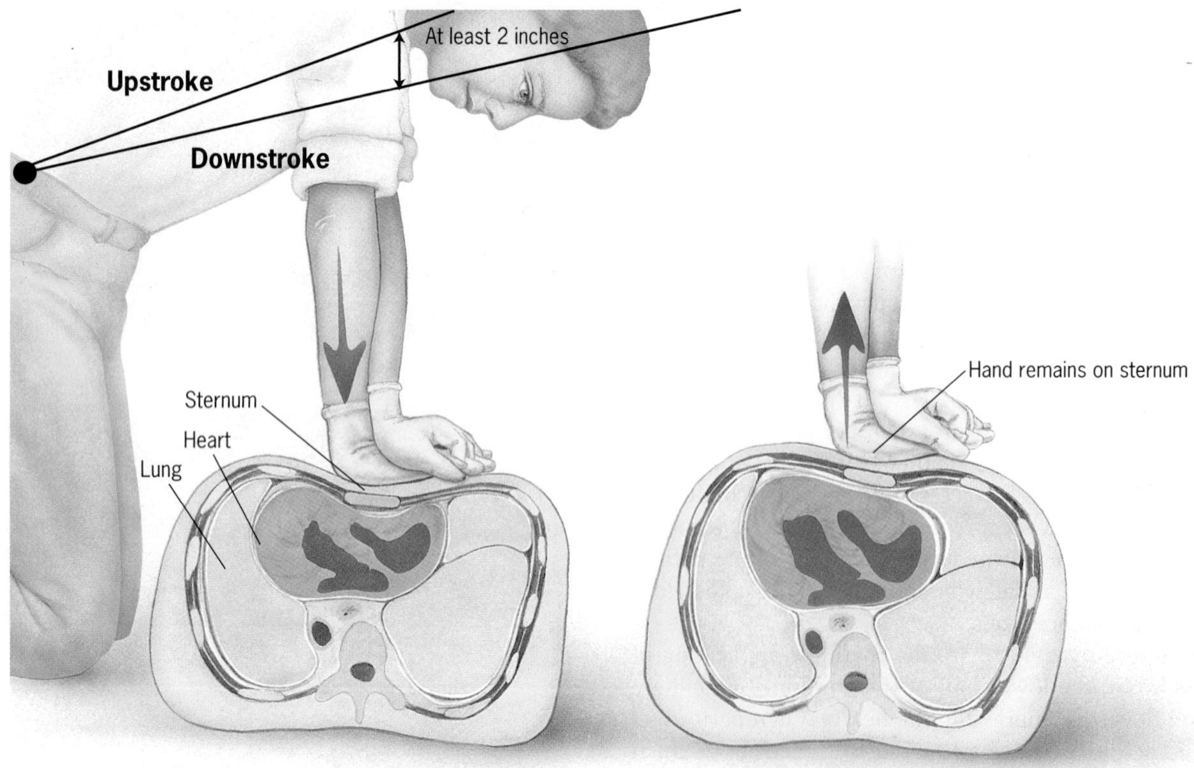

FIGURE 20–14 Body position for chest compressions. The hands remain on the sternum but allow complete chest recoil between compressions.

turn cause lacerations of the lungs. Elderly patients, patients on chronic steroids, or patients with calcium deficiencies are the most susceptible to these injuries. If cracking of the ribs is felt or heard, the rescuer doing compressions should check his or her hand position, make corrections if necessary, and continue to compress as quickly as possible. Another complication of closed chest compression is the formation of fat emboli, which may occur without evidence of overt fractures. Compressing bones such as the rib cage and sternum may lead to microfractures within the medulla of the ribs and sternum and an increase in marrow pressure. Fat may enter the venous circulation from the marrow. Cerebral fat emboli can cause mental deterioration after successful resuscitation of a patient who has suffered an arrest.[33]

When doing chest compressions at a rate of at least 100 per minute, it is important to press hard and fast and then to quickly take your weight off your arms after each compression. This relieves the pressure on the chest wall, allowing it to recoil and the heart to refill with blood before the next compression.[34,35] The effectiveness of chest compressions should be evaluated by a second person who palpates the carotid or femoral arteries for a pulse. Studies have shown that in the absence of an arterial pulse the second rescuer may palpate a venous pulse during CPR.[36] The evidence suggests that blood flow is optimal when the recommended chest compression force is used and a compression rate of at least 100 compressions per minute is maintained.

Resuscitators should make every effort to minimize interruptions in chest compressions. If interruptions are necessary (e.g., for intubation, defibrillation, moving the patient), they should be limited to less than 10 seconds when possible. Remember, there is no blood flow to the brain and heart when a rescuer is not performing compressions. The rescuer should perform five cycles of compressions and ventilations (30 compressions to two breaths) until the defibrillator arrives and is attached to the patient. If the rescuer is alone, CPR can be interrupted to get the automated external defibrillator.

Automated External Defibrillation

There is a strong relationship between the speed with which defibrillation is administered and the survival of patients requiring defibrillation. The length of time from which a patient collapses to the time he or she is electrically defibrillated is one of the most important determinants of survival from cardiac arrest for the following reasons. When a patient has a witnessed sudden cardiac arrest, the most common initial rhythm is ventricular fibrillation.[37] When the heart is in VF it physically quivers and does not pump blood to the other vital organs of the body. The most effective treatment for VF is to deliver an electrical shock to the heart (electrical defibrillation) to momentarily stop the heart and allow it to regain a more normal pacing. The electrical current is passed through the heart in an attempt to eliminate the chaotic asynchronous activity of the heart that causes the ventricular fibrillation. If the defibrillation is successful, the cardiac cells will depolarize and then repolarize in a uniform manner with the resumption of a more coordinated cardiac contraction. If VF is not treated quickly or the defibrillation is not successful, the heart's electrical rhythm quickly deteriorates to asystole.[37] Providing good CPR until electrical defibrillation can be done improves the patient's chances for survival from ventricular fibrillation and cardiac arrest.[38]

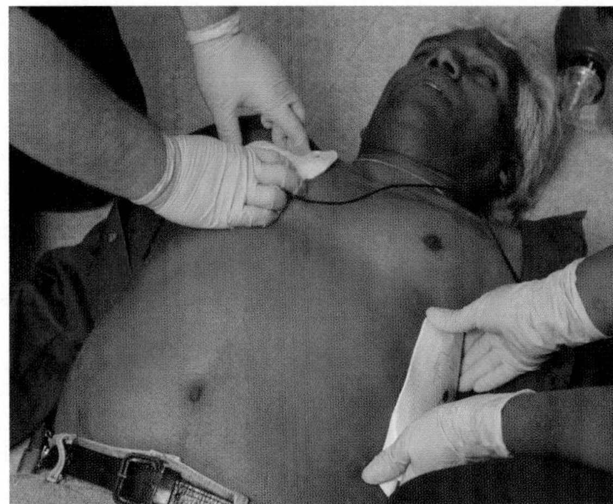

FIGURE 20–15 Pad placement for automated external defibrillation.

The **automated external defibrillator (AED)** is a computerized device that is attached to a breathless, pulseless patient's chest with adhesive pads and delivers an electrical shock to the patient's heart if the computer recognizes a heart rhythm that can be treated with electricity (**Figure 20–15**). The defibrillator then incorporates the rhythm recognition and analysis function with either fully automated or semiautomated shock delivery. When using the AED, it is useful to remember the mnemonic P-A-I-D:

Power on: The first step is to turn on the power. This will usually activate voice prompts for all subsequent steps. With some of the newer AEDs the power will automatically come on when the case or lid is opened.

Attach leads: The first voice prompt is to attach the leads. Choose the correct-size electrode pads (child or adult) for the patient and peel the protective backing from the pads. Quickly wipe the patient's chest if it is wet with water or sweat, attach one electrode pad to the patient's upper-right chest in the area to the right of the sternum and just below the collarbone, and attach the second electrode pad on the left of the nipple and just below the left armpit.

Interpret/analyze: The second voice prompt indicates the beginning of the analysis of the patient's cardiac rhythm. This instructs you to make sure no one is touching or moving the patient, allowing the AED's internal computer to analyze the patient's cardiac rhythm without the interference of chest compressions or ventilation by rescuers. The analysis process will usually take 5 to 15 seconds; afterward, the AED's third voice prompt will instruct you whether analysis of the patient's cardiac rhythm indicates that a shock is indicated.

Defibrillate: If the AED advises that a shock is indicated, the next prompt will be for you to make sure the patient is "clear" to avoid injury to yourself and other rescuers. You should loudly state "clear" and visually check to ensure that others are not touching or manually bagging the patient before you press the Shock button. Immediately after the shock produces a sudden contraction of the patient's skeletal muscles, the rescuers should restart chest compressions.[39,40] After a period of 2 minutes (five sets of 30 compressions and two breaths), the AED should be used to reanalyze the patient to determine whether subsequent shocks are indicated.

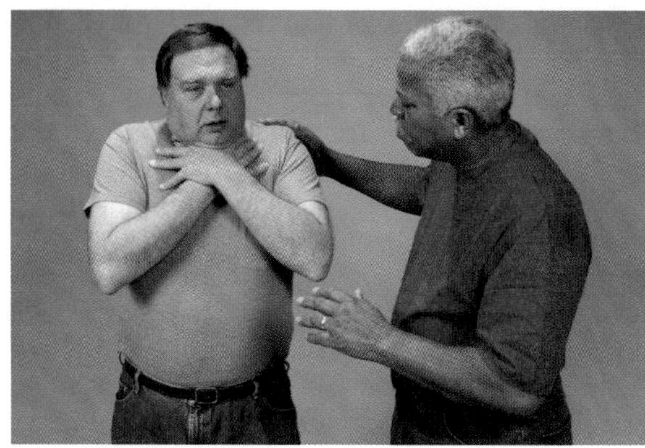

FIGURE 20–16 Universal choking sign.

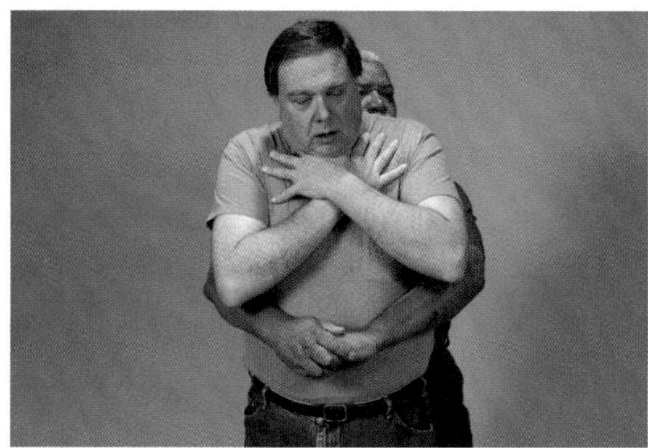

FIGURE 20–17 Heimlich maneuver.

Relief for a Choking Adult

Aspiration of a foreign body can cause mild, severe, or total airway obstruction, which results in a patient's inability to breathe and eventually in death if not quickly alleviated. This is an uncommon but preventable cause of death.[41] The key to helping a choking adult patient is early recognition of airway obstruction and taking quick steps to correct the patient's situation. The signs and symptoms of choking include inability to breathe, poor or ineffective air exchange, a high-pitched sound while the patient is inhaling or the patient being unable to make any sounds or speak, possible cyanosis, and the universal sign of choking, in which patients use their own hands to clutch their neck (**Figure 20–16**).

If patients are choking, their own coughing is the most effective way for their airway to be cleared. If they are coughing, allow them to continue. If their coughing is weak or ineffective, however, the rescuer can assist the patient using the Heimlich maneuver (abdominal thrust) on adults and children. To successfully relieve an airway obstruction may require the rescuer to repeat the Heimlich maneuver several times. Performing the abdominal thrust improperly or with too much force can result in damage to internal organs. It has been reported that approximately 50% of all choking episodes caused by airway obstruction were not relieved by a single abdominal thrust, and that the likelihood of success was increased when a combination of back blows, abdominal thrusts, and chest thrusts were used.[41] It is important to assess for possible damage to the patient if any of these methods have been used to relieve the airway obstruction.

> **RESPIRATORY RECAP**
>
> **Choking Adult**
>
> » Coughing is the most effective way to clear the airway.
>
> » Heimlich maneuvers are used on adults and children.
>
> » Do not perform blind sweeps of the airway.

To perform the Heimlich maneuver, the rescuer should stand behind the adult patient and wrap his or her arms around the patient's waist, making a fist with one hand and placing the thumb side of the fist against the patient's middle abdomen slightly above the navel but well below the breastbone, then grasp the fist with the other hand and, using a quick upward thrust, press their fists into the patient's abdomen and quickly release the pressure (**Figure 20–17**). This is repeated until the object is expelled from the airway or the patient becomes unresponsive. The possibility that a cardiac arrest or unresponsiveness will be caused by an unsuspected foreign body airway obstruction is very low.[42] However, if the patient's airway cannot be cleared and the patient becomes unconscious and unresponsive, the rescuer should support the patient to the ground (**Figure 20–18**).

If the patient becomes unresponsive or is found unresponsive, the rescuer should activate his or her

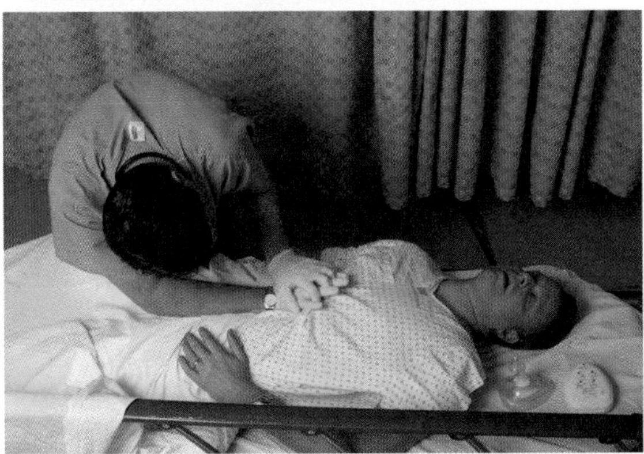

FIGURE 20–18 Abdominal thrust for foreign body airway obstruction.

emergency response system, open the airway, and, if the obstruction is seen in the oropharynx, remove it and begin basic life support. Each time the rescuer provides a breath for the patient, the rescuer should open the patient's mouth, look to see whether the obstruction is now visible, and if possible remove it. Remember, if the airway is blocked, the breaths will not enter the lungs or cause a rise and fall of the chest. In the past, guidelines have recommended using a blind finger sweep for relieving airway obstructions. Case study reports have reported harm to the patient[43,44] or rescuer with blind sweeps, so they are no longer done.[14,45]

Cardiopulmonary Resuscitation for a Child

The major causes of pediatric cardiopulmonary arrest are often respiratory failure, sudden infant death syndrome (SIDS), sepsis, neurologic diseases, and trauma.[46] Attempts to prevent injury can reduce childhood death and disability, especially when prevention strategies are geared toward the six most common types of severe childhood injuries: motor vehicle passenger injuries, pedestrian injuries, bicycle injuries, submersion injuries, fire- and burn-related injuries, and firearm injuries.[47] Even after 20 years of educational efforts to prevent such injuries, studies found that when compared with white children, American Indian/Alaskan Native and African American children consistently have a higher rate of injury deaths. Hispanic children have comparable rates of injury-related deaths, and Asian/Pacific Islanders have a significantly lower rate of death than white children.[48]

> **RESPIRATORY RECAP**
>
> **Child CPR**
>
> » Begin CPR with pulse below 60 beats/min
> » Compression-to-breath ratio of 30 compressions to two breaths for one rescuer and 15 compressions to two breaths for two rescuers
> » Chest compressions at midsternum between the nipples
> » Fast and hard compressions

The authors of the 2005 AHA and ECC guidelines made a consensus decision regarding age delineation for the ease of teaching and practicing BLS and ACLS. Because there is no one anatomic or physiologic characteristic that distinguishes a child from an adult, patients from 1 year of age to the onset of puberty (about 12 to 14 years of age) are considered children. The resuscitation guideline for patients does not come in a one-size-fits-all model, although there are both basic similarities and major differences between the method of BLS for an adult, child, or infant. The main differences are the rate of compressions and the use of defibrillation for specific groups.

When resuscitating a child, just as with an adult, the rescuer begins with a quick assessment of the child for responsiveness. If the patient is found to be unresponsive, the rescuer should activate the emergency system, call for an AED, and then check for breathing. If apneic, the next step is to perform 30 chest compressions, followed by two ventilations. The sequence should be CABD. "Look, listen, and feel for breathing" was removed in the 2010 guidelines.

The rescuer should then check for the pulse for less than 10 seconds (same as adult), at the carotid or femoral arteries. In the 2010 guidelines, however, there is de-emphasis of the pulse check. Chest compressions are performed at midsternum between the nipples at a depth of one-third of the anterior-posterior diameter of the chest; about 2 inches (5 cm) in most children. The compression-to-breath ratio for a child is 30 compressions to two breaths if there is only one rescuer and 15 compression to two breaths if there are two rescuers.[1] When doing the compressions, the rescuer should push fast and hard, making sure that any interruptions, including those for the two breaths, are kept shorter than 10 seconds.

> **AGE-SPECIFIC ANGLE**
>
> Most cardiac arrests in children are *not* caused by ventricular arrhythmias.

Most cardiac arrests in children are *not* caused by ventricular arrhythmias. The time necessary for using an AED (attaching the leads to the patients and analyzing the rhythm) delays or interrupts the vitally important rescue breathing and chest compressions.[49] If the child's arrest occurs outside of the hospital or is unwitnessed, the AED should be placed on the child after rescuers have completed five cycles of 15 compressions and two breaths, which should take about 2 minutes. However, if the child's arrest occurs inside a hospital or is witnessed, the AED should be placed on the child as soon as available and used appropriately for the child.

If the AED is designed for both adults and children, change to the appropriate adult or child shock dose. When the child is younger than 8 years, the rescuer should use electrode pads designated for children and select the appropriate child shock dose. However, if the child is older than 8 years, this shock may not be sufficient for the desired effect.[49] For children older than

8 years, the rescuer should use the adult shock dose and the adult electrode pads.[49] If a shock is indicated, immediately after the shock is delivered the rescuers should begin chest compressions for 2 minutes and then recheck for a pulse.

Relief for a Choking Child

The most common causes of a child choking are balloons, small objects, and food such as hot dogs, round candies, nuts, and grapes.[50] The treatment for a child older than 1 year who is choking is similar to that for an adult. While evaluating the child, the rescuers should try to determine whether the obstruction is mild or severe.

AGE-SPECIFIC ANGLE

The treatment for a child older than 1 year who is choking is similar to that for an adult.

The signs of mild **foreign body obstruction (FBO)** include a sudden onset of respiratory distress associated with coughing, stridor, or unilateral wheezing. When possible, the rescuer should allow the child to clear his or her own airway by coughing. However, the patient with severe obstruction may not be able to cough or make sounds. In this situation it is imperative that rescuers be able to recognize the difference and be prepared to intervene if necessary. Subdiaphragmatic abdominal thrusts (Heimlich maneuvers) are recommended for relief of airway obstruction in children. The sequence of intervention used to treat a child with an obstructed airway is similar to that for an adult.[51,52] When abdominal thrusts are delivered to a child who is unconscious or who becomes unconscious, the heel of one hand is used rather than a two-handed fist.

The exception to use of the Heimlich maneuver is a situation in which the rescuer is alone and the child becomes unresponsive. If this should occur, the rescuer should open the airway and remove the object if it is seen. If the object cannot be removed from the airway, or if the child does not start breathing after the object has been removed, the rescuer should begin basic life support. He or she should then do five cycles of compressions and breaths and activate the emergency response system if the rescuer has not already done so.

Cardiopulmonary Resuscitation for an Infant

Infants and children who develop cardiac arrest usually do so secondary to pulmonary disease or pulmonary arrest. According to the AHA, the term *infant* refers to neonatal patients from the time they leave the delivery room until they are 12 months old. Again, as with the adult or child, first determine whether the infant needs resuscitation, then activate the emergency response system and place the patient on a firm, flat surface.[53] The next step is to perform 30 chest compressions. The sequence should be compressions—airway—breathing. "Look, listen anf feel for breathing" was removed in the 2010 guidelines. Then open the infant's airway using the head tilt–chin lift method, being careful not to press the fingers too deeply into the soft tissue underneath the infant's chin. The most common structure causing airway obstruction for an infant is the tongue, which becomes flaccid and falls backward into the throat. Improper opening of the infant's airway by a rescuer is the most common cause of inadequate ventilation during resuscitation.[54] If the rescuer tilts the infant's head back more than what would resemble a neutral or sniffing position, the infant's airway may become blocked. The rescuer may need to reposition the head several times using the head tilt–chin lift maneuver to deliver two effective breaths.

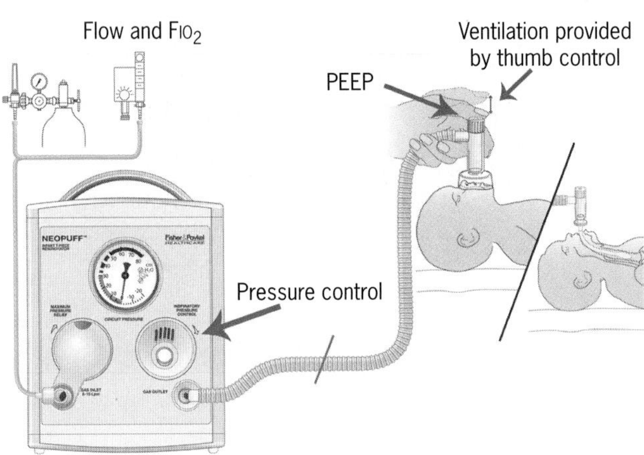

FIGURE 20–19 Neopuff for neonatal resuscitation. Courtesy of Fisher & Paykel Healthcare, Inc.

A bag-mask device or a T-piece resuscitator (Neopuff) can be used to give rescue breaths to an infant. This resuscitator needs a compressed gas source and a tight face mask seal (**Figure 20–19**). Only trained clinical professionals should use the T-piece resuscitator because it is a flow-controlled, pressure-limited manual ventilator.[55] The T-piece resuscitator has six parts: gas inlet, gas outlet, inspiratory pressure control, patient T-piece with positive end-expiratory pressure (PEEP) cap, circuit pressure gauge, and maximum pressure-relief control.[56] Advantages of the T-piece resuscitator include its ability to deliver a consistent pressure and a reliable concentration of 100% oxygen, with no fatigue for rescuers from bagging. Some disadvantages include the need for a readily available compressed gas source, the need for a tight face seal, the time necessary for the rescuers to set pressure prior to use, and the time necessary for changing pressures while the resuscitator is in use. Whenever the T-piece resuscitator is being used, rescuers should make sure a backup self-inflating bag is available.

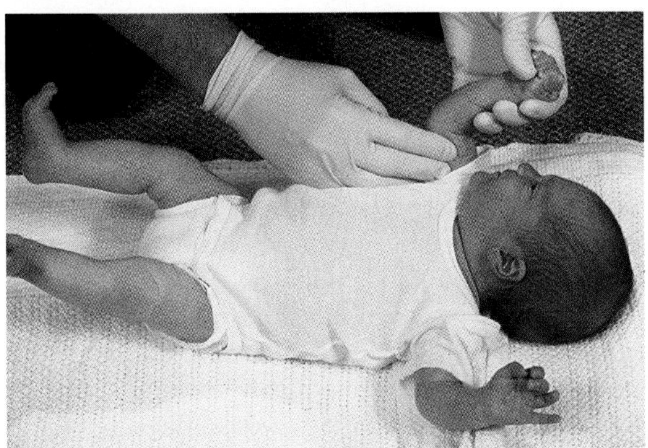

FIGURE 20–20 Brachial pulse check.

When delivering a breath using a bag and mask, it is important that the rescuer take the time to choose the appropriate-sized bag and mask. The face mask should be able to cover the patient's mouth and nose completely without covering the eyes or without extending beyond the infant's chin. The patient's airways should be opened using the head tilt–chin lift maneuver, the mask pressed against the face, making sure to protect the eyes, and the jaw lifted to create a seal. The mask should not be pressed down onto the infant's face to create the seal.

The rescuer should check for the brachial pulse by placing his or her index and middle fingers on the inside of the infant's upper arm (**Figure 20–20**). The size of the neck in an infant younger than 1 year makes palpation of the carotid artery very difficult. In the 2010 guidelines, however, there is de-emphasis of the pulse check. The infant is considered to be in a cardiac arrest if the infant's heart rate is absent or less than 60 beats/min and the infant shows signs of poor perfusion (i.e., cyanosis, pallor) despite oxygenation and ventilation.[1]

The rescuer should perform compressions by placing the tips of two fingers between the nipple line and compressing approximately one-third of the anterior-posterior diameter of the chest.[57,58] An alternative to the two-finger compression technique is the two-thumb compression technique, in which the rescuer encircles the infant's chest with both hands and compresses the chest using his or her thumbs (**Figure 20–21**). The compression-to-breath ratio for an infant is 30 compressions to two breaths if there is only one rescuer and 15 compressions to two breaths if there are two rescuers. It is important for rescuers to keep the tips of their fingers on the infant's chest after each compression and to make sure they release the pressure on the sternum to allow for recoil of the chest. There is no recommendation for use of an AED for an infant younger than 1 year.[49]

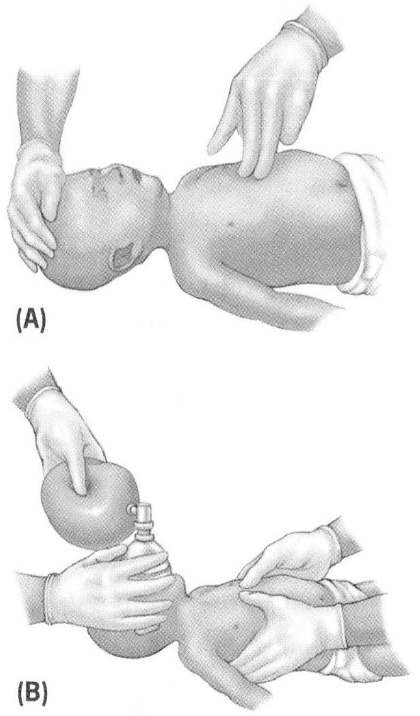

FIGURE 20–21 (**A**) Two-finger chest compressions. (**B**) Two-thumb chest compressions.

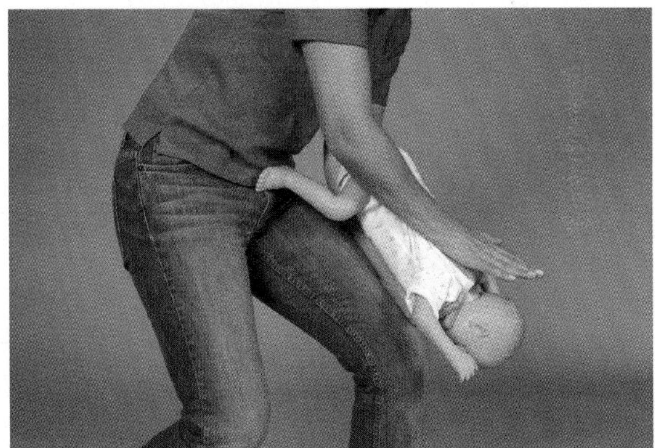

FIGURE 20–22 Back blows in infant foreign body obstruction.

Relief for a Choking Infant

Liquids are the most common cause of an infant choking.[51] The abdominal thrusts used on an adult and child are not used on a choking infant; instead, rescuers use a series of back slaps and chest thrusts (**Figure 20–22**). If the infant is responsive, the rescuer should kneel or sit with the infant in his or her lap and then place the infant in a prone position with the head slightly lower than the chest resting on the rescuer's forearm and hand, while being careful not to compress the soft tissues of the infant's throat. The rescuer should provide five forceful back blows using the heel of his or her hand to the middle of the infant's back in the area located between the infant's shoulder blades. If this does not dislodge the obstruction, the rescuer should place his or her free hand under the infant's back and neck, using the palm to support the head, and turn the infant onto his or her back, keeping the head slightly lower than the trunk, and then provide five quick downward chest thrusts to the same area as used for compressions. Rescuers should provide sequences of five back slaps followed by five chest thrusts until the object is removed or the infant becomes unresponsive.

If the obstruction cannot be removed using back blows and chest thrusts and the infant becomes unresponsive, rescuers should begin basic life support. Because the chest compressions may have dislodged the obstruction, rescuers should open the infant's airway and look for the object each time they open the airway to deliver a breath. If they see an object, they should remove it before breath delivery. If the emergency response system has not been activated, the rescuer should do so after five cycles of breaths to compressions (approximately 2 minutes).

Summary of Basic Life Support

Basic life support and cardiopulmonary resuscitation include the primary management of airway breathing and circulation during the resuscitative effort for an adult, child, or infant patient (**Table 20–1**). Respiratory therapists' knowledge of guidelines and good assessment skills make them an ideal part of most hospital resuscitation teams. After a patient succumbs to a cardiopulmonary arrest, the most important determinant of the patient's survival is the presence of a trained rescuer who is ready, willing, and able to do basic life support. The 2010 American Heart Association recommendations are simple guidelines that will not apply to all patients in all situations. Members of resuscitation teams must use their knowledge, experience, and skills to adapt these guidelines to each patient's unique situation. Basic life support is usually followed by advanced cardiovascular life support. Together they provide a comprehensive outline that can be followed by teams during highly stressful events such as a patient's cardiopulmonary arrest and resuscitation.

Advanced Cardiovascular Life Support

Most respiratory therapists now are required to become certified in ACLS as part of their work. However, BLS is still the foundation for all ACLS algorithms, and nothing in ACLS is as important as maintaining good BLS throughout the resuscitation. Typically, ACLS skills include recognition of the cardiac rhythm and determining which algorithm should be followed, insertion and management of advanced airways, insertion of intravenous or intraosseous lines,

TABLE 20–1 Comparison of Basic Life Support Techniques for Adults, Children, and Infants

Maneuver	Adolescent and Older	1 Year to Adolescent	Infant Younger Than 1 Year
Pulse check (≤ 10 seconds)	Carotid	Carotid	Brachial or femoral
Compression landmarks	Lower half of sternum, between nipples	Lower half of sternum, between nipples	Just below nipple line (lower half of sternum)
Compression method (push hard and fast; allow complete recoil)	Heel of one hand, other hand on top, fingers interlaced	Heel of one hand or as for adults	Two or three fingers, or two thumbs with hands encircling the infant's chest
Compression depth	At least 2 inches	Approximately one-third the depth of the chest	
Compression rate	At least 100/minute		
Compression-to-ventilation ratio	30:2 (one or two rescuers)	30:2 (single rescuer); 15:2 (two rescuers)	
Airway	Head tilt–chin lift (with suspected spinal trauma, use jaw thrust)		
Breathing			
Initial	2 breaths at 1 second/breath		
With advanced airway	8 to 10 breaths/minute (approximately)		
Foreign body airway obstruction	Abdominal thrusts	Abdominal thrusts	Back slaps and chest thrusts
Defibrillation			
AED	Use adult pads; do not use child pads	Use AED after five cycles of CPR (out of hospital)	Not recommended

CPR, cardiopulmonary resuscitation; AED, automated external defibrillator. *Note*: The correct sequence is compressions—airway—breathing.

> **RESPIRATORY RECAP**
>
> **Advanced Life Support**
>
> » Use of airway and ventilation equipment
> » ECG monitoring
> » Insertion of intravenous lines
> » Drug therapy

knowledge of cardiac pharmacology, and the ability to make a differential diagnosis to determine and reverse the cause of cardiopulmonary arrest. Four different cardiac rhythms can produce a pulseless cardiac arrest: ventricular fibrillation, pulseless rapid ventricular tachycardia (VT), pulseless electrical activity (PEA), and asystole (**Algorithm 20–2**, **Algorithm 20–3**, to **Algorithm 20–4**). **Table 20–2** lists drugs commonly administered during CPR.

Airway Management

Although the most recent recommendations for cardiopulmonary resuscitation place a greater emphasis on chest compressions, successful management of the airway, oxygenation, and ventilation is still an important part of the resuscitation process. It is important for all respiratory therapists to be trained and skilled in airway management. Because the placement of advanced airways requires an interruption in chest compressions, the skills necessary to manage the airway using less invasive methods have gained importance given the 2005 AHA guidelines. The rescuer's use of effective bag-mask ventilation during the first few minutes of resuscitation will facilitate uninterrupted chest compressions and defibrillation until an advanced airway is placed.

The rescuer should open the airway using a chin lift or jaw thrust, insert a nasopharyngeal or oropharyngeal airway if necessary, and deliver two breaths using a volume of ventilation that is sufficient to produce a chest rise (approximately 6 to 7 mL/kg, or 500 to 600 mL).[59] Each breath is delivered during a very brief pause in compressions and takes less than 1 second. If not used appropriately, bag-valve ventilation can result in air trapping. Patients with obstructive lung disease are very susceptible to this problem because of their increased airway resistance. This can further reduce cardiac output. If the patient develops hypotension during bag-valve ventilation, ventilation should be stopped for 20 to 30 seconds. If blood pressure is restored during this period of apnea, it suggests the presence of air trapping, and ventilation should be resumed less aggressively. To prevent air trapping, rescuers should deliver a slow respiratory rate (6 to 8 breaths/min), which allows more

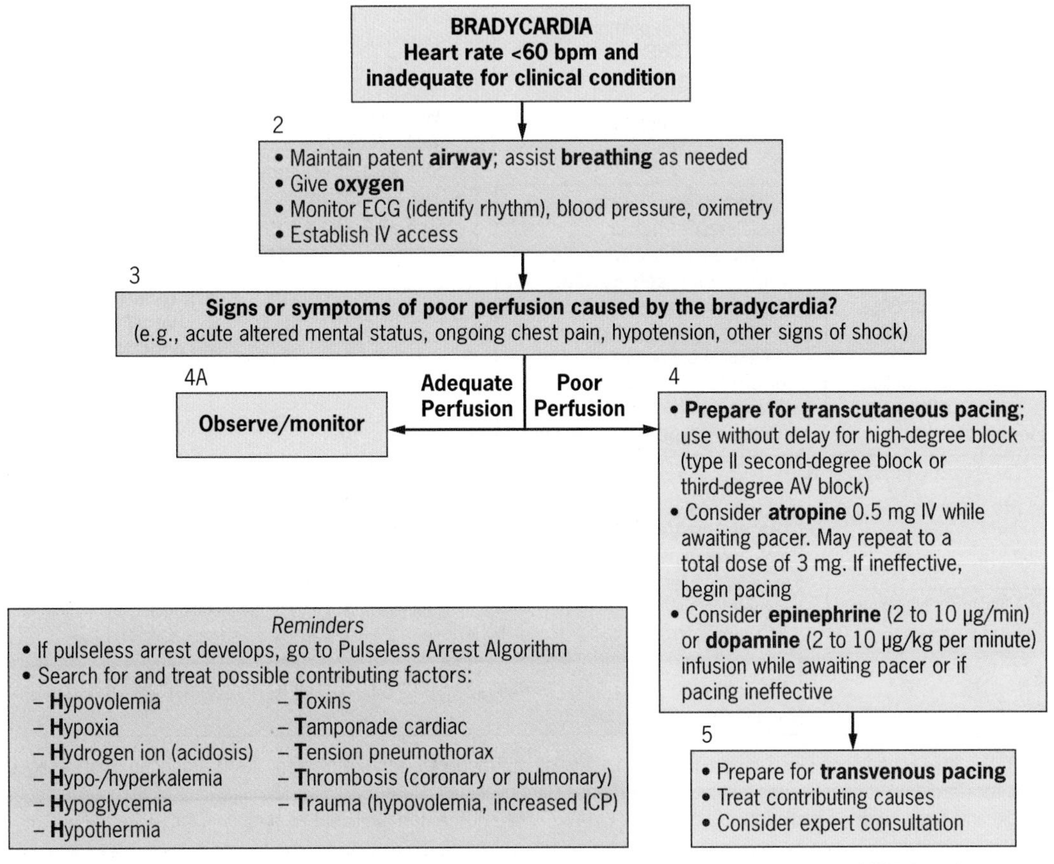

ALGORITHM 20–2 Advanced Life Support Bradycardia Algorithm. Reprinted with permission. 2005 American Heart Association Guidelines for Cardiopulmonary Resuscitation and Emergency Cardiovascular Care. Part 7.3: Management of Symptomatic Bradycardia and Tachycardia. *Circulation*. 2005;112:IV-67–IV-77. © 2005 American Heart Association, Inc.

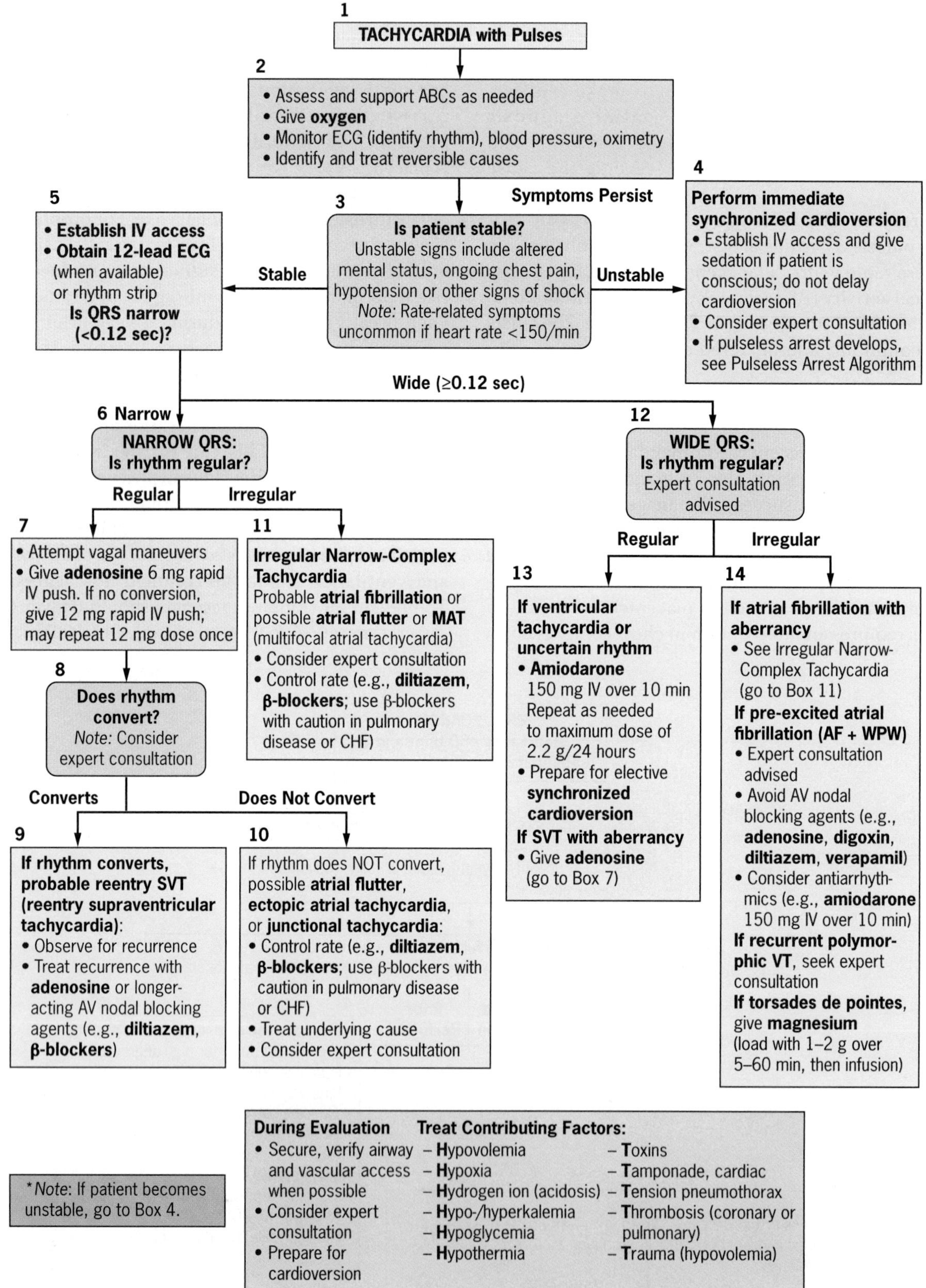

1
TACHYCARDIA with Pulses
2
• Assess and support ABCs as needed
• Give oxygen
• Monitor ECG (identify rhythm), blood pressure, oximetry
• Identify and treat reversible causes
Symptoms Persist
3
Is patient stable?
Unstable signs include altered mental status, ongoing chest pain, hypotension or other signs of shock
Note: Rate-related symptoms uncommon if heart rate <150/min
Stable
Unstable
4
Perform immediate synchronized cardioversion
• Establish IV access and give sedation if patient is conscious; do not delay cardioversion
• Consider expert consultation
• If pulseless arrest develops, see Pulseless Arrest Algorithm
5
• Establish IV access
• Obtain 12-lead ECG (when available) or rhythm strip
Is QRS narrow (<0.12 sec)?
Wide (≥0.12 sec)
6 Narrow
NARROW QRS: Is rhythm regular?
Regular
Irregular
7
• Attempt vagal maneuvers
• Give adenosine 6 mg rapid IV push. If no conversion, give 12 mg rapid IV push; may repeat 12 mg dose once
8
Does rhythm convert?
Note: Consider expert consultation
Converts
Does Not Convert
9
If rhythm converts, probable reentry SVT (reentry supraventricular tachycardia):
• Observe for recurrence
• Treat recurrence with adenosine or longer-acting AV nodal blocking agents (e.g., diltiazem, β-blockers)
10
If rhythm does NOT convert, possible atrial flutter, ectopic atrial tachycardia, or junctional tachycardia:
• Control rate (e.g., diltiazem, β-blockers; use β-blockers with caution in pulmonary disease or CHF)
• Treat underlying cause
• Consider expert consultation
11
Irregular Narrow-Complex Tachycardia
Probable atrial fibrillation or possible atrial flutter or MAT (multifocal atrial tachycardia)
• Consider expert consultation
• Control rate (e.g., diltiazem, β-blockers; use β-blockers with caution in pulmonary disease or CHF)
12
WIDE QRS: Is rhythm regular?
Expert consultation advised
Regular
Irregular
13
If ventricular tachycardia or uncertain rhythm
• Amiodarone 150 mg IV over 10 min Repeat as needed to maximum dose of 2.2 g/24 hours
• Prepare for elective synchronized cardioversion
If SVT with aberrancy
• Give adenosine (go to Box 7)
14
If atrial fibrillation with aberrancy
• See Irregular Narrow-Complex Tachycardia (go to Box 11)
If pre-excited atrial fibrillation (AF + WPW)
• Expert consultation advised
• Avoid AV nodal blocking agents (e.g., adenosine, digoxin, diltiazem, verapamil)
• Consider antiarrhythmics (e.g., amiodarone 150 mg IV over 10 min)
If recurrent polymorphic VT, seek expert consultation
If torsades de pointes, give magnesium (load with 1–2 g over 5–60 min, then infusion)
*Note: If patient becomes unstable, go to Box 4.
During Evaluation
• Secure, verify airway and vascular access when possible
• Consider expert consultation
• Prepare for cardioversion
Treat Contributing Factors:
– Hypovolemia
– Hypoxia
– Hydrogen ion (acidosis)
– Hypo-/hyperkalemia
– Hypoglycemia
– Hypothermia
– Toxins
– Tamponade, cardiac
– Tension pneumothorax
– Thrombosis (coronary or pulmonary)
– Trauma (hypovolemia)

ALGORITHM 20–3 Advanced Life Support Tachycardia Algorithm. Reprinted with permission. 2005 American Heart Association Guidelines for Cardiopulmonary Resuscitation and Emergency Cardiovascular Care. Part 7.3: Management of Symptomatic Bradycardia and Tachycardia. *Circulation.* 2005;112: IV-67–IV-77. © 2005 American Heart Association, Inc.

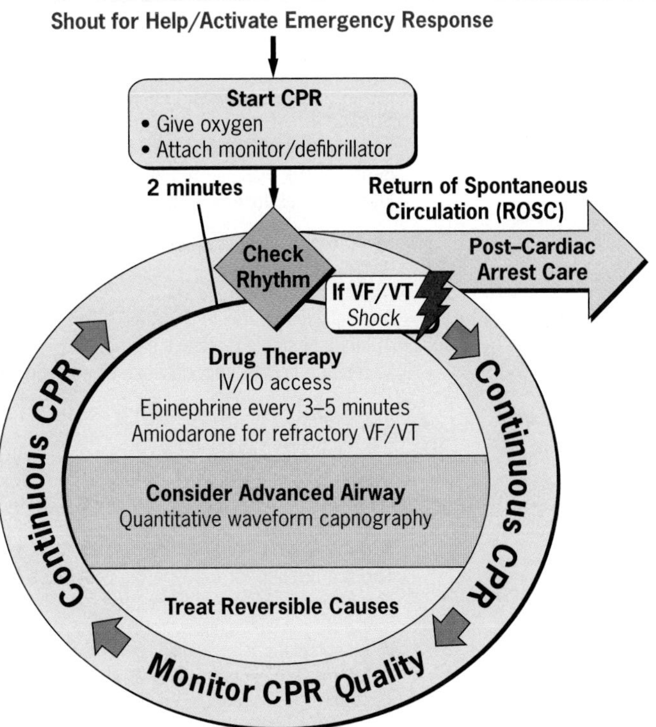

CPR Quality

- Push hard (≥2 inches [5 cm]) and fast (≥100/min) and allow complete chest recoil
- Minimize interruptions in compressions
- Avoid excessive ventilation
- Rotate compressor every 2 minutes
- If no advanced airway, 30:2 compression–ventilation ratio
- Quantitative waveform capnography
  - If P_{ETCO_2} <10 mm Hg, attempt to improve CPR quality
- Intra-arterial pressure
  - If relaxation phase (diastolic) pressure <20 mm Hg, attempt to improve CPR quality

Return of Spontaneous Circulation (ROSC)

- Pulse and blood pressure
- Abrupt sustained increase in P_{ETCO_2} (typically ≥40 mm Hg)
- Spontaneous arterial pressure waves with intra-arterial monitoring

Shock Energy

- *Biphasic:* Manufacturer recommendation (120–200 J); if unknown, use maximum available. Second and subsequent doses should be equivalent, and higher doses may be considered.
- *Monophasic:* 360 J

Drug Therapy

- *Epinephrine IV/IO Dose:* 1 mg every 3–5 minutes
- *Vasopressin IV/IO Dose:* 40 units can replace first or second dose of epinephrine
- *Amiodarone IV/IO Dose:* First dose: 300 mg bolus, second dose: 150 mg

Advanced Airway

- Supraglottic advanced airway or endotracheal intubation
- Waveform capnography to confirm and monitor ET tube placement
- Eight to 10 breaths/min with continuous chest compressions

Reversible Causes

– **H**ypovolemia	– **T**ension pneumothorax
– **H**ypoxia	– **T**amponade, cardiac
– **H**ydrogen ion (acidosis)	– **T**oxins
– **H**ypo-/hyperkalemia	– **T**hrombosis, pulmonary
– **H**ypothermia	– Thrombosis, coronary

ALGORITHM 20–4 Circular ACLS Algorithm. Reprinted with permission. Highlights of the 2010 American Heart Association Guidelines for Cardiopulmonary Resuscitation and Emergency Cardiovascular Care. Part 8: Advanced Cardiovascular Life Support. *Circulation.* 2010;122:S729–S767. © 2010 American Heart Association, Inc.

TABLE 20-2 ALS Drug Therapy

Drug	Indication	Dosage
Epinephrine	Shock, refractory VF and pulseless VT, asystole, PEA	*Cardiac arrest* 1 mg IV push (10 mL of 1:10,000 solution) Repeat 1 mg every 3–5 minutes Endotracheal dose = 2 to 2.5 times intravenous dose *Symptomatic bradycardia* 2–10 μg/minute
Vasopressin	VF/pulseless VT, asystole, PEA	*Any pulseless patient* 40 units IV single dose—1 time only To replace first or second dose of epinephrine
Atropine	Symptomatic bradycardia	*Bradycardia* 0.5 mg every 3–5 minutes Repeat to total dose of 0.04 mg/kg Endotracheal dose = 2 to 2.5 times IV dose
Amiodarone	VF/pulseless VT	300 mg IV push in cardiac arrest (VF/VT) 150 mg IV push for tachycardia with pulse (give over 10 minutes); can repeat *one* dose of 150 mg in 5 minutes
Lidocaine	VT (with pulse—stable), VF/pulseless VT	*VF or pulseless VT* 1–1.5 mg/kg; repeat at 0.5–0.75 mg/kg in 3–5 minutes, for total dose of 3 mg/kg *VT with pulse* 0.5–0.75 mg/kg; repeat in 3–5 minutes, for total dose of 3 mg/kg
Procainamide	Stable monomorphic VT, SVT, tachycardia of unknown origin	20 mg/minute IV infusion; in urgent situations, up to 50 mg/minute (max 17 mg/kg)
Magnesium	Cardiac arrest only if torsades is present or low magnesium is suspected	1–2 g per 10 mL D5W over 1–2 seconds
Adenosine	Stable SVT, undefined stable narrow complex tachycardia	6 mg IV over 1–3 seconds followed by 20 mL saline flush, then elevate arm; repeat 12 mg IV rapid push
Sodium bicarbonate	Preexisting hyperkalemia, drug overdose, known ketoacidosis, prolonged cardiac arrest with adequate ventilation	1 mmol/kg IV bolus

ALS, advanced life support; VF, ventricular fibrillation; VT, ventricular tachycardia; PEA, pulseless electrical activity; SVT, supraventricular tachycardia; D5W, 5% dextrose in water.

time for the patient to exhale. Once an advanced airway has been placed, the rescuer should deliver 10 to 12 breaths/min, and there is no longer the need to pause compressions to deliver the breaths.

Several different types of advanced airway adjuncts can be used during resuscitation. In field studies, it has been reported that 6% to 14% of endotracheal tubes were misplaced when postmortem exams were done.[60–62] In part because of these studies, the AHA stresses training prehospital providers to use several different advanced airways and suggests that it is important to remember that there is no evidence that placing an advanced airway in a prehospital situation improves survival.[59] It is equally important for the individual managing the airway to use multiple techniques to verify that the placement is correct. The 2010 AHA Guidelines recommends quantitative waveform capnography as a means to confirm and monitor endotracheal tube placement and CPR quality.

Endotracheal Tubes

The indications for emergency endotracheal intubation include the inability of the rescuers to adequately ventilate with a bag-mask device, the inability of a patient to protect his or her own airway (i.e., an unconscious patient), and the presence of a rescuer who is adequately trained to do the procedure. The advantages of inserting an endotracheal tube include securing the airway from aspiration, keeping the airway patent, permitting the suctioning of the lower airway, and providing an alternative route for administration of some resuscitative drugs.[63] Complications include trauma to the oropharynx, interruption of compressions and ventilations, and failure of the rescuer

RESPIRATORY RECAP

Equipment for Emergency Airway Management

- Endotracheal tube
- Oropharyngeal airway
- Nasopharyngeal airway
- Esophageal-tracheal Combitube
- Laryngeal mask airway

to recognize the misplacement of a tube. The interruption in compressions for intubation should be only during the time the rescuer needs to visualize the vocal cords. If the first attempt to intubate is unsuccessful, the rescuer doing the intubation should stop the procedure, provide ventilation and oxygenation, and allow time for others to do compressions before attempting intubation again.

Esophageal-Tracheal Combitubes

Esophageal-tracheal Combitubes are relatively easy to place compared with an endotracheal tube. They are more effective than a face mask at isolating the airway and reducing the risk of aspiration, and enable rescuers to provide ventilation and oxygenation.[60] Another advantage of using a Combitube is the ease of training healthcare providers to insert the tube. Complications associated with the Combitube include esophageal trauma, lacerations, bruising, and fatalities that may occur when the position of the tube is not confirmed by the rescuers.[64–66]

Laryngeal Mask Airway

A laryngeal mask airway provides a more secure and reliable means of ventilation than the bag-mask device.[64,65] The advantages of using a laryngeal mask are its relative ease of insertion, simpler training for rescuers (rescuers do not have to visualize the vocal cords), better protection against aspiration than with a face mask, and the ability to insert the airway when a patient has the possibility of an unstabilized neck injury.

Impedance Threshold Valve

The **impedance threshold valve (ITV)** increases the negative intrathoracic pressure in the chest by creating a vacuum pressure that essentially "pulls" venous blood back into the chest during expansion of the chest after compression, thereby enhancing venous return and cardiac output (**Figure 20–23**).[66] During resuscitation, cardiac output is dependent on both the amount of venous return to the heart and the physical compression of the heart. Venous return is partially dependent on the degree of negative intrathoracic pressures. This device is contraindicated in patients with pulmonary edema or congestive heart failure because it can exacerbate these conditions.

The ITV attaches to a resuscitator bag and limits air entry into the chest during chest recoil between each chest compression. This reduces the intrathoracic pressures and thereby increases venous return to the heart during the chest decompression phase of compressions. In several studies it has been successfully used with a laryngeal mask airway, cuffed endotracheal tube, and even a face mask if the rescuers can maintain a tight seal with the mask.[67–71]

Research in a laboratory setting found that during a cardiac arrest, use of the impedance threshold valve decreased intrathoracic pressures by 6 to 8 mm Hg.[70] When the valve is used during active compression–decompression resuscitation, it has resulted in a greater than 50% increase in coronary perfusion pressures, improved 24-hour patient survival, and improved neurologic function following cardiac arrest.[72,73]

Because the ITV reduces negative intrathoracic pressures during recoil of the chest following compressions, there are concerns about the possibility of an increase in the work of breathing, especially for patients who are using the valve with a mask to treat orthostatic

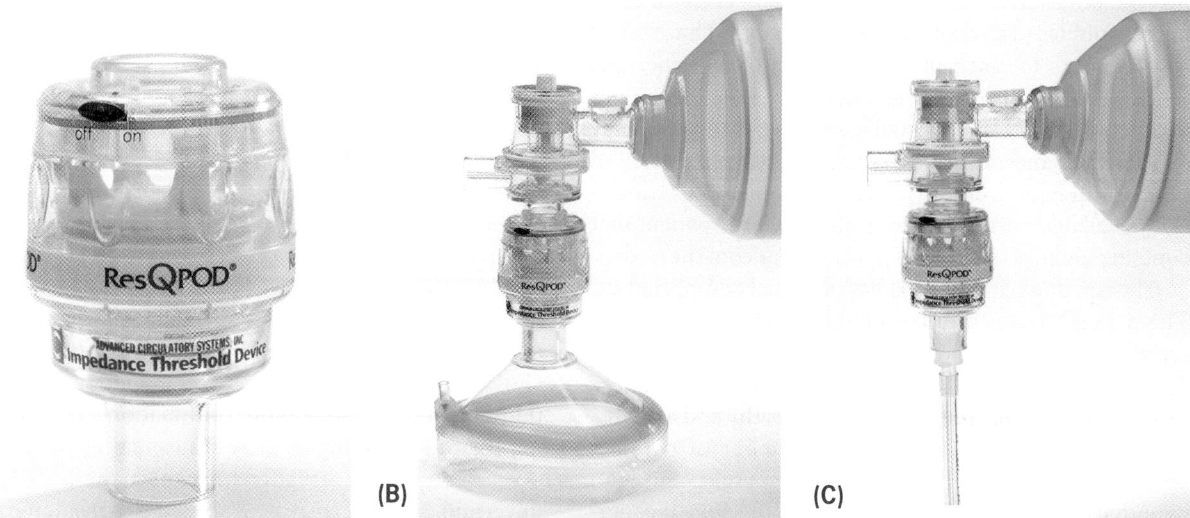

FIGURE 20–23 **(A)** Impedance threshold valve device (ITV). **(B)** ITV attached to mask. **(C)** ITV between bag-valve resuscitator and endotracheal tube.

hypotension.[74] In healthy individuals, the imposed work of breathing was increased but not excessive.[66,74]

Supporting the Patient After Resuscitation

The postresuscitation period is a period of time during which multiorgan dysfunction can occur. Most postresuscitation deaths occur during the first 24 hours.[75] These patients require respiratory support, management of cardiac arrhythmias, monitoring and management of hemodynamic instability using mechanical or pharmacologic agents or both, and monitoring and management of metabolic abnormalities.[1] According to the 2010 AHA guidelines, survival for victims of cardiac arrest who are admitted to the hospital can be improved by implementing a comprehensive, structured, integrated, and multidisciplinary system of post-cardiac arrest care. The key issues to be addressed in this post-cardiac care are (1) optimize cardiopulmonary function and vital organ perfusion after return of spontaneous circulation; (2) transport/transfer to an appropriate hospital or critical care unit with a comprehensive post-cardiac arrest treatment system of care; (3) identify and treat ACS and other reversible causes; (4) control temperature to optimize neurologic recovery; and (5) anticipate, treat, and prevent multiple organ dysfunction, which includes avoiding excessive ventilation and hyperoxia. Clinicians should try to identify the precipitating cause of the arrest, prevent the recurrence of the arrest, and optimize cardiopulmonary functions and systemic perfusion (especially to the brain) to improve long-term survival with neurologic function intact.[76]

Studies have indicated that a mild degree of therapeutic hypothermia may play an important role in the postresuscitative period. In these studies, patients were cooled to a range of 33° C to 34° C for 12 to 24 hours after resuscitation from ventricular fibrillation or pulseless electrical activity or asystole rhythms.[75–79] It is suggested that only a subset of cardiopulmonary arrest patients may befit from induced hypothermia at this time. In the future, others may benefit as well.[80] In some older studies, external cooling techniques (e.g., cooling blankets, ice bags) have taken several hours to reach the desired level of hypothermia; the newer studies suggest that internal cooling techniques (e.g., cold saline, endovascular cooling catheters) may also be used and result in less time to reach the desired temperatures and better patient outcomes.[81] Commercially available devices use pads placed on the patient that contain channels of circulating water that cool the body.

Therapeutic hypothermia has potential complications. The patient's temperature should be continuously monitored, and clinicians should watch for these complications very closely during this period. If the patient's temperature drops below the desired range, coagulopathy and arrhythmias may develop. An increased number of patients develop pneumonia and/or sepsis and hyperglycemia with hypothermia.[81] During therapeutic hypothermia, the temperature on the humidifier of the ventilator should be set at the target core temperature of the patient.[82]

Normal blood gas values should be maintained during the postresuscitation period. Studies have determined that during this time, hyperventilation of the patient, increased airway pressures, and intrinsic positive end-expiratory pressures may cause increased cerebral vasoconstriction, increased intracranial pressures, increased cerebral ischemia, and ultimately ischemic brain injury.[83,84]

Summary of Advanced Cardiovascular Life Support

The successful resuscitation of patients suffering from cardiopulmonary arrest requires teams of rescuers with advanced skills and knowledge. The role of respiratory therapists working on these teams is determined by the institutions where they work. The 2005 and 2010 AHA guidelines provide algorithms to determine appropriate actions for a variety of different situations. However, there are no guidelines that detail the actions necessary to be taken for each and every individual patient. Good assessment skills, airway management skills, a sufficient knowledge base, and the ability to learn new skills helps prepare therapists to function in a range of situations from preventive early response teams to postarrest support teams when managing cardiopulmonary arrest patients.

Ethical Concerns

Healthcare providers are expected to initiate CPR as part of their duty to respond unless there are obvious clinical signs of irreversible death, attempts to perform CPR would place the rescuer at risk of physical injury, or the patient or his or her surrogate has indicated with an advance directive (do-not-resuscitate order) that resuscitation is not desired.[85] Respiratory therapists have a responsibility to know the resuscitation status of patients under their care. Unlike other medical interventions, CPR is initiated without a physician's order, based on implied consent for emergency treatment. A physician's order is necessary to withhold CPR. A physician may also determine that continued care is futile, such as in the case of patients in whom CPR would not restore effective circulation. Noninitiation of resuscitation and discontinuation of life-sustaining treatment during or after resuscitation are ethically equivalent, and in situations in which the prognosis is uncertain, a trial of treatment should be considered while further information is gathered to help determine the likelihood of survival and expected clinical course.

> **RESPIRATORY RECAP**
>
> **Initiation of CPR**
>
> » Healthcare providers are expected to initiate CPR as part of their duty to respond unless there are obvious clinical signs of irreversible death, attempts to perform CPR would place the rescuer at risk of physical injury, or the patient or the patient's surrogate has indicated with an advance directive that CPR is not desired.

All patients in cardiac arrest should receive CPR unless the patient has a valid do-not-resuscitate order, the patient has signs of irreversible death (e.g., rigor mortis, decapitation, decomposition, dependent lividity), or no physiologic benefit can be expected because vital functions have deteriorated despite maximal therapy (e.g., progressive septic, cardiogenic shock). The decision to terminate resuscitative efforts rests with the treating physician in the hospital and is based on consideration of many factors, including time to CPR, time to defibrillation, comorbid disease, prearrest state, and initial arrest rhythm.

KEY POINTS

- Factors related to resuscitation outcomes after CPR include the initial rhythm, time elapsed before initiation of CPR, time elapsed before defibrillation of ventricular fibrillation or pulseless ventricular tachycardia, duration of CPR, and whether arrest was witnessed.
- The primary CABD survey consists of circulation, airway, breathing, and defibrillation.
- Masks, face shields, or bag-mask devices should be used for emergency ventilation.
- With two-rescuer CPR, one person performs chest compressions and the other person performs ventilation and assesses cardiopulmonary function.
- The abdominal thrust maneuver is recommended to relieve airway obstruction.
- In airway management, there is no substitute for tracheal intubation.
- Manual ventilation with a bag-valve-mask device may not provide adequate tidal volumes if performed incorrectly.
- During cardiac arrest, it is important to administer the highest oxygen concentration possible.
- When intravenous access is delayed, some drugs can be administered through the tracheal tube.
- With defibrillation, an electrical current is passed through the heart to eliminate the chaotic asynchronous activity of ventricular fibrillation.
- The impedance threshold valve may improve cardiac output during low flow states.
- Therapeutic hypothermia should be considered after resuscitation from ventricular fibrillation, pulseless electrical activity, or asystole rhythms.

REFERENCES

1. 2005 American Heart Association guidelines for cardiopulmonary resuscitation and emergency cardiovascular care. *Circulation.* 2005;112:IV-19–IV-29.
2. International Liaison Committee on Resuscitation. 2005 international consensus on cardiopulmonary resuscitation and emergency cardiovascular care science with treatment and recommendations. *Circulation.* 2005;112:III-I–III-136.
3. Highlights of the 2010 American Heart Association Guidelines for Cardiopulmonary Resuscitation and Emergency Cardiovascular Care. Part B: Advanced Cardiovascular Life Support. *Circulation.* 2010;122:S729–S767.
4. Azar D, Chamberlain D, Colquhoun M, et al. Randomized controlled trials of staged teaching for basic life support: skill acquisition at bronze stage. *Resuscitation.* 2004;5:7–15.
5. Heidenreich JW, Higdon TA, Kern KB, et al. Single-rescuer cardiopulmonary resuscitation: "two quick breaths"—an oxymoron. *Resuscitation.* 2004;62:283–289.
6. Rea TD, Eisenberg MS, Sinibaldi G, White RD. Incidence of EMS-treated-out-of-hospital cardiac arrest in the United States. *Resuscitation.* 2004:63:17–24.
7. Fredriksson M, Herlitz J, Nichol G. Variations in outcome in studies of out-of-hospital cardiac arrest: a review of studies conforming to the Utstein guidelines. *Am J Emerg Med.* 2003;21:276–281.
8. Nichol G, Stiell IG, Laupacis A, et al. A cumulative meta-analysis of the effectiveness of defibrillator-capable emergency medical services for victims of out-of-hospital arrest. *Ann Emerg Med.* 1999;34(pt 1):517–525.
9. Nichol G, Detsky AS, Stiell IG, et al. Effectiveness of emergency medical services for victims of out-of-hospital cardiac arrest; a metaanalysis. *Ann Emerg Med.* 1996;27:700–710.
10. Caffrey SL, Willoughby PF, Pepe PE, Becker LB. Public use of automated external defibrillators. *N Engl J Med.* 2002:347:1242–1247.
11. Hazinski MF. Is pediatric resuscitation unique? Relative merits of early CPR and ventilation versus early defibrillation for young victims of prehospital cardiac arrest. *Ann Emerg Med.* 1995;25:540–543.
12. Ruppert M, Reith WM, Windmann JH, et al. Checking for breathing: evaluation of the diagnostic capability of emergency medical services personnel, physicians, medical students, and medical laypersons. *Ann Emerg Med.* 1999;34:720–729.
13. Hackl W, Hausberger K, Sailer R et al. Prevalence of cervical spine injuries in patient with facial trauma. *Oral Surg Oral Med Oral Pathol Oral Radiol Endod.* 2001;92:370–376.
14. Elam JO, Greene DG, Schneider AM, et al. Head-tilt method of oral resuscitation. *JAMA.* 1960;172:812–815.
15. Idris AH, Gabrielli A, Caruso L. Smaller tidal volume is safe and effective for bag-valve ventilation, but not for mouth-to-mouth ventilation: an animal model for basic life support. *Circulation.* 1999;100(suppl I):I-644.
16. American Heart Association in collaboration with International Liaison Committee on Resuscitation. Guidelines 2000 for cardiopulmonary resuscitation and emergency cardiovascular care: international consensus on science, part 3: adult basic life support. *Circulation.* 2000;102(suppl I):I-22–I-59.
17. Baskett P, Nolan J, Parr M. Tidal volumes which are perceived to be adequate for resuscitation. *Resuscitation.* 1996;31:231–234.
18. Wenzel V, Idris AH, Banner MJ, et al. The composition of gas given by mouth-to mouth ventilation during CPR. *Chest.* 1994:106:1806–1810.
19. Safar P, Escarraga LA, Chang F. Upper airway obstruction in the unconscious patient. *J Appl Physiol.* 1959;14:760–764.
20. Mejicano GC, Maki DG. Infections acquired during cardiopulmonary resuscitation: estimating the risk and defining strategies for prevention. *Ann Intern Med.* 1998;129:813–828.
21. Tendrup TE, Warner DA. Infant ventilation and oxygenation by basic life support providers: comparison of methods. *Prehospital Disaster Med.* 1992;7:35–40.
22. Hess D, Ness C, Oppel A, Rhodes K. Evaluation of mouth-to-mask ventilation devices. *Respir Care.* 1989;34:191–195.
23. Simmons M, Deao D, Moon L, et al. Bench evaluation: three face-shield CPR barrier devices. *Respir Care.* 1995;40:618–623.
24. Barnes TA. Emergency ventilation techniques and related equipment. *Respir Care.* 1992;37:673–694.
25. Elam JO. Bag-valve-mask O_2 ventilation. In: Safar P, Elam JO, eds. *Advances in Cardiopulmonary Resuscitation; The Wolf Creek Conference on Cardiopulmonary Resuscitation.* New York: Springer-Verlag; 1977:73–79.

26. Elling R, Politis J. An evaluation of emergency medical technicians' ability to use manual ventilation devices. *Ann Emerg Med.* 1983;12:765–768.
27. Hess D, Hirch C, Marquis-D'Amico C, et al. Imposed work and oxygen delivery during spontaneous breathing with adult disposable manual ventilators. *Anesthesiology.* 1994;81:1256–1263.
28. Selleck BA. Cricoid pressure to control regurgitation of the stomach contents during induction of anesthesia. *Lancet.* 1962;2:404.
29. Moule P. Checking the carotid pulse: diagnostic accuracy in students of healthcare professions. *Resuscitation.* 2000;44:195–201.
30. Paradis NA, Martin GB, Goetting MG, et al. Simultaneous aortic, jugular bulb, and right atrial pressures during cardiopulmonary resuscitation in humans: insight into mechanisms. *Circulation.* 1989;80:361–368.
31. Aufderheide TP, Sigurdsson G, Pirrallo RG, et al. Hyperventilation-induced hypotension during cardiopulmonary resuscitation. *Circulation.* 2004;109:1960–1965.
32. Kern KB, Hilwig RW, Berg RA, et al. Importance of continuous chest compressions during cardiopulmonary resuscitation: improved outcomes during a simulated single lay-rescuer scenario. *Circulation.* 2003;108:2575–2594.
33. Handley AJ. Teaching hand placement for chest compressions—a simpler technique. *Resuscitation.* 2002;53:29–36.
34. Aufderheide TP, Pirrallo RG, Yannopoulos D, et al. Incomplete chest wall decompression: a clinical evaluation of CPR performance by EMS personnel and assessment of alternative manual chest-compression-decompression techniques. *Resuscitation.* 2005;64:353–362.
35. Yannopoulos D, McKnite S, Aufderheide TP, et al. Effects of incomplete chest wall decompression during cardiopulmonary resuscitation on coronary and cerebral perfusion pressures in a porcine model of cardiac arrest. *Resuscitation.* 2005;64:363–372.
36. Halperin HR, Tsitlik JE, Guerci AD, et al. Determinants of blood flow to vital organs during cardiopulmonary resuscitation in dogs. *Circulation.* 1986;73:539–550.
37. Bayes de Luna A, Coumel P, Leclercq JF. Ambulatory sudden cardiac death: mechanisms of production of fatal arrhythmia on the basis of data from 157 cases. *Am Heart J.* 1989;117:151–159.
38. Wik L, Hansne TB, Fylling F, et al. Delaying defibrillation to give basic cardiopulmonary resuscitation to patients with out-of-hospital ventricular fibrillation: a randomized trial. *JAMA.* 2003;289:1389–1395.
39. Rea TD, Shah S, Kudenchuk PF, et al. Automated external defibrillators: to what extent does the algorithm delay CPR? *Ann Emerg Med.* 2005;46:132–141.
40. Yu T, Weil MH, Tang W, et al. Adverse outcomes of interrupted precordial compressions during automated defibrillation. *Circulation.* 2002;106:368–372.
41. Redding JS. The choking controversy: critique of evidence on the Heimlich maneuver. *Crit Care Med.* 1979;7:475–479.
42. Fingerhut LA, Cox CS, Warner M. International comparative analysis of injury mortality: findings from the ICE on injury statistics. International Collaborative Effort on Injury Statistics. *Adv Data.* 1998;1–20.
43. Hartrey R, Bingham RM. Pharyngeal trauma as a result of blind finger sweeps in the choking child. *J Accid Emerg Med.* 1995;12:52–54.
44. Kabbani M, Goodwin SR. Traumatic epiglottis following blind finger sweep to remove a pharyngeal foreign body. *Clin Pediatr (Phila).* 1995;34:495–497.
45. Ruben HM, Elam JO, Ruben AM, Greene DG. Investigation of upper airway problems in resuscitation, 1: studies of pharyngeal x-rays and performance by laymen. *Anesthesiology.* 1961;22:271–279.
46. Centers for Disease Control and Prevention. Web-Based Injury Statistics Query and Reporting System (WISQARS) [Online]. National Center for Injury Prevention and Control, Centers for Disease Control and Prevention (producer). Available at: http://www.cdc.gov/noipi/wisqars.
47. Centers for Disease Control and Prevention. Fatal injuries to children—United States, 1986. *JAMA.* 1990;264:952–953.
48. Centers for Disease Control and Prevention. *Injury Fact Book.* Atlanta, GA: U.S. Department of Health and Human Services; 2006.
49. Samson R, Berg R, Bingham R, Pediatric Advanced Life Support Task Force ILCoR. Use of automated external defibrillators for children: an update. An advisory statement from the Pediatric Advanced Life Support Task Force, International Liaison Committee on Resuscitation. *Resuscitation.* 2003;57:237–243.
50. Morley RE, Ludemann JP, Moxham JP, et al. Foreign body aspiration in infants and toddlers: recent trends in British Columbia. *J Otolaryngol.* 2004;33:37–41.
51. Vilke GM, Smith AM, Rau LU, et al. Airway obstruction in children aged less than 5 years: the prehospital experience. *Prehosp Emerg Care.* 2004;8:196–199.
52. Heimlich HJ. A life-saving maneuver to prevent food-choking. *JAMA.* 1975;234:398–401.
53. Orlwski JP. Optimum position for external cardiac compression in infants and younger children. *Ann Emerg Med.* 1986;15:667–673.
54. Day RL, Crelin ES, DuBois AB. Choking: the Heimlich abdominal thrust vs back blows—an approach to measuring of inertial and aerodynamic forces. *Pediatrics.* 1982;70:113–119.
55. Braner DAV, Denson SE, Ibsen LM, eds. *Textbook of Neonatal Resuscitation.* 5th ed. Dallas, TX: American Heart Association; 2000.
56. Finer NN, Rich W, Craft A, Henderson C. Comparison of methods of bag and mask ventilation for neonatal resuscitation. *Resuscitation.* 2001;49:299–305.
57. Clemets F, McGowan J. Finger position for chest compression in cardiac arrest in infants. *Resuscitation.* 2000;44:43–46.
58. Phillips GW, Zideman DA. Relation of infant's heart to sternum; its significance in cardiopulmonary resuscitation. *Lancet.* 1986;1:1024–1025.
59. Dorges V, Ocker H, Hagelberg S, et al. Smaller tidal volumes with room-air are not sufficient to ensure adequate oxygenation during bag-valve mask ventilation. *Resuscitation.* 2000;44:37–41
60. Jones JH, Murphy MP, Dickerson RL, et al. Emergency physician–verified out-of-hospital intubations: miss rates by paramedics. *Acad Emerg Med.* 2004;11:707–709
61. Sayre MR, Sakles JC, Mistler AF, et al. Field trail of endotracheal intubation by basic EMTs. *Ann Emerg Med.* 1998;31:228–233.
62. Katz SH, Falk JL. Misplaced endotracheal tubes by paramedics in an urban emergency medical services system. *Ann Emerg Med.* 2001;37:32–37.
63. Pepe PE, Compass MK, Joyce TH. Prehospital endotracheal intubation: rationale for training emergency medical personnel. *Ann Emerg Med.* 1985;14:1085–1092.
64. Stone BJ, Chantler PJ, Baskett PJ. The incidence of regurgitation during cardiopulmonary resuscitation: a comparison between the bag valve mask and the laryngeal mask airway. *Resuscitation.* 1998;38:3–6.
65. Martens P. The use of the laryngeal mask airway by nurses during cardiopulmonary resuscitation: the result of a multicenter trial. *Anesthesia.* 1994;49:3–7.
66. Ahamed HI, Convertino VA, Ratliff DA, et al. Imposed power of breathing associated with use of an impedance threshold device. *Respir Care.* 2007;52:177–183.
67. Plaisance P, Lurue JG, Payen D. Inspiratory impedance during active compression-decompression cardiopulmonary resuscitation: a randomized evaluation in patients in cardiac arrest. *Circulation.* 2000;101:989–994.
68. Plaisance P, Soleil C, Lurie KG, et al. Use of an inspiratory impedance threshold device on a face mask and endotracheal tube to reduce intrathoracic pressures during the decompression

phase of active compression-decompression cardiopulmonary resuscitation. *Crit Care Med.* 2005;33:990–994.

69. Wolcke BB, Mauer DK, Schoefmann MF, et al. Comparison of standard cardiopulmonary resuscitation versus the combination of active compression–decompression cardiopulmonary resuscitation and an inspiratory impedance threshold device for out-of-hospital cardiac arrest. *Circulation.* 2003;108:2201–2205.
70. Aufderheide TP, Pirrallo RG, Provo TA, Lurie KG. Clinical evaluation of an inspiratory impedance threshold device during standard cardiopulmonary resuscitation in patients with out-of-hospital cardiac arrest. *Crit Care Med.* 2005;33:734–740.
71. Pirrallo RG, Aufderheide TP, Provo TA, Lurie KG. Effect of an inspiratory impedance threshold device on hemodynamics during conventional manual cardiopulmonary resuscitation. *Resuscitation.* 2005;66:13–20.
72. Lurie KG, Voelckel WG, Zielinski T, et al. Improving standard cardiopulmonary resuscitation with an inspiratory impedance threshold valve in a porcine model of cardiac arrest. *Anaesth Analg.* 2001;90(3):649–655.
73. Lurie KG, Zeilinski T, McKnite S, et al. Use of an inspiratory impedance valve improves neurologically intact survival in a porcine model of ventricular fibrillation. *Circulation.* 2002;105:124–129.
74. Concertion VA, Ratliff DA, Crissey J, et al. Effects of inspiratory impedance on hemodynamic responses to a squat-stand test in human volunteers: implications for treatment of orthostatic hypotension. *Eur J Appl Physiol.* 2005;94:392–399.
75. Negovsky VA. The second step in the resuscitation: the treatment of the "post-resuscitation disease." *Resuscitation.* 1972;1:1–7.
76. 2005 American Heart Association guidelines for cardiopulmonary resuscitation and emergency cardiovascular care. Part 7.5: postresuscitation support. *Circulation.* 2005;112:IV-84–IV-88.
77. Hypothermia After Cardiac Arrest Study Group. Mild therapeutic hypothermia to improve the neurological outcomes after the cardiac arrest. *N Engl J Med.* 2002;346:549–556.
78. Bernard SA, Gray TW, Buist MD, et al. Treatment of comatose survivors of out-of- hospital cardiac arrest. *N Engl J Med.* 2002;346:549–556.
79. Hachimi-Idressi S, Corne L, Ebinger G, et al. Mild hypothermia induced by helmet device: a clinical feasibility study. *Resuscitation.* 2001;51:275–281.
80. Langhelle A, Tyvold SS, Lexow K, et al. In-hospital factors associated with improved outcomes after out-of-hospital cardiac arrest: a comparison between four regions in Norway. *Resuscitation.* 2003;56:247–263.
81. Bernard S, Buist M, Monteiro O, Smith K. Induced hypothermia using large volume, ice-cold intravenous fluid in comatose survivors of out-of hospital cardiac arrest: a preliminary report. *Resuscitation.* 2003;56:9–13.
82. Lellouche F, Qader S, Taille S, et al. Under-humidification and over-humidification during moderate induced hypothermia with usual devices. *Intensive Care Med.* 2006;32:1014-1021.
83. Ausina A, Baguena M, Nadal M, et al. Cerebral hemodynamic changes during sustained hypocapnia in severe head injury: can hyperventilation cause cerebral ischemia? *Acta Neurochir Suppl.* 1997;17:1–4.
84. Yudt KD, Diringer MN. The use of hyperventilation and its impact on cerebral ischemia in the treatment of traumatic brain injury. *Crit Care Med.* 1997;13:163–184.
85. 2005 American Heart Association guidelines for cardiopulmonary resuscitation and emergency cardiovascular care. Part 2: ethical issues. *Circulation.* 2005;112;IV-6–IV-11.

CHAPTER 21

Mechanical Ventilators: Classification and Principles of Operation

Robert L. Chatburn
Teresa A. Volsko

OUTLINE

Basic Concepts
Input Power
Power Transmission and Conversion
Control System
Control Variables
Phase Variables
Modes of Ventilation
Targeting Scheme
Output
Effects of the Patient Circuit
Ventilator Alarm Systems

OBJECTIVES

1. Discuss the basic design features of mechanical ventilators.
2. Describe the major drive mechanisms and output control valves of mechanical ventilators.
3. Describe the equation of motion and how it relates to ventilator classification.
4. Compare open- and closed-loop control of mechanical ventilators.
5. Discuss the differences among pressure, volume, and flow control.
6. Define control variables, phase variables, and conditional variables.
7. Draw the pressure, volume, and flow curves for rectangular pressure output and for rectangular, ramp, and sinusoidal flow output.
8. Describe the major modes of ventilation in terms of the control and phase variables for mandatory and spontaneous breaths.
9. Define mandatory and spontaneous breaths. Compare various targeting schemes used during mechanical ventilation.
10. Describe the effects of patient circuit compliance and resistance on ventilator output.
11. Compare input power alarms, control circuit alarms, and output alarms.

KEY TERMS

alarm event
assisted breath
closed-loop control
control circuit
control variable
cycle time
cycle
expiratory flow time
expiratory pause time
expiratory phase
expiratory time
inspiratory flow time
inspiratory pause time
inspiratory phase
inspiratory time
mandatory breath
mode of ventilation
open-loop control
passive expiration
percent cycle time
phase variable
positive end-expiratory pressure (PEEP)
spontaneous breath
target
targeting scheme
time constant
transrespiratory pressure
trigger
ventilatory period

INTRODUCTION

Mechanical ventilators are more than simple machines designed to support the work of the respiratory system and improve or stabilize gas exchange.[1] These machines have evolved significantly over the past three decades[1] and are now complex computers with sophisticated software and artificial intelligence. Their complex design and advanced monitoring capabilities make it possible to deliver mechanical breaths from conventional to high-frequency rates, administer specialty gas therapy such as heliox and nitric oxide, and monitor lung mechanics. In the United States alone, more than 30 different critical care ventilators and at least two dozen transport and home care ventilators are used by clinicians in a variety of healthcare settings. Many different modes of ventilation are currently available on these sophisticated machines. Therefore, it is essential for respiratory therapists to thoroughly understand ventilator design and how different ventilators work in order to safely and effectively match a ventilator's capability to the patient's physiologic need. This chapter presents mechanical ventilation terminology and outlines the basic principles of ventilator design.[2–5]

Basic Concepts

A ventilator is a machine with a system of related elements designed to alter, transmit, and direct applied energy in a predetermined manner to perform useful work.[6] Energy is put into the ventilator in one of two ways, either in the form of compressed gas or electricity. That energy is transmitted or transformed by the ventilator's drive mechanism in a predetermined manner (by the **control circuit**) to assist or replace the patient's muscles in performing the work of breathing. To fully appreciate how to use sophisticated mechanical ventilators, the clinician must first understand their four basic components (**Table 21–1**):

- Input power
- Power transmission and conversion
- Control system
- Output (pressure, volume, and flow waveforms)

Input Power

All ventilators require a source of power that can be used to perform some or all of the work of breathing. The two most common forms of input power are electric and pneumatic. Input power should not be confused with the power for the control circuit. For example, many ventilators use pneumatic input power to drive inspiration but use electricity to power the control circuit. During the inter- or intrafacility transport of mechanically ventilated patients with electrically (battery) or pneumatically powered ventilators, always check the battery power or gas source prior to transport and ensure that the calculated power needs for the transport can be met. A bag-valve resuscitator should be available to manually ventilate the patient in the event of an input power source failure.

RESPIRATORY RECAP

Input Power

» Electric
» Pneumatic

Electric

A common electrical line outlet can be used to power the drive mechanism of electrically powered ventilators. In the United States, this line voltage is typically 110 to 115 volts AC (60 Hz). The AC voltage also is reduced and converted to power electronic microprocessor control circuits.

Some ventilators are designed with internal rechargeable batteries or can adapt to rechargeable external batteries. Internal and external batteries provide a temporary alternative power source when the usual AC current is unavailable. This capability makes them useful in the transport of ventilator-dependent patients within and between healthcare facilities. In the home care setting, the internal battery backup is an essential feature. The power conversion from AC to DC or battery power will occur automatically, so that there is no interruption

TABLE 21–1 Ventilator Classification System

I. Input
   A. Pneumatic
   B. Electric
      1. AC
      2. DC (battery)
II. Power conversion and transmission
   A. External compressor
   B. Internal compressor
   C. Output control valves
III. Control scheme
   A. Control circuit
      1. Mechanical
      2. Pneumatic
      3. Fluidic
      4. Electric
      5. Electronic
   B. Control variables
      1. Pressure
      2. Volume
      3. Flow
      4. Time
   C. Phase variables
      1. Trigger
      2. Target
      3. Cycle
      4. Baseline
   D. Conditional variables
   E. Modes of ventilation
IV. Output
   A. Pressure waveforms
      1. Rectangular
      2. Exponential
      3. Sinusoidal
      4. Oscillating
   B. Volume waveforms
      1. Ascending ramp
      2. Sinusoidal
   C. Flow waveforms
      1. Rectangular
      2. Ascending ramp
      3. Descending ramp
      4. Sinusoidal
V. Alarms
   A. Input power alarms
      1. Loss of electric power
      2. Loss of pneumatic power
   B. Control circuit alarms
      1. General systems failure
      2. Incompatible ventilator settings
      3. Warnings (e.g., inverse I:E)
   C. Output alarms (high/low conditions)
      1. Pressure
      2. Volume
      3. Flow
      4. Time
         a. Frequency
         b. Inspiratory time
         c. Expiratory time
      5. Inspired gas
         a. Temperature
         b. F_{IO_2}

I:E, inspiration-to-expiration ratio.

in delivery of pressure, volume, and flow to the patient. Typically, electrically powered ventilators will alert the clinician or home caregiver with a visual and audible alarm when this transition occurs. Internal batteries have a limited lifespan of from 60 minutes to a several hours and are typically designed to allow the clinician sufficient time to find a power source of longer duration.

The Pulmonetic Systems LTV 800 (CareFusion, Minneapolis, Minn.) is an example of a home care ventilator that has an internal battery life of approximately 60 minutes when fully charged.[7] External battery power on this type of ventilator makes it possible for electrically powered ventilators to operate from DC power for longer periods of time. Many electrically powered ventilators have options for the size as well as the life of external batteries. The LTV 800 has the ability to adapt to a small or large external battery, providing approximately 3 to 4 or 8 hours of battery life, respectively.[7] The use of an external battery provides ventilator-dependent patients the ability to participate in social, educational, or professional activities outside the home for an extended period of time. These alternative power sources are not only lifesaving, as in the uninterrupted provision of assisted ventilation during an unexpected power outage or during transport, but can also improve the quality of life for patients with long-term mechanical ventilatory needs.

Pneumatic

Compressed gas is used to power pneumatically powered ventilators. Ventilators operated by pressurized gas typically have internal reducing regulators so that the normal operating pressure is lower than the source pressure. This feature permits uninterrupted operation from piped gas sources in hospitals, which are usually regulated to 50 pounds per square inch (psi) but are subject to periodic fluctuations. The use of compressed gas as a power source makes a ventilator useful in situations in which no electrical power is available, such as during transport of patients, or in locations where electricity use is undesirable, such as near magnetic resonance imaging (MRI) equipment.

Because compressed air and oxygen are in abundant supply in acute care hospitals, intensive care unit (ICU) ventilators are designed to use the energy stored in pressurized gas. Most ICU ventilators also depend on electrical energy, which is needed to support their computerized control mechanisms. The control mechanisms of pneumatically powered transport ventilators may also depend on electricity to function. The MVC100 (Allied Healthcare Products, St. Louis, Miss.) is a ventilator designed for mass casualty use in individuals weighing more than 44 kg. During transport or when AC power is not available, an internal battery is used to power this ventilator's control circuit, which lasts up to 20 hours if fully charged when the power conversion transpires.[8]

Power Transmission and Conversion

The power transmission and conversion system of mechanical ventilators is composed of two mechanisms. The drive mechanism provides the force needed to deliver gas under pressure. The second mechanism, the output control, consists of one or more valves that regulate gas flow to the patient.

Drive Mechanism

The drive mechanism converts input power to output work. The type of drive mechanism a ventilator uses will, in part, determine the characteristic flow and pressure patterns the ventilator produces. Drive mechanisms create driving pressure either with an internal compressor (e.g., piston, blower) or from a source of compressed gas (e.g., oxygen tank, hospital compressed gas plumbing system).

Output Control Valve

The output control valve shapes the flow of gas from the drive mechanism to the patient. Commonly used output control valves include the pneumatic diaphragm, electromagnetic poppet/plunger valve, and the proportional valve. This valve may be a simple on/off exhalation valve. The Newport HT50 (Newport NMI Ventilators, Newport Medical Instruments, Newport Beach, Calif.) is an example of a ventilator that uses this type of output control valve. Alternatively, the output control valve can shape the output waveform, as in the Maquet Servo-I (Maquet, Bridgewater, N.J.).

Control System

To learn how a ventilator can be operated to perform all or some of the work of breathing, it is necessary to have a thorough understanding of the mechanics of breathing. Specifically, this knowledge involves the pressure necessary to cause a flow of gas to enter the airway and increase the volume of the lungs. The study of respiratory mechanics relies on simple models. The relatively complex respiratory system can be represented by a simple physical model (e.g., straw connected to a balloon). This simple model is similar to electrical circuits: compliance is analogous to capacitance, flow resistance is analogous to electrical resistance, and pressure is analogous to voltage. The similarity between the physical and electrical models makes it possible to borrow mathematic models from electrical engineering, substituting pressure, volume, and flow for voltage, charge, and current, respectively (**Figure 21–1**). The result is known as the *equation of motion* for the respiratory system. A simplified version is as follows:[9]

$$P_{mus} + P_{vent} = (E \times V) + (R \times \dot{V}) + \text{Auto-PEEP}$$

In this simplified form of the equation, muscle pressure, P_{mus}, is the **transrespiratory pressure** (i.e., airway pressure minus body surface pressure) generated by the ventilatory muscles to expand the thoracic cage and lungs. Ventilator pressure, P_{vent}, is the transrespiratory pressure generated by the ventilator during inspiration. The combination of muscle pressure and ventilator pressure causes volume, V, and flow, $\dot{V}$, to be delivered to the patient. Pressure, volume, and flow change with time and hence are *variables*. Elastance, E, and resistance, R, are assumed to remain constant and are called *parameters*; their combined effect constitutes the load experienced by the ventilator and ventilatory muscles. *Elastance* is defined as the ratio of pressure change to volume change (i.e., the reciprocal of compliance), and *resistance* is defined as the ratio of pressure change to flow change. The elastic load is the pressure necessary to overcome the elastance (or compliance) of the respiratory system, and the resistive load is the pressure necessary to overcome the flow resistance of the airways along with lung and chest wall tissue resistance. Resistive load also includes the resistance to flow imposed by artificial airways. The term *parameter* also may refer to a particular aspect of a variable, such as the peak or mean value.

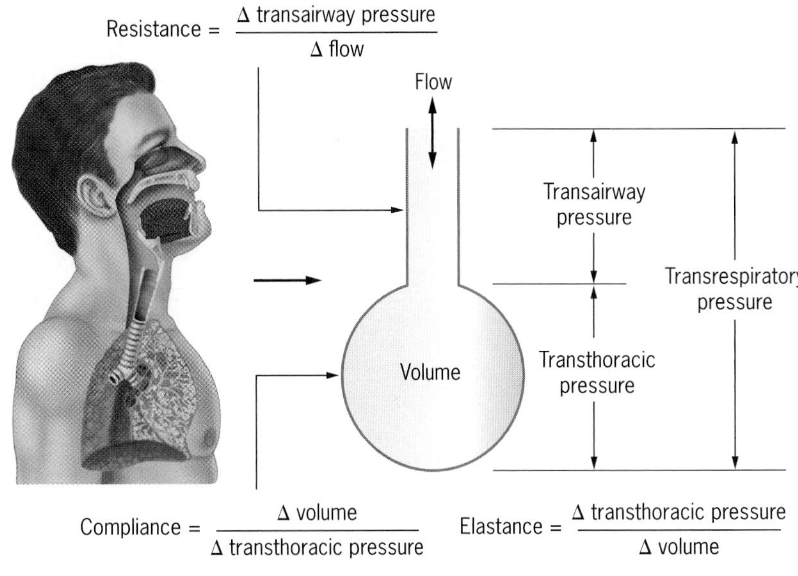

FIGURE 21–1 The study of respiratory system mechanics is based on graphical and mathematical models. The respiratory system can be modeled as a single-flow conducting tube connected to a single elastic compartment. This physical model can be described as mathematical model called the equation of motion for the respiratory system, where pressure, volume, and flow are variables (i.e., functions of time) while resistance and compliance are constants.

Note that pressure, volume, and flow are all measured relative to their baseline values (i.e., their values at end-expiration). This means that the pressure to cause inspiration is measured as the change in airway pressure relative to the pressure at the start of inspiration, that is, above positive end-expiratory pressure (PEEP). Volume is measured as the change in lung volume above end-expiratory lung volume, and the change in lung volume during the inspiratory period is defined as the *tidal volume.* Flow is measured relative to its end-expiratory value (usually zero unless auto-PEEP is nonzero).

The auto-PEEP term in the equation of motion indicates that if auto-PEEP is present, more force is required by the ventilator or the muscles, or both, to generate a given tidal volume and flow. Thus, for volume control ventilation, where the terms E × V and E × $\dot{V}$ are constant because of the preset values of tidal volume and inspiratory flow, as auto-PEEP increases, peak inspiratory pressure increases. On the other hand, for pressure control ventilation, the airway pressure waveform is constant because of the preset value of inspiratory pressure. Thus, as auto-PEEP increases, both inspired tidal volume and peak inspiratory flow decrease.

When pressure, volume, and flow are plotted as functions of time, characteristic waveforms for volume control ventilation and pressure control ventilation are produced (**Figure 21–2**). Common units of measure are cm H_2O for pressure, mL or L for volume, and L/min or L/s for flow; the waveforms are often called *scalar* waveforms, as opposed to loop waveforms, which show one variable (e.g., flow) plotted against another (e.g., volume).

Notice in Figure 21–2 that the expiratory volume and flow waveforms are the same shape (i.e., they show exponential decay). This describes **passive expiration** (i.e., no muscular effort), in which the respiratory system is responding to a sudden release of inspiratory pressure. This characteristic waveform is sometimes referred to in the literature as a "decelerating" flow waveform.[10] It is also interesting to note that for passive inspiration, with a rectangular pressure waveform, inspiratory flow and volume also are exponential. Because the exponential waveform is so common, the convention used to describe it is the **time constant**, which is a measure of the time required for the passive respiratory system to respond to abrupt changes in ventilatory pressure. It has units of time (usually seconds) and is calculated as the product of resistance and compliance.[11] **Figure 21–3** shows inspiratory and expiratory time constants marked on exponential curves.

The time constant equals the time necessary for the lungs to passively empty 63% of the inspired tidal volume (V_T). We can demonstrate this mathematically by the following equation, which sets expiratory time, T_E, equal to the time constant, R × C:

$$P_{lung} = \frac{V_T}{C} e^{-T_E/RC} = \frac{V_T}{C} 2.72^{-1} = \frac{V_T}{C} 0.37$$

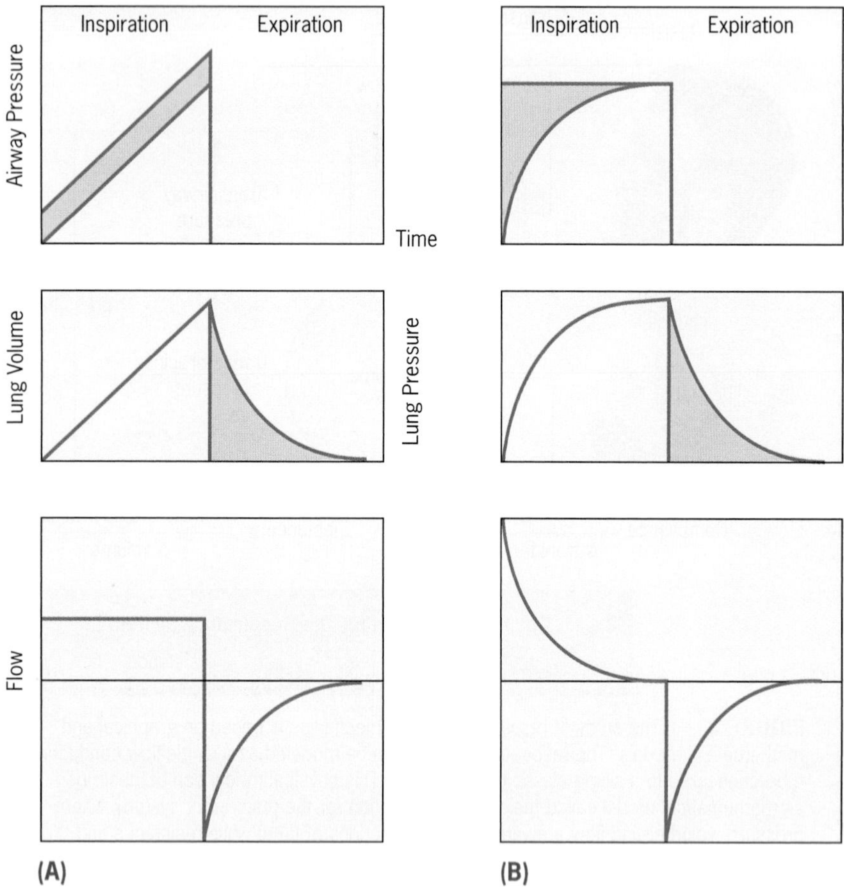

FIGURE 21–2 Theoretical inspiratory output waveforms for volume control ventilation with a rectangular flow waveform (**A**) compared with pressure control ventilation with a rectangular pressure waveform (**B**). The order of presentation is pressure, volume, and flow, according to the order specified by the equation of motion. Note that the volume waveform has the same shape as the transthoracic or lung pressure waveform (i.e., pressure due to elastic recoil). The flow waveform has the same shape as the transairway pressure waveform (i.e., pressure due to airway resistance). The origin of the airway pressure waveform is the end-expiratory pressure; the origins of the volume and flow waveforms both are zero. The shaded areas represent pressures due to flow resistance; the open areas represent pressure due to elastic recoil.

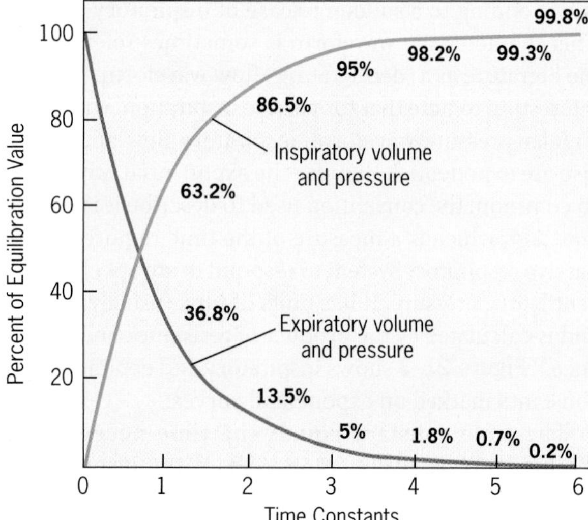

FIGURE 21–3 Time constant is a measure of how long it takes the respiratory system to achieve equilibration with a sudden change in transrespiratory pressure. It is calculated as the product of resistance and compliance (R × C) and is expressed in units of time, usually seconds.

This expression shows that after an expiratory time equal to one time constant (63% change), only 37% of the lung pressure is left. After two time constants (i.e., t = 2RC), exhalation is 86% completed; after three time constants, exhalation is 95% complete. Exhalation is considered to be 100% complete after five time constants (refer to Figure 21–3).

A similar expression can be derived for passive inhalation:

$$P_{lung} = \frac{V_T}{C}\left(1 - e^{-t/RC}\right)$$

This is the equation for lung pressure during inspiration for pressure control ventilation (refer to Figure 21–2).

It is important to understand the concept of time constants in order to make appropriate ventilator setting adjustments. For example, it is clinically important to minimize gas trapping during any form of ventilatory support. To accomplish this, the expiratory time should be at least five time constants long. Similarly, during pressure control ventilation, it may be imperative to obtain the maximum tidal volume from the set pressure gradient. Therefore, inspiratory time (for passive inspiration) should be at least five time constants long.

There are instances in which the patient's ventilatory muscles are not functioning. Patients with respiratory muscle paralysis due to a traumatic spinal cord injury or pharmacologic intervention have no ventilatory muscle effort. The muscle pressure in this situation is zero, and the ventilator must generate all the pressure required to deliver the tidal volume and inspiratory flow. Conversely, if ventilator pressure equals zero (i.e., airway pressure does not rise above baseline during inspiration), no ventilatory support is present. Between these two extremes are an infinite variety of combinations of muscle pressure (patient effort) and ventilator support that are theoretically possible for partial ventilatory support.

The concept of muscle pressure is important for another reason. Many ventilators and bedside pulmonary function monitors provide the clinician with estimates of respiratory system compliance and resistance based on transrespiratory system pressure (i.e., ventilator pressure), volume, and flow. All of them make calculations based on the equation of motion but assuming that $P_{mus} = 0$. If the patient makes an inspiratory effort during an assisted breath (i.e., $P_{mus} > 0$), this effort adds an unmeasured amount of driving pressure to that generated by

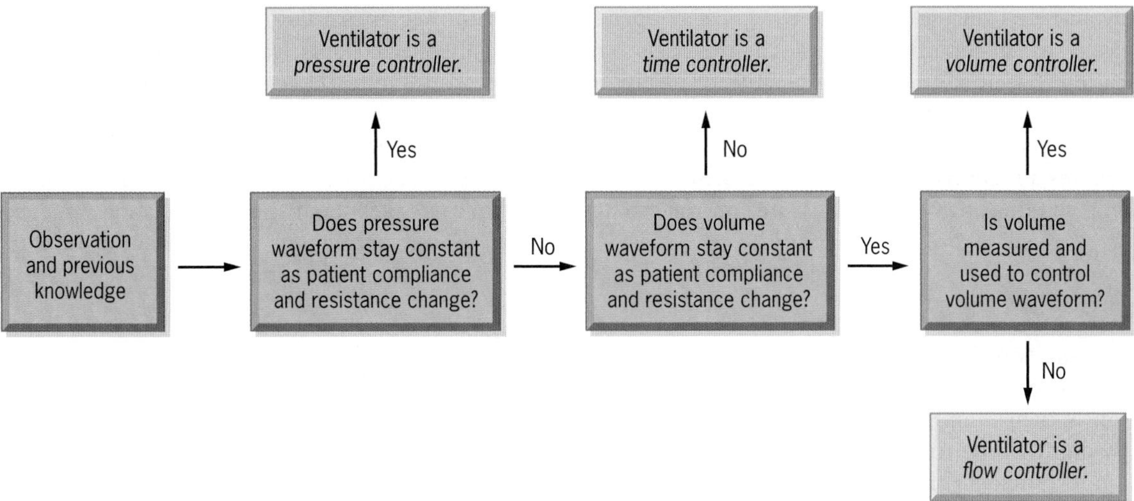

FIGURE 21–4 Criteria for determining the control variables during a ventilator-assisted inspiration.

the ventilator. Thus, elastance and resistance based only on the ventilator's airway pressure sensor measurements underestimate the true values.

Analysis of ventilator–patient interaction based on a mathematic model suggests the proper use of the word *assist*, which is another frequently confused concept. *The American Heritage Dictionary* defines *assist* as "to help; to aid; to give support."[12] From the perspective of the equation of motion, whenever airway pressure (i.e., ventilator pressure) rises above baseline during inspiration, the ventilator performs work. Thus the breath is said to be *assisted*, independent of other breath characteristics (i.e., whether the breath is classified as spontaneous or mandatory). Do not confuse this meaning of the word *assist* with specific names of modes of ventilation (e.g., assist/control). Confusion regarding ventilator terms is quite common. Ventilator manufacturers often coin terms for modes with marketing appeal in mind. The names for ventilator modes are thus often conceived without regard to consistency or theoretic relevance.

Control Variables

In the equation of motion, pressure, volume, and flow are all changeable variables, measured relative to their baseline or end-expiratory values. When expressed as functions of time, any one of these three variables can be predetermined, making it the independent variable and the other two dependent variables. This idea is precisely analogous to the way ventilators operate. During pressure control ventilation, pressure is the independent variable, and the shapes of the volume and flow waveforms depend on the shape of the pressure waveform and the resistance and compliance of the respiratory system. Conversely, during volume control ventilation, the ventilator sets the shape of the volume waveform, making volume the independent variable, and the shape of the flow waveform depends on the shape of the volume waveform. During volume control ventilation, the shape of the pressure waveform depends on the volume waveform, as well as the resistance and compliance of the respiratory system.

> **RESPIRATORY RECAP**
>
> **Pressure Control Versus Volume Control Ventilation**
>
> » During pressure control ventilation, pressure is the independent variable. The shapes of the volume and flow waveforms depend on the shape of the pressure waveform and the characteristics of the patient's lungs.
>
> » During volume control ventilation, volume is the independent variable. The shape of the flow and pressure waveforms depends on the shape of the volume waveform and the characteristics of the patient's lungs.

This concept provides a theoretic basis for the classification of ventilators as pressure, volume, or flow controllers. **Figure 21–4** illustrates the criteria used to determine which variable is controlled (i.e., which variable is the independent variable). Note that if the waveforms for all three variables are not predetermined (i.e., none of the variables can be considered independent), then the ventilator is considered to control only the timing of the inspiratory phase and expiratory phase and is called a *time controller*.

Pressure

The equation of motion states that if the ventilator is an ideal pressure controller, then the left side of the equation (i.e., ventilator pressure as a function of time) is determined by the ventilator settings and remains unaffected by changes in parameter values on the right side (i.e., compliance and resistance).

If the **control variable** is pressure, the ventilator can control either the airway pressure (causing it to rise above body surface pressure for inspiration) or the pressure on the body surface (causing it to fall below airway opening pressure for inspiration). This idea is the basis for classification of ventilators as either positive or negative pressure types. For example, the Newport Wave ventilator would be classified as a positive pressure controller that generates a rectangular pressure waveform, and the Emerson Iron Lung as a negative pressure controller that produces a sinusoidal pressure waveform.

Volume

If the pressure waveform varies as the load imposed by the patient's respiratory system changes, the volume waveform is then examined. However, the observation that the volume waveform remains unchanged is a necessary but not sufficient condition to warrant classification as a volume controller, because the same holds true for a flow controller. The reason is that once the volume waveform is specified, the flow waveform is determined, because they are inverse functions of each other (volume being the integral of flow and flow being the derivative of volume). Therefore, if changes in compliance and resistance do not change the volume waveform, they do not affect the flow waveform, and vice versa.

> **RESPIRATORY RECAP**
>
> **Control Variables**
>
> » Pressure
> » Volume
> » Flow
> » Time
>
> Only one variable can be controlled at a time and is referred to as the *independent variable*.

To qualify as a volume controller, a ventilator must maintain a consistent volume waveform in the presence of a varying load, measure volume, and use the signal to control the volume waveform. Volume can be measured directly only by the displacement of a piston or bellows or similar device. With a piston or bellows, control of the excursion of the device automatically controls the volume waveform. Alternatively, a volume signal could be derived by integration of a flow signal. Although some ventilators, such as the Siemens Servo 900C, the NPB 7200, the Bear 5, and the Hamilton Veolar, display volume readings, they all actually measure and control flow and calculate volume for displays. Thus, they are all flow controllers unless they are operated in a pressure control mode (e.g., during pressure-support ventilation). An examination of a ventilator's schematic diagrams and operator's manual should provide the information necessary to decide whether volume or flow is being measured.

Flow

If the volume change (i.e., tidal volume) remains consistent when compliance and resistance are varied, and if volume change is not measured and used for control, the ventilator is classified as a flow controller. The simplest example of open-loop flow control in a ventilator consists of a pressure regulator supplying gas to a flow meter, such as is found in infant ventilators. An infant ventilator becomes a flow controller rather than a pressure controller if the airway pressure does not reach the set pressure limit.[13] However, the flow meter is usually not back-pressure compensated and varies its output slightly in the presence of a changing load. In contrast, the Servo 900C measures flow and adjusts the output control valve (i.e., the inspiratory scissors valve) accordingly. It can maintain a more consistent inspiratory flow waveform as the load changes.

Time

Supposing that both pressure and volume are affected substantially by changes in lung mechanics, then the only form of control is that in which the ventilatory cycle is defined, or that involving alternation between inspiration and expiration. Therefore, the only variables being controlled are the inspiratory and expiratory times. This situation arises in some forms of high-frequency ventilation, when even the designation of an inspiratory and expiratory phase becomes somewhat obscure.

Phase Variables

Once the control variables and the associated waveforms are identified, more detail can be obtained through examination of the events that take place during a ventilatory cycle (i.e., the period of time between the beginning of one breath and the beginning of the next). Mushin and colleagues proposed that this time span be divided into four phases: (1) the change from expiration to inspiration, (2) inspiration, (3) the change from inspiration to expiration, and (4) expiration.[1] A particular variable is measured and used to start, sustain, and end the phase. In this context, pressure, volume, flow, and time are referred to as **phase variables**.[14] **Figure 21–5** defines the criteria used to determine phase variables.

> **RESPIRATORY RECAP**
>
> **Phase Variables**
>
> » Trigger
> » Target
> » Cycle

Trigger

All ventilators measure one or more of the variables associated with the equation of motion (i.e., pressure, volume, flow, time). Inspiration is started when one of these variables reaches a preset value. Thus, the variable of interest is the initiating, or **trigger**, variable. The most common trigger variables are time (the ventilator initiating a breath according to a set frequency, independent of the patient's spontaneous efforts), pressure (the ventilator sensing the patient's inspiratory effort in the form of a drop in baseline pressure and starting inspiration independent of the set frequency), and flow (the ventilator sensing the patient's inspiratory effort as a drop in the baseline flow through the patient

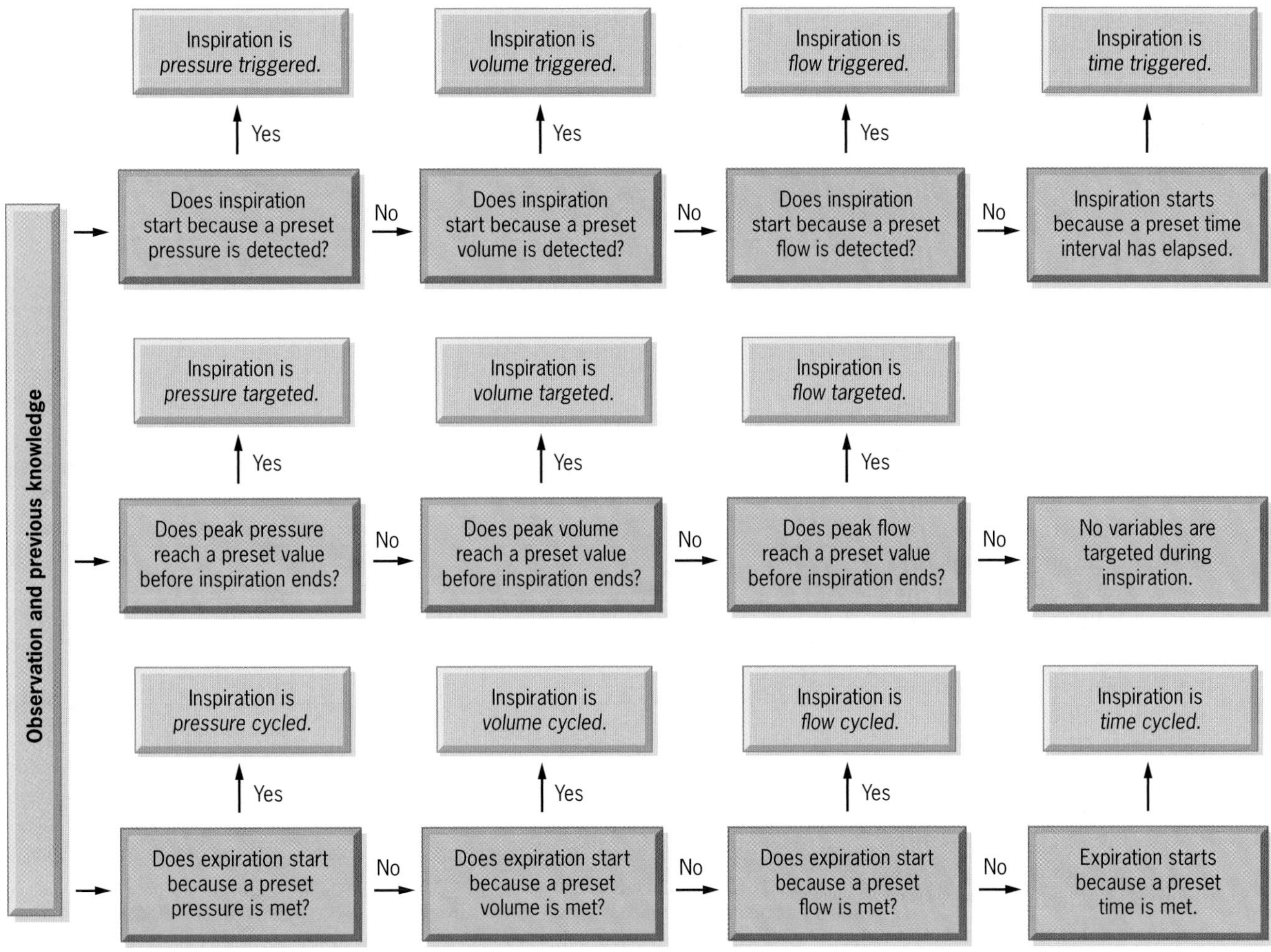

FIGURE 21–5 Criteria for determining the phase variables during a ventilator-assisted breath.

circuit or sensing inspiratory flow directly with a sensor at the patient's airway opening). Any variable that can be measured can potentially be used to trigger inspiration. For example, the Sechrist SAVI system senses inspiration as a change in chest impedance. Of course, manual triggering of inspiration is relatively simple.

Triggering on flow has been shown to reduce the work the patient must perform to trigger inspiration[15,16] because work is proportional to the volume the patient inspires multiplied by the change in baseline pressure necessary for triggering. Most ICU ventilators allow the clinician to select flow or pressure for the trigger variable. Pressure triggering requires some pressure change and hence an irreducible amount of work to trigger. With flow or volume triggering, however, baseline pressure need not change and theoretically the patient need not perform work on the ventilator to trigger a response. At least one ventilator, the Drager Babylog, can be volume triggered. The possible advantage of volume triggering over flow triggering is that when the flow signal is integrated to obtain volume, much of the noise in the signal (e.g., condensate in the patient circuit) is removed and the likelihood of false triggering reduced. A possible disadvantage of this method is the increased delay from signal processing and the phase lag between flow and volume signals.

The amount of patient effort required to trigger inspiration is determined by the ventilator's sensitivity setting. The smaller the change in signal (e.g., pressure change below baseline) required to trigger inspiration to begin, the greater the sensitivity. Many ventilators indicate sensitivity adjustments qualitatively (e.g., min, max). Alternatively, a ventilator may specify a trigger threshold quantitatively. For example, to make a pressure-triggered ventilator more sensitive, the trigger threshold might be adjusted from 2 to 1 cm H_2O below the baseline pressure. There are clinical consequences to the inappropriate adjustment of the trigger sensitivity. If the trigger threshold is set too high, it will be difficult for the patient to trigger a breath when needed. Ineffective triggering has been shown to contribute to prolonged duration of ventilatory support and to increased ICU and hospital lengths of stay.[17,18] Conversely, if the threshold is set too low, the patient may receive breaths

> **RESPIRATORY RECAP**
>
> **Trigger Variables**
>
> » Ventilator (time)
>
> » Patient (e.g., pressure or flow)

without any muscle effort at all (auto-triggering). As a result, patient–ventilator asynchrony may occur and in this case contributes to excessive levels of ventilatory support.[19]

Target

During the **inspiratory phase**, pressure, volume, and flow increase above their end-expiratory values. The inspiratory phase is quantified by specification of the **inspiratory time**, defined as the time interval from the start of inspiratory flow to the start of expiratory flow. Inspiratory hold (or pause) time is included in the inspiratory time. Distinguishing the **inspiratory flow time** as the interval from the start of inspiratory flow to the end of inspiratory flow and the **inspiratory pause time** as the interval from the end of inspiratory flow to the start of expiratory flow sometimes is helpful. This distinction is useful because no standardized method exists to set these intervals on ventilators, and the terminology that manufacturers use may be confusing. For example, on one ventilator, inspiratory flow time may be indirectly set through setting of tidal volume and flow, whereas pause time may be directly set (in seconds), thus indirectly increasing inspiratory time. On another ventilator, inspiratory time may be set directly, with no provision for direct setting of inspiratory pause time. On yet another ventilator, inspiratory time may be set with the Rate and Percent Cycle Time controls and then inspiratory flow time changed via a change in the Percent Inspiration control. Finally, inspiratory flow time must be distinguished from inspiratory time to understand the way Pmax works on the Evita 4 ventilator.

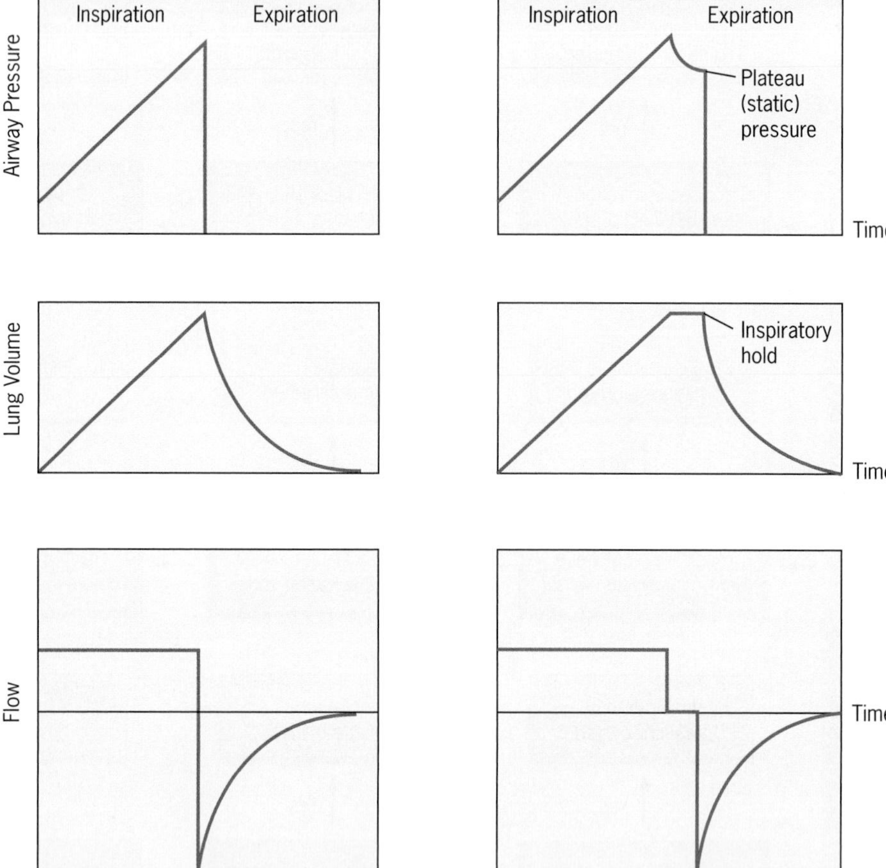

FIGURE 21–6 Importance of distinguishing between *target* and *cycle*. (**Left**) Flow is targeted, but volume is not, and inspiration is volume cycled. (**Right**) Both volume and flow are targeted (because they reach preset values before end inspiration), and inspiration is time cycled (after the preset inspiratory pause time).

Cycle time (or total cycle time) is another name for **ventilatory period**, the reciprocal of ventilatory frequency expressed in seconds. The **percent cycle time** is the ratio of inspiratory time to total cycle time expressed as a percentage. The percent inspiratory time is the inspiratory flow time expressed as a percentage of total cycle time. The percent pause time is the pause time expressed as a percentage of total cycle time. An inspiratory pause is important in estimation of lung pressures and calculation of respiratory system mechanics.

If one (or more) of the inspiratory variables rises no higher than some preset value, the variable is a **target** variable. (This variable was previously described as a limit variable in the literature[2–5] and textbooks.[20] However, the International Standards Organization [ISO] recommends that the term *limit* be used to refer only to alarm conditions and not to control settings.) The target variable must be distinguished from the variable that is used to end inspiration (the **cycle** variable). Therefore, the additional criterion is imposed that inspiration is not terminated because a variable has met its preset target value. In other words, a variable is described as targeted if it increases to a preset value before inspiration ends. **Figure 21–6** illustrates the criteria used to distinguish the terms *target* and *cycle*. For example, in volume control ventilation, flow is a preset target variable. Inspiration proceeds at the preset flow until a preset volume (the cycle variable) terminates the inspiratory time. If an inspiratory hold is added to the breath, then both the volume and flow become target values, and the cycle variable is the time (i.e., the preset inspiratory hold time).

Another potentially confusing issue is that, by convention, peak airway pressure and baseline pressure are measured relative to atmospheric pressure, whereas inspiratory pressure is sometimes measured relative to atmospheric pressure and sometimes relative to PEEP.

Failure to recognize this fact can lead to over- or underventilation when switching a patient from one ventilator to another, or even from one mode to another within the same ventilator.

Cycle

Inspiration always ends or is cycled off because some variable has reached a preset value. The variable that is measured and used to terminate inspiratory time and begin expiratory time is called the *cycle variable.* The cycle variable can be volume, pressure, time, or flow. Deciding which variable is used to cycle off inspiration for a given ventilator can be confusing. For a variable to be used as a feedback signal (in this case a cycling signal), it must first be measured. Most current-generation adult ventilators allow the operator to set a tidal volume and inspiratory flow rate, which would lead the operator to believe that the ventilator is volume cycled. However, closer inspection reveals that these ventilators do not measure volume, which is consistent with their all being flow controllers. Rather, they set the inspiratory time necessary to achieve the set tidal volume with the set inspiratory flow rate, making them time cycled. The tidal volume dial can be thought of as an inspiratory time dial calibrated in units of volume rather than time.

With pressure cycling, the ventilator delivers flow until a preset pressure is reached. When the set pressure is achieved, inspiration stops and expiratory flow begins. Pressure cycling is typically used for alarm settings. During volume control ventilation, a breath may be pressure cycled if a patient coughs and generates enough inspiratory pressure to violate the set high-pressure alarm. Pneumatically or electrically powered machines used to deliver intermittent positive pressure breathing (IPPB) therapy are considered pressure cycled machines.

A ventilator may be set to flow cycle. During flow cycling the ventilator delivers flow until a preset level is met, and then flow stops and expiration begins. The most frequent application of flow cycling is in the pressure support mode. In this mode, the control variable is pressure, and the ventilator provides the flow necessary to meet the inspiratory pressure target. Flow begins at a relatively high value and decays exponentially. When flow has decreased to a relatively low value, such as 25% of peak flow, inspiration is cycled off. Many ICU ventilators allow for adjustable flow cycle thresholds. Manufacturers often set the ventilator's default value for the cycle threshold slightly above zero flow to avoid prolonged inspiratory times and patient–ventilatory asynchrony.

Time cycling occurs when expiratory flow starts because a preset time interval has elapsed. During inspiration, there are several time intervals of interest, including inspiratory flow time and inspiratory hold (or pause) time. Inspiratory flow time is the period during which inspiratory flow is delivered to the patient. During inspiratory hold time, inspiratory flow ceases, but expiratory flow is not yet allowed. The sum of these two intervals is the inspiratory time. Therefore, when inspiratory time ends, time cycling occurs. During mechanical ventilation, an inspiratory hold time may not always be used. When it is used, it may be set directly, or it may occur indirectly if the set inspiratory time is longer than the inspiratory flow time (determined by the set tidal volume and flow; time = volume/flow).

Baseline

The variable controlled during the expiratory time is the baseline variable. **Expiratory time** is defined as the time interval from the start of expiratory flow to the start of inspiratory flow. As with inspiratory time, distinguishing the components of expiratory time is helpful: **expiratory flow time**, defined as the interval from the start of expiratory flow to the end of expiratory flow, and **expiratory pause time**, defined as the interval from the end of expiratory flow to the start of inspiratory flow.

Pressure is the most common baseline variable, which is used by all modern ventilators. Pressure is measured relative to atmospheric pressure, which is zero. Zero end-expiratory pressure is the default baseline pressure value used by ventilator manufacturers. When the baseline pressure is zero, the baseline pressure is equal to atmospheric pressure. No additional baseline pressure is applied to the airways during mechanical ventilatory support. As exhalation begins, the ventilator's expiratory valve opens to the atmosphere, exposing the patient's airway to a relative pressure of zero. Exhalation occurs naturally because alveolar pressure exceeds airway pressure. Gas moves from a greater pressure gradient, within the alveoli, to that of a lesser pressure, out to the atmosphere. During exhalation the lungs and thorax passively recoil down to resting volume, or functional residual capacity (FRC).

The clinician may change the baseline value to one that is above atmospheric. **Positive end-expiratory pressure (PEEP)** is the application of pressure above atmospheric pressure at the airway throughout expiration. The application of PEEP elevates a patient's FRC and can help improve oxygenation by preventing collapse of alveolar units that are made unstable by lack of surfactant or disease.

Pulmonary disease processes that result in uneven emptying of lung units or increased airway resistance may lead to air trapping at the end of expiration. This may also result from operator error, in which inspiratory time is set in a manner that does not permit the expiratory time to be at least three expiratory time constants long. When air is trapped and dynamic hyperinflation occurs within the lung at the end of the **expiratory phase**, there is a positive difference between end-expiratory alveolar pressure and the end-expiratory airway pressure (PEEP or continuous positive airway pressure [CPAP]) that the clinician selected. This phenomenon is known as auto-PEEP. An expiratory pause time is often initiated to measure auto-PEEP.

Modes of Ventilation

The main objective of mechanical ventilation is to ensure that the patient receives the minute volume of appropriate gases required to satisfy respiratory needs while not damaging the lungs, impairing circulation, or increasing the patient's discomfort. A **mode of ventilation** is the specification of the ventilatory pattern with which a ventilator achieves this objective.[6] A mode can be defined by specifying a combination of:

- Control variable (i.e., pressure or volume)
- Breath sequence (i.e., the pattern of mandatory and spontaneous breaths)
- **Targeting scheme** (i.e., the feedback control scheme used to shape the breath and determine the breath sequence)

Table 21–2 outlines the classification scheme for ventilator modes. The scheme is scalable and describes a mode in increasing detail using the first (breath sequence), second (control variable), or all three levels (control variable, breath sequence, and targeting scheme) as appropriate for the situation. These three basic components make up a complete classification for any mode of ventilation.

The key to understanding modes of ventilation is to define terms in a simple, standardized way and then link the terms to build descriptions of varying complexity. This is much more practical than trying to memorize the marketing names that manufacturers create to attract clinicians to promotional ventilator features.

The first component of a mode specification is the control variable, either pressure or volume. The second component is the breath sequence. A breath is defined as an inspiration paired with an expiration of the same relative size. This definition allows the superimposition of a spontaneous breath on a mandatory breath (defined herein), or vice versa. The flow baseline is taken at end-expiration and is traditionally equal to zero. However, because one or more breaths can be superimposed on existing flow in various circumstances (e.g., high-frequency ventilation), the inspiratory and expiratory movements of gas must be judged relative to the level of flow existing when these movements occur. Typically, inspiration immediately precedes expiration, but not necessarily. An example of this would be unrestricted spontaneous breathing during a mandatory pressure control breath. Here, a relatively large mandatory inspiration is followed by one or more relatively small spontaneous inspirations and expirations and then by the mandatory expiration. This feature has become more prominent since the development of the active exhalation valve and is marketed in features such as airway pressure release ventilation (APRV).[21–23]

A **spontaneous breath** is a breath for which the patient controls the timing of inspiration, meaning that the patient triggers and cycles the breath. Spontaneous breaths may be assisted or unassisted (**Figure 21–7**). An **assisted breath** is a breath during which all or part of flow (inspiratory or expiratory) is generated by the ventilator doing work for the patient. An unassisted breath

TABLE 21–2 Ventilation Mode Classification Scheme

1. Control variable
   a. Pressure
   b. Volume
2. Breath sequence
   a. Continuous mandatory ventilation (CMV)
      i. Spontaneous breaths **are not allowed** between mandatory breaths
      ii. Preset backup rate is the maximum value in case of apnea
         1. Actual rate may be higher depending on patient trigger events
   b. Intermittent mandatory ventilation (IMV)
      i. Spontaneous breaths **are allowed** between mandatory breaths
      ii. Preset backup rate is the minimum value in case of apnea
         1. Actual rate may be lower or higher depending on patient trigger events and targeting scheme
   c. Continuous spontaneous ventilation (CSV)
      i. All breaths are spontaneous
3. Targeting scheme (feedback control algorithms)
   a. Setpoint (e.g., Assist/Control)
   b. Dual (e.g., CMV + pressure-limited, flow-adaptive volume control)
   c. Servo (e.g., proportional assist)
   d. Adaptive (e.g., pressure regulated volume control)
   e. Optimal (e.g., adaptive support ventilation)
   f. Intelligent (using artificial intelligence; e.g., SmartCare)

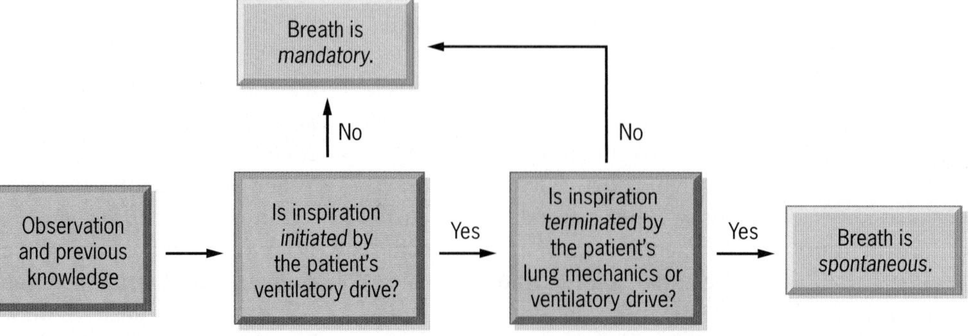

FIGURE 21–7 Algorithm defining spontaneous and mandatory breaths. If inspiration is both triggered and cycled by the patient, then the breath is spontaneous. If inspiration is triggered or cycled by the ventilator, then the breath is mandatory.

is one in which the ventilator provides no work to support the patient's inspiratory effort. Continuous positive airway pressure is an example of unassisted spontaneous breathing. The patient provides all of the work of breathing and controls the initiation, tidal volume, and end of inspiration at a baseline pressure set by the clinician.

A **mandatory breath** is a breath for which the machine controls the timing of inspiration (refer to Figure 21–7). That is, the machine triggers or cycles the breath, or both. All mandatory breaths are, by definition, assisted. The three possible breath sequences are as follows:

- *Continuous mandatory ventilation (CMV)*: All breaths are mandatory.
- *Continuous spontaneous ventilation (CSV)*: All breaths are spontaneous.
- *Intermittent mandatory ventilation (IMV)*: Breaths can be either mandatory or spontaneous.

CMV represents continuous mandatory ventilation. In this breath sequence, all breaths are mandatory and are delivered by the ventilator at a preset volume or pressure, breath rate, and inspiratory time or flow. The ventilator will deliver a patient-triggered breath if the patient has a spontaneous breathing effort. When patient effort is absent, the ventilator will deliver time-triggered mandatory breaths at the preset rate. Because every breath is a mandatory breath, as long as the patient continues to trigger breaths at a consistent respiratory rate, a decrease in the set ventilatory rate will not affect the level of ventilatory support. For example, suppose the patient has a set tidal volume of 0.5 L and a set mandatory rate of 8. The patient has spontaneous respiratory efforts, and the total number of breaths the ventilator delivers is 12. The minute ventilation delivered to the patient is equal to 0.5 L $\times$ 12, or 6.0 L. If the respiratory therapist decreases the mandatory rate to 4, and the total rate remains at 12 because the patient's spontaneous efforts continue, no change in minute ventilation will occur. The mandatory rate is therefore often regarded as a safety "backup" rate in the event of apnea. CMV is considered a method of full ventilatory support. CMV can be either volume control CMV (VC-CMV) or pressure control CMV (PC-CMV).

Intermittent mandatory ventilation (IMV) is a combination of mandatory and spontaneous breaths. IMV is a partial ventilatory support mode, which allows or requires the patient to sustain some of the work of breathing. During IMV, mandatory breaths are delivered at a set rate. On ventilators that offer synchronized pressure control IMV, the start, and perhaps the end, of inspiration may be synchronized with the patient's ventilatory efforts. Thus, it is possible that both the inspiratory and expiratory times may be shorted and, at any given time, the actual ventilatory rate may be slightly higher than the preset rate. Conversely, there are forms of IMV that allow the patient to suppress the preset mandatory breaths so long as the spontaneous trigger rate is high enough (e.g., Dräger's Mandatory Minute Ventilation, Respironics' BiPAP S/T modes). Between the mandatory breaths, spontaneous breathing can occur at the patient's own tidal volume and respiratory rate. The mandatory breaths can be volume control (VC-IMV) or pressure control (PC-IMV). If the mandatory breaths are synchronized to patient effort, this is called synchronized IMV (SIMV).

Technological advances in ventilator design allow for maximal synchrony of patient effort with the timing of the mandatory breath. The development of the active exhalation valve made it possible for the patient to breathe spontaneously during a mandatory pressure control breath. This feature is designed to ensure synchrony between the ventilator and patient when mandatory breath parameters such as preset inspiratory time, pressure, volume, or flow do not match the patient's inspiratory demands. An example of this would be if an operator set a mandatory rate of 12 and an inspiratory time of 3.0 seconds. The total cycle time would be 5 seconds (60 seconds per minute divided by 12 breaths per minute). A patient's comfort and synchrony may be compromised if the patient is forced to breathe at a set inspiratory time of 3 seconds and an expiratory time of 2 seconds. However, the active exhalation valve allows the ventilator to deliver the mandatory breaths at the operator-set cycle times for inspiration and expiration. The patient, by virtue of the active exhalation valve, may breathe spontaneously at any time in the breathing cycle.

There has been no consistent abbreviation created to signify a breathing pattern composed of all spontaneous breaths. However, the logical progression would be from CMV to IMV to CSV (continuous spontaneous ventilation). Spontaneous breath modes include those in which all inspirations are initiated or triggered and ended or cycled by the patient. The level of support this mode of ventilation provides determines the amount of work of breathing the patient will ultimately assume. For patients who do not require full ventilatory support, pressure control CSV (PC-CSV) may be used to reduce the work of breathing and/or to improve or stabilize oxygenation by reducing alveolar derecruitment.[24–26] Pressure support ventilation and CPAP are examples of PC-CSV. Pressure support ventilation is a form of PC-CSV that assists the patient's inspiratory efforts. Pressure support ventilation (PSV) is effective in unloading the work of breathing the ventilator circuitry imposes on the respiratory muscles.[27,28] As pressure support levels are increased, the ventilator assumes more of the work of breathing and at maximal levels may assume all of the work of breathing.[29] High levels of pressure support result in a reduction in respiratory rate, muscle activity, and fatigue, as well as an improvement or stabilization of spontaneous tidal volumes and reduction in oxygen consumption.[30] Regardless of the level of support provided, the patient has primary control over the breath rate and the inspiratory time and flow rate delivered during PSV.

CPAP provides no ventilatory assist or inspiratory muscle unloading. Low levels of CPAP (3–5 cm H_2O)

prevent alveolar collapse at end-expiration.[31] If CPAP is set too high, air trapping and alveolar overdistension results.[31] Circulatory impairment may also result from a decrease in left ventricular stroke volume. Cardiac output and arterial blood pressure are compromised, which inhibits adequate oxygen delivery.[32]

Targeting Scheme

There are two general ways to control a variable: open-loop control and closed-loop control.[33] **Open-loop control** is essentially no control. Early high-frequency ventilators are an example of open-loop control. Pulses of gas flow were generated by the ventilator without measurement or control of pressure, volume, or flow. Flow into the patient was a function of the relative impedances of the respiratory system and the exhalation manifold. Any disturbance in the system, such as changing lung mechanics, leaks, or a change in the patient's ventilatory efforts, affected tidal volume delivery and airway pressures. Conversely, delivered pressure, volume, and flow can be measured with **closed-loop control** and used as feedback information to control the driving mechanism. Inspiratory volumes, flows, and pressures can be made to match or follow operator-set values and are not affected by disturbances such as minor leaks in the system or changes in patient load.

The basic concept of closed-loop control has evolved into several different ventilator control systems, which form the foundation that makes possible several dozen apparently different modes of ventilation. Once one understands how setpoint, dual, servo, adaptive, optimal, and intelligent control work, many of the apparent differences are seen to be similarities. This will also clear the confusion surrounding ventilator marketing and provide a better appreciation of the true clinical capabilities of different ventilators.

Setpoint Control

Setpoint control means that the output is manipulated to match a constant preset input, making standard volume or pressure control breaths possible. The operator either sets a fixed pressure or flow target, and the ventilator then maintains a consistent pressure or flow waveform output. This type of control is analogous to cruise control on an automobile.

Dual Control

Dual control is a more advanced version of setpoint control. It allows the ventilator to switch between volume and pressure control during a given inspiration according to operator-set priorities. The breath may start out in volume control and automatically switch to pressure control. The Dräger Evita 4 uses auto-setpoint control with the Pmax feature. Conversely, inspiration may start out in pressure control and switch to volume control, as with volume-assured pressure support (VAPS).

Servo Control

Servo control is dynamic and able to track a moving input, much like power steering on an automobile. The ventilator's output follows and amplifies the patient's own flow pattern. This control type enables the ventilator to support the abnormal load imposed by disease or in artificial airway adjuncts such as endotracheal tubes, while the patient's own muscles handle a normal load due to the respiratory system's natural resistance and compliance. Servo control makes possible proportional assist ventilation[34] and tube compensation.[35]

Adaptive Control

Adaptive control allows automatic adjustment of one target over several breaths to maintain a different operator-selected target. This control type provides the ventilator with the capability to determine a target level independent of the operator. Whereas setpoint control operates within breaths, adaptive control introduces another feedback loop that operates between breaths. Pressure-regulated volume control (PRVC), a feature on the Servo 300 ventilator, is one of the earliest examples of the use of adaptive control. The ventilator monitors patient's lung mechanics and volume on a breath-by-breath basis during PRVC. Should tidal volume fall below or rise above the operator-set target value, the ventilator will automatically adjust the set pressure limit, over the course of several breaths, to bring the patient's exhaled volume closer to the set target volume. The VersaMed iVent uses adaptive control schemes during volume control to maintain a constant inspiration-to-expiration ratio of 1:2 independent of the patient's breathing frequency.

Optimal Control

Optimal control is an advanced form of adaptive control. The term *optimum* refers to the automatic selection of parameters to either minimize or maximize some performance variable. The Hamilton G5 ventilator uses such a scheme to set the frequency and inspiratory pressure of mandatory breaths during PC-IMV. The optimal control algorithm seeks to achieve a ventilatory pattern that minimizes the work rate of breathing.[36] However, the clinician must set other parameters, such as PEEP, F_{IO_2}, and alarm settings.

Intelligent Control

The term *intelligent control* refers to automatic control strategies that make use of artificial intelligence. Ventilator control systems using fuzzy logic[37,38] and rule-based expert systems[39] have been reported. To date, the only commercial system available as a mode of ventilation is SmartCare (Dräger Evita XL ventilator). SmartCare continuously enacts a weaning protocol in pressure support mode based on measurements of respiratory rate, tidal volume, and the partial pressure of end-tidal carbon dioxide. The algorithm aims

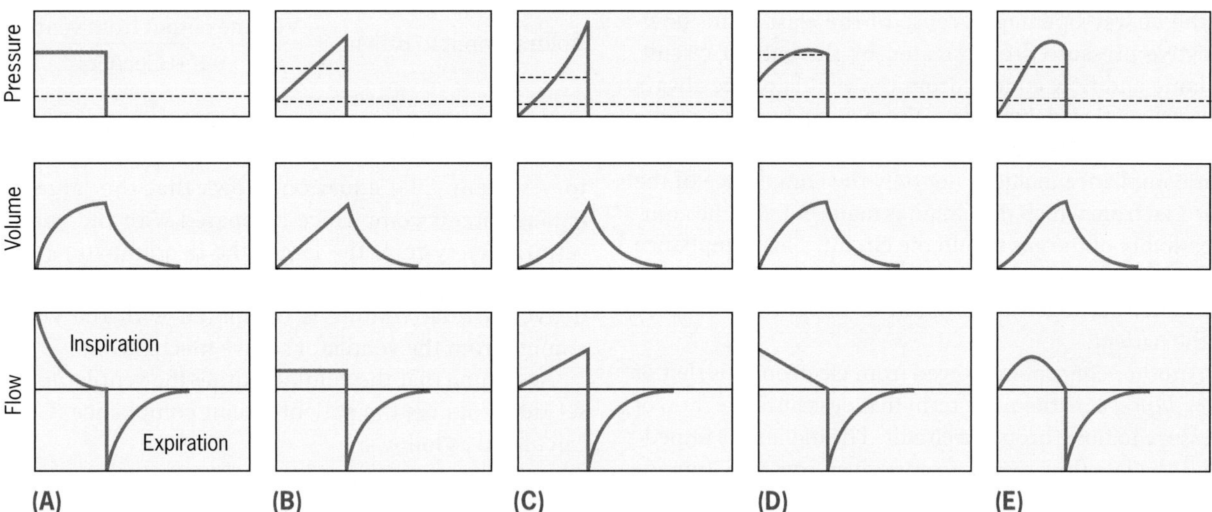

FIGURE 21–8 Typical pressure, volume, and flow waveforms for pressure control (rectangular pressure waveform) and volume control (various flow waveforms) ventilation. The curves show pressure, volume, and flow as functions of time in accordance with the equation of motion (where muscle pressure is 0). The upper dotted line represents mean inspiratory pressure while the lower dotted line represents mean airway pressure measured over one ventilatory period. (**A**) Pressure control ventilation with a rectangular pressure waveform. Mean inspiratory pressure is equal to peak inspiratory pressure. (**B**) Volume control ventilation with a rectangular flow waveform. (**C**) Volume control ventilation with an ascending ramp flow waveform. (**D**) Volume control ventilation with a descending ramp flow waveform. (**E**) Volume control ventilation with a sinusoidal flow waveform.

to maintain patients in a "comfort zone" of respiration by adapting the inspiratory pressure and automatically initiates a spontaneous breathing trial when patients meet predefined criteria.[40] A multicenter trial has provided evidence that SmartCare can reduce the duration of mechanical ventilation and intensive care unit length of stay compared with a physician-controlled weaning process.[41,42]

Output

The study of ventilator operation requires the examination of output waveforms. The waveforms of interest are pressure, volume, and flow waveforms. For each control variable, a limited number of waveforms commonly are used by currently available ventilators. These waveforms can be idealized as shown in **Figure 21–8** and can be grouped into four basic categories: rectangular (pulse), exponential, ramp, and sinusoidal. A rectangular volume waveform is theoretically impossible because volume cannot change instantaneously from zero to some preset value as can pressure and flow.

Characteristic idealized ventilator output waveforms, shown in **Table 21–3**, are precisely defined by mathematic equations and are meant to characterize the operation of the ventilator's control system. As such, they do not show the minor deviations or "noise" often seen in waveforms recorded during actual ventilator use. These waveform imperfections can be caused by a variety of extraneous variables, such as vibration and turbulence, and the appearance of the waveform is affected by the scaling of the time axis. The waveforms also do not show the effects of the resistance of the expiratory side of the patient circuit because this factor varies depending on the ventilator and type of circuit.

RESPIRATORY RECAP

Ventilator Output Waveforms

- » Rectangular
- » Exponential
- » Ramp
- » Sinusoidal

No ventilator is an ideal controller, and ventilators are designed only to approximate a particular waveform. Idealized, or standard, waveforms are nevertheless helpful because they are common in other fields (e.g., electrical engineering), which permit the use of mathematic procedures and terminology that have already been developed. For example, a standard mathematic equation is used to describe the most common waveforms for each control variable. This known equation may be substituted into the equation of motion, which is then solved to obtain the equations of the other two variables. Once the equations for pressure, volume, and flow are known, they are easily graphed (refer to Figure 21–8).

Effects of the Patient Circuit

The pressure, volume, and flow measured inside the ventilator are never the same as pressure, volume, and flow measured at the patient's airway opening. The reason, of course, is that the patient circuit has its own compliance (actually, the compliance of the tubing material plus the compressibility of the inspired gas) and resistance. Therefore, the pressure measured inside the ventilator on the inspiratory side (e.g., on older ventilators such as the Bennett MA-1) is always higher than the pressure at the airway opening because of the elastic and flow-resistive pressure drops created by the patient circuit. Volume and flow coming from the ventilator are always more than that delivered to the patient because of the effective compliance of the patient circuit. Patient circuit compliance includes not only the compliance of the material from which the circuit is made but also the compressibility of the gas within the circuit. This compliance effect absorbs both volume and flow. Compliance and resistance act together to retard or impede gas delivery to the patient.

Another concept borrowed from electronics is that of *impedance,* a mathematic term that describes the ratio of pressure to flow through a circuit. The higher the impedance, the less flow results from a given pressure. Impedance is directly proportional to resistance and elastance and inversely proportional to compliance. Table 21–3 illustrates the effects of the patient circuit on rectangular pressure and flow waveforms.

Using an analogy to electrical circuits, compliance of the delivery circuit can be shown to be connected in parallel with the compliance of the respiratory system (i.e., both elements sharing the same driving pressure). Pneumatic compliance is analogous to electrical capacitance, and pneumatic resistance is analogous to electrical resistance.[11] Therefore, the total compliance of the ventilator–patient system is simply the sum of the two compliances. Similarly, the resistance of the delivery circuit is connected in series with the respiratory system resistance (i.e., both elements sharing the same flow) so that the total resistance is the sum of the two. From these assumptions, the relation between the volume input to the patient (at the point of connection to the patient's airway opening) and the volume output from the ventilator (at the point of connection to the patient circuit) can be shown to be described by the following equation:

$$\text{Volume input to patient} = \frac{\text{Volume output from ventilator}}{1 + \text{Cpc/Crs}}$$

where Cpc is the compliance of the patient circuit, and Crs is the total compliance of the patient's respiratory system. The equation shows that the larger the patient circuit compliance compared with the patient's respiratory system, the larger the denominator on the right-hand side of the equation. Hence, the smaller the delivered tidal volume is compared with the volume coming from the ventilator's drive mechanism.

Assuming that the volume exiting the ventilator is the set tidal volume, the patient circuit compliance (Cpc) is calculated as follows:

$$\text{Cpc} = \frac{\text{Set tidal volume}}{\text{Pplat} - \text{PEEP}}$$

where Pplat is the pressure measured during an inspiratory hold maneuver with the Y piece of the patient circuit occluded (patient not connected), and PEEP is end-expiratory pressure (i.e., baseline pressure). The use of peak airway pressure (PAP) for Pplat in this equation is acceptable but may lead to a slight underestimation of patient circuit compliance. Pplat is slightly lower than PAP because of the flow-resistive pressure drop of the patient circuit if pressure is not measured at the Y piece. This difference is greatest in small-bore, corrugated patient circuit tubing but is probably insignificant.

The effects of patient circuit compliance are most troublesome during volume control ventilation. For example, in neonatal ventilation the patient circuit compliance can be as much as three times that of the respiratory system, even with small-bore tubing and a small-volume humidifier. Thus, in an attempt to deliver a preset tidal volume, the volume delivered to the patient may be as little as 25% of that exiting the ventilator, whereas 75% is compressed in the patient circuit.

During pressure control ventilation, the compliance of the patient circuit has the effect of rounding the leading edge of a rectangular pressure waveform (refer to Table 21–3), which could reduce the volume delivered to the patient. This effect is prevented if the pressure limit is maintained for at least five time constants of the respiratory system.

For both pressure control and volume control ventilation,

TABLE 21–3 The Effects of Loading (by Patient Circuit and Lung Mechanics) on Ventilator Output

Ventilator Type	Respiratory System Impedance	Load Effect	Desired Waveform	Actual Waveform
Pressure controller	Low	Large		
	High	Small		
Volume controller	Low	Small		
	High	Large		

the patient circuit compliance and resistance, along with the resistance of the exhalation valve (in series with the patient circuit and respiratory system resistance), increase the expiratory time constant. Thus, a large circuit compliance coupled with a short expiratory time can lead to inadvertent or auto-PEEP.

In summary, the set values for pressure, volume, and flow may be different from the output (from the ventilator) values due to calibration errors, and may be different from the input (to the patient) values due to the effects of the patient circuit. Thus, two general sources of error cause discrepancies between the desired and actual patient values.

Ventilator Alarm Systems

The ventilator classification scheme described previously centers on the basic functions of input, control, and output. If any of these functions fails, a life-threatening situation may result. Therefore ventilators are equipped with various types of alarms, which may be classified in the same manner as the other major ventilator characteristics.

Day and MacIntyre have stressed that the goal of ventilator alarms is to warn the operator of events.[43,44] They define an **alarm event** as any condition or occurrence that requires the clinician's awareness or action. Technical events are those involving an inadvertent change in the ventilator's performance; patient events are those involving a change in the patient's clinical status that can be detected by the ventilator.[45] A ventilator may be equipped with any conceivable vital sign monitor, but the scope of this discussion is limited to the ventilator's mechanical/electronic operation and those variables associated with the mechanics of breathing (i.e., pressure, volume, flow, time). Because the ventilator is in intimate contact with exhaled gas, analyses of exhaled oxygen and carbon dioxide concentrations are included as possible variables to monitor.

RESPIRATORY RECAP

Ventilator Alarms:
- » Input power alarms
- » Control circuit alarms
- » Output alarms

Alarms may be audible, visual, or both, depending on the seriousness of the alarm condition. Visual alarms may be as simple as colored lights or as complex as alphanumeric messages to the operator indicating the exact nature of the fault condition. Specifications for an alarm event should include (1) the conditions that trigger the alarm, (2) the alarm response in the form of audible and/or visual messages, (3) any associated ventilator response, such as termination of inspiration or failure to operate, and (4) whether the alarm must be manually reset or will reset itself when the alarm condition is rectified. Alarm categories are based on the ventilator classification scheme and are detailed in the following discussion.

Input Power Alarms

Most ventilators have some sort of battery backup in the case of electrical power failure, even if the batteries only power alarms. Ventilators typically have alarms that are activated if the electrical power is cut off while the machine is still switched on (e.g., if the power cord is accidentally pulled from the wall socket). If the ventilator is designed to operate on battery power (e.g., transport ventilators), an alarm usually is designed to warn of a low-battery condition.

Ventilators that use pneumatic power have alarms that are activated if either the oxygen or air supply is cut off or reduced below some specified driving pressure. In some cases, the alarm is activated by an electronic pressure switch (e.g., the Puritan-Bennett 7200), but in other cases the alarm is pneumatically operated as a part of the blender (e.g., the Servo 900C).

Control Circuit Alarms

Control circuit alarms are those that either warn the operator that the set control variable parameters are incompatible (e.g., inverse inspiration-to-expiration ratio) or indicate that some aspect of a ventilator self-test has failed. In the latter case, something may be wrong with the ventilator control circuitry itself (e.g., a microprocessor failure), and the ventilator generally responds with some generic message such as "ventilator inoperative."

Output Alarms

Output alarms are those triggered by an unacceptable state of the ventilator's output. More specifically, an output alarm is activated when the value of a control variable (i.e., pressure, volume, flow, time) falls outside an expected range (**Table 21-4**). Because ventilators are designed to control the mechanical results of exhalation, they may be easily adapted to the analysis of exhaled gas composition, and alarms may be set for the following specific parameters:

- *Exhaled carbon dioxide tension*: End-tidal carbon dioxide monitoring may reflect arterial carbon dio-xide tension and thus indicate the level of ventilation. Calculation of mean expired carbon dioxide tension along with minute ventilation measurements could provide information about carbon dioxide production and contribute to the calculation of the respiratory exchange ratio and the ratio of the tidal volume–to–dead space ratio.
- *Exhaled oxygen tension*: Analysis of end-tidal and mean expired oxygen tension may provide information about gas exchange and could be used along with carbon dioxide data to calculate the respiratory exchange ratio.[46]

TABLE 21-4 Output Alarms

Pressure Alarms • *High and low peak airway pressure*: These alarms occur when a possible endotracheal tube obstruction or leak in the patient circuit, respectively, occurs. • *High and low mean airway pressure*: These alarms indicate a possible leak in the patient circuit or a change in ventilatory pattern that might lead to a change in the patient's oxygenation status. That is, within reasonable limits, oxygenation is roughly proportional to mean airway pressure, or the average pressure (relative to atmospheric pressure) that is applied to the airway during a breath. • *High and low baseline pressure*: These alarms indicate a possible patient circuit or exhalation manifold obstruction (or inadvertent PEEP) and disconnection of the patient from the patient circuit, respectively. • *Failure to return to baseline*: Failure of airway pressure to return to the baseline level within a specified period indicates a possible patient circuit obstruction or exhalation manifold malfunction.
Volume Alarms • *High and low expired volume*: These alarms indicate changes in respiratory system time constant during pressure control ventilation, leaks around the endotracheal tube or from the lungs, or possible disconnection of the patient from the patient circuit.
Flow Alarms • *High and low expired minute ventilation*: These alarms indicate hyperventilation (or possible machine self-triggering) or possible apnea or disconnection of the patient from the patient circuit.
Time Alarms • *High or low ventilatory frequency*: When these alarms activate, hyperventilation (or possible machine self-triggering) or apnea may be happening. • *Inappropriate inspiratory time*: A too-long inspiratory time indicates a possible patient circuit obstruction or exhalation manifold malfunction. A too-short inspiratory time indicates that adequate tidal volume may not be delivered (in a pressure controlled mode) or that gas distribution in the lungs may not be optimal. • *Inappropriate expiratory time*: A too-long expiratory time may indicate apnea, whereas a too-short expiratory time may warn of alveolar gas trapping. That is, expiratory time should be at least five time constants of the respiratory system.
Inspired Gas Alarms • High/low inspired gas temperature • High/low F_{IO_2}
Expired Gas Alarms

KEY POINTS

- The equation of motion can be used to describe the pressure required to move a flow of gas into the lungs and produce a tidal volume during mechanical ventilation.
- During pressure control ventilation, pressure is the independent variable, and the shapes of the volume and flow waveforms depend on the shape of the pressure waveform and the resistance and compliance of the respiratory system.
- During volume control ventilation, volume is the independent variable, and the shape of the flow waveform depends on the shape of the volume waveform, with the pressure waveform depending on the flow waveform and on the resistance and compliance of the respiratory system.
- A ventilator can directly control only one variable at a time: pressure, volume, or flow.
- A ventilator can be classified as either a pressure, volume, or flow controller.
- The trigger variable initiates the inspiratory phase, which can be initiated either by the ventilator (i.e., time) or by the patient (e.g., pressure, flow).
- The ventilator may target pressure, volume, or flow during the inspiratory phase.
- The variable that is measured and used to terminate the inspiratory phase is the cycle variable.
- Mandatory breaths are machine triggered, machine cycled, or both; spontaneous breaths are patient triggered and patient cycled.
- Pressure control occurs when the ventilator attempts to maintain a set airway pressure waveform during inspiration; volume control occurs when the ventilator attempts to maintain a preset volume or flow waveform during inspiration.
- Output control waveforms on ventilators are rectangular, exponential, ramp, and sinusoidal.
- The compliance, compressibility, and resistance of the ventilator circuit affect gas delivery between the ventilator and the patient.
- Ventilator alarms can be classified as input power alarms, control circuit alarms, and output alarms.

REFERENCES

1. Mushin M, Rendell-Baker W, Thompson PW, et al. *Automatic Ventilation of the Lungs*. Oxford: Blackwell Scientific Publications; 1980:62–166.
2. Colice GL. Historical perspective on the development of mechanical ventilation. In: Tobin MJ, ed. *Principles and Practice of Mechanical Ventilation*. 2nd ed. New York: McGraw-Hill; 2006:1–36.

3. Consensus statement on the essentials of mechanical ventilators 1992. *Respir Care.* 1992;37:1000–1008.
4. Chatburn RL. Classification of mechanical ventilators. *Respir Care.* 1992;37:1009–1025.
5. Branson RD, Chatburn RL. Technical description and classification of modes of ventilator operation. *Respir Care.* 1992;37:1026–1044.
6. Chatburn RL. Classification of ventilator modes: update and proposal for implementation. *Respir Care.* 2007;52(3):301–323.
7. Viasys Healthcare. LTV 800 ventilator. Available at: http://www.viasyshealthcare.com/prod_serv/prodDetail.aspx?config=ps_prodDtl&prodID=111. Accessed December 28, 2009.
8. Allied Healthcare Products. Mass casualty ventilator models: MCV100 and MCV100-B. Available at: http://www.alliedhpi.com/images/mcv100_instruction_manual.pdf. Accessed December 28, 2009.
9. Otis AB, McKerrow CB, Bartlett RA, et al. Mechanical factors in distribution of pulmonary ventilation. *J Appl Physiol.* 1956;8:427–443.
10. Muniz J, Guerrero JE, Escalante JL, Palomino R, DeLaCalle B. Pressure-controlled ventilation versus controlled mechanical ventilation with a decelerating inspiratory flow. *Crit Care Med.* 1993;21(8):1143–1148.
11. Chatburn RL, Primiano FP Jr. Mathematical models of respiratory mechanics. In: Chatburn RL, Craig KC, eds. *Fundamentals of Respiratory Care Research.* Stamford, CT: Appleton & Lange; 1988.
12. *The American Heritage Dictionary.* New York; Dell Publishing Company; 1983.
13. Hess D, Lind L. Nomograms for the application of the Bourns Model BP200 as a volume-constant ventilator. *Respir Care.* 1980;25:248–250.
14. Desautels DA. Ventilator performance evaluation. In: Kirby RR, Smith RA, Desautels DA, eds. *Mechanical Ventilation.* New York: Churchill Livingstone; 1985:120.
15. Sassoon CSH, Giron AE, Ely EA, et al. Inspiratory work of breathing on flow-by and demand-flow continuous positive airway pressure. *Crit Care Med.* 1989;17:1108–1114.
16. Branson RD. Flow-triggering systems. *Respir Care.* 1994;42:138.
17. Sassoon CS, Foster GT. Patient–ventilator asynchrony. *Curr Opin Crit Care.* 2001;7:28–33.
18. De Wit M, Miller KB, Green DA, et al. Ineffective triggering predicts increased duration of mechanical ventilation. *Crit Care Med.* 2009;37(10):2740–2745.
19. Thille AW, Rodriguez P, Cabello B, Lellouche F, Brochard L. Patient-ventilator asynchrony during assisted mechanical ventilation. *Intensive Care Med.* 2006;32(10):1515–1522.
20. Chatburn RL. *Fundamentals of Mechanical Ventilation.* Cleveland Heights, OH: Mandu Press; 2004.
21. Stock MC, Downs JB, Frolicher DA. Airway pressure release ventilation. *Crit Care Med.* 1987;15(5):462–463.
22. Baum M, Benzer H, Putensen C, Koller W, Putz G. Biphasic positive airway pressure (BIPAP)—a new form of augmented ventilation [in German]. *Anaesthesist.* 1989;38(9):452–458.
23. MacIntyre NR. Respiratory function during pressure support ventilation. *Chest.* 1986;89:677.
24. Migliori C, Çavazza A, Motta M, Chirico G. Effect on respiratory function of pressure support ventilation versus synchronised intermittent mandatory ventilation in preterm infants. *Pediatr Pulmonol.* 2003;35(5):364–367.
25. el-Khatib MF, Chatburn RL, Potts DL, Blumer JL, Smith PG. Mechanical ventilators optimized for pediatric use decrease work of breathing and oxygen consumption during pressure-support ventilation. *Crit Care Med.* 1994;22(12):1942–1948.
26. Brochard L, Pluskwa F, Lemaire F. Improved efficacy of spontaneous breathing with inspiratory pressure support. *Am Rev Respir Dis.* 1987;136:411.
27. Chittawatanarat K, Thongchai C. Spontaneous breathing trial with low pressure support protocol for weaning respirator in surgical ICU. *J Med Assoc Thai.* 2009;92(10):1306–1312.
28. MacIntyre NR. Pressure support ventilation: effects on ventilatory reflexes and ventilatory muscle workload. *Respir Care.* 1987;32:447.
29. Shikora SA, MacDonald GF, Bistrian BR, Kenney PR, Benotti PN. Could the oxygen cost of breathing be used to optimize the application of pressure support ventilation? *J Trauma.* 1992;33(4):521–526.
30. Tunsmann G, et al. Alveolar recruitment strategy improves arterial oxygenation during general anesthesia. *Br J Anaesth.* 1999;82:8.
31. Klerk AM, Klerk RK. Nasal continuous positive airway pressure and outcomes for preterm infants. *Neonatal Intensive Care.* 2001;14:58.
32. Dinger J, et al. Effect of positive end expiratory pressure on functional residual capacity and compliance in surfactant-treated preterm infants. *Neonatal Intensive Care.* 2001;14:26.
33. Chatburn RL. Computer control of mechanical ventilation. *Respir Care.* 2004;49(5):507–515.
34. Younes M. Proportional assist ventilation, a new approach to ventilatory support: theory. *Am Rev Respir Dis.* 1992;145:121–129.
35. Haberthür C, Lichtwarck-Aschoff M, Guttmann J. Continuous monitoring of tracheal pressure including spot-check of endotracheal tube resistance. *Technol Health Care.* 2003;11:413–424.
36. Brunner JX, Iotti GA. Adaptive support ventilation (ASV). *Minerva Anesthesiol.* 2002;68:365–368.
37. Nemoto T, Hatzakis GE, Thorpe CW, Olivenstein R, Dial S, Bates JH. Automatic control of pressure support mechanical ventilation using fuzzy logic. *Am J Respir Crit Care Med.* 1999;160:550–556.
38. Bates JH, Hatzakis GE, Olivenstein R. Fuzzy logic and mechanical ventilation. *Respir Care Clin North Am.* 2001;7:363–377.
39. Dojat M, Brochard L. Knowledge-based systems for automatic ventilatory management. *Respir Care Clin North Am.* 2001;7:379–396.
40. Burns KE, Lellouche F, Lessard MR. Automating the weaning process with advanced closed-loop systems. *Intensive Care Med.* 2008;34:1757–1765.
41. Lellouche F, Mancebo J, Jolliet P, et al. A multicenter randomized trial of computer-driven protocolized weaning from mechanical ventilation. *Am J Respir Crit Care Med.* 2006;174:894–900.
42. Wysocki M, Brunner JX. Closed-loop ventilation: an emerging standard of care? *Crit Care Clin.* 2007;23:223–240.
43. Day S, MacIntyre NR. Ventilator alarm systems. *Probl Respir Care.* 1991;4:118–126.
44. MacIntyre NR, Day S. Essentials for ventilator-alarm systems. *Respir Care.* 1992;37:1108–1112.
45. Russell DF, Ross DG, Manson HJ. Fluidic cycling devices for inspiratory and expiratory timing in automatic ventilators. *J Biomed Eng.* 1983;5:227–234.
46. Weingarten M. Respiratory monitoring of carbon dioxide and oxygen: a ten-year perspective. *J Clin Monit.* 1990;6:217–225.

CHAPTER 22

Mechanical Ventilation

Dean R. Hess
Neil R. MacIntyre

OUTLINE

OBJECTIVES

1. List the indications for and complications of mechanical ventilation.
2. Discuss issues related to ventilator-associated lung injury.
3. Select appropriate ventilator settings.
4. List parameters that should be monitored during mechanical ventilation.
5. Discuss issues related to liberation from mechanical ventilation.

KEY TERMS

adaptive pressure control
adaptive support ventilation (ASV)
airway pressure release ventilation (APRV)
auto-PEEP
compressible volume
continuous mandatory ventilation (CMV)
continuous positive airway pressure (CPAP)
flow triggering
high-frequency oscillatory ventilation (HFOV)
intermittent mandatory ventilation
lung-protective ventilator strategy
mean airway pressure ($\bar{P}aw$)
neurally adjusted ventilatory assist (NAVA)
oxygen toxicity
patient–ventilator asynchrony
peak inspiratory pressure (PIP)
permissive hypercapnia
plateau pressure
positive end-expiratory pressure (PEEP)
pressure control ventilation (PCV)
pressure support ventilation (PSV)
pressure triggering
proportional assist ventilation (PAV)
spontaneous breathing trial (SBT)
synchronized intermittent mandatory ventilation (SIMV)
transpulmonary pressure
ventilator-induced lung injury (VILI)
volume control ventilation (VCV)
weaning parameters

INTRODUCTION

Mechanical ventilation is an important life support technology that is an integral component of critical care. Mechanical ventilation can be applied as negative pressure to the outside of the thorax (e.g., the iron lung) or, most often, as positive pressure to the airway. The desired effect of positive pressure ventilation is to maintain adequate levels of Pa_{O_2} and Pa_{CO_2} while also unloading the inspiratory muscles. Mechanical ventilation is a life-sustaining technology, but recognition is growing that when used incorrectly, it can increase morbidity and mortality. Positive pressure ventilation is provided in intensive care units (ICUs), subacute facilities, long-term care facilities, and the home. Positive pressure ventilation can be invasive (i.e., with an endotracheal tube or tracheostomy tube) or noninvasive (e.g., with a face mask). This chapter addresses invasive positive pressure ventilation as it is applied in adults with acute respiratory failure. Modern ventilators used in the intensive care unit are microprocessor controlled and available from several manufacturers (**Figure 22–1** and **Figure 22–2**).

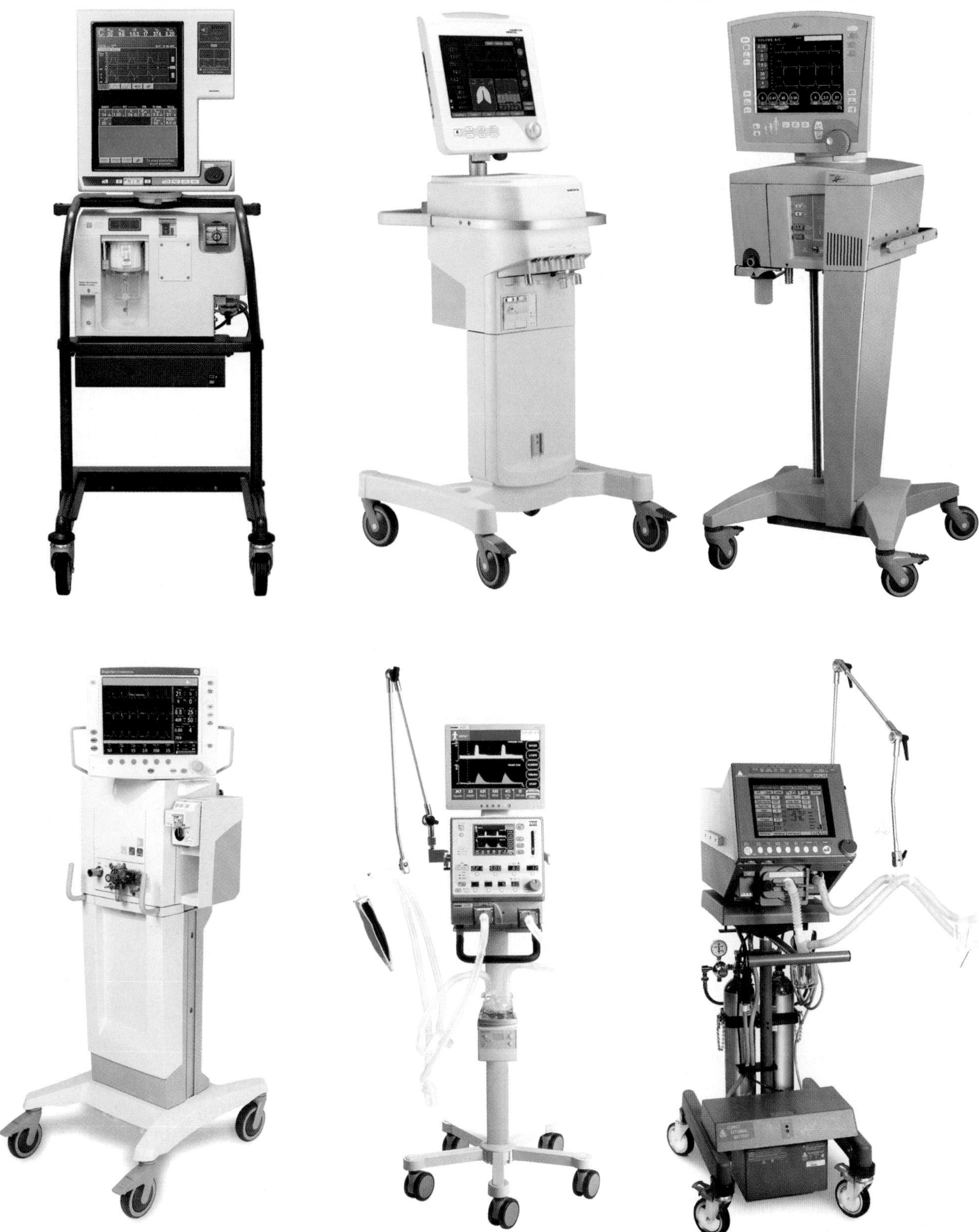

FIGURE 22–1 Examples of mechanical ventilators commonly used in critical care in the United States.

The Equation of Motion

Positive pressure, when applied at the airway opening, interacts with respiratory system (lung and chest wall) compliance, airways resistance, respiratory system inertance, and tissue resistance to produce gas flow into the lung. Inertance and tissue resistance are small and their effects are usually ignored. The interactions of airway pressure (Paw), respiratory muscle pressure (Pmus), flow, and volume with respiratory system mechanics can be expressed as the equation of motion:

$$\text{Paw} + \text{Pmus} = (\text{Flow} \times \text{Resistance}) + (\text{Volume}/\text{Compliance})$$

For spontaneous breathing, Paw = 0 and all of the pressure required for ventilation is provided by the respiratory muscles. For full ventilatory support, Pmus = 0 and all of the pressure required for ventilation is provided by the ventilator. For partial ventilatory support, both the ventilator and the respiratory muscles contribute to ventilation.

For full ventilatory support, the ventilator controls either the pressure or the flow and volume applied to the airway. The equation of motion predicts that Paw will vary for a given resistance and compliance if flow and volume are controlled (volume-targeted ventilation). The equation of motion also predicts that flow and volume will vary for a given resistance and compliance if Paw is controlled (pressure-targeted ventilation).

An important point to remember in considering the equation of motion is that in the setting of high minute ventilation, long inspiratory-to-expiratory time ratios, and prolonged expiratory time constants (e.g., as seen in obstructive lung disease), the lungs may not return to the baseline circuit pressure during exhalation. This creates **auto-PEEP**, which must be counteracted by Pmus and Paw in the equation of motion to affect flow and volume delivery.

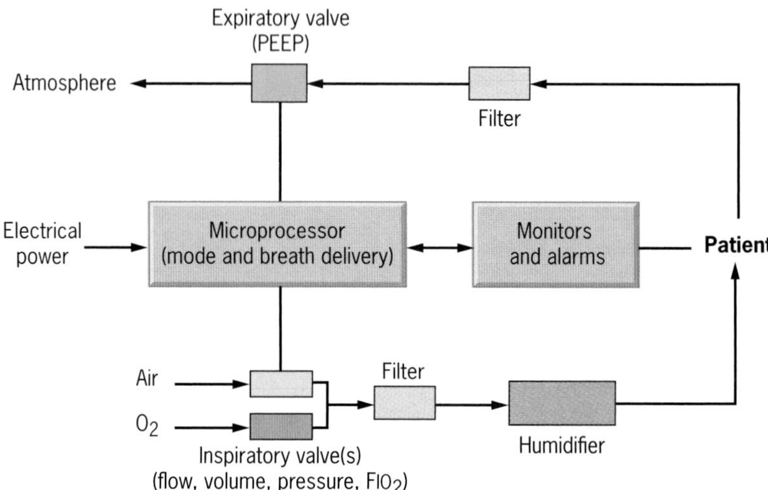

FIGURE 22–2 Modern ventilators are electronically and pneumatically controlled. The inspiratory valves control flow, pressure, and FIO_2 to the patient. The expiratory valve is closed during the inspiratory phase and the inspiratory valve is closed during the expiratory phase. The expiratory valve controls positive end-expiratory pressure (PEEP). The inspiratory and expiratory valves are controlled by the microprocessor. Sensors measure pressure and flow, which are displayed as numeric and graphic data and determine when an alarm condition is generated.

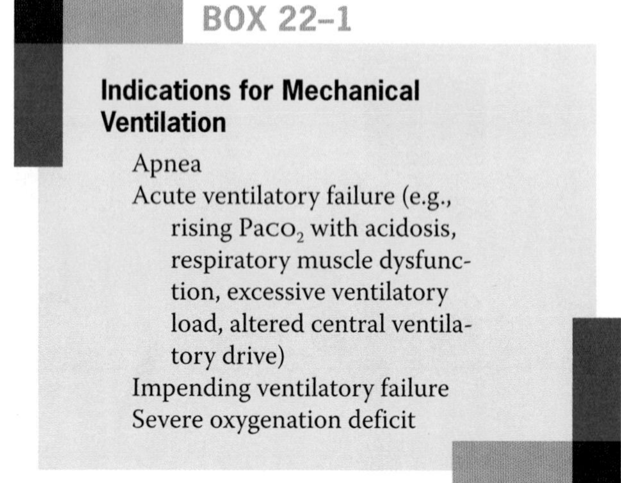

BOX 22–1

Indications for Mechanical Ventilation

- Apnea
- Acute ventilatory failure (e.g., rising $PaCO_2$ with acidosis, respiratory muscle dysfunction, excessive ventilatory load, altered central ventilatory drive)
- Impending ventilatory failure
- Severe oxygenation deficit

Indications for Mechanical Ventilation

Mechanical ventilation is indicated in many situations (**Box 22–1**).[1] Goals of mechanical ventilation are shown in **Box 22–2**. Although these conditions are useful in the determination of whether mechanical ventilation is needed, clinical judgment is as important as strict adherence to absolute guidelines. One indication for mechanical ventilation is imminent acute respiratory failure; in such cases, initiating mechanical ventilation may prevent overt respiratory failure and respiratory arrest. On the other hand, depression of respiratory drive from drug overdose or from anesthesia involved with major surgery is an indication that does not involve primary respiratory system failure. In short, mechanical ventilation is required when the patient's capabilities to ventilate the lung and/or effect gas transport across the alveolocapillary interface is compromised to the point that the patient's life is threatened.

Complications of Mechanical Ventilation

Mechanical ventilation is not a benign therapy, and it can have major effects on the body's homeostasis (**Box 22–3**).[2] In addition to the serious complications reviewed here associated with positive pressure applied to the lungs,[3] intubated mechanically ventilated patients also are at risk for complications associated with the use of artificial airways,[4] the most serious being accidental disconnection and the development of pneumonia from compromised natural airway defenses. Mechanically ventilated patients are also at risk for gastrointestinal bleeding[5] and often are given antacids, proton pump inhibitors, or histamine (H_2) blockers to prevent this complication. The nutritional needs of mechanically ventilated patients play an important role in preventing or promoting complications.[6] Undernourished patients are at risk for respiratory muscle weakness and pneumonia. An excessive caloric intake, on the other hand, may increase carbon dioxide (CO_2) production, which can markedly increase the patient's ventilatory requirements. Sleep deprivation in mechanically ventilated patients has recently become recognized.[7]

BOX 22-2

Goals of Mechanical Ventilation

Provide adequate oxygenation
Provide adequate alveolar ventilation
Avoid alveolar overdistension
Maintain alveolar recruitment
Promote patient–ventilator synchrony
Avoid auto-PEEP
Use the lowest possible F_{IO_2}
When choosing appropriate goals of mechanical ventilation for an individual patient, consider the risk of ventilator-induced lung injury.

Ventilator-Induced Lung Injury

The application of positive pressure to the airways can create lung injury under a variety of circumstances. Pulmonary barotrauma (e.g., subcutaneous emphysema, pneumothorax, pneumomediastinum) is one of the most serious complications of excessive pressure and volume delivery to the lung and is a consequence of alveolar overdistention to the point of rupture (**Figure 22-3**).[3] However, even when the lung is not distended to the point of rupture, excessive transpulmonary stretching pressures

RESPIRATORY RECAP

Types of Ventilator-Induced Lung Injury

» Volutrauma
» Atelectrauma
» Biotrauma
» Oxygen toxicity

BOX 22-3

Complications of Mechanical Ventilation

Airway Complications
Laryngeal edema
Tracheal mucosal trauma
Contamination of the lower respiratory tract
Loss of humidifying function of the upper airway

Mechanical Complications
Accidental disconnection
Leaks in the ventilator circuit
Loss of electrical power
Loss of gas pressure

Pulmonary Complications
Ventilator-induced lung injury
Barotrauma
Oxygen toxicity
Atelectasis
Nosocomial pneumonia
Inflammation
Auto-PEEP
Asynchrony

Cardiovascular Complications
Reduced venous return
Reduced cardiac output
Hypotension

Gastrointestinal and Nutritional Complications
Gastrointestinal bleeding
Malnutrition

Renal Complications
Reduced urine output
Increase in antidiuretic hormone (ADH) and decrease in atrial natriuretic peptide (ANP)

Neuromuscular Complications
Sleep deprivation
Increased intracranial pressure
Critical illness weakness

Acid–Base Complications
Respiratory acidosis
Respiratory alkalosis

beyond the normal maximum (i.e., 30 to 35 cm H_2O) can produce a parenchymal lung injury not associated with extra-alveolar air (**ventilator-induced lung injury [VILI]**).[8] Importantly, it is the physical stretching and distention of alveolar structures that causes the injury. This concept has been demonstrated in numerous animal models in which limiting alveolar expansion (e.g., with chest strapping) prevents lung injury even in the face of very high applied airway pressures.[8]

Clinical trials have confirmed these animal observations and indicate that ventilator strategies exposing injured human lungs to **transpulmonary pressures** in excess of 30 to 35 cm H_2O are associated with lung injury.[9–12] Of note is that this injury may be more than simply the result of excessive end-inspiratory alveolar stretch. Excessive tidal stretch (i.e., repetitive tidal volumes greater than 9 mL/kg), even in the setting of maximal transpulmonary pressures less than 30 cm H_2O, may contribute to VILI.[9,10,13] This provides the rationale for using **lung-protective ventilator strategies** that limit tidal volume and end-inspiratory distending pressures.

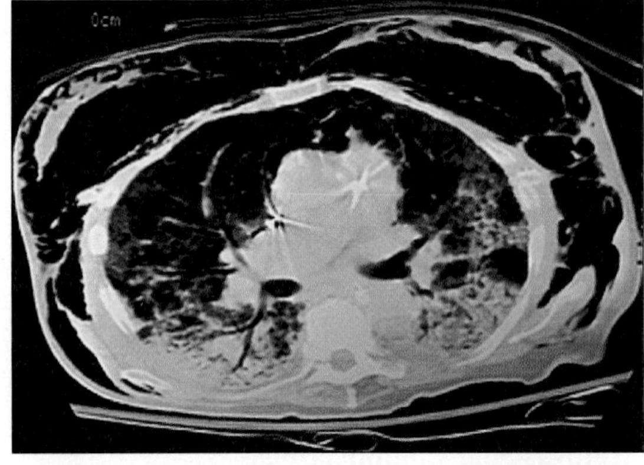

FIGURE 22-3 Computed tomography scan of the thorax of a mechanically ventilated patient with severe barotrauma. Note the presence of pneumothorax, pneumomediastinum, and subcutaneous emphysema.

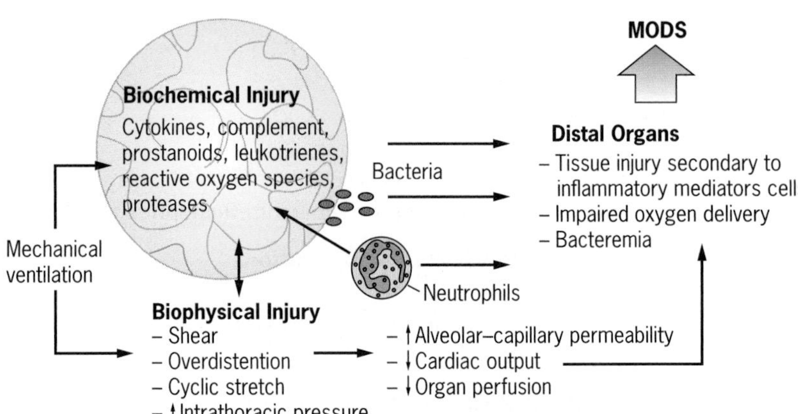

FIGURE 22–4 Mechanical ventilation can result in biochemical and biophysical injury to the lungs, which may result in multisystem organ failure. MODS, multiple organ dysfunction syndrome. Adapted from Slutsky AS, Trembly L. Multiple system organ failure: is mechanical ventilation a contributing factor? *Am J Respir Crit Care Med.* 1998;157:1721–1725.

Importantly, this approach may require acceptance of less than normal values for pH and Pa_{O_2} in exchange for lower (and safer) distending pressures.

VILI also can result from the cyclical opening of an alveolus during inhalation and closure during exhalation (cyclical atelectasis producing atelectrauma).[14,15] Indeed, pressures at the junction between an open and a closed alveolus may exceed 100 cm H_2O during this process.[16] This injury is reduced with the use of smaller tidal volumes and may be ameliorated by optimal lung recruitment and an expiratory pressure that prevents alveolar derecruitment. **Positive end-expiratory pressure (PEEP)**, however, can be a two-edged sword. If an increase in PEEP results in an increase in alveolar recruitment, then the stress (distribution of pressure) in the lungs is reduced. If, on the other hand, an increase in PEEP increases end-inspiratory transpulmonary pressure, then the strain (change in size of the lungs during inflation) on the lungs is increased.[17] Other ventilatory pattern factors may also be involved in the development of VILI. These include frequency of stretch[18] and the acceleration or velocity of stretch.[19] Vascular pressure elevations may also contribute to VILI.[20]

VILI is manifest pathologically as diffuse alveolar damage,[7,8,15] and it increases inflammatory cytokines in the lungs (biotrauma).[21–24] VILI is also associated with systemic cytokine release and bacterial translocation[24] that are implicated in the systemic inflammatory response with multiorgan dysfunction that increases mortality. The way in which the lungs are ventilated may therefore play a role in systemic inflammation (**Figure 22–4**).

Oxygen Toxicity

Oxygen concentrations approaching 100% are known to cause oxidant injuries in airways and lung parenchyma.[25] Much of the data supporting the concept of **oxygen toxicity**, however, have come from animals that often have quite different tolerances to oxygen than humans. It is unclear what the safe oxygen concentration or duration of exposure is in sick humans, such as those with acute lung injury (ALI) or acute respiratory distress syndrome (ARDS). Many authorities have argued that a fraction of inspired oxygen (F_{IO_2}) less than 0.4 is safe for prolonged periods of time and that a F_{IO_2} greater than 0.80 should be avoided. However, VILI may be more important clinically than oxygen toxicity. In one large study (ARDSnet), survival was greater in patients with ALI/ARDS who were ventilated with a lower tidal volume, presumably avoiding significant VILI, despite the fact that the required F_{IO_2} was higher in the group receiving the lower tidal volumes.

Ventilator-Associated Pneumonia

The natural laryngeal mechanism that protects the lower respiratory tract from aspiration is compromised by an endotracheal tube. This permits oropharyngeal debris to leak into the airways. The endotracheal tube also impairs the cough reflex and serves as a potential portal for pathogens to enter the lungs. The underlying disease process makes the lungs prone to infection. Finally, heavy antibiotic use in the ICU and the presence of very sick patients in close proximity to each other are risk factors for antibiotic-resistant infection.

Preventing ventilator-associated pneumonia (VAP) is important because it is associated with morbidity and mortality.[26] VAP prevention has become an important priority in the mechanically ventilated patient.[26–29] Hand washing, elevating the head of the bed, and carefully choosing antibiotic regimens can have important preventive effects. Circuit changes only when visibly contaminated appear to be helpful.[30] Endotracheal tubes that provide continuous drainage of subglottic secretions, endotracheal tubes with specialized cuff designs, and endotracheal tubes made with antimicrobial materials are other ways of reducing lung contamination with oropharyngeal material. However, these tubes are more expensive and their cost-effectiveness is controversial.[31]

Auto-PEEP

Auto-PEEP (also known as intrinsic PEEP or air trapping) is the result of the lungs not returning to the baseline proximal airway pressure at end-exhalation. The determinants of auto-PEEP are high minute volume, long inspiratory-to-expiratory time relationships, and long expiratory time constants (i.e., obstructed airways and high-compliance alveolar units). Auto-PEEP raises all intrathoracic pressures, which can affect gas delivery, hemodynamics, end-inspiratory distention (and thus VILI), and patient breath triggering. Although sometimes desired in long inspiratory time ventilatory strategies, auto-PEEP is generally to be avoided because it is difficult to recognize and to predict its effects.

Hemodynamic Effects of Positive Pressure Ventilation

Because positive pressure ventilation increases intrathoracic pressure, it can reduce venous return, which may result in decreased cardiac output and a drop in arterial blood pressure. Fluid administration and drug therapy (such as with vasopressors and inotropes) may be necessary to maintain cardiac output, blood pressure, and urine output under these circumstances. Mechanical ventilation also can cause an increase in plasma antidiuretic hormone (ADH) and a decrease in atrial natriuretic peptide (ANP), which may reduce urine output and promote fluid retention.[32]

As intrathoracic pressure increases with positive pressure ventilation, right ventricular filling decreases and cardiac output decreases. This is the rationale for using volume repletion to maintain cardiac output in the setting of high intrathoracic pressure. The effect of reduced cardiac filling on cardiac output may be partially counteracted by better left ventricular function due to elevated intrathoracic pressures, which reduce left ventricular afterload.[33] In patients with left heart failure, the reduced cardiac filling and reduced left ventricular afterload effects of elevated intrathoracic pressure may actually improve cardiac function such that intrathoracic pressure removal may produce left ventricular failure if positive pressure ventilation is removed.[34]

> **RESPIRATORY RECAP**
>
> **Indications for and Complications of Mechanical Ventilation**
>
> » Mechanical ventilation is indicated to support oxygenation and ventilation of patients with acute respiratory failure.
>
> » A number of complications are possible with mechanical ventilation, and efforts must be made to minimize these conditions.

Intrathoracic pressure can also influence distribution of perfusion, as described by the West model of pulmonary perfusion. In the supine human lung, blood flow is greatest in zone 3. As intra-alveolar pressure rises, there is an increase in zone 2 and zone 1 (dead space) regions, creating high ventilation-perfusion ($\dot{V}/\dot{Q}$) units. Dyspnea, anxiety, and discomfort associated with inadequate ventilatory support can lead to stress-related catecholamine release, with increases in myocardial oxygen demands and risk of dysrhythmias.[34] In addition, coronary blood vessel oxygen delivery can be compromised by inadequate gas exchange from the lung injury coupled with low mixed venous P_{O_2} due to high oxygen consumption demands by the inspiratory muscles.

Ventilator Settings

Volume Control Versus Pressure Control

With **volume control ventilation (VCV)**, the ventilator controls the inspiratory flow (**Figure 22–5**). The tidal volume is determined by the flow and the inspiratory time. In practice, however, the flow and tidal volume are set on the ventilator. With VCV the tidal volume is delivered regardless of resistance or compliance, and the peak airway pressure varies (**Box 22–4**). VCV should be used whenever a constant tidal volume is important in the

> **RESPIRATORY RECAP**
>
> **Volume Control Versus Pressure Control Ventilation**
>
> » *Volume control*: Ventilation remains constant with changes in respiratory mechanics, but airway and plateau pressures can fluctuate.
>
> » *Pressure control*: Ventilation fluctuates with changes in respiratory mechanics, but pressure is limited to the peak pressure set on the ventilator.

maintenance of a desired Pa_{CO_2}, such as with an acute head injury. The principal disadvantage of VCV is that it can produce a high peak alveolar pressure and areas of overdistention in the lungs. Also, because the inspiratory flow is fixed, VCV can cause **patient–ventilator asynchrony**, particularly if the inspiratory flow is set too low. With VCV, the set flow can be constant or a descending ramp. A descending ramp flow pattern produces a longer inspiratory time unless the peak flow is increased.

With **pressure control ventilation (PCV)** (**Figure 22–6**), the airway pressure is set and remains constant despite changes in resistance and compliance. **Box 22–5** lists factors that affect the tidal volume with PCV. The principal advantage of PCV is that it prevents

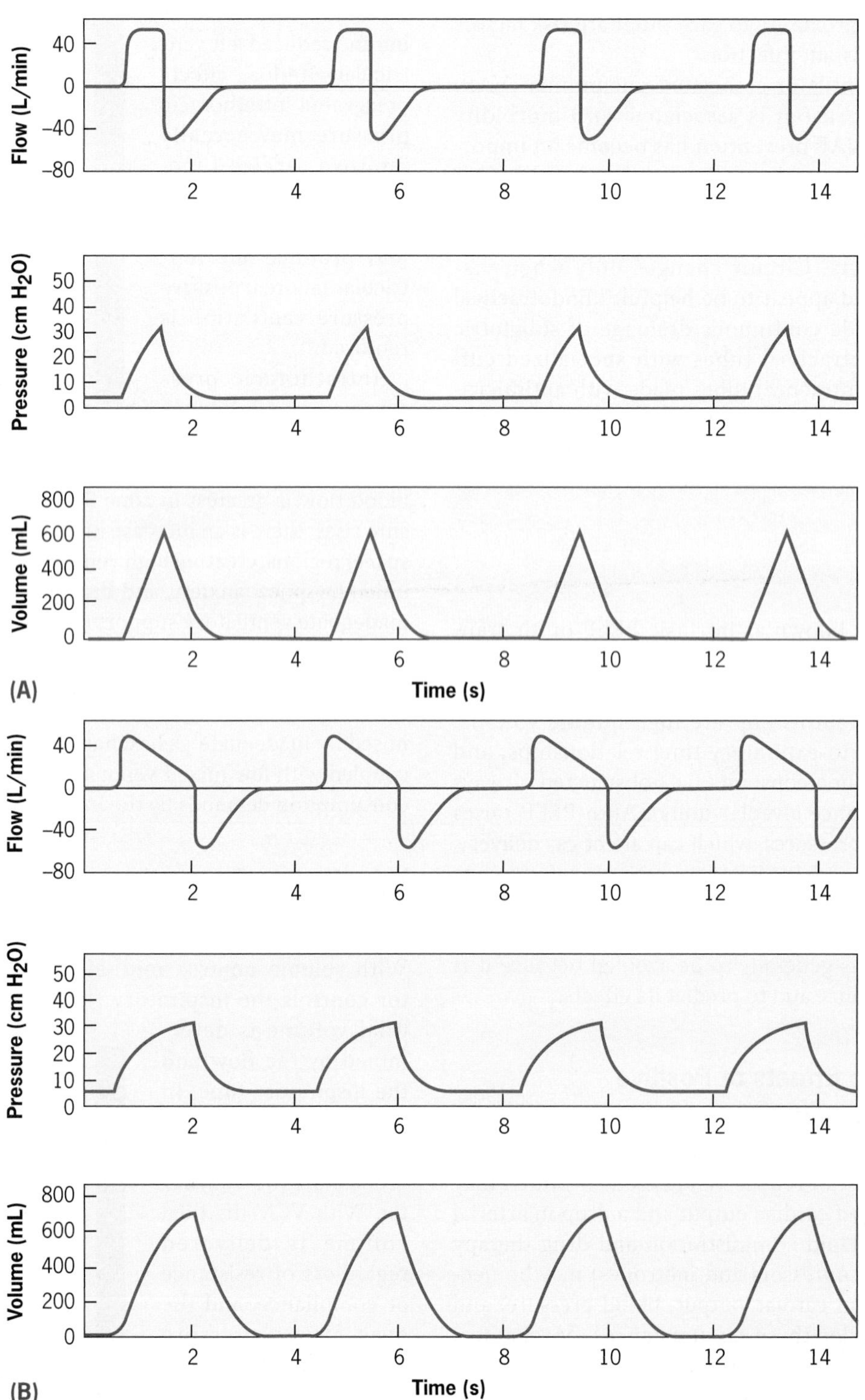

FIGURE 22–5 (**A**) Constant-flow (square wave) volume control ventilation. (**B**) Descending ramp-flow volume control ventilation.

localized alveolar overdistention with changes in resistance and compliance; the peak alveolar pressure cannot be greater than the pressure set on the ventilator. Because the flow can vary with PCV, this mode may improve patient–ventilator synchrony.[35,36] The choice of VCV or PCV often is determined by clinician or institutional bias, and both modes have advantages and disadvantages (**Table 22–1**).[37]

BOX 22–4

Factors That Affect Peak Inspiratory Pressure (PIP) with Volume Control Ventilation

Peak inspiratory flow setting: A higher flow setting increases the PIP.

Inspiratory flow pattern: PIP is lower with descending ramp flow.

Positive end-expiratory pressure (PEEP): An increase in PEEP increases the PIP.

Auto-PEEP: Auto-PEEP increases the PIP.

Tidal volume (VT): An increase in VT results in a higher PIP.

Resistance: Greater airways resistance results in a higher PIP.

Compliance: Decreased compliance results in a higher PIP.

BOX 22–5

Factors That Affect Tidal Volume (VT) with Pressure Control Ventilation

Driving pressure: A higher driving pressure (difference between peak inspiratory pressure and PEEP) increases the VT.

Auto-PEEP: An increase in auto-PEEP reduces the VT.

Inspiratory time: An increase in inspiratory time increases the VT if inspiratory flow is present; after flow decreases to zero, further increases in the time do not affect the VT.

Compliance: Decreased compliance decreases the VT.

Resistance: Increased resistance decreases the VT; after flow decreases to zero, resistance no longer affects the delivered VT.

Patient effort: Greater inspiratory effort by the patient increases the VT.

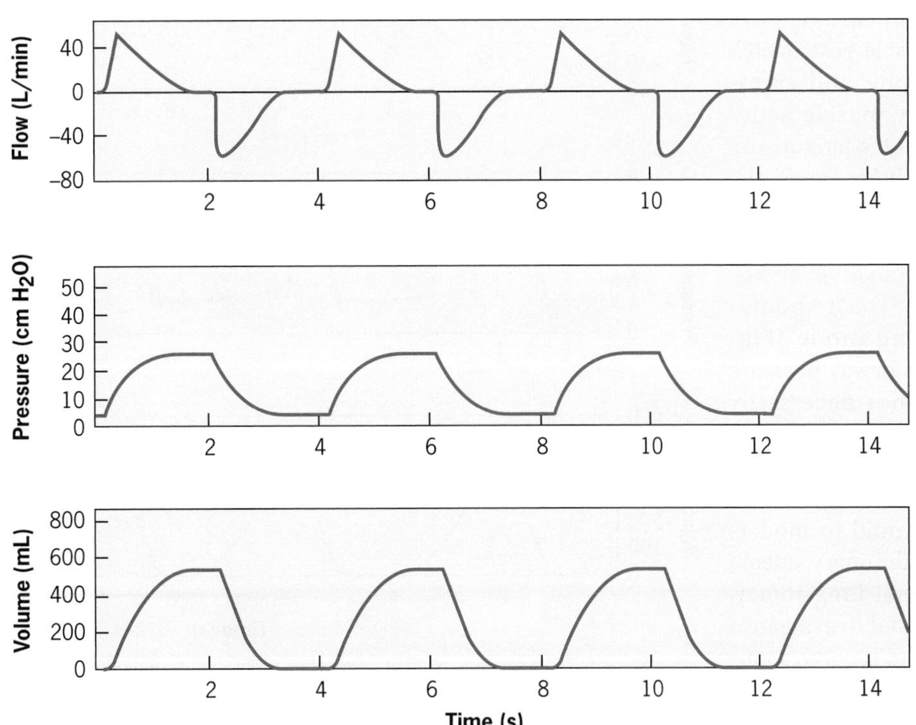

FIGURE 22–6 Pressure control ventilation.

Ventilator Mode

Options for breath delivery are referred to as *modes of ventilation*.[38–41] Traditional modes include continuous mandatory ventilation (CMV), also called assist/control (A/C), synchronized intermittent mandatory ventilation (SIMV), and pressure support ventilation (PSV). The choice of mode often is based on institutional policy or the clinician's bias. No one mode is clearly superior; each has its advantages and disadvantages (**Table 22–2**).

> **RESPIRATORY RECAP**
>
> **Ventilator Modes**
>
> » Continuous mandatory ventilation (CMV)
> » Synchronized intermittent mandatory ventilation (SIMV)
> » Pressure support ventilation (PSV)
> » Continuous positive airway pressure (CPAP)
> » Adaptive pressure control (APC)
> » Adaptive support ventilation (ASV)
> » Airway pressure release ventilation (APRV)
> » Tube compensation (TC)
> » Proportional assist ventilation (PAV)
> » Neurally adjusted ventilatory assist (NAVA)
> » High-frequency oscillatory ventilation (HFOV)

Continuous mandatory ventilation (CMV) (or assist/control ventilation) delivers a set volume or pressure and a minimum respiratory rate (**Figure 22–7**). The patient can trigger additional breaths above the minimum rate, but the set volume or pressure remains constant. When mechanical ventilation is begun, it often is best to use CMV (assist/control) to produce nearly complete respiratory muscle rest (i.e., full ventilatory support). Regardless of the mode used, the goal is to strike a balance between excessive respiratory muscle rest, which promotes atrophy, and excessive respiratory muscle activity, which promotes fatigue—or, put more simply, to avoid the extremes of too much rest and too much exercise.

Continuous positive airway pressure (CPAP) is a spontaneous breathing mode (**Figure 22–8**). The airway pressure is usually but not necessarily greater than atmospheric pressure. CPAP is commonly used as a means of maintaining alveolar recruitment in mild to moderate forms of pulmonary edema and parenchymal lung injury. CPAP often is used to evaluate a patient's ability to breathe spontaneously before extubation.

Pressure support ventilation (PSV) (**Figure 22–9**) is a spontaneous breathing mode in which patient effort is augmented by a clinician-determined level of pressure during inspiration.[42] Although the clinician sets the level of pressure support, the patient sets the respiratory rate, inspiratory flow, and inspiratory time. The V_T is determined by the level of pressure support, the amount of patient effort, and the resistance and compliance of the patient's respiratory system.

TABLE 22–1 Advantages and Disadvantages of Volume Control and Pressure Control Ventilation

Type	Advantages	Disadvantages
Volume control ventilation	Constant tidal volume (V_T) with changes in resistance and compliance Type of ventilation familiar to most clinicians	Increased plateau pressure (Pplat) with decreasing compliance (alveolar overdistention) Fixed inspiratory flow may cause asynchrony
Pressure control ventilation	Reduced risk of overdistention with changes in compliance. Variable flow improves synchrony in some patients	Changes in V_T with changes in resistance and compliance Less familiar type of ventilation for most clinicians

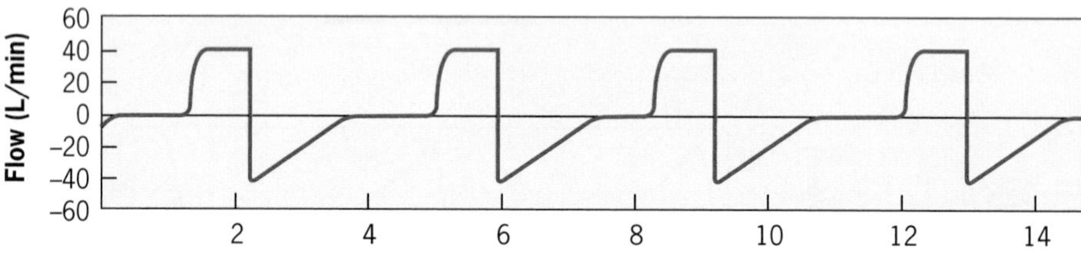

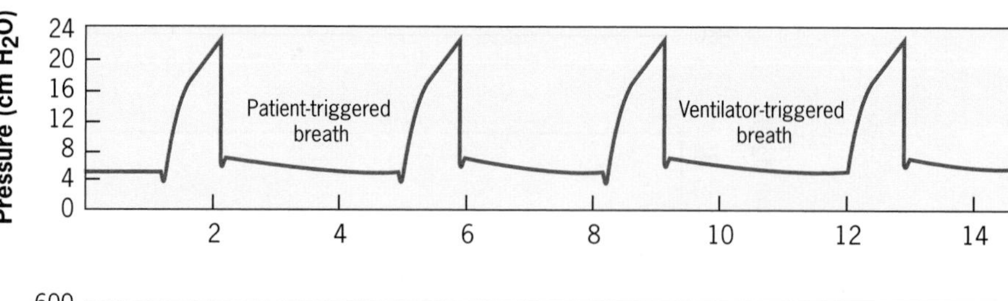

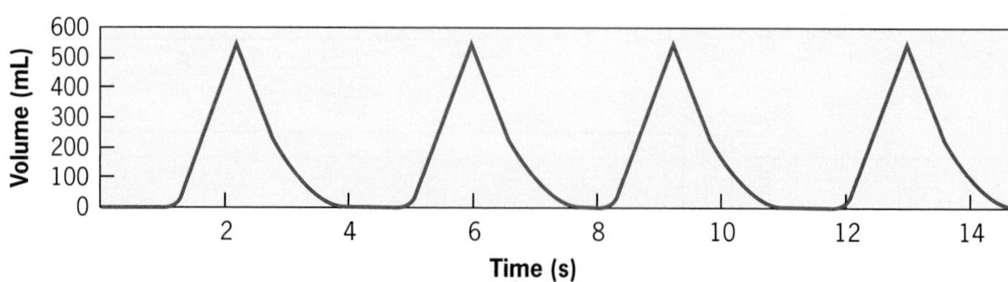

FIGURE 22–7 Continuous mandatory ventilation illustrating ventilator-triggered and patient-triggered breaths.

Pressure support ventilation is a frequently used mode of mechanical ventilation. However, because it is patient triggered, PSV is not an appropriate mode for patients who do not have an adequate respiratory drive. PSV normally is flow cycled, with secondary cycling mechanisms of pressure and time. Although PSV often is considered a simple mode of ventilation, it can be quite complex (**Figure 22–10**). First, the ventilator must recognize the patient's inspiratory effort, which depends on the ventilator's trigger sensitivity and the amount of auto-PEEP. Second, the ventilator must deliver an appropriate flow at the onset of inspiration. A flow that is too high can produce a pressure overshoot, and a flow that is too low can result in patient flow starvation and asynchrony. Third, the ventilator must appropriately cycle to the expiratory phase without the need for active exhalation.

The flow at which the ventilator cycles to the expiratory phase during PSV can be a fixed absolute flow, a flow based on the peak inspiratory flow, or a flow based on peak inspiratory flow and elapsed inspiratory time. Several studies have reported asynchrony with PSV in individuals with airflow obstruction, such as chronic obstructive pulmonary disease (COPD).[43,44] With airflow obstruction, the inspiratory flow decreases slowly during PSV, and the flow necessary to cycle may not be reached; this course of action stimulates active exhalation to pressure cycle the breath. The problem increases with higher levels of PSV and with higher levels of airflow obstruction. On newer ventilators, the termination flow can

TABLE 22–2 Advantages and Disadvantages of Common Modes of Mechanical Ventilation

Mode of Ventilation	Advantages	Disadvantages
Continuous mandatory ventilation (CMV)	Guaranteed volume (or pressure) with each breath Low patient workload if sensitivity and inspiratory flow set correctly	High mean airway pressure Respiratory alkalosis and auto-PEEP if patient triggers at rapid rate Respiratory muscle atrophy possible
Synchronized intermittent mandatory ventilation (SIMV)	Lower mean airway pressure Prevents respiratory muscle atrophy	Asynchrony if rate set too low High work of breathing with older ventilators
Pressure support ventilation (PSV)	Variable flow may improve synchrony in some patients Overcomes tube resistance Prevents respiratory muscle atrophy	Requires spontaneous respiratory effort Fatigue and tachypnea with PSV too low Activation of expiratory muscles with PSV too high
Adaptive pressure control	Ventilator maintains tidal volume with changes in respiratory system mechanics Variable flow may improve synchrony in some patients	Does not precisely control tidal volume Support is taken away if the patient's tidal volume consistently exceeds target
Adaptive support ventilation (ASV)	Ventilator adapts settings to patient's physiology	May not precisely control tidal volume
Airway pressure release ventilation (APRV)	Allows spontaneous breathing at any time during the ventilator cycle May improve ventilation to dependent lung zones May improve oxygenation in patients with ALI or ARDS	May be uncomfortable for some patients May result in large tidal volumes, depending on P_{high}–P_{low} difference May be large transpulmonary pressure swings during spontaneous breathing
Tube compensation (TC)	Overcomes resistance through artificial airway	Effect is usually small and may not affect patient outcomes
Proportional assist ventilation (PAV)	Pressure applied to the airway is determined by respiratory drive and respiratory mechanics	Not useful with weak drive or weak respiratory muscles Clinician has little control over tidal volume or respiratory rate
Neurally adjusted ventilatory assist (NAVA)	Pressure applied to the airway is determined by diaphragm activity	Requires insertion of special gastric tube to measure diaphragm EMG Not useful with weak respiratory drive or motor neuron disease

PEEP, positive end-expiratory pressure; P_{high}, high airway pressure setting; P_{low}, pressure release level; ALI, acute lung injury; ARDS, acute respiratory distress syndrome; EMG, electromyelogram.

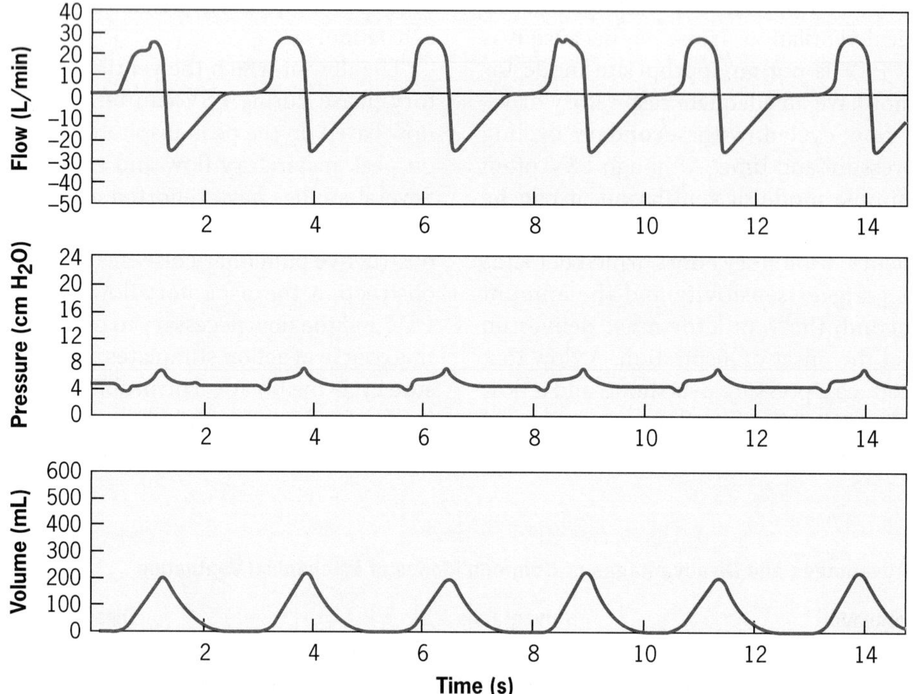

FIGURE 22-8 Continuous positive airway pressure.

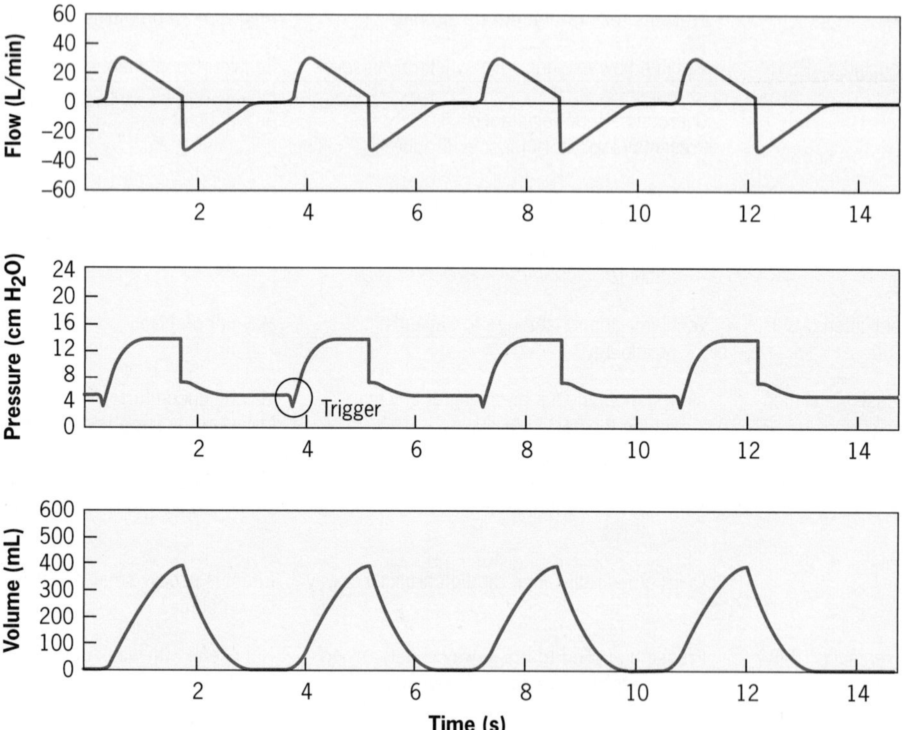

FIGURE 22-9 Pressure support ventilation.

be adjusted to a level appropriate for the patient (**Figure 22-11**).

Another concern with PSV is leaks in the system, such as with a bronchopleural fistula, uncuffed airway, or mask leak with noninvasive ventilation. If the leak exceeds the termination flow at which the ventilator cycles, either active exhalation occurs to terminate inspiration, or a prolonged inspiratory time is applied. With a leak, either PCV or a ventilator that allows an adjustable termination flow should be used. Another option is to

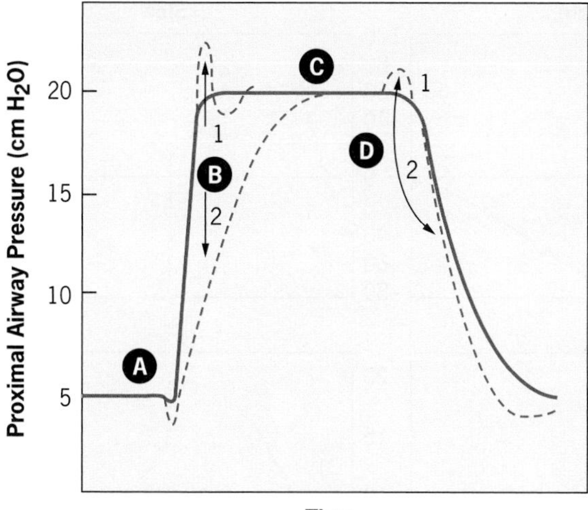

FIGURE 22–10 Design characteristics of a pressure-supported breath. In this example, baseline pressure (i.e., PEEP) is set at 5 cm H_2O and pressure support is set at 15 cm H_2O (PIP 20 cm H_2O). The inspiratory pressure is triggered at point A by a patient effort resulting in an airway pressure decrease. Demand valve sensitivity and responsiveness are characterized by the depth and duration of this negative pressure. The rise to pressure (line B) is provided by a fixed high initial flow delivery into the airway. Note that if flows exceed patient demand, initial pressure exceeds set level (B1), whereas if flows are less than patient demand, a very slow (concave) rise to pressure can occur (B2). The plateau of pressure support (line C) is maintained by servo control of flow. A smooth plateau reflects appropriate responsiveness to patient demand; fluctuations would reflect less responsiveness of the servo mechanisms. Termination of pressure support occurs at point D and should coincide with the end of the spontaneous inspiratory effort. If termination is delayed, the patient actively exhales (bump in pressure above plateau) (D1); if termination is premature, the patient will have continued inspiratory efforts (D2). Modified from MacIntyre N, et al. The Nagoya conference on system design and patient-ventilator interactions during pressure support ventilation. *Chest.* 1990;97:1463–1466.

set a maximum inspiratory time during PSV such that the breath can be time cycled at a clinician-determined setting. This secondary cycle typically has been fixed at a prolonged time to prevent untoward effects of long inspiratory times. Some new ventilators allow both the flow cycle and time cycle to be set.

The flow at the onset of the inspiratory phase may also be important during PCV or PSV. This is called *rise time* and refers to the time required for the ventilator to reach the set pressure at the onset of inspiration. Flows that are too high or too low at the onset of inspiration can cause asynchrony. Most ventilators allow adjustment of the rise time during PSV (**Figure 22–12**). The rise time should be adjusted to the patient's comfort, and ventilator graphics may be useful as a guide to this setting. However, a high inspiratory flow at the onset of inspiration may not be beneficial.[45] If the flow is higher at the onset of inspiration, the inspiratory phase may be prematurely terminated during PSV if the ventilator cycles to the expiratory phase at a flow that is a fraction of the peak inspiratory flow.

Sleep fragmentation may be more likely during PSV than during CMV because there is no backup rate.[46] Central apnea during PSV results in an alarm, which awakens the patient. The pattern of awakening and breathing with sleeping and apnea results in periodic breathing and sleep disruption. This complication of PSV can be addressed by switching to CMV or by using a lower level of pressure support. With CMV, there is a minimum respiratory rate set. With a lower level of pressure support, Pa_{CO_2} will likely be greater, and the associated respiratory drive will decrease the risk of apnea.

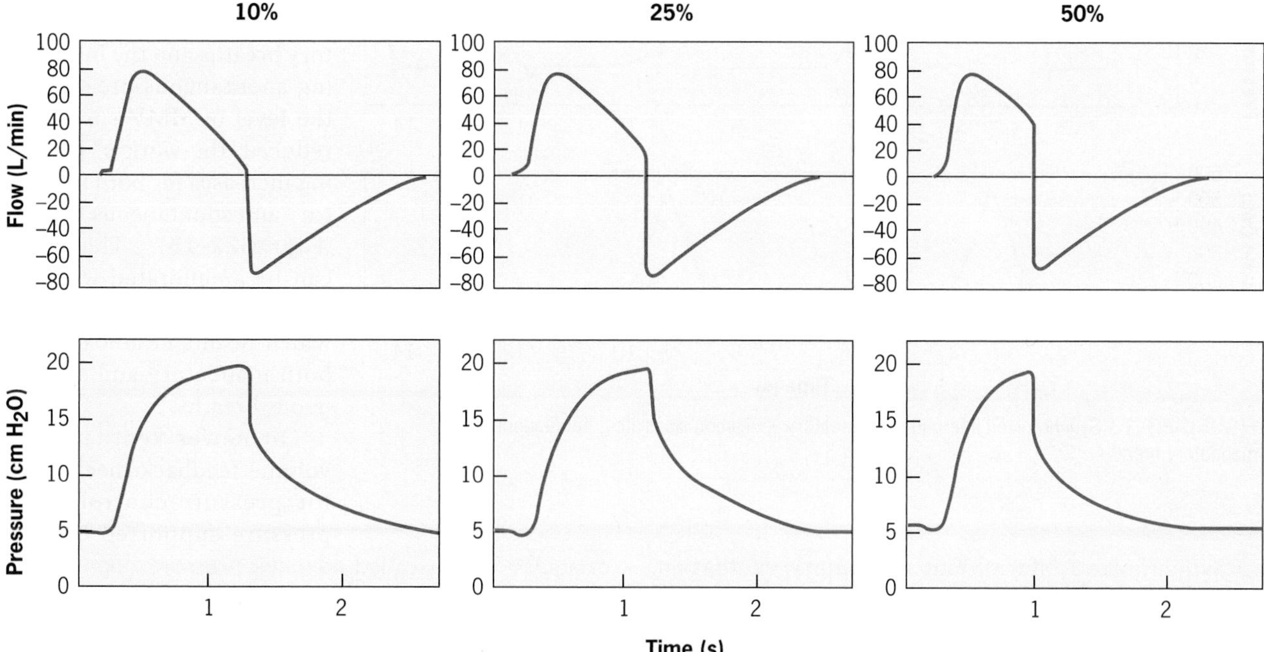

FIGURE 22–11 Effect of changing the flow termination criteria (cycle off flow as a percentage of peak flow) during pressure support ventilation. Note the effect on inspiratory time.

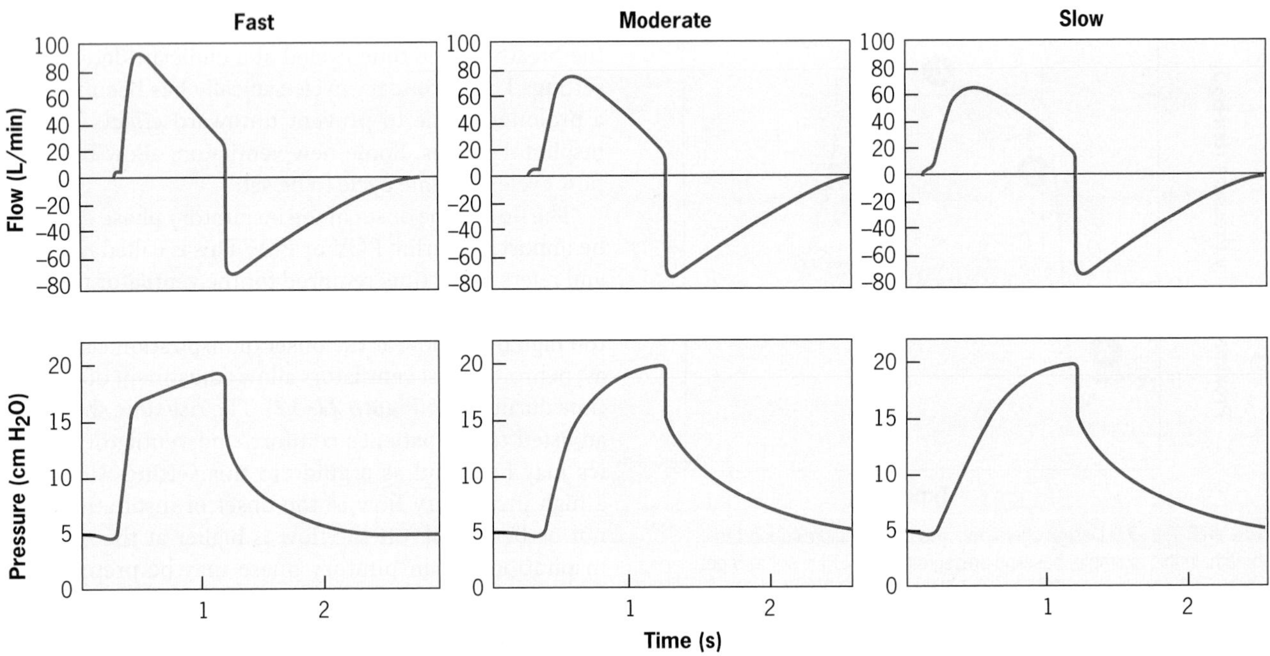

FIGURE 22–12 Effect of changing rise time during pressure support ventilation. Note the effect on peak flow.

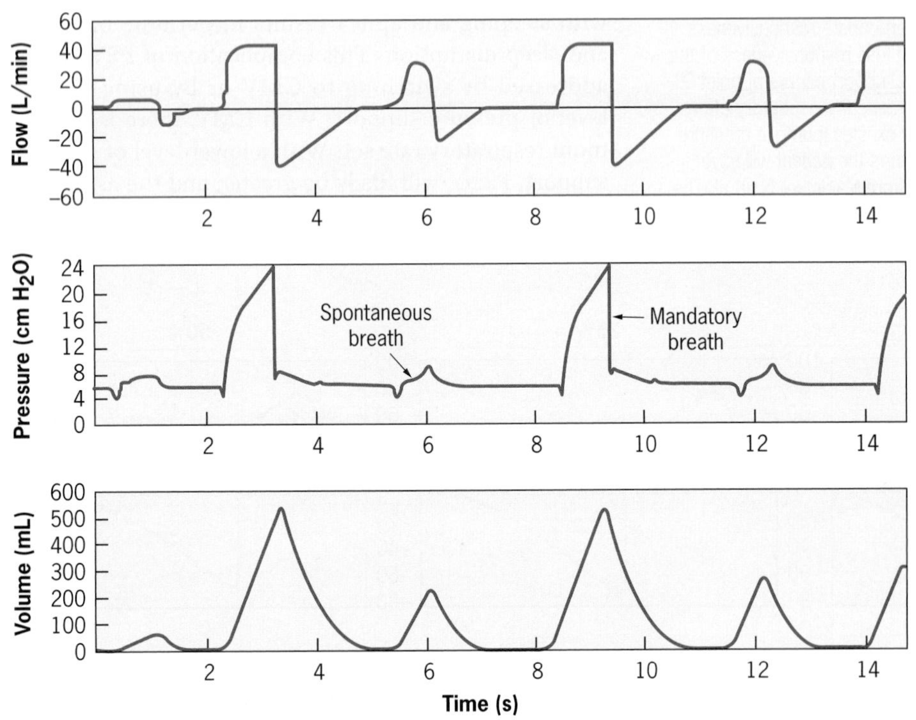

FIGURE 22–13 Synchronized intermittent mandatory ventilation illustrating spontaneous and mandatory breaths.

Synchronized intermittent mandatory ventilation (SIMV) (**Figure 22–13**) provides mandatory breaths (VCV or PCV) that are interspersed with spontaneous breaths. The mandatory breaths are delivered at the set rate, and the spontaneous breaths may be pressure supported (**Figure 22–14**). The intent is to provide respiratory muscle rest during mandatory breaths and respiratory muscle exercise with the intervening breaths. However, it has been shown that considerable inspiratory effort occurs with both the mandatory breaths and the intervening spontaneous breaths. As the level of SIMV support is reduced, the work of breathing increases for both mandatory and spontaneous breaths (**Figure 22–15**).[47] This effect can be ameliorated with the addition of pressure support, which results in unloading of both mandatory and spontaneous breaths.[48]

On newer ventilators, a volume feedback mechanism for pressure-controlled or pressure-supported breaths exists.[49,50] This is called **adaptive pressure control**. The desired tidal volume is set on the ventilator, but the breath type is actually pressure control or pressure support. The ventilator then adjusts the inspiratory

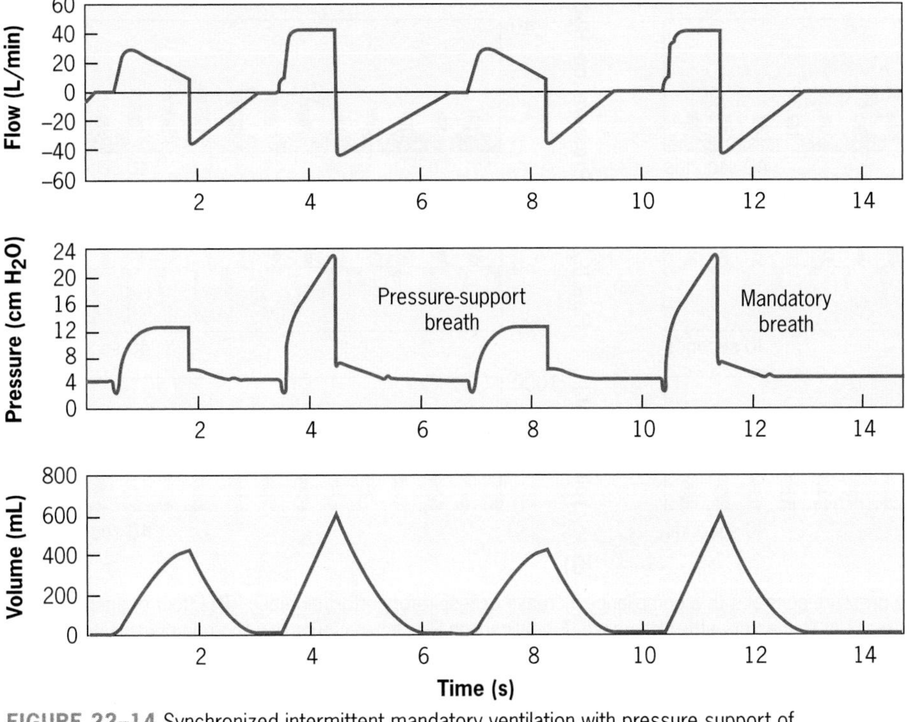

FIGURE 22–14 Synchronized intermittent mandatory ventilation with pressure support of spontaneous breaths.

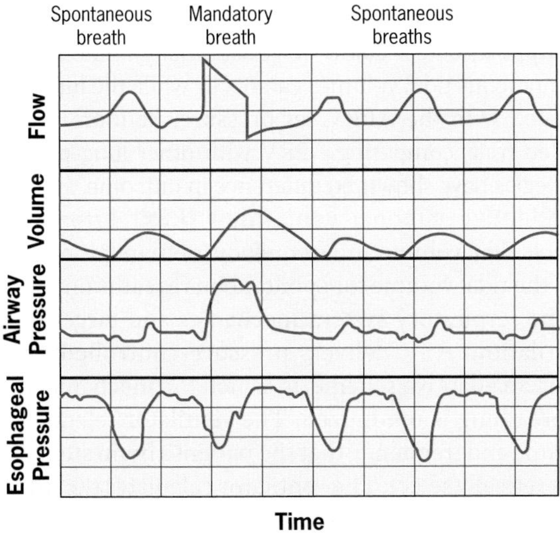

FIGURE 22–15 Synchronized intermittent mandatory ventilation. Note that the esophageal (i.e., pleural) pressure change for the mandatory breath is nearly as great as that for the spontaneous breaths.

pressure to deliver the set minimal target tidal volume (**Figure 22–16**). If tidal volume increases, the machine decreases the inspiratory pressure, and if tidal volume decreases, the machine increases the inspiratory pressure. This mode goes by the following names: pressure regulated volume control (Maquet Servo-i), AutoFlow (Dräger), adaptive pressure ventilation (Hamilton Galileo), volume control plus (Puritan Bennett), and volume targeted pressure control or pressure controlled volume guaranteed (General Electric). Volume support is a volume feedback mode in which the breath type is only pressure support.[50]

Because breath delivery during these volume feedback modes is pressure controlled, tidal volume will vary with changes in respiratory system compliance, airway resistance, and patient effort. If changes in lung mechanics cause the tidal volume to change, the ventilator adjusts the pressure setting in an attempt to restore the tidal volume. However, it is important to realize that providing a volume guarantee negates the pressure-limiting feature of a clinician-set pressure control level (i.e., worsening respiratory system mechanics will increase the applied pressure). Another potential problem with these approaches is that if the patient's demand increases and produces a larger tidal volume, the pressure level will diminish, a change that may not be appropriate for a patient in respiratory failure.

Airway pressure release ventilation (APRV) is a time-cycled, pressure-controlled mode of ventilatory support.[51] It is a modification of SIMV with an active exhalation valve that allows the patient to breathe spontaneously throughout the ventilator-imposed pressures (with or without PSV). Because APRV is often used with a long inspiratory-to-expiratory timing pattern, most of the spontaneous breaths will occur during the long lung inflation period (**Figure 22–17**). APRV is available under a variety of proprietary trade names: APRV (Dräger), BiLevel (Puritan Bennett), BiVent (Siemens), BiPhasic (Avea), PCV+ (Dräger), and DuoPAP (Hamilton).[50]

APRV uses different terminology to describe breath delivery phases. Lung inflation depends on the high airway pressure setting (P_{high}). The duration of this inflation is termed T_{high}. Oxygenation is thus heavily influenced by P_{high}, T_{high}, and F_{IO_2}. The magnitude and duration of lung deflation is determined by the pressure release level (P_{low}) and the release time (T_{low}). The ventilator-determined tidal volume is thus dependent on lung compliance, airways resistance, and the duration and timing of this pressure release maneuver. The timing and magnitude of this tidal volume coupled with the patient's spontaneous breathing determine alveolar ventilation (Pa_{CO_2}). As noted earlier, T_{high} is

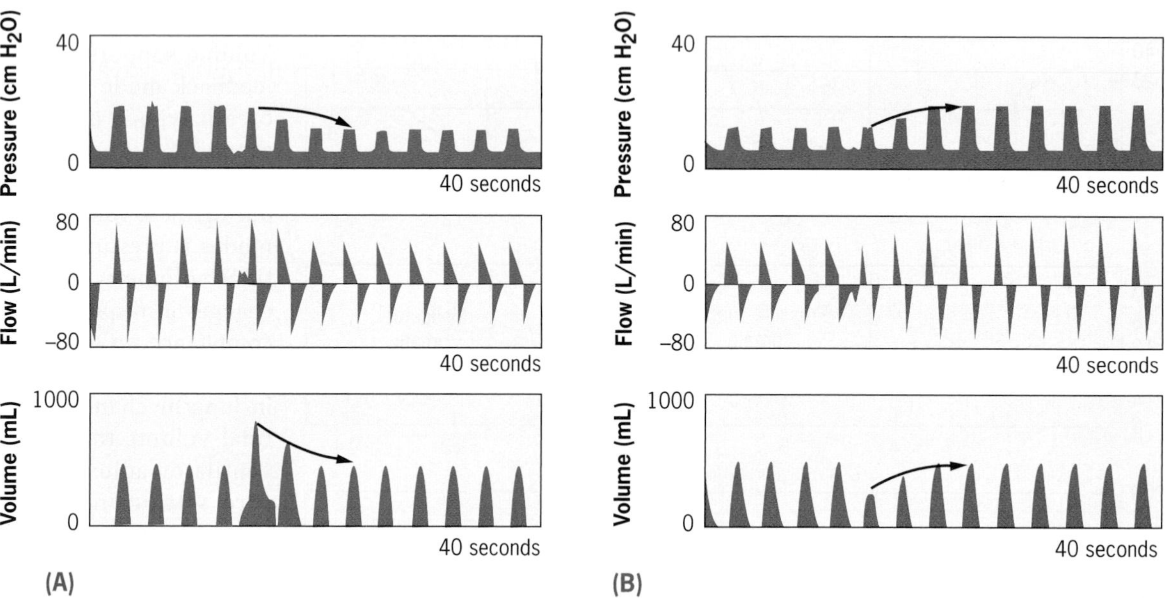

FIGURE 22–16 (**A**) Effect of adaptive pressure control with a compliance increase or respiratory effort increase. (**B**) Effect of adaptive pressure control with a compliance decrease or respiratory effort decrease. From Branson RD, Johannigman JA. The role of ventilator graphics when setting dual-control modes. *Respir Care.* 2005;50:187–201. Reprinted with permission.

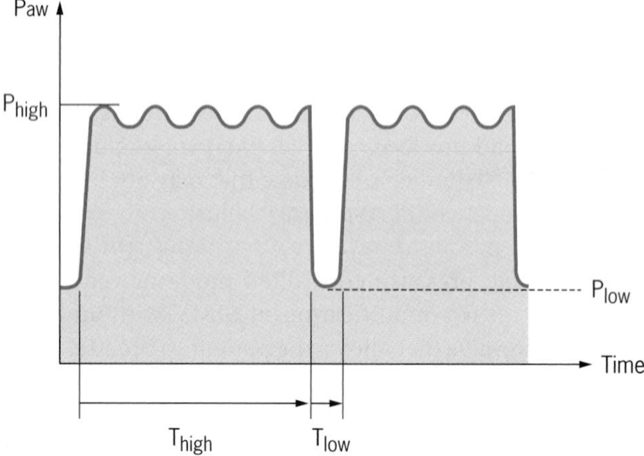

FIGURE 22–17 Airway pressure release ventilation.

usually much greater than T_{low}; thus, in the absence of spontaneous breathing, APRV is functionally the same as pressure-controlled inverse ratio ventilation. To sustain optimal recruitment with APRV, the greater part of the total time cycle (80% to 95%) usually occurs at P_{high}, whereas in order to minimize derecruitment, the time spent at P_{low} is brief (0.2–0.8 second in adults). If T_{low} is too short, exhalation may be incomplete and intrinsic PEEP may result.

Spontaneous breathing during APRV results from diaphragm contraction, which should result in recruitment of dependent alveoli, thus reducing shunt and improving oxygenation. The spontaneous efforts also may enhance both recruitment and cardiac filling as compared with other controlled forms of support. The long inflation phase also recruits more slowly, filling alveoli and raises mean airway pressure without increasing applied PEEP. Improved gas exchange, often with lower maximal set airway pressures than CMV, has been demonstrated with APRV.[51] However, the end-inspiratory alveolar distention in APRV is not necessarily less than that provided during other forms of support, and it could be substantially higher, because spontaneous tidal volumes can occur while the lung is fully inflated with the APRV set pressure. Randomized controlled trials comparing APRV with other lung-protective strategies have shown no difference in outcome.[52,53]

Adaptive support ventilation (ASV) automatically selects tidal volume and frequency for mandatory breaths and the tidal volume for spontaneous breaths on the basis of the respiratory system mechanics and target minute ventilation. ASV delivers pressure-controlled breaths using an adaptive scheme, in which the mechanical work of breathing is minimized. The ventilator selects a tidal volume and frequency that the patient's brain stem would theoretically select. The ventilator calculates the required minute ventilation based on the patient's ideal body weight and estimated dead space volume (2.2 mL/kg). The clinician sets a target percentage of minute ventilation that the ventilator will support; for example, higher than 100% if the patient has increased ventilatory requirements (e.g., because of sepsis or increased dead space), or less than 100% during ventilator liberation. The ventilator measures the expiratory time constant and uses this along with the estimated dead space to determine an optimal breathing frequency in terms of the work of breathing. The target tidal volume is calculated as the minute ventilation divided by the frequency, and the pressure limit is adjusted to achieve an average delivered tidal volume equal to the target. The ventilator also adjusts the inspiration-to-expiration (I:E) ratio to avoid air trapping. ASV has been shown to supply reasonable ventilatory support in a variety of patients with respiratory failure.[54–58] However, outcome studies in patients with acute respiratory failure comparing ASV with conventional lung-protective strategies have not been reported.

Tube compensation (TC) is designed to overcome the flow-resistive work of breathing imposed by an endotracheal tube or tracheostomy tube.[58–61] It measures the resistance of the artificial airway and applies a pressure proportional to that resistance. The clinician can set the fraction of tube resistance for which compensation is desired (e.g., 50% compensation rather than full compensation). Although it has been shown that TC can effectively compensate for resistance through the artificial airway, it has not been shown to improve outcome.[61]

Proportional assist ventilation (PAV) is a positive-feedback control mode that provides ventilatory support in proportion to the neural output of the respiratory center.[50] The ventilator monitors respiratory drive as the inspiratory flow of the patient, integrates flow to volume, measures elastance and resistance, and then calculates the pressure required from the equation of motion. Using this calculated pressure and the tidal volume, the ventilator calculates work of breathing (WoB): WoB $= \int P \times V$. These calculations occur every 5 ms during breath delivery, and thus the applied pressure and inspiratory time vary breath by breath and within the breath (**Figure 22–18**). The ventilator estimates resistance and elastance (or compliance) by applying end-inspiratory and end-expiratory pause maneuvers of 300 ms every 4 to 10 seconds. The clinician adjusts the percentage of support (from 5% to 95%), which allows the work to be partitioned between the ventilator and the patient. Typically, the percentage of support is set so that the work of breathing is in the range of 0.5 to 1.0 joules per liter. If the percentage of support is high, patient work of breathing may be inappropriately low and excessive volume and pressure may be applied (runaway phenomenon). If the percentage of support is too low, patient work of breathing may be excessive.

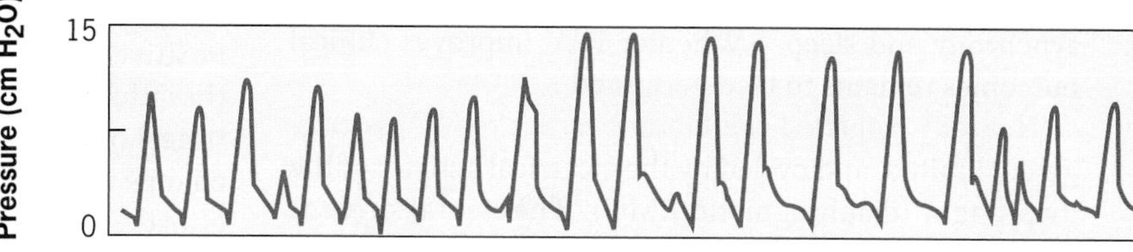

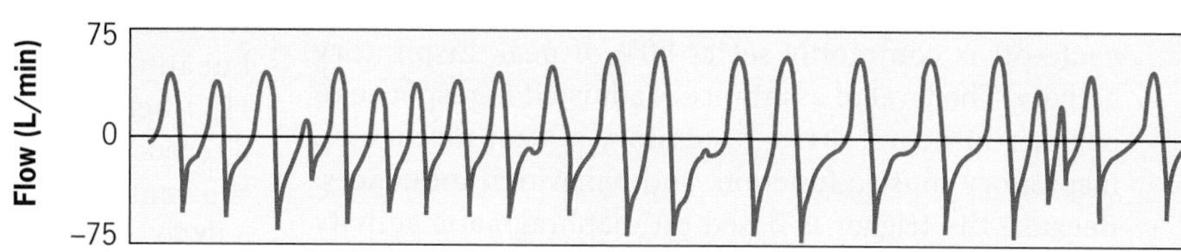

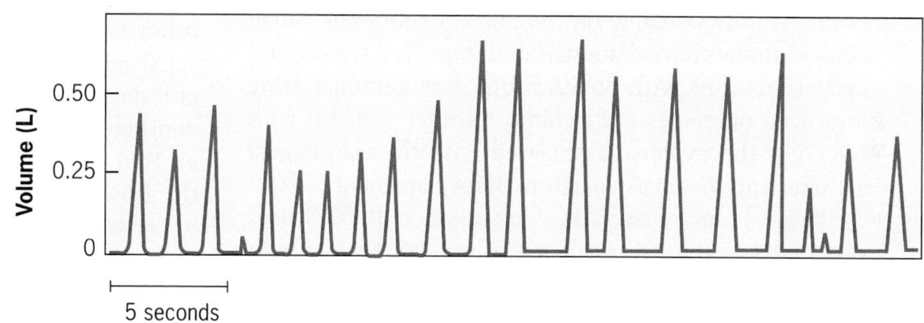

FIGURE 22–18 Proportional assist ventilation. From Marantz S, Patrick W, Webster K, et al. Response of ventilator-dependent patients to different levels of proportional assist. *J Appl Physiol.* 1996;80:397–403. Reprinted with permission.

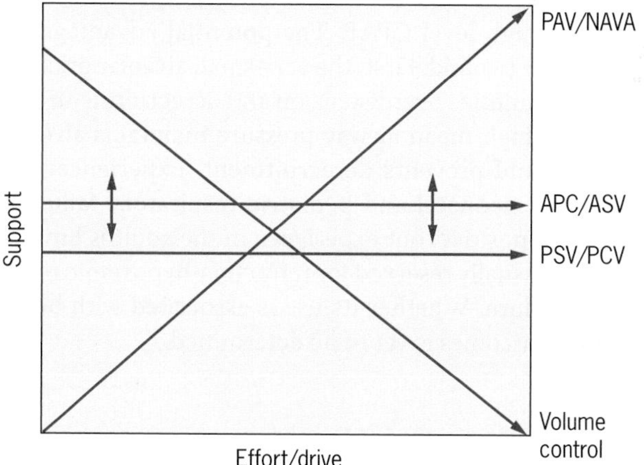

FIGURE 22–19 Effect of patient effort on the amount of support provided with various ventilator modes.

PAV applies a pressure that will vary from breath to breath depending upon changes in the patient's elastance, resistance, and flow demand. This differs from PSV or PCV, in which the level of applied pressure is constant regardless of demand, and from VCV, in which the level of pressure decreases when demand increases (**Figure 22–19**).[62] The cycle criterion for PAV is flow and is adjustable by the clinician, similar to pressure support ventilation. PAV requires the presence of an intact ventilatory drive and a functional neuromuscular system. PAV is only available on one ventilator in the United States (PAV+, Puritan Bennett 840) and cannot be used with noninvasive ventilation because leaks prevent accurate determination of respiratory mechanics. PAV may be more comfortable compared with other modes,[63] and it may be associated with better patient–ventilator synchrony and sleep.[64] Whether PAV improves clinical outcomes remains to be determined.

Neurally adjusted ventilatory assist (NAVA) is triggered, limited, and cycled by the electrical activity of the diaphragm (diaphragmatic EMG). The neural drive is transformed into ventilatory output (neuro-ventilatory coupling). The diaphragmatic EMG is measured by a multiple-array esophageal electrode, which is amplified to determine the support level (NAVA gain). The cycle-off is commonly set at 80% of peak inspiratory activity. The level of assistance is adjusted in response to changes in neural drive, respiratory system mechanics, inspiratory muscle function, and behavioral influences. Because the trigger is based on diaphragmatic activity rather than pressure or flow, triggering is not adversely affected in patients with flow limitation and auto-PEEP. NAVA is only available on the Servo-i ventilator. Small clinical studies have demonstrated improved trigger and cycle synchrony with NAVA,[65] but data demonstrating improved outcomes are lacking. Another concern with NAVA is the expense associated with the esophageal catheter and the invasive nature of its placement.

High-frequency oscillatory ventilation (HFOV) uses very high breathing frequencies[66] (up to 900 breaths/min in the adult) coupled with very small tidal volumes to provide gas exchange in the lungs. HFOV literally vibrates a bias flow of gas delivered at the proximal end of the endotracheal tube and effects gas transport through complex nonconvective gas transport mechanisms. At the alveolar level, the substantial mean pressure functions as high-level CPAP. The potential advantages to HFOV are twofold. First, the very small alveolar pressure swings minimize overdistension and derecruitment. Second, the high mean airway pressure maintains alveolar patency and prevents derecruitment. Experience with HFOV in neonatal and pediatric respiratory failure is generally positive, but experience in the adult is limited. Its use is usually reserved for refractory hypoxemic respiratory failure. Whether its use is associated with better patient outcomes is yet to be determined.

Breath Triggering

Positive pressure breaths can be either time triggered (breaths delivered according to a clinician-set rate or timer) or patient triggered (breaths triggered by either a change in circuit pressure or flow resulting from patient effort). The patient effort required to trigger the ventilator is an imposed load for the patient. **Pressure triggering** occurs because of a pressure drop in the system (**Figure 22–20**). The pressure level at which the ventilator is triggered is set so that the trigger effort is minimal but auto-triggering is unlikely (typically this is 1 to 2 cm H_2O below the PEEP or CPAP). **Flow triggering** is an alternative to pressure triggering. With flow triggering the ventilator responds to a change in flow rather than a drop in pressure at the airway. With some ventilators, a pneumotachometer is placed between the ventilator circuit and the patient to measure inspiratory flow. In other ventilators, a background or base flow and flow sensitivity are set. When the flow in the expiratory circuit decreases by the amount of the flow sensitivity, the ventilator is triggered. For example, if the base flow is set at 10 L/min and the flow sensitivity is set at 3 L/min, the ventilator triggers when the flow in the expiratory circuit drops to 7 L/min (the assumption is that the patient has inhaled at 3 L/min). Flow triggering has been shown to reduce the work of breathing with CPAP.[67] However, it may not be superior to pressure triggering with pressure-supported breaths or mandatory breaths.[68] Neither pressure triggering nor flow triggering may be effective if significant auto-PEEP is present. Regardless of whether pressure triggering or flow triggering is used, the current generation of ventilators is more responsive to patient effort, and differences between pressure and flow triggering are minor.[69]

> **RESPIRATORY RECAP**
>
> **Types of Ventilator Triggering**
>
> » Ventilator self-triggers when a set time is reached.
>
> » Patient triggers the ventilator through changes in pressure or flow.

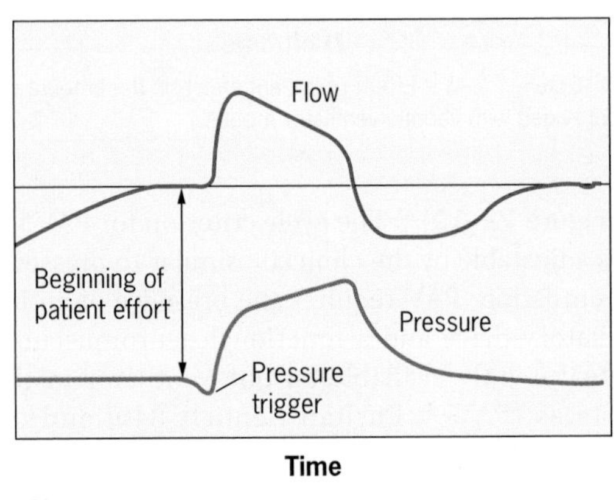

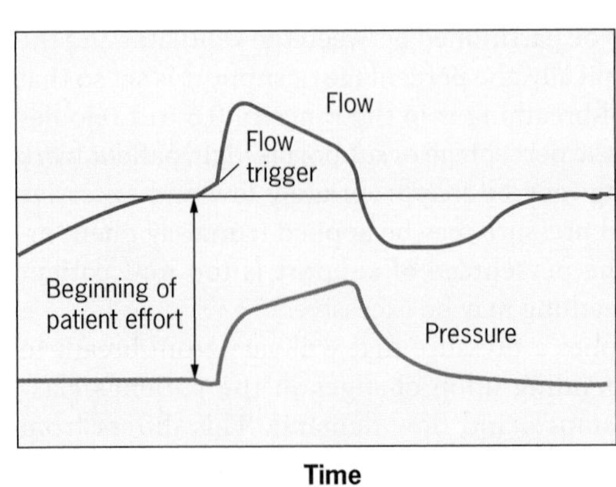

FIGURE 22–20 **(A)** Pressure-triggered breath. **(B)** Flow-triggered breath.

Tidal Volume

Tidal volume is selected to provide an adequate $Paco_2$ but avoid alveolar overdistention, decreased cardiac output, and auto-PEEP.[70] Tidal volume is directly set in VCV but is determined by the driving pressure and inspiratory time in PCV and PSV. As noted earlier, large tidal volumes increase mortality in patients with ALI or ARDS and increase the risk of developing ALI or ARDS in patients with previously normal lungs.[10,71] A tidal volume should be chosen that maintains **plateau pressure** (Pplat) below 30 cm H_2O (assuming a near-normal chest wall compliance), or perhaps higher if chest wall compliance is severely reduced (e.g., morbid obesity, anasarca, ascites). Tidal volume should be selected based on predicted body weight (PBW), which is determined by height and sex:

Male patients: PBW = 50 + 2.3 × [Height (inches) − 60]

Female patients: PBW = 45.5 + 2.3 × [Height (inches) − 60]

A reasonable starting point for most patients with respiratory failure is 6 mL/kg PBW.

Respiratory Rate

A respiratory rate is chosen to provide an acceptable minute ventilation, as follows:

$$\dot{V}_E = V_T \times f$$

where f is the respiratory rate, $\dot{V}_E$ is the minute ventilation, and V_T is the tidal volume. A rate of 15 to 25 breaths/min is used when mechanical ventilation is initiated. If a smaller tidal volume is selected to prevent alveolar overdistention, a higher respiratory rate may be required (25 to 35 breaths/min). The respiratory rate may be limited by the development of auto-PEEP. The minute ventilation that produces a normal $Paco_2$ without risk for lung injury or auto-PEEP may not be possible, and the $Paco_2$ thus is allowed to increase (**permissive hypercapnia**).

Inspiratory Time

For patient-triggered mandatory breaths, the inspiratory time should be short (1.5 seconds or less) to improve ventilator–patient synchrony. A shorter inspiratory time requires a higher inspiratory flow, which increases the **peak inspiratory pressure (PIP)** but does not greatly affect the Pplat. Increasing the inspiratory time increases the **mean airway pressure ($\bar{P}aw$)**, which may improve oxygenation in some patients with ARDS. When long inspiratory times are used (over 1.5 seconds) and spontaneous breaths are not permitted, paralysis or sedation (or both) often is required. Long inspiratory times also can cause auto-PEEP and may result in hemodynamic instability because of the elevated $\bar{P}aw$ or the auto-PEEP. Although inverse ratio ventilation has been advocated to improve oxygenation, unless it is coupled with the ability to spontaneously breathe (see the discussion of APRV earlier in this chapter), this extreme (and potentially hazardous) form of ventilation is seldom necessary to achieve adequate oxygenation.

> **RESPIRATORY RECAP**
>
> **Settings for Tidal Volume, Respiratory Rate, and Inspiratory Time**
>
> » *Tidal volume*: Set to avoid overdistention
> » *Respiratory rate*: Set for desired partial pressure of arterial carbon dioxide ($Paco_2$)
> » *Inspiratory time*: Set to avoid auto-PEEP and hemodynamic compromise

The I:E ratio is the relationship between inspiratory time and expiratory time. For example, an inspiratory time of 2 seconds with an expiratory time of 4 seconds produces an I:E ratio of 1:2 and a respiratory rate of 10 breaths/min. With VCV, the peak inspiratory flow, flow pattern, and tidal volume are the principal determinants of inspiratory time and the I:E ratio. With PCV, the inspiratory time, I:E ratio, or percentage inspiratory time are set directly. In both VCV and PCV, the principal determinant of expiratory time is the respiratory rate.

Inspiratory Flow Pattern

For VCV, the inspiratory flow pattern can be constant or descending ramp. For the same inspiratory time, the PIP is greater with constant flow than with descending ramp flow; the $\bar{P}aw$ is greater with ramp flow than with constant flow; and gas distribution is better with a descending ramp flow pattern. Because the flow is greater at the beginning of inspiration, patient–ventilator synchrony may be better with a descending ramp flow pattern. Although the choice of flow pattern often is based on clinician bias or the capabilities of a specific ventilator, descending ramp flow may be desirable compared with other inspiratory flow patterns. An end-inspiratory pause can be set to improve distribution of ventilation, but this prolongs inspiration and may have a deleterious effect on hemodynamics and auto-PEEP.

The inspiratory flow decreases exponentially with PCV and PSV. The peak flow and rate of flow decrease depend on the driving pressure, airways resistance, lung compliance, and patient effort. With high resistance, flow decreases slowly. With a low compliance and long inspiratory time, flow decreases more rapidly, and a period of zero flow may be present at end-inhalation (**Figure 22–21**).

Positive End-Expiratory Pressure

Because critical care patients are often immobile and supine, with compromised cough ability, it is common to use low-level PEEP (3 to 5 cm H_2O) with all mechanically ventilated patients to prevent atelectasis. In patients with ALI or ARDS, more substantial levels of PEEP may be required to maintain alveolar recruitment. An appropriate PEEP level to maintain alveolar recruitment is

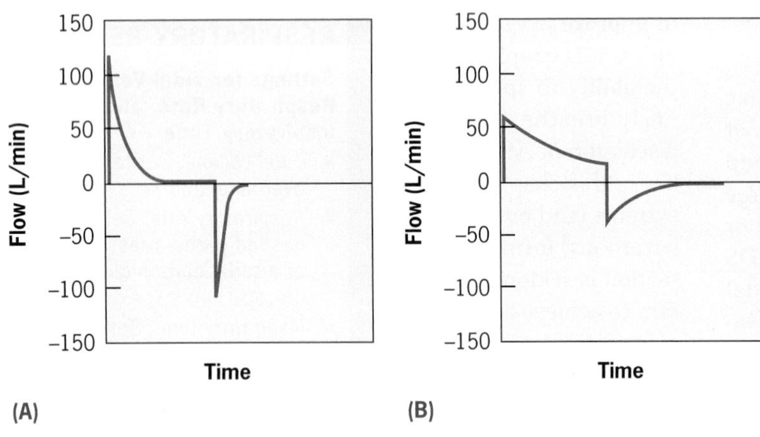

FIGURE 22–21 Flow waveforms during pressure control ventilation: low resistance and low compliance (**A**), and high resistance and high compliance (**B**).

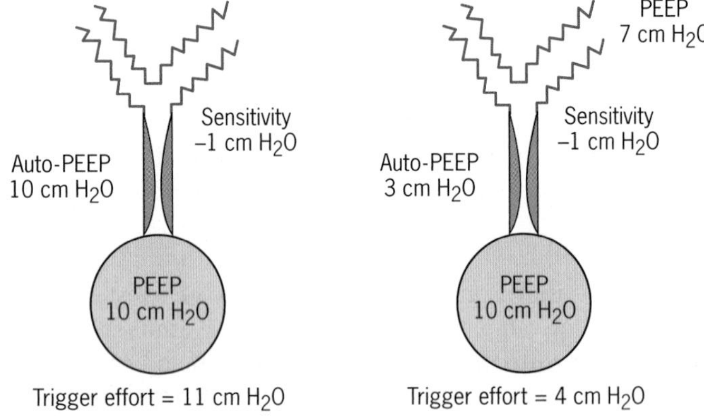

FIGURE 22–22 Trigger effort is increased when auto-PEEP is present. To trigger the ventilator, the patient's effort must first overcome the level of auto-PEEP that is present. Increasing the set PEEP level may raise the trigger level closer to the total PEEP, thus improving the ability of the patient to trigger the ventilator. However, this method should not be used if raising the set PEEP level results in an increase in the total PEEP.

RESPIRATORY RECAP

Uses of Positive End-Expiratory Pressure

» Maintain alveolar recruitment
» Counterbalance auto-PEEP
» Reduce preload and afterload
» Pneumatic splinting of the airway
» Facilitation of leak speech

also part of a lung-protective strategy. PEEP should be used cautiously in patients with unilateral disease, because it may overdistend the more compliant lung, causing shunting of blood to the less compliant lung.

PEEP also may be useful to improve triggering by patients experiencing auto-PEEP.[72–75] Auto-PEEP functions as a threshold pressure that must be overcome before the pressure (or flow) decreases at the airway to trigger the ventilator. Increasing the set PEEP to a level near the auto-PEEP may improve the patient's ability to trigger the ventilator (**Figure 22–22**). Whenever PEEP is used to overcome the effect of auto-PEEP on triggering, PIP and Pplat must be monitored to ensure that increasing the set PEEP does not contribute to further hyperinflation.

Other uses of PEEP include preload and afterload reduction in the setting of left heart failure, pneumatic splinting in the setting of airway malacia, and facilitation of leak speech with cuff deflation in patients with a tracheostomy.[76]

Mean Airway Pressure

Across all modes, oxygenation and cardiac effects of mechanical ventilation often correlate best with the mean airway pressure ($\bar{P}aw$). Indeed, $\bar{P}aw$ is a key component of the oxygenation index (OI = $100 \times [\bar{P}aw \times FIO_2]/PaO_2$) that often is used as a more accurate reflection of gas transport impairment. Factors that affect the $\bar{P}aw$ during mechanical ventilation are the PIP, PEEP, I:E ratio, respiratory rate, and inspiratory flow pattern. Most patients can be managed with mean P values less than 15 to 20 cm H_2O.

Recruitment Maneuvers

A recruitment maneuver (RM) is an intentional transient increase in transpulmonary pressure to promote reopening of unstable collapsed alveoli and thereby improve gas exchange.[77] However, although use of the maneuver is physiologically reasonable, there have been no randomized controlled trials demonstrating an outcome benefit from this improvement in gas exchange. RMs are probably best reserved for the setting of refractory hypoxemia in patients with ARDS.[78] A variety of techniques have been described as recruitment maneuvers (**Table 22–3**). It is uncertain whether any one approach is superior to the others. After performing an RM, it is important to set PEEP to a level that retains recruitment. If the lungs are already maximally recruited as the result of PEEP, the benefits of an RM are likely minimal.

TABLE 22–3 Different Lung Recruitment Maneuvers

Recruitment Maneuver	Method
Sustained high-pressure inflation	Sustained inflation delivered by increasing PEEP to 30–50 cm H_2O for 20–40 seconds
Intermittent sigh	Periodic sighs with a tidal volume reaching Pplat of 45 cm H_2O
Extended sigh	Stepwise increase in PEEP by 5 cm H_2O with a simultaneous stepwise decrease in tidal volume over 2 minutes leading to a CPAP level of 30 cm H_2O for 30 seconds
Intermittent PEEP increase	Intermittent increase in PEEP from baseline to higher level
Pressure control + PEEP	Pressure control ventilation of 10–15 cm H_2O with PEEP of 25–30 cm H_2O to reach a peak inspiratory pressure of 40–45 cm H_2O for 2 minutes

Importantly, an RM can produce injury in the form of hemodynamic compromise and barotrauma.

Inspired Oxygen Concentration

An F_{IO_2} of 1.0 is commonly used when mechanical ventilation is initiated. Pulse oximetry (Sp_{O_2}) is useful to guide titration of the F_{IO_2} (and PEEP) provided periodic blood gas measurements are obtained to confirm the pulse oximetry results. A target Sp_{O_2} of 88% or higher usually provides a partial pressure of arterial oxygen (Pa_{O_2}) of 60 mm Hg or higher. Although it is common practice to wait 20 to 30 minutes after the F_{IO_2} is changed before arterial blood gas measurements are obtained, 10 minutes may be adequate unless the patient has obstructive lung disease, which requires a longer equilibration time.[79]

> **RESPIRATORY RECAP**
>
> **Setting the Fractional Inspired Oxygen Concentration**
>
> » Initiate mechanical ventilation with 100% oxygen.
>
> » Titrate the F_{IO_2} to maintain an acceptable arterial oxygen saturation as measured by pulse oximetry.

Sigh

Some ventilators are capable of providing periodic sigh volumes.[80] The rationale for use of sighs is that the periodic hyperinflation reduces the risk of atelectasis. Indeed, a sigh is actually a very brief RM. For many years the use of sighs during mechanical ventilation was not considered important. However, several studies of patients with ARDS have reported improved alveolar recruitment with the use of sighs.[81,82]

Alarms

It is particularly important that all alarms be correctly set on the ventilator. The most important alarm is the patient-disconnect alarm, which can be a low pressure alarm or a low exhaled volume alarm (or both). A sensitive alarm should detect not only disconnection but also leaks in the system. The ability to detect a leak depends on the site where the volume is measured (**Figure 22–23**). Other alarms set on the ventilator include those for high pressure, I:E ratio, F_{IO_2}, and loss of PEEP. To detect changes in resistance and compliance, the peak airway pressure alarm is important with VCV, and the low exhaled volume alarm with PCV or PSV.

Circuit

Because of the gas compression in the ventilator circuit and the compliance of the ventilator circuit tubing, as much as 3 to 5 mL/cm H_2O can be compressed in the ventilator circuit. In other words, at an airway pressure of 25 cm H_2O above PEEP, about 100 mL of the gas delivered from the ventilator is not delivered to the patient. If the ventilator is set to deliver 500 mL, only 400 mL is delivered to the patient. For patients ventilated with a small tidal volume, the compressible gas volume can greatly affect alveolar ventilation. Some ventilators adjust for the effects of **compressible volume** such that the volume chosen by the clinician is the actual delivered V_T after correction for the effect of compressible volume. The effects of compressible volume on the delivered V_T, auto-PEEP, plateau pressure, and mixed exhaled partial pressure of carbon dioxide ($P\bar{E}_{CO_2}$) are shown in **Equation 22–1**.

The mechanical dead space of the circuit should also be considered. *Mechanical dead space* is that part of the ventilator circuit through which the patient rebreathes and thus becomes an extension of the patient's anatomic dead space. Alveolar ventilation is zero if the sum of the volume loss in the circuit and the mechanical dead space is greater than the V_T set on the ventilator.

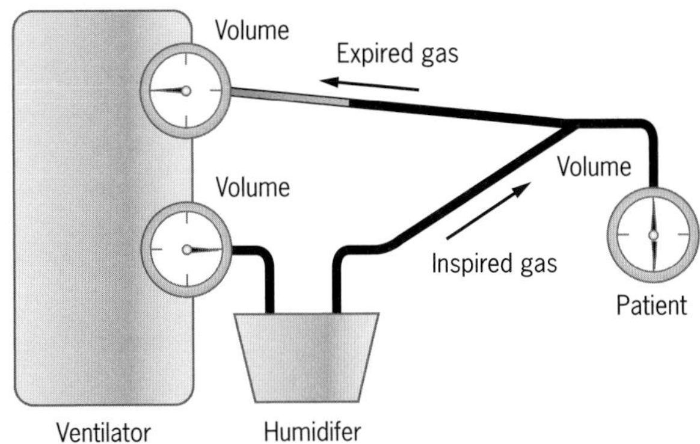

FIGURE 22–23 The ability to detect a leak depends on the site where volume is measured. If the volume on the inspiratory limb is greater than the volume on the expiratory limb, then there is a leak in the system (circuit or patient). If the inspired volume at the patient is greater than the expired volume at the patient, there is a leak in the patient (e.g., around the cuff of the endotracheal tube or a bronchopleural fistula).

Humidification

Because the function of the upper airway is bypassed when endotracheal and tracheostomy tubes are used, the inspired gas must be filtered, warmed, and humidified before delivery to the patient. All ventilator circuits include a filter in the inspiratory limb and an active or passive humidifier. An active humidifier typically humidifies the inspired gas by passing it over or bubbling it through a heated water bath. When an active humidifier is used, the ventilator circuit may be heated to prevent excessive condensation in the circuit. A passive humidifier uses an artificial nose (heat and moisture exchanger) to collect heat and humidity from the patient's exhaled gas and returns that to the patient on the next inhalation. Regardless of the humidification technique used, condensation should be seen in the inspiratory ventilator circuit or the proximal endotracheal tube or both, which indicates that the inspired gas is fully saturated with water vapor.

EQUATION 22–1

Effects of Compressible Volume

The effect of compressible volume on the delivered tidal volume (VT) can be expressed as follows:

$$VTpt = \frac{1}{1 + (Cpc/Crs)} \times VTvent$$

where:

VTpt = Tidal volume delivered to the patient

Cpc = Compliance of the ventilator circuit

Crs = Compliance of the respiratory system

VTvent = Tidal volume from the ventilator circuit

The effect of compressible volume on auto-PEEP (positive end-expiratory pressure) can be expressed as follows:

$$\text{Auto-PEEP} = \frac{Crs + Cpc}{Crs} \times \text{Measured Pplat}$$

where auto-PEEP is the patient's actual auto-PEEP (positive end-expiratory pressure).

The effect of compressible volume on the Pplat (plateau pressure) can be expressed as follows:

$$Pplat = \frac{Crs + Cpc}{Crs} \times \text{Measured auto-PEEP}$$

where Pplat is the patient's actual plateau pressure.

The effect of compressible volume on the mixed exhaled partial pressure of carbon dioxide ($P\bar{E}CO_2$) can be expressed as follows:

$$P\bar{E}CO_2 = P\bar{E}CO_{2(vent)} \times \frac{VTvent}{VTpt}$$

where:

$P\bar{E}CO_2$ = Patient's actual $P\bar{E}CO_2$

$P\bar{E}CO_{2(vent)}$ = $P\bar{E}CO_2$ from the ventilator circuit

VTvent = Tidal volume from the ventilator circuit

VTpt = Tidal volume delivered to the patient

Monitoring the Mechanically Ventilated Patient

It is important to monitor the function of the mechanical ventilator frequently, including checking the ventilator settings and alarm systems, the humidifier and circuitry, and the patient's airway.

Physical Assessment

Asymmetric chest motion may indicate main stem (endobronchial) intubation, pneumothorax, or atelectasis. Paradoxical chest motion may be seen with flail chest or respiratory muscle dysfunction. Retractions may occur if the inspiratory flow or sensitivity is inappropriately set or if the airway is obstructed. If the patient is not breathing in synchrony with the ventilator (i.e., is bucking the ventilator), the settings on the ventilator may not be appropriate or the patient may need sedation or analgesia or both. A patient respiratory rate greater than the trigger rate on the ventilator may indicate the presence of auto-PEEP compromising triggering. In conjunction with inspection, the chest can be palpated to assess the symmetry of chest movement. Palpation of the tracheal position can help detect pneumothorax. Crepitation indicates subcutaneous emphysema. Percussion can be useful in the detection of unilateral hyperresonance or tympany with a pneumothorax. Unilateral decreased breath sounds may indicate bronchial intubation, pneumothorax, atelectasis, or pleural effusion. An end-inspiratory squeak over the trachea usually indicates insufficient air in the artificial airway cuff.

RESPIRATORY RECAP

Methods of Humidification with Mechanical Ventilation

- *Active humidification*: Heated humidifier
- *Passive humidification*: Artificial nose
- The presence of condensate in the inspiratory circuit near the patient indicates adequate humidification.

Blood Gas Measurements

The earliest indicators of hypoxemia often are changes in the patient's clinical status (e.g., restlessness and confusion, changes in level of consciousness, tachycardia or bradycardia, changes in blood pressure, tachypnea, bucking the ventilator, cyanosis). The most commonly used assessment of oxygenation is the partial pressure of arterial oxygen. A low PaO_2 indicates hypoxemia

RESPIRATORY RECAP

Monitoring Required During Mechanical Ventilation

- Physical examination
- Blood gas measurements
- Lung mechanics
- Hemodynamics
- Patient–ventilator synchrony
- Sedation

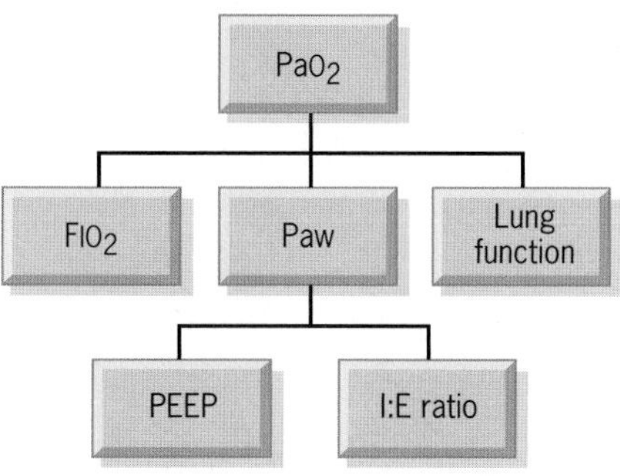

FIGURE 22–24 Factors affecting Pa_{O_2} during mechanical ventilation.

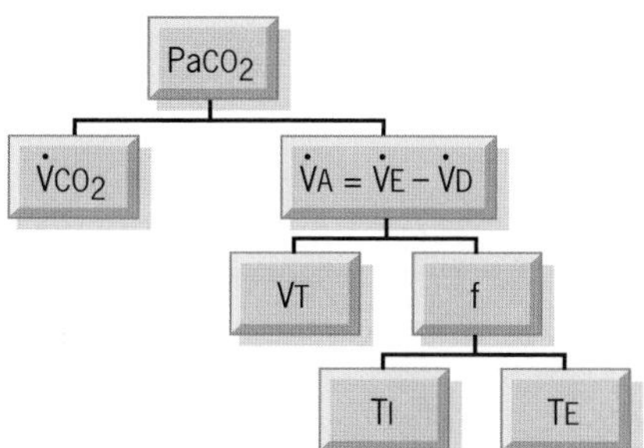

FIGURE 22–25 Factors affecting Pa_{CO_2} during mechanical ventilation.

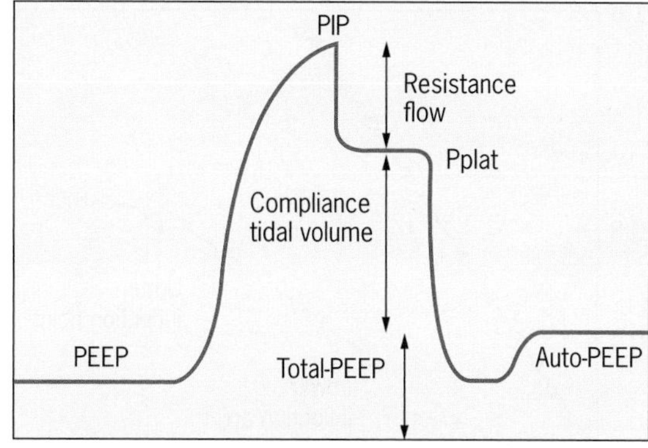

FIGURE 22–26 Airway pressure waveform during volume control ventilation. An end-inspiratory and an end-expiratory breath hold is applied to measure plateau pressure and auto-PEEP. Note that the difference between peak inspiratory pressure and plateau pressure is determined by the flow setting on the ventilator and airways resistance. Note that the difference between plateau pressure and total PEEP is determined by the tidal volume setting on the ventilator and the total level of PEEP (including auto-PEEP).

and a dysfunction in the lungs' ability to oxygenate arterial blood. The Pa_{O_2} must always be interpreted in relation to the F_{IO_2} (and often the mean airway pressure). In mechanically ventilated patients, a number of factors can affect the Pa_{O_2}, such as a change in the F_{IO_2}, the PEEP level, or the patient's lung function (**Figure 22–24**).

The mixed venous oxygenation ($P\bar{v}_{O_2}$ or $S\bar{v}_{O_2}$) is a better indicator of tissue oxygenation. A $P\bar{v}_{O_2}$ less than 35 mm Hg (or $S\bar{v}_{O_2}$ less than 70%) indicates tissue hypoxia. The Pa_{CO_2} is determined by carbon dioxide production ($\dot{V}_{CO_2}$) and the alveolar ventilation ($\dot{V}_A$). If the $\dot{V}_{CO_2}$ is constant, the Pa_{CO_2} varies inversely with the $\dot{V}_A$. The minute ventilation ($\dot{V}_E$) affects the Pa_{CO_2} indirectly because of the relationship between the $\dot{V}_E$ and the $\dot{V}_A$. An increase in the $\dot{V}_E$ decreases the Pa_{CO_2}, and a decrease in the $\dot{V}_E$ increases the Pa_{CO_2}. This is illustrated by the following relationship:

$$Pa_{CO_2} = (\dot{V}_{CO_2} \times 0.863) / (\dot{V}_E \times [1 - V_D/V_T])$$

where Pa_{CO_2} is the partial pressure of arterial carbon dioxide, $\dot{V}_{CO_2}$ is carbon dioxide production, $\dot{V}_E$ is minute ventilation, and V_D/V_T is the ratio of dead space to tidal volume. **Figure 22–25** shows the factors that determine the Pa_{CO_2} during mechanical ventilation.

The use of noninvasive monitors may reduce the need for arterial blood gas determinations, because they allow continuous assessment between blood gas measurements. Pulse oximetry can be used to titrate an appropriate F_{IO_2} and PEEP. Continuous pulse oximetry has become the standard of care in mechanically ventilated patients. End-tidal P_{CO_2} is used to monitor carbon dioxide levels noninvasively. In patients with normal lungs, end-tidal P_{CO_2} closely approximates the Pa_{CO_2}. However, in patients with an elevated V_D/V_T, there can be a large and inconsistent gradient between the Pa_{CO_2} and the end-tidal P_{CO_2}. For this reason, monitoring end-tidal P_{CO_2} is of limited value for the assessment of the Pa_{CO_2} during mechanical ventilation. End-tidal P_{CO_2} is useful to differentiate tracheal intubation from esophageal intubation.

Lung Mechanics

Monitoring of the peak pressure, Pplat, and auto-PEEP is particularly important. Pplat is measured by application of an end-inspiratory pause of 0.5 to 1.5 seconds, and auto-PEEP is determined by application of an end-expiratory pause of 0.5 to 1.5 seconds (**Figure 22–26**). During PCV the inspiratory flow often decreases to a no-flow period at end-inspiration. In this case, the peak pressure and Pplat are equivalent. Both Pplat and auto-PEEP can be accurately measured only when the patient is not exerting effort.

To avoid overdistention and lung injury, the goal is to maintain Pplat below 30 cm H_2O (and lower if possible). To assist in this and to minimize unnecessary cardiac effects and triggering difficulties, auto-PEEP should be as low as possible, preferably zero. Importantly, these circuit measurements of respiratory system pressures all assume normal chest wall compliance in order for them to be a reasonable estimate of transpulmonary pressures (i.e., a normal chest wall compliance will have little effect on the measured airway pressures). In the setting of abnormal, very low chest wall compliance (e.g., obesity, ascites), these airway pressure

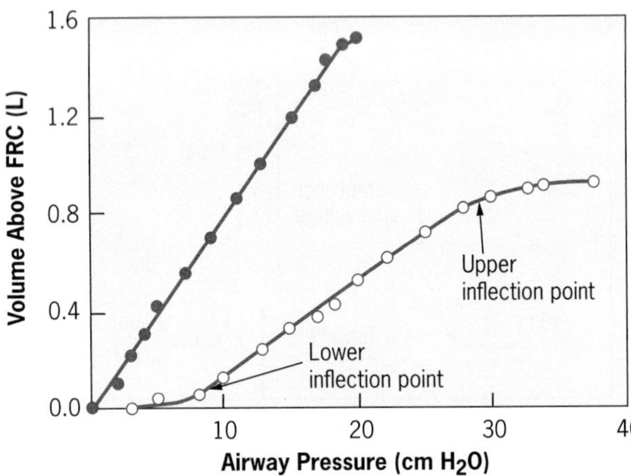

FIGURE 22–27 Pressure–volume curve for normal lungs (solid circles) and ARDS (open circles). Note the presence of a lower and upper inflection point on the pressure–volume curve for ARDS.

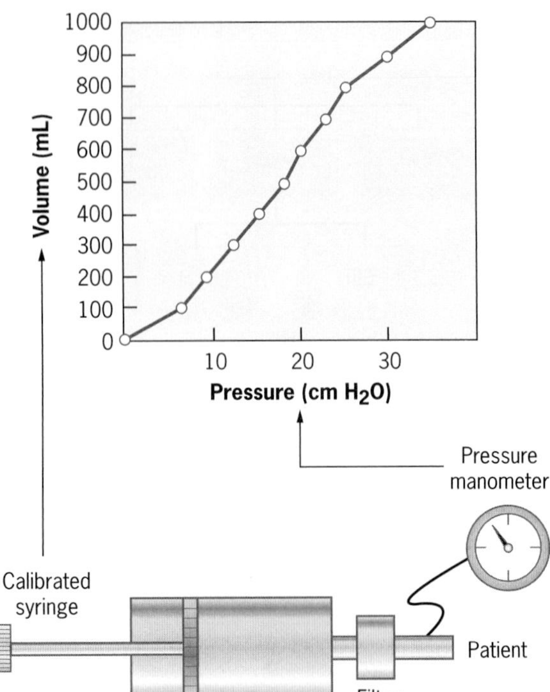

FIGURE 22–28 Super syringe technique to measure pressure–volume curve.

measurements may be profoundly affected by chest wall stiffness and these effects need to be subtracted from the airway pressure to determine true transpulmonary pressure. This can be done directly with an esophageal pressure measurement or estimated by an experienced clinician. The use of esophageal pressures for both estimating true transpulmonary pressures and assessing the triggering loads from auto-PEEP is described in more detail next.

Auto-PEEP has other manifestations that can be monitored. The patient's breathing pattern can be observed; if exhalation is still occurring when the next breath is delivered, auto-PEEP is present. Inspiratory efforts that do not trigger the ventilator suggest the presence of auto-PEEP. From the flow graphics on the ventilator, it can be observed that expiratory flow does not return to zero before the subsequent breath is delivered when auto-PEEP is present.

The inflation pressure–volume (PV) curve of the respiratory system can be used to set the ventilator.[83] For patients with ARDS, the PV curve is sigmoidal (**Figure 22–27**). A lower inflection point presumably represents the pressure at which a large number of alveoli are recruited, or opened. An upper inflection point presumably represents the pressure at which a large number of alveoli are overdistended. Therefore, it would seem reasonable to set the PEEP above the lower inflection point and the Pplat below the upper inflection point. Because there is hysteresis in the PV curve (i.e., it is shifted leftward during deflation), some argue that the ideal PEEP setting should be determined during the deflation phase of the PV plot.

The traditional PV curve is measured as a series of plateau pressures during small incremental changes in inspiratory and expiratory volumes from a super syringe (**Figure 22–28**). The inflation PV curve can also be measured when a slow (e.g., 5 to 10 L/min), constant flow is set on the ventilator and the ventilator display of the PV curve is observed. This slow flow effectively eliminates the effects of resistance on the pressure measurement. The role of the PV curve in setting the ventilator currently is unclear. Although its use is physiologically attractive, more experience is needed with these measurements before the PV curve can be recommended for routine use in setting the ventilator.

The stress index is a method to assess the level of PEEP to avoid overdistension and underrecruitment (**Figure 22–29**).[84] This approach uses the shape of the pressure–time curve during constant-flow tidal volume delivery. If the compliance is worsening as the lungs are inflated (upward concavity, stress index > 1), this suggests overdistension, and the recommendation is to decrease PEEP or tidal volume. If the compliance is improving as the lungs are inflated (downward concavity, stress index < 1), this suggests further potential for recruitment, and the recommendation is to increase PEEP. The ideal stress index is 1, in which there is a linear increase in pressure with constant-flow inflation of the lungs.

Esophageal pressure is measured from a thin-walled balloon, which contains a small volume of air ($<$1 mL), placed into the lower esophagus (**Figure 22–30**).[85] Esophageal pressure changes reflect changes in pleural pressure, but the absolute esophageal pressure does not reflect absolute pleural pressure. Changes in esophageal pressure can be used to assess respiratory effort and patient work of breathing during spontaneous breathing and patient-triggered modes of ventilation, to assess chest wall compliance during full ventilatory support, and to assess auto-PEEP during spontaneous breathing

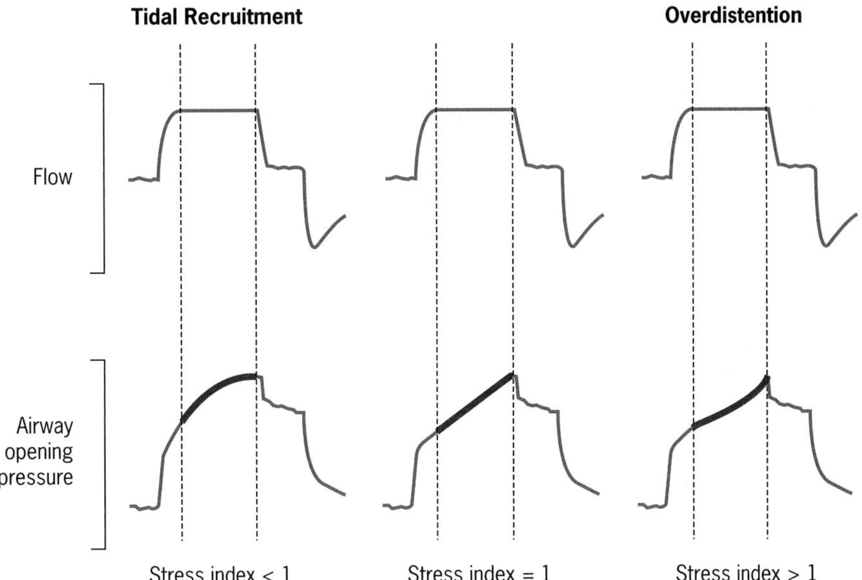

FIGURE 22–29 Stress index concept during constant-flow volume control ventilation. For a stress index less than 1, the airway pressure curve presents a downward concavity, suggesting a continuous decrease in elastance and tidal recruitment. For a stress index higher than 1, the curve presents an upward concavity, suggesting a continuous increase in elastance and overdistention. For a stress index equal to 1, the curve is straight, suggesting the absence of tidal variations in elastance. Reprinted with permission of the American Thoracic Society. Copyright © American Thoracic Society. Grasso S, Stripoli T, De Michele M, et al. ARDSnet ventilatory protocol and alveolar hyperinflation: role of positive end-expiratory pressure. *Am J Respir Crit Care Med.* 2007;176:761–767. Official Journal of the American Thoracic Society; Diane Gern, Publisher.

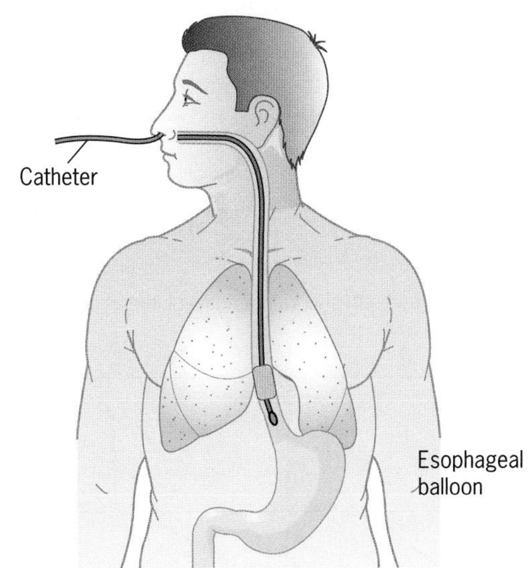

FIGURE 22–30 Position of esophageal balloon to measure changes in intrapleural pressure.

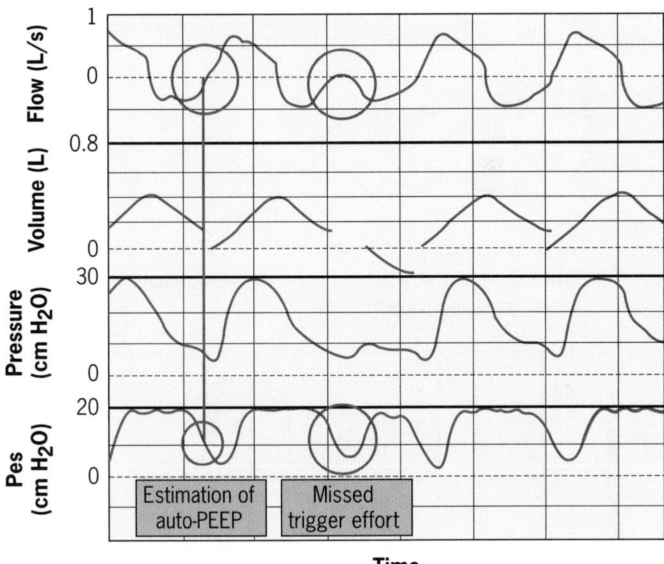

FIGURE 22–31 Auto-PEEP. Note the amount of effort required to trigger the ventilator, represented by the amount of decrease in esophageal pressure required for triggering. Also note the presence of an inspiratory effort that does not trigger the ventilator.

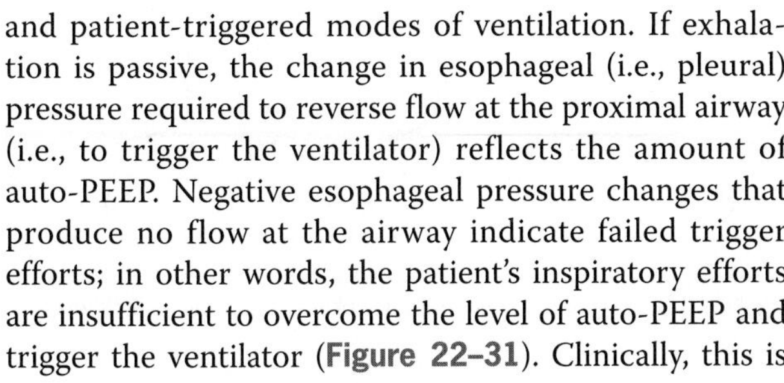
and patient-triggered modes of ventilation. If exhalation is passive, the change in esophageal (i.e., pleural) pressure required to reverse flow at the proximal airway (i.e., to trigger the ventilator) reflects the amount of auto-PEEP. Negative esophageal pressure changes that produce no flow at the airway indicate failed trigger efforts; in other words, the patient's inspiratory efforts are insufficient to overcome the level of auto-PEEP and trigger the ventilator (**Figure 22–31**). Clinically, this is recognized as a patient respiratory rate (observed by inspecting chest wall movement) that is greater than the trigger rate on the ventilator.

The increase in esophageal pressure (ΔPes) during passive inflation of the lungs can be used to calculate chest wall compliance (**Figure 22–32**):

$$C_{CW} = V_T/\Delta Pes$$

Changes in esophageal pressure, relative to changes in alveolar pressure, can be used to calculate transpulmonary pressure (lung stress). This may allow more precise setting of tidal volume (and Pplat) in patients with reduced chest wall compliance. In this case, transpulmonary pressure (difference between Pplat and Pes) is targeted at less than 27 cm H_2O.

The use of an esophageal balloon has been advocated to allow more precise setting of PEEP.[86] If pleural pressure is high relative to alveolar pressure (i.e., PEEP), then there may be a potential for derecruitment. With this approach, PEEP is increased until the transpulmonary pressure is positive (i.e., PEEP is greater than esophageal pressure) (**Figure 22-33**). This is most likely with a decrease in chest wall compliance, such as occurs with abdominal compartment syndrome, pleural effusion, or obesity. In this case, it is desirable to keep PEEP greater than pleural pressure. Unfortunately, artifacts in esophageal pressure, especially in supine critically ill patients, make it very difficult to measure absolute pleural pressure accurately.[87,88] In patients with abdominal compartment syndrome, bladder pressure may be useful to assess intra-abdominal pressure, the potential collapsing effect on the lungs, and the amount of PEEP necessary to counterbalance this effect.[89]

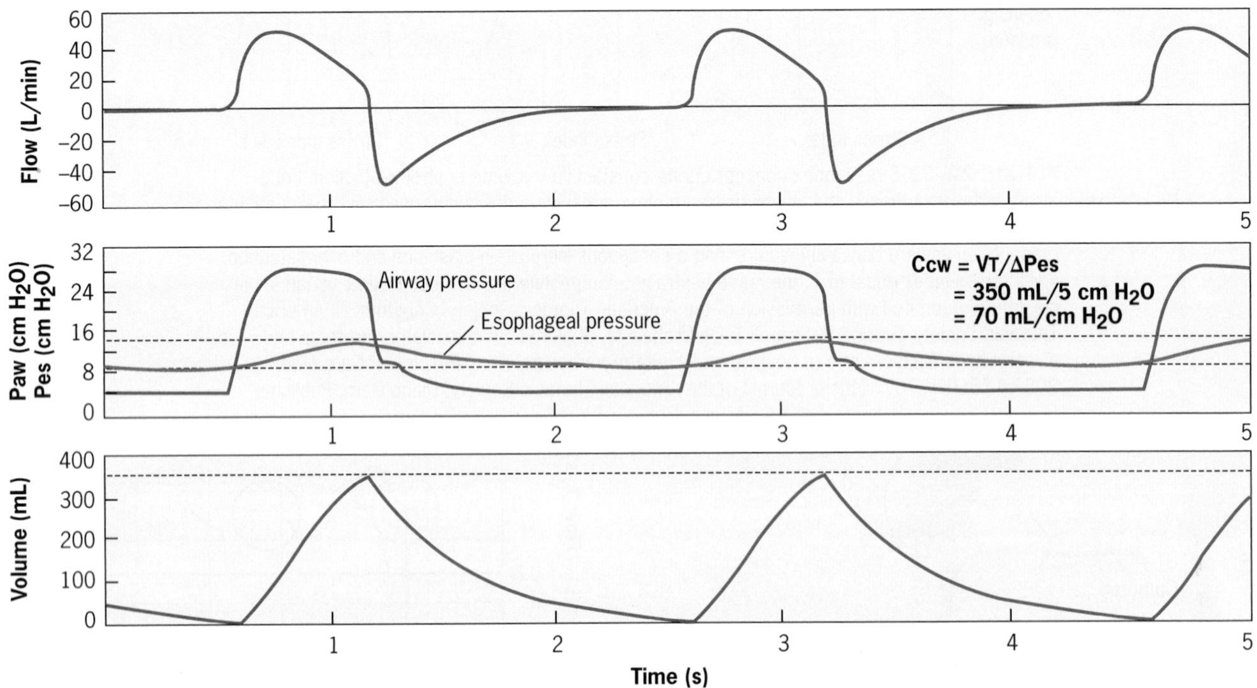

FIGURE 22-32 Calculation of chest wall compliance. The esophageal pressure increases by 5 cm H_2O with a tidal volume of 350 mL in a passively ventilated patient.

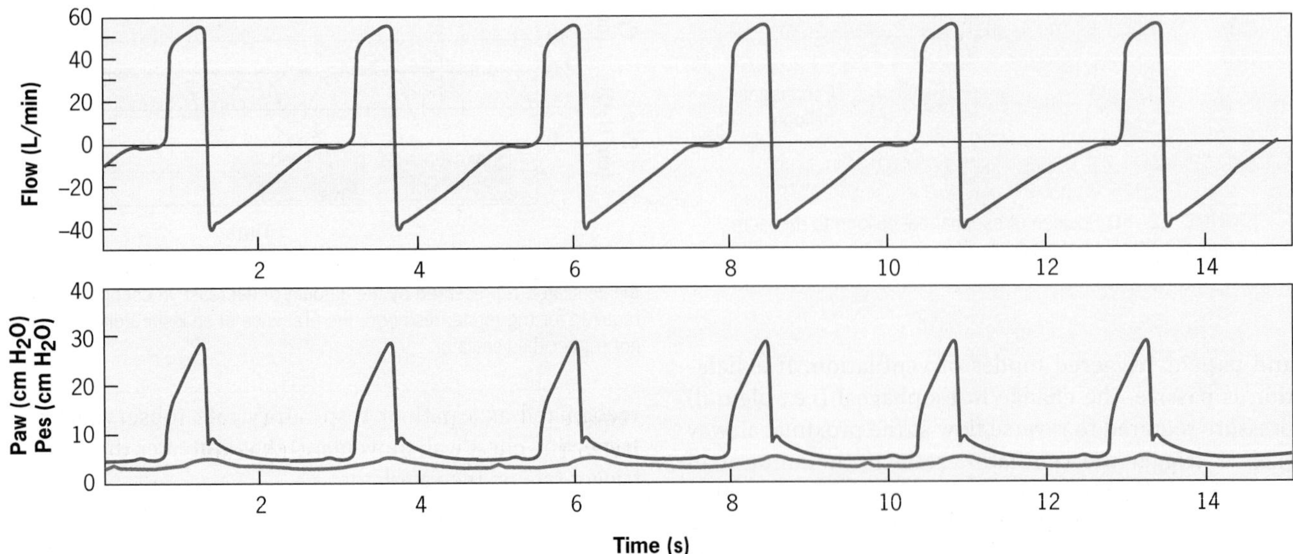

FIGURE 22-33 Airway and esophageal pressures in a passively ventilated patient. In this case, the transpulmonary pressure during exhalation is positive because PEEP is greater than the esophageal pressure.

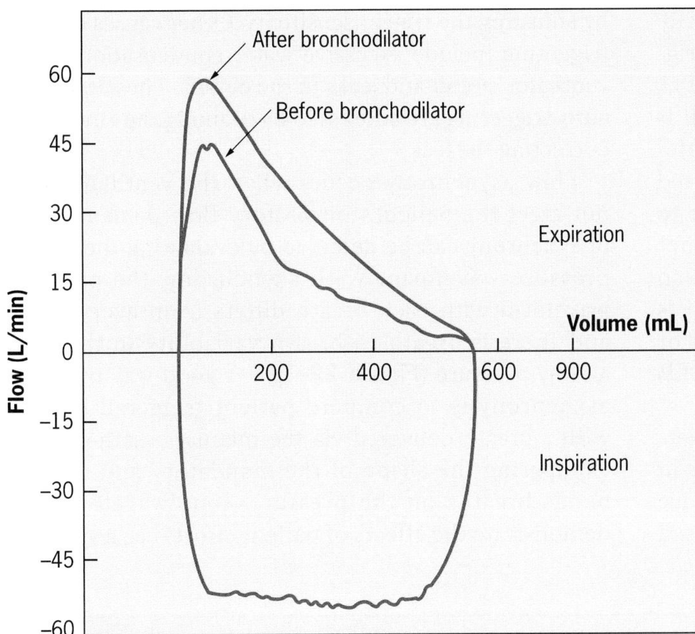

FIGURE 22–34 Flow–volume loops showing a response to bronchodilator administration. The expiratory limb of the curve is concave in patients with expiratory flow limitation. Administration of a bronchodilator aerosol leads to improvement in expiratory flow. From MacIntyre NM, Branson RD. *Mechanical Ventilation.* WB Saunders; 2001:17.

In patients with obstructive lung disease, it may be useful to monitor the flow–volume curve during mechanical ventilation (**Figure 22–34**). The flow–volume curve may provide insight into the severity of airflow obstruction and response to bronchodilator administration.[90]

Hemodynamics

Because positive pressure ventilation can affect cardiac function, it is important to assess hemodynamics during mechanical ventilation. At a minimum, the arterial blood pressure and heart rate should be measured frequently. When the high airway pressures needed to support oxygenation adversely affect cardiac performance, hemodynamics may need to be supported with fluid, inotropes, and pressors. The role of the pulmonary artery catheter in mechanical ventilation is unclear, and its use has declined in recent years.

It is important to appreciate the effect of positive pressure ventilation on hemodynamic assessments. During positive pressure ventilation, pleural pressure increases during inhalation by an amount determined by lung compliance and chest wall compliance:[89]

$$\Delta Ppl/\Delta Pplat = C_L / (C_L + Ccw)$$

where ΔPpl is the change in pleural pressure, ΔPplat is the change in alveolar pressure, C_L is lung compliance, and Ccw is chest wall compliance. By convention, hemodynamic measurements are made at end-exhalation (i.e., when transpulmonary pressures are lowest) to account for the respiratory variation in pleural pressure. At end-exhalation, measurements such as the pulmonary artery wedge pressure, pulmonary artery pressure, and central venous pressure are affected by the amount of PEEP transmitted to the pleural space, which is determined by lung compliance and chest wall compliance. In patients with normal chest wall compliance (over 150 mL/cm H_2O) and decreased lung compliance (under 50 mL/cm H_2O), less than one-fourth of the alveolar pressure is transmitted to the pleural space.

In addition to esophageal pressure measurements, changes in the pleural pressure can also be estimated through observation of the respiratory variation in the thoracic vascular catheter pressure measurements (i.e., the central venous pressure, pulmonary artery pressure, and pulmonary artery occlusion pressure). With a stiff chest wall, the esophageal pressure or vascular pressure shows greater fluctuation during the respiratory cycle, and greater effects of positive pressure ventilation on hemodynamics can be expected.

Patient–Ventilator Interactions: Synchrony and Asynchrony

During any patient-triggered breath, the patient's effort must interact with the ventilator's gas delivery algorithm. These interactions are considered synchronous when ventilator flow is in phase with patient effort. In contrast, asynchronous interactions occur when these processes are out of phase. At its worse, asynchrony appears as if the patient is fighting or bucking the ventilator. However, asynchrony often is much more subtle. Failure of the patient to breathe in synchrony with the ventilator decreases patient comfort and increases both the work of breathing and the oxygen cost of breathing. Asynchrony often leads to increased sedation needs and has been associated with longer time on mechanical ventilation.[91,92] Asynchrony can be categorized as trigger asynchrony, flow asynchrony, cycle asynchrony, and mode asynchrony.

Trigger asynchrony occurs when the patient has difficulty triggering the ventilator or the ventilator auto-triggers. The ventilator trigger sensitivity should be as sensitive as possible without causing auto-triggering. Inability of the patient to trigger can be caused by an insensitive trigger setting on the ventilator, which can be corrected by reduction of the pressure or flow required for the patient to trigger the ventilator. Inability to trigger also can be due to respiratory muscle weakness. Perhaps the most common cause of failure to trigger is auto-PEEP in patients with obstructive airway disease. As noted earlier, auto-PEEP can be reduced by lowering minute ventilation, shortening the I:E ratio, or reducing airway obstruction through administration of bronchodilators and clearing of secretions. Using PEEP to counterbalance auto-PEEP and thus reduce the triggering load can be effective for patients with COPD, but this technique is not effective if the auto-PEEP is primarily the result of a high minute ventilation and insufficient expiratory time. Whenever PEEP is used to counterbalance auto-PEEP, care must be taken to avoid hyperinflation with the PEEP. When the attempt is to counterbalance auto-PEEP with PEEP, the clinician should monitor the peak inspiratory pressure as PEEP is increased. If the PIP rises above the desired threshold or increases by a value greater than the increase in PEEP, overdistention should be suspected.

Another form of trigger asynchrony is auto-triggering. Auto-triggering causes the ventilator to trigger in response to an artifact. One artifact that can produce auto-triggering is cardiac oscillations.[93] This is addressed by adjusting the trigger sensitivity. Other causes of auto-triggering include excessive water condensation in the ventilator circuit and leaks in the circuit. These causes of auto-triggering are addressed by draining the circuit and correcting the leak.

Flow asynchrony occurs when the ventilator does not meet the patient's inspiratory flow demand. Lack of synchrony can be detected by evaluating the airway pressure waveform. With asynchrony, the pressure waveform with each breath differs from every other, and there is breath-to-breath variability in the peak airway pressure (**Figure 22–35**). A good way to detect asynchrony is to compare patient-triggered breaths with a breath delivered via the manual breath control. Comparing the shape of the mandatory and spontaneous breaths on the pressure–time waveform can demonstrate the effects of patient effort (i.e., a vigorous

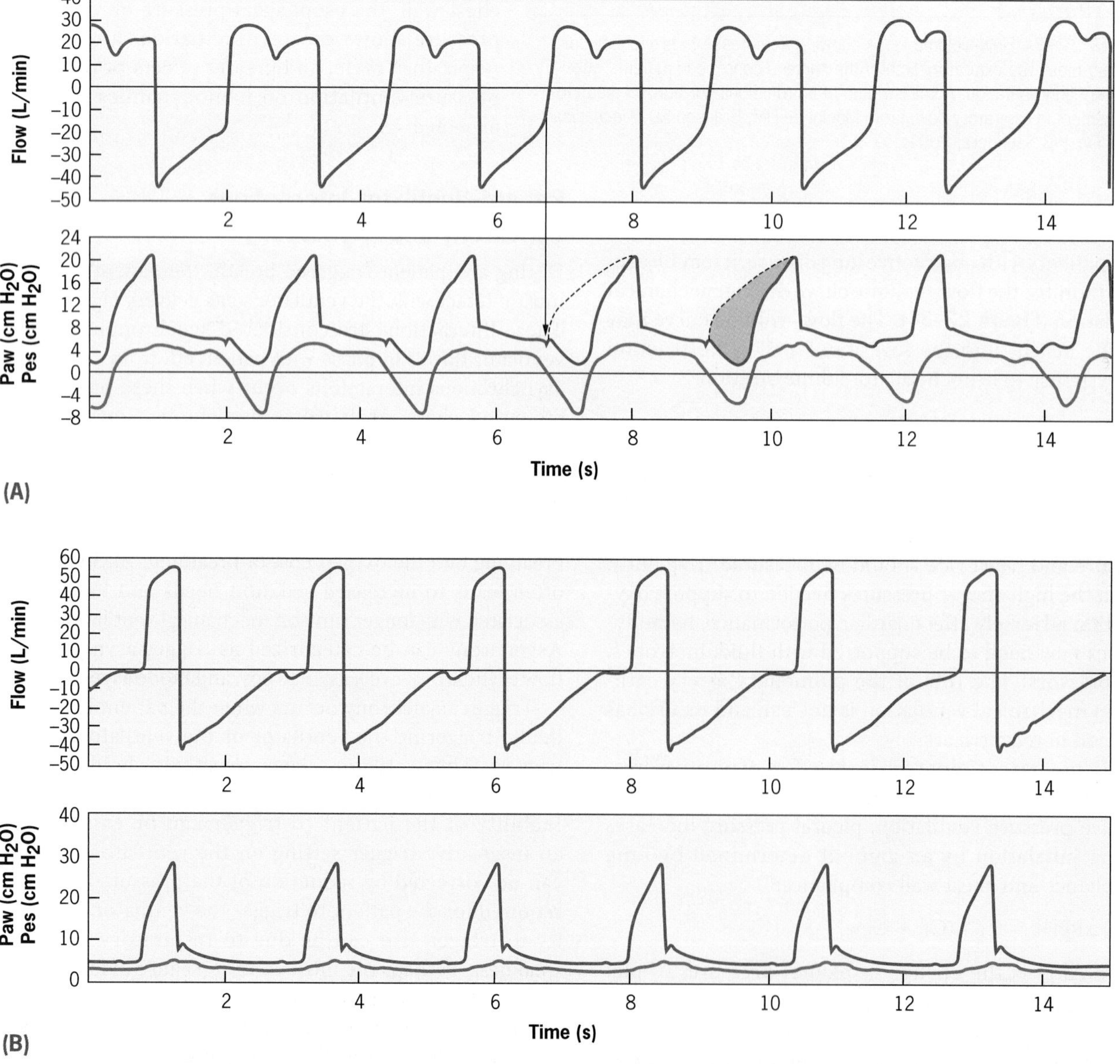

FIGURE 22–35 (**A**) The inspiratory effort of the patient is not met by fixed flow from the ventilator during pressure control ventilation. The dashed line represents the airway pressure curve that would result from passive inflation, and the shaded area represents the work done by the patient against the insufficient flow from the ventilator. (**B**) When the flow setting of the ventilator is increased, the patient is more synchronous with the ventilator.

patient effort literally sucks the airway pressure graphic downward). Clinical signs of asynchrony include tachypnea, retractions, and chest-abdominal paradox. Flow asynchrony can be corrected by an increase in the flow setting or change in the inspiratory flow pattern during VCV, by changing from VCV to PCV,[35,36,94] or by an increase in the pressure setting or the rise time setting during PCV or PSV. However, asynchrony can also occur with PCV (**Figure 22–36**).[95] For patients who have a high respiratory drive because of anxiety or pain, flow asynchrony may be improved by appropriate use of sedation or analgesia.[95]

Cycle asynchrony occurs when the neural inspiratory time of the patient does not match the inspiratory time setting on the ventilator. If the inspiratory time is too short, the patient might double-trigger the ventilator (**Figure 22–37**). During volume control ventilation, this can cause breath stacking, such that the patient is effectively receiving a tidal volume twice what is set. If the inspiratory time is too long, the patient will actively exhale against the ventilator-delivered breath. Cycle asynchrony can occur during PSV in patients with obstructive lung disease or when a leak is present. Cycle asynchrony during PSV can be corrected by lowering the pressure support level, by an increase in the termination flow setting on newer-generation ventilators, or by use of pressure control instead of pressure support (pressure control causes inspiration to be time cycled rather than flow cycled). Cycle asynchrony is recognized as activation of the expiratory (abdominal) muscles during the inspiratory phase; this can be detected clinically by palpation of the patient's abdomen. Cycle asynchrony can also be detected by observation of the ventilator graphics (**Figure 22–38**).

Mode asynchrony occurs when the ventilator delivers different breath types. With SIMV, for example, some breath types are mandatory and others are spontaneous. Because the patient's respiratory center cannot adapt to varying breath types, asynchrony can develop between the patient and the ventilator. Another form of mode asynchrony occurs with adaptive pressure control, in which the ventilator reduces support when the patient's efforts result in a tidal volume that exceeds the set tidal volume.[49,97]

Sedation

Anxiety is a common cause of failure to breathe in synchrony with the ventilator. In these cases pharmacologic support may be necessary in the form of analgesics (narcotics), sedatives (benzodiazepines), or (rarely) paralyzing agents. When short-term sedation is necessary to bring a patient into synchrony with the ventilator, propofol may be useful. When ventilation requires long inspiratory times and high airway pressures, pharmacologic control of the patient's breathing is almost always necessary.

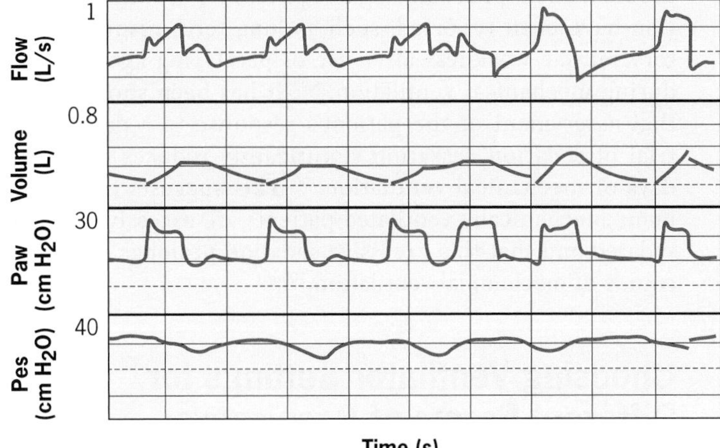

FIGURE 22–36 Patient–ventilator asynchrony in a patient receiving pressure control ventilation. From Kallet RH, Campbell AR, Dicker RA, et al. Work of breathing during lung-protective ventilation in patients with acute lung injury and acute respiratory distress syndrome: a comparison between volume and pressure-regulated breathing modes. *Respir Care.* 2005;50:1623–1631. Reprinted with permission.

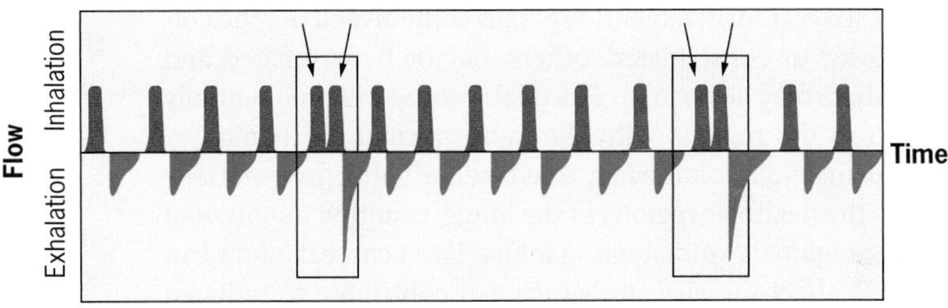

FIGURE 22–37 Double-triggering. Note that the patient receives two breaths in rapid succession. Adapted from Pohlman MC, et al. Excessive tidal volume from breath stacking during lung-protective ventilation for acute lung injury. *Crit Care Med.* 2008;36:3019–3023.

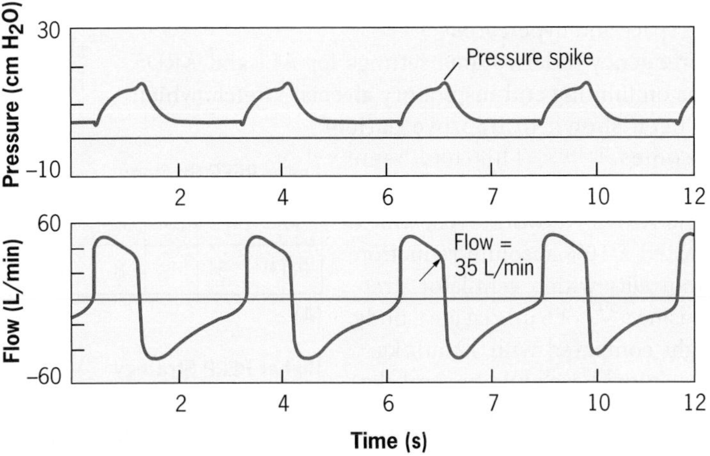

FIGURE 22–38 Airway pressure and flow waveforms illustrating active exhalation during pressure support ventilation. Note that the flow does not decelerate to the flow termination criterion of the ventilator (5 L/min for this specific ventilator). Also note the presence of a pressure spike at the end of each inspiration, indicating that the ventilator is pressure cycling rather than flow cycling. Modified from Branson RD. Modes of ventilator operation. In: MacIntyre NR, Branson RD, eds. *Mechanical Ventilation.* Philadelphia: WB Saunders; 2000. Copyright Elsevier 2000.

It must be remembered that all forms of respiratory suppression are associated with adverse side effects. It is most important that disconnect alarms be properly set when the patient's ability to breathe spontaneously is pharmacologically suppressed. Significant problems with pharmacologic suppression of respiration have been reported, such as long-term respiratory muscle weakness after use of paralyzing agents during mechanical ventilation.[98,99] It has been shown that assessment of the patient's response to a daily trial of sedation cessation significantly reduces the days of mechanical ventilation.[100] This suggests that many mechanically ventilated patients are excessively sedated and that this excessive sedation prolongs the course of mechanical ventilation.[100,101]

Choosing Ventilator Settings for Different Forms of Respiratory Failure

ALI and ARDS (Parenchymal Lung Injury)

With ALI and ARDS, lung compliance is low and lung volume is decreased. It is important to realize, however, that there are often marked regional differences in the degree of alveolar involvement. Whereas some alveoli may be collapsed or consolidated, others may be hyperinflated and others may be normal. The tidal volume will preferentially go to the regions with the more normal mechanics. A normal tidal volume may thus be distributed preferentially to the healthier regions of the lungs, resulting in potential for regional overdistention injury. Parenchymal injury can also affect the airways, which can contribute to reduced regional ventilation to injured lung units. Gas exchange abnormalities with ALI and ARDS are a consequence of alveolar flooding and/or collapse, resulting in $\dot{V}/\dot{Q}$ mismatching and shunts. The low-$\dot{V}/\dot{Q}$ regions result in hypoxemia, and the high-$\dot{V}/\dot{Q}$ regions result in increased dead space and hypercarbia.

Frequency–tidal volume settings for ALI and ARDS focus on limiting end-inspiratory alveolar stretch, which has been shown to improve patient outcomes.[10–18,102] This has been most convincingly demonstrated by the ARDS Network Trial, which reported a 10% absolute reduction in mortality with a ventilator strategy using a V_T of 6 mL/kg ideal body weight compared with 12 mL/kg.[12] Thus, initial V_T should be 6 mL/kg. Moreover, strong consideration should be given to further reducing the V_T if Pplat, adjusted for the effect of excessive chest wall stiffness, exceeds 30 cm H_2O. The V_T can be increased to as much as 8 mL/kg if there is marked asynchrony or severe acidosis, provided that the Pplat does not exceed 30 cm H_2O. Respiratory rate is adjusted to control pH. The potential for air trapping in parenchymal lung injury is low if the breathing frequency is less than 35 breaths/min. An increased inspiratory time, and even inverse ratio ventilation (e.g., APRV), can be used to increase Pa_{O_2} with refractory hypoxemia. The mechanisms for improved oxygenation with inverse ratio ventilation include longer gas mixing time, recruitment of slowly filling alveoli, and development of auto-PEEP.

Although imaging or mechanical techniques to guide proper PEEP settings have physiologic appeal, they are technically challenging and not practical for routine use. Thus, most clinicians rely on various gas exchange criteria to guide PEEP and F_{IO_2} titrations. This involves the use of algorithms designed to provide adequate oxygenation (Pa_{O_2} 55 to 80 mm Hg or Sp_{O_2} of 88% to 95%) while minimizing F_{IO_2}. An example would be the National Institutes of Health's ARDS Network PEEP/F_{IO_2} algorithm (**Figure 22-39**).[12,103] Note that this PEEP/F_{IO_2} algorithm attempts to balance pressure administration (PEEP) with Sp_{O_2} or Pa_{O_2} and with F_{IO_2}. Randomized controlled trials have compared various gas exchange strategies for setting PEEP in conjunction with low V_T strategies and have reported that both aggressive (i.e., 13 to 15 cm H_2O PEEP) and conservative (i.e., 7 to 9 cm H_2O) approaches have comparable outcomes.[103–105] In terms of hospital survival, however, a recent meta-analysis of these studies suggests that higher levels of PEEP may be beneficial for patients with ARDS ($Pa_{O_2}/F_{IO_2} \leq 200$ mm Hg), whereas higher levels of PEEP are not beneficial (and may produce harm) in patients with ALI ($Pa_{O_2}/F_{IO_2} > 200$ mm Hg).[105,106]

Some mechanical approaches to setting PEEP are practiced in ICUs where the staff has considerable experience managing ALI and ARDS (**Box 22-6**). These include titration to the highest compliance,[107] titration to a pressure greater than the lower inflection point of the pressure–volume curve,[83] and the best stress index.[84] PEEP should be avoided that results in a Pplat above 30 cm H_2O. Higher levels of PEEP should be reserved for cases where

Lower PEEP Strategy

F_{IO_2}	0.3	0.4	0.4	0.5	0.5	0.6	0.7	0.7	0.7	0.8	0.9	0.9	0.9	1.0
PEEP	5	5	8	8	10	10	10	12	14	14	14	16	18	18–24

(A)

Higher PEEP Strategy

F_{IO_2}	0.3	0.3	0.3	0.3	0.3	0.4	0.4	0.5	0.5	0.5–0.8	0.8	0.9	1.0	1.0
PEEP	5	8	10	12	14	14	16	16	18	20	22	22	22	24

(B)

FIGURE 22-39 **(A)** Low-PEEP strategy used in the ARDSnet study. **(B)** High-PEEP strategy used in the ARDSnet study. In each case, combinations of PEEP and F_{IO_2} were used to maintain a Pa_{O_2} of 55 to 80 mm Hg or Sp_{O_2} of 88% to 95%.

lung recruitment can be demonstrated. In the setting of refractory hypoxemia, recruitment maneuvers may be used, followed by a level of PEEP to maintain alveolar recruitment. When setting PEEP in patients with ALI or ARDS, the hemodynamic effects of the increased intrathoracic pressure should also be monitored.

Obstructive Lung Disease

Respiratory failure from airflow obstruction is due to increases in airway resistance. This increases the pressure required for airflow, which may overload inspiratory muscles, producing a ventilatory pump failure with spontaneous minute ventilation inadequate for gas exchange. In addition, the narrowed airways create regions of lung that cannot properly empty, and auto-PEEP is produced. These regions of overinflation create dead space and put inspiratory muscles at a substantial mechanical disadvantage, which further worsens muscle function. Overinflated regions may also compress more healthy regions of the lung, impairing $\dot{V}/\dot{Q}$ matching. Regions of air trapping and intrinsic PEEP also function as a threshold load to trigger mechanical breaths.

Noninvasive ventilation (NIV) is standard first-line therapy in patients with COPD and has been shown to improve outcomes by reducing the need for endotracheal intubation and improving survival in this patient population.[108] NIV has also been used in other forms of obstructive lung disease (e.g., asthma, cystic fibrosis), but there is less evidence for better outcomes in these patient populations. Invasive ventilatory support is usually reserved for those who fail NIV or in those in whom NIV is contraindicated.

Tidal volume should be sufficiently low (e.g., 6 mL/kg) to ensure that Pplat values are below 30 cm H_2O. The set rate is used to control pH. However, the elevated airways resistance and the low elastic recoil pressure with emphysema increase the potential for air trapping, and this limits the range of breath rates available. Permissive hypercapnia may be an appropriate trade-off to limit overdistention. The inspiratory time in obstructive lung disease is set as low as possible to minimize the development of air trapping. As noted earlier, judicious application of PEEP (up to 75% to 85% of auto-PEEP) can counterbalance auto-PEEP to facilitate triggering.[109] Use of a low-density gas (e.g., helium–oxygen mixtures [heliox]) is another technique that can be used to decrease auto-PEEP.

BOX 22-6

Methods for Selecting PEEP

Incremental PEEP: This approach uses combinations of PEEP and F_{IO_2} to achieve the desired level of oxygenation or the highest compliance.

Decremental PEEP: This approach begins with a high level of PEEP (e.g., 20 cm H_2O), after which PEEP is decreased in a stepwise fashion until derecruitment occurs, typically with a decrease in Pa_{O_2} and decrease in compliance.

Stress index measurement: The pressure–time curve is observed during constant-flow inhalation for signs of tidal recruitment and overdistention.

Esophageal pressure measurement: This method estimates the intrapleural pressure by using an esophageal balloon to measure the esophageal pressure and subsequently determine the optimal level of PEEP required.

Pressure–volume curve guidance: PEEP is set slightly greater than the lower inflection point.

Neuromuscular Disease

The risk of VILI is generally less in a patient with neuromuscular failure, because lung mechanics are often near normal and regional overdistention is thus less likely to occur. Higher tidal volumes may thus be used to improve comfort, maintain recruitment, prevent atelectasis, and avoid hypercarbia that may adversely affect central nervous system function. However, tidal volume should not exceed 10 mL/kg, and Pplat should be kept below 30 cm H_2O.[110] Low levels of PEEP are often beneficial for preventing atelectasis. If patients with neuromuscular disease develop ALI or ARDS, they should be managed using ventilator strategies incorporating lower tidal volumes and higher levels of PEEP.

Ventilatory Support Involves Trade-Offs

To provide adequate support yet minimize VILI, mechanical ventilation goals must involve trade-offs. The need for potentially injurious ventilating pressures, volumes, and supplemental O_2 must be weighed against the benefits of better gas exchange. Accordingly, pH goals as low as 7.15 and Pa_{O_2} goals as low as 55 mm Hg are often considered acceptable if necessary to protect the lungs from VILI.[111] Ventilator settings are thus selected to provide an adequate, but not necessarily normal, level of gas exchange while meeting the goals of enough PEEP to maintain alveolar recruitment and avoidance of a PEEP–tidal volume combination that unnecessarily overdistends alveoli at end-inspiration.[103–106] This has led to ventilatory strategies such as permissive hypercapnia, permissive hypoxemia, and permissive atelectasis.

Liberation from Mechanical Ventilation

An important aspect of the management of patients receiving mechanical ventilation is recognizing when the patient is ready to be liberated from the ventilator and extubating the patient at that point. Evidence-based clinical practice guidelines have been published related to liberation from mechanical ventilation; **Box 22–7** lists the recommendations from these guidelines.[112]

Respiratory Muscles

For successful liberation from the ventilator, the load placed on the respiratory muscles must be balanced by the muscles' ability to meet that load (**Figure 22–40**). Respiratory muscle fatigue occurs if the load placed on the muscles is excessive, if the muscles are weak, or if the duty cycle (the inspiratory time relative to total cycle time) is too long. Common causes of a high load are high airways resistance, low lung compliance, and high minute ventilation. In addition, malposition of the diaphragm from air trapping compromises inspiratory muscle function. Diminished respiratory muscle function may also be the result of disease, disuse, malnutrition, hypoxia, or electrolyte imbalance. The clinical signs of respiratory muscle fatigue are tachypnea, abnormal respiratory movements (respiratory alternans and abdominal paradox), and an increase in Pa_{CO_2}.[113]

Because the maximum inspiratory pressure (PImax) is a good indicator of overall respiratory muscle strength, a low PImax may predict respiratory muscle fatigue. The PImax is measured by attachment of an aneroid manometer to the endotracheal or tracheostomy tube. The patient then forcibly inhales after maximum exhalation. When the PImax is measured, it is recommended that a unidirectional valve be used and that the airway be completely obstructed for 20 to 25 seconds (**Figure 22–41**). A PImax more negative than –20 cm H_2O suggests adequate inspiratory muscle strength. However, if the patient has high airways resistance or

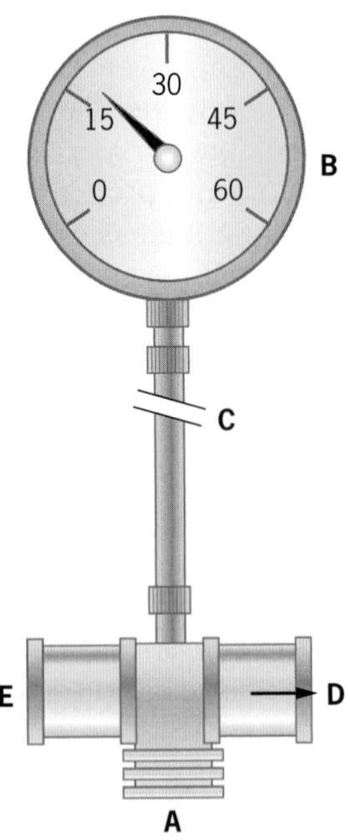

FIGURE 22–41 The one-way valve system used to measure maximum inspiratory pressure. The patient is connected at A, the manometer (B) is connected at C, and the patient exhales through D. Port E is occluded during the measurement. In this way, maximum inspiratory pressure is measured at functional residual capacity. From Kacmarek RM, Cycyk-Chapman MC, Young PJ, Romagnoli DM. Determination of maximal inspiratory pressure: a clinical study literature review. *Respir Care.* 1989;34:868–878. Reprinted with permission.

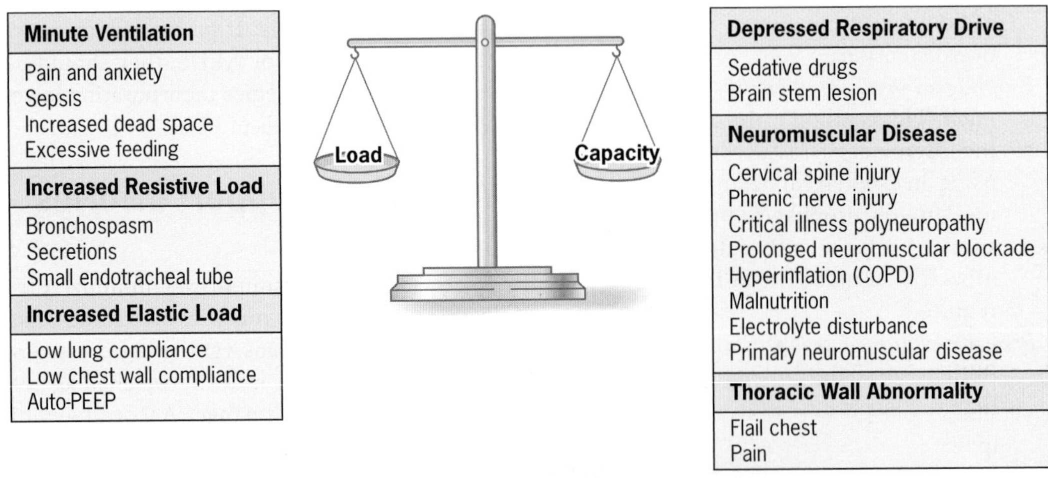

Minute Ventilation
Pain and anxiety
Sepsis
Increased dead space
Excessive feeding
Increased Resistive Load
Bronchospasm
Secretions
Small endotracheal tube
Increased Elastic Load
Low lung compliance
Low chest wall compliance
Auto-PEEP
Load
Capacity
Depressed Respiratory Drive
Sedative drugs
Brain stem lesion
Neuromuscular Disease
Cervical spine injury
Phrenic nerve injury
Critical illness polyneuropathy
Prolonged neuromuscular blockade
Hyperinflation (COPD)
Malnutrition
Electrolyte disturbance
Primary neuromuscular disease
Thoracic Wall Abnormality
Flail chest
Pain

FIGURE 22–40 Respiratory muscle performance is determined by the balance between the load that is placed on the respiratory muscles and the ability of the muscles to meet that load.

BOX 22–7

Evidence-Based Guidelines for Discontinuing Ventilatory Support

Recommendation 1: In patients requiring mechanical ventilation for more than 24 hours, a search for all the causes that may be contributing to ventilator dependence should be undertaken. This is particularly true in the patient who has failed attempts at withdrawing the mechanical ventilator. Reversing all possible ventilatory and nonventilatory issues should be an integral part of the ventilator discontinuation process.

Recommendation 2: Patients receiving mechanical ventilation for respiratory failure should undergo a formal assessment of discontinuation potential if the following criteria are satisfied: (1) evidence for some reversal of the underlying cause for respiratory failure, (2) adequate oxygenation and pH, (3) hemodynamic stability, and (4) the capability to initiate an inspiratory effort.

Recommendation 3: Formal discontinuation assessments for patients receiving mechanical ventilation for respiratory failure should be performed during spontaneous breathing rather than while the patient is still receiving substantial ventilatory support. An initial brief period of spontaneous breathing can be used to assess the capability of continuing onto a formal spontaneous breathing trial (SBT). The criteria with which to assess patient tolerance during SBTs are the respiratory pattern, the adequacy of gas exchange, hemodynamic stability, and subjective comfort. The tolerance of SBTs lasting 30 to 120 minutes should prompt consideration for permanent ventilator discontinuation.

Recommendation 4: The removal of the artificial airway from a patient who has successfully been discontinued from ventilatory support should be based on assessments of airway patency and the ability of the patient to protect the airway.

Recommendation 5: Patients receiving mechanical ventilation for respiratory failure who fail an SBT should have the cause for the failed SBT determined. Once reversible causes for failure are corrected, subsequent SBTs should be performed every 24 hours.

Recommendation 6: Patients receiving mechanical ventilation for respiratory failure who fail an SBT should receive a stable, nonfatiguing, comfortable form of ventilatory support.

Recommendation 7: Anesthesia/sedation strategies and ventilator management aimed at early extubation should be used in postsurgical patients.

Recommendation 8: Weaning/discontinuation protocols that are designed for nonphysician healthcare professionals should be developed and implemented by intensive care units. Protocols aimed at optimizing sedation also should be developed and implemented.

Recommendation 9: Tracheostomy should be considered after an initial period of stabilization on the ventilator when it becomes apparent that the patient will require prolonged ventilator assistance. Tracheostomy then should be performed when the patient appears likely to gain one or more of the benefits ascribed to the procedure. Patients who may derive particular benefit from early tracheostomy are the following: those requiring high levels of sedation to tolerate a translaryngeal tube; those with marginal respiratory mechanics (often manifested as tachypnea) in whom a tracheostomy tube having lower resistance might reduce the risk of muscle overload; those who may derive psychological benefit from the ability to eat orally, communicate by articulated speech, and experience enhanced mobility; and those in whom enhanced mobility may assist physical therapy efforts.

Recommendation 10: Unless there is evidence for clearly irreversible disease (e.g., high spinal cord injury or advanced amyotrophic lateral sclerosis), a patient requiring prolonged mechanical ventilatory support for respiratory failure should not be considered permanently ventilator dependent until 3 months of ventilator liberation attempts have failed.

Recommendation 11: Critical care practitioners should familiarize themselves with facilities in their communities, or units in hospitals they staff, that specialize in managing patients who require prolonged dependence on mechanical ventilation. Such familiarization should include reviewing published peer-reviewed data from those units, if available. When medically stable for transfer, patients who have failed ventilator discontinuation attempts in the intensive care unit should be transferred to those facilities that have demonstrated success and safety in accomplishing ventilator discontinuation.

Recommendation 12: Ventilator liberation strategies in the prolonged mechanical ventilation patient should be slow paced and should include gradually lengthening self-breathing trials.

Modified from MacIntyre NR, Cook DJ, Ely EW Jr, et al. Evidence-based guidelines for weaning and discontinuing ventilatory support: a collective task force facilitated by the American College of Chest Physicians; the American Association for Respiratory Care; and the American College of Critical Care Medicine. *Chest.* 2001;120:375S–396S low compliance, a PImax of –20 cm H_2O may not be adequate for unassisted breathing.

The respiratory muscles should be rested if fatigue occurs, and a rest period of 24 hours or longer may be required.[114] Respiratory muscle rest usually is provided by ventilatory support high enough to provide patient comfort and still allow some inspiratory efforts. Importantly, total rest (i.e., no inspiratory muscle activity with controlled mechanical ventilation) can also be harmful, because muscle atrophy has been shown to develop in as little as 24 hours under these conditions.[98] If respiratory muscle fatigue is the result of an excessive load, the load should be reduced before attempts are made to liberate the patient from the ventilator. This is done with provision of therapy that can increase lung compliance or reduce airways resistance.

The tension–time index has been used to predict diaphragmatic fatigue (**Figure 22–42**).[115] The tension–time index is calculated as the product of the contractile force (Pdi/Pdi–max) and contraction duration (duty cycle, TI/Ttot). This requires measurement of the mean transdiaphragmatic pressure (Pdi), the transdiaphragmatic pressure with maximum inhalation (Pdi–max), the inspiratory time (TI), and the total respiratory cycle time (Ttot). A tension-time index over 0.15 is predictive of respiratory muscle fatigue. Measurement of the transdiaphragmatic pressure requires esophageal and gastric pressure measurements, which are almost never performed in mechanically ventilated patients. A simpler form of tension-time index is the pressure–time index (PTI),[116] which can be determined more readily with equipment available in the critical care unit. It is calculated as follows:

$$PTI = (Pbreath/PImax) \times (TI/Ttot)$$

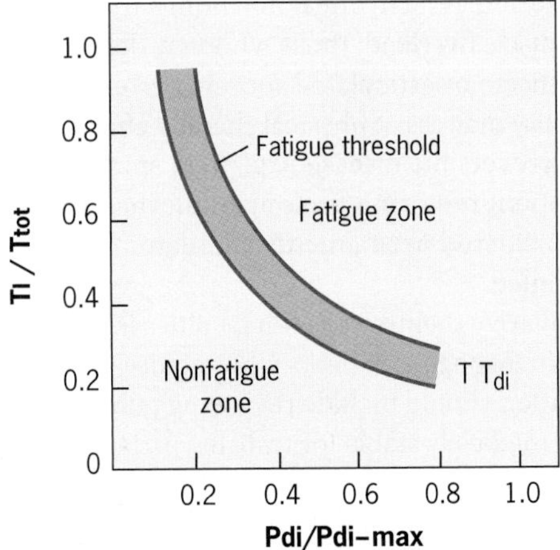

FIGURE 22–42 Tension-time index; note that the fatigue threshold is a tension-time index of about 0.15 to 0.18. From Grassino A, Macklem PT. Respiratory muscle fatigue and ventilatory failure. *Ann Rev Med.* 1984;35:625–647. Reprinted with permission.

where Pbreath is the pressure required to generate a spontaneous breath. The Pbreath can be determined with esophageal balloon measurements during a short trial of spontaneous breathing.

Assessing Readiness for Liberation

A number of factors should be improved before an attempt is made to liberate the patient from the ventilator (**Box 22–8**). **Weaning parameters**[117,118] often are used to assess liberation potential and are divided into two categories: parameters affected by lung mechanics, and gas exchange parameters. The spontaneous VT (> 5 mL/kg), respiratory rate (< 30 breaths/min), minute ventilation (< 12 L/min), vital capacity (> 15 mL/kg), and the PImax (< –20 cm H_2O) have been used as predictors of success. The rapid shallow breathing index (RSBI)[119] is calculated by division of the spontaneous respiratory rate by the VT (in liters). An RSBI less than 105 has been used as predictive of successful ventilator liberation, and an RSBI greater than 105 has been used to predict failure. An increase in VD/VT (which should be less than 0.6) and an increase in $\dot{V}CO_2$ and $\dot{V}O_2$ imply an increased ventilatory requirement.

Despite the many weaning parameters that have been reported, however, no criterion is better at predicting extubation readiness than a **spontaneous breathing trial (SBT)** with an integrated assessment focusing on the respiratory pattern, gas exchange, hemodynamics, and comfort. In fact, overreliance on weaning parameters

BOX 22–8

Criteria Assessed to Determine Readiness for Ventilator Discontinuation (Liberation)

- Evidence for some reversal of the underlying cause for respiratory failure
- Adequate oxygenation (e.g., PaO_2/FIO_2 ratio > 150 to 200; PEEP 5 to 8 cm H_2O; $FIO_2 \leq 0.4$ to 0.5) and pH (e.g., > 7.25)
- Hemodynamic stability, as defined by the absence of active myocardial ischemia and the absence of clinically significant hypotension (i.e., requiring no vasopressor therapy or therapy with only low-dose vasopressors)
- The capability to initiate an inspiratory effort

may result in prolonged stay on the ventilator.[120] It also is important to reduce or temporarily discontinue sedation in preparation of ventilator liberation; this has been reported to decrease both days of ventilation and mortality.[100,121]

Approaches to Liberation

Two prospective, randomized, controlled trials compared SIMV weaning (i.e., gradual reduction in mandatory breath rate), PSV weaning (i.e., gradual reduction in the level of PSV), and daily (or twice daily) SBT.[122,123] In these studies, after meeting screening criteria, an SBT was performed. Both studies reported that the majority of patients were successfully extubated after the first SBT. In those who failed the initial SBT, no difference in outcome (duration of ventilation) was seen between the T piece and PSV methods. However, both the SBT and PSV methods were superior to SIMV in both studies. Although newer-generation ventilators feature modes intended to facilitate weaning (e.g., SmartCare, adaptive support ventilation, volume support), evidence is lacking that these modes hasten ventilator liberation compared with use of a daily SBT.

The traditional approach to an SBT uses a T piece, in which the patient is removed from the ventilator, and humidified supplemental oxygen is provided. Humidified gas typically is provided as a heated or cool aerosol of water from a large-volume nebulizer. For patients with reactive airways, this aerosol may induce bronchospasm. In such cases a humidification system that does not generate an aerosol should be used, such as a heated passover humidifier. Passive humidifiers (e.g., artificial noses, heat and moisture exchangers) should be avoided because of their dead space and resistive workload.

RESPIRATORY RECAP

Liberation from Mechanical Ventilation

- » Regularly assess for liberation readiness.
- » Perform a spontaneous breathing trial to assess readiness for extubation.
- » If a spontaneous breathing trial is not tolerated, assess for causes of failure.
- » Do not use synchronized intermittent mechanical ventilation (SIMV) as a weaning mode.
- » Use protocols to improve successful liberation.

The SBT can be conducted without removal of the patient from the ventilator, and this approach has several advantages. No additional equipment is required, and if the patient fails the SBT, ventilatory support can be quickly reestablished. All the monitoring functions and alarms on the ventilator are available during the SBT, which may allow prompt recognition that the patient is failing the SBT. Most of the literature related to ventilator liberation studies using a traditional SBT, although several studies allowed performance of the SBT with the patient attached to the ventilator.[124–126]

The SBT can be performed with no positive pressure applied to the airway, with a low level of CPAP (5 cm H_2O), or with a low level of PSV (5 to 8 cm H_2O). Proponents of the CPAP approach argue that this maintains functional residual capacity at a level similar to that after extubation. It is argued that, in a patient with obstructive lung disease, this low level of CPAP maintains airway patency if the patient cannot control exhalation because of the presence of the artificial airway. In patients with marginal left ventricular function, however, a low level of positive intrathoracic pressure may support the failing heart. Such patients may tolerate a CPAP trial but then develop congestive heart failure when extubated.[34] Also, a low level of CPAP may counterbalance auto-PEEP in patients with COPD, resulting in a successful SBT, but respiratory failure soon after extubation.

Proponents of the low-level PSV approach argue that this overcomes the resistance to breathing through the artificial airway. However, this argument fails to recognize that the upper airway of an intubated patient typically is swollen and inflamed, such that, at least in one study, the resistance through the upper airway after extubation was similar to that seen with the endotracheal tube in place.[127] Resistance through the artificial airway is affected by many factors, including the patient's inspiratory flow, the inner diameter of the tube, whether the tube is an endotracheal or tracheostomy tube, and the presence of secretions in the tube. This makes it difficult to choose an appropriate level of pressure support to overcome tube resistance. However, one study reported similar outcomes when the SBT was performed with a T piece and with 7 cm H_2O PSV.[128] Similar outcomes of an SBT have also been reported with or without the use of tube compensation during an SBT.[62]

Similar outcomes are likely with a 2-hour SBT or a 30-minute SBT.[129] In the acute care setting, tolerance of an SBT of 30 minutes to 2 hours duration should prompt consideration for extubation. For chronically ventilator-dependent patients with a tracheostomy, the length of each SBT is increased, with alternating periods of ventilatory support and SBT. In this case, the goal may be daytime liberation with nocturnal ventilation.

Recognition of a Failed Spontaneous Breathing Trial

A failed SBT is discomforting for the patient and may induce significant cardiopulmonary distress. Commonly listed criteria for discontinuation of an SBT include tachypnea (respiratory rate over 35 breaths/min for 5 minutes or longer); hypoxemia (Spo_2 below 90%); tachycardia (heart rate over 140 beats/min or a sustained increase above 20%); bradycardia (sustained decrease in the heart rate of over 20%); hypertension (systolic blood pressure over 180 mm Hg); hypotension (systolic blood pressure under 90 mm Hg); and agitation, diaphoresis, or anxiety. In some patients the last three factors are not caused by SBT failure and can be appropriately treated with verbal reassurance or pharmacologic support. When SBT failure is recognized, ventilatory support should be promptly reestablished.

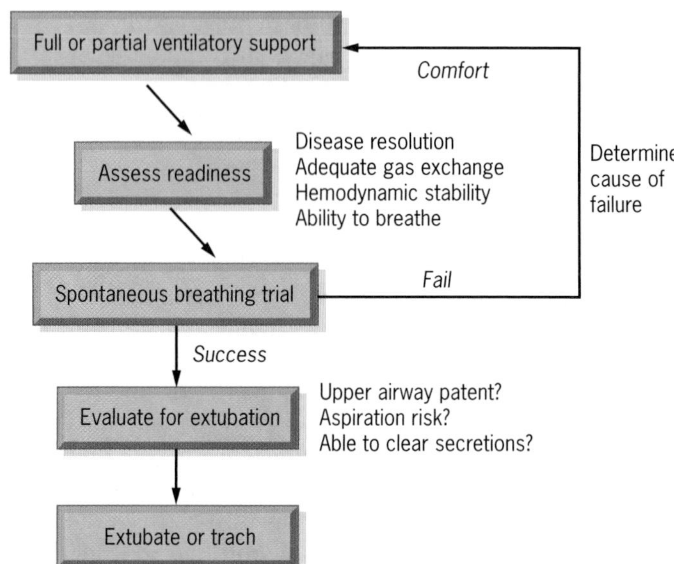

FIGURE 22–43 An evidence-based approach to ventilator discontinuation and extubation.

Causes of Spontaneous Breathing Trial Failure

When an SBT fails, the reason should be identified and corrected before another SBT is performed. There are a variety of physiologic and technical reasons why patients fail an SBT. An excessive respiratory muscle load may be the cause. High airways resistance and low compliance contribute to the increased effort necessary to breathe. Auto-PEEP may delay liberation in patients with COPD, because it increases the pleural pressure needed to initiate inhalation. Electrolyte imbalance may cause respiratory muscle weakness. Inadequate levels of potassium, magnesium, phosphate, and calcium impair ventilatory muscle function. Appropriate nutritional support often improves the ventilator discontinuation process, but care should be taken to avoid overfeeding, because excessive caloric ingestion elevates carbon dioxide production. Failure of any major organ system can result in failure to liberate the patient from the ventilator. Fever and infection are of particular concern because they increase both oxygen consumption and carbon dioxide production, resulting in an increased ventilatory requirement. Cardiac dysfunction can delay liberation until appropriate management of cardiovascular status has occurred.

Once the patient has been judged to no longer need mechanical ventilatory support, attention then turns to the need for the artificial airway. This requires a different set of assessments that focus on the patient's ability to protect the natural airway. Key parameters include cough strength and the need for suctioning (i.e., suctioning requirements exceeding every 2 hours should preclude extubation). Although the ability to follow commands is desirable before extubation, it is not essential in patients otherwise able to protect the airway.

In appropriately selected patients (e.g., those recovering from a COPD exacerbation), extubation to NIV may reduce the duration of mechanical ventilation.[130–132] Extubation to NIV can also be considered to prevent extubation failure in patients at risk, such as those with COPD, cardiac disease, or others at risk for extubation failure. However, NIV is generally not recommended to rescue a failed extubation.[133,134] If the patient fails extubation, consideration should be given to emergent reintubation.

Ventilator Discontinuation (Weaning) Protocols

Ventilator discontinuation (weaning) protocols have become increasingly popular in recent years, and these protocols typically are implemented by respiratory therapists and nurses. Studies have reported improved outcomes when protocols are used.[124–126,134,135] **Figure 22–43** presents the elements of an effective protocol. From these elements incorporating best evidence, a specific protocol can be developed that meets the local culture of the ICU. Note that the use of an SBT is central to the protocol.

KEY POINTS

- Efforts should be made to avoid complications during mechanical ventilation.
- Forms of ventilator-induced lung injury include alveolar overdistention and repetitive opening and closing.
- Volume control ventilation maintains minute ventilation but allows airway pressure and plateau pressure to fluctuate.
- Pressure control ventilation allows minute ventilation to fluctuate, but airway pressure is limited to the peak pressure set on the ventilator.
- Modes on modern ventilators include continuous mandatory ventilation, synchronized intermittent mandatory ventilation, pressure support ventilation, continuous positive airway pressure, adaptive pressure control, adaptive support ventilation, airway pressure release ventilation, tube compensation, proportional assist ventilation, neurally adjusted ventilatory assist, and high-frequency oscillatory ventilation.
- The tidal volume should be set to avoid overdistention lung injury: 6 mL/kg PBW is a suggested initial setting.
- The respiratory rate and I:E ratio are set to control the $Pa{CO_2}$ and to avoid hemodynamic compromise and auto-PEEP.

- The F_{IO_2} initially should be set at 1 and then weaned per pulse oximetry to maintain an Sp_{O_2} over 88%.
- PEEP should be set to avoid alveolar derecruitment for patients with ARDS and to counterbalance auto-PEEP in patients with COPD.
- The following should be monitored in the mechanically ventilated patient: physical signs and symptoms, blood gas measurements, lung mechanics, hemodynamics, patient–ventilator synchrony, and sedation.
- The most important aspect of liberation from mechanical ventilation is assessment for readiness.
- A spontaneous breathing trial identifies most patients who are ready for liberation from mechanical ventilation.
- The poorest outcomes from the ventilator discontinuation process have been reported with SIMV.
- For patients who do not tolerate a spontaneous breathing trial, ventilatory support should be reestablished and the cause of the failure identified.

REFERENCES

1. Pierson DJ. Indications for mechanical ventilation in adults with acute respiratory failure. *Respir Care.* 2002;47:249–265.
2. Matlu GM, Factor P. Complications of mechanical ventilation. *Respir Care Clin North Am.* 2000;6:213–252.
3. Pierson DJ. Alveolar rupture during mechanical ventilation: role of PEEP, peak airway pressure, and distending volume. *Respir Care.* 1988;33:472–484.
4. Stauffer JL. Complications of endotracheal intubation and tracheostomy. *Respir Care.* 1999;44:828–843.
5. Ali T, Harty RF. Stress-induced ulcer bleeding in critically ill patients. *Gastroenterol Clin North Am.* 2009;38:245–265.
6. Oltermann MH. Nutrition support in the acutely ventilated patient. *Respir Care Clin North Am.* 2006;12:533–545.
7. Parthasarathy S, Tobin MJ. Sleep in the intensive care unit. *Intensive Care Med.* 2004;30:197–206.
8. Dreyfuss D, Savmon G. Ventilator induced lung injury: lessons from experimental studies *Am J Respir Crit Care Med.* 1998;157:294–323.
9. Jia X, Malhotra A, Saeed M, et al. Fisk Factors for ARDS in patients receiving mechanical ventilation for > 48 h. *Chest.* 2008;133:853–861.
10. Yilmaz M, Keegan MT, Iscimen R, et al. Toward the prevention of acute lung injury: protocol-guided limitation of large tidal volume ventilation and inappropriate transfusion. *Crit Care Med.* 2007;35:1660–1666.
11. Villar J, Kacmarek RM, Perez-Mendez L, Aguirre-Jaime A. A high positive end-expiratory pressure, low tidal volume ventilatory strategy improves outcome in persistent acute respiratory distress syndrome: a randomized, controlled trial. *Crit Care Med.* 2006;34:1311–1318.
12. NIH ARDS Network. Ventilation with lower tidal volumes as compared with traditional tidal volumes for acute lung injury and the acute respiratory distress syndrome. *N Engl J Med.* 2000;342:1301–1308.
13. Hager DN, Krishnan JA, Hayden DL, Brower RG, ARDS Clinical Trials Network. Tidal volume reduction in patients with acute lung injury when plateau pressures are not high. *Am J Respir Crit Care Med.* 2005;172:1241–1245.
14. Webb HJH, Tierney DF. Experimental pulmonary edema due to intermittent positive pressure ventilation with high inflation pressures: protection by positive end-expiratory pressure. *Am Rev Respir Dis.* 1974;110:556–565.
15. Crotti S, Mascheroni D, Caironi P, et al. Recruitment and derecruitment during acute respiratory failure. *Am J Respir Crit Care Med.* 2001;164:131–140.
16. Mead J, Takishima T, Leith D. Stress distribution in lungs: a model of pulmonary elasticity. *J Appl Physiol.* 1970;28:596–608.
17. Chiumello D, Carlesso E, Cadringher P, et al. Lung stress and strain during mechanical ventilation for acute respiratory distress syndrome. *Am J Respir Crit Care Med.* 2008;178:346–355.
18. Vaporidi K, Voloudakis G, Priniannakis G, et al. Effects of respiratory rate on ventilator-induced lung injury at a constant Pa_{CO_2} in a mouse model of normal lung. *Crit Care Med.* 2008;36:1277–1283.
19. Rich BR, Reickert CA, Sawada S, et al. Effect of rate and inspiratory flow on ventilator induced lung injury. *J Trauma.* 2000;49:903–911.
20. Marini JJ, Hotchkiss JR, Broccard AF. Bench-to-bedside review: microvascular and airspace linkage in ventilator-induced lung injury. *Crit Care (London).* 2003;7:435–444.
21. Trembly L, Valenza F, Ribiero SP, Li J, Slutsky AS. Injurious ventilatory strategies increase cytokines and C-fos M-RNA expression in an isolated rat lung model. *J Clin Invest.* 1997;99:944–952.
22. Ranieri VM, Suter PM, Tortorella C, et al. Effect of mechanical ventilation on inflammatory mediators in patients with acute respiratory distress syndrome: a randomized controlled trial. *JAMA.* 1999;282:54–61.
23. Slutsky AS, Trembly L. Multiple system organ failure: is mechanical ventilation a contributing factor? *Am J Respir Crit Care Med.* 1998;157:1721–1725.
24. Nahum A, Hoyt J, Schmitz L, et al. Effect of mechanical ventilation strategy on dissemination of intertracheally instilled *E coli* in dogs. *Crit Care Med.* 1997;25:1733–1743.
25. Durbin CG, Wallace KK. Oxygen toxicity in the critically ill patient. *Respir Care.* 1993;38:739–753.
26. Kollef MH. Prevention of hospital-associated pneumonia and ventilator-associated pneumonia. *Crit Care Med.* 2004;32:1396–1405.
27. Wip C, Napolitano L. Bundles to prevent ventilator-associated pneumonia: how valuable are they? *Curr Opin Infect Dis.* 2009;22:159–166.
28. Zilberberg MD, Shorr AF, Kollef MH. Implementing quality improvements in the intensive care unit: ventilator bundle as an example. *Crit Care Med.* 2009;37:305–309.
29. Kollef MH. Prevention of hospital-associated pneumonia and ventilator-associated pneumonia. *Crit Care Med.* 2004;32:1396–1405.
30. Han J, Liu Y. Effect of ventilator circuit changes on ventilator-associated pneumonia: a systematic review and meta-analysis. *Respir Care.* 2010;55:467–474.
31. Gentile MA, Siobal MS. Are specialized endotracheal tubes and heat-and-moisture exchangers cost-effective in preventing ventilator associated pneumonia? *Respir Care.* 2010;55:184–196.
32. Perreault T, Gutkowska J. Role of atrial natriuretic factor in lung physiology and pathology. *Am J Respir Crit Care Med.* 1995;151:226–242.
33. Pinsky MR, Summer WR, Wise RA, et al. Augmentation of cardiac function by elevation of intrathoracic pressure. *J Appl Physiol.* 1983;54:450–455.
34. Lemaire F, Teboul JL, Cinotti L, et al. Acute left ventricular dysfunction during unsuccessful weaning from mechanical ventilation. *Anesthesiology.* 1988;69:171–179.
35. Cinnella G, Conti G, Lofaso F, et al. Effects of assisted ventilation on the work of breathing: volume-controlled versus pressure-controlled ventilation. *Am J Respir Crit Care Med.* 1996;153:1025–1033.

36. MacIntyre NR, McConnell R, Cheng KG, et al. Patient-ventilator flow dyssynchrony: flow-limited versus pressure-limited breaths. *Crit Care Med.* 1997;25:1671–1677.
37. MacIntyre NR, Sessler CN. Are there benefits or harm from pressure targeting during lung-protective ventilation? *Respir Care.* 2010;55:175–180.
38. Branson RD, Chatburn RL. Technical description and classification of modes of ventilator operation. *Respir Care.* 1992;37:1026–1044.
39. Chatburn RL. Classification of mechanical ventilators. *Respir Care.* 1992;37:1009–1025.
40. Chatburn RL. Classification of ventilator modes: update and proposal for implementation. *Respir Care.* 2007;52:301–323.
41. Chatburn RL, Primiano FP Jr. A new system for understanding modes of mechanical ventilation. *Respir Care.* 2001;46:604–621.
42. Hess DR. Ventilator waveforms and the physiology of pressure support ventilation. *Respir Care.* 2005;50:166–186.
43. Jubran A, Van de Graaff WB, Tobin MJ. Variability of patient-ventilator interaction with pressure support ventilation in patients with chronic obstructive pulmonary disease. *Am J Respir Crit Care Med.* 1995;152:129–136.
44. Parthasarathy S, Jubran A, Tobin MJ. Cycling of inspiratory and expiratory muscle groups with the ventilator in airflow limitation. *Am J Respir Crit Care Med.* 1998;158:1471–1478.
45. Jubran A. Inspiratory flow: more may not be better. *Crit Care Med.* 1999;27:670–671.
46. Parthasarathy S, Tobin MJ. Effect of ventilator mode on sleep quality in critically ill patients. *Am J Respir Crit Care Med.* 2002;166:1423–1429.
47. Marini JJ, Smith TC, Lamb VJ. External work output and force generation during synchronized intermittent mechanical ventilation: effect of machine assistance on breathing effort. *Am Rev Respir Dis.* 1988;138:1169–1179.
48. Leung P, Jubran A, Tobin MJ. Comparison of assisted ventilator modes on triggering, patient effort, and dyspnea. *Am J Respir Crit Care Med.* 1997;155:1940–1948.
49. Branson RD, Chatburn RL. Controversies in the critical care setting. Should adaptive pressure control modes be utilized for virtually all patients receiving mechanical ventilation? *Respir Care.* 2007;52:478–488.
50. Mireles-Cabodevila E, Diaz-Guzman E, Heresi GA, Chatburn RL. Alternative modes of mechanical ventilation: a review for the hospitalist. *Cleve Clin J Med.* 2009;76:417–430.
51. Habashi NM. Other approaches to open-lung ventilation: airway pressure release ventilation. Crit Care Med. 2005;33(3 suppl):S228–S240.
52. Varpula T, Valta P, Niemi R, et al. Airway pressure release ventilation as a primary ventilatory mode in acute respiratory distress syndrome. *Acta Anaesth Scand.* 2004;48:722–731.
53. Varpula T, Valta P, Markkola A, et al. The effects of ventilatory mode on lung aeration assessed with computer tomography: a randomized controlled study. *J Intensive Care Med.* 2009;24:122–130.
54. Gruber PC, Gomersall CD, Leung PE, et al. Randomized controlled trial comparing adaptive-support ventilation with pressure-regulated volume-controlled ventilation with automode in weaning patients after cardiac surgery. *Anesthesiology.* 2008;109:81–87.
55. Tassaux D, Dalmas E, Gratadour P, Jolliet P. Patient-ventilator interactions during partial ventilatory support: a preliminary study comparing the effects of adaptive support ventilation with synchronized intermittent mandatory ventilation plus inspiratory pressure support. *Crit Care Med.* 2002;30:801–807.
56. Jaber S, Sebbane M, Verzilli D, et al. Adaptive support and pressure support ventilation behavior in response to increased ventilatory demand. *Anesthesiology.* 2009;110:620–627.
57. Sulemanji D, Marchese A, Garbarini P, et al. Adaptive support ventilation: an appropriate mechanical ventilation strategy for acute respiratory distress syndrome? *Anesthesiology.* 2009;111:863–870.
58. Guttmann J, Haberthür C, Mols G, Lichtwarck-Aschoff M. Automatic tube compensation (ATC). *Minerva Anesthesiol.* 2002;68:369–377.
59. Cohen JD, Shapiro M, Grozovski E, et al. Extubation outcome following a spontaneous breathing trial with automatic tube compensation versus continuous positive airway pressure. *Crit Care Med.* 2006;34:682–686.
60. Elsasser S, Guttmann J, Stocker R, et al. Accuracy of automatic tube compensation in new-generation mechanical ventilators. *Crit Care Med.* 2003;31:2619–2626.
61. Haberthür C, Mols G, Elsasser S, et al. Extubation after breathing trials with automatic tube compensation, T-tube, or pressure support ventilation. *Acta Anaesthesiol Scand.* 2002;46:973–979.
62. Marantz S, Patrick W, Webster K, et al. Response of ventilator-dependent patients to different levels of proportional assist. *J Appl Physiol.* 1996;80:397–403.
63. Gay PC, Hess DR, Hill NS. Noninvasive proportional assist ventilation for acute respiratory insufficiency. Comparison with pressure support ventilation. *Am J Respir Crit Care Med.* 2001;164:1606–1611.
64. Bosma K, Ferreyra G, Ambrogio C, et al. Patient-ventilator interaction and sleep in mechanically ventilated patients: pressure support versus proportional assist ventilation. *Crit Care Med.* 2007;35:1048–1054.
65. Sinderby C. Neurally adjusted ventilatory assist (NAVA). *Minerva Anesthesiol.* 2002;68:378–380.
66. Fessler HE, Hess DR. Respiratory controversies in the critical care setting. Does high-frequency ventilation offer benefits over conventional ventilation in adult patients with acute respiratory distress syndrome? *Respir Care.* 2007;52:595–608.
67. Branson RD, Campbell RS, Davis D, et al. Comparison of pressure and flow triggering systems during continuous positive airway pressure. *Chest.* 1994;106:540–544.
68. Goulet RL, Hess D, Kacmarek RM. Flow versus pressure triggering in mechanically ventilated adult patients. *Chest.* 1997;111:1649–1653.
69. Aslanian P, El Atrous S, Isabey D, et al. Effects of flow triggering on breathing effort during partial ventilatory support. *Am J Respir Crit Care Med.* 1998;157:135–139.
70. MacIntyre NR. Is there a best way to set tidal volume for mechanical ventilatory support? *Clin Chest Med.* 2008;29:225–231.
71. Gajic O, Dara SI, Mendez JL, et al. Ventilator-associated lung injury in patients without acute lung injury at the onset of mechanical ventilation. *Crit Care Med.* 2004;32:1817–1824.
72. MacIntyre NR, McConnell R, Cheng KC. Applied PEEP reduces the inspiratory load of intrinsic PEEP during pressure support. *Chest.* 1997;1111:188–193.
73. Smith TC, Marini JJ. Impact of PEEP on lung mechanics and work of breathing in severe airflow obstruction. *J Appl Physiol.* 1988;65:1488–1499.
74. Petrof BJ, Lagare M, Goldberg P, et al. Continuous positive airway pressure reduces work of breathing and dyspnea during weaning from mechanical ventilation in severe chronic obstructive pulmonary disease. *Am Rev Respir Dis.* 1990;141:281–289.
75. Tobin MJ, Lodato RF. PEEP, auto-PEEP, and waterfalls. *Chest.* 1989;96:449–451.
76. Hoit JD, Banzett RB, Lohmeier HL, et al. Clinical ventilator adjustments that improve speech. *Chest.* 2003;124:1512–1521.
77. Hess DR, Bigatello LM. Lung recruitment: the role of recruitment maneuvers. *Respir Care.* 2002;47:308–318.
78. Fan E, Wilcox ME, Brower RG, et al. Recruitment maneuvers for acute lung injury: a systematic review. *Am J Respir Crit Care Med.* 2008;178:1156–1163.
79. Hess D, Good C, Didyoung R, et al. The validity of assessing arterial blood gases 10 minutes after an FIO_2 change in mechanically

ventilated patients without chronic pulmonary disease. *Respir Care.* 1985;30:1037–1041.

80. Branson RD, Campbell RS. Sighs: wasted breath or breath of fresh air? *Respir Care.* 1992;37:462–468.
81. Pelosi P, Cadringher P, Bottino N, et al. Sigh in acute respiratory distress syndrome. *Am J Respir Crit Care Med.* 1999;159:872–880.
82. Badet M, Bayle F, Richard JC, Guérin C. Comparison of optimal positive end-expiratory pressure and recruitment maneuvers during lung-protective mechanical ventilation in patients with acute lung injury/acute respiratory distress syndrome. *Respir Care.* 2009;54:847–854.
83. Harris RS. Pressure-volume curves of the respiratory system. *Respir Care.* 2005;50:78–99.
84. Grasso S, Stripoli T, De Michele M, et al. ARDSnet ventilatory protocol and alveolar hyperinflation: role of positive end-expiratory pressure. *Am J Respir Crit Care Med.* 2007;176:761–767.
85. Benditt JO. Esophageal and gastric pressure measurements. *Respir Care.* 2005;50:68–77.
86. Talmor D, Sarge T, Malhotra A, et al. Mechanical ventilation guided by esophageal pressure in acute lung injury. *N Engl J Med.* 2008;359:2095–2104.
87. Hager DN, Brower RG. Customizing lung-protective mechanical ventilation strategies. *Crit Care Med.* 2006;34:1554–1555.
88. Talmor DS, Fessler HE. Are esophageal pressure measurements important in clinical decision-making in mechanically ventilated patients? *Respir Care.* 2010;55:162–172.
89. Hess DR, Bigatello LM. The chest wall in acute lung injury/acute respiratory distress syndrome. *Curr Opin Crit Care.* 2008; 14:94–102.
90. Dhand R. Ventilator graphics and respiratory mechanics in the patient with obstructive lung disease. *Respir Care.* 2005;50:246–261.
91. de Wit M, Miller KB, Green DA, et al. Ineffective triggering predicts increased duration of mechanical ventilation. *Crit Care Med.* 2009;37:2740–2745.
92. Thille AW, Rodriguez P, Cabello B, et al. Patient-ventilator asynchrony during assisted mechanical ventilation. *Intensive Care Med.* 2006;32:1515–1522.
93. Imanaka H, Nishimura M, Takeuchi M, et al. Autotriggering caused by cardiogenic oscillation during flow-triggered mechanical ventilation. *Crit Care Med.* 2000;28:402–407.
94. Yang LY, Huang YC, Macintyre NR. Patient-ventilator synchrony during pressure-targeted versus flow-targeted small tidal volume assisted ventilation. *J Crit Care.* 2007;22:252–257.
95. Kallet RH, Campbell AR, Dicker RA, et al. Work of breathing during lung-protective ventilation in patients with acute lung injury and acute respiratory distress syndrome: a comparison between volume and pressure-regulated breathing modes. *Respir Care.* 2005;50:1623–1631.
96. Hess DR, Thompson BT. Patient-ventilator dyssynchrony during lung protective ventilation: what's a clinician to do? *Crit Care Med.* 2006;34:231–233.
97. Branson RD, Johannigman JA. The role of ventilator graphics when setting dual-control modes. *Respir Care.* 2005;50:187–201.
98. Levine S, Nguyen T, Taylor N, et al. Rapid disuse atrophy of diaphragm fibers in mechanically ventilated humans. *N Engl J Med.* 2008;358:1327–1335.
99. Hermans G, De Jonghe B, Bruyninckx F, Van den Berghe G. Clinical review: critical illness polyneuropathy and myopathy. *Crit Care.* 2008;12:238.
100. Girard TD, Kress JP, Fuchs BD, et al. Efficacy and safety of a paired sedation and ventilator weaning protocol for mechanically ventilated patients in intensive care (Awakening and Breathing Controlled trial): a randomised controlled trial. *Lancet.* 2008;371(9607):126–134.
101. Strøm T, Martinussen T, Toft P. A protocol of no sedation for critically ill patients receiving mechanical ventilation: a randomised trial. *Lancet.* 2010;375:475–480.
102. Amato MB, Barbas CSV, Medievos DM, et al. Effect of a protective ventilation strategy on mortality in ARDS. *N Engl J Med.* 1998;338:347–354.
103. Brower RG, Lanken PN, MacIntyre N, et al. Higher versus lower positive end-expiratory pressures in patients with the acute respiratory distress syndrome. *N Engl J Med.* 2004;351:327–336.
104. Meade MO, Cook DJ, Guyatt GH, et al. Ventilation strategy using low tidal volumes, recruitment maneuvers, and high positive end-expiratory pressure for acute lung injury and acute respiratory distress syndrome: a randomized controlled trial. *JAMA.* 2008;299:637–645.
105. Briel M, Meade M, Mercat A, et al. Higher vs lower positive end-expiratory pressure in patients with acute lung injury and acute respiratory distress syndrome: systematic review and meta-analysis. *JAMA.* 2010;303:865–873.
106. Mercat A, Richard JC, Vielle B, et al. Positive end-expiratory pressure setting in adults with acute lung injury and acute respiratory distress syndrome: a randomized controlled trial. *JAMA.* 2008;299:646–655.
107. Suter PM, Fairley HB, Isenberg MD. Optimic end expiratory pressure in patients with acute pulmonary failure. *N Engl J Med.* 1975;292:284–289.
108. Nava S, Hill N. Non-invasive ventilation in acute respiratory failure. *Lancet.* 2009;374:250–259.
109. Medoff BD. Invasive and noninvasive ventilation in patients with asthma. *Respir Care.* 2008;53:740–750.
110. Mascia L, Zavala E, Bosma K, et al. High tidal volume is associated with the development of acute lung injury after severe brain injury: an international observational study. *Crit Care Med.* 2007;35:1815–1820.
111. Hickling KG, Walsh J, Henderson S, Jackson R. Low mortality rate in adult respiratory distress syndrome using low-volume, pressure-limited ventilation with permissive hypercapnia: a prospective study. *Crit Care Med.* 1994;22:1568–1578.
112. MacIntyre NR, Cook DJ, Ely EW Jr, et al. Evidence-based guidelines for weaning and discontinuing ventilatory support: a collective task force facilitated by the American College of Chest Physicians; the American Association for Respiratory Care; and the American College of Critical Care Medicine. *Chest.* 2001;120(6 suppl):375S–395S.
113. Cohen CA, Zagelbaum G, Gross D, et al. Clinical manifestations of inspiratory muscle fatigue. *Am J Med.* 1982;73:308–316.
114. Laghi F, D'Alfonso N, Tobin MJ. Pattern of recovery from diaphragmatic fatigue over 24 hours. *J Appl Physiol.* 1995;79:539–546.
115. Stoller JK. Physiologic rationale for resting the ventilatory muscles. *Respir Care.* 1991;36:290–296.
116. Jabour ER, Rabil DM, Truwitt JD, et al. Evaluation of a new weaning index based on ventilatory endurance and the efficiency of gas exchange. *Am Rev Respir Dis.* 1991;144:531–537.
117. Epstein SK. Weaning parameters. *Respir Care Clin North Am.* 2000;6:253–301.
118. Meade M, Guyatt G, Cook D, et al. Predicting success in weaning from mechanical ventilation. *Chest.* 2001;120(6 suppl):400S–424S.
119. Yang KL, Tobin MJ. A prospective study of indices predicting the outcome of trials of weaning from mechanical ventilation. *N Engl J Med.* 1991;324:1445–1450.
120. Tanios MA, Nevins ML, Hendra KP, et al. A randomized, controlled trial of the role of weaning predictors in clinical decision making. *Crit Care Med.* 2006;34:2530–2535.
121. Kress JP, Pohlman AS, O'Connor MF, et al. Daily interruption of sedative infusions in critically ill patients undergoing mechanical ventilation. *N Engl J Med.* 2000;342:1471–1477.
122. Esteban A, Frutos F, Tobin MJ, et al. A comparison of four methods of weaning patients from mechanical ventilation. *N Engl J Med.* 1995;6:345–350.
123. Brochard L, Rauss A, Benito S, et al. Comparison of three methods of gradual withdrawal from ventilatory support during

weaning from mechanical ventilation. *Am J Respir Crit Care Med.* 1994;150:896–903.

124. Ely EW, Baker AM, Dunagan DP, et al. Effect of the duration of mechanical ventilation on identifying patients capable of breathing spontaneously. *N Engl J Med.* 1996;335:1864–1869.
125. Ely EW, Bennett PA, Bowton DL, et al. Large-scale implementation of a respiratory therapist-driven protocol for ventilator weaning. *Am J Respir Crit Care Med.* 1999;159:439–446.
126. Robertson TE, Mann HJ, Hyzy R, et al. Multicenter implementation of a consensus-developed, evidence-based, spontaneous breathing trial protocol. *Crit Care Med.* 2008;36:2753–2762.
127. Straus C, Louis B, Isabey D, et al. Contribution of the endotracheal tube and the upper airway to breathing workload. *Am J Respir Crit Care Med.* 1998;157:23–30.
128. Esteban A, Alia I, Gordo F, et al. Extubation outcome after spontaneous breathing trials with T-tube or pressure-support ventilation. *Am J Respir Crit Care Med.* 1997;156:459–465.
129. Esteban E, Alia I, Tobin MJ, et al. Effect of spontaneous breathing trial duration on outcome of attempts to discontinue mechanical ventilation. *Am J Respir Crit Care Med.* 1999;159:512–518.
130. Girault C, Daudenthun I, Chevron V, et al. Noninvasive ventilation as a systematic extubation and weaning technique in acute on chronic respiratory failure: a prospective, randomized, controlled study. *Am J Respir Crit Care Med.* 1999;160:86–92.
131. Nava S, Ambrosino N, Clini E, et al. Noninvasive mechanical ventilation in the weaning of patients with respiratory failure due to chronic obstructive pulmonary disease: a randomized, controlled trial. *Ann Intern Med.* 1998;128:721–728.
132. Esteban A, Frutos-Vivar F, Ferguson ND, et al. Noninvasive positive-pressure ventilation for respiratory failure after extubation. *N Engl J Med.* 2004;350:2452–2460.
133. Keenan SP, Powers C, McCormack DG, Block G. Noninvasive positive-pressure ventilation for postextubation respiratory distress: a randomized controlled trial. *JAMA.* 2002;287:3238–3244.
134. Marelich GP, Murin S, Battistella F, et al. Protocol weaning of mechanical ventilation in medical and surgical patients by respiratory care practitioners and nurses: effect on weaning time and incidence of ventilator-associated pneumonia. *Chest.* 2000;118:459–467.
135. Ely EW, Meade MO, Haponik EF, et al. Mechanical ventilator weaning protocols driven by nonphysician health-care professionals: evidence-based clinical practice guidelines. *Chest.* 2001;120(6 suppl):454S–463S.

CHAPTER 23

Noninvasive Ventilation and Continuous Positive Airway Pressure

Dean R. Hess

OUTLINE

Interfaces
Noninvasive Positive Pressure Ventilation
Continuous Positive Airway Pressure
Negative Pressure Ventilation, Rocking Beds, and Pneumobelts

OBJECTIVES

1. Compare noninvasive positive pressure ventilation, negative pressure ventilation, and continuous positive airway pressure.
2. Describe interfaces and ventilators for noninvasive ventilation (NIV) and continuous positive airway pressure (CPAP).
3. List selection criteria for noninvasive positive pressure ventilation (inclusion and exclusion).
4. Discuss acute care applications of CPAP.
5. Discuss the use of CPAP to treat obstructive sleep apnea.
6. Discuss the role of humidification in the application of NIV and CPAP.
7. Discuss issues of compliance with CPAP for treatment of obstructive sleep apnea.
8. Describe the operation and use of auto-positive airway pressure devices.
9. Describe the principles of negative pressure ventilation, rocking beds, and pneumobelts.

KEY TERMS

auto-positive airway pressure (APAP)
continuous positive airway pressure (CPAP)
cuirass
expiratory positive airway pressure (EPAP)
helmet
inspiratory positive airway pressure (IPAP)
iron lung
nasal mask
nasal pillows
negative pressure ventilation
noninvasive ventilation (NIV)
oronasal mask
pneumobelt
rocking bed
total face mask

INTRODUCTION

Noninvasive ventilation (NIV) provides ventilatory support without an endotracheal tube or tracheostomy tube. Both positive pressure and negative pressure approaches can be used to provide NIV. With **continuous positive airway pressure (CPAP)**, a pressure greater than atmospheric pressure is applied to the airway throughout the respiratory cycle. This chapter covers the clinical and technical aspects of the application of CPAP and NIV.

Interfaces

The interface is what separates invasive from noninvasive ventilation. Similar interfaces are used for CPAP and NIV.[1] **Figure 23–1** compares NIV and CPAP. The interface has a major impact on patient comfort and compliance during NIV. A poorly fitting interface decreases clinical effectiveness and patient compliance. A number of interfaces are available, each of which has advantages and disadvantages (**Table 23–1**). The most commonly used interfaces are **oronasal** and **nasal masks**; other interfaces include **nasal pillows**, mouthpieces, **total face masks**, hybrid masks, and helmets (**Figure 23–2**). A variety of sizes and designs are commercially available. Desirable features of a

> **RESPIRATORY RECAP**
>
> **Interfaces**
> » Nasal mask
> » Oronasal mask
> » Total face mask
> » Nasal prongs
> » Hybrid
> » Mouthpiece
> » Helmet

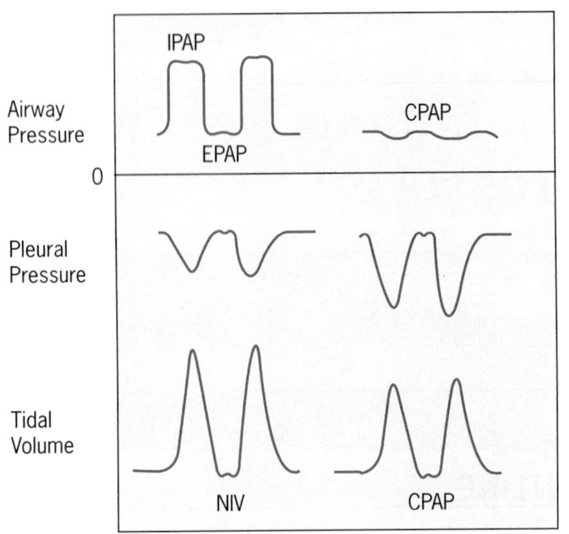

FIGURE 23–1 A comparison of the physiologic effects of NIV and CPAP. Both increase airway pressure, but NIV, unlike CPAP, also provides respiratory muscle unloading.

TABLE 23–1 Advantages and Disadvantages of Various Types of Interfaces for Noninvasive Ventilation

Interface	Advantages	Disadvantages
Nasal mask	Less risk for aspiration Easier secretion clearance Less claustrophobia Easier speech May be able to eat Easy to fit and secure Less dead space	Mouth leak Higher resistance through nasal passages Less effective with nasal obstruction Nasal irritation and rhinorrhea Upper airway dryness with mouth leak
Nasal pillows	Lower profile allows wearing eye glasses Less facial skin breakdown Simple headgear Easy to fit	Mouth leak Higher resistance through nasal passages Less effective with nasal obstruction Nasal irritation and rhinorrhea Upper airway dryness with mouth leak
Oronasal mask	Better oral leak control More effective in mouth breathers	Increased dead space Claustrophobia Increased aspiration risk Increased difficulty speaking and eating Asphyxiation with ventilator malfunction
Mouthpiece	Less interference with speech Very little dead space May not require headgear	Less effective if patient cannot maintain mouth seal Usually requires nasal or oronasal interface at night Nasal leak Potential for orthodontic injury
Hybrid	Eliminates mouth leak Lower profile allows wearing eye glasses Less facial skin breakdown	Increased aspiration risk Increased difficulty speaking and eating Asphyxiation with ventilator malfunction
Total face mask	May be more comfortable for some patients Easier to fit Less facial skin breakdown	Potentially greater dead space Potential for drying of the eyes Cannot deliver aerosolized medications
Helmet	May be more comfortable for some patients Easier to fit (one size fits all) Less facial skin breakdown	Rebreathing Poorer patient–ventilator synchrony Less respiratory muscle unloading Asphyxiation with ventilator malfunction Cannot deliver aerosolized medications

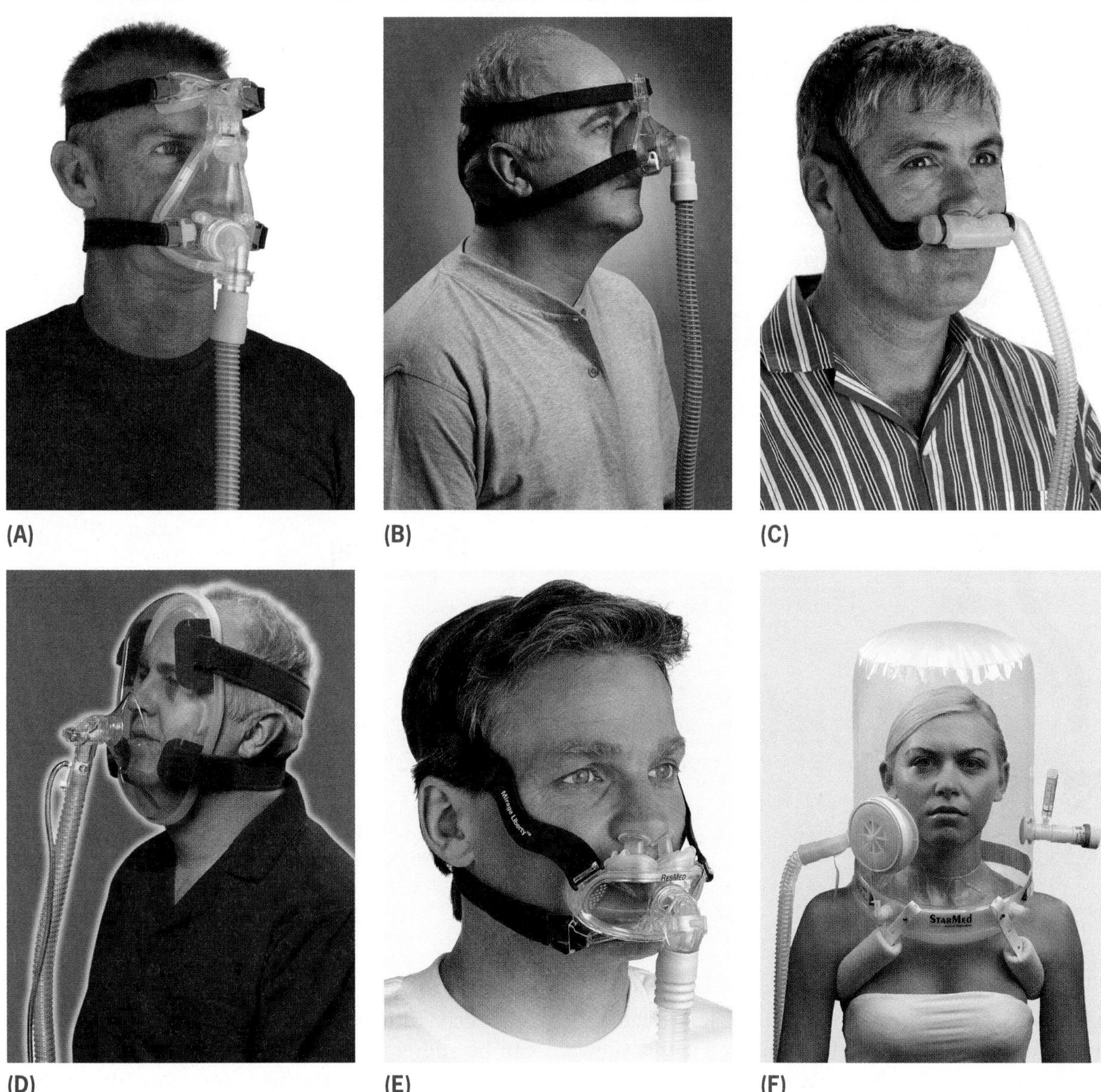

FIGURE 23–2 Interfaces for NIV and CPAP. (**A**) Oronasal mask. (**B**) Nasal mask. (**C**) Nasal pillows. (**D**) Total face mask. (**E**) Hybrid. (**F**) Helmet.

mask include low dead space, transparency, light weight, being easy to secure, having an adequate seal with low facial pressure, being disposable or easy to clean, being nonirritating to the skin, and low cost.

The mask cushion produces the seal between the mask and the patient (**Figure 23–3**). Although it should minimize air leakage, small leaks are common and may not necessarily compromise the effectiveness of CPAP or NIV. Nasal or oronasal masks designed specifically for NIV often use an open cushion with an inner lip, in which pressure inside the mask pushes the cushion against the face. The mask cushion should be soft and malleable to the facial anatomy. Anesthesia and resuscitation masks are not desirable for NIV. Some masks have an inflatable cushion, and some masks are gel filled. A correctly sized mask minimizes leak, improves comfort, and improves effectiveness. Masks for use with a bilevel ventilator or CPAP machine may incorporate a leak port and an anti-asphyxia port that opens if flow is lost from the ventilator (**Figure 23–4**). Masks used with a conventional ventilator have a standard elbow without a leak port. Commercial oronasal masks also have quick-release features so that the mask can be removed quickly if necessary. The hybrid interface is a combination of nasal pillows and a mask that fits over the mouth. The total face mask fits over the entire face of the patient.

The **helmet**, a transparent, latex-free polyvinyl chloride cylinder linked by a metallic ring to a soft collar that seals the helmet around the neck, has been proposed as an effective alternative to conventional face masks for NIV in patients with acute respiratory failure. One concern with the use of the helmet is the risk of rebreathing.

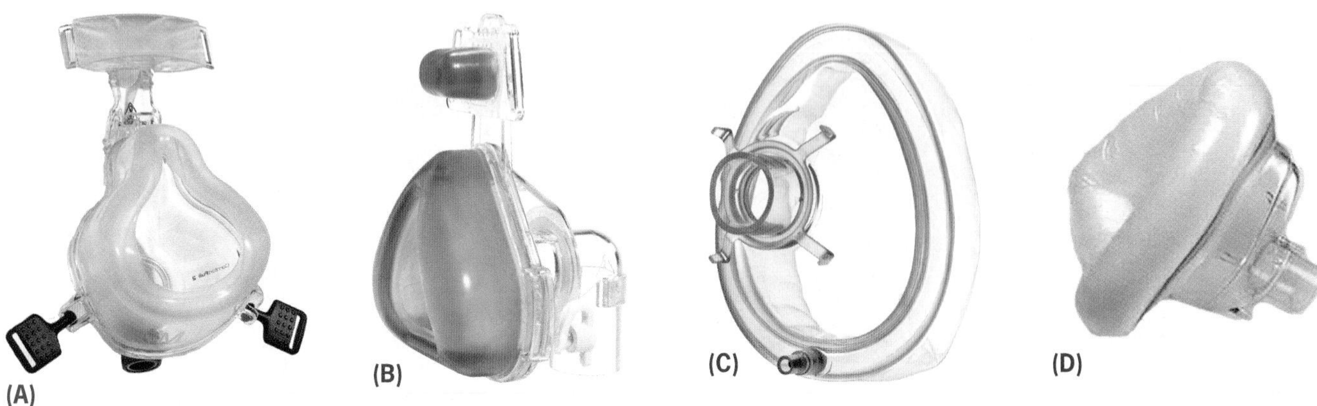

FIGURE 23–3 Styles of cushions on masks for NIV and CPAP. (**A**) Inner flap. (**B**) Gel. (**C**) Air-filled. (**D**) Foam-filled.

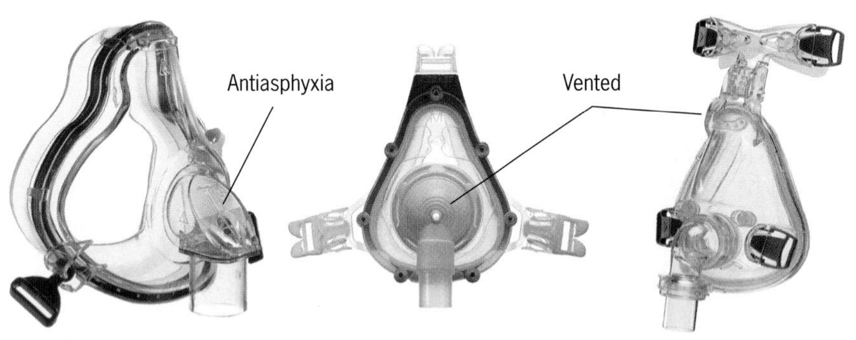

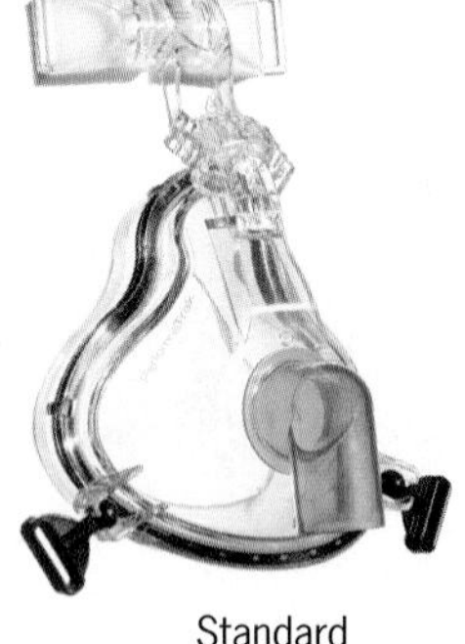

FIGURE 23–4 Masks with antiasphyxia valve, vented leak ports, and standard elbow.

The helmet has also been shown to be less effective in unloading inspiratory muscles compared with a standard face mask and has been associated with patient–ventilator dyssynchrony.

The nasal mask should fit just above the junction of the nasal bone and cartilage, directly at the sides of the nares, and just below the nose above the upper lip. The oronasal mask should fit just above the junction of the nasal bone and cartilage to just below the lower lip. Sizing gauges are available to properly fit masks. These are mask specific and cannot be interchanged between manufacturers or different mask styles of the same manufacturer. A common mistake is to choose a mask that is too large. This results in leaks, decreased effectiveness, and patient discomfort. Leaks through the mouth are common when using a nasal mask. Unsuccessful NIV has been associated with mouth leak. When mouth leak interferes with the effectiveness of ventilation with a nasal mask, a chin strap can be tried. Upper airway dryness may occur with use of a nasal mask and mouth leak. This can be addressed by using an oronasal mask or heated humidification, but a heat and moisture exchanger should not be used with NIV. For many patients with acute respiratory failure, the oronasal mask is better tolerated than a nasal interface.

> **RESPIRATORY RECAP**
>
> **Choosing an Interface**
>
> » Use the proper interface for the patient.
>
> » Avoid an interface that is too large.
>
> » Avoid strapping the mask too tightly.

Appropriate headgear is needed to maintain correct position of the mask. Elastic straps with holes that attach to hooks are commonly used with oronasal masks. The hooks on oronasal masks can be either on the outer edge of the mask or near the center of the mask. Attachment of the headgear to the outer edge of the mask may better distribute the pressure of the mask and facilitate a seal. Most masks designed specifically for NIV and CPAP use cloth straps and Velcro to secure the mask. The cloth straps fit through attachments at the sides and top of the mask. Use of Velcro to secure the mask allows nearly infinite adjustments of the headgear. A common mistake is to fit the headgear too tightly. It should be possible to pass one or two fingers between the headgear and the face. Fitting the headgear too tightly may not improve the fit and always decreases patient comfort and compliance. The design of most masks for NIV is such that the top of the mask is secured on the

BOX 23–1

Strength of Evidence Supporting Use of Noninvasive Ventilation for Acute Respiratory Failure

COPD exacerbations: NIV is first-line therapy and standard of care.

Acute cardiogenic pulmonary edema: NIV or CPAP is first-line therapy and standard of care.

Prevention of extubation failure: Accumulating evidence supports extubating patients directly to NIV who are at risk for extubation failure.

Transplantation, immunocompromise: Evidence supports the use of NIV in patients who develop respiratory failure following transplantation and in those who are immunocompromised.

Respiratory failure following lung resection: Evidence supports the use of NIV in patients who develop respiratory failure following lung resection surgery.

Acute hypoxemic respiratory failure: Evidence does not support the use of NIV for patients with acute hypoxemic respiratory failure, such as those with acute lung injury or acute respiratory distress syndrome.

Asthma: The role of NIV in acute asthma is unclear because there have been few high-level studies for this application.

Patients with Do Not Intubate or Do Not Resuscitate orders: In this patient population, NIV may be indicated in patients with COPD or cardiogenic pulmonary edema; it is not useful for malignancy except for patients in whom it is used for palliation.

Failed extubation: The results of high-level studies do not support the use of NIV to prevent reintubation in patients who fail a planned extubation.

COPD, chronic obstructive lung disease; NIV, noninvasive ventilation; CPAP, continuous positive airway pressure.

forehead rather than at the bridge of the nose. Forehead spacers and an adjustable bridge on the mask are used to decrease pressure on the bridge of the nose.

Pressure sores on the bridge of the nose are a common complaint during NIV. Fortunately, ulceration and skin breakdown are avoided in many patients. Measures to reduce pressure injury should be taken as soon as signs of soreness occur at the bridge of the nose. Correct mask fit and size should be reassessed. The tension of the headgear should be reduced. A different mask style may be tried, such as a hybrid mask or total face mask. A wound care dressing such as DuoDERM can be applied.

Noninvasive Positive Pressure Ventilation

Acute Care Applications

NIV is commonly used in the treatment of patients with acute respiratory failure (**Box 23–1**).[2–4] In appropriately selected patients, NIV decreases the need for endotracheal intubation, decreases the risk of nosocomial pneumonia, and improves survival. The strongest evidence supportive of the use of NIV has been seen in patients with COPD exacerbation and acute cardiogenic pulmonary edema. NIV is also useful in patients with respiratory failure following solid organ transplantation and in those who are immunocompromised.

Box 23–2 lists inclusion and exclusion criteria for NIV. The initial response to NIV may predict success or failure. A more rapid decrease in $Paco_2$ occurs in patients for whom NIV is successful. Unsuccessful nasal NIV has been associated with greater severity of illness, greater mouth leak, and increased difficulty acclimating to NIV.[5] Greater mouth leak has been associated with patients who are edentulous, have excess secretions, and use pursed-lip breathing. Success of NIV also has been reported to be greater for patients with higher baseline pH levels, perhaps because low pH was considered a marker of more severe illness.[6] A good level of consciousness also has been associated with successful responses to NIV for patients with COPD and acute hypercapnic respiratory failure.[7] If a patient does not improve on NIV within 1 to 2 hours of initiation, alternative therapy such as intubation should be considered. Consideration should also be given to transfer of the patient using NIV to a monitored unit such as an intensive care unit (ICU). **Figure 23–5** presents an algorithm for use of NIV.

RESPIRATORY RECAP

Benefits of NIV for Acute Respiratory Failure

- » Decreased intubation rate
- » Improved survival
- » Decreased pneumonia rates

Aerophagia commonly occurs with NIV, but this is usually benign because the airway pressures are less than the esophageal opening pressure. Therefore, a gastric tube is not routinely necessary for mask ventilation. In fact, a gastric tube may interfere with the effectiveness of mask ventilation in several ways. It may be more difficult

BOX 23–2

Selection of Appropriate Patients for Noninvasive Ventilation

Step 1: Patient needs mechanical ventilation, such as

Respiratory distress with dyspnea, use of accessory muscles, abdominal paradox
Respiratory acidosis; pH < 7.35 with $Pa_{CO_2} > 45$ mm Hg
Tachypnea; respiratory rate > 25 breaths/min
Diagnosis shown to respond well to noninvasive ventilation (e.g., chronic obstructive pulmonary disease, cardiogenic pulmonary edema)

Step 2: No exclusions for noninvasive ventilation, such as

Airway protection: respiratory arrest, unstable hemodynamics, high aspiration risk, copious secretions
Unable to fit mask: facial surgery, craniofacial trauma or burns, anatomic lesion of upper airway
Uncooperative patient; anxiety
Patient wishes

BOX 23–3

Clinical Indications for Noninvasive Positive Pressure Ventilation in Chronic Respiratory Failure

Restrictive Thoracic Disorders

Examples: Sequelae of polio, spinal cord injury, neuropathies, myopathies and dystrophies, amyotrophic lateral sclerosis (ALS), chest wall deformities, kyphoscoliosis
Symptoms: Fatigue, dyspnea, morning headache
Physiologic criteria: $Pa_{CO_2} \geq 45$ mm Hg, nocturnal oximetry demonstrating oxygen saturation $\leq 88\%$ for 5 consecutive minutes, maximal inspiratory pressure > -60 cm H_2O or forced vital capacity $< 50\%$ of predicted

Chronic Obstructive Pulmonary Disease

Examples: Chronic bronchitis, emphysema, bronchiectasis, cystic fibrosis
Symptoms: Fatigue, dyspnea, morning headache
Physiologic criteria: $Pa_{CO_2} \geq 55$ mm Hg, Pa_{CO_2} of 50 to 54 mm Hg and nocturnal oximetry demonstrating oxygen saturation $\leq 88\%$ for 5 consecutive minutes while receiving oxygen therapy ≥ 2 L/min, Pa_{CO_2} of 50 to 54 mm Hg and hospitalization related to recurrent episodes of hypercapnic respiratory failure

Data from Clinical indications for noninvasive positive pressure ventilation in chronic respiratory failure due to restrictive lung disease, COPD, and nocturnal hypoventilation—a consensus conference report. *Chest.* 1999;16:521–534.

to achieve a mask seal if a gastric tube is present. Compression of the gastric tube against the face by the mask may increase the likelihood of facial skin breakdown. A nasogastric tube will increase resistance to nasal gas flow, which may decrease the effectiveness of mask ventilation—particularly nasal ventilation.

Chronic Applications

NIV is used for chronic respiratory failure resulting from restrictive lung disease, COPD, and nocturnal hypoventilation. In many patients receiving chronic NIV, however, the therapy is administered only at night. Common goals of this therapy are to improve symptoms (e.g., fatigue, morning headache), to decrease Pa_{CO_2}, and to decrease the degree of nocturnal arterial oxygen desaturation. **Box 23–3** lists recommended clinical indications for the use of NIV in chronic applications.[8] Chronic use of NIV is most common with neuromuscular respiratory failure, where it is used as an alternative to tracheostomy and can be used

RESPIRATORY RECAP

Goals of Chronic Use of NIV

» Improve symptoms
» Decrease Pa_{CO_2}
» Decrease degree of nocturnal oxygen desaturation

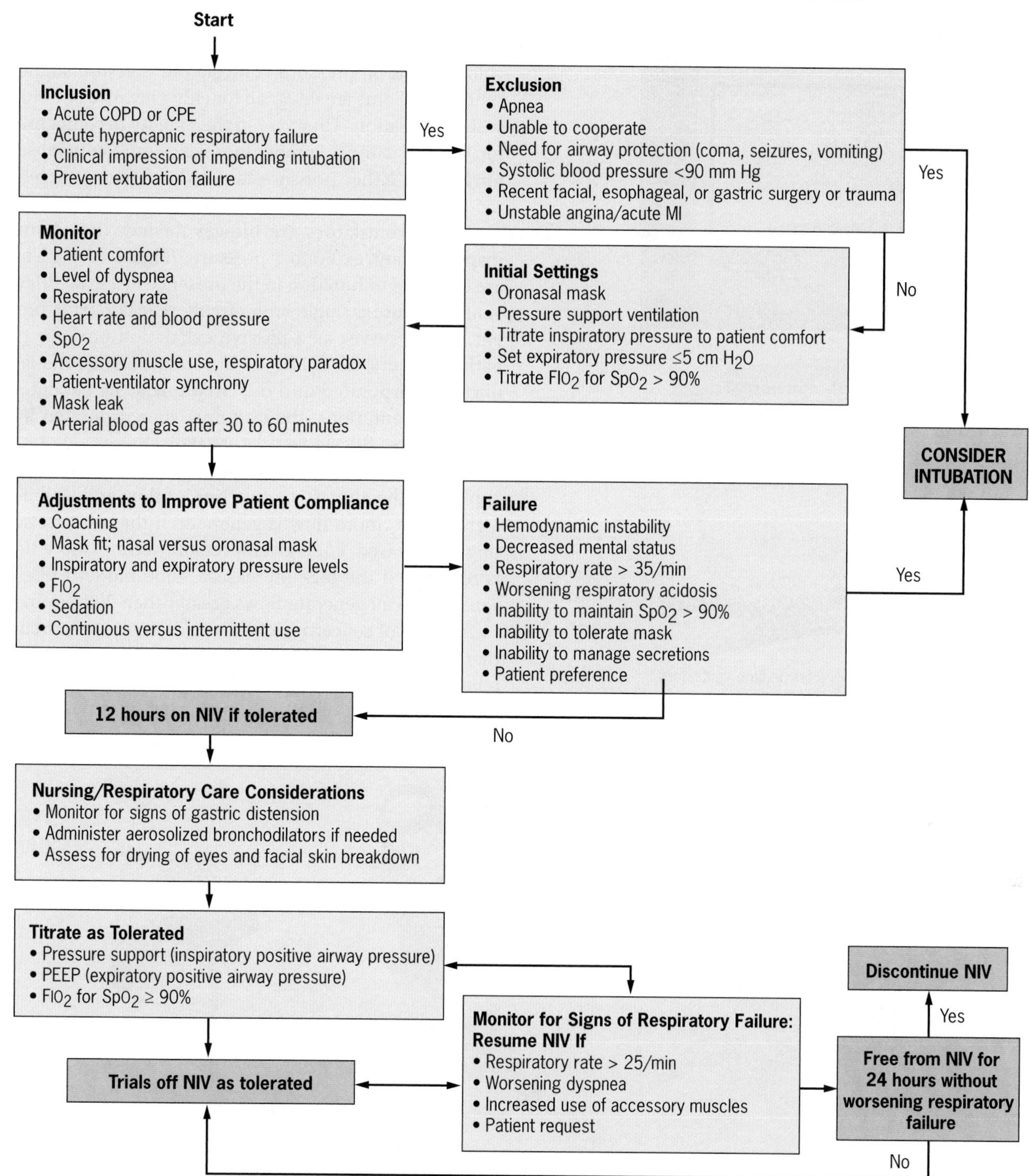

FIGURE 23-5 Clinical algorithm for application of NIV in the acute care setting.

for full-time ventilatory support. Some patients with neuromuscular disease can use a mouthpiece during the daytime and a mask at night. The use of NIV for chronic stable COPD is controversial and is not common.

Ventilators for Noninvasive Positive Pressure Ventilation

Critical care ventilators are designed primarily for invasive ventilation, but can be used for NIV. An issue with the use of critical care ventilators for NIV is that many are leak intolerant. However, newer generations of critical care ventilators feature NIV modes, and some compensate well for leaks.[9,10] Intermediate ventilators are typically used for patient transport or home care ventilation (**Figure 23-6**). Older generations of these ventilators only provided volume control continuous mandatory ventilation and were used for nasal, oronasal, or mouth-piece ventilation. Early studies of nocturnal NIV

RESPIRATORY RECAP

Ventilators for NIV

» Critical care ventilators
» Intermediate ventilators
» Bilevel ventilators

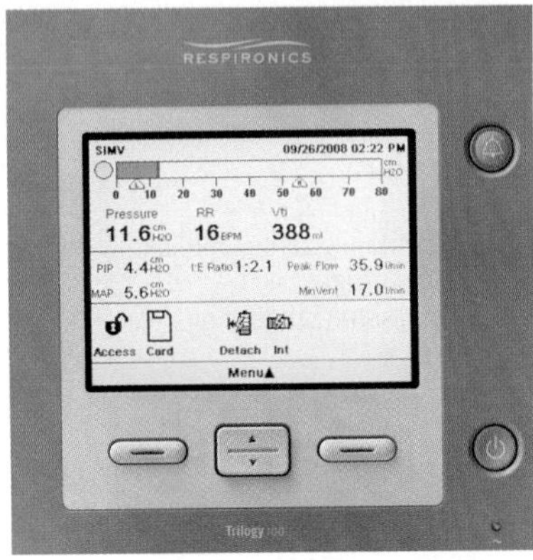

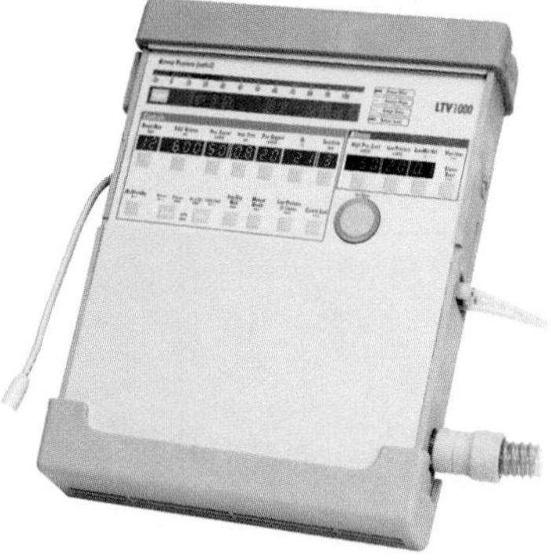

FIGURE 23–6 Intermediate ventilators that can be used for NIV.

in patients with neuromuscular disease typically used these ventilators.[11] Newer generations of these ventilators provide volume control, pressure control, and pressure support ventilation. Some are designed for either invasive or noninvasive ventilation. They vary in their ability to compensate for leaks, but most compensate well; some compensate for leaks in either pressure-targeted or volume-targeted modes. Most have internal batteries.

Bilevel ventilators are blower devices that deliver inspiratory and expiratory pressures (**Figure 23–7**). They are designed to function in the presence of a leak. Bilevel ventilators use a single limb circuit. A leak port is present, which serves as a passive exhalation port for the patient (**Figure 23–8**). In some configurations, the leak port is incorporated into the circuit near the patient. In other configurations, the leak port is incorporated into the interface. Bilevel ventilators typically provide pressure support or pressure control ventilation. Pressure applied to the airway is a function of flow and leak. For a given leak, more flow is generated if the pressure setting is increased. For a given pressure setting, more flow is required if the leak increases. Some modern bilevel ventilators can generate flows greater than 200 L/min.

An issue of concern with the use of single limb circuits that have a passive exhalation port is the potential for rebreathing. If the expiratory flow of the patient exceeds the flow capacity of the leak port, then it is possible to

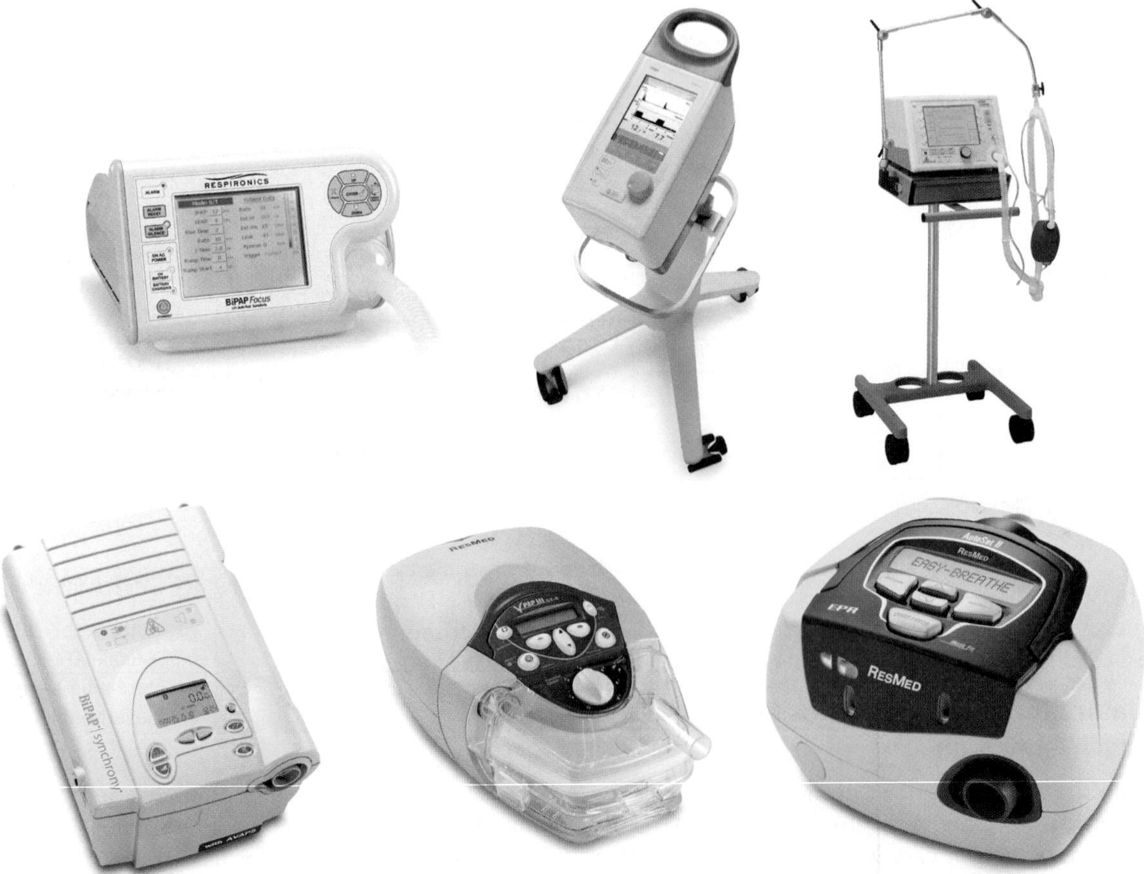

FIGURE 23–7 Bilevel ventilators that can be used for NIV.

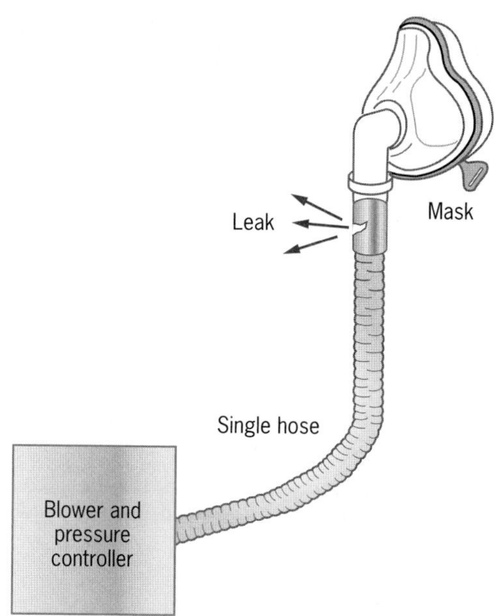

FIGURE 23–8 Schematic drawing of a single limb bilevel ventilator to provide NIV.

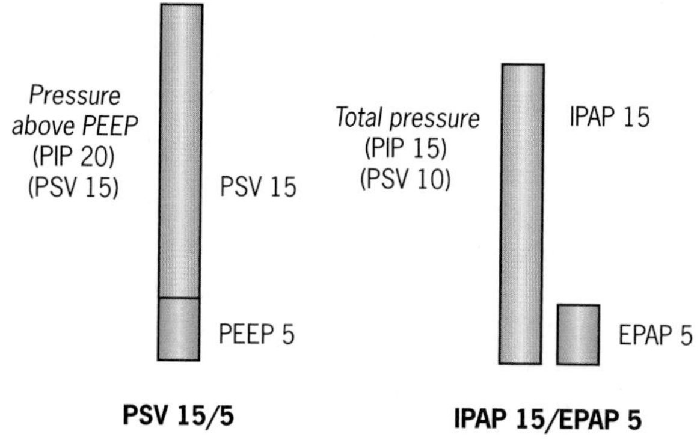

FIGURE 23–9 Comparison of pressure support, such as with a critical care ventilation, and inspiratory positive airway pressure (IPAP) with a bilevel ventilator. Note that the IPAP is the peak inspiratory pressure (PIP) and includes the expiratory positive airway pressure (EPAP), whereas pressure support is provided on top of the positive end-expiratory pressure (PEEP).

exhale into the single limb circuit and rebreathe on the subsequent inhalation. Several steps can be taken to minimize this risk. Rebreathing is decreased if the leak port is in the mask rather than the hose,[12,13] if oxygen is titrated into the mask rather than into the hose,[14] with a higher level of expiratory pressure,[15] and with a plateau exhalation valve.[15] Major determinants of rebreathing are the expiratory time and the flow through the circuit during exhalation. Increasing the expiratory pressure requires greater flow and thus decreases the amount of rebreathing. It is for this reason that the minimum expiratory pressure setting on many bilevel ventilators is 4 cm H_2O. Opening the ports on the interface increases leak, which increases the compensatory flow through the hose and more effectively flushes the hose and decreases rebreathing. Although it effectively decreases rebreathing, the plateau exhalation valve may increase the imposed expiratory resistance.[16]

Some ventilators are able to detect unintentional leak (e.g., leak due to a poorly fitting interface) and adjust flow to accommodate the leak. Some bilevel ventilators allow the user to enter the interface that will be used to allow more precise identification of the unintentional leak. This approach, however, requires the use of an interface provided by the manufacturer of the ventilator. Other bilevel ventilators allow the user to test the leak port as part of the pre-use procedure.

If the leak is great, the patient may breathe from the leak rather than producing a flow or pressure change that will trigger the start of the breath. On the other hand, the leak could produce a pressure or flow drop that produces auto-triggering. Leaks also can affect the ventilator's ability to cycle to exhalation. Unintentional leaks should be minimized, and use of a ventilator with good leak compensation is ideal. All ventilators have a maximum inspiratory time during pressure support (typically 3 seconds), and the maximum inspiratory time is adjustable on some ventilators. Some ventilators allow the flow cycle criteria to be adjusted, which may be useful if a leak is present.

For acute care applications, it is desirable to use a ventilator with a blender allowing precise F_{IO_2} administration from 0.21 to 1.0. Bilevel ventilators used outside the acute care setting generally do not have a blender, but rather provide supplemental oxygen by titration into the circuit or interface.[17] This results in a delivered oxygen concentration that is variable, and only modest concentrations can be achieved (e.g., <60%). With oxygen titration, the F_{IO_2} is not easily predictable and is affected by the site of the oxygen titration, type of exhalation port, ventilator settings, oxygen flow, breathing pattern, and leak.

Pressure support ventilation is used most commonly for NIV.[18] With a critical care ventilator, the level of pressure support is applied as a pressure above the baseline positive end-expiratory pressure (PEEP). However, the approach is different with bilevel ventilators, in which an **inspiratory positive airway pressure (IPAP)** and **expiratory positive airway pressure (EPAP)** are set. In this configuration, the difference between the IPAP and EPAP is the level of pressure support (**Figure 23–9**). With pressure support, the pressure applied to the airway is fixed for each breath, but there is no backup rate or fixed inspiratory time. Rise time (pressurization rate) is the time required to reach the inspiratory pressure at the onset of the inspiratory phase with pressure support or pressure control ventilation.[19] This can be adjusted on many ventilators used for NIV. With a fast rise time, the inspiratory pressure is reached quickly, whereas with a slow rise time it takes longer to reach the inspiratory pressure. A faster rise time may better unload the respiratory muscles of patients with COPD, but this may be accompanied by substantial air leaks and poor tolerance.[20] In patients with neuromuscular disease, a slower rise time is often better tolerated. Rise time should be set to maximize patient comfort.

Pressure control ventilation is similar to pressure support in that the ventilator applies a fixed level of support with each breath. Trigger and rise time are similar in pressure support and pressure control.[21] The primary differences between pressure control and pressure support are that (1) there is a backup rate with pressure control, and (2) the inspiratory time is fixed with pressure control. The backup rate is theoretically beneficial in the setting of apnea or periodic breathing, which may occur with pressure support. The fixed inspiratory time of pressure control is beneficial when the inspiratory phase is prolonged during pressure support due to leak or lung mechanics (e.g., COPD).[22–24]

Bilevel ventilators typically provide pressure support with a mode called *spontaneous*. In the spontaneous mode, IPAP and EPAP are set, but there is no backup rate. For safety, a backup rate should be provided. This is the case with the spontaneous/timed mode on bilevel ventilators. The patient receives pressure support ventilation if the rate is greater than the set rate. However, if the patient becomes apneic, the ventilator will deliver flow-cycled or time-cycled breaths at the rate set on the ventilator. For critical care ventilators set for pressure support, the backup ventilation rate and alarms occur if the patient becomes apneic. A backup rate is also important to prevent periodic breathing. Central apnea is more prevalent with pressure support in normal subjects using a nasal mask,[25] in intubated patients,[26] and in patients being evaluated in an outpatient sleep laboratory.[27] For these reasons, a backup rate is recommended during NIV, particularly with nocturnal applications. Some bilevel ventilators have a timed mode. With this mode, the ventilator is triggered and cycled by the ventilator at the set rate and inspiratory time. This mode provides little interaction between the patient and the ventilator.

RESPIRATORY RECAP

Bilevel Ventilators for NIV

- » Use blower devices
- » Allow adjustment of IPAP and EPAP to produce pressure support ventilation
- » Typically have modes such as spontaneous, spontaneous/timed, and timed
- » Some have new modes such as AVAPS and adaptive servo-ventilation
- » Use a single limb circuit with potential for rebreathing
- » Some have a blender; others provide FIO_2 by titration

With volume control ventilation, the ventilator delivers a fixed tidal volume and inspiratory flow with each breath. Volume control has been used during NIV primarily in the home setting.[28–31] Volume control for home NIV is provided with an intermediate ventilator. NIV with volume control uses a nonvented interface. Volume control has also been used to provide mouthpiece ventilation.[32–34] A low-pressure alarm is prevented during mouthpiece ventilation by producing enough circuit back pressure with sufficient peak inspiratory flow against the restrictive mouthpiece according to the set tidal volume.[35] The ventilator rate is also set at a low level to prevent an apnea alarm. Breath stacking maneuvers can be provided with volume control ventilation, but not with pressure control or pressure support ventilation. **Table 23–2** lists the advantages and disadvantages of pressure-targeted versus volume-targeted ventilation during NIV.

TABLE 23-2 Comparison of Volume Ventilators and Bilevel Pressure Ventilators for Noninvasive Ventilation

Volume Ventilators	Pressure Ventilators
More complicated to use	Simple to use
Wide range of alarms	Limited alarms
Constant tidal volume	Variable tidal volume
Breath stacking possible	Breath stacking not possible
No leak compensation with older models	Leak compensation
Can be used without PEEP	PEEP (EPAP) always present
Rebreathing minimized	Rebreathing possible

PEEP, positive end-expiratory pressure; EPAP, expiratory positive airway pressure.

Average volume assured pressure support (AVAPS) is a feature available on the latest generation of Respironics bilevel ventilators. It helps patients maintain a tidal volume equal to or greater than the target tidal volume by automatically controlling the pressure support. The IPAP level is varied between the minimum and maximum IPAP settings. AVAPS averages tidal volume over time and changes the IPAP gradually over several minutes. If patient effort decreases, AVAPS automatically increases IPAP to maintain the target tidal volume. On the other hand, if patient effort increases, AVAPS will reduce IPAP. AVAPS functions much like adaptive support modes such as volume support.

A feature on the ResMed bilevel ventilator is adaptive servo-ventilation (adapt SV). With adapt SV, the algorithm uses three factors to achieve synchronization between pressure support and the patient's breathing: the patient's average respiratory rate; the direction, magnitude, and rate of change of the patient's airflow; and a backup respiratory rate of 15 breaths/min. When central apnea or hypopnea occurs, support initially continues to reflect the patient's breathing pattern. If apnea or hypopnea persists, the ventilator uses the backup respiratory rate. When breathing resumes and ventilation exceeds the target, pressure support is reduced to the minimum of 3 cm H_2O.

Ramp is used to reduce the pressure and then gradually increase it to the pressure setting. A ramp is used primarily in patients receiving CPAP or bilevel ventilation for sleep apnea, the objective being to allow the patient to fall asleep more comfortably. The role of a ramp during NIV is unclear. Particularly for acute care applications, this feature may be undesirable because it delays application of therapeutic pressure setting.

A feature on the Respironics bilevel ventilators, Bi-Flex, inserts a small amount of pressure relief during the latter

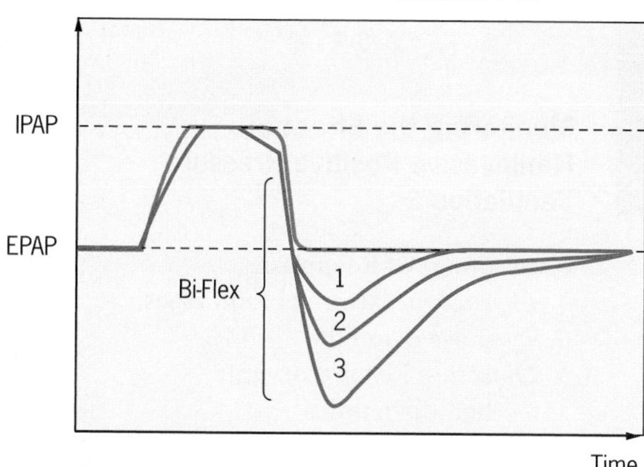

FIGURE 23–10 Bi-Flex mode inserts a small pressure relief during the latter stages of inspiration and at the beginning of exhalation. Adapted from Philips Respironics, Murrysville, Penn.

stages of inspiration and the beginning part of exhalation (**Figure 23–10**). High level evidence supporting the use of Bi-Flex with NIV is lacking. A similar feature on ResMed bilevel ventilators is expiratory pressure relief.

Use of alarms during NIV is a balance between patient safety and annoyance. The extent of alarms necessary depends on the underlying condition of the patient and the ability of the patient to breathe without support. For example, consider the patient with neuromuscular disease receiving near full support by NIV. This patient is unable to reattach the interface or circuit should it become disconnected. In this case, disconnect alarms and alarms indicating large leaks or changes in ventilation are desirable. Similar alarms are desirable in a patient with acute respiratory failure receiving NIV. On the other extreme, in the case of a patient using daytime mouthpiece ventilation, alarms may be an annoyance, and techniques have been described to outsmart these alarms.[35] When there is a question of the extent of alarms necessary, one should err on the side of patient safety. Ventilators for NIV have increasing capability to monitor the patient's breathing. Display of tidal volume, respiratory rate, and leak is useful for titrating settings. Many ventilators also display waveforms of pressure, flow, and volume. These waveforms can be useful in titrating settings to improve patient–ventilator synchrony.

Ventilators for NIV can be battery powered for safety and increased portability. Some have an internal battery, whereas others can be powered with a battery or uninterruptible power supply. Many bilevel ventilators can be powered with a direct current (DC) converter. This allows the ventilator to be powered by the auxiliary power source in a vehicle. Bilevel ventilators can also be powered by a lead-acid battery such as a deep cycle or marine battery. In this case, an inverter is used to convert battery power into mains power. The duration of the battery is determined by the size of the battery, ventilator settings, amount of leak, and whether or not a humidifier is used. When using a battery, it is generally best not to use a humidifier if possible, as this will extend the life of the battery. It is also best to avoid use of the humidifier when the bilevel ventilator is made portable to avoid accidentally spilling water into the ventilator.

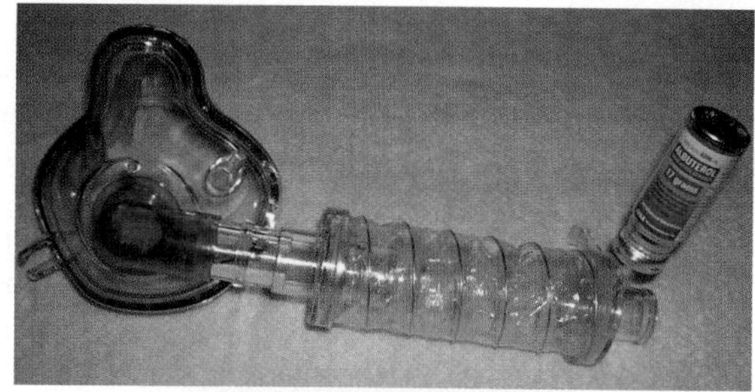

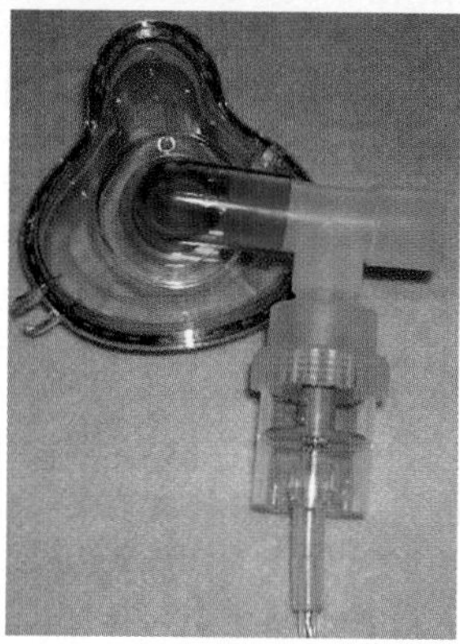

FIGURE 23–11 Insertion site for nebulizer and inhaler for use with a bilevel ventilator during NIV.

Humidity is added by placement of a humidifier between the ventilator and the patient interface. A cool, ambient-temperature, passover humidifier chamber adds a small amount of water vapor to the air flowing to the patient. However, because of the velocity and volume of airflow, the limited surface area of the water chamber, and the evaporative cooling effect, the water content of the air being delivered to the patient increases only slightly. For some patients this may be enough to minimize nasal mucous membrane drying. For others a heated humidifier may be necessary. Heating the water in the reservoir counters the effects of evaporative cooling and raises the temperature of the air passing through the humidifier, allowing it to carry more water content.

Inline aerosol therapy also can be provided during NIV by nebulizer or metered dose inhaler (**Figure 23–11**). To improve drug delivery, the nebulizer should be placed near the mask rather than at the outlet of the ventilator during NIV. A metered dose inhaler should be used with a spacer. Although the amount of aerosol that penetrates the upper airway may be reduced during NIV, a sufficient quantity is delivered to the lungs to produce a physiologic response.[36] Care must be taken to ensure an adequate mask fit so that aerosol is not directed into the eyes of the patient.

Clinical Application

The application of NIV requires caregiver patience and skills with both the technical aspects of mechanical ventilation and patient coaching to adapt to the mask and ventilator. In many cases the appropriate settings for NIV are determined largely by trial and error, with appropriate feedback from the patient. The primary goal in the initiation of NIV is patient comfort and not an improvement in arterial blood gas values per se. An improvement in blood gas values usually follows if patient comfort and respiratory muscle unloading are achieved. Important steps in the clinical application of NIV are as follows:

1. Select patients for NIV who are most likely to benefit (e.g., those experiencing a COPD exacerbation or acute cardiogenic pulmonary edema).
2. Choose a ventilator capable of meeting patient needs.
3. Choose the correct interface; avoid a mask that is too large.
4. Explain the therapy to the patient.
5. Silence alarms and choose low settings.
6. Initiate NIV while holding mask in place.
7. Secure mask, avoiding a tight fit.
8. Titrate inspiratory pressure to patient comfort.
9. Titrate F_{IO_2} to Sp_{O_2} greater than 90%.
10. To minimize gastric insufflation, avoid inspiratory pressure above 20 cm H_2O.
11. Titrate expiratory pressure per trigger effort and Sp_{O_2}.
12. Continue to coach and reassure patient; make adjustments to improve patient compliance.

Complications of NIV are usually minor and include leaks, mask discomfort, eye irritation, facial skin breakdown, sinus congestion, oropharyngeal drying, patient–ventilator dyssynchrony, gastric insufflation, and hemodynamic compromise.[37,38] **Box 23–4** lists parameters that should be monitored during NIV. For acute care applications, NIV should be provided in a setting where the patient can be adequately monitored. If the patient does not improve within 1 to 2 hours after initiation of NIV, endotracheal intubation should be considered. The best approach to weaning from NIV is unclear. In many cases the patient requests removal of the mask after several hours of therapy. If the patient's condition deteriorates after removal of the mask, then the therapy should be resumed.

Continuous Positive Airway Pressure

CPAP has applications in both the acute care and chronic care of patients. In acute care, noninvasive (mask) CPAP is used to administer intermittent lung expansion therapy, to treat acute hypoxemic respiratory failure, and to treat acute cardiogenic pulmonary edema. In chronic care, CPAP is used to treat obstructive sleep apnea (OSA).

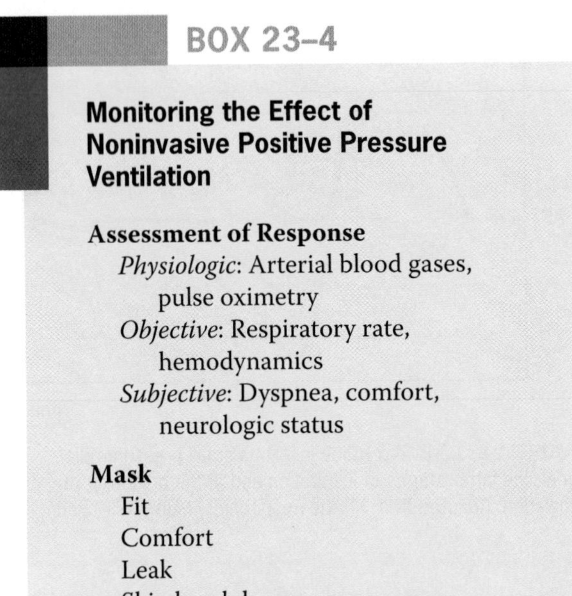

BOX 23–4

Monitoring the Effect of Noninvasive Positive Pressure Ventilation

Assessment of Response
- *Physiologic*: Arterial blood gases, pulse oximetry
- *Objective*: Respiratory rate, hemodynamics
- *Subjective*: Dyspnea, comfort, neurologic status

Mask
- Fit
- Comfort
- Leak
- Skin breakdown

Respiratory Muscle Unloading
- Accessory muscle use
- Thoracoabdominal paradox

Abdomen
- Gastric distention
- Expiratory muscle activation

Acute Care Applications

Mask CPAP can be an effortless, painless type of respiratory care to prevent postoperative atelectasis.[39] It has been used in patients with acute hypoxemic respiratory failure to improve Pa_{O_2}.[40] However, although mask CPAP can produce an initial improvement in Pa_{O_2}, it may not improve important outcomes such as intubation rate or hospital mortality. The strongest evidence for the use of mask CPAP is for patients with acute cardiogenic pulmonary edema. In these patients the increase in intrathoracic pressure decreases preload, decreases afterload, improves lung compliance, decreases intrapulmonary shunt, and increases Pa_{O_2}. A typical CPAP level of 5 to 10 cm H_2O is used. Mask CPAP, similar to NIV, decreases the intubation rate and improves survival rate in patients with acute cardiogenic pulmonary edema.[41]

RESPIRATORY RECAP

Acute Care Applications of Mask CPAP
- » Postoperative pulmonary complications
- » Hypoxemic respiratory failure
- » Cardiogenic pulmonary edema

A bilevel ventilator set to the CPAP mode is commonly used to provide mask CPAP for acute care applications. Otherwise, a CPAP circuit can be used. The CPAP circuit (**Figure 23–12**) consists of a high-flow gas source and an expiratory valve that maintains pressure

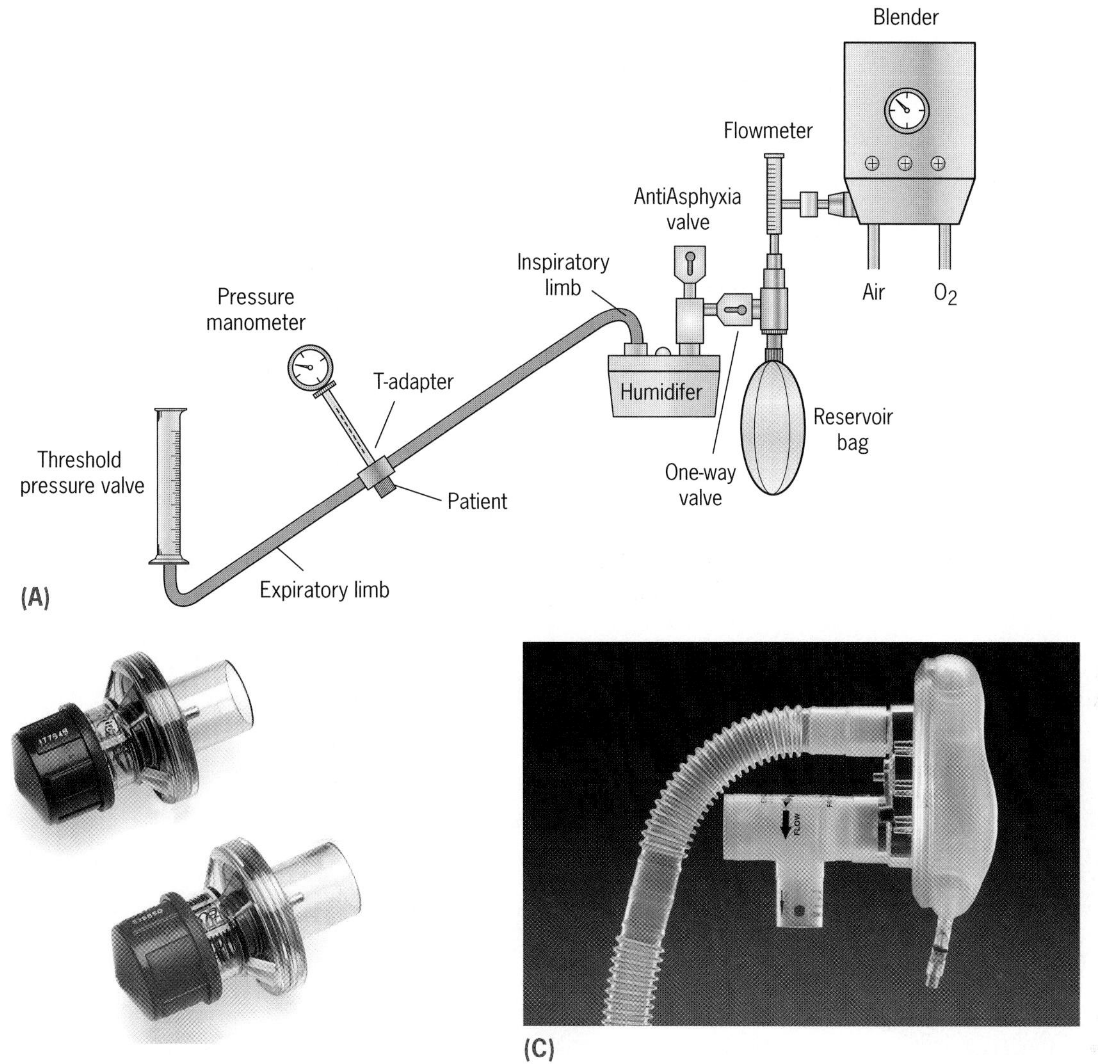

FIGURE 23–12 **(A)** CPAP circuit for acute respiratory failure. **(B)** Commercially available CPAP/PEEP valves. **(C)** Commercially available system for CPAP. **(A)** Adapted from Branson RD. Spontaneous breathing systems: IMV and CPAP. In: Branson RD, Hess DR, Chatburn RL, eds. *Respiratory Care Equipment*. 2nd ed. JB Lippincott; 1999.

in the circuit at the desired level (5 to 20 cm H_2O). CPAP requires a relatively high gas flow to maintain the desired positive airway pressure.

CPAP valves are classified as threshold resistors or fixed orifices. Threshold resistors maintain a constant pressure in the circuit, regardless of flow. A pressure exceeding the threshold opens the valve and allows expiration, whereas pressures below threshold allow the valve to close, sealing the circuit and stopping the flow of gas. Commonly used threshold resistor devices use spring tension to produce CPAP (**Figure 23–13**). With the fixed-orifice device, a restricted opening of a fixed size is placed at the end of the expiratory limb of a breathing circuit. The resistance through the fixed orifice produces back pressure, which is CPAP pressure produced in the circuit. For a given flow, a higher pressure is generated with a smaller orifice. Expiratory pressure is flow dependent, so pressure decreases as flow decreases. The fixed-orifice resistor has been abandoned in adult respiratory care but remains in use in neonatal care.

CPAP for Obstructive Sleep Apnea

Obstructive sleep apnea is a serious, potentially life-threatening condition characterized by repeated collapse of the upper airway during sleep, with subsequent hypopnea and cessation of breathing. The most widely prescribed noninvasive treatment for OSA is CPAP therapy. When applied at the appropriate pressure setting, CPAP eliminates the soft tissue obstruction of the upper airway. With the mechanical cause of obstruction alleviated, the symptoms and effects of OSA quickly vanish. With CPAP, air flows through the nasopharynx and oropharynx at a preset pressure to maintain a constant positive pressure within the upper airway. This action has the effect of splinting the soft tissue, preventing its collapse into the airway during sleep and the subsequent obstruction. The CPAP pressure is prescribed after a

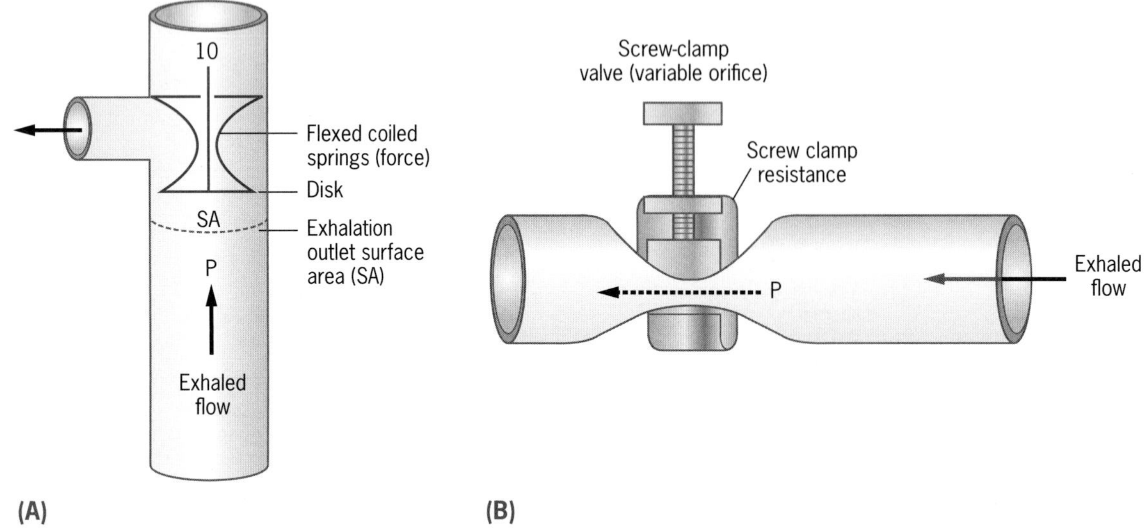

FIGURE 23–13 (**A**) Threshold resistor CPAP valve. (**B**) Fixed-orifice CPAP valve. Adapated from Banner MJ, Lampotang S. Expiratory pressure valves. In: Branson RD, Hess DR, Chatburn RL, eds. *Respiratory Care Equipment*. 2nd ed. JB Lippincott; 1999.

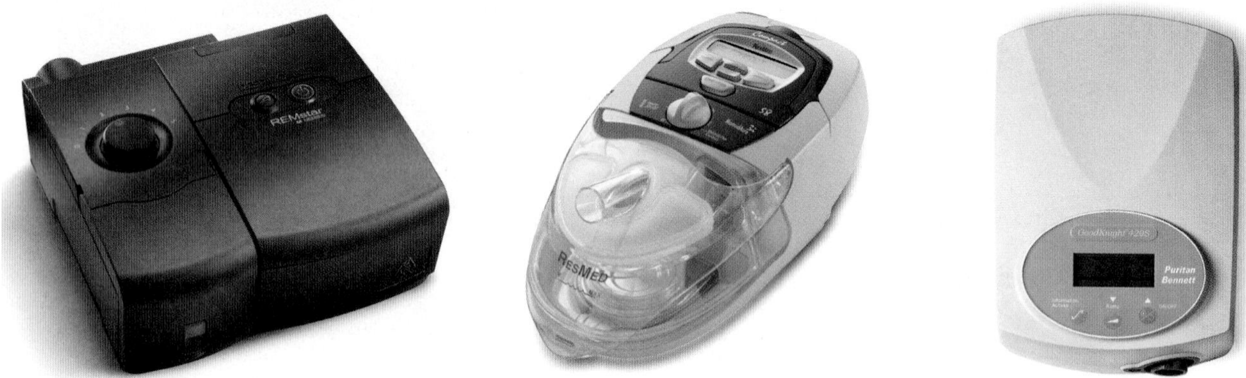

FIGURE 23–14 CPAP machines used in the treatment of obstructive sleep apnea.

sleep study during which the pressure is slowly increased (titrated) until the pressure necessary to significantly eliminate the apneas and hypopneas has been achieved.

CPAP Equipment for OSA

The patient interface used for nocturnal CPAP therapy is the same as that used for NIV. Selecting the most appropriate interface and the correct size for each individual patient is one of the most important factors determining whether a patient will be successful in long-term use of CPAP therapy. Inappropriate selection of the interface and its size, or incorrect selection, fitting, or adjustment of the headgear, results in air leaks around the mask (especially around the bridge of the nose at the corners of the eyes) and skin irritation, which can lead to tissue breakdown and ulceration.

Numerous brands and models of CPAP machines are commercially available (**Figure 23–14**). The basic models are relatively simple devices consisting of an electrically operated flow generator (fan or turbine) that draws in room air through a particulate filter (a gross particulate filter to remove dust, lint, and other large airborne matter) and a secondary filter (to capture smaller particles, such as pollen and spores). The prescribed pressure is entered, usually through digital electronics, into the unit's microprocessor, which causes the flow generator to deliver the flow of air necessary to maintain the prescribed pressure. CPAP systems, similar to ventilators for NIV, are designed to operate with a built-in leak in the circuit. This leak port usually is found in the mask or between the tubing and mask. Because the system is designed to automatically compensate for this leak and to maintain the designated pressure, it also accommodates other small to moderate leaks that occur at the various patient interfaces.

The pressure settings on most CPAP units are in the range of 3 to 20 cm H_2O. Most units also have an adjustable setting referred to as *ramp* or *delay*. When the prescribed pressure is greater than 10 cm H_2O, some

TABLE 23–3 Common Problems During the Use of CPAP for Obstructive Sleep Apnea

Problem	Cause	Solution
Nasal irritation, congestion, or rhinorrhea	Dry air Chronic rhinitis Nasal allergies	Heated humidification Nasal decongestants Nasal steroids Antihistamines
Dry throat and/or mouth	Dry air Mouth leak	Heated humidification Chin strap Oronasal or full-face interface
Painful pressure in ears	High airway pressure Nasal congestion	Verify CPAP level Decrease CPAP level Trial on auto or bilevel mode Nasal decongestants Nasal steroids
Gastric bloating and/or chest discomfort	Air swallowing High airway pressure	Decrease CPAP level Trial on auto or bilevel mode
Claustrophobia	Anxiety Interface	Desensitization Anxiolytics Optimize interface fit
Nasal pressure sores	Poor interface fit	Readjust head gear Change interface size or style Apply skin protection Reassess patient education on interface fit
Eye irritation	Interface air leak	Readjust headgear Change interface size or style Reassess patient education on interface fit
Skin creases	Improperly adjusted headgear	Readjust headgear Change interface size or style Reassess patient education on interface fit
Skin irritation	Sensitivity to interface Improperly adjusted headgear Heat rash	Trial using nasal pillows Readjust headgear Lower temperature on humidifier Trial using nasal pillows or skin protector
Air leaks	Excessive interface/headgear wear Poor interface fit Improperly adjusted headgear Excessive air pressure Facial hair interference	Replace interface and/or headgear Change interface Readjust headgear Verify pressure setting Consider pressure change Consider auto or bilevel mode Trial with nasal pillows Shave

CPAP, continuous positive airway pressure.

From Allen KY, Bollig S, Selecky PA, Smalling T. *The Clinician's Guide to PAP Adherence*. Irving, TX: American Association for Respiratory Care; 2009. Reprinted with permission from the American Association for Respiratory Care.

CPAP users find it difficult to fall asleep, bothered by the high airflow. Because obstructive episodes do not occur until the patient has been asleep for a period of time, the patient, after putting on the interface and adjusting for any leaks, can activate the ramp/delay feature. This activation causes the pressure to drop to 4 to 6 cm H_2O, a more tolerable level, while the patient falls asleep. The ramp feature can be preset to range from 5 to 45 minutes. The unit's microprocessor divides the set prescribed pressure by the number of ramp minutes and delivers an increasing pressure until the prescribed level is reached.

Improving Patient Compliance with CPAP for OSA

Table 23–3 lists common problems, and usual solutions, associated with the use of CPAP for OSA.[42] Respiratory therapists commonly encounter patients with OSA who use CPAP and should be able to assist such patients with

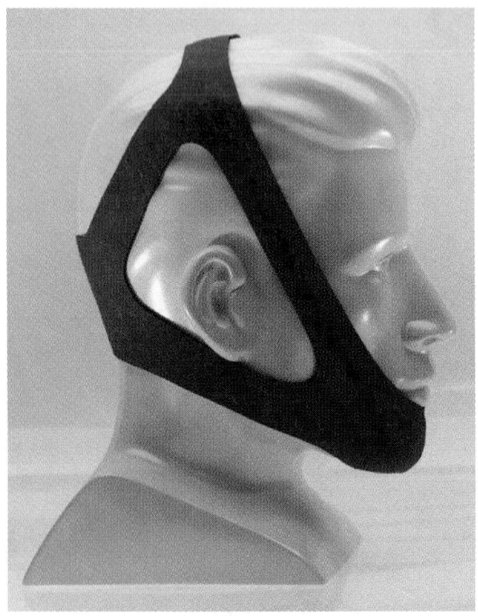

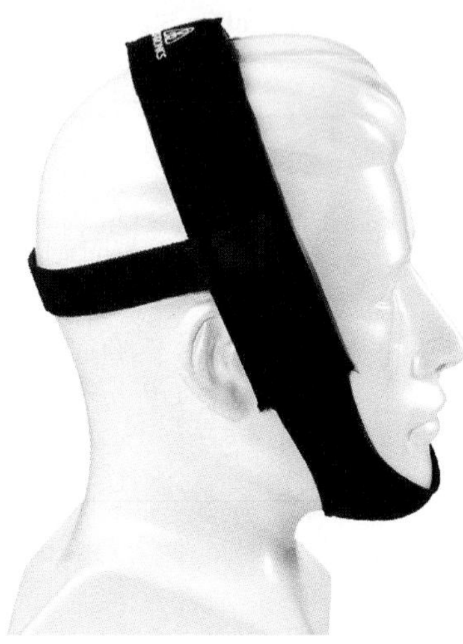

FIGURE 23–15 Chin straps used to prevent mouth leak.

> **RESPIRATORY RECAP**
>
> **Factors Affecting CPAP Compliance**
>
> » Poor patient education and understanding
> » Improper interface size, selection, and fit
> » Drying of nose and mouth
> » High inward flow during exhalation

these problems. Patients should be reminded of the benefits of CPAP in the setting of OSA. Some patients have difficulty adjusting to their interface and/or therapeutic pressure after their CPAP titration in the sleep lab. These patients may benefit from desensitization. CPAP can be applied with a lower than therapeutic CPAP to help the patient adjust to the pressure. When the patient has adapted to the lower pressure, the pressure is gradually increased to the prescribed level. The patient can be encouraged to continue acclimation exercises by performing practice breathing sessions with the interface and pressure for short periods during a distraction such as watching television, listening to music, or reading a book. Patients should use CPAP when they take a nap and should be encouraged to use it during the first 4 to 5 hours of sleep, with the ultimate goal of using CPAP throughout the night.

Upper airway discomforts of dryness of the nasal passages and/or the mouth, epistaxis, nasal congestion, and rhinitis are frequent complaints of CPAP users. The flow of air through the nasal passages during CPAP therapy, especially when high pressures are required, leads to drying and inflammation of the mucous membranes. The inflamed nasal mucosa restricts airflow, increasing nasal airway resistance, which is especially problematic in patients who sleep with their mouths open. The use of a chin strap (**Figure 23–15**) to help keep the mouth closed may be helpful to lessen this problem in some patients. Heated humidification during CPAP therapy improves comfort and compliance.

A number of manufacturers have incorporated into their units the capability to record and hold in memory data, such as the date, time on and off, time at pressure, leak, and use of a ramp. The stored data can be retrieved by downloading to a computer. The data are uploaded to a computer program that displays the data in various graphic and tabular formats. This information is valuable to the equipment provider, referring physician, sleep laboratory, and insurer because it provides details of ongoing patient compliance and helps identify problems requiring intervention.

Some patients find exhaling against the CPAP pressure difficult, creating a feeling of discomfort and anxiety. Bilevel positive airway pressure systems are an alternative for individuals unable to tolerate CPAP therapy. With a bilevel device, the IPAP and EPAP are adjusted independently. The IPAP level is set at a point that eliminates the sleep-disordered breathing (apneas, hypopneas, snoring). The EPAP is set at a lower pressure to allow the patient to exhale against less resistance yet maintain airway splinting and patency. The use of bilevel therapy causes the mean airway pressure to be lower, which may increase comfort and tolerance.

The pressure required to prevent airway collapse varies in most patients from night to night and from hour to hour throughout any night because of changes in body position, level and stage of sleep, ingestion of alcohol or caffeine, and airway congestion. Several CPAP devices actively monitor one or more airway variables during sleep and respond to upper airway changes by automatically adjusting the pressure within a range of 4 to 20 cm H_2O.[43] These devices are called auto-CPAP, **auto-positive airway pressure (APAP)**, or auto-titrating devices. One or more of the following parameters are monitored: pharyngeal wall vibration (snoring), inspiratory flow limitations, hypopneas, and apneas. The APAP algorithms used by different manufacturers are proprietary and may vary greatly in their response to respiratory events. The system responds automatically when it senses an impending respiratory event by slowly increasing the CPAP pressure in a stepwise pattern until airway patency is reestablished. After a few minutes the pressure slowly decreases to the lowest pressure possible to maintain airway stability. APAP devices are potentially useful for patients who require different pressures in different sleep positions or sleep stages or for patients who have weight loss or return of daytime sleepiness and require assessment of their CPAP settings. The use of APAP devices is controversial, particularly if used in lieu of a formal sleep study, and guidelines for the appropriate use of these devices have been published (**Box 23–5**).[44]

Expiratory pressure relief (C-Flex), similar to the Bi-Flex mode described earlier, has been shown to be associated with similar outcomes to standard CPAP, but this

BOX 23–5

Recommendation for the Use of Auto-Positive Airway Pressure (APAP) from the Standards of Practice Committee of the American Academy of Sleep Medicine

Positive airway pressure (PAP) devices are not recommended to diagnose obstructive sleep apnea (OSA).

Patients with congestive heart failure; patients with significant lung disease, such as chronic obstructive pulmonary disease (COPD); patients expected to have nocturnal oxygen desaturation due to conditions other than OSA (e.g., obesity hypoventilation syndrome); patients who do not snore (either naturally or as a result of palate surgery); and patients who have central sleep apnea syndromes are not candidates for APAP titration or treatment.

APAP devices are not currently recommended for split-night titration.

Certain APAP devices may be used during attended titration with polysomnography to identify a single pressure for use with standard continuous positive airway pressure (CPAP) for treatment of moderate to severe OSA.

Certain APAP devices may be initiated and used in the self-adjusting mode for unattended treatment of patients with moderate to severe OSA without significant comorbidities (congestive heart failure [CHF], COPD, central sleep apnea syndromes, or hypoventilation syndromes).

Certain APAP devices may be used in an unattended way to determine a fixed CPAP treatment pressure for patients with moderate to severe OSA without significant comorbidities (CHF, COPD, central sleep apnea syndromes, or hypoventilation syndromes).

Patients being treated with fixed CPAP on the basis of APAP titration or being treated with APAP must have close clinical follow-up to determine treatment effectiveness and safety.

A reevaluation and, if necessary, a standard attended CPAP titration should be performed if symptoms do not resolve or the APAP treatment otherwise appears to lack efficacy.

From Morgenthaler TI, Aurora RN, Brown T, et al. Practice parameters for the use of autotitrating continuous positive airway pressure devices for titrating pressures and treating adult patients with obstructive sleep apnea syndrome: an update for 2007. An American Academy of Sleep Medicine report. *Sleep*. 2008;3(1)141–147. Reprinted with permission.

feature improved adherence for those patients with low compliance.[45] This type of embellishment allows for a slight decrease in pressure at the beginning of exhalation. Although the feature is primarily designed to address the patient's comfort level and perception that exhalation against a positive pressure is difficult, the actual amount of pressure decrease varies from one manufacturer to another.

Negative Pressure Ventilation, Rocking Beds, and Pneumobelts

Negative pressure ventilation (body ventilators) provide intermittent subatmospheric pressure around the thorax and abdomen.[46,47] Typically the patient is partially enclosed in a chamber, with the ventilator providing negative pressure to the area between the chamber and the chest wall. This subatmospheric pressure is transmitted to the pleural space, which promotes gas flow into the lungs. The prototype negative pressure ventilator was the **iron lung** (or tank ventilator), which was popular during the 1952 polio epidemic and remains in limited use today (**Figure 23–16**). The **cuirass** (also called the chest shell or turtle shell) consists of a lightweight rigid dome that fits over the anterior chest wall (**Figure 23–17**) and connects to a negative pressure generator. Other versions of negative pressure ventilators include wrap devices (ponchos,

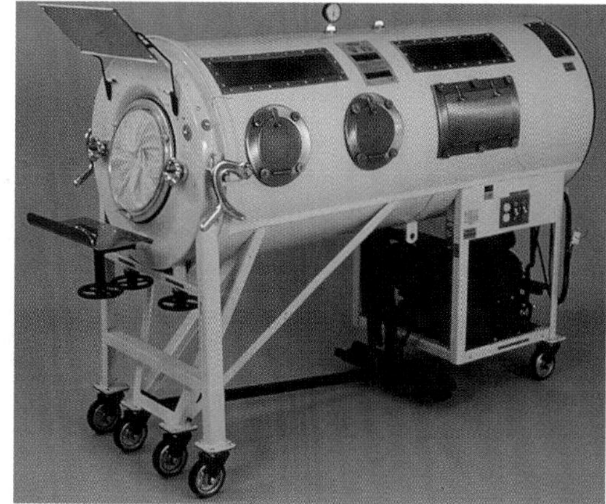

FIGURE 23–16 Iron lung.

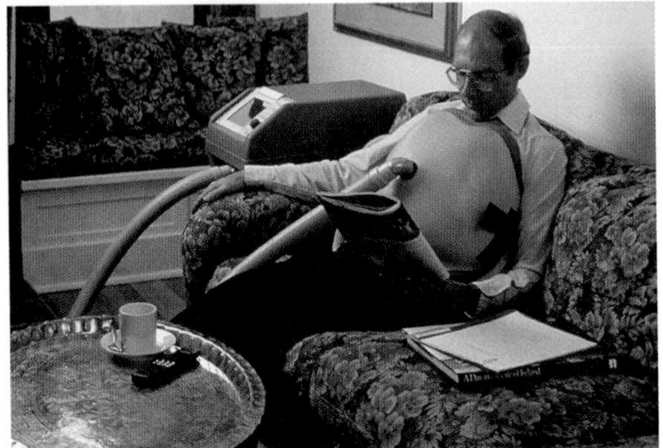

(A)

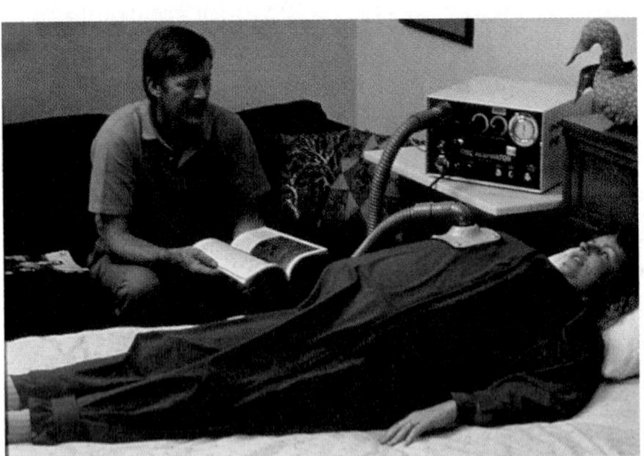

(B)

FIGURE 23–17 (A) Chest shells (cuirasses) to provide negative pressure ventilation. (B) Pneumosuit.

TABLE 23–5 Typical Settings for Body Ventilators

Ventilator	Rate (breaths/min)	Pressure (cm H_2O)
Iron lung	12 to 24	−10 to −35
Porta lung	12 to 24	−10 to −35
Wrap	14 to 28	−15 to −45
Shell	14 to 28	−15 to −45
Pneumobelt	12 to 24	+15 to +50
Rocking bed	12 to 24	40° tilt

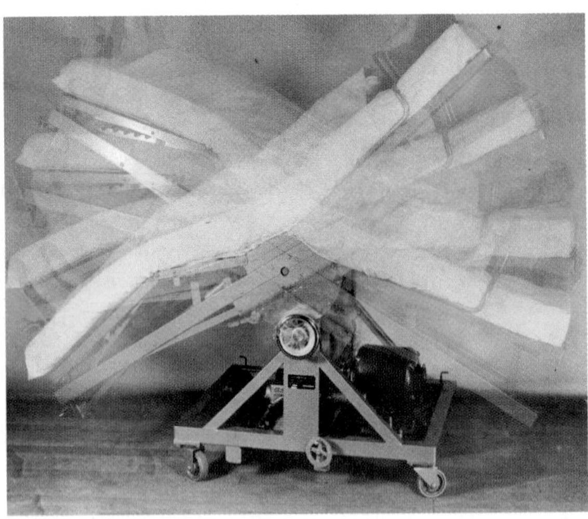

FIGURE 23–18 Rocking bed.

TABLE 23–4 Selection Criteria for Body Ventilators

Considerations	Possible Solutions
Patient Preference	
Portability	Wrap, cuirass, pneumobelt
Convenience	Rocking bed, cuirass
Freedom of hands and face	Rocking bed, pneumobelt
Efficiency and reliability	Iron lung
Diagnosis	
Bilateral diaphragm paralysis	Rocking bed, pneumobelt
High spinal cord lesion	Pneumobelt
Obstructive sleep apnea	Noninvasive positive pressure ventilation
Body Habitus	
Marked kyphoscoliosis or obesity	Noninvasive positive pressure ventilation, iron lung

body suits, and pneumosuits) that fit over the patient, surround a semicylindric grid, and attach to a negative pressure generator.

Given the increased popularity of NIV, negative pressure devices are no longer in common use. However, they provide a treatment option for patients who cannot use NIV. Negative pressure devices are more complex and bulky than NIV devices. In addition, negative pressure devices can produce upper airway obstruction and thus are contraindicated in patients with obstructive sleep apnea. **Table 23–4** outlines selection criteria for body ventilators; **Table 23–5** lists typical settings.

An unconventional ventilation device is the **rocking bed** (**Figure 23–18**). The action of the rocking bed has been compared to a piston in a cylinder. As the patient's head moves down, the pistonlike viscera and diaphragm slide cephalad within the cylinderlike chest wall, assisting exhalation. In the foot-down position the abdominal contents and diaphragm slide caudad, assisting inhalation. Another unconventional ventilation device is the **pneumobelt** (**Figure 23–19**). It consists of an inflatable rubber bladder held over the abdomen by an adjustable corset and assists diaphragmatic motion by causing pistonlike motions of the abdominal viscera.

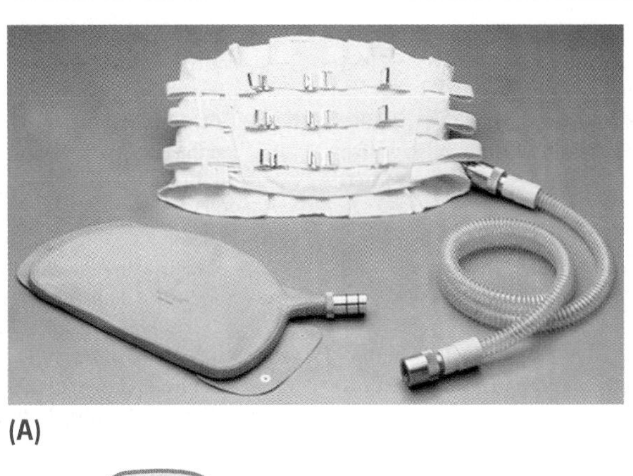
(A)

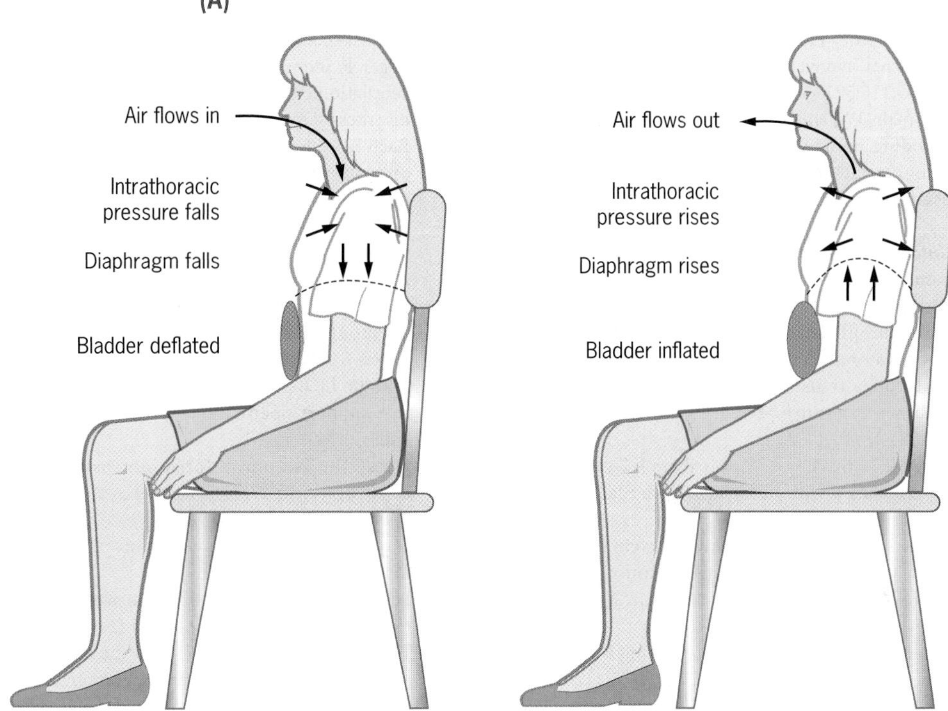

FIGURE 23–19 (**A**) Pneumobelt. (**B**) Mode of action of pneumobelt. (**B**) Adapted from Gilmartin ME. Body ventilators. Equipment and techniques. *Respir Care Clin North Am.* 1996;2:195–222.

KEY POINTS

- Noninvasive ventilation (NIV) for acute respiratory failure has been demonstrated to decrease intubation rate, decrease pneumonia rate, and increase survival rates.
- Some patients—particularly those with neuromuscular disease—may benefit from chronic nocturnal NIV.
- Nasal and oronasal interfaces are available for NIV.
- Any ventilator can be used to provide NIV, but bilevel ventilators are most commonly used.
- The choice of interface, ventilator, and ventilator mode for NIV is determined primarily by clinician and patient preference.
- Mask continuous positive airway pressure (CPAP) can be used in acute care applications to prevent postoperative pulmonary complications and to treat cardiogenic pulmonary edema.
- Mask CPAP is used to treat obstructive sleep apnea.
- CPAP compliance can be improved by the use of an appropriate interface, by humidification of the gas flow, by use of the ramp function, by the use of expiratory pressure relief, and by use of bilevel therapy.
- Auto-CPAP units vary pressure by monitoring changes in upper airway obstruction.
- Negative pressure devices are no longer in common use.

REFERENCES

1. Nava S, Navalesi P, Gregoretti C. Interfaces and humidification for noninvasive mechanical ventilation. *Respir Care.* 2009;54:71–84.
2. Hess DR. The evidence for noninvasive positive-pressure ventilation in the care of patients in acute respiratory failure: a systematic review of the literature. *Respir Care.* 2004;49:810–829.
3. Nava S, Hill N. Non-invasive ventilation in acute respiratory failure. *Lancet.* 2009;374:250–259.

4. Keenan SP, Mehta S. Noninvasive ventilation for patients presenting with acute respiratory failure: the randomized controlled trials. *Respir Care.* 2009;54:116–126.
5. Soo Hoo GW, Santiago S, Williams AJ. Nasal mechanical ventilation for hypercapnic respiratory failure in chronic obstructive pulmonary disease: determinants of success. *Crit Care Med.* 1994;22:1253–1261.
6. Ambrosino N, Folgio K, Rubini F, et al. Non-invasive mechanical ventilation in acute respiratory failure due to chronic obstructive pulmonary disease: correlates for success. *Thorax.* 1995;50:755–757.
7. Anton A, Guell R, Gomez J, et al. Predicting the result of noninvasive ventilation in severe acute exacerbations of chronic airflow limitation. *Chest.* 2000;117:828–833.
8. Clinical indications for noninvasive positive pressure ventilation in chronic respiratory failure due to restrictive lung disease, COPD, and nocturnal hypoventilation: a consensus conference report. *Chest.* 1999;116:521–534.
9. Ferreira JC, Chipman DW, Hill NS, Kacmarek RM. Bilevel vs ICU ventilators providing noninvasive ventilation: effect of system leaks: a COPD lung model comparison. *Chest.* 2009;136:448–456.
10. Vignaux L, Tassaux D, Jolliet P. Performance of noninvasive ventilation modes on ICU ventilators during pressure support: a bench model study. *Intensive Care Med.* 2007;33:1444–1451.
11. Leger P, Bedicam JM, Cornette A, et al. Nasal intermittent positive pressure ventilation. Long-term follow-up in patients with severe chronic respiratory insufficiency. *Chest.* 1994;105:100–105.
12. Schettino GP, Chatmongkolchart S, Hess DR, Kacmarek RM. Position of exhalation port and mask design affect CO_2 rebreathing during noninvasive positive pressure ventilation. *Crit Care Med.* 2003;31:2178–2182.
13. Saatci E, Miller DM, Stell IM, Lee KC, Moxham J. Dynamic dead space in face masks used with noninvasive ventilators: a lung model study. *Eur Respir J.* 2004;23:129–135.
14. Thys F, Liistro G, Dozin O, Marion E, Rodenstein DO. Determinants of FIO_2 with oxygen supplementation during noninvasive two-level positive pressure ventilation. *Eur Respir J.* 2002;19:653–657.
15. Ferguson GT, Gilmartin M. CO_2 rebreathing during BiPAP ventilatory assistance. *Am J Respir Crit Care Med.* 1995;151:1126–1135.
16. Lofaso F, Brochard L, Hang T, Lorino H, Harf A, Isabey D. Home versus intensive care pressure support devices. Experimental and clinical comparison. *Am J Respir Crit Care Med.* 1996;153:1591–1599.
17. Schwartz AR, Kacmarek RM, Hess DR. Factors affecting oxygen delivery with bi-level positive airway pressure. *Respir Care.* 2004;49:270–275.
18. Hess DR. Noninvasive ventilation in neuromuscular disease: equipment and application. *Respir Care.* 2006;51:896–912.
19. Hess DR. Ventilator waveforms and the physiology of pressure support ventilation. *Respir Care.* 2005;50:166–186.
20. Prinianakis G, Delmastro M, Carlucci A, Ceriana P, Nava S. Effect of varying the pressurisation rate during noninvasive pressure support ventilation. *Eur Respir J.* 2004;23:314–320.
21. Williams P, Kratohvil J, Ritz R, Hess DR, Kacmarek RM. Pressure support and pressure assist/control: are there differences? An evaluation of the newest intensive care unit ventilators. *Respir Care.* 2000;45:1169–1181.
22. Hotchkiss JR Jr, Adams AB, Stone MK, Dries DJ, Marini JJ, Crooke PS. Oscillations and noise: inherent instability of pressure support ventilation? *Am J Respir Crit Care Med.* 2002;165:47–53.
23. Hotchkiss JR, Adams AB, Dries DJ, et al. Dynamic behavior during noninvasive ventilation: chaotic support? *Am J Respir Crit Care Med.* 2001;163:374–378.
24. Adams AB, Bliss PL, Hotchkiss J. Effects of respiratory impedance on the performance of bi-level pressure ventilators. *Respir Care.* 2000;45:390–400.
25. Parreira VF, Delguste P, Jounieaux V, et al. Effectiveness of controlled and spontaneous modes in nasal two-level positive pressure ventilation in awake and asleep normal subjects. *Chest.* 1997;112:1267–1277.
26. Parthasarathy S, Tobin MJ. Effect of ventilator mode on sleep quality in critically ill patients. *Am J Respir Crit Care Med.* 2002;166:1423–1429.
27. Johnson KG, Johnson DC. Bilevel positive airway pressure worsens central apneas during sleep. *Chest.* 2005;128:2141–2150.
28. Benditt JO. Full-time noninvasive ventilation: possible and desirable. *Respir Care.* 2006;51:1005–1012.
29. Fauroux B, Boffa C, Desguerre I, Estournet B, Trang H. Long-term noninvasive mechanical ventilation for children at home: a national survey. *Pediatr Pulmonol.* 2003;35:119–125.
30. Kerby GR, Mayer LS, Pingleton SK. Nocturnal positive pressure ventilation via nasal mask. *Am Rev Respir Dis.* 1987;135:738–740.
31. Leger P, Jennequin J, Gerard M, et al. Home positive pressure ventilation via nasal mask for patients with neuromusculoskeletal disorders. *Eur Respir J.* 1989;7(suppl):640s–644s.
32. Bach JR, Alba AS, Bohatiuk G, et al. Mouth intermittent positive pressure ventilation in the management of postpolio respiratory insufficiency. *Chest.* 1987;91:859–864.
33. Bach JR, Alba AS, Saporito LR. Intermittent positive pressure ventilation via the mouth as an alternative to tracheostomy for 257 ventilator users. *Chest.* 1993;103:174–182.
34. Toussaint M, Steens M, Wasteels G, Soudon P. Diurnal ventilation via mouthpiece: survival in end-stage Duchenne patients. *Eur Respir J.* 2006;28:549–555.
35. Boitano LJ, Benditt JO. An evaluation of home volume ventilators that support open-circuit mouthpiece ventilation. *Respir Care.* 2005;50:1457–1461.
36. Hess DR. The mask for noninvasive ventilation: principles of design and effects on aerosol delivery. *J Aerosol Med.* 2007;20(suppl 1):S85–S99.
37. Gay PC. Complications of noninvasive ventilation in acute care. *Respir Care.* 2009;54:246–258.
38. Hill NS. Complications of noninvasive positive pressure ventilation. *Respir Care.* 1997;42:432–442.
39. Ferreyra GP, Baussano I, Squadrone V, et al. Continuous positive airway pressure for treatment of respiratory complications after abdominal surgery: a systematic review and meta-analysis. *Ann Surg.* 2008;247:617–626.
40. Delclaux C, L'Her E, Alberti C, Mancebo J, et al. Treatment of acute hypoxemic nonhypercapnic respiratory insufficiency with continuous positive airway pressure delivered by a face mask: a randomized controlled trial. *JAMA.* 2000;284:2352–2360.
41. Peter JV, Moran JL, Phillips-Hughes J, et al. Effect of non-invasive positive pressure ventilation (NIPPV) on mortality in patients with acute cardiogenic pulmonary oedema: a meta-analysis. *Lancet.* 2006;367:1155–1163.
42. Allen KY, Bollig S, Selecky PA, Smalling T. *The Clinician's Guide to PAP Adherence* [Online]. American Association for Respiratory Care; 2009. Available at: http://www.aarc.org/education/pap_adherence.
43. Brown LK. Autotitrating CPAP. *Chest.* 2006;130;312–314.
44. Morgenthaler TI, Aurora RN, Brown T, et al. Practice parameters for the use of autotitrating continuous positive airway pressure devices for titrating pressures and treating adult patients with obstructive sleep apnea syndrome: an update for 2007. An American Academy of Sleep Medicine report. *Sleep.* 2008;31:141–147.
45. Pepin JL, Muir JF, Gentina T, et al. Pressure reduction during exhalation in sleep apnea patients treated by continuous positive airway pressure. *Chest.* 2009;136:490–497.
46. Hill NS. Use of negative pressure ventilation, rocking beds, and pneumobelts. *Respir Care.* 1994;39:532–549.
47. Hill NS. Clinical applications of body ventilators. *Chest.* 1986;90:897–905.

CHAPTER 24

Neonatal and Pediatric Respiratory Care

Melissa K. Brown
Steven C. Mason

OUTLINE

OBJECTIVES

1. Identify and describe some of the risk factors for developing respiratory distress syndrome.
2. List the five components of the Apgar score.
3. Identify and describe the signs of respiratory distress in the neonate.
4. Describe the hazards associated with oxygen use in premature infants.
5. Describe oxygen administration techniques for infants and children.
6. Compare the use of flow-inflating and self-inflating manual ventilation devices.
7. Describe the proper position for oral endotracheal tubes in neonates and children.
8. Describe the use of nasal continuous positive airway pressure in neonates.
9. Discuss issues related to artificial airway care of neonates and children.
10. List indications for mechanical ventilation of neonates and children.
11. List the usual settings for conventional mechanical ventilation of neonates and children.
12. List the hazards and complications of conventional neonatal and pediatric mechanical ventilation.
13. Discuss approaches to weaning neonates and children from mechanical ventilation.
14. Compare the four general types of high-frequency ventilation of neonates and children.
15. Discuss issues related to surfactant administration, inhaled nitric oxide, and extracorporeal life support of neonates and children.

KEY TERMS

Apgar score
bronchopulmonary dysplasia (BPD)
extracorporeal life support (ECLS)
flow-inflating bag
hertz (Hz)
high-frequency flow interrupter ventilation (HFFIV)
high-frequency jet ventilation (HFJV)
high-frequency oscillatory ventilation (HFOV)
high-frequency positive pressure ventilation (HFPPV)
high-frequency ventilation (HFV)
lecithin-to-sphingomyelin (LS) ratio
mean airway pressure
nasal continuous positive airway pressure (NCPAP)
neutral thermal environment
pressure amplitude
retinopathy of prematurity (ROP)
self-inflating bag
surfactant

INTRODUCTION

Neonates and children may require respiratory therapy for a variety of reasons. Regardless of the pathologic condition, the goal is to achieve adequate gas exchange while minimizing risks and complications. Many factors influence the respiratory management of neonates and children, and no single approach is ideal for all patients. Maintaining adequate support of ventilation and oxygenation by continual reassessment is essential to prevent complications.

Neonatal Assessment

Awareness and understanding of maternal risk factors is crucial for the identification of newborns at risk for life-threatening complications in the perinatal period (**Box 24–1**). Clinicians must be prepared to resuscitate infants with serious problems at birth or soon after. One of the most common problems other than congenital birth defects is preterm birth (prior to 38 weeks' gestation). Infants born prematurely are at risk of developing respiratory distress syndrome (RDS).

Laboratory tests have been developed to assist with the assessment of lung maturity. By assessing the amniotic fluid for the **lecithin-to-sphingomyelin (LS) ratio**, lung maturity can be determined. Lecithin (dipalmitoyl phosphatidylcholine) is the most plentiful phospholipid found in surfactant. Generally, babies with an LS ratio of more than 2:1 are considered to have mature lungs. Usually, the LS ratio will approach 2:1 at approximately 34 to 35 weeks' gestation. Babies with ratios of less than 2:1 are considered at higher risk for developing RDS. Infants of diabetic mothers may develop RDS even with LS ratios greater than 2:1. Phosphatidylglycerol (PG) is the second most plentiful phospholipid in surfactant. Levels of PG increase as a baby gets closer to term. When PG is also present in the amniotic fluid, the infant is less likely to develop RDS.

> **RESPIRATORY RECAP**
>
> **Neonatal Assessment**
>
> » Infants with LS ratios of less than 2:1 are considered at higher risk for RDS.
>
> » The Apgar score evaluates heart rate, respiratory effort, muscle tone, reflex irritability, and color.
>
> » When breathing stops for longer than 20 seconds, it is called apnea.
>
> » Signs of respiratory distress include expiratory grunting, retracting, nasal flaring, and tachypnea.
>
> » Capillary blood gas values are a less invasive way to measure the pH and P_{CO_2} of an infant.

The maternal history and laboratory test results may prepare you for what to expect in the delivery room, but once the baby is born a thorough assessment must be done. The American Academy of Pediatrics Neonatal Resuscitation Program (NRP) outlines a specific sequence of events (**Figure 24–1**).[1] The infant should be dried and warmed, and the airway should be opened and cleared of secretions. The baby should respond to stimulation with adequate depth and rate of respirations. Infants with absent or ineffective ventilations should immediately receive positive pressure ventilation. After evaluation of respirations, the heart rate should be assessed by either feeling the infant's pulse by holding the base of the umbilical cord or by listening with a stethoscope to the apical pulse. If the newborn has adequate respirations and a heart rate of at least 100 beats/min, the newborn's color should be assessed. Many newborns tend to have acrocyanosis (blue extremities) in the first few minutes of life as a result of poor circulation. If central cyanosis persists with adequate ventilation and a heart rate greater than 100, then free-flow oxygen is indicated.

Apgar Score

The **Apgar score**, introduced in 1952 by Virginia Apgar, evaluates five factors: heart rate, respiratory effort, muscle tone, reflex irritability, and color (**Table 24–1**). The score is assigned at 1 and 5 minutes of life. Therapeutic interventions should not be delayed in order to assign the 1-minute score. The 1-minute score is intended to provide an immediate evaluation of the infant and guide appropriate intervention. When the score is less than 7 at 5 minutes, an additional score is usually assigned at 10 minutes. If the Apgar score remains 0 after 10 minutes of resuscitation, it is unlikely the infant will survive.[2]

The Apgar score is not as useful for babies who are born prematurely. Three of the assessment criteria—muscle tone, respiratory effort, and reflex irritability—are a function of the neonate's developmental maturity. Muscle tone may be absent and respiratory effort may be poor in neonates of less than 28 weeks' gestation.

BOX 24–1

Maternal Risk Factors for Perinatal Complications

Preterm birth	Diabetes mellitus
Postterm birth	Infectious diseases
Multiple birth	Premature rupture of the membranes
Maternal tobacco, alcohol, or drug abuse	Placenta and umbilical cord abnormalities
Hypertension	Breech or cesarean delivery
Polyhydramnios (too much amniotic fluid volume)	Oligohydramnios (too little amniotic fluid volume)

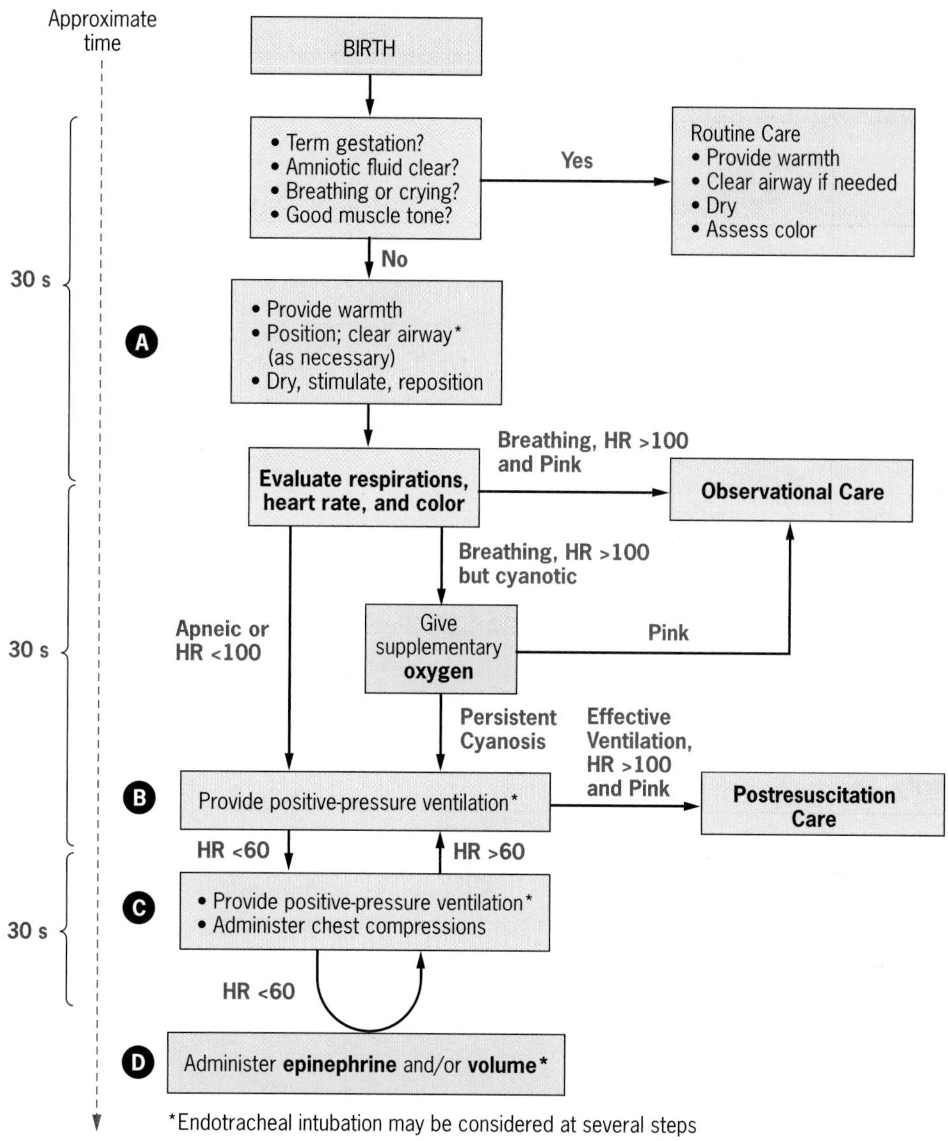

FIGURE 24–1 Algorithm for resuscitation of the neonate. HR, heart rate (beats per minute). From Neonatal resuscitation guidelines. *Circulation.* 2005;112(suppl I):IV-188–IV-195. Reprinted with permission.

TABLE 24–1 Apgar Scoring

Parameter	Points 0	1	2
Heart rate	None	<100 beats/min	>100 beats/min
Respiratory effort	None	Weak, irregular	Strong cry
Color	Pale blue	Body pink, extremities blue	Completely pink
Reflex (irritability to suction)	No response	Grimace	Cry, cough, or sneeze
Muscle tone	Limp	Some flexion	Well flexed

Gestational Age

Gestational age should be assessed by the time the infant is 12 hours old. Gestational age is assessed using several factors: the mother's last menstrual cycle, prenatal ultrasound findings, and postnatal physical and neurologic findings, which are included in the Ballard score (**Figure 24–2**). After gestational age assessment, the newborn's weight, length, and head circumference are plotted on a grid. An infant whose weight is below the 10th percentile is considered small for gestational age (SGA); an infant above the 90th percentile is considered large for gestational age (LGA). Infants born weighing less than 2500 grams are considered low birth

Neuromuscular Maturity

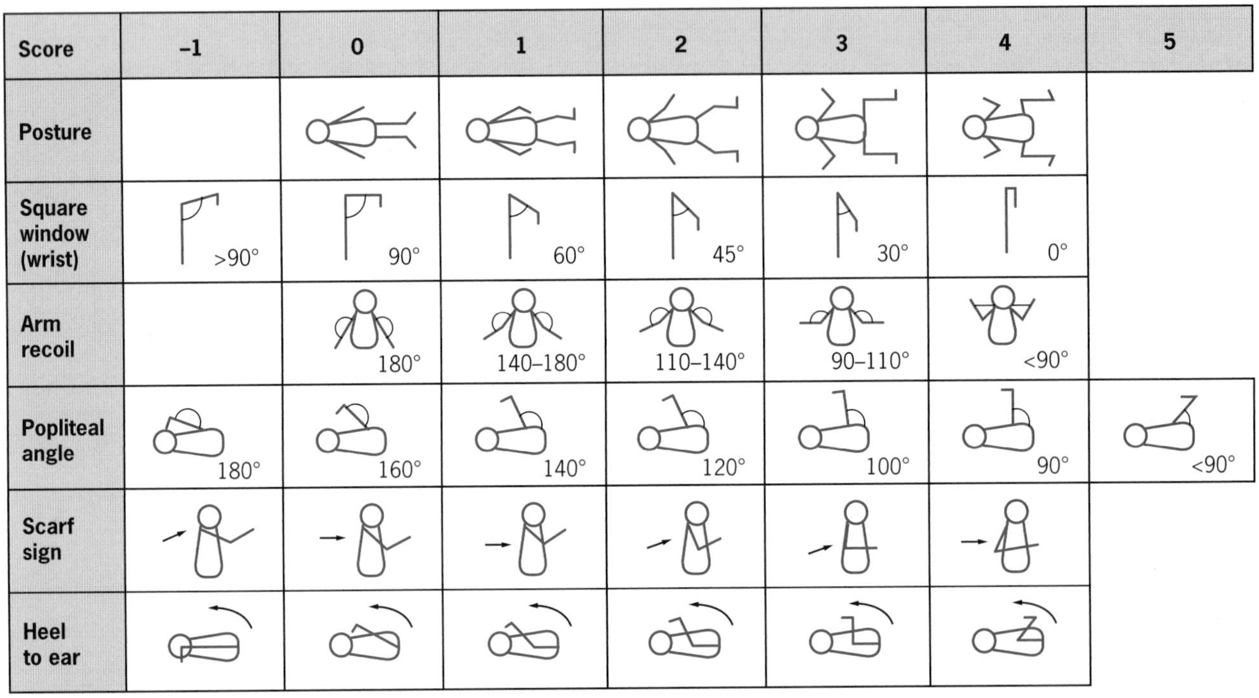

Score	−1	0	1	2	3	4	5
Posture							
Square window (wrist)	>90°	90°	60°	45°	30°	0°	
Arm recoil		180°	140–180°	110–140°	90–110°	<90°	
Popliteal angle	180°	160°	140°	120°	100°	90°	<90°
Scarf sign							
Heel to ear							

Physical Maturity

Skin	Sticky, friable, transparent	Gelatinous, red, translucent	Smooth, pink; visible veins	Superficial peeling and/or rash; few veins	Cracking, pale areas; rare veins	Parchment, deep cracking; no vessels	Leathery, cracked, wrinkled
Lanugo	None	Sparse	Abundant	Thinning	Bald areas	Mostly bald	
Plantar surface	Heel-toe 40–50 mm: −1 < 40 mm: −2	> 50 mm, no crease	Faint red marks	Anterior transverse crease only	Creases anterior 2/3	Creases over entire sole	
Breast	Imperceptible	Barely perceptible	Flat areola, no bud	Stippled areola, 1–2 mm bud	Raised areola, 3–4 mm bud	Full areola, 5–10 mm bud	
Eye/Ear	Lids fused loosely: −1 tightly: −2	Lids open; pinna flat; stays folded	Slightly curved pinna, soft slow recoil	Well curved pinna, soft but ready recoil	Formed and firm, instant recoil	Thick cartilage, ear stiff	
Genitals (male)	Scrotum flat, smooth	Scrotum empty, faint rugae	Testes in upper canal, rare rugae	Testes descending, few rugae	Testes down, good rugae	Testes pendulous, deep rugae	
Genitals (female)	Clitoris prominent, labia flat	Clitoris prominent, small labia minora	Clitoris prominent, enlarging minora	Majora and minora equally prominent	Majora large, minora small	Majora cover clitoris and minora	

Maturity Rating

Score	Weeks
−10	20
−5	22
0	24
5	26
10	28
15	30
20	32
25	34
30	36
35	38
40	40
45	42
50	44

FIGURE 24–2 New Ballard score for estimating gestational age to include extremely premature infants. From Ballard JL. New Ballard score, expanded to include extremely premature infants. *J Pediatr*. 1991;119:417–423. Reprinted with permission.

weight (LBW), those less than 1500 grams are very low birth weight (VLBW), and those less than 1000 grams are extremely low birth weight (ELBW). Neonates who fall into one of these categories are more likely to be at risk for disease and death.

Physical Assessment

The normal infant heart rate is between 120 to 170 beats/min. An infant under stress from overstimulation or pain may have a heart rate greater than 200, temporarily. During deep sleep, the heart rate of a term

TABLE 24-2 Normal Neonatal Vital Signs

Birth Weight (g)	Systolic/Diastolic Blood Pressure (mm Hg)	Mean Blood Pressure (mm Hg)
>600	42/20	25
>1000	48/25	35
>2000	50/30	40
>3000	50/35	45
>4000	65/40	50
Neonate older than 12 hours	75/50	60

Respiratory rate: 30–60 breaths/min; heart rate: 120–170 beats/min.

TABLE 24-3 Normal Respiratory Rates in Awake Children

Age	Mean (breaths/min)	Range (breaths/min)
6–12 months	64	58–75
1–2 years	35	30–40
2–4 years	31	23–42
4–6 years	26	19–36
6–8 years	23	15–30
8–10 years	21	15–31
10–12 years	21	15–28
12–14 years	22	18–26

infant may drop to 80 to 90 beats/min. Right-to-left shunting from a patent ductus arteriosis (PDA) can result in bounding peripheral pulses. **Table 24–2** lists normal ranges for neonatal vital signs. All newborns display an irregular respiratory breathing pattern, but the respiratory rate of a term newborn usually averages 40 to 60 breaths/min. It is common for premature infants to display periodic breathing, which consists of intermittent respiratory pauses that last longer than 5 seconds. When breathing stops for longer than 20 seconds or for shorter periods in combination with bradycardia, cyanosis, or pallor, it is called *apnea*. As children mature, their normal respiratory rates decline until they become teenagers, at which point their respiratory rates mimic those of adults (**Table 24–3**).[3]

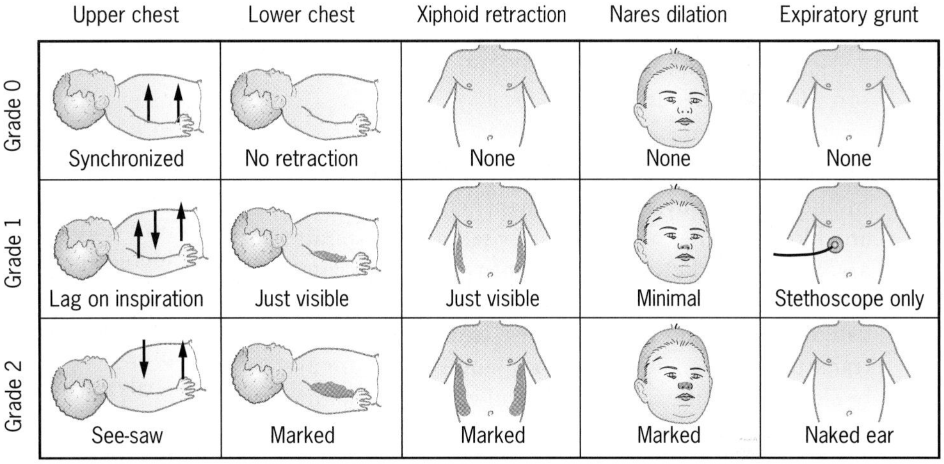

FIGURE 24–3 Silverman score for assessing the magnitude of respiratory distress. Reproduced with permission from *Pediatrics*, Vol. 17, Page 1–6, © 1956 by the AAP.

The Silverman scoring system assesses the magnitude of the respiratory distress of the infant (**Figure 24–3**). Signs of respiratory distress include expiratory grunting, retracting, nasal flaring, and tachypnea. Expiratory grunting is caused by the closing of the glottis during expiration in an attempt to maintain lung volume and expand alveoli. It is a common sign of RDS. Retractions are a visible sinking in of the chest wall on inspiration. Retractions are usually a sign of decreased chest compliance, but can also be a sign of airway obstruction. They are usually observed between the ribs (intercostal), in the area above the collarbone (superclavicular), below the xiphoid process (substernal), and below the ribcage (subcostal). Retractions are more commonly observed in neonates than in adults due to the soft, pliable chest wall and thoracic cage of the neonate. See-saw respirations are when the chest moves in and the abdomen pushes out on inspiration and are indicative of severe respiratory distress. In order to draw more air into the lungs and decrease the resistance to air entry, infants may exhibit nasal flaring. Tachypnea is usually one of the first signs of respiratory distress. Infants and children have difficulty increasing their tidal volume and instead will increase their respiratory rate in order to increase their minute ventilation.

Auscultation of infants and small children can be complicated. Their chests are small, and sounds sometimes transmit from one lung region to another. Infants and children often cry and hold their breath during examination, making assessment difficult. Symmetric assessment from left to right is crucial and will help identify asymmetric disease such as a pneumothorax or a poorly positioned endotracheal tube. Rhonchi are coarse breath sounds that come from air moving through fluid in the large airways. Usually, suctioning will eliminate the secretions and the rhonchi. Crackles, also known as rales, are indicative of fluid in the small airways and alveoli and are commonly heard on inspiration in infants with RDS, pneumonia, or pulmonary edema, and in normal infants soon after birth. Wheezes are high-pitched musical sounds that can be heard on inspiration or expiration and are caused by a narrowing of the conducting airways. Wheezes are most commonly heard in children with asthma. Wheezing over an isolated segment can indicate foreign body aspiration. Stridor is a high-pitched squeaking sound heard on inspiration. Stridor indicates a large upper airway obstruction as can occur in patients with croup, tracheomalacia, and postextubation laryngeal edema. Stridor can be easily distinguished from other sounds by placing the stethoscope over the neck region and isolating the sound. Neonates with RDS, atelectasis, and pulmonary interstitial edema (PIE) may also have diminished breath sounds. In the neonate, transillumination of the chest wall can be used to identify a suspected pneumothorax. A fiberoptic light source is placed on the chest wall in a darkened room. A large pneumothorax will glow, or seem very pink and illuminated, in comparison with the other areas of the chest.

Noninvasive and Hemodynamic Monitoring

In addition to physical assessment, chest radiography and blood gas measurements are vital in the respiratory assessment of the patient. Noninvasive monitoring of both oxygenation and ventilation is widely used in the care of infants and children. Pulse oximetry (Spo_2) and transcutaneous monitoring ($Ptco_2$ and $Ptcco_2$) are used to closely track the oxygenation and ventilation status of patients and are correlated with blood gas values when appropriate.

Blood gas samples can be obtained from umbilical artery catheters (UACs) or umbilical venous catheters (UVCs) in neonates and from peripheral arterial lines in older children. Capillary blood gases are a less invasive way to measure the pH and Pco_2 of an infant, but are not always reliable in determining oxygenation. Poor sampling technique can greatly influence the results of capillary blood gases. Umbilical cord blood gases are often drawn after the birth of the child to document whether the infant was in severe distress in utero. The cord blood gas values are not used to treat the infant after birth. **Table 24–4** provides normal blood gas values.

TABLE 24–4 Normal Cord, Neonatal, and Pediatric Blood Gas Values

Parameter	Umbilical Artery	Umbilical Vein	Newborn	Infant to Toddler	Child to Adult
pH	7.24	7.32	7.3–7.4	7.3–7.4	7.35–7.45
$Paco_2$ (mm Hg)	49	38	30–40	30–40	35–45
Po_2 (mm Hg)	16	27	60–90	80–100	80–100
HCO_3 (mmol/L)	19	20	20–22	20–22	22–24

UACs and arterial lines can also be used for blood pressure monitoring. The UVC or central venous catheter is primarily used for the administration of fluids and drugs to the central circulation and for central venous pressure (CVP) monitoring. CVP monitoring allows for continuous measurement of the right atrial pressure and assessment of the patient's fluid volume. Normal CVP is 2 to 7 mm Hg. Pulmonary artery catheters are used to assess left ventricular function, fluid status, and pulmonary artery pressure (PAP). Normal mean PAP is 10 to 20 mm Hg.

Oxygen Therapy

Indications

The goal of oxygen therapy is to prevent or correct hypoxemia and to provide oxygen to the tissues with the lowest possible concentration of oxygen. Preterm babies, term babies, and children have different oxygen requirements depending on their gestational age or disease state. Children and term infants with a Pao_2 below 80 mm Hg and an oxygen saturation of less than 95% are generally considered to have hypoxemia. In preterm infants, Pao_2 and oxygen saturation goals are lower than those for term babies and are based on corrected gestational age.

RESPIRATORY RECAP

Oxygen Therapy

- » Oxygen therapy directed toward Pao_2 goals of 50 to 80 mm Hg is usually considered safe.
- » Excessive oxygen use could lead to retinopathy of prematurity and bronchopulmonary dysplasia in the premature infant.
- » Fio_2 should be adjusted to meet oximetry goals for the patient based on gestational age.

Hazards

The hazards of oxygen therapy for the preterm infant include **retinopathy of prematurity (ROP)**. ROP is a potentially blinding disease caused by the abnormal development of the retina in premature infants. Generally, babies that are born weighing less than 1500 grams or at less than 32 weeks' gestational ages are monitored for ROP. Oxygen therapy directed toward Pao_2 goals of 50 to 80 mm Hg is usually considered safe.[4] Other factors that contribute to the severity of ROP include gestational age, low birth weight, blood transfusion, respiratory distress, PDA, and the overall health of the infant. Excessive use of oxygen also can lead to the development of **bronchopulmonary dysplasia (BPD)**, which is generally defined as the need for supplemental oxygen at 36 weeks' postmenstrual age or 28 days of life.[5]

The delivery of 100% oxygen can lead to absorption atelectasis as alveolar nitrogen is replaced by oxygen. There also can be cardiovascular effects from the delivery of high concentrations of oxygen, such as pulmonary vasodilation and the constriction of the ductus arteriosus. In patients with hypoplastic left heart disease, the increase in pulmonary blood flow that occurs with oxygen therapy can flood the lungs with blood and decrease systemic circulation. The closing of the PDA can further decrease the flow of blood to the systemic circulation and create a life-threatening situation.

Delivery Devices

Supplemental oxygen can be delivered using many different devices. The best device to use is the one that most closely suits the needs of the individual patient. The clinician should contemplate several factors before choosing an oxygen delivery device, including what fraction of inspired oxygen (F_{IO_2}) is required, whether a precise F_{IO_2} is required, what gas temperature and humidity is needed, how the equipment will affect the nursing care and handling of the infant or child, and what will make the patient the most comfortable. Oxygen therapy should be administered according to the Sp_{O_2} goal. If the patient consistently requires more than 50% oxygen, additional respiratory support may be indicated.

In the neonatal intensive care unit (NICU), special low-flow meters are commonly used, with flow rates that span 25 mL/min to 3 L/min. In most cases, these flow meters should be connected to a 100% oxygen source and flows titrated to meet oximetry goals. On neonatal patients requiring high flow rates, such as 2 L/min, an air–oxygen blender should be used and the F_{IO_2} should be adjusted to meet the Sp_{O_2} goal for the patient. The most frequently used oxygen delivery devices include the conventional nasal cannula, high-flow nasal cannula, entrainment mask, oxygen hood, and incubator; each of which has advantages and disadvantages (**Table 24–5**).

Mechanical Ventilation

Regardless of the pathologic condition, the goal is to achieve adequate gas exchange while minimizing the risks and complications associated with mechanical ventilation. Many factors influence the respiratory management of neonates and children, and no single approach is ideal for all. Maintaining adequate support of ventilation and oxygenation by continual reassessment of the patient and adjustment of the ventilator is essential to prevent complications. Mechanical ventilation in the intensive care environment is an art form. It is practiced differently throughout the world, and the method chosen depends on the strategies adopted by the institution.

Manual Ventilation

Positive pressure ventilation (PPV) usually begins as manual bag-mask ventilation (BMV), often in the delivery room. Immediately after birth, the infant is placed under a warmer and is dried, positioned, and provided with tactile stimulation. BMV is indicated if the infant is apneic or gasping or has a heart rate below 100 beats/min. Appropriate use of positive pressure can make a significant difference in the infant's course. During the initial resuscitation, administration of 100% oxygen is indicated. Once the infant's condition has been stabilized, with improved color and adequate blood pressure, the oxygen concentration is reduced via pulse oximetry and clinical assessment. Once pulse oximetry is initiated, both the high and low Sp_{O_2} alarms should be set to reduce the risks of hyperoxia and hypoxia.

Manual resuscitators are classified as self-inflating or flow-inflating bags (**Figure 24–4**).[6] A **self-inflating bag** inflates automatically and does not need an external gas source to provide positive pressure. These bags usually have a reservoir to deliver 100% oxygen with a flow of

TABLE 24-5 Supplemental Oxygen Delivery Devices

Device	Patient Age	Oxygen Delivered	Advantages	Disadvantages
Nasal cannula	Premature infant to pediatric	Flows of 25 mL/min to 2 L/min	Comfortable, good access to patient, easy to apply	F_{IO_2} not precise
High-flow nasal cannula	Premature infant to pediatric	>2 L/min	Comfortable, good access to patient, easy to apply	F_{IO_2} not precise, possible inadvertent PEEP, low relative humidity unless heated and humidified
Air entrainment mask	Children	Up to 100%	High F_{IO_2}, precise F_{IO_2}	Confining, uncomfortable, low relative humidity
Oxygen hoods (tot huts, care cubes)	Premature infants to 6 months	21% to 100%	Precise F_{IO_2}, heated and humidified	Poor access to patient, excessive noise, must maintain flow to wash out CO_2, gas layering
Incubators	Neonates	21% to 40%	Neutral thermal environment	Poor access to patient, difficult to maintain precise F_{IO_2}

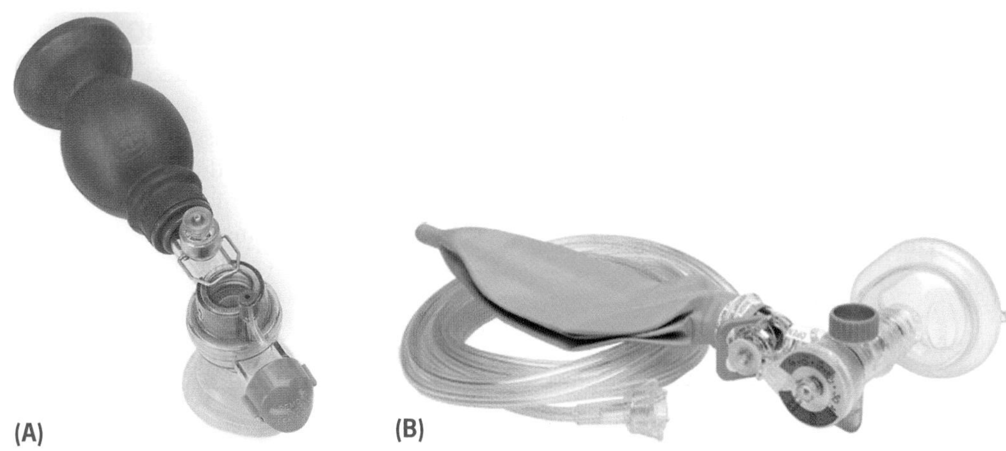

FIGURE 24–4 (**A**) Self-inflating neonatal resuscitation bag. (**B**) Flow-inflating neonatal resuscitation bag.

5 to 10 L/min. Most self-inflating bags incorporate a pressure-limiting device, a pop-off valve, that releases pressure at a preset level. The pop-off valve reduces the risk of excessive pressure being applied, but it can be manually overridden when delivery of high pressures is indicated. Self-inflating bags generally do not allow maintenance of positive end-expiratory pressure (PEEP) unless an external PEEP valve is added.

A **flow-inflating bag** requires a continuous flow from an external gas source. Pressure is determined by the flow and the pressure release valve. Wide ranges of peak inspiratory pressure (PIP) and PEEP are attainable with flow-inflating bags. Continuous flow at the patient connection makes the device suitable for the delivery of continuous positive airway pressure (CPAP) and a convenient method to deliver oxygen short term to spontaneously breathing infants. Flow-inflating bags are well suited to the needs of neonates. Clinicians responsible for resuscitating neonates should be familiar with self-inflating and flow-inflating bags and with the specific characteristics of the bags used in their institution.

RESPIRATORY RECAP

Neonatal Manual Resuscitators

- » Self-inflating bags inflate automatically.
- » Flow-inflating bags require a continuous gas flow.

BMV is ineffective if the mask is not the correct size. A variety of masks are available that fit infants of all sizes. The mask should fit over the infant's nose and mouth, with the edge of the infant's chin resting on the rim of the mask. As the mask is applied to the face, a seal is created by encircling the mask with the thumb and index finger and applying a gentle pressure (**Figure 24–5**). The infant's face should be pulled into the mask to open the airway. The ring finger can be used to hold the chin in the mask. Positioning of the infant is critical to achieve effective BMV; slight extension of the neck, often accomplished by placement of a roll under the shoulders, aligns the airway to allow effective ventilation.

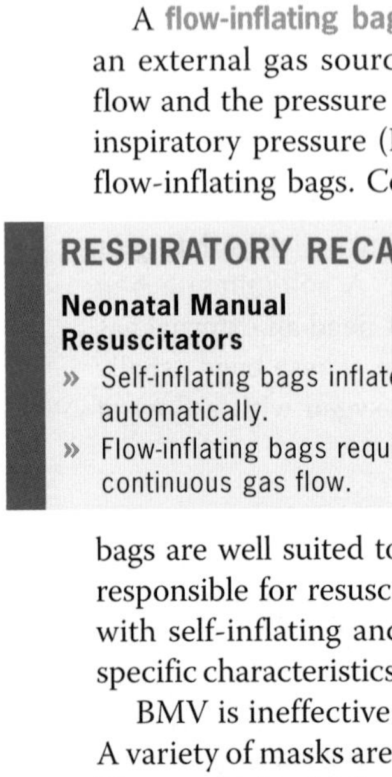

FIGURE 24–5 Positioning of the mask for bag-mask ventilation.

Knowledge of the infant's gestational age and prenatal history may be helpful during initiation of BMV. Premature infants are likely to need higher ventilating pressures (more than 35 cm H_2O) during the initial breaths to overcome the surface tension in surfactant-deficient lungs. Depending on lung maturity, successive breaths may require less pressure as lung volume is established. The pressure used to ventilate should be that needed to cause the infant's chest wall to rise. Maintaining PEEP throughout the respiratory cycle aids in the maintenance of lung volume. Observing chest movement while the bag is being squeezed is essential for correct application of pressure. Common reasons for poor chest movement are an inadequate mask seal, airway obstruction caused by improper head position, secretions in the airway, fingers on the patient's neck, or inadequate ventilating pressure. Inadequate pressure leads to low lung volume, inability to oxygenate, and hemodynamic compromise. Excessive pressure can result in pneumothorax and further respiratory and hemodynamic compromise. An in-line pressure manometer should be used to monitor the applied peak airway pressure and PEEP levels. A disposable carbon dioxide detector can be placed between the resuscitation bag and mask to verify the presence of exhaled carbon dioxide. **Table 24–6** lists factors to consider with BMV.

An apneic or distressed infant typically requires a respiratory rate of 40 to 60 breaths/min with an inspiratory time of 0.4 to 0.5 second. Administration of 100% oxygen during the initial resuscitative effort is indicated. Improvement in the skin color, heart rate, and hemodynamics should be apparent after a brief period. If the patient shows no sign of improvement, the adequacy of the delivery system should be reviewed. Oxygen disconnection or inadequacy of the gas source, mask seal, or head position should be considered.

TABLE 24-6 Bag-Mask Ventilation of the Neonate

Problem	Solutions
No seal between mask and face	Reposition mask; consider different mask size.
No chest movement	Check head position; do not overextend neck or push head forward with mask pressure. Check for secretions in airway. Check for fingers on the neck.
Pressure too low (flow-inflating bag)	Check flow; adjust flow meter; check manometer connections.
Pressure too low (self-inflating bag)	Ensure pop-off valve is active; consider need to override the valve.

Infants with evidence of meconium below the vocal cords, and who are not vigorous at birth, should be intubated and the meconium cleared before they receive positive pressure ventilation. A vigorous infant is one that has a heart rate above 100 beats/min, strong respiratory efforts, and good muscle tone. Intubation with the largest possible endotracheal tube is recommended. Clearing of meconium is attempted with a meconium aspirator. The aspirator is attached to the endotracheal tube, suction is applied at 100 mm Hg, and the endotracheal tube is withdrawn. Reintubation is performed with a new tube, and the process is repeated until no particulate meconium is present. After the meconium has been cleared, positive pressure ventilation can be provided by BMV or through an endotracheal tube. Insertion of a gastric tube to clear meconium from the stomach may reduce the risk of further meconium aspiration.

Mask positive pressure ventilation is contraindicated in infants who have or are suspected of having a congenital diaphragmatic hernia. BMV can promote the entry of air into the gastrointestinal tract and further impair gas exchange. These infants should be intubated and ventilated through an endotracheal tube.

Airway Management

Oral and nasal airways can be used to assist with maintaining an open airway. Oral airways are generally used only in unconscious patients who do not have a gag reflex. The clinician must select an oral airway large enough to keep the tongue from obstructing the pharynx but not so large that the tube itself is an airway obstruction. Nasal airways are generally better tolerated and can be used in awake patients, but they can become occluded with secretions or cause nasal trauma with insertion or removal.

Endotracheal Intubation

After initiating manual ventilation, the clinician reassesses the infant's condition to determine whether intubation is necessary. In some cases, brief periods of manual ventilation can stabilize the infant's condition, making intubation unnecessary. Improved skin color, spontaneous respiratory efforts, and a stable heart rate are indications for withdrawal of manual ventilation. As the bag and mask are withdrawn, free-flowing oxygen can be placed near the infant's face and the infant reassessed. Infants who do not respond to brief periods of manual ventilation or who require prolonged ventilatory support require intubation.

TABLE 24-7 Suggested Neonatal Endotracheal Tube Size Based on Body Weight

Weight (g)	Tube Size*
Less than 1000	2.5
1000 to 2000	3.0
2000 to 3000	3.5
More than 3000	3.5 to 4

*Tube size is given as the inside diameter in millimeters.

TABLE 24-8 Suggested Endotracheal Tube Size Based on Gestational Age

Gestational Age (Weeks)	Tube Size*
Less than 30	2.5
30 to 35	3.0
More than 35	3.5

*Tube size is given as the inside diameter in millimeters.

Oral endotracheal tubes are most commonly used to intubate neonates and children. Nasal intubation is generally more hazardous and is not frequently used. The appropriate tube size (**Table 24-7**) and the distance of insertion can be estimated based on the infant's weight. If the infant's weight is not immediately available, gestational age also is a reliable predictor for tube size (**Table 24-8**).

Unlike adults and large children, the narrowest point of an infant's airway is at the cricoid cartilage; this characteristic allows the use of uncuffed airways. Although a complete seal is not always obtained, the cricoid cartilage provides a functional cuff. Despite some leakage, adequate ventilation can be achieved with an appropriate-sized uncuffed endotracheal tube. Also, use of an uncuffed tube prevents cuff-related tracheal injury in these patients. For these reasons, cuffed tubes are rarely used in neonates.

The correct endotracheal tube (ETT) size for children 1 to 10 years old can be estimated by using the child's age:

Endotracheal tube size (mm internal diameter) =
(Age in years/4) + 4

The clinician should have an ETT one-half size larger and smaller than the estimated size available if needed.

ETT size can also be estimated by using a child's length. Length-based tapes are available and are generally considered useful for children up to 35 kg.

> **RESPIRATORY RECAP**
>
> **Endotracheal Intubation**
>
> » Oral tubes are most commonly used in neonates and children.
>
> » Neonatal tubes are uncuffed.
>
> » Pediatric tubes are sometimes cuffed.

Cuffed ETTs can be just as safe as uncuffed tubes for infants and children in the hospital setting.[7] There are circumstances in which a cuffed ETT is useful, such as when lung compliance is low and high airway pressures are needed. When cuffed ETT tubes are used, cuff inflation pressures should be kept below 20 cm H_2O.[8]

The approximate distance to insert the ETT, measured from the infant's lips, can be estimated by the addition of 6 cm to the infant's weight in kilograms. In children this can estimated by adding 10 to the child's age. These formulas can be used to estimate initial tube placement, but bilateral auscultation of the chest is essential. A disposable CO_2 detector can be placed between the outer end of the resuscitation device and the endotracheal tube and is a quick and easy way to confirm that the ETT is in the trachea. Because false positives and negatives are possible with the device, when bilateral breath sounds are noted, the tube should be secured and its position confirmed by chest radiograph. The tube then can be cut to minimize additional dead space and reduce the risk of inadvertent extubation. In addition, a gastric tube should be inserted and suction applied to decompress the stomach of air inadvertently delivered during mask ventilation.

Suctioning

Suctioning of an intubated neonate or child should be performed secondary to clinical assessment and not as a routine procedure. Suctioning can cause hypoxia, atelectasis, infection, tissue damage, and changes in the heart rate, blood pressure, and intracranial pressure. The need for suctioning is generally related to the underlying pathologic condition. Infants intubated because of respiratory distress syndrome, persistent pulmonary hypertension, or apnea require less suctioning than infants with meconium aspiration, sepsis, or pulmonary hemorrhage. Indications for suctioning include evidence of secretions in the endotracheal tube, diminished breath sounds, decreased tidal volume (during pressure ventilation), or increased peak inspiratory pressure (during volume ventilation). An obstructed airway or endotracheal tube should always be considered when acute desaturation occurs, particularly in infants with meconium aspiration, pulmonary hemorrhage, or pneumonia. Increases in carbon dioxide may also be a sign that the airway is obstructed and suctioning should be attempted. Providing adequate humidity can reduce the risk of tube obstruction, but plugging of artificial airways in infants with thick or abundant secretions is always a concern given the small internal diameter of the tube.

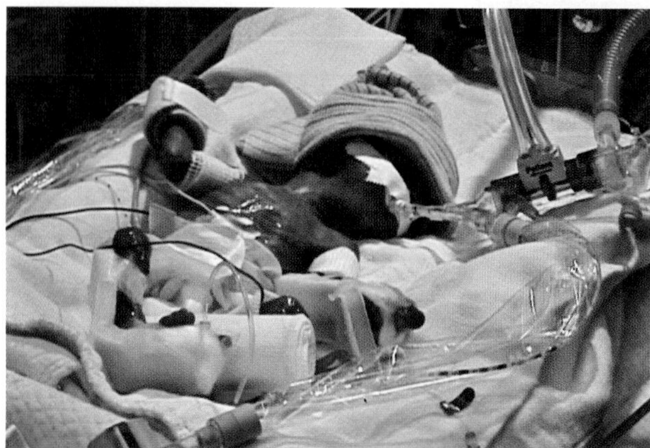

FIGURE 24–6 Neonatal in-line suction catheter.

Oral or nasopharyngeal suctioning of infants is most often accomplished with a bulb syringe or other noninvasive technique to minimize airway trauma and edema. For the intubated patient, an in-line suction catheter (Figure 24–6) offers several advantages over single-use catheters, and their use has become a routine practice in intensive care units (ICUs). With the in-line catheter, the child can be suctioned without ventilator disconnection. Maintaining a closed system can reduce the risk of lung volume loss during suctioning. An in-line catheter that connects directly to the ETT with minimum dead space is ideal.

> **RESPIRATORY RECAP**
>
> **Suctioning**
>
> » The recommended suction level is as low as will effectively remove secretions.
>
> » Select a catheter with a French size two times the size of the inner diameter (in millimeters) of the endotracheal tube.

Selection of the suction catheter size is based on the size of the ETT. A common rule of thumb is to select a catheter with a French size two times the size of the inner diameter (in millimeters) of the ETT. The distance the catheter is inserted should be determined before the procedure to avoid airway trauma.[9,10] With the ETT in proper position, the distance is measured from the lips to the tip of the in-line catheter fully withdrawn. The catheter is then inserted 0.5 cm farther than this distance. The recommended suction level is no greater that 75 to 100 mm Hg for infants (some recommend 60 to 80 mm Hg) and 100 to 125 mm Hg for children (some recommend 80 to 100 mm Hg). The suction pressure should be limited to the lowest level that effectively removes secretions and should be applied intermittently during withdrawal of the catheter. In neonates, an increase in F_{IO_2} of 0.1 to 0.2 prior to and during the suction procedure is generally needed to maintain arterial oxygen saturation. For larger pediatric patients, the use of 100% oxygen to preoxygenate is considered safe.

The patient must be assessed throughout the procedure. Decreases in the heart rate or significant arterial oxygen desaturation during suctioning are indications to remove the catheter and support the child as needed. If further suctioning is indicated, additional oxygen may be required before the procedure continues. After the procedure is completed, reassessment of the heart rate, oxygen saturation, color, chest expansion, and breath sounds is indicated. Ventilator adjustments and changes in the oxygen concentration may be needed to keep the oxygen saturation within the desired range.

Nasal Continuous Positive Airway Pressure

Infants who show adequate spontaneous efforts but whose clinical presentation indicates the potential for low lung volumes and associated hypoxemia may benefit from **nasal continuous positive airway pressure (NCPAP)**. NCPAP can be applied via a variety of different nasal prongs and masks and with different pressure-generating devices (**Figure 24–7**). It can serve as an oxygen delivery source and aid in lung recruitment. NCPAP also is used to minimize airway collapse in patients with tracheomalacia.[11,12]

The CPAP level is started at 4 to 6 cm H_2O, and the child is reevaluated with pulse oximetry, transcutaneous monitoring, and arterial, venous, or capillary blood gas measurements. An appropriately sized nasal prong is needed to achieve the desired benefit. Prongs that are too large can cause skin breakdown at the nares, and prongs that are too small allow the infant to breathe around the device, making continuous airway pressure difficult to maintain. Nasal masks are also available and can be used with some CPAP devices. Nasal masks can be a good alternative to nasal prongs when skin breakdown is an issue and for larger children. The CPAP flow rates must be adequate to meet the patient's inspiratory demand, but not so large as to create significant work of breathing. Insertion of an orogastric tube is strongly advised to minimize air accumulation in the gastrointestinal tract. The circuit used to deliver NCPAP must be heated and humidified, because it becomes the major portion of the child's inspired air. Inadequately humidified gas can increase the risk of airway obstruction, and inadequately heated gas may result in difficulty in maintaining the infant's neutral thermal environment.

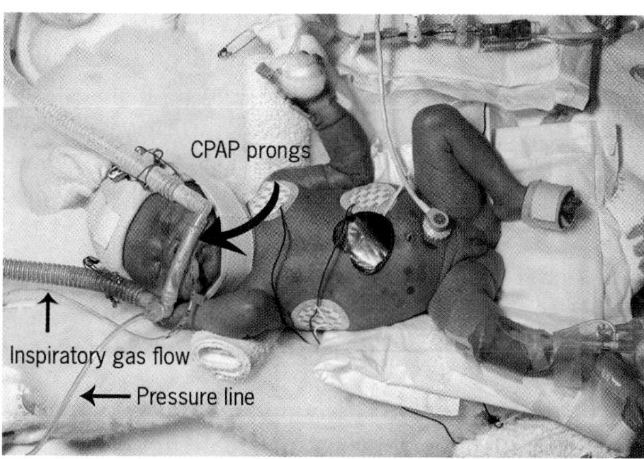

FIGURE 24–7 Setup for neonatal nasal continuous positive airway pressure (NCPAP) therapy.

Currently, nasal cannulas, variable-flow nasal CPAP generators, bubble CPAP setups, and nasal prongs and masks in conjunction with a conventional mechanical ventilator are the primary devices being used to provide NCPAP in neonatal and pediatric ICUs in the United States. All these devices have advantages, disadvantages, and attendant difficulties. Some of the problems of delivering nasal CPAP, no matter which device is used, include difficulty in obtaining a seal and maintaining pressure, tubes becoming blocked and preventing pressure from being delivered to the lungs, and nasal trauma and breakdown. Some of the devices also have issues regarding inaccurate or absent pressure monitoring and increased work of breathing due to the design of the device.

Nasal cannulas are primarily used to deliver supplemental oxygen. In many hospitals, high-flow nasal cannulas (HFNCs) are being used as substitute NCPAP devices. Although there is not complete agreement as to what constitutes high flow, cannulas with flows of at least 1 to 8 L/min are frequently described as HFNCs in the neonatal environment.[13] An air–oxygen blender is used in combination with the cannula to titrate the F_{IO_2} delivered to the patient. The advantages of using nasal cannulas as nasal CPAP devices are that they are low in cost, easy to set up, readily available, and usually well tolerated by neonates. Unlike conventional nasal CPAP devices, however, nasal cannulas do not have a mechanism to monitor or regulate the generation of positive airway pressure. Due to variability in cannula sizes, patient sizes, and disease processes, it is difficult to predict what, if any, airway pressure is being delivered. There are also doubts about whether infants who use HFNCs have a comparable outcome to those infants who use other delivery devices.[14]

Variable-flow nasal CPAP devices, sometimes called flow drivers (FDs), generate CPAP at the airway, unlike continuous-flow CPAP devices such as bubble CPAP. One example of this type of device (**Figure 24–8**) uses the Bernoulli effect and dual injector jets directed toward each nasal passage to maintain a constant pressure. If the infant needs more flow, the Venturi action of the jets will entrain additional flow. The infant can exhale without added work because the expiratory flow is shunted out the expiratory outlet that is open to ambient air. Continuous positive pressure is maintained throughout the respiratory cycle by residual gas pressure. The nasal prongs used can be of a much larger diameter than traditional prongs. They are made of a thin, soft material that flares out during inspiration, increasing the internal diameter and decreasing

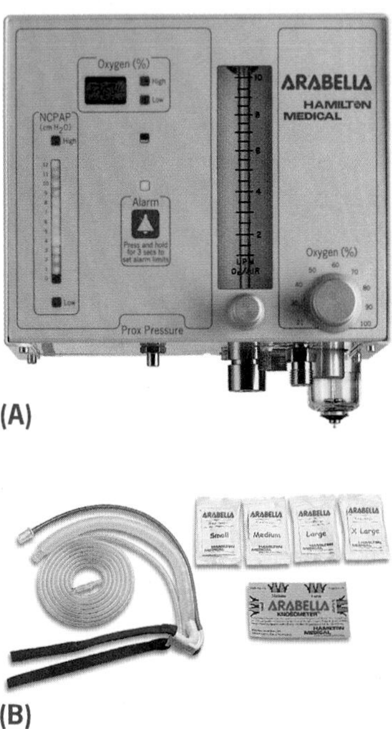

FIGURE 24–8 (**A**) The Arabella continuous positive airway pressure system. (**B**) The Arabella Universal Generator and nasal prongs.

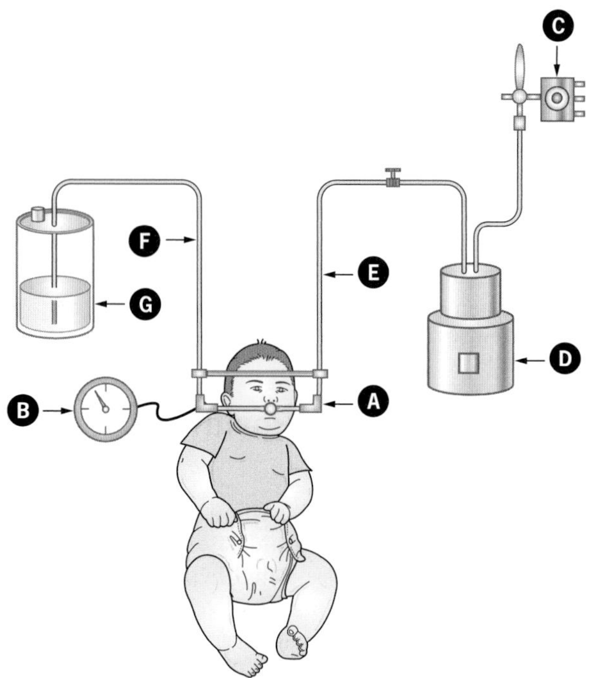

FIGURE 24–9 Schematic of bubble NCPAP delivery system. (**A**) Nasal prongs. (**B**) Manometer. (**C**) Oxygen blender with flowmeter. (**D**) Heated humidifier. (**E**) Inspiratory tubing. (**F**) Expiratory tubing. (**G**) Underwater bubble chamber. Adapted from Liptsen E, et al. Work of breathing during nasal continuous positive airway pressure in preterm infants: a comparison of bubble vs variable-flow devices. *J Perinatology*. 2005;25:453–458.

the leaking around them. No mechanical valves are used, and the intranasal airway pressure can be continuously monitored. The variable-flow capability of the FD assists with spontaneous breathing and creates more stable pressure delivery, which leads to enhanced functional residual capacity (FRC). NCPAP has demonstrated that it creates less work of breathing, and the infant using NCPAP has less thoracoabdominal asynchrony.[15]

Homemade bubble CPAP systems are popular in the United States (**Figure 24–9**). These systems comprise a heater/humidifier, a fresh gas source at a flow of up to 10 L/min, a separate inspiratory and expiratory length of tubing, a nasal prong interface, a pressure manometer, and a water seal column of sterile H_2O plus 0.25% acetic acid. Most of this equipment can be found in any respiratory therapy department. The CPAP level is set by submerging the end of the expiratory tubing under the surface of the liquid to a depth in centimeters that is marked on the side of the column.[16] The pressure delivered is measured in centimeters of water (cm H_2O). The amount of pressure delivered is also influenced by the amount of flow through the system, so a pressure manometer should be placed as close to the nasal interface as possible.[17,18] Some suggest that the oscillations that come from bubble CPAP may improve gas exchange, whereas others dispute this.[17]

Noninvasive Positive Pressure Ventilation

Mechanical ventilation can also be provided without an artificial airway, called noninvasive positive pressure ventilation (NIV). One of the main advantages of NIV is the ability to provide mechanical support for patients without exposing them to the risks involved with intubation. In addition, support can be provided for a short period of time, intermittently as needed, or for longer periods of time if necessary. The patient interface can be either a nasal mask, an oronasal mask, or nasal prongs for infants. The patient interface can be connected to either a noninvasive mechanical ventilator or a standard mechanical ventilator. Although CPAP can be delivered, more frequently this type of ventilation is used in a bilevel mode that combines positive pressure breaths with PEEP. The goals of NIV include mechanical stenting of the airway with tracheal malacia and treatment of acute respiratory failure. NIV is frequently used for obstructive sleep apnea, RDS, and postextubation respiratory failure.[17,19,20] It is also used in acute asthma and with respiratory failure associated with cystic fibrosis. The patient must be monitored for facial skin breakdown due to excessive pressure from the mask or prongs.

Conventional Infant and Pediatric Ventilation

Indications

Mechanical ventilation is required for a variety of clinical presentations in neonates and children (**CPG 24–1**).[21] Full-term infants who require mechanical ventilation can have complex presenting symptoms that often include intrapulmonary and intracardiac shunting. Infants with

CLINICAL PRACTICE GUIDELINE 24–1

Neonatal Time-Triggered, Pressure-Limited, Time-Cycled Mechanical Ventilation

Indications

- Apnea
- Respiratory or ventilatory failure, despite the use of continuous positive airway pressure (CPAP) and supplemental oxygen (i.e., $F_{IO_2} \geq 0.60$)
- Respiratory acidosis with a pH < 7.20–7.25
- $Pa_{O_2} < 50$ mm Hg
- Increased work of breathing demonstrated by grunting, nasal flaring, tachypnea, and sternal and intercostal retractions
- Alterations in neurologic status that compromise the central drive to breathe
- Intracranial hemorrhage
- Congenital neuromuscular disorders
- Impaired respiratory function due to decreased lung compliance and/or increased airways resistance

Hazards and Complications

- Air leak syndromes due to barotrauma and/or volume overinflation (i.e., volutrauma), including pneumothorax, pneumomediastinum, pneumopericardium, pneumoperitoneum, subcutaneous emphysema, pulmonary interstitial emphysema
- Chronic lung disease associated with prolonged positive pressure ventilation and oxygen toxicity (e.g., bronchopulmonary dysplasia)
- Airway complications associated with endotracheal intubation
- Laryngotracheobronchomalacia
- Damage to upper airway structures
- Malpositioning of endotracheal tube
- Partial or total obstruction of endotracheal tube
- Unplanned extubation
- Subglottic stenosis
- Main stem intubation
- Nosocomial pulmonary infection
- Decreased cardiac output
- Increased intracranial pressure leading to intraventricular hemorrhage
- Ventilator failure
- Ventilator circuit and/or humidifier failure
- Ventilator alarm failure
- Loss of or inadequate gas supply
- Patient–ventilator asynchrony

Assessment of Outcome

- Establishment of neonatal assisted ventilation should result in improvement in patient condition and/or reversal of indications such as a reduction in work of breathing or improved gas exchange.
- Ability to maintain a $Pa_{O_2} \geq 50$ torr with $F_{IO_2} < 0.60$ or to reverse respiratory acidosis and maintain a pH > 7.25.

Modified from AARC clinical practice guideline: neonatal time-triggered, pressure-limited, time-cycled mechanical ventilation. *Respir Care.* 1994;39(8):808–816. Reprinted with permission.

congenital heart disease have particularly complex circulatory alterations. Some of these patients depend on the fetal blood flow that normally occurs only in utero. Maintaining patency of a ductus arteriosus or septal defect may save a life. During mechanical ventilation, abrupt changes in hemodynamics, normoxia, and hyperoxia can be fatal to these infants. Blood flow through these shunts is sometimes the primary means to maintain blood flow to the systemic circulation. Until corrective procedures can be performed, oxygen concentrations at or below room air can alter intracardiac shunts and ensure the patient's survival. An understanding of various cardiac anomalies is essential for appropriate ventilator management.

Providing adequate oxygenation and ventilation in conditions such as pneumonia, meconium aspiration, and congenital diaphragmatic hernia often is difficult. Nonhomogeneous lung disease increases the risk of barotrauma because the most compliant alveoli become overdistended. These underlying conditions often cause difficulty in the maintenance of adequate oxygenation and ventilation and lead to pulmonary vasoconstriction and significant pulmonary hypertension. As a result, shunting occurs through a patent ductus arteriosus or patent foramen ovale, making oxygenation more difficult.

Persistent pulmonary hypertension of the neonate (PPHN) can appear as a primary condition and be extremely difficult to manage. In infants with PPHN, either the pulmonary vasculature has increased tone and abnormal responsiveness to vasodilators or the pulmonary arteries are muscularized, with a decreased cross-sectional area. In either condition blood flow is restricted, pulmonary artery pressure increases, and intracardiac shunting occurs. Because limited blood flow reaches the pulmonary vasculature to participate in gas exchange, ventilator adjustments in this population have little effect. Deoxygenated blood is shunted through a patent foramen ovale or a patent ductus arteriosus, making it difficult to achieve an adequate arterial oxygen saturation. The pulmonary vasculature responds to hypoxia with further vasoconstriction, creating the possibility of greater amounts of blood being shunted and worsening oxygenation. Definitive diagnosis of PPHN generally is done by cardiac ultrasound. Clinically, right-to-left shunting is detected when oxygen saturation by Spo_2 is monitored at a site receiving preductal blood (generally the right arm) and compared with a simultaneously monitored postductal site (left arm or right or left lower extremity). A difference in the oxygen saturation values from these two sites (preductal value higher than the postductal value) indicates right-to-left shunting, often a result of pulmonary hypertension.

RESPIRATORY RECAP

Preductal and Postductal Spo_2 Monitoring

- Used to detect right-to-left shunting
- Preductal site: Generally the right arm
- Postductal site: Left arm or either lower extremity

Infant Ventilators

Infant ventilators fall into two major categories: conventional ventilators and high-frequency ventilators. A conventional ventilator offers a variety of modes, alarms, and other options. Selection of the appropriate mode and other ventilator options is based on the infant's underlying condition and the desired effect of ventilatory support during both spontaneous and ventilator-initiated breaths.

Historically, a neonatal ventilator has been continuous flow, time cycled, and pressure limited. This is very similar to pressure control ventilation, with the rapid rise of gas flow and pressurization of the circuit leading to very early tidal volume delivery and then decelerating flow.[22] The first ventilators of this type did not allow for patient triggering. Current infant-only ventilators offer volume-limited and pressure-limited options, as well as patient-triggered and non-patient-triggered modes. Most modern mechanical ventilators have the ability to ventilate all patient types: premature infants, pediatric patients, and adults. These are called cradle-to-grave ventilators. Most ICU ventilators can be set up for neonates or children such that the trigger sensitivity and delivered pressures and volumes are suitable to respond to these patient populations. ICU ventilators evaluated in a 2009 study were capable of responding to neonatal inspiratory efforts and providing initial gas as effectively as traditional infant ventilators.[23]

TABLE 24-9 Initial Ventilator Settings for Conventional Ventilation

Setting	Instructions for Use
Peak inspiratory pressure (PIP)	As needed to provide a tidal volume of 4 to 6 mL/kg
Positive end-expiratory pressure (PEEP)	4 to 6 cm H_2O
Respiratory rate	20 to 40 breaths/min
Inspiratory time	0.3 to 0.5 second
Fractional inspired oxygen concentration (Fio_2)	As needed to maintain Spo_2 based on gestational age
Flow	6 to 12 L/min

When initiating ventilation, the clinician must select a pressure and/or tidal volume, respiratory rate, ventilator mode, inspiratory time or inspiration-to-expiration (I:E) ratio, PEEP, flow rate, and fractional inspired oxygen concentration. **Table 24-9** shows initial ventilator settings.

Pressure Limit and Tidal Volume

In neonatal time-cycled, pressure-limited ventilation, the clinician selects a pressure limit and inspiratory time that result in the delivery of a desired tidal volume. The tidal volume varies depending on the PIP, inspiratory time, and lung compliance. For example, if the lungs are less compliant, as in RDS, a higher PIP is needed to obtain a desired tidal volume. On the other hand, a lower PIP is needed if the lungs are more compliant. It should also be noted that, unlike most adult ventilators, the pressure set on a neonatal ventilator is the PIP—not the pressure above PEEP. Thus, the tidal volume is determined by the difference between the set pressure and PEEP. For this reason, an increase in PEEP may reduce the tidal volume unless the pressure limit is increased by an equivalent amount.

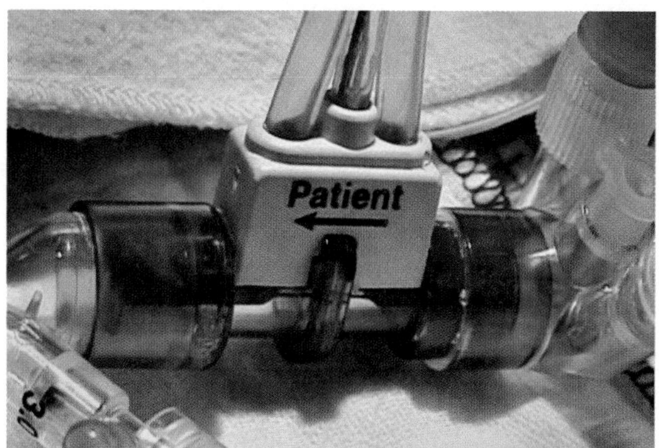

FIGURE 24–10 Flow sensor at airway to measure delivered tidal volume.

In the volume-targeted mode, the delivered tidal volume is preset and the PIP varies. The maximum amount of pressure delivered also is preset by the clinician. Volume ventilation has been found to reduce ventilator days and decrease the risk of pneumothorax and grades 3 and 4 intraventricular hemorrhage, and has shown a trend toward a reduced incidence of BPD.[24] Monitoring of the delivered tidal volume at the airway opening is essential to assess the effect of leaks (**Figure 24–10**). The uncuffed endotracheal tube can be a concern in volume ventilation in neonates because leaks of greater than 60% can limit the effectiveness of volume ventilation. The placement of an appropriate-sized endotracheal tube is key for success with volume-targeted ventilation for neonates.

RESPIRATORY RECAP

Neonatal and Pediatric Ventilator Settings

» Ventilator mode
» Pressure or tidal volume (or both)
» Respiratory rate
» Inspiratory time or inspiration-to-expiration (I:E) ratio
» Positive end-expiratory pressure (PEEP)
» Flow rate
» Fractional inspired oxygen concentration (F_{IO_2})

Pressure-limited ventilation with a target tidal volume is a common approach to neonatal and pediatric ventilation. Whether volume-limited, pressure-limited, or dual ventilation control is selected, a tidal volume of 4 to 6 mL/kg is generally targeted for neonates. For children, 6 to 8 mL/kg is acceptable.[25] As changes in tidal volume occur, clinical assessment determines the best intervention (**Table 24–10**). Adaptive pressure control (APC) can also be used. With APC, the clinician sets a target tidal volume. The ventilator uses either pressure control or pressure support ventilation, but the pressure is increased or decreased as necessary to achieve the target tidal volume.

A practical issue with the ventilation of neonates is the effect of circuit compliance and compressible volume. These can substantially reduce the tidal volume available, particularly with volume ventilation. For this reason, a noncompliant, low-volume circuit typically is used. Because of the high resistance through this smaller-bore tubing, it is important to monitor airway pressure and flow directly at the Y piece of the ventilator circuit.[24]

TABLE 24–10 Changes in Tidal Volume During Pressure Ventilation

Tidal Volume Change	Possible Causes	Solutions
Increase	Increased compliance, decreased resistance, decreased PEEP, increased inspiratory time, decreased leak	Reduce peak inspiratory pressure.
Decrease	Decreased compliance, increased resistance, decreased peak inspiratory pressure, increased PEEP, decreased inspiratory time, increased leak	Suction airway. Reposition infant. Administer surfactant. Increase inspiratory pressure. Perform transillumination to check for pneumothorax. Auscultate to detect pneumothorax or main stem intubation. Obtain chest radiograph. Check tube position.

Respiratory Rate

After a tidal volume is established, the respiratory rate becomes the primary adjustment for the achievement of a desired minute ventilation. Spontaneously breathing neonates normally take 40 to 60 breaths/min to maintain a normal partial pressure of arterial carbon dioxide (Pa_{CO_2}). During mechanical ventilation, delivery of a larger than normal tidal volume (>4 to 6 mL/kg) at a lower respiratory rate can be more effective at eliminating carbon dioxide because a greater percentage of each tidal volume participates in gas exchange. Higher rates at lower tidal volumes result in a higher percentage of dead space ventilation and may result in less effective ventilation.

The ventilator rate should target a desired Pa_{CO_2}. The required rate depends on the target Pa_{CO_2}, the degree of lung disease (i.e., the amount of dead space), carbon dioxide production, the ventilator mode, and the amount of spontaneous breathing.

Mode

In continuous mandatory ventilation (CMV or assist/control) mode, a minimum respiratory rate is set. Each spontaneous respiratory effort triggers a ventilator-assisted breath, and the preset pressure or volume is delivered. The inspiratory time is preset, and the total respiratory rate above the set rate is determined by the patient.

In synchronized intermittent mandatory ventilation (SIMV) mode, a minimum respiratory rate is set. Between the mandatory breaths the patient can breathe spontaneously. Spontaneous efforts are unassisted, and the rate, inspiratory time, and tidal volume are determined by the patient. The patient's inspiratory efforts trigger the mandatory breaths. The mandatory breaths may be pressure or volume limited. If the patient becomes apneic, the SIMV rate is delivered. Intermittent mandatory ventilation (IMV) mode is similar to SIMV except that the mandatory breaths are not synchronized to patient effort. This mode is almost never used anymore because of the large number of complications that can result from the patient's lack of synchrony with the ventilator.

With pressure-support ventilation (PSV), all breaths are triggered by the patient. A pressure limit is set to achieve a target tidal volume. The total rate, inspiratory time, expiratory time, and tidal volume are determined by the patient. Because inspiration normally is flow cycled with PSV, leaks around the endotracheal tube can prolong inspiratory time unless the ventilator has a mechanism to terminate flow in leak situations. Most ventilators offer mechanisms to adjust the flow cycle, preventing prolonged inspiratory times with a leak. Pressure support may improve patient–ventilator synchrony in some patients by allowing flow rates and inspiratory times more consistent with the infant's needs. Improved patient–ventilator synchrony can lead to greater patient comfort, reduce the need for sedation, and potentially reduce the time the infant stays on mechanical ventilation.[20,21] Frequent apnea and periodic breathing are contraindications to this mode.

Inspiratory Trigger and Expiratory Cycle

Patient effort may trigger a breath in two primary ways. Depending on the ventilator, the patient-initiated breaths may be flow triggered, pressure triggered, or volume triggered. The signal for neonatal flow triggering typically occurs from a pneumotachometer positioned close to the infant's airway. A change in flow through the pneumotachometer triggers the ventilator. The amount of flow change required to trigger the ventilator is called the flow-trigger sensitivity, which is set by the clinician at a level that allows the least trigger effort without autotriggering. Pressure triggering occurs with a change in the baseline pressure. The amount of pressure change required to trigger the ventilator is the pressure-trigger sensitivity, set in centimeters of water. At a sensitivity of 1 cm H_2O, a patient effort that reduces the baseline system pressure by 1 cm H_2O below PEEP will trigger a breath. The specifics of the trigger mechanism vary from ventilator to ventilator. Some ventilators will flow trigger in one mode and pressure trigger in other modes. Volume triggering uses the integral of the flow signal for triggering. Because this is an averaging of the flow signal over time, signal noise is reduced. This gives volume triggering a theoretic advantage over flow triggering.

An adjustable expiratory flow cycle is incorporated into some patient-triggered, pressure-limited modes. The expiratory flow cycle is based on a percentage of the peak flow. This cycle produces a variable inspiratory time, much like pressure support, which may reduce ventilator dyssynchrony. Familiarity with the inspiratory trigger and expiratory cycle mechanisms of the ventilator is essential to determine the appropriate settings for an individual patient.

Inspiratory Time

The inspiratory time is set in conjunction with the respiratory rate. The inspiratory time and the respiratory rate determine the I:E ratio. For example, if the respiratory rate is 30 breaths/min, each breathing cycle takes 2 seconds. If the inspiratory time is 0.5 second, the I:E ratio is 1:3. Ventilator graphics should be used to determine the best inspiratory time for each patient's current clinical condition.[26]

An inspiratory time that is too short can compromise both oxygenation and ventilation. The **mean airway pressure** is affected by the inspiratory time. A lower mean airway pressure may result in a loss of lung volume or inability to establish lung volume, causing a decrease in the Pao_2. Decreased ventilation, resulting in less carbon dioxide elimination and a higher $Paco_2$, occurs if a shortened inspiratory time reduces the delivered tidal volume.

An inspiratory time that is too long may shorten the expiratory time and result in auto-PEEP, which may cause alveolar overdistention, increasing the risk of pneumothorax. Alveolar overdistention may also interfere with pulmonary blood flow, increase dead space ventilation, and reduce carbon dioxide elimination. Inspiratory times that are too long can also cause a patient to perform a forced exhalation maneuver, potentially causing excessive pressure, poor tidal volume delivery, and ventilator asynchrony (**Figure 24–11**). A typical inspiratory time with conventional positive pressure ventilation for the neonate is 0.3 to 0.5 of a second. Pediatric patients will have longer inspiratory times, frequently as long as 1 second. Monitoring the expiratory flow with graphics (**Figure 24–12**) or expiratory flow rate monitors and adjustment of the respiratory rate and inspiratory time can help prevent complications related to the I:E ratio such as air trapping and auto-PEEP.

Positive End-Expiratory Pressure

PEEP is routinely set in all ventilator modes to prevent alveolar collapse during expiration. PEEP usually is started at 4 to 6 cm H_2O. In the neonate, lung volumes are assessed by chest radiograph, with the ideal lung volume expansion being to eight or nine ribs bilaterally. PEEP and PIP are adjusted if the lungs appear underinflated or overinflated. Higher PEEP levels may be indicated for patients with a persistently low lung volume. Low levels of

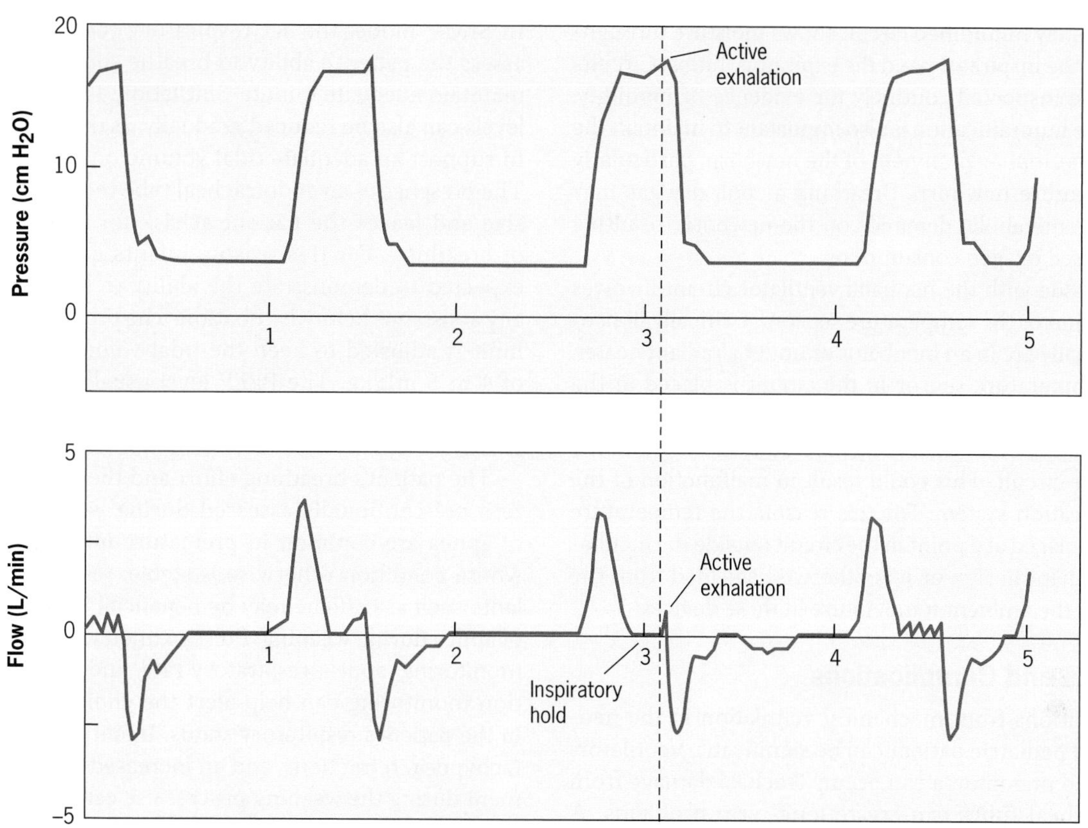

FIGURE 24–11 The inspiratory time is too long, and this causes a spiked appearance at the completion of each breath. This patient is forcibly exhaling. From Waugh, Jonathan B.; Deshpande, Vijay M.; Brown, Melissa K.; Harwood, Robert. *Rapid Interpretation of Ventilator Waveforms, 2nd edition,* © 2007. Printed and electronically reproduced by permission of Pearson Education, Inc., Upper Saddle River, New Jersey.

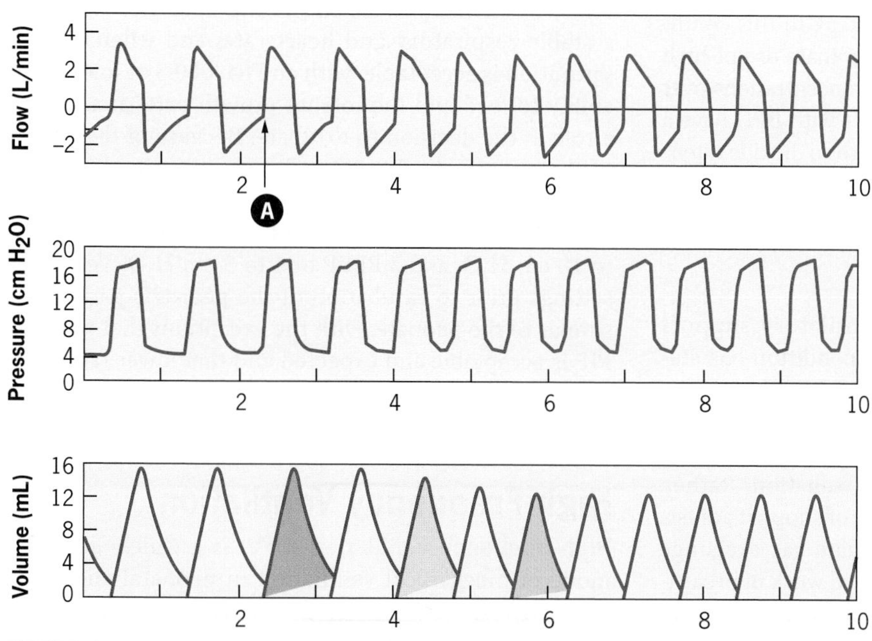

FIGURE 24–12 A ventilator rate set too high can cause breath stacking to occur, resulting in air trapping or auto-PEEP. Point A shows how the flow does not reach baseline before the next breath is delivered. Notice how tidal volumes are decreasing due to air trapping. From Waugh, Jonathan B.; Deshpande, Vijay M.; Brown, Melissa K.; Harwood, Robert. *Rapid Interpretation of Ventilator Waveforms, 2nd edition,* © 2007. Printed and electronically reproduced by permission of Pearson Education, Inc., Upper Saddle River, New Jersey.

PEEP are indicated with evidence of pulmonary interstitial emphysema or persistent air leakage after barotraumas. The delivered tidal volumes should be assessed when PEEP levels are adjusted. In pressure-limited ventilation, the change in the PEEP setting may result in a change in the delivered tidal volume. The pressure limit may need to be adjusted to maintain the volume target.

Humidification

Adequate humidification of the inspired gas is critical to the maintenance of airway patency. A decrease in humidity can lead to dried secretions and atelectasis and may result in partial or complete airway obstruction. This risk is particularly high in neonates because of their small airways. An appropriately humidified circuit shows moisture throughout both the inspiratory and the expiratory limbs. Circuits should be inspected routinely for evidence of humidity. Adequate humidification is also important to maintain the **neutral thermal environment** of the newborn, particularly the premature newborn. Breathing a cool, dry gas may stress the metabolic demands on the newborn, resulting in increased oxygen consumption.

One issue with the neonatal ventilator circuit involves the position of the temperature sensor.[27] Critically ill neonates usually are in an incubator or under a radiant heater. If the temperature sensor in the circuit is placed in the incubator or under the radiant heater, it may be affected by a temperature other than the temperature of the gas in the ventilator circuit. This could result in malfunction of the humidification system. For this reason, the temperature sensor is placed at a point in the circuit outside the incubator or radiant heater, or it is otherwise shielded from the effects of the ambient temperature in these devices.

Hazards and Complications

Complications from mechanical ventilation in the neonatal and pediatric patient can be significant. Ventilator-associated pneumonia can occur. Tracheal damage from endotracheal tubes can create long-term problems. A neuropathologic consequence of reduced cerebral blood flow known as periventricular leukomalacia (PVL) has been associated with ventilator-induced hypocarbia in preterm infants.

Some neonates who survive the newborn course are left with varying degrees of chronic lung disease, a condition called bronchopulmonary dysplasia. The contribution of mechanical ventilators and oxygen therapy to this condition is not entirely known, but indiscriminate use of high pressure and exposure to high oxygen concentrations over time are thought to be factors. Neonates with BPD have a chronic oxygen requirement, chronic carbon dioxide retention, and pulmonary hypertension. These neonates also have an increased susceptibility to pulmonary infections.[5,20]

Weaning

Consideration of weaning from ventilatory support should begin as soon as the patient's condition has stabilized from the disorder that required support. The patient's hemodynamic, pulmonary, neurologic, and nutritional status must be assessed. Also, weaning must not be confused with readiness for extubation. Rather, weaning should be an ongoing process of support adjustment to a level that maintains adequate gas exchange without requiring significantly increased work of breathing. No single approach to weaning can be applied to all patients. The goal is to provide appropriate support by continuous assessment of the patient's total needs and recognizing when weaning is indicated.

In infants and children, weaning is generally done in the SIMV or a PSV mode or a combination of both. In SIMV mode, the set respiratory rate is lowered to assess the patient's ability to breathe spontaneously and maintain adequate minute ventilation. Pressure-support levels can also be reduced gradually, as the patient is able to support an adequate tidal volume on his or her own. The presence of an endotracheal tube reduces the airway size and leaves the patient at risk for increased work of breathing. For this reason, infants generally are not expected to demonstrate the ability to breathe without any assistance before extubation. The pressure or volume limit is adjusted to keep the tidal volume in the range of 4 to 6 mL/kg. The PEEP level usually is maintained at a minimum of 4 to 6 cm H_2O to prevent loss of lung volume.

The patient's breathing effort and the ventilatory pattern are continually assessed during weaning. Periods of apnea are common in premature infants. In infants whose condition otherwise is stable, respiratory stimulants such as caffeine may be beneficial in the reduction of apnea during weaning. Pulse oximetry, transcutaneous monitoring, apnea, respiratory rate, and minute ventilation monitoring can help alert the clinician to changes in the patient's respiratory status. Infants with persistent tachypnea, retractions, and an increased oxygen requirement during the weaning process use calories needed for normal growth and development. Adequate gas exchange may be achieved, but the caloric expense to the patient can be far greater than the benefit. Continual assessment of the patient's tolerance for weaning from a multisystem perspective is essential throughout the weaning process.

Extubation is considered when no contraindications exist from the neurologic or other nonrespiratory systems, when the patient shows the ability to maintain a stable respiratory and heart rate, and when oxygen saturation is acceptable, with an F_{IO_2} of 0.3 or lower. The ability to feed and the infant's growth pattern also play a role in the decision to extubate. Because of the effects of the endotracheal tube on lung volume and work of breathing, extubation of the neonate often occurs with ventilator settings of 10 to 20 breaths/min, a PIP of 10 to 18 cm H_2O, and a PEEP of 4 to 5 cm H_2O. Ventilator settings prior to extubation of the pediatric patient are similar to the neonate, with the exceptions that a higher PIP is acceptable and expected and that lower rates may be tolerated. Readiness for extubation should be assessed daily in all ventilated patients.

High-Frequency Ventilation

High-frequency ventilation (HFV) is a widely accepted mode of mechanical ventilation in neonatal and pediatric critical care. Although it is categorized as nonconventional ventilation, many centers now consider it a conventional mode for the treatment of respiratory failure and pulmonary barotrauma. HFV is defined as positive pressure ventilation at a respiratory rate more than 150 breaths/min and tidal volumes approximating anatomic dead space.[28] The advantage of this technique over conventional mechanical ventilation is its ability to deliver an adequate minute ventilation with a lower airway pressure, often when conventional mechanical ventilation has failed. Treatment with a high mean airway pressure often is better tolerated with HFV than with conventional mechanical ventilation. With conventional mechanical ventilation, the alveolar volume is the difference between tidal volume and the dead space volume. Tidal volumes near the dead space volume produce little alveolar ventilation. The fact that gas exchange occurs with HFV, at times more efficiently than with CMV, is intriguing. HFV is used daily throughout the country, but the exact mechanism by which it accomplishes adequate gas exchange is not completely understood.

Classification

The four general types of HFV are high-frequency positive pressure ventilation, high-frequency jet ventilation, high-frequency flow interrupter ventilation, and high-frequency oscillatory ventilation.

High-frequency positive pressure ventilation (HFPPV) is conventional positive pressure ventilation at a high respiratory rate (more than 150 breaths/min) and small tidal volumes.[29] The inspiratory time is short to facilitate the increased respiratory rate. Exhalation is passive. The use of airway graphics to closely monitor changes in mean airway pressure is essential with HFPPV. Although HFPPV laid the foundation for modern high-frequency ventilation, its use has declined with the availability of high-frequency ventilators.

High-frequency jet ventilation (HFJV) delivers short pulses of gas directly into the trachea through a narrow-bore cannula or jet injector. Jet ventilators can maintain oxygenation and ventilation over a wide range of patient sizes. These systems have negligible compressible gas volume and operate effectively at rates of 150 to 600 breaths/min. Exhalation is passive. The tidal volume often is equal to or slightly less than the dead space volume. The high-flow jet pulse produces a jet mixing effect that creates an area of negative pressure and entrains additional gas into the airway. The high gas velocities and gas mixing effects make pressure monitoring difficult. Jet ventilators are used with a conventional ventilator that provides PEEP, entrained gas, and intermittent sighs.

High-frequency flow interrupter ventilation (HFFIV) delivers inspiratory flow to the patient in short bursts by means of a rotating ball valve or microprocessor-controlled solenoid valve. These ventilators produce breath rates of 2 to 22 Hz (1 **hertz [Hz]** equals 60 breaths/min). HFFIV is similar to high-frequency oscillatory ventilation in that inspiration and exhalation are both active. Active exhalation is defined as a drop in airway pressure during exhalation to accelerate exhaled gas flow.[30] Background mechanical breaths may or may not be used to maintain lung volume.

High-frequency oscillatory ventilation (HFOV) essentially uses airway vibrators, usually with piston pumps or vibrating diaphragms that operate at frequencies ranging from 400 to 2400 breaths/min.[31] During HFOV, inspiration and expiration are both active. Oscillators produce little if any bulk gas delivery. A continuous flow of fresh gas (bias flow) provides inspired gas and clears carbon dioxide from the system. Pressure oscillations in the airway produce tiny tidal volumes around a constant mean airway pressure. The tidal volume is determined by the amplitude of airway pressure oscillations, determined by the stroke of the device producing the oscillations.

> **RESPIRATORY RECAP**
>
> **Categories of High-Frequency Ventilation**
> - » High-frequency positive pressure ventilation (HFPPV)
> - » High-frequency jet ventilation (HFJV)
> - » High-frequency flow interrupter ventilation (HFFIV)
> - » High-frequency oscillatory ventilation (HFOV)

Gas Transport Theories

Several theories have been proposed to explain gas transport at high respiratory frequencies. The mechanisms of gas exchange during HFV are not completely understood, and several effects interact during HFV.[32]

In *spike formation* (**Figure 24–13**), a high-energy wave impulse of gas penetrates the center of the airway, enhancing bulk flow of gas in the upper airway and providing a more expansive area of gas mixing in the more distal lung. In the more compliant airway of the premature infant, spike formation is less effective. It is possible that turbulence increases with a more compliant airway, limiting spike effectiveness.

Helical diffusion (**Figure 24–14**), a variant of the spike theory, also may play a role in HFV. Fresh gas enters the lung through a spike generated in the center of the airway while gas exits the lung circumferentially along the periphery of the airway (coaxial flow).[33] This theory assumes that carbon dioxide removal occurs in a spiral fashion, producing a whirlpool effect, whereby fresh gas moves through the center of the airway while gas simultaneously exits the lungs.

Taylor dispersion (**Figure 24–15**) is the augmented diffusion of gas in situations of parabolic gas flow resulting

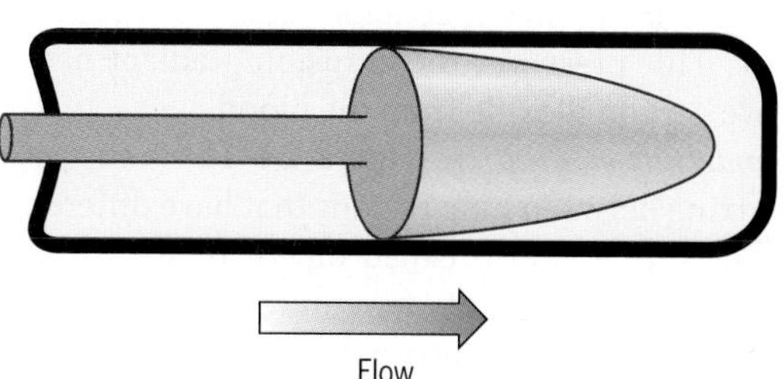

FIGURE 24–13 Spike formation in the airway during high-frequency ventilation.

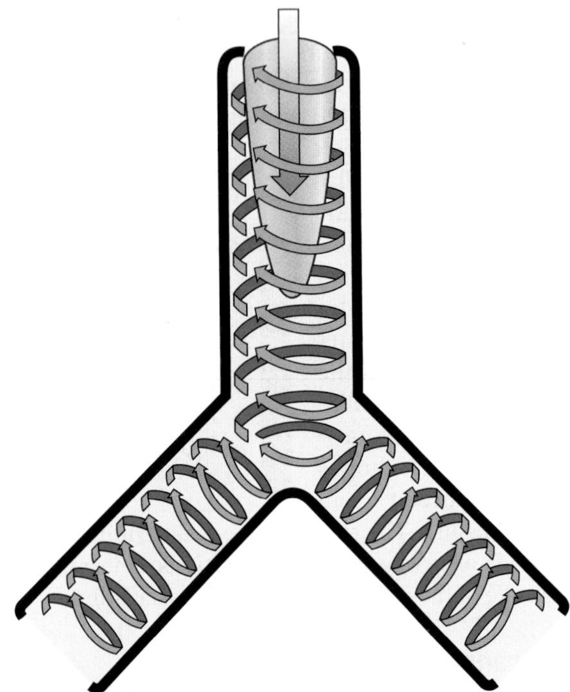

FIGURE 24–14 Helical diffusion during high-frequency ventilation. Adapted from Karp TB, et al. High frequency ventilation: a neonatal nursing perspective. *Neonatal Network*. 1986;4(5):43.

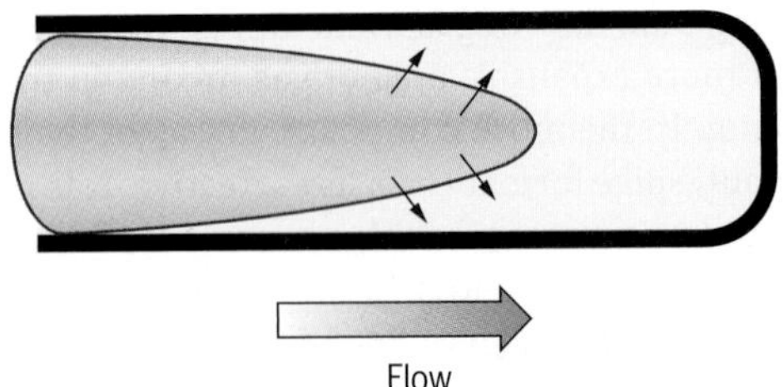

FIGURE 24–15 Taylor dispersion during high-frequency ventilation.

in high energy spikes.[34] This augmented diffusion can occur wherever two gas streams meet, such as in coaxial flow in larger airways and convective streaming more distal in the lung. This diffusion process is facilitated by the increased surface area between two gas streams during HFV. These high-energy jet spikes probably result in the delivery of more total fresh gas to distal respiratory units before significant contamination of the inflow gas occurs. This preserves the diffusion gradient needed to remove carbon dioxide from the blood.

Pendelluft ventilation (**Figure 24–16**) is the result of gas mixing between lung regions that have different time constants; this is also called out-of-phase ventilation. When parallel lung units have different time constants, resistance tends to dominate the rate of filling and emptying at rapid respiratory rates.[32] At the end of a rapid inspiration, gas flows from the fast unit, which is beginning to empty, to the slow unit, which is still filling. This

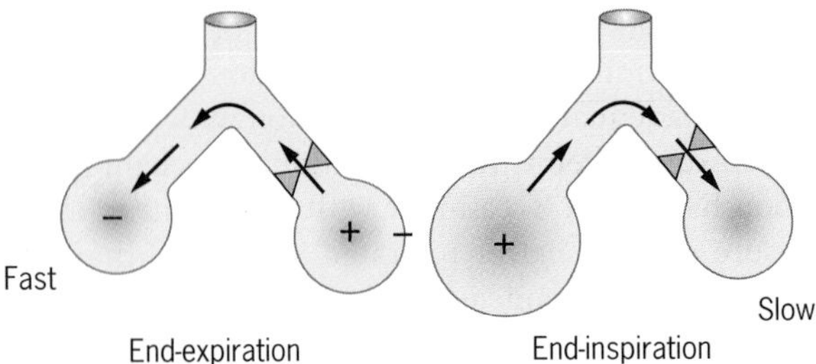

FIGURE 24–16 Pendelluft during high-frequency ventilation.

motion of gas between two neighboring units during phasic ventilation is called pendelluft.[32]

Molecular diffusion is a transport mechanism derived from random thermal oscillation of a molecule. So long as the molecules have a constant temperature, molecular diffusion always occurs. Molecular diffusion is responsible for gas exchange at the level of the alveolocapillary membrane.[32] Molecular diffusion is altered during HFV. The rapid kinetic motion of oxygen and carbon dioxide molecules during HFV and the process of gas exchange at the alveolar level are speculative at this time.

Patient Selection

Specific strategies for the use of HFV depend on the institution. Therefore, the question of when to use HFV in neonatal and pediatric patients is not easily answered. Should HFV be implemented early in the treatment of respiratory failure, or should conventional ventilation be used first and HFV applied only if this approach fails? Some centers are very aggressive and institute HFV without trying conventional ventilation, seeking to protect the patient from pulmonary barotrauma at the onset of ventilation. Others try conventional ventilation before HFV.

Use of HFV should be considered in the following situations:

- Preterm infants with severe hyaline membrane disease requiring a PIP of more than 30 cm H_2O and children with acute respiratory distress syndrome (ARDS) requiring a PIP of more than 40 cm H_2O
- Infants with severe meconium aspiration syndrome and persistent pulmonary hypertension that does not respond to maximum ventilatory support with a PIP of more than 35 cm H_2O
- Infants and children with air leak syndrome, including progressive pulmonary interstitial emphysema, recurring pneumothorax, and pneumopericardium
- Infants with congenital diaphragmatic hernia or pulmonary hypoplasia who have failed conventional ventilation
- Infants and children with severe parenchymal lung disease, such as group B streptococci pneumonia, who require high levels of ventilatory support
- Any of the above disease states that may preclude the use of conventional ventilation and that indicate the need to institute HFV as an initial point of care

High-Frequency Ventilators

The Bunnell Life Pulse jet ventilator (**Figure 24–17**) is a microprocessor-controlled system capable of delivering and monitoring 240 to 660 breaths/min. It is used in conjunction with a conventional ventilator that provides a source of continuous gas flow, PEEP, and low-rate IMV. The Life Pulse ventilator is approved for clinical use in neonates and infants. It appears to be most effective in disorders in which hypercarbia is the major problem. With HFJV, carbon dioxide removal is achieved at lower airway pressures than with other types of high-frequency ventilators. When managed properly, HFJV can acutely improve oxygenation and the oxygen index in infants with PPHN and other associated pulmonary conditions.

The patient box is an integral component of the Life Pulse ventilator. This box contains the pressure transducer and inhalation pinch valve necessary for operation. The patient box is placed close to the patient's head to provide accurate monitoring and delivery of gas to the patient. The pinch valve regulates gas flow. The Life Pulse controls the PIP, respiratory rate, jet valve on-time (inspiratory time), and on/off ratio (I:E ratio). The jet ventilator delivers short pulses of pressurized gas directly into the airway through a narrow-bore cannula or jet injector. The system has negligible compressible volume, and exhalation is always passive. The tidal volume is difficult to measure but is equal to or slightly greater than the dead space volume. Gas surrounding the injector is entrained into the airway with each jet pulse. Airway pressure must be measured far enough downstream from the jet injector to minimize errors caused by air entrainment effects.

A special triple-lumen endotracheal tube (Hi-Lo Jet) can be used for HFJV. In addition to the standard endotracheal tube lumen, this tube has a pressure monitoring port at its distal tip and a jet injector port in the tube wall approximately 7 cm upstream from the pressure monitoring port. A triple-lumen endotracheal tube adapter (**Figure 24–18**) has been designed to allow jet ventilation without the use of a special tube, which eliminates the need to reintubate the infant solely for use of HFJV. This adapter houses the jet injector port and the pressure monitoring port.

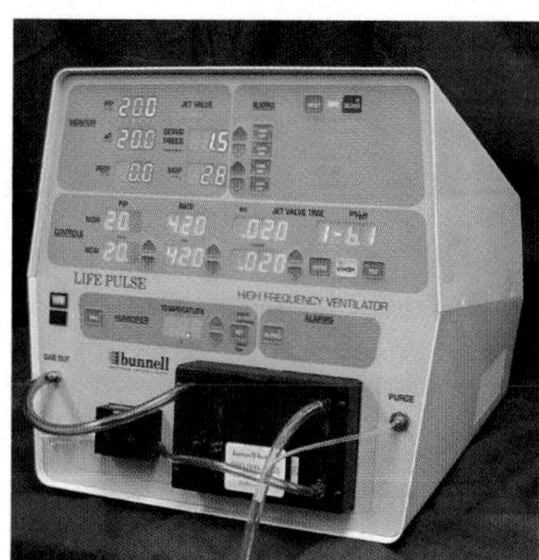

FIGURE 24–17 Bunnell Life Pulse jet ventilator.

The Life Pulse ventilator delivers its jet pulse into the endotracheal tube through the injector port. It then servo controls the driving pressure to the jet to maintain a constant predetermined pressure at the endotracheal tube tip. A unique feature of the Life Pulse ventilator is its ability to monitor and display the jet servo pressure. This allows automatic detection of changes in the infant's lung compliance and airway resistance. Servo pressure is proportional to the lung volume being ventilated. For example, as lung compliance or airway resistance (or both) improves, servo pressure increases. This is typically used as an indicator to begin weaning the patient from high-frequency ventilation. Conversely, a decrease in servo pressure indicates that lung compliance or airway resistance has worsened, the endotracheal tube has become obstructed, a tension pneumothorax has developed, or the patient requires suctioning. Respiratory therapists and other clinicians find servo pressure helpful for assessing the patient's pulmonary status.

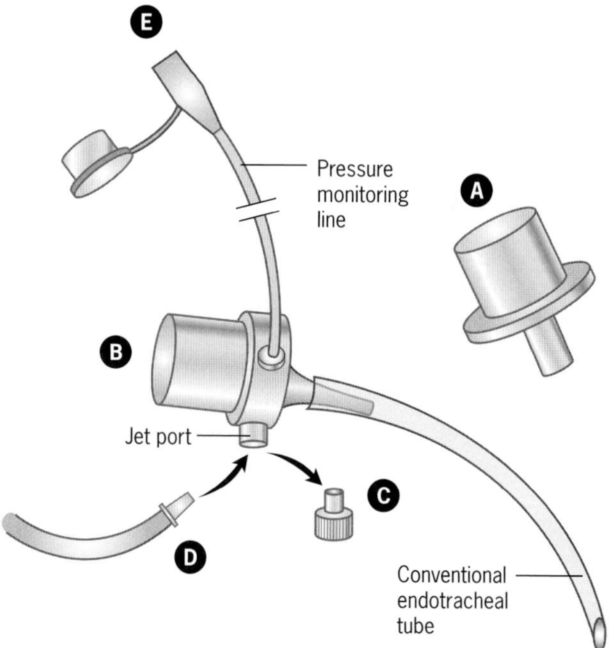

FIGURE 24–18 Triple lumen endotracheal tube adapter for use with the Bunnell Life Pulse jet ventilator. The 15 mm endotracheal tube adapter (**A**) is replaced with the Life Pulse adapter (**B**). The cap on the jet port (**C**) is removed and the luer fitting of the Life Pulse circuit (**D**) is attached to the jet port. The pressure monitoring connector from the jet patient box is attached to the pressure monitoring line (**E**). The conventional ventilator circuit is attached to the 15 mm port of the Life Pulse adapter. Modified from Aloan CA, Hill TV. *Respiratory Care of the Newborn and Child.* 2nd ed. Lippincott Williams & Wilkins; 1997.

The SensorMedics 3100A (CareFusion, San Diego, Calif.) is an electronically controlled oscillatory ventilator (**Figure 24–19**). Its 365-mL oscillatory driver is a diaphragmatically sealed piston with adjustable displacement, frequency, and I:E ratio. It produces 3- to 15-Hz pressure waves superimposed on an adjustable level of mean airway pressure. The SensorMedics 3100A is distinguished from other types of high-frequency ventilators by its active expiratory phase. It is used for ventilatory support and for treatment of respiratory failure and barotrauma in neonates and small pediatric patients.

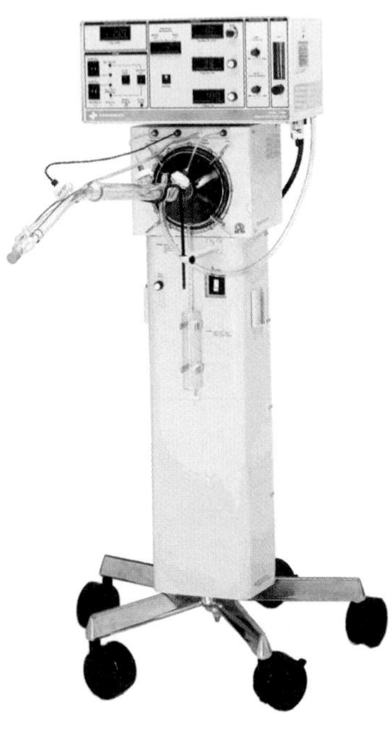

FIGURE 24–19 SensorMedics 3100A.

The primary therapeutic effects are obtained with just two controls: the oscillatory **pressure amplitude** (ΔP) and the mean airway pressure. In some cases, changing the frequency (hertz) or the percent inspiratory time or both may provide additional benefits to those patients who do not respond to initial standard settings.

End-expiratory lung volume is determined by the mean airway pressure and remains relatively constant during the respiratory cycle. The SensorMedics 3100A does not require use of a special endotracheal tube. It has fewer control settings than other high-frequency ventilators, and once the patient's condition has been stabilized, the ventilator settings are changed infrequently.

The mean airway pressure on the SensorMedics 3100A can be adjusted from 3 to 45 cm H_2O. The mean airway pressure limit can be operated in two modes. In the safety limit mode, the mean airway pressure limit is set to a level higher than the range of normal mean airway pressures to protect the patient from accidental overpressure. In the controlled mode, the mean airway pressure limit is set to a level below that which would otherwise exist through the adjustment of the mean pressure control. In this mode, the mean airway pressure remains constant regardless of changes in bias flow, the percent inspiratory time, or frequency settings. With HFOV the mean airway pressure is the most important determinant of oxygenation. It dictates whether the patient can be weaned from the potentially harmful effects of an elevated F_{IO_2}. The mean airway pressure is maximized initially, with close attention paid to hyperinflation and monitoring of the chest radiograph to maintain lung volume at the level of ribs T8 to T9.

RESPIRATORY RECAP

High-Frequency Ventilators

- » Bunnell Life Pulse jet ventilator
- » SensorMedics 3100A

Bias flow is necessary to maintain oxygenation, the mean airway pressure, and an oscillatory waveform. The system must be charged with flow to operate effectively. Standardized bias flow settings are 10 to 20 L/min. A common rule of thumb is that the smaller the child, the lower the bias flow. Manipulations of the Pa_{CO_2} level are made primarily with the amplitude or power control (ΔP). Increasing the amplitude increases displacement of the bellows, which increases tidal volume delivery. This is measured as an increased pressure amplitude at the airway opening and results in a lower Pa_{CO_2}. Frequent arterial blood gas measurements or monitoring of the transcutaneous P_{CO_2} is necessary to titrate the Pa_{CO_2}.

The respiratory rate on the SensorMedics 3100A is measured in hertz. The concept of active inspiration and active expiration allows the delivery of very rapid respiratory rates without air trapping. The rate can be set from 3 to 15 Hz. The higher the respiratory rate, the smaller the tidal volume, partly because of the short cycle time at the higher rate. Conversely, the lower the rate, the larger the tidal volume because of the longer cycle time and the ability to move more volume through the circuit. The respiratory therapist must recognize that the delivered tidal volumes are very small and are equal to or less than the dead space volume. As a rule of thumb, larger babies (more than 2 kg) fall into the lower rate category (8 to 10 Hz), whereas smaller infants (less than 2 kg) fall into the smaller tidal volume requirement category and hence require a higher rate (12 to 15 Hz).

The inspiratory time on the SensorMedics 3100A is nearly always set at 33%, which has been determined to be the standard inspiratory time setting for this ventilator. Only in extreme cases (e.g., with a large patient with a severely elevated physiologic dead space) is the percent inspiratory time increased to improve carbon dioxide elimination. As with slowing of the respiratory rate, an increase in the percent inspiratory time allows a longer inspiratory phase, thus increasing the delivered tidal volume. The inspiratory time can be adjusted from 33% to 50% in 1% increments.

Management Strategies

Management strategies are divided into two categories: high lung volume and low lung volume. Most patients fall into the high lung volume management category. This means that the ventilator parameters are maximized at the clinician's discretion. The only disease that would preclude this approach is air leak syndrome. Establishing lung volume and restoring it to an acceptable level is a critical component of HFV. Because the delivered tidal volumes are small, the mean lung volume does not change dramatically during inspiration. PEEP is the primary contributor to mean airway pressure and end-expiratory lung volume during HFV.

The Bunnell Life Pulse HFV is used with a conventional ventilator. **Table 24–11** shows general management strategies for high-frequency jet ventilation. The conventional ventilator is responsible for controlling the PEEP level. Hence the mean airway pressure is controlled by the conventional ventilator, and the PIP, respiratory rate, inspiratory time, and I:E ratio are controlled by the HFJV. Once the infant's condition has stabilized, efforts are made to reduce the mean airway pressure. The PIP may be reduced gradually and the respiratory

TABLE 24–11 Patient Management Guidelines for Life Pulse High-Frequency Ventilation

1. HFV ΔP (PIP–PEEP) is the primary determinant of $Paco_2$. High-frequency ventilation (HFV) rate is secondary.
2. Resting lung volume (FRC supported by set PEEP) and mean airway pressure are crucial determinants of Pao_2.
3. Avoid hyperventilation and hypoxemia by using optimal PEEP.
4. Minimize IMV at all times using very low rates (typically 0–3 breaths/min) unless IMV is being used to dilate airways or *temporarily* recruit collapsed alveoli. In general, keep IMV PIP 10–30% < HFV PIP.
5. To overcome atelectasis, IMV rates up to 5 breaths/min can be used for 10–30 min. Thereafter, IMV rate should be decreased to 0–3 breaths/min. In general, keep IMV inspiratory time at 0.4–0.6 s.
6. If lowering IMV rate worsens oxygenation, PEEP is probably too low. Higher PEEP and lower IMV rates reduce the risk of lung injury.
7. Decrease Fio_2 before PEEP when until Fio_2 is less than 0.4.

Setting	Usual	When to Raise	When to Lower
HFV PIP	Whatever produces desired $Paco_2$	To lower $Paco_2$	To increase $Paco_2$ (increase PEEP simultaneously to keep $\bar{P}aw$ and Pao_2 constant)
HFV rate	420 breaths/min (neonates) or 300 breaths/min (children)	To decrease $Paco_2$ in *smaller* patients or to increase $\bar{P}aw$ and Pao_2	To eliminate inadvertent PEEP or hyperinflation by lengthening exhalation time or to increase $Paco_2$
HFV inspiratory time	0.02 s	To enable jet to reach PIP at low HFJV rates in *larger* patients (> 15 kg)	Keep at the minimum of 0.02 s in almost all cases
IMV rate	0–3 breaths/min	To reverse atelectasis or dilate restricted airways (3–5 breaths/min)	To minimize volutrauma (especially when air leaks are present) or decrease hemodynamic compromise
IMV PIP	PIP necessary to get adequate chest rise	To reverse atelectasis or dilate airways; PIP may be greater or less than HFJV PIP	To minimize volutrauma (especially when air leaks are present) or decrease hemodynamic compromise
IMV inspiratory time	0.4 s	To reverse atelectasis or dilate airways	To minimize volutrauma (especially when air leaks are present) or decrease hemodynamic compromise
PEEP	7–12 cm H_2O (neonates) or 10–15 cm H_2O (children)	To improve oxygenation and decrease hyperventilation; to find optimal PEEP increase PEEP until Spo_2 stays constant when switching from IMV to CPAP	Lower PEEP only when it appears that cardiac output is being compromised or when oxygenation is adequate and when decreasing PEEP does not decrease Pao_2
Fio_2	< 0.60	Increase as needed after optimizing PEEP	Lower Fio_2 in preference to PEEP when weaning until Fio_2 < 0.4

Special air leak considerations: (1) Minimize IMV by using HFV + adequate CPAP, and (2) if oxygenation is compromised, increase PEEP even if the lungs appear to be over-distended on chest radiograph. PIP, peak inspiratory pressure; PEEP, positive end-expiratory pressure; CPAP, continuous positive airway pressure; Fio_2, fraction inspired oxygen; HFV, high-frequency ventilation; HFJV, high-frequency jet ventilation; IMV, intermittent mandatory ventilation; $\bar{P}aw$, mean airway pressure.

Modified with permission from materials courtesy of Bunnell, Inc., Salt Lake City, Utah.

rate dropped to 250 to 300 breaths/min. The PEEP may also be decreased if the Pao_2 is acceptable and the patient tolerates the change.

Management of the infant on HFOV is more straightforward than with HFJV. **Table 24–12** shows general management strategies for HFOV. HFOV decouples (separates) ventilation and oxygenation. The mean airway pressure and Fio_2 control oxygenation, whereas amplitude, the percent inspiratory time, and respiratory rate determine ventilation. This simplistic approach to HFOV benefits both clinician and patient. Initially, the mean airway pressure and Fio_2 are maximized. Ventilation may be more difficult to control because the patient's size and disease determine what settings are chosen. The smaller the patient, the higher the rate setting; the percent inspiratory time is set at 33%. Amplitude (ΔP) is a more discretional setting, and the respiratory therapist must be judicious in determining it. Amplitude is what ventilates or moves the chest with HFOV. Although the setting of ΔP is arbitrary, what happens to the patient is not. The higher the amplitude setting, the more vigorously the chest wall moves or wiggles; this is called the chest wiggle factor. The clinician must determine what degree of chest wiggle is acceptable for the patient. The patient's compliance determines how aggressive the clinician is with ΔP.

One of the differences between HFOV and HFJV is that higher rather than lower mean airway pressures are required to maintain oxygenation with HFOV. Higher mean airway pressure settings are used early in the ventilatory course and weaned as tolerated when the Pao_2 level is acceptable. In HFOV the mean airway pressure is increased in increments of 1 to 2 cm H_2O, provided there is no air leak, until the Spo_2 rises above 95%, which indicates adequate lung recruitment. A chest radiograph must be obtained to ensure that inflation is adequate,

TABLE 24-12 General Guidelines for Use of High-Frequency Oscillatory Ventilation

Clinical Indicators	Therapeutic Intervention	Treatment Rationale
F_{IO_2} below 0.70		
High Pa_{CO_2} with:		
Pa_{O_2} satisfactory	Increase ΔP	Increase ΔP to achieve optimum Pa_{CO_2}
Pa_{O_2} low	Increase $\bar{P}$aw, ΔP, F_{IO_2}	Adjust $\bar{P}$aw and F_{IO_2} to improve O_2 delivery
Pa_{O_2} high	Increase ΔP; decrease F_{IO_2}	Decrease F_{IO_2} to minimize O_2 exposure
F_{IO_2} below 0.70		
Normal Pa_{CO_2} with:		
Pa_{O_2} satisfactory	Take no action	Take no action
Pa_{O_2} low	Increase $\bar{P}$aw, F_{IO_2}	Adjust $\bar{P}$aw and F_{IO_2} to improve O_2 delivery
Pa_{O_2} high	Decrease F_{IO_2}	Decrease F_{IO_2} to minimize O_2 exposure
F_{IO_2} below 0.70		
Low Pa_{CO_2} with:		
Pa_{O_2} satisfactory	Decrease ΔP	Decrease ΔP to achieve optimum Pa_{CO_2}
Pa_{O_2} low	Increase $\bar{P}$aw, F_{IO_2}; decrease ΔP	Adjust $\bar{P}$aw and F_{IO_2} to improve O_2 delivery
Pa_{O_2} high	Decrease F_{IO_2}, ΔP	Decrease F_{IO_2} to minimize O_2 exposure
F_{IO_2} above 0.70		
High Pa_{CO_2} with:		
Pa_{O_2} satisfactory	Increase ΔP	Increase ΔP to achieve optimum Pa_{CO_2}
Pa_{O_2} low	Increase F_{IO_2}, ΔP	Increase F_{IO_2} to improve Pa_{O_2}
Pa_{O_2} high	Increase ΔP; decrease $\bar{P}$aw	Decrease $\bar{P}$aw to reduce Pa_{O_2}
F_{IO_2} above 0.70		
Normal Pa_{CO_2} with:		
Pa_{O_2} satisfactory	Take no action	Take no action
Pa_{O_2} low	Increase F_{IO_2}	Increase F_{IO_2} to improve Pa_{O_2}
Pa_{O_2} high	Decrease $\bar{P}$aw, F_{IO_2}	Decrease $\bar{P}$aw and F_{IO_2} to reduce Pa_{O_2}
F_{IO_2} above 0.70		
Low Pa_{CO_2} with:		
Pa_{O_2} satisfactory	Decrease ΔP	Decrease ΔP to achieve optimum Pa_{CO_2}
Pa_{O_2} low	Increase F_{IO_2}; decrease ΔP	Increase F_{IO_2} to improve Pa_{O_2}
Pa_{O_2} high	Decrease $\bar{P}$aw, ΔP	Decrease $\bar{P}$aw and F_{IO_2} to minimize O_2 exposure

F_{IO_2}, fractional inspired oxygen concentration; Pa_{CO_2}, partial pressure of arterial carbon dioxide; Pa_{O_2}, partial pressure of arterial oxygen; ΔP, pressure amplitude; $\bar{P}$aw, mean airway pressure.

to the level of the eighth to the ninth rib. Hyperinflation can adversely affect hemodynamics, and the mean airway pressure should be reduced if hyperinflation occurs.[28] Hyperinflation also poses an increased risk of air leakage. As the patient on HFOV improves, the F_{IO_2} should be weaned to 0.6 before the mean airway pressure is reduced, unless hyperinflation is noted by chest radiograph. When the mean airway pressure has been reduced 10 to 12 cm H_2O, the clinician should consider transferring the patient back to CMV or continue weaning to extubation on HFOV.

Complications

Complications associated with HFV include tracheal injury, atelectasis, pulmonary overdistention, acute respiratory alkalosis, hypotension, decreased cardiac output, and a displaced or disconnected endotracheal tube.[35] In early uses of HFV, tracheal injury was reported in some cases, but improved humidification has eliminated this complication. Atelectasis may occur as a result of mucous plugging or low airway pressures leading to alveolar collapse, which can be prevented through maintenance of an adequate mean airway pressure. Pulmonary overdistention and cardiac compromise can result from failure to wean excessive mean airway pressures. Overdistention can cause acute lung injury, pneumothorax, and increased physiologic shunt. Patients must be monitored closely for signs of decreased systemic perfusion when HFV is initiated. A high mean airway pressure may not be tolerated. If myocardial dysfunction occurs, inotropic therapy may be indicated. Minimizing the adverse effects of an increased intrathoracic environment is an essential component of the care of the child on HFV.

An issue related to HFV is the noise caused by the ventilator, which contributes to the noise level in the neonatal and pediatric intensive care unit.[36] Newer models have been designed to operate more quietly, so this should be less of an issue as hospitals acquire new equipment.

Adjuncts to Neonatal and Pediatric Mechanical Ventilation

Preterm infants (those less than 34 weeks of gestational age) have varying degrees of lung maturity, and the respiratory needs of these infants may be significantly different than those of a full-term infant with mature lungs. Infants born at less than 35 weeks' gestation often have a surfactant deficiency. Surfactant production begins about week 23 of gestation, and the fetal lungs reach maturity at week 35. Between weeks 23 and 35, lung maturity may be enhanced in utero by administration of corticosteroids. Corticosteroids often are given to mothers at risk for premature delivery. Infants who receive corticosteroids in utero are likely to have greater lung maturity than infants of similar gestational age who were not treated with steroids in utero. However, many infants are born prematurely with either partial treatment or no treatment with steroids and have a surfactant deficiency.

Surfactant Administration

Surfactant is a combination of lipoproteins found in mature alveoli that reduces surface tension at the alveolar air–fluid interface.[37] Alveoli with low surface tension require less pressure to stabilize lung volume and avoid alveolar collapse. Infants with a surfactant deficiency often show signs of respiratory distress syndrome. The clinical findings associated with RDS are tachypnea, intercostal and sternal retractions, nasal flaring, expiratory grunting, decreased compliance, and an oxygen requirement. The typical chest radiograph of an infant with RDS has a ground glass appearance and low lung volumes. Administration of exogenous surfactant has been shown to prevent and treat RDS (**Table 24–13**). Surfactant can be given as a rescue therapy after clinical signs of RDS have developed, or prophylactic surfactant can be given in the delivery room to try to prevent the development of RDS or minimize its effects (**CPG 24–2**).[38] The evidence favors giving infants of less than 31 weeks' gestation prophylactic surfactant treatment.[39]

Surfactant is given endotracheally (**Box 24–2**). In infants at risk and those with clinical signs of RDS, intubation and early administration of surfactant are recommended. Before the surfactant is administered, the infant's compliance is reduced significantly. It may be necessary to use high pressures to ventilate a surfactant-deficient infant. Reassessment of the infant's ventilatory needs after administration of surfactant is vital. Adjustments to the ventilator are indicated as compliance increases and oxygenation improves. Maintenance of a delivered tidal volume of 4 to 6 mL/kg is achieved by a reduction in the PIP or volume setting. The F_{IO_2} must be adjusted to keep the arterial oxygen saturation in the desired range. Attention to these details is essential to reduce the risk of ventilator-induced complications.

TABLE 24–13 Commercial Surfactant Preparations

Surfactant	Description	Route of Administration	Dose (mL/kg)
Survanta	Bovine lung extract	Endotracheal	4.0
Curosurf	Isolated from minced pig lungs	Endotracheal	2.5
Infrasurf	Calf lung surfactant	Endotracheal	3.0

Inhaled Nitric Oxide

Administration of inhaled nitric oxide (iNO) has been shown to improve oxygenation in neonates with hypoxemia and pulmonary hypertension.[40,41] The primary mechanism is thought to be lowering of pulmonary vascular resistance by vasodilation of the pulmonary vasculature, resulting in decreased right-to-left shunting of blood. Inhaled NO is selective to the pulmonary vasculature and has not been associated with a lowering of systemic blood pressure. Inhaled NO can be administered with either a conventional or high-frequency ventilator. Although the optimum dose of iNO is not entirely clear, 20 ppm or less usually is sufficient. Because administration of iNO can cause methemoglobinemia, this value should be monitored during therapy.

NO and oxygen can combine to produce nitrogen dioxide (NO_2). The NO and NO_2 levels should be monitored during therapy, but a high NO_2 level usually

BOX 24–2

Administration of Surfactant

1. Determine the surfactant preparation to be used and the dose.
2. Allow the drug to reach room temperature.
3. Confirm the position of the endotracheal tube.
4. Instill the drug directly into the endotracheal tube.
5. Continuously monitor the heart rate and oxygen saturation as measured by pulse oximetry (Sp_{O_2}) during administration; also monitor for endotracheal tube obstruction.
6. Monitor tidal volume and Sp_{O_2} immediately after dose is given.
7. Adjust ventilator support as compliance changes.

CLINICAL PRACTICE GUIDELINE 24–2

Surfactant Replacement Therapy

- Surfactant can be extracted from animal lung lavage and from human amniotic fluid or produced from synthetic materials, and administered by trained personnel in delivery rooms and neonatal intensive care units. Two basic strategies for surfactant replacement have emerged: (1) prophylactic or preventive treatment, in which surfactant is administered at the time of birth or shortly thereafter to infants who are at high risk for developing respiratory distress syndrome (RDS) and (2) rescue or therapeutic treatment, in which surfactant is administered after the initiation of mechanical ventilation in infants with clinically confirmed RDS.

Indications

- Prophylactic administration may be indicated in infants at high risk of developing RDS because of short gestation (< 32 weeks) or low birth weight (< 1300 g), both of which strongly suggest lung immaturity.
- Infants in whom there is laboratory evidence of surfactant deficiency, such as a lecithin-to-sphingomyelin ratio less than 2:1 or the absence of phosphatidylglycerol.
- Rescue or therapeutic administration is indicated in preterm or full-term infants who require endotracheal intubation and mechanical ventilation because of increased work of breathing or increasing oxygen requirements mandating an increase in F_{IO_2}.
- Those with clinical evidence of RDS, including a chest radiograph characteristic of RDS.
- Mean airway pressure greater than 7 cm H_2O to maintain an adequate Pa_{O_2}, Sa_{O_2}, or Sp_{O_2}.

Contraindications

- Relative contraindications to surfactant administration are the presence of congenital anomalies incompatible with life beyond the neonatal period and respiratory distress in infants with laboratory evidence of lung maturity.

Hazards and Complications

- Procedural complications resulting from the administration of surfactant include plugging of the endotracheal tube (ETT) by surfactant
- Hemoglobin desaturation and increased need for supplemental O_2
- Bradycardia due to hypoxia
- Tachycardia due to agitation with reflux of surfactant into the ETT
- Pulmonary hemorrhage
- Marginal increase in retinopathy of prematurity
- Barotrauma resulting from increase in lung compliance following surfactant replacement and failure to change ventilator settings accordingly

Assessment of Outcome

- Reduction in F_{IO_2} requirement
- Reduction in work of breathing
- Improvement in lung volumes and lung fields as indicated by chest radiograph
- Improvement in pulmonary mechanics (e.g., compliance, tidal volume)
- Reduction in ventilator requirements (PIP, PEEP, Paw)

PIP, positive inspiratory pressure; PEEP, positive end-expiratory pressure; Paw, mean airway pressure.

Modified from AARC clinical practice guideline: surfactant replacement therapy. *Respir Care.* 1994:39(8):824–829. Reprinted with permission.

can be prevented with proper delivery equipment. The NO concentration is reduced once oxygenation is stable. Continuous monitoring with pulse oximetry as the NO concentration is reduced is essential. Before NO is discontinued, the F_{IO_2} can be increased by 10% to 20% to prevent a rebound effect. During the administration of NO, the manual resuscitation bag at the bedside should be adapted to provide NO in the event manual ventilation is required to avoid abrupt withdrawal of NO and rebound. NO should not flow into the reservoir of the resuscitation bag until needed to avoid production of NO_2.

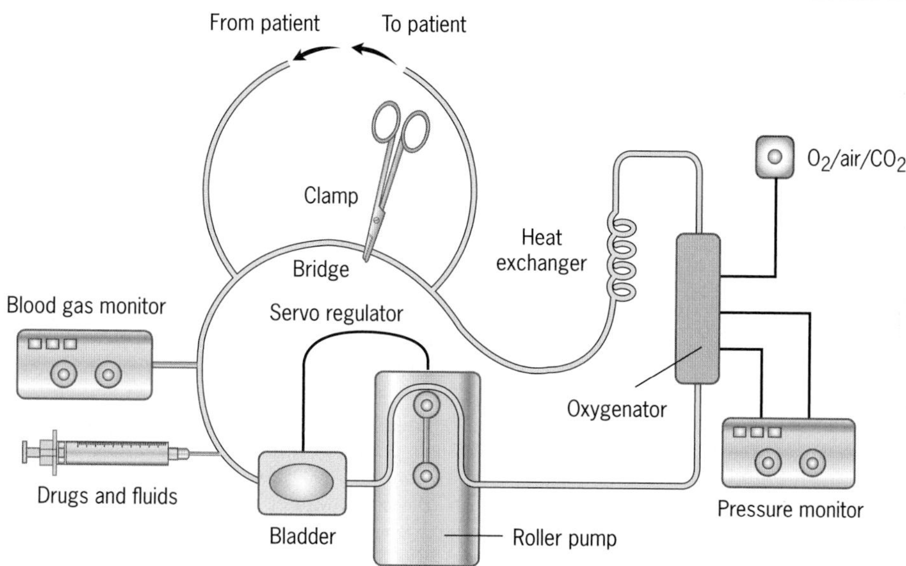

FIGURE 24–20 Schematic drawing of an extracorporeal membrane oxygenation (ECMO) system. Adapted from English PA, Hess DR. Extracorporeal life support. In: Branson RD, Hess DR, Chatburn RL, eds. *Respiratory Care Equipment.* 2nd ed. Lippincott Williams & Wilkins; 1999.

TABLE 24–14 Neonatal Cases by Diagnosis

Diagnosis	Number of Patients Receiving ECLS	Percentage of Patients Surviving
MAS	7513	94
CDH	5821	51
Sepsis	2600	75
PFC/PPHN	3793	78
RDS	1474	84
Other	2294	63

ECLS, extracorporeal life support; CDH, congenital diaphragmatic hernia; MAS, meconium aspiration syndrome; PPHN, persistent pulmonary hypertension of the newborn; RDS, respiratory distress syndrome.

Courtesy of the Extracorporeal Life Support Organization (ELSO). July 2009 International Summary. Ann Arbor, Michigan.

Extracorporeal Life Support

Extracorporeal life support (ECLS) can support neonatal and pediatric patients and reduce mortality during severe respiratory failure (**Table 24–14**).[41,42] Approximately 77% of the more than 28,000 neonatal and pediatric patients treated with ECLS have survived.[43] ECLS requires cannulation of the right heart. Blood is drained from this cannula into a circuit containing a membrane oxygenator and a pump (**Figure 24–20**). Oxygen circulates through one side of the membrane, and blood is pumped through the other side. The difference in partial pressures causes oxygen diffusion into the blood and elimination of carbon dioxide from the blood. The oxygenated blood is warmed and returned to the infant. The blood can be reinfused through a separate lumen of the drainage cannula (venovenous support) or through an additional cannula placed in the carotid artery (venoarterial support). Both methods of ECLS improve delivery of oxygen to the tissues.

Although ECLS does not specifically treat the underlying condition, it allows time for conditions to improve by reducing the risk of further lung damage from high airway pressures and high oxygen concentrations. While the patient is receiving ECLS, ventilator support generally is minimized with lung rest strategies. PEEP is applied to maintain the functional residual capacity with an occasional positive pressure breath (usually 6 to 10 breaths/min), but ventilation and oxygenation are primarily achieved from the extracorporeal support. Additional treatments aimed at the underlying cause of respiratory failure are continued. For example, pulmonary hygiene for an infant with meconium aspiration and antibiotics for a septic infant help improve native gas exchange, and ECLS generally is discontinued after 5 to 7 days.

A disadvantage of ECLS is that systemic anticoagulation is required to reduce the risk of clot formation as the blood is circulated through various circuit components. Intracranial, pulmonary, and surgical site bleeding, as well as air embolization and circuit complications, have been associated with ECLS. Because of the need for anticoagulation with the increased risk of intracranial hemorrhage, premature infants generally are not considered candidates for ECLS.

KEY POINTS

- Awareness and understanding of maternal risk factors is crucial for the identification of newborns at risk for life-threatening complications.
- A specific sequence of events for neonatal resuscitation is outlined in the American Academy of Pediatrics Neonatal Resuscitation Program (NRP).
- Excessive use of oxygen could lead to retinopathy of prematurity and bronchopulmonary dysplasia in the premature infant.
- Positive pressure ventilation usually begins with bag-mask ventilation.
- Nasal CPAP and NIV are used to aid lung recruitment and to minimize airway collapse.
- Uncuffed oral endotracheal tubes are most commonly used in neonates.

- Infant ventilators are either conventional or high-frequency ventilators.
- Traditional conventional neonatal ventilators are continuous flow, time cycled, and pressure limited.
- High-frequency ventilators are classified as high-frequency positive pressure ventilation, high-frequency jet ventilation, high-frequency flow interrupter ventilation, and high-frequency oscillatory ventilation.
- High lung volume and low lung volume management styles are used for high-frequency ventilation.
- Adjuncts to neonatal mechanical ventilation include surfactant administration, inhaled nitric oxide, and extracorporeal life support.

REFERENCES

1. Neonatal resuscitation guidelines. *Circulation.* 2005;112 (suppl I):IV-188–IV-195.
2. Thebaud B, Mercier JC, Dinh-Xuan AT. Congenital diaphragmatic hernia: a cause of persistent pulmonary hypertension of the newborn which lacks an effective therapy. *Biol Neonate.* 1998:74(5):323–336.
3. Iliff A, Le VA. Pulse rate, respiratory rate, and body temperature of children between two months and eighteen years of age. *Child Dev.* 1952;23:237.
4. American Academy of Pediatrics, American College of Obstetricians and Gynaecologists. *Guidelines for Perinatal Care.* 4th ed. Elk Grove Village, IL; 1997.
5. Deakins KM. Bronchopulmonary dysplasia. *Respir Care.* 2009;54(9):1252–1262.
6. Mondolfi AA, Grenier BM, Thompson JE, et al. Comparison of self-inflating bags with anesthesia bags for bag-mask ventilation in the pediatric emergency department. *Pediatr Emerg Care.* 1997;13:312–316.
7. Pediatric advanced life support. *Circulation.* 2005;112 (suppl I):IV-167–IV-187.
8. Parwani VHI-H, Hsu B, Hoffman RJ. Experienced emergency physicians cannot safely or accurately inflate endotracheal tube cuffs or estimate endotracheal tube cuff pressure using standard technique. *Acad Emerg Med.* 2004;11:490–491.
9. Bailey C, Kattwinkel J, Teja K, et al. Shallow versus deep endotracheal suctioning in young rabbits: pathologic effects on the tracheobronchial wall. *Pediatrics.* 1988;82:746–751.
10. Hess DR. Managing the artificial airway. *Respir Care.* 1999;44:759–772.
11. Davis S, Jones M, Kisling J, et al. Effect of continuous positive airway pressure on forced expiratory flows in infants with tracheomalacia. *Am J Respir Crit Care Med.* 1998;158:148–152.
12. Panitch HB, Allen JL, Alpert BE, et al. Effects of CPAP on lung mechanics in infants with acquired tracheobronchomalacia. *Am J Respir Crit Care Med.* 1994;150:1341–1346.
13. Walsh BK, Brooks TM, Grenier BM. Oxygen therapy in the neonatal care environment. *Respir Care.* 2009;54(9):1193–1202.
14. Finer NN, Mannino FL. High-flow nasal cannula: a kinder, gentler CPAP? *J Pediatr.* 2009;154:160–162.
15. Gupta S, Sinha S, Tin W, Donn S. A randomized controlled trial of post-extubation bubble continuous positive airway pressure versus infant flow driver continuous positive airway pressure in preterm infants with respiratory distress syndrome. *J Pediatr.* 2009;154:645–650.
16. Diblasi RM. Nasal continuous airway pressure (CPAP) for the respiratory care of the newborn infant. *Respir Care.* 2009;54(9):1209–1235.
17. Courtney SE, Barrington KJ. Continuous positive airway pressure and noninvasive ventilation. *Clin Perinatol.* 2007;34:73–92.
18. Kahn DJ, Habib RH, Courtney SE. Effects of flow amplitudes on intraprong pressures during bubble versus ventilator generated nasal continuous positive airway pressure in premature infants. *Pediatrics.* 2008;122:1009–1013.
19. Loh LE, Chan YH, Chan I. Noninvasive ventilation in children: a review. *J Pediatr (Rio J).* 2007;83(2 suppl):S91–99.
20. Ramanathan R. Optimal ventilatory strategies and surfactant to protect the preterm lungs. *Neonatology.* 2008;93:302–308.
21. AARC clinical practice guidelines: neonatal time-triggered, pressure-limited, time-cycled mechanical ventilation. *Respir Care.* 1994;39:808–816.
22. Donn SM, Boon W. Mechanical ventilation of the neonate: should we target volume or pressure? *Respir Care.* 2009;54:1236–1243.
23. Marchese AD, Chipman D, de la Oliva P, Kacmarek RM. Adult ICU ventilators to provide neonatal ventilation: a lung simulator study. *Intensive Care Med.* 2009;35:631–638.
24. McCallion N, Davis PG, Morley CJ. Volume-targeted versus pressure-limited ventilation in the neonate. *Cochrane Database Syst Rev.* 2005;3:D003666.
25. Cheifetz IM. Invasive and noninvasive pediatric mechanical ventilation. *Respir Care.* 2003;48:442.
26. Waugh JB, Deshpande VM, Brown MK, Harwood RJ. *Rapid Interpretation of Ventilator Waveforms.* 2nd ed. Upper Saddle River, NJ: Pearson, Prentice Hall; 2007.
27. Chatburn RL. Physiologic and methodologic issues regarding humidity therapy. *J Pediatr.* 1989;114:416–420.
28. Courtney SE, Asselin JM. High-frequency jet and oscillatory ventilation for neonates: which strategy and when? *Respir Care Clin North Am.* 2006;12(3):453–467.
29. Sjostrand UH. Review of the physiological rationale for and development of high-frequency positive pressure ventilation. *Acta Anaesthesiol Scand.* 1977;64:7–27.
30. Hess D, Mason S, Branson R. High-frequency ventilation design and equipment issues. *Respir Care Clin North Am.* 2001;7:577–598.
31. Smith R. Ventilation at high respiratory frequencies. *Anaesthesia.* 1982;37:1011.
32. Chunk HK. Mechanisms of gas transport during ventilation by high-frequency oscillation. *J Appl Physiol.* 1984;56:553.
33. Fredberg JJ, Glass GM, Boynton BR, et al. Features influencing mechanical performance of neonatal high-frequency ventilators. *J Appl Physiol.* 1987;62:2485–2490.
34. Taylor GI. Dispersion of matter in turbulent flow through a pipe. *Proc R Soc Lond B Biol Sci.* 1954;223:446–448.
35. Boros SJ, Mammel MC, Lewullen PK, et al. Necrotizing tracheobronchitis: a complication of high-frequency ventilation. *J Pediatr.* 1986;109:95.
36. Hoehn T, Busch A, Krause ME. Comparison of noise levels caused by four different high-frequency ventilators. *Intensive Care Med.* 2000;26:84–87.
37. Been JV, Zimmermann LJI. What's new in surfactant? *Eur J Pediatr.* 2007;166:889–899.
38. AARC clinical practice guidelines: surfactant replacement therapy. *Respir Care.* 1994:39(8):824–829.
39. Halliday HL. Surfactants: past, present and future. *J Perinatol.* 2008;28:S47–S56.
40. Neonatal Inhaled Nitric Oxide Study Group. Inhaled nitric oxide in full-term and nearly full-term infants with hypoxic respiratory failure. *N Engl J Med.* 1997;336:597–604.
41. Roberts JD Jr, Fineman JR, Morin FC III, et al. Inhaled nitric oxide and persistent pulmonary hypertension of the newborn: the Inhaled Nitric Oxide Study Group. *N Engl J Med.* 1997;336:605–610.
42. Betit P, Craig N. Extracorporeal membrane oxygenation for neonatal respiratory failure. *Respir Care.* 2009;54(9);1244–1251.
43. Conrad SA, Rycu PT. The ELSO registry. In: Van Meurs K, Lally KP, Peek G, Zwischenberger JB, eds. *ECMO: Extracorporeal Cardiopulmonary Support in Critical Care.* 3rd ed. Ann Arbor, MI: Extracorporeal Life Support Organization; 2005.

CHAPTER 25

Pulmonary Rehabilitation

Neil R. MacIntyre

OUTLINE

OBJECTIVES

1. Define pulmonary rehabilitation.
2. List the team members that compose a pulmonary rehabilitation program.
3. Compare intensive programs, maintenance programs, and perioperative programs.
4. Identify candidates for a pulmonary rehabilitation program.
5. Describe the components of patient assessment in a comprehensive pulmonary rehabilitation program.
6. Describe the role of education in a pulmonary rehabilitation program.
7. Discuss the benefits of upper and lower extremity exercise training in a pulmonary rehabilitation program.
8. Explain the guidelines used to prescribe an exercise training program.
9. Discuss the roles of the following in a pulmonary rehabilitation program: psychological therapies, physical therapy, individualized instruction, nutrition counseling, and pharmacologic therapy.

KEY TERMS

Borg Scale of Perceived Exertion	exertional dyspnea
breathing retraining	healthcare utilization
chronic lung disease	intensive program
exercise assessment	maintenance program
exercise capacity	perioperative program
exercise training	pulmonary rehabilitation

INTRODUCTION

Comprehensive **pulmonary rehabilitation** is a concept that has evolved steadily over the last 50 years.[1–4] Prior to that time, the standard therapy for patients with **chronic lung disease** was rest and avoidance of physical activity. In the early 1960s, however, studies challenged this standard therapy by demonstrating that exercise training in patients with chronic obstructive pulmonary disease (COPD) not only resulted in training effects similar to those observed in normal subjects but also promoted a state of well-being.[5–9] Numerous investigations followed that supported these initial findings. Almost universally, the early investigations supported three conclusions:

1. Exercise training in patients with COPD increases **exercise capacity**.
2. Exercise training improves the patient's psychological state.
3. Exercise training *does not* improve pulmonary function.

As a consequence of these developments, the American College of Chest Physicians (ACCP) in 1974 and the American Thoracic Society (ATS) in 1981 both formally recognized the effectiveness of pulmonary rehabilitation and offered the following definition:

> Pulmonary rehabilitation may be defined as an art of medical practice wherein an individually tailored multidisciplinary program is formulated, which, through accurate diagnosis, therapy, emotional support, and education, stabilizes or reverses both the physio- and psychopathology of pulmonary diseases and attempts to return the patient to the highest possible functional capacity allowed by his pulmonary handicap and overall life situation.[1]

Since the 1970s, there has been a steady growth in the number of pulmonary rehabilitation programs. These programs have become increasingly multidisciplinary and comprehensive, incorporating psychological, nutritional, and vocational support; oxygen therapy; bronchial hygiene; education; and, of course, exercise. Along with this growth has come the development of professional societies (e.g., the American Association of Cardiovascular and Pulmonary Rehabilitation [AACVPR]), professional standards, accreditation and certification programs, and ongoing efforts to obtain proper third-party reimbursement.[2–4]

Mechanisms of Functional Deterioration in Patients with Chronic Lung Disease

Without a sudden event to stimulate a change in lifestyle, chronic pulmonary disease patients, unlike cardiac patients, generally have a long, slow, downhill course. Chronic lung disease progressively damages lung tissue and airways and, over a period of years, ultimately results in a depletion of ventilatory reserves.[10] Complicating this physiologically are abnormalities in gas exchange and elevations in pulmonary vascular pressures that lead to right ventricular dysfunction. Finally, data have demonstrated that an ongoing systemic inflammatory process from chronic disease can impair skeletal muscle function.[11] All these factors contribute to the sensation of dyspnea and the resultant limitation on physical activity.

> **RESPIRATORY RECAP**
>
> **Pulmonary Rehabilitation**
>
> » Pulmonary rehabilitation is a multidisciplinary, multifaceted approach to chronic lung disease management.
>
> » Pulmonary rehabilitation has been endorsed by all of the major respiratory societies.

As dyspnea and exercise capacity worsen, the need for medical care increases and the patient's ability for self-care decreases; a confusing combination of functional limitations, complex medical regimens, and dependence on others is thrust on the patient. The net effect is a profound sense of loss of control, with consequent depression and anxiety.[10]

These factors are further worsened by the vicious cycle of inactivity (**Figure 25–1**). The cycle begins when the patient starts to associate **exertional dyspnea** with the disease and no longer recognizes dyspnea as a normal response to exertion. In this setting, exertional dyspnea promotes increased levels of anxiety, depression, and fear of exertion, all of which generally lead to an "exertion phobia" and a reduction in physical activity. The lack of exercise, in turn, leads to both central and peripheral deconditioning and, ultimately, to decreased endurance and weakness, and often to muscular atrophy. As a result of deconditioning, the patient experiences greater dyspnea, an even greater intolerance to exertion, and further loss of functional capacity. As the cycle continues, the patient's exercise capacity spirals progressively downward while the levels of fear, anxiety, and depression increase unabated. As the patient becomes progressively more physically and psychologically incapacitated, the consumption of medical resources increases dramatically. The progressive loss of exercise capacity resulting from the vicious cycle of inactivity is superimposed on the underlying functional reduction caused by the lung disease.

> **RESPIRATORY RECAP**
>
> **Goal of Pulmonary Rehabilitation**
>
> » Functional loss in chronic lung disease is multifactorial and involves respiratory dysfunction as well as cardiovascular, skeletal muscle, and metabolic factors.
>
> » The goal of pulmonary rehabilitation is to improve functional capacity by addressing all of these factors.

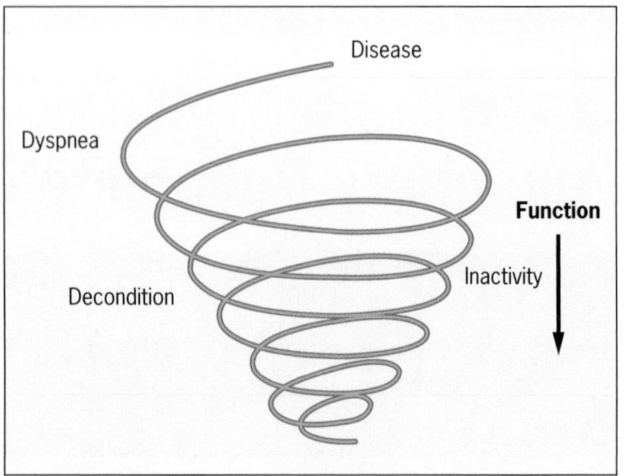

FIGURE 25–1 The downward spiral of functional loss induced by lung disease and accelerated by resulting inactivity.

The goal of pulmonary rehabilitation is to improve the quality of life of patients with chronic lung disease by increasing their functional capacity and sense of well-being. Central to achieving this goal is to break this cycle of inactivity with the institution of a life-long exercise program. The comprehensive nature of pulmonary rehabilitation facilitates this fundamental lifestyle change not only by directing and encouraging formal exercise but also by maximizing all aspects of chronic lung disease management.

Program Structure

The basic elements of today's pulmonary rehabilitation program were first outlined by the 1981 ATS statement on pulmonary rehabilitation[1] and later formalized in the AACVPR guidelines and program certification process.[4] Even within these established guidelines, however, the potential exists for diversity in the structure of pulmonary rehabilitation programs. This potential diversity results from consideration of several factors at the time the pulmonary rehabilitation program is under development, including the patient population, the available physical facilities, and the available pool of health professionals.

The pulmonary rehabilitation team is usually a multidisciplinary team that consists of a pulmonary physician and a number of other health professionals that can include respiratory therapists, physical therapists, psychologists, nutritionists, occupational therapists, social workers, chaplains, and respiratory nurses, among others. Although this implies the necessity for a large, diverse team, the recommended services for pulmonary rehabilitation may be provided by far fewer personnel if the individuals are appropriately trained in the evaluation

> **RESPIRATORY RECAP**
>
> **Pulmonary Rehabilitation Programs**
>
> » Pulmonary rehabilitation programs are based on exercise training, education, and psychosocial support.
>
> » Pulmonary rehabilitation is a life-long process, with formal programs usually being either several week-long intensive programs or life-long maintenance programs.
>
> » In recent years, pulmonary rehabilitation programs focusing on perioperative patients have emerged.

and management of pulmonary disease patients. The ultimate provider of the essential services depends on the health professionals available to the program and the size of the facility and will likely vary from program to program.

Pulmonary rehabilitation programs often provide two types of programs: a short-term, intensive program that provides an intense focus on pulmonary rehabilitation; and a long-term maintenance program that is less time consuming.

Intensive Programs

Intensive programs generally provide two to five sessions per week for periods of 4 to 12 weeks. The emphasis of the intensive program is on exercise training, education, medication optimization, bronchial hygiene, and psychosocial support. In addition to respiratory therapists, other healthcare specialists who contribute regularly to the program through the educational component could include an exercise physiologist, a clinical pharmacist, a nutritionist, a pulmonary nurse clinician, a physical therapist, and an occupational therapist. Individual consultations with specialists in nutrition, psychology, and smoking cessation are common. The intense focus of this program produces recognized benefits sooner than less intensive programs—a factor that enhances patient motivation.

Maintenance Programs

Maintenance programs serve primarily as medically supervised facility- or home-based programs for pulmonary disease patients who reside locally. Enrollment is usually limited to patients who have successfully completed the intensive program. Programs are generally open daily, and participants select their own schedules. Although program emphasis is on exercise conditioning, all intensive program services are available to these participants as needed. Long-term social interaction with peers and the formation of support groups are major advantages of the maintenance program.

Perioperative Programs

In recent years, another type of program has emerged in some centers that focuses on the perioperative management of patients receiving lung volume reduction surgery or lung transplantation.[12] In **perioperative programs**, the preoperative period functions much like the intensive program described earlier and is designed to optimize a patient's functional status prior to surgery. In the postoperative period, these programs are designed to restore and improve function as the patient recovers from the surgery.

The Process of Pulmonary Rehabilitation

Patient Selection

Any patient with stable chronic respiratory disease who is symptomatic and experiences dyspnea on exertion should be considered a candidate for pulmonary rehabilitation. In addition, candidates must be free of acute illness (including unstable other medical conditions such as ischemic coronary disease) and motivated to lead a more active life.

The clinical description of patients who potentially may benefit from pulmonary rehabilitation has broadened over the years. In the original position statement published by the ATS in 1981, the section on patient selection mentioned only patients with COPD.[1] Recent evidence, however, has demonstrated that multidisciplinary pulmonary rehabilitation programs are also of value in the management of patients with restrictive and other pulmonary diseases.[12,13] These findings should encourage acceptance of patients with non-COPD pulmonary diseases as well as those with COPD into pulmonary rehabilitation programs.

The observation that patients with limited ventilatory capacity may be unable to exercise with sufficient intensity to receive a training effect has raised concern over whether they could derive benefits from a comprehensive pulmonary rehabilitation program. Although evidence of a true training effect in this group of patients remains controversial, at a minimum they can benefit from a program designed to improve coordination, muscle strength, suppleness, and state of well-being. Even exercise capacity may be improved in patients with limited ventilatory capacity, since the standard training effect is only one of several ways in which exercise capacity is known to increase.[6,14]

Concern that exercise might precipitate respiratory failure by overloading weakened respiratory muscles leads to speculation that exercise training might be contraindicated in hypercapnic COPD patients. It has been shown, however, that hypercapnic COPD patients with severe ventilatory impairment and respiratory muscle weakness tolerate exercise and benefit significantly from intensive pulmonary rehabilitation.[5–8] Similarly, exercise hypoxemia has been considered by some to be a contraindication to an exercise program. However, appropriate supplemental oxygen and proper monitoring (e.g., oximetry) allow such patients to participate fully in all aspects of the exercise program.[15]

Patient Assessment

A comprehensive patient evaluation is essential to attaining the goals of pulmonary rehabilitation and is the foundation on which the individually tailored program is constructed. Any condition or attitude that potentially limits the patient's ability to perform desired activities or grasp essential information must be identified by the healthcare team, assessed, and ultimately addressed. All members of the rehabilitation team are vital participants in the process of gathering and evaluating information from patient questionnaires, interviews, and a variety of clinical evaluations.

The first step in this assessment is to make an accurate diagnosis of the patient's pulmonary problem and any complicating medical problems. The diagnosis should be substantiated by history, physical examination, pulmonary function testing, and, as needed, chest roentgenography and other laboratory tests. Other diseases or medical problems that may have a potential impact on the rehabilitation process also must be identified. These include rhinitis/sinusitis, hypertension, gastrointestinal conditions, and arrhythmias or coronary artery disease. Other potentially complicating diseases include diabetes, obesity, osteoporosis, and stroke. Once proper diagnoses are made, an appropriate medication regimen can be established.

Exercise assessment is a critical component of participants prior to entering a rehabilitation program. These assessments perform two functions: they quantitate the level of disability and provide information for setting initial exercise loads (see below) and program expectations, and they provide insight into the various cardiorespiratory factors that are involved in the functional disabilities. This permits focused therapies to be done. For instance, detecting exercise hemoglobin desaturation would lead to oxygen therapy, whereas detecting exercise bronchospasm would lead to better bronchodilator therapy, and detecting exercise cardiac dysrhythmias would prompt a more thorough cardiovascular exam. Moreover, subjects who reach a maximal predicted heart rate without reaching ventilatory or gas exchange limits can be expected to derive particular benefit from the cardiovascular training effects of exercise.

In the Duke University program, symptom-limited maximal exercise assessment is performed on all incoming pulmonary rehabilitation patients.[14] Over the years, these tests have detected hemoglobin desaturation with exercise in 34% of patients. In the non-oxygen-requiring patients, ventilation limitations (exercise ventilation/maximal ventilatory volume > 70% or rising $Pa{CO_2}$) were present in 27%, and cardiovascular limitations (maximum heart rate > 80% of predicted maximum) were present in 37%. These data illustrate the wide variety of physiologic derangements of these patients and the importance of designing exercise therapy regimens appropriate to the patient's limitations.

Because psychological disturbances are common in patients with chronic lung disease, psychosocial assessment is important prior to participation in a pulmonary rehabilitation program.[16,17] The most common emotional consequences of COPD are depression and anxiety, which can further reinforce social isolation and inactivity. Cognitive function has also been shown to be impaired in these patients, perhaps as a consequence of chronic hypoxemia. Medications and psychotherapy can be provided as necessary.

Other assessments necessary prior to beginning pulmonary rehabilitation include physical therapy evaluations, nutritional evaluations, occupational therapy evaluations (especially activities of daily living), and an educational assessment for the patient's knowledge and understanding of the disease process and its management. ACCP/AACVPR guidelines[4] also recommend electrocardiograms, complete blood counts, and serum electrolyte levels. A particularly important assessment is tobacco usage. Although it is reasonable to allow current smokers to participate in a rehabilitation program, formal efforts should be made to persuade the patient to discontinue smoking.

Education

A primary purpose of the educational component of pulmonary rehabilitation is to provide the framework for self-care. Through an educational process of instruction, supervision, and practice, patients can acquire an awareness of their disease and its management that allows them to take responsibility for their own care. A spouse, family member, or close friend who participates in the educational activities can provide familial understanding of the disease process and can reinforce the recommended self-care techniques in the home setting.

The educational process usually consists of a combination of lectures, discussions, demonstrations, and practice sessions. During all program activities, the patient's knowledge and ability to perform self-management techniques are continually reinforced. Topics typically covered in formal lectures and discussion sessions include the anatomy and physiology of the lung, the pathophysiology of chronic lung disease, pulmonary medications, nutrition, physiologic responses to exercise, sexual concerns, travel concerns, coping with chronic lung disease, early recognition and management of infections and exacerbations, and psychosocial issues.

Medication management is a critical component of the educational process. The array of inhaled medication options can be bewildering to patients. This bewilderment is further amplified by the complexity of aerosol delivery systems associated with proprietary medications. Considerable education time may be required to ensure that patients have a good working knowledge of their medication regimens.

Another key educational component is the management of COPD exacerbations.[18,19] The cost of treating exacerbations is the single most expensive aspect of caring for the COPD patient. Importantly, patients can be taught to recognize signs and symptoms of an exacerbation developing. An action plan under these circumstances can include transient increased dosing of bronchodilators, prompt initiation of antibiotics, and pulse steroid therapy. Aborting an exacerbation early can lead to reduced need for hospitalizations and a faster return to baseline function.

Respiratory therapy and physical therapy techniques are more appropriately presented in either individual or group demonstrations and in practice sessions. These topics include cleaning and care of equipment; proper use of metered dose inhalers and spacers; relaxation techniques; clearing of secretions using techniques of controlled coughing, postural drainage, percussion, and vibration; and supplemental oxygen therapy. Educational material in the form of pamphlets, booklets, and books is available from a multitude of sources, including the American Lung Association. This additional information should be used to support and reinforce the information the patient receives in the lectures, discussions, and demonstrations.

Breathing retraining traditionally has been a key aspect of the educational component of a pulmonary rehabilitation program. Pursed-lip breathing and diaphragmatic breathing are commonly used concomitantly to reduce shortness of breath and improve gas exchange. By using pursed-lip breathing, patients may be able to maintain adequate oxygenation without supplemental oxygen.

The success of the program's educational process may be assessed by providing testing on didactic information before and after instruction and by requiring each patient to satisfactorily demonstrate the recommended management techniques.

Exercise

In general, the **exercise training** experience provided by the pulmonary rehabilitation program should expose the patient to a balance of three types of exercise: stretching and flexibility exercises, strengthening exercises, and endurance exercises. Stretching and flexibility exercises are usually part of a floor exercise routine that develops suppleness, improves range of motion, and helps provide a general warm-up. Strength training may be obtained as part of the floor exercise routine by performing exercises with dumbbells, cuff weights, or a stretch band. Pulmonary patients also do well with free weights and weight machines for strength training. Strength exercises require a stimulus of high intensity and low frequency. General endurance training involves exercises that produce a cardiopulmonary stress that results in elevated heart rate (HR) and ventilation. Such exercises include walking, rowing, swimming, water aerobics, cycling (arm or leg), stair climbing, and so on, provided that the exercise intensity produces sufficient cardiopulmonary stress. Compared with strength training, endurance training is of lower intensity and higher frequency.

The benefits of exercise training are, for the most part, specific to the muscles and tasks involved in training.[5–7] For instance, a walking program will produce significant improvement in walking performance but not in swimming or biking performance. It is important, therefore, to consider the particular mode of exercise in conjunction with the needs and goals of the patient. If a patient has a stated goal that requires improvement in stair climbing, this should be one of the modes of exercise in the prescription. Walking is generally considered an essential exercise because of its prevalence in daily activities; probably for that reason, most exercise training prescriptions use predominantly lower extremity exercises.

Many patients with chronic airway obstruction experience marked shortness of breath when they use their arms for even simple tasks. Arm exercise may contribute to the dyspnea by contributing to ventilatory muscle fatigue, by placing a load on an already stressed system, and by placing a nonventilatory demand on shoulder girdle muscles that have been recruited to act as accessory muscles of respiration. Improvement in upper extremity function as a result of specific upper extremity exercises has been demonstrated in patients with COPD. Improvement in upper extremity function has been observed to carry over to self-care, leisure, and other arm activities. Combining arm and leg exercises in a training program for patients with chronic airway obstruction has been shown not only to increase exercise performance in both upper and lower extremities but also to significantly improve patients' state of well-being, which was greater in the combined training than in either arm or leg training alone. The conclusion is that leg and arm exercise should be combined in exercise programs for patients with chronic airway obstruction.

Upper extremity exercise training may be accomplished through simple games or activities that use the arms above shoulder height (e.g., passing an object overhead) or gravity-resistive exercises (e.g., performing arm circles at shoulder height, walking with exaggerated arm movement with hand weights). Upper extremity strength training may be achieved by performing exercises with free weights, pulley systems, or weight machines. Arm endurance training may be accomplished with an arm ergometer, rowing machine, combined arm/leg bicycle, or cross-country ski machine.

Well-established guidelines exist for prescribing the intensity of endurance exercise for normal subjects as well as for cardiac patients. These guidelines are based on target exercise heart rates expressed as a percentage of the predicted maximum HR. Application of these guidelines, however, may not always be appropriate to pulmonary patients because the ventilatory impairment may prevent the patient from reaching the predicted maximum HR.[6,7]

The initial load prescription should be of sufficiently low intensity that it can be accomplished by the patient without discomfort. Nothing destroys a patient's motivation faster than failure to complete the initial exercise or experiencing significant discomfort during or after the first exercise session. The initial loads used by the Duke University Pulmonary Rehabilitation Program for the stationary bicycle and arm ergometer are based on the maximum workload reached during the exercise stress test (W_{max}). The initial bicycle workload (W_{bike}) is set at 50% of the maximum workload ($0.5 \times W_{max}$). This value is based on data suggesting that an individual can be expected to work for 8 hours at 50% of maximum work capacity without undue fatigue. The initial load prescription for arm exercise is 30% of W_{max} (or 60% of W_{bike}) and is based on studies showing that the aerobic power of the arms ranges from 50% to 70% of the maximum power output of the legs.[6,7]

Workloads must be reassessed each exercise session and adjusted according to the patient's progress. Following the initial settings, the appropriate intensity for subsequent target workload (the desired training load) has been an area of controversy. Work from Cassaburi and colleagues suggests that training intensity should be pushed to a training effect (i.e., up to 70% to 80% predicted maximal HR) if at all possible.[7] Even patients with ventilatory or gas exchange limitations who cannot reach these target heart rates also appear to benefit from higher rather than lower levels of exercise. Thus, strategies using target intensities reaching the highest level attained on the initial exercise stress test should be the ultimate goal.

> **RESPIRATORY RECAP**
>
> **The Process of Pulmonary Rehabilitation**
>
> » Patients appropriate for pulmonary rehabilitation are those with chronic lung disease and resulting functional impairment.
>
> » Patient assessment should include a general physical exam, a medication review, an exercise test, a psychosocial assessment, and a search for comorbidities that would impair exercise training.
>
> » Program content should include comprehensive educational services (e.g., lectures, demonstrations, practice sessions), intensive exercise training (with careful monitoring), psychosocial support sessions, and the availability of consultative services such as psychology and nutrition.

To accomplish the transition from the relatively low initial loads to the higher target loads, the **Borg Scale of Perceived Exertion** is used as a measure of perceived stress (**Figure 25–2**), and the exercise heart rate as a measure of cardiopulmonary stress.[20] If the Borg rating of the previous exercise session is less than 15 and the HR during exercise is less than the HR achieved during the assessment exercise test, consideration is given to increasing the exercise intensity. Whenever the patient is capable of performing a given load for the duration of the exercise session, the load is increased by 0.25 kilopond for the bicycle ergometer (about 12.5 watts) and 50 kilopond/min for the arm ergometer (about 9 watts). After approximately six exercise sessions, most patients will have attained an exercise level representing a high percentage of the target workload.

Rating	Perception of Effort
6	
7	Very, very light
8	
9	Very light
10	
11	Fairly light
12	
13	Somewhat hard
14	
15	Hard
16	
17	Very hard
18	
19	Very, very hard
20	

FIGURE 25–2 The Borg Scale of Perceived Exertion.

Whenever the patient experiences significant symptoms of fatigue or dyspnea, instead of stopping exercise, the load is reduced while the patient is encouraged to complete the exercise if possible. When the initial load is already the lowest possible, the patient stops until the symptoms subside and then continues the exercise to completion. The duration of the rest period is considered part of the exercise period. The short-term goal then becomes reducing the number of rests during the exercise period.

The recommended minimum duration and frequency of endurance exercise is no less than 20 minutes three times per week.[3,4] Increasing the duration and frequency beyond this minimum must take into consideration the motivation and goals of the patient, and balance the time spent in training against the benefits derived from a more intense training regimen. The primary benefits of spending additional time on training are faster and greater improvement in physical capacity.

All exercise training should be performed under conditions of adequate arterial oxygenation ($Pa_{O_2} > 55$ mm Hg, $Sp_{O_2} > 88\%$).[3,4] If the initial patient assessment has determined that the resting oxygenation is low or that significant desaturation occurs with exertion, supplemental oxygen must be provided to the patient to maintain adequate oxygen saturation. Usually, oxygen delivered at 2 L/min via nasal cannula is sufficient. In some cases, however, it may be difficult to provide adequate oxygenation during exertion with even a partial rebreathing system. When adequate oxygenation cannot be maintained, either the intensity of the exercise must be reduced or the patient must be instructed to stop exercising until oxygenation is again adequate. Besides reducing the medical risk associated with low oxygenation, supplemental oxygen often allows the patient who needs oxygen to exercise for a longer duration at a higher intensity, thereby enhancing the beneficial effects of the exercise.

An interesting additional application for supplemental oxygen may be in patients who have some degree of rest or exercise hemoglobin desaturation but who do not fall to critical levels that impair cardiac function or oxygen delivery (i.e., they remain above Pao_2 values of 60 mm Hg or Spo_2 values above 90%). In this group, oxygen therapy will have little impact on cardiac function or oxygen delivery but may reduce carotid body (i.e., oxygen receptor) output, thereby reducing dyspnea and allowing exercise training at a higher level.[15] This concept needs further study.

Other Interventions

Other focused interventions often depend on the individual patient. Patients with clinically important depression or anxiety may need focused psychological therapies; patients with orthopedic impairments may benefit from physical therapy; patients with specific educational needs (e.g., medication understanding, equipment operation, chest physical therapy procedures) may need individualized instruction; patients with nutritional issues may need nutrition counseling.

Physician review of the medication regimen is particularly important. Chronic medical therapy for COPD and other chronic lung diseases is constantly evolving, and the array of medications (e.g., short- and long-acting beta agonists, short- and long-acting anticholinergics, inhaled and oral steroids, oxygen) can be very confusing to chronically ill patients. As noted previously, patients should also be instructed on an action plan in the event of an exacerbation.

Outcomes from a Pulmonary Rehabilitation Program

In 1997, the ACCP/AACVPR published a landmark comprehensive evidence-based review on the effectiveness of pulmonary rehabilitation.[21] Ten years later, over 1000 new publications were reviewed, and recommendations were updated.[4] In addition, the widely referenced Global Obstructive Lung Disease (GOLD) Initiative has been publishing updated evidence-based recommendations, with the most recent in 2008.[22] In all of these reports, conclusions and recommendations were graded on the strength of the evidence: Grade A conclusions were based on scientific evidence provided by well-designed, well-conducted, controlled trials with statistically significant and consistent findings. Grade B conclusions were based on scientific evidence provided by observational studies or by controlled trials with less consistent results. Grade C conclusions were based on expert opinions because available scientific evidence did not present consistent results or was lacking.

Evidence supporting the benefits of exercise training in chronic lung disease is compelling and received Grade A (lower extremity) and Grade B (upper extremity) support in the most recent GOLD review.[22] Lower extremity exercise programs consistently improved walk distance (6% to 33%) and maximal work load (10% to 102%) in all studies reviewed. Proposed mechanisms of improvement include improved aerobic capacity (in those who can reach cardiovascular training levels), increased motivation, desensitization to the sensation of dyspnea, improved ventilatory muscle function, and improved techniques of performance. Data from upper extremity exercise programs were less extensive but did support the concept that upper extremity exercise might improve the thoracic cage muscles of ventilation and improve activities of daily living.

Evidence supporting the effectiveness of pulmonary rehabilitation in reducing dyspnea also received a Grade A rating in the 2008 GOLD report.[22] This was a consistent finding using any number of dyspnea grading scales (e.g., visual analogue scales, baseline dyspnea index, transitional dyspnea index, other respiratory questionnaires). The mechanisms of reduced dyspnea are no doubt multifactorial but would include better exercise tolerance (and reduced ventilation for a given load), better breathing patterns, better medications, and a better comprehension by the patient of his or her disease and how it can be effectively managed.

Many studies have demonstrated that improved psychosocial function occurs as a result of pulmonary rehabilitation.[16,17] Much of this benefit, however, may come from improved exercise tolerance, reduced dyspnea, informal patient support groups and interactions, and a better understanding of the disease process and management by the patient. Indeed, the recent GOLD report could only give a Grade C rating for the evidence supporting routine, formal psychosocial components in a pulmonary rehabilitation program. However, this should not be interpreted as evidence stating that psychosocial support through less formal processes is unimportant or that selected patients would not benefit from focused therapies or medications.

Quality of life (QOL) indicators have consistently shown benefit from pulmonary rehabilitation. Recent evidence has raised this to a Grade A rating in the 2008 GOLD report.[22] Like improvements in dyspnea and psychosocial function, the mechanisms for improved QOL following pulmonary rehabilitation are probably multifactorial.

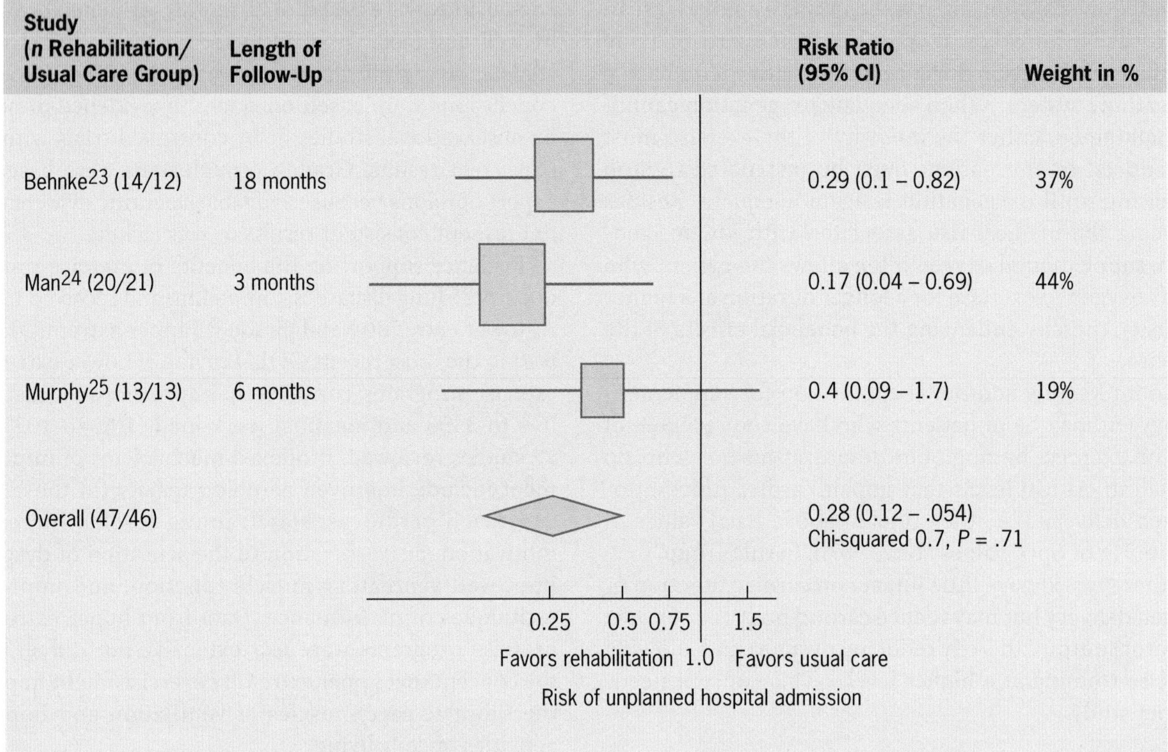

Study
(n Rehabilitation/ Usual Care Group)
Length of Follow-Up
Risk Ratio (95% CI)
Weight in %
Behnke23 (14/12)
18 months
0.29 (0.1 – 0.82)
37%
Man24 (20/21)
3 months
0.17 (0.04 – 0.69)
44%
Murphy25 (13/13)
6 months
0.4 (0.09 – 1.7)
19%
Overall (47/46)
0.28 (0.12 – .054)
Chi-squared 0.7, P = .71
0.25
0.5 0.75
1.5
Favors rehabilitation 1.0 Favors usual care
Risk of unplanned hospital admission

FIGURE 25–3 A meta-analysis depicting significant reductions in exacerbations of COPD from pulmonary rehabilitation. Reproduced from Puhan MA, Scharplatz M, Troosters T, et al. *Respir Res.* 2005;6:54. © 2005 licensee BioMed Central Ltd. Coutesy of Milo A. Puhan, Johns Hopkins Bloomberg School of Public Health.

An important benefit of pulmonary rehabilitation would be a reduction in **healthcare utilization** and costs. Several recent trials supporting this concept have resulted in a Grade A rating by the 2008 GOLD report (**Figure 25–3**).[22–25]

Finally, evidence supporting a survival benefit for pulmonary rehabilitation is largely inferential.[26] This potential effect thus only received a Grade B rating in the GOLD report.[22] This should not be surprising, because the goals of pulmonary rehabilitation are not to reverse the disease process but rather to improve the patient's functional capabilities within the constraints of the reduced lung function.

The outcome benefits noted earlier are largely evaluated at the conclusion of short-term programs (i.e., up to 12 weeks).[27–31] Important questions remain involving the durability of these benefits over time and the role (if any) of maintenance programs in preserving beneficial effects.[23,32,33] Long-term studies are few, but most point to a gradual deterioration in function over time. Continued adherence to regular exercise can forestall this deterioration, but adherence can be difficult in a chronic disease that is punctuated by exacerbations and the development or worsening of comorbidities. Interestingly, despite functional loss, QOL benefits from pulmonary rehabilitation appear more durable.[33] Refresher programs, regular maintenance programs, and even simple routine follow-up encouragement phone calls may help,[23,31] although none of these approaches has been well studied.

Reimbursement Issues

Obtaining proper reimbursement for pulmonary rehabilitation is an ongoing challenge. Until recently, pulmonary rehabilitation was not a specifically identified Medicare benefit and thus funding programs had to be done as incident to physician services. This led to considerable ambiguity and variability in reimbursement rules around the United States. In 2003, the National Emphysema Treatment Trial evaluating lung volume reduction surgery (partially funded by Medicare) required perioperative pulmonary rehabilitation. This opened the doors to three new Medicare G billing codes (**Table 25–1**) that were used for a number of years to fund many programs. In 2008, pulmonary rehabilitation was finally added as an official Medicare benefit, which provides opportunities for more appropriate levels of reimbursement both from Medicare and other third parties, who often follow Medicare practices. Under these new rules the billing code is G0424 for a session of pulmonary rehabilitation.

RESPIRATORY RECAP

Outcomes of Pulmonary Rehabilitation

» A growing body of evidence supports that pulmonary rehabilitation improves exercise tolerance, dyspnea, and quality of life and reduces healthcare costs.

» Evidence-based reviews have all given this growing evidence base the highest ratings.

TABLE 25-1 Medicare G Codes for Pulmonary Rehabilitation Billing

Code	Description
G0237	Therapeutic procedures to increase strength or endurance of respiratory muscles, 1:1, 15 minutes
G0238	Therapeutic procedures to improve respiratory function, 1:1, 15 minutes
G0239	Therapeutic procedures to improve respiratory function, group, 15 minutes

This code represents a bundled service (including physician supervision) and can be used a maximum of twice daily. One session must be at least 30 minutes in duration, two sessions on the same day must be at least 90 minutes in duration. Importantly, this new billing code applies only to patients with COPD at the present time. Pulmonary rehabilitation services for patients with other lung diseases must still be billed using the codes in Table 25–1.

SUMMARY

Both scientific rationale and abundant clinical evidence support physiologic and psychological mechanisms that explain the functional benefits derived from pulmonary rehabilitation. Incorporating these principles into structured programs has repeatedly been shown to improve exercise tolerance and quality of life and reduce the healthcare costs associated with chronic lung disease. Indeed, pulmonary rehabilitation is actually a form of comprehensive disease management. All of the important professional societies have endorsed these concepts. However, regulatory and political barriers persist for proper reimbursement. Continued political advocacy is required to ensure access to these important services for all patients limited by chronic lung disease.

KEY POINTS

- Pulmonary rehabilitation programs are comprehensive and multidisciplinary.
- The goal of pulmonary rehabilitation is to improve quality of life and increase functional capacity and sense of well-being.
- Individuals with stable chronic respiratory disease who are symptomatic, experience dyspnea on exertion, are free from acute illness, and are motivated to lead a more active life are candidates for a pulmonary rehabilitation program.
- Patient education and self-care are critical components of a pulmonary rehabilitation program.
- Exercise training generally entails the enhancement of upper and lower extremity function.
- In the establishment of an exercise training prescription, the initial load should be of sufficiently low intensity that the patient can accomplish it without discomfort.
- Both rationale and evidence exist for consideration of physiologic and psychologic mechanisms for the functional benefits derived from pulmonary rehabilitation.

ACKNOWLEDGMENT

The author is grateful to Nelson Leatherman, PhD, a cofounder of the Duke University pulmonary rehabilitation program, for his invaluable help in developing the original version of this chapter.

REFERENCES

1. American Thoracic Society. ATS official statement: pulmonary rehabilitation. *Am Rev Respir Dis.* 1981;124:663–666.
2. Ries AL. Position paper of the American Association of Cardiovascular and Pulmonary Rehabilitation: scientific basis of pulmonary rehabilitation. *J Cardiopulm Rehabil.* 1990;10: 418–441.
3. Nici I, Donner C, Wouters E, et al. American Thoracic Society/European Respiratory Society statement on pulmonary rehabilitation. *Am J Respir Crit Care Med.* 2006;173:1390–1413.
4. Ries AL, Bauldoff GS, Carlin BW, et al. Pulmonary rehabilitation: joint ACCP/AACVPR evidence-based clinical practice guidelines. *Chest.* 2007;131(5 suppl):4S–42S.
5. Belman MJ. Exercise in patients with COPD. *Thorax.* 1993; 48:936–946.
6. Ries AL, Archibald CJ. Endurance exercise training at maximal targets in patients with chronic obstructive pulmonary disease. *J Cardiopulm Rehabil.* 1987;7:594–601.
7. Cassaburi R, Petessio A, Ioli F, et al. Reductions in exercise lactic acidosis and ventilation as a result of training in patients with obstructive lung disease. *Am Rev Respir Dis.* 1991;143:9–18.
8. Lacasse Y, Wong E, Guyatt GH, et al. Meta-analysis of respiratory rehabilitation in COPD. *Lancet.* 1996;348:1115–1119.
9. O'Donnell DE, McGuire M, Samis L, et al. The impact of exercise reconditioning on breathlessness in severe chronic airflow limitation. *Am J Respir Crit Care Med.* 1995;152(6 pt 1):205–213.
10. MacIntyre NR. Muscle dysfunction associated with COPD. *Respir Care.* 2006;51:840–848.
11. American Thoracic Society and European Respiratory Society Task Force. Skeletal muscle dysfunction in chronic obstructive pulmonary disease. A statement of the American Thoracic Society and European Respiratory Society. *Am J Respir Crit Care Med.* 1999;159:S1–40.
12. Foster S, Thomas HM III. Pulmonary rehabilitation in lung disease other than chronic obstructive pulmonary disease. *Am Rev Respir Dis.* 1990;141:601–604.
13. Palmer SM, Tapson VF. Pulmonary rehabilitation in the surgical patient. Lung transplantation and lung volume reduction surgery. *Respir Care Clin North Am.* 1998;4:71–83.
14. Plankeel JF, McMullen B, MacIntyre NR. Exercise outcomes after pulmonary rehabilitation depend on the initial mechanism of exercise limitation among non-oxygen-dependent COPD patients. *Chest.* 2005;127:110–116.
15. Emtner M, Porszasz J, Burris M, et al. Benefits of supplemental oxygen in exercise training in nonhypoxemic chronic obstructive pulmonary disease patients. *Am J Respir Crit Care Med.* 2003;169(9):1034–1042.
16. Emery CF, Leatherman NE, Burker EJ, et al. Psychological outcomes of a pulmonary rehabilitation program. *Chest.* 1991;100:613–617.

17. Ries AL, Kaplan RM, Linberg TM, et al. Effects of pulmonary rehabilitation on physiological and psychological outcomes in patients with COPD. *Ann Intern Med.* 1995;122:823–832.
18. Bourbeau J, Julien M, Maltais F, et al. Reduction of hospital utilization in patients with chronic obstructive pulmonary disease: a disease-specific self-management intervention. *Arch Intern Med.* 2003;163:585–591.
19. Puhan MA, Scharplatz M, Troosters T, et al. Respiratory rehabilitation after acute exacerbation of COPD may reduce risk for readmission and mortality—a systematic review. *Respir Res.* 2005;5:54.
20. Borg GA. Psychophysical bases for perceived exertion. *Med Sci Sports Exerc.* 1982;14:377–381.
21. ACCP/AACVPR Pulmonary Rehabilitation Guidelines Panel. Pulmonary rehabilitation: evidence based guidelines. *Chest.* 1997;112:1363–1396.
22. Global Initiative for Chronic Obstructive Lung Disease. *Global Strategy for the Diagnosis, Management, and Prevention of Chronic Obstructive Pulmonary Disease.* 2008. Available at: http://www.goldcopd.com/GuidelineItem.asp?intid=2175. Accessed April 1, 2009.
23. Behnke M, Taube C, Kirsten D, et al. Home-based exercise is capable of preserving hospital-based improvements in severe chronic obstructive pulmonary disease. *Respir Med.* 2000;94:1184–1191.
24. Man WD, Polkey MI, Donaldson N, Gray BJ, Moxham J. Community pulmonary rehabilitation after hospitalisation for acute exacerbations of chronic obstructive pulmonary disease: randomised controlled study. *BMJ.* 2004;329:1209.
25. Murphy N, Bell C, Costello RW. Extending a home from hospital care programme for COPD exacerbations to include pulmonary rehabilitation. *Respir Med.* 2005;99(10):1297–1302.
26. Troosters T, Gosselink R, Paepe KD. Pulmonary rehabilitation improves survival in COPD patients with a recent severe acute exacerbation. *Am J Respir Crit Care Med.* 2002;165:A16.
27. Goldstein RS, Gort EH, Stubbing D, et al. Randomized controlled trial of respiratory rehabilitation. *Lancet.* 1994;344(8934):1394–1397.
28. Foglio K, Bianchi L, Bruletti G, et al. Long-term effectiveness of pulmonary rehabilitation in patients with chronic airway obstruction. *Eur Respir J.* 1999;13(1):125–132.
29. Young P, Dewse M, Fergusson W, et al. Improvements in outcomes for chronic obstructive pulmonary disease (COPD) attributable to a hospital-based respiratory rehabilitation programme. *Aust N Z J Med.* 1999;29(1):59–65.
30. Finnerty JP, Keeping I, Bullough I, et al. The effectiveness of outpatient pulmonary rehabilitation in chronic lung disease: a randomized controlled trial. *Chest.* 2001;119(6):1705–1710.
31. Griffiths TL, Phillips CJ, Davies S, et al. Cost effectiveness of an outpatient multidisciplinary pulmonary rehabilitation program. *Thorax.* 2001;56:779–784.
32. Foglio K, Bianchi L, Ambrosino N. Is it really useful to repeat outpatient pulmonary rehabilitation programs in patients with chronic airway obstruction? A 2-year controlled study. *Chest.* 2001;119:1696–1704.
33. Ries AL, Kaplan RM, Myers R, et al. Maintenance after pulmonary rehabilitation in chronic lung disease: a randomized trial. *Am J Respir Crit Care Med.* 2003;167:880–888.

CHAPTER 26

Home Respiratory Care

Angela King
Robert McCoy

OUTLINE

Home Care Services
Goals of Home Care
The Medicare Program
Requirements for Home Medical Equipment Companies
The Respiratory Therapist as Home Care Provider
The Initial Home Visit
Bag Technique
Home Environment Evaluation
Long-Term Oxygen Therapy
Home Mechanical Ventilation

OBJECTIVES

1. Discuss factors leading to the increase in home respiratory care.
2. Describe the role of the home medical equipment company.
3. Discuss the reimbursement system for home care in the United States.
4. Discuss issues related to home oxygen administration.
5. Compare home oxygen administration systems.
6. Compare mechanical ventilation in the hospital to that provided in the home.
7. List key safety considerations for the ventilator-assisted individual.

KEY TERMS

backup ventilator
bag technique
clinical respiratory services
compressed gas system
continuous-flow oxygen (CFO)
demand delivery device
durable medical equipment (DME) companies
emergency plan
equipment management services
go-bag
ground circuit detector
home medical equipment (HME) companies
home respiratory care
intermittent-flow device
intermittent-flow oxygen
liquid oxygen (LOX) storage system
long-term oxygen therapy (LTOT)
Medicaid
Medicare
oxygen concentrator
oxygen-conserving device (OCD)
portable oxygen concentrator (POC)
pulse flow
remote alarms
transtracheal oxygen

INTRODUCTION

The American Association of Respiratory Care defines **home respiratory care** as "[t]hose prescribed respiratory care services provided in a patient's personal residence." Prescribed respiratory care services may include patient assessment and monitoring, such as listening to breath sounds; observing the patient's respiratory rate, chest excursion, and skin tone; and evaluating the patient's sputum. Respiratory care services may involve diagnostic and therapeutic modalities, such as observing the patient's pulse oximetry and transcutaneous carbon dioxide (CO_2) values, and performing airway clearance therapy. Importantly, home respiratory care services may include providing education regarding respiratory equipment, disease management, and health-promoting behaviors for the patient and the family caregiver(s). This chapter covers issues related to home respiratory care, with specific emphasis on home oxygen (O_2) therapy and home mechanical ventilation.

Home Care Services

The patient's home may be a single-family residence, a multifamily dwelling, an assisted living facility or group home, a retirement community, or a skilled nursing facility.[1] There are four types of home care services: home medical equipment services, episodic home health care, hospice home health care, and chronic home care services.[2]

Depending on the equipment ordered, **home medical equipment (HME) companies**, also called **durable medical equipment (DME) companies**, can provide service by a technician, respiratory therapist (RT), or a qualified nurse. A hospital bed would most likely be set up by a technician, whereas a suction machine and a mechanical ventilator would be set up by an RT. Episodic home health care is often ordered for the time period immediately following the patient's hospital stay, and is usually provided for a finite period of time. Hospice care is provided for the terminally ill and provides palliative end-of-life care. Chronic home care services, sometimes referred to as *private duty*, are typically provided on an hourly basis and may involve nurses, health aides, chore providers, and companions.

RESPIRATORY RECAP

Individuals Providing Services for DME Companies

- Technician
- Respiratory therapist
- Qualified nurse

Improved medical equipment has resulted in an increase in home respiratory care. The Medicare prospective payment system encourages earlier hospital discharge.[3] Modern therapies for the treatment of newborns have resulted in more infants and pediatric patients requiring home O_2 and home mechanical ventilation.[4] Another factor driving the increase in home care is the proportion of the population older than 65 years, which is projected to increase to 19.6% of the total population in 2030.[5] In the United States, approximately 80% of all persons over age 65 have at least one chronic condition, and 50% have at least two. Since the early 1990s, accumulating data have supported the cost-effectiveness of home care for respiratory patients (**Table 26–1**).[6,7] Medicare and other healthcare providers began encouraging the transition of technology-dependent patients from the acute care setting to less costly environments of care.[8] In addition to technological advances, changing demographics, and economic pressures, another key factor increasing home respiratory care is that most patients prefer to be cared for at home if possible.

RESPIRATORY RECAP

Goals of Home Care

- Achieve the optimum level of patient function
- Educate patients and their caregivers
- Administer diagnostic and therapeutic services
- Conduct disease management and promote health

Goals of Home Care

The goals of home respiratory care are to achieve the optimum level of patient function through goal setting, educate patients and their caregivers, administer diagnostic and therapeutic modalities and services, conduct disease management, and promote health.[1] The general goals of home care for individuals with respiratory disorder are to increase survival, decrease morbidity, improve function and quality of life, support independence and self-management, encourage positive health behaviors, and, for children with lung disease, to promote optimal growth and development; for patients with a terminal illness, the goals are to provide physical and psychological comfort and to make it possible for the patient to die at home.[2]

The Medicare Program

As part of the Social Security Amendments of 1965, **Medicare** was established to provide a health insurance program for aged persons to complement the retirement, survivors, and disability insurance benefits under Title II of the Social Security Act. The Medicare program began on July 1, 1966. In 1973, persons who were entitled to Social Security or Railroad Retirement disability benefits for at least 24 months, persons with end-stage renal disease, and certain other persons became eligible for Medicare benefits. Persons with amyotrophic lateral sclerosis (ALS) were allowed to waive the 24-month waiting period after passage of Public Law 106-554, the Medicare, Medicaid, and SCHIP Benefits Improvement and Protection Act of 2000.

Hospital insurance is known as Medicare Part A. Part A covers inpatient care, skilled nursing facility care, and hospice care. Supplementary medical insurance is known as Part B. Most people have to pay a premium for Part B coverage. Part B includes medical services typically delivered in the outpatient setting and includes

TABLE 26-1 Hospital Cost Versus Home Care Cost, Per Patient, Per Month

Condition	Hospital Cost	Home Care Cost	Savings
Adult, ventilator dependent*	$21,570	$7050	$14,520
Pediatric, oxygen dependent†	$12,090	$5250	$6840

*Data from Bach JR. The ventilator-assisted individual: cost analysis of institutional vs. rehabilitation and in-home management. *Chest.* 1992;101:26–30.

†Data from Field AI. Home care cost-effectiveness for respiratory technology-dependent children. *Am J Dis Child.* 1991;145:729–733.

Adapted from National Association for Home Care and Hospice. *Basic Statistics About Home Care: Updated 2008.* Washington, DC: The National Association for Home Care and Hospice; 2008.

tests, lab services, and various health screenings. Part B also includes home health services, which are defined as medically necessary, reasonable, and part-time care and services such as skilled nursing care, home health aide services, physical and occupational therapies, speech and language pathology therapy, and medical social services. Part B also includes certain prescribed medical supplies and durable medical equipment, such as wheelchairs, hospital beds, home O_2 devices and mechanical ventilators, and related equipment. The Medicare Advantage program, also known as Part C, was established by Public Law 105-33, the Balanced Budget Act of 1997, which expanded options for beneficiaries to participate in private-sector healthcare plans. In most cases, Part C is a lower-cost alternative to the original Medicare plan, and Part C providers usually offer extra benefits to beneficiaries. The newest part of Medicare is prescription drug coverage, also known as Part D. This legislation was authorized by the Medicare Prescription Drug Improvement and Modernization Act of 2003. It provides seniors and people with disabilities a prescription drug benefit.

To qualify for Medicare skilled nursing services, the patient must (1) be under the care of a physician; (2) receive services under a plan of care established and periodically reviewed by a physician; (3) be in need of skilled nursing care, physical therapy, occupational therapy, and/or speech and language pathology therapy on an intermittent basis; and (4) be homebound, meaning that the patient is confined to the home or that leaving the home is a major effort that is seldom undertaken. For example, the patient may leave the home to get therapeutic or psychosocial care or to attend a funeral, graduation, or other infrequent event. Skilled nursing services must be provided by a registered nurse or by a licensed practical nurse under the supervision of a registered nurse. Unfortunately, respiratory therapists are not included in the Medicare home health services benefit.

RESPIRATORY RECAP

Medicare Benefits

- Part A: hospital insurance
- Part B: supplementary medical insurance
- Part C: low-cost alternative to Medicare
- Part D: prescription drug coverage

Medicare Part B covers medically necessary durable medical equipment such as O_2 concentrators, nebulizer compressors, and mechanical ventilators, but there is no separate reimbursement for the respiratory therapist's professional expertise. Twenty years ago, a patient with chronic obstructive pulmonary disease (COPD) who was prescribed home O_2 would have received a home safety evaluation and equipment instruction, as well as periodic respiratory assessments, from a home care respiratory therapist. Unfortunately, as Medicare reimbursement for home O_2 has steadily declined over the years, the number of DME providers using technicians, as opposed to respiratory therapists, to set up and monitor the home respiratory equipment has increased dramatically. The majority of home O_2 patients today do not receive in-home clinical monitoring from a therapist. In addition, because many patients on home O_2 therapy leave the home frequently to attend religious services or social outings or to go shopping, they do not qualify for Medicare skilled nursing services either.

Medicaid Coverage for Home Medical Equipment

Many patients who need respiratory-related durable medical equipment but who are not eligible for Medicare may receive DME through the **Medicaid** program. For example, a child on a mechanical ventilator whose parents do not have private medical insurance will most likely receive coverage from the Medicaid program. In many cases, the DME provider must obtain prior authorization from the Medicaid program to determine whether a specific piece of equipment is covered. The coverage determination criteria for a given piece of respiratory equipment within the Medicaid program can vary by state. For example, one northeastern state does not cover a noninvasive ventilator used with a mouthpiece for a patient with Duchenne muscular dystrophy (DMD), but covers that same ventilator if the patient undergoes a tracheostomy. The best strategy to help the home patient obtain coverage for a given item is to proactively work with the Medicaid case worker, offering relevant educational materials and a detailed letter of medical necessity from the patient's physician. In many cases, appealing a negative coverage decision and presenting additional supporting documentation will result in a favorable outcome. In the case of the patient with DMD mentioned earlier, the Medicaid program did agree to cover the ventilator upon appeal after receiving information about the increased life expectancy of DMD patients when ventilated with noninvasive ventilation and presented with data showing that noninvasive ventilation was a more cost-effective alternative than a tracheostomy.

Requirements for Home Medical Equipment Companies

Depending on state respiratory care laws and regulations, and depending on the types of services offered, an HME company may require some or all of the following: retail license, HME license, a bedding supplier license, and an O_2 manufacturer/distributor license and possibly other licenses/permits as required by the state. Medicare also requires that all HME companies obtain a surety bond of at least $50,000. A surety bond is issued by an entity on behalf of a second party. It guarantees that the second party will fulfill an obligation to a third party. In the event that the obligation is not met, the third party will recover its losses via the bond. Medicare also requires all HME companies to have liability insurance.

BOX 26–1

Medicare Home Medical Equipment Supplier Standards

1. A supplier must be in compliance with all applicable federal and state licensure and regulatory requirements.
2. A supplier must provide complete and accurate information on the DMEPOS supplier application. Any changes to this information must be reported to the National Supplier Clearinghouse within 30 days.
3. An authorized individual (one whose signature is binding) must sign the application for billing privileges.
4. A supplier must fill orders from its own inventory, or must contract with other companies for the purchase of items necessary to fill the order. A supplier may not contract with any entity that is currently excluded from the Medicare program, any state health care programs, or from any other federal procurement or nonprocurement programs.
5. A supplier must advise beneficiaries that they may rent or purchase inexpensive or routinely purchased durable medical equipment, and of the purchase option for capped rental equipment.
6. A supplier must notify beneficiaries of warranty coverage and honor all warranties under applicable state law, and repair or replace free of charge Medicare-covered items that are under warranty.
7. A supplier must maintain a physical facility on an appropriate site.
8. A supplier must permit Centers for Medicare and Medicaid Services (CMS) or its agents to conduct on-site inspections to ascertain the supplier's compliance with these standards. The supplier location must be accessible to beneficiaries during reasonable business hours, and must maintain a visible sign and posted hours of operation.
9. A supplier must maintain a primary business telephone listed under the name of the business in a local directory or a toll free number available through directory assistance. The exclusive use of a beeper, answering machine, or cell phone is prohibited.
10. A supplier must have comprehensive liability insurance in the amount of at least $300,000 that covers both the supplier's place of business and all customers and employees of the supplier. If the supplier manufactures its own items, this insurance must also cover product liability and completed operations. Failure to maintain required insurance at all times will result in revocation of the supplier's billing privileges retroactive to the date the insurance lapsed.
11. A supplier must agree not to initiate telephone contact with beneficiaries, with a few exceptions allowed. This standard prohibits suppliers from calling beneficiaries in order to solicit new business.
12. A supplier is responsible for delivery and must instruct beneficiaries on use of Medicare-covered items, and maintain proof of delivery.
13. A supplier must answer questions and respond to complaints of beneficiaries, and maintain documentation of such contacts.

(continues)

Beginning in September 2009, Medicare began requiring all HME companies to be accredited by an approved agency. **Box 26–1** lists the Medicare supplier standards.

Accreditation of Home Medical Equipment Companies

Home care providers must be accredited by one of several accreditation agencies approved by the Medicare program, similar to accreditation for hospitals. There are generally two types of accreditation: Equipment Management Services and Clinical Respiratory Services. Accreditation in Clinical Respiratory Services includes everything required for accreditation in equipment management, plus additional requirements governing actual hands-on patient care and clinical personnel qualifications and requirements.

RESPIRATORY RECAP

Accreditation of Home Medical Equipment Companies

» Equipment Management Services
» Clinical Respiratory Services

Not all home medical equipment companies are accredited for Clinical Respiratory Services, and that specific accreditation is not required by Medicare to participate in the program. However, if a company provides hands-on patient care such as performing patient assessment, administering treatment, providing disease management education, and/or monitoring respiratory status, it must be accredited for Clinical Respiratory Services.[9] Several accreditation agencies are approved by Medicare, including the Joint Commission (formerly known as the Joint Commission on Accreditation of Healthcare Organizations), Community Health Accreditation Program

Box 26–1 *(continued)*

14. A supplier must maintain and replace at no charge or repair directly, or through a service contract with another company, Medicare-covered items it has rented to beneficiaries.
15. A supplier must accept returns of substandard (less than full quality for the particular item) or unsuitable items (inappropriate for the beneficiary at the time it was fitted and rented or sold) from beneficiaries.
16. A supplier must disclose these supplier standards to each beneficiary to whom it supplies a Medicare-covered item.
17. A supplier must disclose to the government any person having ownership, financial, or control interest in the supplier.
18. A supplier must not convey or reassign a supplier number; i.e., the supplier may not sell or allow another entity to use its Medicare Supplier Billing Number.
19. A supplier must have a complaint resolution protocol established to address beneficiary complaints that relate to these standards. A record of these complaints must be maintained at the physical facility.
20. Complaint records must include: the name, address, telephone number and health insurance claim number of the beneficiary, a summary of the complaint, and any actions taken to resolve it.
21. A supplier must agree to furnish CMS any information required by the Medicare statute and implementing regulations.
22. All suppliers must be accredited by a CMS-approved accreditation organization in order to receive and retain a supplier billing number. The accreditation must indicate the specific products and services, for which the supplier is accredited in order for the supplier to receive payment of those specific products and services (except for certain exempt pharmaceuticals).
23. All suppliers must notify their accreditation organization when a new DMEPOS location is opened.
24. All supplier locations, whether owned or subcontracted, must meet the DMEPOS quality standards and be separately accredited in order to bill Medicare.
25. All suppliers must disclose upon enrollment all products and services, including the addition of new product lines for which they are seeking accreditation
26. Must meet the surety bond requirements specified in 42 C.F.R. 424.57(c).

Note: This list is an abbreviated version of the application certification standards that every Medicare DMEPOS supplier must meet in order to obtain and retain their billing privileges. These standards, in their entirety, are listed in 42 C.F.R. pt. 424, sec 424.57(c) and were effective on December 11, 2000.

DMEPOS, durable medical equipment, prosthetics, and orthotics supplies.

From Centers for Medicare and Medicaid Services. *Medicare Enrollment Application: Durable Medical Equipment, Prosthetics, and Orthotics Supplies (DMEPOS) Suppliers, Form CMS-855S.* Available at: http://www.cms.hhs.gov/cmsforms/downloads/cms855s.pdf.

(CHAP), and Accreditation Commission for Health Care (ACHC). The accreditation survey is normally repeated every 3 years, but the interval may vary based on the accrediting agency.

Equipment Management Services Versus Clinical Respiratory Services

Equipment management services are not hands-on patient care services. In other words, the patient is not touched by the RT for the purpose of providing care. The RT checks the home medical equipment, such as the percent oxygen from the O_2 concentrator or the ventilator settings and alarms, makes prescribed setting changes, delivers additional supplies, and performs similar equipment-related duties. The therapist does not perform diagnostic or therapeutic procedures. Equipment management services require a physician's order for the home medical equipment and settings. If the RT provides professional services in the home beyond that of a service technician, the RT is performing **clinical respiratory services**, which include performing clinical assessments and diagnostic procedures, administering treatments or medications, providing patient education, and monitoring the patient's respiratory status. If patient education involves more than education on the use of the equipment, the RT is considered to be providing clinical respiratory services.

RESPIRATORY RECAP

Types of Respiratory Care Services

» Equipment management services
» Clinical respiratory services

TABLE 26–2 Key Characteristics Required of the Home Care Respiratory Therapist

Objective Requirements	
Licensed or certified (as applicable per state)	All reputable DME providers hire only licensed/certified therapists. Note: If the therapist will visit patients in multiple states, a current license is required for each state.
Driver's license	Most DME providers will obtain an annual copy of the therapist's driving record, and employment is often contingent upon maintaining a clean driving record.
Automobile insurance	Most DME providers will require proof that the therapist has adequate automobile insurance coverage.
Subjective Requirements	
Highly skilled at patient assessment	The therapist often is the only clinician visiting the patient's home, or the patient may be seen by other clinicians only sporadically. The respiratory therapist must be skilled at respiratory assessment for patients ranging from preterm infants to geriatric patients.
Highly skilled at home safety assessment	The therapist often will be the only clinician assessing the patient's home for safety and the proper use of the medical equipment.
Excellent critical thinking ability	On occasion, the therapist will need to call the patient's physician or protective services on an emergent basis. The therapist requires excellent judgment and decision-making skills in order to appropriately handle such situations.
Good teacher	The bulk of the home care therapist's job is to teach patients and families. Most DME providers offer equipment and service to a wide variety of patient populations, from preterm infants to geriatric patients; thus, the therapist must be skilled at teaching diverse patient populations.
Respects people from other cultures and socioeconomic backgrounds	The home care therapist will most likely be visiting patients from a variety of backgrounds, with diverse belief systems and ways of doing things. The therapist must keep in mind that he or she is a guest in the patient's home and treat all patients and families with respect.
Good communication skills	The therapist will need good communication skills, both verbal and written, to work with a wide variety of patients, families, coworkers, other home care providers (e.g., nursing, PT, OT, SLP, MSW, HHA), and physicians.
Intrinsically motivated	The home care therapist will most often be working without direct supervision.
Good organizational skills	The home care therapist must be organized regarding prioritizing and planning home visits, ensuring that all required equipment and supplies are ordered and stocked in his or her vehicle, and that all required paperwork is completed in a timely fashion.

DME, durable medical equipment; PT, physical therapist; OT, occupational therapist; SLP, speech language pathologist; MSW, master of social work; HHA, home health aide.

Orders for Clinical Respiratory Services

Orders for clinical respiratory services are considered a part of the care plan and should be included in the HME company's care plan as well as the home health agency's nursing care plan, if applicable. The home care RT should coordinate the care plan with that of the home health agency's personnel (nursing; physical, occupational, or speech therapy) to encourage a collaborative approach. The plan of care describes the planned treatments, education, and services and must be approved and signed by the patient's physician.

The Respiratory Therapist as Home Care Provider

By virtue of education, training, and competency testing, the respiratory therapist is the most competent healthcare professional to provide home respiratory care. Home respiratory care, particularly for ventilator-assisted individuals, can be highly complex; therefore, the risk of a negative outcome is great if the services are not performed by a highly skilled professional.[1]

Requirements for the Respiratory Therapist Providing Home Respiratory Care

Table 26–2 lists some of the key characteristics required of the home care respiratory therapist. The ability to assess many different aspects of the patient is probably the most important skill for a home care therapist.[10] The RT must be able to assess respiratory and overall physical status. The home RT is often the first to note a deterioration in the patient's physiologic condition. He or she also needs to evaluate the patient's and family caregiver's ability to learn and retain new information and maintain the prescribed medical equipment. The home care RT teaches pediatric, adult, and geriatric patients and their families, and must be able to work with patients from diverse cultures and economic backgrounds. The RT must be able to assess the family and social support available as well as the safety and appropriateness of the patient's home environment. The RT must also be aware of the requirements of insurance coverage for commonly prescribed home medical equipment. Organizational skills are important because coverage of a large geographic area means that making a trip back to the office to retrieve a forgotten item is often impossible.

The daily routine of a home care RT is much different from that of a hospital-based therapist. Although home care RTs see a variety of patients and families each day, they do not enjoy the same camaraderie with their coworkers as experienced by RTs working in a hospital. The home care RT often is on call 24 hours a day, 7 days a week. On the positive side, the home care therapist often develops long-term relationships with patients and their families.

The Initial Home Visit

The tasks completed during the initial home visit vary depending on the equipment and services ordered (clinical respiratory services versus equipment management services) and on the policies and procedures of the HME company. For a patient on a ventilator at home, the initial home visit must not be the first time the therapist makes face-to-face contact with the patient. The home environment evaluation should always be done prior to discharge, so that any safety issues or inadequacies are identified and corrected prior to the patient's return home. Equipment can be set up in the home days prior to discharge, but billing for the equipment cannot be started prior to the patient's discharge to the home.

During the initial home visit, the RT has several important tasks to complete:

- Establish a rapport with the patient and family.
- Evaluate the home environment.
- Complete the equipment setup and instruction.
- Perform any ordered patient assessments and diagnostic or therapeutic procedures.
- Determine if there are unmet needs and make a plan for addressing those needs.
- Communicate, as appropriate, with other professional caregivers (e.g., home health nurse, physical therapist, physician).
- Complete the required admission paperwork.

The RT should have a company photo identification card visible to allay any security concerns. The RT should address the patient and family using the appropriate titles (e.g., Mrs., Ms., Mr.) unless invited to do otherwise. RTs must keep in mind that, although performing a professional role in the patient's home, they also are guests in the home. The RT should ask where to wash his or her hands or should use an alcohol-based hand sanitizer in view of the patient and family caregivers.

The patient rights and responsibilities document explains to the patient the right to refuse service, the right to make a complaint without fear of retaliation, and the right to know how much the services being provided are going to cost. In addition, this document explains the patient's responsibilities for open and honest communication, likes and dislikes with regard to treatment and services being provided, using the equipment in the manner prescribed, voicing grievances or complaints regarding treatment or services, and paying any deductible or copayment as required by regulation or law or the terms of an insurance contract.

The patient should also receive a copy of the company's complaint procedure form. This form outlines the procedure the patient needs to follow in order to file a complaint and lists contact numbers the patient can call to issue a complaint, including Medicare, Medicaid, and the accreditation agency by which the company is accredited. The document also includes an overview of the actions the company will take to resolve the issue.

If the patient has not already completed an advance directive, he or she should be given written information about advance directives and an explanation. Obtaining a copy of the patient's advance directive for the medical record is crucial so that the RT, or any other caregiver in the home, knows how to respond to a cardiopulmonary arrest.

The patient must receive information on the HME company's methods for ensuring Health Insurance Portability and Accountability Act (HIPAA) compliance. This document will inform the patient about how his or her medical information will be stored by the company and who will have access to it.

If the patient qualifies for Medicare, the advance beneficiary notice (ABN) and the assignment of benefits (AOB) forms must be completed. The ABN form is to help patients make an informed choice about whether or not they want to receive items or services, knowing that there might be an additional personal cost if the items and services are not covered by their insurance plan. The AOB gives the patient's authorization to the HME company to assign Medicare, Medicaid, or insurance benefits to the company for all covered medical equipment and supplies; for direct billing to Medicare, Medicaid, or other insurers; and for release of personal health information (PHI) to Medicare, Medicaid, or other valid insurance companies and to other healthcare providers.

The home environment must be evaluated specific to the type of home medical equipment being provided. For example, if the patient will be receiving home O_2, the RT will need to ensure there are no sources of open flame in the home when O_2 is being used and that a working smoke detector is installed. If the patient will be receiving postural drainage therapy, the RT must evaluate the home to determine whether there is a suitable bed to perform the therapy.

The RT may provide the patient and family with additional information, such as a list of community resources. This resource list may include agencies and services such as the American Lung Association (ALA), Better Breather's Clubs, Meals on Wheels, the Area Agency on Aging, hospice services, free or reduced-cost medical clinics in the area, domestic violence hotline information, poison control hotline information, and the closest ALS or muscular dystrophy clinic.

If home medical equipment has been prescribed, the therapist will set up the equipment and instruct the patient and family caregivers in the proper use and care of the equipment. The instructional checklist should include common troubleshooting tips and maintenance requirements for the equipment delivered. The instructional checklist may also include instructions for the patient to follow to order additional O_2 or supplies, as well as what to do in the event of home medical equipment failure or patient emergency.

All insurance companies, Medicare, and Medicaid require proof of delivery of the equipment and supplies.

Generally, the delivery ticket lists the patient's name and demographic information and specifies the quantity, manufacturer, and serial number (if applicable) of the home medical equipment provided. For some high-tech equipment, such as mechanical ventilators, it is crucial that the serial number be properly recorded and tracked in the event there is a recall of the equipment.

After assessing the home environment and teaching the patient and caregivers about the equipment, the RT will have an idea of the patient's needs and goals. If the patient is receiving only equipment management services, information can be documented on a progress note or any other document that can be incorporated into the patient's medical record. Alternatively, if the patient is on a home ventilator and is receiving clinical respiratory services, a goal might be for the patient to be able to speak. The therapist would document this goal on the patient's plan of care, which must be signed by the physician. For example, the therapist may request an order to determine the patient's ability to tolerate cuff deflation, and, if successful, attempt the use of a speaking valve.

Bag Technique

It is important for home care RTs to determine whether **bag technique** should be incorporated into their routine.[11] Most home care RTs carry a bag containing their hand wash, stethoscope, blood pressure cuff, pulse oximeter, CO_2 monitor, peak flow meter, and other necessary implements. Because the RT will be traveling from home to home, it is prudent that the therapist minimize the likelihood of disease transmission. Stethoscopes and other items can be contaminated with various pathogens.[12] It is also important for patients receiving both nursing and RT visits to receive the same standard of care from each discipline.

Bag technique means keeping the bag and its contents as clean as possible. The bag should not rest on an unclean area, such as the floor or on the patient's unmade bed. Depending on the space available in the home environment, it may be easiest for the therapist to use a barrier, such as a blue pad or sheet of newspaper, to serve as a clean resting place for the bag. Using a blue pad also helps protect the patient's furniture from damage, which communicates that the RT is respectful of the patient's home. The RT should wash his or her hands before reaching into the bag. Everything needed for the visit should be removed at one time, prior to beginning patient care. When the visit is finished, anything that may have been soiled should be wiped clean before being replaced in the bag.

Home Environment Evaluation

The home care RT is responsible for evaluating the home environment to ensure that it is appropriate for the planned equipment and services. Some components of the home environment evaluation apply to all patients, such as ensuring that there are adequate means of egress and no fall hazards.

Environmental Issues for Patients on Home Oxygen Therapy

Patients who receive O_2 at home are exposed to the risk of improper storage and handling of O_2 cylinders, unsafe usage of O_2 in the kitchen or workshop, improper transfer of liquid O_2, inadequate ventilation, and smoking or other unsafe flames.[13] It is important for the RT to evaluate whether there are smoking materials and other fire safety risks, such as candles or open flames, in the home and whether the home has functional smoke detectors.[14] Patients receiving O_2 may also be exposed to risk from not securing portable O_2 properly while driving or riding in an automobile. It is crucial that the cylinders be secured in the event the car brakes suddenly or is involved in an accident.

Environmental Issues for Patients on Home Mechanical Ventilation

If the patient will receive a home ventilator, the environment evaluation should include verifying the adequacy of the home electrical system. Home medical equipment that is double insulated generally does not require grounding. However, most home medical equipment companies do not have a biomedical engineer on staff to verify the electrical safety of each piece of medical equipment; therefore, it is prudent for the therapist to ensure that the electrical outlets used for home medical equipment are properly grounded.[14] Most hardware stores stock a **ground circuit detector** that can be purchased inexpensively. These devices typically use red and amber bulbs to indicate the outlet status, although the therapist must read the instructions for the particular brand of ground circuit detector being used. In the case of the ground circuit detector shown in **Figure 26–1**, the outlet is properly grounded if the two amber bulbs illuminate. If the red bulb or a single amber bulb illuminates, there is a problem with the outlet that must be remedied before that outlet can be safely used.

RESPIRATORY RECAP

Environmental Issues

- Safe storage of oxygen
- Electrical safety
- Backup electrical/battery power
- Emergency plan
- Alarms and communication
- Local EMS and firefighters

Another important aspect of electrical safety in the home is ensuring that the electrical circuit is not overloaded. Most ventilator patients have several pieces of electrical equipment (e.g., ventilator, heated humidifier, nebulizer, O_2 concentrator, suction machine) within the

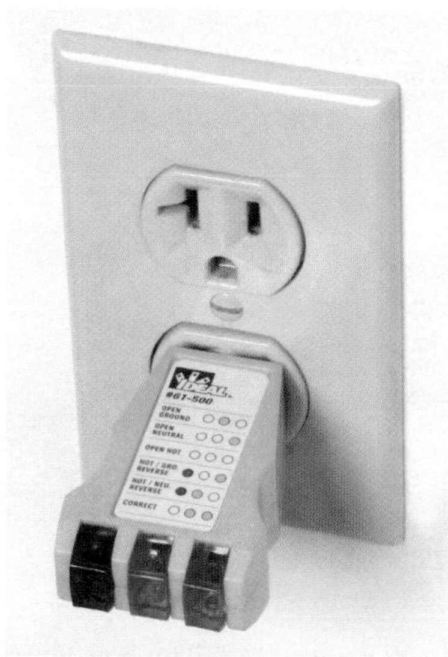

FIGURE 26–1 Two LEDs indicating a properly grounded outlet.

Formula

$$\frac{\text{Power consumption of vent in watts} \times \text{Hours per day of use}}{1000} = \textbf{Kilowatts per day}$$

$$\text{Kilowatts per day} \times \text{Cost per kilowatt} \times \text{30 days} = \textbf{Cost per month}$$

Sample Calculation

Note: Get ***watts*** *from the ventilator manufacturer; get* ***cost per kilowatt*** *from the local electric company.*

$$\frac{\text{50 watts} \times \text{24 hours per day}}{1000} = \textbf{1.2 kilowatts per day}$$

$$\text{1.2 kilowatts per day} \times \text{0.124 per kilowatt} \times \text{30 days} = \textbf{\$4.46 per month}$$

FIGURE 26–2 Estimating the cost of electricity for a home ventilator. Data from Turner J. *Handbook of Adult and Pediatric Respiratory Home Care.* Mosby; 1994.

same room in addition to the standard household items. It is easy to overload the electrical circuit. Sometimes the homeowner will have a diagram detailing which outlets are on the same circuit, but usually testing must be done. To determine which outlets are on the same circuit, turn off the circuit breaker for that room and then insert the ground circuit detector into each outlet. If the outlet circuit detector does not illuminate (no bulbs light), that outlet is controlled by the circuit breaker that was turned off. If the bulbs on the outlet circuit detector illuminate, that outlet is on a different circuit. The therapist should be careful not to plug too many devices into the same circuit. If concerned, the therapist can total the amperes of each item he or she intends to plug into a particular circuit and compare that total to the rated amperage of the circuit breaker. This information can usually be found in the operator's manual for each piece of equipment. Note that some ventilators draw more current on startup and then drop back after the ventilator is operating.[15]

The therapist should avoid the use of extension cords for the home medical equipment if at all possible. However, in practical application, there will be times when an extension cord is needed. If an extension cord must be used, ensure that the cord is of high quality, is in good condition, and includes three prongs rated appropriately to carry the anticipated amperage. Of course, the extension cord must be plugged into an outlet that the therapist has already tested with the ground circuit detector. Some new extension cords include a ground fault interrupter (GFI), which can add an additional measure of safety when properly used. Of course, when there is any concern about the home's electrical system, it is imperative that a licensed electrician provides the final word on the home's electrical safety.

Some patients who are on home O_2 and/or a home mechanical ventilator will be concerned about the anticipated increase in their electric bill. If the patient expresses a significant concern about the bill, the RT can help the patient estimate the additional electric consumption and the increased cost.[16] See **Figure 26–2** for a sample calculation.

Some communities allow patients who are dependent on a mechanical ventilator to be placed on a priority restoration service in the event of a power failure. If the patient's electric company offers this service, the therapist should forward a letter to the electric company including the patient's name, address, and reason for the priority designation along with a request signed by the patient and physician. However, even if priority designation is granted, the patient must be cautioned that it is not always possible for the electric company to restore service promptly, and alternate plans must be put into place for whenever electrical power is interrupted.

The RT must work with the patient and family to determine the optimal **emergency plan** for handling a power failure. Some families choose to obtain a generator. Generators vary in complexity of operation. Some generators automatically turn on when necessary, and even perform self-tests at scheduled intervals. However, some generators are difficult to start, and may require physical strength and agility to pull-start. It is imperative that this type of generator be started periodically, per the manufacturer's guidelines. It is wise for the family to identify and train several people who are usually available and able and willing to start the generator should the need arise.

All patients who depend on a ventilator should have a battery system in case of emergency and for mobility purposes.[17] Each patient's need for battery duration

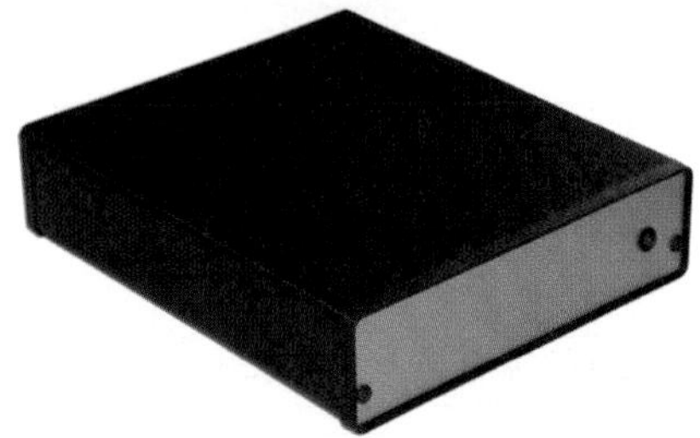

FIGURE 26–3 The PowerTech Vent Power Center.

must be evaluated individually. For example, a patient who has no spontaneous breathing capability and who lives in an area with frequent power outages will require much longer battery duration than a patient capable of spontaneous ventilation who uses a ventilator only at night. All home ventilator manufacturers offer various battery types and sizes. Richardson Products (Frankfort, Ill.) makes a product called the PowerTech Vent Power Center that allows the patient to operate the ventilator from a power wheelchair battery (**Figure 26–3**). Many patients also have a DC power cord; in an absolute emergency, the patient could use the ventilator in the car. In some communities, the local fire department may allow the patient to wait out a power outage at the fire station if it has power. Firefighter personnel may also help operate the patient's generator if previous arrangements have been made. Determining the optimal plan for handling power outages requires an understanding of the patient's needs, the family's capabilities, and the community services available.

An important aspect of the home environmental assessment is to ensure that the ventilator alarms can be heard by the caregiver in all areas of the home.[18] It is not uncommon for the alarms to be inaudible in the basement, or even in the main living areas if a dishwasher or window air conditioner unit is running. Most ventilator manufacturers offer **remote alarms** that can be placed strategically to ensure that the ventilator alarm is heard throughout the home. Because these alarms work in conjunction with the ventilator, the patient and caregiver can be confident that the alarm has been tested thoroughly. Some families also use commercially available baby monitors in order to hear the patient and ventilator alarms in another room. Some of the latest monitors allow visual observation as well as auditory monitoring of the patient and ventilator. These have served some patients and caregivers well.[19]

A caregiver's direct visual observation of the patient offers the most security for the home mechanical ventilator patient; however, it is not always practical or even preferable. Caregivers sometimes need to use the restroom, and patients often prefer their privacy. Therefore, it is crucial that the patient be able to summon assistance if needed.[17] Although ventilator alarms usually activate appropriately, there can be conditions in which the alarm does not sound. Additionally, the patient may have a problem or need that is not ventilator related; therefore, the patient needs a mechanism for calling the caregiver.

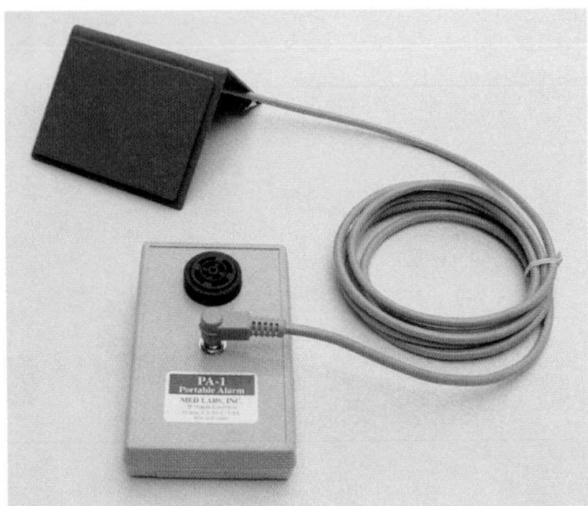

FIGURE 26–4 E-Z Call and PA-1.

Finally, the patient needs a means to call for help if something happens to the caregiver. Ideally, patients should have a means of summoning a caregiver who is in the home with them as well as a means of summoning 911 services. It may be especially important for patients on mouthpiece ventilation to have a means of calling for help because these patients often do not have a low-pressure or disconnect alarm set on their ventilator because the mouthpiece is not in the mouth all of the time.

It is important for the RT to recognize that there is no single communication system that will work for all patients. Some patients are able to shout for help, whereas others cannot speak, or more often, cannot speak loudly enough to be heard in another room. Part of the RT's assessment of the patient should include evaluating what method or methods may work reliably for the patient. Some patients may be able to use a wireless doorbell to summon the caregiver, placing the button with the patient and the chimer with the caregiver. It is important to test the range of the device. Other patients use a cellular phone that is programmed to dial their own home land-line telephone so that the home phone will ring, alerting the caregiver,[19] although this method is dependent on the cellular phone battery being properly charged, having sufficient service, and having a good signal. Unfortunately, both of these methods require a degree of finger strength and dexterity.

The E-Z Call and the PA-1 portable alarm (Med Labs, Goleta, Calif.) are available for the patient who has very limited movement or strength (**Figure 26–4**). The E-Z Call can be connected to a hospital call system or can be used in conjunction with the PA-1 portable alarm. The E-Z Call features a square pad that can be placed on the patient's tray-table. The pad is very sensitive, so that a very light tap on the pad will trigger the PA-1 alarm. If the patient can move only his or her head, the alarm pad can be clipped to the pillow. The PA-1 alarm will sound by pressing the head onto the pad. Another model, called the Bite-or-Puff, uses a strawlike device that the patient bites or puffs into in order to trigger an alarm.

Most DME companies require the family of home-ventilated patients to have a land-line telephone system

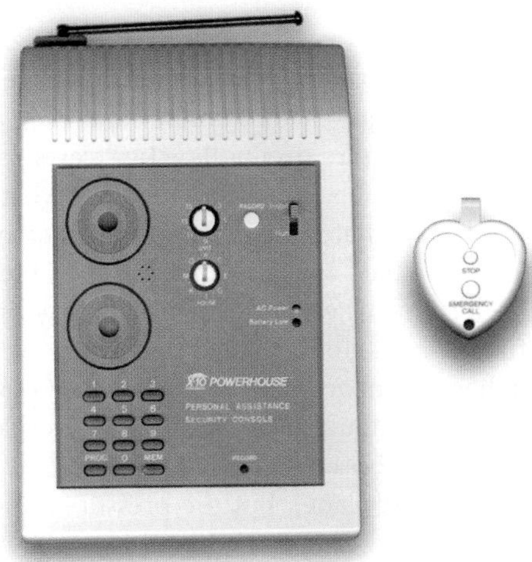

FIGURE 26–5 X10 Personal Assistance Voice Dialer

instead of, or in addition to, a cellular phone.[17] The rationale is that caregivers will most likely take the cell phone with them if they leave the patient in the care of the nurse, potentially leaving the home nurse without a means to summon emergency services should the need arise. Another important reason for the requirement of a landline is that most emergency services providers may be able to more quickly pinpoint the address and location of the individual calling for help when the call comes from a land line.

X10 (Renton, Wash.) makes a relatively inexpensive product called the Personal Assistance Voice Dialer that may be helpful for some patients (**Figure 26–5**). It consists of a base unit connected to the home telephone. It can be activated by pressing a button that can be mounted on the patient's wheelchair tray or worn like a wristwatch or pendant. When activated, the device flashes its lights, sounds a siren alarm, and dials up to four preprogrammed telephone numbers. When the dialed party answers, the Personal Assistance Voice Dialer plays the prerecorded outgoing voice message and then allows the dialed party to listen into the patient's home.

Working with Local Emergency Medical Services and Firefighters

It is a good idea for some home care patients, particularly O_2 and ventilator patients, to meet with their local emergency medical services (EMS) personnel or firefighters before there is any type of emergency. In most communities, EMS personnel or firefighters will visit the patient's home, free of charge, to help perform the home environment evaluation. This visit also allows them to learn where the patient's home is, to note if the house numbers are sufficiently visible, and to learn about any special conditions or needs. If the patient has a do-not-resuscitate order, it should be discussed with the EMS squad during the visit. In some communities, the EMS squad may ask that a copy of the order be taped over the patient's bed, placed on the refrigerator, or worn on an alert bracelet so that it is easily visible should they be called to the home in an emergency situation.

The Physician Order

The initial order for home respiratory equipment often comes to the DME company on a prescription from a physician's pad or on a discharge note from the hospital. If the patient is in the Medicare program, an additional document called a certificate of medical necessity (CMN) may be required. If the patient is to receive clinical respiratory services, a concise description of the planned services must be documented and signed for by the physician. Some therapists refer to these physician-signed orders as a *care plan*, which is the same terminology used by home health nurses. Other therapists refer to the signed orders as a *plan of treatment*, and still others refer to the orders as *the prescription*. Unfortunately, there is no standardized terminology across all home care disciplines.

In recent years, guided self-management has become more commonplace.[20] Guided self-management means that patients or caregivers have appropriate knowledge or are adequately trained so that they know when they can make adjustments to the treatment plan, what adjustments they can make, and when they need to seek medical attention.[21] For the patient who is mechanically ventilated at home, it is now relatively common for a range of ventilator settings to be prescribed by the physician, allowing the patient or caregiver to make adjustments within the prescribed range in order to meet the patient's changing needs.

Long-Term Oxygen Therapy

The Evidence Supporting Home Oxygen Therapy

Oxygen therapy in the home or alternate-site healthcare facility is indicated for the treatment of hypoxemia and has been shown to significantly improve survival in hypoxemic patients with COPD.[22] The Nocturnal Oxygen Therapy Trial (NOTT) and Medical Research Council (MRC) multicenter studies created the foundation for studies showing that continuous use of O_2 improves survival.[23,24] A later review of the NOTT study (**Figure 26–6**) reported that home **long-term oxygen therapy (LTOT)** reduced healthcare costs by reducing hospitalizations.[25]

Key Issues in Oxygen Therapy

The goal for efficient O_2 delivery is proper arterial O_2 saturation at all activity levels.[26] The degree of pulmonary disease is the major determinant of a patient's inspired O_2 requirement. It is important to note that saving O_2 is considered accomplished only *after* the patient is adequately oxygenated and is a secondary objective for device performance. Even if an O_2 delivery device is providing consistent O_2 delivery, results can vary for an individual patient from moment to moment, and between groups of patients using similar devices.

Increased respiratory rate will shorten inspiratory time and may reduce the amount of O_2 a patient will receive (**Figure 26-7**). In the past, the general rule of thumb was to double the patient's flow rate (e.g., from 2 L/min to 4 L/min) during exercise. Any change in respiratory rate or pattern may affect the patient's oxygenation. The lack of attention to this variable in the past has created the misperception that some O_2 delivery devices, especially conserving devices, are not effective. Oxygen-dependent patients should be tested on their O_2 system at different activity levels reflecting real-life conditions—sleep, rest, and exercise, as well as at altitude. A titration test is the standard method of measuring patients' O_2 needs with exercise. There is no standard for O_2 titration. Most clinicians use a simple method that only requires an oximeter and exercise. If a patient will be doing more strenuous activity, every attempt should be made to simulate that activity to see whether the device properly oxygenates the user. Overnight oximetry is strongly recommended for intermittent-flow O_2 delivery devices to determine whether the device is triggering with each breath and maintaining patient Spo_2.[22]

> **RESPIRATORY RECAP**
>
> **Long-Term Oxygen Therapy**
>
> » The goal is to maintain adequate arterial O_2 satuation.
>
> » Studies show that O_2 therapy is life prolonging in patients with chronic obstructive pulmonary disease.
>
> » Respiratory rate affects the amount of O_2 the patient receives.

Altitude has an impact on the pressure of O_2 and not necessarily on the amount of O_2. Oxygen delivery devices deliver approximately the same volume of O_2 at higher altitudes (or in an airplane), but the pressure at different altitudes may have an impact on blood oxygenation. It is important to understand that if an O_2 system is able to meet a patient's O_2 needs at a lower altitude, it is possible that that same system may not be able to meet the patient's needs at a higher altitude. It is generally unfeasible to test patients on their O_2 systems at pressures that they would be experiencing at varying altitudes. A common practice is to double the setting when the patient is at altitude. However, if the O_2 system the patient is using is already running at or near its top setting at a lower altitude, another system should be considered for use at higher altitudes.

By selecting one breathing pattern and one breath rate, a delivered dose volume of O_2 can be made equivalent to the volume taken in during continuous flow of O_2.[27] As a result, manufacturers select a volume of O_2 for a given oxygen conserving device setting that they feel would be equivalent to **continuous-flow oxygen (CFO)** and make that the flow setting on their device. However, this only works if the patient never changes his or her breathing pattern. Most oxygen-conserving devices have a number on the selector dial and, though they claim to deliver O_2 equivalently to CFO at that same setting, are not equivalent to CFO, let alone another conserving device at that setting (**Figure 26-8**). There is a wide variety in FiO_2, and no device can be considered to have delivered therapy equivalent to CFO.

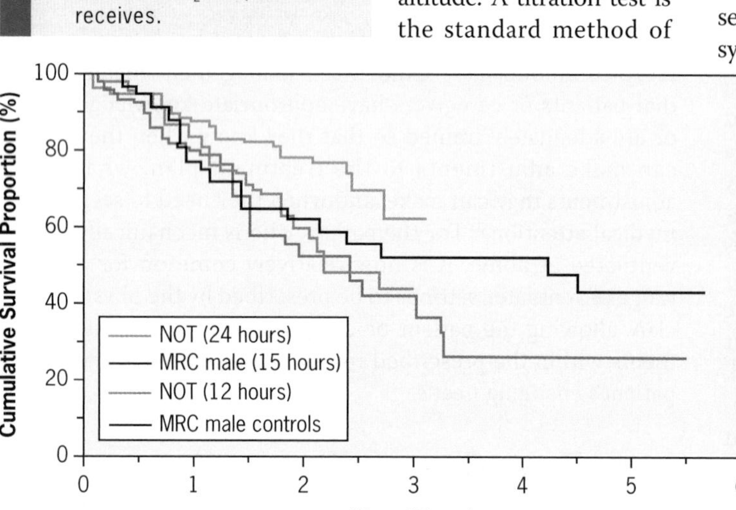

FIGURE 26-6 Nocturnal Oxygen Therapy Trial study results. From Petty TL, McCoy RW, Doherty DE. Long Term Oxygen Therapy (LTOT) History, Scientific Foundations, and Emerging Technologies: Sixth Oxygen Consensus Conference Recommendations. National Lung Health Education Program; August 2005.

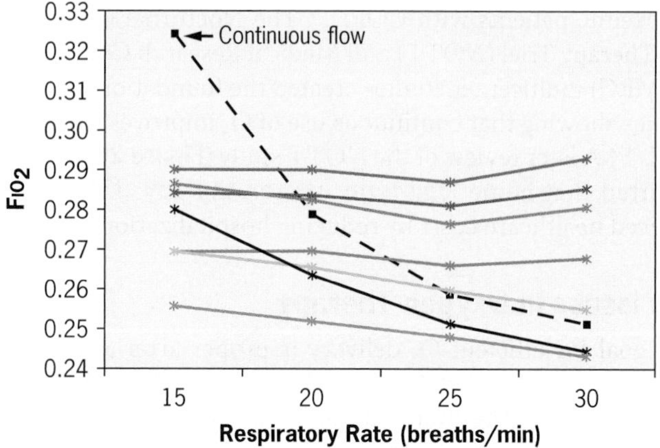

FIGURE 26-7 An example of the impact increased respiratory rate has on FIO_2 between continuous flow and a variety of oxygen-conserving devices.

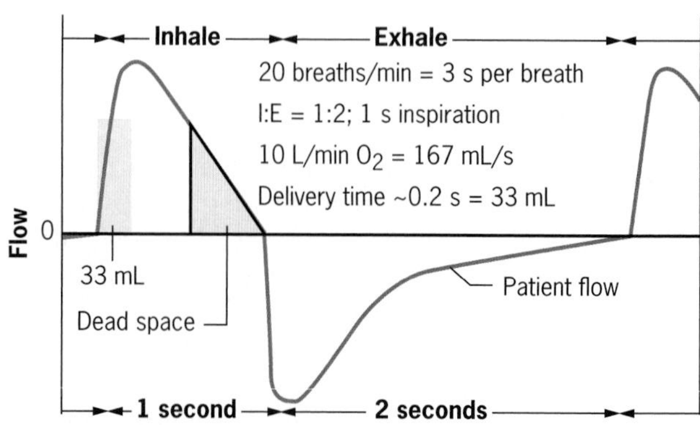

FIGURE 26-8 Increasing peak flow on an oxygen-conserving unit can provide more gas delivery to useful sections of the lung, preventing delivery of oxygen to dead space.

Patients on home O_2 therapy need to stay active to maintain a healthy lifestyle and prevent complications associated with a sedentary lifestyle.[25] Activity is important to health, yet patients requiring supplemental O_2 are challenged by the need to carry or transport the O_2 necessary to maintain proper oxygenation. In the hospital, patients are requested to stay in their beds, and when transportation is necessary, an assistant carries the O_2 and moves patients to their destinations within the hospital. In the home, this is not possible or practical, so patients will need to be provided an O_2 system that is both light enough to transport and capable of providing the required O_2 to meet their needs with activity. In the NOTT study, patients who were high walkers with 12 hours of O_2 had a higher survival than low walkers on 24 hours of O_2 (**Figure 26–9**). This finding indicated that activity had a greater impact on survival than continuous-flow O_2 delivery.

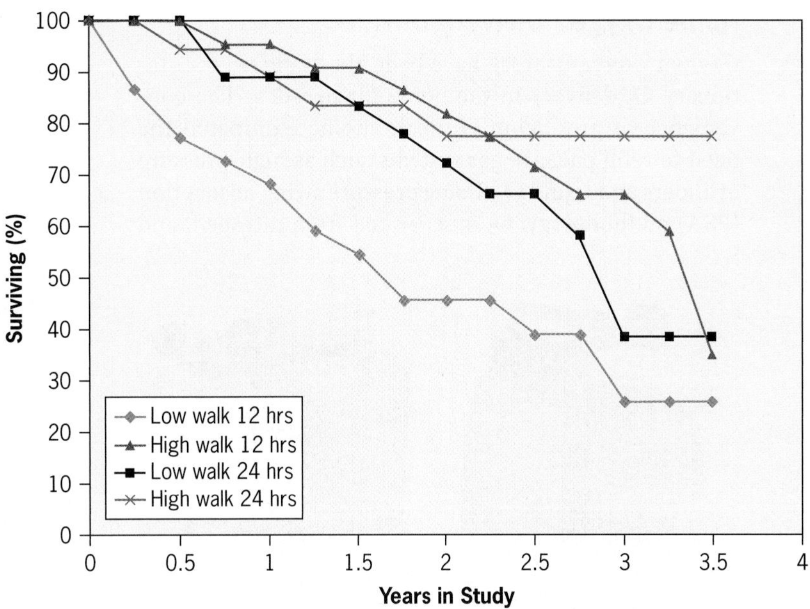

FIGURE 26–9 A retrospective analysis of the Nocturnal Oxygen Therapy Trial data shows the value of exercise to the survival of patients on long-term oxygen therapy. Eighty patients matched for age, treatment group, and FEV_1. They were split into activity groups by walking level measured by pedometer at baseline study. No oxygen during 1-week trial. Medial level was 0.68 miles per day. From Petty TL, McCoy RW, Doherty DE. Long Term Oxygen Therapy (LTOT) History, Scientific Foundations, and Emerging Technologies: Sixth Oxygen Consensus Conference Recommendations. National Lung Health Education Program; August 2005.

Methods of Oxygen Delivery

Continuous-flow O_2 delivery is the standard for O_2 delivery in the hospital and in institutional settings with unlimited O_2 supply, typically from an industrial liquid O_2 source. This is the simplest form of O_2 delivery because the only requirements are a device to meter the flow of O_2 and a patient interface. With an unlimited supply of O_2, simply increasing flow when patient O_2 demands increase is a viable solution. With a limited supply of O_2, however, alternatives are required. In the home, stationary O_2 from a concentrator (**Figure 26–10**) can be thought of as unlimited because the O_2 source is dependent only on electricity, which is usually available. If a packaged gas is used, such as liquid oxygen or compressed gas, refill and distribution issues as well as cost become a consideration.

Intermittent-flow oxygen was a technical challenge until the mid-1980s, when the first intermittent-flow O_2 delivery system was introduced.[28] Sensing a patient's inspiratory effort and triggering a dose of O_2 at the beginning of the patient's inspiratory cycle was an engineering challenge because technology had not evolved to accomplish the objective. Fluidic amplifiers and sensitive pressure switches were included in the first intermittent-flow devices, and the technology has evolved to a high level of sophistication at this time. The challenge to provide a device that is as sensitive as possible to trigger consistently, yet not too sensitive to cause the device to auto-trigger, continues. At this time, all intermittent-flow devices sense breathing through a nasal cannula.

RESPIRATORY RECAP

Methods of Oxygen Delivery
- » Continuous flow
- » Intermittent flow

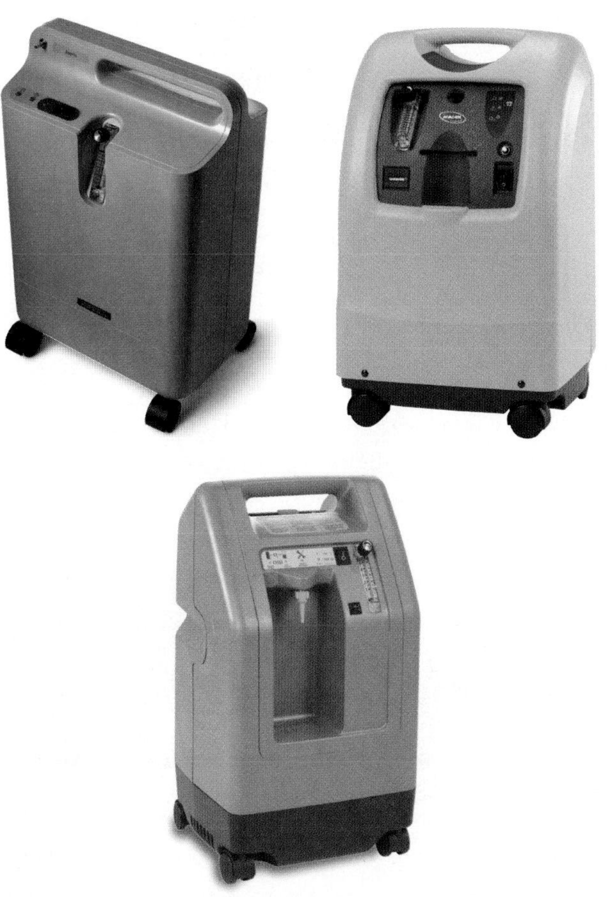

FIGURE 26–10 Example of three stationary oxygen concentrators.

Home Oxygen Delivery Devices

Oxygen concentrators have been the standard for stationary O_2 delivery in the home for decades. The convenience of producing O_2 in the home eliminated the need to refill package gas systems such as high-pressure cylinders and liquid O_2. Using pressure swing adsorption (PSA) methodology, O_2 is separated from nitrogen, and the net result is an F_{IO_2} of 0.93 ± 0.03. Over the years these systems have become more reliable and smaller, and consume less electricity than previous models. Today's typical home stationary O_2 concentrator weighs about 35 pounds (16 kg) and can provide up to 5 L/min continuous-flow O_2. These smaller systems produce less noise and heat, which had been an issue in years past. Stationary concentrators have become the anchor for most home O_2 programs, yet for an ambulatory patient, a portable O_2 system must be provided.

> **RESPIRATORY RECAP**
>
> **Home Oxygen Delivery Devices**
> - » Oxygen concentrators
> - » Compressed gas systems
> - » Liquid oxygen systems
> - » Concentrators that fill compressed gas systems
> - » Portable oxygen concentrators

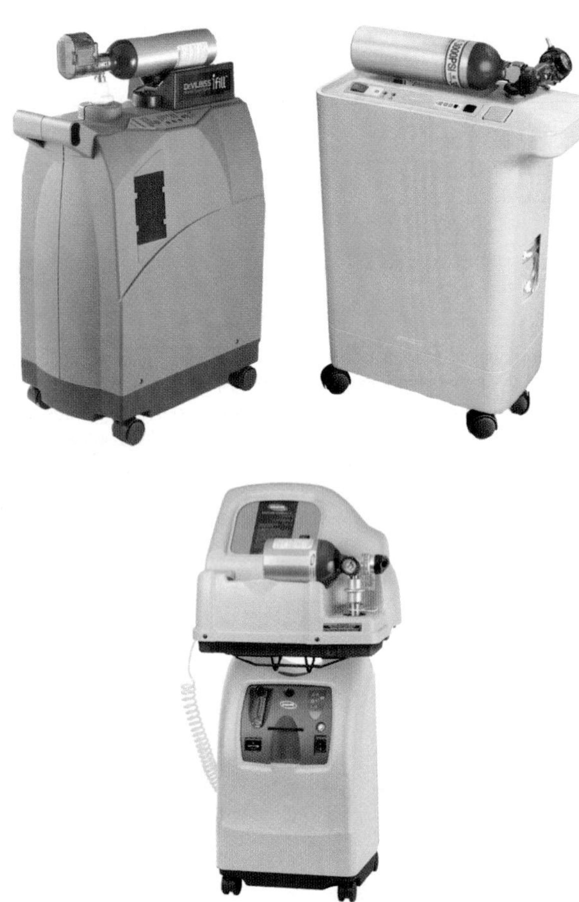

FIGURE 26–11 Transfilling concentrators.

Compressed gas systems were the standard for home O_2 therapy until other options became available. Large cylinders were used in both the hospital and the home as the only source of O_2. When concentrators and liquid oxygen systems became available for the home, cylinder usage decreased. Small cylinders are still used with stationary O_2 when appropriate and in conjunction with a concentrator transfilling system (**Figure 26–11**). Small cylinders come in a variety of sizes and shapes designed to provide the lightest system for the patient, along with the greatest operating range. A typical fill pressure for a cylinder is 2000 psig, yet 3000 psig is available for newer cylinders designed for that operating pressure. Cylinders that are transfilled from a home concentrator will be at a purity equal to the source concentrator, which typically produces 93% ± 3% O_2. Cylinders filled at an industrial gas supplier are at 99% purity.

Liquid oxygen (LOX) storage systems have the greatest storage capacity for O_2 (**Figure 26–12**). Most hospitals use large cryostats to supply the large volume

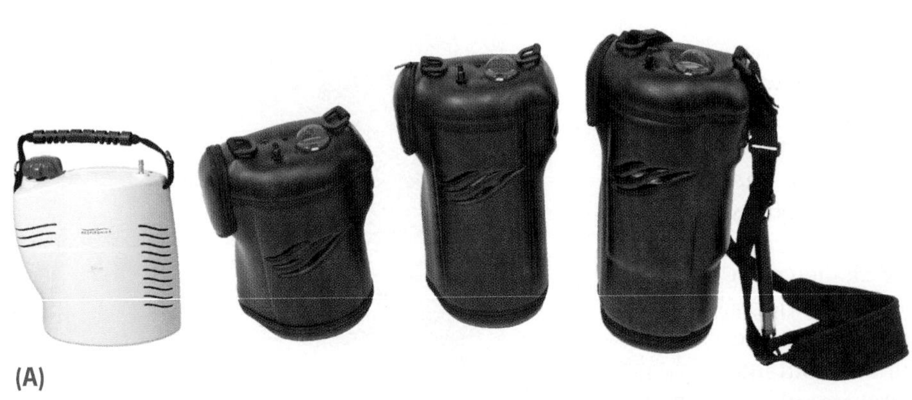

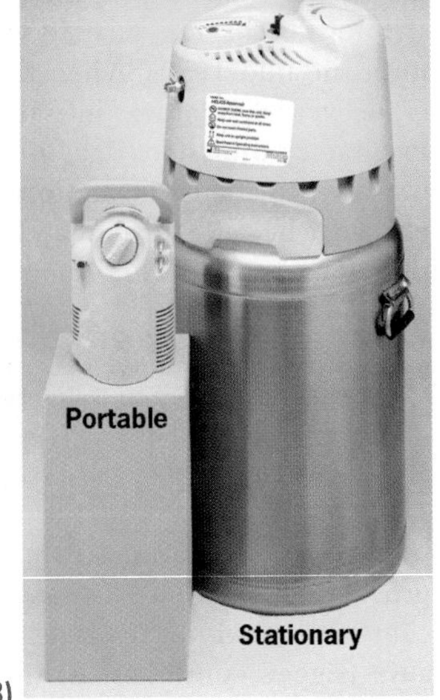

FIGURE 26–12 (**A**) Portable liquid oxygen units. (**B**) A liquid oxygen base unit with a portable.

of O_2 gas required by the hospital. Home LOX systems became available in the mid-1960s when Union Carbide introduced the first home LOX system. The benefit of the home LOX system is the ability to transfill a smaller, lightweight, portable O_2 system. Liquid O_2 has an 860:1 expansion ratio, so 1 liter of LOX will expand to 860 liters of gaseous O_2 with more efficiency and greater weight-to-operating-time ratio than packaged gas. LOX became the choice for patients who were highly ambulatory and required more functionality from their portable O_2 system. Limitations of a LOX system are that it has a finite amount of gas and requires refilling from a larger base unit. Both the base units and portable units come in a variety of sizes, allowing for refilling options for both patients and O_2 distributors.

Concentrators that fill compressed gas cylinders in the home entered the market a few years ago. Models differ among manufacturers, but the principles remain the same. A concentrator generates O_2 and then transfers the O_2 as compressed gas to the portable cylinder. O_2 monitoring equipment ensures gas purity. This allows patients to refill cylinders themselves, and it saves the home care provider from visiting patients' homes to exchange cylinders. Concentrators that fill LOX portables have just become available for commercial use. The concentrator generates O_2 for the portable, but rather than pressurizing the gas, it is liquefied and transfills to the portable. This allows patients the advantage of both a lightweight and long-term-use portable.

O_2 purity in the portable that is transfilled, with both compressed gas and LOX, is about 94% due to the concentrator being the source gas. The variable with these systems is often the conserving device used with the portable because the source gas for all the systems is similar. Options available for a transfilling system are interchangeable regulators with post valve cylinders, pressure ranges that affect operating times with 2000- and 3000-psig fill pressures, and an option for a combined or separate gas pumping unit for cylinders.

Portable oxygen concentrators (POCs) manufacture O_2; they do not store O_2 (**Figure 26–13**). This requires the POC to produce enough O_2 per minute to allow for an acceptable dose of O_2 to the patient with each breath. POC O_2 production is similar to the larger stationary systems, used in the home since the mid-1970s, that use PSA technology to generate O_2. POC manufacturers have been able to reduce the size of the sieve bed, improve compressor performance, utilize O_2-conserving technology, and integrate sophisticated battery systems to make these systems as small as possible. Each manufacturer has determined how much O_2 the device will produce, which determines maximum O_2 delivery, weight, and operating time.[29] These differences will have an impact on patient therapy, and the clinician needs to know the capabilities of a POC to determine the appropriate device to use for the patient. Patient needs vary as much as the POCs, so there is no one right POC for all patients. Knowing the capabilities of

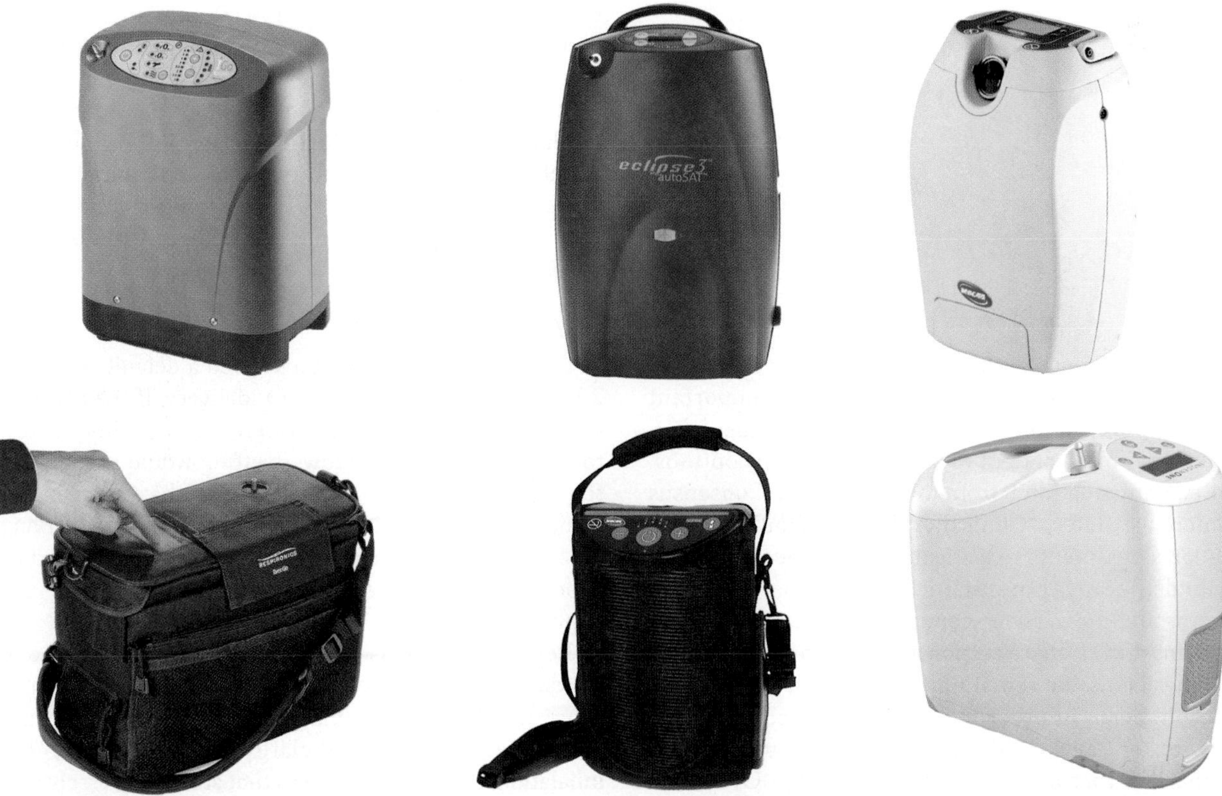

FIGURE 26–13 Portable oxygen concentrators. The units on top are greater than 10 lbs, and the units on the bottom are less than 10 lbs.

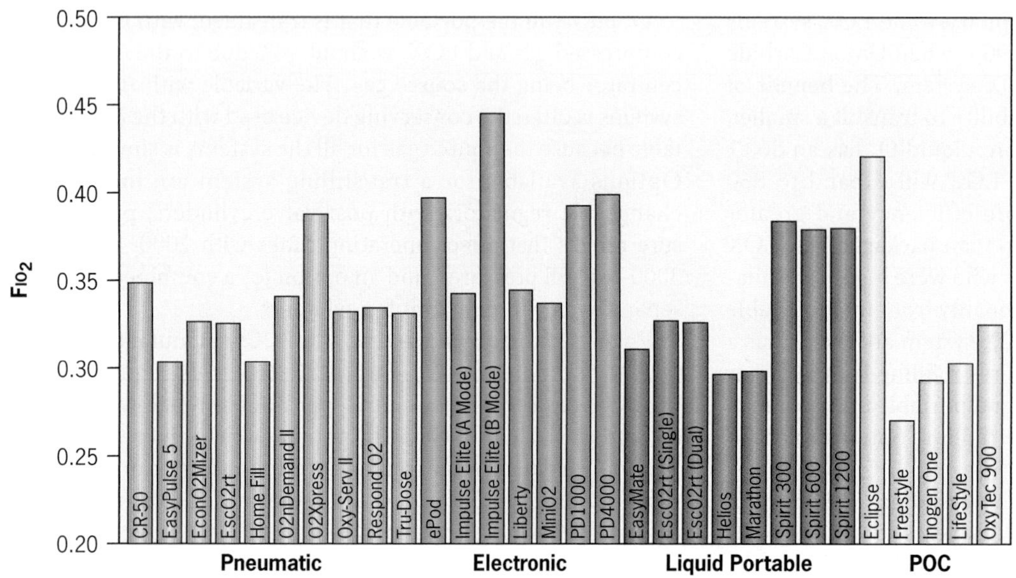

FIGURE 26–14 Maximum FIO_2 delivery at 20 breaths per minute among a variety of home portable oxygen systems.

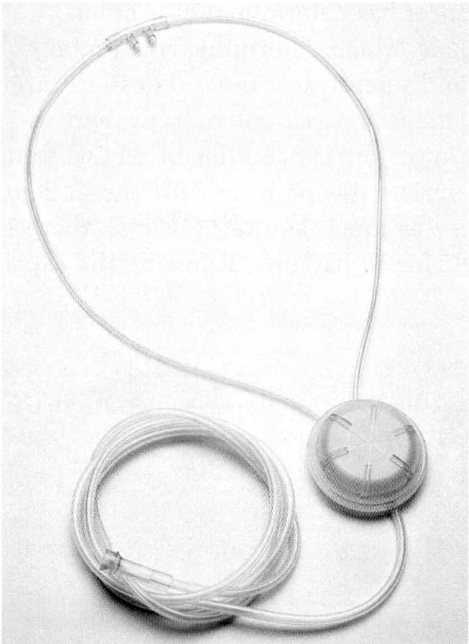

FIGURE 26–15 Reservoir cannula.

the POC, the needs of the patient, and the activities the patient will be doing while using the POC are important points of information for the clinician to consider when working with the patient to determine therapy options.

Recommendation 8 from the 1987 LTOT Consensus Conference states, "Clinical evaluation should include regular assessments of patients' compliance with prescribed therapy, potential complications, potential hazards and the need for continued education. Patients receiving LTOT share responsibility with the prescribing physicians for remaining in communication with their physician in order to assure continued appropriate care for their condition."[30] This recommendation emphasizes that patients be titrated on the O_2 system they will be using at all activity levels at which they will be using the device. Portable O_2 concentrators have the potential to be used at rest, exercise, sleep, and altitude. Each one of these situations needs to be evaluated with the patient and the specific POC.

Portable O_2 concentrators provide the benefit of making O_2 rather than storing it, which allows patients to use electricity to charge batteries so as to use the concentrator when they travel from home. These advantages are tempered by other constraints on the system's operation. Portable O_2 concentrators use the same technology as stationary O_2 concentrators, only in smaller sizes. That means that the maximum O_2 produced and the dosing of the O_2 differ by concentrator. These two variables restrict the system because the concentrator cannot make more O_2 than it was originally intended to produce. If the patient increases the demand with a higher dose setting or respiratory rate, either delivered dose, O_2 purity, or both will decrease.[31] These limitations must be considered when prescribing and monitoring patients on this system, as well as any portable O_2 system, due to the limited maximum amount of O_2 that can be provided (**Figure 26–14**). Systems weighing less than 10 pounds (4.5 kg) only use oxygen-conserving technology and therefore are suitable for use in a car, airplane, or wheelchair (patient seated); they may have variable effectiveness with exercise. Systems weighing more than 10 pounds (4.5 kg) are capable of continuous-flow and O_2-conserving and can be used for most purposes, including exercise and sleep.

Oxygen-Conserving Devices

In the past, patients were prescribed a default setting of 2 L/min continuous flow for O_2 delivery. If the patient's O_2 levels were appropriate, rarely did the clinician test to determine whether a lower setting would accomplish the same objective. Doing so would have conserved some O_2.[32] With the introduction of **oxygen-conserving devices (OCDs)**, regular CFO therapy from O_2 cylinders is being used much less than in the past for home care applications.

Reservoir cannulas, often referred to as moustache or pendant cannulas depending on the design and use characteristics, have approximately 20 mL of reservoir space that stores O_2 during exhalation (**Figure 26–15**). On inhalation, the patient receives that stored O_2, essentially adding a bolus volume to the ongoing continuous-flow delivery. These devices are simple, effective, and, when used properly, can allow a patient to receive the same therapy at a lower CFO flow rate, thus conserving O_2. Although they are effective, their appearance has been a limiting factor.

Intermittent-flow devices operate by turning O_2 delivery on during some portion of inhalation and off for the balance of the breathing cycle. In this way, O_2 that would otherwise be wasted as the patient exhales is conserved. This often allows a supply of O_2 to last two to four times as long as it would if it were delivered continuously. One benefit of the use of intermittent-flow conserving devices is that a smaller O_2 supply may be carried. With intermittent-flow devices, the way in which O_2 is delivered to the patient differs greatly from one device to another, and no device delivers O_2 in the same way as continuous-flow devices. Intermittent-flow devices can be separated into two broad categories, pulse and demand, and within these categories there are many variants.

Pulse flow is defined as the device responding to the patient's inspiratory effort and terminating flow at a predetermined time that is controlled electronically.[33] Pulse delivery devices deliver O_2 in the form of a relatively high flow rate bolus beginning early in inhalation. Some pulse delivery devices vary the dose of O_2 by changing the duration of the bolus. Others increase the peak flow rate at which the dose is delivered as the user increases the setting number. Some devices do a combination of both. Most pulse delivery devices deliver volumes at a given setting regardless of the breathing rate. As respiratory rate increases, the volume of O_2 inhaled from a CFO device over time does not change. With a typical pulse delivery device, however, the bolus volume is always the same, and so the O_2 volume inhaled per minute increases as the breath rate increases (assuming the entire bolus volume is inhaled; at high rates and/or high settings this may not be the case). As a patient moves from rest to activity and his or her breath rate increases, a pulse device operating in this manner may maintain oxygenation better than a continuous-flow or a demand device. However, this has not been proven clinically and it is impossible to say that pulse-type delivery is equivalent to continuous-flow delivery across a wide variety of breathing patterns. Device manufacturers, however, label their products with the same setting numbers used for continuous flow (1, 2, 3, etc.), and so there is often confusion about why a conserving device set at 2 is not oxygenating a patient like a continuous-flow device at 2 L/min. Pulse systems typically need a power source, so batteries are a factor to consider.

RESPIRATORY RECAP

Oxygen-Conserving Devices

- » Reservoir cannulas
- » Intermittent-flow devices
- » Pulse-flow devices
- » Demand delivery devices
- » Transtracheal oxygen

Demand delivery devices have evolved from the initial idea of creating an oxygen-conserving device that uses the patient's breathing to turn on the device during inhalation and off during exhalation. Demand flow senses the patient's inspiratory effort, yet flow is terminated on exhalation. The amount of O_2 delivered will vary with inspiratory time. These units are not as efficient as pulse-flow devices in utilization of O_2, yet have the advantage of not requiring batteries. Most demand systems use a dual-lumen cannula, with one channel of the cannula sensing inspiration and the other channel delivering O_2. A set rate of O_2 is delivered over the entire inhalation cycle only. These devices are sometimes called hybrids because they act like both a pulse and demand device, delivering a fixed pulse volume at the onset of inhalation and then continuing to deliver O_2 until the device senses the beginning of exhalation.

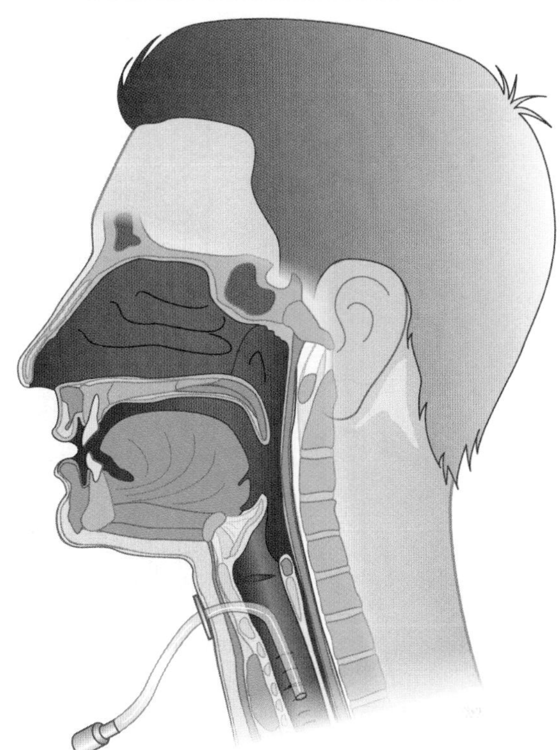

FIGURE 26–16 Transtracheal placement of oxygen delivery catheter.

Transtracheal oxygen (**Figure 26–16**) uses a catheter that is placed during a surgical procedure to bypass the upper airway.[34] The catheter is placed through a small hole made in the front of the neck and into the trachea. O_2 conservation is achieved because the patient is usually able to be given the equivalent of CFO therapy with nasal breathing at a lower continuous-flow setting. A single-lumen intermittent-flow conserving device can be used with transtracheal delivery, but the O_2 savings are about the same as using nasal breathing with that same intermittent-flow device. A benefit of transtracheal O_2 therapy is an increase in patient compliance with therapy because it is hidden from others to see the catheter.

With the manufacturers focusing on O_2 savings rather than patient oxygenation, OCDs have

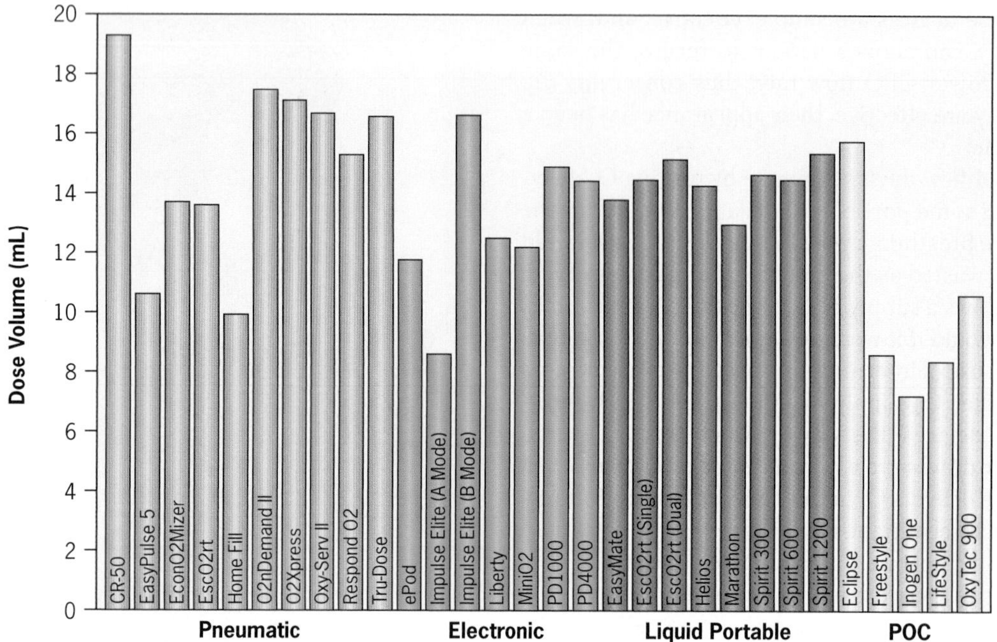

FIGURE 26–17 The average dose volume per setting at 20 breaths per minute for a variety of oxygen-conserving devices, indicating the high variability of dose volume among products.

had an acceptance problem.[35] Because the devices differ in dose delivery (**Figure 26–17**), patients should be tested on the unit they will be using in the home and at the activity levels at which they will use the device. Clinicians need to be informed about the performance capabilities of each piece of equipment that a patient uses. A respiratory-rate-regulated OCD monitors the patient's respiratory rate and has an algorithm that switches the dose setting to a higher dose with a higher respiratory rate. As the patient breathes faster, the dose will increase; as the patient breathes slower, the dose will return to a lower setting. This technique allows the patient to increase the dose of O_2 with demand without manually changing the dose setting. An oximeter-regulated OCD monitors the patient's Spo_2. An algorithm in the device changes the O_2 dose based on Spo_2. There is an approved product with this feature, but it is not currently commercially available. A motion-regulated OCD senses movement and changes the O_2 dose to a higher setting. When movement stops, the OCD then switches back to the lower dose setting. An approved product featuring this ability to change dose setting as a result of movement is currently on the market.

High-Flow Oxygen Delivery in the Home

Typically, home O_2 therapy is provided in a range of 1 to 6 L/min, yet flows of up to 10 L/min are possible from some O_2 concentrators. Home LOX systems can provide up to 15 L/min with units designed for that flow. Industrial LOX units can be used for flows higher than 15 L/min. Home portable O_2 systems can operate at higher flows, yet for a very short time. Patients requiring high-flow portable O_2 typically use a LOX system for the efficient operation. Special delivery tubing and cannulas need to be used for higher-flow systems to compensate for the resistance to the higher flows.

Diagnostics Systems for Long-Term Oxygen Therapy

Personal oximeters are used to assess a patient's Spo_2. Small, simple-to-operate units can be used by patients to assess their O_2 status. Patients' ability to understand the oximeter values and the variability of both the oximeter and the O_2 delivery system have caused some concern, yet many patients are purchasing personal oximeters. Education is key to the safe and effective use of a personal oximeter, and clinicians should take every opportunity to reinforce the issues related to their use.

Home care providers check continuous-flow units with devices that monitor O_2 concentration and flow. A simple liter meter can verify flow in the home and determine whether the O_2 delivery device is providing the flow correctly or whether extended O_2 supply tubing has created a drop in flow. There is a device that monitors both flows and O_2 concentrations. Basic O_2 monitors are also used for doing routine checks on home O_2 equipment. Pulse-dose O_2 delivery from an oxygen-conserving device requires a test unit that can measure volume rather than flow. These O_2 systems deliver a specific amount (mL) of O_2 that can be measured to determine whether the device is operating within specifications. Each oxygen-conserving device provides a different volume of O_2 at a specific setting, so the manufacturer's specific value is needed to determine whether the device is working within the specifications.

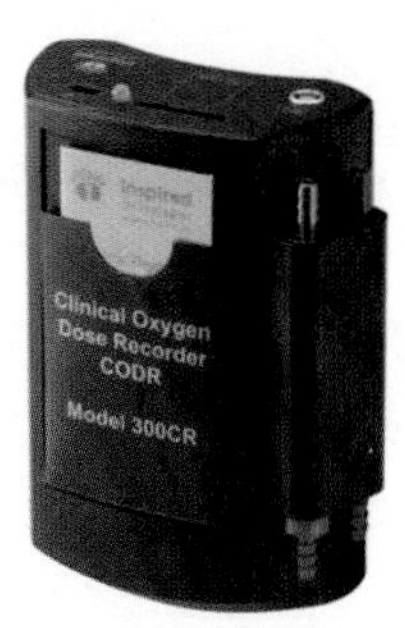

FIGURE 26–18 Clinical Oxygen Dose Recorder system.

A system has been developed that can monitor both the O_2 delivery device and the patient (**Figure 26–18**). This unit can determine the delivery capabilities of the O_2 system and how the patient is responding. Given the great variability of performance in portable O_2 systems, this unit can help clinicians determine which home O_2 system should be used based on patient requirements.

Oxygen Delivery Accessory Items

Carts have helped patients be more mobile with their O_2 systems. Originally O_2 carts were the same as those used in the hospital, with weight and aesthetics being an issue. Now lightweight functional carts are available for the home O_2 patient's use. Backpacks became a request of patients who wanted to have more free use of their hands. A user-friendly backpack allows for more mobility for an active LTOT patient performing the activities of daily living than is typically possible with a shoulder strap. Shoulder straps have also evolved to more comfortable, aesthetically pleasing options. Some shoulder straps are made of elastic material that can act as a shock absorber for the pressure transferred to the shoulder.

Liter meters are devices that are used to spot-check the continuous flow from a low-flow O_2 device. These devices are used by home care providers to check the accuracy of the flow setting, yet patients can do the same spot check with proper training and availability of the tool. Pulse meters are devices that check the pulse volume of a pulse-style intermittent-flow device. These products are used by home care providers yet are more expensive than a liter meter, so may not be an option for patient purchase and use.

Batteries are an option for POCs because the operation time of a POC away from an AC or DC source is determined by the use time of the battery. If necessary, additional batteries can extend use time and are an important factor for air travel. Pulse-style conserving devices have a set battery life, so extra batteries should be available for the system as a backup.

Patient Delivery Interface Devices

The nasal cannula has been the standard for low-flow O_2 delivery. Cannula options have included multiple lengths for specific applications, different materials (e.g., plastic, silicone) different-diameter nasal prong lumens, and accessories for comfort. Lumen size and tubing length have an impact on O_2 delivery, and if the cannula is changed to a different capability, the flow and patient oximetry should be checked. Single-lumen cannulas are typical and account for the majority of cannula options. Dual-lumen cannulas are used with demand flow-conserving devices and can be used for other gas monitoring, such as CO_2 monitoring.

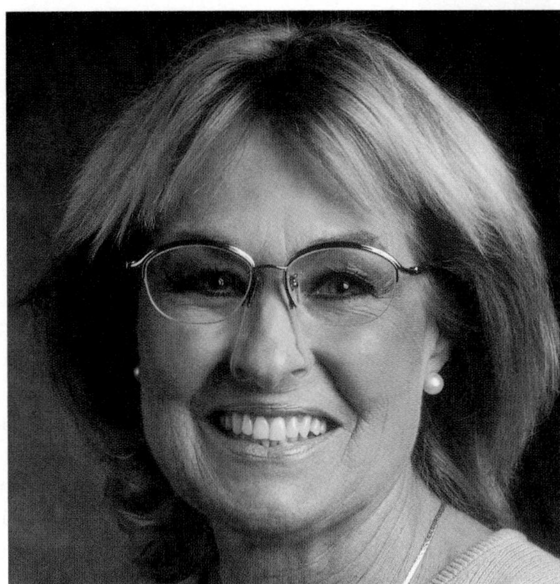

FIGURE 26–19 Oxy-View glasses.

Headset low-flow O_2 delivery was originally designed to provide an alternative to the cannula putting pressure on the ears and cheeks. Headsets are used with prolonged phone use, so they appear to be a good option for patients using home O_2. Oxygen glasses have the same potential as the headset (**Figure 26–19**). The oxygen glasses also add an aesthetic value because often patients using these devices are not known to be wearing oxygen.

Nasal masks are an alternative to the cannula. The nasal mask cups O_2 around the nose to eliminate the prongs entering the nose. If the nasal cannula prongs are causing irritation, the nasal mask can be used as an option. The nasal mask must be used with continuous-flow O_2 because the conserving-type systems would not be able to sense an inspiration and function properly.

Home Mechanical Ventilation

There is no general agreement on the definition of a home mechanical ventilator. Some clinicians refer to a bilevel flow-generator that includes a backup rate, known in Medicare parlance as a *respiratory assist device* (RAD), as a mechanical ventilator. Other clinicians reserve the term *mechanical ventilator* for devices that include an exhalation valve (as opposed to a passive exhalation port) and the ability to set a breath rate and alarms. The Medicare program has categorized devices with exhalation valves, adjustable breath rates, and alarms as mechanical ventilators and places them in the group of devices requiring frequent and substantial service. Medicare will rent a mechanical ventilator for qualified patients as long as medical necessity exists. However, Medicare

TABLE 26–3 FDA Classification of Home Mechanical Ventilators

FDA Code	FDA Definitions	Common Use Description
CBK	Continuous facility use	Life support ventilator for patients with respiratory failure
NOU	Continuous home use	Life support ventilator for patients with respiratory failure
MNS	Continuous, non–life supporting; non-active exhalation valve	Non–life support, for patients with respiratory insufficiency or obstructive sleep apnea

places respiratory assist devices in the capped rental category. For capped rental equipment, the DME provider receives a monthly rental fee for 13 months, after which the ownership of the equipment is transferred to the Medicare beneficiary. It is imperative for the home care RT to periodically reevaluate patients receiving any type of home ventilation, including those who are using respiratory assist devices. Some patients with deteriorating conditions such as ALS or Duchenne muscular dystrophy who are using a respiratory assist device may ultimately need to transition to a mechanical ventilator appropriate for life-support ventilation. The plan for managing the patient's respiratory needs throughout the disease process should be discussed in advance with the patient and the physician, as well as the patient's family when appropriate.

The Food and Drug Administration (FDA) classifies mechanical ventilators as described in **Table 26–3**. Note that all of the home ventilators classified by the FDA as life-support ventilators have been placed in the Medicare category that requires frequent and substantial service. In the United States, individuals who have a tracheostomy and need home mechanical ventilation have traditionally been placed on a CBK device. The FDA has recently created a new code, NOU, for home mechanical ventilators. The new code's purpose is to clarify that home mechanical ventilators must be tracked by the home medical equipment company so that, in the event of a recall, the device can be located. The FDA broadly defines the intended use of each device; individuals who need noninvasive home mechanical ventilation for respiratory insufficiency are often placed on a CBK, NOU, or MNS device, depending on the acuity of the patient's condition and the expected course of the disease, and the physician's preference.

An accurate count of the number of individuals receiving home mechanical ventilation in the United States is unknown. Unlike many European countries, the United States does not have a central registry or database tracking individuals receiving either invasive or noninvasive home mechanical ventilation. In 1998 there were an estimated 10,000 to 20,000 patients on home mechanical ventilation.[19] Using Medicare claims data from 2005, a rough estimate of 3100 patients can be derived. Based on the estimated number of Medicare home ventilator patients, the actual number of invasively ventilated patients at home is likely close to 10,000. Medicare claims data for 2005 for noninvasive positive pressure ventilation (NIV) suggests there are approximately 7600 patients using NIV with a backup rate.[8]

Diagnoses and Indications for Home Mechanical Ventilation

A number of medical conditions and indications may result in the need for home mechanical ventilation (**Box 26–2** and **Box 26–3**). Note in particular that the indication for invasive ventilation (as opposed to noninvasive ventilation) for individuals requiring more than 20 hours of ventilatory support per day is not a hard and fast rule. Some individuals can be successfully ventilated with noninvasive methods for 24 hours per day for many years.[36] However, some patients prefer invasive ventilation if the need for support is continuous or almost continuous. Also note that the indications listed are similar to, but not exactly the same as, the Centers for Medicare and Medicaid Services (CMS) requirements for coverage of respiratory assist devices. The American Association of Respiratory Care and the American College of Chest Physicians both have drafted goals for the management of mechanical ventilation in the home (**Table 26–4**).

Discharge Planning for the Patient Going Home with a Mechanical Ventilator

If a hospitalized patient is prescribed home mechanical ventilation, a comprehensive team approach to discharge planning is required (**CPG 26–1**). Most home care RTs

TABLE 26–4 Goals for Home Mechanical Ventilation

American College of Chest Physicians	American Association for Respiratory Care
Provide an environment that enhances the individual's potential Improve physical and physiologic function Reduce morbidity Extend life Provide cost-effective care	Sustain and extend life Enhance the quality of life Reduce morbidity Improve or sustain physical and psychological function of all VAIs and enhance growth and development in pediatric VAIs Provide cost-effective care

VAI, ventilator-assisted individual.

Adapted from Make BJ, Hill NS, Goldberg AI, et al. Mechanical ventilation beyond the intensive care unit: report of a consensus of the American College of Chest Physicians. *Chest.* 1998;113:5(suppl):289S–344S.

BOX 26–2

Medical Conditions That May Be Appropriate for Home Mechanical Ventilation

Central Nervous System Disorders

- Arnold-Chiari malformation
- Central nervous system trauma
- Cerebrovascular disorders
- Congenital and acquired central control of breathing disorders
- Myelomeningocele
- Spinal cord traumatic injuries

Neuromuscular Disorders

- Amyotrophic lateral sclerosis
- Guillain-Barré syndrome
- Muscular dystrophies
- Myasthenia gravis
- Phrenic nerve paralysis
- Polio and postpolio sequelae
- Spinal muscle atrophy
- Myotonic dystrophy

Skeletal Disorders

- Kyphoscoliosis
- Thoracic wall deformities
- Thoracoplasty

Cardiovascular Disorders

- Acquired and congenital heart disease

Respiratory Disorders

- Upper airway
  - Pierre-Robin syndrome
  - Tracheomalacia
  - Vocal cord paralysis
- Lower airway
  - Bronchopulmonary dysplasia
  - Chronic obstructive pulmonary disease
  - Cystic fibrosis
  - Complications of infectious pneumonias
  - Pulmonary fibrotic diseases

Adapted from Make BJ, Hill NS, Goldberg AI, et al. Mechanical ventilation beyond the intensive care unit: report of a consensus of the American College of Chest Physicians. *Chest.* 1998;113(5 suppl):289S–344S.

BOX 26–3

Indications for Home Mechanical Ventilation

Indications for Noninvasive Ventilation

Patient has chronic stable or slowly progressive respiratory failure:

- Significant CO_2 retention ($\geqq$50 mm Hg) with appropriately compensated pH *or*
- Mild daytime nocturnal CO_2 retention (45 to 50 mm Hg) with symptoms attributable to hypoventilation (e.g., morning headaches, restless sleep, nightmares, enuresis, daytime hypersomnolence)
- Significant nocturnal hypoventilation or oxygen desaturation

The following conditions have been met:

- Patient has had optimal medical therapy for underlying respiratory disorders
- Patient is able to protect airway and adequately clear secretions
- Patient's reversible contributing factors have been treated (e.g., obstructive sleep apnea, congestive heart failure, severe electrolyte disturbance)

The diagnosis is appropriate.

Indications for Invasive Ventilation

Patient meets indications for noninvasive ventilation and has the following:

- Uncontrollable airway secretions despite use of noninvasive expiratory aids *or*
- Impaired swallowing leading to chronic aspiration and repeated pneumonias

Patient has persistent symptomatic respiratory insufficiency and fails to tolerate or improve with noninvasive ventilation.

Patient needs round-the-clock (>20 hours per day) ventilatory support because of severely weakened or paralyzed respiratory muscles (e.g., high spinal cord injury or end-stage neuromuscular disease) and patient or provider prefers invasive ventilation.

Adapted from Make BJ, Hill NS, Goldberg AI, et al. Mechanical ventilation beyond the intensive care unit: report of a consensus of the American College of Chest Physicians. *Chest.* 1998;113(5 suppl):289S–344S.

CLINICAL PRACTICE GUIDELINE 26–1

Oxygen Therapy in the Home or Alternate-Site Healthcare Facility

Indications

- Long-term oxygen therapy (LTOT) in the home or alternate-site healthcare facility is normally indicated for the treatment of hypoxemia. LTOT has been shown to significantly improve survival in hypoxemic patients with chronic obstructive pulmonary disease (COPD). LTOT has been shown to reduce hospitalizations and lengths of stay.
- Laboratory indications: Documented hypoxemia in adults, children, and infants older than 28 days as evidenced by (1) Pao_2 less than or equal to 55 mm Hg or Sao_2 less than or equal to 88% in subjects breathing room air or (2) Pao_2 of 56 to 59 mm Hg or Sao_2 or Spo_2 less than or equal to 89% in association with specific clinical conditions (e.g., cor pulmonale, congestive heart failure, erythrocythemia with hematocrit above 56).
- Some patients may not demonstrate a need for oxygen therapy at rest (normoxic) but will be hypoxemic during ambulation, sleep, or exercise. Oxygen therapy is indicated during these specific activities when the Sao_2 is demonstrated to fall to 88% or below.
- Oxygen therapy may be prescribed by the attending physician for indications outside of those noted above or in cases where strong evidence may be lacking (e.g., cluster headaches) on the order and discretion of the attending physician.
- Patients who are approaching the end of life frequently exhibit dyspnea with or without hypoxemia. Dyspnea in the absence of hypoxemia can be treated with techniques and drugs other than oxygen. Oxygen may be tried in these patients at 1 to 3 liters per minute, to obtain subjective relief of dyspnea.
- All oxygen must be prescribed and dispensed in accordance with federal, state, and local laws and regulations.

Contraindications

- No absolute contraindications to oxygen therapy exist when indications are present.

Precautions and Possible Complications

- There is a potential in some spontaneously breathing hypoxemic patients with hypercapnia and chronic obstructive pulmonary disease for oxygen administration to lead to an increase in $Paco_2$.
- Undesirable results or events may result from noncompliance with physicians' orders or inadequate instruction in home oxygen therapy.
- Complications may result from use of nasal cannulas or transtracheal catheters.
- Fire hazard is increased in the presence of increased oxygen concentrations.
- Bacterial contamination associated with certain nebulizers and humidification systems is a possible hazard.
- Possible physical hazards can be posed by unsecured cylinders, ungrounded equipment, or mishandling of liquid oxygen. Power or equipment malfunction and/or failure can lead to an interruption in oxygen supply.

Modified from AARC clinical practice guideline: oxygen therapy in the home or alternative site health care facility. *Respir Care.* 2007;52:1063–1068. Reprinted with permission.

suggest a minimum of 2 weeks of preparation to ensure that the home environment is appropriate and that all required education has been performed. Most home care companies require that a minimum of two family or lay caregivers be identified and trained prior to discharge of the home mechanically ventilated patient. Appropriately trained lay caregivers must be able to explain and demonstrate the proper use, troubleshooting, and routine maintenance of the ventilator and all related equipment (**Table 26–5**). The caregiver must know how and when to order supplies, and must be able to maintain good infection control processes. Importantly, the caregiver must verbalize and demonstrate the proper response to emergencies such as power failures, equipment failures, or serious patient events such as accidental decannulation.[37]

Ideally, the home care RT works with the appropriate hospital staff to jointly complete an instructional checklist to ensure that the patient and family are properly trained (**Table 26–6**). Education of the patient and of family caregivers should promote positive interactions in a low-key manner.[38] Depending on the patient's

TABLE 26-5 Common Home Medical Equipment and Supplies for a Patient Ventilated at Home

Home Medical Equipment		
Bedside ventilator and wheelchair ventilator	Oxygen concentrator	Enteral pump
Power wheelchair	Portable oxygen cylinder system (regulator, cart, or carry bag)	Special mattress surface (to promote skin integrity and to avoid pneumonia)
Heated humidifier	Nebulizer compressor and/or 50-psi compressor	Cough assist device
Portable suction machine (stationary suction machine optional)	Hospital bed	Intermittent percussive ventilator (IPV)
External battery and charger or universal power supply (UPS)	Portable battery and charger	Lymphedema pump
Oximeter	End-tidal CO_2 monitor	Remote ventilator alarm and/or patient monitoring system
Supplies		
Oxygen tubing	Suction tubing and canister	Nebulizer cups
Oximeter probe	End-tidal CO_2 tubing and connector	Gloves
Tracheostomy tubes and inner cannulas (patient size and one size down)	Syringes (for cuff maintenance)	Suction catheters
Flex tubing (tracheostomy tube to ventilator circuit)	Ventilator circuits	Speaking valve
Tracheostomy care kits	Tracheostomy ties	Elbows (tracheostomy tube to flex tubing)
Heat and moisture exchangers	Humidifier chambers	Distilled or sterile water for humidifier (per prescription)
Bacterial filters for ventilator and cough assist	Tubing for cough assist	IPV circuit
Water traps (if not using heated tubing)	Enteral pump sets	Lymphedema stockings

TABLE 26-6 Predischarge Joint Instructional Plan for Home Mechanical Ventilation

Instructions for form completion: 1. List the topic that will be covered. 2. Jointly determine whether the hospital RN, hospital RT, or home care RT is responsible for instruction of each topic. 3–6. Record the instructor's name, the date(s) of the verbal instruction, and the date(s) of the demonstration. Record your initials and date in column 5 if the patient/family demonstrated with verbal assistance and in column 6 if patient/family demonstrated skill completely independently.

1. Topic	2. Person Responsible for Instruction	3. Verbal Instruction Provided *(Also note "WM" if written materials provided)*	4. Demonstration Provided	5. Patient/Family Performed Satisfactory Demonstration with Verbal Assistance	6. Patient/Family Performed Satisfactory Demonstration Without Assistance
Use of resuscitation bag • When to use • Connect to O_2 • Adjusting O_2 flow • How hard to squeeze bag • Rate of squeeze					
Suctioning • Check suction pressure • Supplies used at home (glove[s], kit) • When to suction • Preoxygenation • Remove from ventilator • Insert catheter • Remove catheter • Number of passes • Back on ventilator					

condition and on family caregiver availability, it helps if each educational session is limited to 30- to 60-minute time periods over several days. These sessions may be taught by the RT and reinforced by the hospital nursing staff, or vice versa. It is also crucial that patients (when able), as well as family caregivers, perform return demonstrations without prompting. Home care RTs usually recommend a minimum 24-hour live-in demonstration, during which the family caregivers perform all of the patient's care without help from the RT or hospital staff,

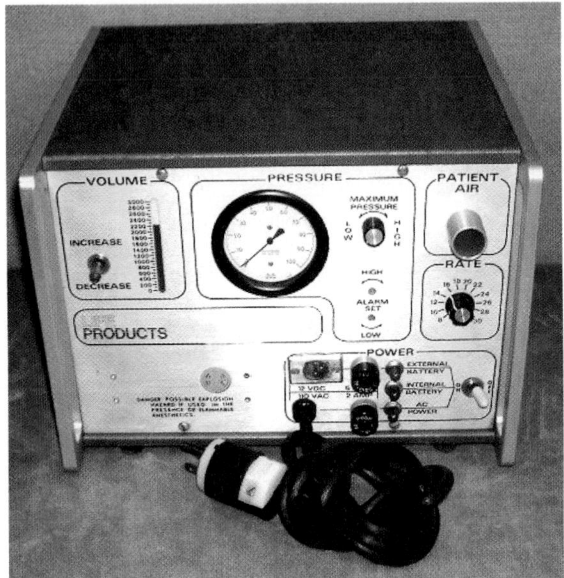

FIGURE 26–20 Life Products LP-3.

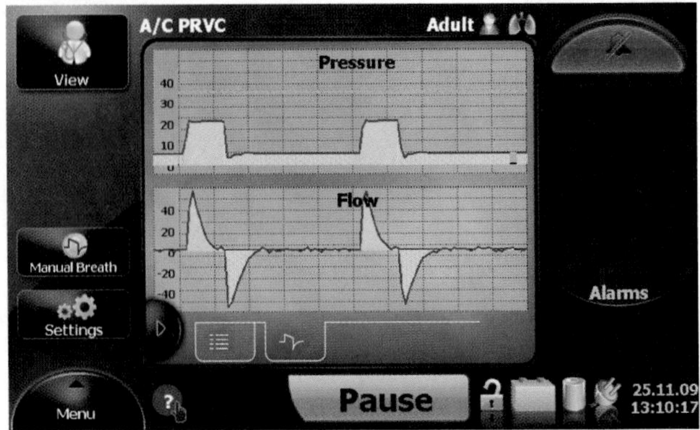

FIGURE 26–21 User interface showing A/C PRVC (assist/control, pressure-regulated volume control mode) on the iVent 101.

as the final indication that the patient and family are ready for discharge.

Evolution of Positive Pressure Home Mechanical Ventilators

The first generation of positive pressure home care ventilators were piston driven and offered volume-controlled breaths only (**Table 26–7**). These ventilators weighed over 30 pounds (14 kg) and had very limited internal battery duration. First-generation devices had few options for external batteries other than large, sealed lead acid batteries. Bulky external positive end-expiratory pressure (PEEP) valves also contributed to the lack of easy portability. First-generation home care ventilators included the Life Products LP-3 (**Figure 26–20**) and Lifecare Services PLV-100 portable ventilators. Many patients still use first-generation devices.

With a few exceptions, the second generation of home ventilators switched from piston driven to turbine driven. Another major difference between first- and second-generation ventilators was the addition of modes such as pressure control, pressure support, and synchronized intermittent mandatory ventilation (SIMV). The second-generation ventilators also offered significant improvements in battery options, as well as enhanced portability. Most of the second-generation ventilators allow supplemental O_2 to be connected to a port directly on the ventilator rather than titrated into the patient circuit. Additionally, most of the second-generation devices changed from using an external PEEP control to a PEEP control integrated into the ventilator. There are many patients using second-generation devices.

> **RESPIRATORY RECAP**
>
> **Home Mechanical Ventilators**
>
> » First-generation ventilators were piston driven and offered only volume-controlled breaths.
>
> » Second-generation ventilators switched from piston driven to turbine driven and offered a variety of modes.
>
> » Third-generation ventilators are turbine driven and include significant advances in portability and features.

All of the third-generation ventilators are turbine driven and include significant advances in portability and features. Some allow the use of both passive circuits (such as found on a traditional bilevel device) and active circuits (which include an exhalation valve rather than an exhalation port). Some third-generation ventilators allow both single-limb active circuits and dual-limb active circuits. Generally, the dual-limb circuit offers exhaled volume monitoring. Additionally, the portability of the third-generation ventilators has increased significantly, and the first hot-swappable battery was introduced. The iVent 101 (GE Healthcare, Waukesha, Wisc.) is the first ventilator to offer pressure-regulated volume control for home patients. The latest home ventilators also feature graphics (**Figure 26–21**) and allow various reports to be downloaded and printed, including waveforms, ventilator settings, alarm history, patient compliance data, and summary reports (**Figure 26–22**). These additional data are quite helpful for the RT when troubleshooting ventilator problems.

Backup Ventilator and Emergency Supplies

There is wide variation across the United States with regard to when a **backup ventilator** is provided to the patient. The Medicare system generally does not pay for a backup ventilator, but may pay for a secondary ventilator when medically indicated.[39] Generally, in order for Medicare to consider coverage for a secondary ventilator, there must be documentation from the physician stating that the patient cannot maintain spontaneous ventilation for 4 or more hours, that a ventilator is required on the patient's wheelchair or mobility device as part of the patient's rehabilitation plan, or that the expected response time from emergency services is greater than 2 hours. Unfortunately, lack of reimbursement often means that patients who have a clearly demonstrated clinical requirement for a second ventilator do not receive one.

TABLE 26-7 Evolution of Positive Pressure Home Mechanical Ventilators

	Generation 1		Generation 2					Generation 3		
Name	LP-3 to LP-20	PLV Series	T-Bird Series	LTV Series	HT 50	Achieva	iVent 201	PB 540	Trilogy 100	iVent 101
Current manufacturer	Covidien (Boulder, CO)	Phillips Respironics (Murrysville, PA)	CareFusion (San Diego, CA)	CareFusion (San Diego, CA)	Newport Medical (Costa Mesa, CA)	Covidien (Boulder, CO)	GE Healthcare (Madison, WI)	Covidien (Boulder, CO)	Philips Respironics (Murrysville, PA)	GE Healthcare (Madison, WI)
Weight (lb)	34	28.9	34	14.5	15	32	22	9.9	11.5	14.7
Dimensions (in.)	9.75 × 14.5 × 13.25	9 × 12.25 × 12.25	13.0 × 11.0 × 13.5	3.25 × 10.5 × 13.5	10.63 × 7.87 × 10.24	10.75 × 13.30 × 15.60	13 × 9.5 × 10.3	6.0 × 9.2" × 12.4	4.5 × 6.88 × 9.5	13.70 × 4.72 × 11.42
Flow generator	Piston	Piston	Turbine	Turbine	Dual pistons	Piston	Turbine	Turbine	Turbine	Turbine
FDA approval date	1977	10/20/83	5/3/96	10/30/98	8/4/00	10/18/00	7/18/01	10/31/08	3/13/09	11/23/09
FDA code	CBK	CBK	CBK	CBK	CBK	CBK	CBK	CBK	CBK	CBK, NOU
Minimum patient weight (kg)	Not specified	Not specified	10	5	10	5	5	5	5	5
Modes	A/C vol; A/C vol. with press. limit; SIMV vol.; SIMV vol. with press. limit; press. cycle	Control vol.; A/C vol.; SIMV vol.	Control (vol. or pres.); A/C (vol. or pres.); SIMV (vol. or pres.); CPAP; pressure support	A/C (vol. or press.); SIMV (vol. or pres.), pressure support, CPAP	A/C (vol. or press.); SIMV (vol. or press.); spontaneous	A/C (vol. or pres.); SIMV (vol. or press.); spontaneous, CPAP, PS+CPAP	A/C (vol. or pres.); SIMV (vol. or pres); adaptive bilevel; CPAP; pressure support	CPAP; PSV, A/C (vol. or pres.); SIMV (vol. or pres.)	Pres. modes: CPAP ; S ; S/T ; T ; PC ; PC-SIMV Vol. modes: A/C; SIMV + PS; CV	A/C (vol. or pres.); SIMV (vol. or pres.); adaptive bilevel; CPAP; PRVC
Single-limb passive	No	No	No	No	No	No	No	Yes	Yes	Yes
Single-limb valve	Yes	Yes	No	No	Yes	Yes	No	Yes	Yes	Yes
Dual-limb valve	No	No	Yes	Yes	No	No	Yes	Yes	No	Yes
Tidal volume (mL)	100–2200	200–3000	50–2000	50–2000	100–2200	50–2200	50–2000	50–2000	50–2000	100–2500
Breath rate (breaths/min)	1–38	2–40	2–80	0–80	1–99	1–80	1–80	1–60	1–60	4–40
Pressure control (cm H_2O)	No	No	1–100	1–99	5–60	No	5–80	0–60	4–50	4–50
Pressure support (cm H_2O)	No	No	1–60	1–60	0–60	0–50	0–60	5–55	0–30	0–40
Inspiratory time	0.5– 5.5 s	10–120 L/min	?	0.3–9.9 s	1.1–3.0 s	02–5.0 s	0.3–3.0 s	0.3–6.0 s	0.3–5.0 s	0.3–5.0 s
Trigger	Pressure	Pressure	Flow	Flow	Pressure	Flow and pressure	Flow and pressure	Pressure	Flow	Flow and pressure

A/C, assist/control; SIMV, synchronized intermittent mandatory ventilation; CPAP, continuous positive airway pressure; PSV, pressure support ventilation; S, spontaneous; S/T, spontaneous-timed; T, timed; PC, pressure control; CV, control ventilation; PRVC, pressure-regulated volume control; VCV, volume control ventilation; PCV, pressure control ventilation.

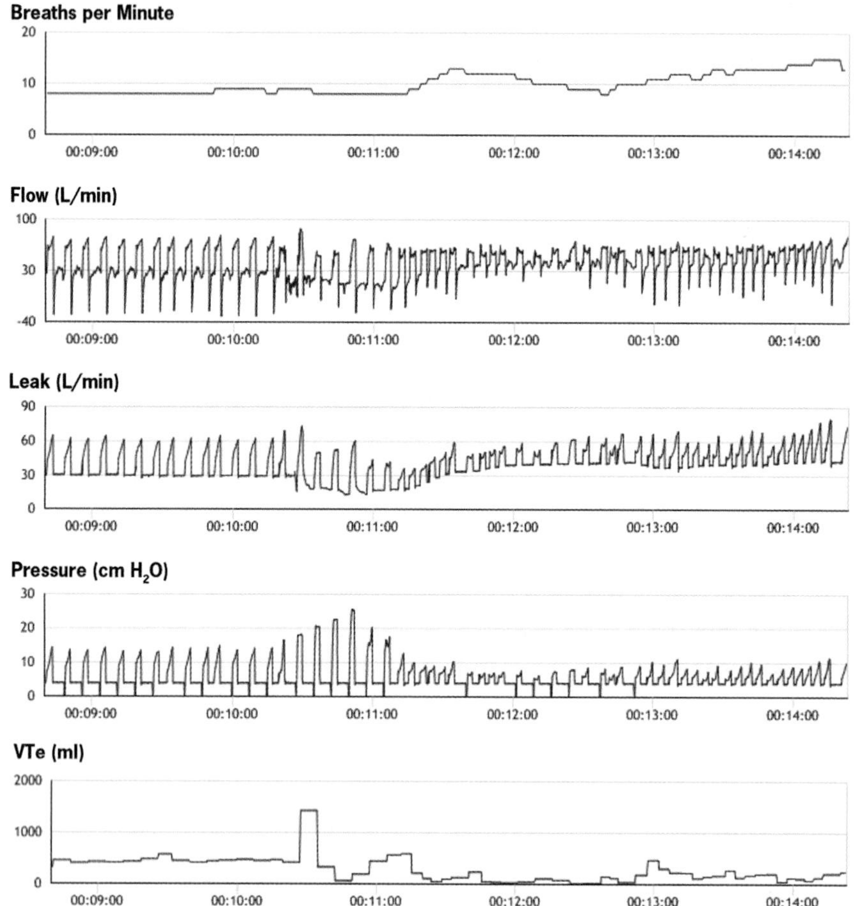

FIGURE 26–22 Sample report downloaded and printed from the Trilogy ventilator.

All home mechanically ventilated patients should have a **go-bag** prepared to accompany them on any trips outside the home. The detail-oriented RT should include a check of the go-bag during each visit to the patient's home. The most important item in the go-bag is a manual resuscitation bag. It must be stressed to the patient and family that the resuscitation bag *always* goes with the patient. Other important items for the go-bag may include the following:

For Patients Receiving Invasive or Noninvasive Ventilation

- Copy of prescription
- Copy of important phone numbers, including referring physician
- Second power supply for ventilator (external battery or DC power cord)
- Hand wash gel
- Flashlight
- Ventilator circuit (including metered dose inhaler and/or nebulizer port)
- Extra patient interface and headgear (if noninvasive)
- Cylinder wrench (if on O_2)
- O_2 tubing (if on O_2)
- Battery-operated nebulizer and medications
- Inhaler(s)

For Patients Receiving Invasive Ventilation

- Spare tracheostomy tube (one size smaller)
- Tracheostomy ties and gauze
- Syringes for cuff inflation/deflation
- Spare heat and moisture exchangers
- Battery-operated suction machine and catheters
- Normal saline vials
- Nebulizer circuit adapter

Setting Ventilator Alarms

Unfortunately, patients sometimes die at home from accidental ventilator disconnections, even patients who have been home for a long period of time and presumedly have experienced caregivers.[40] Continuous visual monitoring of the home mechanically ventilated patient is best, but there are times when the family caregiver must rely on the audible alarms. One of the most important and problematic tasks faced by the RT is determining appropriate alarm settings. Some RTs may simply duplicate the alarm settings that were in use at the hospital prior to the patient's discharge. However, this method of alarm setting may not be adequate at home. While in the hospital, the patient's Spo_2, respiratory rate, and heart rate were undoubtedly monitored via a central monitoring system that added another layer of protection above and beyond the ventilator alarms. Many payers do not cover a home continuous-use pulse oximeter, however.

RTs may think that because the doctor signed off on the ventilator settings, the therapist is not responsible for the alarm settings. Realistically, the physician cannot be expected to know the intricacies of every home ventilator. Clearly the RT is the expert on the ventilator and must make appropriate recommendations to the physician if the proper orders are not received.

Particularly for pediatric patients, there has been a move toward the use of pressure control ventilation. While in the hospital, if the patient partially decannulates, the low Spo_2 alarm and the high respiratory rate alarm will alert the staff, even if the ventilator did not sound a low-pressure alarm. Many of the second- and third-generation home ventilators

RESPIRATORY RECAP

Setting Ventilator Alarms

» A balance between safety and nuisance should be maintained.

» The RT should test ventilator alarms, with special caution for pediatric pressure ventilation.

have superior flow capabilities and are able to reach the pressure control setting even in the face of significant leaks. At home, a patient who decannulates in pressure ventilation, particularly if the diameter of the tracheostomy tube is small, may not trigger a low-pressure ventilator alarm because the ventilator will most likely be able to achieve the prescribed pressure control setting. In this situation, a properly set low exhaled volume alarm, low exhaled minute volume alarm, high inspired volume alarm, or high inspired minute volume alarm would most likely sound.

Another problematic situation can occur for patients who are prone to mucous plugging and who are on pressure control ventilation at home. If the patient develops a mucous plug that occludes a significant portion of the lung, or even a plug that completely blocks the tracheostomy tube, a high-pressure alarm will not sound. The same situation can develop if the heat and moisture exchanger becomes occluded, or if the patient rolls over on the ventilator circuit.[41] In these situations, a properly set low exhaled volume alarm, low exhaled minute volume alarm, low inspired volume alarm, or low inspired minute volume alarm would most likely sound.

The RT should test the ventilator alarms per the manufacturer's instructions during every home visit, but some additional tests beyond the manufacturer's recommendations may be prudent. Many pediatric patients use uncuffed tracheostomy tubes with varying leaks, which complicates the use of exhaled volume alarms. Especially for pediatric patients on pressure control ventilation, the vigilant RT can simulate an accidental decannulation using a tracheostomy tube one size smaller than the patient's usual tube to ensure that an alarm will sound if the tube accidentally comes out and remains attached to the Y piece of the circuit. If indicated for the patient's clinical condition, the RT may simulate a mucous plug by occluding the Y-piece and observing whether an alarm sounds. If an alarm does not sound, it is crucial that the RT obtain the proper order to take one or more of the following actions, as appropriate: adjust the alarm settings, change the ventilator settings, change the ventilator to one that has the necessary alarm, or provide a pulse oximeter with audible alarms. When there is no insurance coverage for a pulse oximeter, the RT must become a vigorous advocate for the patient's safety. Often a letter to the insurance company describing the potential safety issues, signed by the physician and the respiratory therapist, may help the family obtain the needed device.

Safety Tips

It is important that the RT make frequent and regular visits to the ventilator patient's home to check the ventilator and related equipment. These visits are especially important for pediatric patients because they provide an opportunity to observe the patient's growth and development and how that may affect the respiratory care plan. For example, most ventilator-dependent infants are placed in a crib while sleeping for the first several months of life. Typically, a heated humidifier rests on a table near the crib. One possible safety hazard can occur when parents allow the infant to play and crawl while on the floor. The vigilant therapist needs to make sure the parents understand that the baby should never be placed below the heated humidifier. Similarly, as the infant becomes stronger, care must be taken to prevent the infant from pulling the ventilator down off a table or bureau, perhaps sustaining an injury in the process or damaging the ventilator.

Toddlers are often fascinated by the lighted O_2 concentrator flow meter, as well as the lights and buttons on the front of the ventilator, and inadvertent setting changes can be the result. Another safety hazard for the pediatric patient is accidental decannulation as the toddler tries to walk beyond the length of the ventilator circuit. Note that some ventilator manufacturers offer longer circuits to allow increased physical activity for the patient. Also, most parents know they have to secure the pediatric patient in a car seat while in a vehicle, but parents also need to be taught that they must secure the ventilator as well.

There are some safety considerations for school-aged children as well. A resuscitation bag should always travel with the patient, including on the school bus. Some schools may allow the patient to keep an extra power cord and/or battery and charger at the school, rather than carry them back and forth each day. It may be helpful for the therapist to offer to visit the child's classroom to give a simple talk on what the ventilator is and how it helps the patient. The school nurse may appreciate a brief overview of the ventilator as well.

Older children who hang their ventilator on the back of their wheelchair must be cautioned not to hang a heavy backpack over their ventilator and not to allow the backpack to block the ventilator's air intake. Older children may also appreciate a longer circuit, which allows them to shower while keeping the ventilator a safe distance away. Note that special ventilator covers can be purchased to protect the ventilator from moisture (Freedom Vent Systems, West End, N.C.). Care must be taken to prevent water from entering into or around the tracheostomy tube. A tracheostomy mask or sheet of plastic wrap placed over the area may be helpful. Active children may have trouble with their ventilator circuit disconnects from the tracheostomy tube. A number of commercial products are available to secure the circuit. **Figure 26–23** shows one patient's ingenuity. Each day she chooses a grosgrain ribbon, color-coordinated with her outfit, to secure her circuit.

Caregiver Burden

There is a high incidence of depression among family caregivers.[42] The home care RT should be mindful that the family caregiver may be at risk for depression and may consider discussing with the physician the use of a depression screening tool for caregivers, such as the Center for Epidemiological Studies Depression Screening Index (CES-D). When appropriate, the RT may consider querying the caregiver about his or her quality and amount of sleep to determine whether nuisance ventilator alarms are interrupting sleep. The

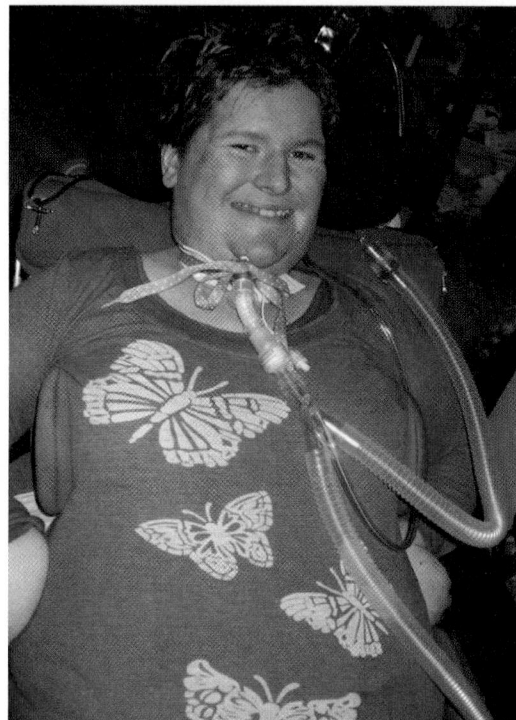

FIGURE 26–23 Example of patient and caregiver ingenuity: MJ uses a color-coordinated ribbon to secure her trach tube.

RT should also be knowledgeable about local respite programs, daycare facilities that accept ventilator patients, camps for ventilator-dependent children, or other agencies that may provide some respite for the family caregiver.

Ventilator User's Quality of Life

Many healthcare workers underestimate the ventilator user's quality of life.[36] In a report of 621 ventilator users with neuromuscular conditions, it was found that about one-third of patients were employed; a few others reported they were active on a daily basis as volunteers or students. Healthcare professionals underestimated the satisfaction of severely disabled, ventilator-assisted people. The RT who has internalized that ventilator-dependent patients can have meaningful, productive lives can have a significant positive impact on the patient and family's quality of life (**Figure 26–24**).

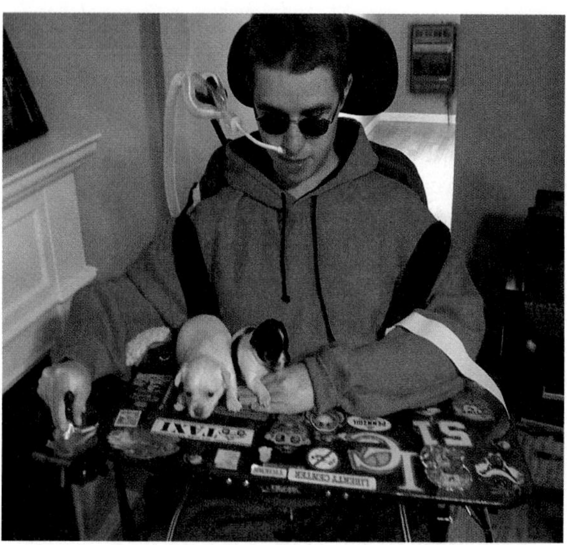

FIGURE 26–24 This young adult uses mouthpiece ventilation all day, and mask ventilation at night. He works part time and enjoys raising puppies.

KEY POINTS

- Depending on the equipment ordered, durable medical equipment (DME) companies can provide service by a technician, respiratory therapist, or qualified nurse.
- The goals of home respiratory care are to achieve the optimum level of patient function through goal setting, educate patients and their caregivers, administer diagnostic and therapeutic modalities and services, conduct disease management, and promote health.
- Unfortunately, respiratory therapists are not included in the Medicare home health services benefit.
- A DME or home medical equipment (HME) company may be required to have a retail license, HME license, a bedding supplier license, an O_2 manufacturer/distributor license, and/or possibly other licenses/permits as required by the state.
- There are generally two types of accreditation for a DME or HME: Equipment Management Services and Clinical Respiratory Services.
- The respiratory therapist is the most competent healthcare professional to provide home respiratory care.
- The home environment must be evaluated specific to the type of home medical equipment.
- Bag technique means that the respiratory therapist's bag and its contents must be kept as clean as possible.
- Patients who receive O_2 at home are exposed to the risk of improper storage and handling of O_2 cylinders, unsafe usage of O_2, improper transfer of O_2, inadequate ventilation, and smoking or other unsafe flames.
- The environmental evaluation should verify the adequacy of the home electrical system for patients with a home ventilator.
- An important aspect of the home environmental assessment is to ensure that alarms can be heard by the caregiver in all areas of the home.
- It is a good idea for some home care patients, particularly O_2 and ventilator patients, to meet with their local EMS personnel and/or firefighters before there is any type of emergency.
- For patients with COPD, long-term O_2 therapy prolongs life and decreases overall cost of care.
- The goal for efficient O_2 delivery is proper arterial O_2 saturation at all activity levels.

- Methods of O_2 delivery in the home include continuous-flow oxygen and intermittent-flow oxygen.
- Home O_2 delivery devices include oxygen concentrators, compressed gas systems, liquid O_2 systems, concentrators that fill compressed gas systems, and portable O_2 concentrators.
- Oxygen-conserving devices include reservoir cannulas, intermittent-flow devices, pulse-flow devices, demand delivery devices, and transtracheal O_2.
- Medicare categorizes devices with exhalation valves, adjustable breath rates, and alarms as mechanical ventilators.
- The indication for invasive ventilation (rather than noninvasive ventilation) for individuals requiring more than 20 hours per day of support is not a hard and fast rule.
- A comprehensive team approach to discharge planning is required.
- The first generation of positive pressure home care ventilators were piston driven and offered only volume-controlled breaths.
- The second generation of home ventilators switched from piston driven to turbine driven and offered additional modes.
- All of the third-generation ventilators are turbine driven and include significant advances in portability and features.
- One of the most important and problematic tasks faced by the respiratory therapist is determining appropriate alarm settings.
- There is a high incidence of depression among family caregivers of patients ventilated at home.
- Many healthcare workers underestimate the ventilator user's quality of life.

REFERENCES

1. American Association for Respiratory Care. Position statement: home respiratory care services. Available at: http://www.aarc.org/resources/position_statements/hrcs.html. Published December 14, 2000. Updated December 2007.
2. American Thoracic Society Documents. Statement on home care for patients with respiratory disorders. *Am J Respir Crit Care Med.* 2005;171(12):1443–1464.
3. Gay EG. Increasing home health services referrals, boon or bane? *Home Health Care Serv Q.* 1994;14:49–67.
4. Halliday H. History of surfactant from 1980. *Biol Neonate.* 2005; 87:317–322.
5. U.S. Census Bureau. International data base, Table 94. Midyear population by age and sex. Available at: http://www.census.gov/population/www/projections/natdet-D1A.html.
6. Bach JR, Intintola P, Alba AS, Holland IE. The ventilator-assisted individual. Cost analysis of institutionalization vs. rehabilitation and in-home management. *Chest.* 1992;101:26–30.
7. Field AI, Rosenblatt A, Pollack MM, Kaufman J. Home care cost-effectiveness for respiratory technology-dependent children. *Am J Dis Child.* 1991;145:729–733.
8. Lewarsksi JS, Gay PC. Current issues in home mechanical ventilation. *Chest.* 2007;132:671–676.
9. The Joint Commission. *2010 Standards for Home Medical Equipment, Rehabilitation Technology Services, and Clinical Respiratory Services.* Oakbrook Terrace, IL: Joint Commission; 2009.
10. Dunne PJ, McInturff SL. *Respiratory Home Care: The Essentials.* Philadelphia: FA Davis; 1998.
11. Posey SC, Aaltonen PM, DePalma RA, Femea P. Use of the public health nursing bag reexamined. *Public Health Nursing.* 2007;4:111–113.
12. Merlin MA, Wong ML, Pryor PW, et al. Prevalence of methicillin-resistant *Staphylococcus aureus* on the stethoscopes of emergency medical services providers. *Prehosp Emerg Care.* 2009;13: 71–74.
13. Wolf A. When health care moves home. *NFPA.* 1998;92(1). Available at: http://findarticles.com/p/articles/mi_qa3737/is_199801/ai_n8773480/?tag=content;col.
14. ECRI Institute. Medical device safety report. Leaving ventilator-dependent patients unattended. *Health Devices.* 1986;15(4): 102–103.
15. Pulmonetic Systems. *LTV 1000 Operator's Manual.* Minneapolis, MN: Pulmonetic Systems; 2005.
16. Turner J, McDonald GJ, Larter NL. *Handbook of Adult and Pediatric Respiratory Home Care.* St. Louis, MO: Mosby; 1994.
17. American Association for Respiratory Care. Clinical practice guideline: long-term invasive mechanical ventilation in the home. *Respir Care.* 2007;52:1056–1062.
18. Make BJ, Hill NS, Goldberg AI, et al. Mechanical ventilation beyond the intensive care unit: report of a consensus of the American College of Chest Physicians. *Chest.* 1998;113:289S–344S.
19. Stuban S. Safety issues generate practical solutions. *Ventilator-Assisted Living.* 2007;21(2).
20. Dunbar H, Wensley D. Guided self-management. In: Silverman M, O'Callaghan C, eds. *Practical Paediatric Respiratory Medicine.* London: Arnold; 2001:265–274.
21. Partridge MR. Self-management plans: uses and limitations. *Br J Hosp Med.* 1996;55:120–122.
22. AARC clinical practice guideline: oxygen therapy in the home or alternate site health care facility—2007 revision and update. *Respir Care.* 2007;52:1066–1068.
23. Nocturnal Oxygen Therapy Trial Group. Continuous or nocturnal oxygen therapy in hypoxemic chronic obstructive lung disease: a clinical trial. *Ann Intern Med.* 1980;93:391–398.
24. Report of the Medical Research Council Working Party: long-term domiciliary oxygen therapy in chronic hypoxic cor pulmonale complicating chronic bronchitis and emphysema. *Lancet.* 1981;1:681–686.
25. Petty TL, Bliss PL. Ambulatory oxygen therapy, exercise and survival with advanced COPD (the Nocturnal Oxygen Therapy Trial revisited). *Respir Care.* 2000;45:204–213.
26. Doherty DE, Petty TL, Bailey W, et al. Recommendations of the 6th Long-Term Oxygen Therapy Consensus Conference. *Respir Care.* 2006;51:519–525.
27. Bliss PL, McCoy RW, Adams AB. A bench study comparison of demand oxygen delivery systems and continuous flow oxygen. *Respir Care.* 1999;44:925–931.
28. Dunne PJ. The clinical impact of new long term oxygen therapy technology. *Respir Care.* 2009;54:1100–1111.
29. McCoy B, Gay P, Petty T, et al. Portable oxygen concentrating device comparison during exercise. Abstract 556; ATS International Conference, 2007.
30. Further recommendations for prescribing and supplying long-term oxygen therapy. Summary of the Second Conference on Long-Term Oxygen Therapy held in Denver, Colorado, December 11–12, 1987. *Am Rev Respir Dis.* 1988;138:745–747.
31. Diesem R, Voss G, McCoy R. A bench study to compare the performance characteristics of portable oxygen concentrators [Abstract]. *Respir Care.* 2007;51(11):1327.
32. McCoy R. Oxygen-conserving techniques and devices. *Respir Care.* 2000;45:95–103.

33. Valley Inspired Products. *Your 2007 Guide to Understanding Oxygen Conserving Devices.* Apple Valley, MN: Valley Inspired Products; 2007.
34. Christopher KL, Spofford BS, Goodman JR. A program for transtracheal oxygen delivery, assessment of safety and efficacy. *Ann Intern Med.* 1987;6:802–808.
35. Block AJ. Intermittent flow oxygen devices—technically feasible, but rarely used [Editorial]. *Chest.* 1984;86:657–658.
36. Bach JR, Tzeng AC. *Guide to the Evaluation and Management of Neuromuscular Disease.* Philadelphia: Hanley & Belfus; 1999:134–137.
37. Tearl DK, Hertzog JH. Home discharge of technology-dependent children: evaluation of a respiratory therapist driven family education program. *Respir Care.* 2007;52:171–176.
38. Stegmaier J. The role of patient education in compliance. *Focus: J Respir Care Sleep Med.* 2005;22(Winter):85.
39. Hanna S. Working down denials: EO463 pressure support ventilator. *HomeCare,* October 16, 2009.
40. Gilgoff RL, Gilgoff IS. Long-term follow-up of home mechanical ventilation in young children with spinal cord injury and neuromuscular conditions. *J Pediatr.* 2003;142:476–480.
41. Kun SS, Nakamura CT, Ripka JF, et al. Home ventilator low-pressure alarms fail to detect accidental decannulation with pediatric tracheostomy tubes. *Chest.* 2001;119:562–564.
42. Gelinas D, O'Connor P, Miller RG. Quality of life for ventilator-dependent ALS patients and their caregivers. *J Neurol Sci.* 1998;160:S134–136.

CHAPTER 27

Disaster Management

Richard D. Branson

OUTLINE

OBJECTIVES

1. Define mass casualty respiratory failure.
2. List the most likely disaster scenarios likely to result in mass casualty respiratory failure.
3. Describe the requirements of devices required to provide ventilation in mass casualty respiratory failure.
4. Describe issues related to respiratory consumables and oxygen in mass casualty respiratory failure.
5. Discuss the role of the respiratory therapist in a disaster.
6. Justify a system for triage of patients based on severity of illness in a mass casualty respiratory failure event.

KEY TERMS

automatic resuscitator
chemical agent
critical care ventilators
disaster management plan
electrically powered portable ventilator
EMS portable ventilator
epidemic
mass casualty respiratory failure (MCRF)
noninvasive ventilator
personal protective equipment (PPE)
pneumatically powered portable ventilator

INTRODUCTION

Recent history is rife with natural disasters, the threat of terrorism, and outbreaks of severe febrile respiratory illness, including H1N1 influenza and severe acute respiratory syndrome (SARS). These real and perceived threats have focused healthcare planners, hospitals, and communities on how to care for large numbers of critically ill patients. Planning requires not only space for the care of patients, but also adequate equipment and staff.[1] This chapter focuses specifically on the concerns related to and requirements for **mass casualty respiratory failure (MCRF)**, which is defined as an event resulting in patients requiring mechanical ventilation in excess of the space to care for them and devices to provide ventilatory support.[2–4]

History

Mass casualty respiratory failure has an interesting, yet mostly unimpressive past. History's most illuminating instance occurred in the 1950s during the European poliomyelitis epidemic. The care of patients at a hospital in Copenhagen at the height of the epidemic is instructive.[5] During the summer of 1952, the hospital owned five ventilators, all negative pressure devices. In the same time frame the hospital had over 100 patients requiring mechanical ventilation. This surge of patients relative to available ventilators had never been seen in modern times. The hospital staff devised a clever solution to their problem. Instead of negative pressure ventilation with an iron lung, they performed tracheostomy and enlisted medical students to perform manual ventilation in 4-hour shifts. Using a non-self-inflating bag and carbon dioxide absorber, they were able to use very low flows of oxygen to sustain ventilation and oxygenation. Interestingly, manual ventilation was also used following Hurricane Katrina, when electricity failed at Charity Hospital in New Orleans.[6]

Terrorist attacks using nerve agents have been attempted, but in each case the number of patients requiring mechanical ventilation was fewer than 10 individuals. The SARS epidemic was an example of a natural febrile respiratory illness that resulted in significant morbidity and mortality. SARS highlighted the impact of international travel on the spread of disease and the importance of caregiver protection. In Toronto, a number of patients with SARS were nurses and respiratory therapists who had cared for early cases. In 2009, while the world awaited an anticipated H5N1 (avian flu) outbreak, a novel H1N1 virus originated in Mexico. The resulting pandemic taxed intensive care units (ICUs) around the world with severe respiratory failure in pediatric, obese, and obstetric patients. The H1N1 epidemic is a lesson in the unpredictability of viruses. H1N1 did not overwhelm hospitals, but did result in ICUs full of critically ill patients. There were no reports of ventilator or bed shortages, but the severity of adult respiratory distress syndrome (ARDS) associated with H1N1 infection spurred a renewed interest in rescue therapies for refractory hypoxemia.[7]

Fortunately for the U.S. population, neither natural nor human-made events has resulted in a surge of critically ill patients requiring mechanical ventilation and exceeding the capacity for space, stuff, or staff. Alternatively, each small event provides lessons from which we can learn. What seems clear is that whatever mass casualty event occurs, it is likely to be unexpected and unpredictable.

The Threat

In the United States, the Department of Homeland Security's *National Planning Guidelines* coordinates and prioritizes emergency preparedness efforts at all response levels. Contained within the guidelines are 15 national planning scenarios; at least two-thirds of these may result in MCRF.[8]

The medical impact of a mass casualty event will depend on the disaster's characteristics (e.g., lethality of exposure, numbers of persons exposed) and interaction with the exposed population's and medical response systems' capabilities and vulnerabilities. Only in disasters likely to result in exposed victims developing ARDS will mechanical ventilation potentially be a limiting factor for survival. Disaster characteristics that may influence the demand for ventilators include the number of victims, the time from exposure to development of ARDS, and the duration of ARDS. It is possible that victims requiring mechanical ventilation may far outnumber normal mechanical ventilator capacity. If this were to occur, many patients with potentially reversible disease would likely die. Each scenario considers the expected number of victims requiring mechanical ventilation, the time from injury until need for mechanical ventilation, the pathophysiology necessitating mechanical ventilation, and the geographic area affected.

> **RESPIRATORY RECAP**
>
> **Disasters Causing Mass Casualty Respiratory Failure**
> » Traumatic injury
> » Chemical weapons
> » Epidemics and febrile respiratory illness

Traumatic Injury

Traumatic injury may result on a local level from fire, explosion, or terrorist attack. These events typically result in fewer than 100 casualties. The Israeli experience with homicide bombers suggests that most incidents result in 20 to 30 casualties, with half of these patients being hospitalized and half admitted to ICUs, the majority of those for life-saving mechanical ventilation. Traumatic injury also may result from a natural disaster such as an earthquake or tsunami. These events occur over a wider area, damaging infrastructure and impeding response. Mechanical ventilation may be required following near drowning, crush injuries, and chest trauma.[8]

- *Expected number of victims*: In a local explosion or fire, typically fewer than 100 victims require hospitalization and fewer require mechanical ventilation.
- *Time from injury to need for mechanical ventilation*: The severity of trauma may require immediate mechanical ventilation for survival (e.g., head injury, blast lung injury), whereas others only require ventilation after operative repair.
- *Pathophysiology*: Traumatic injuries resulting in a need for mechanical ventilation include closed head injury, hemothorax, pneumothorax, pulmonary contusion, flail chest, traumatic amputation, blood loss, and blast injury.

- *Area affected:* In an explosion or fire, the affected area is usually finite. The result is a defined local area in which casualties are limited and local infrastructure can handle the surge in patients easily. A larger natural event may affect greater numbers of patients and result in damage to hospitals and transportation systems. In these instances, critically ill victims at the scene are likely to expire.

Chemical Weapons

Injuries following exposure to chemical weapons vary with the agent. **Chemical agents** are classified as lung-damaging agents, blood agents, blister agents, and nerve agents. These agents include chlorine, phosgene, and ammonia, all of which are commonly used in industrial processes and readily available. Nerve agents causing paralysis have been used recently. Mustard gas is perhaps the best-known blister agent, and cyanide is the most likely blood agent.

- *Expected number of victims*: Under the appropriate environmental conditions, population density, and dispersion, chemical agents may result in thousands of victims. Despite this prediction, however, to date the number of victims has been in the hundreds and the number of victims requiring mechanical ventilation has been less than a dozen.
- *Time from injury to need for mechanical ventilation*: The time until respiratory failure requires mechanical ventilation varies with the agent and exposure. Pulmonary agents can cause sudden death as a result of laryngeal obstruction or severe respiratory failure days after exposure. Nerve agents causing paralysis may require ventilation to be performed at the scene. Historically, those patients who survive exposure to nerve agents require only short-term mechanical ventilation (<8 hours).[9]
- *Pathophysiology*: Chemical weapons enter the body through the respiratory system and skin. Blistering agents and coking agents result in bronchospasm and, over time, ARDS. Cyanide poisons mitochondria and prevents cellular respiration, resulting in death from cellular hypoxia. Nerve agents result in flaccid paralysis and apnea, but also produce significant bronchorrhea and bronchospasm. Thus, although patients exposed to nerve agents may have normal lung compliance, airway resistance may be elevated.
- *Area affected*: The optimum effectiveness of these agents as a weapon requires exposure of a large number of victims in a closed space. Therefore, these exposures are limited to a small geographic area.

Epidemics and Febrile Respiratory Illness

Epidemics and febrile illness may result from both natural and human-made causes. SARS and pandemic flu are good examples of diseases that traveled around the world in short order. Anthrax and botulism exposure are most likely to be the result of bioterrorism, although botulism poisoning can occur from improperly preserved foods. Anthrax, caused by the bacillus *Anthracis*, has been used in the United States as a weapon, infecting 22 people and killing 5. Anthrax, however, is not contagious.

- *Expected number of victims*: Epidemics have the possibility of involving people from all over the world, affecting tens of thousands of people. Weaponized botulism and anthrax have the ability to infect similar numbers of people.
- *Time from injury to need for mechanical ventilation*: Epidemics are likely to result in the greatest number of casualties, and typically the time from exposure until respiratory failure develops is prolonged (days to weeks). In these cases, patients will likely arrive at the hospital with early signs of respiratory distress.
- *Pathophysiology:* Pandemic flu and SARS result in ARDS in the worst cases. Botulism results in neuromuscular ventilatory failure from paralysis and may require prolonged mechanical ventilation. Anthrax results in hemorrhagic mediastinitis, hemoptysis, sepsis, profound hypoxemia, and acute respiratory failure.
- *Area affected*: Natural epidemics and bioterrorism agents in this class have the ability to infect entire regions, depending on the length of the incubation period and the continued presence of the contagion. These events may be limited to a municipality or may include an entire city. In the case of pandemic flu, entire portions of a country may be affected.

Planning for Mass Casualty Respiratory Failure

Respiratory therapists play an important role during disasters, and even more so during MCRF scenarios. This role includes managing staff, providing personal protective equipment, assuming additional duties, ensuring an adequate supply of disposables (e.g., ventilator circuits, suction catheters, heat and moisture exchangers), arranging for appropriate oxygen reserves, and devising a plan for additional mechanical ventilators—all this in addition to normal duties.

Staffing

Any MCRF scenario will result in an exponential need for mechanical ventilation and will dramatically increase the need for ICU nurses, respiratory therapists, and physicians. This is a particular challenge considering that many current ICUs have lost beds due to staffing shortages. In an MCRF scenario the respiratory therapist will be overwhelmed by responsibility. Staffing will be based on patient acuity and caregiver availability. A plan for respiratory extenders has been developed, but has

RESPIRATORY RECAP

Planning for Mass Casualty Respiratory Failure

- » Staffing
- » Personal protective equipment
- » Oxygen
- » Disposables
- » Ventilators

yet to be put to use. The major issue is identifying the appropriately trained people. Occupational and physical therapists, veterinarians, and prehospital providers have all been discussed. Additionally, the duties these individuals would be assigned is unclear.[10] On the other hand, in the event of a mass casualty incident not involving large numbers of patients with respiratory failure, the respiratory therapist should be prepared to aid physicians, nurses, and others professionals in duties not normally in the scope of respiratory care.

The respiratory therapy department should be involved in the community and hospital **disaster management plan**. A plan for notifying department members via text, email, or phone is essential. Disaster planning cannot be done in isolation.

Personal Protective Equipment

Several of the febrile respiratory illnesses associated with MCRF are highly contagious. **Personal protective equipment (PPE)** is a critical component of mass casualty care in this setting. Availability of PPE is important because it allows caregivers to feel safe during patient interactions. In the absence of sufficient PPE, concerns about personal and family health may lead to employees avoiding the workplace. Adequate supplies are not enough, however; proper use of PPE must be taught and evaluated. The risk of secondary transmission is likely greater in the ICU as a result of the number of interventions causing aerosolization of infectious material. Procedures such as endotracheal intubation, open circuit suctioning, and bronchoscopy are associated with increased risk of secondary transmission. The risk associated with procedures such as noninvasive ventilation, administration of medications by nebulizer, and manual ventilation is unclear. Some have advocated higher levels of respiratory protection for those engaging in high-risk interventions such as use of powered air-purifying respirators for bronchoscopy.

The SARS experience showed that correct use of recommended PPE among healthcare workers is highly efficacious in limiting disease spread. Ensuring correct use of PPE, however, especially during a prolonged response, remains a challenge. Reports from the SARS outbreak reveal that compliance with PPE regimens was below 70% in Hong Kong and U.S. healthcare workers caring for infected patients.[11]

The use of filters in the ventilator circuit on the inspired or expired side, or both, or inside a heat and moisture exchanger (HME) appears to be suggested by common sense, but data are lacking. Ventilators that use room air for gas delivery to the patient should have a filter on the inspiratory inlet. Filters are used in the expiratory limb of the ventilator circuit to protect the delicate, expensive flow and pressure monitoring components rather than for infection control. It is unknown whether there is any risk of secondary infection in caregivers from expired gas from intubated patients. The use of an HME with a filter (HMEF) has not been shown to reduce the rate of ventilator-associated pneumonia or to alter contamination of the environment. The presence of a filter in the HME, however, increases the risk of airway obstruction. If used, filters in the expiratory limb of the circuit should be inspected frequently for signs of obstruction to avoid complications secondary to air trapping (barotrauma, hypotension).

Oxygen

Oxygen is readily available in liquid form at most hospitals. Under normal circumstances the liquid system of a hospital can provide gas for approximately 3 weeks. In part because of the threat of disaster, most hospitals request that the liquid oxygen vessel never be allowed to fall below half-full. Systems are typically filled at night to prevent interference with workflow and reduce the risk of accidents. A typical liquid system has 6000 to 9000 gallons of liquid oxygen, which evaporates to nearly 30,000,000 gaseous liters of oxygen. It has been estimated that a 500-bed hospital uses 1.5 million liters of oxygen per day.[12]

Oxygen can also be supplied by cylinders, portable liquid systems, and concentrators. Note that most concentrators are only capable of producing 93% oxygen from room air. Most hospitals do not have space to house sufficient numbers of cylinders to prove useful in a disaster. Concentrators can provide low-flow oxygen, but are little help for the critically ill ventilated patient. Liquid systems are the standard, and portable, truck-mounted systems are available for emergencies, assuming the roads are passable.

During a disaster, oxygen conservation can be helpful. This includes use of reservoir or pendant cannulas, turning off flow to manual resuscitators, switching from heated aerosols to HMEs, and accepting lower levels of oxygen saturation in patients.

Disposables

A frequently overlooked aspect of MCRF is availability of disposable equipment. Ventilators require circuits, HMEs or humidifiers, and suction catheters. Oxygen requires delivery tubing, cannulas, masks, and other appliances. In keeping with cost containment, these devices are commonly kept at a level sufficient for several weeks of supply. In MCRF, most experts suspect that the disposables will be among the first supplies to run out. Reuse of circuits has been suggested, but this should only be considered as a last resort.

Ventilators

Ventilators may be needed following a disaster in three distinct scenarios: (1) in the field to move patients from the scene of an accident to definitive care, (2) between facilities (decompressing a localized event), and (3) for in-hospital care of critically ill and injured patients. The movement of patients from the scene may be accomplished with oxygen, manual ventilation, or use of a portable ventilator under the purview of the emergency medical services (EMS) director. In scenarios such as pandemic flu, patients are likely to seek relief of flu symptoms long before they require mechanical ventilation. In these cases, the need for large numbers of EMS ventilators will be unnecessary.

The second and third scenarios involve the care of critically ill patients with respiratory failure and ARDS requiring mechanical ventilation. Ventilators used for interfacility transport and ICU care are under the purview of the critical care team, including an intensivist and respiratory therapist. Evidence-based management of the patient with ARDS is founded in the success of the Adult Respiratory Distress Syndrome Network (ARDSnet) trial.[13] The principles of ARDS management are straightforward:

- Low tidal volume (6–8 mL/kg) of predicted body weight based on height
- Ability to give a constant tidal volume
- Plateau pressures (Pplat) less than or equal to 30 cm H_2O
- Stable inspired oxygen concentration (FIO_2) from 0.21 to 1.0
- Continuous mandatory ventilation (CMV)
- Positive end-expiratory pressure (PEEP) to maintain alveolar recruitment

On the first day of the ARDSnet trial, the patients in the low-tidal-volume arm of the trial received a PEEP of 6 to 13 cm H_2O, an FIO_2 of 0.35 to 0.75, and a minute ventilation of 10 to 16 L/min. On day 7, PEEP was reduced to an average of 8 cm H_2O and FIO_2 to 0.50, and minute ventilation averaged about 14 L/min. These data provide standard requirements for the functional performance of ventilators to be stockpiled for use in MCRF. Ventilators for MCRF should be capable of setting PEEP from 6 to 13 cm H_2O, FIO_2 from 0.35 to 0.75, and a minute ventilation of 10 to 18 L/min. Assuming predicted body weights of 62 to 90 kg (males with a height of 65 inches and 77 inches, or 5 feet 5 inches to 6 feet 5 inches), tidal volumes of 375 to 540 mL (6 mL/kg) must be capable of being set. It is important to note that the desired tidal volume is based on predicted patient weight, not lung compliance or actual weight.

There are many opinions about what kind of ventilator should be stockpiled for MCRF, ranging from a minimalist approach of just replacing the manual resuscitator to the ICU approach that every possible option must be available. At a minimum, ventilators stockpiled for MCRF *must* be capable of delivering a respiratory frequency of 6 to 35 breaths/min, a tidal volume of 350 to 600 mL (the adjustment of respiratory rate and tidal volume must be separate), an FIO_2 of 0.35 to 0.75, and a PEEP of 5 to 15 cm H_2O. Ventilators that are unable to produce these settings at a minimum are not suitable for in-hospital MCRF. **Figure 27–1** shows examples of suitable ventilators.

Ventilator Performance Characteristics

Operational characteristics of ventilators for MCRF have been suggested by the American Association for Respiratory Care (AARC).[14] Some explanation and clarification of these characteristics are in order.[15,16] **Table 27–1** lists the desirable characteristics of ventilators for MCRF. The optimal ranges for operation remain to be determined, but represent the minimum required characteristics as well as characteristics that might provide added benefit. Physical characteristics of ventilators for MCRF, which are more difficult to quantify, are clearly just as important. A ventilator for MCRF should be rugged, portable, withstand shock and vibration, and continue to operate if dropped. There is a military specification for these characteristics, but it is unclear whether ventilators for MCRF must meet this standard. Clearly, meeting the military standard would be desirable. Portability is important. A weight of less than 10 kg is often the goal. A portable device is one that a respiratory therapist or nurse can pick up with one hand (with or without a carrying case) and move without difficulty.

> **RESPIRATORY RECAP**
>
> **Performance Characteristics of a Ventilator for Mass Casualty Respiratory Failure**
>
> » Rugged
> » Portable
> » Low gas consumption
> » Adequate battery life
> » Minimal imposed work of breathing

Ideally, a ventilator for MCRF should have low gas consumption. That is, oxygen should not be wasted. Gas consumption of ventilators can be affected by pneumatic or fluidic control, continuous flow for triggering, pressure relief from mechanical blenders, and internal leaks. Although this has not been well studied, ideally 90% of the gas entering the ventilator should go to the patient as part of the minute ventilation. Equally important is battery life. Battery life is affected by age of the battery, temperature, and the battery's charging history regardless of the ventilator. Ventilator characteristics that decrease battery life include the mode of ventilation, FIO_2, and PEEP. Patient characteristics can also affect battery life: the greater the load (lower compliance, higher airway resistance), the shorter the duration of operation.

The ventilator should be easy to trigger and have an acceptable imposed work of breathing. Most current-generation portable ventilators meet this requirement.

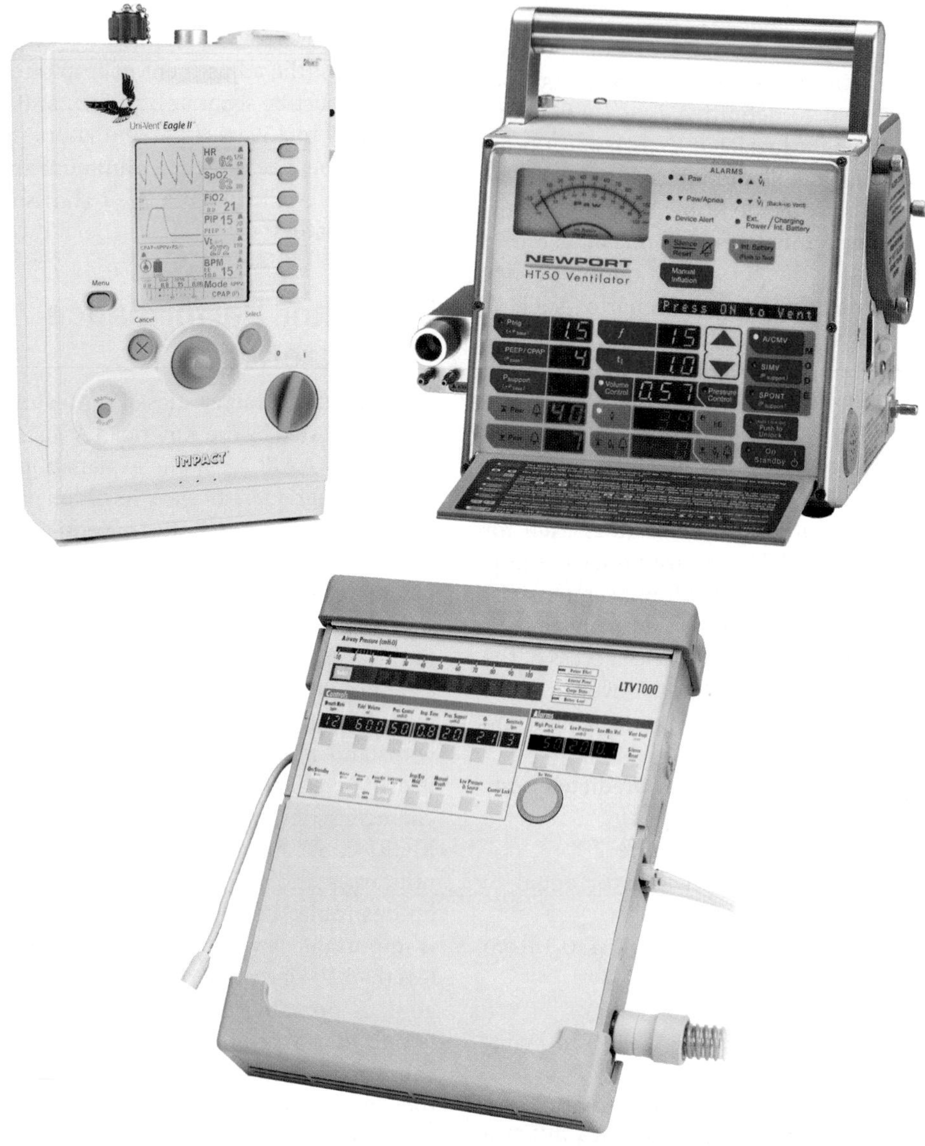

FIGURE 27–1 Examples of ventilators that might be used in the setting of mass casualty respiratory failure.

Cost should be less than $10,000. In large purchases, such as those made by the government for mass casualty care, significant price reductions can be realized. The ventilator should be intuitive and easy to use. In addition, the manufacturer should provide training in person and via multimedia (DVD or Web based). Maintenance, including battery charging and replacement, is also an important issue. Ventilator maintenance should be able to be accomplished by trained technicians on site, and requirements for battery charging should be explicitly detailed.

Finally, vendor support and longevity is critical. The manufacturer should have a technical support line that operates all day, every day of the year. There is some advantage to purchasing ventilators made in the United States because in a pandemic situation both shipping times and the loyalty of foreign manufacturers may create a problem.

Ventilators for Mass Casualty Respiratory Failure

For the purposes of describing ventilators for MCRF, their operation and application leads to categorization based on functional characteristics. These categories include automatic resuscitators, emergency medical services (EMS) ventilators, pneumatically powered portable ventilators, electrically powered portable ventilators,

RESPIRATORY RECAP

Ventilators for Mass Casualty Respiratory Failure

- » Automatic resuscitators
- » EMS ventilators
- » Pneumatically powered portable ventilators
- » Electrically powered pneumatic ventilators
- » Critical care ventilators
- » Noninvasive ventilators

TABLE 27–1 Suggested Performance Characteristics of Ventilators for Mass Casualty Respiratory Failure

Characteristic	Rationale	Mandatory and Desirable Characteristics	
		Mandatory	*Desirable*
FDA approved for adults and pediatrics	Natural disasters, pandemics, and chemical/bioterrorism attacks will also affect children	Ventilate 10-kg patient	Ventilate 5-kg patient
Ability to operate without 50-psig compressed gas	The redundancy for electrical power in hospitals far exceeds oxygen stores and redundancy In the absence of high-pressure oxygen, low-flow oxygen from a flow meter can be used to increase F_{IO_2}	Operate without 50-psig input F_{IO_2} from 0.21 to 1.0	Operate with or without 50-psig input alone
Battery life of 4 hours or greater	Allow for transport from facility to facility Provide continuous support during intermittent power failure	4 hours of operation at nominal settings	Greater than 4 hours operation at nominal settings
Constant volume delivery	Meet guidelines for tidal volume delivery as dictated by ARDSnet protocol Reduce potential for ventilator-induced lung injury Provide age-appropriate settings	Volume control ventilation (350 to 600 mL)	Pressure control and volume control ventilation
Mode	Meet ARDSnet guidelines Ensure minimum ventilation in a situation of multiple patients and a shortage of caregivers	CMV	CMV, IMV, and pressure support
Positive end-expiratory pressure (PEEP)	Meet ARDSnet guidelines Prevent ventilator-induced lung injury Reverse hypoxemia	Adjustable from 5 to 15 cm H_2O	Adjustable from 5 to 20 cm H_2O
Separate controls for respiratory rate and tidal volume	Meet ARDSnet guidelines Ensure minute ventilation in apneic patients	Respiratory rate from 6 to 35 breaths/min	Respiratory rate from 6 to 75 breaths/min (for pediatric patients)
Monitor airway pressures and tidal volume	Meet ARDSnet guidelines Provide assessment of patient's lung compliance Patient safety (prevent overdistension)	Monitor peak inspiratory pressure and delivered tidal volume	Monitor plateau pressure and patient tidal volumes
Alarms	Patient safety Improve ability to monitor large numbers of patients with reduced staff	Alarms for: • Circuit disconnect • High airway pressure • Low airway pressure (leak) • Loss of electric power • Loss of high-pressure source gas	Alarms for: • High tidal volume in pressure modes • Low minute ventilation • Remote alarms

ARDSnet, Adult Respiratory Distress Syndrome Network; CMV, continuous mandatory ventilation; IMV, intermittent mandatory ventilation.

full-feature critical care ventilators, and noninvasive ventilators.

Automatic Resuscitators

An **automatic resuscitator** is designed to replace the need for manual ventilation. These devices are predominantly pneumatically powered and pressure cycled. Automatic resuscitators have few to no alarms, cannot provide a constant tidal volume, cannot set rate and tidal volume separately, and commonly provide 100% source gas or a lower concentration with the use of a Venturi. Most manuals of automatic resuscitators start with the warning "Do not leave the patient unattended," which is problematic in a scenario in which there are too many patients and not enough caregivers. These devices are inexpensive, but fail to meet the demands of patients with ARDS and are not suitable for stockpiling to treat MCRF.

EMS Portable Ventilators

An **EMS portable ventilator** is used in patient transport, typically in emergency care via ambulance. These devices are more reliable, rugged, and have greater functionality than automatic resuscitators. The functionality and cost in this group of ventilators are variable. Some devices set tidal volume and respiratory rate via a single control. Others have separate controls for both settings. PEEP is usually set on an external valve. F_{IO_2} is commonly provided by 100% O_2 source gas or a single lower concentration with use of an air entrainment system. Most of these devices are pneumatically powered, with or without electronic control. Monitoring and alarms are limited. These devices require a 50-psig input; this, along with the limited alarms and monitoring, limits their usefulness in the stockpile.

Pneumatically Powered Portable Ventilators

Sophisticated **pneumatically powered portable ventilators** have the ability to provide continuous mandatory ventilation (CMV) and intermittent mandatory ventilation (IMV), set PEEP, have a low imposed work of breathing, and allow separate control of tidal volume and respiratory rate. These devices meet most of the performance characteristics for MCRF. The limitations of these devices are related to the pneumatic power source. In the absence of a 50-psig gas source, these devices cannot operate. F_{IO_2} is typically limited to 100% source gas, which wastes oxygen. Few alarms are also a weakness.

Electrically Powered Portable Ventilators

Electrically powered portable ventilators often are used for home care and for in-hospital transport. Electrically powered, sophisticated portable ventilators meet the performance characteristics required of a ventilator for MCRF. There is some significant difference in the weight of these devices (ranging from 5 to 15 kg). Battery life and gas consumption vary depending on the driving system of the ventilator. A number of commercially available ventilators in this category have been stockpiled by the Centers for Disease Control and Prevention and by state disaster management teams for MCRF.

Critical Care Ventilators

Critical care ventilators are capable of managing all types of respiratory failure. These devices have not been recommended for MCRF because of their large size, cost (over $30,000), and complexity. The plethora of modes and options provided by a critical care ventilator is an advantage in routine use by critical care respiratory therapists and intensivists, but becomes a liability in a mass casualty situation.

Noninvasive Ventilators

Noninvasive ventilation (NIV) is a standard of care for respiratory failure in patients with chronic obstructive pulmonary disease (COPD) under normal circumstances. The use of NIV in MCRF, however, has significant limitations.

- NIV is not the treatment of choice for ARDS, commonly seen in MCRF.
- The significant time commitment (1–2 hours) spent by the respiratory therapist at the bedside at initiation is impractical in MCRF.
- NIV failure may require emergency intubation, which is a more difficult scenario when there are too many patients and too few caregivers.
- In infectious disease, the ability of the patient to cough and the high flows associated with NIV may spread infectious agents into the ambient air.

Noninvasive ventilators tend to be inexpensive and smaller than many invasive devices, but have limitations that preclude recommendation for stockpiling, such as lack of battery backup, limited monitoring, limited alarms, and inability to provide volume control (most devices provide pressure-targeted ventilation). Despite the limitations of noninvasive ventilators, many hospitals have these devices available. In an MCRF situation, noninvasive ventilators can be repurposed for use as invasive ventilators. **Table 27–2** lists possible sources of additional ventilators during an MCRF scenario.

TABLE 27–2 Sources of Additional Ventilators for a Mass Casualty Respiratory Failure Scenario

Source	Method	Problems
Affected hospital	Cancel elective surgeries Repurpose anesthesia workstations as mechanical ventilators and ICU monitors (during nontrauma disasters)	Numbers of anesthesia machines are limited. If the duration of mechanical ventilation is prolonged, anesthesia machines will be needed when surgeries and other procedures are reinitiated.
Unaffected hospitals	Redistribution of available equipment from unaffected hospitals to those in need	There are few extra available ventilators at most hospitals even during usual conditions. Delayed situational awareness may reduce the willingness of unaffected hospitals to share equipment.
Mechanical ventilator rental services	Provision of additional ventilators by a rental company	The same company may have contracts with a number of affected hospitals, so the total number of additional ventilators may be limited. Logistical delays may be encountered when sending ventilators from distant geographic areas.
Strategic national stockpile	Deployment of mechanical ventilators to states or cities in need	Delay in distribution may occur because most states still have limited capacity to distribute equipment from the strategic national stockpile. It is unclear how distribution will be prioritized when multiple hospitals are requesting ventilators at the same time.

Triage

No discussion of MCRF is complete without mentioning triage of ventilators. This is an ethical dilemma that the modern world has not yet had to face. In MCRF, all patients will receive care based on the likelihood of survival. These systems are being developed by national societies to allow the most good to be done for the most patients with the best possible outcome. All patients will receive care in a mass casualty situation, even if it is only comfort care.

KEY POINTS

- At least two-thirds of potential disasters result in mass casualty respiratory failure (MCRF).
- Traumatic injury may result on a local level from fire, explosion, or terrorist attack.
- Chemical agents are classified as lung-damaging agents, blood agents, blister agents, and nerve agents.
- Epidemics and febrile illness may result from both natural and human-made causes.
- Personal protective equipment is a critical component of mass casualty care in the disaster setting.
- During a disaster, oxygen conservation can be helpful.
- Ventilators may be needed following a disaster in three distinct scenarios: (1) in the field to move patients from the scene of an accident to definitive care, (2) between facilities (decompressing a localized event), and (3) for in-hospital care of critically ill and injured patients.
- Operational characteristics of ventilators for MCRF have been suggested by the American Association for Respiratory Care.
- Ventilators for MCRF include automatic resuscitators, EMS ventilators, pneumatically powered portable ventilators, electrically powered portable ventilators, critical care ventilators, and noninvasive ventilators.
- Respiratory therapists play an important role during disasters, and even more so during MCRF.

REFERENCES

1. Hotchkin DL, Rubinson L. Modified critical care and treatment space consideration for mass casualty critical illness and injury. *Respir Care.* 2008;53:67–74.
2. Rubinson L, Nuzzo JB, Talmor DS, et al. Augmentation of hospital critical care capacity after bioterrorist attacks or epidemics: recommendations of the Working Group on Emergency Mass Critical Care. *Crit Care Med.* 2005;33:2393–2403.
3. Rubinson L, O'Toole T. Critical care during epidemics. *Crit Care.* 2005;9:311–313.
4. Rubinson L, Branson RD, Pesik N, Talmor D. Positive-pressure ventilation equipment for mass casualty respiratory failure. *Biosecur Bioterror.* 2006;4:183–194.
5. Lassen HCA. *Management of Life-Threatening Poliomyelitis. Copenhagen, 1952–1956, with a Survey of Autopsy-Findings in 115 Cases.* Edinburgh: Livingstone; 1956.
6. deBoisblanc BP. Black Hawk, please come down: reflections on a hospital's struggle to survive in the wake of Hurricane Katrina. *Am J Respir Crit Care Med.* 2005;172:1239–1240.
7. Tang JW, Shetty N, Lam TT. Features of the new pandemic influenza A/H1N1/2009 virus: virology, epidemiology, clinical and public health aspects. *Curr Opin Pulm Med.* 2010;16:235–241.
8. Homeland Security. *National Preparedness Guidelines.* October 2007. Available at: http://www.dhs.gov/xlibrary/assets/National_Preparedness_Guidelines.pdf. Accessed April 24, 2010.
9. Muskat P. Mass casualty chemical exposure and implications for respiratory failure. *Respir Care.* 2008;53:58–63.
10. Hanley ME, Bogdan GM. Mechanical ventilation in mass casualty scenarios. Augmenting staff: project XTREME. *Respir Care.* 2008;53:176–188.
11. Daugherty E, Branson RD, Desai A, Rubinson L. Infection control in mass respiratory failure: preparing to respond to H1N1. *Crit Care Med.* 2010;38(4 suppl):e103–109.
12. Ritz RH, Privitera JE. Oxygen supplies during a mass casualty situation. *Respir Care.* 2008;53:215–224.
13. NIH ARDS Network. Ventilation with lower tidal volumes as compared with traditional tidal volumes for acute lung injury and the acute respiratory distress syndrome. *New Engl J Med.* 2000;342:1301–1308.
14. American Association for Respiratory Care. *Guidelines for Acquisition of Ventilators to Meet Demands for Pandemic Flu and Mass Casualty Incidents.* Available at: http://www.aarc.org/headlines/ventilator_acquisitions/vent_guidelines.pdf. Accessed April 14, 2008.
15. Branson RD, Johannigman JA, Daugherty EL, Rubinson L. Surge capacity mechanical ventilation. *Respir Care.* 2008;53:78–90.
16. Daugherty EL, Branson RD, Rubinson L. Mass casualty respiratory failure. *Curr Opin Crit Care.* 2007;13:51–56.

CHAPTER 28

Respiratory Care of the Elderly

Helen M. Sorenson

OUTLINE

OBJECTIVES

1. Discuss the importance of gerontology and geriatric principles in respiratory care practice.
2. Explain how the demographics of aging will affect healthcare professionals.
3. Describe the age-associated changes in pulmonary anatomy and physiology.
4. Compare the components of a physical assessment and a comprehensive geriatric assessment in elderly individuals.
5. Explain some of the reasons why older patients may not present with typical complaints when ill and list some of the more common atypical symptoms.
6. Elaborate on the issues surrounding medication management in older adults.
7. Discuss the adverse consequences of miscommunication with elderly patients.
8. Compare and contrast symptoms of asthma and chronic obstructive pulmonary disease in older adult patients.
9. Describe the beneficial effects of the aging population adhering to healthy lifestyle choices.

KEY TERMS

baby boomers
clubbing
frailty
glycosuria
goiter
hepatosplenomegaly
hypoglycemia
hypothermia
immunosenescense
life expectancy
life span
obesity
orthopnea
orthostatic hypotension
polydipsia
polyphagia
polyuria
sarcopenia
turgor

INTRODUCTION

The incorporation of geriatrics into respiratory care publications and the educational curricula has been gradual. The American Association for Respiratory Care (AARC) position statement on respiratory care of the geriatric patient was penned many years ago. In addition, the AARC held two educational consensus conferences in the early 1990s. The first identified aging of the population as a major trend affecting the profession,[1] and the second stated that programs should better prepare students in geriatrics and gerontology, among other areas.[2] Aging issues have been on the radar screen for well over a decade. Although the desire and intent to follow up on the recommendations were strong, many factors, including already crowded curricula, forestalled the entrance of geriatric education into existing programs.

Perhaps another mitigating factor is that respiratory therapists (RTs), by virtue of what we do and for whom we care, have always provided therapy to older adults. Thirty years ago, it is likely that less than 50% of our pulmonary patients were over the age of 65 years. Today there is a much larger pool of prospective older patients who suffer from both acute and chronic disease. Many RTs have cared for patients who are in their 70s, 80s, or 90s, and even some who were older than 100 years. Unfortunately, the tidal wave of elderly is approaching the shore and we, as a profession, may not be prepared. "Almost no one reaches the age of sixty-five without some disease or associated illness."[3]

Respiratory problems, both chronic and acute, multiple comorbidities, and adverse drug events are more common in the elderly. Pneumonia is a leading cause of morbidity and mortality in older adults. Fragile bones, thin skin, altered thermoregulatory mechanisms, weaker immune systems, and age-related changes in organ systems all affect patient care. This chapter provides information on some of the essentials of geriatric respiratory care. Although reading this will not make you a gerontologist or geriatric specialist, it is hoped that it will help you understand that our older patients are not just 40-year-old adults who got older. Older adults are unique in many ways and deserve care that is customized to their advanced age.

The Demography of Aging

The projected increase in older adults will rise sharply in 2011 when the **baby boomers** (defined as those born between 1946 and 1964) officially enter the old-age category. Given the potential of 10,000 adults per day turning 65 years of age for a period of 12 to 15 years, the growth in the older adult population will be unprecedented. This boom in the aging population, often referred to as the "graying of America," is not just a national phenomenon. Among both developed and undeveloped nations, in America and worldwide, the older population is growing (**Table 28–1**). The U.S. Census Bureau has compiled actual and projected growth charts for the aging population.[4] Adults over the age of 85 years are the fastest-growing segment of the population in the United States. Global projected populations of adults over age 65 years have also been compiled by the U.S. Census Bureau (**Table 28–2**).[4]

Another way of understanding the magnitude of change in the older population is to view a chart of the projected population change of adults over age 85 years in the United States (**Figure 28–1**). Reviewing the changes in the growing elderly population in the United States and globally is essential when considering the quality of care for our older patients. Almost every medical specialty will be affected by this phenomenon. The leading causes of morbidity and mortality in adults over the age of 65 are cardiac, cerebrovascular, and pulmonary diseases and malignancy. Five of the six leading causes of death among older adults are chronic in nature. Given the role of RTs in acute care, chronic care, and home care, understanding the delivery of healthcare to older adults will be a necessity. The terms *life expectancy and life span* often are interchanged both in conversation and in printed materials, but they are decidedly different concepts. **Life expectancy** is defined as the average number of years an individual is expected to live, either from birth or the number of years remaining at

> **AGE-SPECIFIC ANGLE**
>
> Adults over the age of 85 are the fastest-growing segment of the U.S. population.

TABLE 28–1 Aging Population in United States, 1900–2050 (Projected)

	1900	1950	2000	2050 (Projected)
Total population (in millions)	76.0	150.7	276.2	392.0
Percentage of population age 65 years and older	4.1%	8.1%	12.8%	20.4%
Percentage of population age 85 years and older	0.2%	0.4%	1.6%	4.8%

TABLE 28–2 Percentage of Adults Over the Age of 65 Years

	Europe	North America	Latin America	Asia
2000	15.5%	12.6%	5.5%	6%
2030 (projected)	24.3%	20.3%	11.6%	12%

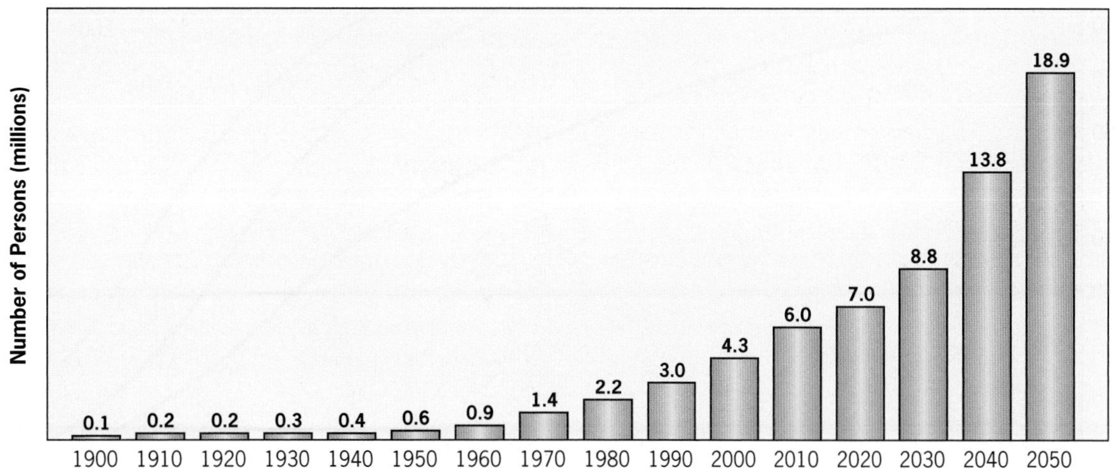

FIGURE 28–1 Projections of the U.S. population aged 85 years and older. Data from U.S. Census Bureau. *Current Population Reports: Special Studies, 65+ in the United States* (P23–190). Washington, DC: U.S. Government Printing Office. Available at: http://www.census.gov/prod/1/pop/p23-190/p23-190.pdf.

AGE-SPECIFIC ANGLE

Five of the six leading causes of death among older adults are chronic in nature.

any given age. A 1-year-old female in the United States is expected to live to about age 83 years. A 1-year-old male in the United States is expected to live about 7 years less, or to age 76 years. The life expectancy of a female who is 63 years of age is about 20 additional years. **Life span**, on the other hand, is species specific and defined as the typical length of time a species is expected to live. The life span of a housefly is about 21 days, and that of a mouse is 3 to 4 years. The life span of humans is currently considered to be 122 years, based on the age to which Jean Calment survived in France.

One way to compare these two values is to see them in a chart form (**Figure 28–2**), which clearly demonstrates the rectangularization of the survival curve. Note that in 1900, 95% of infants were alive at age 5 years, and in 2004 nearly 100% had survived. Also note that by age 50 years, the percentage surviving in 1900 was only about 60%, as compared with about 94% at age 50 years in 2004. This clearly shows that life expectancy is increasing. However, note that at age 100 years there is little difference in survivability between 1900 and 2004, demonstrating that life span has not changed appreciably in the last century.

Aging Pulmonary Anatomy and Physiology

Like other organ systems, the lungs, surrounding muscles, pulmonary vessels, and bony structure are all affected by age. Although the changes are not major, some subtle changes in structure and function occur that affect ventilation, perfusion, and diffusion in the elderly.

The lungs and the chest wall both have elastic properties. The thorax has the tendency to pull outward, and the lungs are inclined to recoil inward. Normally these opposing forces balance each other. With age the chest wall becomes stiffer, due in part to costal cartilage calcification, osteoporosis, changes in rib–vertebral articulations, and narrowing of the intervertebral disk,[5] often resulting in settling of the vertebrae with age, and loss in height. While the chest wall is becoming stiffer, the lungs are becoming more compliant as a result of reduced elastic recoil pressure. The net effect is an overall decrease in compliance, which increases the work of breathing for older adults. Realistically, a 70-year-old adult will have a 50% increase in work of breathing compared with a 20-year-old.[6] The alterations in the lungs and chest wall also effect the anterior–posterior (A-P) chest configuration. A normal A-P chest wall diameter is 1:2; with advanced age, the A-P chest wall diameter approaches 1:1.

Respiratory muscle strength declines with age. **Sarcopenia**, the age-related loss of muscle mass, starts to develop somewhere between ages 40 and 60 years for both sexes. Longitudinal studies have established the rate of decline to be between 1% and 3% per year after age 50 years.[7] In a study comparing transdiaphragmatic pressure (Pdi-max) among young (19 to 28 years) and older (65 to 75 years) men at a variety of lung volumes, the average Pdi-max

AGE-SPECIFIC ANGLE

Sarcopenia, the age-related loss of muscle mass, starts to develop somewhere between the ages of 40 and 60.

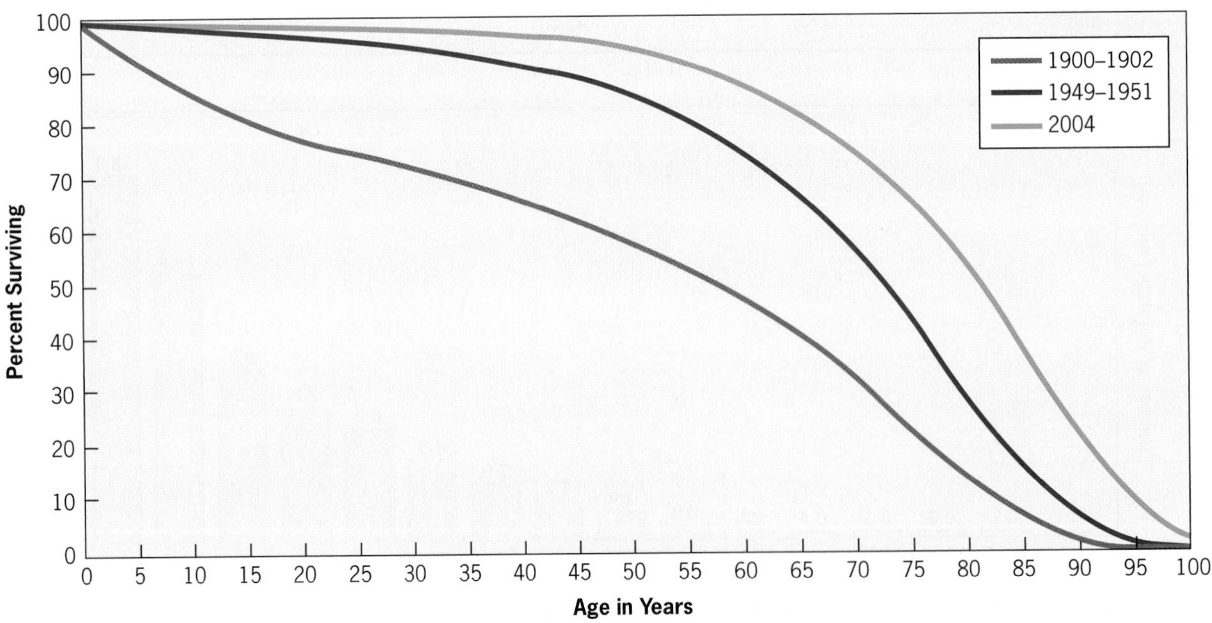

FIGURE 28–2 Percentage of persons surviving by age, 1900–2004. Modified from Arias E. *Natl Vital Stat Report.* 2007;56(9):6. Available at: http://www.cdc.gov/nchs/data/nvsr/nvsr56/nvsr56_09.pdf.

TABLE 28-3 Age-Associated Changes in Pulmonary Function Values in Healthy Elders

Value	Age-Related Change
Pulmonary Function	
Total lung capacity (TLC)	Relatively stable over time
Forced vital capacity (FVC)	Decreases 20–30 mL/year after age 20 years
Forced expiratory volume in 1 second (FEV_1)	Decreases
Functional residual capacity (FRC)	Increases (as a result of increased residual volume)
Residual volume (RV)	Increases
RV/TLC ratio	Increases from 20% to roughly 40% in old age
Peak expiratory flow (PEF)	Decreases
Diffusing capacity of lung for carbon monoxide (D_{LCO})	Decreases
Arterial Blood Gases and Oxygenation	
pH	Relatively stable
$Paco_2$	Relatively stable
Pao_2	Decreases slightly (<70 mm Hg is abnormal in otherwise healthy adults regardless of age) Supine Pao_2 5 mm Hg less than seated Pao_2
Spo_2	Relatively stable (<94% is abnormal in otherwise healthy adults; <90% in COPD patients should be treated)
$P(A - a)o_2$	Increases slightly

in the older subjects was significantly lower than in the younger men.[8] Because all of the respiratory muscles, including inspiratory and expiratory accessory muscles, go through age-associated decremental change, many pulmonary flows, volumes, and capacities are altered with age (**Table 28–3**).

An additional change in the pulmonary system notable in the elderly is a reduction in the alveolar gas exchange surface area. Alveoli dilate and the pores of Kohn become larger, likely due to changes in elasticity in the parenchyma. Less surface area reduces the diffusion of pulmonary gases. The central and peripheral chemoreceptors are less responsive to changes in Pao_2 and $Paco_2$. The adaptation to low oxygen or high carbon dioxide in terms of ventilatory response in a 75-year-old is almost half of that noted in a 25-year-old adult.[9]

There are many reasons why understanding normal age-related physiologic changes in the pulmonary system is important to RTs. Well over half the patients seen by RTs are older than 65 years. Our patients not only have age-associated decremental change but also almost always have a disease process that we are treating. RTs must be able to distinguish age-related decline from pathology. Most notable is the tendency to falsely presume that older adults with a 1:1 A-P chest diameter and enlarged alveoli have "senile emphysema."

AGE-SPECIFIC ANGLE

Over half the patients seen by the average respiratory therapist are over the age of 65 years.

RESPIRATORY RECAP

Primary Age-Related Pulmonary Changes

» Loss of elasticity
» Loss of muscle strength
» Loss of alveolar gas exchange surface area
» Decreased responsiveness of the chemoreceptors

The implications for RTs may be more critical when caring for older adults in the intensive care unit. A weaker diaphragm, reduced vital capacity, and compromised cough mechanism must be taken into consideration postextubation. Older patients may need closer monitoring and hyperinflation therapy to prevent atelectasis. Unfortunately, because of age-associated physiology, older adults are more likely to become ventilator dependent and to suffer the consequences associated with long-term mechanical ventilation. Liberating older patients from the ventilator in less than 48 hours is optimal. This may be facilitated by extubation to noninvasive ventilation.

Geriatric Patient Assessment

Physical Assessment

Physical assessments include all systems, vital signs, skin, chest and back, sensory and motor function, mental acuity, and nutritional status. Consider this scenario: You walk into an elderly patient's room early morning to deliver therapy. You listen to lung sounds, gather vital signs, ask the patient a few questions, and ask if he or she can sit up in bed for you. While listening to lung sounds on the posterior thorax, you note that the scapulas are uneven and there is significant kyphosis. You also notice that the patient's skin is very dry and lacking the normal tension or fullness known as **turgor**. These are signs of a restrictive disease process and possible dehydration. How will this affect the patient's breathing? The lung sounds are decreased and you hear crackles in the bases, but you also note that the patient is using accessory muscles to breathe. While auscultating the right upper lobe, you hear wheezes. Which of these findings are normal in an older adult? Because of an increased A-P chest diameter, the lung sounds may be decreased. Crackles in the bases are not uncommon in older adults; this signifies some atelectasis, which often clears if you can get the patient to take a few good deep breaths. The use of accessory muscles to breathe and the wheezes, however, are likely associated with pathology.

Did the patient complain of dizziness or lightheadedness when he or she sat up in bed? Changing position from being supine to being seated or standing can occasionally cause a drop in blood pressure. A decrease in systolic pressure of 20 mm Hg upon change in position is diagnostic for **orthostatic hypotension**. Although this may not affect a patient's pulmonary system, it will increase his or her risk of falling.

While checking the identification band on the patient's wrist, look to see whether clubbing is present. **Clubbing**, an enlargement of the terminal aspect of the fingers, is neither age related nor normally associated with either chronic bronchitis or emphysema. If clubbing is present in your patient with chronic obstructive pulmonary disease (COPD), suspect an additional comorbidity such as bronchiectasis, bronchogenic cancer, or asbestosis. Renal and cardiac disease have also been associated with clubbing.[10]

RESPIRATORY RECAP

Physical Assessment Findings in the Elderly

- » Increased A-P chest diameter
- » Decreased lung sounds
- » Atelectasis in the bases
- » Increased pulse pressure
- » Respiratory rate a little faster (16–24 breaths/min)
- » Heart rate normal or a little slower
- » Bounding pulses (due to atherosclerotic change in blood vessels)
- » Lower body temperature (decreased metabolism and decreased muscle mass)

In less than 1 or 2 minutes, you have made a cursory assessment of the patient for breath sounds, dehydration, restrictive disease, orthostatic hypotension, and clubbing (comorbidities). Continuing on with the assessment, asking an open-ended question such as "How did you sleep last night?" or "What did you order for breakfast?" is instructive. The patient's response will give you information about his or her level of cognition and possibly some insight into nutritional or other habits.

Heart rate does not change appreciably with age. In sedentary older adults, it may be a little lower. RTs may notice stronger or "bounding" pulses in older patients, likely an effect of atherosclerotic changes in blood vessels. There is an age-associated decrease in the number of pacemaker cells in the sinoatrial node, which may lead to symptomatic bradyarrhythmias.[11] To get an accurate heart rate in elderly patients, it may be necessary to count their pulse for a full minute.

While palpating for the pulse, note whether the patient feels extremely warm or cold. Body temperature is often a little lower in older adults due in part to decreased metabolism. The thermoregulatory mechanism is also blunted with age, making older patients more susceptible to changes in environmental temperatures. How would a cold room (<65° F) affect your COPD patient? **Hypothermia**, defined as a core temperature of 95° F (35° C) or less, can develop in rooms where the temperature is maintained at 60° to 65° F. A pulmonary consequence of accidental hypothermia may be bradypnea, which can lead to hypoxemia or hypercapnia or both. Hypothermia that develops as a consequence of a surgical procedure can also affect immunity. Even mild hypothermia (core temperature decrease by 1° C) can cause significant alteration to the normal immune response.[12]

Do not assume that an afebrile patient is infection free. Fever may be blunted 20% to 30% of the time in a patient with an infection, which unfortunately contributes to diagnostic delays.[13] If elderly patients do have a fever, it is likely to be associated with a more serious viral or bacterial infection than fever in a younger adult.

Respiratory rate is stable across the adult life span. It is advisable to measure respiratory rate prior to starting therapy. When patients are actively involved in nebulizer or hyperinflation therapy, their respiratory rate will be altered. A normal respiratory rate in adults over age 65 years remains in the range of 16 to 24 breaths per minute despite physiologic changes in the lungs. Dyspnea, however, is rarely normal. If patients have a resting respiratory rate greater than 25 years, there is likely some pathology associated with the increased work of breathing.

Comprehensive Geriatric Assessment

A comprehensive geriatric assessment (CGA) does not generally fall under the duties of a RT. Normally conducted by a geriatrician or family practitioner, this is a comprehensive systems assessment with a goal of uncovering treatable health problems or issues in community-dwelling older adults. The process involves screening select patients (often those older than 75 to 80 years) for functional ability, geriatric syndromes, specific medical conditions, medication management, and support systems.

Frailty

Frail elderly, a Medline medical subject heading (MeSH) term since 1991, has been defined as "older adults who are lacking in general strength and are unusually susceptible to disease or other infirmity."[14] **Frailty** has attracted increased attention in the medical literature recently, likely corresponding with the increased numbers of frail individuals being admitted to healthcare institutions. In addition to assessing activities of daily living (ADLs) and instrumental activities of daily living (IADLs), the CGA involves screening for a myriad of potential disabilities. The Mini-Mental Status Exam (MMSE), clock-drawing test, Geriatric Depression Scale (GDS), Mini-Nutritional Assessment (MNA), Snellen eye test, whispered voice test, Functional Assessment Staging (FAST), and the Hearing Handicap Inventory for the Elderly (HHIE) are just a few of the available instruments. In addition, the Caregiver Burden Interview may be valuable in heading off potential elder abuse before it becomes a reality. (See **Appendix 28–1** at the end of this chapter.)

TABLE 28–4 Normal Age-Related Changes in Various Organ Systems

Cardiac	Cardiac muscle thickens, leading to enlarged left ventricle. Arterial walls stiffen with age; aorta becomes dilated and elongated. Aortic knob calcification (crescent-shaped ring on top of aorta) is noted in about 30% of older adults but has no pathologic significance. Systolic blood pressure increases more than diastolic, leading to increased pulse pressure and isolated systolic hypertension.
Pulmonary	Diaphragm loses strength, up to 25% by age 75–80 years. At age 20 years, alveolar surface area is about 70 m^2; at age 70 years, it is reduced to about 60 m^2.
Brain/central nervous system	Cell loss in some areas of the brain is stable; profound loss in other areas. The weight of the brain gradually decreases with age (approximately 10% from age 30 years to age 90 years).
Kidneys	Renal mass slowly diminishes (from about 250–270 g in young adults to about 180–200 g in adults older than 80 years).

RESPIRATORY RECAP

Comprehensive Geriatric Assessment

- ADLs and IADLs
- Vision and hearing (Snelling eye test, HHIE, and whisper voice test)
- Mental status (MMSE and clock-drawing test)
- Geriatric Depression Scale (GDS)
- Nutrition (MNA) and nutritional health assessment
- Functional Assessment Staging (FAST)
- Caregiver Burden Interview (possible need for assistance)

Chronological age is sometimes used as a marker of frailty (e.g., only screening adults over the age of 75 or 80 years); however, there is a wide range of function in the older adult population. In an effort to find a simple and useful marker of frailty, a cross-sectional study comparing hand-grip strength and 10 additional aging markers was conducted in the United Kingdom on 717 individuals between the ages of 64 and 74 years. The results showed that hand-grip strength in both men and women was associated with more markers of frailty than chronological age within the narrow range studied.[15]

As the aging population continues to grow and expand, RTs who see the need for additional assessments in elderly pulmonary patients may need to take the lead in recommending a comprehensive assessment for the patient. Home care RTs may be in the best position to recommend screening services for their elderly patients.

Atypical Disease Presentation

Atypical or nonspecific clinical presentation of disease in the elderly is much like the diversity common in the whole population of older adults. There are no hard and fast specifics, but there are generalities about which healthcare professionals should be knowledgeable. In older adults, the first signs of an acute illness or an exacerbation of a chronic disease may be functional decline, cognitive impairment, or both. Because symptoms are not always typical, older adults may not recognize subtle changes as being associated with a disease process. Atypical symptoms may be ignored, may be denied, often out of fear, or may simply be regarded as one of the joys of aging. Well elders are more likely to present with fewer atypical symptoms. Nonspecific symptoms, which are more difficult to diagnose, are much more common in frail elders, in particular women over the age of 80 years.

Unfortunately, the lines between aging and ailing are often blurred. Aches and pains may be caused by chronic osteoarthritis, overexertion, exercise, the weather, lack of activity, medications, or pathology. A change in gait or new onset of tripping or running into furniture may be related to infection, medications, or dehydration. A new onset of confusion in a formerly cognitive, sapient individual may be related to infection or hypoxemia. Weak nonproductive coughing may be a side effect of drugs (e.g., angiotensin-converting enzyme inhibitors) or a pulmonary disorder. Other causes of a cough may be gastroesophageal reflux disease (GERD), aspiration associated with dysphagia,[16] a stroke or transient ischemic attack (TIA), laryngeal dysfunction, or an endobronchial tumor.[17] RTs are accustomed to looking for usual symptoms, such as pain, fever, cough, dyspnea, and nausea/vomiting, in patients as signs of illness. In the elderly, it may be better to ask about dizziness, syncope, abdominal pain, and fatigue.

Two major reasons why symptoms in the elderly are not typical are age-associated changes in the immune system and normal age-related change in various organ systems (**Table 28–4**). The reasons why older adults do not present with classic symptoms are poorly understood but are likely multifactorial. Age-associated changes in physiology, a reduced response to hypoxemia and hypercapnia, and alterations in the cardiac conduction system are all likely contributors. Also suggested is a decreased peripheral sensitivity that can reduce the sensation of pain.[18] The immune system undergoes age-related functional decline. The thymus gland decreases in size and function. The T-lymphocyte response to antigens decreases. **Immunosenescense**, defined as aging of the immune system, progresses as we grow older, reducing both cell-mediated and humoral immunity. These factors combined may be the reason why elderly persons are susceptible to respiratory infections from all causes.[3]

The presentation of symptoms may also be disproportionate to the severity of illness, causing further diagnostic confusion. A temperature of 99.6° F (38° C) in an older adult may be recorded and noted as a little elevated, but not associated with disease. Consider, however, that this same patient had a core body temperature of 96.8° F (37° C) and that his or her temperature is now elevated three degrees. Would this justify an intervention? The importance of monitoring body temperature on a regular basis in the elderly cannot be overstated. Early intervention is needed if we are to keep our older patients from suffering repeated exacerbations of chronic or acute disease.

Atypical Symptoms

Some of the more common diseases and disorders that present atypically in older adults are pneumonia, urinary tract infection, myocardial infarction, congestive heart failure (CHF), tuberculosis, hyperthyroidism, depression, diabetes, and alcoholism. The atypical symptoms and important age-related considerations for each are presented here.

> **AGE-SPECIFIC ANGLE**
>
> Pneumonia is a leading cause of morbidity and mortality in older patients.

Pneumonia[3]

- Patients may present with weakness, confusion, altered mental status, a decrease in appetite, and lethargy.
- Fever and chills are present 50% of the time in adults older than 75 years.
- Older adults have fewer complaints of cough and dyspnea.
- Signs of more serious disease: respiratory rate > 24, C-reactive protein > 10 mg/dL.
- Diagnostic tests recommended: chest x-ray, sputum Gram stain and culture, two sets of blood cultures.
- Chest x-ray may not show abnormalities if patient is dehydrated. Rehydrate and get follow-up chest x-ray.

Urinary Tract Infections[18]

- Incontinence, increased confusion, falls

Myocardial Infarction[19,20]

- Patients may present with syncope, confusion, palpitations, stroke, vertigo, nausea.
- Dyspnea is the most common symptom.
- In women, the most common prodromal (>1 month prior) symptoms are unusual fatigue, sleep disturbance, and shortness of breath. Acute chest pain was absent in 43% of older women.
- Chest pain in adults younger than 65 years occurs 89% of the time.
- Chest pain in adults older than 65 years occurs 66% of the time.
- Chest pain in adults older than 85 years occurs 33% of the time.
- Silent presentation is not uncommon.

Congestive Heart Failure[18,21]

- New-onset pulmonary edema (a classic sign of CHF) may be confounded by comorbid conditions.
- **Orthopnea** (difficulty breathing in a flat position) may be hidden if the patient has a habit of sleeping on two to three pillows.
- Dyspnea on exertion may be absent in older adults who have little exertion on a daily basis.
- Patients may present with complaints of tiredness, decreased appetite, weight gain of 2 to 3 pounds (0.9 to 1.4 kg), fatigue and generalized weakness, and/or a nonproductive cough and complaints of poor sleep.

Tuberculosis[22]

- Adults older than 65 years are much less likely to present with typical symptoms of hemoptysis, fever, or night sweats.
- Older adults may present with **hepatosplenomegaly** (enlarged liver and spleen), weight loss, abnormal liver function tests, and/or anemia.
- A high index of suspicion is recommended if a patient presents with cough or pneumonia unresponsive to conventional therapy.
- Tuberculosis infection is four times higher for nursing home residents than for community-dwelling older adults.
- Mortality rates from tuberculosis are highest in the elderly.

Hypothyroidism[18]

- **Goiter**, enlargement of the thyroid gland, is present in 94% of younger adults but present in only 50% of older adults.
- 80% of older patients present with unexplained weight loss.
- 50% of older patients present with palpitations and tremor.

> **RESPIRATORY RECAP**
>
> **Diseases That May Present Atypically in Older Adults**
>
> » Pneumonia
> » Urinary tract infection
> » Myocardial infarction
> » Congestive heart failure
> » Tuberculosis
> » Hyperthyroidism
> » Depression
> » Diabetes (type 2)
> » Alcoholism

- In the elderly, new-onset atrial fibrillation, weight loss, proximal muscle weakness, and confusion may be presenting symptoms.

Depression[18]

- Depression is the most commonly occurring mental health problem for the older adult population.
- The ageist attitude that older adults usually complain of feeling sad, tired, or depressed may make depression hard to recognize.
- Screening for depression in high-risk groups is recommended, including alcoholics; drug addicts; and adults with dementia, stroke, cancer, hip fracture, myocardial infarction, COPD, or Parkinson disease.
- The Geriatric Depression Scale is a useful instrument.

Diabetes (Type 2)[9,18]

- The diagnosis is usually made in an asymptomatic older patient during a routine physical exam.
- **Polyuria** (excessive urination), **polydipsia** (excessive thirst), and **polyphagia** (increased food consumption) may not be present.
- Dehydration, confusion, and incontinence may develop due to **glycosuria**, the presence of sugar in the urine.
- Confusion is an early symptom of **hypoglycemia** (low blood sugar).
- Occasionally, peripheral neuropathy may be the initial manifestation of type 2 diabetes.

Alcoholism[23]

- The signs and symptoms of alcoholism are often attributed to aging.
- Chronic pancreatitis is associated with alcoholism.
- Abuse of alcohol is often overlooked unless it is very obvious.
- Signs of alcohol abuse include falls, confusion, memory loss, gait changes, and hostile behavior.
- Estimates are that 40% of older adults use alcohol, and 5% to 10% abuse it.

To help identify alcoholism, ask patients the following four questions (the CAGE questionnaire):

C Do you need to cut down on drinking?
A Are you annoyed by criticism of drinking?
G Do you feel guilty about drinking?
E Do you need an early-morning eye-opener drink?

Two positive answers on the CAGE questionnaire can identify 75% of alcoholics with 95% specificity.

Geriatric Pharmacotherapy

Medication management in older adults is becoming a major public health issue. As a result of their increased incidence of both acute and chronic illness, older adults are the highest users of medication compared with all other age groups. Although the elderly make up on average 12% to 13% of the total population of the United States, they consume about 33% of all prescription drugs and about 25% of all over-the-counter drugs. Among the issues related to geriatric pharmacotherapy are medication safety, adverse drug events, inappropriate medication use, underprescribing and overprescribing, and the rising cost of drugs.

Medication Safety

Medication safety has long been on the radar screen of medical professionals. Almost 30 years ago, it was stated that "there is ample biological basis . . . for concern by legislators, regulators and the general public over drug use in older adults."[24] Some of the biological reasons why older adults are more likely than younger adults to have adverse drug reactions are as follows: smaller body size and different body composition (reduced lean muscle mass), a reduced ability of the kidneys and liver to metabolize and clear drugs out of the body, a decrease in gastric motility, and a decline in gastric pH.

To fully understand the effect age-associated physiology has on drugs, it is instructive to look at the half-life of drugs. The liver is the primary site of drug metabolism. With age, the liver volume, mass, and blood flow all decline. Hepatic metabolism of drugs decreases up to 25% over the life span.[9] The duration of drug action is determined by the metabolic rate and is measured in terms of half-life. Consider the following:

- The half-life of diazepam (Valium) in a younger adult is about 24 hours.
- The half-life of diazepam (Valium) in an older adult is about 82 hours.
- The half-life of flurazepam (Dalmane) in a younger adult is about 74 hours.
- The half-life of flurazepam (Dalmane) in an older adult is about 106 hours.

If the dosing is not adjusted, significant amounts of drug can accumulate in the body.

Despite the fact that drug safety is a concern, newer medications have saved countless lives, and few would argue against their benefit. In older adult patients, however, caution must be exercised. The often-repeated advice "Start low and go slow" regarding dosing of medications for the elderly is a wise and prudent course of action.

> **AGE-SPECIFIC ANGLE**
>
> Whereas the half-life of Valium in a 20-year-old is approximately 24 hours, in an 80-year-old the half-life is approximately 82 hours.

Adverse Drug Reactions

Adverse drug reactions (ADRs) are common in the elderly, but what is most concerning is that many are preventable. A 2002 meta-analysis found that up to 88%

AGE-SPECIFIC ANGLE

Adverse drug reactions (ADRs) are common in the elderly; one study found that older adults were four times more likely to be hospitalized with an ADR than younger adults. Many ADRs are preventable.

of ADRs that resulted in hospitalizations were preventable. This study also revealed that older adults were four times more likely to be hospitalized with an ADR than younger adults.[25] Another concern is the prescribing of potentially inappropriate drugs to older adults when there are safer alternatives. A drug that will effectively treat a 40-year-old patient may not be indicated for an 80-year-old patient. Drugs that are successful in treating a specific disease process may not be appropriate for an older patient who is already on multiple drugs for other comorbidities. The more medication an individual takes, the greater the potential for an adverse effect.

Unfortunately, few drug studies are done on healthy elders, so prescribing appropriately for sick elders can sometimes be a challenge. One excellent resource is *Beers Criteria for Determining Potentially Inappropriate Medication Use by the Elderly*. First published in 1991, and again in 1997, the criteria were updated in 2003.[26] The final criteria include 48 individual medications or classes of medications that should be avoided in older adults. The guidelines (in a table format) list the drug, the reason for concern, and whether the risk is high or low. Although beyond the scope of this chapter, anyone who works with older adults would be well advised to print out the tables in the guidelines as a reference.[26] It should also be noted that with all the new drugs being approved by the Food and Drug Administration (FDA) and marketed, revisions of the Beers criteria will likely be available every 3 to 4 years in the future.

Medication Undertreatment and Overtreatment

Medication undertreatment in the elderly is another troubling reality in many long-term care facilities. A multicenter survey of a stratified random sample of 193 residential care and assisted living facilities in four states (2104 residents older than 65 years) revealed the following: of 328 subjects with CHF, 204 (62%) were not receiving an angiotensin-converting enzyme inhibitor; of 172 subjects with a prior history of myocardial infarction, 60.5% were not receiving aspirin and 76% were not receiving beta blockers; and of 435 subjects with a prior history of stroke, only 37.5% were receiving an anticoagulant or antiplatelet agent.[27] Although drugs must be given judiciously to older adults, failure to prescribe appropriate drugs whose value in decreasing morbidity has been established in clinical trials is also inappropriate.

The self-medication habits of older adults, although harder to track, have some commonalities. Many older adults continue to take medications and consume alcohol at the same time. Healthcare literacy issues may be a factor, but willful noncompliance with recommended dosing instructions is also a reality. Many older adults regularly depend on over-the-counter cold medicine, pain relievers, and vitamins. They do not always perceive these to be real medicine and thus continue to self-dose while on prescription medications. Sources of information about over-the-counter medication use are received at best from the container label, the physician, or the pharmacist only 54% of the time.[28] Even recommendations by the pharmacist regarding whether to take medications with or without food are often ignored.

Drug Expenditures

Prescription drug costs have risen exponentially in the past few years. Older adults on fixed incomes or with incomes that have dwindled due to the changes in the economy are finding it harder to afford medications. Medicare Part D offers some help, as do other prescription drug plans, but not all older adults have coverage. Compounding the problem is the fact that prescription drugs may cost more in poor areas. Although chain pharmacies are often less expensive, they are not always located in poor areas. Prescription drugs can cost up to 15% more from independent pharmacies in poor zip codes.[29] Although there are independent pharmacies in poor zip codes that do not inflate costs, issues of finances, transportation, and health literacy limit consumers from shopping around. When older adults cannot access medication, and thus cannot control their disease process, they will end up in emergency departments, adding to the burden of escalating healthcare costs (**Figure 28–3**).

Communicating with Older Adults

Most RTs have encountered frustrating situations in which communication with the patient seems nonexistent. Language barriers, hearing deficits, poststroke aphasia, Alzheimer disease, and even patients on mechanical ventilators pose a challenge. Knowing that patient cooperation will increase the effectiveness of therapy makes communication more important in any of these situations. Taking the time to establish some measure of mutual understanding, however, is not always possible. In today's healthcare environment, time constraints create barriers to effective communication. When busy, the amount of time spent with each patient decreases, and communication gets lost in the hustle. What is important to remember, though, is that effective communication benefits more than just the patient. RTs who sense that their encounter with a patient was

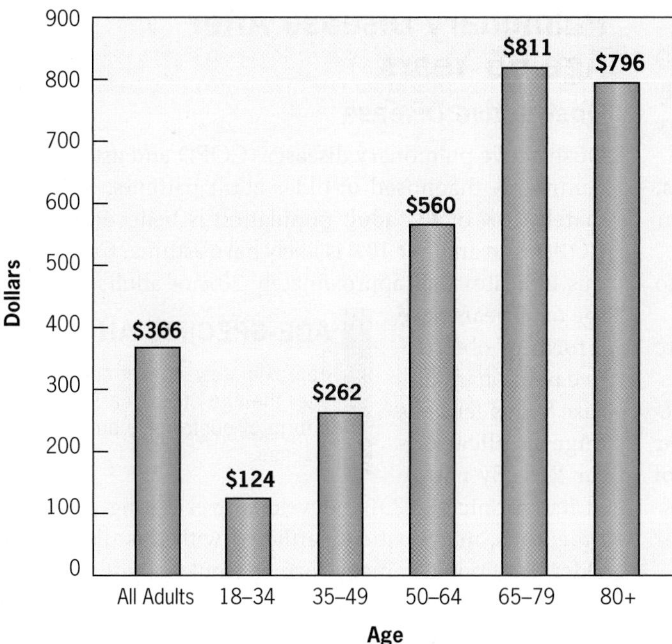

FIGURE 28–3 Increase in prescription drug expenditures. Reproduced from Ihara E, Summer L, Shirey L; Center on an Aging Society, Georgetown University. Data profile: prescription drugs—challenges for the 21st century. *Chronic and Disabling Conditions*. 2002;5. Available at: http://ihcrp.georgetown.edu/agingsociety/pdfs/rxdrugs.pdf. Reprinted with permission.

successful will feel that they have accomplished something and will be more rewarded by the whole process.

Communication Defined

Communication implies two things: a message delivered and a message understood. Although some people appear to be better at relaying information than others, most can be taught this skill; thus, we often refer to it as the "art of communication." Communication is a dynamic, two-way process of imparting data or information between two or more individuals. Communication can be verbal or nonverbal, in written or sign language. Transferral of data likewise can be formal or informal. What is essential is that the information desired to be delivered has been received and comprehended. Talking to patients in a language foreign to them is delivering the message, but if they do not understand, there has been no communication.

> **RESPIRATORY RECAP**
>
> **Communication Is Dependent on Two Variables**
>
> » Message delivered
>
> » Message understood

Effective Communication

Successful transfer of information with an elderly patient is challenging at times. Actually, effective communication often starts with attitude. A RT who is tired and frustrated at the end of his or her shift may not communicate well with an older patient. Nonverbal communication may interfere. An observation attributed to Ralph Waldo Emerson states, "Who you are speaks so loudly, I can't hear what you're saying." When dealing with older adults, RTs must be careful not to send mixed messages. Sitting in a chair reading a paper while a patient is taking a treatment devalues both the patient and the therapy you are delivering.

Another useful tactic in effective communication is the expression of empathy instead of sympathy to patient concerns. Although saying "I'm sorry" appears to be kind, it may be better to try to understand what the patient is going through. A statement such as "I can see that this is really distressing for you" does not imply that you can fix anything, just that you acknowledge the patient's feelings. Often this is enough to calm the patient down a little.

Patient Scenarios

The Angry Patient

Barney Towne, an 82-year-old patient with COPD, is angry much of the time. Staff members have come to accept the fact that he can be grumpy and difficult to handle. Today when you enter his room to deliver his medication, he snarls, "I don't need that, and I don't need you bothering me today either." How will you respond? Your choices are as follows:

1. "Yes you do need this medicine, and if I don't give it to you, who will?"
2. "What's the matter, Mr. Towne?"
3. "I'm just following the doctor's orders and he wants you to take this medicine."
4. Turn and walk angrily out of the room without responding.

Depending on the time of day and the existing patient load, RTs may be inclined to say or do any of the above. What is important to remember, however, is that most likely the patient's mood is not about us. Patients often lash out at caregivers when they are struggling with something that has nothing to do with other people. In this situation, perhaps the best response is to just say, "What's the matter Mr. Towne?" He may or may not share his problem with you, but at the very least you have not caused an escalation of the situation.

Contrary to what we are accustomed to hearing, "Don't just do something, stand there" may be an effective way of communicating. Giving patients time to collect their thoughts and tell you what is bothering them, or giving them time to rethink the angry words they have spoken, may open doors to more effective communication.

The Verbally Abusive Patient

You are delivering therapy to Mr. Lawson, a COPD patient with Alzheimer disease (AD) who is continually cursing at you. How will you respond? Your choices are as follows:

1. Curse back at him and let him know how it feels.
2. Respond by saying, "You need to change your nasty behavior—let's work on it together."
3. Say, "I'm sorry you feel like this, but I don't care to be spoken to in that manner."
4. Step back, look out the window, and say, "It sure is nice today."

One unfortunate characteristic of patients with AD is that dementia robs them of the ability to control their behavior. When AD begins to develop, the frontal part of the brain is damaged, and subsequently destroyed, causing lack of impulse control. Thus, AD patients may swear and use words that make us uneasy.[30]

When caring for patients with dementia, sometimes there are no effective solutions, but the therapy still needs to be delivered. If faced with a situation like this, remain calm and do not attempt to argue or correct such patients. Back off a little, perhaps try to distract them, and continue to proceed with the task at hand. The Alzheimer's Association offers these communication tips for caregivers:[31]

- Identify yourself, approach the person from the front, and call him or her respectfully by name.
- Speak slowly and distinctly, using short simple words and sentences. Avoid vague words and confusing expressions.
- Avoid sudden movements, maintain eye contact, and smile.
- Ask one question at a time and give the person time to respond. Offer a guess if the person used the wrong word and cannot find the right one.
- Give one-step directions and simple explanations.
- Be patient and supportive. Avoid criticism and support positive behavior.
- If the patient seems agitated, back up; he or she may feel threatened.

One final issue deals with communication of symptoms in patients with dementia. Decreased communication skills have been well documented in AD.[32] Patients who cannot accurately report symptoms are at increased risk for developing more serious complications from a disease process. Asking questions may not always generate accurate information, especially if they are yes-or-no questions. Patients with AD may answer yes or no without understanding the question.[33] RTs need to be aware that a change in behavior such as restlessness, decreased activity, decreased appetite, or anything out of the ordinary for the patient may be a clue of physical impairment or illness.

Pulmonary Disease After Age 65 Years

Obstructive Disease

Obstructive pulmonary diseases (COPD and asthma) are commonly diagnosed in older adult patients. Approximately 10% of the adult population is believed to have COPD, and another 10% is likely have asthma. Combined, this indicates that approximately 20% of adults over the age of 65 years have a form of obstructive pulmonary disease.[3] This fact has huge implications for RTs. By nature of its chronicity, COPD develops over a long period of time; thus, many patients afflicted with this disease are older. Additionally, many former smokers who have the disease may never be diagnosed until age-associated decline is coupled with tobacco-related damage, making the disease process more obvious. Because both diseases present with similar symptoms, and some symptoms present simultaneously, it is sometimes difficult to determine whether the patient has asthma, COPD, or both. Because the diseases are treated differently, it is important to try to determine the primary problem. **Table 28–5** may be helpful in differentiating asthma from COPD.[34]

AGE-SPECIFIC ANGLE

Approximately 20% of adults over the age of 65 years have a form of obstructive pulmonary disease.

An increased IgE level is often used to distinguish asthma from COPD; however, the serum IgE levels and antigen-specific IgE production both decline with aging, making this marker less useful.[35]

Geriatric patients admitted to the hospital with COPD and either chronic mucus hypersecretion (CMH) or an acute respiratory infection, or both, should be given special attention. The presence of either CMH or an acute respiratory infection places the COPD patient at increased risk for a more complicated hospital stay. Infection control measures, although always important, are imperative in hospitalized elders. A 2003 study showed that chronic mucus production was a strong predictor of the incidence of respiratory infection and was also a strong predictor of death from COPD.[36] Based on both disease- and age-associated physiologic changes in the lungs, hospitalized elders with COPD must be considered extremely susceptible to adverse events and should be monitored closely. Many of our regular patients with COPD—those "known well to pulmonary services"—may not desire special attention and may resist monitoring. To treat them the same as younger adults, however, would be a mistake. Their lives may depend on our diligence. Once the acute phase of their disease is controlled and the patient has stabilized, the focus needs to be on disease management. Smoking cessation, nutrition, exercise (pulmonary rehabilitation), a review of their medications and

TABLE 28-5 Differentiation of Asthma Versus COPD in Older Adults

Likely Asthma if Patient Is/Has	Likely COPD if Patient Is/Has
Under age 40 years	Over age 40 years
A nonsmoker	A smoker
History of allergies	No history of allergies
Symptoms at night (or anytime)	Symptoms with exertion
Higher room air Pa_{O_2} (mean 65 mm Hg)	Lower room air Pa_{O_2} (mean 55 mm Hg)
Lower room air Pa_{CO_2} (mean 39 mm Hg)	Higher room air Pa_{CO_2} (mean 45 mm Hg)
$FEV_1 > 15\%$ postbronchodilator	$FEV_1 < 15\%$ postbronchodilator

Adapted from Petty TL, Seebass JS, eds. *Pulmonary Disorders of the Elderly*. Philadelphia: American College of Physicians; 2007; and Sin BA, Akkoca Ö, Öner F, et al. Differences between asthma and COPD in the elderly. *J Invest Allerg Clin Immunol*. 2006;16(1):44–50.

delivery devices, recognition of the signs and symptoms of an exacerbation, and social support networks are all important aspects of patient education. RTs should take the time to review these with every patient with COPD prior to discharge, regardless of how many admissions and discharges the patient has had.

Elderly patients with asthma, likewise, are at risk for developing complications. Unfortunately, asthma is often underdiagnosed or misdiagnosed as COPD, CHF, or GERD, and thus not managed appropriately. Although only 2% to 3% of older adults with asthma require hospitalization, 10% to 12% of those days are spent in the intensive care unit.[37] Elderly patients with asthma may also have a more severe form of the disease or may be affected more seriously. Despite better medications, asthma action plans, and a better understanding of the pathophysiology of the disease, mortality is still increasing. According to a 1999 survey, the death rate from asthma was 11 times higher in the over-65 population as compared with individuals aged 18 to 35 years.[38] Asthma in the elderly is not a benign disease, and care must be taken to ensure appropriate disease management.

Pharmacotherapy for adult asthmatics depends on the severity of the disease. Inhaled corticosteroids remain the medication of choice for persistent asthma. For moderate and severe persistent asthma, the addition of a long-acting beta agonist (LABA) in addition to inhaled corticosteroids is recommended. Unfortunately, the guidelines are not always followed. One study found that only 30% of elderly patients with asthma received inhaled corticosteroids.[39]

The Salmeterol Multicenter Asthma Research Trial (SMART) study questioned the safety of LABAs as first-line therapy for asthma caused concern in many patients with COPD who were already using the drug.[40] In many instances the solution is a matter of educating patients with COPD that the publication was not questioning the use of LABAs in COPD. The long-acting anticholinergic tiotropium is useful for many patients with COPD.

Restrictive Disease

Many disease processes are capable of contributing to less compliant lungs in older adults. Restrictive disease is characterized by smaller lungs, reduced total lung compliance, and reduced volumes. The precipitating factors may be an alteration in the lung parenchyma or pathology in the pleura, chest wall, or neuromuscular function. If the cause is parenchymal lung disease, as in asbestosis, diffusion of gases will also be impaired. Because airflows and airway resistance are relatively normal, pulmonary function testing will show a restrictive pattern: FEV_1/FVC normal or above normal, with all lung volumes reduced. Causes of pulmonary restrictive disease in the elderly can be divided into three categories: intrinsic lung disease, extrinsic disorders, and idiopathic fibrotic disease.

Intrinsic lung diseases comprise the largest number of etiologic factors. The prevalence of intrinsic pulmonary disease in adults aged 35 to 44 years is 2.7 cases per 100,000 individuals. In adults over age 75, the prevalence exceeds 175 cases per 100,000 individuals.[41] Included in the intrinsic category are collagen vascular diseases; diseases caused by certain drugs, organic dust exposure, or inorganic dust exposure; and unclassified diseases. The collagen vascular diseases most often associated with the development of a restrictive pulmonary component are scleroderma, polymyositis, dermatomyositis, systemic lupus erythematosus, ankylosing spondylitis, and perhaps the most common, rheumatoid arthritis. The pharmaceutical agents implicated in the development of intrinsic lung disease are drugs such as amiodarone, bleomyocin, and methotrexate, which damage lung tissue. Organic dust exposure over time may cause restrictive lung disease, and is usually occupation related.

Byssinosis (cotton worker's disease) and farmer's lung disease are but two examples of the pulmonary diseases caused by organic dusts. Inorganic dusts such as silicon, asbestos, and hard metal dust are causative agents in the development of fibrosis, and their inhalation may also be occupation related. The final category of intrinsic lung disease includes unclassified diseases such as sarcoidosis, alveolar proteinosis, and bronchiolitis obliterans with organizing pneumonia (BOOP).

The extrinsic category of restrictive pulmonary diseases includes both primary and secondary kyphoscoliosis, postpolio syndrome, pleural effusions, and morbid obesity (defined as more than 130% of desired weight),[9] all of which cause a restrictive component.

Idiopathic fibrotic disorders are a challenge. The rate of disease progression is highly variable, and disease does not always respond to therapy. The prognosis for older adults who do not respond to therapy is poor. Lung transplantation is an optional therapy but is not always available to the elderly (those younger than 65 years usually qualify). The scope of this chapter does not allow for a full explanation of treating the myriad of intrinsic and extrinsic disorders; however, corticosteroids are often prescribed. Because treatment differs, however, it is important on diagnosis to determine, based on pulmonary function values, whether the disorder is intrinsic or extrinsic.

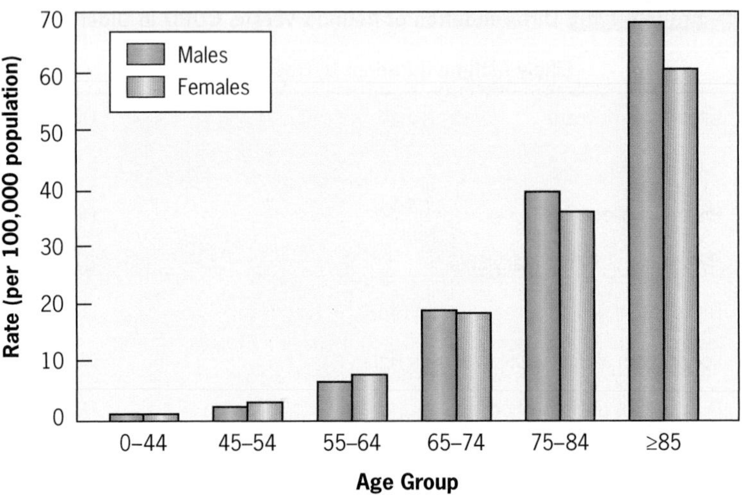

FIGURE 28–4 Age-specific death rate among decedents with pulmonary hypertension by sex and age group: United States, 2000–2002. Modified from Hyduk A, Croft JB, Ayala C, et al. *MMWR*. 2005;54(SS05):1–28.

Pulmonary Hypertension

Pulmonary hypertension (PHTN) in older adults often accompanies COPD, interstitial lung disease, and sleep apnea.[42] Diseases that result in systolic or diastolic dysfunction account for many diagnoses of pulmonary venous hypertension, as do pulmonary emboli, true idiopathic hypertension, and congenital heart disease. Because it is sometimes difficult to separate out PHTN associated with disorders of the respiratory system, hypoxemia, and cardiac failure, treatment is controversial. The use of sildenafil, inhaled prostacyclin, and iloprost in older patients with PHTN secondary to pulmonary fibrosis has shown some benefit without worsening ventilation-perfusion matching, but without large-scale randomized trials that specifically target pulmonary hypertension associated with COPD, no recommendations can be made at this time.[42–44]

Pulmonary rehabilitation is an option, however. A study published in 2005 discussed the advantages and disadvantages of pulmonary rehabilitation in a small cohort of adults (mean age 68 years) with PHTN associated with lung disease. The 6-minute walk distance improved after rehabilitation, as did the items measured by the Chronic Respiratory Disease Questionnaire (CRDQ).[45] More research is indicated regarding the care of elderly patients with pulmonary hypertension, because the mortality rate in adults over age 75 years is significant (**Figure 28–4**).

Healthy Aging Strategies

Most of the advertisements targeted at the elderly are selling youth with the right diet, the appropriate exercises, the newest antiaging serums, or cosmetic surgery. Many older adults, however, are not all that concerned about looking or acting younger. Issues such as paying the bills, dealing with their chronic diseases, finding transportation, and caring for younger family members often take precedence. Having time to do things that are enjoyable and being able to spend time with family and friends are important to most older adults; thus, maintaining adequate health to allow for these activities is the goal of many.

Biological aging is a process of change and does take its toll on tissues and organs. Functional decline is a factor of advanced age, even in the absence of disease, but can be slowed down. Healthy lifestyle choices or the avoidance of health-damaging behaviors may ultimately result in preserved functionality for an extended period of time. Although the human life span is currently 120 years, two renowned scientists are betting that in the year 2150, someone will be alive at either 130 years (Olshansky's bet) or 150 years (Austad's bet). The heirs of the scientist who wins the bet will collect the prize, estimated to be about $500 million in 2150. The scientists are basing their claims on the progress in aging research, including cloning technology, and stem cell research. They both agree that better understanding of the fundamental processes of aging, newer pharmaceuticals, and gene therapy may be able to combat aging within the next few decades.[46]

Health-Damaging Behaviors

According to 2008 statistics, tobacco use is associated with 5 million deaths per year worldwide and is a leading cause of premature death.[47] Although the incidence of smoking is lower in older adults, there are still an estimated 3 million geriatric smokers in the United States.[48] Older adults who have smoked for a long time will often refuse to even consider quitting, arguing that "the damage has been done, so why quit now?" Smoking has become so much of a habit that many have no desire to quit or, having tried, find they are sad and depressed and thus resume smoking. This is more often the case when they try to quit cold turkey. Nicotine works as an antidepressant, and in its absence, addicted smokers suffer.

> **AGE-SPECIFIC ANGLE**
>
> Healthy lifestyle choices or the avoidance of health damaging behaviors may ultimately result in preserved functionality for an extended period of time.

Smoking has many negative effects that can exacerbate already existing comorbidities in older adults. The two main components of tobacco smoke are tar and nicotine. The nicotine causes an increase in blood pressure and an increase in the incidence of arrhythmias. The myriad of chemicals in tar, many of which are known to cause cancer, are associated with an increase in damage to the arteries and malignancy. Smoking cessation programs specifically designed to help older adults exist; information regarding them can be found at http://www.nicotine-anonymous.org or http://www.tobaccofreeafter50.com.

As with any patient who smokes, always ask older patients who smoke whether they have considered stopping smoking. In March 2005, the Centers for Medicare and Medicaid Services determined that there was sufficient evidence to support Medicare coverage for smoking or tobacco use cessation counseling. As of January 2006, the Medicare prescription drug benefit also covers smoking cessation treatments.[49] Effective programs should include behavioral modification techniques, support systems, nicotine replacement therapy, bupropion if indicated, and possibly varenicline (Chantix). Because elderly patients are more likely to have decreased renal function, dosage may need to be reduced, and it may be useful to monitor renal function.

> **AGE-SPECIFIC ANGLE**
>
> Although the incidence of smoking is lower in older adults, there are still an estimated 3 million geriatric smokers in the United States.

Alcohol abuse, as mentioned previously, is another health-damaging behavior that is not uncommon in the elderly population. Loneliness, depression, and loss of a spouse are all contributing factors. If asked, many older adults will deny that they have a problem and may even become quite defensive. Approaching alcohol use from a healthcare standpoint and not addressing drinking as a moral issue may be more productive. Adverse complications of excessive alcohol consumption that may affect the pulmonary system are pulmonary edema, esophageal varices, altered electrolyte levels, and decreased hemoglobin. Additionally, the immune system is weakened and malnutrition is more likely in alcoholics. Lack of medication compliance (under- or overdosing) is a dangerous consequence of alcohol consumption, and when drugs are taken with alcohol, the effects or side effects of the drugs may be altered, leading to disastrous results.

Physical activity, although recommended for every age group, is of particular importance in older adults. Regular exercise can help prevent or delay the onset of chronic conditions and can improve endurance, strength, and flexibility, all of which decrease the incidence of falls. Lack of activity today is partly a result of social change in the past 50 years. Computers, television, remote controls, cars, and desk jobs have all had a part in engineering routine daily physical activity out of the lives of many. By age 75 years, few older adults engage in regular physical activity. Many health-related organizations have recommended walking programs for seniors as a means of increasing physical activity. It should be noted that previously sedentary older adults should consult with a physician prior to starting an exercise program. Once the go-ahead is given, recruiting friends to participate in activities may provide the support and encouragement needed to keep active. Many communities have senior centers or a local YMCA that may have specially designed programs for well elders.

The importance of nutrition in older adults cannot be overemphasized, in particular, older adults with COPD. It has been estimated that as many as 25% to 30% of patients with COPD are malnourished.[50] Malnutrition is not just a factor of being underweight; it also can be applied to individuals who are grossly overweight. In both cases, nutrition is poor. Being underweight with COPD can make symptoms worse and further reduce the effectiveness of the immune system. Older adults with COPD are advised to eat small, frequent meals with nutrient-dense foods that are easy to prepare in the microwave. Nutritional supplements are also recommended, not to replace meals but rather as a supplement after or between meals to add calories.

Obesity in older adults has risen dramatically in the past 20 years and is associated with functional decline, ill health, dependency, and a reduced quality of life. **Obesity** is defined as a body mass index (BMI) of greater than 30. It is now estimated that about 40% of individuals between the ages of 60 to 69, and 30% of individuals between the ages of 70 to 79 years, are obese (**Figure 28–5**).[51] Obesity in the elderly must be approached carefully and monitored to prevent major nutrient loss and worsening of existing comorbidities. Given the already marginal health status of many older adults, health-damaging behaviors will add to the incidence of exacerbations and frequency of hospitalizations and will be an increased drain on the already strained healthcare budget.

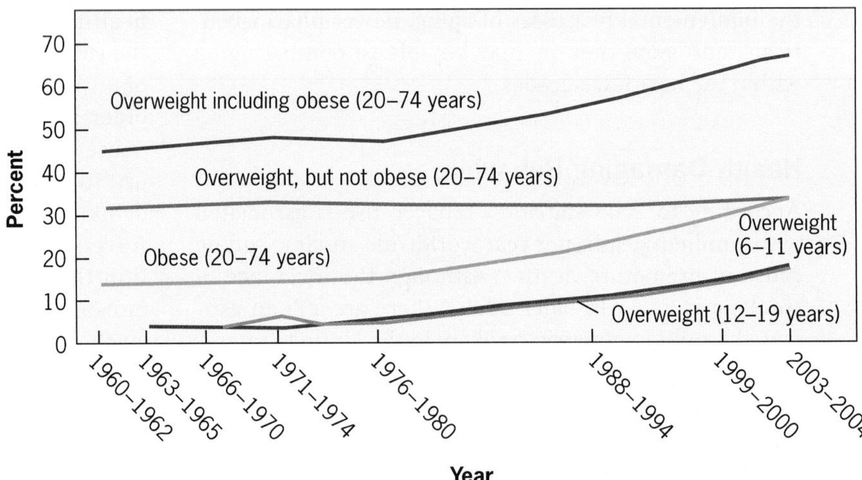

FIGURE 28–5 Increased incidence of overweight and obesity, by age: United States, 1960–2004. Reproduced from National Center for Health Statistics. *Health, United States, 2006. With Chartbook on Trends in the Health of Americans*. Available at: http://www.cdc.gov/nchs/data/hus/hus06.pdf.

Considering that 100 million older adults are likely to enter the Medicare system over the next 25 years, the potential benefits of interventions are huge. Effectively controlling hypertension could reduce healthcare spending by $890 trillion and add 75 million disability-adjusted life years (DALYs). Controlling or eliminating diabetes could add 90 million life-year equivalents at a cost of $2661 per DALY. Reducing obesity would have little effect on mortality but would have a huge effect on morbidity, with a cost savings of over $1 trillion.[52] Unfortunately, there is an underutilization of preventive services in the elderly population. Whether because of cost, transportation, or healthcare literacy, older adults do not always have access to the preventive screenings and educational interventions that would be useful. To find out which disease-specific screenings are currently recommended for older adults, search specific diseases in the U.S. Preventive Services Task Force guidelines (available at http://odphp.osophs.dhhs.gov/pubs/guidecps).

AGE-SPECIFIC ANGLE

Obesity, which is defined as a body mass index (BMI) of greater than 30, is estimated to represent approximately 40% of individuals between the ages of 60 to 69 and 30% of individuals between the ages of 70 to 79.

KEY POINTS

- Geriatrics is a vital component of the respiratory care curriculum and the practice of respiratory care.
- The elderly population is projected to rise sharply with the aging of the baby boom generation in 2011, with the potential of 10,000 adults per day turning 65 years of age.
- Five of the six leading causes of death among the elderly are chronic in nature, and thus the role of the RT will be significant and will demand a richer, deeper understanding of this elderly population.
- Physical assessments in older adults may take a few minutes longer, but they are extremely important to do accurately.
- Hypothermia (core temperatures below 95° F or 35° C) can develop in room temperatures of 60° to 65° F (16 to 18° C) in older frail adults.
- Hand-grip strength may be a marker of frailty in the oldest-old.
- The immune system weakens are we grow older.
- Confusion is an early symptom of many diseases in the elderly.
- Depression is the most commonly occurring mental health problem in older adults.
- Although the elderly make up (on average) about 13% of the total U.S. population, they consume 33% of prescription drugs and 25% of all over-the-counter drugs.
- Up to 88% of adverse drug reactions in the elderly that resulted in hospitalization were preventable.
- Elderly patients with asthma are often misdiagnosed or underdiagnosed, resulting in inappropriate treatment in both cases.
- Pulmonary hypertension in the elderly is often a comorbidity with COPD, interstitial lung disease, and sleep apnea.

REFERENCES

1. Douce HF. A critical analysis of respiratory care scope of practice and education: past, present and future. In: American Association for Respiratory Care. *Delineating the Educational Direction for the Future Respiratory Care Practitioners: Proceedings of a National Consensus Conference on Respiratory Care Education.* Dallas, TX: AARC; 1992.

2. American Association for Respiratory Care. *An Action Agenda: Proceedings of the Second National Consensus Conference on Respiratory Care Education.* Dallas, TX: Author; 1993.
3. Petty TL, Seebass JS, eds. *Pulmonary Disorders of the Elderly.* Philadelphia: American College of Physicians; 2007.
4. U.S. Census Bureau. Numeric growth: changes in age population. Available at: http://www.census.gov/prod/1/pop/p23190/p23190-f.pdf. Accessed February 3, 2009.
5. Janssens JP, Pache JC, Nicod LP. Physiological changes in respiratory function associated with aging. *Eur Respir J.* 1999;13(1):197–205.
6. Turner JM, Mead J, Wohl ME. Elasticity of the human lung in relation to age. *J Appl Physiol.* 1968;25:664–671.
7. Doherty TJ. Aging and sarcopenia. *J Appl Physiol.* 2003; 95:1717–1727.
8. Tolep K, Higgins N, Criner G, et al. Comparisons of diaphragm strength between healthy adult elderly and young men. *Am J Respir Crit Care Med.* 1995;152(2):677–682.
9. Beers MH, Jones TV, eds. *The Merck Manual of Geriatrics* [Online]. 3rd ed. Available at: http://www.merck.com/mkgr/mmg/home.jsp.
10. Finesilver C. Pulmonary assessment: what you need to know. *Prog Cardiovasc Nursing.* 2003;18(2):83–92.
11. Sebastian JL, Pfeifer KJ. Cardiac disorders. In: Duthie EH, Katz PR, Malone ML, eds. *Practice of Geriatrics.* 4th ed. Philadelphia: Saunders-Elsevier; 2007.
12. Harris SN. Anesthetic considerations for geriatric surgery. In: Rosenthal RA, Zenilman ME, Katlic MR, eds. *Principles and Practices of Geriatric Surgery.* New York: Springer-Verlag; 2000.
13. Normal DC. Fever in the elderly. *Clin Infect Dis.* 2000;31:148–151.
14. Bergman H, Ferrucci L, Guralnik J, et al. Frailty: an emerging research and clinical paradigm—issues and controversies. *J Gerontol Med Sci.* 2007;62A(7):731–737.
15. Syddall H, Cooper C, Martin F, et al. Is grip strength a useful single marker of frailty? *Age Aging.* 2003;32:650–656.
16. Smyrnios NA, Irwin RS, Curley FJ, et al. From a prospective study of chronic cough: diagnostic and therapeutic aspects in older adults. *Arch Intern Med.* 1998;158:1222–1228.
17. Hammond CS. Evaluating cough; the role of dysphagia and aspiration: when should aspiration be suspected in a patient with cough? *J Respir Dis.* 2008;29(7):263.
18. Amella EJ. Presentation of illness in older adults: if you think you know what you're looking for, think again. *Am J Nursing.* 2004;104(10):40–51.
19. McSweeney JC, Cody M, O'Sullivan P, et al. Women's early warning symptoms of acute myocardial infarction. *Circulation.* 2003;108:2619–2623.
20. Woon VC, Lim KH. Acute myocardial infarction in the elderly—the differences compared with the young. *Singapore Med.* 2003;44(8):414–418.
21. Emmett KR. Nonspecific and atypical presentation of disease in the older patient. *Geriatrics.* 1998;53(2):50–52, 58–60.
22. Chmura K, Chan ED. Tuberculosis in the elderly: keep a high index of suspicion. *J Respir Dis.* 2006;27(7):307–315.
23. Ewing JA. Detecting alcoholism: the CAGE questionnaire. *JAMA.* 1984;252:1905–1907.
24. Avorn JL, Lamy PP, Vestal RE. Prescribing for the elderly safely. *Patient Care.* 1982;16(12):14–62.
25. Beijer HJ, deBlacey CJ. Hospitalizations caused by adverse drug reactions (ADR): a meta-analysis of observational studies. *Pharm World Sci.* 2002;24:46–54.
26. Fick DM, Cooper JW, Wade WE, et al. Updating the Beers criteria for potentially inappropriate medication use in older adults. *Arch Intern Med.* 2003;163(27):2716–2724.
27. Sloane PD, Gruber-Baldini AL, Zimmerman S, et al. Medication undertreatment in assisted living settings. *Arch Intern Med.* 2004;164(18):2031–2037.
28. Neafsey PJ, Shellman J. Adverse self-medication practices of older adults with hypertension attending blood pressure clinics. *Internet J Nursing Pract.* 2001;5(1). Available at: http://www.ispub.com/ostia/index.php?xmlFilePath=journals/ijfp/vol2n1/self.xml. Accessed February 19, 2009.
29. Gellad WF. Variation in drug prices at pharmacies: are prices higher in poorer areas? *Health Services Res.* 2008. Available at: http://www.hbns.org/getDocument.cfm?documentID=1800. Accessed February 19, 2009.
30. Ahrendsen CO, Snow T. Alzheimer's disease, family caregivers and Faith in Action in North Carolina. *NC Medical Journal.* 2005;66(1):69–71.
31. Wagenaar DO. Communicating with the elderly. *Dialogue Diagnosis.* 2007;19–21.
32. Murdoch BE, Chenery HJ, Wilks V, Boyle RS. Language disorders in dementia of the Alzheimer's type. *Brain Language.* 1987;31:122–137.
33. Hamilton HE. *Conversations with an Alzheimer's Patient.* Cambridge, England: Cambridge University Press; 1994.
34. Sin BA, Akkoca Ö, Saryal S, Öner F, et al. Differences between asthma and COPD in the elderly. *J Invest Allerg Clin Immunol.* 2006;16(1):44–50.
35. Vignola AM, Scichilone N, et al. Aging and asthma: pathophysiologic mechanisms. *Allergy.* 2003;58(3):165–182.
36. Pistelli R, Lange P, Miller DL. Determinants of prognosis of COPD in the elderly: mucus hypersecretion, infections, cardiovascular comorbidity. *Eur Respir J.* 2003;21(suppl 40):10S–14S.
37. Cydulka RK, McFadden ER, Emerman CL, et al. Patterns of hospitalization in elderly patients with asthma and chronic obstructive pulmonary disease. *Am J Respir Crit Care Med.* 1997;156:1807–1812.
38. Maninno DM, Homa DM, Akinbami LJ, et al. Surveillance for asthma—United States 1980–1999. *MMWR.* 2002;51(1):1–13.
39. Enright PL, McClelland RL, Newman AB, et al. Underdiagnosis and undertreatment of asthma in the elderly. *Chest.* 1999;116:603–613.
40. Nelson HS. Is there a problem with inhaled long-acting beta-agonists? *J Allergy Clin Immunol.* 2006;117:3–16.
41. Sharma S. Restrictive lung disease. eMedicine. June 2006. Available at: http://emedicine.medscape.com/article/301760-print. Accessed March 3, 2009.
42. McArdle JR, Trow TK, Lerz, KL. Pulmonary hypertension in older adults. *Clin Chest Med.* 2007;28(4):713–733.
43. Ghofrani HA, Wiedemann R, Rose F, et al. Sildenafil for treatment of lung fibrosis and pulmonary hypertension: a randomized controlled trial. *Lancet.* 2002;360(9337):895–900.
44. Olschewski H, Ghofrani HA, Walmrath D. Inhaled prostacyclin and iloprost in severe pulmonary hypertension secondary to lung fibrosis. *Am J Respir Crit Care Med.* 1999;160(2):600–607.
45. Carrillo M, Szymanski CA, Truesdell SK, et al. Efficacy and safety of pulmonary rehabilitation in patients with pulmonary hypertension: preliminary results. *Chest.* 2005;128:366.
46. Gresh LH, Weinberg RE. *The Science of Supervillains.* Hoboken, NJ: Wiley & Sons; 2005:120–121.
47. Hatsukami DK, Stead LF, Gupta PC. Tobacco addiction. *Lancet.* 2008;371:2027–2038.
48. Appel DW, Aldrich TK. Smoking cessation in the elderly. *Clin Geriatr Med.* 2003;19:77–100.
49. Centers for Medicare and Medicaid Services. Overview: smoking cessation. Available at: http://www.cms.hhs.gov/SmokingCessation. Accessed March 9, 2009.

50. Rennard SI. Patient information: chronic obstructive pulmonary disease (COPD) treatments. UpToDate. Available at: http://www.uptodate.com. Last updated February 26, 2008.
51. U.S. Department of Health and Human Services. *National Health and Nutritional Examination Survey (NHANES) 1999–2000.* Hyattsville, MD: National Center for Health Statistics; 2002.
52. Goldman DP, Cutler DM, Shang B, Joyce GF. The value of elderly disease prevention. *Forum Health Econ Policy.* 2006;9(2). Available at: http://www.bepress.com/fhep/biomedical_research/1.

APPENDIX 28–1

Resources for Screening Tests in the Elderly

Test	Website
Hearing Handicap Inventory for the Elderly (HHIE)	http://www.audiologyonline.com
Mini-Nutritional Assessment (MNA)	http://www.mna-elderly.com/mna_forms.html
Functional Assessment Staging (FAST)	http://www.ec-online.net/Knowledge/articles/alzstages.html

The following instruments can be accessed on the University of Iowa's Geriatric Education website (http://www.medicine.uiowa.edu/igec/tools/default.asp):

- Snellen eye test (visual acuity)
- Whispered voice test (hearing loss)
- Nutritional health assessment
- Clock-drawing test
- Geriatric Depression Scale (GDS)
- Mini-Mental Status Exam (MMSE)
- Activities of daily living (ADL)
- Instrumental activities of daily living (IADL)
- Caregiver Burden Interview

CHAPTER 29

Medical Information Management and Patient Safety

Thomas Malinowski

OUTLINE

Medical Information Management
Electronic Medical or Health Records
Appropriate Handling of Patient Information
Patient Safety
Safety Initiatives and Respiratory Care Applications

OBJECTIVES

1. Define medical information management.
2. Describe the rationale for documenting respiratory care activities.
3. List the elements of a patient medical record.
4. Identify medical record documentation standards.
5. List respiratory care information commonly recorded in the medical record.
6. Describe a properly transcribed verbal order.
7. Explain medical record authentication.
8. Describe the rationale for the electronic medical or health record.
9. Explain the legal implications of the medical record.
10. Describe the guidelines for medical record retention.
11. Explain the concept of patient confidentiality.
12. Explain the issues of patient safety, including the concepts and characteristics of high-reliability organizations, a culture of safety, root-cause analysis, and the process for incident reporting.
13. Explain safety initiatives as they apply to the practice of respiratory care, including rapid response teams, medication reconciliation, report handoffs and rounds, the Universal Protocol, discharge education and planning, and healthcare-associated infections.

KEY TERMS

active errors
authentication
confidentiality
cryptography
culture of safety
electronic health record (EHR)
electronic medical record (EMR)
electronic signature
handoff
hard stops
healthcare-associated infections (HAIs)
Health Insurance Portability and Accountability Act (HIPAA)
high-reliability organizations (HROs)
HITECH Act
incident report
interoperability
latent errors
medical information management
medical record
medication reconciliation
National Committee for Quality Assurance (NCQA)
root-cause analysis (RCA)
SBAR
sentinel event
Universal Protocol

INTRODUCTION

Medical information management and patient safety are critical issues in the practice of respiratory care. Medical information is obviously needed for the information gathering, data analysis, and therapeutic decision-making process. Without such information, the respiratory therapist would be working in a vacuum and would be unable to provide effective and efficient care. Patient safety issues have gained increased attention and importance in recent years. Regrettably, numerous documented examples of unsafe practices and patient harm have resulted in reports and directives from the National Institutes of Health, the Joint Commission, and other organizations.

This chapter provides a detailed account of medical information and patient safety as these concepts apply to the practice of respiratory care. It specifically addresses the rationale and standards of medical information management; the electronic medical record; appropriate handling of patient records; legal issues related to confidentiality; and safety issues, including high-reliability organizations, the creation of a culture of safety, root-cause analysis, and incident reporting. Additionally, safety initiatives related to the practice of respiratory care are addressed, specifically, rapid response teams; medication reconciliation; reports, handoffs, and rounds; discharge education and planning; and healthcare-associated infections.

Medical Information Management

Medical information management is defined as the acquisition, storage, and transfer of data or details pertinent to the care of the patient. Traditional definitions center around the **medical record**, but information is not only written or captured; often it is transferred verbally, such as during reports or rounds.

Rationale

Documentation within the medical record serves many purposes, but its primary function is to describe information pertinent to the patient (e.g., assessment, history, diagnostics, response to care) and provide for continuity in information about the patient's medical treatment. The patient's medical record is a permanent document, intended for use both inside and outside the hospital. Other key uses of the medical record include the following: a method for evaluating the quality of care provided; a basis for financial reimbursement to hospitals, healthcare providers, and patients; a tool for evaluating resource allocation (e.g., staffing, supplies, equipment); and a legal document for use in other legal proceedings.

Some respiratory therapists may consider documentation to be a burden or an afterthought, but documentation is an essential element of the provision of care. Documentation provides a reference on the status of the patient's condition prior to intervention, a record of key steps associated with the provision of care, an account of the effectiveness of care, an opportunity to record recommendations or modifications to the care, and a record of the educational materials provided to the patient, along with his or her ongoing needs and the discharge plan.

Elements of a Patient Medical Record

The medical record includes documentation of commonly used clinical data, including the patient assessment, problem identification, care plans, treatments, and outcomes. Technologic options include the use of multiple forms of digital media, including images and recordings. Healthcare providers should only document factual and objective information from their own treatment or observation of the patient. When documenting information derived from other sources (e.g., other healthcare providers, other medical records, or entries in the same medical record), be sure to reference the source of that information. **Table 29–1** includes examples of

TABLE 29–1 Elements of a Patient Medical Record

Elements	Examples
Progress notes	Notes of daily assessment and progress by physician or other members of the healthcare team
Physician orders	All medical orders written by physician or recorded as verbal orders by authorized individuals
Discharge summary	Summary of patient condition on discharge, postdischarge instructions, and care plan
Flow sheets/graphic sheets	Input and output records, daily graph of vital signs, mechanical ventilation records, and therapy records
Laboratory reports	Clinical laboratory reports and pulmonary function laboratory reports
Medication administration	Medication log
Photographs	Digital images, photographs from specific procedures, such as ultrasound or bronchoscopy
Videotapes/audio recordings	Digital recordings, tapes from procedures, such as sleep studies or bronchoscopy
Radiology reports	Radiographs, scans, and images
Monitoring strips	Electrocardiogram strips
Admissions sheet	Demographics, pertinent patient information, admitting diagnosis, and physician information
History and physical	Body system review by physician and all pertinent history information
Consultation sheet	Review, impressions, and recommendations of patient by specialists consulted
Consent forms	Forms signed by patient or representative for special procedures, such as surgery or bronchoscopy
Surgical records	Recording of all events occurring immediately before, during, and after surgery

Adapted from Care First Blue Choice. *Medical Records Documentation Standards*. Available at: http://www.carefirst.com/providers/attachments/BOK5129.pdf. Accessed February 9, 2010.

BOX 29–1

Medical Record Documentation Standards

1. Elements of the record are organized.
2. Records are stored and maintained in a way to protect safety and confidentiality of information.
3. Patient name and ID appear on each page.
4. The record is legible to others.
5. All entries are dated.
6. All entries contain the author's identification (written or electronic signature).
7. Personal biographical data are included.
8. Contributory past medical history, family, and birth history are noted as appropriate.
9. Medication allergies and adverse reactions are prominently noted.
10. Personal habits—including smoking, alcohol, and substances history and sexual behavior—are noted.
11. Significant illnesses/medical conditions are indicated on the problem list.
12. Chief complaint or reason for visit is noted.
13. The history and physical examination identify appropriate information pertinent to patient's complaints and a working diagnosis consistent with the findings.
14. Treatment plans are consistent with diagnoses.
15. Medical record shows clear justification for diagnostic tests and therapies.
16. Unresolved problems from previous office visits are addressed in subsequent visits.
17. Follow-up care is noted when indicated.
18. Current medications are documented; long-term medications are reviewed at least annually.
19. Healthcare education is provided, noted, and updated as appropriate.
20. Immunization record (for children) is up to date or there is an appropriate history.
21. Evidence that preventive screening and services have been offered is noted.
22. Consultation requests are justified by medical records evidence.
23. Laboratory and diagnostic results reflect practitioner review.
24. Patients are notified of abnormal diagnostic results and recommended to follow up.
25. Evidence of continuity of care between primary care and specialist providers is noted.

Adapted from Care First Blue Choice. *Medical Records Documentation Standards.* Available at: http://www.carefirst.com/providers/attachments/BOK5129.pdf. Accessed January 29, 2010.

elements of the medical record and the types of media that may be considered part of such a record.[1]

Medical Record Documentation Standards

Consistent, current, and complete documentation in the medical record is an essential component of quality patient care. Regulatory and standards organizations have developed guidelines for the essential elements a medical record should contain.[1] **Box 29–1** reflects a set of commonly accepted standards for medical record documentation. Organizations use these standards to audit the quality and thoroughness of medical record documentation.

Essentials for Respiratory Care Documentation

Respiratory charting should represent the key elements of patient interventions and data. It should be organized and integrated into the other areas of the medical record. It is primarily designed to reflect the presentation and status of the patient, yet it also needs to meet the needs of other end users of information. It should be structured in an organized manner that lends itself to ease of entry and of interpretation and analysis. Information should be organized for rapid access and presentation to be used to its fullest. Consequently, the respiratory care section of the medical record should be systematically designed to record the information clinically appropriate for the patient's presentation.

Respiratory therapists must possess the necessary skills to document, manage, and access patient information if they are to be effective clinicians. They also must remain informed about the various medical, ethical, legal, and financial roles that documentation and medical information play. Careless or insufficient documentation may result in misinterpretation and patient harm, penalties, lawsuits, and financial consequences. Departments should describe in policy and procedure manuals the key charting requirements for the various activities

TABLE 29–2 Respiratory Care Information Commonly Recorded in the Medical Record

Category	Examples of Data Recorded
Patient demographics	Patient identification, institution, medical record number, accession (hospital visit) number
Date/time	Date and time of assessment, therapeutic intervention, and documentation
Interview and respiratory history	Pulmonary history, contributory health, smoking history
Vital signs	Pulse, respiratory rate, blood pressure, temperature
Physical examination	Breath sounds, head and neck, thorax
Laboratory and blood gases	Blood gas values, hematology, chemistry, microbiology
Pulmonary function testing	FVC, SVC, IC, FEV_1, peak expiratory flow
Radiographic diagnostic information	Chest radiograph, CT, MRI
Essential monitoring data	Pulse oximetry; capnometry; ventilator settings; flow, volume, and pressure information; minute ventilation; cuff pressure; tube position
Medication administration	Aerosolized, airway instilled, intravenous
Risk assessment, severity, and triage scores	Mild to severe, ALI/ARDS risk, sepsis score
Therapeutic interventions	Aerosol, bronchial hygiene, lung inflation, ventilatory care
Other systems information	Nutritional, hemodynamic, neurologic
Therapeutic effectiveness/readiness to progress	Response to applied adjuncts, readiness to wean, extubate
Adverse reactions/actions taken	Unforeseen consequences, actions taken when identified
Patient education/discharge planning	Discharge asthma education instruction, tobacco cessation

FVC, forced vital capacity; SVC, slow vital capacity; IC, inspiratory capacity; FEV_1, forced expiratory volume in 1 second; CT, computed tomography; MRI, magnetic resonance imaging; ALI/ARDS, acute lung injury/adult respiratory distress syndrome.

performed. **Table 29–2** describes respiratory care information commonly recorded in the medical record.

Patient name and identification number
Date
Perform lung volumes and airways resistance today 4 hours after MDI administration with albuterol.
v.o. T. Smith, MD
Mary Jane Jones, RRT, RPFT
2-25-11 10:12 AM

FIGURE 29–1 Example of a transcribed verbal order.

Orders

Physician-directed orders drive the course of care for all patients. Each healthcare system has specific policies and procedures governing who may write orders, who may accept verbal orders, and the procedure used to document the order in the medical record. All medical orders, whether written or verbally accepted, must be recorded accurately to ensure patient safety and accurate care.

The Joint Commission specifies standards for all medical orders. Verbal orders may be accepted by authorized individuals and transcribed by qualified personnel identified by title or category in the medical staff rules and regulations.[2] Respiratory therapists meet this requirement, but nonlicensed respiratory therapy students are not qualified to accept verbal orders; consequently, students require licensed respiratory therapists to take and transcribe orders during their clinical experiences. Qualified individuals must strictly follow the institution's procedure for recording of verbal orders. Respiratory therapists providing any clinical care of patients should understand and review the institution's procedures for acceptance and recording of verbal orders. **Figure 29–1** provides an example of a transcribed verbal order.

Medical Record Authentication

Authentication is the process used to verify that an entry being made to the medical record is complete, accurate, and final. Authentication is essential for history and physical exams, operative reports, consultations, and discharge summaries. Accrediting organizations, state laws, and other bodies specify authentication requirements for medical records. The healthcare delivery system must comply with various requirements to maintain accreditation, meet legal standards, and receive reimbursement. The level of authentication of each entry in a medical record varies, depending on the regulatory agency.

As healthcare delivery systems change and ambulatory care increases, the requirements for medical records will continue to change. Respiratory therapists working in alternative settings or managed care organizations may be subject to other requirements through quality initiatives. One example of a quality initiative is the **National Committee for Quality Assurance (NCQA)**, which accredits managed care plans. The NCQA evaluates how well a healthcare plan manages all parts of its delivery system, including physicians, hospitals, other providers, and administrative services. The NCQA standards for ambulatory records require provider identification and dating on each medical record entry, but not authentication.[3] The requirements for medical record entries may be vastly different based on the setting, and each therapist should review the policies and procedures for each clinical site or setting.

Electronic Medical or Health Records

Electronic medical record (EMR) and **electronic health record (EHR)** are two terms used synonymously to describe computerized systems that track and record patient information electronically. The premise of the EMR is that electronic capture of information speeds entry, improves the storage and retrieval of patient information, and subsequently improves the provision of care. The transition from paper to electronic records provides an extraordinary opportunity to reduce risk, improve quality and efficiency, and affect outcome. Properly designed and applied EMR systems can be robust tools to help with all manner of clinical applications and can be a great advantage to the respiratory therapist for respiratory charting, work assignments, triaging, and the application of clinical guidelines, protocols, or pathways.

The EMR allows providers to review health information or interventions that may have occurred from multiple patient visits. Another advantage of the EMR is its ability to store records under a single unique identifier. The single information repository increases a department's effectiveness and quality. **Figure 29–2** illustrates an integrated centralized electronic medical record repository and how other users may access data.

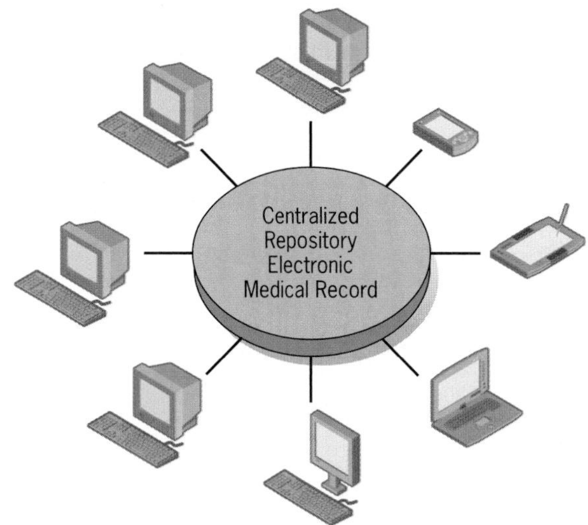

FIGURE 29–2 Centralized electronic medical record (EMR). The centralized EMR is available to multiple users with multiple hardware configurations. Various users may include physicians, therapists, nurses, laboratory staff, and admitting and financial departments.

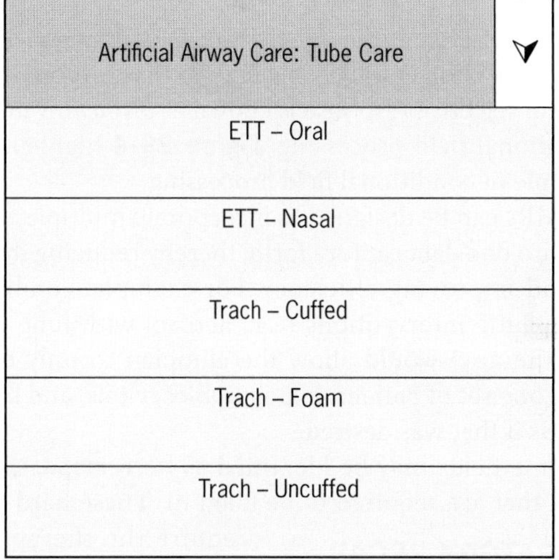

FIGURE 29–3 Drop-down table. Only one selection may be chosen. This example includes options for both endotracheal and tracheostomy tubes.

The EMR is typically designed to guide the clinician through an activity from start to finish and incorporates data that are critical to the provision or evaluation of response to care. (The American Association for Respiratory Care's clinical practice guidelines serve as templates to describe commonly applied respiratory activities.) The EMR can be designed to provide the clinician the opportunity to select from a drop-down list of activities or choices. These drop-down lists help limit errors in data entry, provide consistency, and speed up the selection process. **Figure 29–3** provides an example of how drop-down lists or tables may be used in charting the type of artificial airway selected. Depending on the

Any Unintended Consequences?	✓
☐ Clear All	
☐ None Observed	
☐ Nausea and/or Vomiting	
☐ Tremors	
☐ Increased Heart Rate from Baseline	
☐ Decreased Heart Rate from Baseline	
☐ Decreased SpO_2% from Baseline	
☐ Other	

FIGURE 29–4 Example of branching logic or conditional field processing. In this example, if the patient demonstrated any unintended consequences during care, the practitioner is directed by the charting system to select the observed response. The Clear All option provides the practitioner an opportunity to clear all the responses in the selection and start again. Multiple selections can be chosen (e.g., tremors and decreased SpO_2%).

Action Taken for Unintended Consequences	✓
☐ Clear All	
☐ Provided Supplemental Oxygen	
☐ Monitored Patient Until Status Returned to Baseline	
☐ Notified MD	
☐ Notified Bedside RN	
☐ Stopped Intervention	
☐ Additional Intervention Required (see comment)	

FIGURE 29–5 Hard stops. Hard stops are fields that require entry. This example shows the choices that would be presented for selection if the Unintended Consequences box had been previously selected. The electronic documentation system will not allow the practitioner to complete the record or commit it to being saved unless at least one of the boxes shown here is selected. Multiple boxes may be selected. Note how each of the responses takes action or escalates communication about the event.

response selected, the drop-down lists may generate a new set of choices applicable only to that response. This form of selective response is known as *branching logic* or conditional field processing. **Figure 29–4** highlights an example of conditional field processing.

EMRs can be designed to incorporate multiple activities into one data capture form, thereby reducing duplicity and improving efficiency. For example, combining therapeutic interventions (e.g., aerosol with lung inflation therapy) would allow the clinician to only document one set of patient demographics, vitals, and breath sounds if that was desired.

Some fields may be identified as **hard stops**, that is, fields that are required to be filled in. These hard stops require the therapist to enter data or complete the required field selection prior to progressing or committing the record to the EMR. **Figure 29–5** describes the application of a hard stop. Hard stops are helpful in reminding the therapist to complete an important documentation entry (e.g., patient identification, time care was administered, adverse reactions, alarms set).

RESPIRATORY RECAP

Drop-Down Lists and Hard Stops

» Drop-down lists allow the therapist to choose from a list of activities or choices and are designed to limit errors, provide consistency, and speed up the selection process.
» Hard stops require the therapist to fill in the various fields before continuing and are helpful in reminding the therapist to complete an important documentation entry.

Health systems that are fully integrated, using an EMR in all areas of the hospital, are rare. Most health systems are hybrids, using different computer systems or some form of paper record. A typical hospital may have as many as 200 stand-alone information systems used throughout the institution (e.g., patient registration, laboratory, pharmacy, respiratory care, patient billing, admissions, physical therapy). The difficulties often lie in integrating the systems. **Interoperability** is a term that describes the capacity for different information technology systems and software applications to communicate, exchange data, and use the information that has been exchanged in various formats and applications.

Respiratory therapists will continue to see refinements and increases in the utilization of the EMR. The 2009 economic stimulus package (**HITECH Act**) passed by the U.S. Congress will increase the incentives to promote physician and hospital adoption of the EMR.

Electronic Signature

An **electronic signature** is a method to allow practitioners to sign off on care rendered. Electronic signatures may be used not only in hospitals but also in ambulatory care, long-term care, and mental health, but only by the practitioners authorized to use it. The Joint Commission outlines specific requirements for the use of electronic signatures, including reviewing before sign-off.[4]

Appropriate Handling of Patient Information

Legal Implications of the Record

The medical record is a crucial element in preventing and minimizing potential adverse consequences. It also serves as a primary source of information for describing what transpired when an event occurred, and the subsequent actions taken. This is particularly important

RESPIRATORY RECAP

Legalities of the Medical Record

» Medical records that are poorly maintained, incomplete, inaccurate, or illegible or altered increase liability risk for the hospital and healthcare provider.

when performing root-cause and risk analysis. Medical records that are poorly maintained, incomplete, inaccurate, or illegible or altered create questions of fact regarding the treatment given to a patient and increase the liability risk for a hospital or healthcare provider.

The medical record is a legal document that, when properly completed, represents an accounting of the assessment and care provided to a patient. When used haphazardly or inconsistently, it becomes a source of ambiguity, question, and error. In a courtroom setting, it may be likened to a witness whose memory is never lost. It serves to correlate, for all involved, important patient information regarding the treatment rendered and the patient's treatment plan and is the means by which a level of communication is achieved among all healthcare providers involved in the patient's care.

Securing Medical Records Information

Three types of controls are used in information security: management controls, operational controls, and technical controls. Management controls focus on the management of the information security program and risk. Operational controls include contingency planning, user awareness and training, physical and environmental protections, computer support and operations, and handling of security breaches. Technical controls in-clude user identification and authentication, access control, audit trails, and **cryptography**. Authentication validates the identity of the user or other system authorized to access the healthcare information. Authentication usually is verified via a user password during log-in. Access control determines the content of information that may be entered or viewed based on the user's identification, and an audit trail identifies each log-in into the system.

RESPIRATORY RECAP

Securing Information

» Information security should protect the integrity, availability, and confidentiality of computer-based information and the resources used to enter, store, process, and communicate medical information.

Healthcare organizations should develop a set of technical and organizational policies, practices, and procedures to protect patient-identifiable healthcare information. These safeguards help prevent corruption of the data and breaches in security. Threats include equipment failure, disgruntled employees, malicious codes, hackers, theft, errors, omissions, and browsing. Employees should be assigned a unique and individual password. To decrease risks, a system should be in place to change the password at defined intervals. When an employee is terminated or retires, the identification should be immediately inactivated. Security also can be improved through deactivation of identification for individuals on prolonged leaves, such as with disability.

Retention of Medical Records

Healthcare systems also have guidelines for medical record retention, including a schedule for the length of retention. The guidelines should address the type of information to be kept, the time period for which the information should be kept, and the storage medium in which such information should be retained. The Medicare conditions of participation for hospitals require medical records and radiology service films, scans, and images to be kept for at least 5 years. The conditions of participation for other care sites vary, and respiratory therapists should be aware of the requirements for the healthcare delivery site at which they work.

Healthcare facilities are unable to maintain individual patient health information indefinitely, which requires the development and implementation of retention and destruction policies and procedures. Destruction of patient information should be carried out in accordance with federal and state laws according to the written retention and destruction policy of the healthcare facility.

Patient Confidentiality Issues

Confidentiality is the right of an individual to have personal, identifiable medical information kept private. Medical information should be available only to the physician of record and other healthcare and insurance personnel as necessary. Patient confidentiality is protected by federal statute, namely, by the passage of the **Health Insurance Portability and Accountability Act (HIPAA)**.[5] HIPAA is intended to ensure the privacy and protection of personal records and data in an environment of electronic medical records and third-party insurance payers. HIPAA provides a uniform set of guidelines that apply to all providers and organizations.

All healthcare systems must have policies and procedures to protect patient confidentiality. Employees must be familiar with their system's information security plan, which outlines steps governing access to medical information. Practitioners should refrain from discussing patients in the hallways, cafeterias, and elevators. Practitioners should not review the confidential information of any patient unless

RESPIRATORY RECAP

Confidentiality

» The Health Insurance Portability and Accountability Act (HIPAA) is a federal mandate that ensures patient confidentiality. Respiratory therapy students and clinicians should carefully follow policies and procedures to protect patient confidentiality.

TABLE 29-3 Characteristics of Highly Reliable Organizations (HROs)

Characteristic	Description
Preoccupation with failure	HROs do not focus on broadcasting successes; in fact, they continually look for failures or problems and implement ways to resolve them. They realize there are always areas to improve, and they relentlessly seek out these difficulties.
Reluctance to simplify interpretations	HROs recognize the complexity of the issues being dealt with, and do not oversimplify. They seek out differences in perspectives and avoid the pitfalls of groupthink.
Sensitivity to operations	HROs focus on unexpected events and *latent failures*, a term that describes loopholes in safeguards or a system's defenses. Latent failures are often only identified after a safety event has occurred. Latent failures are often attributable to training, process, or management deficiencies.
Commitment to resilience	HROs know that any operation is not perfect, but respond to errors without overreacting or becoming paralyzed or disabled.
Deference to expertise	Diversity brings different perspectives, which helps identify complexity and consequently aids problem solving. Problem identification and solution move to those individuals most familiar and expert and are not dependent on hierarchy or rank.

Adapted from Weick KE, Sutcliffe KM. *Managing the Unexpected: Assuring High Performance in an Age of Complexity.* San Francisco: Jossey-Bass; 2001:10–17.

it is directly essential to the provision of care. Engaging in discussions outside the care setting is unprofessional behavior and breaches patient confidentiality.

The release of patient information should always ensure confidentiality as the first premise. Patients must authorize the release of their health information in most situations. If the patient is unable to authorize release of information, other guidelines apply. The medical records department should be able to answer queries about whether a signed release is necessary.

Releasing only the specific medical information that is requested and authorized, and no more, is a good practice. Hospital departments generally involved with the release of medical information include medical records, risk management, quality management, and utilization management. These departments may coexist or be organized under a health information management division. Corporate offices or headquarters may serve as the institutional authority for an entire healthcare network within a state, regional, national, or international network.

Patient Safety

Medical errors have been implicated in the premature deaths of 98,000 patients per year, accounting for between $17 and $29 billion in costs annually.[6] Respiratory therapists play an essential role in preventing or reducing errors and improving overall healthcare quality. Learning and practicing safe respiratory care is therefore extremely important for all respiratory therapists. A practitioner's decision to practice safe care is a choice and is influenced by the present circumstance or situation as well as his or her knowledge, skills, and previous experiences.

RESPIRATORY RECAP

Medical Errors

» Medical errors have been implicated in the premature deaths of 98,000 patients per year, accounting for between $17 and $29 billion in costs annually.

High-Reliability Organizations

The concept of a **culture of safety** originated outside healthcare, in what are described as **high-reliability organizations (HROs)**—organizations that consistently minimize adverse events despite carrying out intrinsically complex and hazardous work (e.g., air traffic control, nuclear power generating plants, aircraft carriers). HROs adjust quickly to changing situations and are adept at building safeguards against failure of high-risk processes and solutions for possible failures. Five characteristics of HROs are their preoccupation with failure, reluctance to simplify interpretations, sensitivity to operations, commitment to resilience, and deference to expertise.[7] **Table 29-3** lists the characteristics of HROs and briefly describes each of them.

Culture of Safety

A purposeful and appropriate goal for any provider or department is to continually strive to achieve a highly reliable level of safety practice and to help others achieve the same goal. Organizations that embrace this safety philosophy create a culture of safety. Safe cultures are relentless in their pursuit of fewer errors and critical events. They also are realistic about the complexity of the work environment and the inevitability of the occurrence of errors. They recognize that many problems are process oriented, and work to resolve those issues.

The following characteristics are commonly seen in highly engaged safety cultures and serve as a foundation for establishing a safety-focused culture within a respiratory department:

- Recognition of the high-risk nature of an organization's activities and the determination to achieve consistently safe operations (high risk/high reliability)
- An environment in which individuals are able to report errors or near misses without fear of reprimand or punishment (safe harbor)
- Collaboration within and between disciplines to seek solutions to patient safety problems (teamwork)
- Organizational commitment to addressing safety issues (commitment)

High Risk/High Reliability

Respiratory care by its very nature requires operation in high-risk environments (e.g., transport, rapid response teams, resuscitation, emergency care, trauma) as well as areas of lower urgency. Our actions and behaviors in these environments often determine the success of the outcome. Practitioners need to be continually diligent, for errors and mistakes can occur with the most basic and simplistic tasks (e.g., connecting a cannula to an air flow meter in lieu of an oxygen flow meter for a newly admitted patient in a dark room at 3:00 AM) as well as the more critical tasks, such as initiating inhaled nitric oxide for the first time in 5 months. Safe cultures initiate process improvements that reduce the probability of error. In the night-shift nasal cannula example, two practitioners (a respiratory therapist and registered nurse) might be used to verify the proper connection of oxygen, or a "lights on for safety" policy might be used for all night admissions. For the infrequent application of nitric oxide, mock drills conducted every 4 to 6 weeks would help maintain skill sets and confidence.

Safe Harbor

A culture of blame can impair the advancement of a culture of safety. Some circumstances are a result of individual accountability, but more often safety events occur as a result of breakdown in processes. Practitioners should be rewarded for good catches, that is, identification of situations or events that could have been a problem. Staff should be encouraged to describe problems that they have observed and should be solicited for solutions. In addition, these problems should be highlighted to all staff, through methods such as bulletin boards and start-of-shift huddles.

This is not to say that practitioners are not responsible for their actions. When organizations focus on identifying and understanding the causes of unsafe behavior and simultaneously hold individuals accountable for reckless behavior, they develop a just culture. In a just culture, the response to an error or near miss is predicated on the type of behavior associated with the error, not the severity of the event. For example, reckless behavior such as refusing to perform a duplicate patient ID check prior to performing an arterial blood gas assessment or assisting with a bronchoscopy would merit punitive action, even if no patients were harmed.

Teamwork

Safe healthcare requires highly trained individuals with differing perspectives to act together for the common interest of the patient. Communication barriers across hierarchies, failure to acknowledge human fallibility, and lack of situational awareness combine to cause poor teamwork, which can lead to clinical adverse events.

Teamwork training is intended to minimize the potential for error by training each team member to respond appropriately in acute situations. Teamwork training focuses on respect, responsibility, and communication. It is intended to enhance cohesion among team members and to create an atmosphere in which all personnel feel comfortable speaking up when they suspect a problem. Team members are trained to cross-check each other's actions, offer assistance when needed, and address errors in a nonjudgmental fashion. Debriefing and providing feedback, particularly after critical incidents, is an important part of teamwork training.

Respiratory care departments can apply the principles of teamwork training in multiple areas of clinical training and practice. Applications include all aspects of departmental orientation, start-of-shift safety huddles, transport teams, rapid response teams, and shift report or transfer of care to other providers. Many departments are using more structured reporting methods such as SBAR (situation, background, assessment, recommendation) to standardize the report process. SBAR is discussed in more detail later in this chapter.

Commitment

Fundamentally, in order to improve the safety culture, the underlying problem areas must be identified and solutions constructed to target each specific problem. Although many organizations measure safety culture at the institutional level, significant variations in safety culture may exist within an organization. For example, the perception of a culture of safety may be high in one unit within a hospital and low in another unit, or high among management and low among frontline workers. These variations likely contribute to the mixed record of interventions intended to improve safety climate and reduce errors.

Root-Cause Analysis

Root-cause analysis (RCA) is a structured method used to identify underlying problem issues or to analyze serious adverse events. The process was initially developed

TABLE 29–4 Examples of Latent Error Factors in Respiratory Care

Type of Factor	Example
Organizational/management	A respiratory student detects a medication error, but the preceptor therapist discourages the student from reporting it.
Work environment	Lacking appropriate gas storage space, medical gases are kept in the same storage location as nonmedical gas. A gas cylinder of acetylene was found mixed in the heliox gas cylinders transferred to an intensive care unit location.
Team environment	A pulmonologist insists on continuing with a bronchoscopy even though the consent form has not been completed. The patient has already received a sedative and the physician does not want to reschedule the procedure.
Staffing	A department had three sick calls for the shift, and no additional staff members are available to call in. A therapist makes a decision to triage care without having assessed a patient, and the patient has a history of severe asthma.
Task related	A respiratory therapist fails to follow proper procedure and complete the transport checklist prior to departing with a ventilator patient to obtain an MRI. The patient self-extubates during transfer in the imaging room, and no resuscitator mask is available to bag the patient prior to intubation.
Patient characteristics	An elderly patient with COPD fails to follow proper directions and is taking his long-acting beta-agonist medication six times a day.

MRI, magnetic resonance imaging; COPD, chronic obstructive pulmonary disease.

to help analyze industrial accidents but now is widely used in healthcare to analyze errors. RCA is used to get to the source of a problem. RCA can identify both **active errors** (errors occurring when practitioners apply processes) and **latent errors** (hidden problems that increase the probability of error). The reason to use RCA is to prevent future harm by eliminating the active and latent errors that frequently are the cause of adverse events. The Joint Commission has mandated use of RCA to analyze **sentinel events**.

RCAs generally follow a protocol that begins with data collection and reconstruction of the event in question through record review and participant interviews. A multidisciplinary team is often assembled to analyze the sequence of events leading to the error, with the goals of identifying how the event occurred (through identification of active errors) and why the event occurred (through systematic identification and analysis of latent errors). **Table 29–4** describes examples of latent errors in respiratory care.

Incident Reports

When an untoward event occurs, an **incident report** may be filed to initiate tracking of the event. For example, an incident report should be completed when a patient receives an incorrect medication or when a patient accidentally falls when getting out of bed. The individual who observes or discovers the incident should begin the documentation process. An occurrence report may include specifics such as patient name and identification number; date, time, and description of the incident; the immediate action taken; and the signature of the reporting employee and additional individuals involved in the incident.

A supervisor should always be notified when an untoward incident is observed, and the written reporting procedure should address how and to whom incident reports should be routed. The process includes an evaluation of the incident and follow-up action. Some state laws protect incident reports from discovery in litigation and address the state's protection of the report if it is qualified or limited in any way. Access to patient-identifiable incident report information is limited to designated individuals.

Safety Initiatives and Respiratory Care Applications

The Joint Commission has described a series of safety initiatives that, if fully implemented, would profoundly improve the quality of patient care. These initiatives have become national patient safety goals and are monitored by the Joint Commission when performing surveys of care.[8] **Table 29–5** lists the Joint Commission's National Patient Safety Goals and provides examples of respiratory therapy applications. The following subsections provide more information on specific applications for some of the goals, namely, implementation of rapid response teams; medication reconciliation; reporting, handoffs, and rounds; discharge education and planning; and healthcare-associated infections.

Rapid Response Teams

Rapid response teams are designed to intervene during the critical prearrest period when patients often demonstrate clinical warning signs of pending demise. When summoned to the bedside, the rapid response team

TABLE 29–5 2010 National Patient Safety Goals as Applied to Respiratory Services

National Patient Safety Goal	Practical Respiratory Therapy Examples
Improve accuracy of patient identification	Use two patient identifiers before initiating care (ask patient name, check patient ID band)
Improve effectiveness of communication among caregivers	Use SBAR; read-back of verbal orders; verification of ventilator alarms during report
Improve safety of using medications	Pharmacy review of all new orders
Reduce risk of healthcare-associated infections	Hand hygiene surveillance; ventilator-associated pneumonia prevention initiatives
Reconcile medications across the continuum of care	Discharge medication review; note action to take for exacerbation of symptoms
Reduce risk of patient harm resulting from falls	Bed rails up upon leaving patient room
Identify safety risks inherent to the patient population	Initiate quarterly skills fairs for infrequently applied procedures or equipment; perform mock inhaled nitric oxide drills on a monthly basis to compensate for infrequent use
Universal Protocol for prevention of wrong site, wrong person, wrong procedure incidents	Preprocedure verification process and time-out for diagnostic bronchoscopy

Adapted from the Joint Commission. NPSG chapter outline and overview: hospital. In: 2010 National Patient Safety Goals. Available at: http://www.jointcommission.org/NR/rdonlyres/CEE2A577-BC61-4338-8780-43F13279610/0/NPSGChapterOutline_FINAL_HAP_2010.pdf. Accessed January 29, 2010.

immediately assesses and treats the patient with the goal of preventing intensive care unit transfer, cardiac arrest, or death. Team composition varies from institution to institution, but often includes a respiratory therapist, a critical care nurse, and occasionally a house physician. **Figure 29–6** describes model criteria for the composition and activation of a rapid response team.

Rapid response teams were identified in 2008 and 2009 as a Joint Commission National Patient Safety Goal. Bedside staff—and, at some hospitals, patients or family members—are encouraged to activate the team response when certain clinical signs or symptoms are present. In spite of the absence of clear outcomes benefit (mortality, length of stay), most hospitals have embraced the rapid response system and incorporate it into their daily clinical response models.

Model	Personnel	Duties
Rapid response team	Critical care nurse, respiratory therapist, and physician (critical care or hospitalist) backup	• Respond to emergencies • Follow up on patients discharged from ICU • Proactively evaluate high-risk ward patients • Educate and act as liaison toward staff
Any staff member may call the team if one of the following criteria is met: • Heart rate over 140 beats/min or less than 40 beats/min • Respiratory rate over 28 breaths/min or less than 8 breaths/min • Systolic blood pressure greater than 180 mm Hg or less than 90 mm Hg • Oxygen saturation less than 90% despite supplementation • Acute change in mental status • Urine output less than 50 cc over 4 hours • Staff member has significant concern about the patient's condition • Chest pain unrelieved by nitroglycerin • Threatened airway • Seizure • Signs of stroke		

FIGURE 29–6 Typical rapid response staffing model and activation criteria.

Medication Reconciliation

When patients are admitted for exacerbation of their conditions, they may receive new medications or use aerosol delivery methods different from their preexisting home medications. As a result, the new medication regimen prescribed at the time of discharge may inadvertently omit needed medications that patients have been receiving for some time.

Such unintended inconsistencies in medication regimens may occur at any point of transition in care (e.g., transfer from an intensive care unit to a general ward), not just at hospital admission or discharge. More than 50% of patients discharged have an unintended medication discrepancy.[9] **Medication reconciliation** is reviewing the patient's complete medication regimen at the time of admission, transfer, and discharge and comparing it with the regimen being considered for the new setting of care.

Medication reconciliation was named a 2005 National Patient Safety Goal by the Joint Commission across the continuum of care. Respiratory therapists most commonly deal with reconciliation issues on a patient's admission to the facility or during discharge education. It is important that the medications and delivery systems explained to the patient be the same that the patient will receive on discharge.

Reports, Handoffs, and Rounds

Patients are inevitably cared for by different providers during their hospitalization. Respiratory therapists and nurses may change shifts every 8 to 12 hours, and physicians (particularly hospitalists) typically change service coverage as well. These shift changes create opportunities for error when clinical information is not accurately transferred between providers.

> **RESPIRATORY RECAP**
>
> **Handoffs**
> » Transitions in care from one provider to another
> » Involve the transfer of information, primary responsibility, and authority between providers

A **handoff**, or transition in a patient's care from one provider to another, involves the transfer of information, primary responsibility, and authority between providers. In hospitals, handoffs take place in multiple activities and locations, such as on admission, during shift and unit changes, before and after procedures, and at discharge.

Communication problems cause almost 70% of sentinel events in accredited healthcare organizations, and at least 50% of communication breakdowns take place during handoffs.[10] Care handoff has been identified by the World Health Organization and the Joint Commission as a risk factor associated with increased errors, and consequently has been a National Patient Safety Goal since 2007.[11,12] Respiratory care is not immune from this area of potential errors. The seemingly straightforward act of communicating important information beyond a treatment-due time is not uniformly practiced in most facilities.

Current report mechanisms may vary from department to department or from area to area (e.g., the intensive care unit vs. general care floors). Guidelines for safe reporting recommend standardizing the report process. **SBAR** is an acronym (situation, background, assessment, recommendation) that is used to describe key points about a patient and the present environmental context in which the patient is being treated. It has become widely accepted not only as a sign-out tool but also as a structured method for all communications between providers. **Figure 29–7** provides an example of an SBAR report process for respiratory care.

Other guidelines have been equally effective in helping improve communication; examples include ensuring that communication is interactive (e.g., reading back an order), limiting interruptions (e.g., pagers, phones), providing a processes for verification (e.g., making rounds on ventilators during report time to verify), and providing an opportunity to review historical data (chart review).

SBAR (Situation, Background, Assessment, Recommendation)
Situation: A patient has been on the ventilator for 3 days, and is slated to go to CT today for a scan between 10 AM and 12 noon.
Background: The patient meets ALI/ARDS criteria, and we have been using lung-protective strategies to guide a low-tidal-volume ventilator strategy and PEEP. He has been extremely agitated for 2 days, requiring frequent boluses for sedation. Blood pressure has been labile and requiring pressors to maintain > 60 mm Hg mean. The patient is very PEEP-dependent and desaturates rapidly when disconnected from the vent, turned, or moved.
Assessment: This patient is very unstable and a transport today, while necessary, will be difficult and require careful attention by experienced staff.
Recommendation: Contact the team leader and let them know about the transport so they may help you prior to your arrival. Make sure the most experienced RT travels with the patient. Use the transport check-off list. Use the capnograph, pulse oximeter, and a transport ventilator with PEEP capability.

FIGURE 29–7 Example of an SBAR report process for respiratory care.

> **RESPIRATORY RECAP**
>
> **Guidelines Effective in Improving Communication**
> » Ensuring that communication is interactive
> » Limiting interruptions
> » Providing a process for verification
> » Providing an opportunity to review historical data

Universal Protocol

The **Universal Protocol** was created to address the continuing occurrence of wrong site, wrong procedure, and wrong person surgery. It is used to verify the correct procedure, for the correct patient, at the correct site. When possible, it should involve the patient in the verification process. It should also use a standardized list to verify the availability of items for the procedure. The Universal Protocol is required for procedures such as diagnostic bronchoscopy or a tracheostomy tube change. However, it is not required for minor procedures such as arterial puncture.

An invasive procedure should not be started until all questions or concerns are resolved. A time-out should be conducted immediately before starting the procedure. A designated member of the team starts the time-out, which involves all immediate members of the procedure team, including the respiratory therapist as appropriate. All relevant members of the procedure team, including the respiratory therapist, actively communicate during the time-out. During the time-out, the team members agree, at a minimum, on the correct patient identity, correct site, and the procedure to be done. Completion of the time-out must be documented.

Discharge Education and Planning

Safe care transitions (e.g., from hospital to home) require a systematic approach. One of the most problematic areas is discharge education and management for chronic respiratory conditions (e.g., chronic obstructive pulmonary disease, asthma) in the event of symptom escalation. Proper discharge education ensures a higher probability of compliance, which reduces readmissions and untoward safety events. The respiratory therapist can assist the healthcare team by reviewing three key areas prior to discharge:

- *Medication reconciliation*: Review the patient's medications to ensure that maintenance and rescue medications are appropriate.
- *Structured discharge communication*: Inform the patient of medication changes, pending tests and studies, and follow-up appointments. Communicate with outpatient physician offices whenever possible.
- *Patient education*: Patients and their families must understand their diagnosis, medications, equipment and techniques, and steps to take in case of exacerbation of symptoms after discharge.

Healthcare-Associated Infections

Healthcare-associated infections (HAIs) are the most common complication of hospital care. According to the Centers for Disease Control and Prevention (CDC), nearly 1.7 million HAIs occur yearly, leading to approximately 99,000 deaths every year.[13] Recent efforts have demonstrated that relatively simple measures can prevent the majority of common HAIs. Four specific infections together account for more than 80% of all HAIs: surgical site infections (SSIs), catheter-associated urinary tract infections (CAUTIs), central venous catheter–related bloodstream infections (CRBSIs), and ventilator-associated pneumonia (VAP).[14] Although all of these are important to the respiratory therapist, VAP is an especially prominent concern.

Reducing the risk of HAI is one of the Joint Commission's National Patient Safety Goals.[8] The goal specifically requires adherence to hand hygiene practices and also considers death or serious disability due to HAI to be a sentinel event. Appropriate hand hygiene, influenza vaccination for healthcare workers, and prevention of VAP, CRBSI, and SSI are among the National Quality Forum's Safe Practices for Better Healthcare.[15]

HAIs have resulted in considerable regulatory attention. The Centers for Medicare and Medicaid Services recently announced that it will not reimburse hospitals for the costs of care associated with certain HAIs, including SSIs, CRBSIs, and CAUTIs.[16] One important challenge in using public reporting and payment policies to catalyze efforts to decrease HAIs is that the definitions are complex and may be subject to interpretation. For example, the utility of VAP as a quality measure is hampered by the lack of standardized diagnostic criteria. Bronchoalveolar lavage has not demonstrated superiority to standard nonquantitative culture techniques.[17] Nonetheless, the respiratory therapist must be diligent in the care of such patients and adhere to accepted practices.

> **RESPIRATORY RECAP**
>
> **Safe Practices for Better Healthcare**
>
> » Appropriate hand hygiene
> » Influenza vaccination for healthcare workers
> » Prevention of central venous catheter–related bloodstream infections, ventilator-associated pneumonia, catheter-associated urinary tract infections, and surgical site infections

The respiratory therapist is expected to practice the art of respiratory care with knowledge, skill, and a continuously professional attribute. It is equally important that the therapist understand that information, and the manner in which they impart and record that information, affects the safety and sequential care the patient receives. All documentation and communication must be provided in a manner consistent with institutional and regulatory standards for accuracy, clarity, and confidentiality. Technologic advances will continue to drive many of the changes in the development, maintenance, and transfer of medical information over the next few years. The challenge of each respiratory practitioner is to understand the basic principles and to apply them in the future to improve safe, effective patient care through better information management.

KEY POINTS

- Medical information management is a comprehensive concept that deals with the acquisition, storage, and transfer of data and information.
- Medical documentation serves many purposes: as a method to evaluate quality of care, a basis for financial reimbursement, a means to evaluate resources, and as a legal document.
- Regulatory and standards organizations have guidelines identifying essential elements of medical documentation.
- Respiratory charting should not be taken lightly because if it is careless or insufficient, it could result in patient harm, penalties, lawsuits, and financial consequences.
- Requirements for medical record entries vary based on setting and institution, but therapists

must be knowledgeable about the policies and procedures for their respective clinical settings.

- The electronic medical record is gaining popularity: it speeds entry, improves storage and retrieval, and improves the provision of care.
- Confidentiality is the fundamental right for patients to have personal, identifiable medical information kept private and is protected by a federal statue known as HIPAA.
- Institutions strive to create a culture of safety in which high risk/high reliability, a safe harbor, teamwork, and commitment are focal points.
- An incident report should be filed whenever an untoward event occurs.
- Rapid response teams have become commonplace in healthcare and are designed to encourage early intervention for adverse signs, symptoms, or conditions.
- Medication reconciliation is designed to pick up inconsistencies or discrepancies in a patient's medication regimen.
- Reports, handoffs, and rounds are the source of many medical errors in care.
- A time-out should be conducted immediately before starting an invasive procedure.
- Proper discharge education ensures a higher probability of compliance and reduces readmission and untoward safety events.
- Healthcare-associated infections continue to be the source of numerous medical problems and complications, and regulatory interventions are exerting significant influence on healthcare institutions to reduce their incidence.

REFERENCES

1. Care First Blue Choice. *Medical Records Documentation Standards.* Available at: http://www.carefirst.com/providers/attachments/BOK5129.pdf. Accessed August 5, 2009.
2. Joint Commission Resources, Accreditation Manager Plus, Edition v1.5.5.2. *Hospital Accreditation Requirements; Record of Care, Treatment of Services.* RC.02.03.07. Available at: http://amp:jcrinc.com/Frame.aspx. Accessed August 5, 2009.
3. American Health Information Management Association. *Practice Brief: Authentication of Health Record Entries (Updated).* March 2000. Available at: http://library.ahima.org/xpedio/groups/public/documents/ahima/bok1_000040.hcsp?dDocName=bok1_000040. Accessed August 5, 2009.
4. Joint Commission Resources, Accreditation Manager Plus, Edition v1.5.5.2. *Hospital Accreditation Requirements; Record of Care, Treatment of Services.* RC.01.02.01. Available at: http://amp:jcrinc.com/Frame.aspx. Accessed August 5, 2009.
5. U.S. Department of Health and Human Services. *Understanding HIPPA Privacy for Covered Entities.* Available at: http://www.hhs.gov/ocr/privacy/hipaa/understanding/coveredentities/index.html. Accessed August 5, 2009.
6. Kohn LT, Corrigan JM, Donaldson MS, eds. *To Err Is Human: Building a Safer Health System.* Washington, DC: National Academies Press; 2000.
7. Weick KE, Sutcliffe KM. *Managing the Unexpected: Assuring High Performance in an Age of Complexity.* San Francisco: Jossey-Bass; 2001:10–17.
8. The Joint Commission. *2009 National Patient Safety Goals Hospital Program.* Available at: http://www.jointcommission.org/NR/rdonlyres/CEE2A577-BC61-4338-8780-43F132729610/0/NPSGChapterOutline_FINAL_HAP_2010.pdf. Accessed February 8, 2010.
9. Wong JD, Bajcar JM, Wong GG, et al. Medication reconciliation at hospital discharge: evaluating discrepancies. *Ann Pharmacother.* 2008;42:1373–1379.
10. Greenberg CC, Regenbogen SE, Studdert DM, et al. Patterns of communication breakdowns resulting in injury to surgical patients. *J Am Coll Surg.* 2007;204:533–540.
11. Joint Commission, International Center for Patient Safety. Improving handoff communications: meeting National Patient Safety Goal 2E. September 2006. Available at: http://www.jcipatientsafety.org/15427/. Accessed August 5, 2009.
12. World Health Organization for Patient Safety Initiatives. *Communication During Patient Handovers.* 2007. Available at: http://www.ccforpatientsafety.org/common/pdfs/fpdf/presskit/PS-Solution3.pdf. Accessed August 5, 2009.
13. Klevens RM, et al. Estimating health care associated infections and deaths in U.S. hospitals, 2002. *Public Health Rep.* 2007;122:160–166.
14. Centers for Disease Control and Prevention. Estimates of healthcare associated infections. Available at: http://www.cdc.gov/ncidod/dhqp/hai.html. Accessed February 8, 2010.
15. National Quality Forum. *Safe Practices for Better Healthcare: 2009 Update.* Available at: http://www.qualityforum.org/Search.aspx?keyword=safe+practices. Accessed February 8, 2010.
16. Centers for Medicare and Medicaid Services, Department of Health and Human Services. Medicare program: changes to the hospital inpatient prospective payment systems and fiscal year 2008 rates. *Fed Register.* 2007;72:47129–48175.
17. Canadian Critical Care Trials Group. A randomized trial of diagnostic techniques for ventilator associated pneumonia. *N Engl J Med.* 2006;355:2619–2630.

SECTION III

Respiratory Diseases

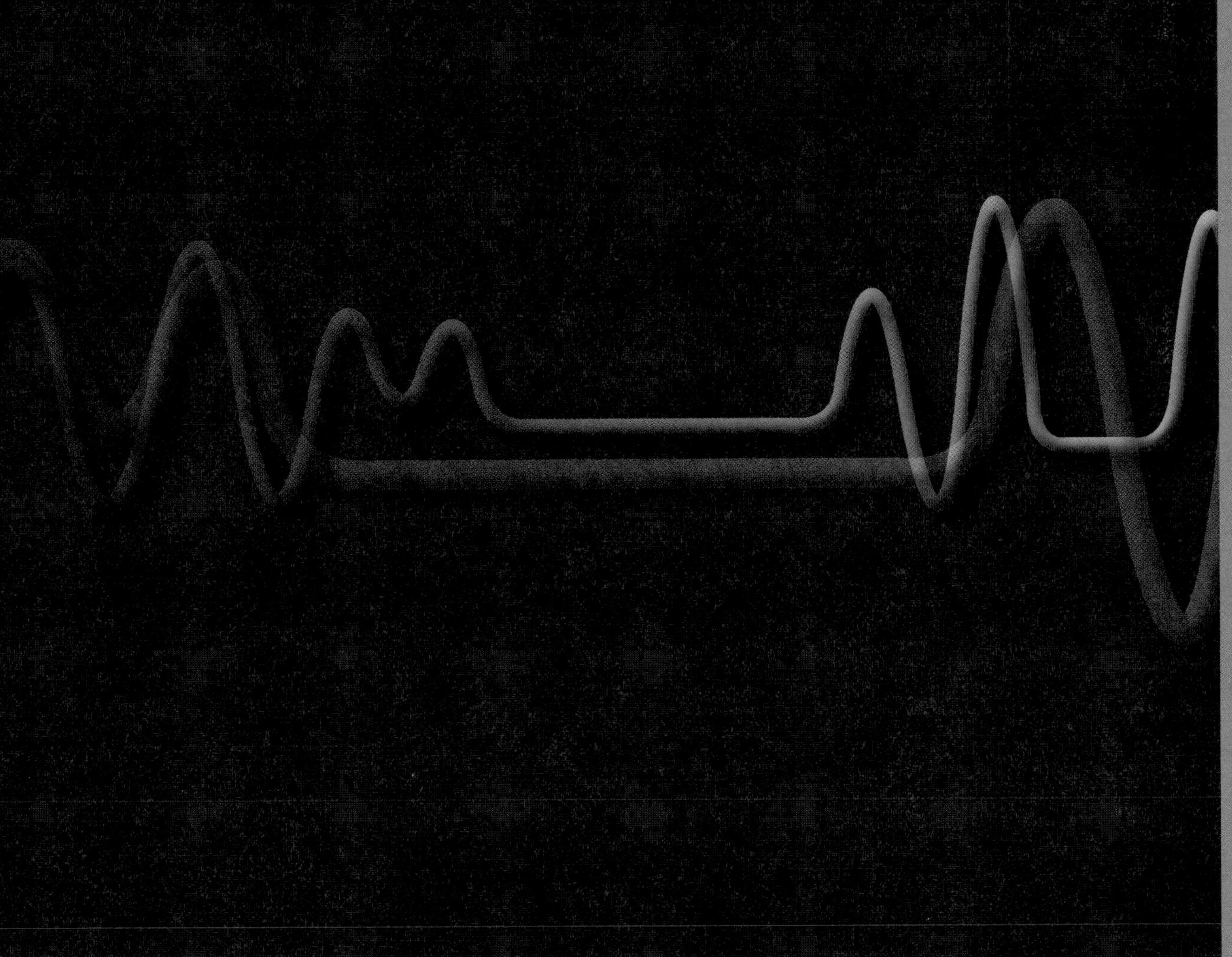

CHAPTER 30

Principles of Disease Management

William F. Galvin

OUTLINE

Forces Driving Disease Management
History and Evolution of Disease Management
Terms, Factors, and Concepts Associated with Disease Management
Goals of Disease Management
Basic Principles of Disease Management
Diseases Targeted for Disease Management Programs
Steps to Develop a Disease Management Program
Barriers and Opportunities
Respiratory Therapists as Disease Managers

OBJECTIVES

1. Identify the forces driving disease management and the new mind-set in managing disease.
2. Explain the history and evolution of the disease management movement.
3. Define disease management and terms associated with care management.
4. Explain the difference between case management and disease management.
5. Identify the core components of disease management.
6. Explain the goals of disease management.
7. Describe the concept of health value as it pertains to disease management.
8. List and explain the basic principles of disease management.
9. Identify the diseases best suited for disease management programs.
10. Identify and explain the steps used to develop a disease management program.
11. List and explain the barriers and opportunities of disease management.
12. Explain the roles of respiratory therapists with regard to disease management.

KEY TERMS

care management
case management
component management
demand management
disease management
evidence-based medicine
pathways
protocols

INTRODUCTION

Disease management is a term that has been around for many years. Anecdotal conversations as well as a review of the literature reflect an increased emphasis on the issues of chronicity and the importance of providing care across the healthcare continuum. This chapter addresses the forces driving disease management; the history and evolution of the disease management movement; defines the terms associated with disease management; addresses the goals, principles, and specific cardiopulmonary diseases targeted for disease management programs; explains the steps in the development of a disease management program; and focuses on the barriers and opportunities for disease management. The chapter concludes with an explanation of the role of the respiratory therapist as a disease manager.

Forces Driving Disease Management

The primary forces driving disease management are cost (**Figure 30–1**) and the changing pattern of disease (**Table 30–1**), specifically, the increase in chronic, debilitating disease. The healthcare cost component of the gross domestic product (GDP) shifted from 5.2% in 1960 to over 16% in 2008.[1] This escalating increase in the healthcare component of the GDP is at the heart of efforts to reform and restructure the healthcare system.

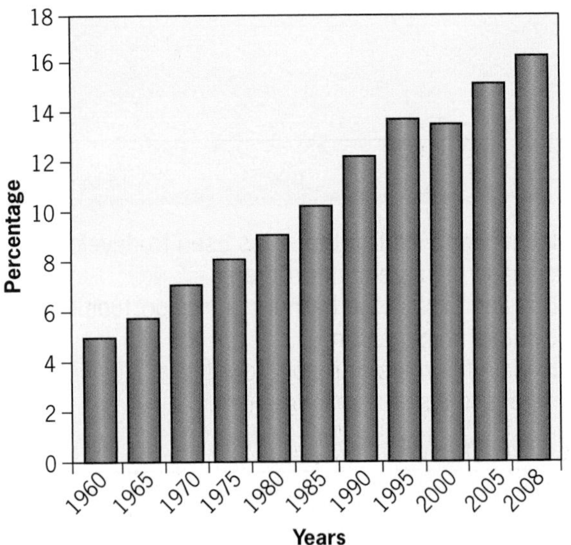

FIGURE 30–1 Healthcare expenditure as a percentage of gross domestic product. Data from Centers for Medicare and Medicaid Services. National health expenditures aggregate, per capita amounts, percent distribution, and average annual percent growth, by source of funds: selected calendar years 1960–2008. Available at: http://www.cms.hhs.gov/NationalHealthExpendData/downloads/tables.pdf.

TABLE 30–1 Changing Patterns of Disease: 1900–2006*

1900	2006
Pneumonia	Heart disease
Tuberculosis	Cancer
Diarrhea and enteritis	Stroke (cerebrovascular diseases)
Heart disease	Chronic lower respiratory diseases
Stroke	Accidents (unintentional injuries)
Liver disease	Diabetes
Injuries	Alzheimer's disease†
Cancer	Influenza and pneumonia
Senility	Nephritis, nephrotic syndrome, and nephrosis
Diphtheria	Septicemia

*Diseases listed are in order of prevalence, from most prevalent to least prevalent for the time spans stated.

†Preliminary data show Alzheimer's disease positioned to go to sixth position and diabetes to seventh position.

1900 data from Centers for Disease Control and Prevention. Control of infectious diseases, 1900–1999. *MMWR.* 1999;48:621–629; 2006 data from Heron M, Hoyert DL, Murphy SL, et al. *Deaths: final data for 2006.* Hyattsville, MD: National Center for Health Statistics; 2009.

The infectious diseases prevalent in 1900 had given way to chronic, lifestyle diseases by the year 2006. This issue of chronicity is especially important because it is currently estimated that about 125 million Americans have one or more chronic disease, one-half of whom have two or more chronic illnesses.[2] Additionally, the Centers for Medicare and Medicaid Services (CMS) indicate that patients with five or more chronic conditions account for 23% of its beneficiaries but 68% of its spending. The conditions cited are primarily heart disease, diabetes, glaucoma, asthma, chronic obstructive pulmonary disease, and cancer. Of particular concern is the projection that by 2020 the aging baby boomers will raise the percentage of Americans having multiple chronic conditions to 25%, with associated care costs projected at $1.07 trillion.[3]

It is interesting to note that of the four determinants of one's healthcare status, lifestyle, which is reflected in an individual's health behaviors, clearly reflects the largest percentage of an individual's health status. It accounts for about 50% of an individual's health status (**Figure 30–2**) and is associated with every leading cause of death in the United States.[4] Its impact is even more pronounced when one views the leading causes of death from the perspective of the behavioral causes of death (**Table 30–2**). Of particular note is that tobacco use is at the top of the list, representing 18.1% of total deaths, and that poor diet and physical inactivity is at second position at 16.6%, with a strong likelihood of overtaking tobacco as the leading behavioral cause of death.[5]

These forces have given rise to the adoption of a new mind-set in the way we perceive health.[6] This new mind-set is the impetus behind the disease management movement and is the theme of this chapter. The disease management movement has lead to a new direction in the delivery of healthcare (**Table 30–3**).

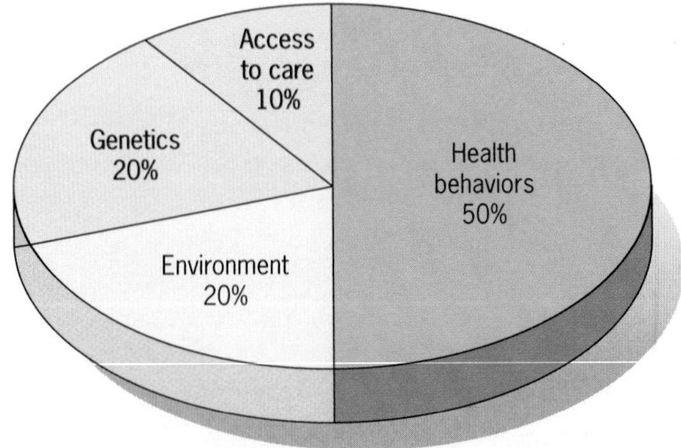

FIGURE 30–2 Determinants of health. Data from Centers for Disease Control and Prevention. *Ten Leading Causes of Death in the United States, 1975.* Atlanta, GA: CDC; 2000.

TABLE 30-2 Behavioral Causes of Death in the United States in 2000

Cause	Number of Total Deaths	Percentage of Total Deaths
Tobacco use	435,000	18.1
Diet/activity patterns	400,000	16.6
Alcohol	85,000	5.0
Microbial agents	75,000	3.1
Toxic agents	55,000	2.2
Firearms	29,000	1.2
Sexual behavior	20,000	<1.0
Motor vehicles	43,000	1.8
Illicit use of drugs	17,000	<1.0
Total	1,159,000	Approximately 50

Adapted from Mokdad AH, Marks JS, Stroup DF, Gerberding JL. Actual causes of death in the United States, 2000. *JAMA.* 2004;291(10):1238–1245.

TABLE 30-3 Trends and Directions in Health Care Delivery

Illness → Wellness
Acute care → Primary care
Inpatient → Outpatient
Individual health → Community well-being
Fragmented care → Managed care
Independent institutions → Integrated systems
Service duplication → Continuum of services

From Shi L, Singh D. *Delivering Health Care in America: A Systems Approach.* 3rd ed. Sudbury, MA: Jones & Bartlett Learning; 2004:19.

History and Evolution of Disease Management

The origin and evolution of disease management are rooted in the desire to improve healthcare quality and contain healthcare costs. Disease management first became popular in 1993 when the Boston Consulting Group introduced the term in its study of the pharmaceutical industry.[7] Since that time, every healthcare-related group or entity has been involved in some way with the evolution, development, and implementation of disease management (**Table 30-4**). Two groups in particular are considered responsible for spearheading the popularity of disease management: managed care organizations and the pharmaceutical industry. Their goals are to optimize profits, contain healthcare costs, and provide quality patient care.

TABLE 30-4 Selected List of Participants in the Disease Management Movement

Parent Group	Specific Organizations
Managed care organizations	Aetna U.S. Healthcare, Group Health Care of Puget Sound
Pharmaceutical firms	Merck, Smith Kline Beecham, Glaxo Wellcome
Integrated delivery systems	Lovelace Health System, Henry Ford Health System, Mayo Clinic
Specialty centers	National Jewish Center for Immunology and Respiratory Diseases, Memorial Sloan Kettering
Academic health centers/ systems	University of Pennsylvania Health System, Johns Hopkins Health System
Multihospital chains	Columbia HCA, Tenet, Intermountain Health Care
Employers and coalitions	Xerox, GTE, Digital, Business Health Care Action Group
Pharmaceutical benefit companies	Medco, PCS, DPS, Caremark, Value Rx
Independent disease management companies	Greenstone Health Care, Stuart Disease Management, AirLogix

From Couch JB. *The Physician's Guide to Disease Management.* Gaithersburg, MD: Aspen; 1997:2.

Large pharmaceutical corporations purchased pharmaceutical benefits companies with the initial intention of capturing market distribution channels for managed care organizations and leveraging resources and contacts to develop state-of-the-art programs to manage the various diseases of these large populations.[8] Although pharmaceutical companies do not provide direct treatment, they do have extensive databases and can use them to influence the industry. Local pharmacies have a distinct advantage: they are strategically placed in the community and have access to the databases of both physicians and patients. This allows them to provide advice, guidance, and support; identify adverse drug interactions; adjust dosages and schedules; employ utilization review; and document compliance through knowledge of the refill and usage patterns of their customers.[9] Disease management provides them with an opportunity to demonstrate how appropriately selected and administered drug and device interventions may result in improved outcomes, patient satisfaction, and financial rewards.

The impetus for use of disease management programs by managed care organizations comes from two sources: the employment benefits consultant community and the employer coalition community. The people who write the request for proposals (employee benefits managers) drive the market. The employer coalition community is bringing enormous numbers of employees to managed care, which serves to shape thought and acceptable standards.[10] Managed care organizations have strong motivation and strong financial incentives to cut resource consumption at all provider sites, and they tend to move aggressively to this end. They are at the forefront of adopting this approach because the shift from discounted fees to a prepaid per-member formula for enrollees drives demand to increase efficiencies, ensuring that providers are uniformly using the most effective procedures, drugs, and supplies.[11]

Disease management has become a way for pharmaceutical firms to sell more products, for managed care organizations to contain costs, and for healthcare professionals (e.g., respiratory therapists) to improve patient outcomes.[9] For disease management to be effective, a partnership must exist between the patient, health plan, and provider.

Terms, Factors, and Concepts Associated with Disease Management

Care Management

Care management is a general term for the coordination of patient interventions. It is an umbrella term under which many loosely related terms are gathered. The more popular terms associated with care management are *component management, demand management, case management,* and *disease management.* Respiratory therapists must have an understanding of these terms because efforts are continuously under way to institute measures aimed at the coordination of the care and management of respiratory diseases.

Component Management

Component management is the opposite of disease management.[12] Component management is the predominant method that has been used to control healthcare costs since the 1980s. Its focus is cost control through limitation of the use of resources or services such as therapeutic procedures, diagnostic tests, medications, or hospital lengths of stay. Unfortunately, component management often results in lower quality of care and poorer clinical outcomes and is an ineffective way to truly control costs.

The problem with component management is that each aspect of care—emergency room visits, physician services, medications—is managed separately and services are not integrated. In the case of the patient with asthma, all health plans cover emergency room visits, inpatient hospital stays, and physician services. Medications may or may not be covered. However, few provide coverage for patient education and counseling. Consequently, the limited coverage for medications and patient education leads to significantly higher costs in the form of more emergency room visits, inpatient hospitalizations, and physician office visits. When respiratory therapy departments were revenue generators, component care approaches allowed them to flourish. However, component management is flawed: it is episodic, uncoordinated, emphasizes treatment instead of prevention, and provides little incentive to treat the entire disease.[12]

Demand Management

Demand management entails any organized effort or program designed to guide healthcare consumers into the most appropriate level of healthcare service by involving them in their own care.[13] It reduces the need for and use of costly, often unnecessary, medical services and arbitrary managed care interventions. The tools of demand management consist of patient **protocols**, clinical **pathways**, case management, and disease management. These tools were developed to enable clinicians to achieve better outcomes by making it easier to give patients what they need when they need it. The intention is to weed out inappropriate and unnecessary care.[14]

Case Management

Case management is defined as a collaborative process that assesses, plans, implements, coordinates, monitors, and evaluates the options and services required to meet an individual's health needs, using communication and available resources to promote quality, cost, and effective outcomes.[15] It is generally employed for the high-risk, high-cost patient who suffers repeated admissions, encounters significant variances, is unpredictable, and may be socioeconomically disadvantaged.[14] Case management was built on the notion that 20% of patients were responsible for 80% of costs. The rationale was that focusing on the care of the 20% would reduce this 80% cost. Traditional case management is one-on-one care and is expensive.[16] Case managers focus on an individual patient and assist in acquiring equipment and services, work with schools and other community-based organizations, provide technical support, conduct patient education, and identify and remove barriers to effective implementation of the care plan.[14]

Disease Management

Disease management is one of the most innovative and exciting concepts in the healthcare delivery system. Numerous synonyms are associated with the concept; some of the more popular are *disease state management, system-based disease management, total health management, medical management, population-based management, best practices, care mapping,* and *outcomes management.* The different terminology attempts to capture or highlight one or more of the numerous principles that drive the disease management movement.

Definitions for disease management are numerous and diverse, as shown by the following examples:

- A clinical management process of care that spans the continuum of care from primary prevention to ongoing long-term health maintenance for individuals with chronic health conditions or diagnoses[10]
- An approach to identify a specific subpopulation of patients at high risk for undesirable outcomes and intervene to modify that risk[17]
- The cure to high-cost conditions[10]
- An ongoing, comprehensive case management program for specific chronic diseases that is based on clearly defined, well-established best practices of care[14]

For purposes of this chapter, the definition provided by the Disease Management Association of America (DMAA) will be used: disease management is a system of coordinated healthcare interventions and communications for populations with conditions in which patient self-care efforts are significant.[18]

RESPIRATORY RECAP

Synonyms for Disease Management

» Disease state management
» System-based disease management
» Total health management
» Medical management
» Population-based management
» Best practices
» Care mapping
» Outcomes management

Often the difference between case management and disease management is not apparent. **Table 30–5** compares conventional case management and disease management.

Core Components of Disease Management

According to the DMAA, there are six core components of a full-service disease management program (**Box 30–1**). Programs consisting of fewer than these six components are considered disease management support services.

Goals of Disease Management

The purpose of disease management is to take what was learned in epidemiology and research and incorporate that knowledge into everyday practice, while measuring the results and attempting to make improvements. The plan is never really finished but rather is under continuous quality improvement.[11] The challenge is to apply a gradation of resources to members of the population in question so that each does not get too little (low quality) or too much (poor cost containment), but just the right amount of resources (high value).[16] In short, disease management attempts to achieve better control of the episodic cost of care, reduce mortality, improve functional status, improve patient and physician satisfaction, acquire meaningful outcomes data (e.g., medication

TABLE 30-5 Comparison of Conventional Case Management and Disease Management

Traditional or Catastrophic Case Management	Disease Management
Emphasis is on single patient	Emphasis is on population with a chronic illness
Early identification of people with acute catastrophic conditions (known high cost or known diagnoses that lead to high cost in the near term)	Early identification of all people with targeted chronic diseases (20–40) whether mild, moderate, or severe
Acuity level of catastrophic cases is high; acuity level of traditional cases is high to moderate	Acuity level is moderate
Applies to 0.5% to 1% of commercial membership	Applies to 15% to 25% of commercial membership
Value relies heavily on price negotiations and benefit flexing	Value is result of member and provider behavior change that results in improved health status
Requires plan design manipulation	Requires no need to change plan design
Primary objective is to arrange for care using the least restrictive, clinically appropriate alternatives	Primary objective is to avoid hospitalization *and* modify risk factors, lifestyle, and medication adherence to improve health status
Episode is 60 to 90 days	Intervention is 365 days for most conditions
Site of interaction is primarily hospital, hospice, subacute facility, or home health care	Sites of interaction include work, school, and home
Driven by need for arrangement of support services, community resources, transportation	Driven by nonadherence to medical regimens
Outcome metrics are single-admission length of stay and cost per case	Outcome metrics are annual cost per diseased member and disease-specific functional status

From Kongstvedt P. *Essentials of Managed Health.* 5th ed. Sudbury, MA: Jones & Bartlett Learning; 2007. Reprinted with permission.

BOX 30–1

Core Components of a Disease Management Program

Population identification processes
Evidence-based practice guidelines
Collaborative practice models to include physician and support-service providers
Patient self-management education (may include primary prevention, behavior modification programs, and compliance/surveillance)
Process and outcomes measurement, evaluation, and management
Routine reporting/feedback loop (may include communication with patient, physician, health plan and ancillary providers, and practice profiling)

Reprinted with permission of DMAA: The Care Continuum Alliance. Copyright by DMAA: The Care Continuum Alliance, 2010. http://www.dmaa.org/dm_definition.asp.

compliance), and develop an improved ability to bear financial risk for services.[15]

Health Value

Although the goal of disease management is reduction of cost and improvement in quality, the overriding goal of healthcare is value.[8,16] *Value* is defined as quality of outcomes per unit of cost to the stakeholders (**Equation 30–1**).[8] Outcomes can be of a clinical, economic, service, or humanistic nature. Clinical outcomes can entail rates of mortality, morbidity, complications, or infection. Economic outcomes can be measured in terms of overall costs for hospitalization; emergency room visits; outpatient-, physician-, and pharmaceutical-related services; and member-per-month costs. Service outcomes are generally subjective and include patient perception of care, patient and provider satisfaction, and health plan enrollment rates. Humanistic outcomes can include overall perception of health status; physical, role, and social functioning; and levels of pain.

EQUATION 30–1

Healthcare Value

$$\text{Heathcare value} = \frac{\text{Quality of clinical, economic, service, and humanistic outcomes}}{\text{Overall costs, time, resources, and hassles to all stakeholders}}$$

Costs are the total of all costs involved in healthcare delivery and include time, resources, and hassles. Controlling costs entails appropriate choice of equipment, personnel, and services and using all three of these in a timely fashion. Efficiency and effectiveness minimize absenteeism and losses in productivity. All stakeholders (purchasers, payers, providers, and patients) experience hassles, such as submitting claims and securing referrals. Stakeholder concerns about hassles are real and should not be taken lightly.[8]

RESPIRATORY RECAP

Goals of Disease Management

- Achieve control of episodic cost of care
- Reduce morbidity
- Improve functional status
- Improve patient and physician satisfaction
- Acquire more meaningful outcomes data
- Develop an improved ability to bear financial risk for services

Basic Principles of Disease Management

Understanding the five underlying principles that characterize disease management will provide a deeper appreciation of the disease management movement. **Box 30–2** lists the five principles; a brief description of each follows.[17]

BOX 30–2

Principles Characterizing Disease Management

Understanding of the disease's natural course, causes, and cost drivers
Diagnosis and treatment based on the disease process rather than on reimbursement patterns
Patient education and compliance programs for chronic disease management
Management of treatment that cuts across care settings and provides full continuity of care
Directing resources toward the best and most cost-effective treatments and comparing outcomes among plans and treatments

Adapted from Zitter M. Disease management: a new approach to health care. *Med Interface.* 1994;7:70–76.

Natural Course, Causes, and Cost Drivers of Disease

One of the more important principles of disease management is understanding the natural course of the disease, the causes of the disease, and the factors that typically drive costs.[19] The course and causes of most cardiopulmonary disease are fairly predictable and straightforward. However, the factors that drive the cost of disease may not be obvious. Cost drivers of disease are compliance, prevention, rapid resolution, acute flare-ups, and the 80/20 rule.[19]

Tuberculosis is an example of a respiratory disease in which noncompliance with long-term pharmacologic management results in ineffective treatment, lack of resolution of the disease process, and risk of exposure and transmission to the public. Patients with tuberculosis typically require a regimen of multiple medications for a prolonged period of time (6 to 12 months). However, patients often feel better shortly after initial treatment and stop taking their medications. The result is a lack of eradication of the disease and potentially serious health consequences for the individual and the public. In short, compliance with the care plan results in a significant impact on cost containment.

RESPIRATORY RECAP

Cost Drivers of Disease

- » Compliance
- » Prevention
- » Rapid resolution
- » Acute flare-ups
- » The 80/20 rule

With regard to prevention, many patients with acquired immune deficiency syndrome (AIDS) could be spared disease by practicing safe sex. In other words, the high cost of treatment could have been prevented if the individuals had engaged in a healthy lifestyle practice. About 85% of managed care organizations' disease management efforts are focused on treatment rather than prevention. In the future this is likely to shift: efforts will be directed at prevention rather than treatment.[10]

Rapidly resolving the disease or condition curtails healthcare costs. For example, a patient who develops a serious case of pneumonia should receive immediate treatment with antibiotics. Ideally, the invading organism is identified, the appropriate antibiotic ordered, and the patient adheres to the therapeutic care plan. Delays in a patient's seeking medical attention or inaccurate assessment and diagnosis will result in a more serious affliction and a condition that is protracted or sustained. A prolonged illness can result in an increase in the number and intensity of additional services, an increased length of stay, and ultimately increased healthcare costs. Efforts should always be directed at rapidly resolving the disease or condition.

Asthma often is characterized by acute exacerbation of the disease. These acute flare-ups are preventable by identification of triggers, education on the action and use of medications, and instruction in the proper use of medication delivery devices. Hospitalization and frequent emergency room visits are extremely costly. Efforts directed at curtailing these acute flare-ups result in significant reduction of healthcare costs.

The 80/20 rule indicates that a high percentage of healthcare costs are represented by a relatively small number of conditions. A report states that in a typical employee group, 10% of employees make up 70% of the group's healthcare costs, whereas just 1% consume 30% of total expenditures.[20] With regard to specific diseases, approximately 10% of asthmatics account for 44% of the total medical costs of treating this condition.[21] Using the 80/20 rule and targeting the at-risk population for prevention and treatment is an effective and efficient means to control cost drivers.[19]

Diagnosis and Treatment Based on Disease Rather than Reimbursement Patterns

Fragmentation is a major problem within the healthcare system. The critically important functions of the provision of care and reimbursement for services rendered are fragmented and disharmonious. The provider network made up of physicians and other care providers is interested primarily in quality of care issues, whereas the payer network is concerned almost exclusively with the costs of services and the method and amount of reimbursement. The two seem to be going in different directions. Under a disease management program, the system is integrated and the primary focus is on diagnosing and treating the disease process, with emphasis on preventive measures.

Patient Education and Compliance Programs for Chronic Disease Management

With regard to disease management, strong patient education skills and abilities take on new meaning. Failure to achieve desired results from noncompliance reportedly averages 40%, depending on the condition being treated. The rate for asthma is approximately 20%, whereas the rate for arthritis is 71% and that for hypertension is approximately 40%.[22] About 10% of all hospitalizations and 23% of all nursing home admissions are attributed to nonadherence.[23] The cost of nonadherence in the United States has been estimated at more than $100 billion each year.[24] The problem of noncompliance is monumental; thus, there is a critical need for patient education through scheduled inpatient sessions at the bedside, counseling, telephone and mail prompts, home visits, or a combination of these. Disease management programs emphasize and employ many of these measures on a more concerted basis.

Empowering the patient and stressing the importance of self-management of the disease process are emphasized. The patient needs to be more knowledgeable and better informed. In addition, patients must be held accountable for their actions. This often is difficult;

however, patient involvement is key because one of the major measures of quality is patient satisfaction.

Management of Treatment Across the Full Continuum of Care

Disease management programs have the ability to coordinate all aspects of care across all elements of the healthcare delivery system and to individualize that care to the specific needs of the patient. Coordinating care across the continuum implies that healthcare settings are no longer confined to the hospital or the physician's office. Delivery settings have proliferated in response to the changing configuration of economic incentives, and disease management programs treat disease in a broader array of settings that include extended care (skilled nursing homes), acute care (hospitals), ambulatory care (physician offices and outpatient clinics), home care (hospice, durable medical equipment, home health visits), outreach (screening, information and referrals, telephone contact), wellness and health promotion (educational and exercise programs, support groups), and housing (assisted living, retirement communities). Acute care is clearly the most expensive form of care, whereas home care and self-care are significantly cheaper. This is especially true in the critical care areas, in which significant human and technologic resources are expended. In addition, most patients prefer the home care setting because it offers the added advantages of comfort, familiarity, and proximity to the family.

Funding for the Most Powerful Interventions

Disease management entails funding of the most powerful and successful interventions. It calls for physicians to discard their old, autonomous way of making decisions and substitute new group-tested approaches for the treatment of common conditions. It swaps medicine's tradition of independence for "group think."[11] The notion of group think has given rise to the term **evidence-based medicine**, an approach to practice and teaching that integrates pathophysiologic rationale, caregiver experience, and patient preferences with valid and current clinical research evidence.[25] It entails precise definition of the patient problem, proficient searching and critical appraisal of relevant information from the literature, and subsequent incorporation of that information into medical practice.[26] This prevents common conditions from spiraling out of control and creates a clinical road map for each targeted condition.[11]

BOX 30–3

Characteristics of the Ideal Illness for a Disease Management Program

High incidence of preventable complications
Improper prescribing that can be addressed through physician education
A chronic nature that lends itself to management
A large patient population
Highly visible costs
The ability to lower costs through patient education
The ability to measure outcomes

From Dubbs WH. Disease management: a proven strategy for reducing costs, enhancing care. *AARC Times.* 1996;20(12):30–32. Reprinted with permission.

Diseases Targeted for Disease Management Programs

A number of diseases and conditions are ideally suited for a disease management program. The Disease Management Association of America identifies what it considers the "big five" as follows: ischemic heart disease, diabetes, chronic obstructive pulmonary disease (COPD), asthma, and heart failure.[18] Many of the cardiorespiratory diseases are considered ideal illnesses for implementation of a disease management intervention.[27] **Box 30–3** provides a short list of characteristics of the ideal illness for a disease management program.

RESPIRATORY RECAP

Conditions Targeted for Disease Management: The Big Five

» Ischemic heart disease
» Diabetes
» COPD
» Asthma
» Heart disease

The following factors make specific diseases especially well suited for a disease management intervention:[15]

- A high rate of preventable complications (with the goal of a reduction in emergency department visits and hospital readmissions)
- A short time frame during which alterations in natural history can show a measurable impact (e.g., 1 to 3 years)
- Chronic, outpatient-focused conditions that are common, low technology, and nonsurgical
- High rate of variability in patterns of therapeutics from patient to patient and from physician to physician
- High rates of patient noncompliance with the therapeutic regime (amenable to change by education directed at patients, family members, and physicians)

- Existence of or development of practice guidelines on optimal treatment
- Achievable consensus on what constitutes good quality, which outcomes to measure, and how to improve them

Steps to Develop a Disease Management Program

Numerous approaches exist for the development of a disease management program.[8,26] This chapter addresses three: the work of Ellrodt and colleagues,[25] the work of Lamb and Zazworsky,[28] and the work of Kongstvedt.[3]

The approach suggested by Ellrodt and colleagues is of particular value because it is evidence based and well suited for respiratory care. The Ellrodt model includes the following characteristics: a multidisciplinary team of healthcare workers to define the problem; a process to search, select, appraise, and summarize the relevant literature to develop practice guidelines, pathways, and algorithms; implementation of the guidelines, pathways, and algorithms; and development of a method to measure and report process and outcome measures that inform the quality improvement exercise (**Box 30–4**).[25]

The first step taken to create a disease management program in this model is to define the clinical and economic scope of the condition. What is the economic cost to society? How large a population is affected? Which patients should be included in the program? What critical interventions are likely to improve clinical and economic outcomes? What is the problem and what are the realistic goals or desired outcomes of the disease management process? Additionally, team composition is crucial, and involvement of all relevant caregivers should be ensured. Typically, the team includes a physician, a nurse, a respiratory therapist, a financial and actuarial professional, and individuals with marketing and communications expertise.

After the scope is defined and the team assembled, data must be garnered on current practice patterns, patient outcomes, and resource utilization. Ascertaining prevailing practices and accurately measuring the impact of the program is important. At this point in the process, the team needs to develop questions regarding clinical and economic measures related to the condition. In the case of asthma, what medications are appropriate? What mode of medication delivery is most effective? Which medications are most cost-effective? Critical and insightful questions must be asked.

The next step is literature reviews that are systematic, comprehensive, and rigorous. The results of the search require critical appraisal and finally a summary of the findings. The summary should include a description of the design, population, intervention, and outcomes of each study. The conclusions and recommendations are graded to indicate the quality of the evidence. After the summary, the team considers the anticipated benefits, harm, and costs in light of local practice and administrative constraints. In the absence of high-quality research, patient values are considered.

The team then attempts to gain consensus on the results of the effort and to format the findings into practice guidelines. The guidelines should reflect the best scientific evidence (from controlled clinical trials, the medical literature, and outcome-validated databases) concerning which clinical processes have achieved the best results for the best expenditure of resources. The guidelines and protocols should be user friendly and widely disseminated. The practice guidelines are converted to pathways that become timed and sequenced events. Algorithms entail conditional responses and are generally if-then statements.

The impact of the effort should be measured and a system of reporting the results determined. Key questions must be addressed. What will be measured? Who will do the measuring? Who will report the findings? How will it be reported? The intention is to compare the actual outcomes measured after the intervention with the original goals.

BOX 30–4

Steps in the Development of a Disease Management Program

1. Formulate a clear definition of the disease, its scope, and its impact over time using a multidisciplinary team.
2. Develop comprehensive baseline information to understand current healthcare delivery and resource utilization.
3. Generate specific clinical and economic questions and search the literature.
4. Critically appraise and synthesize the evidence.
5. Evaluate the benefits, harms, and costs.
6. Develop evidence-based practice guidelines, clinical pathways, and algorithms.
7. Create a system for process and outcome measurement and reporting.
8. Implement the evidence-based guidelines, pathways, and algorithms.
9. Complete the quality improvement cycle.

Another step in the development of a disease management program entails facilitation of the implementation of the guidelines, pathways, and algorithms into clinical practice. The intention is to communicate the intervention (guidelines, pathways, and algorithms) in a manner most likely to change clinical decision making. This step is often underrated. The most important variables are message content, the media for delivery, and feedback. Even the most rigorously validated evidence-based guidelines must be recast into an appropriate format to influence the clinical decision-making behavior of clinicians and patients.

Clinicians prefer to receive short manuals, executive summaries of guideline recommendations, or a synopsis of the supporting evidence and quantification of the expected benefits. Involving respected peers and opinion leaders is an important consideration used to gain acceptance and compliance; this has proven to be an effective way to change practice patterns.

Steps are essential to ensure compliance with the evidence-based practice guidelines. Compliance can be undermined for a number of reasons. Clinicians may be unaware of the guidelines, they may lack confidence in the recommendations because of controversy or divergence in the literature, or inefficiencies or barriers in the system may preclude their use. Updated literature searches and feedback on outcome measures should be periodically provided.

A second approach to disease management, known as the FAST approach, was proposed by Lamb and Zazworsky,[28] who identified four components of disease management. The FAST approach is action oriented and based on the assumption that to effectively care for at-risk populations, there must be a system in place for rapid identification, triage, monitoring, and communication.[29] The four components are find, assess, stratify, and treat/train/track.

RESPIRATORY RECAP

The FAST Approach to Disease Management

» Find
» Assess
» Stratify
» Treat/train/track

The first component is to identify high risk, high-volume populations using multiple sources, including service use data, pharmacy data, and easy-access referral forms in physician offices. The second component is to conduct a brief assessment to determine the risk for hospitalization, severe complications of chronic illness, and skilled facility placement. The third component is stratification, in which the disease manager matches patients to clinical interventions according to risk level. The fourth component is to treat, train, and track. The disease manager should determine the appropriate treatment regimens as well as train patients to care for themselves and track the progression or regression of their condition. The FAST approach has been heralded as a systematic, organized, and simple process to follow in the implementation of a disease management program.[29]

The work of Kongstvedt[3] indicates that there are basically two primary delivery options in disease management: in-house programs and outsourced programs. Outsourced programs represent a larger market segment. The essential elements common to most programs are condition prioritization, participant identification, recruitment and engagement, interaction and management, documentation, information technology support, and reporting.

Condition prioritization entails claims analysis and understanding which major diagnostic categories are the largest drivers of claims. Feasibility analysis is performed and entails treatment decisions that are evidence based and assurance that behavior modification can be accomplished at an acceptable overhead cost. Participant identification occurs by applying algorithms that identify candidates projected to become high cost. The resulting candidates are screened by disease managers, and a plan for intensity of outreach resources is developed. Recruitment and engagement occur either through an opt-in model, in which the candidate initiates enrollment, or an opt-out method, in which enrollment is automatic based on an algorithm, but the candidate can decline to participate.

Interaction and management are considered the most important activities of the disease manager. These elements entail a call center professional who interviews patients and motivates them to adhere to their medical regimen. The interaction and management phase can involve calls or mailings to participants or physicians, or both. Additionally, it could entail home monitoring and medication adherence technology. The documentation phase entails documenting each participant's risk stratification and establishing a level of severity to determine call frequency. Information technology support is critical and entails creation of automated care plans, the disease manager's ability to view claim history, and the participants' electronic medical records. The final phase is reporting, in which disease managers produce fulfillment reports, which include activity and participation (e.g., call frequencies, mailings).

Box 30–5 lists the essential elements common to most disease management programs.

Barriers and Opportunities

Box 30–6 lists the major barriers to implementation of disease management,[30] and **Box 30–7** provides opportunities as identified by the Disease Management Association of America.[31] We will elaborate on the opportunities.

In *Managing Disease: A Comprehensive Guide*, Lisa Greenberg alludes to national opportunities as well as industry-specific opportunities for disease management. One of the national opportunities entails linking financial rewards to performance and doing so at all levels, such physicians, consumers, health plans, and government.

BOX 30–5

Essential Elements Common to Most Disease Management Programs

Condition prioritization
Participant identification
Recruitment and engagement
Interaction and management
Documentation
Information technology support
Reporting

From Kongstvedt P. *Essentials of Managed Care.* 5th ed. Sudbury, MA: Jones & Bartlett Learning; 2007:235–239. Reprinted with permission.

BOX 30–6

Barriers to the Implementation of Disease Management

Fragmented reimbursement
Short-term orientation
Fragmented delivery
Physician resistance
Patient indifference
Inadequate information technology

Data from Institute for the Future. *Health and Healthcare 2010: The Forecast, The Challenge.* San Francisco: Jossey-Bass; 2000.

She speculates that physicians will be rewarded through pay for performance (P4P), adopted to incentivize the physician community to engage more effectively in chronic care management. Consumers are more likely to be engaged through health savings accounts, designed to encourage consumers to use healthcare services more wisely. The government's role is encouraged through the Medicare Health Support pilot programs, which are designed to reach out to high-need consumers, such as the elderly, poor, and racial and ethnic minorities.

A second national level opportunity is the development of an interoperable health information infrastructure as the platform for integrated, coordinated, and more effective healthcare delivery. Simply stated, communicating information in real time across different providers of care—such as hospitals, ambulatory care, and disease management organizations—will have a huge impact to the disease management movement and to the realization of an effective healthcare delivery system.

BOX 30–7

Opportunities for Disease Management

Linking financial rewards to performance at all levels
Developing an interoperable healthcare information infrastructure as the platform for integrated, coordinated, and more effective healthcare delivery
Expanding comorbidity management and wellness programs
Increasing use of decision support information, monitoring, and behavioral change approaches
Adopting systems-based approaches for improving quality and reducing disparities

Data from Disease Management Association of America. *Managing Disease: A Comprehensive Guide.* Washington, DC: DMAA; 2007.

Industry-specific opportunities entail expanding comorbidity management and wellness programs; increasing the use of decision support information, monitoring, and behavioral change approaches; and adopting systems-based approaches to improving quality and reduce disparity. The former issue is best represented by recognizing that diseases (such as COPD) are frequently coupled or accompanied with mental diseases (such as depression), so it is critical to integrate physical and behavioral medicine to address such conditions. With regard to the second industry-specific opportunity, it should be noted that consumers will increasingly be required to make independent decisions about their care. They need to be better informed and, thus, disease management can provide this much-needed information, allowing the consumer to make better and more accurate decisions regarding effective and appropriate management of their condition. The final industry-specific opportunity entails tying evidence-based medicine, rather than ability to pay or other factors, into the provision of care. Disease managers can continue to create and employ best techniques for reaching out to and supporting sustainable behavioral change to improve quality to all consumers especially the underserved population.[31]

Respiratory Therapists as Disease Managers

Respiratory therapists are bedside specialists in the care and treatment of the patient with cardiopulmonary disease. Their experience and expertise make them the ideal professionals to engage in cardiopulmonary disease management and care coordination. An opportunity exists for them to position themselves for such a role, and they would be wise to embrace the merits of the disease management movement.

KEY POINTS

- The two major forces driving disease management are escalating healthcare costs and the changing patterns of cardiopulmonary diseases.
- The origin and evolution of the disease management movement are rooted in the pharmaceutical industry and managed care organizations.
- *Care management* is an umbrella term for component management, demand management, case management, and disease management.
- Component management is episodic, uncoordinated, and focuses on treatment versus prevention.
- The tools of demand management are patient-driven protocols, clinical pathways, case management, and disease management.
- Case management focuses on an individual patient and is expensive.
- Disease management focuses on subpopulations of patients and emphasizes coordinated comprehensive care along the continuum of disease and across healthcare delivery systems.
- The challenge of disease management is to apply a gradation of resources to members of the population so that each does not get too little (low quality) or too much (high cost), but just the right (high quality) amount of care.
- The goal of healthcare is to provide value, defined as quality outcomes per unit of cost.
- The principles of disease management include an understanding of the course, cause, and cost drivers of a disease; diagnoses and treatment based on the disease process; emphasis on patient education and compliance for chronic disease management; management across care settings with full continuity of care; and direction of resources to proven methodologies.
- The cost drivers of a disease are compliance, prevention, rapid resolution, acute flare-ups, and the fact that 80% of the costs are produced by 20% of diseases.
- Disease management programs entail assembly of a multidisciplinary team to define the problem, an extensive search of the literature, development of guidelines and protocols, implementation of the guidelines and protocols, and assessment of the process and outcomes measures.

REFERENCES

1. Centers for Medicare and Medicaid Services. National health expenditures aggregate, per capita amounts, percent distribution, and average annual percent growth, by source of funds: selected calendar years 1960–2008. Available at: http://www.cms.hhs.gov/NationalHealthExpendData/downloads/tables.pdf.
2. Geyman JP. Disease management: panacea, another false hope, or something in between? *Ann Fam Med*. 2007;5:257–260.
3. Kongstvedt P. *Essentials of Managed Care*. 5th ed. Sudbury, MA: Jones & Bartlett Learning; 2007:234.
4. McGinnis JM, Foege WH. Actual causes of death in the United States. *JAMA*. 1993;270:2208.
5. Mokdad AH, Marks JS, Stroup DF, Gerberding JL. Actual causes of death in the United States, 2000. *JAMA*. 2004;291:1238–1245.
6. Shi L, Singh D. *Delivering Health Care in America: A Systems Approach*. 3rd ed. Sudbury, MA: Jones & Bartlett Learning; 2004.
7. Boston Consulting Group. *The Changing Environment for Pharmaceuticals*. Boston: Boston Consulting Group; 1993.
8. Couch JB. *The Physician's Guide to Disease Management*. Gaithersburg, MD: Aspen; 1997.
9. Phillips L. Disease management: the next step in managed care depends on information sharing. *J AHIMA*. 1996;67:44–46.
10. Johnson SK. The state of disease state management. *Case Rev*. Fall 1996:53–55.
11. Lumsdon K. Disease management: the heat and heartaches of retooling patient care create hard labor. *Hosp Health Networks*. April 5, 1995:34–42.
12. Patterson R. Disease management. *Case Rev*. Fall 1995.
13. Ward M, Rieve J. Disease management: case management's return to patient-centered care. *Care Management*. 1995;1:8.
14. Bunch D. Demand management tools help providers lower costs of care. *AARC Times*. 1996;20(12):24–27.
15. Kongstvedt P. *Essentials of Managed Health Care*. 2nd ed. Gaithersburg, MD: Aspen; 1997.
16. O'Brien K. Asthma management: a new paradigm. *Case Rev*. March/April 1998:16, 18, 59, 60.
17. Durbin CG. The role of the respiratory care practitioner in the continuum of disease management. *Respir Care*. 1997;42:159–165.
18. Disease Management Association of America. DMAA definition of disease management. Available at: http://www.dmaa.org/dm_definition.asp.
19. Zitter M. Disease management: a new approach to health care. *Med Interface*. August 1994:70–76.
20. Meyer LC, Rohl B. An innovative approach to treating chronic disabling asthma. *Case Manager*. 1993;4:54–69.
21. Buxton MJ. The economics of asthma: an introduction. *Eur Respir Rev*. 1995;6:105–107.
22. Greenberg RN. Overview of patient compliance with medication dosing: a literature review. *Clin Ther*. 1984;6:592–599.
23. McKenny JM, Harrison TL. Drug-related hospital admissions. *Am J Hosp Pharm*. 1976:33:792–795.
24. Muma RD, Lyons BA. *Patient Education: A Practical Approach*. 2nd ed. Sudbury, MA: Jones & Bartlett Learning; 2012.
25. Ellrodt G, Cook D, Lee J, et al. Evidence-based disease management. *JAMA*. 1997;278:1687.
26. Evidence-Based Working Group. Evidence-based medicine: a new approach to teaching the practice of medicine. *JAMA*. 1992;268:2420–2425.
27. Dubbs WH. Disease management: a proven strategy for reducing costs, enhancing care. *AARC Times*. 1996;20(12):30–33.
28. Lamb GS, Zazworsky D. Improving outcomes fast: the FAST approach to disease management. *Adv Providers Post-Acute Care*. 2000;3(11):28–29.
29. Cesta TG. *Survival Strategies for Nurses in Managed Care*. St. Louis: Mosby; 2002:392.
30. Institute for the Future. *Health and Healthcare 2010: The Forecast, the Challenge*. San Francisco: Jossey-Bass; 2000.
31. Disease Management Association of America. *Managing Disease: A Comprehensive Guide*. Washington, DC: DMAA; 2007.

CHAPTER 31

Patient Education

William F. Galvin

OUTLINE

OBJECTIVES

1. State the rationale for patient education in the practice of respiratory care.
2. Define patient education and related terms, using several sources.
3. List the goals of patient education from the patient's perspective and that of the provider (i.e., the respiratory therapy educator).
4. Identify the four major components of the patient education process.
5. Assess the learning needs of a patient.
6. Identify the factors that can adversely affect learner readiness.
7. Discuss the planning phase of the patient education process, specifically, the development of goals and objectives, use of learning domains, content development, and evaluation.
8. Identify and explain the appropriate use of various teaching strategies in patient education.
9. Identify and discuss the nine basic principles of adult learning.
10. Discuss the evaluation phase of the patient education process, namely, evaluation as a process and evaluation of individual learning.
11. Explain how patient education can be incorporated into asthma education, pulmonary rehabilitation, and smoking cessation.

KEY TERMS

affective domain
assessment
behavioral contracting
behavior modification
client education
clinical practice guidelines
cognitive domain
consumer education
disease prevention
documentation
evaluation
health belief model
health promotion
illness/wellness continuum
implementation
locus of control
motivation
motivational interviewing (MI)
patient education
planning
PRECEDE-PROCEED model
prevention
programmed instruction
psychomotor domain
self-instructional
teaching moment
wellness

INTRODUCTION

Patient education plays an important role in the delivery of healthcare. The goal of this chapter is to better prepare respiratory therapists to assist patients and caregivers in assuming an effective role in prevention, care, rehabilitation, and health promotion. The focus of the chapter is the increasing importance of self-care and the need to help patients develop the ability to care for themselves. Today's patients must be knowledgeable and self-sufficient; therefore, healthcare providers must effectively transfer to them the necessary knowledge, skills, and attitudes.

The following sections provide an overview of all aspects of patient education. The areas addressed include definitions of patient education terminology; an explanation of the purpose, goals, objectives, and rationale for patient education; and a detailed discussion of the four major components of the patient education process. Emphasis is placed on assessment of a patient's needs, planning for instruction, identification and removal of barriers to teaching and learning, implementing teaching/learning strategies, and acquisition of an understanding of the basic principles of adult learning. The chapter concludes with a brief description of how patient education can be incorporated into asthma education, pulmonary rehabilitation, and smoking cessation.

Making the Case for Patient Education

Self-Management and Self-Empowerment

The traditional view of healthcare was rather paternalistic: the healthcare provider was considered the expert and the only one capable of determining the care and management of the patient. This provider, usually a physician, was considered to know what was best for patients, was solely responsible for making decisions, and did not share information with or involve patients in their own care or treatment except as recipients. Simply stated, the patient was outside the healthcare system and was not involved in the process. Patients were controlled by the experts—by the system.

Although much of the practice of medicine clearly is the responsibility of the healthcare expert, more-contemporary thinking supports the idea that there are many stakeholders in the provision of healthcare. Perhaps the most crucial stakeholders are the patients themselves. Patients must be educated and equipped to assume greater control over their health and well-being. They must come to understand that the healthcare system of the future requires personal responsibility, ownership, and a greater degree of self-empowerment. In short, healthcare requires self-control rather than other-control.

RESPIRATORY RECAP

The Need for Patient Education

- The healthcare system of the future requires personal responsibility, accountability, ownership, and a greater degree of self-empowerment.
- In short, healthcare requires a greater degree of self-management.

Forces Affecting the Patient Education Movement

Enabling patients to assume greater responsibility for their healthcare is a theme that has taken on increasing importance over the years. Patient education programs are the fastest-growing component of the healthcare system. In 1970 about 50 hospitals in the United States had patient education programs; now almost all healthcare institutions engage in some form of patient education activity.[1] This increasing emphasis has been driven by economic, social, demographic, regulatory and legal, philosophic, and practical considerations (**Box 31–1**).

The current system clearly is driven by economic incentives to curtail costs and reduce a healthcare budget that is spiraling out of control. In 2006, healthcare expenditures in the United States represented 15.5% of the gross domestic product, over $2.1 trillion, and $7,026 per person.[2] More and more, costs and risk are being shifted to the consumer and away from employers, insurers, and providers.

BOX 31–1

Rationale for Patient Education in Respiratory Care

Economic incentive: Reimbursement requirements are shifting to an emphasis on greater patient involvement and patient accountability.

Social incentive: The consumer education movement and a well-informed public have demanded such education.

Demographic incentive: Given the "graying of America," the number of people requiring healthcare has risen, and the use of informal caregivers (families and friends) has increased.

Regulatory and legal incentives: Patient education is a requirement of the Joint Commission.

Philosophic incentive: The wellness model of healthcare has become more popular than the traditional healthcare model, and self-management of one's own health has become an important issue.

Practical incentives: Patients prefer to care for themselves, and it is more sensible and easy for them to participate in their own care.

Demographic factors mean that an increasing number of people, namely those of the baby boom generation, are approaching their retirement years, often developing chronic, debilitating diseases that create significant healthcare needs. This places considerable economic tension on a healthcare delivery system that is already strained. The care and treatment of this elderly population will come from a variety of sources, among them informal caregivers, assisted living providers, and unskilled healthcare extenders. These new providers will require a more sophisticated understanding of the conditions and diseases affecting the elderly population.

From legislative and social perspectives, more emphasis is being placed on consumer education. The public is becoming better informed and is demanding more information about the consequences of unhealthy lifestyle behaviors. Regulatory agencies, such as the Joint

Commission, have established policies and requirements for patient education and have withheld accreditation for serious neglect of such programs.

Philosophically and practically, **disease prevention** and **health promotion** appear to be logical, cost-effective ways to curtail healthcare costs. Adoption of a disease prevention and health promotion philosophy helps instill in patients some degree of responsibility for and ownership of their health and **wellness**. Assuming individual responsibility for and having a greater degree of involvement in one's own healthcare is simply good medicine. Likewise, increasing the number of well-informed patients and caregivers goes a long way toward improving the efficiency and effectiveness of healthcare in the United States. With these points in mind, it seems only logical that effective patient education should be considered an integral component of the healthcare system.

Role of the Respiratory Therapist

Bedside clinician, astute diagnostician, resourceful technical expert, and troubleshooter are the well-established roles of the respiratory therapist. The more contemporary view includes the roles of patient advocate, care coordinator, counselor, and patient educator.

The role of patient educator has been often de-emphasized, frequently misunderstood, seldom appreciated, and not uncommonly absent from the array of duties and responsibilities of today's respiratory therapist. However, as discussed previously, patient education is assuming new prominence and will be of paramount importance in future healthcare practice. Healthcare providers with sophisticated teaching skills and a savvy ability to assess patients' educational needs will be held in high esteem. Equally important will be the ability to develop educational goals, communicate accurately and effectively, and ensure that patients have an understanding of their disease and comply with treatment.

> **RESPIRATORY RECAP**
>
> **Roles of Respiratory Therapists in Patient Education**
>
> » Bedside clinician
> » Diagnostician
> » Technical expert
> » Troubleshooter
> » Patient advocate
> » Care coordinator
> » Counselor
> » Patient educator

Respiratory therapists are considered the nonphysician experts in cardiorespiratory care. Their continual presence at the patient's bedside enables them to assume greater responsibility for effective patient education. Respiratory therapists must recognize that patient education is not a game of show-and-tell. It requires three important attributes: (1) savvy, sophisticated skills and knowledge of the teaching and learning process; (2) an understanding of motivational theory and what makes people tick; and (3) an appreciation of the principles of adult learning. Respiratory therapists must develop a greater appreciation for the significant role they play in the patient education movement.

Definition of Terms

Client Education, Consumer Education, and Patient Education

Patient education is more than the provision of information about a disease or condition.[3] It also is more than simple identification of common signs and symptoms and explanations of therapeutic interventions. Patient education is a process with succinct, discrete steps that must be followed to engage the patient effectively in the important function of self-management.[3] Before describing this process, this discussion focuses on terminology, clarifies discrepancies, and provides working definitions of the key components of patient education.

A number of terms frequently are associated with patient education. Two particularly important ones are *client education* and *consumer education*. **Client education** has been defined as the use of the educational process for individuals who are partners in the health education effort.[4] Inherent in this definition is the notion that the teacher and learner work together to identify the issues to be taught and the manner in which the teaching is to be carried out. The term implies that the learner has some degree of autonomy and is self-directed.

> **RESPIRATORY RECAP**
>
> **Definitions Used in Patient Education**
>
> » *Client education*: the use of the educational process to aid individuals who are partners in the health education effort
> » *Consumer education*: the use of the educational process by a person or a group of people who are independent decision makers
> » *Patient education*: the use of the educational process to aid individuals, their families, and other significant persons when they become dependent on the healthcare system for diagnosis, treatment, or rehabilitation

The term **consumer education** is closely related to client education but differs in that it involves a person or a group of people who are independent decision makers; they identify the health learning need and initiate the learning process. The teacher facilitates the learning process.[4]

Patient education has been defined in a number of ways, and authors emphasize or highlight different components of their definitions. For example, one author defines it as the use of the educational process to aid individuals, their families, and other significant persons when they become dependent on the healthcare system for diagnosis, treatment, or rehabilitation.[4]

The three terms can be distinguished on the basis of the amount of teaching assistance that learners require to

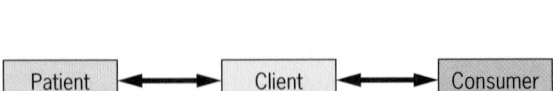

FIGURE 31–1 Level of learner dependency. From Boyd MD, et al. *Health Teaching in Nursing Practice: A Professional Model.* 3rd ed. Appleton & Lange. © 1998. Electronically reproduced by permission of Pearson Education, Inc., Upper Saddle River, New Jersey.

make behavioral changes. As shown in **Figure 31–1**, consumers are highly independent and capable of exercising considerable self-responsibility, whereas patients are more dependent and require more teaching assistance; clients fall somewhere in between.

In both consumer and client education, the healthcare provider or professional serves as a facilitator, assists in decision making, acts as a resource person, and gives encouragement and support to ideas the individual already has. In patient education, the learner is highly dependent on the healthcare provider or professional and frequently has little if any knowledge of the content to be learned. In such situations the healthcare provider or professional may well need to direct the teaching process almost entirely.

Illness/Wellness Continuum

Another view of patient education is the **illness/wellness continuum** proposed by Travis and Ryan.[5] In this model, health is viewed both from a medical perspective and from a wellness perspective (**Figure 31–2**). The left side of the continuum represents the medical model of health; it starts at the neutral point, the center of the continuum. The neutral point represents the absence of any physical disease; at this point, the individual is considered healthy. On moving to the left, the individual is exposed to certain risks, which become signs and symptoms. If left untreated, they lead to disability and eventually to premature death.

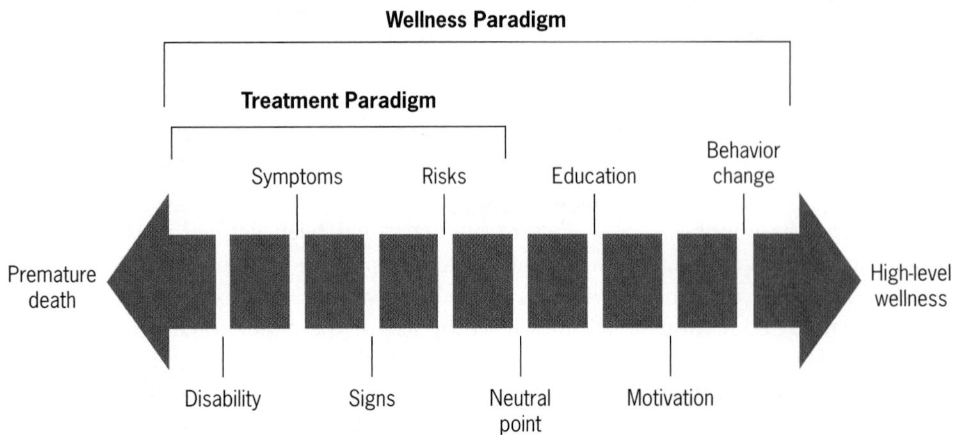

FIGURE 31–2 Illness/wellness continuum. Adapted with permission from Illness/Wellness Continuum in *Wellness Workbook, 3rd edition*, by John W. Travis, MD, and Regina Sara Ryan (Celestial Arts, 2004). © 1981, 1988, 2004 by John W. Travis. www.wellnessworkbook.com

The entire continuum reflects a wellness model of health. It signifies that health is more than the absence of disease; rather, it is a state of high-level wellness over which the individual has considerable control. The person can choose to follow a lifestyle that incorporates health promotion and disease prevention principles and measures. The individual who adopts the wellness model would become knowledgeable about healthy lifestyle practices, would be sufficiently motivated to incorporate such practices into his or her daily routine, would use **behavior modification** techniques as needed, and ultimately would enjoy a higher level of wellness and well-being.

An example from respiratory disease may help clarify the importance of this continuum. The traditional view of health holds that the absence of disease exists at the neutral point. A man who begins smoking has moved to the left and incurred a risk factor for chronic obstructive pulmonary disease (COPD). Continued use of cigarettes could lead to increased production of mucus and shortness of breath (i.e., the signs and symptoms of the disease—another move to the left). Continued and unabated use of cigarettes could lead to the man's inability to walk up a single flight of stairs, at which point he becomes a pulmonary cripple, having a disability, which is yet another move left. Progression of this process ultimately leads to premature death. Rather than living to age 75, the normal life expectancy of men in the United States,[6] this man might die at age 65.

> **RESPIRATORY RECAP**
>
> **Wellness and Education**
>
> » The critical step in the wellness model is education.

In contrast to this scenario, let's say the individual as a boy or young man is taught that smoking is harmful to his health. If he accepts this and is motivated to ban smoking from his lifestyle, along with following other healthy practices, he will attain a state of well-being and ultimately high-level wellness. Furthermore, he can benefit even if he quits after several years of smoking. One study showed that men who quit smoking at age 40 lived just 1 year less than those who never smoked.[7] Men who stopped at 50 increased their life expectancy by 6 years, and men who stopped at 60 added an average of 3 years to their life. The point is that if our hypothetical individual is educated about the ill effects of smoking and is motivated to eliminate this unhealthy lifestyle behavior by modifying his behavior, he is likely to enjoy a more favorable, lengthy, and healthy existence. The critical step in the wellness model is education.

It is vital that patients be educated about their condition and about the ill effects of unhealthy lifestyle behaviors. Effective patient education can go a long way toward effectively engaging the patient in self-management, fostering a healthy lifestyle, and addressing health concerns.

Clinical Practice Guidelines

The American Association for Respiratory Care (AARC) defines patient education through **clinical practice guidelines** (**CPG 31-1** and **CPG 31-2**).[8,9] According to these guidelines, patient and caregiver training is a process initiated by the healthcare provider to help patients or caregivers acquire knowledge and skills that will help

CLINICAL PRACTICE GUIDELINE 31-1

Training the Healthcare Professional for the Role of Patient and Caregiver Educator

The process of training the healthcare professional as a patient or caregiver educator involves addressing and ensuring adequate knowledge, skills, and attitude mastery to allow both the development of patient rapport and effective teaching.

The ultimate goal of the process is to provide patients and caregivers with an education that equips them with the knowledge, skills, and attitudes to better understand the patient's condition and participate more fully in healthcare.

Modified from AARC clinical practice guideline: training the health care professional for the role of patient and caregiver educator. *Respir Care*. 1996;41:654–657. Reprinted with permission.

CLINICAL PRACTICE GUIDELINE 31-2

Providing Patient and Caregiver Training

Indications

- The presence of a patient population with the need to:
  - Increase knowledge and understanding of health status, disease pathophysiology, and therapy
  - Improve skills necessary for safe and effective healthcare (i.e., inability to perform needed therapy)
  - Foster a positive attitude, stronger motivation, and increase adherence to therapeutic modalities
  - Know the answers to "Ask Me 3:" What is my main problem?, What do I need to do?, and Why is it important for me to do this?

Contraindications

- There are no contraindications to patient and caregiver training when a need exists.

Hazards and Complications

- Omission of essential steps in care, inconsistency in information presented, or failure to validate the learning process can lead to untoward results
- Lack of cultural competence, materials in plain language, and information appropriate to the language needs of the patient and/or caregiver (including languages other than English and American sign language), which result in less than desirable outcomes
- Lack of trust by the patient, family or care provider of the medical team, institution, or individual instructor

Limitations

- Patient limitations:
  - Lack of motivation or interest in acquiring knowledge or skills
  - Impairment (e.g., in hearing or vision, poor dexterity, decreased energy, strength, learning defects or stamina, age-specific, pain, medication adverse effects)

(continues)

Clinical Practice Guideline 31–2 *(continued)*

- Inability to comprehend or lack of awareness due to factors such as anxiety, depression, hypoxemia, or substance abuse, which may include denial
    - Negative response to past educational experiences or encounters
    - Lack of health literacy, despite level of education completed, which may include functional illiteracy in dealing with the healthcare process
    - A mindset that leads to misapplication, misinterpretation, or rejection of instruction as irrelevant
    - Language that is different than that of the healthcare provider
    - Conflict of religious beliefs and/or cultural practices with material presented or manner in which it is presented
- Healthcare provider limitations:
    - Lack of positive attitude or adaptability
    - Limited understanding of knowledge or skill to be taught
    - Inadequate assessment of patient's need or readiness to learn as well as inability to individualize the instructional approach to the patient, including age-specific needs
    - Multiple patient needs and training goals to be met in the allotted time
    - Inappropriate or inadequate communication skills (e.g., unnecessary use of medical terminology, lack of listening skills)
    - Lack of documentation or discussion with other team members or inconsistency in information presented
    - Inadequate knowledge of cultural or religious practice that may affect educational process, communication, or adherence to the plan of care
    - Inadequate teaching skills of the healthcare provider/respiratory therapist conducting the training
- System limitations:
    - Hospital stay too brief
    - Absence of interdisciplinary cooperation and communication
    - Inconsistency in information provided
    - Failure to coordinate the assistance of family or community-based interpreters
    - Education and training started too late in the discharge planning process
- Psychosocial limitations:
    - Absence of support system
    - Reimbursement issues
- Environmental limitations:
    - Inadequate lighting, poor temperature control, uncomfortable seating, or inadequate space for demonstrations
    - Interruptions, distractions, and noise that interrupt the learning environment
    - Failure to use trained interpreters
    - Failure to provide translated vital materials for language groups meeting the numerical threshold
    - Poorly chosen resources, including inappropriate reading level and vocabulary

Recommendations

- The following recommendation is made following the Grading of Recommendations Assessment, Development, and Evaluation (GRADE) criteria:
    - Level 1. It is suggested that respiratory therapists take an active role in educating patient, family, and caregivers in the management of their cardiopulmonary disease state.

Modified from AARC clinical practice guideline: providing patient and caregiver training. *Respir Care.* 2010;55(6):765–769. Reprinted with permission.

them understand the patient's medical condition and participate in its management. This training process should occur with every encounter.[8]

Teaching and Learning Aspects of Patient Education

Although patient education can be defined in numerous ways, it always entails teaching. Teaching, whether done formally or informally, is a process that facilitates learning. Learning is the process of acquiring new knowledge, skills, and attitudes, which are synthesized to bring about a change in an individual's behavior.[10] This change in behavior ultimately results in patients living longer and more productively.

Unfortunately, too often healthcare providers think that teaching a patient or family member means telling them about the diagnosis or condition and what can be done about it. Certainly, explaining the facts about a diagnosis or condition is important, but it is not likely by itself to produce a change in the patient's behavior. Furthermore, this type of teaching generally is done hurriedly and at the convenience of the provider, not that of the patient or family members. Often little regard is shown for privacy or comprehension of the subject matter. The provider receives no assurance that learning has occurred.

> **RESPIRATORY RECAP**
>
> **Learning**
>
> » Teaching facilitates learning.
>
> » The foundation for learning is behavior change.

Patient education should be viewed as an orderly, sequential process, whether done in the formal setting of a classroom or in an informal manner at the bedside. Healthcare educators must rid themselves of the notion that simply informing patients of their disease and the appropriate therapeutic interventions is effective patient education. Effective patient education can occur only when learning has occurred, resulting in a change in the patient's behavior. For learning to occur, teaching must entail a logical set of steps.

Indications and Goals in Patient Education

Although the indications for patient education are rather obvious and clear-cut, the goals should be considered from two distinct perspectives—those of the patient or informal caregiver and those of the healthcare professional. The caregiver usually is a person who plays a crucial role in the patient's life; this often is a family member or significant other, although the caregiver may not be legally related to the patient.[8] Important to note is that in most cases caregivers are not healthcare professionals; they usually are laypeople who are genuinely interested in the patient's health and well-being but who may not have a sophisticated understanding of the patient's disease or condition. The healthcare professional, on the other hand, does have an extensive knowledge of the particular health condition and has established some degree of competence in providing healthcare. The goals of these participants are different.

> **RESPIRATORY RECAP**
>
> **Goals of the Patient or Informal Caregiver**
>
> » To obtain accurate information about the patient's condition
>
> » To develop the ability to make appropriate health decisions
>
> » To learn skills and attitudes that foster self-care and appropriate use of health services
>
> » To alleviate anxiety and increase satisfaction in health matters and healthcare

The goals of the patient and caregiver are to (1) obtain accurate information about the condition, (2) develop the ability to make appropriate health decisions, (3) learn skills and attitudes that foster self-care and appropriate use of health services, and (4) alleviate anxiety and increase satisfaction with health matters and healthcare.[10]

The goals of the healthcare provider or professional are to (1) provide more effective and efficient healthcare, (2) improve patient compliance, (3) increase the patient's satisfaction with healthcare, (4) obtain informed consent when necessary, and (5) meet professional practice requirements.[10]

These two sets of goals work together toward the ultimate goal of the patient education process, that is, to equip the patient and caregiver with the knowledge, skills, and attitudes to better understand the patient's condition and to more fully participate in healthcare.[9] Teaching therefore is intended to foster change in the patient's adaptation to illness; it is a planned activity that is individualized to the learner's abilities, needs, resources, and support systems.[11]

> **RESPIRATORY RECAP**
>
> **Goals of the Healthcare Provider**
>
> » To provide more effective and efficient healthcare
>
> » To improve the patient's compliance with the therapeutic regimen
>
> » To increase the patient's satisfaction with healthcare
>
> » To obtain informed consent when necessary
>
> » To fulfill professional practice requirements

Process of Patient Education

Most resource materials on patient education describe it as a process. The parts vary somewhat, but most sources note four major components: assessment, planning, implementation, and evaluation. The acronym A PIE can be used as a mnemonic to better recall these four elements (**Figure 31–3**).

Overview: A PIE

Assessment is the process of collecting information to help plan and implement teaching activities. The healthcare provider must assess both the need for patient education and the readiness of the patient, or learner, to

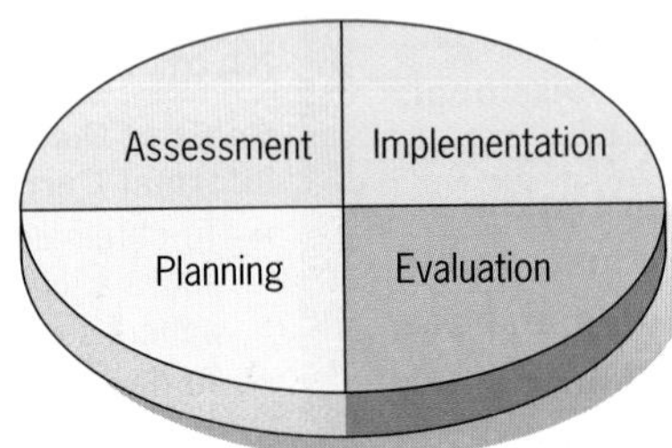

FIGURE 31–3 Major components of the patient education process.

benefit from it. Assessment requires extensive collection of data, including information about (1) the learner's readiness and ability to learn, (2) the learner's current knowledge of the subject, (3) what the learner wants to know about the subject, (4) any incorrect information or misconceptions the learner may have, and (5) the educational needs of both the learner and the family.[11]

Planning is the next step in the process and involves construction of an individualized patient education program. Planning involves identification of goals, development of objectives, addressing of the learning domains, and creation, development, and refining of the information to be covered.

Implementation is the third major component. It is the actual process of teaching and requires the use of a variety of teaching methods and tools.

Evaluation, the last of the four major components, enables the teacher to determine whether learning has occurred. It basically is a feedback loop set up by the method of evaluation developed during the planning stage.

Box 31–2 presents a more detailed outline of the four components and specific steps involved in each. The way in which the process is used varies from practitioner to practitioner, and seldom does an orderly, sequential flow come about. In their zeal to jump in and get started, respiratory therapy educators often skip from one component to another. More often than not the assessment component is overlooked, and the educator consequently becomes frustrated and discouraged when obstacles to learning are uncovered later in the process. Gross errors in the practice of patient education occur with some regularity. One author noted that such errors probably are made in the following order: omission of assessment of the patient's need to learn, followed by omission of a particular step (e.g., assessment of readiness, setting of goals, systematic evaluation of learning).[1] The actual implementation component rarely is omitted.

Completion of each component is critical to successful and effective patient education. The respiratory care educator should resist the temptation to take immediate action without proper assessment, planning, and evaluation and should be vigilant in thoroughly addressing each step.

BOX 31–2

Major Components of the Patient Education Process

Assessment

Assess the need for patient education.

Assess the readiness of the learner for patient education.

Planning

Establish goals and objectives.

Determine use of learning domains (cognitive, psychomotor, and affective).

Select content.

Implementation

Choose teaching methods.

Establish types of learning.

Ensure therapeutic use of time.

Determine learning needs of staff members.

Evaluation

Evaluate patient education process.

Evaluate individual learning:

- Written tests
- Teaching checklist
- Oral questioning
- Observational checklist
- Documentation
- Interdisciplinary patient education/family education record

Assessment

No reputable physician would prescribe a therapeutic intervention before performing a thorough diagnostic evaluation. It is equally important for the respiratory therapy educator to assess the patient's educational needs before launching into a detailed and elaborate discussion of the disease and its treatment. Assessment, the first component of the patient education process, addresses two distinct issues—the need for patient education and the patient's readiness to learn.

Assessment of the need for patient education is directed at identification of the specific content to be covered in the teaching process. Need identification can be complicated because the educator must distinguish between a real educational need and a felt need, something the person or persons concerned regard as necessary. A real educational need refers to a lack of specific knowledge, skills, and attitudes that the patient needs to attain a more desirable condition.[10] A real educational need is one that can be met by means of a learning experience. In other words, the patient must have a deficit in understanding, performance, or feelings

BOX 31-3

Common Assessment Questions

1. Do you understand your symptoms?
2. How did you first respond to the symptom?
3. Why do you think these symptoms have occurred?
4. Are you aware of any previous illness or conditions?
5. Are you aware of any family history or previous illnesses?
6. Are you aware of how your symptoms relate to your various laboratory, radiographic, and diagnostic tests?
7. What is your psychological state with regard to this condition?
8. How do you typically respond to worsening of your condition?
9. How has your illness affected family and friends?
10. Have you been provided with previous education about this condition? If so, by whom?
11. Have you responded to suggestions and recommended treatments?
12. What are your social habits?
13. Do you smoke?
14. Do you drink alcohol? If so, how much? How often?
15. Has your condition affected your employment?
16. Can you read and write?
17. What is your highest level of education?
18. Do you understand the illness and its treatment?
19. Is English the primary language spoken in your home?
20. Are your beliefs or practices affected by any particular cultural influences?
21. Do you have adequate medical coverage?

If the patient is too young or is unable to answer any or all of these questions, the caregiver may provide the answers.

about the health condition, testing, procedures, treatment, or prognosis. The assessment process addresses these issues, and the information derived helps in the planning and development of the lesson plan and learning objectives.

Assessment can be accomplished through direct questioning of the patient, consultation with family members, collaboration with other healthcare professionals, and review of medical records and patient information sources. Conferring directly with the patient or a family member is a technique that should not be taken lightly, because many variables influence the communication process, as is addressed in Chapter 60.

The educator must assess the deficits in the patient's understanding of the disease and its manifestations, progression, and resolution, a process best done systematically with some type of standardized document. **Box 31–3** presents a list of questions that can be used in the patient assessment process. The list is fairly extensive, yet additional questioning may be necessary and appropriate, depending on the patient's disease or condition.

A standardized document also can be used to assess the educator's capabilities and limitations. The sample rating form for a patient education session shown in **Figure 31–4** identifies some critical points used to evaluate the respiratory therapist as a patient educator. Parts 1, 5, and 6 list some of the key factors to be addressed during the opening interview and the use of appropriate counseling techniques. Parts 2, 3, and 4 focus on the educator's assessment of the patient's awareness and understanding of the medical condition.

In discussing the issues on this checklist with the patient, the educator essentially is covering the presenting signs and symptoms; the patient's health history; the physical assessment; laboratory, radiographic, and diagnostic tests; evidence of any previous patient education; evidence of compliance or noncompliance; and the patient's sociocultural and economic status. This checklist is quite useful to assess the performance of the respiratory therapy as a patient educator, but more detailed evaluation points could be added.

Any program, survey, checklist, or questionnaire that helps the respiratory therapy educator perform a thorough assessment is a valuable tool; omitting this first and crucial step can be catastrophic. A thorough assessment prevents backpedaling during the implementation phase, contributes to the development of an effective action plan, and aids the effort to have patients assume responsibility for their care.

Directions: Rate the patient educator's performance in each of the following areas. Using the scale below, place the appropriate number in the space next to each item. Comments and suggestions should be noted to allow for improvement where necessary.

Weak <---> **Outstanding**

1 2 3 4 5 6 7 8 9 10

1. Opening of the interview
   - Ability to put the patient at ease
   - Use of social amenities
   - Use of eye contact
   - Professional demeanor
   - Layout of plan
2. Discussion of disease
   - Assessment of what patient wants
   - Assessment of patient's attitudes/feelings
   - Reporting of laboratory findings
   - Explanation of pathophysiology
   - Use of vocabulary appropriate to patient
   - Correctness of information
   - Assessment of patient's final understanding
3. Treatment
   - Presentation of complete plan
   - Presentation of treatment goals
   - Explanation of side effects/complications
   - Treatment individualized to patient
   - Assessment of patient compliance
   - Correctness of information
   - Assessment of patient's final understanding
4. Assessment of patient's understanding of disease and condition
   - Assessment of patient's overall understanding of disease and treatment
   - Assessment of patient's attitudes
   - Time allowed for questions
   - Flexibility in presentation
5. Appropriate use of counseling techniques
   - Attempts to clarify patient's statement
   - Reassurance and empathy
   - Appropriate use of silence
   - Appropriate vocabulary
   - Use of open-ended questions
   - Facilitation of behavior
   - Use of notes
   - Use of educational aids
   - Flexibility
   - Good use of probes
   - Good transitions
   - Appropriate pacing
   - Good use of summaries
   - Overall physical appearance
   - Nonverbal language
   - Appropriate use of patient's background
   - Clarification of the next step for patient
   - Request for questions
6. Overall effectiveness of patient counseling
   - Rapport building
   - Discussion of disease
   - Treatment program
   - Assessment of patient's understanding of disease and treatment
   - Use of counseling techniques
7. Comments and suggestions for improvement

FIGURE 31–4 Sample rating form for patient education session. From Muma RD, Lyons BA. *Patient Education: A Practical Approach.* 2nd ed. Jones & Bartlett Learning; 2012.

Readiness to Learn

Assessing the patient's readiness to learn can be a bit tricky. Some patients may mask their denial of the need for education and training or their unwillingness to accept it. Other patients may be willing but physically or mentally incapable of learning. The educator's time limitations may compound these problems. Factors that can adversely affect learner readiness are lack of awareness of the diagnosis, previous knowledge and experience of the disease, intellectual ability, motivational level, physical condition, psychological state, and lack of a perceived need to learn.[3] Other experts have identified similar problems of the learner, including lack of readiness, physical obstacles, emotional obstacles, language barriers, and lack of **motivation**.[11]

> **RESPIRATORY RECAP**
>
> **Factors That Adversely Affect Learner Readiness**
>
> » Lack of awareness of the diagnosis
> » Previous knowledge and experience of the disease
> » Intellectual ability
> » Motivational level
> » Physical condition
> » Psychological state
> » Lack of a perceived need to learn

Patients must always be assessed to determine what they know about their condition. Healthcare educators should not assume that patients understand the nature of their disease. For example, patients with COPD often simply say that they have something wrong with their lungs. They may or may not fully understand the source and extent of their condition. A wise healthcare educator always starts with an open-ended question that allows patients to state what they know about the illness. Such a question might be, "What have you been told about your illness?"

> **RESPIRATORY RECAP**
>
> **Common Problems of the Learner**
>
> » Lack of readiness
> » Physical obstacles
> » Emotional obstacles
> » Language barriers
> » Lack of motivation

The educator also should question patients closely about any previous knowledge or experience with the illness or condition. The educator might ask, "Did any family members have a similar problem? What do you remember about their experiences? Were they able to work? Were they hospitalized frequently? Were they severely debilitated?" These factors are likely to have influenced the way the patient views the condition and the way in which he or she deals with it.

The respiratory therapy educator also should take into account the patient's intellectual level, which affects the ability to comprehend the illness and determines the teaching approach. A plumber with COPD who needs frequent suctioning might be more responsive if the situation is compared to the clogging of a pipe, with the resultant drainage problem and obstruction of water flow. Asking a family member to breathe through a straw for a minute or so can be quite effective in having that person live the experience of severe bronchoconstriction. Most people do not understand the complicated jargon used to describe medical conditions; therefore, the teaching approach must match the patient's intellectual level.

Health Literacy

Walking into a physician's office or through the doors of the emergency department does not ensure access to healthcare. For healthcare to be truly effective, the patient must understand what is being said and must be engaged in his or her care. Until recently, this lack of understanding and disengagement on the part of the patient had gone largely unrecognized. However, numerous articles, surveys, reports, and publications have brought attention to this disturbing and alarming problem, resulting in a call to action and interest in the topic of health literacy.

Health literacy is the ability to obtain, process, and understand basic health information and services needed to make appropriate healthcare decisions and follow instructions for treatment.[12] The genesis of the health literacy issue dates back to 1993, with the federal government's release of the landmark report *Adult Literacy in America*. This report surveyed approximately 26,000 adults in the United States, asking them to perform tasks such as identifying a particular intersection on a street map, finding an expiration date on a license, or simply demonstrating the ability to sign one's name. Participants were categorized into literacy levels, and the results demonstrated that 49.5% (almost 50%) were either functionally illiterate or marginally illiterate; approximately 90 million Americans were estimated to have limited literacy skills.[13]

> **RESPIRATORY RECAP**
>
> **Definition of Health Literacy**
>
> » The ability to obtain, process, and understand basic health information and services needed to make appropriate healthcare decisions and follow instructions for treatment.

A sequel to this survey was performed in 2002 and entitled the National Assessment of Adult Literacy.[14] This survey consisted of approximately 19,000 individuals and was based on a comprehensive set of tasks to measure an individual's ability to read and understand text (prose literacy), interpret numbers (numeracy literacy), and interpret documents (document literacy). The findings were similarly categorized and the results equally alarming, with some 36% of the group categorized at the basic or below basic level and considered by the surveyors to be problematic.

> **RESPIRATORY RECAP**
>
> **Adult Literacy in America**
>
> » This landmark 1993 federal government report demonstrated that 49.5% (almost 50%) of adults in the United States were functionally or marginally illiterate.

In 2003 the American Medical Association (AMA) and the AMA Foundation released a report entitled *Health Literacy: A Manual for Clinicians*.[15] The results of this report were equally alarming and quite revealing. Of particular note was the identification of risk factors for limited literacy as well as behaviors and responses that may indicate limited literacy, or what the authors call "red flags." **Box 31–4** lists the key risk factors for limited literacy, and **Box 31–5** lists the behaviors and responses that indicate limited literacy.

> **RESPIRATORY RECAP**
>
> **National Assessment of Adult Literacy**
>
> » A sequel to the 1993 survey demonstrated equally alarming results: 36% of individuals surveyed were at the basic or below basic level and considered to have serious literacy problems.

The sequel to this first AMA/AMA Foundation publication was a 2007 publication entitled *Health Literacy and Patient Safety: Help Patients Understand*.[16] This document further substantiated the fact that we need to be more cognizant of the health literacy problem and more vigilant in our interaction with our patients, especially with regard to providing patient education.

The severity and magnitude of the health literacy problem caught the attention of the accreditation and regulatory agencies. In 2007, the Joint Commission published its own white paper, entitled "What Did the Doctor Say? Improving Health Literacy to Protect Patient Safety." The paper was considered a call to action for

BOX 31–4

Key Risk Factors for Limited Literacy

- Elderly
- Low income
- Unemployment
- Did not finish high school
- Minority ethnic group
- Recent immigrant to United States who does not speak English
- Born in United States but English is second language

Reprinted from Weiss B. *Help Patients Understand: A Manual for Clinicians.* 2nd ed. © 2007 American Medical Association Foundation and American Medical Association.

BOX 31–5

Behaviors and Responses That Indicate Limited Literacy

Patient registration forms that are incomplete or inaccurately completed
Frequently missed appointments
Noncompliance with medication regime
Lack of follow-through with test results or referrals to consultants
Aloofness or seeming disinterest
Patient indicates s/he is taking medications but lab tests and/or physiologic parameters do not reflect expected outcomes
Statements such as, "I forgot my glasses. I'll read this when I get home," "I forgot my glasses. Can you read this to me?" or "Let me bring this home so I can discuss it with my children"

Reprinted from Weiss B. *Help Patients Understand: A Manual for Clinicians.* 2nd ed. © 2007 American Medical Association Foundation and American Medical Association.

those who influence, develop, or carry out policies that lead the way to resolution of these issues.[17] Additionally, the Commission assembled a roundtable of experts, charging them with framing the issues that underlie the health literacy problem. The findings of these experts culminated in the development of the three recommendations highlighted in **Box 31–6**. The Commission indicated that effective communication is a cornerstone of patient safety and that Commission standards underscore the fundamental right and need for patients to receive information—both orally and written—about their care in a way in which they can understand.[17]

RESPIRATORY RECAP

Health Literacy and Patient Safety: Help Patients Understand

» This 2007 AMA publication that substantiated the health literacy problem and the need for more diligence and vigilance in patient education.

A final report of considerable note was the publication *Ask Me 3*, developed by the Partnership for Clear Health Communication.[18] The purpose of the document was to aid physicians and other clinicians in gaining access to information, resources, and practical tools designed to enhance communication between patients and providers. The key point was to encourage patients to understand the answers to three key questions: What is my main problem? What do I need to do? and Why is it important for me to do this?

BOX 31–6

Three Recommendations of the Joint Commission That Underlie the Focus on the Health Literacy Problem

Make effective communications an organizational priority to protect the safety of patients.
Address patients' communication needs across the continuum of care.
Pursue policy changes that promote improved practitioner–patient communications.

Adapted from The Joint Commission. *"What Did the Doctor Say?" Improving Health Literacy to Protect Patient Safety.* Oakbrook Terrace, IL: The Joint Commission; 2007.

The literature suggests numerous solutions—some related to the patient, some to the provider, and some to the health literature or information provided. Although all three should be considered, there are six strategies that appear to be most effective in improving interpersonal communication with patients: slow down, use plain or nonmedical language, show or draw pictures, limit the amount of information provided and repeat it, use the teach-back or show-me technique, and create a shame-free environment.[15]

RESPIRATORY RECAP

Ask Me 3

» What is my main problem?
» What do I need to know?
» Why is it important for me to do this?

The first suggestion may seem simple; however, it is extremely profound. Slowing down is particularly important because many patients may be overwhelmed concerning their condition and require additional time to not only hear but to comprehend what is being said. Providers often find themselves repeating the same information over and over from patient to patient. This constant repetition can create a situation in which the provider goes on automatic pilot and repeats directives or information much like a recording. Patients' need may not be met, and true understanding left unsatisfied. The provider simply needs to slow down and be more deliberate in his or her delivery.

The second strategy is to use plain, nonmedical language. This is another one of those simple and yet often overlooked issues. As respiratory therapists, we have our own unique vocabulary—our own language. Terms and language commonly understood between healthcare providers, such as PRN, STAT, qid, and so on, are not typically known or understood by the layperson. Virtually every discipline, whether it be accounting, computer science, or engineering, has its own jargon or discipline-specific terminology. It is imperative that we refrain from using such language when conversing with our patients.

A third strategy entails the use of drawings, pictures, charts, tables, brochures, and even video clips (such as on YouTube) to teach or illustrate a concept, principle, technique, or procedure. The old adage that "a picture is worth a thousands words" is particularly relevant when imparting knowledge, a skill, or a belief. Whereas some individuals may like to read the book, others may like to listen to the audiotape, and still others view the movie. This third strategy speaks to the learning style of the patient, and using multiple-sense learning is clearly more effective than any single-sense strategy.

The fourth strategy is to limit the amount of information provided at any one sitting and to repeat this information, especially the critical elements. It should be obvious that individuals can only absorb so much information at a time. The amount will vary from person to person but nonetheless will be limited to a certain amount. It is best to focus on what patients need to *do* rather than what they need to *know*. Clearly there are concepts that the patient should know; however, it is far more critical that they leave the session being able to perform the necessary tasks or procedures. Practitioners may be well intentioned in their effort to teach virtually every portion of the topic at hand. However, an extensive knowledge and understanding of the anatomy, physiology, and pathology of the respiratory system is not appropriate for the initial encounter. It is far more effective to provide such information in bits and pieces and to spread such a discussion and elaboration over a period of sessions. Additionally, spaced repetition—that is, constant repetition and reinforcement—is extremely effective in imparting a more thorough and comprehensive understanding of the information.

> **RESPIRATORY RECAP**
>
> **Six Strategies to Improve Interpersonal Communication with Patients**
>
> » Slow down
> » Use plain, nonmedical language
> » Show or draw pictures
> » Limit the amount of information provided and repeat it
> » Use the teach-back or show-me technique
> » Create a shame-free environment

A fifth strategy is the teach-back or show-me technique. This is also known as return demonstration and simply means that once the information, technique, or concept is taught, the patient is required to give it back to the therapist educator to confirm the degree of understanding or mastery of the subject at hand. Therapist educators will frequently ask, "Do you understand?" which is often followed by an abrupt or quick transition to the next issue at hand. We seldom take the time to stop, listen, and truly engage in a dialogue that allows for confirmation or assurance of understanding. This technique is frequently employed in our respiratory care programs in the form of competency assessment. Respiratory care programs are mandated to prepare competent respiratory therapists. Program and clinical faculty will often begin by teaching the theory, follow this with a show and tell or laboratory demonstration, which is followed by observation, practice, and reinforcement, finally culminating in a summative clinical evaluation or competency assessment. The teach-back or show-me technique entails requiring the patient to demonstrate mastery and can be expressed by statements such as, "I explained and demonstrated the correct way to use your metered dose inhaler (MDI). There will obviously be occasions for you to use your MDI without the aid of the instruction booklet or the presence of your therapist. So, I would like you to show me how to use your MDI correctly and independently."

An anecdotal story associated with this technique concerns the renowned medical missionary Dr. Albert Schweitzer, who was often described as demanding that his patients repeat back to him the directions, instructions, or advice given by him in the care and management of their condition. Dr. Schweitzer recognized the value of this technique because he often experienced the poor and marginalized patients' unfamiliarity with modern medicine and the critical need for them to self-manage their condition. Simply stated, return demonstration ensures better understanding and greater likelihood of treatment compliance for the low-literate or less educated patient.

The sixth and final strategy is perhaps the most important: it is to create a shame-free environment. Personal experience, as well as documented evidence in the literature, suggests that patients may be ashamed and embarrassed by their lack of understanding of written materials, professional advice, guidance, or direction. Their hidden secret is known by few and may in fact never be shared with anyone, perhaps not even their spouse or family. They may feel stupid and will mask this inadequacy by feigning understanding, providing excuses, or modeling expected behaviors or conformity. The respiratory therapy educator must demonstrate patience, sensitivity, care, and compassion. It is best to use statements such as, "I teach the use of the MDI to many people and often find that it can be difficult to master. I understand this and want you to know how hard it can be to learn. I want you to feel comfortable in asking me questions about this. I will help you master this procedure."

Simply stated, patients need to know that it is all right not to know something and acceptable to ask questions regardless of how seemingly simple or ridiculous the questions may seem. You as the respiratory therapy educator may be the first and only person who truly allowed them to express their feeling of inadequacy. Wouldn't it be morally wrong, callous, and extremely insensitive to say, "Boy, are you stupid" or "I can't believe you don't know how to take a simple breathing treatment"? An insightful quotation hangs in my office that says, "People don't care how much you know, until they know how much you care." It is important that we establish a rapport with our patients. If we are to address the issue of health literacy, we must build a relationship by demonstrating sensitivity, compassion, empathy, and cultivation of trust.

Locus of Control

Educators also should determine whether patients are interested in changing any undesirable behaviors associated with their condition. Are they motivated to learn the best ways to deal with the condition? If so, what provides that motivation? For patients who want to quit smoking, is it because they want to prolong life, save money, live to see their grandchildren, or increase their physical activities (or all of those)? Is their motivation internal or external? Do they feel they have control over their actions, or do they believe they are helpless creatures of society or fate? These questions get at the issue of **locus of control** and reflect whether patients are willing to assume responsibility for their actions.

> **RESPIRATORY RECAP**
>
> **Health Belief Model of Intrinsic Motivation**
>
> Disease prevention and the taking of action depend on a person's perception of the following factors:
>
> » The person's level of susceptibility to the condition
> » The severity of the consequences of developing the condition
> » The possible benefits of the health action in preventing or reducing susceptibility
> » Barriers or costs related to starting or continuing the proposed behavior

Many people are of the mind-set that their condition is the result of fate or happenstance. They believe that they are literally at the mercy of others, of the environment, or of the system. These people have an *external locus of control*. They may make little effort to watch their salt intake, for example, because they believe that there is nothing they can do about the condition or believe that they can indulge in an unhealthy practice and simply take a magic pill later to counteract any ill effects. They may not have an interest in preventing the problem or from practicing healthy lifestyle behaviors. These individuals simply do not take ownership of their conditions, and they feel that they can do little to influence them. Individuals with an *internal locus of control* believe they can direct their destiny; they therefore are more likely to assume responsibility for their actions and comply with recommended treatments and interventions. This concept obviously is centered on the notion of self-care, and a number of health models deal with the issue.

Health Models

One of the more frequently cited theories of intrinsic motivation is the **health belief model**. This model proposes that **prevention** of disease and the taking of action depends on a person's perception of four issues: the person's level of susceptibility to the condition, the severity of the consequences of developing the condition, the possible benefits of the health action in preventing or reducing susceptibility, and the barriers or costs related to starting or continuing the proposed behavior.[4]

> **RESPIRATORY RECAP**
>
> **The PRECEDE-PROCEED Model**
>
> **PRECEDE**
> » **P**redisposing
> » **R**einforcing
> » **E**nabling
> » **C**onstructs
> » **E**ducational/environmental
> » **D**iagnosis
> » **E**valuation
>
> **PROCEED**
> » **P**olicy
> » **R**egulatory
> » **O**rganizational
> » **C**onstructs
> » **E**ducational
> » **E**nvironmental
> » **D**evelopment

An equally popular health model that deals more with planning and focuses on extrinsic motivation is the **PRECEDE-PROCEED model**.[19] The acronym *PRECEDE* stands for predisposing, reinforcing, and enabling constructs in educational/environmental diagnosis and evaluation. *PROCEED* stands for policy, regulatory, and organizational constructs in educational and environmental development. This model, which is widely used in health promotion, focuses on factors external to the individual that shape healthcare behavior.

A person's physical or psychological state also can have a major bearing on readiness to learn. Many patients are simply too sick to engage in any meaningful patient education or training. The respiratory therapy educator may have every good intention to inform, train, and educate, but patients may be too ill to absorb what is being said. They may be in pain, groggy from sedation, or just too weak or too tired. The educator must be adept at recognizing such situations and postpone intervention to a more appropriate time.

A mix of emotions also is likely to be a factor. Such feelings could include anxiety, fear, anger, or depression, or all of these. Given such a state of mind in a patient, attempts to teach may be met with rejection or hostility. The respiratory therapy educator must be astute at recognizing a need to learn. If the patient is unreceptive to the need to learn, any attempt

> **RESPIRATORY RECAP**
>
> **Assessment of Readiness to Learn**
>
> » An aroused interest or motivation
> » Relevant preparatory training
> » Physiologic maturity

to educate will fail. Simply stated, the patient must *want* to learn.

In short, readiness to learn depends on three major factors: an aroused interest or motivation, relevant preparatory training, and physiologic maturity.[20] Respiratory therapy educators must not only be experts on the subject matter but also must be able to read the patient effectively and follow the subtle cues provided to ensure that the patient learns.

Planning

After assessing the need for patient education and determining the individual's readiness to learn, the respiratory therapy educator can move on to planning, the second phase of the patient education process. Planning involves establishment of goals or learning outcomes and crafting of more specific learning objectives. It also requires an understanding and appropriate use of learning domains, the development of content and subject matter, and preliminary design and development of evaluation strategies. Although evaluation is the final major step in the patient education process, its framework should be developed earlier. The planning phase is an appropriate starting point for this step, and soliciting feedback from the patient and family members during the planning phase ensures harmony among all parties.

Goals

Goals are general statements of the expected outcomes of the teaching and learning process. The expected learning outcomes are tied to the real educational need identified during the assessment phase. The goal statement must center on the learner. Each learning goal should be tailor-made for the individual patient. Also important is that the patient and family members participate in the process of goal establishment. This collaboration promotes cooperation and buying in from all parties and is more likely to produce the desired change in behavior that drives the patient education activity. Goals give direction to the teaching and learning process. **Box 31–7** presents an example of a goal.

Objectives

Objectives are stated more specifically than goals and allow for fine-tuning; they are smaller steps along the path to goal achievement.

SMART Objectives

A good objective can be characterized as "SMART": specific, measurable, attainable, relevant, and having timelines. General statements, such as "I will lose weight," are far too vague and should be avoided. Much better is the specification of an actual value, such as "I will lose 10 pounds." Measurability is important because it allows the educator to determine whether the objective has been reached, and attainability ensures that the objective is reasonable and possible. Losing 30 pounds in 1 week is hardly likely, let alone healthy or desirable.

Relevancy simply means that the objective must relate to the goal. For example, losing weight and quitting smoking are two separate behaviors, even though a person may gain weight after quitting smoking. These are distinct behaviors and should be approached separately.

Timelines are an important part of an objective because they establish closure or an end point to the process.

RESPIRATORY RECAP

SMART Objectives

- » **S**pecific
- » **M**easurable
- » **A**ttainable
- » **R**elevant
- » **T**imelines

ABCDs of Objectives

In addition to characteristics, a well-written objective has elements that can be expressed as the ABCDs of objective development (**Table 31–1**).[4]

BOX 31–7

Example of a Goal

The goal of the National Asthma Education and Prevention Program Expert Panel Report 3 is to help people with asthma control their asthma so that they can be active all day and sleep well at night.

From National Heart, Lung, and Blood Institute. *National Asthma Education and Prevention Program: Guidelines for the Diagnosis and Management of Asthma*. Bethesda, MD: National Health Institutes; October 2007. NIH Publication 08-5846.

TABLE 31–1 ABCDs of Objective Development

Acronym Letter	Word	Definition	Meaning
A	Audience	The "who"	Patient, family member, or informal caregiver
B	Behavior	The "what"	Action to be achieved
C	Condition	The "givens"	Any condition that must be present or met for the objective to be completed correctly (possibly also entailing timelines)
D	Degree	How well or by when	Degree to which the action or task must be done

Modified from Boyd M, Graham B, Gleit C, et al. *Teaching in Nursing Practice: A Professional Model*. 3rd ed. Stamford, CT: Appleton & Lange. © 1998. Electronically reproduced by permission of Pearson Education, Inc., Upper Saddle River, New Jersey.

TABLE 31–2 Use of the ABCDs of Objective Development

Who (A)	What (B)	Under What Condition (C)	How Well or By When (D)
John Doe	Will administer the medication in his metered dose inhaler	After correctly assembling the device	By following all steps identified in the patient education packet; taking the medication twice daily

Modified from Boyd M, Graham B, Gleit C, et al. *Teaching in Nursing Practice: A Professional Model.* 3rd ed. Stamford, CT: Appleton & Lange. © 1998. Electronically reproduced by permission of Pearson Education, Inc., Upper Saddle River, New Jersey.

A stands for audience and should reflect the "who" in the objective. The audience is the patient, the family member, or the informal caregiver. *B* is the behavior and signifies the "what," or the action to be achieved. An action word (e.g., *list, explain, apply, perform, express*) is the hallmark of this part of the objective. *C* stands for condition, which means any specific condition that must be present or met to complete the objective correctly. This part of the objective might be stated with phrases such as *after gathering the appropriate equipment, after viewing the tape*, or *from the handouts provided*. Conditions also could involve timelines in a phrase such as *at the end of the teaching session* or *by the end of the semester*. *D* stands for degree of performance or accuracy. It states how well the action or task is to be done, with phrases such as *with 100% accuracy, as specified in the policy and procedure manual*, or *identify at least three indications*. **Table 31–2** presents an example of an objective segmented according to the four elements listed.

Learning Domains

The respiratory therapy educator must be familiar with the three learning domains: cognitive, psychomotor, and affective. The **cognitive domain** involves *knowing*, the **psychomotor domain** involves *doing*, and the **affective domain** involves *feeling*. When planning an individualized patient education program, the educator must consider using learning objectives from each of these three domains to obtain the desired learning outcome.

> **RESPIRATORY RECAP**
>
> **Learning Domains**
> - » Cognitive = knowing
> - » Psychomotor = doing
> - » Affective = feeling

For example, an asthma education program clearly entails the use of all three domains. In teaching the patient about the signs, symptoms, pathophysiology, mechanism of action of medications, and adverse effects of the asthmatic condition, the respiratory therapy educator might best establish objectives that fall into the cognitive domain, because this is largely information that the patient must *know*.

When teaching the use of a metered dose inhaler, the educator is using the psychomotor domain and therefore should develop objectives that engage the patient in the actual performance of the maneuver; the patient must *do*.

Finally, when a family member is asked to show compassion, patience, or understanding for what the patient is experiencing, that person is exhibiting an affective quality, expressing *feelings*. Many patient educators are somewhat uncomfortable in dealing with the affective domain because it focuses on values, attitudes, and emotions. Although such issues are difficult to discuss, the key to writing affective objectives is to focus on measurable behaviors. For example, the educator can observe a person placing a hand on the patient's shoulder in an attempt to console and comfort; such a display represents affective behavior and is clearly measurable.

Content and Subject Matter

Obviously, content and subject matter vary according to the topic. A vast amount of material is available on almost every cardiorespiratory condition. The respiratory therapy educator should focus on the goals and objectives already determined and develop the specific content from these points. Programs such as Open Airways,[21] which was developed by the American Lung Association, and those described in the *Guidelines for the Diagnosis and Management of Asthma*,[22] written by a panel of experts under the guidance of the National Institutes of Health, are excellent models that can be used to plan and identify the detailed content of a patient education program.

Implementation

The third phase of the patient education process is implementation. In this phase, respiratory therapy educators can roll up their sleeves and get down to the business of putting the teaching plan into action. However, as mentioned previously, the educator should not jump in too quickly; simply providing an explanation of the disease and its treatment does not constitute effective patient education or ensure understanding and compliance. Various teaching and learning strategies should be considered, and sending the message does not ensure reception, let alone understanding or adherence to the treatment plan.

Implementation of a teaching plan requires a dynamic, interactive encounter between the respiratory therapy educator and the patient, family member, or caregiver. Numerous techniques can be used. Some of the more popular ones are the lecture, the modified lecture or guided discussion, the demonstration, use of printed materials, case studies or simulations, role playing, problem solving, self-instructional materials or programmed instruction, drills, and behavioral contracting. Combining techniques can have a synergistic effect that can enhance the learning process.

Teaching Techniques

Lecture

Perhaps the single most popular teaching method is the lecture, which is also referred to as simply "talking to" or "talking at" the patient. The advantages of such an approach are that a considerable amount of material can be presented at one time, the presentation time can be controlled to the minute, many instructors can be used, topics can be specialized, additional questions and discussion can be elicited, and a certain degree of spontaneity and instantaneous modification of the subject matter can occur. Disadvantages include the potential for passivity on the part of the audience or recipient; the need for preparation on the part of the presenter; the need to avoid a lengthy, preachy approach that can result in boredom and resentment; and the risk that the patient simply will not use the information provided. The respiratory therapy educator must be astute in identifying problems and modifying this approach to better engage the patient in the learning process.

> **RESPIRATORY RECAP**
>
> **Teaching Strategies for Patient Education**
>
> » Lecture
> » Modified lecture (guided discussion)
> » Demonstration
> » Printed materials
> » Case studies or simulations
> » Role playing
> » Problem solving
> » Self-instructional materials and programmed instruction
> » Drills
> » Behavioral contracting

Demonstration

Another popular approach is the demonstration. Demonstrations allow the patient both to see and to hear the necessary information. More important, demonstrations allow the patient to engage in more active learning. Information can be provided simultaneously, and discussion and questioning can be enhanced.

Demonstrations can be more time consuming and resource dependent than lectures. They should follow a planned sequence, and dividing the tasks into smaller components generally results in a more successful encounter.

Of considerable importance is the return demonstration, which requires the learner to repeat for the instructor predetermined steps essential to the proper performance of the procedure in question. Demonstration should be followed by practice and skill refinement. Frequent repetition of the procedure, coupled with remediation and feedback, leads to a higher degree of competency.

Printed Materials

The use of printed materials—in the form of books, pamphlets, brochures, or handouts—is an especially effective teaching strategy. The use of such materials is especially valuable when the respiratory therapy educator has a limited amount of time. Printed materials can address a wide variety of topics at a variety of reading levels. They also can serve as reinforcement for other teaching strategies. The limitations of printed materials lie in the reading level and ability of the patient and in their expense, the lack of social contact and interaction between the educator and patient, and the need to evaluate the huge amount of material available.

Case Studies, Role Playing, and Problem Solving

Although they are used less often, case studies, role playing, and problem solving all have a place in patient education. They generally are effective in urging patients to think critically about problems and situations that could arise because of their condition. These techniques are inexpensive, usually take little time to implement, and require direct interaction with others. **Self-instructional** materials and **programmed instruction** allow patients to learn at their own pace, are helpful in clarifying complex issues, and require little time on the part of the instructor. Many of these materials provide direct feedback and reinforcement of critical information. Their limitations are that they require a motivated, disciplined patient; can be boring; may require resources; and are extremely impersonal.

Drills

Drills are valuable in that they are a quick way to learn sequences of a required skill or procedure, allow for repetition and reinforcement of tasks, and generally break down the specific elements of a task into separate elements. The disadvantages are that they require a high degree of patient cooperation and may require the continual presence of additional resources and equipment.

Behavioral Contracting

Behavioral contracting is a highly accountable technique. It can create a higher level of responsibility and call on the patient's integrity and autonomy. It has an added advantage of identifying expectations up front and creating a strong alliance between patient and instructor. However, some patients might refuse to use this technique or may be reluctant to assume responsibility for behavior change.

Aligning Teaching Strategies and Learning Domains

The respiratory therapy educator should make an effort to identify the teaching strategies that might be more effective for a particular learning domain. For example, if the educator is attempting to teach a cognitive objective, he or she could employ the lecture, group discussion, or printed materials, or a combination of these or other techniques. **Table 31–3** matches the teaching strategy or methodology with the learning domain of the objective. Additionally, it lists general characteristics of the learner's role and the teacher's role as well as the advantages and limitations of these strategies or methodologies.

TABLE 31-3 General Characteristics of Teaching Strategies or Instructional Methodologies

Method	Domain	Learner Role	Teacher Role	Advantages	Limitations
Lecture	Cognitive	Passive	Presents information	Cost effective Targets large groups	Not individualized
Group discussion	Cognitive Affective	Active—if learner participates	Guides and focuses discussion	Stimulates sharing ideas and emotions	Shy or dominant member High levels of diversity
One-to-one instruction	Cognitive Psychomotor Affective	Active	Presents information and facilities individualized learning	Tailored to individual's needs and goals	Labor intensive Isolates learner
Demonstration	Cognitive	Passive	Models skill or behavior	Preview of exact skill/behavior	Small groups needed to facilitate visualization
Return demonstration	Psychomotor	Active	Individualizes feedback to refine performance	Immediate individual guidance	Labor intensive to view individual performance
Gaming	Cognitive Affective	Active—if learner participates	Oversees pacing Referees Debriefs	Captures learner enthusiasm	Environment too competitive for some learners
Simulation	Cognitive Psychomotor	Active	Designs environment Facilitates process Debriefs	Practice reality in safe setting	Labor intensive Equipment costs
Role playing	Affective	Active	Designs format Debriefs	Develops understanding of others	Exaggeration or underdevelopment of role
Role modeling	Cognitive Affective	Passive	Models skills or behavior	Helps with socialization to role	Requires rapport
Self-instruction	Cognitive Psychomotor	Active	Designs package Gives individual feedback	Self-paced Cost effective Consistent	Procrastination Requires literacy
Computer-assisted instruction	Cognitive	Active	Purchases or designs program Provides individual feedback	Immediate and continuous feedback Private Individualized	Costly to design or purchase Must have hardware
Distance learning	Cognitive	Passive	Presents information Answers questions	Targets learners who are at varying distances from expert	Lack of personal contact Accessibility

From Bastable SB. *Nurse as Educator*. Sudbury, MA: Jones & Bartlett Learning; 1997:278.

Common Problems of the Provider

Like patients, educators face obstacles in the teaching and learning process (**Box 31–8**).[23] One of the more important problems, inadequate assessment, can arise for a number of reasons. It may be as simple as a burning desire on the part of educators to jump in and get started without acquainting themselves with patient or family conditions. Clinicians often assume that they know what is best for the patient and what needs to be taught. They fail to individualize the teaching program and to center it on the specific needs of the patient. They may overlook social or environmental issues, such as a broken family or cramped living conditions in the home. They may use poor communication skills or poor observational techniques and miss important information. The value of a thorough, complete assessment cannot be overstated. Vigilance in this first step is essential and goes a long way toward prevention of later problems.

Another problem cited by respiratory therapy educators is the financial limitations imposed by the institution, a form of inadequate support. A number of healthcare administrators and decision makers consider patient education a nonessential or at least less essential healthcare service. However, the Joint Commission and the consumer movement do not concur. Managed care organizations are demanding better patient outcomes. Patient education has been cited as a means to increase patient compliance and to reduce costs, the length of

BOX 31–8

Common Problems of the Provider

Inadequate assessment
Cost limitations
Inadequate support
Time limitations
Environmental limitations
Sociocultural differences between teacher and learner
Inadequate evaluation

Modified from Bopp A, Lubkin I. *Chronic Illness: Impact and Interventions.* 2nd ed. Sudbury, MA: Jones & Bartlett Learning; 1990.

TABLE 31–4 Levels of Patient Education

Level	Time Constraints	Teaching Method
1	Only a few hours available before patient is discharged	Provide literature, fact sheets, and teaching guides and discuss with patient to the extent possible.
2	A few days available for teaching	Provide literature and reinforce with an instructional videotape.
3	A considerable amount of time available for teaching	Use four-step process (assess, plan, implement, and evaluate). Use counseling skills (active listening, coaching, clarifying, summarizing).

Modified with permission from Winthrop E. *Patient Teaching Tips*. St. Louis: Mosby; 1995.

the hospital stay, and the need for more expensive acute care. The Joint Commission has developed standards that require patient education in all healthcare institutions; most institutions designate a department to ensure that the requirements are met. These mandates and the emergence of a savvier healthcare consumer likely will change the perception of patient education in the future and promote more widespread acceptance.

Environmental limitations, sociocultural differences, and inadequate evaluation are related to the educator's ability to function successfully as a teacher. Environmental limitations involve issues such as privacy, room temperature, lighting, noise, and distractions. Privacy can be dealt with if the educator shows sensitivity and awareness. Patients are not likely to share their innermost thoughts without some degree of privacy, confidence, and confidentiality. Sociocultural differences also must be recognized and require a caring, nonjudgmental demeanor on the part of the educator. Inadequate evaluation is always a concern because patient educators must be astute enough in their observations to note nonverbal and verbal cues that indicate the patient does not understand or accept the material.

Perhaps the most frequently cited problem of patient educators is the serious time limitation imposed by the high treatment load expected of healthcare providers. This is a recurrent theme and a product of the times. Healthcare administrators are constantly reminding their workforce of the need to do more with less. Direct patient care will always win out over education, but greater appreciation is needed of the value of effective patient teaching. A strong argument can be made that effective patient education is cost effective because a well-informed, motivated patient places fewer demands on the healthcare system, especially emergency room visits. Ultimately, patient education can curtail the use of healthcare services and reduce healthcare costs.

Levels of Patient Education

When the respiratory therapy educator is faced with the problem of time limitations, the teaching plan can be modified according to the three levels of education (**Table 31–4**).[24]

Level 1 education is used in cases in which the educator is informed that the patient is leaving in 2 hours and must be educated about the condition. In such cases the teaching method is limited to literature in the form of a well-written fact sheet. This fact sheet must be written in language comfortable for the patient, and the educator must read it in advance so as to circle or highlight key points and address questions before the patient is discharged.

Level 2 education is used when the educator has a few days to accomplish the teaching plan. It involves literature and reinforcement of the written material by some other means, such as a videotape. Educators should preview such material so that they or other members of the healthcare team can highlight key points and follow up with a discussion of the material.

Level 3 education is used when the educator has considerable time for the program. This optimal situation allows for the incorporation of all four major components of the patient education process. Level 3 education includes a counseling role and is more likely to result in a successful intervention.

Principles of Adult Learning

The basic principles of adult learning are important elements of any patient teaching program. Numerous courses, books, and articles have been written on this topic, but a useful and meaningful delineation has been provided by Kroehnert,[25] who uses the mnemonic RAMP-2-FAME to represent nine critical principles of adult learning.

R stands for recency, which means that the principles or concepts taught last are most likely to be remembered best. This stems from human beings' tendency to remember material that was addressed most recently; this also is affected by the order in which material is presented (see information on primacy that follows). The implication for respiratory therapy educators is that they should plant important information in the patient's mind just before leaving the room. Keeping sessions short and summarizing often helps the patient remember essential information.

The second letter in the mnemonic, *A*, stands for appropriateness and signifies that learners engage in the learning process only if the material presented has meaning and relevance for their needs. Explaining the biochemistry of leukotriene inhibitors in the discussion of medication for the treatment of airway obstruction would be inappropriate and futile. Equally inappropriate would be a discussion of detailed respiratory anatomy, such as the pores of Kohn. A more appropriate discussion would be to explain the inflammatory reaction as being similar to a sunburn or to describe bronchoconstriction as similar to breathing through a narrow straw. Such everyday examples have more meaning and more relevance. They are more likely to be received favorably.

RESPIRATORY RECAP

Principles of Adult Learning: RAMP-2-FAME

» **R**ecency
» **A**ppropriateness
» **M**otivation
» **P**rimacy
» **2**-way communication
» **F**eedback
» **A**ctive learning
» **M**ultiple-sense learning
» **E**xercise

The *M* stands for motivation. Patients must be moved to take action; they must want to learn. Imparting a sense of urgency or a strong need to learn the subject matter can create this motivation. For example, a parent whose child had recently experienced a serious asthmatic attack while playing soccer would be greatly motivated to learn the correct use of the child's metered dose inhaler. Patient educators must find the motivating factors and push those buttons to get the point across and engage the patient or family member in patient education.

The fourth letter, *P*, stands for primacy, meaning that the information the patient learns first is usually learned best. As with recency, patients are more attentive at both the beginning and end of a presentation, thus there is an emphasis on increased learning at these stages. Primacy gets at the issue of first impressions and the need to deliver the most important information first. More often than not, the respiratory therapy educator has a receptive audience at the first meeting with the patient because the patient is curious about what the educator has to say. This is a golden opportunity for educators to put their best foot forward and make their case.

The numeral *2* in the mnemonic signifies the need for two-way communication. The conversation should be *with*, not *at* the patient. Interaction should be encouraged.

The *F* stands for feedback, which should be given both to the patient and to the educator. People simply need to know how they are doing. Feedback provides the opportunity for both parties to validate their roles and their understanding of the interaction.

The second *A* stands for active learning, which entails participation in the learning process. This point is extremely important because patient passivity progresses to boredom, loss of concentration, and ultimately, to very little learning.

The second *M* stands for multiple-sense learning, one of the most important points. Whenever another sense is brought into the learning process, the amount of material that will be remembered has been estimated to double. People learn in different ways, and educators should use as many different techniques as possible. Although explaining a procedure to patients may be effective, showing them a picture and letting them touch or handle the equipment adds considerable value to the learning experience; it clearly results in a heightened sense of understanding and ultimately to subject mastery.

The last letter, *E*, is exercise and refers to the value of the educator's repeating the new information over and over to better ensure retention. The repetition of the times tables in elementary school is a classic example of the power of repetition. The more often patients repeat the material, the more likely they are to remember it.

Teaching Principles for Children Through the Elderly

In addition to these adult learning principles, respiratory therapy educators should become knowledgeable about the unique learning needs of all age groups (infants and toddlers through older adults). Whereas the teaching/learning process for infants and children will generally require more parental involvement, relatively shorter sessions, and techniques that are more concrete and interactive, the elderly have more sensory deficits and will generally require more involvement in the planning and decision-making process. **Table 31–5** notes age-related considerations across the population.

The Teaching Moment

The respiratory therapy educator must take advantage of the **teaching moment**, that is, any opportunity to impart meaningful information to a captive audience. Such an opportunity likely will occur only after a certain degree of trust, comfort, and mutual respect has been established between patient and educator. It behooves the respiratory therapy educator to establish this relationship as soon as possible and to be prepared to take advantage of teaching moments.

RESPIRATORY RECAP

Teaching Moment

» Any opportunity to impart meaningful information to a captive audience

TABLE 31–5 Age-Related Considerations in Patient Teaching

Patient's Age	Teaching Considerations
Infant or toddler	Involvement of parents (key players) is important. Parents should be present to alleviate separation anxiety. Educator must establish a relationship with patient and caregiver (trust). Story reading, pictures, and puppets are useful tools. Terminology should be kept simple (concrete, nonthreatening). Familiar surroundings are comforting. Session should be kept short (2 to 5 minutes). Teaching session should be held close to the occurrence of the event. Activity should be incorporated into learning.
Preschool	Child may participate in planning. If possible, a choice between two options should be allowed. A group size of five to eight is best. Physical and visual stimuli are better than verbal stimuli. Neutral, concrete, and action-oriented words should be used whenever possible. A safe, secure environment for learning should be created. Sessions should be kept short (15 minutes or less) and slow paced; the focus should be present oriented. Tangible rewards work well and should be given immediately.
School age	Participation in activities is important. Repetition and summarizing are useful methods. This age group is responsive to modeling and to peer-group and mass-media influence. Decision making is based on simple scientific knowledge of cause and effect. Groups of friends of the same age are important. Safety and security are less important than with preschoolers. Sessions can be longer (15 to 30 minutes). Careful listening is important. This age group can be assisted to move from the concrete (how) to the abstract (why). These children often have misconceptions that may need clarification. Time is needed to clarify, validate, and expand the child's knowledge. Privacy is important. Praise is very effective.
Adolescent	Cognitive abilities allow for greater participation in learning and planning. Patient can begin to process future health implications. Written information is more meaningful and useful. Privacy is also important. Learning can be enhanced by use of group methods. Issues may need to be clarified. Reinforcement through recognition is a valuable motivator.
Adult	Independence in self-care and decision making should be promoted. Actions may be influenced by experience, economics, sociocultural factors, and values. Learning needs should be determined. Readiness to learn should be recognized. Relevancy should be maintained. Connecting to patient's knowledge and experience is important. Analogies can be used for complex ideas. Patient should be involved in planning and decision making.
Older adult	Distinct, large configurations should be used in visual aids. Good lighting and high-contrast colors are helpful. Educator should speak clearly, adjusting the rate and loudness as necessary. Short learning sessions involving a small amount of material work best. Adequate response time should be allowed. Repetition aids learning. Goals should be mutually established and reachable. New learning should be integrated with previously established information. Patient should be encouraged to participate in planning and decision making. Family involvement should be encouraged.

Modified from Boyd M, Graham B, Gleit C, et al. *Teaching in Nursing Practice: A Professional Model.* 3rd ed. Stamford, CT: Appleton & Lange.

Evaluation

Evaluation, the last major component of the patient education process, involves measurement and documentation of the results of the interventions. It is the culmination of all the effort that has been expended throughout the patient–educator interaction. The evaluation component can be divided into two subcategories: process evaluation and evaluation of learning.

Process Evaluation

Process evaluation is a continuous reassessment of the effectiveness of all components of the teaching/learning interaction. Respiratory therapy educators must constantly ask themselves, "Did I gather all the information needed during the assessment phase? Did I achieve my goals and objectives? Was my decision to use a demonstration technique the right one? Did I use appropriate language?" and "Did I progress too quickly?"

Evaluation of Learning

Evaluation of learning requires the respiratory therapy educator to take a step back and look at each component of the teaching/learning interaction individually, with a view to corrective intervention and remediation. It often requires educators to ask themselves, "What did the patient learn?" or "How can I enhance teaching or learning?"

Evaluation of the patient's learning involves measurement of the learner's achievement, a task easily performed through rephrasing of the learning objectives as a series of oral questions or as questions on a written test, teaching checklist, or observational checklist that the patient completes. This evaluation must be as objective as possible, and judgments must be determined against an accepted standard. **Figure 31–5** is an example of a teaching checklist used to evaluate a patient's use of an inhaler.[22]

1.__ Remove the cap and hold the inhaler upright.
2.__ Shake the inhaler.
3.__ Tilt your head back slightly and breathe out slowly.
4.__ Position the inhaler.
5.__ Press down on the inhaler to release medication as you start to breathe in slowly.
6.__ Breathe in slowly (3 to 5 seconds).
7.__ Hold your breath for 10 seconds to allow the medicine to reach deep into your lungs.
8.__ Repeat puff as directed. Waiting 1 minute between puffs may permit a second puff to penetrate your lungs better.
9.__ Spacers/holding chambers are useful for all patients. They are particularly recommended for young children and older adults and for use with inhaled corticosteroids.

FIGURE 31–5 Example of a teaching checklist for use of an inhaler. From U.S. Department of Health and Human Services, National Institutes of Health, National Heart, Lung, and Blood Institute. *Practical Guide for the Diagnosis and Management of Asthma.* National Institutes of Health; 1997. NIH Publication 97-4051.

Documentation

Documentation of the patient education process is crucial and serves a number of purposes, including cataloguing the respiratory therapist's involvement in teaching; demonstrating a systematic, planned approach to teaching; serving as a means of communication among healthcare professionals; satisfying legal and regulatory requirements; reflecting patients' levels of understanding or misunderstanding of the subject matter; and providing patients the opportunity to express their responses to the intervention.[4]

Documentation can take many forms. Some institutions use electronic documentation, whereas others use such techniques as anecdotal chart entries, checklists, and standardized forms. An informal survey of a variety of institutions showed that almost all believed that documentation of patient education should be included as part of the patient's permanent record and that such documentation should be interdisciplinary. The following five key components were identified:

1. Date and time of the intervention
2. Initials of the healthcare provider
3. Subject matter or content addressed
4. Method of instruction
5. Response of the learner or the results of the learning

Figure 31–6 shows a sample interdisciplinary patient education/family education record that includes some of the points identified previously.

For ease of charting, some institutions use a coded checklist. For example, under method of instruction, the educator would check off *E* for explanation, *D* for demonstration, *P* for printed materials, or *V* for video. Under response of the learner, *1* might stand for communicates understanding, *2* for return demonstration provided, *3* for requires reinforcement, *4* for referral indicated, or *5* for refused interaction. Almost all methods of documentation include a section for educator comments, and some have a more elaborate section for factors noted at the initial assessment, such as barriers to learning and the patient's motivational level and learning preferences.

Above all, respiratory therapy educators must be mindful of the need to constantly update and refine their teaching skills. Observation of colleagues, formal training through academic and professional courses and programs, and practice can help the patient educator attain this goal and become a more effective teacher.

Examples of Patient Education Programs

It should be obvious that multiple opportunities for patient education abound within the profession of respiratory care. Three areas of practice are particularly applicable for intervention, namely, asthma education, pulmonary rehabilitation, and tobacco cessation. Although some redundancy occurs in the respective

Interdisciplinary Patient Education/Family Education Record

Patient's name:____________________

Date:____________________ Time of intervention:____________________

Subject matter/content addressed:____________________

Method of instruction:____________________

Response of learner/results of learning:____________________

Initials/signature of healthcare provider: ____________________

FIGURE 31–6 Sample of an interdisciplinary patient education/family education record.

sections for these topics, a brief but pointed treatise is provided here as to how patient education can be incorporated within these topical areas.

Asthma Education

Asthma education represents one of the best examples of how respiratory therapists can incorporate their knowledge, skills, and abilities in fulfilling their role as patient educators. The landmark and most authoritative reference for the management of asthma is the NIH report entitled *National Asthma Education and Prevention Program, Expert Panel Report 3: Guidelines for the Diagnosis and Management of Asthma*. Embedded within this document is a detailed account of the four components of care for an asthma disease management program, namely, assessment and monitoring, education, control of environmental factors and comorbid conditions, and medications. **Table 31–6** provides an overview of the four components of care as well as the key clinical activities and action steps identified in the guidelines.[26] The four components addressed in this document are quite similar in design to the four components addressed in previous literature and expressed through the acronym ACME: assess, control, medicate, and educate. Incorporating the principles and concepts of patient education within the area of asthma management entails the theme of "Education for a Partnership in Care."[26]

> **RESPIRATORY RECAP**
>
> **Theme of Patient Education**
>
> » The theme of patient education as it relates to asthma education is "Education for a Partnership in Care."

An asthma education program using these guidelines stresses self-management, development of a written action plan, and the integration of education into all points of care. To be successful, the therapist must follow the educational process. We provide some commentary here on how respiratory therapy educators can incorporate these concepts into their teaching.

As previously noted, when the respiratory therapy educator begins the education process, it is critical that he or she avoid the temptation to jump right into the teaching/learning process by *telling* the patient about his or her asthma. Rather, the four components of the teaching process—assessment, planning, implementation, and evaluation (A PIE)—should be followed. Assessment entails determining what patients know about their condition and, more important, assessing what they need to know. Where are the gaps in their knowledge and understanding of their asthma? What is needed in order for them to care for themselves?

Armed with this knowledge, the therapist educator develops a plan, often referred to as an asthma action plan, that is tailored to the unique needs of the patient.[22] **Figure 31–7** provides an example of an asthma action plan for schools and families. The action plan should address the goals of asthma care as well as specific objectives to achieve these goals. The respiratory therapy educator must be mindful that there are concepts that should be known and understood (cognitive objectives) as well as procedures and therapies that patients must be able to perform (psychomotor objectives) and beliefs or feelings that patients must possess (affective objectives) in order for them to effectively care for their asthma. In short, there are objectives that the patient should *know*, *do*, and *believe* or *feel*.

Development of the action plan is followed by implementation of the plan and the actual teaching and learning strategy. This could include a one-on-one

TABLE 31–6 Four Components of Care for an Asthma Disease Management Program

Clinical Issue	Key Clinical Activities	Action Steps
Assessment and monitoring	Assess asthma severity to initiate therapy. Assess asthma control to monitor and adjust therapy. Schedule follow-up care.	Use severity classification chart, assessing both domains of impairment and risk, to determine initial treatment. Use asthma control chart, assessing both domains of impairment and risk, to determine whether therapy should be maintained or adjusted (step up if necessary; step down if possible). Asthma is highly variable over time, and periodic monitoring is essential. In general, consider scheduling patients at 2- to 6-week intervals while gaining control; at 1- to 6-month intervals, depending on step of care required or duration of control, to monitor if sufficient control is maintained; at 3-month intervals if a step down in therapy is anticipated. Assess asthma control, medication technique, written asthma action plan, and patient adherence and concerns at every visit.
Control environmental factors and comorbid conditions	Recommend measures to control exposure to allergens and pollutants or irritants that make asthma worse. Treat comorbid conditions.	Determine exposures, history of symptoms in presence of exposures, and sensitivities (in patients who have persistent asthma, use skin or in vitro testing to assess sensitivity to perennial indoor allergens). Advise patients on ways to reduce exposure to those allergens and pollutants or irritants to which the patient is sensitive. Multifaceted approaches are beneficial; single steps alone are generally ineffective. Advise all patients and pregnant women to avoid exposure to tobacco smoke. Consider allergen immunotherapy, by specifically trained personnel, for patients who have persistent asthma and when there is clear evidence of a relationship between symptoms and exposure to an allergen to which the patient is sensitive. Consider especially allergic bronchopulmonary aspergillosis, gastroesophageal reflux, obesity, obstructive sleep apnea, rhinitis and sinusitis, and stress or depression. Recognition and treatment of these conditions may improve asthma control. Inhaled corticosteroids are the most effective long-term control therapy. When choosing among treatment options, consider domain of relevance to the patient (impairment, risk, or both), patient's history of response to the medication, and patient's willingness and ability to use the medication.
Medications	Select medication and delivery devices to meet patient's needs and circumstances.	Use stepwise approach to identify appropriate treatment options. Inhaled corticosteroids (ICSs) are the most effective long-term control therapy. When choosing among treatment options, consider domain of relevance to the patient (impairment, risk, or both), patient's history of response to the medication, and patient's willingness and ability to use the medication.
Education	Provide self-management education. Develop a written asthma action plan in partnership with patient. Integrate education into all points of care where health professionals interact with patients.	Teach and reinforce: • Self-monitoring to assess level of asthma control and signs of worsening asthma (either symptom or peak flow monitoring shows similar benefits for most patients). Peak flow monitoring may be particularly helpful for patients who have difficulty perceiving symptoms, a history of severe exacerbation, or moderate or severe asthma. • Using written asthma action plan (review differences between long-term control and quick-relief medication). • Taking medication correctly (inhaler technique and use of devices). • Avoiding environmental factors that worsen asthma. Tailor education to literacy level of patient. Appreciate the potential role of a patient's cultural beliefs and practices in asthma management. Agree on treatment goals and address patient concerns. Provide instructions for (1) daily management (long-term control medication, if appropriate, and environmental control measures) and (2) managing worsening asthma (how to adjust medication, and knowing when to seek medical care). Involve all members of the healthcare team in providing/reinforcing education, including physicians, nurses, pharmacists, respiratory therapists, and asthma educators. Encourage education at all points of care: clinics (offering separate self-management programs as well as incorporating education into every patient visit), emergency departments and hospitals, pharmacies, schools and other community settings, and patients' homes. Use a variety of educational strategies and methods.

From National Heart, Lung and Blood Institute. *National Asthma Education and Prevention Program, Expert Panel Report 3: Guidelines for the Diagnosis and Management of Asthma*. Bethesda, MD: National Institutes of Health; August 2007. NIH Publication 07-4051.

School Information | **Asthma Action Plan for Schools and Families** | Health Care Provider Information

Last Name: ____ First Name: ____

Date of Birth (mm/dd/yyyy): ____ Medical Record #: ____

School Name: ____ School Contact Phone #: ____

Parent/Guardian Name: ____ Parent/Guardian Phone #: ____

Emergency Contact: ____ **Emergency Phone #:** ____

Health Care Provider Name: ____ Health Care Provider Phone #: ____

To be completed by health care provider: **Asthma Severity:** ☐ Intermittent ☐ Mild Persistent ☐ Moderate Persistent ☐ Severe Persistent

Attention Parent/Guardian/School Personnel: ANY student with asthma (of any severity) can have a severe asthma attack.

Asthma symptoms are triggered by: ☐ **Exercise** ☐ **Dust** ☐ **Animal dander** ☐ **Strong Odors or Fumes** ☐ **Mold** ☐ ____

Green Zone **Personal Best Peak Flow (PF)** ____ Date: ____
Peak flow is between ____ (80% of personal best) and ____ (100% of personal best)

1. Take CONTROLLER medication(s) (at home) EVERY DAY:

Take ____ (Name of Medicine) inhaler ____ (How much) puffs ____ (How often) times/day.

Take ____ (Name of Medicine) inhaler ____ (How much) puffs ____ (How often) times/day.

If asthma is triggered by exercise (at school or home), take ☐ Albuterol or ____ (Name of Medicine) inhaler ____ (How much) puffs at least ____ minutes before exercise. Restrictions or activity limitations: ____

Yellow Zone-Caution! **DO NOT LEAVE STUDENT ALONE!**
Peak flow is between ____ (50% of personal best) and ____ (80% of personal best).

1. Begin QUICK RELIEF medication (at school or home) **right NOW:**

Take ☐ Albuterol or ____ (Name of Medicine) inhaler ____ (How much) puffs **OR** ____ (Name of Medicine) solution ____ (How much) ml by nebulizer.

- If symptoms are better or if the peak flow is improved within ☐ 15 minutes/____ minutes, THEN repeat QUICK RELIEF MEDICATION (as listed above in 1) every ____ (Number) hours for ____ (Number) days.
- If symptoms are **NOT** better or if the peak flow is **NOT** improved, go to Red Zone.
  ☐ **Attention School: Call Parent/Guardian when quick relief medication has been administered by student and/or staff.**

2. Attention Parent/Guardian (Home Instructions):
   ☐ Call your child's Health Care Provider
   ☐ Continue to take CONTROLLER medication (at home) everyday as written above in *Green Zone* instructions.
   ☐ Increase CONTROLLER medication:
   Take ____ (Name of Medicine) inhaler ____ (How much) puffs ____ (How often) times/day for ____ (Number) days.

Red Zone-Medical Alert! **Get Help! DO NOT LEAVE STUDENT ALONE!** **Peak flow is below** ____ (50% of personal best).

1. Take QUICK RELIEF medication (at school or home) right NOW:

Take ☐ Albuterol or ____ (Name of Medicine) inhaler ____ (How much) puffs **OR** ____ (Name of Medicine) solution ____ (How much) ml by nebulizer and **REPEAT EVERY 20 MINUTES UNTIL PARAMEDICS ARRIVE!**

- **Call 9-1-1 immediately and call Parent/Guardian**

2. Attention Parent/Guardian (Home Instructions):
   ☐ Call your child's Health Care Provider. ☐ Continue CONTROLLER medication (at home):
   Take ____ (Name of Medicine) inhaler ____ (How much) puffs ____ (How often) times/day for ____ (Number) days.
   ☐ And ADD ____ (Name of Medicine) ____ (How much) mg orally once daily for ____ (Number) days.

Authorization and Disclaimer from Parent/Guardian: I request that the school assist my child with the above asthma medications and the Asthma Action Plan in accordance with state laws and regulations. Yes ☐ No ☐
My child may carry and self-administer asthma medications and I agree to release the school district and school personnel from all claims of liability if my child suffers any adverse reactions from self-administration of asthma medications: Yes ☐ No ☐

____ Parent/Guardian Signature ____ Date

Health Care Provider: My signature provides authorization for the above written orders. I understand that all procedures will be implemented in accordance with state laws and regulations. Student may carry and self-administer asthma medications: Yes ☐ No ☐ (This authorization is for a maximum of one year from signature date.) ____ Healthcare Provider Signature ____ Date

1-24-07 California Asthma Public Health Initiative, California Department of Health Services

Using Symptoms and/or Peak Flow to Know Your Zone

Green Zone 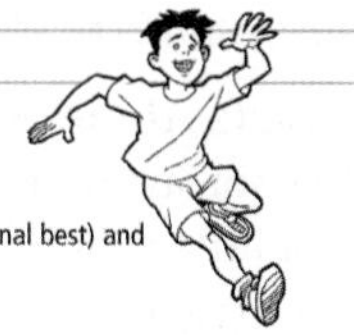
✔ No cough or wheeze at day or night.
✔ No chest tightness.
OR
✔ **Peak flow** is between ____ (80% of personal best) and ____ (100% of personal best).

Yellow Zone - Caution! 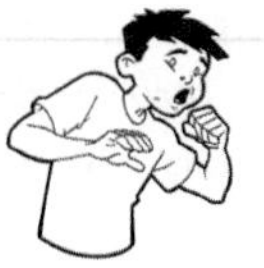
Any asthma symptoms:
✔ Cough or wheeze at day or night.
✔ Chest tightness.
✔ Problems playing.
✔ Waking at night with asthma symptoms.
OR
✔ **Peak flow** is between ____ (50% of personal best) and ____ (80% of personal best).

Red Zone - Medical Alert! 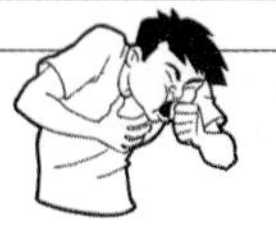
Any asthma symptoms:
✔ Persistent cough or wheeze.
✔ Severe chest tightness.
✔ Can not walk, talk, or move well.
✔ Blue skin color around lips or nails.
OR
✔ **Peak flow is below** ____ (50% of personal best).

AUTHORIZATION FOR USE OR DISCLOSURE OF HEALTH INFORMATION TO SCHOOL DISTRICTS

Completion of this document authorizes the disclosure and/or use of individually identifiable health information, as set forth below, consistent with Federal laws (including HIPAA) concerning the privacy of such information. Failure to provide all information requested may invalidate this authorization.

USE AND DISCLOSURE INFORMATION:

Patient/Student Name: ____ Last ____ First ____ MI / ____ Date of Birth

I, the undersigned, do hereby authorize (name of agency and/or health care providers):

(1) ____ (2) ____

to provide health information from the above-named child's medical record to and from:

____ School District to Which Disclosure is Made ____ Address / City and State / Zip Code

____ Contact Person at School District ____ Area Code and Telephone Number

The disclosure of health information is required for the following purpose:

Requested information shall be limited to the following: ☐ All health information; **or**
☐ Disease-specific information as described:

DURATION:
This authorization shall become effective immediately and shall remain in effect until ____ *(enter date)* or for one year from the date of signature, if no date entered.

RESTRICTIONS:
Law prohibits the Requestor from making further disclosure of my health information unless the Requestor obtains another authorization form from me or unless such disclosure is specifically required or permitted by law.

YOUR RIGHTS:
I understand that I have the following rights with respect to this Authorization: *I may revoke this Authorization at any time. My revocation must be in writing, signed by me or on my behalf, and delivered to the health care agencies/persons listed above. My revocation will be effective upon receipt, but will not be effective to the extent that the Requestor or others have acted in reliance to this Authorization.*

RE-DISCLOSURE:
I understand that the Requestor (School District) will protect this information as prescribed by the Family Equal Rights Protection Act (FERPA) and that the information becomes part of the student's educational record. The information will be shared with individuals working at or with the School District for the purpose of providing safe, appropriate, and least restrictive educational settings and school health services and programs.

I have a right to receive a copy of this Authorization. Signing this Authorization may be required in order for this student to obtain appropriate services in the educational setting.

APPROVAL: ____ Printed Name ____ Signature ____ Date

____ Relationship to Patient/Student ____ Area Code and Telephone Number

10/13/04

FIGURE 31–7 Asthma action plan for schools and families. From California Asthma Public Health Initiative. *Asthma Action Plan for Schools and Families*. Available at: http://www.betterasthmacare.org. Courtesy of the California Asthma Public Health Initiative.

presentation, a demonstration, and/or a group session. During the teaching session, the therapist educator must be mindful of learning styles and barriers to learning. Once the actual teaching has occurred, the therapist educator evaluates the effectiveness of the learning, perhaps through a quick question and answer session or through a return demonstration. It is critical that the therapist educator follow the process and equally important that he or she address the key teaching points. **Box 31–9** includes key teaching messages from the National Asthma Education and Prevention Program's guidelines that should be taught and reinforced at every opportunity.[26]

Pulmonary Rehabilitation

Pulmonary rehabilitation is another area within the profession of respiratory care where patient education skills have a significant role. Perhaps the most obvious and prominent condition associated with pulmonary rehabilitation is COPD. COPD is addressed quite extensively in Chapter 35, and thus this section simply refers to the patient education components of the topic.

One of the more authoritative publications related to pulmonary rehabilitation is the clinical practice guidelines jointly developed by the American College of Chest Physicians and the American Association of Cardiovascular and Pulmonary Rehabilitation entitled "Pulmonary Rehabilitation: Joint ACCP/AACVPR Evidence-Based Clinical Practice Guidelines." Among the many recommendations in this document is the statement that education should be an integral component of pulmonary rehabilitation and should include information

BOX 31–9

Key Educational Messages for Asthma Education

Basic Facts About Asthma

The contrast between airways of a person who has and a person who does not have asthma; the role of inflammation

What happens to the airways in an asthma attack

Roles of Medications: Understanding the Difference Between the Following

Long-term control medications: prevent symptoms, often by reducing inflammation. Must be taken daily. Do not expect them to give quick relief.

Quick-relief medications: short-acting beta-2 agonists relax muscles around the airway and provide prompt relief of symptoms. Do not expect them to provide long-term asthma control. Using quick-relief medication on a daily basis indicates the need for starting or increasing long-term control medications.

Patient Skills

Taking medications correctly

- Inhaler technique (demonstrate to patient and have the patient return the demonstration)
- Use of devices, such as prescribed valved holding chamber (VHC), spacer, nebulizer

Identifying and avoiding environmental exposures that worsen the patient's asthma (e.g., allergens, irritants, tobacco smoke)

Self-monitoring

- Assess level of asthma control
- Monitor symptoms and, if prescribed, peak flow
- Recognize early signs and symptoms of worsening asthma

Using written asthma action plan to know when and how to

- Take daily actions to control asthma
- Adjust medication in response to signs of worsening asthma
- Seek medical care as appropriate

From National Heart, Lung and Blood Institute. *National Asthma Education and Prevention Program, Expert Panel Report 3: Guidelines for the Diagnosis and Management of Asthma.* Bethesda, MD: National Institutes of Health; August 2007. NIH Publication 07-4051.

on collaborative self-management and on the prevention and treatment of exacerbations.[27] Additionally, the *Guidelines for Pulmonary Rehabilitation Programs,* prepared by the American Association for Cardiovascular and Pulmonary Rehabilitation, support the use and value of pulmonary rehabilitation.[28] These guidelines indicate that three key steps are essential in the education process: assessing the patient's educational needs, determining how the patient learns best, and selecting the approach or style that most benefits the patient.

The respiratory therapy educator must first determine the gaps in the patient's knowledge and understanding of his or her condition and contemplate a teaching plan. Assessing gaps in the patient's knowledge or understanding is best accomplished through a series of straightforward but nonthreatening questions. In developing the teaching plan, the therapist educator must be mindful of the patient's demographic characteristics, such as age, cultural background, language, educational level, and previous life experiences. Active rather than passive participation should be stressed, and the use of repetition and reinforcement of key messages emphasized. Variation in presentation methods, meaning multiple-sense approaches in the form of visual, auditory, and tactile teaching techniques, is more effective. There is considerable value in providing patients written material to take home and share with their family and support persons. Ensuring coverage of key educational content is critical to the success of the patient education program. **Box 31–10** lists key educational topics for pulmonary rehabilitation.[28] Clinical competency guidelines for professionals engaged in the assessment and intervention stages of education and training have also been identified.[29]

RESPIRATORY RECAP

Three Key Steps in Teaching Pulmonary Rehabilitation

1. Assessing the patient's educational needs
2. Determining how the patient learns best
3. Selecting the approach or style that most benefits the patient

BOX 31–10

Key Educational Topics for a Pulmonary Rehabilitation Program

- Normal pulmonary anatomy and physiology
- Chronic lung disease
- Description and interpretation of medical tests
- Breathing retraining
- Bronchial hygiene
- Medications
- Benefits of exercise
- Activities of daily living
- Eating right
- Irritant avoidance/Prevention and control of respiratory infections
- Leisure activities
- Coping with chronic lung disease and end-of-life planning

Adapted with permission from American Association for Cardiovascular and Pulmonary Rehabilitation. *Guidelines for Pulmonary Rehabilitation Programs.* 3rd ed. Champaign, IL: Human Kinetics; 2004:23.

Tobacco Cessation

Clearly, one of the more exciting opportunities for respiratory therapists to have an impact and to practice as a patient educator involves tobacco cessation. The definitive document for tobacco cessation is the government's clinical practice guideline entitled *Treating Tobacco Use and Dependence: 2008 Update.*[30] Driving this need and opportunity for respiratory therapists' involvement is a directive from the Joint Commission that mandates that all patients diagnosed with acute myocardial infarction, heart failure, or pneumonia must receive some form of smoking cessation counseling. This counseling must be medically documented and can be in the form of advice, a brochure or handout, an aid (e.g., nicotine patch, gum), or the viewing of a video.[31] Just how seriously clinicians take this mandatory requirement is highly questionable, and the earnestness of interventions has been subjected to considerable criticism. Although the effectiveness of intervention is debatable, it is apparent that opportunity abounds for someone to take this mandate seriously and boldly move the antitobacco agenda forward. Respiratory therapists are well positioned and well qualified to take on this role and make a huge impact in the tobacco cessation movement.

RESPIRATORY RECAP

Tobacco Cessation Movement

- » One driving force is a directive from the Joint Commission mandating that all patients diagnosed with acute myocardial infarction, heart failure, or pneumonia must receive some form of smoking cessation counseling.

The clinical practice guidelines provide guidance and direction for tobacco cessation by addressing such issues as the rationale for smoking cessation, patient readiness, and various strategies for effective intervention. **Box 31–11** outlines the ten key findings from the clinical practice guidelines that therapists should use in treating tobacco use and dependence. The guidelines also indicate that tobacco use presents a rare confluence of circumstances; that is, it is a highly significant health threat, there is a disinclination among clinicians to intervene consistently, and there exist highly effective interventions.[30]

Of profound importance is the fact that smoking tobacco is the leading cause of preventable morbidity and mortality in the United States. Tobacco use is no longer considered merely a habit but rather an addiction. This latter point is particularly critical because it reflects the need for both a behavioral and a pharmacologic intervention. The patient must be motivated to change, and thus stages of readiness have been identified, with intervention strategies associated with each stage. **Table 31–7** lists the stages of readiness as well as their characteristics and appropriate intervention techniques. Behavioral approaches entail individual, group, and telephone counseling; the literature indicates that effectiveness increases with treatment intensity.[30]

RESPIRATORY RECAP

Unique Considerations Related to Tobacco Cessation

- » Smoking poses a highly significant health threat.
- » There is a disinclination among clinicians to intervene consistently.
- » Highly effective interventions exist.

Clinicians specializing in tobacco cessation counseling can adopt a behavioral technique known as **motivational interviewing (MI)**. The overall spirit of motivational interviewing has been described as collaborative, evocative, and honoring of patient autonomy.[32] It is collaborative in that instead of an uneven power relationship in which the clinician assumes a superior position and directs the care, the patient assumes a more active role and participates with the clinician in the decision-making process. The MI process is evocative in that it seeks to motivate the patient to align his or her goals, dreams, desires, and aspirations with health behaviors that are in the patient's best interest. Finally, the MI process strives to honor the autonomy of the patient. Patients inherently strive for self-determination and freedom of choice. The MI process avoids being paternal and judgmental and is

BOX 31–11

Ten Key Findings of *Treating Tobacco Use and Dependence: 2008 Update*

1. Tobacco dependence is a chronic disease that often requires repeated intervention and multiple attempts to quit. Effective treatments exist, however, that can significantly increase rates of long-term abstinence.
2. It is essential that clinicians and healthcare delivery systems consistently identify and document tobacco use status and treat every tobacco user seen in a healthcare setting.
3. Tobacco dependence treatments are effective across a broad range of populations. Clinicians should encourage every patient willing to make a quit attempt to use the recommended counseling treatments and medications in the guideline.
4. Brief tobacco dependence treatment is effective. Clinicians should offer every patient who uses tobacco at least the brief treatments shown to be effective in the guideline.
5. Individual, group, and telephone counseling are effective, and their effectiveness increases with treatment intensity. Two components of counseling are especially effective and clinicians should use these when counseling patients making a quit attempt:
   - Practical counseling (problem-solving/skills training)
   - Social support delivered as part of treatment
6. There are numerous effective medications for tobacco dependence, and clinicians should encourage their use by all patients attempting to quit smoking, except when medically contraindicated or with specific populations for which there is insufficient evidence of effectiveness (i.e., pregnant women, smokeless tobacco users, light smokers, adolescents).
   - Seven first-line medications (five nicotine and two nonnicotine) reliably increase long-term smoking abstinence rates: bupropion SR, nicotine gum, nicotine inhaler, nicotine lozenge, nicotine nasal spray, nicotine patch, and varenicline.
   - Clinicians should also consider the use of certain combinations of medications identified as effective in the guideline.
7. Counseling and medication are effective when used by themselves for treating tobacco dependence. However, the combination of counseling and medication is more effective than either alone. Thus, clinicians should encourage all individuals making a quit attempt to use both counseling and medication.
8. Telephone quit line counseling is effective with diverse populations and has broad reach. Therefore, clinicians and healthcare delivery systems should both ensure patient access to quit lines and promote quit line use.
9. If a tobacco user is currently unwilling to make a quit attempt, clinicians should use the motivational treatments shown in the guideline to be effective in increasing future quit attempts.
10. Tobacco dependence treatments are both clinically effective and highly cost effective relative to interventions for other clinical disorders. Providing coverage for these treatments increases quit rates. Insurers and purchasers should ensure that all insurance plans include the counseling and medication identified as effective in the guideline as covered benefits.

From Fiore MC, Jaén CR, Baker TB, et al. *Treating Tobacco Use and Dependence: 2008 Update. Quick Reference Guide for Clinicians.* Rockville, MD: U.S. Department of Health and Human Services; April 2009.

respectful of the patient's freedom to make choices and to self-manage his or her health.

Motivational interviewing entails four guiding principles: (1) resisting the righting reflex, (2) understanding and exploring the patient's own motivations, (3) listening with empathy, and (4) empowering the patient, encouraging hope and optimism.[32] Resisting the righting reflex simply means to avoid telling people what they should do. Although telling the patient what to do is admirable and seemingly the right thing to do, it will typically result in resistance from the patient and can be destructive to the relationship. The patient will likely defend his or her behavior and attempt to minimize or justify his or her actions. It is imperative that one avoid arguing. Little progress can occur when feelings of hostility are present, and thus it is more effective to express empathy and attempt to understand what motivates the patient's behavior. One should first *listen* to what patients have to say and elicit from them what they

RESPIRATORY RECAP

Motivational Interviewing

» Collaborative
» Evocative
» Honoring of patient autonomy

TABLE 31–7 Stages of Readiness: Characteristics and Intervention Techniques

Stage	Characteristics	Intervention Techniques
Precontemplative	Uninterested, unaware, or unwilling to make a change May be in denial	Best to avoid arguing. Maintain a positive relationship. Demonstrate empathy. Ask thought-provoking questions such as, "What would have to happen for you to know there is a problem with your smoking?" Well-phrased questions will leave patients pondering and will move them along the process to change.
Contemplative	Considering a change Ambivalent about change	Continue to demonstrate empathy, praise, and encouragement. Consider having the patient weigh the benefits and costs of behavior change. Ask questions such as, "Why do you want to change?", "What are reasons for not changing?", and "What are the barriers that keep you from change?"
Preparation	Preparing to make a specific change	Continue to assist with problem-solving barriers. Strategies should shift from motivational to behavioral skills. Encourage small changes, such as switching to a different brand of cigarette.
Action	Practicing new behaviors Taking definitive action	Ask about successes and difficulties. Continue to provide praise and admiration.
Maintenance	Involves incorporating the new behavior over the long haul	Continue to ask about successes and difficulties. Continue to provide praise and admiration.
Relapse	Resumption of old behaviors May feel demoralized	Recognize that this is common. Explain that, despite relapses, they have learned something new about themselves, such as that it is best to avoid smoke-filled environments. Evaluate triggers. Focus on the successful part of the plan. Be supportive, and re-engage their efforts.

Data from Zimmerman G, Olsen C, Bosworth M. A "Stage of Change" approach to help patients change behavior. *Am Fam Physician.* 2000; 61:1409–1416.

desire. In other words, actively listen with the intention of eliciting discrepancy (a gap) between desired behavior versus actual behavior. This can take the form of reflective and respectful listening in which one reserves judgment and avoids criticism. More often then not, the proper and appropriate actions are known and desired by the patient.

Finally, it is critical that the patient be empowered to actively come to the right choice and to essentially *own* his or her decision. The therapist should invite new perspectives and not impose his or her desires. Thus, the patient must be the source of finding answers and solutions. Patients must believe in the possibility of change and that they are *in control* and *have control* over their actions. The therapist's role is to affirm this view as well as provide assistance in appropriate interventions. **Table 31–8** provides some interviewing strategies that pertain to each of the four guiding principles. These techniques are often represented in brief by the acronym RULE: resist, understand, listen, and empower.[32]

> **RESPIRATORY RECAP**
>
> **Guiding Principles of Motivational Interviewing: RULE**
>
> » **R**esist the righting reflex.
> » **U**nderstand and explore the patient's own motivations.
> » **L**isten with empathy.
> » **E**mpower the patient.

The practice guidelines provide considerable guidance regarding the steps to follow for the patient who is willing to change as well as the patient who is unwilling to change. **Table 31–9** provides a detailed account of the action and strategies for implementation of the five steps to follow for the patient willing to change. These five steps are also known as the five As and consist of the following: ask, advise, assess, assist, and arrange. **Figure 31–8** depicts the model for the treatment of

> **RESPIRATORY RECAP**
>
> **Critical Components of the Mayo Clinic Smoking Cessation Program**
>
> » A comprehensive tobacco use assessment
> » Personalized treatment plans and educational materials appropriate for the patient's stage of readiness to change
> » Different interventions at various stages of behavior change
> » Individual counseling sessions
> » Information on local support groups
> » Relapse prevention strategies
> » Cessation resources
> » Outcome measurement and assessment
> » Oversight and distribution of nicotine replacement therapy

TABLE 31-8 Selective Examples of Interviewing Strategies from the Four Guiding Principles of Motivational Interviewing

Guiding Principle	Interviewing Strategies	Statements Supporting Strategies
Resist the righting reflex	Back off and use reflection when the patient expresses resistance Express empathy Ask permission to provide information	"Sounds like you are feeling pressured about your smoking." "You are worried about how you would manage withdrawal symptoms." "Would you like to hear about some strategies that can help you address that concern when you quit?"
Understand your patient's motivations	Highlight the discrepancy between the patient's present behavior and expressed priorities, values, and goals Reinforce and support "change talk" and "commitment" language Build and deepen commitment to change	"It sounds like you are very devoted to your family. How do you think your smoking is affecting your children?" "So, you realize how smoking is affecting your breathing and making it hard to keep up with your kids." "It's great that you are going to quit when you get through this busy time at work." "There are effective treatments that will ease the pain of quitting, including counseling and many medication options." "We would like to help you avoid a stroke like the one your father had."
Listen with empathy	Use open-ended questions to explore: • The importance of addressing smoking or other tobacco use • Concerns and benefits of quitting Use reflective listening to seek shared understanding: • Reflect words or meaning • Summarize Normalize feelings and concerns Support the patient's autonomy and right to choose or reject change	"How important do you think it is for you to quit smoking?" "What might happen if you quit?" "So do you think smoking helps you to maintain your weight?" "What I have heard so far is that smoking is something you enjoy. On the other hand, your boyfriend hates your smoking, and you are worried you might develop a serious disease." "Many people worry about managing without cigarettes." "I hear you saying you are not ready to quit smoking right now. I'm here to help you when you are ready."
Empower the patient	Help the patient to identify and build on past successes Offer options for achievable small steps toward change: • Call the quit line (1-800-QUIT-NOW) for advice and information • Read about quitting benefits and strategies. • Change smoking patterns (e.g., no smoking in the home) • Ask the patient to share his or her ideas about quitting strategies	"So you were fairly successful the last time you tried to quit."

Modified from Fiore MC, Jaen CR, Baker, TB, et al. *Treating Tobacco Use and Dependence: 2008 Update. Clinical Practice Guideline*. Rockville, MD: U.S. Department of Health and Human Services; May 2008:58.

TABLE 31–9 The Five Steps of a Tobacco Cessation Program for Patients Willing to Quit (the 5 As)

Strategy	Action	Strategies for Implementation
1. Ask	Implement an officewide system that ensures that, for every patient at every clinic visit, tobacco use is queried and documented.	Expand the vital signs to include tobacco use, or use an alternative universal identification system.
2. Advise	In a clear, strong, and personalized manner, urge every tobacco user to quit.	Advice should be: • *Clear:* "It is important that you quit smoking (or using chewing tobacco) now, and I can help you." "Cutting down while you are ill is not enough." "Occasional or light smoking is still dangerous." • *Strong:* "As your clinician, I need you to know that quitting smoking is the most important thing you can do to protect your health now and in the future. The clinic staff and I will help you." • *Personalized:* Tie tobacco use to current symptoms and health concerns, and/or its social and economic costs, and/or the impact of tobacco use on children and others in the household. "Continuing to smoke makes your asthma worse, and quitting may dramatically improve your health." "Quitting smoking may reduce the number of ear infections your child has."

3. Assess	Assess every tobacco user's willingness to make a quit attempt at this time.	Assess patient's willingness to quit: "Are you willing to give quitting a try?"
		• If the patient is willing to make a quit attempt at this time, provide assistance.
		  • If the patient will participate in an intensive treatment, deliver such a treatment or link/refer to an intensive intervention.
		  • If the patient is a member of a special population (e.g., adolescent, pregnant smoker, racial/ethnic minority), consider providing additional information.
		• If the patient clearly states that he or she is unwilling to make a quit attempt at this time, provide an intervention shown to increase future quit attempts.

4. Assist	Help the patient with a quit plan. Recommend the use of approved medication, except when contraindicated or with specific populations for which there is insufficient evidence of effectiveness (e.g., pregnant women, smokeless tobacco users, light smokers, adolescents). Provide practical counseling (problem-solving/skills training). Provide intratreatment social support. Provide supplementary materials, including information on quit lines. For the smoker unwilling to quit at this time	A patient's preparations for quitting: • **S**et a quit date. Ideally, the quit date should be within 2 weeks. • **T**ell family, friends, and coworkers about quitting, and request understanding and support. • **A**nticipate challenges to the upcoming quit attempt, particularly during the critical first few weeks. These include nicotine withdrawal symptoms. • **R**emove tobacco products from your environment. Prior to quitting, avoid smoking in places where you spend a lot of time (e.g., work, home, car). Make your home smoke-free. Recommend the use of medications found to be effective in this guideline. Explain how these medications increase quitting success and reduce withdrawal symptoms. The first-line medications include bupropion SR, nicotine gum, nicotine inhaler, nicotine lozenge, nicotine nasal spray, nicotine patch, and varenicline; second-line medications include clonidine and nortriptyline. There is insufficient evidence to recommend medications for certain populations (e.g., pregnant women, smokeless tobacco users, light smokers, adolescents). *Abstinence.* Striving for total abstinence is essential. Not even a single puff after the quit date. *Past quit experience.* Identify what helped and what hurt in previous quit attempts. Build on past success. *Anticipate triggers or challenges in the upcoming attempt.* Discuss challenges/triggers and how the patient will successfully overcome them (e.g., avoid triggers, alter routines). *Alcohol.* Because alcohol is associated with relapse, the patient should consider limiting/abstaining from alcohol while quitting. (Note that reducing alcohol intake could precipitate withdrawal in alcohol-dependent persons.) *Other smokers in the household.* Quitting is more difficult when there is another smoker in the household. Patients should encourage housemates to quit with them or to not smoke in their presence. Provide a supportive clinical environment while encouraging the patient in his or her quit attempt. "My office staff and I are available to assist you." "I'm recommending treatment that can provide ongoing support." *Sources:* Federal agencies, nonprofit agencies, national quit line network (1-800-QUIT-NOW), or local/state/tribal health departments or quit lines. *Type:* Culturally, racially, educationally, and age-appropriate for the patient. *Location:* Readily available at every clinician's workstation. See Table 31–10.
5. Arrange	Arrange for follow-up contacts, either in person or via telephone. For smokers unwilling to quit at this time	*Timing:* Follow-up contact should begin soon after the quit date, preferably during the first week. A second follow-up contact is recommended within the first month. Schedule further follow-up contacts as indicated. *Actions during follow-up contact:* For all patients, identify problems already encountered and anticipate challenges in the immediate future. Assess medication use and problems. Remind patients of quit line support (1-800-QUIT-NOW). Address tobacco use at next clinical visit (treat tobacco use as a chronic disease). For patients who are abstinent, congratulate them on their success. If tobacco use has occurred, review circumstances and elicit recommitment to total abstinence. Consider use of or link to more intensive treatment. See Table 31–10.

Modified from Fiore MC, Jaen CR, Baker, TB, et al. *Treating Tobacco Use and Dependence: 2008 Update. Clinical Practice Guideline.* Rockville, MD: U.S. Department of Health and Human Services; May 2008:40–43.

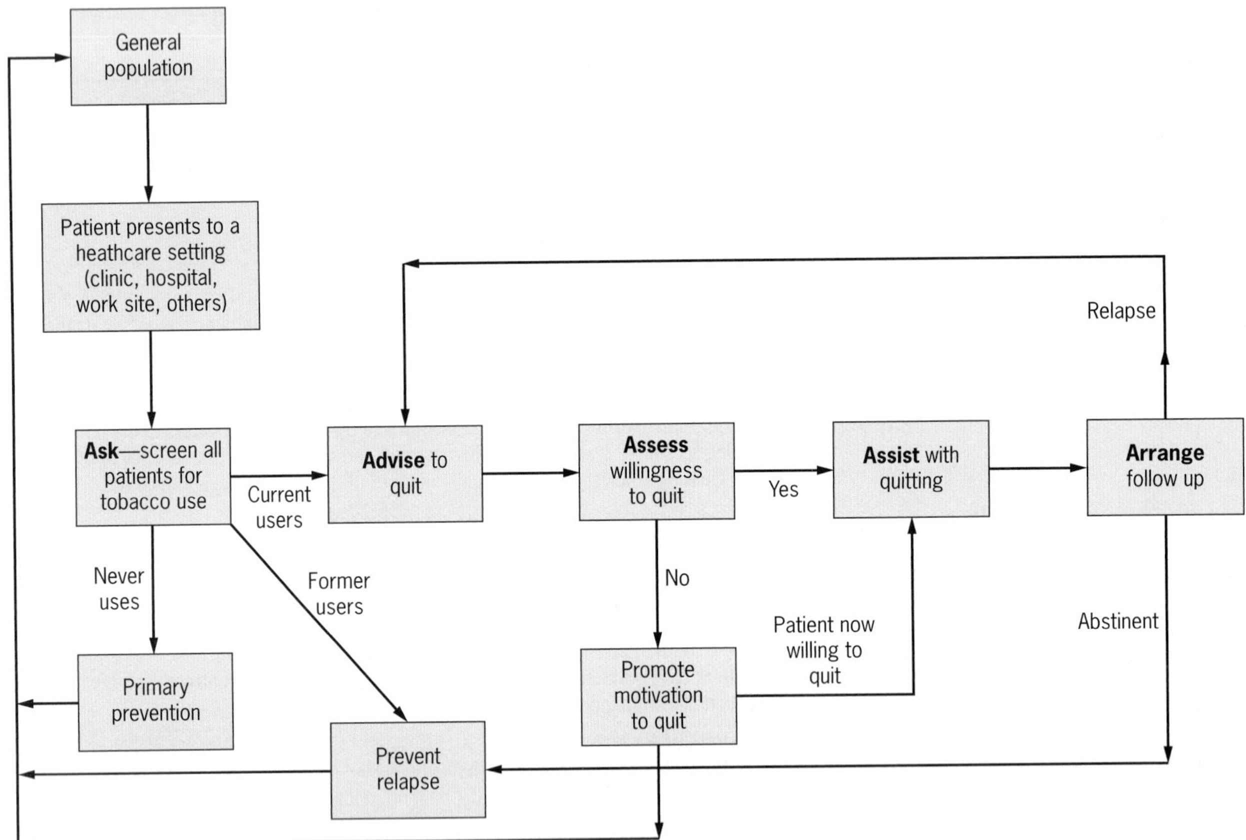

FIGURE 31–8 Model for the treatment of tobacco use and dependence. From Fiore MC, et al. *Treating Tobacco Use and Dependence: 2008 Update*. U.S. Department of Health and Human Services; 2009.

tobacco use and dependence and demonstrates how these five steps can be employed in a tobacco cessation program.[30]

In the event the patient is not motivated or is unwilling to change, the guidelines recommend the use of the five Rs: relevance, risk, rewards, roadblocks, and repetition. **Table 31–10** provides a detailed account of the five Rs.

The practice guidelines also are helpful with regard to pharmacologic support. The guidelines recommend seven approved, first-line medications for the treatment of tobacco cessation. The seven consist of the five nicotine replacement therapies (NRTs)—nicotine gum, nicotine inhaler, nicotine lozenge, nicotine nasal spray, and the nicotine patch—as well as two non-nicotine-based products, bupropion SR and varenicline. The actions of each group are different. NRTs are intended to satisfy the craving for nicotine by replacing the nicotine provided by cigarettes with nicotine in the various forms just identified. The nicotine levels are gradually reduced in the body; in essence, the patient is weaned from nicotine by methodically and systematically decreasing the dose delivered.

Bupropion was the first nonnicotine drug. It is marketed as Wellbutrin as an antidepressant and as Zyban as a smoking cessation aid. It is considered to function by blocking the neuronal reuptake of dopamine and norepinephrine and by blockade of nicotinic acetylcholinergic receptors. Varenicline, marketed as Chantix, is also an antidepressant that was found to reduce the cravings for nicotine. Varenicline is said to work in two ways: it targets nicotine receptors in the brain, attaches to them, and blocks nicotine from reaching them. The blocking of nicotine results in reduction of craving, and thus smokers find little if any satisfaction in smoking and discontinue the smoking habit.

Finally, relapse is a serious issue related to success, and variables associated with abstinence have been identified. **Table 31–11** provides examples of variables associated with both high as well as low abstinence.

Although there are numerous smoking cessation programs, perhaps one of the most popular and authoritative is the program model developed at the Mayo Clinic. What brings considerable notoriety to the Mayo Clinic program is its comprehensive nature. It consists of the

TABLE 31-10 The Five Steps of a Tobacco Cessation Program for Patients Unwilling to Quit (the 5 Rs)

Step	Explanation
1. Relevance	Encourage the patient to indicate why quitting is personally relevant, being as specific as possible. Motivational information has the greatest impact if it is relevant to a patient's disease status or risk, family or social situation (e.g., having children in the home), health concerns, age, gender, and other important patient characteristics (e.g., prior quitting experience, personal barriers to cessation).
2. Risk	The clinician should ask the patient to identify potential negative consequences of tobacco use. The clinician may suggest and highlight those that seem most relevant to the patient. The clinician should emphasize that smoking low-tar/low-nicotine cigarettes or use of other forms of tobacco (e.g., smokeless tobacco, cigars, pipes) will not eliminate these risks. Examples of risks are as follows. • *Acute risks:* Shortness of breath, exacerbation of asthma, increased risk of respiratory infections, harm to pregnancy, impotence, infertility. • *Long-term risks:* Heart attacks and strokes, lung and other cancers (e.g., larynx, oral cavity, pharynx, esophagus, pancreas, stomach, kidney, bladder, cervix, acute myelocytic leukemia), chronic obstructive pulmonary diseases (e.g., chronic bronchitis, emphysema), osteoporosis, long-term disability, and need for extended care. • *Environmental risks:* Increased risk of lung cancer and heart disease in spouses; increased risk for low birth weight, sudden infant death syndrome (SIDS), asthma, middle ear disease, and respiratory infections in children of smokers.
3. Rewards	The clinician should ask the patient to identify potential benefits of stopping tobacco use. The clinician may suggest and highlight those that seem most relevant to the patient. Examples of rewards follow. • Improved health • Food will taste better • Improved sense of smell • Saving money • Feeling better about oneself • Home, car, clothing, and breath will smell better • Setting a good example for children and decreasing the likelihood that they will smoke • Having healthier babies and children • Feeling better physically • Performing better in physical activities • Improved appearance, including reduced wrinkling/aging of skin and whiter teeth
4. Roadblocks	The clinician should ask the patient to identify barriers or impediments to quitting and provide treatment (e.g., problem-solving counseling, medication) that could address barriers. Typical barriers might include the following. • Withdrawal symptoms • Fear of failure • Weight gain • Lack of support • Depression • Enjoyment of tobacco • Being around other tobacco users • Limited knowledge of effective treatment options
5. Repetition	The motivational intervention should be repeated every time an unmotivated patient visits the clinic setting. Tobacco users who have failed in previous quit attempts should be told that most people make repeated quit attempts before they are successful.

Modified from Fiore MC, Jaen CR, Baker, TB, et al. *Treating Tobacco Use and Dependence: 2008 Update. Clinical Practice Guideline.* Rockville, MD: U.S. Department of Health and Human Services; May 2008:59–60.

following components: a comprehensive tobacco use assessment, personalized treatment plans and educational materials appropriate for the patient's stage of readiness to change, different interventions at various stages of behavior change, individual counseling sessions, information on local support groups, relapse prevention strategies, cessation resources, outcome measurement and assessment, and oversight and distribution of NRT.[33]

TABLE 31-11 Variables Associated with Higher and Lower Tobacco Abstinence

Variable	Examples
Higher Abstinence Rates	
High motivation	Tobacco user reports a strong motivation to quit.
Ready to change	Tobacco user is ready to quit within a 1-month period.
Moderate to high self-efficacy	Tobacco user is confident in his or her ability to quit.
Supportive social network	A smoke-free workplace and home; friends who do not smoke in the quitter's presence.
Lower Abstinence Rates	
High nicotine dependence	Tobacco user smokes heavily (≥20 cigarettes per day), and/or has first cigarette of the day within 30 minutes after waking in the morning.
Psychiatric comorbidity and substance use	Tobacco user currently has elevated depressive symptoms, active alcohol abuse, or schizophrenia.
High stress level	Stressful life circumstances and/or recent or anticipated major life changes (e.g., divorce, job change).
Exposure to other smokers	Other smokers in the household.

Modified from Fiore MC, Jaen CR, Baker, TB, et al. *Treating Tobacco Use and Dependence: 2008 Update. Clinical Practice Guideline*. Rockville, MD: U.S. Department of Health and Human Services; May 2008:81.

The clinical practice guidelines stress two basic and minimal components of any effective smoking cessation program, namely, behavioral counseling and pharmacologic intervention. However, the guidelines also make a compelling case that a successful tobacco dependence treatment strategy must be tied to the healthcare system in which it is embedded.[30] It must include clinicians, administrators, insurers, and purchasers. One can clearly see that the role of the respiratory therapist as the front-line patient educator, patient advocate, and clinician is central to the smoking cessation movement.

KEY POINTS

- Patient education plays an increasingly important role in healthcare delivery.
- Regulatory, social, demographic, economic, philosophic, and practical incentives drive patient education.
- The healthcare system must better prepare patients and informal caregivers to engage in preventive, maintenance, and restorative healthcare measures.
- Respiratory therapists must be aware of the highly dependent nature of patients.
- The goals and indications of patient education focus on the creation of behavior change.
- Patient education is a detailed, sequential process.
- Assessment is the first step; it involves determination of the patient's learning needs and readiness to learn.
- The planning phase involves development of goals and well-written objectives and addressing of the three learning domains.
- The implementation phase involves actual teaching, which requires a variety of strategies and techniques.
- Common barriers to learning include lack of readiness, physical and emotional obstacles, language barriers, and lack of motivation.
- The nine principles of adult learning produce the mnemonic RAMP-2-FAME: recency, appropriateness, motivation, primacy, two-way communication, feedback, active learning, multiple-sense learning, and exercise.
- Evaluation, the last phase in patient education, should be a continual process encompassing evaluation of the entire teaching process and of the effectiveness of the patient's learning.
- Respiratory therapy educators should always be alert to take advantage of the teaching moment.
- Examples of programs in which patient education skills can be incorporated within the practice of a respiratory therapist are asthma education, pulmonary rehabilitation, and smoking cessation programs.
- Patient education for a partnership is one of the four key components of asthma care.
- One of the major goals of any pulmonary rehabilitation program is teaching the patient how to care for himself or herself and to improve his or her quality of life.
- The Joint Commission mandates that all patients with certain conditions receive medically documented smoking cessation counseling.
- Effective smoking cessation entails behavioral counseling as well as pharmacologic intervention.
- Respiratory therapists possess the skill set to effectively serve as patient educators and should continue to endorse and welcome this critical role.

REFERENCES

1. Redman BK. *The Practice of Patient Education*. 9th ed. St. Louis: Mosby; 2001.
2. National Center for Health Statistics. *Health, United States, 2009: With Special Feature on Medical Technology*. Hyattsville, MD: U.S. Government Printing Office. Available at: http://www.cdc.gov/nchs/data/hus/hus09.pdf#123.
3. DuBrey SR, Jean R. *Promoting Wellness in Nursing Practice: A Step-by-Step Approach in Patient Education*. St. Louis: Mosby; 1982.

4. Boyd M, Graham B, Gleit C, et al. *Health Teaching in Nursing Practice: A Professional Model.* 3rd ed. Stamford, CT: Appleton & Lange; 1998.
5. Travis J, Ryan RS. *Wellness Workbook.* 2nd ed. Berkeley, CA: Ten Speed Press; 1988.
6. U.S. Census Bureau. Expectation of life at birth, 1970 to 2005, and projections, 2010 to 2020. Available at: http://www.census.gov/compendia/statab/2009/tables/09s0100.pdf.
7. Doll R, Peto R, Boreham J, Sutherland I. Mortality in relation to smoking: 50 years' observations on male British doctors. *BMJ.* 2004;328:1519.
8. American Association for Respiratory Care. Clinical practice guideline: providing patient and caregiver training. *Respir Care.* 2010;55(6):765–769.
9. American Association for Respiratory Care. Clinical practice guideline: training the health-care professional for the role of patient and caregiver educator. *Respir Care.* 1996;41:654–657.
10. Chatham MAH, Knapp BL. *Patient Education Handbook.* Bowie, MD: Robert J Brady; 1982.
11. Lubkin IM. *Chronic Illness: Impact and Intervention.* 7th ed. Sudbury, MA: Jones and Bartlett; 2008.
12. Committee on Health Literacy, Institute of Medicine; Nelsen-Bohlman LN, Panzer AM, Kindig DA, eds. *Health Literacy: A Prescription to End Confusion.* Washington, DC: National Academies Press; 2004.
13. Kirsch I, Jungeblut A, Jenkins A. *Adult Literacy in America: A First Look at the Results of the National Adult Literacy Survey (NALS).* Washington, DC: National Center for Education Statistics, U.S. Department of Education; September 1993.
14. Kutner M, Greenberg E, Jin Y, Paulsen C. *The Health Literacy of America's Adults: Results from the 2003 National Assessment of Adult Literacy.* Washington, DC: National Center for Education Statistics, U.S. Department of Education; 2006.
15. American Medical Association Foundation. *Health Literacy: A Manual for Clinicians.* Chicago: American Medical Association Foundation and American Medical Association; 2003.
16. Weiss B. *Health Literacy and Patient Safety: Help Patients Understand.* Chicago: American Medical Association Foundation and American Medical Association; 2007.
17. The Joint Commission. "What Did the Doctor Say?" Improving Health Literacy to Protect Patient Safety. Oakbrook Terrace, IL: The Joint Commission; 2007.
18. Partnership for Clear Health Communication. *Ask Me 3: Program Implementation Guide for Health Care and Information Providers.* Available at: http://www.npsf.org/askme3/pdfs/Ask_Me_Implem_Guide.pdf.
19. McKenzie J, Smeltzer J. *Planning, Implementing and Evaluating Health Promotion Programs: A Primer.* 2nd ed. Boston: Allyn & Bacon; 1997.
20. Babcock D, Mary M. *Client Education: Theory and Practice.* St. Louis: Mosby; 1994.
21. National Heart, Lung, and Blood Institute. *Open Airways: Asthma Self-Management Program.* Bethesda, MD: National Institutes of Health; 1984. NIH Publication 84-2365.
22. National Heart, Lung and Blood Institute. *National Asthma Education and Prevention Program, Expert Panel Report 3: Guidelines for the Diagnosis and Management of Asthma.* Bethesda, MD: National Institutes of Health; August 2007. NIH Publication 07-4051. Available at: http://www.nhlbi.nih.gov/guidelines/asthma/asthgdln.htm.
23. Bopp A, Lubkin I. *Chronic Illness: Impact and Interventions.* 2nd ed. Sudbury, MA: Jones & Bartlett Learning; 1990.
24. Winthrop E. *Patient Teaching Tips.* St. Louis: Mosby; 1995.
25. Kroehnert G. *Basic Training for Trainers: A Handbook for Trainers.* 2nd ed. New York: McGraw-Hill; 1995.
26. National Heart, Lung and Blood Institute. *National Asthma Education and Prevention Program, Expert Panel Report 3: Guidelines for the Diagnosis and Management of Asthma—Summary Report.* Bethesda, MD: National Institutes of Health; October 2007. NIH Publication 08-5846. Available at: http://www.nhlbi.nih.gov/guidelines/asthma/asthsumm.htm.
27. Ries AL, Bauldoff GS, Carlin BW, et al. Pulmonary rehabilitation: joint ACCP/AACVPR evidence-based clinical practice guidelines. *Chest.* 2007;131(5 suppl):4S–42S.
28. American Association for Cardiovascular and Pulmonary Rehabilitation. *Guidelines for Pulmonary Rehabilitation Programs.* 3rd ed. Champaign, IL: Human Kinetics; 2004:21.
29. Nici L, Limberg T, Hilling L, et al. Clinical competency guidelines for pulmonary rehabilitation professionals. *J Cardiopulm Rehabil Prev.* 2007;27:355–358.
30. Fiore MC, Jaén CR, Baker TB, et al. *Treating Tobacco Use and Dependence: 2008 Update. Quick Reference Guide for Clinicians.* Rockville, MD: U.S. Department of Health and Human Services; April 2009. Available at: http://www.surgeongeneral.gov/tobacco/treating_tobacco_use08.pdf.
31. Tobacco Free Nurses. Tobacco Free Nurses fact sheet on the Joint Commission on Accreditation of Healthcare Organization's (JCAHO) smoking cessation counseling performance measures. Available at: http://tobaccofreenurses.org/media/documents/facts01print.pdf.
32. Rollnick S, Miller WR, Butler CC. *Motivational Interviewing in Health Care: Helping Patients Change Behavior.* New York: Guilford Press; 2008.
33. Mayo Clinic Health Solutions. Mayo Clinic Tobacco Quitline: program components. Available at: http://www.mayoclinichealthsolutions.com/products/Tobacco-Quitline-Program-Components.cfm.

CHAPTER 32

Decision Making and the Role of Respiratory Therapists as Consultants

Shelley C. Mishoe
Laura H. Beveridge

OUTLINE

OBJECTIVES

1. Describe the evolving role of respiratory therapists as decision makers and consultants.
2. Define clinical practice guidelines (CPGs), respiratory care protocols, critical pathways, and other key words.
3. Discuss the design, implementation, and evaluation of CPGs, respiratory care protocols, and critical pathways.
4. Discuss the advantages and limitations of CPGs, protocols, and critical pathways.
5. Describe outcomes evaluation.
6. Define variance and the ways to track it.
7. Describe evidence-based medicine.
8. Describe internal consulting and how it can improve organizational effectiveness.
9. Elaborate on the roles and skills of internal consultants.
10. Make the case that respiratory therapists can function as consultants.

KEY TERMS

algorithm
benchmarking
clinical practice guidelines (CPGs)
critical pathway (CP)
evidence-based medicine (EBM)
managed care
multidisciplinary
outcomes evaluation
respiratory care protocol
variance

INTRODUCTION

This chapter describes the role of respiratory therapists as decision makers and consultants. Expanding roles are possible with the use of clinical practice guidelines, respiratory care protocols, and critical pathways. This chapter discusses strategies for using these tools. The ultimate goal is to improve the outcomes of respiratory care. Respiratory therapists as consultants can improve the allocation and effectiveness of care. The consultant role requires motivated respiratory therapists who are well prepared.

The Evolving Role of Respiratory Therapists as Decision Makers and Consultants

Longer life expectancies have increased the use and costs for healthcare.[1] Providing healthcare at a decreased cost requires many changes. The roles, skills, and traits of healthcare professionals have changed. There is a continued need to support the role of respiratory therapists as decision makers and consultants.[2] Respiratory therapists must possess expanded knowledge beyond technical training. Technical knowledge alone does not assure competence.

Throughout the evolution of the profession, there have been efforts to prepare for the future. A Delphi study funded by the American Association for Respiratory Care (AARC) in the late 1980s looked at the desired attributes of future respiratory therapists and suggested curriculum needs for graduates. The AARC also held two consensus conferences, the first in 1992 and another in 1993. These conferences further evaluated the needs in healthcare and the profession. It was agreed that respiratory therapists should be critical-thinking, multiskilled, and flexible. The 1993 conference focused on a plan to improve and standardize educational outcomes.[3–5]

The AARC established a task force to look ahead to 2015 and beyond. The goal was to analyze the future roles of respiratory therapists. The task force looked specifically at new responsibilities. Evolving changes in healthcare include rising costs and an aging population, leading to increased attention on chronic disease management. Technology is changing rapidly, and there is increased involvement by consumers. The 2015 task force agreed that evidence-based medicine will continue to grow in importance and that biomedical inventions will mandate that respiratory therapists be more sophisticated.[6]

In the past, respiratory therapists were technicians valued for their technical skills. The profession was called *inhalation therapy*. Their role in the 1940s included giving treatments. They used special equipment, which included oxygen tanks and aerosol generators. They also used ventilators. Early practitioners assisted nursing staff. Most respiratory care departments were a part of the nursing department.

Separate respiratory therapy departments developed to support the demand. They performed procedures and therapies ordered by physicians under a fee for service. This was defined as retrospective payment. There was little incentive to evaluate effectiveness. No one questioned the traditional model, even when it resulted in poor utilization of services.[7] Healthcare based its practices on individual judgment, much of which was based in turn on anecdotal information.

Beginning in the 1980s it became clear that respiratory therapy was overutilized. Reducing the number of procedures did not have negative effects on healthcare outcomes.[8] By the early 1990s, poor allocation of respiratory care was described. Reports indicated that some patients were receiving unneeded respiratory therapy whereas others were not getting the care they needed.[9] Poor use of respiratory care services occurs for many reasons. One is insufficient knowledge by those who prescribe the care. Another is the changing needs of patients when physicians are unavailable.[10]

Respiratory therapists achieved the registered respiratory therapist (RRT) credential and developed into experts. RRTs were capable of using protocols. By the 1990s, protocol-based respiratory care was being used, which improved the effectiveness of care. These protocols included infection control to minimize ventilator-acquired pneumonia[11,12] and protocols for chest physiotherapy.[13] The clinical use of arterial blood gases[14] and oxygen therapy[15] also was described. Additional protocols on inhaled bronchodilator administration were described.[16–18] And, protocols for weaning from mechanical ventilation were introduced,[19,20] as were protocols for daily breathing trials[21] and team-driven extubation.[22] Many protocols were designed to reduce medical care costs.[23] They also unburdened physicians from tasks. Most important, they improved patient outcomes.[23] Protocols or practice guidelines are important to standardize medical practices.

Technology and costs have placed respiratory therapists into positions as consultants. As consultants, RRTs are decision makers. Respiratory therapists also are involved in patient education. They deliver and evaluate patient education, which can improve quality of life. Patients and therapists work together to design treatment plans.

Studies have shown that respiratory therapists can successfully prescribe and carry out standardized respiratory care.[8,15,18–20,23–28] Randomized controlled trials compared care from respiratory therapists and from physicians. These studies found better agreement with the care plan when respiratory therapists directed the care. They also found lower costs and no adverse events.[2] Studies also have documented physicians' positive views regarding a respiratory therapy consult service.[29]

Rapid response teams, also called rapid assessment teams (RATs), were developed. RATs identify, assess, and quickly act to prevent a patient from deteriorating into a full code. Respiratory therapists have shown consultant strengths as part of these multidisciplinary teams.

Respiratory therapy continues to function under medical direction. Today, medical direction is best provided in the form of guidelines, pathways, or protocols. These allow independent assessment and require judgment and decision making. **Box 32–1** lists examples of protocols.[2] In these roles, respiratory therapists function as physician extenders. They might be compared with physician assistants.

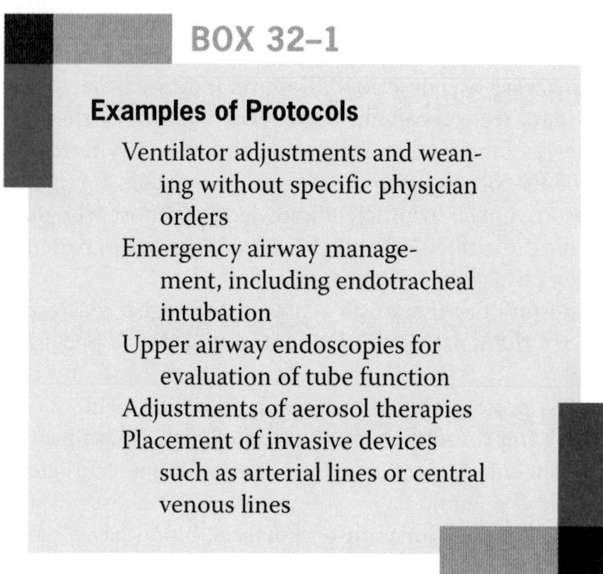

BOX 32–1

Examples of Protocols

Ventilator adjustments and weaning without specific physician orders
Emergency airway management, including endotracheal intubation
Upper airway endoscopies for evaluation of tube function
Adjustments of aerosol therapies
Placement of invasive devices such as arterial lines or central venous lines

Centralized respiratory care departments remain important, because equipment management requires high expertise. Skills documentation is also required. Continuing education and credentialing are other reasons to maintain a respiratory care department. Respiratory therapists must continue to work closely with physicians. These helpful relationships can achieve better patient care and better education. Using protocols increases the role of therapists as consultants. Outcomes assessment and evidence-based medicine (EBM) are other factors. Administrators must recognize the cost effectiveness of care by well-trained respiratory therapists.

Introduction to Guidelines, Protocols, and Pathways

Clinical guidelines, protocols, and critical pathways are developed to standardize care. Standardized care can improve efficiency, reduce costs, and document effectiveness. This section provides a brief overview of these terms and examines the advantages, limitations, and strategies of each concept.

Clinical Practice Guidelines

Clinical practice guidelines (CPGs) are statements that suggest healthcare for specific situations.[30] CPGs are developed by professional associations and by clinical groups. They address the appropriateness of healthcare using the best evidence; specify indications for tests, procedures, and treatments; and describe how to treat certain conditions. CPGs also describe the use of modalities.

The American Association for Respiratory Care initiated the development of CPGs in 1990. CPGs standardize care from one hospital to another, as well as from one geographic region to another.[31] The first five CPGs were published in *Respiratory Care*, the scientific journal. By 1999, almost 50 CPGs had been published. In 2009 there were 63 guidelines posted on the AARC website. Two were evidence based, 47 from expert panels, 1 a combination of evidence based and expert panel, and 13 CPGs were from a variety of organizations. Many of these are regularly updated by AARC members and other invited experts.

RESPIRATORY RECAP

Clinical Practice Guidelines

- » Specify indications for tests, procedures, and/or treatments
- » Determine appropriateness of care
- » Specify treatment plans, protocols, and algorithms
- » Describe "how to" in brief, generic language
- » Are developed by the profession who will use them
- » Are voluntary guidelines that evolve as the profession changes

CPGs provide clinical indicators for performance improvement (PI). They also support the enhanced role of respiratory therapists.[32] CPGs have helped in establishing protocols. They provide flexibility in designing care for patients. Healthcare organizations have incorporated CPGs into policy and procedure manuals.

Development

CPGs are practical documents that address specific respiratory care procedures. They help standardize healthcare and can improve quality. All CPGs follow a specific format to answer similar questions (**Table 32–1**).

Working groups develop a CPG by carefully reviewing the literature, considering surveys of current practice, and using group expertise. Many revisions and edits are made. When the working group is satisfied with the draft, a steering committee distributes the CPG for peer review. The working group carefully considers all comments. Following this process, *Respiratory Care* publishes the CPG. The journal widely distributes CPGs as reprints.[33] This textbook provides many examples of CPGs and protocols throughout.

Advantages

Institutions gain many benefits from using clinical practice guidelines. CPGs have been excellent tools for designing protocols and consult services.[24–27,34,35] CPGs provide a basis for therapist–physician interactions and help respiratory therapists meet physicians' expectations. CPGs are also useful for guiding physicians to meet the expectations of respiratory therapists. CPGs improve the consistency and appropriateness of care. CPGs can help in developing triage systems and also can guide education and research.[34] The adoption of CPGs has resulted in lower malpractice premiums[36] and significant cost savings.[37]

TABLE 32-1 Format Used in the Development of Clinical Practice Guidelines

Section	Description
Procedure	Common names by which the procedure is known
Description or definition	Describes or defines the procedure in the context of the guideline
Setting	Places where the procedure can be appropriately performed
Indications	Recognized objectives or indications for the procedure
Contraindications	Relative and absolute conditions when it is not safe to use or employ the procedure
Hazards/complications	Hazards and complications that are associated with the procedure
Limitations	Limitations of which the practitioner should be aware
Need	Determination that a procedure is indicated
Outcomes	Benefit (or lack thereof) derived from the procedure
Resources	Equipment or personnel required to perform the procedure
Monitoring	Issues related to specific monitoring that is needed
Frequency	Statements related to determination of how often the procedure should be performed
Infection control	Issues related to specific infection control considerations
References	Studies that support the recommendations

From Hess D. The AARC clinical practice guidelines. *Respir Care.* 1991; 36:1398–1401. Reprinted with permission.

Limitations

CPGs are usually brief and nonspecific. Therefore, they serve as a basis to establish protocols. They are also a basis for critical pathways. Institutions can tailor CPGs to meet the needs of their specific organizations. A major limitation is that often there is not enough evidence to support current practices. Establishing CPGs is sometimes done though the consensus of experts. This major limitation of CPGs has demonstrated the need for specific outcomes research to establish the effectiveness of therapies.

Respiratory Care Protocols

Respiratory care protocols were first described in 1981.[26] Since then, respiratory care protocols have become very important. Clinicians often refer to respiratory care protocols as *therapist-driven protocols* (TDPs); others call them *patient-driven protocols* (PDPs). They often are simply called *protocols*. Protocols are patient care plans. They are created and implemented by respiratory therapists. Protocols provide flexibility because they can be modified to the individual patient's needs.

Development

The main purpose of protocols is to standardize decision making. Physicians often develop protocols, but respiratory therapists can also develop them. Medical staff and hospital administration approve the protocols, after which they are adopted. Each protocol has a title and purpose and describes the type of patient to whom it applies. The protocols contain indications, contraindications, and outcomes and describe when it is appropriate to reduce or discontinue therapy.

Respiratory care protocols can take several forms, including narratives, worksheets, or **algorithms**. Protocols may be specific to a patient, diagnosis, or symptom. Patient-specific protocols are generic protocols. Diagnosis-specific protocols are part of a patient's critical path of care. Examples include protocols for cystic fibrosis or asthma care. Symptom-specific protocols follow a patient with a particular problem. Such problems might be wheezing or chest pain. Using CPGs typically generates respiratory care protocols.

Once a protocol is ordered, the respiratory therapist has the authority to evaluate, initiate, adjust, discontinue, or restart respiratory care procedures. This is done on a shift-by-shift or hour-to-hour basis. Successful use of protocols requires each respiratory therapist to have a strong cardiopulmonary knowledge base. In addition, respiratory therapists must be competent in patient assessment. This includes gathering data, formulating an assessment, and treating the patient appropriately. Assessment and communication skills are important. Protocols require extra time for patient assessment, treatment, thorough communication with others, and documentation.[38]

Advantages

Hospitals implement protocols for many reasons. A major advantage is that protocols are institution specific. They guide clinical decision making. Protocol development considers the competencies of the staff as well as the needs of patients. Numerous other variables can also be incorporated.

Many advantages of protocols have been documented. These include improvements in allocation of respiratory care services and in triage of care, as well as objective criteria for initiation of respiratory care. Protocols help determine when to discontinue therapies. They can help achieve decreased costs of care without adverse effects. Protocol use also can help achieve improvements in patient care outcomes.[15–20,23–27]

Additional advantages include recruitment of better therapists. These therapists enjoy the challenging

RESPIRATORY RECAP

Respiratory Care Protocols

- » Institution-specific patient care plans
- » Not standing orders
- » Approved by the medical staff and hospital administration
- » Each protocol has a title, purpose, and description of patients to whom it applies
- » Each protocol has indications, contraindications, and outcomes
- » Provide guidelines and criteria for initiating the care plan
- » Provide guidelines for when it is appropriate to reduce or discontinue therapy

work environment and increased job satisfaction.[38] Cost containment is achieved because patients receive appropriate care. For instance, if a patient is very ill, a protocol order can achieve continuous therapy with assessment. Therapy can be decreased to every 2 hours, then every 4 hours, and then twice daily as the patient improves. Tremendous cost savings can be realized when respiratory therapists discontinue therapy at appropriate times. Healthcare organizations regularly update their protocols to incorporate changes in technology and new research. Ongoing updates should be part of the process. Updates should have few or no negative effects on the overall program. The AARC website (http://www.aarc.org) has a link to guidelines for preparing respiratory care protocols.

Limitations

There are no inherent disadvantages to respiratory care protocols. However, successful use requires a dedicated effort. Protocols must be regularly updated to optimize approaches. They must not interfere with therapists' ability to alter practices using clinical judgment. There must also be sufficient numbers of respiratory therapists.[23,39,40] Staff competency and compliance may be barriers for effective implementation.

Increased protocol use and decision making by respiratory therapists depends on environmental factors and the organizational culture.[23,41,42] The institution must create the right culture; responsibility then falls on each respiratory therapist. The consultant role does not evolve simply because a protocol is implemented. Success depends on a partnership with physicians. These physicians should respect respiratory therapists.[2,3]

Critical Pathways

A **critical pathway (CP)** describes a probable sequence of events during a patient's course of care. It outlines all the tests, procedures, and education during a length of stay (LOS).[43] Other terms used to describe critical pathways include *critical paths, clinical algorithms, care maps, care paths, collaborative plans of care, multidisciplinary action plans* (MAPS), *practice plans, anticipated recovery paths,* and *clinical paths* among others.

RESPIRATORY RECAP

Common Names for Critical Pathways

- » Care plans
- » Critical paths
- » Practice plans
- » Care maps
- » Clinical algorithms
- » Collaborative plans of care
- » Anticipated recovery paths
- » Multidisciplinary action plans

CPs define the optimal sequence or timing of the key interventions performed by every discipline involved in patient care. The CP applies to a particular diagnosis, procedure, or symptom.[44] Another interpretation of a CP is as the sequence of events in a process that takes the greatest length of time.[13]

Some institutions are reluctant to use the term *critical pathway* because it may scare some patients to learn they are on a "critical pathway." Patients might mistakenly think that their condition is critical and requires some special pathway. Some dislike the term *pathway* because it implies that there is one best way. It may suggest that any other approach is substandard. Regardless of the terms used, success comes from the use of CPs. Clinicians can use CPs in any setting across the continuum of healthcare.

Development

Critical pathways originated in construction and manufacturing, where CPs were developed as tools to identify and manage rate-limiting steps in production processes.[45] Their purpose has been to maximize the efficiency of production. To develop a CP, all activities to be accomplished during a process are identified and timed. Techniques include the critical path method (CPM) and the program evaluation review technique (PERT). Gantt charts are also used. Activities are sequenced according to projected times of completion. By definition, a critical path is the key sequence of events that drives the timeline of the project.

In healthcare, a critical pathway is an optimal sequencing of events. It is also the timing of each event. These pathways are for a particular diagnosis or procedure. Critical pathways are designed to minimize delays and to use the least amount of resources. They also can maximize the quality of care.[44] Initially, nurses in hospitals developed CPs for nursing care.[15] Eventually multidisciplinary teams began to develop pathways for all aspects of care.[46] A basic assumption is the 80/20 rule. This means that 80% of patients follow a predictable path 100% of the time. An additional 20% of patients stray from that pathway. A portion of that 20% deviate far from the original pathway.[43]

The health professionals who will use CPs should be the ones to develop them. The most effective CP teams include a wide range. Members can offer varied input through meetings, documents, and pathway reviews. Respiratory therapists are important members of the team and process.

CPs are available for specific diagnoses or procedures.[47] Some organizations, such as the AARC, provide critical pathways for a fee.[48] Although it may seem like a simple solution, this approach does not provide a chance for health professionals to learn from the process. Adopting CPs developed elsewhere does not allow the time needed to work through the specific organization's problems and needs.

CP team members gain valuable insight into their special contributions to patient care. In addition, they develop greater understanding of others' roles. It is common for a physician or nurse to chair the group. Teams should include people from hospital administration and quality management. Pharmacy and ancillary services are often represented. Respiratory therapists are usually responsible for the development of CPs on respiratory care. These might include ventilator weaning or mechanical ventilation.

It is wise to spend time at the beginning securing buy-in. Committing all staff members to CPs is possibly the greatest challenge. Practitioner input in their development and implementation is also important for buy-in. Achieving buy-in requires a chance for the staff to express and resolve concerns. Like any change, there will be some disagreement. A carefully chosen critical pathway team can increase the success of the resulting CP.

Advantages

Critical pathways have become an important part of case management. Case management is a process in which healthcare professionals assess, plan, and implement care. They also coordinate, monitor, and evaluate choices that can meet an individual's health needs.[43] Case management incorporates critical pathways. The goals of case management include better utilization of resources and the promotion of quality outcomes at the lowest cost.

Critical pathways are implemented to provide a **multidisciplinary** approach. Pathways coordinate care. They incorporate the entire team in providing the best healthcare. Hospitals achieve immediate benefits. They frequently use CPs as a part of a performance improvement (PI) plan. CPs outline daily triggers used to identify variations in the response to a planned intervention.[49] The daily triggers are a reminder that anything out of the ordinary can have a negative impact on outcomes.

For example, a patient with cystic fibrosis may develop wheezing after an intestine blockage. This event is a trigger that an unexpected event has occurred. The wheezing varies from the planned course. Another example is the presence of atelectasis after surgery. The presence of atelectasis triggers a variance that requires attention. Respiratory therapists can use triggers to assist in their responses.

Limitations

It is a mistake to approach CPs without sufficient thought. CPs require preparation and communication. CPs can promote a change in institutional culture. CPs are intended to reduce cost and LOS. They can also improve quality and patient satisfaction. Without a firm commitment from leaders, CPs will not achieve these goals. Significant overlap exists with the use of CPGs, protocols, and pathways. These three tools are appropriate to use in certain situations at specific times. For example, your organization might develop a respiratory care protocol by using a specific CPG. In addition, your organization might incorporate the protocol into a CP for a specific disease.

Care bundles are a recent concept in critical care. Bundles are grouping of evidence-based interventions that come under one protocol.[50] They have strengthened evidence-based practice and have been shown to improve outcomes. For example, the ventilator-associated pneumonia bundle addresses at least five aspects of care, as shown in **Box 32–2**. The success of this bundle is due to interaction among the critical care team, which includes the respiratory therapist.[51]

Healthcare organizations usually develop CPs primarily for high-volume procedures. They are also developed for most common hospital diagnoses. CPs provide the most efficient combination of sequencing and timing of staff actions. Despite the rapid dissemination of CPs, uncertainties about their use remain.[52]

RESPIRATORY RECAP

Critical Pathways

- » Focus on efficiency and effectiveness of treatment decisions
- » Represent the completion of the protocol or guideline that results in the accomplishment of critical pathway events
- » Describe "when to" via specific timelines for the accomplishment of events
- » Affected by any delays or complications in treatment plans
- » Are multidisciplinary in their development and implementation
- » Employ healthcare practitioners' discipline-specific and professional skills earlier in the patient care process
- » Become part of the medical record in most instances

BOX 32–2

Bundles for Ventilator-Acquired Pneumonia

Elevation of the head of the bed
Daily sedation aimed at quicker extubation
Peptic ulcer prophylaxis
Deep venous thrombosis prophylaxis

Each organization must evaluate its outcomes when using these tools. **Outcomes evaluations** should include patient care outcomes, institutional outcomes, and care provider outcomes. Length of stay is a key clinical outcome. Other clinical outcomes include benchmarking, compliance with regulatory agencies, patient adherence, patient education, marketing, clinical operations management, and research. Healthcare outcomes have the potential to change practice over time.

Outcomes Evaluation and Evidence: What Do the Data Show?

Patient Outcomes

Morbidity and mortality rates are the most common indicators of patient outcomes. Additional indicators include complications, patient satisfaction, improved quality of life (QOL), increased longevity, improved functionality, and improved emotional health. Examples of improved QOL include self-care and health-promoting behaviors, having a positive outlook, and a decrease in stress level. Questions to ask to determine which patient outcomes to measure include the following: Is the patient better off because of this treatment? Has the patient's quality of life been improved or maintained, or has it declined? Is the patient able to manage his or her own disease and demonstrate health-promoting behaviors?

Patient satisfaction has gained in importance. It is monitored by third-party payers, affects public relations, and influences marketing—all of which are important in the competitive healthcare industry. Therefore, healthcare organizations pay special attention to this outcome.

Institutional Outcomes

Costs and quality of care are the most common outcomes evaluated related to the facility. These are often called institutional outcomes. LOS correlates directly with the cost of healthcare. To decrease institutional costs, healthcare organizations strive for the shortest LOS possible without creating adverse effects. Therefore, LOS is the number one variable in preserving revenue. Some studies show that the majority of healthcare costs occur within the first few days of a patient's stay.

Quantifying quality of care is much more difficult than determining LOS. Patient education to achieve understanding might be one outcome. If a patient follows directions, LOS can be reduced. Therefore, it is important to document what the patient actually learned, which is more important than what was taught. For example, patient education in a pathway for asthma may include understanding the role and use of bronchodilators. This would include knowing the step-up approach. The institutional outcome may be that the patient understands when to contact the physician. The office should thus follow the patient after discharge to document whether the patient notifies the physician before going to the emergency department. Evaluation of progress on the pathway or protocols becomes a verification of an institutional outcome.

Care Provider Outcomes

Studies have shown that positive care provider outcomes lead to better patient outcomes. In a study of nine critical care units, reduced mortality was demonstrated in units with certain characteristics, including a patient-centered focus; strong leadership as evidenced by shared visions and supportive, visible leaders; a collaborative approach to problem solving by all members of the healthcare team; and effective communication.[43] Care provider outcomes include greater autonomy in clinical practice, participation in decision making, increased satisfaction, and reduced staff turnover. Managers who are leaders work to create a culture of teamwork and effective problem solving. Innovative healthcare organizations look for these attributes during recruitment of new graduates. They also look for these attributes in experienced healthcare professionals.

> **RESPIRATORY RECAP**
>
> **Types of Outcomes**
>
> » *Patient outcomes*: patient satisfaction, functionality, quality of life
>
> » *Institutional outcomes*: LOS, morbidity, complications, costs of care
>
> » *Provider outcomes*: low staff turnover, role in decision making, greater autonomy in clinical practice, job satisfaction

Variance Tracking

One definition of a **variance** is "the difference between desired outcomes and what actually happened." Variance is simply the difference between what you expect and what you find. What you expect are good patient, institutional, and provider outcomes. Variance describes any deviation from what you hoped to achieve. Variances reflect issues that can impact patient outcomes.[53] A variance occurs when a patient does not progress as anticipated, and when an expected outcome is not achieved.[54] Variances can alert healthcare providers to the need for action. Variances serve as a database for PI. There are at least four categories of variances: patient and family variances, caregiver or clinician variances, hospital or system variances, and community variances.

Guideline, pathways, and protocols help the healthcare team to reduce variance as part of the general improvement process.[54] For example, achieving an outcome earlier than expected provides clues for more cost-effective care. Timely recognition is the most important step for achieving success. Addressing problems early is important. The PI format also ensures delivery of quality patient care. Variance tracking is essential in transforming CPGs into protocols and pathways. Continuous quality improvement, CPGs, CPs, and protocols work together. These integrated systems are desirable in building effective organizations.

There are many useful formats for collecting and analyzing variance, including notations written directly on the protocol document; retrospective chart reviews; variance data collection instruments; and computerized systems. Generally, numeric data and statistical methods are used. Qualitative methods are also used to analyze nonnumeric data.

Once the outliers are known, variance analysis explains the reasons for the variance. Cause-and-effect relationships can be established. Such relationships may involve medical conditions, treatment variables, or resource utilization issues. Data from care plans can be compared to standard performance indicators. Changes can be made for maximum patient benefit. In most cases, the practitioner will alter the treatment in real time, which can prevent over- or underutilization of resources.

RESPIRATORY RECAP

Variance Tracking

» *Purpose*: Track differences between what is expected and what happens.
» *Methods*: Written notations written on the CP or protocol, retrospective chart review, variance data collection sheet, and/or computerized systems.
» *Results*: Establishes cause-and-effect relationships among medical condition, treatment variables, and resource utilization; guides continuous quality improvement process.
» *Pitfalls*: May inhibit individual judgments.
» NIH, AHCPR, AARC have research funding to promote outcomes research.
» Outcomes research provides evidence to guide clinical practice.

Another reason variances are analyzed is to compare the effectiveness of provider plans.[43] This process of peer comparison, or **benchmarking**, is key in the standardization of healthcare. It is also important in maximizing the benefits of healthcare delivery. The term *benchmark* is a general one for the most medically appropriate utilization per diagnosis.[43]

Variance tracking requires timely intervention to achieve desired outcomes. Ideally, the design of the variance tracking will catch deviations as they occur. This is important in helping individual patients. If healthcare providers do not track variances in a timely manner, outcome measurements will not help that particular patient but will only benefit future patients as problems are addressed over time. Disadvantages of tracking variances sometimes result from the audit process. Clinicians may be hesitant to implement changes in processes because of concern that the change will show up as a variance.[40] After the data are collected, analysis and reporting are the next tasks.

Case managers use a quality improvement process for any recurrent variances. By keeping track of variance data, administrators are able to document the effectiveness of the care. In addition, the quality improvement process should reduce complications and reduce LOS. Several organizations have funded proposals to study patient outcomes. These include the National Institutes of Health (NIH), the Agency for Healthcare Research and Quality (AHRQ), and the AARC. Published outcome data promote particular strategies that provide the most effective healthcare with the best outcomes.

Evidence-Based Medicine

This chapter describes how organizations use outcomes to evaluate the effectiveness of healthcare. **Evidence-based medicine (EBM)** expresses what we know about healthcare, based on scientific evidence and outcomes data. EBM also is called evidence-based healthcare (EBH) or evidence-based practice (EBP). The volume and accessibility of medical information influenced the development of EBM, which requires specific criteria, including analysis of strong scientific data, to support approaches to healthcare. EBM evaluates outcomes research using methods to increase the general application of findings. EBM is the "conscientious, explicit and judicious use of current best evidence in making decisions about the care of individual patients."[55] You could say that EBM is a comprehensive approach to systematically document achievable healthcare outcomes.[56,57]

Research in EBM involves the methodical collection of studies that meet strict quality criteria. All or portions of these studies can then be merged, distilled, and interpreted. Meta-analysis is used. The "discoveries" in EBM are reviews and practice guidelines. These are developed from conservative evaluation of the effect and effectiveness of care.

The Grades of Recommendations, Assessment, Development, and Evaluation (GRADE) system is an evidence-based system that has been endorsed by many professional societies and organizations, including the American College of Chest Physicians (ACCP), the American Thoracic Society (ATS), the European Respiratory Society (ERS), and the American Association of Respiratory Care (AARC) among others. It is used in the development of many practice guidelines. It is simply a system that grades the quality of evidence used in the development of CPGs. Evidence falls into four grades of quality: high, moderate, low, and very low. This system does not rely on study design alone. It provides a more transparent look at evidence strength.[58]

The Cochrane Library is one organization that has adopted GRADE. It currently maintains five databases. These include controlled trials, review methodologies, health technology assessment, systematic reviews of the effects of care, and critical assessments of effectiveness.[56,59] The Cochrane Library regularly updates its databases, which are designed to make evidence available so that clinicians can make informed healthcare decisions. A bimonthly publication, *Evidence-Based Medicine*, reports on recent reviews and commentaries from EBM.

RESPIRATORY RECAP

Levels of Evidence

- *Level 1*: from a multisite randomized, controlled study or several single-site controlled trials.
- *Level 2*: from a variety of quasi-experimental studies.
- *Level 3*: includes correlational or descriptive studies.
- Examining the levels of evidence does not provide an indication of the quality of a study or the overall strength of the body of evidence.

EBM categorizes research evidence into three levels, based on the design of the study. Level 1 evidence comes from a multisite, randomized clinical trial or several single-site, randomized control trials. Level 2 evidence comes from a variety of quasi-experimental studies. Level 3 evidence includes correlational or descriptive studies.

Examining the levels of evidence does not provide an indication of the quality of a study or the overall strength of the evidence. However, examining the levels of evidence is useful to address the effectiveness of a study design to establish cause and effect. The Cochrane Library and other EBM databases provide guidance for respiratory therapists. Using EBM, respiratory therapists can be valuable consultants. Applying levels of evidence is imperative when developing, implementing, and evaluating CPGs, protocols, and pathways. **Figure 32–1** illustrates pathway examples used in research-based practice.

Shape clinical question → Obtain several reports of potentially relevant studies → Focus or broaden the clinical question → (a) Locate a state-of-the-science report → Appraise the findings of the state-of-the-science summary; (b) Identify and retrieve all relevant reports → Appraise collective evidence from two or more studies / Appraise the findings of a single study → Decide whether or not to change practice → Plan and make the change in practice → Evaluate if change has benefitted patients

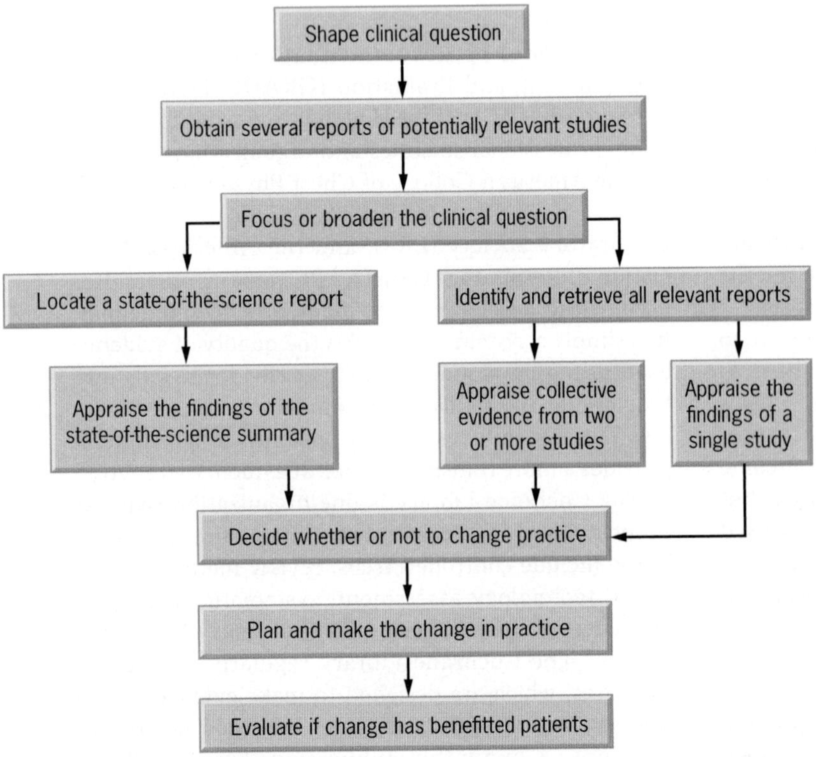

FIGURE 32–1 Possible pathways for research-based practice. This article was published in *Knowledge for Health Care Practice: A Guide to Using Research Evidence*. Brown SJ. Copyright Elsevier (WB Saunders) 1999.

Public health agencies, hospitals, and payers have accelerated the development of EBM. Respiratory therapists should use EBM in clinical practices. This should include evaluating CPGs, CPs, and protocols. One caveat is that EBM is not about cookbook medicine or cost-cutting strategies. Evidence-based practice provides a consistent framework for evaluation of current healthcare. EBM also facilitates better evaluation of methods of care. This can improve effectiveness without ignoring the needs of individual patients.

Consultation Skills for Healthcare Professionals

Previous sections discussed the role of respiratory therapists as decision makers. The following sections address the roles of internal consultants.

What Is Internal Consulting?

Healthcare is composed of labor-intensive organizations filled with high-tech individuals. These individuals are dependent on working together. They must consult with each other. Internal consulting defines an effective helping relationship that leads to effective outcomes.[60] The more effective the internal consulting skills, the more effective the healthcare organization. The Joint Commission (TJC) specifies accreditation standards that support teamwork. It requires organizations to improve quality of care. Improving organizational effectiveness demands the highest productivity. Human resources accounts for the major portion of the operating budget of any healthcare organization.

Internal consultants include direct patient caregivers, support groups who assist care teams, and the administration. Support group consultants include human resources, education, marketing, planning, environmental services, public relations, business, and others. Direct patient caregivers include physicians, nurses, respiratory therapists, social workers, physical therapists, and many others.

How Internal Consulting Can Increase Organizational Effectiveness

Internal consulting does not happen in a vacuum. It occurs within the culture of an organization. The focus is on effectiveness and efficiency. True consultants are able to think beyond the needs and functions of individual departments. They work to assist others across the organization. Technical skills combined with internal consulting skills can lead to effective problem identification and

Case 3. "Convince Me: Why Should Respiratory Therapists Be Internal Consultants?"

You are the department manager at the local community hospital, which includes acute care, subacute care, home care, and rehabilitation. The respiratory therapy staff has good rapport with the pulmonologists, allergists, sleep specialists, and emergency department physicians. The neurologists and cardiologists are less supportive. They rely more on the nursing staff. How will you convince your administration, physicians, nursing staff, and other professionals that respiratory therapists should function as internal consultants? Will your plan also convince them that organizational effectiveness will improve? Will your plan demonstrate how to limit costs? Where will you start and why? The following is one approach, but you are encouraged to make up your own mind. Develop a strategy that you believe in and can pursue!

As the manager, you must convince upper management that respiratory therapists have technical and process expertise. They offer services at the patient's bedside, in the lab, in the home, and across the continuum of care. In my opinion, you should start with your physician allies. Then, shift focus to gaining additional alliances. You must receive buy-in from physicians. They must trust your ability to deliver what you say you will. They also must have confidence in your staff. Only then should you approach administration.

You can elaborate on and document your respiratory therapists' education, expertise, and credentials. You should also convince administration that the respiratory therapy staff is an untapped resource. Remind administrators that respiratory therapists have been able to improve organizational effectiveness as part of critical pathway teams and protocol-based care. The respiratory therapist is the nonphysician expert in the area of cardiorespiratory care. Respiratory therapists have training in cardiopulmonary physiology, pathophysiology, assessment, invasive and noninvasive monitoring, treatment, education, and research. You should elaborate on additional strategies. These may include ideas about how physicians can utilize respiratory therapists as physician extenders using more protocol-based care.

Respiratory therapists are trained to use technology in obtaining data that can enhance decision making. More specifically, they can obtain data that will improve ventilation of the difficult patient. They can use protocols to manage patients who are difficult to wean from mechanical ventilation. In addition, the respiratory therapist's role as educator is a primary area for expanding the consultant role. This educator role could expand in-service education opportunities to other disciplines. The staff can provide advanced life support courses to new critical care nurses. They can provide community outreach in areas of pulmonary rehabilitation, smoking cessation, and asthma education. They can assist with institutional public relations. As the manager, you must explain how the role of respiratory therapists can be extended into alternate care sites. Their services may include airway management in the long-term care site or oxygen service/delivery in the home care environment.

You must convey that respiratory therapists know how the technology works and how it can be best utilized. Respiratory therapists also know patient assessment. They are experts in procedures, monitoring, and treatments to reverse pathophysiology. Finally, respiratory therapists have patient education expertise. They can design and implement age-specific education and can assess and improve patient outcomes. The literature offers a multitude of examples that document problems involving patient adherence to care plans. A patient- and family-centered care approach including education is required to overcome these problems. Respiratory therapists can work with the organization to develop, implement, and evaluate strategies to improve patient education, which will ultimately improve patient and institutional outcomes.

KEY POINTS

- Clinical practice guidelines (CPGs), respiratory care protocols, and critical pathways have emerged in healthcare to standardize care.
- CPGs, protocols, and pathways improve efficiency, reduce costs, and document effectiveness.
- CPGs, protocols, and pathways have contributed to the decision-making role of respiratory therapists.
- Protocol-based respiratory care has been used to improve the effectiveness of respiratory care.
- Protocols have improved the care of patients.
- Many protocols were designed for implementation by respiratory therapists to reduce medical care costs.
- Protocols can unburden physicians from care performed by respiratory therapists to improve patient outcomes.
- Misallocation of respiratory care services occurs for many reasons. Insufficient knowledge of respiratory care by those who prescribe it is one such cause.
- Position statements and letters of support from physician organizations note the important role of respiratory therapists in healthcare.
- Physicians have also published editorials, conference summaries, and original studies supporting protocol-based care by respiratory therapists.
- A growing role for respiratory therapists is as physician extenders.
- Respiratory therapists have the education, opportunity, and potential to play an increasing role as internal consultants.

TABLE 32-2 The Problem-Solving Process

Step	Description
Awareness of a problem	Recognizing that something is not right and that there is a gap between what should happen and what actually is happening.
Problem identification	Determining and then describing the exact nature of the problem. Often, the presenting problem is not the main problem.
Selection of criteria for solutions	Specifying what a solution will look like when it solves the problem. This step may seem easy or obvious, but it takes much communication, thinking, and work to achieve this step of the problem-solving process.
Formulation of alternatives	Describing alternative solutions for resolution.
Selection of strategy	Selecting from the alternatives the strategy that will most likely achieve the desired goals.
Specification of an action plan	Describing how to specifically implement the strategy.
Implementation of the action plan	Putting the developed plan into action.
Monitoring and evaluation	Reviewing to determine whether the action plan was carried out and the problem was corrected. This also is a time to reflect on the selected strategy, the action plan, and the implementation to gain further insight as to their appropriateness for the specific problem.

resolution, which can lead to increased organizational effectiveness.[60]

The stages of internal consulting are as follows: precontracting, contracting, data collection, data analysis, presentation, action planning, evaluation, and termination. Internal consultants must devote attention to each of these stages to be effective in their consulting role. Each stage requires special skills and attributes, described in the next section.

RESPIRATORY RECAP

Internal Consulting

- » Internal consultants can be direct patient caregivers, support personnel, administrators, or a combination of these.
- » Effective healthcare providers have technical expertise as well as professional expertise, including consulting skills and traits.
- » Internal consultants can be technical experts or process experts, or both.
- » Technical skills combined with consultation skills improve problem identification and resolution.
- » Problem resolution contributes to improved organizational effectiveness.
- » Consulting improves the effectiveness and utilization of human resources.

The Roles and Skills of Internal Consultants

Technical skills alone are insufficient. Today's healthcare professionals need interpersonal skills that go beyond technical expertise. Respiratory therapists must have the ability to work with others and to negotiate differences with others. Internal consultants are able to go beyond simple verbal and communication skills. This requires exceptional communication abilities. In addition, internal consultants must be able to determine the needs of the client. Clients include other departments, health professionals, and patients. Internal consultants must identify their role in relation to a department or service, they must agree what steps need to occur, and they need to carry out the steps and evaluate the results.

The consultant can have multiple roles. These roles include being an advocate, information specialist, trainer, educator, joint problem solver, facilitator, and identifier of alternatives. It is also important to be a link to resources, a fact finder, a technical exert, and a process consultant. The approach to consulting will vary depending on whether the consultant is focusing on a process or a procedure. The basic approach to consulting includes problem verification, problem solving, feedback, utilization of research, involvement, relationship to the client, and a systems approach. Many descriptions of the problem-solving process are available. **Table 32-2** describes the basic, generic components of problem solving.

Respiratory Therapists as Healthcare Consultants

Effectiveness can improve if competent respiratory therapists have an increased decision-making role. The word *competent* must be emphasized. An expanded role comes with more responsibility and accountability. Numerous physician organizations support respiratory therapists at their institution. Position statements and letters of support from physician organizations such as the ACCP, the ATS, and the American Society of Anesthesiologists (ASA) have noted the important role of respiratory therapists in healthcare.[57]

In addition, the ACCP has issued a position statement supporting the use of respiratory care protocols.[1] Physicians have published editorials, conference summaries, and original studies supporting respiratory therapists as physician extenders. They have also backed protocol-based care by respiratory therapists.[2,10,15,18–20,23,27,29,34,40,41] There has been some argument that implementation of protocols would interfere with the respiratory care training of medical staff. However, there is evidence to suggest that the use of respiratory care protocols does not interfere with house staff's knowledge of respiratory care and may actually contribute to increased knowledge of how to order respiratory care.[23,29,51,52]

Support from national professional associations has facilitated the expanded role of respiratory therapists as consultants. Several medical directors and many physicians are involved in state and national professional associations for respiratory care. This includes the National Association for Medical Direction of Respiratory Care (NAMDRC). NAMDRC has issued a statement of support for respiratory care practitioners as the caregivers best qualified to render respiratory services.[2] Many physicians have been instrumental in helping state licensure bills become approved by legislatures.

Expanded roles for respiratory care require continued reforms. These reforms include how we educate, manage, and utilize respiratory therapists. We must embrace issues of responsibility and accountability. One such change has been the commissioning of respiratory therapists in the U.S. Public Health Service in 2007. The U.S. Public Health Service is one of the United States' seven uniformed services serving under the management of the Surgeon General. As commissioned officers, respiratory therapists will respond to domestic and international emergencies such as hurricanes, earthquakes, and terrorist attacks.[61]

Respiratory therapists must demonstrate professionalism. Responsibility and accountability are required, and continuing education is essential. Respiratory therapy needs strong institutional support and regulatory support. We continue to need data to document the cost effectiveness of protocol-based care, critical pathways, and CPGs. Our patients must be the strongest advocates for respiratory therapists' role in their quality care. This support is needed to expand professional roles for respiratory therapists.

CASE STUDIES

Case 1. The Crossroads: Are Respiratory Therapists Paid for What They Know or for What They Do?

Mr. Jason Jeffries is the respiratory care manager for a 400-bed teaching hospital within the state university educational system. He has worked in respiratory care for almost 20 years. He has over 6 years' experience in his current position. Recently, the board of regents formed an independent corporation, which will have a board of directors to manage the hospital. This resulted in separation of the hospital and educational portions of this state university. Although the state government continues to own the teaching hospital, it has authorized the board of directors to make decisions. Mr. Jeffries understands that the major goals of the new organization are to decrease the costs of care without jeopardizing patient safety or the respiratory care they need. He must present a plan to upper administration on how he intends to decrease the costs of providing respiratory care services. The policy and procedure manual incorporates clinical practice guidelines. The respiratory therapy department has had limited involvement in critical pathways or protocols. The staff provides respiratory care services within the hospital and outpatient clinics. How should he approach this problem, and what recommendations could he make?

There are several strategies the manager should consider, including decreasing staff size, increasing the efficiency of staff, improving allocation of services, and documenting successful outcomes. The manager should think about his organization and consider whether the respiratory therapists are paid for what they know or for what they do. The primary goal of this manager is to document and communicate strategy to upper administration. This includes demonstration of his staff's cost effectiveness. If he finds that his hospital has been paying respiratory therapy staff primarily for what they do, then he must actively address this limitation. Mr. Jeffries must critically examine how he can influence his own staff, his physician supporters, and upper administration to pay respiratory therapists for what they know.

The manager can decrease staff size by shifting technical tasks to lesser-skilled employees. Technical multitasking makes broader use of the traditional task-oriented practitioner. Little or no assessment is required. Decision making is usually limited to very specific items, which might include device selection and fine-tuning of the therapy. These individuals often have good procedural skills and technical knowledge. It is this technical expertise that makes these practitioners valuable to hospitals. On the other hand, assessment and decision making are not major parts of the job. These individuals often are conceptually grouped by administrators with other task-oriented hospital workers, such as electrocardiographic technicians, radiology technicians, and phlebotomists.

The role of the professional respiratory therapist implies the need for assessment and judgment. A professional is sometimes referred to as "one whose opinion matters."[2] This advanced professional career track still operates under medical direction. However, the medical direction is in the form of guidelines or protocols. This method incorporates independent assessment, judgment, and decision making. In these roles, the advanced respiratory care practitioner is a professional who actually functions as a physician extender. This manager must document that the respiratory care provided is truly needed and that therapy is discontinued when the objectives are met. Variance tracking is critical here.

Mr. Jeffries must maximize the involvement of his staff in the creation of the new organizational climate. He can do this through critical pathway teams and other organizational committees. At the same time, he should ally himself with physicians. The physicians can help the department to develop, implement, and evaluate respiratory care protocols. He should provide current evidence on how protocol-based care can improve allocation of resources, patient objectives, and economic objectives. This must be carried out without jeopardizing educational training of medical students, house staff, and others.

Another strategy is to find less expensive sites than acute care for providing respiratory care. This hospital should transfer patients to subacute care, home care, rehabilitation, and long-term care facilities that affiliate with this teaching hospital.

He also must develop and implement a plan to attract and retain qualified respiratory therapists who can function in this expanded, professional role. Otherwise, implementation of these cost-effective strategies will not be possible. The manager must develop a system for documentation of continuing education, credentials, performance reviews, peer review, and each employee's contributions to institutional and patient outcomes.

The strategies must incorporate short- and long-term action plans. They must also evaluate success. In the interim, everyone must behave competently and professionally at all times. Peer pressure and effective communication are essential. The department must pull together for the benefit of everyone. Staff who either cannot or will not adjust to the changing organization will be a detriment. It is important that the manager nurture, mentor, and promote the right staff. Incompetent staff members are a liability for the department and its future potential. Therefore, accountability and consequences are fundamental components for success.

Case 2. "Where's Respiratory?" The Case of Alternate Site Care

Tracey is a respiratory therapist with over 15 years of experience. She has worked in numerous acute care settings, including coronary care units, neonatal intensive care, and medical intensive care. She is an expert in management of the airway and mechanical ventilation. She has been a member of several critical pathway teams. Others respect her because of her professionalism and interpersonal skills. Yesterday, her department manager presented her with a proposal to develop a long-term acute care facility (LTAC) on the eighth floor of the existing hospital. Her department head explains that with her experience and competencies, she is the ideal person for the job. They want her to work with nursing and administration to develop, implement, and eventually manage the LTAC. How should Tracey deal with this opportunity?

First, Tracey must recognize that this is a
tunity for the department. It is also an opport
professional growth. She must recognize that
ager sees her leadership abilities. The manager i
her toward a management-related position that
allow her to retain hands-on patient care. Sec
must realize that the nature of the work will be r
ferent. She will have more management respon
The clinical work will rely heavily on a team a
The types of patients and their needs will be
Third, she should discuss with the manager v
opportunity means in terms of her work hours,
ments, wages, and fringe benefits. Tracey should
all of these issues with her department head up
a professional manner. Neither Tracey nor her
should make assumptions about their agreeme
aspect should be negotiated. Her job descript
position must be clearly described in writing.

Tracey will need to do research to learn as
possible. For example, she needs to know that
are a form of subacute care. Subacute care attri
growth to the Medicare prospective payment
(PPS), initiated between 1982 and 1986. Manag
sets limits on the amount of payment for care. It a
strict review criteria to make sure that patients n
requirements for acute care. Subacute care has
a feasible alternative that is often a middle step b
the hospital and returning the patient to the hom

LTACs are licensed hospitals that are exemp
the Medicare prospective payment system. This r
that they keep their average patient length of stay
than 25 days. Long-term hospitals receive payme
Medicare on a reasonable-cost basis. LTAC h
usually specialize in patients who have pulmon
complex problems. The patients no longer require
sive diagnostic workups, but need additional t
and nursing support. LTACs usually offer occup
therapy, physical therapy, and respiratory therap
daily basis. If the LTAC has ventilator patients, it
respiratory therapy on a 24-hour basis, 7 days a
Patients usually stay between 10 and 60 days on av
The cost for subacute care is hundreds of dollars p
less than acute care.

Anyone who has worked in respiratory therapy f
time has probably heard loud, frantic calls of "Wh
respiratory?" In an emergency situation, especiall
involving the airway, it is not unusual for someone t
out loudly for "respiratory." This situation happens
though the nurses, physicians, and other clinicians
our names. I suspect this happens sometimes in an e
gency situation because the person calling wants to
no doubt about the expertise needed and the urgen
the request. Just as respiratory therapists have beco
vital component of acute care, our expertise has bec
increasingly important in alternate sites. Calls for "r
ratory" or "Where's respiratory?" should be freq
across the continuum of care.

- Internal consulting defines an effective relationship leading to improved outcomes.
- Internal consultants can be direct patient caregivers, support personnel, or administrators, or a combination of these.
- Internal consultants can be technical experts or process experts, or both.
- Technical skills with consultation skills improve problem identification and resolution.
- Respiratory consultants can improve healthcare and organizational effectiveness.

REFERENCES

1. Stewart KJ. Managing respiratory care: where is the science? *Respir Care.* 2008;53(7):903–907.
2. Mishoe SC, MacIntyre NR. Expanding professional roles for respiratory care practitioners. *Respir Care.* 1997;42(1):71–91.
3. American Association for Respiratory Care. *Delineating the Educational Direction for the Future Respiratory Care Practitioner: Proceedings of a National Consensus Conference on Respiratory Care.* Dallas, TX: AARC; 1992.
4. American Association for Respiratory Care. *An Action Agenda: Proceedings of the Second National Consensus Conference on Respiratory Care Education.* Dallas, TX: AARC; 1993.
5. O'Daniel C, Cullen DL, Douce FH, et al. The future educational needs of respiratory care practitioners: a Delphi study. *Respir Care.* 1992;37(1):65–78.
6. Kacmarek RM, Durbin CG, Barnes TA, et al. Creating a vision for respiratory care in 2015 and beyond. *Respir Care.* 2009;54(3):375–389.
7. Hess DR. Professionalism, respiratory care practice, and physician acceptance of a respiratory consult service. *Respir Care.* 1998;42(7):546–548.
8. Zibrak JD, Rossetti P, Wood E. Effects in reduction of respiratory therapy on patient outcome. *N Engl J Med.* 1986;315(5):292–295.
9. Kester L, Stoller JK. Ordering respiratory care services for hospitalized patients: practices of overuse and under-use. *Cleve Clin J Med.* 1992;59(6):581–585.
10. Stoller JK. The rationale for therapist-driven protocols. *Respir Care Clinic North Am.* 1996;2(1):1–14.
11. Kelleghan SI, Salemi C, Padilla S, et al. An effective continuous quality improvement approach to the prevention of ventilator-associated pneumonia. *Am J Infect Control.* 1993;21(6):322–330.
12. Joiner GA, Salisbury D, Bollin GE. Utilizing quality assurance as a tool for reducing the risk of nosocomial ventilator-associated pneumonia. *Am J Med Qual.* 1996;11(2):100–103.
13. Alexander E, Weingarten S, Mohsenifar Z. Clinical strategies to reduce utilization of chest physiotherapy without compromising patient care. *Chest.* 1996;110(2):430–432.
14. Pilon CS, Leathley M, London R, et al. Practice guidelines for arterial blood gas measurement in the intensive care unit decreases numbers and increases appropriateness of tests. *Crit Care Med.* 1997;25(8):1308–1313.
15. Konschak MP, Binder A, Binder RE. Oxygen therapy utilization in a community hospital: use of a protocol to improve oxygen administration and preserve resources. *Respir Care.* 1999;44(5):506–511.
16. Goldberg R, Chan L, Haley P, Harmata-Booth J, Bass G. Critical pathway for the emergency management of acute asthma: effect on resource utilization. *Ann Emerg Med.* 1998;31(5):562–567.
17. Ford RM, Phillips-Clar JE, Burns DM. Implementing therapist-driven protocols. *Respir Care Clin North Am.* 1996;2(1):51–76.
18. Lierl MB, Pettinichi S, Sebastian KD, Kotagel U. Trial of a therapist-directed protocol for weaning bronchodilator therapy in children with status asthmaticus. *Respir Care.* 1999;44(5):497–505.
19. Wood G, MacLeod B, Moffatt S. Weaning from mechanical ventilation: physician- directed versus a respiratory-therapist-directed protocol. *Respir Care.* 1995;40(3):219–224.
20. Kollef MH, Shapiro SD, Silver P, et al. A randomized-controlled trial of protocol-directed versus physician-directed weaning from mechanical ventilation. *Crit Care Med.* 1997;25(4):567–574.
21. Robertson TE, Sona C, Schallom L, et al. Improved extubation rates and earlier liberation from mechanical ventilation with implementation of a daily spontaneous breathing trial protocol. *J Am Coll Surg.* 2008;206(3):489–495.
22. Chan PKO, Fischer S, Stewart TE, et al. Practising evidence-based medicine: the design and implementation of a multidisciplinary team-driven extubation protocol. *Crit Care.* 2001;5(6):349–354.
23. Kollef MH. Therapist-directed protocols: their time has come. *Respir Care.* 1999;44(5):495.
24. Shrake KL, Scaggs JE, England KR, Henkle JQ, Eagleton LE. Benefits associated with a respiratory care assessment-treatment program: results of a pilot study. *Respir Care.* 1994;39(7):715–724.
25. Walton JR, Shapiro BA, Harrison CH. Review of a bronchial hygiene evaluation program. *Respir Care.* 1983;29(2):174–179.
26. Nielson-Tietsort J, Poole B, Creagh CE, Repsher LE. Respiratory care protocol: an approach to in-hospital respiratory therapy. *Respir Care.* 1981;26(5):420–436.
27. Stoller JK, Haney D, Burkhart J, et al. Physician-ordered respiratory care vs physician-ordered use of a respiratory therapy consult service: early experience at the Cleveland Clinic Foundation. *Respir Care.* 1993;38(11):1143–1154.
28. Torrington KG, Henderson CI. Perioperative respiratory therapy (PORT): a program of perioperative risk assessment and individualized postoperative care. *Chest.* 1988;93(5):946–951.
29. Stoller JK, Michnicki I. Medical house staff impressions regarding the impact of a respiratory therapy consult service. *Respir Care.* 1998;43(7):549–551.
30. Hess D. Clinical practice guidelines—valuable resources. *NBRC Horizons.* 1997;23:1, 6.
31. Brougher P. CPGs 1994: Where are we? Where have we been? Where are we going? *Respir Care.* 1994;39:1146–1148.
32. Hess D. The AARC clinical practice guidelines. *Respir Care.* 1991;36:1398–1401.
33. Hess D. Clinical practice guidelines: why, whence, and whither? *Respir Care.* 1995;40:1264–1267.
34. Komara JJ Jr, Stoller JK. The impact of a postoperative oxygen therapy protocol on use of pulse oximetry and oxygen therapy. *Respir Care.* 1995;40:1125–1129.
35. Orens DK. A manager's perspective on respiratory therapy consult services. *Respir Care.* 1993;38:884–886.
36. McGinn P. Practice standards leading to premium reductions. *AMA News.* 1998;2:1, 28.
37. Thompson RS, Kirz HL, Gold RA. Changes in physician behavior and cost savings associated with organizational recommendations on the use of routine chest x rays and multichannel blood tests. *Prev Med.* 1983;2:385–396.
38. Weber K, Milligan S. Conference summary. Therapist-driven protocols: the state of the art. *Respir Care.* 1994;39:746–756.
39. Thorens JB, Kaelin RM, Jolliet P, Chevrolet JC. Influence of the quality of nursing on the duration of weaning from mechanical ventilation in patients with chronic obstructive pulmonary disease. *Crit Care Med.* 1995;23(11):1807–1815.
40. Ely EW, Bennett PA, Bowton DL, Murphy SM, Florance AM, Haponick EF. Large scale implementation of a respiratory therapist-driven protocol for ventilator weaning. *Am J Respir Crit Care Med.* 1999;159(2):439–446.
41. Clemmer TP, Spuhler VJ. Developing and gaining acceptance for patient care protocols. *New Horizons.* 1998;6(1):12–19.
42. Mishoe SC. Critical thinking in respiratory care practice: a qualitative research study. *Respir Care.* 2003;48(5):500–551.

43. Dykes PC, Wheeler K, eds. *Planning, Implementing and Evaluating Critical Pathways: A Guide for the 21st Century.* New York: Springer; 1997.
44. Coffey R, Richard J, Remmert C, et al. An introduction to critical paths. *Qual Manage Health Care.* 1992;1:45–54.
45. Pearson S D, Goulart-Fisher D, Lee T. Critical pathways as a strategy for improving care: problems and potentials. *Ann Intern Med.* 1995;123:941–948.
46. Hoffman PA. Critical path method. *J Qual Improve.* June 1993:235–246.
47. Ignatavicius DD, Hausaman KA. *Clinical Pathways for Collaborative Practice.* Philadelphia: WB Saunders; 1995.
48. American Association for Respiratory Care, 11030 Ables Lane, Dallas, Texas, 75229.
49. Birdsall C, Sperry S. *Clinical Paths in Medical-Surgical Practice.* St. Louis: Mosby-Year Book; 1997.
50. Fulbrook P, Mooney S. Care bundles in critical care: a practical approach to evidence-based practice. *Nurs Crit Care.* 2003;8(6):249–255.
51. Blamoun J, Alfakar M, Rella ME, et al. Efficacy of an expanded ventilator bundle for the reduction of ventilator-associated pneumonia in the medical intensive care unit. *Am J Infect Control.* 2009;37(2):172–175.
52. Berger JT, Rosner F. The ethics of practice guidelines. *Arch Intern Med.* 1996;156:2051–2056.
53. Schriefer J. Managing critical pathway variances. *Qual Manage Health Care.* 1995;3:30–42.
54. Aronson B, Maljanian R. Critical path education: necessary components and effective strategies. *J Contin Educ Nurs.* 1996;27:215–219.
55. Sackett DL, Rosenberg WMC, Gray MJA, et al. Evidence-based medicine: what it is and what it isn't. *BMJ.* 1996;312:71–72.
56. Brown SJ. *Knowledge for Health Care Practice. A Guide to Using Research Evidence.* Philadelphia: WB Saunders; 1999.
57. Sackett DL, Richardson WS, Rosenberg W, Haynes RB. *Evidence-Based Medicine: How to Practice and Teach EBM.* 2nd ed. Edinburgh: Churchill Livingstone; 2000.
58. Brożek JL, Aki EA, Alonso-Coello P, et al. Grading quality of evidence and strength of recommendations in clinical practice guidelines. *Allergy.* 2009;64(5):669–677.
59. Jones A. Second International Cochrane Colloquium—Official Annual Meeting of the Cochrane Collaboration: a conference report. *Respir Care.* 1995;40(1):171–174.
60. Ulschak FL, SnowAntle SM. *Consultation Skills for Health Care Professionals: How to Be an Effective Consultant Within Your Organization.* San Francisco: Jossey-Bass; 1990.
61. U.S. Department of Health and Human Services. U.S. Public Health Service Commissioned Corps: profession—therapist. October 28, 2008. Available at: http://www.usphs.gov/profession/therapist.

CHAPTER 33

Infection Control Principles

Donna D. Gardner

OUTLINE

Transmission of Infection
Strategies for Infection Control
Regulatory Agencies
Cleaning, Disinfection, and Sterilization
Precautions
Healthcare-Associated Infections Related to Respiratory Care Equipment

OBJECTIVES

1. Define healthcare-associated infection.
2. Compare the different methods of transmitting infections.
3. Describe the strategies for infection control.
4. Discuss the methods for processing equipment.
5. Explain the importance of a regular surveillance and monitoring program.
6. Explain the importance of hand hygiene.
7. Determine the appropriate isolation procedure for preventing transmission of infections.

KEY TERMS

airborne precautions
antisepsis
bactericidal
cleaning
contact precautions
cough etiquette
disinfection
droplet precautions
equipment surveillance
hand hygiene
healthcare-associated infections (HAIs)
infection control
pasteurization
personal protective equipment
standard precautions
sterilization
vehicle transmission

INTRODUCTION

There are at least two million **healthcare-associated infections (HAIs)** each year, with about 100,000 deaths associated with these infections; a third of these infections are preventable.[1] HAIs cost $4.5 to $6.5 billion per year in the United States. HAIs are acquired during the delivery of care in any healthcare setting (e.g., hospital, long-term care facility, ambulatory setting, home care).[1] These infections are commonly known as nosocomial infections, but the Centers for Disease Control and Protection (CDC) replaced the term *nosocomial infection* with *healthcare-associated infections* because patients move among and between different healthcare sites frequently. A number of factors contribute to HAIs. The development of progressive and complex medical procedures, invasive technology, and antimicrobial-resistant bacteria place patients at greater risk for contracting these infections.

Preventing these infections has become a priority in the United States as a result of initiatives led by the Joint Commission, professional organizations, government, legislators, regulators, payers, consumer advocacy groups, and guidelines from the CDC.[2,3] Reports suggest that HAIs can be prevented by implementing evidence-based best practices.[3] Bundling multiple concurrent interventions has synergistic effects in specific settings.[3] The Institute for Healthcare Improvement created the 5 Million Lives campaign to promote practices aimed at preventing HAIs.[4] More than 160 years ago, Semmelweis was able to decrease mortality related to puerperal fever by initiating a systematic hand washing protocol.[5] Hand hygiene remains the most important infection control measure.[5]

This chapter describes issues related to infection control, including methods of infection transmission, principles of infection control, and methods of sterilizing equipment.

Transmission of Infection

For the transmission of infectious agents, three conditions are necessary: (1) a source of infectious agents, (2) a susceptible host with a portal of entry receptive to the agent, and (3) a mode of transmission for the agent. Infections are transmitted during patient care primarily via human contact or inanimate sources. Human sources include patients, healthcare personnel, family members, and visitors. Individuals may have active infections, they may be asymptomatic, or they may be carriers.[1] Individuals also may be colonized and become the source of their own infection. Respiratory care equipment, stethoscopes, bedside tables, and other inanimate objects can also be sources of infection.

A susceptible host is a person who is exposed to an infection and becomes an asymptomatic carrier or develops the disease. Others exposed to the same infection may be immune and will not develop the disease. Factors that can make a person more susceptible to infection include underlying diseases, recent surgery, anesthesia, indwelling catheters, antimicrobial or corticosteroid treatments, immunosuppressive agents, and age. Transplant recipients and patients with acquired immunodeficiency syndrome (AIDS) are immunocompromised hosts; these patients are extremely susceptible to any type of infection.[1] Patients who have their upper airways bypassed with an endotracheal tube or tracheostomy tube are also susceptible hosts. These tubes bypass the normal protective mechanisms of the upper airway, allowing microorganisms to easily gain access to the lower airway. Cross contamination may occur when suctioning artificial airways.[6]

Table 33–1 lists the most common routes for transmitting disease. Direct contact transmission occurs when there is body surface–to–body surface contact between people in which a transfer of microorganisms occurs between a susceptible host and an infected or colonized individual. Transmission by direct transfer can occur during open suctioning of a patient if one is not wearing gloves and touches the secretions. Sexually transmitted infections can be transmitted via secretion transfer as well.[1]

TABLE 33–1 Transmission Routes

Mode of Transmission	Examples
Contact	
Direct contact	HIV
Indirect contact	*Staphylococcus* *Pseudomonas aeruginosa* Hepatitis B and C, HIV
Droplet	Rhinovirus, SARS, rubella
Airborne	Legionellosis, tuberculosis Varicella
Vehicle	Waterborne: cholera Foodborne: salmonellosis and hepatitis
Vector-borne	Ticks: rickettsia, Lyme disease Mosquitoes: malaria

HIV, human immunodeficiency virus; SARS, severe acute respiratory syndrome.

Indirect contact transmission occurs when a susceptible host comes in contact with a contaminated object such as a needle or stethoscope. The hands of healthcare providers who touch a contaminated object or a patient and then touch a different patient are the most common cause of indirect contact transmission in the healthcare setting.

Droplet transmission occurs when droplets larger than 5 μm containing microorganisms are propelled a short distance (about 3 feet) through the air from an infected person when coughing, sneezing, or talking, or during procedures such as suctioning or bronchoscopy, and are deposited on another person's conjunctivae, nasal mucosa, or mouth. These droplets do not remain suspended in the air and therefore cannot be cleared with ventilation systems. The wearing of appropriate masks by healthcare providers is an important barrier to preventing droplet transmission.

> **RESPIRATORY RECAP**
>
> **Routes of Infection Transmission**
>
> » Contact
> » Droplet
> » Airborne
> » Vehicle
> » Vector

Airborne transmission occurs by the spread of evaporated droplet nuclei smaller than 5 μm or of dust particles containing microorganisms that remain suspended in the air for a long period of time. Microorganisms carried in this manner can be dispersed widely by air currents and may be inhaled by individuals within the same room. Preventing this type of transmission requires special handling and ventilation in which there are 12 air exchanges per hour for new construction and 6 air exchanges per hour for existing facilities. Air exhaust is directed to the outside or recirculated through high-efficiency particulate-arresting (HEPA) filtration before return. Two of the most common microorganisms transmitted in this way are the tuberculosis bacillus and the varicella virus. Personal respiratory protection via use of a National Institute for Occupational Safety and Health (NIOSH)–approved N95 (or higher) respirator mask is required to prevent airborne transmission.

Types of airborne transmission of disease include obligate, preferential, and opportunistic.[7] An *obligate airborne transmission* is an infection, such as tuberculosis, acquired under natural conditions via aerosols deposited in the distal lung.[7] *Preferential airborne transmission* occurs through multiple routes but is predominantly via aerosols deposited in the distal airways.[7] Measles and smallpox can be acquired by either preferential or obligate airborne transmission. *Opportunistic airborne transmission* includes those organisms that naturally cause disease through other routes such as the gastrointestinal tract and can also initiate infection through the distal lung.[7] The severe acute respiratory syndrome (SARS) epidemic provided an opportunity for critical reevaluation of aerosol transmission routes of communicable respiratory diseases. An aerosol plume that originated from sewage that was contaminated by the index SARS patient may have been responsible for the SARS outbreak at Amoy Gardens, Hong Kong.[7]

Vehicle transmission occurs when microorganisms are transmitted by contaminated food, water, medications, devices, or equipment. Vector-borne transmission occurs when vectors such as mosquitoes, flies, and other vermin transmit microorganisms.[6]

Strategies for Infection Control

Infection control procedures decrease the spread of infection. Infection control programs in the healthcare setting must have a commitment to patient and healthcare provider safety. Employers and employees must participate in practices to protect patients and healthcare providers by using protective equipment and participating in immunization programs and safety training.

Healthcare providers must be immunized against certain communicable diseases. The Occupational Safety and Health Administration (OSHA) requires that employees provide proof of hepatitis B vaccination and immunity against varicella, rubella, and measles. If the employee is not immune to these microorganisms, the employer must provide the immunizations. It is also recommended that employees receive annual influenza vaccinations.[6]

Spaulding devised a rational approach to disinfection and sterilization of patient care equipment assigned to three levels of concern: critical, semicritical, and noncritical.[8,9] Critical equipment, such as a chest tube, comes directly into contact with sterile tissue such as the pleural space. This equipment *must* be sterile. Semicritical equipment touches mucosal surfaces, where transmission of an infective agent is relatively possible, requiring high-level disinfection of the equipment during processing. Most respiratory care equipment is semicritical. The components of a ventilator circuit have been categorized as semicritical in the Spaulding classification system because they come into direct or indirect contact with mucous membranes but do not ordinarily penetrate body surfaces. An exception is equipment passed through an endotracheal tube in which a protected passage to the lower airways is established that bypasses the relatively unclean upper airway. In this setting, use of sterile supplies such as suction catheters may decrease the infectious load introduced to the lower airways. Noncritical equipment touches only intact skin and must be cleaned only, although disinfection is usually performed.

> **RESPIRATORY RECAP**
>
> **Levels of Equipment Processing**
>
> » *Critical (sterile)*: no viable (living) organisms
> » *Semicritical (disinfected)*: few organisms remaining, with spores and nonlipid viruses possibly remaining viable
> » *Noncritical (clean)*: grossly appreciable organic matter (dirt) removed

Regulatory Agencies

The Environmental Protective Agency (EPA), Food and Drug Administration (FDA), and CDC are the agencies involved in creating the regulations that govern the sale, distribution, and use of disinfectants and sterile agents. The Joint Commission is a nongovernmental agency that devises standards of quality used to accredit hospitals. These standards are varied and include the responsibility of an employer to an employee in regard to employee education, safety, and ethics. The Joint Commission has mandated that all healthcare facilities have an infection control committee. OSHA enforces activities to reduce the occupational risk of bloodborne infections and to promulgate standards on other exposures. One set of standards requires employers to provide hepatitis B vaccinations, personal protective equipment, and postexposure medical evaluation with follow-up. OSHA ensures healthcare facility compliance through periodic inspections.[1,6]

Cleaning, Disinfection, and Sterilization

Cleaning

To prevent cross contamination, respiratory care equipment surfaces are first cleaned and then disinfected or sterilized. Cleaning is part of the daily routine for respiratory therapists in the patient care setting. Equipment processing uses one or a combination of four modalities: cleaning, disinfection, antisepsis, and sterilization. **Cleaning** equipment removes gross contamination such as dirt, secretions, or other visible materials from a surface, reducing the number of microorganisms and removing much of their potential growth medium. Equipment should be cleaned according to the manufacturer's guidelines. Cleaning is generally a prerequisite for the other three modalities. Most respiratory care supplies, however, are disposable.

> **RESPIRATORY RECAP**
>
> **Equipment Processing**
>
> » Cleaning
> » Disinfection
> » Sterilization
> » Monitoring and surveillance

Respiratory care departments should have a designated area in which to clean equipment. This area should separate dirty equipment from clean equipment. In order for equipment to be cleaned, it must be disassembled and examined. It should be placed in a sink or basin filled with hot water, soap, detergent, or enzymatic cleaner. Water alone will not dissolve any secretions or other organic materials. Soap is not **bactericidal**, but many detergents are weakly bactericidal against gram-positive bacteria. Adding a detergent can dissolve substances that are not soluble in water and therefore help to remove contamination. Equipment can be washed with a brush or placed into an ultrasonic washer to remove debris.

Equipment must be rinsed and dried after cleaning. Rinsing the equipment will remove any residue formed from the soap or detergent. Residue can irritate human tissues and may interfere with the sterilization and disinfection processes. Drying is also important to prevent bacterial growth on the equipment. Once the equipment is clean and dry, it should be packaged appropriately for the sterilization or disinfection process or taken to the clean area of the department and reassembled. Prior to reassembling the equipment, hand hygiene is important to prevent recontamination of the equipment.

Disinfection

Disinfection does not remove all microorganisms, but rather reduces the number of potentially infectious organisms by killing most of those present. Spores, mycobacteria, and viruses are the most resistant to being destroyed. The term **antisepsis** is sometimes used synonymously with *disinfection*, but usually describes the use of chemical agents (antiseptics) to inhibit microbial growth. Microbes may not be killed with an antiseptic, but the microbes' ability to replicate and produce toxins is impaired. Disinfection occurs through physical or chemical methods and is affected by several factors, such as prior cleaning of the object, type of contamination, temperature, and the pH of the disinfection solution. **Table 33–2** summarizes disinfecting agents.

Pasteurization is a common technique used to disinfect equipment. A pasteurizer is similar to a kitchen dishwasher. The equipment is immersed in water heated to just below its boiling point for a period of time. Respiratory care equipment is typically immersed in water of about 70° C for 30 minutes. Once the equipment is pasteurized, it is placed in a dryer.[1]

> **RESPIRATORY RECAP**
>
> **Methods of Disinfection**
>
> » Pasteurization
> » Alcohols
> » Glutaraldehyde
> » Hydrogen peroxide
> » Iodophors
> » Ortho-phthalaldehyde (OPA)
> » Acetic acid
> » Peracetic acid
> » Phenolics
> » Quaternary ammonium compounds

Chemical disinfectants are used on the contaminated surface of the equipment. The equipment is immersed in the disinfectant for a period of time. Contact time may range from 20 minutes to 3 hours. Once the time requirement for disinfection is met, the equipment is removed, rinsed in sterile water, and dried. Once the equipment is dried, it must be handled with sterile gloves and towels to prevent recontamination during reassembly and packaging. Examples of disinfectants include alcohol, chlorine, glutaraldehyde, iodophors, phenolics, ammonia compounds, acetic acid, peracetic acid (a mixture of acetic acid and hydrogen peroxide), and hydrogen peroxide.

Ethyl or isopropyl alcohol applied to the skin is used in healthcare settings to disinfect the skin prior to injections or drawing of blood samples. Alcohols can penetrate the cell wall and denature proteins or disrupt the hydrogen bonds. These agents are bactericidal, tuberculocidal, fungicidal, and virucidal. They do not kill spores and therefore are not recommended for sterilizing medical equipment. Alcohols may damage equipment made of rubber and plastic. They may be used to disinfect oral thermometers, pagers, scissors, and stethoscopes. Small alcohol pads are frequently used to disinfect the tops of medication vials.[8]

Chlorine and chlorine compounds are referred to as *hypochlorite* disinfectants. They are contained in the household bleach used in homes. Hypochlorite solutions are antimicrobial, do not leave any toxic residue on equipment, are inexpensive, and are fast acting. The CDC recommends using hypochlorite solutions in a 1:10 dilution of 5.25% concentration in water for routine environmental disinfection of blood spills and in rooms where patients are infected with *Clostridium difficile* after the surfaces are cleaned.[8] It is important to avoid mixing any hypochlorite solution with an acid because of the risk of creating toxic chlorine gas.[8]

Glutaraldehyde (Cidex, Sonacide, Sporicidin, Hospex, Omnicide, Matricide, Wavicide) is a high-level disinfectant. It is a colorless, oily liquid with a sharp pungent odor. It turns green when activated to a pH of 7.5 to 8.5. Glutaraldehyde can disinfect within 20 minutes and sterilize in 6 to 10 hours. Glutaraldehyde is safe to use with metal, rubber, or plastic equipment. It is also used to sterilize bronchoscopes and spirometry tubing. Because glutaraldehyde is toxic, the equipment must be rinsed with sterile water and usually dried. Although its use is limited to immersible equipment, glutaraldehyde is convenient because the solution may be kept in a small container and reused for 14 to 30 days. The solution should be monitored regularly for contamination.

Glutaraldehydes are toxic, and therefore healthcare providers need to use caution when working with this type of solution. Glutaraldehydes should be used in a designated area where there is adequate ventilation and where people and the cleaning process can be monitored. Glutaraldehyde should be stored in a tightly closed, properly labeled container in a cool, secure area. Activated glutaraldehyde is safe to use for 14 to 21 days. Glutaraldehyde can be disposed of with an abundant amount of cold water into a drain connected to a sanitary sewer. It should not be discarded into a septic system.

TABLE 33-2 Disinfecting Agents

Agent	Example of Use	Advantages	Disadvantages
Alcohols	Thermometers, scissors, stethoscopes	Easily accessible.	Damages the shellac mountings of instruments. Swells and hardens rubber and plastic tubing. Discolors rubber and plastic tiles.
Chlorine and chlorine compounds	Spot disinfection, CPR training manikins	Easily accessible.	Pungent odor. Do not mix with acidic solutions.
Glutaraldehyde	Spirometry tubing, anesthesia resuscitation bags	Can be reused for 14 to 20 days after activation. Relatively inexpensive. Excellent materials compatibility.	Respiratory tract irritation. Pungent and irritating odor. Relatively slow mycobactericidal activity. Allergic contact dermatitis. Monitoring recommended. Must use butyl gloves and well-ventilated area.
Hydrogen peroxide	Ventilator surfaces	No activation required. May enhance removal of organic matter. No disposal issues. Does not coagulate blood or fix tissue to surface.	Material compatibility concerns. Serious eye damage with contact.
Iodophors	Hydrotherapy tanks, thermometers	Does not stain. No activation required.	Should not be used to disinfect surfaces.
OPA	Endoscopes	Better than glutaraldehyde because it does not irritate the eyes or nasal passages. Fast acting. No activation required. Odor is not significant. Excellent materials compatibility.	Stains skin, mucous membranes, clothing, and environmental surfaces gray if used improperly. Repeated exposure may result in hypersensitivity in some patients. More expensive than glutaraldehyde. Eye irritation with contact. Slow sporicidal activity.
Peracetic acid	Endoscopes	Rapid sterilization cycle time (30–45 minutes). Low-temperature (50–55° C) liquid immersion sterilization. Environmentally friendly by-products. Fully automated. Single-use system eliminates need for concentration testing. Standardized cycle. May enhance removal of organic materials. No adverse health effects under normal operating conditions. Compatible with many materials and instruments.	Potential materials incompatibility. Used for immersible instruments only. Biological indicator may not be suitable for routine monitoring. Only one scope or a small number of instruments can be processed in a given time; thus, it is more expensive. Serious eye and skin damage is possible. Point-of-use system.
Phenols	Environmental surfaces such as bed rails, tables, and surfaces	Long history of being safe and of use in hospitals.	Do not use in nurseries; hyperbilirubinemia has been found.
Quaternary ammonium compounds	Floors, furniture, and walls; blood pressure cuffs	Long history of being safe and of use in hospitals.	May cause asthma exacerbation.

CPR, cardiopulmonary resuscitation; OPA, ortho-phthalaldehyde.

Modified from Rutala WA, Weber DJ, and the Health Infection Control Practices Advisory Committee. *Guideline for Disinfection and Sterilization in Healthcare Facilities 2008*. November 2008. Available at: http://www.cdc.gov/ncidod/dhqp/pdf/guidelines/Disinfection_Nov_2008.pdf.

Side effects associated with glutaraldehyde exposure include epistaxis, rhinitis, and asthma exacerbations. Dermatitis, skin irritations, and mucous membrane irritation have also been reported with acute and chronic exposures to glutaraldehyde. To prevent these side effects from occurring, exhaust hoods should be used in the room where the agent is kept. Tight-fitting lids should be secured to the immersion baths, and personal protective equipment such as nitrile or butyl rubber gloves or polyethylene and spun-bonded polypropylene-coated gloves should be worn to protect the hands. An isolation gown or lab coat should be worn. Appropriate respirators should be worn to prevent exposure to glutaraldehyde vapors.

Hydrogen peroxide was added to the CDC guidelines for disinfection and sterilization in healthcare facilities as a safe disinfectant agent in a 2008 update.[8] Hydrogen peroxide is germicidal and active against bacteria, fungi, yeasts, and viruses and is available in 7.35%, 3.0%, and 1.0% solutions. Hydrogen peroxide produces destructive hydroxyl free radicals that attack the cell membrane. It is a safe disinfectant used on heat-sensitive medical devices such as bronchoscopes. However, peroxides are oxidizing chemicals and may cause cosmetic and functional damage to the scope.

Iodophor (povidone iodine) solutions or tinctures have been used as antiseptics on skin or tissue. Iodophors are germicidal because they penetrate the cell wall and disrupt protein/nucleic acid structure and synthesis.[8] Iodophors do not stain like the general iodines. This type of agent is reported to be bactericidal, mycobactericidal, and virucidal with long contact times.

Ortho-phthalaldehyde (OPA) has received clearance from the FDA as a high-level disinfectant. It is a clear, pale blue liquid with a pH of 7.5. OPA has advantages over glutaraldehyde in that it is more stable and does not irritate the eyes or nasal passages. OPA does not require exposure monitoring, has a slight odor, and requires no activation. It has excellent material compatibility. Because OPA stains proteins gray, unprotected skin will be stained by exposure. It is important to be trained to use this agent and to wear the proper personal protective equipment, including gown, gloves, and goggles. Exposure time is 12 minutes, and it is important to rinse the equipment with water.[8]

Acetic acid is white household vinegar, which is used exclusively in home care settings. Acetic acid with a pH of 2.0 or greater is bactericidal, lowers a microbe's intracellular pH, and inactivates energy-producing enzymes. The optimal concentration for acetic acid is 1.25%, which is equal to one part 5% white household vinegar and three parts water. Exposure time is 1 hour. It is an effective bactericidal agent against *Pseudomonas aeruginosa*, but its sporicidal and virucidal activity has not been established.

Peracetic acid is acetic acid with an additional oxygen atom. It acts rapidly against all microorganisms. It will inactivate gram-positive and gram-negative bacteria, fungi, and yeasts in less than 5 minutes. An advantage of this agent is that it lacks harmful decomposition products, which enhances the removal of organic material and leaves no residue. Little is known about the mechanism of action of this agent, but it is believed to denature proteins and disrupt cell wall permeability. A 35% peracetic acid solution is diluted to 0.2% with filtered water at 50° C. This method may be more expensive because an automated system requiring training must be installed.

Phenolics have been used in the healthcare settings for years. They are germicidal, antimicrobial, bactericidal, fungicidal, virucidal, and tuberculocidal at recommended dilutions. Phenolics in high concentrations penetrate and disrupt the cell wall, and in low concentrations they inactive the essential enzyme system and leak metabolites from the cell wall. Phenolics are absorbed by porous material, and residual disinfectant can irritate the skin. These agents are used to disinfect environmental surfaces such as bedside tables or bed rails. Phenolics are not recommended in neonatal units because of a reported link to hyperbilirubinemia when phenolics were used to clean bassinets and incubators.[8]

Quaternary ammonium compounds (quats) are cationic detergents that dissolve the cell membranes of microorganisms. Quats are used as disinfectants and cleaning agents. Later-generation quats are considered fungicidal, bactericidal, and virucidal; however, they are not sporicidal.[8] Quats inactivate the enzymes and denature the cell proteins of the cell membrane. They are used to disinfect medical equipment that comes into contact with skin, such as blood pressure cuffs, and to clean floors, furniture, and walls in healthcare settings. In the home care setting, they can be used as an alternative to acetic acid at a dilution of 1 ounce to 1 gallon of sterile or distilled water for at least 10 minutes.

Sterilization

Sterilization is the complete destruction of all microorganisms, including spores. Sterilization prevents the transmission of diseases.[8] Sterilization processes are effective when healthcare providers adhere to the recommendations and instructions on the product labels. There are two types of sterilization: physical and chemical. Physical processes include steam and radiation. Chemical processes include ethylene oxide (ETO), hydrogen peroxide gas plasma, and peracetic acid. **Table 33–3** summarizes sterilization techniques.

As discussed previously, critical items are those medical devices that come in contact with sterile body tissues or fluids. These critical items must be sterilized to prevent any possibility of transmitting diseases. Steam sterilization is recommended for equipment that is heat resistant. Those pieces of equipment that are sensitive to heat and moisture require a low-temperature process such as ETO, hydrogen peroxide gas plasma, or peracetic acid.[8]

TABLE 33–3 Sterilization Techniques and Uses

Agent	Example of Use	Advantages	Disadvantages
Steam (autoclave)	Critical and semicritical items that are heat and moisture resistant; respiratory therapy and anesthesia equipment; hemostats; surgery utensils; laboratory specimens	Nontoxic to patient, staff, and environment. Cycle is easy to control and monitor. Rapidly microbicidal. Least affected by organic/inorganic soils among sterilization processes.	Deleterious for heat-sensitive instruments. Damages microsurgical instruments. Potential for burns.
Hydrogen peroxide gas plasma	Materials that cannot tolerate high temperatures or humidity such as plastics and electrical devices	Safe for the environment. Cycle time is 28–75 minutes. Used for heat- and moisture-sensitive items (temperature <50° C). Simple to operate and install and monitor. Only requires electrical outlet.	Linens, paper, and liquids cannot be processed. Sterilization chamber size varies. Some medical devices with long or narrow lumens will not be processed in this system. Hydrogen peroxide can be toxic.
Ethylene oxide (ETO)	Critical items and some semicritical items that are moisture or heat sensitive and cannot be sterilized by steam sterilization	Penetrates packaging materials, device lumens. Single-dose cartridge and negative-pressure chamber minimize the potential for gas leak and ETO exposure. Simple to operate. Compatible with most medical materials.	Requires aeration time to remove ETO residue. Sterilization chamber size varies. ETO is toxic, carcinogenic, and flammable. ETO emission must be regulated. ETO cartridges must be stored in flammable liquid storage cabinet. Lengthy cycle aeration time.
Peracetic acid	Endoscopes	Rapid cycle time (30–45 minutes). Low-temperature immersion sterilization (50–55° C). Environmentally friendly by-products. Flows through the scopes.	Point-of-use system. No sterile storage. Biological indicator may not be suitable for routine monitoring. Used for immersible instruments only. Some materials incompatibility. Small number of instruments processed in the cycle. Potential for serious eye and skin damage with contact.

Modified from Rutala WA, Weber DJ, and the Health Infection Control Practices Advisory Committee. *Guideline for Disinfection and Sterilization in Healthcare Facilities 2008*. November 2008. Available at: http://www.cdc.gov/ncidod/dhqp/pdf/guidelines/Disinfection_Nov_2008.pdf.

Steam autoclaving kills microorganisms by heat-denaturing microbial proteins. Effective sterilization requires adequate heat and time, but increases in pressure or the addition of moisture enhances and hastens killing. Moist heat in the form of saturated steam under pressure is the most commonly used method for sterilization of equipment. Autoclaves are similar to pressure cookers and range in size from a desktop unit to a walk-in closet. The autoclave is used to expose equipment to direct steam at the required temperature and pressure for a specific time. Therefore, autoclaving has the advantage of being fast (typically 5 to 15 minutes plus cooling time), but it damages some types of equipment.[8]

Autoclaving is nontoxic, inexpensive, rapidly microbicidal, sporicidal, and penetrates fabrics. The four parameters that influence this process are steam, pressure, time, and temperature. The most common temperatures used are 121° C (250° F) and 132° C (270° F).[8] The temperatures must be maintained for a minimum time to kill organisms. All equipment must be cleaned before being placed in the steam sterilization process. The clean equipment is wrapped in linen, muslin, or paper wraps. Equipment exposed to steam heat for 30 minutes at 15 psi and 121° C or for 4 minutes at 15 psi and 132° C should be sterile.[8] The times and temperatures used will be determined by the type of items being sterilized. Air is evacuated and is replaced with steam, which reaches a higher temperature than air. The high-temperature steam can surround and infiltrate the equipment, including all of the crevices.

RESPIRATORY RECAP

Methods of Sterilization

- » Steam (autoclaving)
- » Ethylene oxide
- » Hydrogen peroxide gas plasma
- » Peracetic acid sterilization

The equipment must have time to air dry because water can become trapped in the wrappers or equipment

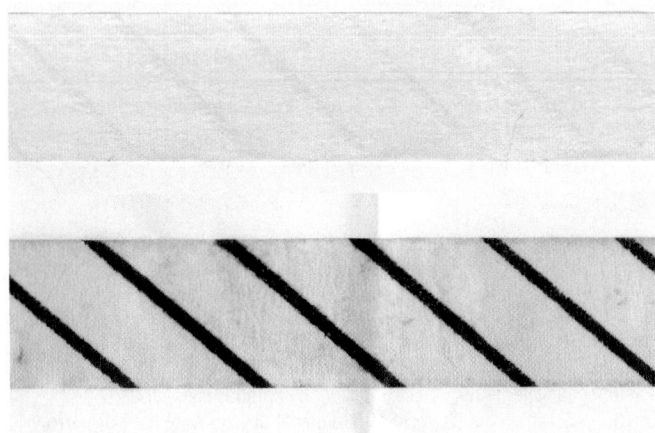

FIGURE 33–1 Indicator strips.

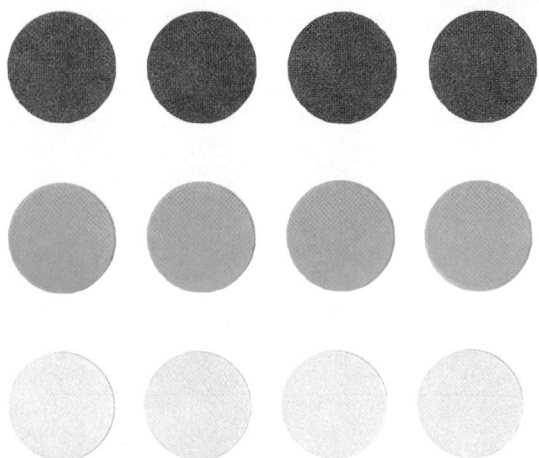

FIGURE 33–2 Indicator strips for sterilization via ethylene oxide, steam, and radiation methods.

itself. Autoclaves should be monitored by mechanical, chemical, and biological indicators. Wrapped packages should have a piece of indicator tape placed on the seal of the wrapper before being placed in the autoclave. The indicator tape will change color when the equipment has been sterilized.

Flash sterilization is a modification of the steam sterilization process in which the flashed item is placed in an open tray at 132° C for 3 minutes at 27 psi.[8] It is not recommended as a routine sterilization method because there is no method for monitoring its performance. This type of process may be useful in surgical suites where this sterilizer is in close proximity to the site of use. It is considered acceptable for processing cleaned patient care items that cannot be packaged, sterilized, and stored before use. This process should not be used for convenience or as an alternative to the previous method discussed.

Low-temperature sterilization at temperatures below 60° C is used on equipment that is sensitive to heat and moisture. ETO, hydrogen peroxide gas plasma, and liquid peracetic acid chemicals all are examples of low-temperature sterilization techniques.

Ethylene oxide is a colorless, flammable, explosive, and toxic gas that has been used since the 1950s. Ethylene oxide is a dry gas that sterilizes without need for heat or moisture. It is used to process equipment that is unable to tolerate autoclaving or immersion. The equipment must be dry when placed in the ETO chamber to prevent ethylene glycol from forming. The equipment must be packaged in a moisture-permeable wrapping made of muslin, paper, or plastic made of polyethylene. Indicator tape similar to the tape used for the autoclave is used and will change color to indicate that proper conditions were met for sterilization (**Figure 33–1** and **Figure 33–2**). The chambers are controlled at temperatures between 50° C and 56° C and humidity between 30% and 70% to ensure optimum conditions for sterilization.[8] Approximately 3 to 4 hours of gas exposure are required, and processed equipment usually requires ventilation for 8 to 24 hours afterward.[8] Chronic exposure to ETO is associated with nausea, headache, dizziness, and airway inflammation. Residue from the ETO on equipment can lead to tissue inflammation and hemolysis. Contact of ethylene oxide with water produces ethylene glycol (antifreeze), which may persist on the equipment as a toxic, sticky residue. ETO also has carcinogenic, mutagenic, and teratogenic effects.

Hydrogen peroxide gas plasma is a new sterilization technology. Gas plasmas are generated in an enclosed chamber under deep vacuum using radio frequency or microwave energy to excite the gas molecules and produce charged free radicals.[8] The free radical production within a plasma field is capable of interacting with cell components and disrupting the metabolism of microorganisms.[8] The sterilization chamber is evacuated, and hydrogen peroxide solution is injected from a cassette and vaporized into the chamber.[8] It vaporizes in the chamber over the surfaces of the equipment, and an electrical field created by a radio frequency is applied to the chamber to create a gas plasma over 50 to 75 minutes.[8] The excess gas is then removed from the chamber, followed by depressurization. This is the preferred choice for sterilizing equipment that cannot tolerate high temperatures and humidity.

Peracetic acid sterilization is usually used on surgical and medical endoscopes. This method uses 35% peracetic acid and an anticorrosive agent in a single-dose container.[8] The container is punctured at the time of use and activated when the lid is closed. The peracetic acid is diluted with filtered water at 50° C and then circulated within the chamber and pumped through the equipment for 12 minutes. Once used, it is discarded into the sewer, and the instruments are rinsed with filtered water.

Ionizing radiation uses cobalt 60 gamma rays or electron accelerators. Radiation can sterilize tissues for transplantation, pharmaceuticals, and medical devices, but it is not an FDA-approved process for use by healthcare facilities.

Dry heat sterilizers should be used for equipment that might be damaged by moist heat or products that are impenetrable to moist heat, such as plastics or rubber. Dry heat is effective and usually used for laboratory glassware, surgical instruments, petroleum products, sharp instruments, and powders. Dry heat is nontoxic and does not harm the environment, yet the process is very time consuming, requiring exposure for 60 minutes at 170° C.

Incineration is the simplest means of destroying microorganisms. Incineration is used when there is no other way of sterilizing equipment.

Equipment Surveillance and Monitoring

Maintaining a regular program of **equipment surveillance** and monitoring is im-portant to ensure that sterile and disinfected equipment is being properly processed to meet the necessary levels of cleanliness. A surveillance program usually includes three components: monitoring equipment-processing procedures, sampling in-use equipment, and microbiologically identifying suspect pathogens.

> **RESPIRATORY RECAP**
>
> **Equipment Surveillance Methods**
>
> » Aspiration
> » Plating
> » Swabbing

Equipment in use can be sampled with a sterile cotton swab or aerosol impaction. The swabs can be used to sample easily accessible surfaces of respiratory care equipment. The microbiology laboratory then identifies the infectious organisms.

Although indicator tapes are regularly placed in autoclaves and gas sterilizers to indicate that proper heat and gas concentrations and duration have been achieved for each run, this action does not ensure that sterilization has actually taken place. Biologic tests also are regularly run in each sterilizer. The tubes containing bacteria in growth media are subsequently cultured to ensure complete killing. Still, this step does not guarantee that the equipment itself is being sterilized. Inadequate cleaning before autoclaving, for example, may allow organisms to survive, requiring that the equipment itself be cultured periodically to verify sterility or to detect low bacterial counts for clean equipment. One of the following three methods is typically used:

- *Aspiration*: A quantity of sterile saline is drawn through the lumen of the equipment to be tested, after which the saline is cultured.
- *Plating*: To culture exterior surfaces, the equipment may be rolled directly onto a culture medium, usually a Petri dish filled with agar (the plate). The culture obtained may be qualitative (measuring only the presence and type of organism) or quantitative (measuring the level of infection by counting the number of colonies that grow on the agar surface).
- *Swabbing*: Irregular surfaces that are not easily rolled onto an agar plate may be rubbed with a sterile swab coated with culture medium. The swab may then be used to inoculate a plate.

Precautions

The healthcare setting is a place where respiratory therapists and other healthcare professionals can be exposed to patients' blood and body fluids. Protecting patients and ourselves against infection requires strict adherence to the standard and transmission-based precautions set out by the *Guideline for Isolation Precautions: Preventing Transmission of Infectious Agents in Healthcare Settings 2007* published by the CDC.[1] The CDC identifies two tiers of precautions to prevent transmission of infectious agents: standard precautions and transmission-based precautions. **Standard precautions** are intended to be applied to the care of all patients in all healthcare settings. Patients who are known or suspected of being infected or colonized with infectious agents require additional control measures in the form of transmission-based precautions.

Standard Precautions

Universal precautions, as defined by the CDC, are a set of precautions designed to prevent transmission of human immunodeficiency virus (HIV), hepatitis B virus (HBV), and other bloodborne pathogens when providing healthcare (**Table 33–4**). Under universal precautions, blood and certain body fluids of all patients are considered potentially infectious for HIV, HBV, and other bloodborne pathogens. Universal precautions involve the use of protective barriers such as gloves, gowns, aprons, masks, and protective eyewear, which reduce the risk of exposure of the healthcare worker's skin or mucous membranes to potentially infective materials. In addition, it is recommended that all healthcare workers take precautions to prevent injuries caused by needles, scalpels, and other sharp instruments or devices. In 1996, the CDC established standard precautions, which synthesized the major features of body substance isolation (a form of isolation precautions used before 1996) and universal precautions to prevent transmission of microorganisms.

> **RESPIRATORY RECAP**
>
> **Standard Precautions**
>
> » Hand hygiene
> » Use of gloves, masks, and eye protection (goggles or face shield), depending on reasonably anticipated exposure to blood and body fluids

Standard precautions include hand hygiene and the use of gloves, gowns, masks, and eye protection (goggles or face shield), depending on reasonably anticipated exposure to

TABLE 33-4 Recommendations for Application of Standard Precautions for All Patients in All Healthcare Settings

Assume *all* patients are potentially infected with an organism that could be transmitted to you, other patients, or other healthcare providers.

Component	Recommendation
Hand hygiene	After touching blood, body fluids, secretions, excretions, contaminated items; immediately after removing gloves; between patient contacts.
Personal protective equipment (PPE)	
Gloves	For touching blood, body fluids, secretions, excretions, contaminated items; for touching mucous membranes and nonintact skin.
Gowns	During procedures and patient care activities when contact of clothing/exposed skin with blood, body fluids, secretions, and excretions is anticipated.
Masks, eye protection, face shields	During procedures and patient care activities likely to generate splashes or sprays of blood, body fluids, or secretions, especially suctioning and endotracheal intubation.
Patient placement	Prioritize for single-patient room if patient is at increased risk of transmission, is likely to contaminate the environment, does not maintain appropriate hygiene, or is at increased risk of acquiring infection or developing adverse outcome following infection.
Patient resuscitation	Use mouthpiece, resuscitation bag, other ventilation devices to prevent contact with mouth and oral secretions.
Soiled patient care equipment	Handle in a manner that prevents transfer of microorganisms to others and to the environment; wear gloves if visibly contaminated; perform hand hygiene.
Textiles and laundry	Handle in a manner that prevents transfer of microorganisms to others and to the environment.
Environmental control	Develop procedures for routine care, cleaning, and disinfection of environmental surfaces, especially frequently touched surfaces in patient care areas.
Needles and other sharps	Do not recap, bend, break, or hand-manipulate used needles; if recapping is required, use a one-handed scoop technique only; use safety features when available; place used sharps in puncture-resistant container.
Respiratory hygiene/cough etiquette (source containment of infectious respiratory secretions in symptomatic patients, beginning at initial point of contact)	Instruct symptomatic persons to cover mouth/nose when sneezing/coughing; use tissues and dispose in no-touch receptacle; observe hand hygiene after soiling of hands with respiratory secretions; wear surgical mask if tolerated or maintain spatial separation >3 feet if possible.

Modified from Siegel JD, Rhinehart E, Jackson M, Chiarello L, and the Healthcare Infection Control Practices Advisory Committee. *Guideline for Isolation Precautions: Preventing Transmission of Infectious Agents in Healthcare Settings 2007*. Atlanta, GA: Centers for Disease Control and Prevention; 2007.

blood and body fluids. This also includes concerns about equipment in the patient environment that may be contaminated with infectious body fluids, which must be handled appropriately to prevent the transmission of diseases. The appropriate precautions to use (standard or transmission based) will be determined by the nature of the healthcare provider, the patient interaction, and the extent of the anticipated blood, body fluid, or pathogen exposure. For some interactions, only gloves are required. For other interactions, gloves, gowns, and eye protection will be required. Standard precautions are recommended in all healthcare settings, including hospitals, long-term acute care settings, rehabilitation hospitals, home care settings, doctor's offices, and clinics. Combining body substance isolation policies and universal precautions will reduce the risk of transmission of infections between patients and healthcare providers.

Hand Hygiene

Hand hygiene is the most important part of standard precautions. It is the single most important measure to reduce the transmission of microorganisms from one person to another or from one site to another on the same patient.[10,11] **Hand hygiene** refers to either hand washing with soap and water for 15 to 20 seconds or the use of alcohol-based gels, foams,

RESPIRATORY RECAP

Hand Hygiene

- » Hand hygiene is the most important factor in the prevention of spread of infection.
- » Alcohol-based hand rubs are an effective form of hand hygiene.
- » Wash hands if soiled by blood, body fluids, or excrement.
- » Hand hygiene effectiveness is reduced with long nails, extenders, and jewelry.

or rubs that do not require water. In the absence of visible soiling of hands, approved alcohol-based products for hand disinfection are preferred over antimicrobial or plain soap and water because of their superior microbicidal activity, reduced drying of the skin, and convenience. Current guidelines for hand hygiene promote the use of alcohol-based antiseptic preparations. Competent hand rubbing requires that a sufficient volume of an alcohol-based rub be applied to cover all surfaces of the hands and fingers and that at least 15 seconds of rubbing be used before the hands are dry. Application of the hand rub can be assisted by placing the bottle in specially designed dispensers (**Figure 33–3**).

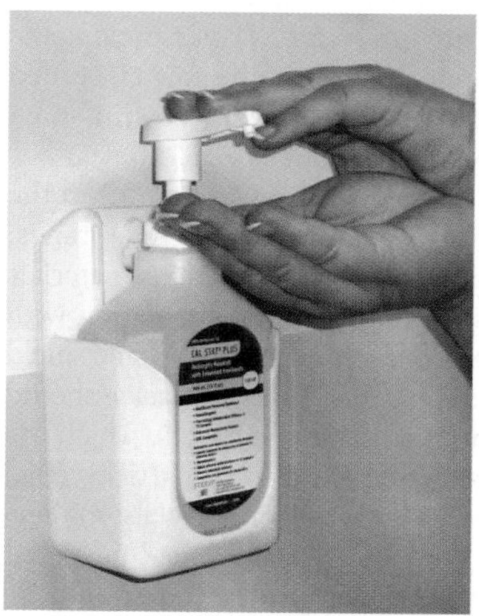

FIGURE 33–3 Hand hygiene dispenser, as found throughout healthcare facilities.

Hands should be washed with soap and warm water if they are soiled with blood, body fluids, or excrement. Hand hygiene effectiveness can be reduced by the type and length of fingernails, extenders, and jewelry. The use of artificial nails, extenders, and jewelry is discouraged for healthcare personnel who have contact with high-risk patients.

Personal Protective Equipment

Personal protective equipment (PPE) for healthcare providers refers to the various barriers and respirators used to protect the mucous membranes, skin, airways, and clothing from contact with infectious agents. The selection of PPE is based on the nature of the patient interaction and possible mode of transmission. Specific PPE includes gloves, eye protection, face protection, gowns, and respiratory masks (**Figure 33–4** and **Figure 33–5**). Hand hygiene is performed after removing PPE. **Box 33–1** describes the order in which PPE is donned and removed.

Gloves are used to protect the patient and healthcare provider from pathogens that may be transmitted by direct contact with blood or body fluids, those who are colonized or infected with pathogens on the hands, and

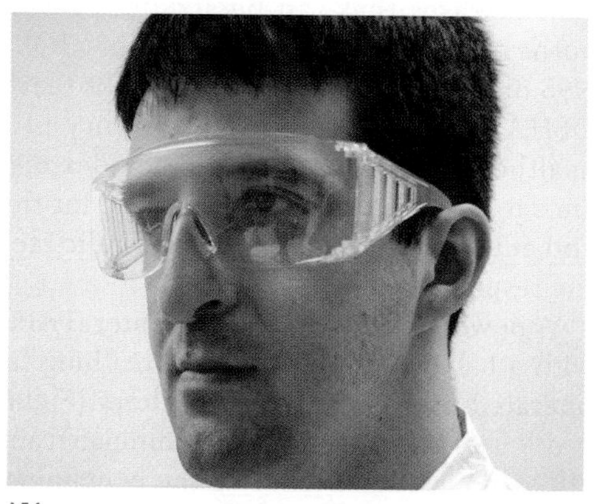

(A)

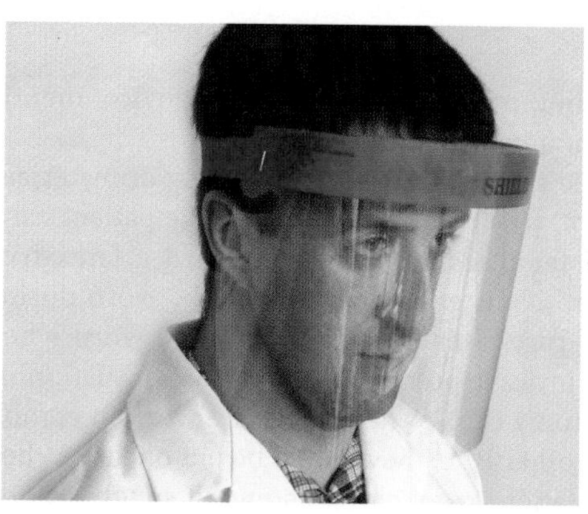

(B)

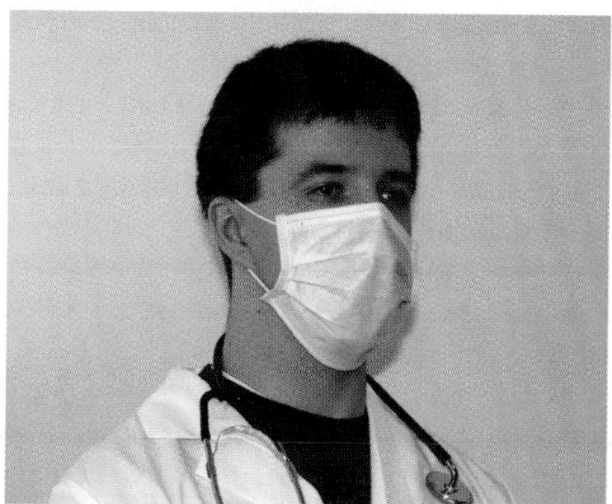

(C)

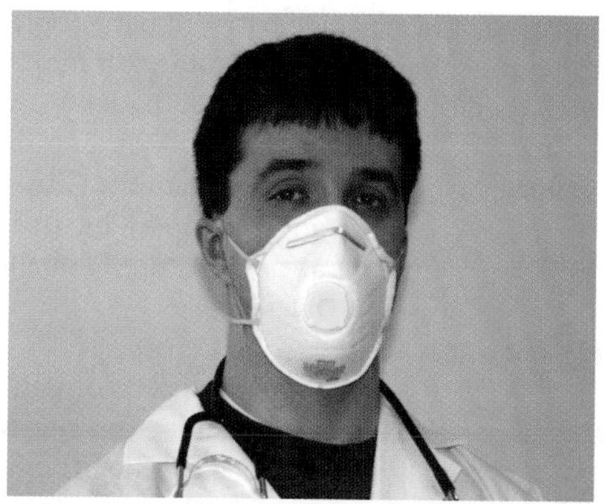

(D)

FIGURE 33–4 Personal protective equipment. (**A**) Goggles. (**B**) Face shield. (**C**) Surgical mask. (**D**) N95 respirator mask.

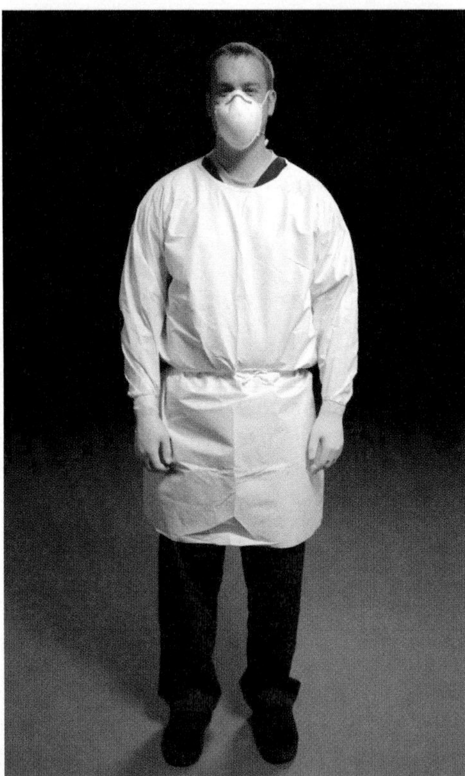

FIGURE 33–5 Mask, gown, and gloves for personal protection.

when handling patient equipment and environmental surfaces contaminated with pathogens.

Nonsterile gloves are made of a variety of materials, such as latex, vinyl, and nitrile for routine patient care. Healthcare facilities are moving toward a latex-free environment. Nonsterile gloves should be worn during any patient care. Sterile gloves should be worn when performing invasive procedures such as open suctioning or tracheostomy care. When gloves are worn in combination with other PPE, they should be put on last. When using an isolation gown, gloves should fit snugly around the wrist to cover the cuff of the gown and provide a more reliable barrier for the wrists and hands.

Gloves may need to be changed between patient procedures and after touching portable computers or mobile equipment. Always discard gloves between patients and perform hand hygiene immediately after discarding the gloves and before caring for the next patient. Gloves should *never* be used as a substitute for hand hygiene.

RESPIRATORY RECAP

Personal Protective Equipment
- » Gloves
- » Eye protection
- » Face protection
- » Gowns
- » Masks

Isolation gowns, aprons, jackets, or pants are used as a barrier to protect the healthcare provider from contamination of the clothes and any exposed body area from blood and body fluids. Selection of the type of isolation gown is based on the nature of the interaction with the patient and the anticipated degree of contact with infectious material or blood and body fluids. Isolation gowns are always worn in combination with gloves and other PPE. Gowns are usually the first PPE to be donned. Isolation gowns should be removed before leaving the patient care area to prevent contamination of the environment outside the patient's room. When removing the gown, the outer contaminated side of the gown is turned inward and rolled into a bundle and the gown is then placed in the correct waste container.

Masks, goggles, or face shields are used to protect the healthcare provider's eyes, skin, mucous membranes, mouth, and nose from contact with infectious materials from patients. Masks can be used in combination with goggles to provide protection for the face. A face shield also can be worn. Masks (such as surgical masks) should not be confused with particulate respirators, which are recommended for protection from small particles (e.g., N95 respirator masks used for airborne isolation). Personal eyeglasses and contact lenses are *not* considered adequate eye protection. Face protection should be donned before entering the patient's room and removed before leaving the patient's room.[12]

Respiratory protection is intended for use to prevent diseases that can be acquired through the airborne route. This includes the use of NIOSH-approved N95 or higher-level respirator masks that fit properly. OSHA broadly regulates respiratory protection for healthcare providers, which includes medical clearance to wear a respirator, fit testing for the respirator, and education on the use and periodic reevaluation of the respirator.[12]

A powered air-purifying respirator (PAPR) is a device with a half- or full-face piece, breathing tube, battery-operated blower, and HEPA filters (**Figure 33–6**). A PAPR uses a blower to pass contaminated air through the HEPA filter, which removes the contaminant and supplies purified air to a face piece. However, it is not a true positive pressure device because it can be overbreathed when inhaling. A face shield may be used in conjunction with a half-mask PAPR respirator for protection against body fluids. The most common use for a PAPR is in the case where an N95 respirator mask does not fit. It can also be used if the healthcare provider has facial hair or facial deformity that interferes with the mask-to-face seal. It might also be used when a N95 respirator mask is unavailable. Some prefer to use a PAPR for high-risk aerosol-generating procedures.

Accidental injuries associated with needle sticks and other sharp objects have been associated with transmission of hepatitis C, HIV, and other pathogens. Prevention of needle sticks and other sharps injuries is a major concern for healthcare providers. Healthcare providers must use caution when handling any and all sharp

BOX 33–1

Sequence for Donning and Removing Personal Protective Equipment

Sequence for Donning Personal Protective Equipment (PPE)

The type of PPE used will vary based on the level of precautions required.

1. Gown
   Fully cover torso from neck to knees, arms to end of wrists, and wrap around the back.
   Fasten in back of neck and waist.
2. Mask or respirator
   Secure ties or elastic bands at middle of head and neck.
   Fit flexible band to nose bridge.
   Fit snug to face and below chin.
   Fit-check respirator.
3. Goggles or face shield
   Place over face and eyes and adjust to fit.
4. Gloves
   Extend to cover wrist of isolation gown.

Sequence for Removing Personal Protective Equipment (PPE)

Except for respirator, remove PPE at doorway or in anteroom. Remove respirator after leaving patient room and closing door.

1. Gloves
   Outside of gloves is contaminated.
   Grasp outside of glove with opposite gloved hand and peel off.
   Hold removed glove in gloved hand.
   Slide fingers of ungloved hand under remaining glove at wrist.
   Peel glove off over first glove.
   Discard gloves in a waste container.
2. Goggles or face shield
   Outside of goggles or face shield is contaminated.
   To remove, handle by headband or ear pieces.
   Place in designated receptacle for reprocessing or in a waste container.
3. Gown
   Gown front and sleeves are contaminated!
   Unfasten ties.
   Pull away from neck and shoulders, touching inside of gown only.
   Turn gown inside out.
   Fold or roll into a bundle and discard.
4. Mask or respirator
   Front of mask/respirator is contaminated; do not touch.
   Grasp bottom and then top ties or elastics and remove.
   Perform hand hygiene immediately after removing all PPE.

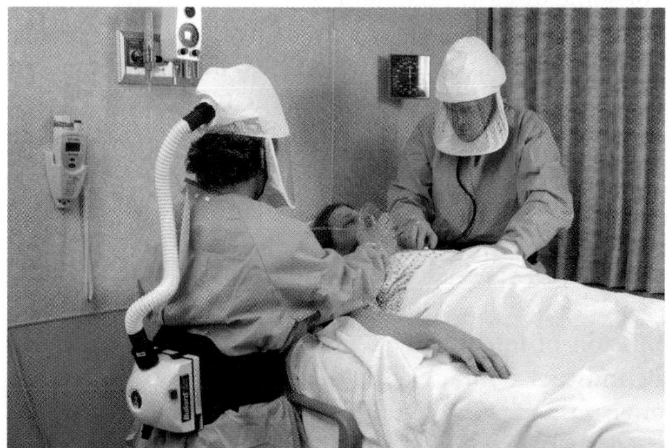

FIGURE 33–6 Powered air-purifying respirator (PAPR).

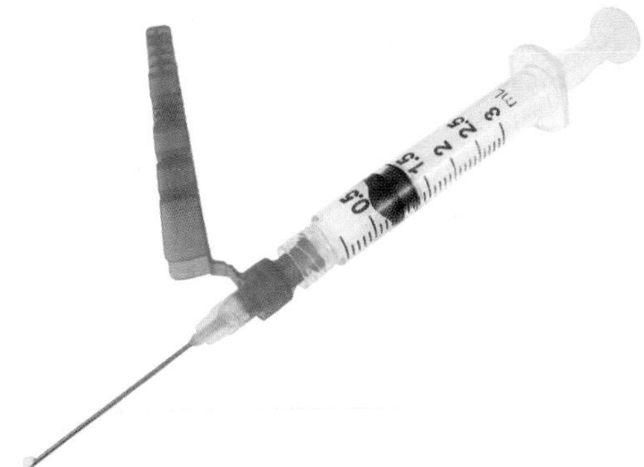

FIGURE 33–7 Syringe with needle guard.

instruments, including needles and syringes. Needle protection devices should be used on arterial blood gas syringes, and a needle-free syringe should be used whenever possible (**Figure 33–7**). Needles should be properly disposed of in an appropriate sharps container (**Figure 33–8**). If a needle stick injury occurs, the area should be immediately washed with soap and water, and the incident should be reported to a supervisor.

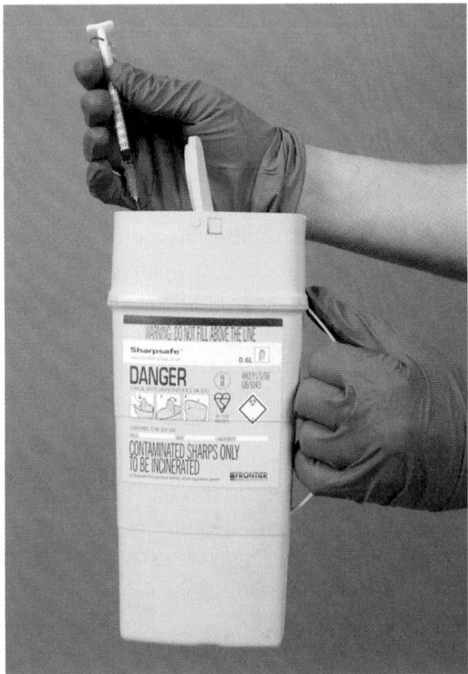

FIGURE 33–8 Sharps container.

Patient Placement

When there is a concern about transmission of an infectious agent, patients should be placed in a single-patient room. Single-patient rooms are indicated for patients requiring airborne isolation and those in need of a protective environment and are preferred for those requiring contact or droplet precautions. However, patients may be placed in the same room if they have the same transmittable disease. Limiting the transport of patients with contagious diseases limits the risk of transmission. When they must be transported, it is imperative the patient wear barrier protection (gown, gloves, or mask) consistent with the route for transmission. An N95 respirator mask is not required for the patient. It is also imperative to notify the healthcare personnel in the area receiving the patient to ensure that precautions are taken to prevent transmission.

Patient equipment that has been contaminated should be placed into an impervious bag before removal from the patient's room. A single bag may be used if the contaminated equipment can be placed in the bag without contaminating the outer surface of the bag. Otherwise, the equipment must be double-bagged. The bags should be clearly labeled and are often colored red. These bags prevent exposure of healthcare providers and the environment to the contaminated equipment. The contaminated equipment should be processed according to OSHA procedures.

The need for respiratory hygiene and **cough etiquette** at the first point of contact became evident after reevaluating the SARS outbreaks, where failure to implement simple source control measures with patients, visitors, and healthcare personnel with respiratory symptoms may have contributed to SARS corona virus (SARS-CoV) transmission. This new strategy is targeted at patients, family members, and friends with undiagnosed transmissible respiratory infections and applies to any person with signs of illness that include cough, congestion, rhinorrhea, or increased production of respiratory secretions. Respiratory hygiene and cough etiquette includes educating staff, patients, and visitors; posting instructions for patients and family members in the appropriate language; source control measures such as covering the mouth and nose with a tissue when coughing and prompt disposal of used tissues; providing surgical masks for persons with a cough; hand hygiene after contact with respiratory secretions; and spatial separation, ideally more than 3 feet, between people with respiratory infection and those in the waiting areas. The main source of control is covering sneezes and coughs and applying a mask to a coughing person. These simple acts have been proven to prevent infected persons from dispersing secretions in the air. Measures such as these are important for infectious diseases such as the H1N1 influenza virus and other highly contagious respiratory infections.

Healthcare providers should observe droplet precautions and hand hygiene when caring for patients with signs and symptoms of respiratory infections. Those healthcare providers who have a respiratory infection are advised to avoid direct patient contact with high-risk patients. If this is not possible, the healthcare provider should wear a mask as well.

Transmission-Based Precautions

For some diseases, standard precautions are not enough to keep them from being spread to others or to other sites on the same patient. Therefore, we must use standard precautions *and* one or more of the transmission-based precautions. Remember that standard precautions are *always* used in the healthcare setting in interactions with all patients. Categories of transmission-based precautions include contact precautions, droplet precautions, and airborne precautions (**Table 33–5**).

Contact precautions are used to prevent the transmission of infectious agents that are spread by direct or indirect contact with the patient or the patient's environment. This includes placing the patient in a single-patient room; if a multipatient room placement is unavoidable, there must be more than 3 feet of separation between beds to reduce the opportunity for sharing of items between the infected/colonized patient and other patients. Healthcare providers should wear a gown and gloves for *all* interactions that may involve contact with the patient or with potentially contaminated areas in the

TABLE 33-5 Isolation Precautions

Type	Selected Patients	Major Specifications
Standard	All patients	Hand hygiene before and after every patient contact. Gloves, gowns, eye protection as required. Safe disposal or cleaning of instruments and linen. Cough etiquette: Patients and visitors should cover their nose or mouth when coughing, promptly dispose of used tissues, and practice hand hygiene after contact with respiratory secretions.
Contact	MRSA, VRE, *C. difficile* Scabies Impetigo Noncontained abscesses or decubitus ulcers (especially for *Staphylococcus aureus* and group A streptococci)	**In addition to standard precautions:** Private room preferred; cohorting allowed if necessary. Gloves required upon entering room. Change gloves after contact with contaminated secretions. Gown required if clothing may come into contact with the patient or environment surfaces, or if the patient has diarrhea. Patient wears gown during transport. Contact precautions plus: Wash hands after removing gown and before hand hygiene. Strict contact precautions: Must wear gown.
Droplet	**Known or suspected:** Influenza Meningococcal disease Epiglottitis (*Haemophilus influenzae*) Diphtheria Pneumonic plague Rubella Mumps Adenovirus Parvovirus	**In addition to standard precautions:** Private room preferred; cohorting allowed if necessary. Wear a surgical mask when within 3 feet of the patient. Patient wears surgical mask during transport. Cough etiquette: Patients and visitors should cover their nose or mouth when coughing, promptly dispose of used tissues, and practice hand hygiene after contact with respiratory secretions.
Airborne	**Known or suspected:** Tuberculosis Smallpox Measles SARS	**In addition to standard precautions:** Place the patient in an AIIR (airborne infection isolation room), a monitored negative-pressure room with at least 6 to 12 air exchanges per hour. Room exhaust must be appropriately discharged outdoors or passed through a HEPA filter. An N95 respirator mask must be worn when entering the room of the patient. Transport of the patient should be minimized; the patient should wear a surgical mask if transported within the hospital. Cough etiquette: Patients and visitors should cover their nose or mouth when coughing, promptly dispose of used tissues, and practice hand hygiene after contact with respiratory secretions.

MRSA, methicillin-resistant *Staphylococcus aureus*; VRE, vancomycin-resistant *Enterococcus*; HEPA, high-efficiency particulate-arresting; SARS, severe acute respiratory syndrome.

Modified from Siegel JD, Rhinehart E, Jackson M, Chiarello L, and the Healthcare Infection Control Practices Advisory Committee. *Guideline for Isolation Precautions: Preventing Transmission of Infectious Agents in Healthcare Settings 2007*. Atlanta, GA: Centers for Disease Control and Prevention; 2007.

patient's environment. The PPE should be put on prior to entering the patient's room and discarded before exiting the patient's room. Examples of patients requiring contact precautions include those with methicillin-resistant *Staphylococcus aureus* (MRSA), vancomycin-resistant enterococci (VRE), herpes simplex, and herpes zoster.

A more strict form of contact precautions is contact precautions plus. This requires hand washing between the steps of removing the gown and hand hygiene with an alcohol-based rub. Contact precautions plus are used if the patient has *Clostridium difficile* diarrhea. Another form of contact precautions is strict contact precautions, used with vancomycin-insensitive *S aureus* (VISA) and vancomycin-resistant *S aureus* (VRSA). With strict contact precautions, a gown is required when entering the room (not just for patient contact).

RESPIRATORY RECAP

Transmission-Based Precautions

» Contact
» Droplet
» Airborne

Droplet precautions are used to prevent the transmission of pathogens spread by close respiratory or mucous membrane contact with respiratory secretions. Coughing and sneezing can generate droplets in the air. These pathogens are not typically transmissible over a distance greater than 3 feet. A single-patient room is preferred. Healthcare providers should wear a mask for all close contact with the patient. An N95 respirator mask is not required; a surgical mask is sufficient. The mask should be put on before entering the room. In the event the patient must be transported outside the room, the patient should wear a surgical mask and follow respiratory hygiene and cough etiquette. Examples of patients requiring droplet precautions include those with influenza, pertussis, adenovirus (in which case contact precautions should also be used), meningococcal disease, and *Haemophilus influenza* epiglottitis.

Airborne precautions are used to prevent the transmission of infectious agents over a long distance when suspended in the air. These patients must be placed in a private room that has monitored negative air pressure. The door must remain closed. Healthcare providers must wear a NIOSH-approved N95 respirator mask that has been fit-tested to ensure that the mask seals appropriately. A surgical mask must be worn by the patient during transport. Examples of patients requiring airborne precautions are those with tuberculosis, measles, smallpox, and hemorrhagic fevers. Another form of airborne precautions is airborne/contact precautions, in which a gown is required if the healthcare provider has contact with the patient or the patient's environment. Airborne/contact precautions are used for chickenpox and herpes zoster if disseminated or in an immunocompromised patient.

> **RESPIRATORY RECAP**
>
> **Precautions**
>
> » Precautions protect both the patient and the caregiver.
> » Apply standard precautions for every patient encounter, assuming everyone is at risk.
> » When body fluids (including significant aerosol) may be encountered, use appropriate barriers, including gloves, mask, eye protection, gowns, and booties.
> » Use hand hygiene before and after contact with each patient.

A protective environment is designed to minimize fungal spore counts in the air and reduce the risk of invasive environmental fungal infections for allogenic hematologic stem cell transplant (HSCT) patients. The air quality for HSCT patients is improved through a combination of environmental controls that include HEPA filtration of incoming air, directed room air flow, positive room air pressure relative to the corridor, well-sealed rooms to prevent the flow of air from the outside, ventilation to provide more than 12 air changes per hour, strategies to reduce dust, and the elimination of dried or fresh flowers and potted plants from the rooms of HSCT patients.[1]

Healthcare-Associated Infections Related to Respiratory Care Equipment

A primary issue in respiratory care is to prevent the introduction of infectious agents into the lungs. Although the majority of nosocomial pneumonia cases arise from microaspiration, respiratory care equipment itself can be a source of infection. Therefore, it is imperative to use single-patient, disposable equipment when available. Otherwise, respiratory therapists must handle reusable equipment cautiously.

Ventilator-Related Issues

The CDC recommends that ventilator circuits *not* be changed routinely, but only when there is visual or known contamination of the circuit. Several studies have shown that less-frequent tubing changes may reduce infection rates, although the optimum frequency for ventilator tubing changes is still considered uncertain.[12,13] Common practice is to fill the humidification chamber of the ventilator with sterile water to prevent the introduction of heat-resistant organisms, such as *Legionella* species, which may contaminate the device despite its high temperatures that inactivate most common respiratory pathogens. The efficacy of this practice has not been validated but appears prudent given the demonstrated danger of *Legionella* presence in hospital tap water. Water condenses and accumulates in the ventilator circuit, which is a potential growth medium for microorganisms. Regardless of the humidification technique used, care should be taken to drain condensate and, when manipulating the tubing, to prevent the condensate from unintentionally pouring into the patient's airway via the endotracheal or tracheostomy tube.[12,13]

> **RESPIRATORY RECAP**
>
> **Healthcare-Associated Sources of Respiratory Infection**
>
> » Ventilator circuit changes
> » Condensate in ventilator tubing
> » Humidifiers
> » Nebulizers
> » Suction catheters
> » Pulmonary function testing equipment

Suction catheters can introduce microorganisms into a patient's lower respiratory tract. The single-use open catheter system requires the therapist to maintain a sterile field while suctioning the patient's airway. The inline closed suction system has an advantage because the circuit does not have to be broken when suctioning the patient. Although inline suction catheters become colonized with organisms originating from the patient's lower respiratory tract, the clinical importance of this is unclear.[12,13]

Nebulizers

Between treatments on the same patient, rinse with sterile water and air-dry small-volume nebulizers. Rinsing the nebulizer between treatments and allowing it to air dry is an acceptable practice. Nebulizers placed in-line in the ventilator circuit can become contaminated by colonized condensate and increase the patient's risk of pneumonia. It is reasonable to use a metered dose inhaler rather than a nebulizer as an infection control measure, given that it is virtually impossible to contaminate the interior of a metered dose inhaler. Nebulizers should be changed every 24 hours because they produce aerosols that can carry microorganisms into the lower respiratory tract.[6] Transmission of infection from contaminated nebulizers is particularly problematic in patients with cystic fibrosis.

Spirometers and Pulmonary Function Testing Equipment

Pulmonary function testing (PFT) equipment is not believed to carry a high risk of infection, although cross contamination between patients is possible. The use of filters between the patient and PFT equipment has been advocated to trap aerosolized microbes.[12,13]

KEY POINTS

- Healthcare-associated infections (HAIs) result in preventable suffering and lost lives.
- The common routes of disease transmission are by contact, vehicle, airborne, and vector routes; the most common routes are contact (direct and indirect), airborne, and vehicle-borne.
- Infection control methods include cleaning, disinfecting, and sterilizing the equipment.
- Isolation precautions assist with preventing the spread of HAIs.
- Primary precautions include hand hygiene, standard precautions, and personal protective equipment.
- The most important way to prevent transmission of infection is hand hygiene before and after patient contact.
- Transmission-based precautions include contact precautions, droplet precautions, and airborne precautions.
- Hospitals are implementing vaccination programs and monitoring as part of infection control programs.

REFERENCES

1. Siegel JD, Rhinehart E, Jackson M, Chiarello L, and the Healthcare Infection Control Practices Advisory Committee. *Guideline for Isolation Precautions: Preventing Transmission of Infectious Agents in Healthcare Settings 2007*. Atlanta, GA: Centers for Disease Control and Prevention; 2007.
2. Yokoe DS, Mermel LA, Anderson DJ, et al. A compendium of strategies to prevent healthcare-associated infections in acute care hospitals. *Infect Control Hosp Epidemiol.* 2008;29(1):S12–S21.
3. Yokoe D, Classen D. Improving patient safety through infection control: a new healthcare imperative. *Infect Control Hosp Epidemiol.* 2008;29(1):S3–S11.
4. Institute for Healthcare Improvement. Protecting 5 million lives from harm. Available at: http://www.ihi.org/IHI/Programs/campaign/campaign.htm?Tabld=2#PreventSrugicaglsiteinfection. Accessed March 30, 2009.
5. Eggimann P, Pittet D. Infection control in the ICU. *Chest.* 2001;120;2059–2093.
6. Sehulster LM, Chinn RYW, Arduino MJ, et al. *Guidelines for Environmental Infection Control in Health-care Facilities. Recommendations from CDC and the Healthcare Infection Control Practices Advisory Committee (HICPAC).* Chicago: American Society for Healthcare Engineering/American Hospital Association; 2004.
7. Ignatius TS, Yuguo L, Tze WW. Evidence of airborne transmission of the severe acute respiratory syndrome virus. *N Engl J Med.* 2004;350(17):1731–1739.
8. Rutala WA, Weber DJ, and the Health Infection Control Practices Advisory Committee. *Guideline for Disinfection and Sterilization in Healthcare Facilities 2008*. November 2008. Available at: http://www.cdc.gov/ncidod/dhqp/pdf/guidelines/Disinfection_Nov_2008.pdf.
9. Rutala WA, Weber DJ. Disinfection and sterilization in health care facilities: what clinicians need to know. *Clin Infect Dis.* 2004;39:702–709.
10. Rupp M, Fitzgerald T, Puumala S, et al. Controlled cross-over trial of alcohol-based hand gel in critical care units. *Infect Control Hosp Epidemiol.* 2008;29(1):8–15.
11. Calfee DP, Salgado CD, Classen D, et al. Strategies to prevent transmission of MRSA in acute care hospitals. *Infect Control Hosp Epidemiol.* 2008;29(1):S62–S80.
12. Centers for Disease Control and Prevention. Guidelines for preventing healthcare-associated pneumonia, 2003. *MMWR.* 2004;55(RR03):1–36.
13. Clinical practice guidelines for respiratory care. Available at: http://www.rcjournal.com/cpgs. Accessed March 30, 2009.

CHAPTER 34

Asthma

Timothy R. Myers
Timothy Op't Holt

OUTLINE

OBJECTIVES

1. Define asthma.
2. Discuss the epidemiology of asthma.
3. Discuss the pathophysiology of asthma.
4. List the risk factors for asthma.
5. Describe the clinical features of nocturnal asthma, exercise-induced asthma, and occupational asthma.
6. Describe the disease severity classification proposed by the National Asthma Education and Prevention Program.
7. Discuss the role of peak flow monitoring in the management of asthma.
8. Compare the role of controller medication and quick-relief medication in the management of asthma.
9. Compare the use of nebulizers, metered dose inhalers, and dry powder inhalers in the delivery of aerosols to the patient with asthma.
10. Discuss the role of alternative treatment modalities in the management of asthma.
11. List the goals of mechanical ventilation of the patient with asthma.
12. Discuss the role of education in the disease management of asthma.

KEY TERMS

airway hyperresponsiveness
airway inflammation
allergen
asthma
asthma education program
asthma trigger
bronchial challenge testing
controller medication
exercise-induced asthma (EIA)
exhaled nitric oxide (eNO)
extrinsic asthma
heliox
intermittent asthma
intrinsic asthma
mild persistent asthma
moderate persistent asthma
National Asthma Education and Prevention Program (NAEPP)
nocturnal asthma
peak flow meter
quick-relief medication
severe persistent asthma

INTRODUCTION

Asthma is one of the most common chronic diseases of the pulmonary system. The third expert panel report (EPR) from the **National Asthma Education and Prevention Program (NAEPP)** of the National Institutes of Health issued this working definition of **asthma**, which remains unchanged from previous EPR guidelines:

> Asthma is a chronic inflammatory disorder of the airways in which many cells and cellular elements play a role: in particular, mast cells, eosinophils, T lymphocytes, macrophages, neutrophils and epithelial cells. In susceptible individuals, this inflammation causes recurrent episodes of wheezing, breathlessness, chest tightness and coughing, particularly at night or in the early morning. These episodes are usually associated with widespread but variable airflow obstruction that is often reversible either spontaneously or with treatment. The inflammation also causes an associated increase in the existing bronchial hyperresponsiveness to a variety of stimuli; reversibility of airflow limitation may be incomplete in some patients with asthma.[1]

This chapter presents issues related to the respiratory care of patients with asthma.

Epidemiology

Asthma is a common chronic disease that is increasing in prevalence and severity. The asthma literature frequently mentions epidemiology, prevalence, and incidence. Webster's ninth *New Collegiate Dictionary* defines *epidemiology* as a branch of medical science that deals with the incidence, distribution, and control of disease in a population. *Prevalence* refers to the number of individuals with a diagnosis at any given time (e.g., in 2010), whereas *incidence* refers specifically to the number of newly diagnosed cases that occur within a specific period of time (e.g., the past century).

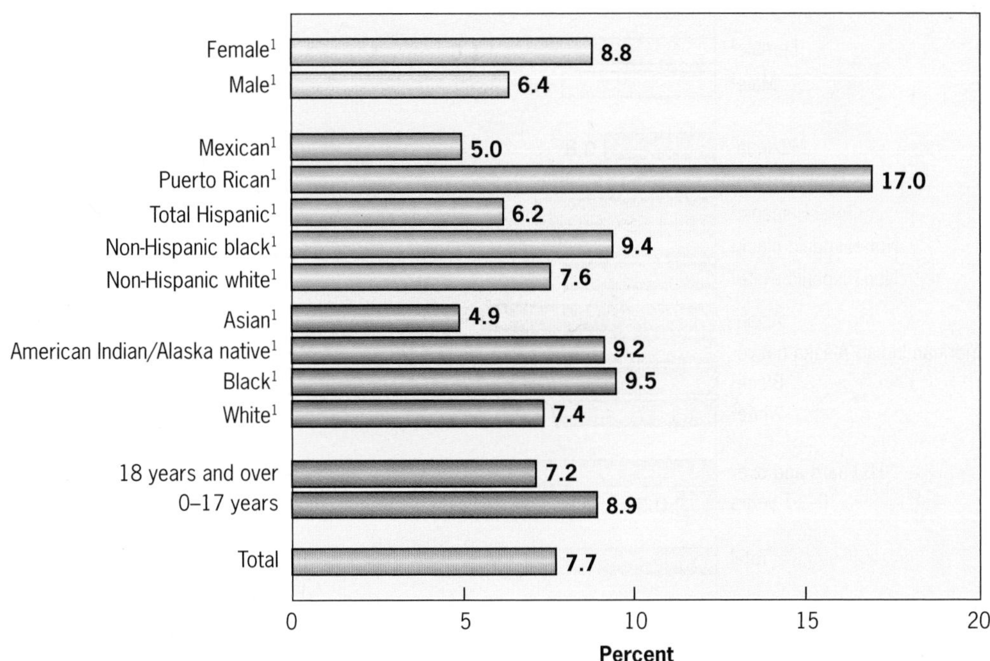

FIGURE 34–1 Asthma prevalence in the United States in 2005. [1]Age adjusted to 2000 U.S. standard population. From National Health Interview Survey, National Center for Health Statistics, Centers for Disease Control and Prevention. Available at: http://www.cdc.gov/nchs/products/pubs/pubd/hestats/asthma03-05/asthma03-05.htm.

The prevalence and incidence of asthma are difficult to estimate because of the inherent problems with surveys and the varying definitions for asthma. Asthma is prevalent in approximately 10% to 12% of the population in different countries. This represents an estimated 300 million cases globally, 22 million of which are in the United States (**Figure 34–1**).[2,3]

Despite recent advances in both pharmacologic and nonpharmacologic management strategies, the prevalence of asthma is increasing, particularly in developing and developed nations. Presently, prevalence in the United States is monitored in terms of prevalence of attacks per year. This increased in the period from 1999 to 2005. Likewise, outpatient and physician office visits increased, but fortunately emergency department visits and deaths decreased (**Table 34–1**).[3]

TABLE 34–1 Changes in Rate (per 100,000) of Attack in the Past Year, Outpatient, Emergency Department Visits, and Deaths Due to Asthma, 1999–2005

	1999	2005
Prevalence	40,700	42,000
Outpatient visits	40,000	50,800
Emergency department visits	7500	6400
Deaths	20	14

Data from Mannino DM, Homa DM, Akinbami LJ, Moorman JE, Gwynn C, Redd SC. Surveillance for asthma—United States, 1980–1999. *MMWR.* 2002;51(SS01):1–13; and Akinbami L. Asthma prevalence, health care use and mortality: United States, 2003–2005. Available at: http://www.cdc.gov/nchs/products/pubs/pubd/hestats/asthma03-05/asthma03-05.htm#fig2.

Although asthma is more prevalent in males, it tends to be more severe in females. African Americans, especially those residing in urban areas, are three times more likely to be diagnosed with asthma in the United States. In the United States, asthma is the third leading cause of preventable hospitalization and resulted in 4055 deaths in 2003.[3]

People with asthma who are Puerto Rican have death rates that are four times higher than those of Caucasians (**Figure 34–2**).[3] Patients who have had frequent hospital admissions or previous life-threatening asthma are the most susceptible to asthma mortality.

Patients classified as having life-threatening asthma have been subgrouped into the following three classes:

- The typical case, a patient who presents with a gradual deterioration over time and experiences a life-threatening episode
- The patient with relatively mild, asymptomatic chronic asthma who suffers an acute episode in a relatively short time frame (referred to as *acute asphyxia asthma*)
- The patient who is a combination of the previous two classes

Misdiagnosis and inadequate treatment by disease severity are significant factors contributing to the increased incidence and prevalence of asthma.

The severity of acute episodes may vary from mild to life threatening within a given patient over the course of the disease or within a given year. In 2003, people with asthma lost 22.9 million school and work days because of their disease.[3] Likewise, there were 497,000 hospitalizations for asthma in 2004.[1]

> **AGE-SPECIFIC ANGLE**
>
> Death rates are greatest for people with asthma aged 18 years and older.

Along with the increasing prevalence of asthma

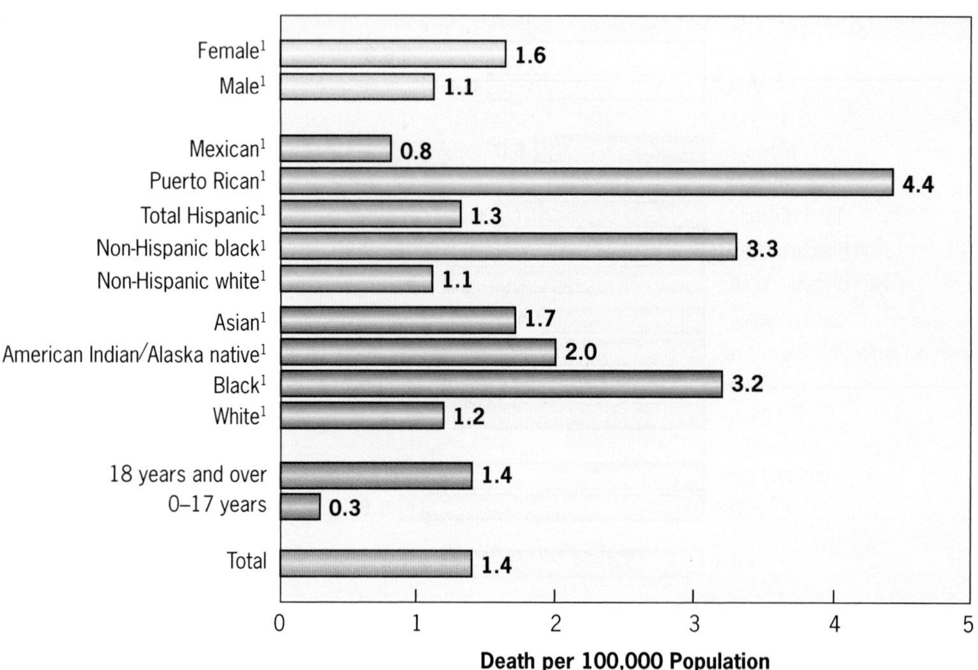

FIGURE 34–2 Asthma deaths per 100,000 population in the United States in 2005. [1]Age adjusted to 2000 U.S. standard population. From National Health Interview Survey, National Center for Health Statistics, Centers for Disease Control and Prevention. Available at: http://www.cdc.gov/nchs/products/pubs/pubd/hestats/asthma03-05/asthma03-05.htm.

is the economic burden that comes with this chronic condition. In the early 1990s, the cost to treat asthma was estimated to be approximately $6 billion per year, with 43% of the cost associated with hospitalizations, emergency department (ED) visits, and death. The cost of ED therapy for asthma in the same year was $270 million, which represented 8% of the total direct cost of caring for asthma.[4] The fastest-growing age segment with asthma is children, a fact that has been reported to have had a staggering impact on the cost to treat asthma. A recent study suggests that the hospitalization costs for children younger than 5 years with asthma reach approximately 74% of their total healthcare costs.[5] The same study reported that the highest sector in the adult population for cost is also associated with hospitalizations (54%). Medications resulted in 16.5% of the total cost to treat asthma in adults, compared with 5.4% in children younger than 5 years.

AGE-SPECIFIC ANGLE

Asthma is increasing at the fastest rate in children younger than 5 years.

The high cost associated with acute care treatment of asthma has led to the implementation of disease management programs.[6–8] Because of the high volume of asthma visits and admissions in most urban areas, disease management programs or clinical practice guidelines can reduce cost by eliminating practice variation in the emergency department or hospital in the treatment of asthma. Eliminating acute treatment that adds cost without degrading the overall quality of care can be an effective tool in the management of asthma.[9,10]

Although asthma is not a curable disease, it can be managed effectively. Asthma mortality, and to a lesser degree morbidity, is largely preventable. Appropriate medications based on disease severity, and patient or caregiver adherence to a written asthma action plan can result in highly effective disease management. Patient education and awareness and control of environmental triggers also play a significant role in the overall management of the disease. Even with overall effective management from an educational, medical, and adherence standpoint, some patients develop severe persistent asthma with frequent exacerbations that may result in ED visits or hospitalizations.

Pathophysiology

The exact underlying cause of asthma is still unknown. Asthma is a multifactorial disease that has been associated with allergenic, hereditary, psychosocial, socioeconomic, environmental, and infectious causes. Asthma is not the only cause of wheezing. **Box 34–1** lists other potential causes or diagnoses associated with wheezing.

Even if the underlying cause of asthma is known in an individual, the trigger stimuli of an exacerbation may change over time. The pathophysiology of the disease is largely related to inflammation, hyperresponsiveness, and obstruction. **Figure 34–3** demonstrates the interrelationship of these three factors in the underlying mechanism of the disease.

RESPIRATORY RECAP

Pathophysiology of Asthma

- » Airway inflammation
- » Airway hyperresponsiveness
- » Airway obstruction

Airway Inflammation

Regardless of the trigger mechanism or the underlying cause of asthma, **airway inflammation** plays an important role. Acute and chronic inflammation affects airway caliber, airflow, and underlying bronchial hyperresponsiveness, which enhances susceptibility to bronchospasm. Chronic inflammation may be associated with a

BOX 34–1

Differential Diagnosis of Wheezing

Small and Large Airway Obstruction

- Asthma
- Airway tumors
- Bronchiolitis (in children)
- Cardiogenic pulmonary edema
- Cystic fibrosis
- Pneumonia; aspiration
- Bronchopulmonary dysplasia

Large Airway Obstruction

- Airway and esophageal foreign bodies
- Pulmonary emboli
- Tumors
- Vascular rings
- Focal pneumonia
- Laryngeal webs or malacia
- Tracheal stenosis
- Lymphadenopathies
- Vocal cord dysfunction

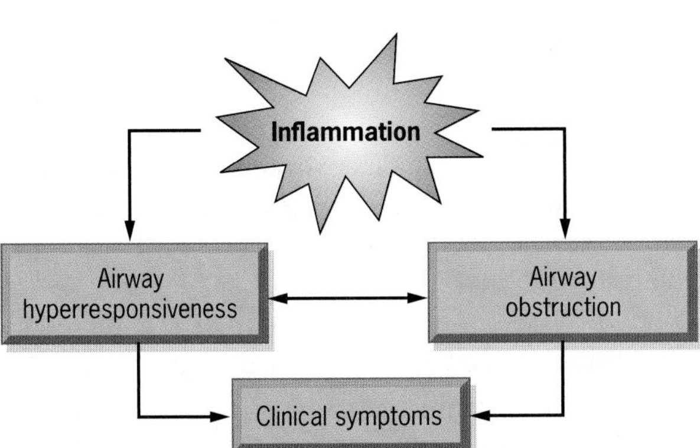

FIGURE 34–3 The interplay and interaction between airway inflammation and the clinical symptoms and pathophysiology of asthma. Modified from National Asthma Education Program, National Heart, Lung and Blood Institute. *Expert Panel Report 3: Guidelines for the Diagnosis and Management of Asthma. Full Report 2007.* Bethesda, MD: National Institutes of Health; 2007. NIH Publication 08-4051.

permanent alteration in airway structure, know as *remodeling*. Once remodeling occurs, the patient's asthma is not responsive to current treatment. Therefore, the control of inflammation is a central feature of asthma therapy.

Inflammatory cells that appear to be the most significant are lymphocytes, dendritic cells, mast cells, eosinophils, macrophages, epithelial cells, and T helper 2 cells. Among the mediators of inflammation are chemokines, nitric oxide, IgE, interleukins, cytokines, histamine, granulocyte macrophage colony-stimulating factor (GM-CSF), and tumor necrosis factor-α (TNF-α). The release of inflammatory mediators results in recurrent exacerbations that manifest as wheezing, progressive shortness of breath, chest tightness, and coughing that may be more persistent nocturnally or in the early mornings.[11] In most patients, these exacerbations are usually self-limiting or resolve rapidly to appropriate asthma treatment.

Airway Hyperresponsiveness

A marker associated with asthma is the increased sensitivity, or **airway hyperresponsiveness**, to both specific and nonspecific factors. These factors have little or no effect on people with normal airways. The Lung Health Study showed that the majority of women and half the men diagnosed with chronic obstructive pulmonary disease (COPD) also have a component of hyperresponsiveness.

Airway hyperresponsiveness is a mechanism in which the airways constrict too easily and frequently, an exaggerated bronchoconstrictor response to a wide variety of stimuli. Factors associated with hyperresponsive airways include environmental factors (both indoor and outdoor), exercise, allergens, and viral infections. The degree or level of airway hyperresponsiveness usually correlates with the clinical severity of the disease.[1] Control of inflammation can reduce airway hyperresponsiveness and improve asthma control.[1]

Bronchial challenge testing with methacholine serves as a measure of responsiveness to general stimuli. Asthma is characterized by the reversibility of airflow obstruction. These challenge tests are usually administered in a pulmonary function laboratory. The methacholine challenge test begins with spirometry. The patient then inhales five breaths of increasing concentrations of methacholine, each time followed by performance of spirometry. The methacholine concentration at which a 20% decrease in FEV_1 (forced expiratory volume in 1 second) occurs ($PC_{20\%}$) is the end point. $PC_{20\%}$ is reached sooner and with a lower dose of methacholine in patients with asthma than in subjects without asthma. The test is followed (usually within 15 minutes) by administration of a short-acting β_2-agonist that should result in a 12% to 15% increase in FEV_1.

Airway Obstruction

The final component in the definition of asthma is airway obstruction, or the limitation of airflow through the airways. Airflow limitation is most commonly caused by the IgE-mediated release of inflammatory mediators into the airways, which come into contact with airway smooth muscles. More specifically, the mediators usually associated with an IgE response include histamine, tryptase, prostaglandin, and leukotrienes. However, when the airways are hyperresponsive, several stimuli can exacerbate bronchoconstriction (**Box 34–2**).

BOX 34-2

Changes That Lead to Airway Obstruction

Acute bronchoconstriction
Chronic mucous plug formation
Airway edema
Airway remodeling

In most patients, the airflow limitation or bronchoconstriction will spontaneously resolve with the administration of a short-acting β_2-agonist. Patients who have persistent disease or who have had asthma for a number of years may develop an incomplete response as a result of airway remodeling. These patients are difficult to separate from the COPD population. Patients who continue to have airway obstruction after initiation of conventional therapy are considered to be in status asthmaticus.

Pathogenesis

The factor that initiates the inflammatory process in the first place is unknown. It is known that the origins of asthma occur early in life, with the interplay of genetic and environmental factors as the immune system develops. This field of study, which emerged after the release of the second EPR, focuses on what has become known as the hygiene hypothesis.[1] Two types of T helper (Th) lymphocytes exist: Th1 and Th2. Th1 lymphocytes produce interleukin-2 and interferon-γ, which are important in response to infection. Th2 lymphocytes generate cytokines that mediate inflammation. At birth, Th2 is favored, and exposure to environmental stimuli such as infections will activate Th1 responses and balance Th1 and Th2. The imbalance in or favoring of Th2 favors the development of asthma. The favoring of Th2 is associated with the Western lifestyle: widespread use of antibiotics, an urban environment, diet, and sensitization to house-dust mites and cockroaches. The favoring of Th1 occurs when the child is exposed to other children or siblings, viral infection, and a rural environment. Thus, our Western obsession with cleaning everything and eliminating microorganisms from the environment may not be doing our children any favors (the hygiene hypothesis). A review can be found elsewhere.[12]

Other factors affecting pathogenesis are genetics (asthma has an inheritable component), gender (asthma predominates in boys until puberty), environmental factors (which are important in the development, persistence, and severity of asthma), allergens (sensitivity and exposure to allergens are important to the development of asthma in children), respiratory infections (see the earlier discussion of the hygiene hypothesis), and other environmental exposures (especially tobacco). This interaction of host and environmental exposures early in life is related to development of asthma.

Risk Factors

The strongest identifiable predisposing factor for the development of asthma is atopy. Atopy is the familial or genetic predisposition to develop an IgE-mediated response to common allergens in the environment. Asthma in childhood is normally linked to atopic factors. Among the many phenotypes of asthma, this is called *atopic, pediatric,* or *allergic asthma.* A study of 6- to 34-year-olds in Tucson, Arizona, found a strong, direct correlation between serum IgE levels and the development or presence of asthma, and a weaker correlation between positive skin test reactions and the development or presence of asthma.

Atopic asthma is diagnosed by skin-prick testing, in which a multitude of known allergens are introduced to the patient's immune system through small pricks in the arms. The most common method of skin testing is a radioallergosorbent test (RAST) that measures antigen-specific IgE. A study of children in eight metropolitan areas indicated that the highest risk factors for atopic asthma in inner-city children were cockroach antigen, animal dander, and dust mites.[13]

RESPIRATORY RECAP

Risk Factors for Asthma

- » Allergens
- » Pollution
- » Food and drug additives
- » Viral agents

Factors that may contribute to or enhance the development of asthma include environmental pollution, low birth weight, tobacco smoke, diet, and viral infections. Asthma has also been associated with sinusitis and gastrointestinal reflux.

Allergens

The majority of asthmatics suffer attacks exacerbated by inhalation of an **allergen**. Many allergens, both indoor (e.g., mold, animal dander, cockroach antigen, dust mites) and outdoor (e.g., grass and tree pollens), may trigger an exacerbation. Other allergens are found in certain foods such as dairy products, shellfish, nuts, mushrooms, and preservatives.

An allergic asthma exacerbation usually has two phases. The first phase is the acute phase. The presence of an **asthma trigger** on a hypersensitive airway causes rupture and degranulation of mast cells. Airway mast cells release mediators (leukotrienes, eosinophil chemotactic factor of anaphylaxis [ECF-A], prostaglandins, and histamine) into the tracheobronchial tree. These mediators all interact with the airway smooth muscle, resulting in bronchoconstriction, edema, vasodilation, and eosinophil release, and also may cause increased secretion production.

The second phase of an asthma attack is the inflammatory phase, occurring several hours after the first phase has resolved. Inflammatory mediators are released into the airway. Evidence suggests that airway inflammation is caused not by one particular type of inflammatory mediator but by an intricate cycle of complex interactions that develop between multiple mediators, inflammatory cells, and other cells and tissues commonly found in the airways. The inflammatory response usually results in the migration of these various inflammatory cells and mediators into the airways, where they cause direct injuries, such as alterations in epithelial integrity, abnormalities in autonomic neural control of airway tone, mucus hypersecretion, change in mucociliary function, and an increase in airway smooth muscle responsiveness.[1] The presence of the second phase of an asthma exacerbation is why a patient should be monitored for 4 to 8 hours after the initial phase has resolved, and why oral corticosteroids are considered for rapid relief in the emergency department for treatment of exacerbation. Oral corticosteroids help to control the severity of the second phase.

Allergens from indoor sources consist mainly of cockroach antigen, domestic dust mites, animal dander, and mold (*Alternaria*) or fungi. Indoor allergens appear to be a main trigger in industrialized, developed countries. In developed countries, insulated housing that has been heated, humidified, cooled, and carpeted is prone to increased levels of indoor allergenic sources.

Dust mites appear to be the major cause of asthma worldwide, especially when infants are exposed to high concentrations in the first 3 to 6 months of life. The predominant domestic mite is *Dermatophagoides* species. The allergens are located in the inhaled microscopic fecal pellets. Dust mites are found in common household products but are especially prominent in bedding, carpet, stuffed animals, and soft furnishings. Dust mites grow best in humid air at temperatures of 22° to 26° C (71.6° to 78.8° F). The best method for eradicating mites is to wash potential breeding material in hot water (>54.4° C [>130° F]). One study indicated cockroach antigen as the leading allergenic cause of inner-city asthma.[14] Cockroach antigen is found in the microscopic excrement and powdered dried bodies of cockroaches and is inhaled by the sensitized patient.

AGE-SPECIFIC ANGLE

Dust mites are a major cause of asthma when infants are exposed to high concentrations in their first 3 to 6 months of life.

Cats are highly allergenic. The principal source of allergen is found in cat excrement. Cat saliva has also been identified as a source of cat antigen. Dog sensitivity is not as well documented but has been found to contribute to allergenic sources.

Fungi and molds also have been identified as allergenic risks in specific individuals with moderate to severe asthma. Fungi are most commonly found to grow extremely well in areas used for heating, cooling, or humidification. Home humidifiers provide a special risk for indoor fungal growth and air contamination.

Outdoor allergen sources are primarily pollens. The sources of these pollens include grasses, trees, flowers, weeds, and fungi. Each season particular outdoor allergen sources appear as major contributing factors for initiating asthma exacerbations. In the early spring, trees are the prominent trigger in pollen-associated asthma attacks. As the temperatures warm in the late spring and early summer, grasses and flowers reign as the initiators. In early fall, weeds play an important role in eliciting asthma exacerbations. The fall season also initiates the mold-induced exacerbations, predominately from *Alternaria* and *Cladosporium* species.

Pollution and Environmental Irritants

The role of indoor and outdoor air pollution in the development or initiation of an asthma attack remains unproved and controversial. Air pollution often has been accused of being a viable source for the increase in prevalence of asthma, but research has failed to produce a direct link to air pollution and asthma. Outdoor types of pollution are mainly associated with industrialized nations that have a large amount of industrial or photochemical smog.

Indoor air pollutants have had a higher association with the development of respiratory symptoms. Maternal smoking during pregnancy results in harmful in utero exposure of the fetus and increases the risk of the child's developing recurrent wheezing in the first 5 years of life. It is well established that exposure to environmental tobacco smoke increases the severity of asthma, increases the risk of asthma-related ED visits and hospitalizations, and decreases the quality of life in both children and adults.[1] Other potential sources of indoor air pollution include nitric oxide, carbon dioxide, carbon monoxides, nitrogen oxides, sulfur dioxides, formaldehydes, cleaning chemicals, solvents and paint, perfumes or aerosol sprays, and biologic sources such as endotoxins.

Temperature changes often have been associated with eliciting asthma exacerbations. Although this appears to be largely unfounded, the roles of humidity in the summer months and cold air during winter months are still a mystery.

Food and Drug Additives

Many patients with asthma who have allergies to specific foods increase their potential to develop exacerbations from intake of these foods. Foods that contain salicylates, some food-coloring agents, food preservatives (e.g., sulfites), and monosodium glutamate are substances known to be associated with asthma exacerbations.

Drugs may be associated with an increased likelihood of exacerbation. The primary risk is with nonsteroidal anti-inflammatory agents and aspirin. Patients who have sensitivity to aspirin have an increased risk of developing asthma later in life.

Viruses

Viral illness seasons (October through December and February through April) coincide with the most prevalent hospitalization periods for asthma in both children and adults. It has been reported that 37% of adult patients with acute asthma admitted over a 12-month period had evidence of recent respiratory tract infection.[15] This phenotype of asthma has been called **intrinsic asthma**, in contrast to **extrinsic asthma**. The inflammatory responses to viral infections (especially in the lower respiratory tract) may start the cascade of symptomatic wheezing from inflammatory debris or excessive mucus production in the airways.

Induced sputum[16] has been used as a marker of the effects of natural colds and influenza on the airways of the lungs. Natural colds (by day 4) cause neutrophilic lower airway inflammation that is greater in people with asthma than in healthy subjects. The greater inflammatory response in people with asthma may be due to the changes associated with trivial eosinophilia or to the different viruses involved. As was stated earlier, exposure to viral infections early in life influences the development of the immune system, promoting a protective function.

The most prominent of these viral infections is respiratory syncytial virus (RSV). The population at highest risk for severe cases of RSV and other lower respiratory tract infections, namely, the indigent inner-city population, also is at high risk for asthma. Infants with RSV early in life who developed high titers of RSV IgE were three times more likely to have recurrent wheezing after 48 months.

> **AGE-SPECIFIC ANGLE**
>
> A relationship exists between respiratory viral infections in early childhood and the development of asthma.

The exact role that early childhood respiratory tract infections play in the development of asthma is unclear. However, respiratory tract infections are a significant risk factor for the initiation of an asthma exacerbation that may or may not result in an individual seeking acute care. Infections should be identified to the patient with asthma as a trigger. Furthermore, written asthma treatment plans should include a component for increasing or stepping up therapy at the onset of symptoms. There is an advantage of hospitalization prevention when families of children with asthma had a written treatment plan that could initiate more aggressive outpatient management with the onset of coldlike symptoms.[17]

Other Asthma Phenotypes

Nocturnal Asthma

Nocturnal symptoms are quite common in people of all ages with asthma and even in patients who have intermittent or mild persistent asthma. Although **nocturnal asthma** is prevalent in up to 75% of all patients with asthma,[18] many do not correlate these nighttime symptoms with asthma. The presence of nocturnal asthma is a marker for uncontrolled or more severe asthma.[19–21]

A variety of mechanisms are interactive when nocturnal asthma is present.[22] The mechanisms seem to revolve around circadian alterations of body temperature, vagal tone, mediators, inflammation, epinephrine, and β_2-receptor function.[23,24] Other variables considered to be potential causes include gastroesophageal reflux, inhalation of cooler or drier air by mouth while sleeping, aspiration, sinusitis, increased mucus production, sleep apnea, and the normal decrease in lung function while sleeping.

An extensive amount of research has been undertaken in an attempt to optimize the treatment of nocturnal asthma. Treatment of nocturnal asthma requires therapy that uses a chronopharmacologic approach, that is, use of medications on a schedule that decreases nocturnal asthma symptoms.[22] An optimal therapeutic regimen should include some or multiple components of sustained-release theophylline, long-acting β-adrenergics, and/or inhaled corticosteroids. Comorbid conditions (e.g., obstructive sleep apnea, gastroesophageal reflux) must also be treated. Nighttime awakenings are a sign of persistence of asthma and loss of control, and are not to be tolerated.

Exercise-Induced Asthma

Exercise-induced asthma (EIA) is characterized by transient airway obstruction, typically occurring 5 to 15 minutes after strenuous exertion. EIA is prevalent in 90% of individuals with asthma. The prevalence of EIA among athletes is estimated to range between 3% and 11%.

There are cases of undiagnosed asthma that suddenly appears in competitive high school athletes.[25] Diagnosis of EIA may be made based on a history of symptoms (cough, wheeze, and chest tightness with exercise challenge testing). More traditionally or for definitive diagnosis, a fall of 10% or more in the FEV_1 or in peak expiratory flow (PEF) rate after exercise is diagnostic. Vocal cord dysfunction is commonly confused with EIA.[1]

The exact etiology of EIA is unclear. Theories range from temperature-related causes to inflammatory mediator release (**Box 34–3**). EIA symptoms typically appear during or after exercise, peak at 8 to 15 minutes after exercise, and eventually spontaneously resolve in about 20 to 30 minutes. Frequently, a refractory period (of up to 3 hours) occurs after initial recovery, during which repeat exercise causes less bronchospasm.

BOX 34–3

Etiologic Theories for Exercise-Induced Asthma

Respiratory heat or water loss (or both) from the bronchial mucosa

Mucosal drying and increased osmolarity stimulating mast cell degranulation

Rapid airway rewarming after exercise, causing vascular congestion, increased permeability, and edema leading to obstruction

Hyperventilation, causing discharge of bronchospastic chemical mediators

Appropriate treatment with anti-inflammatory medication (evidence grade A) reduces airway hyperresponsiveness and is associated with a reduction in the frequency and severity of EIA.[1] Other therapy for EIA includes the use of a short-acting β_2 agonist (SABA) 15 to 20 minutes before exercise; although a long-acting β_2 agonist (LABA) is also appropriate, frequent use may mask poorly controlled persistent asthma. Leukotriene receptor antagonists (LTRAs) can help in 50% of cases of EIA. Cromolyn may be effective but is not as good as SABAs. A warm-up period before exercise and cool-down afterward may help attenuate EIA, as will a mask or scarf over the mouth and nose in cold weather. Coaches should be made aware of EIA in any student so a SABA can be used prior to exercise classes. Although prevention is the main objective in managing EIA, education regarding its nature and management is important.

Occupational Asthma

Occupational asthma is characterized by variable airway hyperresponsiveness in the workplace. The patient typically reports increased symptoms while at work or within several hours of the completion of a shift, with improvement on weekends or during vacations. In addition, the presence of sensitizing agents and the presence of similar symptoms in coworkers are suggestive of occupational asthma. The diagnosis can be made by monitoring peak flows for 2 weeks in the workplace and 1 week away. Both new-onset asthma and exacerbations of preexistent asthma may occur as a result of occupational exposures. Occupational asthma is the most common occupational lung disease in developed countries.

Isocyanates are the most common etiologic agents. Inciting agents are divided into two broad categories: low-molecular-weight chemicals (e.g., trimellitic anhydride, formaldehyde), which require combination of the chemical, which is an incomplete antigen (i.e., a hapten), with a protein conjugate to produce a sensitizing neoantigen; and high-molecular-weight organic materials (e.g., grain dust, avian proteins), which may serve as complete antigens. Cigarette smoking is also an important risk factor for occupational asthma. The asthma educator may work with the onsite healthcare providers to discuss avoidance, ventilation, respiratory protection, and provision of a tobacco smoke-free environment.

Disease Severity Classification

Asthma is classified in terms of severity and control. *Severity* is defined as the intrinsic intensity of the disease process, wherein the patient's frequency and intensity of symptoms is evaluated. *Control* refers to the degree to which the manifestations of asthma are minimized and the goals of therapy are met. Both severity and control include the domains of current impairment (symptoms) and future risk (based on history of exacerbation and use of oral corticosteroids). Preferably, the patient's asthma should be classified before beginning controller therapy. Once classification has occurred, therapy is started based on a stepwise approach, to include recommended SABAs, LABAs, and inhaled corticosteroids. Once a patient has been on the recommended regimen and efforts have been made to control environmental factors, the patient is reevaluated for asthma control.

RESPIRATORY RECAP

Asthma Disease Severity Classification

» Intermittent
» Mild persistent
» Moderate persistent
» Severe persistent

Patients are divided into three age categories by the EPR-3: children aged 0 to 4 years, children aged 5 to 11 years, and children aged 12 and older to adults. For the child 0 to 4 years of age, upon presentation, the child is evaluated for frequency of symptoms, nighttime awakenings, use of SABAs, and interference with normal activity (the elements of impairment) and risk (i.e., the number of exacerbations requiring oral corticosteroids in the past year and the frequency of exacerbations).[1] For the child aged 5 to 11 years, the same factors are used to assess impairment, plus spirometry is added, with particular attention to FEV_1 and the ratio of FEV_1 to percent forced vital capacity (FEV_1/FVC%).[1] The same criteria are used for risk. In all patients older than 12 years, the same criteria are used to assess impairment, with age-specific ranges for FEV_1/FVC%. The same criteria are used for risk as with children.[1]

The NAEPP expert panel has developed a four-tiered system to classify chronic disease severity.[1] The four categories are intermittent, mild persistent, moderate persistent, and severe persistent asthma. A patient may have a higher severity in one area versus another. When classifying the patient's asthma, the level of severity corresponds to the worst level of the patient's impairment or risk. For example, the patient may have symptoms on more than 2 days per week, but not daily, but has an FEV_1 less than 60% of predicted. This patient would be classified as having severe persistent asthma, and treated accordingly.

Therapy is a stepwise approach, according to level of severity. Once the level of severity is established, the clinician selects a therapeutic step (steps 1 through 6, with step 6 being reserved for the most severe cases).

Intermittent

Intermittent asthma is the least severe of the four classes of disease severity. People with asthma in this category experience symptoms two or more times per week. These patients generally are expected to experience nocturnal symptoms of coughing, wheezing, or breathlessness no more than two times per month. They require SABAs no more than twice per week. There is no interference with normal activity. These patients have normal pulmonary function tests between exacerbations, although their exacerbations are generally brief (from a few hours to a few days). They have required zero to one course of oral corticosteroids in the past year.

Routine management of these patients (regardless of age) generally consists of as-needed SABAs. Although these patients may have the chronic component of their disease classified as intermittent, the periodic exacerbations that occur may vary in their intensity. Sometimes, although rarely, these exacerbations result in this class of patients needing to seek ED treatment or resulting occasionally in hospitalization.

Mild Persistent

People with **mild persistent asthma** experience symptoms of coughing or wheezing more than twice per week but less than once per day. These patients generally experience nocturnal symptoms of coughing, wheezing, or breathlessness more than two times per month. These patients may use their SABA more than twice per week, but not daily. These patients have symptoms that cause a minor limitation to normal activities of daily living. Pulmonary function is normal. Exacerbations may be more frequent.

Routine management of these patients generally consists of step 2 therapy: as-needed short-acting β_2-agonist with the addition of a controller medication. In all patients, the recommended controller medication is an inhaled corticosteroid (ICS), whereas in children aged 0 to 4 the options of cromolyn sodium or montelukast are indicated as a potential substitute for inhaled corticosteroids. In children aged 5 to 11, alternatives include cromolyn, montelukast, theophylline, or nedocromil. The alternatives are only used if there is a contraindication to ICS, since the ICS is actually controlling inflammation. The same therapy is used for those aged 12 years and older.

Although these patients may have the chronic component of their disease classified as mild persistent, the periodic exacerbations that occur also vary in their intensity. These exacerbations periodically result in this class of patients needing to seek ED treatment or occasionally result in hospitalization.

Moderate Persistent

People with **moderate persistent asthma** experience symptoms of coughing or wheezing on a daily basis. Moderate persistent asthma patients generally experience nocturnal symptoms of coughing, wheezing, or breathlessness more than once per week. SABA use is daily. These patients have symptoms that cause some interference with normal activities of daily living. Spirometry results show an FEV_1 above 60% but less than 80% of predicted, and FEV_1/FVC% is reduced by 5%.

Management of patients aged 0 to 4 years consists of step 3 or 4 therapy: SABA for exacerbations and medium-dose inhaled corticosteroid (step 3) in addition to LABA or montelukast (step 4) daily. In older children, step 3 therapy consists of low-dose ICS and either LABA, LRTA, or theophylline, or medium-dose ICS. Step 4 therapy is medium-dose ICS with a LABA or medium-dose ICS and either LRTA or theophylline. For those aged 12 and older, step 3 therapy is low-dose ICS and the addition of a LABA, or low-dose ICS with an LRTA or theophylline. Step 4 therapy is medium-dose ICS with a LABA or medium-dose ICS with either LRTA or theophylline. These patients may routinely need to seek ED treatment or require hospitalization secondary to the chronic inflammatory component of their asthma.

Severe Persistent

This category is the highest level of the four classes of disease severity. Patients with **severe persistent asthma** experience symptoms of coughing or wheezing almost continually. Severe persistent asthma patients experience nocturnal symptoms of coughing, wheezing, or breathlessness almost every night. These patients may use their SABA several times daily, a dangerous practice that correlates with an increased incidence of death. These patients have symptoms that cause extremely limited activities of daily living. Spirometry results show an FEV_1 less than 60% of predicted and an FEV_1/FVC% reduced more than 5%.

Management of these patients consists of step 5 or 6 therapy: short-acting β_2-agonist for exacerbations for all age groups. Controller drugs for the 0- to 4-year age group are high-dose ICS in addition to either LABA or montelukast (step 5), or high-dose ICS with LABA or montelukast or oral corticosteroids (step 6). Step 5 therapy for the 5- to 11-year age group consists of high-dose ICS with a LABA, or high-dose ICS and LRTA or theophylline. Step 6 is high-dose ICS and LABA with consideration of oral corticosteroid, or high-dose ICS and LRTA or theophylline plus an oral corticosteroid. For those 12 and older, step 5 therapy is high-dose ICS in combination with a LABA and consideration of omalizumab for those with allergies. In step 6, an oral corticosteroid is added to step 5 therapy and omalizumab is considered. These patients may frequently seek ED treatment and require hospitalization secondary to the chronic inflammatory component of their asthma.

Although patients may be classified in any of the four categories, periodic review of chronic symptoms and adherence is necessary. Quite often asthma is controlled with appropriate medications, and compliance and treatment can be decreased to a lower severity class with a decrease in symptoms. From the opposite perspective, with increasing symptomatic data, it may be necessary to intensify the treatment regimen to address the increase in symptoms.

Assessing Control of Asthma

After initiating therapy according to the stepwise scheme, patients should be evaluated for control of asthma. Just as when initiating therapy, the practitioner evaluates the patient in the domains of impairment and risk, using the same criteria: frequency of symptoms, nighttime awakenings, interference with normal activity, SABA use, lung function (age 5 and older), validated questionnaires about quality of life (adults), number of exacerbations requiring oral corticosteroids, and treatment-related adverse effects.

Asthma is classified as well controlled, not well controlled, or very poorly controlled, according to the worst symptom or finding. If a patient's asthma is well controlled for at least 3 months, consideration is given to stepping therapy down one step. If the asthma is not well controlled, patient adherence is checked and consideration is given to stepping up one step, with reevaluation in 6 weeks. If asthma is very poorly controlled, a short course of oral corticosteroids is considered, as is stepping up one to two steps, in addition to checking adherence and evaluating side effects. In either case, alternative treatment options are considered in the presence of adverse effects.

Status Asthmaticus

Severe attacks of asthma poorly responsive to adrenergic agents and associated with signs or symptoms of potential respiratory failure are referred to as *status asthmaticus*. The mechanisms of airflow obstruction and the principles of treatment for status asthmaticus are similar to those in which the asthma responds promptly to treatment. Although this term has been used for years when referring to a refractory asthma exacerbation, it is not used anywhere in the EPR-3, other than in a few references. Perhaps it is time to refer to this condition as a severe exacerbation or an exacerbation requiring admission to an intensive care unit.

Objective Measurements

One of the primary goals of asthma management and control is to maintain normal (or near normal) lung function. Objective assessment of the degree of variable airflow obstruction, hyperresponsiveness, and airflow reversibility is a fundamental component in the diagnosis of asthma. The precise measurement of airflow changes is important to evaluate the effectiveness of therapeutic maintenance or interventions.

The most familiar ways to diagnose and monitor airflow are pulmonary function testing (spirometry) and peak flow meters. In 1994 the American Thoracic Society (ATS) differentiated between diagnostic and monitoring devices.[26] Diagnostic evaluation by pulmonary function testing includes bronchial challenge, spirometry, lung volumes, and airway resistance. A relatively new diagnostic tool for the inflammatory component of asthma is measurement of exhaled nitric oxide levels.

> **RESPIRATORY RECAP**
>
> **Objective Measurements in Asthma**
>
> » Spirometry
> » Lung volumes and airways resistance
> » Peak flow
> » Exhaled nitric oxide

Spirometry

Studies have demonstrated that children as young as 3 years of age can perform spirometry approximately 20% of the time. The NAEPP recommends diagnostic spirometry at initial diagnosis and at least yearly after initial diagnosis, at the age of 5 or later. The airflow obstructive component of asthma is caused primarily by a decrease in expiratory flows and/or a high airway resistance. The spirometry data of a patient with asthma with airflow obstruction show a normal or slightly decreased FVC, a decreased or normal FEV_1, a decreased or normal PEF, and a decreased percentage of FEV_1/FVC. The ATS has recommended a diagnosis of asthma when airflow reversibility achieves an increase in FEV_1 of 200 mL and 12%.[26] Pre- and postbronchodilator testing is the hallmark intervention to decipher airflow reversibility. Normal spirometry with a suspected history of asthma symptoms may be an indication for bronchial challenge testing. During periods of acute exacerbations, people with asthma may have significant amounts of hyperinflation and air trapping that will suggest a restrictive disease and require the measurement of lung volumes for accurate diagnosis.

Lung Volumes and Airways Resistance

Body plethysmography is the diagnostic tool that is used to achieve measurements of airways resistance (Raw), airway conductance (Gaw), and static lung volumes.

Static lung volumes are the primary test that differentiates restrictive diseases from obstructive diseases. Static lung volumes are useful also to detect the presence of hyperinflation. Raw may be normal in asymptomatic asthma, although Gaw may be decreased. Normally during acute exacerbations, Raw is increased. Bronchodilator effectiveness is accurately evaluated with measurements of Raw during acute exacerbations.

Peak Flow Meters

Peak flow meters (**Figure 34–4**) have been classified by the ATS as monitoring devices for the management of asthma.[26] The EPR-3 recommends that written asthma action plans be based on either symptoms or peak flow measurements.[1] Peak flow monitoring should be considered for patients who have moderate or severe persistent

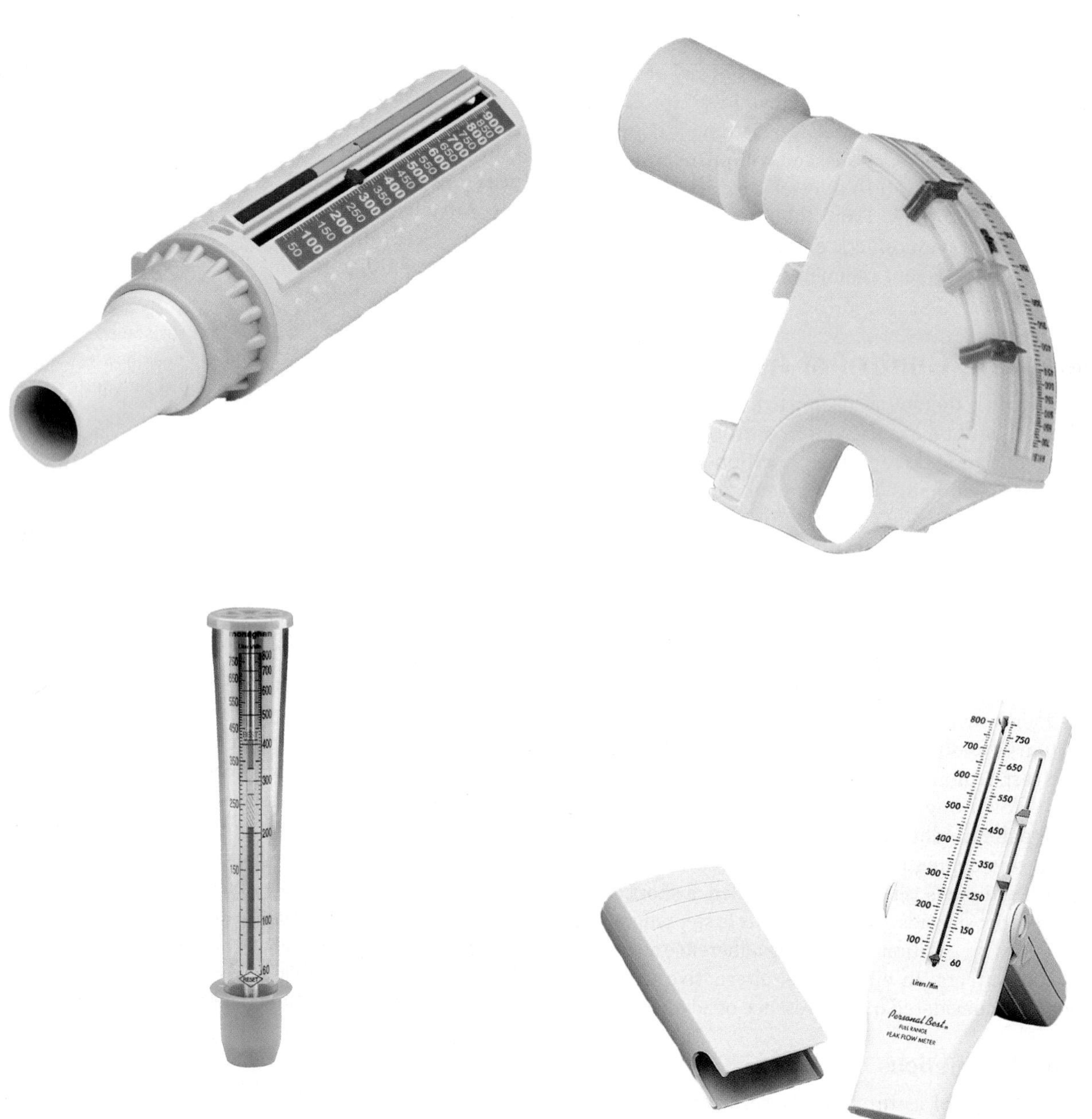

FIGURE 34–4 Commercially available peak flow meters.

asthma, those classified as "poor perceivers," or those with worsening asthma, an unexplained response to environmental or occupational exposures, and others at the discretion of the clinician and the patient. The patient's "personal best" peak flow should be known. The personal best is the highest peak flow of three successive measurements, taken during an asymptomatic period.

The accuracy and reliability of different peak flow meters have been questioned. Variation occurs even within a manufactured brand of peak flow meter. For this reason, a patient should use a specific device for consistent readings. When analyzing peak flow data, one must realize the limitations of the measurements. Peak flow readings are extremely effort dependent and are an indicator of large airway obstruction. Often the mistake is made to attribute all low measurements to poor effort or lack of cooperation when there is airway obstruction present. Sometimes the clinician cannot differentiate between poor data or airway obstruction.

Consensus opinion from the NAEPP committee established a traditional three-zone approach to the management of acute asthma exacerbations: green (>80% of personal best), yellow (50% to 79% of personal best), and red (<50% of personal best) (**Box 34–4**). Most of the predicted normal values or nomograms for peak flow values are based on sex and height in healthy subjects. Most people with moderate to severe asthma could not achieve these predicted values on their best days. This is the rationale to develop a personal best reading for peak flows on an individual-by-individual basis.

Exhaled Nitric Oxide

In 1993, Jorgens and colleagues described the potential significance of measuring **exhaled nitric oxide (eNO)** in disorders of the pulmonary system. Exhaled nitric oxide has been indicated to be a useful marker of airway inflammation in patients with asthma. Unfortunately, varied protocols make it difficult to compare and compile information from early studies on eNO and asthma.

An important issue is standardization of measurement techniques for eNO analysis. Measurement of eNO can be complicated by two factors: contamination by nasal nitric oxide and variable expiratory flow rates. The eNO concentration can be up to 1000 times higher in the nasal cavity and paranasal sinuses than concentrations found in the lower airways. Turbulent gas mixing during exhalation allows nitric oxide contamination from the nasal cavity. The eNO concentration is also highly flow dependent, allowing for measurement difficulty with variable flow rates. With high expiratory flow rates, nitric oxide levels will be lower than with a constant and slow expiratory maneuver. Techniques have been developed for measuring eNO that potentially overcomes these factors.[27]

Exhaled nitric oxide is an important measurement of the inflammatory component of both acute and chronic asthma in both children and adults. People with asthma who suffer from nocturnal asthma have higher eNO levels during the day and night than those who do not suffer from nocturnal symptoms.[28] Given recent efforts to standardize measurement techniques, information concerning the role and degree of inflammation in both acute and chronic asthma should be available. Information regarding the impact of corticosteroids on decreasing or suppressing inflammation should also be readily at hand for clinicians.

The adequacy of asthma control is often, but imperfectly, measured by assessing symptom control, improvement in physical findings, and improvements in pulmonary function, because these outcomes do not track each other consistently.[29] The available evidence supports that the measurement of FeNO is a marker of inflammation, is highly reproducible, is responsive to change in the underlying disease state, and is predictive of response to therapeutic intervention with anti-inflammatory medications. FeNO is elevated in patients with asthma and that the level of FeNO decreases after the administration of either inhaled or systemic corticosteroids. **Table 34–2** summarizes the usefulness of measuring FeNO.

BOX 34–4

Traditional Peak Flow Zones

Green Zone: Normal Zone
Predicted or personal best in the range of 80% to 100%

Yellow Zone: Caution Zone
Predicted or personal best in the range of 50% to 80%

Red Zone: Danger Zone
Predicted or personal best less than 50%

TABLE 34–2 Usefulness of Determining Fraction of Exhaled Nitric Oxide

Establish the correct diagnosis of asthma in corticosteroid-naive patients Chronic cough Exercise-induced bronchospasm Differentiate COPD from asthma Predictive of a favorable response to corticosteroids in subjects with asthma, COPD, or nonspecific respiratory symptoms
Titration of anti-inflammatory medication in patients with asthma
Attainment and maintenance of asthma control
Predictive of impending asthma exacerbation
Monitor asthma medication adherence

COPD, chronic obstructive pulmonary disease.

A FeNO of more than 35 parts per billion (ppb) in a steroid-naive patient presenting with respiratory symptoms is compatible with a diagnosis of asthma; however, the FeNO cannot be used to determine the classification of the asthma. Two devices are presently approved for FeNO measurement by the Food and Drug Administration (FDA). Reimbursement is presently very limited. The reluctance regarding third-party reimbursement was based on a review of several articles that concluded that methodology was heterogeneous and that there were different FeNO cutoffs, differences in definition of outcomes, and conflicting trial conclusions. Presently, FeNO measurement is an adjunct in the diagnosis and management of asthma. Reimbursement remains limited, but the practice is becoming more widespread and cost should become more competitive.

Pharmacologic Therapy

The purpose of pharmacologic therapy in the treatment of asthma is to prevent or control asthma symptoms, or at least to attempt to reduce the frequency or severity of acute exacerbations. Medications for asthma are classified as either long-term controllers or quick relievers in the new guidelines released by the expert panel.[1] The long-term **controller medications** are taken to decrease the degree of inflammatory mediator release in the airways. These medications include anti-inflammatory agents, long-acting bronchodilators, leukotriene modifiers, and immunomodulators.

Quick-relief medications are used to combat acute exacerbations of bronchoconstriction or provide quick, complete resolution of airflow obstruction and its accompanying symptoms of cough, wheezing, and chest tightness. This class of medications includes short-acting β_2-agonists and anticholinergics. Patients in all severity classes of asthma should receive a prescription for quick-relief medications for use during acute exacerbations.

Because the new asthma guidelines stress the importance of the inflammatory component in asthma, the following medication sections start with a description of the controller medications.

Controller Medications

Inhaled Corticosteroids

Corticosteroids are considered the most potent and consistent anti-inflammatory agents currently available by inhaled therapy in the long-term management of the inflammatory component of asthma. Anti-inflammatory medications are now stressed as the first line of treatment in the management of asthma. All asthma severity classes that have a persistent component are most effectively controlled with daily anti-inflammatory therapy.

Corticosteroids have been shown to suppress the release of certain inflammatory mediators. The use of corticosteroids in the management of asthma has been correlated with an overall reduction in asthma symptoms, an increase in lung function (as well as a decrease in the decline of FEV_1 over years of the disease), a decrease in airway hyperresponsiveness, a decrease in the frequency of acute exacerbations, and possibly a decrease in the amount of airway remodeling in both adults and children.[30]

The exact mechanism of action involved with corticosteroids and inflammation is not well understood. Several mechanisms appear to be actively and intimately involved. Corticosteroid therapy has provided evidence of an interference with the production of cytokines or suppression of cytokine release, a depression in the production of leukotrienes, and active recruitment of eosinophils. Clinical effects may take 2 to 3 weeks or more, but some newer agents, such as fluticasone, have demonstrated improvement in a day.

> **RESPIRATORY RECAP**
>
> **Asthma Controller Medications**
>
> » Inhaled corticosteroids
> » Nonsteroidal anti-inflammatory agents
> » Long acting β_2-agonists
> » Methylxanthines
> » Leukotriene modifiers
> » Immunomodulators
> » Oral corticosteroids

Dosage and frequency of corticosteroids can vary, depending on the specific type of product or delivery device (**Table 34–3**). However, dosing to effect is patient and time dependent. The ability to eventually wean patients off corticosteroids also depends on patient physiology. An attempt to decrease the dose of ICS should be made only after asthma has been well controlled for 3 to 6 months. Patients who have moderate to severe persistent asthma often have persistent symptoms and a decline in lung function with attempts to wean or decrease the dose or use of corticosteroids.

The dose and frequency of ICS vary with the corticosteroid to be administered. Adherence is enhanced as the frequency decreases. Most controller preparations are formulated to be given once or twice daily. In cases of uncontrolled asthma or increasing disease severity, the dosage and frequency can be increased. However, it is important to also review the patient's environmental control and medication technique before increasing the ICS dose.

The most common complications associated with the use of corticosteroids are persistent reflex cough, occasional dysphonia, sore throat, and oropharyngeal candidiasis. The majority of these short-term complications can be eliminated or greatly reduced with the use of spacer devices and rinsing the mouth after inhalation. Systemic toxic effects are a rare occurrence with inhaled corticosteroids. The effect of corticosteroids on the linear growth of preadolescents who are taking this class of medications long term is controversial.[31,32] The EPR-3 states the following:[1]

1. ICS are the preferred therapy for initiating long-term control therapy in children of all ages.
2. ICS, especially at low doses, and even for extended periods of time, are generally safe.

3. The potential for the adverse effect of low- to medium-dose ICS on linear growth is usually limited to a small reduction in growth velocity (approximately 1 centimeter in the first year of treatment) that is generally not progressive over time.
4. The potential risks of ICS are well balanced by their benefits.
5. High doses of ICS administered for prolonged periods of time (>1 year), particularly in combination with frequent courses of oral corticosteroid therapy, may be associated with adverse growth effects.

Mast Cell Stabilizers

This class of long-term controller medications is predominantly used in adolescents and children. These medications are an alternative to low-dose ICS in patients who have mild persistent asthma. The two drugs in this category are cromolyn sodium and nedocromil (Table 34-3). Both medications have distinct properties but appear to have similar anti-inflammatory actions.[33] The mechanism of action with these medications appears to be chloride channel blockade, and they modulate mast cell mediator release and promote eosinophil release.[34]

These anti-inflammatories appear to reduce the need for quick-relief medications, reduce bronchial hyperresponsiveness, improve morning peak flows, and decrease the symptoms of nocturnal asthma.[35] Nedocromil may have a broader range of activity in protection of EIA,[36] cough-variant asthma,[37] and cold air–induced bronchospasm.

The side effects of these drugs are practically nonexistent. Both drugs have a strong safety profile with a low adverse event profile. Cromolyn is available as a solution for nebulization. The onset of action for both drugs may be 4 to 6 weeks to determine maximum benefit. Cromolyn and nedocromil in a pressurized metered dose inhaler (pMDI) were phased out in 2010 because they used chlorofluorocarbon propellants.

Long-Acting β_2-Agonists

This class of long-term controller medication is predominantly used to provide a longer duration of airway smooth muscle relaxation. This class of medication is

TABLE 34-3 Long-Term Controller Medications

Medication	Dose Strength	Adult Medium Daily Dose
Corticosteroids		
Metered dose inhalers (MDIs)		
Beclomethasone dipropionate (QVAR)	40 or 80 μg/puff	>240–480 μg
Budesonide (Pulmicort)	90, 180, or 200 μg/puff	>600–1200 μg
Fluticasone propionate (Flovent)	44, 110, or 220 μg/puff	>264–440 μg
Mometasone (Asmanex)	200 μg/puff	400 μg
Ciclesonide (Alvesco)	80 or 160 μg/puff	Starting dose in steroid-naive patients is 160 μg bid
Tablets		
Prednisone	1, 2.5, 5, 10, 20, 25, and 50 mg	40–60 mg/day for 3–10 days for control in exacerbation
Prednisolone	5 mg	40–60 mg/day for 3–10 days for control in exacerbation
Methylprednisolone	2, 4, 8, 16, 24, and 32 mg	7.5–60 mg/day or qod as needed for control
Mast Cell Stabilizer		
Cromolyn sodium (Intal)	20 mg/2-mL ampule	1 ampule qid
Long-Acting β_2-Agonists		
Dry powder inhalers (DPIs)		
Salmeterol (Serevent)	50 μg/puff	bid
Formoterol (Foradil)	12 μg/puff	bid
Methylxanthines (Oral)		
Theophylline (Slo-Bid, Theo-24, Theo-Dur, Uniphyl)	Various, depending on formulation	
Leukotriene Modifiers (Oral)		
Montelukast (Singulair)	10-mg tablets	qd
Combination Products		
Advair DPI or MDI (fluticasone/salmeterol)	100/50, 250/50, 500/50 (DPI) 45/21, 115/21, 230/21 HFA MDI	250/50 bid
Symbicort (budesonide/formoterol)	80/4.5, 160/4.5	160/4.5 bid
Immunomodulatars	Based on 1gE level and weight	
Omalizumab		

bid, twice a day; qid, four times a day; qod, every other day; qd, daily; HFA, hydrofluoroalkane.

not intended for relief of acute bronchospasm or for monotherapy (delivery without an ICS). LABAs have a bronchodilation duration of approximately 12 hours but a longer onset of action than SABAs. Two medications are in this class of controller: salmeterol and formoterol (refer to Table 34–3).

LABAs relax smooth muscle by stimulating the β_2 receptors, thereby increasing cyclic adenosine monophosphate (cAMP). LABAs have a 12-hour duration of effect; the molecule remains bound within the muscle cell wall because it is lipophilic. These medications work well as an adjunct therapy to anti-inflammatory medications in the long-term control of symptoms.[38,39] LABAs appear to work exceptionally well at controlling symptoms that occur at night[40] and at preventing exercise-induced exacerbations.

The complications of long-acting β_2-agonists are still somewhat controversial. There are reports of sudden severe asthma attacks that could have been worsened or initiated with the use of salmeterol.[41] Two studies that looked closely at this issue in a large cohort of patients found more deaths in patients who were taking salmeterol than in those who were not taking salmeterol.[42,43] Based on this data, clinicians need to pay close attention to properly educating patients who are using salmeterol. Salmeterol should be used only as a supplement to inhaled corticosteroids and never as a quick-relief medication.

The EPR-3 recommendations for the use of LABAs are as follows:[1]

1. LABAs are used as an adjunct to ICS therapy for providing long-term control of symptoms.
2. LABAs are not recommended as monotherapy for long-term control of persistent asthma.
3. The use of LABAs is not recommended to treat acute symptoms or exacerbation of asthma.
4. LABAs may be used before exercise to prevent exercise-induced bronchoconstriction, but frequent and chronic use of LABAs for exercise-induced bronchoconstriction may indicate poorly controlled asthma, which should be managed with daily anti-inflammatory therapy.

Methylxanthines

Theophylline is an alternative, but not preferred, therapy in mild to moderate persistent asthma. Slow-release theophylline is used primarily as adjuvant therapy for nocturnal asthma (refer to Table 34–3). The exact mechanism of action of methylxanthines in asthma is not well established.[44,45] Theophylline acts as a nonselective phosphodiesterase inhibitor. This results in an increase in cyclic guanosine monophosphate levels and cAMP levels that inhibit inflammation cells and produce bronchodilation. Recent studies indicate that low serum concentrations of theophylline may act as a mild anti-inflammatory medication.[46] This is possible most likely because of the decreased mediator release from mast cells and reactive oxygen species and the inhibition of neutrophil activity.

Theophylline is relatively safe. However, its use requires frequent monitoring of serum drug levels so that therapeutic, but not toxic, levels are achieved. Serum drug levels are affected by a patient's comorbidities and the presence of smoking and are therefore often difficult or impractical to manage. Potential toxic side effects include tachycardia, nausea and vomiting, central nervous system stimulation, arrhythmias, headache, seizures, hyperglycemia, and hypokalemia. The therapeutic serum range has recently been decreased from 10 to 20 mg/L to 5 to 15 mg/L to limit potential toxic effects. Pay close attention to other medications that patients using theophylline are receiving (e.g., antibiotics, β_2-blockers, quinolones).

Leukotriene Modifiers

Leukotriene modifiers also fall into the class of controller medications. This class of medications acts on the inflammatory cells known as leukotrienes. Leukotrienes are mediators that are released from mast cells, eosinophils, and basophils; they are responsible for airway bronchoconstriction, inflammatory cell recruitment, increased vascular permeability, and secretion production.

Montelukast is a leukotriene receptor antagonist (LTRA) that blocks the receptor sites on inflammatory cells for leukotrienes. Leukotriene receptor antagonists appear to work best in patients who have mild to moderate persistent asthma. Leukotriene receptor antagonists are an alternative, but not preferred, therapy to low- to medium-dose inhaled corticosteroids. Studies demonstrate a greater improvement in lung function and symptom scores with the use of ICS versus LTRA.[47] Regardless, LRTAs improve lung function, diminish asthma symptoms, and decrease the need for short-acting β_2-agonists, particularly in patients with allergies.[48,49]

Immunomodulators

There is currently one immunomodulator drug used for asthma: omalizumab, which has a trade name of Xolair. Omalizumab is a recombinant DNA-derived monoclonal antibody that inhibits the binding of IgE to the IgE receptor on the surface of mast cells and basophils. When the IgE receptors are bound by omalizumab, there is a reduction in surface-bound IgE, and therefore a decrease in the activation of mast cells and a decrease in the release of inflammatory mediators. Omalizumab is an alternate, but not preferred, drug in the treatment of moderate to severe persistent asthma in patients who have a positive skin test to aeroallergens and whose symptoms are inadequately controlled with ICS. It has been approved only for patients 12 years old and older.

Omalizumab is administered subcutaneously, and the dose is based on IgE level and patient weight. Omalizumab must be administered only in a closely observed clinic, because a rare adverse effect is anaphylaxis. The patient is directed to remain in the clinic for a period of observation following injection. Omalizumab has been shown to decrease the incidence of asthma exacerbations and emergency department visits, increase efficacy in patients with severe persistent allergic asthma who are already on high-dose ICS and LABA, and improve quality of life scores. Other than its adverse effects, the other drawback to omalizumab is its cost, which is approximately $1000 per month.[1]

Quick-Relief Medications

Short-Acting β_2-Agonists

This class of quick-relief medication is used predominantly to relieve airway bronchoconstriction and symptoms of cough, chest tightness, and wheezing. Short-acting β_2-agonists are the first-line medications used to treat an acute asthma exacerbation and for preventing exercise-induced bronchoconstriction. Before the 1990s, this was the first line of medications prescribed to result in overall control of asthma symptoms. Given the focus on the role of airway inflammation in the chronic management of asthma, SABAs have become rescue medications. This class of medications includes albuterol, metaproterenol, pirbuterol, and terbutaline (**Table 34–4**).

The mechanism of action is to relax smooth airway muscle and cause quick (15- to 30-minute) resolution to airway obstruction. Bronchodilation occurs primarily through β_2-adrenergic receptor stimulation in bronchial smooth muscle. These receptors are also present in airway epithelium, airway smooth muscle, mucus glands, and mast cells. The onset of action for a short-acting β_2-agonist is approximately 5 to 15 minutes under most circumstances of mild to moderate acute exacerbations.

Complications from SABAs are usually mild and self-limiting upon stopping the medication. Potential side effects include tachycardia, nausea, vomiting, tremors, headache, palpitation, paradoxical bronchospasm, and hypokalemia. Some potential complications from high use or prolonged use over time include subsensitivity (reduction in bronchodilation effect), increased airways hyperreactivity, and life-threatening episodes with overuse. The frequency of SABA use or prescription refills can be used as a marker of disease worsening or to indicate an increased risk of death or near death.

Patients should be cautioned to use SABAs only as needed. If the patient uses a SABA more often than twice per week, this indicates decreased asthma control. A red flag for the practitioner is if the patient uses more than one canister of SABA per month,

RESPIRATORY RECAP

Asthma Quick-Relief Medications

» Short-acting β_2-agonists
» Anticholinergics
» Systemic corticosteroids

TABLE 34–4 Quick-Relief Medications

Medication	Dose	Frequency
Short-Acting β_2-Agonists		
Metered dose inhalers		
Racemic albuterol (Ventolin HFA, Proventil HFA, Pro-Air HFA)	90 μg/puff	prn; q4h–q6h
Levalbuterol (Xopenex HFA)	45 μg/puff	prn, q6h
Pirbuterol (Maxair)	200 μg/puff	prn, q4h–q6h
Nebulization		
Racemic albuterol (Ventolin, Proventil, generic)	2.5 mg (0.5% solution	prn; q4h–q6h
Levalbuterol (Xopenex)	0.31 mg and 0.63 mg	
Metaproterenol (Alupent)	5% solution	
Oral tablets		
Albuterol (Repetabs, Volmax)	2 and 4 mg	prn; q4h–q6h
Metaproterenol	10 and 20 mg	
Terbutaline (Brethaire)	2.5 and 5 mg	
Syrup		
Albuterol	2 mg/5 mL	prn; q4h–q6h
Metaproterenol	10 mg/5 mL	
Subcutaneous injection		
Terbutaline	1 mg/mL injection	prn; q4h–q6h
Anticholinergics		
Metered dose inhalers		
Ipratropium bromide (Atrovent)	18 μg/puff	bid–qid
Nebulization		
Ipratropium bromide (Atrovent)	500-μg solution	bid–qid

HFA, hydrofluoroalkane; prn, as needed; bid, twice a day; qid, four times a day; q4h, every 4 hours; q6h, every 6 hours.

because this indicates that the patient has used his or her SABA approximately three times per day. The need for this much SABA is an indication that the underlying inflammation has worsened. The patient should seek medical attention in this event.

Anticholinergics

This class of quick-relief medication is used predominantly as an adjunct to short-acting β_2-agonists in acute severe exacerbations of airway bronchoconstriction in the emergency department. The mechanism of action of anticholinergics is airway smooth muscle tone relaxation through cholinergic innervation. Ipratropium is the primary asthma medication in the anticholinergic class. Ipratropium is a derivative of atropine without the common side effects of atropine (refer to Table 34–4).

The overall effectiveness of ipratropium bromide in the management of asthma remains controversial.[50–53] Its effectiveness for long-term asthma management has not been demonstrated. Adult patients who have asthma and a component of chronic obstructive pulmonary disease apparently experience some beneficial outcomes.

Studies in children have demonstrated that the use of ipratropium in combination with β_2-agonists in patients with acute exacerbations or severe airway obstruction may be beneficial. However, routine administration of this combination therapy does not appear to be beneficial.[54,55]

Systemic Corticosteroids

Systemic corticosteroids are usually combined with a short-acting β_2-agonist for a quick resolution of airway obstruction in an emergency department or hospital setting.[56] These drugs may be given either orally or intravenously. Normal dosage in this setting is 2 mg/kg (given every 6 hours, up to a maximum dose of 120 mg). The mechanism of action for systemic corticosteroids is the same as inhaled corticosteroids. The administration of a systemic corticosteroid in the ED is used to help prevent or ease the onset of the delayed (phase 2) asthmatic response. This phase 2 response is secondary to the event that led the patient to present to the ED. In the absence of a systemic corticosteroid, the patient may present to the ED again following discharge with more severe bronchospasm and inflammation than during the initial admission.

For outpatient use, systemic corticosteroids are prescribed for short-term burst therapy (once a day for 3 to 10 days). Normal dosing is prescribed at the lowest possible dose (0.5 to 2 mg/kg/day). Maximum dose is normally restricted to 60 mg for outpatient use. If chronic use of systemic corticosteroids is needed, a study has documented improved efficacy when the medication is given at 3 PM instead of in the morning.

Aerosol Therapy

The main routes of delivery for asthma medications are systemic or inhaled. The main routes of systemic delivery are oral (ingested) or parenteral (subcutaneous, intramuscular, or intravenous).[1] Oral medications are mainly in either pill or liquid form. Parenteral medications are usually limited to patients who either are in the emergency department or are admitted to the hospital.

The inhaled route is more convenient and common because of fewer side effects and quicker onset of action. The disadvantages of the inhaled route are associated with the delivery device and the factors that affect drug penetration and deposition in the lungs. The main factors involved in penetration and deposition are physical (sedimentation, inertial impaction, and diffusion) and clinical (particle size, ventilatory pattern, and lung function).[57]

Nebulizers, pressurized metered dose inhalers (pMDIs), and dry powder inhalers (DPIs) are used for inhaled medications. Opinions have varied on the best and most efficient method, but available evidence suggests that all three devices are equally effective in treating an acute exacerbation.[58]

RESPIRATORY RECAP

Aerosol Delivery Devices for Patients with Asthma

- Metered dose inhaler
- Metered dose inhaler with accessory device
- Dry powder inhaler

Nebulizers

The small-volume nebulizer (SVN) is the most common device used to deliver medications to small children and patients requiring hospitalization. Although theoretically aerosol delivery and deposition in an asthmatic airway may be improved with a less dense gas (such as **heliox**),[59–62] there are potential problems with the use of nebulizers powered by heliox.[63] Heliox is best reserved for severe cases refractory to conventional therapy. A number of factors affect an SVN's performance.[58,64–66] The use of nebulizers relies on proper technique. Deposition of appropriate particle size in the lower respiratory tract depends on ventilatory pattern. To ensure optimal particle deposition, a slow breath (through the mouth) to total lung capacity with an end-inspiratory breath hold is ideal. With proper breathing technique, aerosol delivery with an SVN is equally effective with a mask or mouthpiece.

Continuous Aerosols

In a severe asthma attack, aggressive intermittent aerosol therapy may fail to relieve symptoms. Studies have demonstrated that continuous bronchodilator therapy is as effective or more effective than intermittent therapy. Continuous aerosol bronchodilator therapy has become a accepted alternative to intermittent therapy in emergency departments for patients who fail to respond to less aggressive therapy. Current evidence supports the use of continuous bronchodilator administration in patients with severe acute asthma who present to the ED to increase their pulmonary functions and reduce hospitalization.[67] Moreover, it appears to be safe and well tolerated.

Pressurized Metered Dose Inhalers

The pMDI is the most common device used to deliver medications in an ambulatory setting and is rapidly increasing in use in hospitalized and ED treatment. The canister is activated by compressing it into a mouthpiece, which causes a metered dose of the drug to be delivered for inhalation.

A number of factors can affect pMDI performance and drug delivery. A potential factor that can interfere with appropriate metered dose delivery is using medications from one manufacturer with an actuator or accessory device from another manufacturer. Most of the factors that affect optimal delivery involve patient delivery technique; this is especially the case in the very young or elderly. Factors critical in the effectiveness of pMDI performance include timing of actuation, lung volume, pMDI position to the mouth (without spacer), inspiratory flow rate, and the ability to perform a breath hold.[53] An alternative to using a spacer is the breath-actuated MDI. With such a device, the MDI actuates automatically as the patient begins to inhale, thus appropriately timing drug delivery with inspiration.

Compared with pMDIs with CFC as a propellant, pMDIs with hydrofluoroalkane (HFA) propellants have a softer, warmer spray. Each type of pMDI has its own instructions on priming, so it is important for the therapist to read the package insert and learn how many times any given pMDI needs to be primed and how and when to clean the pMDI actuator, so that this information may be taught to the patient.

Chlorofluorocarbon propellant pMDIs are being removed from the market and replaced with hydrofluoroalkane propellants. Some patients who were accustomed to a CFC pMDI may complain that their HFA pMDI does not provide relief because the sensation of the plume in the mouth is different. The asthma educator needs to be aware of this and be prepared to reinforce proper inhaler technique.

Spacers and Valved Holding Chambers

If patients find it difficult to properly use a pMDI or if an ICS pMDI is being used, patients should use a spacer or valved holding chamber to enhance optimal drug delivery. A spacer is a cylindrical or cone-shaped chamber that receives the pMDI actuator on one end and has a mouthpiece on the other. A valved holding chamber is a spacer with a one-way valve at the mouthpiece end that prevents the patient from exhaling into the chamber. Several of these devices also incorporate a flow signal that has an audible sound if the patient is inhaling too fast. With optimal MDI delivery technique, evidence exists (even with children) of no difference in deposition with or without a spacing device.[68]

With an accessory spacing device, a pMDI is actuated into the chamber, and the patient breathes the medication from a mouthpiece or mask attached to the chamber. For optimal medication availability, the valved holding chamber is preferred. This decreases the potential of medication being lost through the device on exhalation. Different spacing devices affect drug delivery,[57,69] and more studies are needed to evaluate new medications and spacing devices.

Another potential factor that may affect the amount of drug delivered with a spacing device is a static charge that occurs from washing the chamber. Antistatic chambers have also been developed. Generally, the device should be disassembled and washed in soapy water, rinsed, and allowed to air dry before use. Manufacturers' instructions should be followed regarding appropriate device cleaning.

Dry Powder Inhalers

Two types of DPI exist: single-dose devices (e.g., Spiriva Handihaler, Foradil Aerolizer), and multidose devices (e.g., Advair discus, Pulmicort Flexhaler).[57] DPIs are breath activated with a high inspiratory flow generated at the mouthpiece. Because of the requirement of a high inspiratory flow for actuation, DPIs are not indicated for use in children younger than 12 years. Several instructions are common to DPIs. The DPI must be kept level during inhalation, it must be kept in a dry location to prevent clumping of the powder, and the patient must not exhale into the DPI. Multidose DPIs have dose counters to alert the patient as to the remaining doses in the device.

Adjunctive Treatments

Oxygen, inhaled β_2-adrenergic agonists, and corticosteroids remain the cornerstones of therapy for asthma. This section discusses four alternative therapies to aerosolized medications in the treatment of a severe asthma exacerbation: helium–oxygen gas mixtures (heliox), magnesium sulfate, noninvasive ventilation, and invasive mechanical ventilation. Because of the risk of immediate respiratory decompensation, these therapies are normally administered in the confines of an intensive care unit or emergency department.

RESPIRATORY RECAP

Adjunctive Treatments for Asthma

- » Heliox
- » Magnesium sulfate
- » Noninvasive ventilation
- » Invasive ventilation

Heliox

Helium is a gas that is less dense than air, which may be beneficial in the treatment of asthma.[63] Heliox is not a stand-alone therapy to treat a severe asthma exacerbation, but rather is supportive therapy before intubation to allow time for bronchodilators and corticosteroids to take effect.[70] A difficulty in the provision of heliox in nonintubated patients is that the available gas mixtures in concentrations may not provide adequate supplemental oxygen to achieve acceptable oxyhemoglobin saturations (80% helium to 20% oxygen or 70% helium to 30% oxygen).

The therapeutic benefits of heliox are controversial. Reports of the therapeutic benefits of heliox are isolated primarily to the management of pediatric asthma[60,61,71] or the management of adult patients who present to the ED with a respiratory acidosis and/or a short duration of symptoms.[72] Some studies have shown that the use of heliox has no effect on FEV_1.[73,74] Given the safety profile of heliox and the short time to achieve a positive response, a brief trial of heliox may serve as a therapeutic bridge until corticosteroid therapy has taken effect. One study documented a rapid resolution (less than 60 minutes) to respiratory acidosis by using heliox, especially in patients who had brief duration of symptoms (less than 24 hours) and a severely acidotic pH (7.20 or less) at presentation.[75] Randomized trials in patients with asthma have reported benefit with the use of heliox.[61,76] The EPR-3 cites a meta-analysis of six studies that did not find a statistically significant improvement in pulmonary function or other measured outcomes in patients receiving heliox compared with oxygen or air.[1] The EPR-3 recommends consideration of heliox-driven albuterol nebulization for patients who have life-threatening exacerbations and for those patients whose exacerbations remain in the severe category after 1 hour of intensive conventional therapy.[1]

Magnesium Sulfate

Administration of magnesium sulfate is an alternative treatment for a severe asthma exacerbation.[77,78] The EPR-3 recommends intravenous magnesium sulfate in patients who have life-threatening exacerbations and in those whose exacerbations remain in the severe category after 1 hour of conventional therapy.[1] The mechanisms of action include calcium-channel blockade in the airway smooth muscle and inhibition of acetylcholine and histamine release. Magnesium may promote bronchodilation that would improve β_2-agonist delivery. A study comparing nebulized magnesium to salbutamol demonstrated a similar response,[79] but nebulized magnesium does not consistently have this bronchodilator effect. Other studies have documented no improvement in FEV_1 in patients who were treated with magnesium intravenously.[80–81]

The dose for intravenous magnesium is 2 g in adults and from 25 to 75 mg/kg up to 2 g in children administered over a half hour. The onset of action for magnesium can occur within minutes of administration. Potential side effects are usually minor (facial warmth and flushing). However, magnesium can be toxic with high serum levels. Signs of magnesium toxicity include hypotension, dysrhythmias, areflexia, and muscle weakness. The use of magnesium sulfate in the treatment of severe exacerbations is not recommended as a first-line therapy. The treatment has no apparent value in exacerbations of lesser severity.[1]

Noninvasive Ventilation

The use of noninvasive positive pressure ventilation (NIV) has taken a role in the management of patients who are at high risk for intubation and mechanical ventilation. NIV offers a viable means of overcoming increased work of breathing without an endotracheal tube. Uncontrolled studies have documented the use of noninvasive ventilation as a viable alternative to mechanical ventilation.[82,83] The key factor in the use of NIV is early initiation of the therapy in conjunction with bronchodilators and corticosteroids. Appropriate inspiratory flow is important to ensure patient comfort and to decrease the work of breathing. Avoiding delivery of excessive minute ventilation is important, because it could lead to hyperinflation and air trapping. The use of aerosolized medications with NIV is feasible.[84] NIV in patients with asthma is supportive and meant to be used in conjunction with established therapies. NIV may be useful in carefully selected patients with a severe exacerbation, even though there have been few trials of NIV in asthma.[85]

Invasive Ventilation

Invasive ventilation of patients with asthma is a treatment of last resort for patients experiencing respiratory failure because of severe airflow obstruction, increased mucus production, and/or severe airway inflammation.[85,86] Asthma resulting in intubation and mechanical ventilation is not a common event, occurring in less than 5% of patients treated. **Box 34–5** lists the general indications for mechanical ventilation in the patient with asthma. The obstructive nature of a severe exacerbation of asthma produces a ventilation-perfusion mismatch and increased work of breathing, but this rarely produces severe hypoxemia. The more difficult issue in the patient with acute asthma is optimizing the pH and Pa_{CO_2} because of bronchoconstriction, air trapping, and increased dead space.[87]

On intubation of a patient with acute asthma, full ventilatory support is usually provided (i.e., no spontaneous breathing by the patient). This allows optimization of the patient–ventilator interface under the best possible conditions. The principal goal of mechanical ventilation of the patient with asthma is to provide acceptable gas exchange while avoiding air trapping (auto-PEEP [positive end-expiratory pressure]). With auto-PEEP, alveolar overdistention may occur with concomitant hypotension and barotrauma.

BOX 34–5

Indications for Mechanical Ventilation of the Patient with Asthma

Pa_{CO_2} > 40 mm Hg (especially if increasing)
Refractory hypoxemia (Pa_{O_2} < 60 mm Hg or $F_{IO_2} \geq 0.5$)
Mental status deterioration
Decrease or loss of breath sounds
Apnea

RESPIRATORY RECAP

Mechanical Ventilation of the Patient with Asthma

- » Avoid strategies that cause air trapping and auto-PEEP.
- » Consider PEEP to counterbalance auto-PEEP.
- » Avoid plateau pressure above 30 cm H_2O.
- » Permissive hypercapnia may be necessary.
- » Inhaled bronchodilators can be administered using nebulizers or pMDIs.

The choice of ventilator mode is often based on clinical preference or institutional bias. Either volume or pressure control modes can be used, and advantages and disadvantages exist for both. With volume control ventilation, auto-PEEP results in increased plateau pressures and alveolar overdistention. With pressure control ventilation, auto-PEEP results in decreased tidal volumes and respiratory acidosis. In patients with asthma with severe airflow obstruction, it may be difficult to deliver an adequate tidal volume with pressure control ventilation. Regardless of the mode chosen, auto-PEEP and plateau pressures must be monitored closely.

The ultimate goal of tidal volume selection in severe asthma exacerbation is to avoid overdistention of the alveoli. Generally, tidal volumes are set in the 5 to 8 mL/kg range and adjusted to minimize overdistention (i.e., to avoid a plateau pressure of more than 30 cm H_2O). This often results in a ventilator strategy of permissive hypercapnia. With permissive hypercapnia, Pa_{CO_2} is allowed to rise and an acidic pH is tolerated. The limits of safe Pa_{CO_2} and pH are debated, but general consensus suggests that Pa_{CO_2} levels of 80 to 100 mm Hg and pH levels of 7.15 to 7.20 are acceptable.[88,89]

The use of positive end-expiratory pressure when ventilating the patient with asthma is controversial. PEEP as a means to prevent atelectasis or collapse is not necessary. PEEP has been used to combat auto-PEEP. The intent is to counterbalance auto-PEEP by applying PEEP so that the patient will be better able to trigger the ventilator. However, care must be taken to avoid increased overdistention with the application of PEEP. PEEP has no role in counterbalancing auto-PEEP in the patient who is not attempting to trigger the ventilator.[90,91]

One study observed that there are three different responses to PEEP in the setting of auto-PEEP. In the biphasic response, expiratory flow and lung volume remained constant during progressive PEEP steps until a threshold was reached, beyond which overinflation ensued. In the classic overinflation response, any increment of PEEP caused a decrease in expiratory flow and overinflation. In the paradoxic response, a drop in functional residual capacity during PEEP application was commonly accompanied by decreased plateau pressures and total PEEP, with increased expiratory flow.[92] Generally, no more than 10 cm H_2O PEEP is used to counterbalance auto-PEEP. Some auto-PEEP that occurs during mechanical ventilation of the patient with asthma may not be measurable in the usual manner because of complete airway closure during the expiratory phase.[92]

The inspiratory-to-expiratory (I:E) ratio in a patient with airflow obstruction is important to avoid air trapping. The I:E ratio is determined by the inspiratory time (flow and tidal volume for volume control ventilation) and respiratory rate. The goal when setting the I:E ratio in patients with asthma is to allow adequate expiratory time to minimize auto-PEEP. Use of prolonged expiratory times requires a low respiratory rate and a shortened inspiratory time in the range of 0.8 to 1.2 seconds (high flow). Typically, a respiratory rate of 15 per minute or less is used.

When aggressive therapy fails to stabilize a patient's asthma and intubation occurs, the need to provide aerosol therapy remains important in the resolution of the acute exacerbation. Aerosol therapy of the intubated patient has been an area of debate.[93] Some support either nebulizers or MDIs as the most effective and efficient method from a clinical and financial standpoint. Aerosol delivery to intubated patients with either nebulizers or MDIs is less effective than when delivered to a spontaneously breathing patient. Many factors in intubated patients affect optimal aerosol delivery and deposition. Higher-than-standard doses may be necessary to elicit a desired response because of potential barriers involved with mechanically ventilated patients. Aerosol administration by both nebulizers and MDIs is an effective means of delivering medication to ventilated patients. Studies using both devices have demonstrated lung deposition efficiency of 5% to 15%.[94] Sufficient attention to detail, including the use of an efficient nebulizer and/

or adapter and proper placement and operating method, is required to provide optimal delivery.

The use of heliox with mechanical ventilation may be beneficial when a patient with asthma is difficult to manage with traditional ventilator manipulations.[95] Caution is warranted because the addition of heliox may result in ventilator malfunction. Many, but not all, of the current-generation ventilators are compatible with heliox. Inhalational anesthetics (e.g., isoflurane, halothane, enflurane) have a bronchodilatory effect and are used rarely in the most severe cases.

Mechanical ventilation of the patient with asthma may be a lifesaving measure, but it can also be associated with significant morbidity and mortality.[92,96–98] The major complications of mechanical ventilation of the patient with asthma include overdistention, pneumothorax, hypotension, air trapping, patient–ventilator asynchrony, and neuromuscular blocking agent–related myopathies.

Education

Asthma education begins at diagnosis and should be reinforced with each visit. The ability to modify morbidity and resource consumption through education has been well documented in asthma. Over the past 20 years, many programs and formats have been designed and implemented to demonstrate that asthma education is a main component of the overall successful management of the disease. The items in **Box 34–6** should be included in **asthma education programs**.[1]

Many studies of educational interventions are available in the literature, covering many different care settings. These include ambulatory clinics, allergy or pulmonary specialty clinics, emergency departments, hospitals, patient homes, and asthma camps. The impact of educational interventions has been evaluated regarding readmission rates, hospitalizations, compliance, ED visits, clinic follow-up rates, test scores, and behavior changes.

The rapid expansion of managed health care in the 1990s led to the study of the financial aspects of providing asthma education. Some of the earlier managed care education interventions assessed patients with asthma determined to be at high risk. Although these programs still exist, asthma educators are looking at ways to target a variety of patients with asthma because of a regression-toward-the-mean concept. The theory of regression toward the mean implies that patients with chronic conditions do not have steady-state healthcare resource consumption year after year. One year's high-resource consumers do not necessarily translate into the next year's high-resource consumers. Therefore, these earliest managed care programs and interventions resulted in a shifting of the costs from group to group or from year to year (**Table 34–5**).

The asthma education program needs to take a proactive approach. An asthma education program should provide education to the patient with asthma and include all potential caregivers (spouses, parents, older children, day-care providers, teachers, coaches, group leaders, and counselors). The National Cooperative Inner City Asthma Study (NCICAS) reported that often a child has several care providers in the home.[99] This pediatric study demonstrated the importance of involving as many caregivers as possible in the asthma education to ensure consistent management. This study also identified that pediatric asthma has additional educational barriers. Often education providers overlook the child to concentrate their educational efforts on the caregivers. However, children as young as 2 years can begin learning about their asthma and its management. As children age, the scope and the depth of the information will need

BOX 34–6

Educational Recommendations of the NAEPP

- Teach basic facts about asthma
- Teach the necessary medication skills (techniques, delivery devices, and dosing regimens)
- Teach self-monitoring skills: symptom-based, peak flow monitoring
- Teach relevant environmental control/avoidance strategies
- Provide a written asthma exacerbation treatment plan

From National Asthma Education Program, National Heart, Lung, and Blood Institute. *Expert Panel Report 3: Guidelines for the Diagnosis and Management of Asthma.* Bethesda, MD: National Institutes of Health; 2007. NIH Publication 07-4051.

AGE-SPECIFIC ANGLE

Children as young as 2 years can begin learning about asthma and its management.

TABLE 34–5 Theoretic Look at Regression Toward the Mean

	Percentage of Resource Cost Consumption			
	Original Percentage of Patients	*Year 1*	*Year 2*	*Year 3*
High-resource consumers	10	80	10	4
Low-resource consumers	90	20	90	96

to continue to grow. As children grow into adolescents, they should receive all asthma information themselves.[100]

Asthma education information should be repeated several times for maximum effect, and educational objectives should be reinforced with written materials targeted for age appropriateness. Asthma self-management education should be modified to the needs of each individual patient. Cultural beliefs and unharmful practices should be approached and discussed with sensitivity and understanding. The education provider should be attentive and document the concerns of the patient and the family regarding medications and asthma management. Addressing concerns and explaining the rationale for treatment may be the overriding factor in patient compliance with chronic asthma management. The asthma educator also must be prepared to intervene and problem solve in the areas of medications, level of treatment, trigger avoidance, compliance, and self-management skills.

One of the indicators of a chronic condition is the ability to modify or reduce morbidity and mortality risks through patient education. Asthma is a chronic disease condition that has demonstrated this ability. An unlimited number of approaches or interventions are readily available to provide effective and efficient asthma education to healthcare providers. Perhaps one method is not truly better than another. The important features are to provide the resources and information at diagnosis and consistently thereafter to each patient with asthma individually.

CASE STUDIES

Case 1. Ambulatory Asthma Management

A 43-year-old woman with asthma presents to an inner-city emergency department with coughing, wheezing, and shortness of breath. She reports a respiratory viral infection within the last week that resolved with over-the-counter medicines in 3 or 4 days. Her initial physical examination reveals the following: respiratory rate of 36 breaths/min, labored; heart rate of 120 beats/min; blood pressure of 120/80 mm Hg; pulse oximetry of 93% in room air; inspiratory and expiratory wheezing upon auscultation; equal air exchange bilaterally; moderate intercostal retractions; and peak expiratory flow (PEF) of 290 L/min (60% of predicted). The initial treatment consists of six puffs of albuterol, administered via an MDI with a holding chamber. Each puff is given with the appropriate technique. Posttreatment PEF is 300 L/min (62% of predicted).

The woman reports that she stopped taking her beclomethasone about 2 months before this visit. The following additional information is acquired:

- *Reported medications*: Beclomethasone two puffs twice a day, and albuterol two puffs as needed and before exercise
- *Treatment before arrival*: None
- *Peak flow meter diary*: None
- *Unscheduled ED/MD visits in the past month*: 0
- *Unscheduled ED/MD visits in the past year*: 3
- *Hospital admissions in the past year*: 1
- *Prior intensive care unit (ICU) admissions*: 0
- *Cough or wheeze frequency*: Two times per week
- *Activity limitations*: Occasionally
- *Nocturnal cough or wheeze*: Two to three times per week
- *Work absenteeism*: 6 days per year

Approximately 20 minutes after the initial treatment, a second treatment is administered with six puffs of albuterol via pMDI and holding chamber as before. The patient is also given 60 mg of prednisolone. Posttreatment assessment reveals a respiratory rate of 24 breaths/min; heart rate of 100 beats/min; oxygen saturation of 95% breathing room air; inspiratory and expiratory wheezing upon auscultation; equal air exchange bilaterally; mild intercostal retractions; and PEF of 315 L/min (65% predicted).

Approximately 20 minutes after the second treatment, a third treatment of albuterol (six puffs) is administered, along with two puffs of Atrovent. Posttreatment assessment reveals a respiratory rate of 16 breaths/min; heart rate of 80 beats/min; oxygen saturation of 95% breathing room air; faint end-expiratory wheezes with auscultation and bilateral equal air exchange; no intercostal retractions; and PEF of 365 L/min (75% predicted).

The woman's next β_2-agonist treatment is withheld, and she is reassessed in 60 minutes. The prior assessment response is sustained upon physical examination, and the woman is readied for discharge. Based on the self-reported asthma history, the woman's chronic asthma is determined to be moderate persistent asthma. She is instructed to continue her albuterol treatments with two puffs every 4 to 6 hours for the next several days. She also is told to resume her beclomethasone therapy of two puffs twice a day for chronic inflammatory control. She is given a peak flow meter and instructed in its proper use. She is also instructed in the use of an asthma action plan with a peak flow diary that illustrates meter readings in three color-coded zones to assist her in self-management. She is also instructed to call her primary care physician and to schedule a follow-up visit in the next week to 10 days.

Case 2. Life-Threatening Asthma Management

A 10-year-old boy with asthma presents to an inner-city ED with dyspnea at rest, talking in phrases, agitated, and dusky in color. The boy's mother reports having administered three nebulizer treatments before arrival in the emergency department. The child's initial physical examination reveals the following: respiratory rate of 48 breaths/min, labored; heart rate of 170 beats/min; blood pressure of 160/100 mm Hg; oxygen saturation of 89% breathing room air; breath sounds muffled to inaudible;

severe intercostal and substernal retractions; and inability to perform a PEF.

The patient is then started on undiluted albuterol that was nebulized with 100% oxygen. An IV is placed and he is given 60 mg methylprednisone. During the aerosol treatment, an asthma history is taken from the boy's mother. She reports that her child had been outside playing basketball with his friends for most of the afternoon. Before this episode, he was in good health. The following information is acquired:

- *Reported medications*: Albuterol two puffs as needed before exercise
- *Treatment before arrival*: Three nebulized treatments with albuterol
- *Peak flow meter diary*: None
- *Unscheduled ED/MD visits in the past month*: 0
- *Unscheduled ED/MD visits in the past year*: 1
- *Hospital admissions in the past year*: 1
- *Prior ICU admissions*: 1 (3 years ago)
- *Cough or wheeze frequency*: With respiratory infections
- *Activity or play limitations*: Always
- *Nocturnal cough or wheeze*: One to two times per week
- *School absenteeism*: Three to four days per year

While receiving continuous albuterol treatments, the child is assessed every 20 minutes. Electrocardiography and pulse oximetry are monitored continuously. After the initial 20 minutes, 0.5 mg of ipratropium is added to the aerosol. Thirty-five minutes after treatment was started, the boy's status is a respiratory rate of 20 breaths/min, labored; heart rate of 80 beats/min; blood pressure of 200/100 mm Hg; oxygen saturation of 88% on continuous nebulizer; inaudible breath sounds; severe intercostal and substernal retractions; inability to perform PEF; and lethargy and drowsiness. Arterial blood gas results are pH 7.29, $Paco_2$ 52 mm Hg, Pao_2 60 mm Hg, HCO_3^- 26 mmol/L, and oxygen saturation of 87%.

The decision is made to intubate the child. After atropine, ketamine, and succinylcholine are administered, he is intubated with a 6.0 mm cuffed endotracheal tube. Upon arrival in the pediatric intensive care unit, the child is placed on the following settings: volume control continuous mandatory ventilation (VC-CMV), tidal volume 350 mL (7 mL/kg), PEEP 3 cm H_2O, mandatory breath rate 10 breaths/min, I:E ratio of 1:5, and Fio_2 0.50. After 1 hour on the ventilator, the arterial blood gas results are pH 7.32, $Paco_2$ 46 mm Hg, Pao_2 120 mm Hg, HCO_3^- 22 mmol/L, and oxygen saturation 99%. The Fio_2 is weaned to 0.4. The patient is ventilated with permissive hypercapnia to prevent auto-PEEP and overdistention. Continuous ventilator waveform analysis is used to detect auto-PEEP, and the flow is increased to allow for a longer expiratory time. The patient is kept moderately sedated, and paralysis is not necessary at this time. The child is given albuterol via MDI through the ventilator circuit with 10 puffs every 30 minutes and 2 puffs of Atrovent every 6 hours. The patient remains on IV methlyprednisone.

After 6 hours of this therapy, the albuterol treatments are changed to a frequency of every hour. After 12 hours of mechanical ventilation and pharmacologic therapy, blood gas results are pH 7.42, $Paco_2$ 33 mm Hg, Pao_2 95 mm Hg on Fio_2 of 0.25, HCO_3^- 24 mmol/L, and oxygen saturation 99%. He is awake and triggering at a rate of 6 to 10 breaths/min above the mandatory rate. A spontaneous breathing trial is successful, he is extubated to a 2 L/min nasal cannula, 5.0 mg nebulized albuterol every hour, and IV methlyprednisone and ipratropium 0.5 mg every 6 hours.

KEY POINTS

- Asthma is a common chronic disease that is increasing in prevalence and severity.
- The pathophysiology of asthma is largely related to inflammation, hyperresponsiveness, and airway obstruction.
- The most identifiable predisposing factor for the development of asthma is atopy.
- Nocturnal symptoms of asthma are common.
- Exercise-induced asthma is characterized by transient airway obstruction after strenuous exercise.
- Occupational asthma is characterized by variable airway hyperresponsiveness in the workplace.
- The NAEPP has developed a four-tiered system to classify asthma disease severity.
- The most common ways to diagnose and monitor airflow obstruction in asthma are spirometry and peak flow meters.
- Asthma medications are classified as either long-term controllers or quick-relief medications.
- Inhaled medications are delivered by nebulizer, metered dose inhaler, or dry powder inhalers.
- Oxygen, inhaled β_2-agonists, and corticosteroids are the cornerstones of therapy for asthma.
- Mechanical ventilation is the treatment of last resort for patients with asthma and respiratory failure.
- Asthma education begins with diagnosis and should be reinforced with each visit.

REFERENCES

1. National Asthma Education Program, National Heart, Lung, and Blood Institute. *Expert Panel Report 3: Guidelines for the Diagnosis and Management of Asthma*. Bethesda, MD: National Institutes of Health; 2007. NIH Publication 07-4051.
2. Mannino DM, Homa DM, Akinbami LJ, Moorman JE, Gwynn C, Redd SC. Surveillance for asthma—United States, 1980–1999. *MMWR*. 2002;51(SS01):1–13.
3. Akinbami L. Asthma prevalence, health care use and mortality: United States, 2003–2005. Available at: http://www.cdc.gov/nchs/products/pubs/pubd/hestats/ashtma03-05/asthma03-05.htm#fig2. Accessed October 30, 2008.
4. Schaubel D, Johansen H, Mao Y, et al. Risk of preschool asthma: incidence, hospitalization, recurrence, and readmission probability. *J Asthma*. 1996;33:97–103.

5. Smith D, Malone D, Lawson K, et al. A national estimate of the economic costs of asthma. *Am J Respir Crit Care Med.* 1997;156:787–793.
6. McFadden ER, Elsanadi N, Dixon L, et al. Protocol therapy for acute asthma: therapeutic benefits and cost savings. *Am J Med.* 1995;99:651–660.
7. Myers TR, Chatburn RL, Kercsmar CM. A pediatric asthma unit staff by respiratory therapists demonstrates positive clinical and financial outcomes. *Respir Care.* 1998;43:22–29.
8. McDowell KM, Chatburn RL, Myers TR, et al. A cost-saving algorithm for children hospitalized for status asthmaticus. *Arch Pediatr Adolesc Med.* 1998;152:977–984.
9. Mayo PH, Weinberg BJ, Kramer B, et al. Results of a program to improve the process of inpatient care of adult asthmatics. *Chest.* 1996;110:48–52.
10. Kwann-Ghett TS, Lozano P, Mullin K, et al. One-year experience with an inpatient asthma clinical pathway. *Arch Pediatr Adolesc Med.* 1997;151:684–689.
11. Global Initiative for Asthma. *Global Strategy for Asthma Management or Prevention. NHLBI/WHO Workshop Report.* Bethesda, MD: National Institutes of Health; 1995:78–79. NIH Publication 95-3659.
12. Liu AH, Murphy JR. Hygiene hypothesis: fact or fiction? *J Allergy Clin Immunol.* 2003;111(3):471–478.
13. Eggleston PA, Rosenstreich D, Lynn H, et al. Relationship of indoor allergen exposure to skin test sensitivity in inner-city children with asthma. *J Allergy Clin Immunol.* 1998;102:563–570.
14. Rosenstreich DL, Eggleston P, Kattan M, et al. The role of cockroach allergy and exposure to cockroach allergen in causing morbidity among inner-city children with asthma. *N Engl J Med.* 1997;336:1356–1363.
15. Teichtahl H, Buckmaster N, Pertnikovs E. The incidence of respiratory tract infection in adults requiring hospitalization for asthma. *Chest.* 1997;112:591–596.
16. Pizzichini MM, Pizzichini E, Efthimiadis A, et al. Asthma and natural colds. Inflammatory indices in induced sputum: a feasibility study. *Am J Respir Crit Care Med.* 1998;158:1178–1184.
17. Lieu TA, Quesenberry CP Jr, Capra AM, et al. Outpatient management practices associated with reduced risk of pediatric asthma hospitalization and emergency department visits. *Pediatrics.* 1997;100:334–341.
18. Martin RJ. Nocturnal asthma and the use of theophylline. *Clin Exp Allergy.* 1998;28:64–70.
19. Meijer GG, Postma DS, Wempe JB, et al. Frequency of nocturnal symptoms in asthmatic children attending a hospital out-patient clinic. *Eur Respir J.* 1995;8:2076–2080.
20. Di Stefano A, Lusuardi M, Braghiroli A, et al. Nocturnal asthma: mechanisms and therapy. *Lung.* 1997;175:53–61.
21. Fix A, Sexton M, Langenberg P, et al. The association of nocturnal asthma with asthma severity. *J Asthma.* 1997;34:329–336.
22. Martin RJ. *Nocturnal Asthma.* Mount Kisco, NY: Futura; 1993.
23. Silkoff PE, Martin RJ. Pathophysiology of nocturnal asthma. *Ann Allergy Asthma Immunol.* 1998;81:378–383.
24. Syabbalo N. Chronobiology and chronopathophysiology of nocturnal asthma. *Int J Clin Pract.* 1997;51:455–462.
25. Kukafka DS, Lang OM, Porter S, et al. Exercise-induced bronchospasm in high school athletes via a free running test: incidence and epidemiology. *Chest.* 1998;114:1613–1622.
26. American Thoracic Society. Standardization of spirometry: 1994 update. *Am J Respir Care Med.* 1995;152:1107–1136.
27. Silkoff PE, McClean PA, Slutsky AS, et al. Marked flow-dependence of exhaled nitric oxide using a new technique to exclude nasal nitric oxide. *Am J Respir Crit Care Med.* 1997;155:260–267.
28. ten Hacken NH, van der Vaart H, van der Malk TW, et al. Exhaled nitric oxide is higher both at day and night in subjects with nocturnal asthma. *Am J Respir Crit Care Med.* 1998;158:902–907.
29. Lim KG, Mottram C. The use of fraction of exhaled nitric oxide in pulmonary practice. *Chest.* 2008;133:1232–1242.
30. Barnes PJ, Pederson S. Efficacy and safety of inhaled corticosteroids in asthma. *Am Rev Respir Dis.* 1993;146:1524–1530.
31. Russell G. Inhaled corticosteroid therapy in children: an assessment of the potential for side-effects. *Thorax.* 1994;49:1185–1188.
32. Wolthers OD, Pederson S. Short-term growth during treatment with inhaled fluticasone propionate and beclomethasone dipropionate. *Arch Dis Child.* 1993;68:673–676.
33. Clark B. General pharmacology, pharmacokinetics, and clinical toxicology of nedocromil sodium. *J Allergy Clin Immunol.* 1993;92:200–202.
34. Alton E, Norris AA. Chloride transport and the actions of nedocromil sodium and cromolyn sodium in asthma. *J Allergy Clin Immunol.* 1994;98:S102–S106.
35. Schwartz HJ, Blumenthal M, Brady R, et al. A comparative study of the clinical efficacy of nedocromil sodium and placebo. *Chest.* 1996;109:945–952.
36. Novembre G, Frongia GF, Veneruso G, et al. Inhibition of exercise-induced asthma (EIA) by nedocromil sodium and sodium cromoglycate in children. *Pediatr Allergy Immunol.* 1994;5:107–110.
37. Lal S, Dorow PD, Venho KK, et al. Nedocromil sodium is more effective than cromolyn sodium for the treatment of chronic reversible obstructive airway disease. *Chest.* 1993;104:438–447.
38. Greening AP, Wind P, Northfield M, et al. Added salmeterol versus higher-dose corticosteroids in asthma patients with symptoms on existing corticosteroids. *Lancet.* 1994;344:219–224.
39. Woolcock A, Lundback B, Ringdal N, et al. Comparison of addition of salmeterol to inhaled steroids with doubling of the dose of inhaled steroid. *Am J Respir Crit Care Med.* 1996;153:1481–1488.
40. Yates DH, Sussman HS, Shaw MJ, et al. Regular formoterol treatment in mild asthma. Effect of bronchial responsiveness during and after treatment. *Am J Respir Crit Care Med.* 1995;152:1170–1174.
41. Clark CE, Ferguson AD, Siddorn JA. Respiratory arrests in young asthmatics on salmeterol. *Respir Med.* 1993;87:227–228.
42. Castle W, Fuller R, Hall J, et al. Serevent nationwide surveillance study: comparison of salmeterol with salbutamol in asthmatic patients who require bronchodilator treatment. *BMJ.* 1993;306:1034–1037.
43. Mann RD, Kubota K, Pearce G, et al. Salmeterol: a study by prescription-event monitoring in a UK cohort of 15,407 patients. *J Clin Epidemiol.* 1996;49:247–250.
44. Weinberger M, Hendeles L. Theophylline in asthma. *N Engl J Med.* 1996;334:1380–1388.
45. Hendeles L, Harman E, Huang D, et al. Theophylline attenuation of airway responses to allergen: comparison with cromolyn metered-dose inhaler. *J Allergy Clin Immunol.* 1995;95:505–514.
46. Kidney J, Dominguez M, Taylor PM, et al. Immunodilation by theophylline in asthma. *Am J Respir Crit Care Med.* 1995;151:1907–1914.
47. Malmstrom K, Rodriguez-Gomez G, Guerra J, et al. Oral montelukast, inhaled beclomethasone, and placebo for chronic asthma. A randomized, controlled trial. Montelukast/Beclomethasone Study Group. *Arch Intern Med.* 1999;130:487–495.
48. Spector SI, Smith LJ, Glass M. Effects of 6 weeks of therapy with oral doses of ICI 204,219, a leukotriene D4 receptor antagonist, in subjects with bronchial asthma. *Am J Respir Crit Care Med.* 1994;150:618–623.
49. Israel E, Cohen J, Dube L, et al. Effects of treatment with zileuton, a 5-lipoxygenase inhibitor, in patients with asthma. *JAMA.* 1996;275:931–936.
50. Karpel JP, Schacter EN, Fanta C, et al. A comparison of ipratropium and albuterol vs albuterol alone for the treatment of acute asthma. *Chest.* 1996;110:611–616.
51. FitzGerald JM, Grunfeld A, Pare PD, et al. The clinical efficacy of combination nebulized anticholinergic and adrenergic bronchodilators vs nebulized adrenergic bronchodilator alone in acute asthma. Canadian Combivent Study Group. *Chest.* 1997;111:311–315.

52. McFadden ER Jr, el Sanadi N, Strauss L, et al. The influence of parasympatholytics on the resolution of acute attacks of asthma. *Am J Med.* 1997;102:7–13.
53. Lanes SF, Garrett JE, Wentworth CE, et al. The effect of adding ipratropium bromide to salbutamol in the treatment of acute asthma: a pooled analysis of three trials. *Chest.* 1998;114:365–372.
54. Ducharme FM, Davis GM. Randomized controlled trial of ipratropium bromide and frequent low doses of salbutamol in the management of mild and moderate acute pediatric asthma. *J Pediatr.* 1998;133:479–485.
55. Qureshi F, Pestian J, Davis P, et al. Effect of nebulized ipratropium on the hospitalization rates of children with asthma. *N Engl J Med.* 1998;339:1030–1035.
56. Connett GJ, Warde C, Wooler E, et al. Prednisolone and salbutamol in the hospital treatment of acute asthma. *Arch Dis Child.* 1993;70:170–173.
57. Hess DR. Aerosol delivery devices in the treatment of asthma. *Respir Care.* 2008;53:699–725.
58. Raimondi AC, Schottlender J, Lombardi D, et al. Treatment of acute asthma with inhaled albuterol delivered via jet nebulizer, metered dose inhaler with spacer, or dry powder. *Chest.* 1997;112:24–28.
59. Kim IK, Saville AL, Sikes KL, Corcoran TE. Heliox-driven albuterol nebulization for asthma exacerbations: an overview. *Respir Care.* 2006;51:613–618.
60. Myers TR. Use of heliox in children. *Respir Care.* 2006;51:619–631.
61. Dolovich MB, Ahrens RC, Hess DR, et al. Device selection and outcomes of aerosol therapy: evidence-based guidelines. *Chest.* 2005;127:335–371.
62. Hess DR, Acosta FL, Ritz RH, et al. The effect of heliox on nebulizer function using a beta-agonist bronchodilator. *Chest.* 1999;115:184–189.
63. Hess DR, Fink JB, Venkataraman ST, et al. The history and physics of heliox. *Respir Care.* 2006;51:608–612.
64. Hoffman L, Smithline H. Comparison of Circulaire to conventional small volume nebulizer for the treatment of bronchospasm in the emergency department. *Respir Care.* 1997;42:1170–1174.
65. Hess D, Fisher D, Williams P, et al. Medication nebulizer performance. Effects of diluent volume, nebulizer flow, and nebulizer brand. *Chest.* 1996;110:498–505.
66. O'Callaghan CO, Barry PW. The science of nebulised drug delivery. *Thorax.* 1997;52:S31–S44.
67. Camargo CA Jr, Spooner CH, Rowe BH. Continuous versus intermittent beta-agonists in the treatment of acute asthma. *Cochrane Database Syst Rev.* 2003;CD001115.
68. Newman SP. Principles of metered-dose inhaler design. *Respir Care.* 2005;50:1177–1190.
69. Barry PW, O'Callaghan C. Inhalational drug delivery from seven different spacer devices. *Thorax.* 1996;51:835–840.
70. Tobias JD. Heliox in children with airway obstruction. *Pediatr Emerg Care.* 1997;13:29–32.
71. Kudukis TM, Manthous CA, Schmidt GA, et al. Inhaled helium-oxygen revisited: effect of inhaled helium-oxygen during the treatment of status asthmaticus in children. *J Pediatr.* 1997;130:217–224.
72. Kass JE, Castriotta RJ. Heliox therapy in acute severe asthma. *Chest.* 1995;107:757–760.
73. Carter ER, Webb CR, Moffitt DR. Evaluation of heliox in children hospitalized with acute severe asthma. A randomized crossover trial. *Chest.* 1996;109:1256–1261.
74. Verbeek PR, Chopra A. Heliox does not improve FEV_1 in acute asthma patients. *J Emerg Med.* 1998;16:545–548.
75. Kass JE, Castratta RJ. Heliox therapy in acute severe asthma. *Chest.* 1995;107:757.
76. Kass JE, Terregino CA. The effect of heliox in acute severe asthma: a randomized controlled trial. *Chest.* 1999;116:296–300.
77. Ciarallo L, Sauer AH, Shannon MW. Intravenous magnesium therapy for moderate to severe pediatric asthma: results of a randomized placebo-controlled trial. *J Pediatr.* 1996;129:809–814.
78. Bloch H, Silverman R, Mancherje N, et al. Intravenous magnesium sulfate as an adjunct in the treatment of acute asthma. *Chest.* 1995;107:1576–1581.
79. Mangat HS, D'Souza GA, Jacob MS. Nebulized magnesium sulphate versus nebulized salbutamol in acute bronchial asthma: a clinical trial. *Eur Respir J.* 1998;12:341–344.
80. Hill J, Britton J. Dose-response relationship and time-course of the effect of inhaled magnesium sulphate on airflow in normal and asthmatic subjects. *Br J Clin Pharmacol.* 1995;40:539–544.
81. Bernstein WK, Khastgir T, Khastgir A, et al. Lack of effectiveness of magnesium in chronic stable asthma. A prospective, randomized, double-blind, placebo-controlled, crossover trial in normal subjects and in patients with chronic stable asthma. *Arch Intern Med.* 1995;155:271–276.
82. Meduir GU, et al. Noninvasive positive pressure ventilation in status asthmaticus. *Chest.* 1996;110:767–774.
83. Teague GW, Fortenberry JD. Noninvasive ventilator support in pediatric respiratory failure. *Respir Care.* 1995;40:86–95.
84. Pollack C, Fleisch K, Dowsey K. Treatment of acute bronchospasm with beta-adrenergic agonist aerosols delivered by a nasal bilevel positive airway pressure circuit. *Ann Emerg Med.* 1995;26:552–557.
85. Medoff BD. Invasive and noninvasive ventilation in patients with asthma. *Respir Care.* 2008;53(6):740–748.
86. Marquette CH, Saulnier F, Leroy O, et al. Long-term prognosis of new fatal asthma. A 6-year follow-up of 145 asthmatic patients who underwent mechanical ventilation. *Am Rev Respir Dis.* 1992;146:76–81.
87. Leatherman J. Life-threatening asthma. *Clin Chest Med.* 1994;15:453–479.
88. Feihl F, Perret C. Permissive hypercapnia: how permissive should we be? *Am J Respir Crit Care Med.* 1994;150:1722–1737.
89. Darioli R, Perret C. Mechanical controlled hypoventilation in status asthmaticus. *Am Rev Respir Dis.* 1984;129:385–387.
90. Ranieri VM, Grasso S, Fiore T, et al. Auto-positive end-expiratory pressure and dynamic hyperinflation. *Clin Chest Med.* 1996;17:379–394.
91. Tuxen DV, Williams TJ, Scheinkestel CD, et al. Use of a measurement of pulmonary hyperinflation to control the level of mechanical ventilation in patient with acute severe asthma. *Am Rev Resp Dis.* 1992;146:1136–1142.
92. Caramez MP, Borges JB, Tucci MR, et al. Paradoxical responses to positive end-expiratory pressure in patients with airway obstruction during controlled ventilation. *Crit Care Med.* 2005;33:1519–1528.
93. Leatherman JW, Ravenscraft SA. Low measured auto-positive end-expiratory pressure during mechanical ventilation of patients with severe asthma: hidden auto-positive end-expiratory pressure. *Crit Care Med.* 1996;24:541–546.
94. Dhand R. Bronchodilator therapy in mechanically ventilated patients: patient selection and clinical outcomes. *Respir Care.* 2007;52:152–153.
95. Douglass JA, Tuxen DV, Horne M, et al. Myopathy in severe asthma. *Am Rev Respir Dis.* 1992;146:517–519.
96. Levy BD, Kitch B, Fanta CH. Medical and ventilatory management of status asthmaticus. *Intensive Care Med.* 1998;24:105–117.
97. Jain S, Hanania NA, Guntupalli KK. Ventilation of patients with asthma and obstructive lung disease. *Crit Care Clin.* 1998;14:685–705.
98. Trautner C, Richter B, Berger M. Cost-effectiveness of a structured treatment and teaching programme on asthma. *Eur Respir J.* 1993;6:1485–1491.
99. Wade S, Weil C, Holden G, et al. Psychosocial characteristics of inner-city children with asthma: a description of the NCICAS psychosocial protocol. National Cooperative Inner-City Asthma Study. *Pediatr Pulmonol.* 1997;24:263–276.
100. Wade SL, Islam S, Holden G, et al. Division of responsibility for asthma management tasks between caregivers and children in the inner city. *Dev Behav Pediatr.* 1999;20:93–98.

CHAPTER 35

Chronic Obstructive Pulmonary Disease

John E. Heffner

OUTLINE

Burden of Chronic Obstructive Pulmonary Disease
Definitions and Staging of Disease
Etiology of Chronic Obstructive Pulmonary Disease
Pathophysiology of Chronic Obstructive Pulmonary Disease
Diagnosis and Clinical Course
Outpatient Care of Stable Chronic Obstructive Pulmonary Disease
Surgery
Overview of Management of Stable Chronic Obstructive Pulmonary Disease
Managing Exacerbations
Palliative and End-of-Life Care
Case Studies

OBJECTIVES

1. Define chronic obstructive pulmonary disease (COPD).
2. Describe the epidemiology, pathogenesis, and pathophysiology of COPD.
3. Compare therapeutic strategies for stable patients and patients experiencing an exacerbation in the ambulatory or inpatient setting.
4. Discuss the surgical approaches to improve lung function in COPD.
5. Identify important aspects of palliative and end-of-life care for patients with COPD.

KEY TERMS

air trapping
α_1-antitrypsin deficiency (AAT)
antibiotics
anticholinergic agent
bullae
bullectomy
chronic bronchitis
chronic obstructive pulmonary disease (COPD)
corticosteroids
dynamic airway compression
dynamic hyperinflation
dyspnea
elastic recoil
emphysema
exacerbation
hyperinflation
intrinsic positive end-expiratory pressure (auto-PEEP)
long-acting β_2-agonists
long-acting muscarinic antagonists (LAMA)
long-term oxygen therapy (LTOT)
lung transplantation
lung volume reduction surgery (LVRS)
methylxanthines
mucokinetic agents
noninvasive positive pressure ventilation (NIV)
pulmonary rehabilitation
short-acting β_2-agonists
sleep apnea hypopnea syndrome (SAHS)
smoking cessation

INTRODUCTION

Chronic obstructive pulmonary disease (COPD) has emerged as a major health condition worldwide, with 80 million people affected. In the United States, more than 12 million people carry a diagnosis of COPD and an equal number have the disease but have not yet been diagnosed.[1]

This chapter provides a general discussion of the diagnosis and care of patients with COPD, with an emphasis on practical elements of management. It centers on the premise that respiratory therapists have the needed expertise to intercede at all stages of COPD to improve patients' functional status, quality of life, and the outcome of their disease.

Burden of Chronic Obstructive Pulmonary Disease

In both the United States and in the world, COPD is the fourth most common cause of death and will increase in prevalence worldwide by 30% within the next 10 years.[2] The estimated prevalence of COPD varies from 7% to 19% in epidemiologic studies.[3] In 2002, the direct and indirect costs of COPD in the United States amounted to $32 billion.[4] Unfortunately, COPD remains underdiagnosed in the United States. Many patients with long-term respiratory symptoms due to COPD first receive a diagnosis when they have far-advanced disease.[5]

Regardless of the stage of the disease, COPD has important effects on health status. Early symptomatic disease decreases exercise capacity, causes work absenteeism, and interferes with vigorous lifestyle pursuits. More advanced COPD increases the risk of pneumonia, heart disease, metabolic syndrome, and lung cancer.[6] The association of COPD with dysfunction of body systems and organs other than the lung has reclassified COPD from a disorder of the lungs to a chronic condition characterized by systemic inflammation and degenerative effects on multiple organs that adversely affect the entire patient.[7] Patients with severe COPD suffer from major limitations in activities of daily living and may experience progressive cachexia. Because of the chronic nature of COPD and its typically relentless progression, few conditions present such long-term and disabling burdens for personal health and well-being.

Definitions and Staging of Disease

The term *chronic obstructive pulmonary disease (COPD)* refers to a group of preventable and treatable disorders characterized by progressive airflow limitation that is not fully reversible by bronchodilator or anti-inflammatory therapy.[8] Airflow limitation is associated with an abnormal inflammatory response of the lungs to noxious particles or gases, especially cigarette smoking.[8] COPD also produces systemic inflammation and important nonpulmonary consequences, such as cachexia, skeletal muscle dysfunction, cardiovascular disease, osteoporosis, depression, fatigue, and cancer. The airflow limitation is caused by a combination of destruction of lung parenchyma (emphysema) and small airways disease (obstructive bronchiolitis), with the relative proportions of each varying in individual patients.[8] Other specific causes of chronic airflow limitation, such as cystic fibrosis, asthma, bronchiolitis obliterans, and bronchiectasis, are not categorized as types of COPD.

RESPIRATORY RECAP

Definition of COPD

- COPD refers to a group of preventable and treatable disorders characterized by progressive airflow limitation that is not fully reversible by bronchodilator or anti-inflammatory therapy.
- The term *chronic bronchitis* is less preferred because it incorrectly limits its focus to inflammatory changes observed in pathologic examinations of central (bronchi) airways.
- Some degree of emphysema occurs in nearly all patients with COPD.
- Expiratory airflow limitation is defined by an FEV_1/FVC less than 0.70.

The broad term *airway disease* is used to define the pathologic and physiologic abnormalities observed in airways of patients with COPD because these changes occur both in central (bronchi) and small (bronchioles) airways. The historical categorical term **chronic bronchitis** is less preferred because it incorrectly limits its focus to inflammatory changes observed in pathologic examinations of central (bronchi) airways. *Chronic bronchitis* presents additional confusion because it defines a clinical condition wherein patients have a productive cough for at least 3 months of the year for 2 or more successive years. Some patients with chronic bronchitis diagnosed clinically may not have spirometric evidence of airflow obstruction and therefore do not fulfill the definition of COPD. The newer terminology of *airway disease* recognizes that mucus hypersecretion occurs in the proximal airways, but that the site of increased airway resistance in COPD is in the peripheral, small airways, where inflammation results in fibrosis and airway distortion.[9] The specific causative factors of airflow limitation in peripheral airways, however, have not been clearly defined, as indicated by the poor correlation between pathologic changes observed in the bronchioles and the degree of measured airflow limitation.

Some degree of **emphysema** occurs in nearly all patients with COPD, although the extent of emphysema observed varies widely between patients. *Emphysema* is a pathologic and not a clinical term. Emphysema is detected by histopathologic examination of lung tissue or by imaging studies, such as high-resolution computed tomography (HRCT), that can detect emphysema-related pathologic changes.[10] It has been defined by an expert panel as "a condition characterized by abnormal enlargement of the airspaces distal to the terminal bronchiole, accompanied by destruction of their walls, and without obvious fibrosis"[11] (**Figure 35–1**). This irreversible airspace enlargement occurs in the alveolar, alveolar duct, and respiratory bronchiolar regions of the lung where gas exchange occurs. Structural abnormalities in these regions cause uneven distribution of ventilation and hypoxemia, hypercapnia, and decreased lung diffusion as measured by the diffusing capacity for carbon monoxide (DLCO). Airspace enlargements larger than 1 cm in diameter are termed **bullae** (**Figure 35–2**). Bullae can progressively enlarge and compress adjacent lung tissue, further impairing respiratory function. Emphysema contributes to airflow limitation by decreasing lung elastic recoil. During exhalation, positive intrathoracic pressure compresses airways that are no longer tethered open by surrounding normal lung tissue. This process is termed **dynamic airway compression**, which results in **air trapping** and **hyperinflation** (**Figure 35–3**).

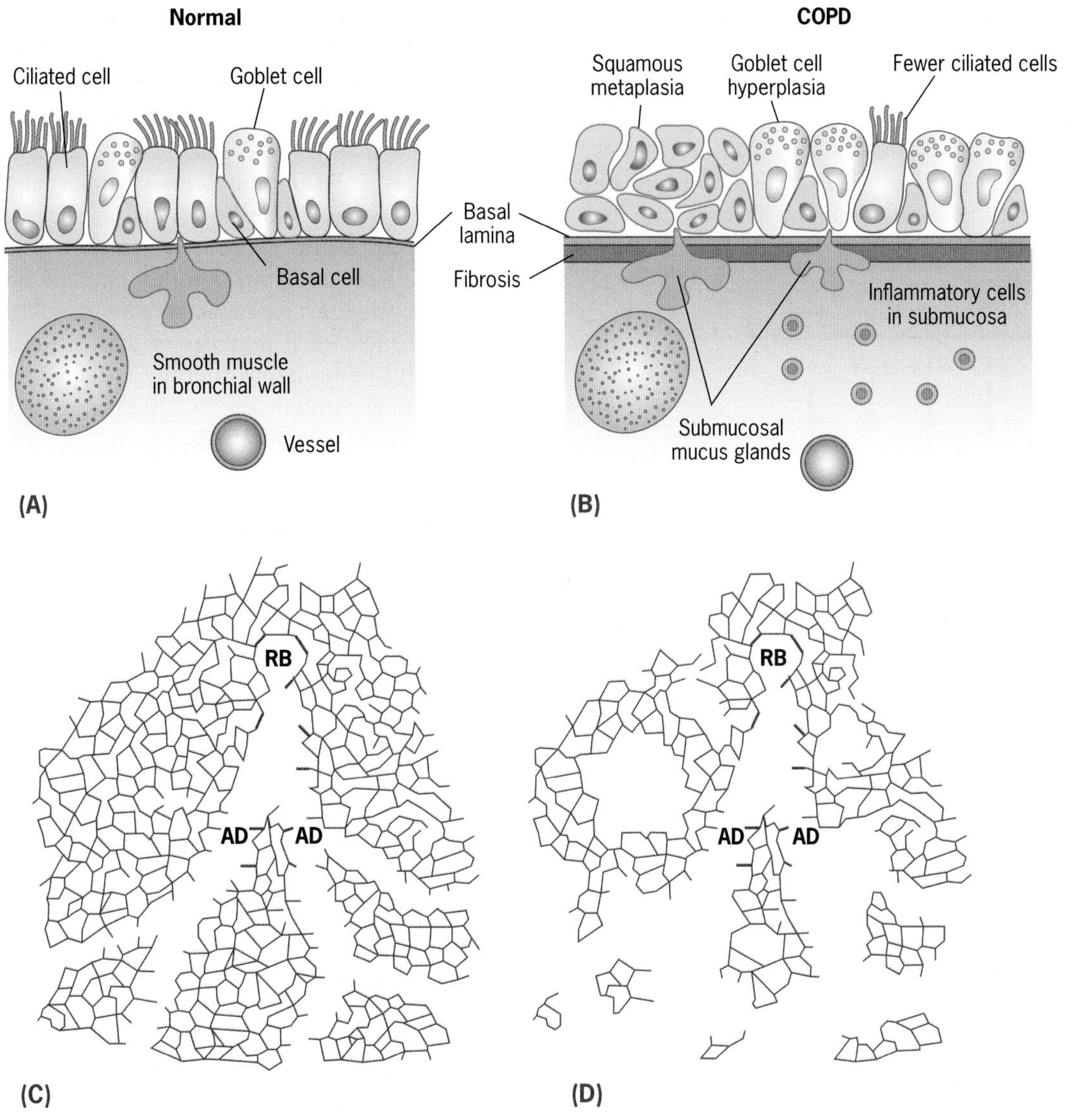

FIGURE 35–1 Schematic models showing the airways and lung parenchyma of normal individuals (**A** and **C**) and patients with COPD (**B** and **D**). Airways in COPD patients are characterized by hyperplasia of surface mucous cells, enlargement of tracheobronchial submucosal glands, excess mucus, loss of cilia and ciliary dyskinesia, and the presence of inflammatory cells. Compared with patients with normal lungs (**C**), patients with COPD have permanently enlarged airspaces distal to terminal bronchioles caused by alveolar wall destruction (**D**). RB, respiratory bronchioles; AD, alveolar ducts.

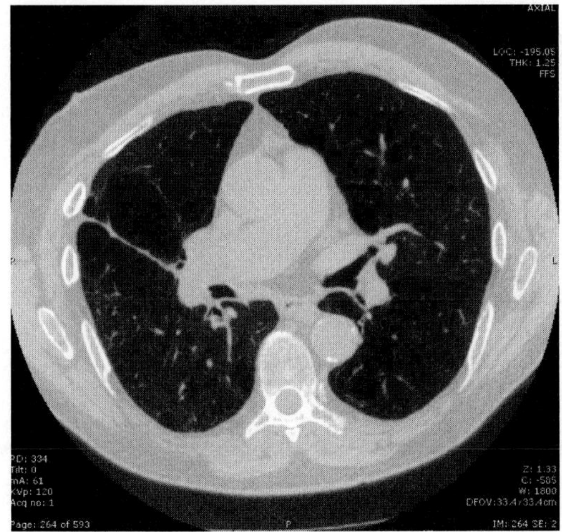

FIGURE 35–2 Computed tomography scan of a patient with severe emphysema. Note the multiple bullae throughout the lung parenchyma, which appears hyperlucent, indicating generalized loss of lung tissue and hyperinflation.

Hyperinflation with increased lung volumes may be apparent on chest radiographs (**Figure 35–4**) and chest computed tomography (CT) scans.

Limitation of maximal expiratory flow rate represents the cardinal abnormality associated with COPD and serves both to diagnose the presence of the disease and stage its severity. Simple spirometric measures of post-bronchodilator forced expiratory volume in the first second of expiration (FEV_1) and the ratio of FEV_1 to forced vital capacity (FEV_1/FVC) provide the best measures of expiratory airflow limitation, with airflow obstruction defined by an FEV_1/FVC less than 0.70,[8] which is an abnormal finding in nearly all age groups. This FEV_1/FVC threshold, however, may overdiagnose COPD in elderly subjects because of the normally observed decrease in lung volumes and airflows with aging. The clinical practice guidelines of the Global Alliance for Chronic Obstructive Pulmonary Disease (GOLD) use spirometric values to classify the severity of COPD into four stages (**Table 35–1**).[8]

Spirometric values of FEV_1 and FVC alone, however, do not correlate well with severity of dyspnea and functional performance, survival, or response to therapy. Because hyperinflation has important effects on lung function, lung volume measurements, such as the ratio of the inspiratory capacity to the total lung capacity, are better predictors of survival than FEV_1. It has recently been recognized that the systemic nonpulmonary manifestations of COPD have important effects on prognosis. Multidimensional measures of dyspnea, body mass, and functional levels, which capture effects of these systemic manifestations, predict survival and response to therapy more accurately than FEV_1. The BODE index (body mass index, airflow obstruction, dyspnea, and exercise capacity) provides clinicians with a multidimensional measure of disease severity, prognosis, and response to therapy (**Table 35–2**).[12] Some experts now combine the BODE index with spirometry to stage COPD (**Table 35–3**).

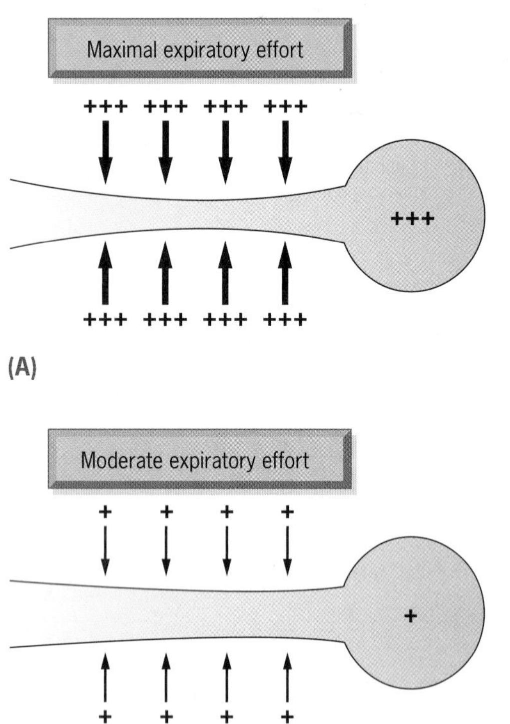

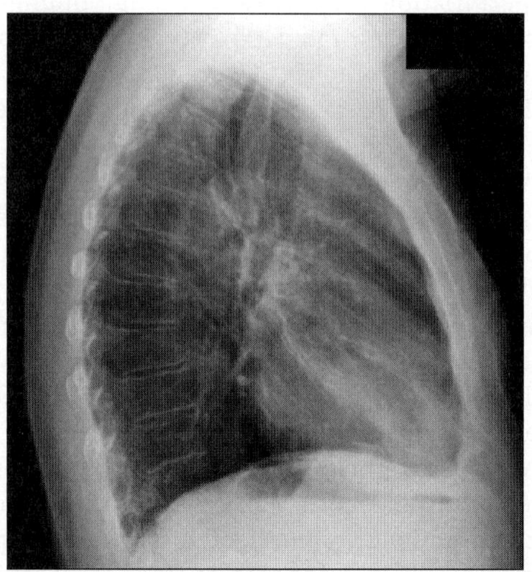

FIGURE 35–3 Schematic model demonstrating the morphologic changes associated with dynamic airway compression in patients with COPD. The loss of parenchymal tethering external to airways causes airway collapse during forced expiration. Maximal expiratory effort (**A**) creates more compressing pressure around airways and produces more dynamic compression as compared with moderate expiratory effort (**B**).

Etiology of Chronic Obstructive Pulmonary Disease

Epidemiologic and experimental evidence demonstrates that smoking is the major cause of COPD.[13] Nonsmokers, however, may also develop COPD when exposed to other risk factors,[14,15] which include passive exposure to cigarette smoke[16] and nontobacco inhalational factors such as occupational dusts and chemicals and both indoor and outdoor air pollution.

Because not all smokers develop clinically apparent COPD, genetic factors must modify risk from tobacco inhalation. The best characterized genetic risk factor for COPD is **α_1-antitrypsin (AAT) deficiency**. This condition is a hereditary defect that occurs almost entirely in whites and results from abnormal function or insufficient production of AAT.[17] Patients with AAT deficiency demonstrate an abnormal antiprotease response to proinflammatory effects of tobacco smoke. The resultant activation of proteases and toxic oxygen metabolites results in accelerated lung destruction and emphysema in early life. Individuals with AAT may remain healthy throughout their lives, but even nonsmokers with AAT

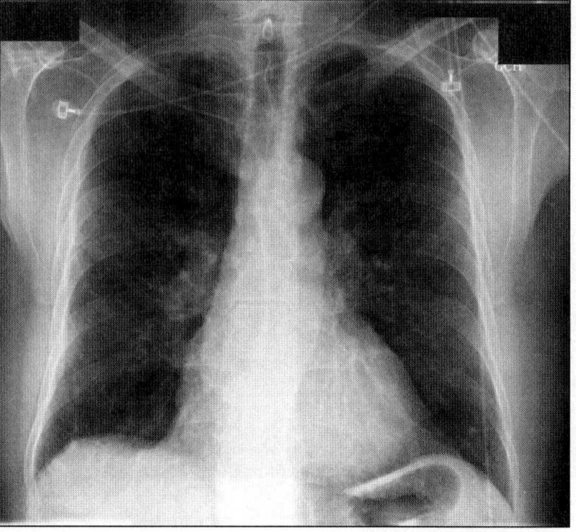

FIGURE 35–4 Chest radiograph of a patient with emphysema showing hyperinflation as evidenced by the flattening of the diaphragms, best observed on the lateral view, and hyperlucent lung fields.

TABLE 35-1 Spirometric Classification of COPD Severity Based on Postbronchodilator FEV_1

Stage I: Mild	$FEV_1/FVC < 0.70$ $FEV_1 \geq 80\%$ predicted
Stage II: Moderate	$FEV_1/FVC < 0.70$ $50\% \leq FEV_1 < 80\%$ predicted
Stage III: Severe	$FEV_1/FVC < 0.70$ $30\% \leq FEV_1 < 50\%$ predicted
Stage IV: Very severe	$FEV_1/FVC < 0.70$ $FEV_1 < 30\%$ predicted *or* $FEV_1 < 50\%$ predicted plus chronic respiratory failure

FEV_1, forced expiratory volume in 1 second; FVC, forced vital capacity. Respiratory failure is defined as a Pa_{O_2} less than 60 mm Hg with or without a Pa_{CO_2} greater than 50 mm Hg while breathing air at sea level.

TABLE 35-2 BODE Index

	Points on BODE Index			
Variable	*0*	*1*	*2*	*3*
FEV_1 (% predicted)	>65	50–64	36–49	≤ 35
Distance walked in 6 minutes (m)	>350	250–349	150–249	≤149
MMRC dyspnea scale*	0–1	2	3	4
Body mass index	>21	<21		

The total possible values range from 0 to 10. *Scores on the modified Medical Research Council (MMRC) dyspnea scale can range from 0 to 4, with a score of 4 indicating that the patient is too breathless to leave the house or becomes breathless when dressing or undressing. FEV_1, forced expiratory volume in 1 second.

TABLE 35-3 Classification of COPD Severity Based on BODE Index and Spirometry

At risk	$FEV_1/FVC < 0.70$ $FEV_1 \geq 80\%$ predicted
Mild	$FEV_1/FVC < 0.70$ $FEV_1 < 80\%$ predicted BODE index 0–2
Moderate	$FEV_1/FVC < 0.70$ $FEV_1 < 80\%$ predicted BODE index 3–4
Severe	$FEV_1/FVC < 0.70$ $FEV_1 < 80\%$ predicted BODE Index 5-6
Very severe	$FEV_1/FVC < 0.70$ $FEV_1 < 80\%$ predicted BODE index 7–10

FEV_1, forced expiratory volume in 1 second; FVC: forced vital capacity; BODE, body mass index, airflow obstruction, dyspnea, and exercise capacity.

Modified with permission from Celli BR. Update on the management of COPD. *Chest.* 2008;133:1451–1462.

deficiency may develop COPD symptoms, usually late in life. The most common abnormal gene for AAT is the Z allele. Normal genes are labeled M. The most common genotype associated with AAT is ZZ (also referred to as PiZ). There are about 100,000 people with the ZZ phenotype in the United States.

Males and females have an equivalent prevalence of COPD, although some studies suggest a greater risk of COPD among women smokers.[18] Prevalence of COPD is greater in smokers with lower socioeconomic status,[19] but this observation may result from associated differences in living conditions, exposure to environmental toxins, or smoking behaviors.[20] Various occupational dusts, including coal and grain dusts; air pollution; indoor air pollution caused by cooking fuels or cigarette smoke; and childhood respiratory infections are additional risk factors for the development of COPD.

Pathophysiology of Chronic Obstructive Pulmonary Disease

Recognition of the pathogenetic importance of impaired antiprotease defenses in AAT deficiency led to the protease–antiprotease theory for the etiology of smoking-related COPD. In this model, smoking and other noxious inhalants overwhelm the lungs' antioxidant and antiprotease defense mechanisms, allowing proteolytic digestion of lung tissue. Recently, different COPD-like phenotypes have been generated in animal models by targeting the immune system or causing disturbances of apoptotic control in pulmonary endothelium.[21] These observations have expanded the pathophysiologic understanding of COPD beyond protease–antiprotease mechanisms to include multiple immunogenetic disturbances that can combine in varying ways to produce unique COPD phenotypes in different patients. The convergence of these different mechanisms may explain why the COPD population has diverse clinical expressions.

The cardinal structural abnormalities that produce respiratory symptoms and functional limitations in COPD occur in the central and peripheral airways and the lung parenchyma. The central airways are the site of most of the increased mucus production in patients who raise excess sputum and carry the clinical diagnosis of chronic bronchitis. Mucous glands below the epithelial basement

RESPIRATORY RECAP

Pathophysiology of COPD

- » Most of the increase in airways resistance occurs in peripheral airways.
- » Loss of pulmonary elasticity is due to destruction of alveolar structures.
- » Decreased diameter of airways lowers the maximum expiratory airflow at all lung volumes.
- » Flow limitation results in dynamic hyperinflation.
- » Lung volume is more closely associated with dyspnea and functional limitation than spirometry.

membrane in central airways secrete mucus that serves in health as a mechanical host defense mechanism against environmental particulate inhalants. Some, but not all, patients with COPD have moderate enlargement of mucous glands,[22] which correlates directly with cough and sputum production. Mucus-secreting goblet cells are nested among epithelial cells along all segments of the conducting airways. Descriptive studies suggest that goblet cells may expand in number in the central airways of patients with COPD and contribute to excess mucus production. Ciliary dyskinesia, loss of cilia, and epithelial metaplasia have also been observed in central airways (refer to Figure 35–1). Inflammation is present in the form of neutrophils, macrophages, and lymphocytes within the epithelium and submucosa of central airways and neutrophils and eosinophils within airway secretions.[23] Eosinophils are found in the airway submucosa during exacerbations of COPD. Nodules rich in both T and B cells develop in regions of abnormal lung tissue, lending support to an immunogenic etiology to COPD.[24] Altered T- and B-cell responses are also observed in the peripheral blood, indicating the systemic nature of the disease and the presence of immunodysregulation in nonpulmonary organs.[25]

In normal lungs, most of the resistance to airflow occurs in peripheral small airways.[26] In COPD, most of the increase in airway resistance similarly occurs in peripheral airways, where multiple pathologic changes occur. Early in the course of COPD, brown-pigmented macrophages aggregate in respiratory bronchioles. As COPD progresses, a low-grade inflammatory response develops in membranous bronchioles, characterized by a modest influx of neutrophils, macrophages, and lymphocytes. In some patients, smooth muscle enlargement, minimal fibrosis, squamous cell metaplasia of airway epithelial cells, and goblet cell metaplasia develop. These changes combined with abnormalities of smooth muscle and connective tissue result in a narrowed caliber of the airway lumen both from a thickening of airway walls and a decrease in cross-sectional total airway diameter.

Although these pathologic abnormalities in peripheral airways contribute to the expiratory airflow limitation observed in COPD, they do not entirely explain the increased airway resistance. Other contributory factors, such as the loss of airway tethering caused by decreased elastic recoil of the lung parenchyma, airway secretions, changes in the properties of airway lining fluid, and smooth muscle contraction, interact in complex and poorly understood ways.[27] Among these factors, loss of elastic recoil plays an important role.

The term **elastic recoil** refers to the lung's natural tendency to deflate after inspiration. It is expressed by plotting lung volume as a function of transpulmonary pressure. **Figure 35–5** shows the comparative pressure–volume curves of a normal adult and a patient with emphysema. With loss of pulmonary elasticity from destruction of alveolar and interstitial structures, the

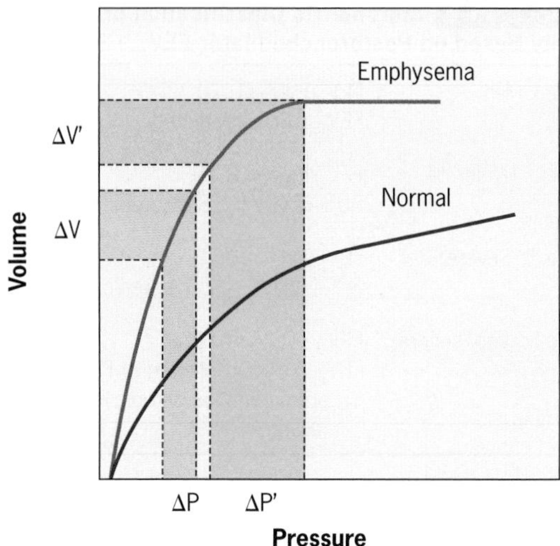

FIGURE 35–5 Volume–pressure relationships of individuals with normal lungs and patients with emphysema. Patients with emphysema experience a small increase in pressure (ΔP) with an increase in volume (ΔV) while breathing at low lung volumes. In contrast, patients with emphysema have large increases in pressure (ΔP′) for a similar change in volume (ΔV′) when breathing at high lung volumes, at which point their lungs become hyperinflated and stiff. Patients with emphysema have heterogeneous distribution of emphysema, so that normal regions of lung follow the normal volume–pressure curve and emphysematous regions follow the emphysema curve.

patient with emphysema has increased lung compliance, as shown by a shift of the pressure–volume curve up and to the left. Increased lung compliance results in an attenuation of the tethering effect that normal lung parenchyma has on airways to resist airway narrowing during expiration. Consequently, the airways of patients with COPD decrease in caliber and resist expiratory airflow to a greater degree than normal (refer to Figure 35–3). Consequently, dynamic airway compression occurs during expiration as patients contract expiratory muscles and increase intrathoracic pressure, which is transmitted to the external walls of conducting airways.

Figure 35–6 shows the effects of dynamic airway compression on expiratory flows in normal and emphysematous lungs. Positive intra-airway pressures relative to negative intrathoracic pressures (external to airways) during inspiration keep airways open and support the normal linear relationship between flow and alveolar pressure for both normal and emphysematous lungs. During forced expiration, however, dynamic airway compression alters this linear relationship and causes expiratory flow to reach a maximal value (plateau) that does not increase with additional expiratory effort. This plateau representing expiratory airflow limitation is reached earlier for patients with emphysema. If they increase expiratory effort further, increases in intrathoracic pressure are applied to external airway walls, decreasing airway caliber and raising airway resistance, which prevents any further increase in airflow.

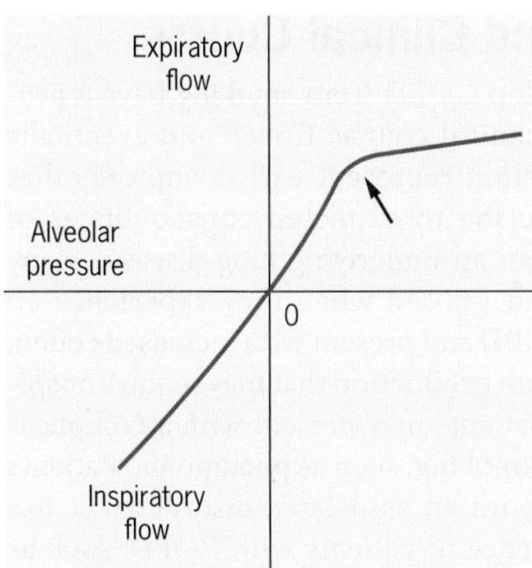

FIGURE 35–6 Relationship of flow to pressure during inspiration and expiration at a given lung volume. This relationship is linear during inspiration, but dynamic airway compression (arrow) causes expiratory flow to reach an early maximal value that does not increase with further increases in alveolar pressure.

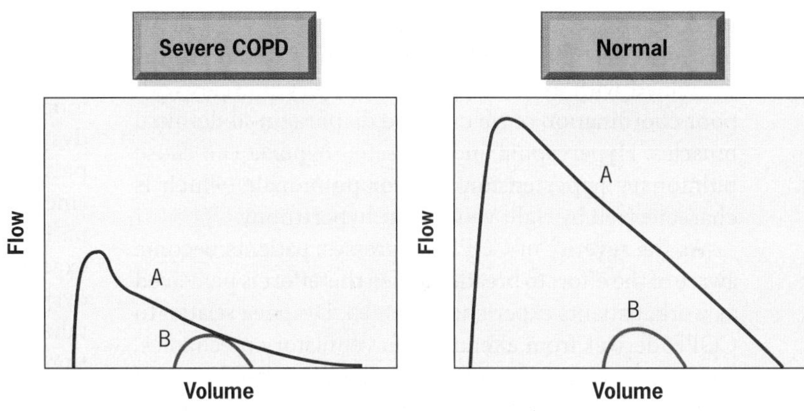

FIGURE 35–7 Expiratory flow–volume curves of a patient with severe COPD compared with an individual with normal lungs. The patient with COPD reaches maximal expiratory airflow during tidal breathing. A, forced vital capacity; B, tidal breathing.

Expiratory flow–volume curves present a visual image of these relationships (**Figure 35–7**). Individuals with normal lung function increase their expiratory airflow during forced expiratory maneuvers until dynamic airway compression occurs, at which point airflow does not increase with increased effort. During tidal breathing, expiratory airflow is much lower than during a maximal, forced expiration, indicating that patients in good health have considerable ventilatory reserve available for increasing minute ventilation ($\dot{V}_E$).

In patients with COPD, decreased diameter of conducting airways lowers the maximal expiratory airflow and airflow at all lung volumes compared with normal individuals. Because of the loss of lung elasticity and the collapsibility of airways in patients with emphysema, dynamic airway compression occurs at lower intrathoracic pressures. In patients with severe COPD, maximal airflow may be reached during minimal exercise and eventually at resting tidal breathing (refer to Figure 35–7). When maximal airflow is reached during tidal breathing, patients faced with increased ventilatory demands from exercise cannot increase airflow to recruit a larger tidal volume (V_T). To respond to exercise demands, therefore, they must raise $\dot{V}_E$ by generating higher respiratory rates. An increased respiratory rate decreases expiratory time, which promotes air trapping and increased intrathoracic pressures and further aggravates dynamic airway compression.[28]

As air trapping progresses, intra-alveolar pressure at end-expiration may remain positive rather than equilibrating with ambient pressure as occurs in healthy patients. This condition is termed **intrinsic positive end-expiratory pressure (auto-PEEP)**. Auto-PEEP places an inspiratory threshold load that increases the work of breathing because patients must contract inspiratory muscles to negate auto-PEEP before they can create the necessary negative alveolar pressure that initiates inspiration. These changes result in patients breathing with a decreased V_T and increased respiratory rates at higher lung volumes. Higher lung volumes at end-expiration increase the inspiratory work of breathing because patients must overcome the increased elasticity of the chest wall and lungs that begin inspiration in an already expanded anatomic configuration.

Hyperinflation is assessed by measuring lung volumes, which demonstrate increased total lung capacity (TLC), functional residual capacity (FRC), and residual volume (RV) in patients with COPD. As FEV_1 and FVC decrease with progressive COPD, a corresponding increase in lung volumes occur that maintains a close correlation.[29]

The severity of emphysema and airflow limitation in small airways varies between different regions of the lung. This heterogeneity causes regional variations in the distribution of ventilation, which results in mismatching of ventilation and perfusion. Although emphysematous regions of the lung are underventilated, perfusion is more severely decreased, so that ventilation-perfusion ratios ($\dot{V}/\dot{Q}$) increase. Consequently, emphysematous regions of the lung have increased dead space that causes hypoxemia and hypercapnia. In other regions of the lung, increased resistance or partial obstruction of airways that ventilate relatively normal alveolocapillary units generates decreased $\dot{V}/\dot{Q}$ ratios that cause venous admixture and hypoxemia. The combination of lung regions with high and low $\dot{V}/\dot{Q}$ alters gas exchange and places demands on the ventilatory capacity of patients, thereby increasing respiratory work.[30] Worsening $\dot{V}/\dot{Q}$ abnormalities eventually result in hypoxemia and, if ventilation is markedly impaired, hypercapnia, both of which are associated with a poor prognosis in patients with COPD. Shunts are notably absent in stable COPD, indicating the efficiency of collateral ventilation and hypoxic pulmonary vasoconstriction and the absence of complete airway obstruction.

Patients with COPD also experience abnormalities in the coordination of respiratory muscle function. During exercise and voluntary hyperventilation, patients demonstrate early fatigue of the exercising muscle groups combined with asynchrony of respiratory muscles with poor coordination of rib cage and diaphragm-abdominal muscles. Hypercapnia and untreated hypoxia can cause pulmonary hypertension and cor pulmonale, which is characterized by right ventricular hypertrophy.

As the severity of COPD progresses, patients become aware of the effort to breathe. When this effort is perceived as work, patients experience **dyspnea**. Dyspnea related to COPD derives from alterations in ventilatory mechanics. Patients with early COPD and mildly increased airflow limitation respond to abnormalities in gas exchange by increasing their respiratory drive and $\dot{V}E$ through recruitment of a larger VT to normalize PCO_2 and PO_2. With more severe disease, increasing VT causes too much work of breathing, so $\dot{V}E$ is maintained through an increase in respiratory rate. To increase respiratory rate, patients must shorten their inspiratory time (TI), resulting in a decreased fractional duration of inspiration (TI/Tot) and an increased mean inspiratory flow rate (VT/TI).

An increased respiratory rate eventually decreases expiratory time to such a degree that airspace emptying cannot occur and further hyperinflation develops. Worsening hyperinflation shifts the pressure–volume curve of emphysematous lung units further upward and to the left, adding a restrictive pulmonary defect to the underlying airflow limitation. This produces the rapid and shallow respiratory pattern commonly observed in patients with severe COPD.

Rapid and shallow breathing places greater demands on respiratory muscles both in terms of the amount of pressure they need to generate for breathing (P_{breath}) and the proportion of the respiratory cycle during which muscle contraction is required to occur (TI/Tot). Progressive dyspnea correlates both with increasing P_{breath} and TI/Tot.[31] As P_{breath} approaches the maximal pressure that respiratory muscles can generate (PImax), patients begin to function near their limits of ventilatory reserve and fatigue threshold. Further demands on respiratory muscles, such as an exacerbation of COPD with increased airway resistance, can overburden compensatory mechanisms and cause acute respiratory failure.

Increasing evidence indicates that lung volumes are more closely associated with dyspnea and functional limitations of patients with advanced disease than spirometric measurements, such as FEV_1. As patients exercise, $\dot{V}E$ increases and expiratory airflow limitations produce **dynamic hyperinflation**, as expressed as the ratio of inspiratory capacity to total lung capacity. This ratio has been shown to predict survival better than FEV_1. Additionally, improvements in exercise capacity and dyspnea produced by inhaled bronchodilators, pulmonary rehabilitation, and lung volume reduction surgery are less closely associated with improvements in FEV_1 and more tightly linked to delaying dynamic hyperinflation.[32]

Diagnosis and Clinical Course

Patients who develop COPD from smoking have a prolonged initial subclinical course. Cough and eventually dyspnea with exertion represent early symptoms that patients often ascribe to expected consequences of smoking rather than an underlying lung disease. Many patients are first diagnosed when they experience an exacerbation of COPD and present with increased cough, dyspnea, and sputum production that may require hospitalization. Other patients may present with a complication of COPD and smoking, such as pneumonia. Patients may also present with an associated disorder that has an increased incidence in patients with COPD, such as cancer or heart disease.

Because early diagnosis helps patients consider smoking cessation and emerging data suggest that therapy may alter the course of the disease,[33] patients over 40 years old with respiratory symptoms (**Box 35–1**) who smoke should undergo spirometry. Once diagnosed by spirometry, patients with COPD follow a variable

BOX 35–1

Symptoms That Suggest a Diagnosis of COPD

Dyspnea that progressively worsens over time, increases with exercise, persists on a daily basis, and feels to the patient like an "increased effort to breathe," "heaviness," or "gasping."

Chronic cough that may be persistent, intermittent, and/or nonproductive.

Chronic sputum production of any pattern or nature of sputum.

History of risk factors of tobacco smoke, occupational dusts or chemicals, and/or smoke from home cooking or heating fuels.

 Modified from Rabe KF, Hurd S, Anzueto A, et al. Global strategy for the diagnosis, management, and prevention of chronic obstructive pulmonary disease: GOLD executive summary. *Am J Respir Crit Care Med.* 2007;176:532–555. Official Journal of the American Thoracic Society. Diane Gern, Publisher.

clinical course. Patients who continue to smoke have an accelerated decline in FEV_1 as compared with nonsmoking, age-matched individuals. Patients with moderate to severe COPD commonly experience exacerbations, each of which risks respiratory failure and a potentially irreversible decrement in lung function. Patients who have COPD with onset in the fifth decade of life or in the absence of a smoking history should be evaluated for AAT deficiency.

Outpatient Care of Stable Chronic Obstructive Pulmonary Disease

An integrated outpatient approach to the management of COPD provides opportunities to reduce symptoms and improve quality of life, slow the decline in lung function, prevent complications, avoid or minimize adverse effects of therapy, and prolong survival. Approaches recommended by clinical practice guidelines incorporate drug therapy, surgical interventions, rehabilitation, education, prophylactic measures, and supplemental oxygen. Chronic disease management models recommend collaborative care wherein clinicians partner with patients to ensure self-reliance and high personal esteem. Preventive care is a cornerstone of therapy that includes immunization with pneumococcal vaccine and yearly influenza vaccinations. Unfortunately, considerable gaps exist in primary care management of patients with COPD, with many patients being both underdiagnosed and undermanaged.

RESPIRATORY RECAP

Outpatient Care of the Patient with COPD

» Smoking cessation is indicated for all smokers.
» Encourage exercise and vaccinations for all patients with airflow limitation.
» Drug therapy is prescribed for all symptomatic patients; additional drugs are added as airflow limitation and functional impairment worsen.
» Long-term oxygen therapy improves survival.
» NIV improves outcomes for exacerbations; the benefit of chronic intermittent use in stable patients is uncertain.
» Sleep-disordered breathing should be considered.
» Pulmonary rehabilitation is beneficial.
» Evaluate patients with advanced disease and functional limitations for surgical options.

Goals of treatment center on preventing deterioration of lung function, enhancing quality of life by diminishing symptoms, managing complications, and prolonging meaningful life. Survival benefits have been demonstrated for smoking cessation,[34] long-term oxygen therapy for hypoxic patients,[35] lung volume reduction surgery for patients with upper lobe emphysema and poor exercise capacity,[36] and **noninvasive positive pressure ventilation (NIV)** during episodes of exacerbations with acute respiratory failure.[37] Drug therapy improves symptoms of cough and dyspnea and lowers the risk of exacerbations. Emerging data suggest that long-acting inhaled beta-agonists and inhaled corticosteroids may improve survival[38] and slow the rate of deterioration of FEV_1.[33] Other therapies, such as lung transplantation and pulmonary rehabilitation, improve functional levels, symptoms, and quality of life for patients with advanced COPD.[39]

Smoking Cessation

Smoking cessation is the only healthcare intervention clearly shown to slow the accelerated annual decline of FEV_1 experienced by patients with COPD. Although most smokers want to quit smoking, they face multiple barriers, which include the lack of training in smoking cessation self-reported by physicians. Respiratory therapists and other caregivers can assist patients in stopping smoking by addressing the issue, providing brief advice, and guiding patients toward smoking cessation resources. Brief interventions during hospitalization, however, have negligible effects.[40] Referral to counseling programs represents an effective tobacco use treatment strategy.[41] While delivering respiratory care to hospitalized patients, respiratory therapists and others should discuss the health benefits that smoking cessation can provide at any patient age (**Box 35–2**). Five-step interventions for promoting smoking cessation are shown in **Table 35–4** and **Box 35–3**.[42] The American College of Physicians has published a review of smoking cessation interventions that provides caregivers with information to guide patients toward available resources.

Combining pharmacotherapy with behavioral therapy and other interventions increases success rates for patients motivated to stop smoking (**Box 35–4**). Nicotine replacement therapy reduces symptoms related

BOX 35–2

Health Benefits of Quitting Smoking

Longer life
Decreased risk for lung cancer and other types of cancer, heart attack, and stroke
Reduction in risk for cardiac events
Improved circulation
Chronic cough improves
Lung function improves within 3 months
Dyspnea improves within 1 to 9 months
Improved sense of smell and taste
Improved functional abilities such as walking and climbing stairs

TABLE 35–4 Five As for Patients Willing to Quit Smoking

Ask about tobacco use	Identify and document tobacco use status for every patient at every visit.
Advise to quit	In a clear, strong, and personalized manner, urge every tobacco user to quit.
Assess willingness to make a quit attempt	Is the tobacco user willing to make a quit attempt at this time?
Assist in quit attempt	For the patient willing to make a quit attempt, offer medication and provide or refer for counseling or additional treatment to help the patient quit. For patients unwilling to quit at the time, provide interventions designed to increase future quit attempts.
Arrange follow-up	For the patient willing to make a quit attempt, arrange for follow-up contacts, beginning within the first week after the quit date. For patients unwilling to make a quit attempt at the time, address tobacco dependence and willingness to quit at next clinic visit.

BOX 35–3

Five Rs to Motivate Patients Unwilling to Quit Smoking

Encourage patient to think of the **relevance** of quitting smoking to their lives.
Assist patients in identifying the **risks** of smoking.
Assist the patient in identifying **rewards** of smoking cessation.
Discuss with patient **roadblocks** or barriers to attempting cessation.
Repeat the motivational intervention at all visits.

to nicotine withdrawal and produces smoking cessation rates of 17% at 6 months as compared with 10% among control groups.[42] Only limited data support combination nicotine replacement therapy as being superior to a single route of nicotine replacement.[43] Other than cost, no differences exist in efficacy between the different forms of nicotine replacement therapy. Bupropion reduces cravings for cigarettes through unknown mechanisms. Insufficient comparative data with nicotine replacement therapy exist, but one study reported a doubling of quit rates at 1 year as compared with the nicotine patch.[44] Varenicline reduces cravings for cigarettes by binding to a nicotine receptor associated with the relaxing effects felt by smoking. Clinical trials of varenicline as compared with placebo or bupropion demonstrated higher abstinence rates for varenicline.[45] Limited evidence of efficacy exists for clonidine, nortriptyline, naltrexone, alprazolam, silver acetate, mecamylamine, and lobeline, and these agents

BOX 35–4

Pharmacologic Interventions to Assist Smoking Cessation

Nicotine Replacement Therapy

Gum: Increases cessation rates about 1.5 to 2 times control at 6 months
24-hour patch: Increases cessation rates about 1.5 to 2 times control at 6 months
Nasal sprays: Increase cessation rates about 1.5 to 2 times control at 6 months
Inhaler: Increases cessation rates about 1.5 to 2 times control at 6 months
Lozenges: Increase cessation rates about 1.5 to 2 times control at 6 months

Bupropion

Oral sustained-release formulation: Increases cessation rates about 2 times control at 1 year

Varenicline

Oral tablet: Increases cessation rates over 3.5 times control and almost 2 times bupropion at 12 weeks

BOX 35–5

Drug Therapy for COPD

First step: Short-acting β_2-agonists, short-acting muscarinic antagonist (anticholinergic), or both in combination as needed for symptoms.
Second step: Add long-acting β_2-agonists or long-acting muscarinic antagonist.
Third step: Use a combination of long-acting β_2-agonists and long-acting anticholinergics.
Fourth step: Add inhaled corticosteroids to the combination of long-acting β_2-agonists and long-acting muscarinic antagonist.
Fifth step: Consider adding theophylline to combination inhaled therapies.
Antibiotics: Use during exacerbations. Patients with coexisting bronchiectasis benefit from chronic or seasonal use of antibiotics to prevent exacerbations.
Systemic corticosteroids: Use only during exacerbations, for 7 to 10 days.

are not FDA approved for smoking cessation. Clonidine and nortriptyline are recommended as second-line therapy for patients who fail first-line therapy or have contraindications to first-line drugs.

Drug Therapy

Symptomatic patients with COPD benefit from pharmacologic therapy. Oral and inhaled medications are directed toward relieving symptoms, improving functional capacity and quality of life, decreasing hyperinflation, and preventing or reversing exacerbations and worsening of lung function. The modern approach to pharmacotherapy in COPD initiates drug therapy in a stepwise manner based on the severity of the disease and the efficacy of different drugs on various outcomes (**Box 35–5**). Mild disease (GOLD stage I) with intermittent symptoms responds to occasional use of short-acting bronchodilators, either a short-acting β_2-agonist (SABA), a short-acting muscarinic agent (an anticholinergic, such as ipratropium), or both. Maintenance bronchodilator therapy with long-acting agents can be used for patients with moderate disease (GOLD stage II), poorly controlled symptoms, or for those who rely on rescue therapy with more than one aerosol canister a month. Available long-acting agents include a once-daily **long-acting muscarinic antagonist (LAMA)** or twice-daily long-acting β_2-agonist (LABA). Evidence suggests that combining drugs from different classes (β_2-agonists, muscarinic antagonists, inhaled corticosteroids) has additive beneficial effects.[8,46]

These recommendations are based on observations that 80% of stable patients with COPD experience improved measured airflow with bronchodilator therapy,[1] and a larger proportion have improved symptoms and exercise capacity even in the absence of measured improvements in airflow due to mechanisms such as decreased air trapping.[32] The inhaled route with a metered dose inhaler (MDI), breath-activated MDI, dry powder inhaler (DPI), or nebulizer is the preferred mode. Effectiveness of therapy is highly dependent on the ability of patients to use MDI or DPI aerosol devices correctly. Because long-acting inhaled bronchodilators are preferred over short-acting agents for maintenance therapy, patients who cannot coordinate use of portable devices may benefit from once-a-day or twice-a-day therapy with a home nebulizer.

Inhaled β_2-agonist drugs promote airway smooth muscle relaxation by stimulating airway β_2-receptors and increasing intracellular cyclic adenosine monophosphate. They also promote mucociliary clearance, inhibit cholinergic neurotransmission, and limit inflammatory mediator release from mast cells and basophils, although the clinical importance of these effects is uncertain.[47] Inhaled β_2-agonists are preferred over oral tablet forms because of a lower incidence of systemic adverse effects. Although these drugs bind preferentially to β_2-receptors, they have minimal binding to β_1-receptors in the heart and can produce hypertension, tachycardia, and other cardiac symptoms in some patients. Rarely, paradoxical bronchospasm has been reported with both oral and inhalational formulations of β_2-agonists.

Short-acting β_2-agonists have a peak bronchodilatory effect within 5 to 15 minutes and abate within 4 to 6 hours. Albuterol is the most commonly used SABA in the United States and comes in an MDI, as a solution for nebulization, and in pill and syrup formulations. The MDI is dosed with two puffs four times a day for management of intermittent symptoms in patients with mild COPD.[8] Levalbuterol is the R-enantiomer of albuterol, which has not been shown to have advantages as compared with albuterol, which comprises both the R- and S-enantiomers in a racemic form. SABAs have been shown to provide temporary improvements in FEV_1, lung volumes, dyspnea, and exercise endurance in COPD.[48] Other SABAs include pirbuterol and terbutaline. Frequent and regular use is discouraged because SABAs can downregulate β_2-receptors, causing tachyphylaxis.

Long-acting β_2-agonists are recommended as twice-a-day maintenance therapy for patients with persistent symptoms and moderate to very severe COPD.[8,49] The available drugs are salmeterol, formoterol, and arformoterol. Salmeterol and formoterol have been shown to temporarily improve FEV_1, decrease lung volumes, improve dyspnea, decrease adverse events, and improve quality of life.[48] One study demonstrated that salmeterol with or without an inhaled corticosteroid slows the annual decline of FEV_1 in patients with COPD.[33] It is unclear whether LABAs reduce the incidence of exacerbations. Salmeterol binds to lipophilic β_2-agonist sites and has a time to onset of effect of 30 to 60 minutes and a duration of effect up to 12 hours. Formoterol binds both to amphiphilic and lipophilic receptor sites and has a rapid onset of action of 5 to 15 minutes and a duration of 12 hours. Salmeterol and formoterol are available as a DPI formulation. Formoterol and arformoterol are available as a solution for nebulization. Initial experience with arformoterol indicates that patients can experience sustained benefit over 12 weeks of taking the drug.[50] Considerable clinical experience with both short-acting and long-acting β_2-agonists demonstrates their safety for patients with COPD.[51]

Anticholinergic agents decrease airflow limitation by blocking muscarinic (M) receptors on airway smooth muscle and submucosal gland cells. Stimulation of these receptors results in bronchoconstriction and increased mucus secretion. As with other inhaled drugs, symptomatic improvement results from a decrease in exercise-related dynamic hyperinflation. Ipratropium is a short-acting and relatively nonselective drug that blocks both M2 and M3 receptors. Blockage of M2 receptors increases acetylcholine release, whereas blockage of M3 causes bronchodilation, which is the dominant effect from ipratropium. Ipratropium has no effect on decreasing mucus secretion. At conventional doses, ipratropium provides greater bronchodilatory potency compared with β_2-agonists, although bioactivity is similar at maximal doses.[52] Ipratropium has been shown to improve FEV_1, reduce lung volumes and dyspnea, decrease adverse events, and improve exercise tolerance.[48] Long-term use does not promote tolerance. Usual doses with an MDI are two to four puffs every 6 or 8 hours, although some patients may tolerate higher doses. Ipratropium is available in an MDI, as a single agent or combined with albuterol, and as a solution for nebulization. Atropine-like adverse effects are typically mild, but patients should be observed for urinary retention, closed angle glaucoma, and constipation. Case-control studies suggest that ipratropium is associated with an increased risk of cardiovascular mortality among patients treated for COPD.[53]

Tiotropium is an inhaled long-acting anticholinergic agent available as a DPI that requires only once-a-day dosing. It blocks M1, M2, and M3 receptors nonselectively, like ipratropium, but disassociates more rapidly from M2 receptors than M1 or M3 receptors. The onset of peak bronchodilation ranges between 1 and 3 hours, so tiotropium is not used for acute relief of bronchospasm. It improves FEV_1, lung volumes, dyspnea, adverse events from COPD, and exercise endurance.[54] In contrast to ipratropium, tiotropium has been shown to improve quality of life and prevent exacerbations.[54] Tiotropium has also been shown to improve the effectiveness of pulmonary rehabilitation.[55] Exacerbation rates have recently been shown to be similar between tiotropium as compared with salmeterol combined with inhaled corticosteroids. Compared with LABAs, tiotropium produces better bronchodilation and greater improvements in dyspnea.[56]

Theophylline is a phosphodiesterase inhibitor that raises intracellular concentrations of cyclic adenosine monophosphate within smooth muscle cells. It has moderate bronchodilatory effects in addition to acting as a diuretic, stimulant of central respiratory drive, enhancer of diaphragmatic contractility, and reliever of diaphragmatic fatigue. It may alter genes that promote airway inflammation in COPD and provide an anti-inflammatory effect, although the clinical importance of this effect is uncertain.[57] It is available in sustained-release formulations for once- or twice-daily dosing. A meta-analysis of 18 primary studies reported that theophylline improves FEV_1 and FVC both during the trough and peak phases of its serum concentrations.

Theophylline has a narrow therapeutic window, however, and can cause serious adverse effects that include cardiac arrhythmias and seizures, which may be the initial manifestations of toxicity. Theophylline is now recommended as third-line therapy for patients with inadequate responses to inhaled bronchodilators and for patients who cannot use inhaler therapy optimally. Target drug serum concentrations are 8 to 13 mg/dL, which is achieved in most patients with a 300 mg dose once daily at bedtime.[8] Theophylline has multiple interactions with other drugs.

Short-term administration of systemic **corticosteroids** for 7 to 14 days has a role in managing patients with exacerbations of COPD, but for patients with stable COPD, no measurable benefit is achieved by long-term use of oral corticosteroids. Moreover, corticosteroid therapy causes multiple adverse effects that include osteoporosis, diabetes, fluid retention, hypertension, cataracts, immunosuppression with risk of infection, integument changes, and redistribution of fat. A trial of oral corticosteroids does not predict which patients with COPD will benefit from inhaled corticosteroids.

Inhaled corticosteroids have anti-inflammatory effects on the airways and provide opportunities to improve symptoms and the clinical course of patients with COPD while avoiding many of the side effects associated with oral corticosteroids. Most multicenter trials have not shown benefit from inhaled corticosteroids in slowing the annual rate of decline of FEV_1 in COPD,[58–60] although reanalysis of data from one trial found a slower rate of decline for patients with moderate to severe COPD treated with inhaled fluticasone.[33] Several studies demonstrate that inhaled corticosteroids lower the rate of progressive loss of quality of life and the frequency of exacerbations among patients with advanced COPD.[58,59,61] Clinical trials and meta-analyses suggest that inhaled corticosteroids in combination with an LABA or alone may decrease mortality.[38] Because of these benefits, clinical guidelines recommend inhaled corticosteroids for patients with severe (GOLD stage III) or very severe (GOLD stage IV) COPD and repeated exacerbations (e.g., three within the previous 3 years).[8]

Inhaled corticosteroids may cause oral thrush but have negligible risks for cataracts, muscle weakness, or osteoporosis. The effect on blood glucose among patients with diabetes is poorly defined. Two studies have noted a higher risk of pneumonia among patients treated with inhaled corticosteroids, but no increase in pneumonia-related deaths.

Combination therapy with inhaled and oral bronchodilators from different drug classes provides additive benefit. Adding theophylline to inhaled albuterol and ipratropium[62] or to salmeterol[63] improves FEV_1 as compared with each individual drug. The combination of salmeterol and ipratropium also has additive effects on spirometric values.[64] Combining once-a-day tiotropium and twice-a-day formoterol improved morning and evening FEV_1 and resting hyperinflation.[65] Additive benefit was also achieved when formoterol was dosed only once a day with tiotropium. Similar additive benefits have been observed with tiotropium combined with salmeterol and fluticasone. Tiotropium combined with a SABA has additive effects, but not when combined with ipratropium.[66] A large multicenter trial (the TORCH trial) demonstrated that salmeterol added to fluticasone improves FEV_1, exacerbation rate, and quality of life as compared with either drug alone, which is consistent with previous studies that examined the effects of adding inhaled corticosteroids to β_2-agonists.[67] A reanalysis of the TORCH trial data determined that the combination of salmeterol and fluticasone slowed the annual decline of FEV_1, although salmeterol had similar benefit in this study when given alone.[33] Guideline approaches for combining inhaled drugs based on severity of disease are presented later in this chapter.

Antibiotics are reserved for patients with COPD exacerbations characterized by fever, leukocytosis, purulent sputum, or chest radiographic changes consistent with bronchitis.[68] Chronic use of antibiotics for stable patients has not been consistently shown to preserve lung function or prevent exacerbations. One study, however, demonstrated benefit in decreasing rates of exacerbations among patients treated with intermittent or continuous antibiotics during at-risk periods if they had a history of frequent exacerbations in the past.[69]

Mucokinetic agents are intended to reduce mucus viscosity and assist with the mobilization of airway secretions. Iodinated glycerol has been demonstrated in a placebo-controlled trial to improve cough symptoms and sense of well-being, although objective markers of airflow limitation did not improve.[70] Because of these marginal benefits, mucokinetic agents are used empirically in occasional patients who have marked difficulty with expectoration of secretions despite maximal therapy. Oral *N*-acetylcysteine has the potential to break sulfhydryl bonds and provide antioxidant effects. The largest study to date, however, did not demonstrate efficacy.[71] Aerosolized surfactant has been shown to improve pulmonary function and ciliary sputum transport in patients with stable chronic bronchitis.[72] Inhaled ribonuclease benefits patients with cystic fibrosis but provides no benefit in COPD.[8]

Long-Term Oxygen Therapy

Long-term oxygen therapy (LTOT) for hypoxemic patients with COPD prolongs survival.[35,73] The mechanisms of benefit are unclear, although patients treated with LTOT for an average of 19 hours per day have a slower progression of pulmonary hypertension compared with those treated with 12 hours per day or less, suggesting a positive effect on pulmonary vasculature as the basis for improved survival.[35] LTOT also decreases dyspnea awareness, oxygen cost of breathing, pulmonary hypertension, disordered sleep, nocturnal dysrhythmias, exercise endurance, strength, and mental alertness.[74]

Patients are selected for oxygen therapy on the basis of specific indications derived from clinical and laboratory findings (**Box 35–6**).[1,8] Demonstration of hypoxemia should occur after a 4-week stable period when patients are receiving full medical therapy and are not smoking. Subsequent monitoring of oxygenation is performed on an individual basis. Up to 40% of patients initiated on LTOT experience improve oxygenation after 1 month of therapy and no longer fulfill the indications for supplemental oxygen.[75]

Vaccinations

Vaccinations are a central preventive measure in the management of patients with COPD. All caregivers interacting with patients should counsel them regarding their annual vaccination with trivalent influenza vaccine. Pneumococcal vaccination is recommended for patients with COPD regardless of age.

Ventilatory Support

The benefit of intermittent noninvasive ventilation (NIV) in the outpatient management of patients with severe stable COPD is not clearly defined. The purpose of ventilator support is to unload respiratory muscles and

BOX 35–6

Indications for Long-Term Oxygen Therapy for Stable COPD

Continuous Oxygen Therapy

$Pao_2 \leq 55$ mm Hg or oxygen saturation $\leq 88\%$ at rest while breathing room air

Pao_2 between 56 to 59 mm Hg or oxygen saturation of 89% at any time during breathing of room air with one or more of the following:

- Polycythemia (Hct > 56%)
- Pulmonary hypertension as evidenced by right heart dysfunction

Noncontinuous Oxygen Therapy

$Pao_2 \leq 55$ mm Hg or oxygen saturation $\leq 88\%$ during exertion or sleep while breathing room air

BOX 35–7

Guidelines for Medicare Reimbursement for Noninvasive Positive Pressure Ventilation in Patients with COPD

1. Symptomatic despite optimal medical therapy.
2. Abnormal gas exchange:
   a. $Paco_2 \geq 52$ mmHg *and*
   b. Nocturnal hypoventilation with $SpO_2 < 89\%$ for ≥ 5 consecutive minutes while breathing usual FIO_2
3. Obstructive sleep apnea excluded at least on clinical grounds. If obstructive sleep apnea exists, CPAP is indicated initially.
4. Repeated hospital admissions for hypercapnic respiratory failure can be considered.

treat or prevent muscle fatigue. Such therapy has been shown to benefit patients with chronic respiratory failure caused by restrictive lung diseases, such as kyphoscoliosis.[76] A systematic review of 15 studies of NIV observed that the 6 available randomized controlled trials (RCTs) demonstrated no improvement in gas exchange, but the 9 non-RCTs did report some other clinical improvements.[77] These improvements included health-related quality of life and dyspnea. The authors of the review concluded that a subset of patients on maximal medical treatment for severe stable COPD may receive benefit from bilevel noninvasive positive pressure ventilation when used as adjunctive therapy. Additional studies are needed, however, before recommending intermittent ventilation as standard therapy. Guidelines exist from Medicare for reimbursement for NIV for patients with COPD (**Box 35–7**).

Management of Sleep-Related Abnormalities

Patients with COPD are at risk for sleep-related disorders characterized by poor sleep quality and worsening hypoxia and hypercapnia at night.[78] Although the prevalence of sleep-related disorders among patients with varying severity of COPD is unknown, studies indicate that 45% of normoxic COPD patients develop significant oxyhemoglobin desaturation during sleep,[79] and 47% of hypercapnic COPD patients experience a 10 mm Hg increment in $Paco_2$ at night.[80] Multiple factors contribute to sleep-related breathing disorders in COPD, but alveolar hypoventilation is the predominant mechanism. Sleep-related increases in upper airway resistance, worsening of $\dot{V}/\dot{Q}$, and changes in oxygen consumption, carbon dioxide production, and cardiac output most likely play contributory roles. Alterations in sleep-related breathing patterns create greater changes in respiratory function for patients with COPD as compared with normal subjects because COPD patients have higher physiologic dead space at baseline. Patients with COPD also have abnormal respiratory system mechanics—with hyperinflation and diaphragmatic flattening—that amplify the effects of altered breathing patterns during sleep.

The coexistence of COPD with **sleep apnea hypopnea syndrome (SAHS)** occurs in approximately 10% of patients with a history of SAHS. Patients with the combined disorders develop more severe hypoxia during sleep as compared with other patients with SAHS.

BOX 35–8

Components of Pulmonary Rehabilitation for the Patient with COPD

Detailed history and physical examination
Measurement of spirometry before and after a bronchodilator drug
Assessment of exercise capacity
Measurement of health status and impact of breathlessness
Assessment of inspiratory and expiratory muscle strength and lower limb strength in patients with muscle wasting
Assessment of patient's advance planning needs

It remains unresolved whether combined disease results from the coincidental occurrence of these two relatively common conditions in the same individual or whether COPD predisposes patients to SAHS. Affected patients may present with greater degrees of polycythemia and lower extremity edema than expected by the severity of their airway obstruction. A sleep study is indicated if patients have these findings or evidence of general symptoms of SAHS, such as daytime sleepiness, heavy snoring, or observed obstructed breathing during sleep.

Respiratory stimulants or other pharmacologic agents have not been shown to improve sleep architecture or reduce nocturnal oxygen desaturation in patients with COPD. Nasal continuous positive airway pressure (CPAP) remains the mainstay of therapy for patients with SAHS with or without COPD, although little data exist demonstrating the outcome of this therapy for patients with COPD.

Pulmonary Rehabilitation

Enrollment of patients with moderate to severe COPD in outpatient **pulmonary rehabilitation** programs provides opportunities to restore patients to the highest possible level of independence and functioning in the community.[81] Components of an effective, multidisciplinary rehabilitation program include exercise training and conditioning, physical therapy, education for patients and family (e.g., nutrition, oxygen use, inhaler techniques), instruction in airway clearance techniques, energy conservation, vocational counseling, and psychological support (**Box 35–8**). The effectiveness of pulmonary rehabilitation has long been debated because of the limited outcomes data available to demonstrate measurable improvements in postrehabilitation endpoints. A systematic review of scientific evidence concluded that pulmonary rehabilitation is beneficial for patients with COPD.[81] Such evidence has resulted in approval by Medicare for payment of pulmonary rehabilitation services.

Surgery

Multiple surgical procedures have been evaluated over the last 50 years to improve lung function in COPD.[82] Presently, only giant bullectomy, lung volume reduction surgery, and lung transplantation have survived scientific scrutiny and demonstrated clinical utility for selected patients with COPD.

Giant Bullectomy

Giant bullae represent an unusual complication of emphysema that can cause pulmonary decompensation as bullae expand and compress adjacent functioning lung tissue. Patients are selected for **bullectomy** by estimating the degree of lung compression and the functional status of the compressed lung to determine the amount of improvement that can be anticipated by bullectomy. Patients with giant bullae who have limited amounts of potentially functioning compressed lung tissue, called "vanishing lung syndrome," gain no benefit from bullectomy. CT scans can assess the size of bullae, the amount of compressed lung, and the severity of diffuse emphysema.[83] Pulmonary function tests (PFTs) determine the severity of underlying emphysema. Appropriate candidates for surgery have a restrictive rather than an obstructive PFT pattern because of lung compression by the bullae (**Table 35–5**). A severe obstructive pattern suggests the presence of advanced diffuse emphysema that will not improve with bullectomy. The gas volume of giant bullae can be calculated by subtracting the total lung volume (TLC) determined by helium dilution (which does not measure the volume of bullae) from the TLC measured by plethysmography (which includes the volume of bullae).

Lung Volume Reduction Surgery

The term **lung volume reduction surgery (LVRS)** refers to surgical procedures that resect the regions of lung tissue most severely affected by emphysema. After removal

TABLE 35–5 Giant Bullectomy Indications, Contraindications, and Ideal Candidate

Indications	Contraindications	Ideal Candidate
Severe functional limitation despite maximal medical therapy Nonsmoker or ex-smoker Little bronchodilator responsiveness Bulla occupies more than one-third of hemithorax Crowding of adjacent lung on CT angiogram Elevated trapped gas (elevated RV) on PFTs Normal or near-normal DLCO Normal Pao_2 and $Paco_2$	Substantial emphysema elsewhere in the lung	All of the preceding indications *and* • Bulla > 50% of hemithorax All of the preceding indications *without* • Chronic bronchitis or recurrent infections • Pulmonary hypertension • Comorbid illness • Older age • FEV_1 < 35% of predicted

CT, computed tomography; RV, residual volume; PFT, pulmonary function test; DLCO, diffusing capacity of the lung for carbon monoxide; FEV_1, forced expiratory volume in 1 second.

From Benditt JO. Surgical options for patients with COPD: sorting out the choices. *Respir Care.* 2006;51:173–182. Reprinted with permission.

TABLE 35–6 Lung Volume Reduction Surgery Indications, Contraindications, and Ideal Candidate

Indications	Contraindications	Ideal Candidate
Severe functional limitation despite maximal medical therapy Nonsmoker for at least 3 months Completed pulmonary rehabilitation (6–12 weeks) Postbronchodilator FEV_1 < 45% of predicted RV > 150% of predicted TLC > 100% of predicted Pao_2 > 45 mm Hg $Paco_2$ < 60 mm Hg Post-pulmonary rehabilitation 6-min walk distance > 140 m	Comorbid illness Substantial untreated cardiac disease Cancer other than basal cell or squamous cell skin cancer within the last 5 years Diseases in other organs increasing surgical risk BMI > 31.1 kg/m² (males) or 32.3 kg/m² (females) FEV_1 < 20% of predicted and either DLCO < 20% of predicted or homogeneous emphysema on CT scan Pulmonary artery hypertension Systolic > 45 mm Hg Mean > 35 mm Hg Prednisone > 20 mg/d	All of the preceding indications *and* • Upper lobe emphysema and cycle-ergometry exercise capacity < 25 watts (women) or < 40 watts (men) while breathing FIO_2 of 0.30 All of the preceding indications *without* • Older age • Comorbid illness • Pulmonary hypertension • Frequent respiratory tract infections or chronic bronchitis

FEV_1, forced expiratory volume in 1 second; RV, residual volume; TLC, total lung capacity; BMI, body mass index; DLCO, diffusing capacity of the lung for carbon monoxide; CT, computed tomography.

From Benditt JO. Surgical options for patients with COPD: sorting out the choices. *Respir Care.* 2006;51:173–182. Reprinted with permission.

of 20% to 30% of an emphysematous lung, the remaining lung expands beyond its previous boundaries and gains increased recoil elasticity. The lung, chest wall, and diaphragm demonstrate improved mechanics, with higher expiratory airflow and less air trapping. The procedure can be performed through a midline sternotomy or by video-assisted thoracotomy, both of which allow stapled resection of tissue.[82]

The National Emphysema Treatment Trial (NETT) demonstrated improved short-term outcomes in carefully selected patients with COPD (**Table 35–6**). Patients with a heterogeneous upper lobe distribution of emphysema and low exercise capacity experienced improved long-term survival following LVRS as compared with continued medical therapy.[36] Patients without these preoperative characteristics did not benefit from LVRS and had either worse or similar survival as compared with medical management. In secondary subgroup analyses, patients with upper lobe distribution of emphysema and poor exercise capacity had improved quality of life and exercise capacity.

The long-term results of LVRS are not completely defined. Most studies report improved lung function and gas exchange for some patients up to 24 to 36 months after surgery.[84] Complications of LVRS include prolonged air leak, pneumonia, respiratory failure, postoperative ileus and colonic or cecal perforation, and cardiac ischemia.[85]

Extensive research is now examining nonsurgical alternatives to LVRS that achieve similar goals of reducing lung volume by deflating lung regions that are most affected by emphysema. Bronchoscopic insertion of one-way valves and biological substances into the airways occlude ventilation to emphysematous regions and allow other lung segments to expand.

Lung Transplantation

COPD is the most common indication for **lung transplantation**. In the absence of contraindications, patients are selected for transplantation if they have advanced COPD with an estimated survival of less than 2 years

TABLE 35–7 Lung Transplant Indications, Contraindications, and Ideal Candidate

Indications	Contraindications	Ideal Candidate
Advanced COPD Symptomatic despite maximal medical therapy High risk of death within 2 to 3 years COPD-specific (one or more) $FEV_1 < 25\%$ to 30% of predicted Pulmonary artery hypertension Right ventricular failure $Paco_2 > 55$ mm Hg Severe functional limitation, but preserved ability to walk Suggested age limitations Age < 55 for heart–lung transplantation candidates Age < 60 for bilateral lung transplantation candidates Age < 65 for single-lung transplantation candidates	Active malignancy within 2 years (except basal or squamous cell skin cancer) Substance addiction within 6 months Substantial dysfunction of extrathoracic organs HIV infection Hepatitis B antigen positive Hepatitis C with biopsy-proven evidence of liver disease	All of the preceding indications *and* • Highly motivated individual • Excellent social support All of the preceding indications *without* • Symptomatic osteoporosis • Oral steroids > 20 mg/day • Invasive mechanical ventilation • Colonization with fungi, resistant organisms, or atypical mycobacteria

LVRS, lung volume reduction surgery; COPD, chronic obstructive pulmonary disease; FEV_1, forced expiratory volume in 1 second; HIV, human immunodeficiency virus.

From Benditt JO. Surgical options for patients with COPD: sorting out the choices. *Respir Care.* 2006;51:173–182. Reprinted with permission.

(**Table 35–7**).[82] It is difficult to estimate the survival of individual patients, but markers of high near-term mortality include an FEV_1 below 25% to 30% of predicted, a rapid decline in lung function, and severe hypoxemia, hypercapnia, and secondary pulmonary hypertension despite maximal medical therapy.[82] Recent Canadian guidelines on lung transplantation include the BODE index for patient selection (**Box 35–9**).[86]

Both single- and double-lung transplantations are performed for COPD, but single-lung procedures are most common because of the limited availability of donor lungs. Similar postoperative exercise functional capacities result from either procedure, but data suggest improved survival with double-lung transplantation. Double-lung transplantation also produces greater improvement in spirometric measures. Coexistence of bronchiectasis with associated purulent airway secretions requires double-lung transplantation to prevent infection of the allograft.[87] Single-lung transplantation is usually performed through a lateral thoracotomy incision. Bilateral lung transplantation is done most often through a median sternotomy or transverse thoracosternotomy "clam shell" incision. Bilateral lung transplantation may require cardiopulmonary bypass in 20% of patients. The selection of patients for lung volume reduction surgery versus lung transplantation is guided by the criteria in **Table 35–8**.

One-year survival for patients undergoing lung transplantation for COPD is 90%, with 5-year survival being 40% to 50%. Although lung transplantation in COPD has not been subjected to randomized trials to determine its effect on survival, analyses of retrospective data controlled for independent risk factors of death indicate improved survival compared with patients with severe COPD who have not received transplants. In contrast, other retrospective analyses reported similar survival between patients who received lung transplants and those who remained on the transplant list.[88] The primary rationale for lung transplantation centers on improvement of functional status and quality of life rather than survival benefits.[82] Nearly all studies demonstrate that patients experience improved pulmonary function,[89] exercise capacity,[90] and quality of life[91] after transplantation.

Complications of lung transplantation include infection, early allograft dysfunction that may progress to acute lung injury, hemorrhage, dehiscence of the bronchial anastomoses, and acute and chronic lung rejection. The development of acute postoperative allograft edema that requires mechanical ventilation in patients who

BOX 35–9

Canadian Guidelines for Transplantation

Patients with a BODE index of 7 to 10 or at least one of the following:

- History of hospitalization for exacerbation associated with acute hypercapnia > 50 mm Hg
- Pulmonary hypertension or cor pulmonale, or both, despite oxygen therapy
- FEV_1 of less than 20% and either DLCO of less than 20% or homogeneous distribution of emphysema

FEV_1, forced expiratory volume in 1 second; DLCO, diffusing capacity of the lung for carbon monoxide.

From Orens JB, Estenne M, Arcasoy S, et al. International guidelines for the selection of lung transplant candidates: 2006 update—a consensus report from the Pulmonary Scientific Council of the International Society for Heart and Lung Transplantation. *J Heart Lung Transplant.* 2006;25:745–755. Reprinted with permission from Elsevier. http://www.sciencedirect.com/science/journal/10532498.

TABLE 35-8 Criteria for Selection of LVRS Versus Lung Transplant in Patients with COPD

Lung Transplant	LVRS	LVRS or Lung Transplant, or LVRS Followed by Lung Transplant
Purulent obstructive disease Bronchiectasis More than ¼ cup of phlegm per day Associated pulmonary artery hypertension and/or right heart failure Absence of hyperinflation: TLC $<$ 100% of predicted or RV $<$ 150% of predicted $FEV_1 < 20\%$ of predicted with either homogenous emphysema or DLCO $<$ 20% of predicted (NETT high-risk subgroup) Non-upper-lobe emphysema with low exercise capacity $Paco_2 > 55$ mm Hg $Pao_2 < 50$ mm Hg 6-min walk distance $<$ 300 feet	Age $>$ 65, with upper lobe emphysema and low exercise capacity Age $>$ 65 with upper lobe disease and high exercise capacity Age $>$ 65, with non-upper-lobe disease and low exercise capacity Age $<$ 65 with FEV 30% to 40% of predicted but disabling symptoms present despite maximal medical therapy	Age $<$ 65 and meets criteria for both transplant and LVRS

LVRS, lung volume reduction surgery; COPD, chronic obstructive pulmonary disease; TLC, total lung capacity; RV, residual volume; FEV_1, forced expiratory volume in 1 second; DLCO, diffusing capacity of the lung for carbon monoxide; NETT, National Emphysema Treatment Trial.

From Benditt JO. Surgical options for patients with COPD: sorting out the choices. *Respir Care.* 2006;51:173–182. Reprinted with permission.

have undergone single-lung transplantation complicates ventilator management. The overexpansion of the highly compliant native lung compared with the low-compliant allograft may necessitate independent lung ventilation with a double-lumen endotracheal tube.

Overview of Management of Stable Chronic Obstructive Pulmonary Disease

Clinical practice guidelines have proposed a stepwise initiation of increasingly more intensive therapy directed by the severity of airflow limitation as measured by FEV_1 (**Figure 35-8**). The introduction of the BODE index has provided a more comprehensive measure of patients' functional limitations from COPD and associated conditions than FEV_1 alone.[12] Clinicians are beginning to include such measures of functional limitations in their decisions for escalating therapeutic interventions. Based on clinical trials that demonstrate added benefit from combined inhaled medications, the stepwise management shown in **Figure 35-9** for patients with progressive disease and functional limitations has been proposed as a clinical approach.[48]

Managing Exacerbations

Patients with COPD are at risk for exacerbations of their airways disease that may require hospitalization. The GOLD guideline defines an **exacerbation** as "a change in a patient's baseline dyspnea, cough, and/or sputum that is beyond day-to-day variations, is acute in onset, and may warrant a change in regular medications."[92] Exacerbations are characterized by lung inflammation, which plays a central etiologic role and may cause irreversible decrements in lung function and functional status after each exacerbation. Bacterial or viral respiratory infections precipitate most exacerbations, although environmental pollutants and other undefined precipitants play a role.[93] Exacerbations may remain mild and respond to outpatient modifications of therapy or become severe and require ventilatory support. The mortality of hospitalized patients with exacerbations is 10%,[94] with 25% of patients requiring admission to the intensive care unit (ICU).

> **RESPIRATORY RECAP**
>
> **COPD Exacerbations**
>
> » Mild exacerbations can be managed at home.
> » Inhaled β_2-agonists are the first-line therapy. Inhaled anticholinergics may be added, but evidence of added benefit is limited.
> » A 7- to 10-day course of systemic corticosteroids is standard practice.
> » Antibiotics are used for patients with increased sputum volume or purulence and/or dyspnea.
> » Oxygen is titrated to maintain an adequate Spo_2 above 90% without aggravating CO_2 retention.
> » NIV is useful in the management of COPD exacerbation.
> » Life-threatening respiratory failure requires intubation and mechanical ventilation.

Mild exacerbations can be managed with home therapy in the absence of severe COPD, clinically important acute or chronic comorbidities, or other factors that present risk of hypercapnic respiratory failure. Patients should be encouraged to maintain adequate fluid intake to avoid dehydration and should monitor their ability to cough and raise secretions. Patients benefit from a written action plan to manage their medications and alert them to when they should contact their physician or go to the emergency department. Inhaled short-acting β_2-agonist bronchodilators should be increased to their maximum dosages. Many

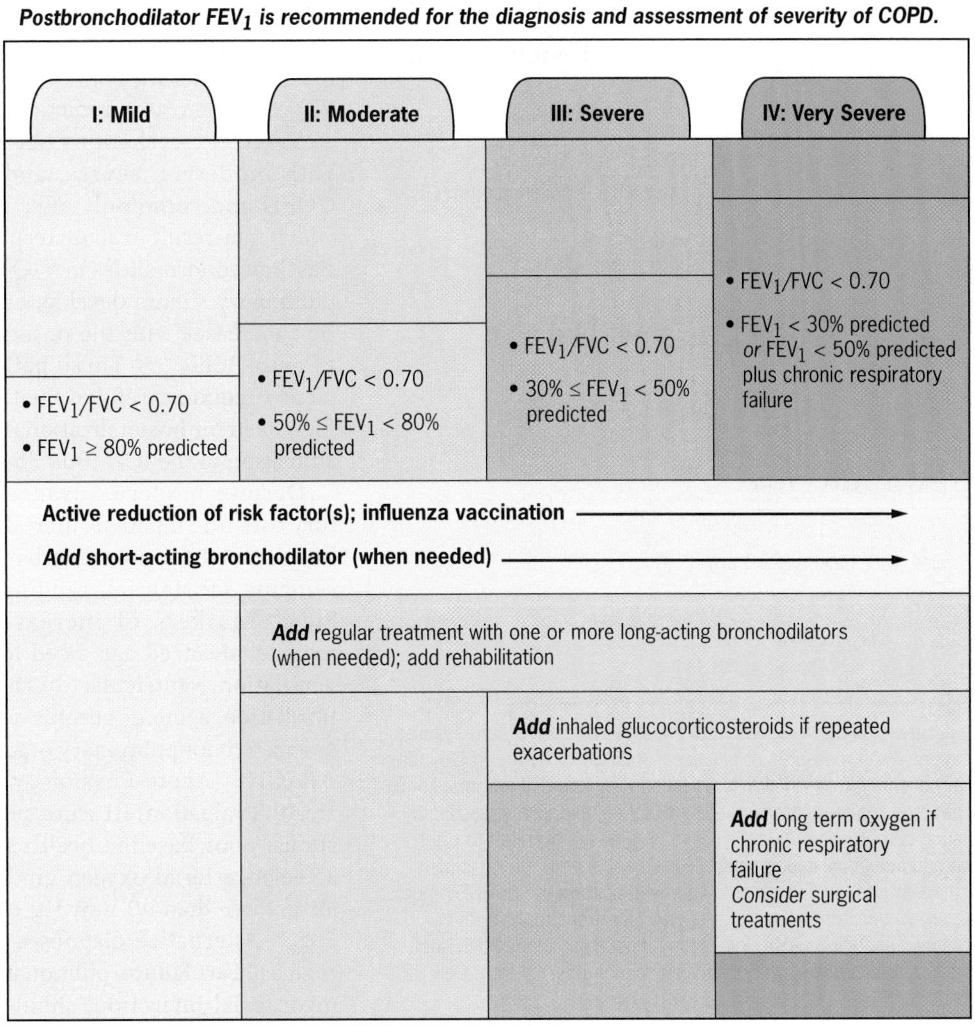

Postbronchodilator FEV_1 is recommended for the diagnosis and assessment of severity of COPD.

I: Mild	II: Moderate	III: Severe	IV: Very Severe
• $FEV_1/FVC < 0.70$ • $FEV_1 \geq 80\%$ predicted	• $FEV_1/FVC < 0.70$ • $50\% \leq FEV_1 < 80\%$ predicted	• $FEV_1/FVC < 0.70$ • $30\% \leq FEV_1 < 50\%$ predicted	• $FEV_1/FVC < 0.70$ • $FEV_1 < 30\%$ predicted *or* $FEV_1 < 50\%$ predicted plus chronic respiratory failure

Active reduction of risk factor(s); influenza vaccination →

***Add* short-acting bronchodilator (when needed)** →

Add regular treatment with one or more long-acting bronchodilators (when needed); add rehabilitation (II–IV)

Add inhaled glucocorticosteroids if repeated exacerbations (III–IV)

Add long term oxygen if chronic respiratory failure *Consider* surgical treatments (IV)

FIGURE 35–8 Therapy for COPD based on the GOLD stages of disease. Reprinted with permission of the American Thoracic Society. Copyright © American Thoracic Society. From Rabe KF, et al. Global strategy for the diagnosis, management, and prevention of chronic obstructive pulmonary disease: GOLD executive summary. *Am J Respir Crit Care Med.* 2007;176:532–555. Official Journal of the American Thoracic Society; Diane Gern, Publisher.

physicians add an inhaled short-acting anticholinergic bronchodilator if the patient is not already taking one, although the evidence of efficacy of combined therapy with ipratropium and a SABA in exacerbations is conflicting.

The role of antibiotics in mild exacerbations remains uncertain because of the heterogeneity of existing clinical trial designs. At least a third of respiratory infections that underlie exacerbations are viral in etiology and would not be expected to respond to antibiotics. Nevertheless, a recent meta-analysis concluded that antibiotics reduce mortality and treatment failures in those patients who require hospitalization.[95] The ATS COPD guidelines recommend the initiation of antibiotics for exacerbations if any two of the following three features are present: increased dyspnea, sputum volume, or sputum purulence.[8] An oral antibiotic is selected with activity against the common pathogens in COPD exacerbations, which are *Streptococcus pneumoniae, Haemophilus influenzae,* and *Moraxella catarrhalis.* Patients with severe COPD are at risk for gram-negative bacteria, including *Pseudomonas aeruginosa.* A systematic review observed equivalent clinical outcomes between drug trials that compared quinolones, macrolides, and amoxicillin-clavulonate.[96] Recently, the length of time after antibiotic therapy during which the patient avoids a subsequent exacerbation (termed *disease-free interval* [DFI]) has been used as an endpoint for studies of antibiotic efficacy. Studies using this endpoint suggest that quin-olones are associated with longer DFIs.[96]

Numerous studies have examined the value of systemic corticosteroids in outpatients with mild exacerbations.[95,97] Thompson and colleagues treated outpatients with 9 days of prednisone versus placebo and observed more rapid and greater degrees of improvement in oxygenation and FEV_1 and fewer treatment failures with prednisone.[98] The

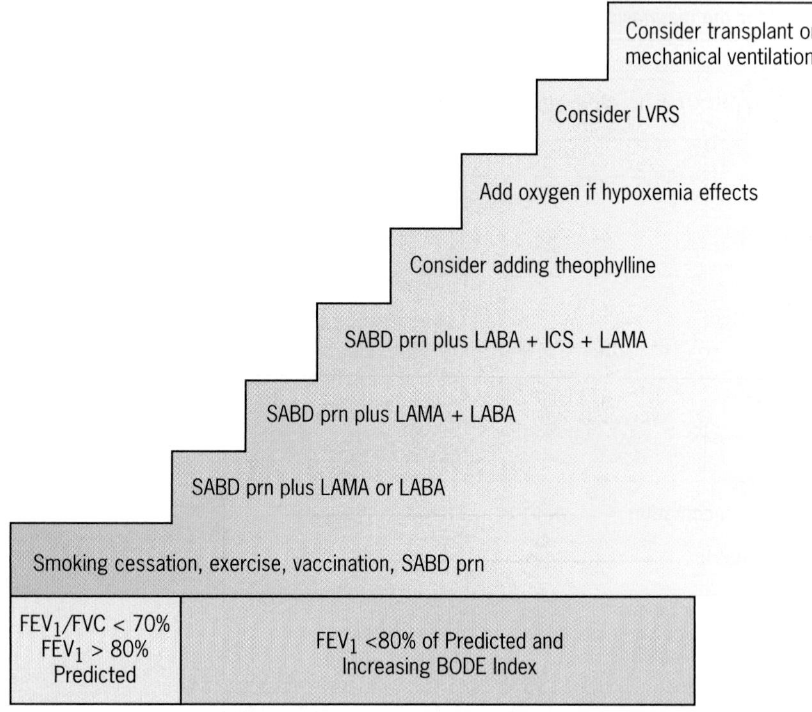

FIGURE 35–9 Stepwise progression of management of patients that combines measures of airflow limitation by spirometry and measures of functional impairment by the BODE index. The first step indicates that patients have mild airflow limitation with some symptoms, such as a cough, but have not become impaired with worsening dyspnea, exercise capacity, or symptoms related to systemic compromise. As the disease progresses from left to right, increasing airflow limitation and functional impairment occur. At each step, the clinician is looking for a response to the new intervention either in improved spirometric or BODE index values. SABD, short-acting bronchodilator such as a β_2-agonist, ipratropium, or both in combination; LABA, long-acting β_2-agonist; LAMA, long-acting muscarinic antagonist, such as tiotropium; LVRS, lung volume reduction surgery. Modified with permission from Celli BR. Update on the management of COPD. *Chest.* 2008;133:1451–1462.

GOLD guidelines recommend a dose of 30 to 40 mg of prednisone per day for 7 to 10 days for outpatients with an exacerbation and an FEV_1 less than 50% predicted.[8]

Severe exacerbations occur in patients with moderate, severe, and very severe COPD and commonly alter gas exchange, which may result in acute respiratory failure. Baseline abnormalities in $\dot{V}/\dot{Q}$ worsen, intrapulmonary shunts develop, and hyperinflation increases with the onset or worsening of auto-PEEP.[99,100] These pathophysiologic factors require careful evaluation of patients for a need for hospitalization (**Box 35–10**) or admission to the ICU (**Box 35–11**).

Despite modern advances in respiratory care, the inpatient mortality of patients hospitalized for an exacerbation of COPD remains substantial, ranging from 6% to 30%.[94] Markers of increased mortality include advanced age, need for mechanical ventilation, ventricular dysrhythmia, atrial fibrillation, acute or chronic cardiac disease, associated nonpulmonary organ failure, high APACHE (Acute Physiology and Chronic Health Evaluation) III score, poor nutritional status, poor baseline health status, and an alveolar–arterial oxygen gradient on room air greater than 40 mm Hg or a low Pa_{O_2}/F_{IO_2}.[94] Alternative diagnoses (**Box 35–12**), such as heart failure, pulmonary emboli, and myocardial infarction, should be carefully

BOX 35–10

Indications for Hospital Assessment or Admission for Exacerbations of COPD

Marked increase in intensity of symptoms, such as sudden development of resting dyspnea
Severe underlying COPD
Onset of new physical signs such as cyanosis, peripheral edema
Failure of exacerbation to respond to initial medical management
Significant comorbidities
Frequent exacerbations
Newly occurring arrhythmias
Diagnostic uncertainty
Older age
Insufficient home support

Reprinted with permission of the American Thoracic Society. Copyright © American Thoracic Society. From Rabe KF, Hurd S, Anzueto A, et al. Global strategy for the diagnosis, management, and prevention of chronic obstructive pulmonary disease: GOLD executive summary. *Am J Respir Crit Care Med.* 2007;176:532–555. Official Journal of the American Thoracic Society; Diane Gern, Publisher.

BOX 35–11

Indications for Intensive Care Unit Admission of Patients with Exacerbations of COPD

Severe dyspnea that responds inadequately to initial emergency therapy
Changes in mental status (confusion, lethargy, coma)
Persistent or worsening hypoxemia ($Pa{O_2} < 40$ mm Hg), and/or severe or worsening respiratory acidosis (pH < 7.25) despite supplemental oxygen and noninvasive ventilation
Need for invasive mechanical ventilation
Hemodynamic instability—need for vasopressors

Reprinted with permission of the American Thoracic Society. Copyright © American Thoracic Society. From Rabe KF, Hurd S, Anzueto A, et al. Global strategy for the diagnosis, management, and prevention of chronic obstructive pulmonary disease: GOLD executive summary. *Am J Respir Crit Care Med.* 2007;176:532–555. Official Journal of the American Thoracic Society; Diane Gern, Publisher.

BOX 35–12

Conditions That May Simulate an Exacerbation of COPD

Pneumonia
Pulmonary emboli
Myocardial infarction or ischemia
Congestive heart failure
Dysrhythmia
Pneumothorax
Aspiration
Neuromuscular weakness
Rib or vertebral body fractures
Metabolic acidosis or other electrolyte disturbance
Pleural effusion
Sedating drugs or beta-blocking drugs
Inappropriate use of oxygen with hyperoxia and retained CO_2
Other organ dysfunction, such as renal failure or gastrointestinal hemorrhage

considered and excluded if suggestive findings exist. Of note, 25% of patients with COPD hospitalized for severe exacerbations of uncertain etiologies have pulmonary emboli.

Severe exacerbations require a prompt acceleration of outpatient therapy. Supplemental oxygen should be administered routinely and titrated to a flow rate to maintain $Pa{O_2}$ above 60 mm Hg and $Sa{O_2}$ above 90% (**Figure 35–10**). Sampling of arterial blood gas values is indicated within 30 to 60 minutes to ensure adequate oxygenation and the absence of progressive hypercapnia. Either a Venturi mask or a nasal cannula is an acceptable oxygen delivery device, depending on patient tolerance.

Because of their rapid onset of action, SABAs represent preferred first-line therapy,[8] although systematic reviews report similar clinical benefit from inhaled ipratropium.[101] SABAs, but not anticholinergic agents, may transiently worsen hypoxia through pulmonary vascular effects.[102] Little evidence supports the combination of SABAs and ipratropium,[101] although this combination is commonly recommended in view of the absence of an increased risk of short-term adverse drug effects.[8]

A meta-analysis of randomized trials does not support the use of methylxanthine bronchodilators, such as aminophylline or theophylline, for the treatment of exacerbations of COPD.[103] Administration of **methylxanthines** was noted to increase adverse events of nausea and vomiting without demonstrated improvement of respiratory endpoints. The GOLD guideline, however, recommends methylxanthines as second-line therapy for patients who have inadequate response to SABAs.[8]

Systematic reviews report that systemic corticosteroids improve respiratory physiologic measures during the first 72 hours of care and reduce risk for 30-day treatment failure, although the incidence of hyperglycemia during steroid treatment is increased. It is currently recommended that all hospitalized patients with exacerbations be treated with corticosteroids.[8] The recommended dose is 30 to 40 mg of oral prednisone or an equivalent dose of methylprednisolone intravenously for 7 to 10 days.[8] A response to corticosteroids during

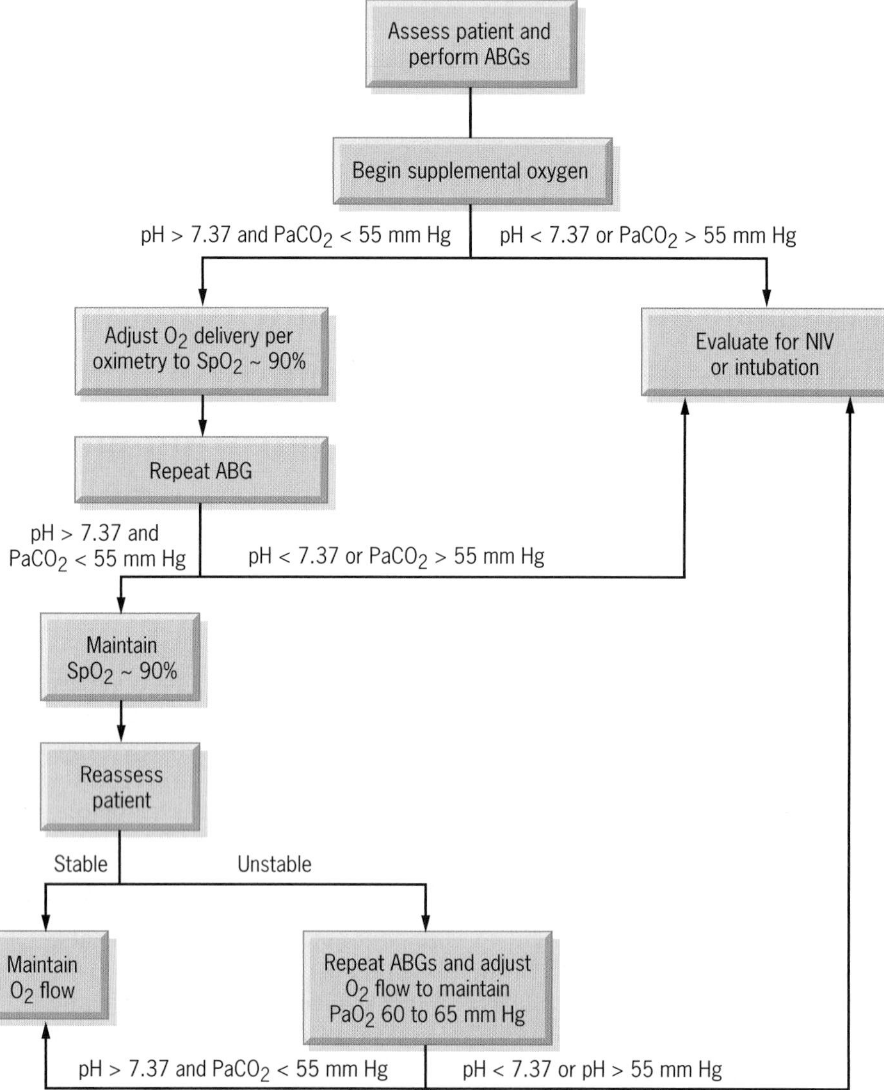

FIGURE 35–10 Algorithm for the management of supplemental oxygen in patients hospitalized for an exacerbation. ABGs, arterial blood gas values; Sp_{O_2}, arterial oxygen saturation by pulse oximetry; Pa_{CO_2}, partial pressure of arterial carbon dioxide.

an acute hospitalization should not be interpreted as an indication for chronic corticosteroid therapy.

Recommendations for antibiotic therapy for patients hospitalized for severe exacerbations are similar to those for mild exacerbations (discussed earlier). Recent guidelines, however, have suggested stratifying patients according to their risk for treatment failure. Patients with worse lung function, increased frequency of exacerbations or office visits, ischemic heart disease, and other comorbidities may benefit from treatment with extended-spectrum antibiotics.

Hospitalized patients with exacerbations may present with acute respiratory failure or develop respiratory failure after a period of initial medical management. The cause of respiratory failure varies between patients, but a common scenario occurs when patients with moderate to severe airway obstruction increase their $\dot{V}_E$ and work of breathing in response to increased airway resistance due to worsening airway inflammation, edema, bronchospasm, and secretions. The increasing respiratory rate shortens expiratory time and causes dynamic hyperinflation and auto-PEEP. Other factors, such as pulmonary hypertension, poor nutrition with muscle weakness, disadvantageous chest wall mechanics from hyperinflated lungs, and baseline hypercapnia, may lower ventilatory reserve. As work of breathing continues to increase, the patient tires and acute respiratory failure ensues.

Patients with acute respiratory failure have fatigued respiratory muscles and benefit from ventilatory assistance. Goals of assisted ventilation include unloading of respiratory muscles to allow recovery from muscle fatigue, reduction of air trapping, and maintenance of Pa_{CO_2} at or near the patient's baseline value. Many patients develop acute respiratory failure in the setting of chronic compensated respiratory acidosis. It is important to adjust ventilatory support to the patient's baseline Pa_{CO_2}, which can be estimated by the patient's serum bicarbonate level at admission or during a previous period of stability. Overventilation to a normal Pa_{CO_2} of 40 mm Hg if the patient is chronically hypercapnic results in renal loss of bicarbonate and uncompensated respiratory acidosis when the patient returns to the baseline level of hypercapnia during discontinuation of ventilatory support.

Ventilatory support can be delivered by invasive or noninvasive mechanical ventilation. NIV avoids potential complications of invasive ventilation, such as airway injury from intubation, requirements for sedation, and ventilator-associated pneumonia. Randomized clinical trials[37,104–111] and meta-analyses[95,112,113] have compared outcomes of NIV with standard care. The meta-analyses established benefit for patients with more severe disease in decreasing mortality and need for intubation.[95,112] A regression analysis of primary studies recommends NIV for patients with a pH less than 7.37 or a Pa_{CO_2} greater than 55 mm Hg.[113]

NIV may be delivered with either an oronasal or nasal mask, but a comfortable mask fit is important for patient acceptance. Most clinical trials have used

NIV, but successful outcomes have been reported with CPAP.[114] Patients managed with NIV require close monitoring because up to 50% of patients may fail and require intubation.

Patients who fail NIV or have immediately life-threatening respiratory failure (severe hypoxemia, hypercapnia, hemodynamic instability, altered mental status, or increased work of breathing with impending apnea) require intubation and mechanical ventilation. Initial ventilator settings should limit the inspiratory effort necessary to trigger the ventilator to reduce work of breathing and allow recovery from respiratory muscle fatigue. The mode of ventilation, V_T, respiratory rate, and inspiratory flow rate should be adjusted to ensure that fatigued respiratory muscles are adequately unloaded and dynamic hyperinflation improved or eliminated.

Invasive ventilation presents the greatest risk in COPD for severe dynamic hyperinflation because the ventilator can deliver a V_T and $\dot{V}_E$ beyond the patient's expiratory capabilities if an insufficient expiratory time is provided (**Box 35–13**). The resulting air trapping and auto-PEEP cause lung overdistension, patient discomfort, and patient–ventilator asynchrony in addition to barotrauma-related complications (e.g., pneumothorax, hemodynamic instability). Hemodynamic instability occurs because auto-PEEP decreases venous return and cardiac output.[115] Overdistension of lung regions can compress functional adjacent lung units and aggravate $\dot{V}/\dot{Q}$ mismatch, which may worsen hypoxia and paradoxically increase Pa_{CO_2} with further increases in $\dot{V}_E$. Additionally, auto-PEEP increases inspiratory effort by increasing the amount of negative intrathoracic pressure necessary to trigger the ventilator.

RESPIRATORY RECAP

Goals of Invasive Mechanical Ventilation in the Patient with COPD

- Unload ventilatory muscles and allow the patient to rest and recover from fatigue
- Provide an adequate expiratory time to avoid auto-PEEP and dynamic hyperinflation
- Prevent overventilation and respiratory alkalosis
- Prevent patient–ventilator asynchrony or excessive effort to trigger the ventilator

The ventilator should be set to avoid dynamic hyperinflation. Respiratory rate, V_T, inspiratory flow waveform, and inspiratory-to-expiratory (I:E) ratio should be set to allow a sufficient expiratory time. Some patients with extreme air trapping may require heavy sedation and paralysis to allow tolerance of a low respiratory rate that provides a longer expiratory time and permits less air trapping. Application of PEEP may improve dynamic hyperinflation by countering airway closure during exhalation. Applied PEEP theoretically stents open airways and increases expiratory flow. Multiple studies demonstrate that applied PEEP in this setting may have no effect, may decrease inspiratory flow, or may increase inspiratory flow with beneficial effects not occurring until applied PEEP approaches 80% of the auto-PEEP.[116] Determining the appropriate PEEP setting for an individual patient to avoid adverse effects remains a challenge with existing methods that employ an airway occlusion technique or an esophageal balloon. Some authorities discount the value of applied PEEP in stenting open airways, although evidence supports that it can reduce triggering effort. Some patients with air trapping may experience decreased auto-PEEP and work of breathing with application of helium–oxygen mixtures.[117]

After starting mechanical ventilation, caregivers should monitor patients for the presence of air trapping. Rising plateau pressures (Pplat), which should be low in patients with emphysema because of high lung compliance, suggest the pressure of auto-PEEP. The flow–time curves can also suggest the presence of auto-PEEP by demonstrating that expiratory flow continues to the initiation of inspiration. Quantifying actual values of auto-PEEP for spontaneously breathing patients remains challenging because minimal inspiratory or expiratory patient efforts have large effects on measured auto-PEEP values.[115]

BOX 35–13

Guidelines for Initial Ventilator Settings for Patients with COPD

Set respiratory rate low, 8–12 breaths/min.

Set initial tidal volume at 6–8 mL/kg.

Start F_{IO_2} initially at 100%, obtain arterial blood gas values, and wean oxygen to provide an oxygen saturation of 90% to 92% with F_{IO_2} goals of 40%.

Adjust PEEP between 0 and 5 cm H_2O to manage ventilator triggering and auto-PEEP.

Set peak flow high to provide adequate expiratory time.

Avoid overventilation and target baseline Pa_{CO_2}.

Monitor auto-PEEP, peak pressure, and plateau pressure to avoid dynamic hyperinflation and barotrauma.

Consider early extubation to noninvasive positive pressure ventilation.

F_{IO_2}, fractional concentration of inspired oxygen; Pa_{CO_2}, partial pressure of arterial carbon dioxide; PEEP, positive end-expiratory pressure.

Respiratory parameters measured at the bedside are poor predictors of extubation readiness.[118] Among patients with COPD who are difficult to liberate from mechanical ventilation, no differences exist between pressure support weaning versus spontaneous breathing trials.[119] Patients who fail a spontaneous breathing trial after 48 hours of ventilation have been shown to benefit from extubation to NIV.[120] In patients who pass a spontaneous breathing trial, extubation directly to NIV may prevent extubation failure.[121] Breathing a helium–oxygen mixture may decrease work of breathing after extubation but has not been shown to prevent extubation failure.[122] Elevation of *N*-terminal pro-brain natriuretic peptide blood levels in difficult-to-wean patients may identify patients with clinically occult heart failure as the cause of extubation failure.[123] Patients treated with corticosteroids for a COPD exacerbation are at risk for critical illness-related neuromuscular disease. One study reported that 9 of 26 patients ventilated for more than 48 hours and treated with more than 240 mg of methylprednisolone a day developed acute quadriplegic myopathy.[124] This respiratory muscle weakness may make ventilator liberation more difficult.

Prolonged weaning failure warrants consideration of a tracheostomy. Conversion of a translaryngeal endotracheal tube to a tracheostomy increases patient comfort, provides easier access for suctioning, enhances patient mobility, and may allow a more aggressive weaning approach.[125] Patients also may have an improved sense of well-being because of the ability to speak with a tracheostomy in place. No data indicate that a tracheostomy must be performed after any specific duration of translaryngeal intubation. Patients with COPD are considered for tracheostomy after an initial 7 days of mechanical ventilation if successful ventilator discontinuation is not imminent. Earlier tracheostomy can be performed if the severity of the illness makes extubation unlikely within a reasonable time. Considering that most of the benefits of tracheostomy are comfort related, it is less compelling to perform an early tracheostomy in patients with depressed mental status who are otherwise tolerating translaryngeal intubation well. The decision regarding tracheostomy should be based on the individual needs of a specific patient rather than general guidelines that direct routine tracheotomy only after 21 days of intubation.[126]

Palliative and End-of-Life Care

Patients with COPD may experience progressively worsening symptoms and quality of life as their disease becomes more severe. Palliative care provides opportunities to prevent and relieve suffering by managing symptoms and providing support to both patients and their families. As defined by the World Health Organization, palliative care is "an approach that improves the quality of life of patients and their families facing the problems associated with life-threatening illness, through the prevention and relief of suffering by means of early identification and impeccable assessment and treatment of pain and other problems, including physical, psychosocial, and spiritual issues."[127] The ATS endorses the concept that palliative care should be available to patients at all stages of their illness and should be individualized based on the needs and preferences of the patient and the patient's family.[128] Caregivers of patients with COPD should have an understanding of palliative care and a willingness to consult with palliative care specialists to assist with special patient needs.

Most patients hospitalized for COPD exacerbations survive to hospital discharge. A subgroup of patients, however, present with acute respiratory failure as the terminal event. Intubation and life support are burdensome for this group of patients and may prolong their dying process. Unfortunately, clinical and laboratory findings available at the time of admission are poor discriminators between those patients who will survive their hospitalization and those who will not recover. In such circumstances, decisions about the withdrawal of life support are aided by clinicians having a clear understanding of their patients' end-of-life wishes. Patients can formulate their own decisions about the acceptability of life support by blending their life goals and values with their physicians' estimates of anticipated outcome from life support interventions. This process centers on a patient's ability to provide informed decision making and requires an ongoing dialogue among patients, families, and caregivers.

Nonphysician educators can supplement physician discussions on end-of-life issues to promote patients' abilities to provide informed decisions.[129] Nurses, for instance, often have heightened sensitivities to their patients' needs and greater opportunities than physicians for discussing emotionally charged issues, such as advance planning. Although not yet studied, end-of-life discussions initiated by respiratory therapists may effectively introduce patients with COPD to topics of life support and advance planning during hospitalizations, home visits, and enrollment in pulmonary rehabilitation. Patients have demonstrated that they are willing to learn about advance planning from a wide range of nonphysician sources.[130] The Society of Critical Care Medicine encourages all members of the healthcare team, physicians and nonphysicians alike, to initiate discussions with their patients about end-of-life issues.[131]

Patients with severe COPD who choose to forego life supportive care in the terminal phases of their disease must be continuously reassured by all caregivers that they will not be medically or emotionally abandoned.[128] Intensive comfort care and close monitoring to detect a need for aggressive pain, anxiety, and dyspnea relief are fundamentally important. In such settings, the principle

BOX 35–14

Parameters to Identify Patients Who Qualify for Hospice Services

Patients will be considered to be in the terminal stage of pulmonary disease (life expectancy of 6 months or less) if they meet the following criteria. The criteria refer to patients with various forms of advanced pulmonary disease who eventually follow a final common pathway for end-stage pulmonary disease. (Criteria 1 and 2 should be present. Criteria 3, 4, and 5 will lend supporting documentation.)

1. Severe chronic lung disease as documented by both a and b:
   a. Disabling dyspnea at rest, poor response or unresponsive to bronchodilators, resulting in decreased functional capacity (e.g., bed-to-chair existence), fatigue, and cough. (Documentation of FEV_1, after bronchodilator, less than 30% of predicted is objective evidence for disabling dyspnea, but is not necessary to obtain.)
   b. Progression of end-stage pulmonary disease, as evidenced by increasing visits to the emergency department or hospitalizations for pulmonary infections and/or respiratory failure or increasing physician home visits before initial certification. (Documentation of serial decrease of $FEV_1 > 40$ mL/yr is objective evidence for disease progression, but is not necessary to obtain.)
2. Hypoxemia at rest on ambient air, as evidenced by PO_2 less than or equal to 55 mm Hg; or oxygen saturation less than or equal to 88% on supplemental oxygen determined either by arterial blood gases or oxygen saturation monitors; OR hypercapnia, as evidenced by $PCO_2 \geq 50$ mm Hg. These values may be obtained from recent (within 3 months) hospital records.
3. Right heart failure secondary to pulmonary disease (cor pulmonale) (e.g., not secondary to left heart disease or valvulopathy).
4. Unintentional progressive weight loss of greater than 10% of body weight over the preceding 6 months.
5. Resting tachycardia > 100/minute.

of “double effect” ethically, morally, and legally allows the administration of sufficient sedatives and analgesics to relieve pain and suffering even if drug therapy accelerates the patient’s death, as long as the intent is to relieve suffering.[128] Alternatives to acute care hospitalization do exist for patients with terminal COPD. COPD is recognized as a condition warranting hospice services by the National Hospice Organization, which has published guidelines to identify patients who qualify for hospice care (**Box 35–14**).

CASE STUDIES

Case 1. Initial Presentation of Chronic Obstructive Pulmonary Disease

During a routine physical examination, a 62-year-old woman complains of increasing shortness of breath with exertion. She has a 40-year smoking history and presently smokes one pack of filtered cigarettes per day. She reports occasional nonproductive cough but denies ever having symptoms compatible with an exacerbation of COPD. Physical examination reveals bilateral breath sounds with no adventitious sounds. Respiratory rate and pattern are normal at rest. No cyanosis or edema is present, and the remainder of the history and physical examination are unremarkable. She is referred to the pulmonary clinic for consultation, pulmonary function testing, and arterial blood gas analysis.

Results of pulmonary function testing are an FVC of 2.10 L (80% predicted), FEV_1 of 1.20 L (65% of predicted), and FEV_1/FVC of 58%. After administration of inhaled β_2-agonist, the FEV_1 increases to 1.35 L (73% of predicted). Lung volumes (residual volume, functional residual capacity, and total lung capacity) reveal mild hyperinflation. Single-breath D_{LCO} is 70% of predicted. Arterial blood gases on the breathing of room air are pH 7.42, $PaCO_2$ 39 mm Hg, and PaO_2 72 mm Hg. A chest radiograph is unremarkable other than giving the suggestion of mild hyperinflation.

The patient is counseled in the office about the importance of stopping smoking and referred to a smoking cessation program. She receives influenza and pneumococcal vaccinations. Albuterol by MDI is prescribed every 4 to 6 hours as needed to relieve symptoms. She is told to use the MDI before exertion if she anticipates dyspnea. She is instructed in the proper use of inhalers with a valved holding chamber. Pulmonary rehabilitation is arranged. She is scheduled for a follow-up at 2 months to evaluate her symptoms and exercise capability after smoking cessation and rehabilitation. If she remains exercise limited, long-acting inhaled bronchodilator therapy will be presented as an opportunity to improve her symptoms and quality of life. The potential benefits of preventing exacerbations and diminishing her decline in lung function by long-acting bronchodilator therapy will also be discussed.

Case 2. Exacerbation of Chronic Obstructive Pulmonary Disease

A 72-year-old man with a history of severe COPD is admitted to the emergency department with progressively increasing dyspnea over the past 48 hours. He uses continuous home oxygen at 2 L/min. He also uses inhaled albuterol, fluticasone (a corticosteroid), and tiotropium by MDI. His sputum became purulent 3 days ago, and his primary care physician prescribed antibiotic therapy (azithromycin). The patient has a respiratory rate of 30 breaths/min with use of accessory muscles and pursed lip exhalation. Breath sounds are distant, but no adventitious sounds are present. The chest is hyperinflated. Mild neck vein distention and ankle edema are present. The electrocardiogram is normal, with the exception of a mild tachycardia (110 beats/min). The patient appears dyspneic, but he cooperates with the physical examination. Arterial blood gas values are obtained with the patient breathing oxygen at 2 L/min: pH 7.28, $Paco_2$ 78 mm Hg, and Pao_2 52 mm Hg.

A nebulizer treatment has been administered with albuterol and ipratropium. Prednisone is given at a dose of 40 mg, and an antibiotic (moxifloxacin) is started. NIV is initiated. An oronasal mask is necessary because of the patient's dyspnea and inability to maintain a closed mouth. After 30 minutes of ventilation, accessory muscle use decreases, respiratory rate improves, and dyspnea is reported by the patient to be better. Inspired oxygen is titrated to maintain a Spo_2 of 88% to 90%. Preparations are made to admit him to the ICU.

Two hours later, the patient is in the ICU. He continues on NIV, but appears more comfortable. Arterial blood gas values at this time are pH 7.36, $Paco_2$ 65 mm Hg, and Pao_2 66 mm Hg. Four hours later, the patient asks to have the mask removed. He initially appears comfortable, but after 1 hour he has increasing dyspnea and accessory muscle use. NIV is resumed at the previous settings, but with the use of a nasal mask instead of the oronasal mask. This pattern of failed attempts to discontinue NIV continues for the next 36 hours, at which time the patient remains comfortable after removal of the mask. Six hours after discontinuation of NIV, his arterial blood gas values breathing 2 L/min of oxygen by nasal cannula are pH 7.37, $Paco_2$ 60 mm Hg, and Pao_2 62 mm Hg. The patient is transferred from the ICU to a general ward.

The following day, he continues to do well, and plans are made for discharge home. Options related to future exacerbations are discussed with the patient and his wife. He decides that NIV may be used for future exacerbations, but he elects not to be intubated or receive other resuscitative measures if he fails NIV. He completes a living will and advance directive for healthcare and ensures that his healthcare providers have future access to this information.

KEY POINTS

- Chronic obstructive pulmonary disease is the fourth most common cause of death in the United States, and its prevalence is increasing worldwide.
- Airflow limitation defines the presence of COPD. Both central and peripheral airways are affected by inflammatory and immunologic changes, but most of the observed increased airway resistance occurs in the peripheral airways.
- Smoking is the cause of COPD in 85% to 90% of patients. The prognosis of this progressive disorder is improved at any age with smoking cessation.
- Although existing clinical practice guidelines stage the severity of COPD by FEV_1, patients' quality of life and prognosis relate more closely to multidimensional measures that assess both respiratory and systemic features of COPD.
- The BODE index (body mass index, airflow obstruction, dyspnea, and exercise capacity) provides clinicians with a comprehensive measure of the severity of disease and response to therapy.
- COPD is a treatable disease. Management is directed toward reducing symptoms and improving quality of life, reducing decline in lung function, preventing complications, preventing or minimizing adverse effects of therapy, and prolonging survival.
- NIV improves outcomes of patients with COPD exacerbation.
- Palliative care and end-of-life planning are important components in the management of patients with all stages of COPD.

REFERENCES

1. National Heart, Lung and Blood Institute. COPD: for healthcare professionals. Available at: http://www.nhlbi.nih.gov/health/public/lung/copd/health-care-professionals/index.htm. Accessed November 3, 2008.
2. World Health Organization. Chronic respiratory diseases: burden. Available at: http://www.who.int/respiratory/copd/burden/en/index.html. Accessed November 3, 2008.

3. Mannino DM, Buist AS. Global burden of COPD: risk factors, prevalence, and future trends. *Lancet.* 2007;370:765–773.
4. National Heart, Lung and Blood Institute. *2007 NHLBI Morbidity and Mortality Chart Book.* Available at: http://www.nhlbi.nih.gov/resources/docs/cht-book.htm. Accessed November 3, 2008.
5. Talamo C, de Oca MM, Halbert R, et al. Diagnostic labeling of COPD in five Latin American cities. *Chest.* 2007;131:60–67.
6. Fabbri LM, Luppi F, Beghe B, Rabe KF. Complex chronic comorbidities of COPD. *Eur Respir J.* 2008;31:204–212.
7. van Eeden SF, Sin DD. Chronic obstructive pulmonary disease: a chronic systemic inflammatory disease. *Respiration.* 2008;75:224–238.
8. Rabe KF, Hurd S, Anzueto A, et al. Global strategy for the diagnosis, management, and prevention of chronic obstructive pulmonary disease: GOLD executive summary. *Am J Respir Crit Care Med.* 2007;176:532–555.
9. Speizer FE. The rise in chronic obstructive pulmonary disease mortality: overview and summary. *Am Rev Respir Dis.* 1989;140:S106–S107.
10. Muller NL, Coxson H. Chronic obstructive pulmonary disease. Part 4: imaging the lungs in patients with chronic obstructive pulmonary disease. *Thorax.* 2002;57:982–985.
11. The definition of emphysema. Report of a National Heart, Lung, and Blood Institute, Division of Lung Diseases workshop. *Am Rev Respir Dis.* 1985;132:182–185.
12. Celli BR, Cote CG, Marin JM, et al. The body-mass index, airflow obstruction, dyspnea, and exercise capacity index in chronic obstructive pulmonary disease. *N Engl J Med.* 2004;350:1005–1012.
13. U.S. Department of Health and Human Services. *The Health Consequences of Smoking: Chronic Obstructive Pulmonary Disease.* Rockville, MD: Author; 1984. DHHS Publication No. (PHS) 84-50205.
14. Celli BR, Halbert RJ, Nordyke RJ, Schau B. Airway obstruction in never smokers: results from the Third National Health and Nutrition Examination Survey. *Am J Med.* 2005;118:1364–1372.
15. Behrendt CE. Mild and moderate-to-severe COPD in nonsmokers: distinct demographic profiles. *Chest.* 2005;128:1239–1244.
16. Eisner MD, Balmes J, Katz PP, Trupin L, Yelin EH, Blanc PD. Lifetime environmental tobacco smoke exposure and the risk of chronic obstructive pulmonary disease. *Environ Health.* 2005;4:7.
17. Stoller JK, Fromer L, Brantly M, Stocks J, Strange C. Primary care diagnosis of alpha-1 antitrypsin deficiency: issues and opportunities. *Cleve Clin J Med.* 2007;74:869–874.
18. Silverman EK, Weiss ST, Drazen JM, et al. Gender-related differences in severe, early-onset chronic obstructive pulmonary disease. *Am J Respir Crit Care Med.* 2000;162:2152–2158.
19. Prescott E, Lange P, Vestbo J. Socioeconomic status, lung function and admission to hospital for COPD: results from the Copenhagen City Heart Study. *Eur Respir J.* 1999; 13:1109–1114.
20. Tao X, Hong CJ, Yu S, Chen B, Zhu H, Yang M. Priority among air pollution factors for preventing chronic obstructive pulmonary disease in Shanghai. *Sci Total Environ.* 1992;127:57–67.
21. Churg A, Wright JL. Animal models of cigarette smoke-induced chronic obstructive lung disease. *Contrib Microbiol.* 2007;14:113–125.
22. Jeffery PK. Comparative morphology of the airways in asthma and chronic obstructive pulmonary disease. *Am J Respir Crit Care Med.* 1994;150:S6–S13.
23. Jeffery PK. Remodeling and inflammation of bronchi in asthma and chronic obstructive pulmonary disease. *Proc Am Thorac Soc.* 2004;1:176–183.
24. Curtis JL, Freeman CM, Hogg JC. The immunopathogenesis of chronic obstructive pulmonary disease: insights from recent research. *Proc Am Thorac Soc.* 2007;4:512–521.
25. Lee SH, Goswami S, Grudo A, et al. Antielastin autoimmunity in tobacco smoking-induced emphysema. *Nat Med.* 2007;13:567–569.
26. Van Brabandt H, Cauberghs M, Verbeken E, Moerman P, Lauweryns JM, Van de Woestijne KP. Partitioning of pulmonary impedance in excised human and canine lungs. *J Appl Physiol.* 1983;55:1733–1742.
27. Di Stefano A, Capelli A, Lusuardi M, et al. Severity of airflow limitation is associated with severity of airway inflammation in smokers. *Am J Respir Crit Care Med.* 1998;158:1277–1285.
28. O'Donnell DE. Ventilatory limitations in chronic obstructive pulmonary disease. *Med Sci Sports Exerc.* 2001;33:S647–S655.
29. Dykstra BJ, Scanlon PD, Kester MM, Beck KC, Enright PL. Lung volumes in 4,774 patients with obstructive lung disease. *Chest.* 1999;115:68–74.
30. Parot S, Miara B, Milic-Emili J, et al. Hypoxemia, hypercapnia, and breathing patterns in patients with chronic obstructive pulmonary disease. *Am Rev Respir Dis.* 1982;126:882–886.
31. Killian K. Dyspnea. *J Appl Physiol.* 2006;101:1013–1014.
32. O'Donnell DE, Sciurba F, Celli B, et al. Effect of fluticasone propionate/salmeterol on lung hyperinflation and exercise endurance in COPD. *Chest.* 2006;130:647–656.
33. Celli BR, Thomas NE, Anderson JA, et al. Effect of pharmacotherapy on rate of decline of lung function in chronic obstructive pulmonary disease: results from the TORCH study. *Am J Respir Crit Care Med.* 2008;178:332–338.
34. Anthonisen NR, Skeans MA, Wise RA, Manfreda J, Kanner RE, Connett JE. The effects of a smoking cessation intervention on 14.5-year mortality: a randomized clinical trial. *Ann Intern Med.* 2005;142:233–239.
35. Nocturnal Oxygen Therapy Trial Group. Continuous or nocturnal oxygen therapy in hypoxemic chronic obstructive lung disease: a clinical trial. *Ann Intern Med.* 1980;93:391–398.
36. Fishman A, Martinez F, Naunheim K, et al. A randomized trial comparing lung-volume-reduction surgery with medical therapy for severe emphysema. *N Engl J Med.* 2003;348:2059–2073.
37. Bott J, Carroll MP, Conway JH, et al. Randomised controlled trial of nasal ventilation in acute ventilatory failure due to chronic obstructive airways disease. *Lancet.* 1993;341:1555–1557.
38. Sin DD, Wu L, Anderson JA, et al. Inhaled corticosteroids and mortality in chronic obstructive pulmonary disease. *Thorax.* 2005;60:992–997.
39. Nici L, Donner C, Wouters E, et al. American Thoracic Society/European Respiratory Society statement on pulmonary rehabilitation. *Am J Respir Crit Care Med.* 2006;173:1390–1413.
40. Rigotti NA, Munafo MR, Murphy MF, Stead LF. Interventions for smoking cessation in hospitalised patients. *Cochrane Database Syst Rev.* 2003;CD001837.
41. Fiore MC, Jaén CR, Baker TB, et al. *Treating Tobacco Use and Dependence: 2008 Update.* Clinical Practice Guideline. Rockville, MD: U.S. Department of Health and Human Services, Public Health Service; May 2008.
42. Silagy C, Lancaster T, Stead L, Mant D, Fowler G. Nicotine replacement therapy for smoking cessation. *Cochrane Database Syst Rev.* 2004;CD000146.
43. Blondal T, Gudmundsson LJ, Olafsdottir I, Gustavsson G, Westin A. Nicotine nasal spray with nicotine patch for smoking cessation: randomised trial with six year follow up. *BMJ.* 1999;318:285–288.
44. Jorenby DE, Leischow SJ, Nides MA, et al. A controlled trial of sustained-release bupropion, a nicotine patch, or both for smoking cessation. *N Engl J Med.* 1999;340:685–691.
45. Gonzales D, Rennard SI, Nides M, et al. Varenicline, an $\alpha 4\beta 2$ nicotinic acetylcholine receptor partial agonist, vs sustained-release bupropion and placebo for smoking cessation: a randomized controlled trial. *JAMA.* 2006;296:47–55.
46. COMBIVENT Inhalation Aerosol Study Group. In chronic obstructive pulmonary disease, a combination of ipratropium

bromide and albuterol is more effective than either agent alone. An 85-day multicenter trial. *Chest.* 1994;105:1411–1419.
47. Nelson HS. β-Adrenergic bronchodilators. *N Engl J Med.* 1995;333:499–506.
48. Celli BR. Update on the management of COPD. *Chest.* 2008;133:1451–1462.
49. Rennard SI, Anderson W, ZuWallack R, et al. Use of a long-acting inhaled β_2-adrenergic agonist, salmeterol xinafoate, in patients with chronic obstructive pulmonary disease. *Am J Respir Crit Care Med.* 2001;163:1087–1092.
50. Hanrahan JP, Hanania NA, Calhoun WJ, Sahn SA, Sciarappa K, Baumgartner RA. Effect of nebulized arformoterol on airway function in COPD: results from two randomized trials. *COPD.* 2008;5:25–34.
51. Rodrigo GJ, Nannini LJ, Rodriguez-Roisin R. Safety of long-acting beta-agonists in stable COPD: a systematic review. *Chest.* 2008;133:1079–1087.
52. Easton PA, Jadue C, Dhingra S, et al. A comparison of the bronchodilating effects of a beta-2 adrenergic agent (albuterol) and an anticholinergic agent (ipratropium bromide), given by aerosol alone or in sequence. *N Engl J Med.* 1986;315:735–739.
53. Lee TA, Pickard AS, Au DH, Bartle B, Weiss KB. Risk for death associated with medications for recently diagnosed chronic obstructive pulmonary disease. *Ann Intern Med.* 2008;149:380–390.
54. Tashkin DP, Celli B, Senn S, et al. A 4-year trial of tiotropium in chronic obstructive pulmonary disease. *N Engl J Med.* 2008;359:1543–1554.
55. Casaburi R, Kukafka D, Cooper CB, Witek TJ Jr, Kesten S. Improvement in exercise tolerance with the combination of tiotropium and pulmonary rehabilitation in patients with COPD. *Chest.* 2005;127:809–817.
56. Rodrigo GJ, Nannini LJ. Tiotropium for the treatment of stable chronic obstructive pulmonary disease: a systematic review with meta-analysis. *Pulm Pharmacol Ther.* 2007;20:495–502.
57. Barnes PJ, Ito K, Adcock IM. Corticosteroid resistance in chronic obstructive pulmonary disease: inactivation of histone deacetylase. *Lancet.* 2004;363:731–733.
58. Burge PS, Calverley PM, Jones PW, Spencer S, Anderson JA, Maslen TK. Randomised, double blind, placebo controlled study of fluticasone propionate in patients with moderate to severe chronic obstructive pulmonary disease: the ISOLDE trial. *BMJ.* 2000;320:1297–1303.
59. The Lung Health Study Research Group. Effect of inhaled triamcinolone on the decline in pulmonary function in chronic obstructive pulmonary disease. *N Engl J Med.* 2000;343:1902–1909.
60. Vestbo J. The TORCH (Towards a Revolution in COPD Health) survival study protocol. *Eur Respir J.* 2004;24:206–210.
61. Calverley P, Pauwels R, Vestbo J, et al. Combined salmeterol and fluticasone in the treatment of chronic obstructive pulmonary disease: a randomised controlled trial. *Lancet.* 2003;361:449–456.
62. Karpel JP, Kotch A, Zinny M, Pesin J, Alleyne W. A comparison of inhaled ipratropium, oral theophylline plus inhaled beta-agonist, and the combination of all three in patients with COPD. *Chest.* 1994;105:1089–1094.
63. ZuWallack RL, Mahler DA, Reilly D, et al. Salmeterol plus theophylline combination therapy in the treatment of COPD. *Chest.* 2001;119:1661–1670.
64. van Noord JA, de Munck DR, Bantje TA, Hop WC, Akveld ML, Bommer AM. Long-term treatment of chronic obstructive pulmonary disease with salmeterol and the additive effect of ipratropium. *Eur Respir J.* 2000;15:878–885.
65. van Noord JA, Aumann JL, Janssens E, et al. Effects of tiotropium with and without formoterol on airflow obstruction and resting hyperinflation in patients with COPD. *Chest.* 2006;129:509–517.
66. Kerstjens HA, Bantje TA, Luursema PB, et al. Effects of short-acting bronchodilators added to maintenance tiotropium therapy. *Chest.* 2007;132:1493–1499.
67. Calverley PM, Boonsawat W, Cseke Z, Zhong N, Peterson S, Olsson H. Maintenance therapy with budesonide and formoterol in chronic obstructive pulmonary disease. *Eur Respir J.* 2003;22:912–919.
68. Anthonisen NR, Manfreda J, Warren CP, et al. Antibiotic therapy in exacerbations of chronic obstructive pulmonary disease. *Ann Intern Med.* 1987;106:196–204.
69. Adams SG, Melo J, Luther M, Anzueto A. Antibiotics are associated with lower relapse rates in outpatients with acute exacerbations of COPD. *Chest.* 2000;117:1345–1352.
70. Petty TL. The National Mucolytic Study. Results of a randomized, double-blind, placebo-controlled study of iodinated glycerol in chronic obstructive bronchitis. *Chest.* 1990;97:75–83.
71. Decramer M, Rutten-van Molken M, Dekhuijzen PN, et al. Effects of *N*-acetylcysteine on outcomes in chronic obstructive pulmonary disease (Bronchitis Randomized on NAC Cost-Utility Study, BRONCUS): a randomised placebo-controlled trial. *Lancet.* 2005;365:1552–1560.
72. Anzueto A, Jubran A, Ohar JA, et al. Effects of aerosolized surfactant in patients with stable chronic bronchitis: a prospective randomized controlled trial. *JAMA.* 1997;278:1426–1431.
73. Long term domiciliary oxygen therapy in chronic hypoxic cor pulmonale complicating chronic bronchitis and emphysema. Report of the Medical Research Council Working Party. *Lancet.* 1981;1:681–686.
74. Criner GJ, Celli BR. Ventilatory muscle recruitment in exercise with O_2 in obstructed patients with mild hypoxemia. *J Appl Physiol.* 1987;63:195–200.
75. Tarpy SP, Celli BR. Long-term oxygen therapy. *N Engl J Med.* 1995;333:710–714.
76. Simonds AK, Elliott MW. Outcome of domiciliary nasal intermittent positive pressure ventilation in restrictive and obstructive disorders. *Thorax.* 1995;50:604–609.
77. Kolodziej MA, Jensen L, Rowe B, Sin D. Systematic review of noninvasive positive pressure ventilation in severe stable COPD. *Eur Respir J.* 2007;30(2):293–306.
78. Krachman S, Minai OA, Scharf SM. Sleep abnormalities and treatment in emphysema. *Proc Am Thorac Soc.* 2008;5:536–542.
79. O'Donohue WJ Jr, Bowman TJ. Hypoxemia during sleep in patients with chronic obstructive pulmonary disease: significance, detection, and effects of therapy. *Respir Care.* 2000;45:188–191; discussion 192–193.
80. O'Donoghue FJ, Catcheside PG, Ellis EE, et al. Sleep hypoventilation in hypercapnic chronic obstructive pulmonary disease: prevalence and associated factors. *Eur Respir J.* 2003;21:977–984.
81. Ries AL, Bauldoff GS, Carlin BW, et al. Pulmonary rehabilitation: joint ACCP/AACVPR evidence-based clinical practice guidelines. *Chest.* 2007;131:4S–42S.
82. Benditt JO. Surgical options for patients with COPD: sorting out the choices. *Respir Care.* 2006;51:173–182.
83. Morgan MD, Denison DM, Strickland B. Value of computed tomography for selecting patients with bullous lung disease for surgery. *Thorax.* 1986;41:855–862.
84. Snyder ML, Goss CH, Neradilek B, et al. Changes in arterial oxygenation and self-reported oxygen use after lung volume reduction surgery. *Am J Respir Crit Care Med.* 2008;178:339–345.
85. Edelman JD, Kotloff RM. Surgical approaches to advanced emphysema. *Respir Care Clin North Am.* 1998;4:513–539.
86. Orens JB, Estenne M, Arcasoy S, et al. International guidelines for the selection of lung transplant candidates: 2006 update—a consensus report from the Pulmonary Scientific Council of the International Society for Heart and Lung Transplantation. *J Heart Lung Transplant.* 2006;25:745–755.

87. Schulman LL. Lung transplantation for chronic obstructive pulmonary disease. *Clin Chest Med.* 2000;21:849–865.
88. Hosenpud JD, Bennett LE, Keck BM, Edwards EB, Novick RJ. Effect of diagnosis on survival benefit of lung transplantation for end-stage lung disease. *Lancet.* 1998;351:24–27.
89. Bavaria JE, Kotloff R, Palevsky H, et al. Bilateral versus single lung transplantation for chronic obstructive pulmonary disease. *J Thorac Cardiovasc Surg.* 1997;113:520–527; discussion 528.
90. Pellegrino R, Rodarte JR, Frost AE, Reid MB. Breathing by double-lung recipients during exercise: response to expiratory threshold loading. *Am J Respir Crit Care Med.* 1998;157:106–110.
91. Gross CR, Savik K, Bolman RMR, Hertz MI. Long-term health status and quality of life outcomes of lung transplant recipients. *Chest.* 1995;108:1587–1593.
92. Fabbri L, Pauwels RA, Hurd SS. Global Strategy for the Diagnosis, Management, and Prevention of Chronic Obstructive Pulmonary Disease: GOLD executive summary updated 2003. *COPD.* 2004;1:105–141; discussion 103–104.
93. Sethi S, Sethi R, Eschberger K, et al. Airway bacterial concentrations and exacerbations of chronic obstructive pulmonary disease. *Am J Respir Crit Care Med.* 2007;176:356–361.
94. Connors AF Jr, Dawson NV, Thomas C, et al. Outcomes following acute exacerbation of severe chronic obstructive lung disease. The SUPPORT (Study to Understand Prognoses and Preferences for Outcomes and Risks of Treatments) investigators. *Am J Respir Crit Care Med.* 1996;154:959–967.
95. Quon BS, Gan WQ, Sin DD. Contemporary management of acute exacerbations of COPD: a systematic review and meta-analysis. *Chest.* 2008;133:756–766.
96. Siempos II, Dimopoulos G, Korbila IP, Manta K, Falagas ME. Macrolides, quinolones and amoxicillin/clavulanate for chronic bronchitis: a meta-analysis. *Eur Respir J.* 2007;29:1127–1137.
97. Niewoehner DE. The role of systemic corticosteroids in acute exacerbation of chronic obstructive pulmonary disease. *Am J Respir Med.* 2002;1:243–248.
98. Thompson WH, Nielson CP, Carvalho P, Charan NB, Crowley JJ. Controlled trial of oral prednisone in outpatients with acute COPD exacerbation. *Am J Respir Crit Care Med.* 1996;154:407–412.
99. Stevenson NJ, Walker PP, Costello RW, Calverley PM. Lung mechanics and dyspnea during exacerbations of chronic obstructive pulmonary disease. *Am J Respir Crit Care Med.* 2005;172:1510–1516.
100. Parker CM, Voduc N, Aaron SD, Webb KA, O'Donnell DE. Physiological changes during symptom recovery from moderate exacerbations of COPD. *Eur Respir J.* 2005;26:420–428.
101. McCrory DC, Brown CD. Inhaled short-acting β2-agonists versus ipratropium for acute exacerbations of chronic obstructive pulmonary disease. *Cochrane Database Syst Rev.* 2001;2.
102. Cazzola M, Spina D, Matera MG. The use of bronchodilators in stable chronic obstructive pulmonary disease. *Pulm Pharmacol Ther.* 1997;10:128–144.
103. Barr RG, Rowe BH, Camargo CAJ. Methylxanthines for exacerbations of chronic obstructive pulmonary disease: meta-analysis of randomised trials. *BMJ.* 2003;327:643.
104. Angus RM, Ahmed AA, Fenwick LJ, Peacock AJ. Comparison of the acute effects on gas exchange of nasal ventilation and doxapram in exacerbations of chronic obstructive pulmonary disease. *Thorax.* 1996;51:1048–1050.
105. Plant PK, Owen JL, Elliott MW. Early use of non-invasive ventilation for acute exacerbations of chronic obstructive pulmonary disease on general respiratory wards: a multicentre randomised controlled trial. *Lancet.* 2000;355:1931–1935.
106. Martin TJ, Hovis JD, Costantino JP, et al. A randomized, prospective evaluation of noninvasive ventilation for acute respiratory failure. *Am J Respir Crit Care Med.* 2000;161:807–813.
107. Dikensoy O, Ikidag B, Filiz A, Bayram N. Comparison of noninvasive ventilation and standard medical therapy in acute hypercapnic respiratory failure: a randomised controlled study at a tertiary health centre in SE Turkey. *Int J Clin Pract.* 2002;56:85–88.
108. Confalonieri M, Potena A, Carbone G, Porta RD, Tolley EA, Umberto Meduri G. Acute respiratory failure in patients with severe community-acquired pneumonia. A prospective randomized evaluation of noninvasive ventilation. *Am J Respir Crit Care Med.* 1999;160:1585–1591.
109. Celikel T, Sungur M, Ceyhan B, Karakurt S. Comparison of noninvasive positive pressure ventilation with standard medical therapy in hypercapnic acute respiratory failure. *Chest.* 1998;114:1636–1642.
110. Barbé F, Togores B, Rubi M, et al. Noninvasive ventilatory support does not facilitate recovery from acute respiratory failure in chronic obstructive pulmonary disease. *Eur Respir J.* 1996;9:1240–1245.
111. Avdeev SN, Tret'iakov AV, Grigor'iants RA, Kutsenko MA, Chuchalin AG. [Study of the use of noninvasive ventilation of the lungs in acute respiratory insufficiency due exacerbation of chronic obstructive pulmonary disease]. *Anesteziol Reanimatol.* 1998;45–51.
112. Keenan SP, Sinuff T, Cook DJ, Hill NS. Which patients with acute exacerbation of chronic obstructive pulmonary disease benefit from noninvasive positive-pressure ventilation? A systematic review of the literature. *Ann Intern Med.* 2003;138:861–870.
113. Peter JV, Moran JL. Noninvasive ventilation in exacerbations of chronic obstructive pulmonary disease: implications of different meta-analytic strategies. *Ann Intern Med.* 2004;141(5):W78–W79.
114. Goldberg P, Reissmann H, Maltais F, Ranieri M, Gottfried SB. Efficacy of noninvasive CPAP in COPD with acute respiratory failure. *Eur Respir J.* 1995;8:1894–1900.
115. Tuxen DV, Lane S. The effects of ventilatory pattern on hyperinflation, airway pressures, and circulation in mechanical ventilation of patients with severe air-flow obstruction. *Am Rev Respir Dis.* 1987;136:872–879.
116. Dambrosio M, Cinnella G, Brienza N, et al. Effects of positive end-expiratory pressure on right ventricular function in COPD patients during acute ventilatory failure. *Intensive Care Med.* 1996;22:923–932.
117. Tassiopoulos AK, Kwon SS, Labropoulos N, et al. Predictors of early discharge following open abdominal aortic aneurysm repair. *Ann Vasc Surg.* 2004;18:218–222.
118. Alvisi R, Volta CA, Righini ER, et al. Predictors of weaning outcome in chronic obstructive pulmonary disease patients. *Eur Respir J.* 2000;15:656–662.
119. Reissmann HK, Ranieri VM, Goldberg P, Gottfried SB. Continuous positive airway pressure facilitates spontaneous breathing in weaning chronic obstructive pulmonary disease patients by improving breathing pattern and gas exchange. *Intensive Care Med.* 2000;26:1764–1772.
120. Nava S, Ambrosino N, Clini E, et al. Noninvasive mechanical ventilation in the weaning of patients with respiratory failure due to chronic obstructive pulmonary disease. A randomized controlled trial. *Ann Intern Med.* 1998;128:721–728.
121. Ferrer M, Sellarés J, Valencia M, et al. Non-invasive ventilation after extubation in hypercapnic patients with chronic respiratory disorders: randomised controlled trial. *Lancet.* 2009;374:1082–1088.
122. Diehl JL, Mercat A, Guerot E, et al. Helium/oxygen mixture reduces the work of breathing at the end of the weaning process in patients with severe chronic obstructive pulmonary disease. *Crit Care Med.* 2003;31:1415–1420.

123. Grasso S, Leone A, De Michele M, et al. Use of *N*-terminal pro-brain natriuretic peptide to detect acute cardiac dysfunction during weaning failure in difficult-to-wean patients with chronic obstructive pulmonary disease. *Crit Care Med.* 2007;35:96–105.
124. Amaya-Villar R, Garnacho-Montero J, Garcia-Garmendia JL, et al. Steroid-induced myopathy in patients intubated due to exacerbation of chronic obstructive pulmonary disease. *Intensive Care Med.* 2005;31:157–161.
125. Heffner JE. The role of tracheotomy in weaning. *Chest.* 2001;120:477S–481S.
126. King C, Moores LK. Controversies in mechanical ventilation: when should a tracheotomy be placed? *Clin Chest Med.* 2008;29:253–263.
127. World Health Organization. Palliative care. Available at: http://www.who.int/cancer/palliative/en. Accessed November 3, 2008.
128. Lanken PN, Terry PB, Delisser HM, et al. An official American Thoracic Society clinical policy statement: palliative care for patients with respiratory diseases and critical illnesses. *Am J Respir Crit Care Med.* 2008;177:912–927.
129. Heffner JE. End-of-life ethical issues. *Respir Care Clin North Am.* 1998;4:541–559.
130. Heffner JE, Fahy B, Barbieri C. Advance directive education during pulmonary rehabilitation. *Chest.* 1996;109:373–379.
131. Task Force on Ethics of the Society of Critical Care Medicine. Consensus report on the ethics of foregoing life-sustaining treatments in the critically ill. *Crit Care Med.* 1990;18:1435–1439.

CHAPTER 36

Interstitial Lung Disease

Kathleen A. Short
Andrew J. Ghio

OUTLINE

Pathophysiology
Classification
Clinical Presentation and Diagnostic Evaluation
Pathology
Prognosis
Management
Associated Diseases

OBJECTIVES

1. Describe the precipitating causes, clinical manifestations, and radiographic, laboratory, and pathophysiologic findings of interstitial lung disease.
2. Describe the diseases associated with pulmonary fibrosis.
3. Describe the management and therapy of interstitial lung disease.
4. Discuss the prognosis of interstitial lung disease.

KEY TERMS

bronchiolitis obliterans with organizing pneumonia (BOOP)
collagen vascular disease
eosinophilic granuloma
idiopathic pulmonary fibrosis (IPF)
interstitial lung disease (ILD)
pulmonary alveolar proteinosis (PAP)
respiratory bronchiolitis
sarcoidosis

INTRODUCTION

Interstitial lung disease (ILD) encompasses approximately 200 distinct diseases in which the interstitium is altered by some combination of inflammation and fibrosis. The interstitium of the lung comprises the alveolar walls (and lumens), pulmonary microvasculature, interstitial macrophages, fibroblasts, myofibroblasts, and matrix components of the lungs (**Figure 36–1**). The inflammatory and fibrotic disorders of ILD can affect any of these components. The resulting infiltration of the acinar region by cellular and extracellular elements may either distort the alveolar and bronchiolar architecture or may cause little associated damage (**Figure 36–2**).

ILD is an extremely diverse group of both acute and chronic disorders. Common clinical, radiographic, and pathophysiologic features form the basis for collective reference to this complex group of disorders as interstitial lung disease (**Box 36–1**). Most often the patient complains of dyspnea; a chest radiograph shows abnormal markings; and lung function tests demonstrate a loss of function, including decreased volumes and reduced diffusing capacity. To make the diagnosis, the clinical presentation, radiographic findings, pulmonary function test results, laboratory values, and lung biopsy findings all must be correlated. In most cases, a definitive diagnosis cannot be made without a biopsy.

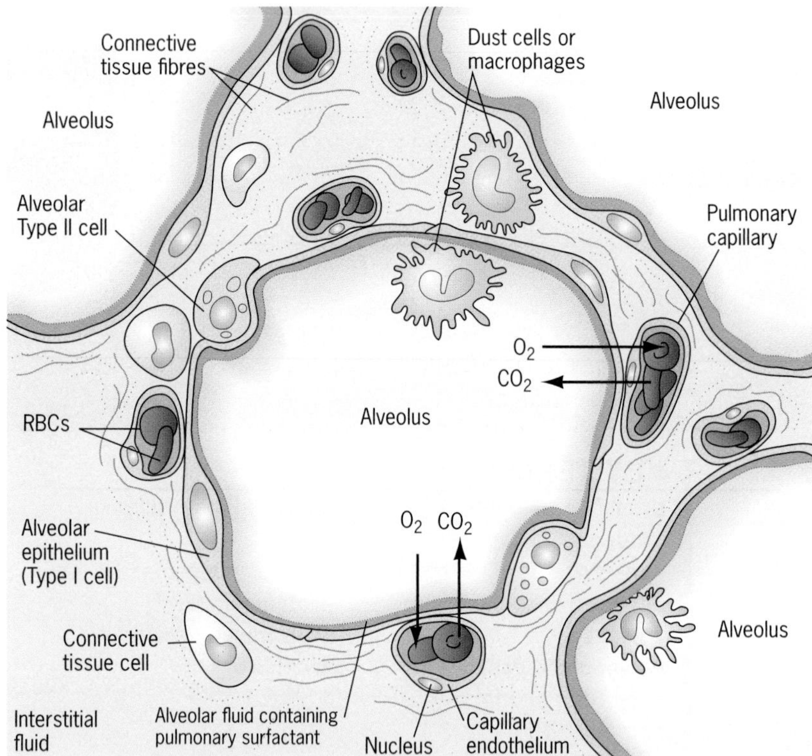

FIGURE 36–1 Schematic of lung illustrating components of the interstitium.

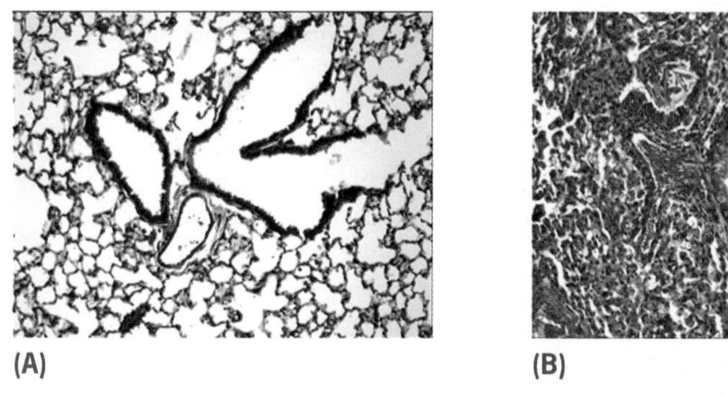

FIGURE 36–2 Micrographs showing **(A)** normal lung and **(B)** interstitial lung disease. In contrast to normal lung, there are alterations in the interstitium with an accumulation of inflammatory cells and subsequent widening. The stain is hematoxylin and eosin at a magnification of approximately 100×.

Pathophysiology

A common sequence of events that results in ILD begins when either a recognized or an unidentified agent induces alveolitis and vasculitis (**Box 36–2**). Persistence of this inflammatory lesion results in alveolar, capillary, and parenchymal cell injury. Abnormal repair leads to proliferation of mesenchymal cells, with the production of excess collagen and other extracellular matrix connective tissue elements. In the later stages of ILD, the normal architecture of the lung is replaced by cystic spaces separated by thick bands of fibrous tissue, a condition called *honeycomb lung.*

Although the end stage of the lung is histologically similar in many types of ILD, the alveolitis stage often is distinctive because of the number and influence of various inflammatory and immune effector cells present, such as neutrophils, eosinophils, and lymphocytes. Oxidants (generated both exogenously and endogenously) and neutrophil proteases (e.g. elastase, collagenase, cathepsins) are assumed to mediate some portion of tissue injury in many of these disorders. The alveolar macrophage was previously considered to coordinate this injury because of its release of reactive oxygen species, chemoattractants for neutrophils, and growth factors for mesenchymal cells, including fibronectin, platelet-derived growth factor, and insulin-like factor 1, which are involved in the progression to fibrosis. However, it has been demonstrated that respiratory epithelial cells have a similar capacity to elaborate these same mediators and coordinate an inflammatory and fibrotic response to numerous agents.

BOX 36–1

Key Diagnostic Features of Interstitial Lung Disease

Dyspnea at rest or with exertion (or in both cases)

Bilateral diffuse interstitial infiltrates on chest radiograph

Physiologic abnormalities of a restrictive lung defect: decreased lung volumes, decreased diffusing capacity for carbon monoxide (DLCO), and abnormal difference between the alveolar and arterial oxygen pressure gradients ($P[A - a]O_2$) at rest and/or with exertion

Histopathologic features of inflammation or fibrosis (or both) of the pulmonary parenchyma

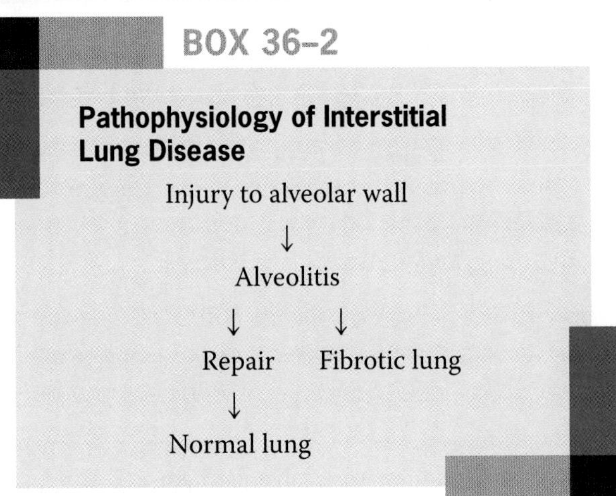
BOX 36–2

Pathophysiology of Interstitial Lung Disease

Classification

As a result of a lack of knowledge regarding etiology, a satisfactory classification system for ILD is not yet available. For practical purposes, it is useful to categorize the disorders by whether the cause is known or unknown (**Box 36–3**). An alternative criterion is the presence or absence of granulomas as a pathologic feature of the inflammatory process. Hypersensitivity pneumonitis, sarcoidosis, eosinophilic granuloma, Wegener granulomatosis, Churg-Strauss syndrome, and silicosis all are associated with the formation of granulomas. Idiopathic pulmonary fibrosis (IPF), connective tissue disorders, asbestosis, and disease caused by drugs, radiation, and toxic gas exposure are not associated with granulomas.

BOX 36–3

Classification of Interstitial Lung Disease

Known Cause

Infection
- Bacteria (*Legionella pneumophila, Bordetella pertussis*)
- Viruses (cytomegalovirus, human immunodeficiency virus, respiratory syncytial virus, adenovirus, influenza, parainfluenza, measles)
- *Mycoplasma* species
- *Mycobacterium* species
- Fungi (*Aspergillus* species)
- Parasites
- *Pneumocystis carinii* pneumonia

Occupational exposure
- Inorganic dusts (silicosis, asbestosis, talcosis, berylliosis, coal worker's pneumoconiosis, siderosis, baritosis)
- Microbial antigens (farmer's lung, humidifier lung, bird fancier's lung)
- Fumes (lung injury from exposure to chlorine gas, sulfuric acid, hydrochloric acid, nitrogen dioxide, or ammonia)

Neoplasm
- Bronchoalveolar carcinoma
- Leukemia
- Hodgkin disease
- Non-Hodgkin lymphoma

Congenital and metabolic causes
- Lipoidoses (Gaucher disease, Niemann-Pick disease)
- Storage disorders (Hermansky-Pudlak syndrome)
- Cystic fibrosis
- Radiation

Drug reactions

Recurrent aspiration

Lipoid pneumonia

Amyloidosis

Microlithiasis

Heart disease (congestive heart failure)

Liver disease (chronic active hepatitis, primary biliary cirrhosis)

Renal disease (renal failure)

(continues)

Box 36–3 *(continued)*

Bowel disease (ulcerative colitis, Crohn disease)
Graft-versus-host disease
Pulmonary veno-occlusive disease
Acute respiratory distress syndrome (ARDS)
Acute eosinophilic pneumonia (parasitic infections, such as with *Strongyloides*, *Ascaris*, and *Ancylostoma* subspecies)

Unknown Cause

Idiopathic pulmonary fibrosis
Sarcoidosis
Vasculitides

- Wegener granulomatosis, Churg-Strauss angiitis, lymphomatoid granulomatosis, alveolar hemorrhage syndromes accompanied by capillaritis, microscopic polyangiitis, Behçet syndrome, Takayasu disease, Henoch-Schönlein purpura

Collagen vascular diseases

- Rheumatoid arthritis, systemic sclerosis, systemic lupus erythematosus (SLE), polymyositis, dermatomyositis, Sjögren syndrome, mixed connective tissue disease, ankylosing spondylitis

Diffuse alveolar hemorrhage syndromes

- Antiglomerular basement membrane antibody disease (Goodpasture syndrome), bleeding in patients with systemic necrotizing vasculitis (Wegener granulomatosis and microscopic polyangiitis) and collagen vascular diseases, hemorrhage in immunocompromised hosts and after administration of exogenous agents (trimellitic anhydride, cocaine, and penicillamine), idiopathic pulmonary hemosiderosis

Eosinophilic granuloma
Chronic eosinophilic pneumonia
Bronchiolitis obliterans with organizing pneumonia
Respiratory bronchiolitis
Pulmonary alveolar proteinosis
Lymphangioleiomyomatosis, tuberous sclerosis, and ataxia telangiectasia
Lymphoid interstitial pneumonitis
Acute interstitial pneumonitis

Clinical Presentation and Diagnostic Evaluation

Symptoms and Signs

The most common presentation of ILD is a slowly progressive onset of dyspnea and a nonproductive cough. The dyspnea may occur on exertion at first but progresses to dyspnea at rest. The history is the most important tool in the identification of the etiology of ILD. A thorough history limits the differential diagnosis and may preclude the need for biopsy. However, even with a detailed history, the causative agent is identified in fewer than 20% to 30% of patients with ILD.[1]

To determine the causative agent of the ILD, the clinician must ask detailed questions and note specific symptoms. A list of all medications the patient has been taking should be compiled to detect drug-related causes of ILD. It should be remembered that patients can be vague about medications they are currently taking or may have been provided in the past. A detailed job history can help define occupational exposures and possible dusts, fumes, and antigens associated with ILD. Hobbies and environmental exposures (e.g., pigeon breeding, home saunas, heating and air conditioning units) should also be noted. Knowledge of the agents that can cause ILD can serve as a guide to the areas that should be emphasized in the occupational and environmental history. Risk factors for infection with the human immunodeficiency virus (HIV) must be explored. A review of systems must include attention to symptoms of fevers, chills, night sweats (e.g., hypersensitivity pneumonitis, vasculitis), arthralgia and myalgia (ILD with connective tissue disorders), sinusitis, hemoptysis (alveolar hemorrhage syndromes), and chest pain (ILD resulting from toxic gas exposure). A past medical history should inquire into episodes of pneumothorax. The family medical history should be reviewed closely to rule out a number of inherited disorders known to cause ILD, such as IPF, tuberous sclerosis, and neurofibromatosis. A history of cigarette smoking is important in the pathogenesis of some interstitial lung diseases, including eosinophilic granuloma, respiratory bronchiolitis, and alveolar hemorrhage syndromes.

The physical examination is frequently less helpful than the history in the determination of a specific diagnosis in ILD (**Table 36–1**). Bilateral, end-inspiratory, basilar crackles are a feature in several ILD diseases, including IPF, ILD with collagen vascular diseases, and asbestosis. Wheezes are rare except in Churg-Strauss syndrome. Other findings on the physical examination can assist in the differential diagnosis. Patients who have had severe disease for a protracted period may show evidence of pulmonary hypertension on the physical examination.

RESPIRATORY RECAP

Clinical History of Interstitial Lung Disease

- Dyspnea on exertion or at rest
- Cough
- Fevers, chills, and night sweats
- Medications taken
- Detailed work history
- Hobbies
- Environmental exposures
- Risk factors for infection with the human immunodeficiency virus (HIV)
- Past medical history of pneumothoraces
- Family medical history of interstitial lung disease
- Cigarette smoking

TABLE 36–1 Physical Examination Findings with Interstitial Lung Disease

Finding	Associated Disease
Digital clubbing	Idiopathic pulmonary fibrosis
Cutaneous lesions	Sarcoidosis, tuberous sclerosis, necrotizing vasculitis, dermatomyositis, collagen vascular diseases
Ocular signs	Sarcoidosis, ILD in systemic vasculitis, ILD with Sjögren syndrome or other connective tissue disorders
Polyarthritis	Sarcoidosis, ILD in systemic vasculitis, ILD with Sjögren syndrome or other connective tissue disorders
Peripheral lymphadenopathy	Sarcoidosis, lymphoid interstitial pneumonitis, ILD with connective tissue disorders
Hepatosplenomegaly	Sarcoidosis, amyloidosis, eosinophilic granuloma, chronic cor pulmonale
Neurologic manifestations	Tuberous sclerosis, systemic vasculitis, sarcoidosis, eosinophilic granuloma

ILD, interstitial lung disease.

Pulmonary Function Changes

The initial evaluation of pulmonary function in the patient with ILD should include spirometry, measurement of lung volumes and diffusing capacity (DLCO), inspiratory effort, maximum voluntary ventilation, arterial blood gas measurements, and exercise oxygen saturation. These studies characteristically reveal restriction with a decreased forced vital capacity (FVC), a decreased forced expiratory volume in the first second (FEV_1), and a normal or increased FEV_1 to FVC ratio. Total lung capacity (TLC) and the DLCO are decreased. The DLCO can sometimes be the most sensitive of the pulmonary function measures and may be abnormal even when lung volumes are preserved.[2]

A mild resting hypoxemia with significant arterial oxygen desaturation after exercise often is seen. The resting hypoxemia is the result of both ventilation-perfusion mismatch and shunt; the worsening of the condition with exercise may reflect diffusion restrictions in addition to mismatch and shunt. In patients with normal lung volumes or spirometry results, desaturation with ambulation may be a clue to the presence of pulmonary fibrosis.[2] A 6-minute walk test with a finger oximeter in place is well tolerated, provides a measure of oxygen requirements, and can be a quantifiable index of disease progression.[3]

Pulmonary function test results reflecting airway obstruction sometimes are seen in sarcoidosis, hypersensitivity pneumonitis, eosinophilic granuloma, Wegener granulomatosis, and lymphangioleiomyomatosis.

Radiographic Findings

The classic findings of ILD on a posteroanterior chest radiograph are those of a diffuse reticular, nodular, or reticulonodular pattern and reduced lung volume (**Figure 36–3**). Upper lobe predominance is seen in sarcoidosis, eosinophilic granuloma, silicosis, coal worker's pneumoconiosis, eosinophilic pneumonia, and ILD with ankylosing spondylitis. Lower lobe predominance is found in IPF, ILD with collagen vascular diseases, and asbestosis. The presentation usually is bilateral and symmetric but may be asymmetric and even unilateral, and alveolar infiltrates may be seen rather than small opacities. If the disorder has been long-standing, pulmonary hypertension may have developed and sometimes can be documented by the chest radiograph. An array of abnormalities can be seen on the chest radiographs of patients with ILD, which sometimes can be helpful in the determination of the differential diagnosis (**Table 36–2**).

High-resolution computed tomography (HRCT) is an important advance in the diagnosis and staging of ILD. Thin sections (1 to 2 mm) are used to portray two distinct patterns of disease: a ground glass increase in attenuation and a reticular pattern. The ground glass appearance is associated with a cellular histologic appearance of that area of lung, whereas the reticular pattern is found in patients whose subsequent lung biopsy confirms fibrosis. HRCT is significantly more sensitive and specific than a chest radiograph in the diagnosis of ILD and in the assessment of both the extent and severity of the disease.[4] It can identify disease before any abnormality is apparent on a chest radiograph. The distribution patterns and variability of involvement in ILD are more evident with HRCT and can be virtually pathognomonic for several forms of ILD, such as eosinophilic granuloma, IPF, lymphangioleiomyomatosis, lymphangitis carcinomatosa, sarcoidosis, and hypersensitivity pneumonitis.[5] HRCT also has prognostic value in that a demonstration of honeycomb cysts indicates end-stage, irreversible fibrosis and loss of alveolar walls. HRCT can also guide parenchymal biopsy sites or direct the surgeon to lymph nodes for biopsy by mediastinoscopy.

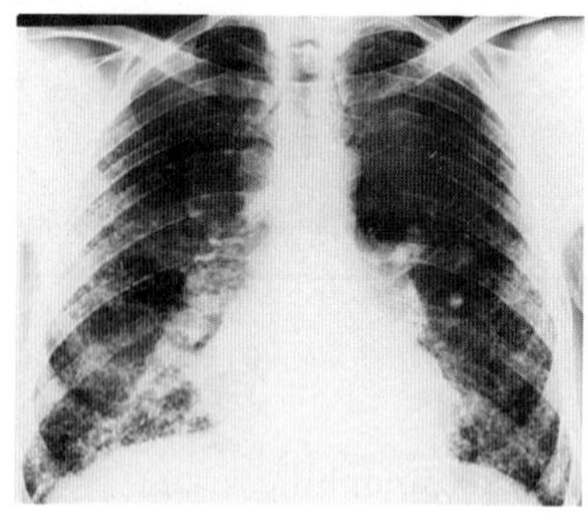

(A)

(B)

FIGURE 36–3 Chest radiographs demonstrating predominantly rounded opacities in the upper lung fields consistent with either silicosis or coal worker's pneumoconiosis (**A**). These are in contrast to the linear markings of asbestosis most commonly observed in the lower lung fields (**B**).

Nuclear scintigraphy with gallium citrate Ga 67 has been proposed as a diagnostic and staging tool in the assessment of patients with ILD, particularly sarcoidosis and IPF. However, gallium uptake is nonspecific, and this procedure has no clinical utility either in the monitoring or prediction of the clinical course of patients with ILD. Similarly, technetium Tc 99m radionuclide scans and positron emission tomography (PET) scans currently have no clinical role in either the diagnosis or staging of ILD.

TABLE 36–2 Radiographic Findings with Interstitial Lung Disease

Finding	Associated Disease
Normal radiograph (10% of ILD cases)	Early IPF, sarcoidosis, and hypersensitivity pneumonitis
Spontaneous pneumothorax	Eosinophilic granuloma and lymphangioleiomyomatosis
Hilar or mediastinal lymphadenopathy	Sarcoidosis, berylliosis, and silicosis
Eggshell calcification	Silicosis
Pleural disease	Asbestos-related ILD, tuberculosis, ILD with collagen vascular disease, malignancies, and lymphangioleiomyomatosis
Honeycombing	IPF, eosinophilic granuloma, collagen vascular diseases, pneumoconioses, sarcoidosis

ILD, interstitial lung disease; IPF, idiopathic pulmonary fibrosis.

RESPIRATORY RECAP

High-Resolution Computed Tomography

» High-resolution computed tomography (HRCT) can aid in the diagnosis of idiopathic pulmonary fibrosis, eosinophilic granuloma, lymphangioleiomyomatosis, sarcoidosis, and hypersensitivity pneumonitis.

Laboratory Findings

Routine blood and serologic test results most often are unremarkable for patients with ILD. Many patients have a mild anemia and elevated erythrocyte sedimentation rate, reflecting inflammation. Serologic tests (including angiotensin-converting enzyme, antinuclear antibody, and antineutrophil cytoplasmic antibody determinations), hypersensitivity pneumonitis screening (serum precipitins), and complement fixation for fungi can be helpful in some patients.

Although nonspecific, laboratory results can support diagnoses and narrow the differential diagnosis in ILD. Evidence of renal insufficiency or hematuria raises the possibility of renal–pulmonary syndromes (e.g., Wegener granulomatosis, Goodpasture syndrome, systemic lupus erythematosus, systematic necrotizing vasculitis), whereas abnormal results on liver function tests and high serum calcium levels are clues to the diagnosis of either sarcoidosis or metastatic malignancy.

Bronchoscopy

With ILD it is unusual to reach a specific diagnosis on the basis of the history, physical examination, pulmonary function test results, chest radiograph, and laboratory studies. The next step is to obtain an HRCT scan, and bronchoscopy with lavage and transbronchial lung biopsy usually follows. The exception to this order of investigation is the patient for whom bronchoscopy is thought to be more diagnostic; in such cases this procedure might be done before HRCT (**Figure 36–4**).

In the United States more than 60% of all patients with ILD undergo bronchoscopy.[1] In the evaluation of ILD, bronchoalveolar lavage samples cells and noncellular material from the lower respiratory tract.[6] Currently the clinical application of lavage in ILD is limited. Although the technique can be diagnostic (e.g., pulmonary alveolar proteinosis and pneumoconiosis), especially when particular cytologic or immunohistologic stains are applied (e.g., eosinophilic granuloma and alveolar hemorrhage syndromes), precise information is not obtained for most ILD disorders. However, lavage can be extremely useful

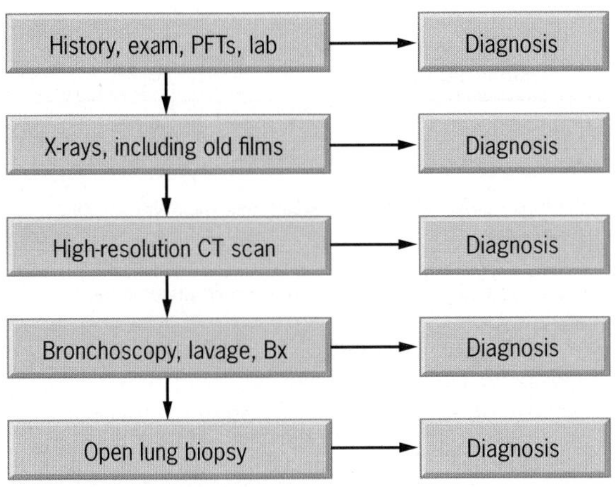

FIGURE 36–4 Approach to the evaluation of a patient with interstitial lung disease.

in the exclusion of specific etiologies and in the provision of supportive data to determine the differential diagnosis. The processing of lavage fluid should include cytologic studies and smears or cultures for acid-fast bacilli, fungi, *Pneumocystis carinii*, and viruses. This allows the clinician to exclude certain malignancies and specific infectious agents.

> **RESPIRATORY RECAP**
>
> **Bronchoalveolar Lavage**
>
> » Bronchoalveolar lavage can assist in the diagnosis of lung infections, alveolar hemorrhage, pulmonary alveolar proteinosis, eosinophilic granuloma, and pneumoconioses.

The cellular profiles obtained through analysis of the lavage fluid may indicate the underlying nature of the ILD. A lymphocytosis can be seen in sarcoidosis, berylliosis, and hypersensitivity pneumonitis. The CD4 (T helper) cells increase in sarcoidosis, with a ratio of CD4 to CD8 (T suppressor) cells of more than 3:5, whereas CD8 cells predominate with hypersensitivity pneumonitis. A lavage sample yielding more than 30% eosinophils supports a diagnosis of chronic or acute eosinophilic pneumonia. Neutrophils abound in several forms of ILD, including IPF and asbestosis.

> **RESPIRATORY RECAP**
>
> **Transbronchial Biopsy**
>
> » Transbronchial biopsy can aid in the diagnosis of sarcoidosis, lung infection, cancer, and hypersensitivity pneumonitis.

Transbronchial biopsy (TBB) is particularly helpful if a primary lung neoplasm, infectious pneumonitis, or sarcoidosis is high in the differential diagnosis. TBB can sometimes diagnose Wegener granulomatosis, rheumatoid lung disease, lymphangioleiomyomatosis, eosinophilic granuloma, eosinophilic pneumonitis, pulmonary alveolar proteinosis, silicosis, hypersensitivity pneumonitis, lymphangitic spread of carcinoma, and Goodpasture syndrome. Several specimens (up to six) should be obtained from both the upper and lower lobes of either the right or the left lung. If lavage and TBB are not diagnostic, surgical lung biopsies should be done unless specific contraindications exist.

> **BOX 36–4**
>
> **Indications for Surgical Lung Biopsy**
>
> Patient younger than 65 years
> History of fevers, weight loss, and sweats
> History of hemoptysis
> Family history of interstitial lung disease
> Symptoms and signs of peripheral vasculitis
> History of pneumothorax
> Normal chest radiograph despite clinical signs
> Atypical radiographic features of idiopathic pulmonary fibrosis
> Unexplained extrapulmonary manifestations
> Unexplained pulmonary hypertension
> Unexplained cardiomegaly
> Rapidly progressive disease

Surgical Lung Biopsy

When lavage and transbronchial biopsy are nondiagnostic, surgical lung biopsies should be done unless specific contraindications exist. Lung biopsy is conventionally regarded as the gold standard used to determine a specific diagnosis for patients with ILD. In the United States, fewer than 50% of patients with ILD have a lung biopsy of some type for diagnostic purposes, although the decision to obtain a surgical lung biopsy must be individualized. There are several indications for surgical lung biopsy (**Box 36–4**). Examination of tissue can allow confirmation of a specific diagnosis, affect the development of a plan of treatment, predict response to therapy, and provide prognostic information.[7] It can present insight into the pathogenesis of the ILD.

Morbidity and mortality rates are low with open biopsy and even lower with thoracoscopic biopsy.[8] Biopsy through video-assisted thoracoscopic surgery (VATS) is tolerated extremely well and results in less pain and fewer complications than the open approach. Subsequently, VATS has replaced open lung biopsy because of its reduced perioperative morbidity and the shorter hospital stay for the patient.[8] Lung specimens obtained through VATS provide equivalent specimen volume and diagnostic accuracy.

TABLE 36–3 Histologic Patterns with Interstitial Lung Disease

Pattern	Associated Disease
Common interstitial pneumonitis	IPF, ILD with collagen vascular disease, asbestosis, sarcoidosis, hypersensitivity pneumonitis, drug reactions, organizing pneumonia
Cellular interstitial pneumonitis	IPF, ILD with collagen vascular disease, idiopathic BOOP, drug reactions, hypersensitivity pneumonitis, lymphocytic interstitial pneumonitis
Desquamative interstitial pneumonitis	IPF, respiratory bronchiolitis, eosinophilic granuloma, drug reactions, lipoid pneumonia
Diffuse alveolar damage	Acute respiratory distress syndrome, cytotoxic drugs, ILD with collagen vascular disease, Hamman-Rich syndrome
Bronchiolitis obliterans with organizing pneumonia	IPF, ILD with collagen vascular disease, drug reactions, radiation, alveolar hemorrhage, eosinophilic pneumonia, hypersensitivity pneumonitis
Diffuse alveolar hemorrhage	Vasculitis, ILD with collagen vascular disease, Goodpasture syndrome, idiopathic pulmonary hemosiderosis
Eosinophilic pneumonia	IPF, drug reactions, allergic granulomatosis of Churg-Strauss, tropical eosinophilia, hypereosinophilic syndrome

IPF, idiopathic pulmonary fibrosis; ILD, interstitial lung disease; BOOP, bronchiolitis obliterans with organizing pneumonia.

Biopsy specimens should be obtained from several sites, including apparently normal lung tissue adjacent to and remote from obviously involved tissue. HRCT can help determine the needed biopsy sites. Alveolar tissue is preferred. Tissue processing requirements include untreated samples for bacteriologic and virologic studies; samples fixed in 10% formalin; samples fixed in Methacarnoys solution for immunofluorescence; samples fixed in glutaraldehyde for electron microscopy; and samples cryopreserved for immunologic and molecular studies.

Pathology

The pathologic findings in ILD are remarkably similar.[9] Alveolitis (granulomatous or nongranulomatous) is initially observed, which may continue for a prolonged period. Eventually collagen is deposited in the interstitium, and fibrosis results. Airways, blood vessels, and pleura may be involved. Different clinical entities may have similar underlying histologic pictures, and several histologic patterns may evolve for one clinical entity (Table 36–3).

Prognosis

The prognosis of ILD depends on the specific diagnosis, and most of the current information results from studies of IPF. Findings in the history, the chest radiograph, the pathology of the disease, and the response to therapy can provide prognostic information. In IPF, factors that predicted a better chance of survival in an untreated group were female gender and a younger age at presentation or at the onset of symptoms; the median survival among these patients was 4.5 years. In a treated group, factors associated with a better chance of survival were a younger age at the time of either presentation or onset of symptoms, less dyspnea, less impairment of carbon monoxide transfer factor, less radiographic abnormality, a more cellular histologic appearance on biopsy, and an early response to corticosteroids. The response to steroids was closely linked with a more cellular appearance on biopsy.

HRCT has been used to predict response to treatment and outcome and is deemed more accurate than a chest radiograph.[10] A ground glass appearance was associated with 100% survival rate at 50 months after diagnosis of IPF, compared with a 50% survival rate for patients with disease that appeared with a more reticular pattern. Bronchoscopy with lavage also can provide prognostic information. An increased number of lymphocytes can be associated with a good response to corticosteroids and a better overall prognosis, compared with an elevated number of eosinophils and neutrophils, which predicts a poorer response to corticosteroids in IPF.

RESPIRATORY RECAP

Factors Indicating an Improved Prognosis in Idiopathic Pulmonary Fibrosis

- Female patient
- Younger age
- Less dyspnea
- Greater cellular response in lavage

Management

Left untreated, the majority of the disorders included in ILD are progressive and result in death that occurs secondary to respiratory insufficiency and cor pulmonale. The most important tenet of therapy is to remove the agent of injury to the lung if possible, which may mean an exhaustive search for a causative agent.

If no agent is found, therapy can be directed toward suppression of inflammatory and cellular immune responses.[11] Agreement has never been reached on guidelines for standards of care and time of treatment for patients with ILD. The natural history of many with ILD is a steady progression and functional deterioration to the point where treatment is warranted. An important and challenging issue is when to start treatment. Many of the drugs used to treat ILD have the potential for serious side effects, which often is a disincentive to their use until no choice remains. By this time the patient has developed unequivocal breathlessness, and a considerable proportion of functional lung capacity has already been lost. It therefore is not surprising that meaningful improvements in lung function are uncommon and that often the best that can be achieved is stabilization of the disease to prevent further deterioration.

In ILD, few diseases are amenable to specific treatments; lavage in pulmonary alveolar proteinosis is an exception. Effective therapy is not available because the etiology or mechanism of disease is not recognized. The alveolitis may be suppressed with either corticosteroids or immunosuppressive agents, but these medications do not cure the disease. Corticosteroids almost always are the initial therapy, but they are associated with many adverse side effects. A few adequately controlled trials have assessed corticosteroid use in ILD. Among IPF patients, half experienced subjective improvement with steroids, yet only 15% to 20% improved by objective measures. The specific steroid regimen varies. Most commonly, therapy is initiated with prednisone 1 mg/kg, which is given for 3 to 6 months and then tapered over 4 to 6 months to 0.25 mg/kg. The efficacy of alternate-day regimens is not known.

Immunosuppressive or cytotoxic agents may be considered for patients for whom corticosteroids appear to have failed or for those who experience adverse side effects or have contraindications to corticosteroids, such as age, morbid obesity, insulin-dependent diabetes mellitus, or severe osteoporosis. Cyclophosphamide and methotrexate have been used in a number of disorders included in ILD. Methotrexate has been used infrequently because pulmonary toxicity can occur in a significant number of patients. Azathioprine also has been used as a corticosteroid-sparing agent in diverse autoimmune disease and as therapy for sarcoidosis, IPF, and ILD with collagen vascular disease. This medication is given orally and is associated with fewer adverse side effects than methotrexate, cyclophosphamide, or alkylating agents.

Meticulous supportive care can improve the quality of life of patients with ILD. Such therapy includes vaccines, antibiotics for episodes of purulent sputum, supplemental oxygen when the partial pressure of arterial oxygen (Pa_{O_2}) drops below 55 mm Hg, bronchodilators for wheezing, psychosocial therapy, and pulmonary rehabilitation. Supplemental oxygen therapy can be used to relieve symptoms of dyspnea at rest and during exercise. A 6-minute walk test can help to determine adequate oxygen flows and concentrations to prescribe. Oxygen therapy may help patients with ILD maintain activities of daily living and help to increase exercise endurance, especially in patients with end-stage disease. Higher oxygen flow rates and oxygen-conserving devices may be needed as the ILD progresses and hypoxia-related complications occur. Bronchodilators may be used to affect an increase in exercise capacity for patients with moderate to severe ILD and to reduce the increased work of breathing and feelings of breathlessness associated with ILD. Coupled with oxygen therapy, bronchodilators may promote physiologic improvements and subsequently improve quality of life among patients with severe symptoms from ILD.

Chronic lung conditions such as ILD can benefit from pulmonary rehabilitation programs. A comprehensive and individualized exercise training and education program can provide long-term health benefits and help to prevent and treat acute exacerbations. Rehabilitation programs can provide psychosocial support for patients, smoking cessation programs, and good nutrition guidance. The goal of individualized rehabilitation programs is to put patients in control of their disease rather than the disease in control of them.

Associated Diseases

Idiopathic Pulmonary Fibrosis

Idiopathic pulmonary fibrosis (IPF) predominantly affects males in the fifth to seventh decade of life.[12] No genetic basis has yet been determined. The pathogenesis is not known but is likely to reflect either an aberrant host response to injury at the alveolar epithelium and endothelium or a protracted response to the same. A history of a gradual onset of dyspnea with exercise is typical. More than 30% of patients experience constitutional symptoms such as weight loss, malaise, and easy fatigability. With progression of the disease, dyspnea at rest, clubbing of the fingers and toes, crackles in lung bases, and evidence of cor pulmonale become more prominent. The chest radiograph correlates poorly with clinical findings. In 10% of patients the radiograph is normal, but a reticulonodular pattern at the lung bases is characteristic in IPF. The distribution and pattern of the lesions are highly distinctive on HRCT scans, which show patchy subpleural and basilar lesions.

Pulmonary function tests show reduced lung volumes and a decrease in diffusing capacity. Laboratory values are nonspecific. Transbronchial biopsy is usually nondiagnostic. Most but not all patients with IPF ultimately require a surgical lung biopsy. Biopsies reveal a mixture of fibrosis and inflammatory cell infiltration in the pulmonary interstitium. IPF has no pathognomonic clinical, biochemical, or pathologic finding and therefore is currently diagnosed by histologic exclusion of other specific

> **RESPIRATORY RECAP**
>
> **Characteristics of Idiopathic Pulmonary Fibrosis**
>
> » Disease predominantly affects men in the fifth to seventh decades of life.
> » History of exertional dyspnea is typical.
> » Chest radiograph correlates poorly with clinical findings.
> » High-resolution computed tomography shows the disease's highly distinctive distribution and pattern of lesions.
> » Transbronchial biopsy usually is not diagnostic.
> » Most patients require a surgical lung biopsy.
> » Disease currently is diagnosed by histologic exclusion of other specific entities.
> » Mortality rate is approximately 50% at 5 years.
> » Initial trial of prednisone (40 to 60 mg given orally once a day for 3 months) is a reasonable treatment choice; continuation of therapy depends on an objective response.

entities. As the lesions progress, the lung architecture is distorted, and respiratory failure ensues within 5 years. The mortality rate approximates 50% at 5 years. The prognosis is worse in men and for patients with honeycombing, severely depressed pulmonary function, and an absence of lymphocytes on lavage.

The decision as to which patients should be treated with steroids and/or cytotoxic agents is difficult. Most would agree in the treatment of patients who have significant gas exchange abnormalities with ILD symptoms. Corticosteroids have been associated with a favorable response in 10% to 30% of these patients. An initial trial of 40 to 60 mg by mouth daily for 3 months is reasonable. Continuation of therapy should depend on an objective response to these agents. Criteria and end points used to document a response are controversial. A 10% or greater increase in the FVC and FEV_1 or a 20% or greater increase in the DLCO is considered a favorable response. Responders should be tapered to 10 to 20 mg by mouth daily within 6 months. The optimum duration of therapy has not been determined. In nonresponders the corticosteroid should be tapered and stopped. Immunosuppressive or cytotoxic agents (cyclophosphamide and azathioprine) should be considered for patients in whom corticosteroids appear to be ineffective or who are at risk of adverse effects from corticosteroids. However, data show a low rate of response to alternative therapies in patients whose condition is resistant to steroids. Single-lung transplantation is an option for younger patients whose condition fails to respond to medical therapy.

Sarcoidosis

Sarcoidosis is a disorder in which multiple organ systems usually demonstrate noncaseating granulomas.[13] It is a common disorder and is the most prevalent ILD of unknown etiology. The prevalence of sarcoidosis in North America is 10 to 20 cases per 100,000 people, and the rate in Scandinavia is approximately 80 per 100,000. The disorder is rare in Africa, South America, and Central America. Most cases occur between 20 and 45 years of age, and the disease is rare in children and the elderly. Sarcoidosis is more common among African Americans relative to Caucasians.

In sarcoidosis the lung is the organ most frequently involved. This high frequency of respiratory tract involvement may represent a response to an inhaled antigen. A significant proportion of individuals with sarcoidosis are asymptomatic (40% to 60%), but the chest radiograph is abnormal in more than 90%. The chest radiograph in sarcoidosis shows one of the following patterns: lymph node enlargement, which most frequently is bilateral and hilar (stage I disease); ILD with lymph node enlargement (stage II); or ILD alone (stage III). HRCT has no routine role in the diagnosis or staging of sarcoidosis. Most patients with stage II or stage III disease demonstrate restrictive results on pulmonary function tests. Some individuals with sarcoidosis may show a pattern of airway obstruction. Laboratories can demonstrate an increased serum concentration of angiotensin-converting enzyme (ACE) and hypercalcemia. The level of ACE may correspond to disease activity, and this measurement has been used as an index of granuloma burden.

> **RESPIRATORY RECAP**
>
> **Characteristics of Sarcoidosis**
>
> » Disease causes noncaseating granulomas in several organ systems.
> » Sarcoidosis is the most common ILD of unknown etiology.
> » Most cases are seen in patients 20 to 45 years old.
> » Disease is common in African Americans.
> » Lung is the organ most frequently involved.
> » Chest radiograph shows bilateral hilar lymph node enlargement (stage I), ILD with lymph node enlargement (stage II), and ILD alone (stage III).
> » Adenopathy and ILD frequently regress spontaneously.
> » Extrapulmonary involvement is common.
> » Transbronchial biopsy demonstrates noncaseating granulomas.
> » Thoracoscopic or open lung biopsy is rarely needed for diagnosis.
> » Steroids are given with functional impairment of one or more organs.

Over time both the adenopathy and the ILD may regress spontaneously in about 60% of all patients (this occurs in 80% of patients in stage I, 40% in stage II, and 10% in stage III sarcoidosis). However, at the other extreme, the interstitial disease may progress to extensive scarring and end-stage lung disease, at which point the patient may have severe respiratory compromise. The course of the disease usually is dictated in the first 24 months, with almost all spontaneous remissions occurring during this time.

Extrapulmonary involvement is common in patients with sarcoidosis. Eye and skin involvement are particularly common manifestations of sarcoidosis, but the disease may also have cardiac, neuromuscular, hematologic, hepatic, endocrine, and peripheral lymph node effects. Mortality from sarcoidosis most often is the result of cardiac involvement.

The diagnosis can be made in several ways. The history, a physical examination, and chest radiography may provide the diagnosis in a young African American woman with bilateral hilar adenopathy. Transbronchial biopsy demonstrates noncaseating granulomas (which have a central core of histiocytes, epithelioid cells, and multinucleated giant cells) in as many as 90% of patients, because this process involves peribronchial and bronchiolar tissue. If bronchoscopy is not diagnostic, mediastinoscopy may be done to sample hilar and mediastinal lymph nodes. Biopsies of other involved tissues (skin, conjunctiva, salivary glands, or liver) can also provide a diagnosis. Thoracoscopic or open lung biopsy is rarely needed for diagnosis.

Treatment of sarcoidosis consists of steroid administration when evidence of progressive functional impairment of one or more vital organs is seen. Treatment of patients with mild symptoms or nonprogressive disease is inappropriate. Severe pulmonary dysfunction, hypercalcemia, and myocardial, nervous system, and eye involvement and disfiguring skin lesions necessitate corticosteroid treatment. The appropriate dose, duration, and tapering of the corticosteroid have not been defined. Response to the treatment is evident within 12 weeks, but the corticosteroid should be continued for at least 12 months at a minimally effective dose, because relapses of sarcoidosis occur often as the corticosteroid is tapered. Immunosuppressive agents (methotrexate and azathioprine) have been used for steroid-resistant cases, for steroid sparing, and for individuals who have contraindications to or who have had adverse effects from steroids. Transplantation has been used in end-stage lung disease with sarcoidosis.

Interstitial Lung Disease with Collagen Vascular Disease

Patients with a **collagen vascular disease** can develop ILD. Specific collagen vascular diseases associated with ILD include progressive systemic sclerosis,[14] systemic lupus erythematosus (SLE),[15] polymyositis and dermatomyositis, Sjögren syndrome, and mixed connective tissue disease. Although progression of ILD with collagen vascular diseases is usually slower, the clinical presentation is comparable to that of IPF. The histopathologic features of ILD in this setting also correspond to those of IPF, with the additional features of lymphoid hyperplasia, cellular interstitial pneumonitis, lymphoid interstitial pneumonitis, diffuse alveolar damage, and bronchiolitis obliterans with organizing pneumonia. The diagnosis is assumed in patients with a known, underlying collagen vascular disease and classic clinical features of ILD (crackles, dyspnea, interstitial infiltrates, and restrictive results on pulmonary function tests). Before aggressive immunosuppressive therapy is begun, bronchoscopy with lavage and TBB should be performed to exclude alternative etiologies such as malignancy and infection. For patients with a deteriorating course, treatment involves administration of corticosteroids or immunosuppressive agents or both.

ILD shows a high association with progressive systemic sclerosis, and most patients with this disorder have ILD at some time during the course of their illness. There is an even greater prevalence of pulmonary hypertension (80% to 95%).

> **RESPIRATORY RECAP**
>
> **Interstitial Lung Disease with Collagen Vascular Disease**
>
> » Progression of ILD with collagen vascular diseases is slow, but the clinical presentation is comparable to that of idiopathic pulmonary fibrosis, as is the histopathology.
>
> » Diagnosis is assumed in patients with a known underlying collagen vascular disease and classic clinical features of ILD.
>
> » Treatment involves administration of corticosteroids or immunosuppressive agents or both.

Eosinophilic Granuloma

Eosinophilic granuloma, also called *Langerhans cell granulomatosis*, was first described in 1953 as a bone disease having characteristics similar to those of Letterer-Siwe disease and Hand-Schüller-Christian disease.[16] Since then, it has been shown to be predominantly a pulmonary disorder. Eosinophilic granuloma is a rare disease that occurs almost exclusively in smokers or former smokers 10 to 40 years old. Although the etiology remains unknown, eosinophilic granuloma probably is an inflammatory response by Langerhans cells to a component of tobacco smoke. Common presenting symptoms are a nonproductive cough, chest pain, and dyspnea on exertion. Weight loss, fever, and hemoptysis occasionally occur. Extrapulmonary features, including involvement of the posterior pituitary gland with the development of diabetes insipidus and lytic bony lesions, have frequently been described (20% of patients).

The physical examination often is unremarkable, but occasional wheezing may be heard. Pulmonary function tests show a decrease in lung volumes and diffusing capacity with normal or reduced expiratory flow rates. Radiographic findings of nodular densities in the upper and midlung fields with sparing of the lung bases are characteristic, but reticular, reticulonodular, and cystic lesions can be observed. Pleural effusions are uncommon. Pneumothorax occurs in approximately 10% of patients. The HRCT scans are highly distinctive, revealing numerous peribronchiolar nodular and cystic lesions.

As the disease progresses, the nodules are replaced by cysts that become confluent. Biopsy shows a mixture of inflammatory, cystic, nodular, and fibrotic lesions

> **RESPIRATORY RECAP**
>
> **Characteristics of Eosinophilic Granuloma**
>
> » Disease also is called Langerhans cell granulomatosis.
> » Eosinophilic granuloma was first described as a bone disease but is now recognized as a predominantly pulmonary disorder.
> » Disease occurs almost exclusively in smokers or former smokers 10 to 40 years old.
> » Etiology is unknown.
> » Common presenting symptoms are a nonproductive cough, chest pain, and dyspnea on exertion.
> » Extrapulmonary features include diabetes insipidus and lytic bony lesions.
> » High-resolution computed tomography scans are highly distinctive.
> » Light microscopy shows the cleft nuclei of the Langerhans cells and stellate pattern of fibrosis in 80% of patients.
> » Spontaneous remissions are the rule.
> » Patient must stop smoking if the disease is to resolve.

centered at or adjacent to bronchioles. Light microscopy shows the cleft nuclei of the Langerhans cells and the stellate pattern of fibrosis in 80% of patients. Aggregates of Langerhans cells can be demonstrated by immunostaining for S-100 protein or OKT6 antigen. Electron microscopy reveals Birbeck granules (X bodies) within these large, mononuclear phagocytes. As the inflammation progresses, alveolar architecture is destroyed and replaced by cysts and fibrosis.

In some cases TBB can provide the diagnosis. Spontaneous remissions are the rule, and no therapy beyond symptomatic and supportive care has been shown to be effective. Cigarette smoking must be stopped. There is progressive loss of pulmonary function in up to one quarter of these individuals, who can die of respiratory failure. Corticosteroids often are used in severe and progressive disease, but no data are available on their efficacy.

Respiratory Bronchiolitis

Respiratory bronchiolitis is a rare disorder that occurs exclusively in cigarette smokers.[17] Most of these individuals are asymptomatic, but they may have a mild cough, dyspnea, and sputum production. Crackles can be detected in some of these patients in the physical examination. The chest radiograph may demonstrate reticulonodular infiltrates at the bases, but it also may be normal. Pathologic studies reveal intracytoplasmic, golden-brown, granular pigment in alveolar macrophages in the respiratory and terminal bronchioles. The disease resolves in almost all patients after the person stops smoking.

Pulmonary Alveolar Proteinosis

Pathologically, **pulmonary alveolar proteinosis (PAP)** is characterized by filling of alveolar spaces with a lipoproteinaceous exudate and interstitial fibrosis.[18] The intra-alveolar phospholipid stains bright pink with periodic-acid Schiff (PAS) reagent. Although some patients are asymptomatic, most have dyspnea and cough, and alveolar infiltrates are seen on the chest radiograph. Laboratory values can verify hypoxemia. The disease spontaneously remits in one-third of patients. Although the mortality rate formerly was high, death is now rare following introduction of whole-lung lavage of 20 to 40 L of saline as the treatment of choice. The etiology remains unknown, but some patients have a history of exposure to silica and hydrocarbons.

Drug-Induced Interstitial Lung Disease

A number of different drugs can result in ILD.[19] The clinical and radiographic features differ depending on the implicated agent. Clinical presentations are specified as syndromes of acute pneumonitis, chronic interstitial pneumonitis, acute alveolar hemorrhage, or noncardiac pulmonary edema. A dose-related toxicity (e.g., as with antineoplastic agents) may be seen but often is not (such as with bleomycin), and the presentation may be that of an idiosyncratic reaction. Agents may be synergistic with each other, with radiation, or with oxygen exposure in the resultant lung toxicity.

A number of mechanisms are involved in drug-induced ILD, including cytotoxicity, hypersensitivity pneumonitis, and noncardiogenic pulmonary edema. Cytotoxic drug injury may occur with bleomycin, alkylating agents, and nitrosoureas. Previous chemotherapy or radiation therapy can amplify the risk of ILD with use of these drugs. The histopathologic features include type II pneumocyte proliferation with cellular atypia (large nuclei, prominent nucleoli, and bizarre chromatin patterns), inflammatory cell incursion, and fibrosis. Cytotoxic lung injury has a significant mortality rate (10% to 50% of patients, depending on the drug). Corticosteroids are most effective if given early, when a cellular rather than a fibrotic histology is present; the response is extremely variable and often negative with established disease. Methotrexate, nitrofurantoin, gold, and sulfasalazine are associated with hypersensitivity pneumonitis. Both acute and subacute forms manifest with fever, chest pain, and interstitial or alveolar infiltrates on the radiograph. The prognosis is good when the medication is stopped. Corticosteroids may hasten resolution. Salicylates, thiazides, narcotics, and cytarabine all can induce a noncardiac pulmonary edema.

Acute Interstitial Lung Disease

A number of interstitial lung diseases manifest in a more acute fashion. They include acute interstitial pneumonitis (Hamman-Rich syndrome), acute **bronchiolitis obliterans with organizing pneumonia (BOOP)**, acute eosinophilic pneumonia, and lymphoid interstitial pneumonitis.[20] The presentation of these diseases mimics an atypical pneumonia, with the patient reporting an unproductive cough, dyspnea, fever, and malaise. It is not unusual for these patients to develop acute respiratory failure that requires mechanical ventilation.

Acute interstitial pneumonitis is a rapidly progressive form of interstitial pneumonitis thought either to exemplify an accelerated phase of IPF or to be a distinct entity of unknown etiology. It has been described as an acute respiratory distress syndrome without an underlying precipitating injury. Acute interstitial pneumonitis is characterized by an epithelial cell injury that results in denudation of the epithelial lining of the alveolus and edema of the alveolar walls (i.e., diffuse alveolar damage). Intra-alveolar fibrin, edema accumulation, mild acute and chronic interstitial inflammation, and formation of intra-alveolar hyaline membranes also are frequently described. Collagen deposition by fibroblasts and honeycomb lung can follow. Hypoxemic respiratory failure is common, and the mortality rate is high. Patients are treated with corticosteroids, but the drugs' effectiveness is not known.

Acute BOOP appears to be a response of the lung to a variety of injuries that affect the smaller airways and alveoli as a unit. These injuries include infections, exposure to toxic gases, radiation therapy, drug toxicity, eosinophilic pneumonia, Wegener granulomatosis, and hypersensitivity pneumonitis. Acute BOOP manifests as an upper respiratory infection with a persistent cough and then dyspnea. Focal alveolar infiltrates are seen on the chest radiograph. Histologically, proliferating fibroblasts are noted in alveolar spaces, and polyps (inflammatory cells and fibrosis) project into the lumina of distal bronchioles. Extrapulmonary involvement does not occur. Treatment is administration of corticosteroids, with most individuals demonstrating good response. The idiopathic form of BOOP is classified as cryptogenic organizing pneumonia (COP) and the secondary form as secondary organizing pneumonia (SOP).[21]

Acute eosinophilic pneumonia is distinguished by fleeting pulmonary infiltrates and peripheral eosinophilia. Simple pulmonary eosinophilia (Löffler syndrome) is most commonly the result of infection with parasites such as *Strongyloides*, *Ascaris*, and *Ancylostoma* species but also can be caused by a drug reaction. The most common symptom is a dry cough. The infiltrates resolve within 2 weeks, and the peripheral eosinophilia is transitory. Treatment is directed at an identifiable underlying cause. Tropical eosinophilia can manifest as an acute eosinophilic pneumonia and is believed to be part of a hypersensitivity reaction to the filarial worm. Cough, fever, myalgia, and dyspnea are common. The histologic appearance is that of a cellular interstitial pneumonia with both infiltration of the interstitium and alveolar spaces by mononuclear cells and eosinophils and areas of BOOP. This can lead to respiratory failure requiring mechanical ventilation.

Various drugs have also been reported to produce acute eosinophilic pneumonia. In these cases the bronchoalveolar lavage shows a predominance of eosinophils. Treatment with corticosteroids cures the disease, and recurrences are unusual.

Allergic bronchopulmonary aspergillosis manifests as an acute eosinophilic pneumonia and is seen in asthmatics. Patients have a productive cough, eosinophilia, and a patchy infiltrate. Treatment is administration of corticosteroids.

Lymphoid interstitial pneumonitis is distinguished by dense lymphocytic infiltrates in the alveolar interstitium and lymphatics. The patient complains of cough and dyspnea. On the radiograph, bilateral reticular and reticulonodular infiltrates, dense alveolar infiltrates, or focal nodules are observed. The disease is considered a lymphoproliferative disorder. Lymphoid interstitial pneumonitis is associated most commonly with HIV infection (especially in children) but also with dysproteinemias, hypogammaglobulinemia, common variable immunodeficiency syndrome, monoclonal gammopathy, SLE, Sjögren syndrome, chronic active hepatitis, primary biliary cirrhosis, and bone marrow transplantation. Treatment is administration of corticosteroids, but no data are available on their effectiveness. The mortality rate for lymphoid interstitial pneumonitis is high.

KEY POINTS

- Interstitial lung disease is a heterogenous group of disorders classified together because of similarities in their clinical and pathologic presentation.
- The most common identifiable causes of interstitial lung disease are related to occupational or environmental exposure.
- A large number of ILD patients have interstitial lung disease of unknown etiology, including idiopathic pulmonary fibrosis and sarcoidosis.
- Treatment of interstitial lung disease most often is supportive.

REFERENCES

1. du Bois RM. Diffuse lung disease. An approach to management. *Br Med J.* 1994;309:175–179.
2. Martinez FJ, Flaherty K. Pulmonary function testing in idiopathic interstitial pneumonias. *Proc Am Thorac Soc.* 2006;3:315–321.
3. Eaton T, Young P, Milne D, Wells AU. Six-minute walk, maximal exercise tests: reproducibility in fibrotic interstitial pneumonia. *Am J Respir Crit Care Med.* 2005;171:1150–1157.
4. Sung A, Swigris J, Saleh A, Raoof S. High-resolution chest tomography in idiopathic pulmonary fibrosis and nonspecific interstitial pneumonia: utility and challenges. *Curr Opin Pulm Med.* 2007;13:451–457.
5. Mueller-Mang C, Grosse C, Schmid K, et al. What every radiologist should know about idiopathic interstitial pneumonias. *Radiographics.* 2007;27:595–615.
6. Nagai S, Handa T, Ito Y, Takeuchi M, Izumi T. Bronchoalveolar lavage in idiopathic interstitial lung diseases. *Semin Respir Crit Care Med.* 2007;28:496–503.
7. Katzenstein AL, Mukhopadhyay S, Myers JL. Diagnosis of usual interstitial pneumonia and distinction from other fibrosing interstitial lung diseases. *Hum Pathol.* 2008;39:1275–1294.

8. Riley DJ, Costanzo EJ. Surgical biopsy: its appropriateness in diagnosing interstitial lung disease. *Curr Opin Pulm Med.* 2006;12:331–336.
9. Lai CK, Wallace WD, Fishbein MC. Histopathology of pulmonary fibrotic disorders. *Semin Respir Crit Care Med.* 2006;27:613–622.
10. Ryu JH, Daniels CE, Hartman TE, Yi ES. Diagnosis of interstitial lung diseases. *Mayo Clin Proc.* 2007;82:976–986.
11. Nathan SD. Therapeutic intervention: assessing the role of the international consensus guidelines. *Chest.* 2005;128(5 suppl 1): 533S–539S.
12. Walter N, Collard HR, King TE Jr. Current perspectives on the treatment of idiopathic pulmonary fibrosis. *Proc Am Thorac Soc.* 2006;3:330–338.
13. Judson MA. Sarcoidosis: clinical presentation, diagnosis, and approach to treatment. *Am J Med Sci.* 2008;335:26–33.
14. Fischer A, Swigris JJ, Groshong SD, et al. Clinically significant interstitial lung disease in limited scleroderma: histopathology, clinical features, and survival. *Chest.* 2008;134:601–605.
15. Cheema GS, Quismorio FP Jr. Interstitial lung disease in systemic lupus erythematosus. *Curr Opin Pulm Med.* 2000;6:424–429.
16. Abbott GF, Rosado-de-Christenson ML, Franks TJ, Frazier AA, Galvin JR. From the archives of the AFIP: pulmonary Langerhans cell histiocytosis. *Radiographics.* 2004;24:821–841.
17. Caminati A, Harari S. Smoking-related interstitial pneumonias and pulmonary Langerhans cell histiocytosis. *Proc Am Thorac Soc.* 2006;3:299–306.
18. Presneill JJ, Nakata K, Inoue Y, Seymour JF. Pulmonary alveolar proteinosis. *Clin Chest Med.* 2004;25:593–613.
19. Camus P, Fanton A, Bonniaud P, Camus C, Foucher P. Interstitial lung disease induced by drugs and radiation. *Respiration.* 2004;71:301–326.
20. Vourlekis JS. Acute interstitial pneumonia. *Clin Chest Med.* 2004;25:739–747.
21. Heffner JE. No matter how you push and squeeze, organizing pneumonia remains more than one disease. *Respir Care.* 2009;54:1020–1023.

CHAPTER 37

Pulmonary Vascular Disease

C. William Hargett
Victor F. Tapson

OUTLINE

OBJECTIVES

1. Describe the physiology of the right ventricle and pulmonary circulation in normal and disease states.
2. Describe the signs and symptoms of pulmonary vascular diseases, including those present in pulmonary embolism (PE), cor pulmonale, and idiopathic pulmonary arterial hypertension (IPAH).
3. Define the role of ventilation-perfusion scanning, computed tomographic angiography, and pulmonary angiography in the diagnosis of PE.
4. Discuss the role of anticoagulation, vena cava filters, and thrombolytic therapy in the management of acute PE.
5. Describe the pathogenesis and treatment of cor pulmonale.
6. Discuss the role of advanced therapies in the management of IPAH.

KEY TERMS

anticoagulation
calcium channel blockers
computed tomographic angiography (CTA)
cor pulmonale
deep vein thrombosis (DVT)
hypoxic pulmonary vasoconstriction
idiopathic pulmonary arterial hypertension (IPAH)
inferior vena cava (IVC) filter
prostacyclin
pulmonary angiography
pulmonary arterial hypertension (PAH)
pulmonary embolism (PE)
pulmonary hypertension (PH)
pulmonary vascular resistance
thrombolytic therapy

INTRODUCTION

Disorders of the pulmonary circulation include a large and heterogeneous group of conditions. Some pulmonary vascular diseases, such as pulmonary thromboembolism, occur quite commonly, whereas others, such as idiopathic pulmonary arterial hypertension, are quite rare. Diseases of the pulmonary circulation occur as a result of intrinsic abnormalities of the pulmonary vessels, of embolic complications from elsewhere in the vascular system, or secondary to underlying cardiac or pulmonary disease. Because the right ventricle (RV) is poorly suited to respond to elevations in pulmonary vascular pressure, similar pathologic consequences occur once pulmonary hypertension develops, regardless of the etiology. In this chapter, the pathophysiology of pulmonary vascular disease is reviewed in light of the normal physiology and function of the RV and pulmonary circulation. Features common to many pulmonary vascular diseases are described, in addition to issues related to the specific diagnosis and management of several common disorders of the pulmonary circulation.

Pathophysiology

Normal Pulmonary Vascular Physiology

The principal function of the pulmonary circulation is gas exchange. Venous blood low in oxygen and rich in carbon dioxide passes through the pulmonary capillaries, where oxygen is absorbed and carbon dioxide is eliminated, thus allowing the left ventricle to return oxygenated blood to the rest of the body. Under normal circumstances, the pulmonary circulation is a low-pressure, high-flow system, providing little resistance to the right ventricular outflow. Mean pulmonary artery pressure and **pulmonary vascular resistance** at rest are approximately one-sixth that of the systemic circulation.[1] Although the RV is sensitive to the pulmonary vascular load, in a classic view the RV serves primarily as a capacitance chamber for blood returning from the systemic veins. As long as pulmonary vascular resistance is normal, blood flows from the right side of the heart through the lungs to the left side of the heart as a result of left heart action. The contraction of the left ventricle and interventricular septum pulls the free wall of the RV against the septum and augments the flow of blood through the pulmonary circulation.[2] The phasic changes in intrathoracic pressure that accompany respiration also direct the forward flow of blood from the RV through the pulmonary circulation.

Normally, the pulmonary vascular bed is able to accommodate large increases in blood flow without much change in pressure, thus effectively preventing RV overload. For example, cardiac output can increase substantially during exercise in normal individuals, with increases of up to fivefold in pulmonary blood flow.[2,3] The thin-walled RV is highly compliant and able to accommodate large volumes and filling pressures. Recruitment of vessels in the poorly perfused upper lung and distention of the compliant vessels in the dependent areas allow the pulmonary circulation to accommodate these increases in cardiac output and pulmonary blood flow.[4,5]

Pulmonary Vascular Pathophysiology

The pulmonary vascular tree is a low-resistance circulation that can absorb large changes in cardiac output without significant increases in pulmonary pressures. However, many pathologic conditions can give rise to **pulmonary hypertension (PH)**, as summarized in **Box 37–1**. PH was originally classified as secondary in the presence of a known cause and primary when no

BOX 37–1

Selected Causes of Pulmonary Hypertension

Disorders of the Pulmonary Arterial Vasculature (Pulmonary Arterial Hypertension)
- Idiopathic and familial pulmonary arterial hypertension
- Connective tissue disease (e.g., scleroderma)
- Portal hypertension
- Human immunodeficiency virus (HIV)
- Congenital heart disease (Eisenmenger syndrome)
- Drugs (e.g., anorexic agents, methamphetamine)
- Pulmonary venoocclusive disease*

Disorders of the Pulmonary Venous Vasculature (Cardiac Disease)
- Left-sided heart failure
- Left-sided valvular heart disease

Disorders of Hypoxemia
- Chronic obstructive pulmonary disease (COPD)
- Interstitial lung disease (e.g., idiopathic pulmonary fibrosis)
- Hypoventilation and sleep-disordered breathing

Disorders of Obstruction of the Pulmonary Vasculature
- Venous thromboembolism
- Other materials (e.g., parasites, tumor, foreign material)

Other Disorders
- Sarcoidosis
- Compression of pulmonary vessels (e.g., mediastinal lymphadenopathy)

*Pulmonary venoocclusive disease starts in the pulmonary veins but ultimately causes pulmonary arterial changes.

underlying etiology or risk factor could be identified.[6] Major advances in our understanding have led to the current classification, in which pulmonary hypertensive diseases are grouped into five categories according to cause and therapeutic strategy, with each category subdivided to reflect diverse underlying etiologies and sites of injury.[7]

Destruction or obliteration of the pulmonary vascular bed is likely to play a key role in patients with pulmonary parenchymal diseases, such as chronic obstructive pulmonary disease (COPD).[8] In contrast, **pulmonary arterial hypertension (PAH)** is characterized by vasoconstriction and vascular remodeling in the precapillary segments of the pulmonary vasculature due to an imbalance between endothelial mediators such as prostacyclin, thromboxane, and endothelin;[9,10] the histopathology may include plexogenic arteriopathy, thrombotic lesions, and medial hypertrophy with intimal fibrosis. Unexplained PAH is designated idiopathic pulmonary arterial hypertension (formerly primary pulmonary hypertension) and is the most well-studied form of PAH. In addition, in many individuals with pulmonary vascular diseases, chronic alveolar hypoxia, and associated hypoxic pulmonary vasoconstriction contribute to the development of PH.

Once PH develops, independent of the inciting event, pulmonary vascular remodeling occurs, leading to medial hypertrophy and intimal fibrosis, which further reduces pulmonary vascular cross-sectional area and exacerbates PH. **Figure 37–1** illustrates vascular changes observed in a patient with PH. As right ventricular afterload increases with worsening PH, right ventricular hypertrophy, dilation, or failure can occur. **Cor pulmonale** is "pulmonary heart failure," that is, right ventricular dysfunction resulting from disorders of the pulmonary circulation, such as PH as a result of pulmonary parenchymal disease. COPD and idiopathic pulmonary fibrosis (IPF) are two diseases commonly associated with the development of cor pulmonale.

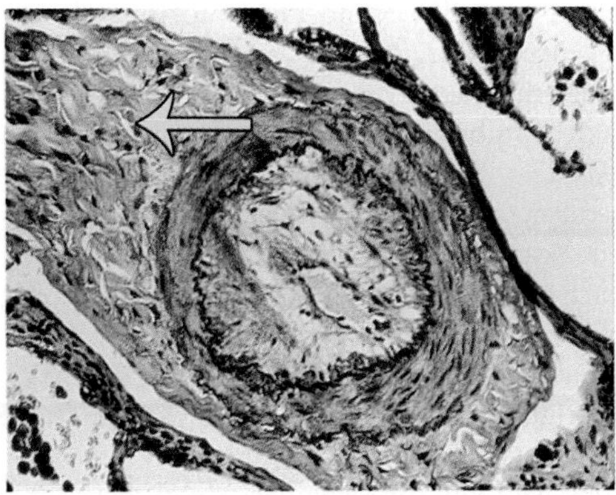

FIGURE 37–1 Arrow shows pulmonary arteriolar smooth muscle cell hypertrophy, with prominent thickening of the medial layer.

Pathophysiology of Acute Pulmonary Embolism

Venous thromboemboli that cause **pulmonary embolism (PE)** usually arise from **deep vein thrombosis (DVT)** in the lower extremities. When emboli acutely obstruct a significant portion of the pulmonary arterial bed, profound hemodynamic alterations occur. Hypoxemia occurs as a result of regions with low ventilation-perfusion ($\dot{V}/\dot{Q}$) ratios and shunting secondary to perfusion of atelectatic areas. The impact of the embolic event depends on the extent of reduction of the cross-sectional area of the pulmonary vasculature and on the presence or absence of underlying cardiovascular disease.[11] With massive emboli, cardiac output is diminished but may be sustained to a certain point. Increased pulmonary vascular resistance impedes right ventricular outflow and reduces left ventricular preload. More than 50% obstruction of the pulmonary arterial bed is usually present before substantial elevation of mean pulmonary artery pressure develops. When the extent of obstruction of the pulmonary circulation approaches 75%, a normal individual cannot generate the right ventriclular systolic pressures in excess of 50 mm Hg required to preserve pulmonary perfusion, and cardiac failure and death will occur.[12] Thus, although supportive measures may sustain a patient with massive PE, any additional increment in embolic burden may be fatal.

Epidemiology

Disorders of the pulmonary circulation include a diverse group of clinical conditions that result in substantial morbidity and mortality. Pulmonary thromboembolism, for example, is recognized as the third most common cause of cardiovascular disease in the United States after ischemic heart disease and stroke.[13] Autopsy studies suggest that more than 600,000 patients in the United States develop DVT or PE or both each year, with over half of these cases not recognized before death. PE probably causes or contributes to the death of at least 100,000 of these patients each year.[12]

In addition, cor pulmonale appears to contribute substantially to mortality in patients with a variety of pulmonary parenchymal diseases, especially COPD. The exact incidence and prevalence of cor pulmonale in COPD is not known, but recent estimates suggest that 10% to 40% of patients with COPD have evidence of right ventricular hypertrophy.[8] Cor pulmonale increases in prevalence with increased severity of lung disease and may occur in over 70% of COPD patients with a forced expiratory volume in the first second of expiration (FEV_1) of less than 0.6 L.[14] The development of cor pulmonale in these patients portends a significantly worse prognosis than in patients with normal right ventricular pressures. In patients with COPD, which causes an estimated 120,000 deaths each year in the United States, overt right heart failure is associated with a 5-year survival of only 30%.[8,15]

In fibrotic lung disease, such as IPF, pulmonary artery pressures are also important predictors of survival.[16,17]

Idiopathic pulmonary arterial hypertension (IPAH) is an uncommon disorder of the pulmonary vessels associated with severe elevation in pulmonary vascular resistance. The incidence of IPAH is unknown but is estimated at 2 to 6 cases per million people in the population.[10,18] IPAH is most common among younger patients (ages 20 to 40 years) and occurs at least three times as frequently in women. IPAH is a devastating disease and has traditionally been associated with poor prognosis, with a 5-year survival of only 34%.[19] Poor survival has been associated with worse functional class (III or IV) and reduced right ventricular hemodynamic function (specifically, elevated mean right atrial pressure, elevated mean pulmonary arterial pressure, and decreased cardiac index). The intensive study and approval by the Food and Drug Administration of seven PAH drugs in three different classes over the past 15 years has greatly facilitated the approach to this disease.

Pulmonary vascular disease clinically and pathologically indistinguishable from IPAH can occur in association with a number of systemic illnesses, such as scleroderma and human immunodeficiency virus (HIV) infection, or in association with certain drugs, including appetite suppressants.[20–22] The appetite suppressants fenfluramine and dexfenfluramine have been found to significantly increase the risk of pulmonary hypertension (odds ratio of greater than 20 with more than 3 months of use).[22] In general, the prognosis for patients with these associated forms of pulmonary hypertension is similar to that in IPAH and remains poor.

BOX 37–2

Important Risk Factors for Pulmonary Embolism

- Recent surgery
- Acute medical illness
- Malignancy
- Pregnancy or postpartum
- Immobilization or paralysis
- Prior history of deep vein thrombosis or pulmonary embolism
- Hypercoagulable states such as:
  - Factor V Leiden mutation
  - Prothrombin gene mutation
  - Protein C or S deficiency
  - Antithrombin deficiency
  - Dysfibrinogenemia
  - Antiphospholipid syndrome
  - Heparin-induced thrombocytopenia

Diagnosis

Pulmonary Embolism

The history, physical exam, arterial blood gas analysis, electrocardiogram (ECG), and chest radiograph often are useful in suggesting the presence or absence of pulmonary embolism. The clinical evaluation alone, however, is not a reliable guide to the diagnosis of PE, as is underscored by the high incidence of unsuspected PE in autopsy series.[23] PE should be considered whenever unexplained dyspnea occurs, but it also should be considered when a patient with another potential explanation for dyspnea, such as underlying cardiopulmonary disease, develops new or worsening symptoms. **Box 37–2** lists common risk factors for PE. The presence of one or more risk factors should increase the clinical suspicion. Unexplained dyspnea in association with pleuritic chest pain or hemoptysis is suggestive of PE. PE must also be considered in the setting of unexplained syncope or sudden hypotension.

The physical examination may be unrevealing in patients with acute PE. Because patients with lower extremity DVT often do not exhibit pain, warmth, erythema, or swelling, the physical exam may not provide clues to the presence of an underlying DVT. An increased pulmonic component of the second heart sound has been reported in massive PE, but the nonspecific findings of tachypnea and tachycardia are the most common physical examination abnormalities described in PE.

Hypoxemia is common in acute PE but is not universally present. Young patients without underlying lung disease may have a normal PaO_2. In a retrospective analysis of hospitalized patients with proven PE, the PaO_2 was more than 80 mm Hg in 29% of patients younger than 40 years, compared with 3% in the older group.[24] The alveolar–arterial difference was abnormal in all patients, however. Thus, the diagnosis of acute PE cannot be excluded based on a normal PaO_2.

Laboratory tests that may be useful include testing for D-dimer, a breakdown product of cross-linked fibrin present in acute DVT and PE. Unfortunately, D-dimer may be present in patients with infections, cancer, and other disorders, rendering it nonspecific for acute venous thromboembolism. However, if suspicion of acute DVT or PE is relatively low, a *negative* D-dimer test is generally considered sensitive enough to rule it out.

Electrocardiographic findings in acute PE are generally nonspecific and include T wave changes, ST segment abnormalities, and left or right axis deviation. Manifestations of acute right heart failure, including the S1 Q3 T3 pattern, right bundle branch block, P wave pulmonale, or right axis deviation, were present in only 32% of patients with massive PE in the Urokinase Pulmonary Embolism Trial (UPET).[25]

The majority of patients with PE have nonspecific abnormalities on chest radiographs, with common

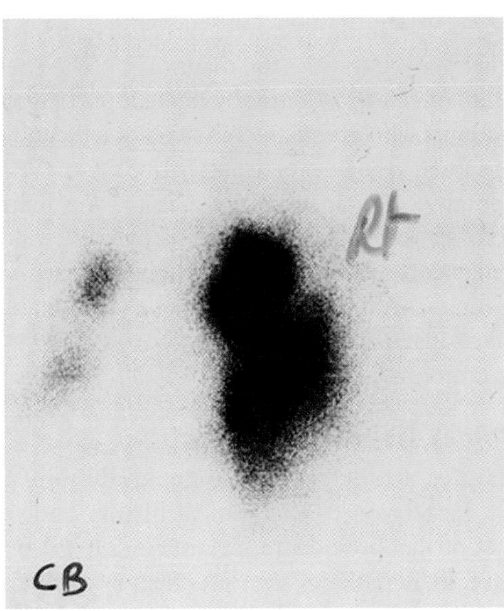

FIGURE 37–2 This perfusion scan (posterior view) reveals extensive pulmonary embolism with essentially absent flow to the left lung and perfusion defect in the right lung. The ventilation scan was normal.

findings including atelectasis, pleural effusion, pulmonary infiltrates, and elevation of a hemidiaphragm.[26] Classic radiographic findings of pulmonary infarction such as wedge-shaped pleural density (Hampton's hump) or decreased vascularity (Westermark sign) are suggestive but infrequent. A normal chest radiograph in the setting of severe dyspnea and hypoxemia without evidence of bronchospasm or cardiac shunt is strongly suggestive of PE. In general, however, the chest radiograph cannot be used to conclusively prove or exclude PE.

Ventilation-perfusion scanning may be performed when PE is suspected. When abnormal, $\dot{V}/\dot{Q}$ scans are conventionally read as showing low, intermediate, or high probability for PE. Normal and high-probability scans are considered diagnostic. **Figure 37–2** illustrates a high-probability $\dot{V}/\dot{Q}$ scan in a patient with PE. In the Prospective Investigation of Pulmonary Embolism Diagnosis (PIOPED) study, the utility of $\dot{V}/\dot{Q}$ scanning combined with clinical assessment of patients with suspected PE was prospectively evaluated in more than 700 patients.[27] Patients with PE had scans that were high, intermediate, or low probability, but so did most patients without PE. Although the specificity of high-probability scans was 97%, the sensitivity was only 41%. Of interest, 33% of patients with intermediate-probability scans and 12% of patients with low-probability scans were diagnosed definitively with PE by pulmonary arteriography. When the clinical suspicion of PE was considered high, PE was found to be present in 96% of patients with high-probability scans, 66% of patients with intermediate-probability scans, and 40% of patients with low-probability scans. Thus, additional diagnostic tests must be pursued when the $\dot{V}/\dot{Q}$ scan is of low or intermediate probability if the clinical scenario is suggestive of PE.

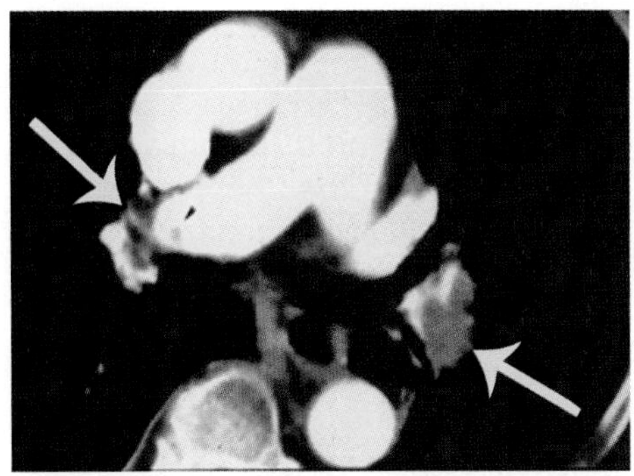

FIGURE 37–3 Computed tomographic angiogram in a patient with bilateral, proximal, acute pulmonary emboli (arrows).

Over the past decade, $\dot{V}/\dot{Q}$ scanning has decreased in favor of contrast-enhanced **computed tomographic angiography (CTA)** of the chest, which may reveal emboli in the main, lobar, or segmental pulmonary arteries. The reported sensitivity and specificity of single-slice helical CTA has ranged from 53% to 100% and from 81% to 100%, respectively, but visualization of segmental and subsegmental pulmonary arteries is substantially better with newer multidetector scanners, as evidenced by the PIOPED II, where the specificity of chest CTA was 95% and the sensitivity 83%.[28,29] **Figure 37–3** illustrates chest CTA identification of a proximal pulmonary artery clot in a patient with PE. **Box 37–3** summarizes advantages and disadvantages of chest CTA in the diagnosis of PE.

In patients requiring additional testing, **pulmonary angiography** can be performed and remains the gold-standard diagnostic technique. **Figure 37–4** illustrates a pulmonary angiogram diagnostic of PE. Serious complications of pulmonary angiography occur infrequently (less than 0.5% incidence in most series), but respiratory failure, renal failure, significant bleeding, and death have been reported.[30] Angiography requires the presence of experienced physicians to perform the test and interpret the results; however, this test is rarely needed because CTA is

RESPIRATORY RECAP

Diagnosis of Pulmonary Embolism

- » The physical exam may be unremarkable.
- » Hypoxemia is common but not universally present.
- » Electrocardiographic findings often are nonspecific.
- » The chest radiograph is often unremarkable; a normal chest radiograph with dyspnea and hypoxemia (and without significant bronchospasm) is suggestive of PE.
- » High-probability $\dot{V}/\dot{Q}$ scans are virtually diagnostic when acute PE is *clinically* likely.
- » Chest computed tomographic angiography is the most common test employed to detect PE and is sensitive and specific.
- » Pulmonary angiography is the most accurate diagnostic test for PE but is invasive.
- » Echocardiography is insensitive for the diagnosis of PE but may play a role in evaluation and risk stratification.

BOX 37–3

Utility of Computed Tomographic Angiography of the Chest in the Diagnosis of Pulmonary Embolism

Advantages

Excellent visualization of pulmonary arteries
Noninvasive
Relative rapidity of procedure
Diagnosis of other (nonvascular) abnormalities

Disadvantages

Experienced radiologist required to interpret results
Adverse reactions to contrast (e.g., anaphylaxis, nephrotoxicity)
Radiation exposure

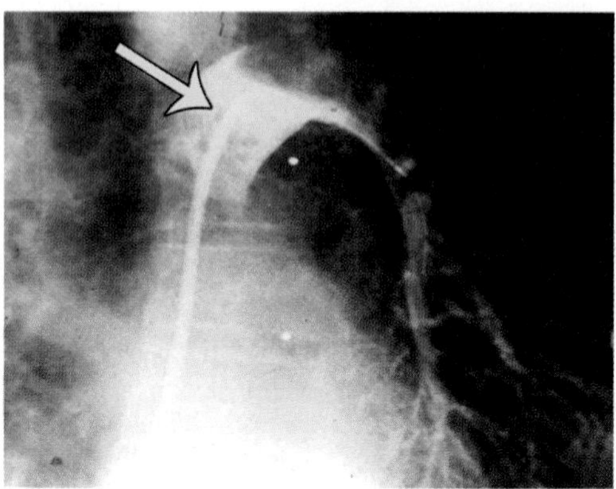

FIGURE 37–4 Pulmonary arteriography reveals a large pulmonary embolus occluding the left pulmonary artery.

very accurate and offers the potential for additional diagnoses. In selected stable patients with suspected acute PE and nondiagnostic lung scans, serial noninvasive lower extremity testing to rule out DVT may be a reasonable alternative approach because a positive lower extremity study requires treatment without further testing.[31]

Echocardiography is insensitive for the diagnosis of PE but may nonetheless play an important role in the evaluation of PE. Transthoracic echocardiographic signs of acute PE include dilation and hypokinesis of the RV, paradoxical motion of the interventricular septum, tricuspid regurgitation, and lack of collapse of the inferior vena cava during inspiration.[32] The McConnell sign (free-wall RV hypokinesis that spares the apex) may be a more specific finding; rarely, direct visualization of a thrombus may guarantee the diagnosis.[33] The speed and portability of echocardiography make it particularly useful in patients who are suspected of having PE and are too unstable for further evaluation with CTA or $\dot{V}/\dot{Q}$ scan. Additionally, echocardiography has proven helpful for risk stratification in patients with proven PE, and serial exams may demonstrate interval change in cardiac function.[34,35] Echocardiography may also be useful in identifying other causes of shock, such as aortic dissection and cardiac tamponade.

Pulmonary Hypertension

The manifestations of PH are generally nonspecific, so careful attention to the clinical history and physical examination can provide important clues to the presence of disease. In all patients, a careful history of current and prior medication use and concomitant medical conditions is essential.

Dyspnea is a common feature, and chest pain may also occur, but these symptoms may often be attributed to other more common conditions such as asthma, deconditioning, weight gain, panic attacks, coronary artery disease, or gastroesophageal reflux disease. This may significantly delay the diagnosis; in fact, patients in the IPAH registry had symptoms from 2 to 5 years prior to a formal diagnosis.[36] Raynaud phenomenon may occur in patients with IPAH but is much more common with PAH associated with connective tissue disease. Exertional presyncope and syncope may be due to the inability to increase cardiac output in response to the increased demand and suggests advanced PH with right heart failure.

Orthopnea is relatively common in patients with severe COPD, although it is not necessarily accompanied by worsening cardiac function. Orthopnea in these patients is believed to be related to hyperinflation of the lungs and the subsequent effects on ventricular function or reduction in venous return, or both. In patients with cor pulmonale and other forms of PH, increased venous and hepatic congestion can occur in advanced disease and lead to the development of early satiety, increasing lower extremity edema and fluid overload.

The presence of a loud pulmonic valve closure sound is a common finding in patients with PH, independent of the cause. It may be accompanied by a parasternal or epigastric lift resulting from a hypertrophied RV. Tricuspid valvular regurgitation also develops because of dilation of the RV, which causes a prominent jugular V wave. Progressive signs of chronic right ventricular dilation and failure include pulmonic valve insufficiency, a right ventricular third heart sound, jugular venous distention, hepatojugular reflux, hepatomegaly, lower extremity edema, ascites, and eventually anasarca.

Patients with cor pulmonale and PH resulting from COPD also invariably have findings associated with their obstructive lung disease, including decreased breath sounds and hyperinflation. Individuals with cor pulmonale secondary to interstitial lung disease often have dry crackles at the lung bases. Auscultation of the lungs in IPAH is generally unremarkable. Clubbing also is a common finding in patients with pulmonary fibrosis, but not in PH alone.

Hypoxemia is frequently observed in patients with significant PH and cor pulmonale. Patients with IPAH may have a normal arterial oxygen content until late in the disease. Pulmonary function tests may sometimes help identify the etiology of pulmonary vascular disease. The presence of significant PH and cor pulmonale with mild abnormalities in pulmonary function tests should suggest a diagnosis of primary pulmonary vascular disease.

In contrast to PE, in which nonspecific ECG changes are commonly observed, right heart strain, including P pulmonale, right axis deviation, and right ventricular hypertrophy, is typically present in patients with advanced pulmonary hypertension or cor pulmonale. For example, evidence of right heart strain ultimately occurs in approximately 80% of patients with IPAH.[36]

Patients with longstanding PH or cor pulmonale have markedly abnormal radiographs that suggest the presence of their disease. Enlarged pulmonary arteries with or without an enlarged RV are often evident. **Figure 37–5** illustrates severe bilateral pulmonary artery and RV enlargement in a patient with IPAH.

RESPIRATORY RECAP

Diagnosis of Pulmonary Hypertension

- » Dyspnea is common but not specific.
- » Chest pain may occur, but generally with more advanced PH.
- » Exertional presyncope or syncope or both may occur with advanced PH.
- » A loud second heart sound (pulmonic valve closure) is common.
- » Hypoxemia is often present in patients with advanced PH.
- » Electrocardiographic findings consistent with right heart strain are commonly observed.
- » Enlarged pulmonary arteries may be seen on the chest radiograph.
- » Echocardiography may help determine the underlying cause of PH.
- » Echocardiography is also useful in determining and following RV size and function.
- » The gold standard for diagnosis of pulmonary hypertension is right heart catheterization.

Echocardiography is quite useful in the diagnosis of PH.[37] The echocardiogram also helps establish secondary causes for PH, such as left ventricular dysfunction, mitral valve abnormalities, or congenital heart disease. Although echocardiography is not foolproof in the detection of mild to moderate PH, it is sensitive in the detection of severe elevations in pulmonary artery pressure. The majority of such patients have tricuspid regurgitation, thereby allowing a reasonably accurate estimate of pulmonary artery systolic pressure. Because echocardiography is noninvasive, it is generally used early to determine the presence and severity of PH in the presence or absence of cor pulmonale. It is also useful for serial monitoring of patients with established PH after therapeutic interventions. For evaluation of a patient with PH, $\dot{V}/\dot{Q}$ scanning is important in excluding chronic thromboembolic disease as a secondary cause of PH.[37]

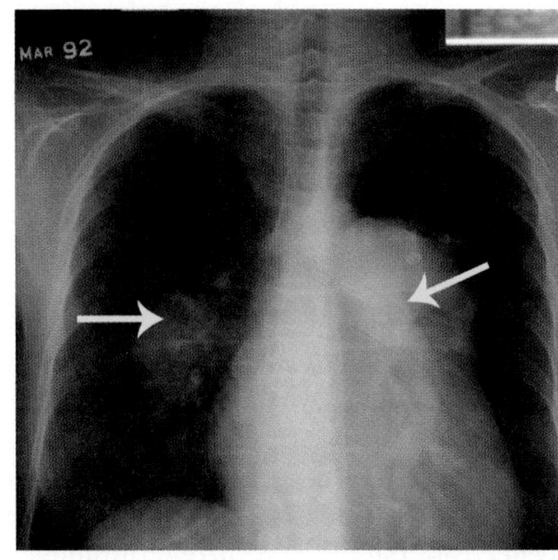

FIGURE 37–5 Chest radiograph in a patient with severe idiopathic pulmonary arterial hypertension reveals severely enlarged proximal pulmonary arteries (arrows) and cardiomegaly. The latter is due to massive right ventricular enlargement.

The gold standard for the diagnosis of PH remains right heart catheterization, which should always be done prior to instituting therapy. This technique utilizes a thermodilution balloon catheter to measure right ventricular, pulmonary artery, and pulmonary capillary wedge pressures.[38] Patients with IPAH have normal wedge pressures. The presence of an abnormal capillary wedge pressure suggests a left-sided cause of PH. In addition, right heart catheterization allows for comparisons between the oxygen saturation in the central veins, right atrium, right ventricle, and pulmonary artery. This determines whether left-to-right or right-to-left shunting is present. Right heart catheterization supplements the echocardiographic data in the diagnosis and evaluation of congenital heart disease. In many centers, exposure to a pulmonary vasodilator is done during cardiac catheterization to assess vascular reactivity.

In summary, in patients in whom PH is suspected based on the clinical history or physical exam, a reasonable diagnostic approach may begin with a chest radiograph and echocardiogram. A $\dot{V}/\dot{Q}$ scan should be performed to exclude PE in patients with evidence of PH. If PH is a high probability, then CTA, pulmonary arteriography, or both should be performed.

Management of Selected Pulmonary Vascular Diseases

Pulmonary Thromboembolism

Anticoagulation has been proven to reduce mortality in acute PE, and it should be immediately instituted unless contraindications are present. Although anticoagulants do not directly dissolve preexisting clots, they prevent thrombus extension and indirectly decrease clot burden by allowing the natural fibrinolytic system to proceed unopposed.[39] When there exists a high clinical suspicion for PE, anticoagulation is appropriate while diagnostic testing is under way unless the risk of therapy is deemed excessive.

Unfractionated heparin (UFH) is usually delivered by continuous IV infusion, and therapy is monitored by measurement of the activated partial thromboplastin time (aPTT). Traditional, or physician-directed, dosing of heparin often leads to subtherapeutic aPTT; validated dosing nomograms are generally favored because they reduce the time to achieve therapeutic anticoagulation and may decrease the risk of recurrent thromboembolic events.[40–42] A heparin regimen consisting of a bolus of 80 μ/kg followed by 18 μ/kg/hr has been recommended, and, following the institution of intravenous UFH, the aPTT should be followed at 6-hour intervals until it is consistently in the therapeutic range of 1.5 to 2.0 times control values.[43] Further adjusting of the heparin dose should be weight based.

Low-molecular-weight heparin (LMWH) is at least as safe and effective as UFH for the treatment of acute venous thromboembolism (VTE) and is now favored for most hemodynamically stable patients[44,45] with acute DVT or PE, except when the much shorter acting heparin is deemed more appropriate. LMWH preparations offer several advantages over UFH, including greater bioavailability, longer half-life, lack of need for an intravenous infusion, more predictable anticoagulant response to weight-based dosing, and a decreased risk of heparin-induced thrombocytopenia (HIT). These preparations can be administered once or twice per day subcutaneously and do not require monitoring of the aPTT. Monitoring of antifactor Xa levels is reasonable in certain settings such as morbid obesity, very small patients (<40 kg), pregnancy, renal dysfunction, or patients with unanticipated bleeding or recurrent VTE despite appropriate weight-based dosing.

Other, newer agents may be useful in the treatment of VTE. Fondaparinux is a heparin-derived synthetic polysaccharide that catalyzes factor Xa activation. Direct thrombin inhibitors such as lepirudin and argatroban have an important niche in the treatment of HIT, but their anticoagulant effect is not readily reversible. Rivaroxaban, apixaban, and dabigatran are newer oral agents that have been studied extensively and could ultimately be approved for use in DVT and PE.

Long-term treatment with warfarin is effective for preventing recurrent VTE, and therapy may be initiated after a heparin preparation or fondaparinux is begun. Initial therapy with warfarin alone may cause a transient hypercoagulable state due to the abrupt decline in vitamin K–dependent coagulation inhibitors and may paradoxically increase the risk of recurrent PE or DVT. Thus, warfarin therapy should be overlapped with therapeutic heparin or fondaparinux for a minimum of 5 days and until two consecutive international normalized ratio (INR) values of 2.0 to 3.0 have been documented at least 24 hours apart.[46] The duration of anticoagulation depends on the presence or persistence of risk factors, but in all cases, documented PE should be treated with anticoagulation for at least 3 months. In some cases, however, with underlying hypercoagulable states (refer to Box 37–2), lifetime anticoagulation may be indicated. Oral warfarin therapy must take into account many drug and food interactions, as well as genetic variations in drug metabolism, and careful monitoring is warranted.

Complications of heparin include bleeding and heparin-induced thrombocytopenia. The rates of major bleeding in trials using heparin by continuous infusion are less than 5%.[47] Heparin-induced thrombocytopenia (defined as a platelet count that drops by greater than 50% or to less than 100,000 mm^3) typically develops 5 to 10 days after the initiation of heparin therapy, occurring in 3% to 5% of patients. The syndrome is caused by heparin-dependent IgG antiplatelet antibodies and can result in either paradoxical thrombosis or bleeding.[48] If a patient is placed on heparin for venous thromboembolism and the platelet count progressively decreases to 100,000/mm^3 or less, heparin therapy should be discontinued. It is important to realize that HIT can occur with a platelet count of higher than 100,000/mm^3. Several anticoagulants have been approved for use in the setting of HIT.

Inferior vena cava (IVC) filter placement can be undertaken to prevent lower extremity thrombi from embolizing to the lungs. These devices have been widely used for nearly two decades. The primary indications for filter placement include contraindications to anticoagulation, significant bleeding complications during anticoagulation, and recurrent embolism while on adequate therapy.[49] Filters are sometimes placed in the setting of massive PE when it is believed that any further emboli might be lethal. A randomized study suggested that filter placement in patients with new DVT reduces the risk of acute PE at day 12 but increases the risk of recurrent DVT at 2 years.[50] A number of filter designs exist, and temporary, removable filters are widely used currently. Filters can be inserted via the jugular or femoral vein. These devices are effective, and complications are unusual but may include perforation of the IVC, filter migration, and IVC obstruction due to filter thrombosis. In general, anticoagulation is continued when a filter is placed unless it is contraindicated.

The National Institutes of Health consensus guidelines for PE thrombolysis issued in 1980 suggested that **thrombolytic therapy** was appropriate for patients with obstruction of blood flow to a lobe or multiple pulmonary segments and for patients with hemodynamic compromise, regardless of the size of the PE.[51] Current guidelines also favor the use of thrombolytic therapy in patients with hemodynamic instability (hypotension) or severely compromised oxygenation. Risk stratification is important in acute PE, and more stable patients with a significant embolic load are considered on an individual basis, with thrombolytic therapy being considered in the absence of absolute or relative contraindications. Such settings might include severe hypoxemia, significant RV dysfunction by echocardiography, elevated troponin values, or a combination of these.

Acceleration of clot lysis in PE with thrombolytic therapy was documented in several trials.[25,52] One trial demonstrated that thrombolysis was accelerated in patients receiving urokinase compared with those on heparin when pulmonary arteriograms and lung perfusion scans were examined 24 hours after treatment. At present, tissue plasminogen activator (100 mg intravenous infusion delivered over 2 hours) may be the most commonly employed protocol when thrombolysis is used in PE.[53] Heparin should be withheld until the thrombolytic infusion is completed.

Some patients deemed candidates for thrombolytic therapy based on the severity of their PE may have contraindications such as bleeding or high risk of bleeding (e.g., recent surgery). In such cases, surgical removal of clot (pulmonary embolectomy) can be considered.

Cor Pulmonale

Cor pulmonale describes RV dysfunction caused by diseases affecting the lung or its vasculature. The treatment of patients with cor pulmonale focuses on treatment of the underlying lung disease, with efforts toward improving oxygenation, decreasing pulmonary vascular resistance, and improving RV function. In the case of COPD, β-receptor agonists (e.g., albuterol, salmeterol) and anticholinergics (e.g., ipratropium, tiotropium) are inhaled bronchodilators used in patients with airflow obstruction. Theophylline is also a bronchodilator, but may offer additional beneficial effects such as improved cardiac contractility, mild pulmonary vasodilation, and enhanced diaphragm endurance. Finally, inhaled or systemic corticosteroids, or both, appear to benefit a subset of patients with COPD.

Because **hypoxic pulmonary vasoconstriction** is thought to contribute to the pathogenesis of PH in patients with cor pulmonale, supplemental oxygen therapy is often employed. Supplemental oxygen reduces hypoxic pulmonary vasoconstriction, thereby reducing pulmonary artery pressures and decreasing the workload of the right ventricle. Two large trials have demonstrated a survival benefit of supplemental oxygen therapy in COPD patients with hypoxemia and cor pulmonale.[54,55] Based on the results of these and other studies, long-term oxygen therapy is recommended in patients with a Pao_2 of 55 mm Hg or less, or in patients with a Pao_2 of 60 mm Hg or less and evidence of cor pulmonale or secondary polycythemia.

There are only limited data regarding the use of inotropic agents or pulmonary vasodilators in cor pulmonale. Digoxin does not improve RV function in patients with COPD and cor pulmonale without concomitant left ventricular failure.[56] Diuretic therapy may improve right heart function by decreasing the RV filling volume in cases of significant volume overload. Traditional pulmonary vasodilators (e.g., hydralazine, calcium channel blockers) have not shown sustained benefits and may be associated with deleterious effects resulting from systemic vasodilation.

More advanced therapy (e.g., sildenafil, epoprostenol) may be considered in selected patients with persistent PH and a poor functional status despite maximal primary therapy. There is little direct evidence, however, supporting advanced therapy in cor pulmonale; thus, this approach remains controversial and should only be considered at specialized centers.

Pulmonary Arterial Hypertension

Initial therapeutic trials in PAH focused on the use of **calcium channel blockers** to treat PH, and an improvement in pulmonary hemodynamics occurs in a minority of treated patients.[57] A sustained improvement is less common, and these agents also may have significant adverse effects such as hypotension. As in patients with cor pulmonale, traditional therapies such as supplemental oxygen and diuretics are useful. However, these forms of therapies for PAH are generally insufficient, and advanced therapies are needed.

Prostacyclin (epoprostenol, PGI_2) is a pulmonary vasodilator that has proven to be the most effective therapy available in the treatment of patients with IPAH. Because prostacyclin has a short half-life and is rapidly inactivated by the low gastric pH, it is given as a continuous intravenous infusion via a permanent indwelling catheter with a portable infusion pump. A large, prospective, randomized, multicenter trial compared prostacyclin plus conventional therapy with conventional therapy alone in patients with class III and IV IPAH.[58] The patients treated with prostacyclin had significant improvements in exercise capacity, hemodynamics, and survival. Long-term benefits are likely due to the vasodilative, antiplatelet, and antiproliferative properties of prostacyclin. Prostacyclin analogues, such as treprostinil and iloprost, are also beneficial in the management of PAH;[59,60] treprostinil has proven effective when delivered via the subcutaneous, intravenous, and inhaled routes, and iloprost is effective via the intravenous or inhaled routes.

Extraordinary advances in the understanding of PH have led to the development of other treatment regimens for PAH. Endothelin is a potent vasoconstrictor and smooth muscle mitogen, and oral endothelin receptor antagonists (bosentan, ambrisentan) have been shown to improve hemodynamics and functional status in patients with PAH.[61,62] Oral phosphodiesterase-5 inhibitors (sildenafil, tadalafil) prolong the vasodilatory effects of endogenous nitric oxide and are also effective therapies.[63,64] There is also emerging evidence that combination therapy is useful in the treatment of PAH. Finally, lung transplantation is appropriate in carefully selected patients with PAH who fail medical therapy.

Because microscopic thrombi and frank VTE are associated with PAH, systemic anticoagulation has been suggested to improve survival in patients with IPAH.[57,65] When warfarin is used, an INR of 1.5 to 2.5 is considered therapeutic. The risk–benefit ratio must be considered on an individual basis when considering anticoagulant therapy.

Other Classes of Pulmonary Hypertension

Other classes of PH should be managed with primary therapy directed at the underlying cause of the PH as described previously. For example, the treatment of PH resulting from cardiac disease is aimed at the treatment of the underlying cardiac defect (i.e., mitral stenosis, left ventricular systolic or diastolic failure, sleep apnea). In general, treatment of any underlying disease that may be contributing to the development of PH and the use of supplemental oxygen to alleviate hypoxic pulmonary vasoconstriction remain important goals of therapy. Following treatment, the severity of PH may be reassessed and more advanced therapy considered on a case-by-case basis by physicians who are experienced in the evaluation and management of PH at a specialized center.

Recent consensus statements by the World Health Organization convening at Dana Point, California, in 2008, as well as the American College of Cardiology, have offered detailed evidence-based recommendations for the treatment of PH. These include having a low threshold to refer patients to PH centers with expertise in treating this disease.[66,67]

CASE STUDIES

Case 1. Acute Right Ventricular Failure

A 50-year-old man with a history of arthritis 5 days after left hip replacement suddenly developed shortness of breath and hypotension. The patient previously had been healthy and well. His postoperative course was uncomplicated, and warfarin had been started for thromboembolism prophylaxis. The patient had just gotten out of bed to go to the bathroom when he suddenly felt short of breath and dizzy. On examination he looked pale and in moderate respiratory distress. Blood pressure was 85 systolic, heart rate 120 beats/min, respiratory rate 30 breaths/min, and oxygen saturation 90% on 15 L/min oxygen via nonrebreathing mask. Physical exam was notable for clear lungs, an elevated jugular venous pressure with a prominent V wave, tachycardia with a prominent S_2 sound, a systolic murmur at the left sternal border, and an S_3 sound that was augmented with inspiration. The left leg was edematous. An arterial blood gas revealed a pH of 7.45, a $Paco_2$ of 28 mm Hg, and a Pao_2 of 59 mm Hg on supplemental O_2 at 15 L/min. An ECG revealed tachycardia with a new right bundle branch pattern, and a chest radiograph disclosed bilateral lower lobe atelectasis.

The patient has had an acute event resulting in hypoxemia, hypotension, and signs of right heart failure. Given his recent hip surgery, the most likely etiology is acute PE. Hypotension is likely from acute right-sided heart failure. This results from an acute rise in the pulmonary vascular resistance leading to a decrement in RV stroke volume and an increase in the RV end diastolic volume. This increase has multiple detrimental effects, including increased oxygen demands resulting in ischemia and decreased left ventricular compliance via ventricular interdependence. The result is decreased cardiac performance and shock.

The approach to this patient will involve prompt, accurate diagnosis and treatment. Diagnostically, the patient could have a $\dot{V}/\dot{Q}$ scan or a chest CTA. Given the instability of the patient, a CTA, the faster test, is preferred. The options for treatment include anticoagulation with UFH or LMWH, anticoagulation plus inferior vena cava filter placement, or fibrinolytic therapy. In the meantime the patient will require transfer to an intensive care unit for hemodynamic and respiratory support. His oxygen requirement is high, and he is hypotensive. Fluids should be administered, and vasopressor therapy should follow if the blood pressure remains low. This patient would meet the indications for thrombolytic therapy, but recent surgery (less than 1 week ago) increases the risk for bleeding complications. A careful assessment of the risks and benefits of fibrinolytic therapy is necessary in this case. Pulmonary embolectomy could be considered if thrombolytics were deemed contraindicated.

Case 2. Idiopathic Pulmonary Arterial Hypertension

A 30-year-old woman developed progressive dyspnea over a 6-month period. The patient had been previously healthy and active until approximately 6 months before presentation, when she noted dyspnea when walking to her third-floor apartment. This was associated with occasional sharp chest pains but no wheezing or fever. The dyspnea had progressed over the next few months such that the patient was getting short of breath after climbing only a few stairs or walking on a hill. An evaluation had disclosed a normal chest radiograph, normal spirometry, a decreased diffusion capacity at 55% of predicted, and an ECG consistent with strain on the right ventricle. An echocardiogram disclosed a dilated, hypokinetic RV with an estimated RV systolic pressure of 76 mm Hg. The left ventricle had normal size and function. No shunts were evident when contrast bubbles were injected.

On presentation, the patient was dyspneic with short walks on a flat surface. She had had a syncopal episode about 1 week before presentation. Further review of the history disclosed no history of prior lung disease, connective tissue disease (or unexplained arthritis or skin abnormalities), diet pill use, exotic travel, or previous thromboembolic disease. She had no history of smoking, and a noncontributory family history. Her oxygen saturation was 89% on room air. She had clear lungs on auscultation. Her cardiac exam was notable for elevated neck veins and a prominent RV heave. On auscultation she had a loud P_2 with a right-sided S_3. A prominent systolic murmur was detectable at the left lower sternal border that increased in intensity with inspiration (tricuspid regurgitation). The patient also had 2+ edema of her lower extremities. A full laboratory evaluation was notable for normal serologies, a negative HIV test, normal coagulation profile, and normal liver function. The chest radiograph was clear with prominent central pulmonary arteries. A $\dot{V}/\dot{Q}$ scan disclosed only small peripheral defects and was considered low probability for PE.

The patient was diagnosed with IPAH and referred to a PH specialist for additional diagnostic workup and consideration for prostacyclin therapy.

KEY POINTS

- The low-pressure pulmonary circulation normally offers little resistance to the flow of blood out of the right ventricle.
- Pulmonary vascular disease leads to increased pulmonary vascular resistance. When sustained over time, elevations in pulmonary vascular resistance lead to right ventricular hypertrophy, dilation, and failure.
- The diagnosis of pulmonary vascular disease based on clinical examination is often difficult because many signs and symptoms are nonspecific. Therefore, when pulmonary embolism (PE) or pulmonary hypertension (PH) is suspected, additional diagnostic testing is indicated.
- Chest computed tomographic angiography (CTA) often is the first diagnostic study employed in patients with suspected PE.
- Anticoagulation with unfractionated heparin or low-molecular-weight heparin is the primary therapy in acute PE, except in cases with hemodynamic instability or severe hypoxemia, where thrombolytic therapy may be indicated.
- Treatment of cor pulmonale is directed at the reduction of hypoxic pulmonary vasoconstriction and the treatment of any underlying pulmonary disease that may be contributing to the PH.
- Prostacyclin decreases pulmonary vascular resistance and improves survival in patients with idiopathic pulmonary arterial hypertension.
- Other new therapies, including endothelin receptor antagonists and phosphodiesterase inhibitors, can be considered for treatment of pulmonary arterial hypertension.

REFERENCES

1. Schulman DS, Matthay RA. The right ventricle in pulmonary disease. *Cardiol Clin.* 1992;10:111–135.
2. Weber KT, Janicki JS, Shroff SG, et al. The right ventricle: physiologic and pathophysiologic considerations. *Crit Care Med.* 1983;11:323–328.
3. Damato AN, Galante JG, Smith WM. Hemodynamic response to treadmill exercise in normal subjects. *J Appl Physiol.* 1966;21:959–966.
4. Epstein SE, Beiser GD, Stampfer M, et al. Characterization of the circulatory response to maximal upright exercise in normal subjects and patients with heart disease. *Circulation.* 1967; 3:1049–1062.
5. Fishman AP. State of the art: chronic cor pulmonale. *Am Rev Respir Dis.* 1976;114:775–794.
6. Hatano S, Strasser T, eds. *Primary Pulmonary Hypertension. Report on a WHO Meeting.* Geneva: World Health Organization; 1975:7–45.
7. Simonneau G, Galie N, Rubin LJ, et al. Clinical classification of pulmonary hypertension. *J Am Coll Cardiol.* 2004;43(12 suppl S): 5S–12S.
8. Klinger JR, Hill NS. Right ventricular dysfunction in chronic obstructive pulmonary disease. Evaluation and management. *Chest.* 1991;99:715–723.
9. Christman BW, McPherson CD, Newman JH, et al. An imbalance between the excretion of thromboxane and prostacyclin metabolites in pulmonary hypertension. *N Engl J Med.* 1992;327:70–75.
10. Rubin LJ. Primary pulmonary hypertension. *N Engl J Med.* 1997;336:111–117.
11. McIntyre KM, Sasahara AA. The ratio of pulmonary arterial pressure to pulmonary vascular obstruction: index of preembolic cardiopulmonary status. *Chest.* 1977;71:692–697.
12. Dalen JE, Alpert JS. Natural history of pulmonary embolism. *Prog Cardiovasc Dis.* 1975;17:259–270.
13. Giuntini C, Di Ricco G, Marini C, et al. Pulmonary embolism: epidemiology. *Chest.* 1995;107(1 suppl):3S–9S.
14. Renzetti AD Jr, McClement JH, Litt BD. The Veterans Administration cooperative study of pulmonary function. 3. Mortality in relation to respiratory function in chronic obstructive pulmonary disease. *Am J Med.* 1966;41:115–129.
15. McFadden E, Brunwald E. Cor pulmonale. In: Braunwald E, ed. *Heart Disease: A Textbook of Cardiovascular Medicine.* 3rd ed. Philadelphia: Saunders; 1988:1597–1616.
16. Bishop JM, Cross KW. Physiological variables and mortality in patients with various categories of chronic respiratory disease. *Bull Eur Physiopathol Respir.* 1984;20:495–500.
17. Behr J, Ryu JH. Pulmonary hypertension in interstitial lung disease. *Eur Respir J.* 2008;31:1357–1367.
18. Humbert M, Sitbon O, Chaouat A, et al. Pulmonary arterial hypertension in France: results from a national registry. *Am J Respir Crit Care Med.* 2006;173:1023–1030.
19. D'Alonzo GE, Barst RJ, Ayres SM, et al. Survival in patients with primary pulmonary hypertension. Results from a national prospective registry. *Ann Intern Med.* 1991;115: 343–349.
20. Petitpretz P, Brenot F, Azarian R, et al. Pulmonary hypertension in patients with human immunodeficiency virus infection.

Comparison with primary pulmonary hypertension. *Circulation.* 1994;89:2722–2727.

21. Brenot F, Herve P, Petitpretz P, et al. Primary pulmonary hypertension and fenfluramine use. *Br Heart J.* 1993;70:537–541.
22. Abenhaim L, Moride Y, Brenot F, et al. Appetite-suppressant drugs and the risk of primary pulmonary hypertension. International Primary Pulmonary Hypertension Study Group. *N Engl J Med.* 1996;335:609–616.
23. Goldhaber SZ, Hennekens CH, Evans DA, et al. Factors associated with correct antemortem diagnosis of major pulmonary embolism. *Am J Med.* 1982;73:822–826.
24. Green RM, Meyer TJ, Dunn M, Glassroth J. Pulmonary embolism in younger adults. *Chest.* 1992;101:1507–1511.
25. The Urokinase Pulmonary Embolism Trial. A national cooperative study. *Circulation.* 1973;47(2 suppl):II1–108.
26. Stein PD, Terrin ML, Hales CA, et al. Clinical, laboratory, roentgenographic, and electrocardiographic findings in patients with acute pulmonary embolism and no pre-existing cardiac or pulmonary disease. *Chest.* 1991;100:598–603.
27. Value of the ventilation/perfusion scan in acute pulmonary embolism. Results of the prospective investigation of pulmonary embolism diagnosis (PIOPED). The PIOPED Investigators. *JAMA.* 1990;263:2753–2759.
28. Rathbun SW, Raskob GE, Whitsett TL. Sensitivity and specificity of helical computed tomography in the diagnosis of pulmonary embolism: a systematic review. *Ann Intern Med.* 2000;132:227–232.
29. Stein PD, Fowler SE, Goodman LR, et al. Multidetector computed tomography for acute pulmonary embolism. *N Engl J Med.* 2006;35:2317–2327.
30. Stein PD, Athanasoulis C, Alavi A, et al. Complications and validity of pulmonary angiography in acute pulmonary embolism. *Circulation.* 1992;85:462–468.
31. Stein PD, Hull RD, Pineo G. Strategy that includes serial noninvasive leg tests for diagnosis of thromboembolic disease in patients with suspected acute pulmonary embolism based on data from PIOPED. Prospective Investigation of Pulmonary Embolism Diagnosis. *Arch Intern Med.* 1995;155:2101–2104.
32. Goldhaber SZ. Echocardiography in the management of pulmonary embolism. *Ann Intern Med.* 2002;136:691–700.
33. McConnell MV, Solomon SD, Rayan ME, et al. Regional right ventricular dysfunction detected by echocardiography in acute pulmonary embolism. *Am J Cardiol.* 1996;78:469–473.
34. Grifoni S, Olivotto I, Cecchini P, et al. Short-term clinical outcome of patients with acute pulmonary embolism, normal blood pressure, and echocardiographic right ventricular dysfunction. *Circulation.* 2000;101:2817–2822.
35. Kucher N, Rossi E, De Rosa M, Goldhaber SZ. Prognostic role of echocardiography among patients with acute pulmonary embolism and a systolic arterial pressure of 90 mm Hg or higher. *Arch Intern Med.* 2005;165:1777–1781.
36. Rich S, Dantzker DR, Ayres SM, et al. Primary pulmonary hypertension. A national prospective study. *Ann Intern Med.* 1987;107:216–223.
37. D'Alonzo GE, Bower JS, Dantzker DR. Differentiation of patients with primary and thromboembolic pulmonary hypertension. *Chest.* 1984;85:457–461.
38. Swan HJ, Ganz W, Forrester J, et al. Catheterization of the heart in man with use of a flow-directed balloon-tipped catheter. *N Engl J Med.* 1970;283:447–451.
39. Hirsh J, Dalen JE, Deykin D, Poller L. Heparin: mechanism of action, pharmacokinetics, dosing considerations, monitoring, efficacy, and safety. *Chest.* 1992;102(4 suppl):337S–351S.
40. Raschke RA, Reilly BM, Guidry JR, et al. The weight-based heparin dosing nomogram compared with a "standard care" nomogram. A randomized controlled trial. *Ann Intern Med.* 1993;119:874–881.
41. Hull RD, Raskob GE, Brant RF, et al. Relation between the time to achieve the lower limit of the APTT therapeutic range and recurrent venous thromboembolism during heparin treatment for deep vein thrombosis. *Arch Intern Med.* 1997;157:2562–2568.
42. Hull RD, Raskob GE, Brant RF, et al. The importance of initial heparin treatment on long-term clinical outcomes of antithrombotic therapy. The emerging theme of delayed recurrence. *Arch Intern Med.* 1997;157:2317–2321.
43. Hull RD, Raskob GE, Rosenbloom D, et al. Optimal therapeutic level of heparin therapy in patients with venous thrombosis. *Arch Intern Med.* 1992;152:1589–1595.
44. van Dongen CJ, van den Belt AG, Prins MH, Lensing AW. Fixed dose subcutaneous low molecular weight heparins versus adjusted dose unfractionated heparin for venous thromboembolism. *Cochrane Database Syst Rev.* 2004;4:CD001100.
45. Quinlan DJ, McQuillan A, Eikelboom JW. Low-molecular-weight heparin compared with intravenous unfractionated heparin for treatment of pulmonary embolism: a meta-analysis of randomized, controlled trials. *Ann Intern Med.* 2004;140:175–183.
46. Kearon C, Kahn SR, Agnelli G, et al. Antithrombotic therapy for venous thromboembolic disease: American College of Chest Physicians Evidence-Based Clinical Practice Guidelines. 8th ed. *Chest.* 2008;133(6 suppl):454S–545S.
47. Clagett GP, Anderson FA Jr, Heit J, et al. Prevention of venous thromboembolism. *Chest.* 1995;108(4 suppl):312S–334S.
48. Kelton JG, Sheridan D, Santos A, et al. Heparin-induced thrombocytopenia: laboratory studies. *Blood.* 1988;72:925–930.
49. Greenfield LJ. Vena caval interruption and pulmonary embolectomy. *Clin Chest Med.* 1984;5:495–505.
50. Decousus H, Leizorovicz A, Parent F, et al. A clinical trial of vena caval filters in the prevention of pulmonary embolism in patients with proximal deep-vein thrombosis. Prevention du Risque d'Embolie Pulmonaire par Interruption Cave Study Group. *N Engl J Med.* 1998;338:409–415.
51. Thrombolytic therapy in thrombosis: a National Institutes of Health consensus development conference. *Ann Intern Med.* 1980;93:141–144.
52. Miller GA, Gibson RV, Honey M, Sutton GC. Treatment of pulmonary embolism with streptokinase. A preliminary report. *Br Med J.* 1969;1(5647):812–815.
53. Goldhaber SZ, Kessler CM, Heit J, et al. Randomised controlled trial of recombinant tissue plasminogen activator versus urokinase in the treatment of acute pulmonary embolism. *Lancet.* 1988;2(8606):293–298.
54. Nocturnal Oxygen Therapy Trial Group. Continuous or nocturnal oxygen therapy in hypoxemic chronic obstructive lung disease: a clinical trial. *Ann Intern Med.* 1980;93:391–398.
55. Long term domiciliary oxygen therapy in chronic hypoxic cor pulmonale complicating chronic bronchitis and emphysema. Report of the Medical Research Council Working Party. *Lancet.* 1981;1(8222):681–686.
56. Mathur PN, Powles P, Pugsley SO, et al. Effect of digoxin on right ventricular function in severe chronic airflow obstruction. A controlled clinical trial. *Ann Intern Med.* 1981;95:283–288.
57. Rich S, Brundage BH. High-dose calcium channel-blocking therapy for primary pulmonary hypertension: evidence for long-term reduction in pulmonary arterial pressure and regression of right ventricular hypertrophy. *Circulation.* 1987;76:135–141.
58. Barst RJ, Rubin LJ, Long WA, et al. A comparison of continuous intravenous epoprostenol (prostacyclin) with conventional therapy for primary pulmonary hypertension. The Primary Pulmonary Hypertension Study Group. *N Engl J Med.* 1996;334:296–302.
59. Tapson VF, Gomberg-Maitland M, McLaughlin VV, et al. Safety and efficacy of IV treprostinil for pulmonary arterial hypertension: a prospective, multicenter, open-label, 12-week trial. *Chest.* 2006;129:683–688.

60. Olschewski H, Simonneau G, Galie N, et al. Inhaled iloprost for severe pulmonary hypertension. *N Engl J Med.* 2002;347:322–329.
61. Rubin LJ, Badesch DB, Barst RJ, et al. Bosentan therapy for pulmonary arterial hypertension. *N Engl J Med.* 2002;346:896–903.
62. Galie N, Olschewski H, Oudiz RJ, et al. Ambrisentan for the treatment of pulmonary arterial hypertension: results of the Ambrisentan in Pulmonary Arterial Hypertension, Randomized, Double-Blind, Placebo-Controlled, Multicenter, Efficacy (ARIES) Study 1 and 2. *Circulation.* 2008;117:3010–3019.
63. Galie N, Ghofrani HA, Torbicki A, et al. Sildenafil citrate therapy for pulmonary arterial hypertension. *N Engl J Med.* 2005;353:2148–2157.
64. Galie N, Brundage BH, Ghofrani HA, et al. Tadalafil therapy for pulmonary arterial hypertension. *Circulation.* 2009;119:2894–2903.
65. Fuster V, Steele PM, Edwards WD, et al. Primary pulmonary hypertension: natural history and the importance of thrombosis. *Circulation.* 1984;70:580–587.
66. Barst RJ, Gibbs JSR, Ghofrani HA, et al. Updated evidence-based treatment algorithm in pulmonary arterial hypertension. *J Am Coll Cardiol.* 2009;54(1 suppl):S78–S84.
67. McLaughlin VV, Archer SL, Badesch DB, et al. ACCF/AHA 2009 expert consensus document on pulmonary hypertension: a report of the American College of Cardiology Foundation Task Force on Expert Consensus Documents and the American Heart Association. *J Am Coll Cardiol.* 2009;53:1573–1619.

CHAPTER 38

Pneumonia

Bekele Afessa

OUTLINE

Definition and Classification of Pneumonia
Diagnostic Workup
Bacterial Causes of Pneumonia
Anaerobic Bacterial Infection
Viral Causes of Pneumonia
Mycobacterial Causes of Pneumonia
Fungal Respiratory Infections
Actinomycosis and Nocardiosis
Community-Acquired Pneumonia
Healthcare-Associated Pneumonia and Hospital-Acquired Pneumonia
Pneumonia in Immunocompromised Patients Without HIV Infection
Pneumonia in Patients with HIV Infection
Pneumonia in Children
Case Studies

OBJECTIVES

1. Define pneumonia.
2. Compare community-acquired and healthcare-associated pneumonia.
3. Describe noninvasive and invasive methods for the diagnosis of pneumonia.
4. List causes of gram-positive bacterial pneumonia, gram-negative bacterial pneumonia, atypical organisms causing pneumonia, anaerobic bacterial pneumonia, viral pneumonia, mycobacterial pneumonia, fungal pneumonia, actinomycosis, and nocardiosis.
5. Discuss the etiology, diagnosis, and treatment of gram-positive bacterial pneumonia, gram-negative bacterial pneumonia, atypical organisms causing pneumonia, anaerobic bacterial pneumonia, viral pneumonia, mycobacterial pneumonia, fungal pneumonia, actinomycosis, and nocardiosis.
6. Discuss the differences among community-acquired, healthcare-associated, hospital-acquired, and ventilator-associated pneumonia.
7. Discuss the etiology, initial management, and prognosis of community-acquired pneumonia.
8. Discuss the epidemiology, etiology, initial management, mortality, prognosis, and prevention of healthcare-associated pneumonia.
9. Discuss the prevention and treatment of ventilator-associated pneumonia.
10. Describe the clinical and radiographic findings, diagnostic procedures, causes, and therapeutic considerations for pneumonia in the immunocompromised host.
11. Describe the management of pneumonia in patients with HIV infection.
12. Discuss the management of pneumonia in children.

KEY TERMS

anaerobic bacterial pneumonia
antigen detection and polymerase chain reaction (PCR)
atypical organisms
atypical pneumonia
bronchoalveolar lavage (BAL)
community-acquired pneumonia (CAP)
fungal respiratory infections
gram-negative bacteria
gram-positive bacteria
Gram stain
hospital-acquired pneumonia (HAP)
human immunodeficiency virus (HIV)
mycobacterial pneumonia
pneumonia
protected specimen brush (PSB)
transbronchial lung biopsy
transthoracic needle aspiration (TTNA)
transtracheal aspiration (TTA)
tuberculosis
typical pneumonia
ventilator-associated pneumonia (VAP)
viral pneumonia

INTRODUCTION

Respiratory infections are among the most common clinical problems respiratory therapists encounter in their practice. In 2004, 1.3 million hospitalized patients in the United States, 800,000 of them aged 65 years or older, had pneumonia as the first listed diagnosis at discharge.[1] The rate of pneumonia as a primary diagnosis was 45.5 per 10,000 population, and it was associated with an average hospital length of stay of 5.5 days and with 72,000 deaths.[1]

Definition and Classification of Pneumonia

Pneumonia is the inflammation and consolidation of lung tissue caused by infectious agents. Aspiration, inhalation, and hematogenous dissemination are the mechanisms by which organisms gain access to the lower respiratory tract and cause pneumonia. Most clinicians base the diagnosis of pneumonia on clinical criteria (**Box 38–1**). Unfortunately, the clinical criteria can lead to underdiagnosis or overdiagnosis of pneumonia, particularly in patients requiring endotracheal tubes and those with acute respiratory distress syndrome (ARDS).

The management of patients with pneumonia requires early diagnosis and administration of empirical antibiotic therapy. This in turn requires good knowledge of the most likely pathogens and the patient's underlying comorbidities. Based on the place of acquisition and presence of certain risk factors, pneumonias are classified as community acquired, hospital acquired, healthcare associated, and ventilator associated (**Table 38–1**). Traditionally, all pneumonias that developed outside the hospital were categorized as **community-acquired pneumonia (CAP)**. However, recent data suggest that the causative pathogens and the clinical outcome of pneumonias that develop in patients who reside in nonhospital healthcare facilities such as nursing homes, those who receive hemodialysis, those who receive wound or infusion therapy as outpatients, those who have been hospitalized for at least 3 days within the past 90 days, and those who are immunocompromised are distinct from those that are truly community acquired.[2] *Healthcare-associated pneumonia* (HCAP) refers to the pneumonia that develops in these groups of patients. Although hospital-acquired, healthcare-associated, and ventilator-associated pneumonias differ from each other in their places of acquisition and underlying risk factors, they are caused primarily by similar pathogens and require similar initial antibiotic therapy.

When evaluating patients with CAP, clinicians must make decisions about antibiotic therapy and site of care. The Infectious Disease Society of America (IDSA) and the American Thoracic Society (ATS) recommend implementing guidelines to improve process-of-care variations and relevant clinical outcomes.[3] Classification of CAP based on severity is important because the management strategies, site of treatment, and type of antibiotic therapy differ according to severity. Severity-of-illness scores, such as the CURB-65 criteria (confusion, uremia, respiratory rate, low blood pressure, age 65 years or greater), or prognostic models, such as the Pneumonia Severity Index (PSI), can be used to identify patients with CAP who may be candidates for outpatient treatment.[3] The IDSA/ATS guidelines for the management of patients with CAP recommend admitting patients to an intensive care unit (ICU) if they meet one of the major or three of the minor criteria for severity (**Box 38–2**).[3]

Given the recent trend of many traditional inpatient services being provided in outpatient settings, the

RESPIRATORY RECAP

Management of Pneumonia

- Vaccinate if possible.
- Differentiate between community-acquired and healthcare-associated pneumonia.
- Identify the infecting organism.
- Administer appropriate antimicrobial therapy.
- Provide supportive care.

BOX 38–1

Clinical Criteria for the Diagnosis of Pneumonia

- Radiographic appearance of new or progressive pulmonary infiltrates
- Fever
- Leukocytosis or increased immature neutrophils or leukopenia
- Purulent tracheal secretions

TABLE 38–1 Classification of Pneumonia

Type	Definition
Community acquired	Acquired in the community in patients who lack risk factors for healthcare-associated pneumonia
Hospital acquired	Acquired after 48 hours of hospitalization
Healthcare associated	Occurs within 48 hours of hospital admission or as an outpatient in patients with one or more of the following risk factors: • Transfer from another healthcare facility, such as a nursing home • Receiving hemodialysis, wound, or infusion therapy as outpatient • Prior hospitalization for at least 3 days within 90 days • Immunocompromised state due to underlying disease or therapy
Ventilator associated	Occurs in invasively ventilated patients after 48 hours of tracheal intubation

Data from Kollef MH, Shorr A, Tabak YP, et al. Epidemiology and outcomes of health-care-associated pneumonia: results from a large US database of culture-positive pneumonia. *Chest.* 2005;128:3854–3862.

boundary between the community and the hospital has become blurred. Invasive medical therapies and parenteral medications, including antibiotics, are now routinely administered in nursing homes and other outpatient settings. Although the frequency of drug resistance in HCAP may not be as high as in **ventilator-associated pneumonia (VAP)**, the pathogens causing infection in nursing home residents and other patient populations at risk for HCAP are different from the pathogens causing CAP and are often multiple-drug resistant.[4] To minimize the inaccuracies associated with the clinical diagnosis of VAP, an international consensus conference recommended several criteria and categories, as listed in **Box 38–3**.[5] The ATS/IDSA guidelines recommend empiric initial antibiotic management of patients with **hospital-acquired pneumonia (HAP)** and HCAP like patients with VAP.[4]

HAP and VAP are further divided into the following two categories: early onset, occurring within less than 5 days of admission, and late onset, occurring 5 days or more after admission. Some have classified hospital-acquired pneumonia into three groups: primary endogenous, secondary endogenous, and exogenous. Primary endogenous pneumonias are community acquired and caused by *Streptococcus pneumoniae* and *Haemophilus influenzae*. Secondary endogenous pneumonias are caused by *Pseudomonas aeruginosa* and *Enterobacter* species, organisms that have replaced the normal pharyngeal population and usually are of hospital origin. Exogenous pneumonias are those caused by organisms from colonized respiratory care equipment.

Diagnostic Workup

Controversy remains regarding aggressive microbiologic workup in the setting of CAP. However, treatment should not be delayed because of diagnostic considerations. It is important to evaluate the local prevalence of respiratory pathogens and the state of resistance and to document the precise microbiologic etiology of each case whenever possible. Etiologic diagnoses can simplify and optimize antibiotic treatment. However, the etiology of CAP may not be determined in more than 40% of cases despite aggressive evaluation.[6]

Noninvasive Diagnostic Methods

Sputum

Sputum is a mixture of lower respiratory secretions with oropharyngeal contamination. Although its reliability is affected by inadequate collection methods and contamination, a **Gram stain** and culture of sputum are the cornerstones of diagnosis of pneumonia. Specimens of lower respiratory secretions should contain 25 or more neutrophils and up to 10 epithelial cells per microscopic field (magnified times 100) before being subjected to a Gram stain. A predominant pathogen identified on a screened sputum sample, yielding 10^6 or more colony-forming units (CFU) per milliliter, is considered positive. Both false-positive and false-negative results complicate the diagnosis of pneumococcal pneumonia. *S pneumoniae* is commonly found in the pharynx of healthy subjects and can give false-positive results. Its growth can be hindered by stronger bacteria such as gram-negative bacilli and in patients pretreated with antibiotics. The

BOX 38–2

IDSA/ATS Criteria for Severe Community-Acquired Pneumonia

Major

- Invasive mechanical ventilation
- Septic shock

Minor

- Respiratory rate ≥ 30 breaths/min
- $Pa_{O_2}/F_{IO_2} \le 250$ mm Hg
- Multilobar infiltrates
- Confusion/disorientation
- Uremia with blood urea nitrogen ≥ 20 mg/dL
- Leukopenia < 4000 cells/mm^3
- Thrombocytopenia with platelet count < 100,000 cells/mm^3
- Hypothermia with core temperature < 36° C
- Hypotension requiring aggressive fluid resuscitation

Data from Mandell LA, Wunderink RG, Anzueto A, et al. Infectious Diseases Society of America/American Thoracic Society consensus guidelines on the management of community-acquired pneumonia in adults. *Clin Infect Dis.* 2007;44(suppl 2):S27–S72.

BOX 38–3

Criteria Used in the Diagnosis of Ventilator-Associated Pneumonia

A. *Definite pneumonia*: New or persistent pulmonary infiltrates and purulent secretions in addition to one of the following:
   1. Radiographic evidence of abscess and positive needle aspirate culture
   2. Pathogenic evidence of pneumonia on histologic examination of lung tissue obtained by open lung biopsy or postmortem plus a positive quantitative culture of lung parenchyma ($>10^4$ CFU/g of lung tissue)

B. *Probable pneumonia*: New or persistent pulmonary infiltrate (in the absence of the above) and one of the following:
   1. The presence of positive quantitative culture by protected specimen brush (PSB) or bronchoalveolar lavage (BAL)
   2. Blood culture positive for the same organisms as respiratory sample
   3. Positive pleural fluid culture as respiratory secretions
   4. Pathologic evidence of pneumonia by open lung biopsy or autopsy

C. *Definitive absence of pneumonia*: One of the following:
   1. No histologic evidence of pneumonia postmortem
   2. Definitive alternate etiology
   3. Cytologic identification of nonpneumonia diagnosis

D. *Probable absence of pneumonia*: Lack of significant growth from reliable specimen in addition to one of the following:
   1. Resolution of fever, infiltrate or radiographic infiltrate without antibiotic, and a definite alternative diagnosis
   2. Persistent fever and infiltrate with alternative diagnosis

Modified from Pingleton SK, Fagon JY, Leeper KV Jr. Patient selection for clinical investigation of ventilator-associated pneumonia. Criteria for evaluating diagnostic techniques. *Chest.* 1992;102:553S–556S.

absence of organisms in a sample with neutrophils favors *Legionella* species or an atypical agent. The presence of antibody-coated bacteria may help in the discrimination between true pathogens and colonizers. New techniques such as **antigen detection and polymerase chain reaction (PCR)** applied to sputum samples can help in the rapid identification of pathogens that may be difficult to culture or of pathogens barely growing because of prior antibiotic treatment.

Induced sputum is helpful in patients unable to produce adequate sputum. It has been used in the diagnosis of *Pneumocystis jiroveci* (formerly *Pneumocystis carinii*) pneumonia (PCP). Before sputum induction, patients brush their teeth and gums and gargle with water to remove any debris. They then inhale 3% saline for 20 minutes from an ultrasonic nebulizer and are encouraged to cough every 5 minutes. β_2-agonist inhalers are administered to patients prone to develop bronchospasm during sputum induction. Cytochemical stains (toluidine blue O, Papanicolaou, Giemsa, methenamine silver nitrate), monoclonal antibody, and PCR are applied to the induced sputum to diagnose PCP.

Antigen detection can be applied to sputum, serum, urine, and body fluids. Pneumococcal antigen detection in sputum has not been proven to be cost effective. Antigen detection for *H influenzae* is possible for strains capable of being typed. Antigen detection has been most valuable in the diagnosis of difficult-to-culture organisms, such as *Mycoplasma pneumoniae, Legionella pneumophila, Chlamydophila* (formerly *Chlamydia*) *pneumoniae,* and viral pneumonias. Direct fluorescent antigen (DFA) detection for *L pneumophila* has high specificity but low sensitivity.

Serology

Serologic testing for atypical bacteria is of minor help in the acute phase. Paired acute and convalescent serologic testing provides a reliable retrospective diagnosis, useful only for epidemiologic studies. Serology is used in *L pneumophila, M pneumoniae, C pneumoniae,* and viral infections.

Blood Culture

The overall positivity of blood culture in CAP is 5%. However, the rate of bacteremia reaches 20% to 30% in pneumococcal pneumonia. Bacteremia complicates around 8% of cases of hospital-acquired pneumonia. Two blood cultures are routinely obtained before antibiotics are initiated in hospitalized patients with pneumonia.

Blood culture has low sensitivity but high specificity in the diagnosis of pneumonia. The presence of bacteremia is associated with high morbidity and mortality.

Pleural Fluid

In patients with a significant amount of pleural effusion, diagnostic thoracentesis is used to exclude empyema or complicated parapneumonic effusion. The pleural fluid should be analyzed for pH, protein, lactate dehydrogenase, and Gram stain and culture.

Urine

Pneumococcal antigen detection has an acceptable sensitivity but is cumbersome. *L pneumophila* antigen detection has a good diagnostic accuracy.

Invasive Diagnostic Methods

In nonintubated patients with CAP and HCAP, the diagnosis of pneumonia relies on clinical and radiologic signs and noninvasive investigations with low risk of misdiagnosis. However, in mechanically ventilated patients, clinical and radiologic signs are poorly specific, and it is not easy to determine whether a patient has pneumonia and what the causative organisms are. Fever and new radiologic infiltrates are seen in many noninfectious conditions.[7] Culture of endotracheal aspirates has high sensitivity but low specificity in intubated patients. Invasive diagnostic techniques are used in such conditions.

Bronchoscopy

Quantitative culture of bronchoscopic specimen has higher specificity than that of tracheal aspirates. However, the sensitivity of **bronchoalveolar lavage (BAL)** and **protected specimen brush (PSB)** in the diagnosis of VAP is 36% to 58%. Because of the lack of data showing that the use of invasive methods in the diagnosis of VAP improves outcome, the use of bronchoscopy in the diagnosis of pneumonia is controversial. Bronchoscopy is rarely performed in nonintubated patients for the diagnosis of bacterial pneumonia.

> **RESPIRATORY RECAP**
>
> **Diagnostic Methods**
>
> » Sputum culture and sensitivity
> » Serology
> » Blood culture
> » Diagnostic thoracentesis
> » Bronchoscopy (bronchoalveolar lavage and protected specimen brush)
> » Nonbronchoscopic bronchoalveolar lavage
> » Transbronchial lung biopsy
> » Transthoracic needle aspiration and transtracheal aspiration
>
> Choice of diagnostic method depends on cost effectiveness, availability, expertise, severity, and likelihood of changing empiric treatment. Diagnostic testing should be performed before antibiotics are started.

The double-lumen brush catheter bypasses the nasopharyngeal and oropharyngeal flora. PSB culture showing 10^3 CFU/mL is used as a cutoff point for positivity. False-positive and false-negative results can be seen with PSB. To eliminate false-positive results, the following actions should be taken: avoid suctioning through the working channel of the bronchoscope before the double-lumen brush catheter is passed to the subglottic airways, avoid injection of lidocaine through the working channel below the vocal cords (lidocaine is bacteriostatic), premedicate the patient with atropine, and place the patient in the supine Trendelenburg or lateral decubitus position with the lung to be sampled upright. In patients with chronic obstructive pulmonary disease (COPD), endobronchial disease, or acute bronchitis, the PSB can recover high counts of pathogens in the absence of pneumonia. To avoid false-negative results, bacterial processing is done within 2 hours of sampling, and antibiotics are not given before sampling.

BAL specimens are contaminated by oropharyngeal flora in nonintubated patients. However, quantitative cultures and direct examination for intracellular bacteria make it a useful diagnostic tool. BAL explores large areas of the lung and is more helpful than PSB in the diagnosis of opportunistic infections. In patients with focal disease, BAL is performed by wedging the bronchoscope in the area of greatest involvement. In patients with diffuse disease, BAL is performed from two lobes, usually the upper lobe and the middle lobe or lingula. Dependent segments such as the anterior or apical segment of the upper lobe are preferred to increase the volume of lavage return. About 100 to 200 mL of sterile normal saline in 20- to 60-mL aliquots is instilled, and a return of 40% to 50% of instilled volume, with a minimum of 50 mL, is considered acceptable. The BAL sample can be processed for Gram stain, bacterial culture, *Pneumocystis* stain, mycobacterial and fungal stains and culture, and cytology. A threshold of 10^4 CFU/mL is used in the diagnosis of bacterial pneumonia.

Transbronchial lung biopsy is taken from the most involved lung segment. The biopsy samples are processed for histology, microbiologic stains, and cultures. Because of potential complications, transbronchial lung biopsies are rarely performed in patients receiving positive pressure ventilation.

Transthoracic Needle Aspiration and Transtracheal Aspiration

Transthoracic needle aspiration (TTNA) has good sensitivity and excellent specificity. **Transtracheal aspiration (TTA)** was used in the past to diagnose pneumonia, especially anaerobic pneumonia. However, TTNA and TTA are rarely performed in clinical practice today.

Choosing Diagnostic Methods

The choice of diagnostic method depends on cost effectiveness, availability, expertise, severity of disease, and likelihood of changing empirical treatment. An attempt should

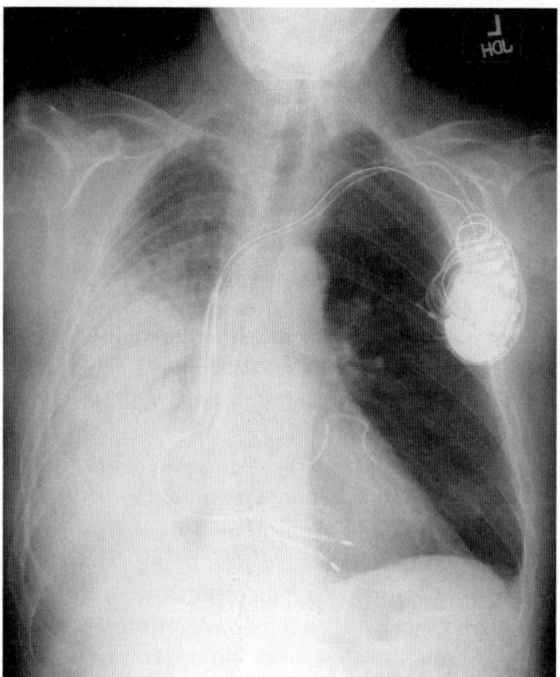
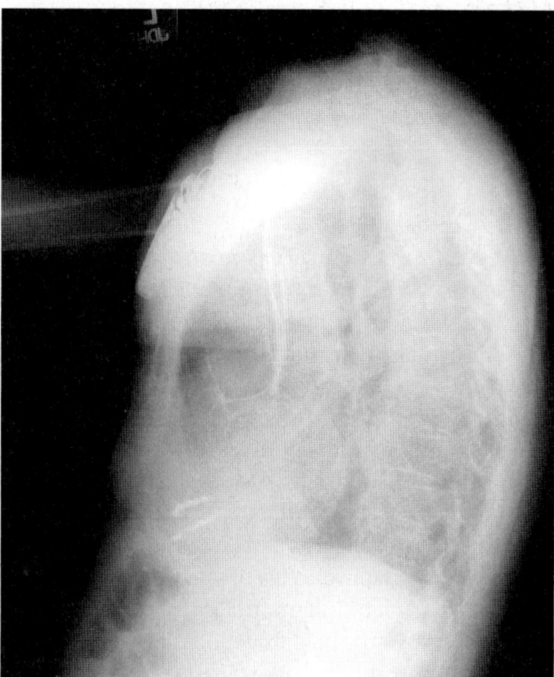

FIGURE 38–1 Posteroanterior and lateral chest radiograph of a patient with pneumococcal pneumonia and empyema showing right lower lobe and right middle lobe consolidation and right pleural effusion.

be made to establish the etiologic diagnosis of pneumonia to permit optimal antibiotic selection and identify pathogens of potential epidemiologic significance.[3,4]

In a patient with mild pneumonia who is treated as an outpatient, a Gram stain of sputum should be performed if possible. In severe and presumed pneumococcal pneumonia, sputum Gram stain, culture, and antibiotic sensitivity testing; two blood cultures; and pleural fluid (if significantly present) Gram stain and culture should be obtained. In severe pneumonia of unknown etiology, sputum Gram stain and cultures (including *Legionella* species), two blood cultures, acute-phase serology for *Legionella* species and atypical agents, urine *Legionella* antigen, and pleural fluid stains and cultures should be performed. In the appropriate clinical setting, a respiratory specimen should be examined for acid-fast bacilli (AFB), *Pneumocystis* stains, and mycobacterial cultures.

Bronchoscopy, TTA, and TTNA can be used to obtain specimens for the diagnostic workup. Many clinicians consider these invasive procedures to be the last step in nonresponding cases, whereas others consider them earlier in the course of treatment, when the patient is not yet in critical condition, in order to have a higher impact on outcome.

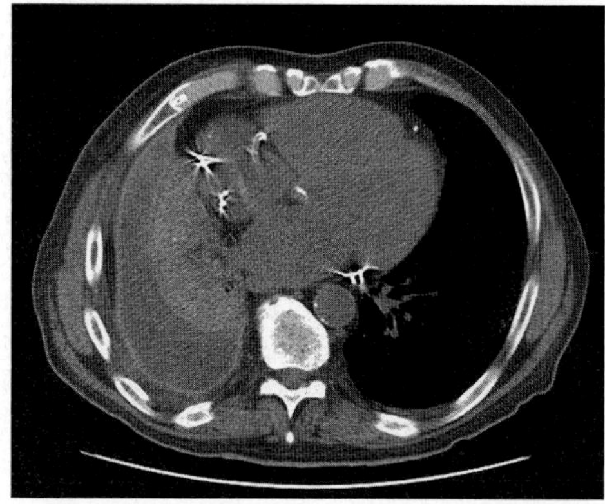

FIGURE 38–2 Computed tomography of the chest of a patient with right-sided pneumococcal empyema.

Bacterial Causes of Pneumonia

Gram-Positive Bacteria

Streptococcus Pneumoniae

Streptococcus pneumoniae is the most common cause of pneumonia. *S pneumoniae* is a lancet-shaped diplococcus, described as a **gram-positive bacterium** because it retains the stain, or resists decolorization, in the Gram staining method. It is found worldwide and causes 40% to 50% of all cases of CAP. Risk factors for pneumococcal disease include anatomic or functional asplenia, **human immunodeficiency virus (HIV)** infection, alcoholism, cirrhosis of the liver, hypogammaglobulinemia, and COPD.

The typical presentation of pneumococcal pneumonia includes fever, rigor, cough productive of rusty sputum, and chest pain. The chest radiograph reveals a unilobar or multilobar infiltrate (**Figure 38–1**). Complications of pneumococcal infection include lung abscesses, empyema (**Figure 38–2**), septic shock, pericarditis, endocarditis, meningitis, and brain abscesses.

Penicillin has been the drug of choice for treatment of *S pneumoniae*. Third-generation cephalosporins, imipenem, and vancomycin are used to treat penicillin-resistant

S pneumoniae. The Centers for Disease Control and Prevention (CDC) recommends the 23-valent pneumococcal vaccine for individuals at increased risk of pneumococcal disease. Revaccination is recommended in 6 years.

Staphylococcus Aureus

Staphylococcus aureus appears as clusters on Gram stain. The incidence of *S aureus* pneumonia has been increasing recently. The risk factors for *S aureus* pneumonia include endotracheal intubation, injection drug use, long-term intravenous catheters, arteriovenous shunts for hemodialysis, burns, infections of the skin, head trauma, chronic pulmonary diseases, quantitative or qualitative neutrophil dysfunction, HIV infection, and viral infections (especially influenza).

The clinical presentation of *S aureus* pneumonia includes fever, cough productive of purulent sputum, and hemoptysis. *S aureus* pneumonia can be complicated with abscess, empyema, hematogenous spread, rash, and septic shock. Neutrophilic leukocytosis is common. The chest radiograph reveals diffuse parenchymal infiltrates, occasionally with focal distribution and cavitation.

The incidence of *S aureus* pneumonia is increased in neurosurgical patients receiving mechanical ventilation. *S aureus* is the organism that most commonly causes pneumonia in critically ill comatose patients. The development of methicillin-resistant *S aureus* (MRSA) has become a growing problem, especially in tertiary and teaching hospitals. Patients with MRSA infection are more likely to have received steroids, to have received antibiotics for more than 48 hours, to have been ventilated for more than 6 days, to be older than 25 years, and to have COPD. Compared with methicillin-sensitive *S aureus* (MSSA), MRSA is associated with more frequent bacteremia, septic shock, and *Pseudomonas* species coinfection and with higher mortality.

The mortality of patients with staphylococcal pneumonia ranges from 30% to 40%. Nafcillin, clindamycin, and the first-generation cephalosporins are the drugs of choice for MSSA pneumonia. Vancomycin and linezolid are used to treat MRSA. Contact isolation and early hospital discharge of patients with MRSA, culture surveillance of staff and patients, and elimination of nasal carriage are necessary to prevent outbreaks of MRSA.

Gram-Negative Bacteria

Haemophilus Influenzae

Haemophilus influenzae is a common inhabitant of human pharyngeal flora. It appears as coccobacilli on Gram stain. This **gram-negative bacterium**, so called because it loses the stain (becomes decolorized by alcohol) in Gram staining, is the most common cause of bacteremia in children. *H influenzae* serotype b is the most significant cause of serious disease. In addition to pneumonia, *H influenzae* can cause meningitis, epiglottitis, arthritis, and bacteremia. Both type b and nontypeable strains of *H influenzae* have been implicated in nosocomial pneumonia. Risk factors for *H influenzae* infection include COPD, defects in B cell function, functional and anatomic asplenia, and HIV infection.

Encapsulated strains of *H influenzae* cause severe pneumonia with acute onset of fever, pleuritic chest pain, productive cough, and hemoptysis. The nonencapsulated strains cause insidious, bronchitis-like disease. The typical chest radiograph finding is bronchopneumonia with small patchy infiltrates. Adults and most children without meningitis recover fully. In patients with severe underlying disease, respiratory and multiple-organ failure may develop.

In cases in which the frequency of β-lactamase-producing *H influenzae* is low, ampicillin and amoxicillin are used for treatment. In cases in which the frequency of β-lactamase-producing *H influenzae* is high, amoxicillin-clavulanate potassium, fluoroquinolones, and second- and third-generation cephalosporins are the preferred treatment. Influenza vaccination protects against *H influenzae* type b.

Moraxella Catarrhalis

Moraxella catarrhalis is a natural inhabitant of the human pharynx. *M catarrhalis* is the third most prevalent cause, following *S pneumoniae* and *H influenzae*, of acute exacerbation of chronic bronchitis in patients with COPD.

Because most patients with *M catarrhalis* pneumonia have underlying lung disease, their clinical presentation is similar to an acute exacerbation of chronic bronchitis. The chest radiograph usually reveals patchy infiltrates. Because most strains of *M catarrhalis* are β-lactamase producing, amoxicillin-clavulanate potassium, ampicillin-sulbactam, fluoroquinolones, macrolides, trimethoprim-sulfamethoxazole, and second- and third-generation cephalosporins are used to treat *M catarrhalis* pneumonia.

Pseudomonas Aeruginosa

Pseudomonas aeruginosa is ubiquitous in a moist environment, and it colonizes the gut, wounds, burns, and catheterized urinary tract. *P aeruginosa* is the gram-negative bacillus isolated most often in VAP and is the leading cause of death among intubated patients with pneumonia. Fewer than 10% of cases of *P aeruginosa* pneumonia are bacteremic. Risk factors for *P aeruginosa* VAP include COPD, HIV infection, neutropenia, mechanical ventilation for more than 8 days, antibiotic use for more than 48 hours, poor nutritional status, and tracheostomy. The crude mortality rate among patients with *P aeruginosa* VAP is 55.5%.

The clinical presentation of *P aeruginosa* pneumonia includes fever, chill, and cough productive of yellow or green sputum. The chest radiograph usually shows diffuse infiltrates. Bacteremic *P aeruginosa* pneumonia is more common in neutropenic patients and has a poor prognosis. Chronic *Pseudomonas* infection, seen in cystic fibrosis and chronic pulmonary disease, has a less severe clinical course.

The treatment of *P aeruginosa* pneumonia includes antipseudomonal penicillin such as piperacillin or a cephalosporin such as ceftazidime combined with aminoglycoside, ciprofloxacin, meropenem, imipenem, or aztreonam. Although instillation of aminoglycosides via endotracheal tube does not improve clinical outcome, it has a higher bacterial eradication rate.

Klebsiella Species

Klebsiella pneumoniae is the most common *Klebsiella* species associated with pneumonia. In addition to nosocomial pneumonia, *Klebsiella* species can cause CAP in alcoholics. Presenting features include fever, productive cough, hemoptysis, and chest pain. Chest radiograph shows lobar consolidation with bulging interlobular fissures.

The antibiotics of choice in the treatment of *Klebsiella* pneumonia include third-generation cephalosporins and the ureidopenicillins, such as piperacillin, and aminoglycosides.

Escherichia Coli

Escherichia coli normally is present in the intestinal tract. It is more commonly the cause of nosocomial pneumonia rather than CAP. Third-generation cephalosporins and fluoroquinolones are used for treatment.

Enterobacter Species

Enterobacter cloacae and *Enterobacter aerogenes* are the species most commonly implicated in pneumonia. Pneumonia caused by *Enterobacter* species is treated with a combination of third-generation cephalosporins and aminoglycosides.

Serratia Species

Serratia species are responsible for about 7% of cases of nosocomial pneumonia. Such pneumonia usually responds to treatment with imipenem, aztreonam, trimethoprim-sulfamethoxazole, or a combination of an extended penicillin and amikacin.

Acinetobacter Species

Acinetobacter species cause pneumonia in ICU patients receiving long-term mechanical ventilation. The clinical features and treatment are similar to *P aeruginosa* pneumonia. *Acinetobacter* species are transmitted on the hands of personnel. Most cases occur after the second week of hospitalization and after the patient has received a long course of broad-spectrum antibiotic therapy. It is associated with high mortality. Risk factors for its development include the severity of the patient's illness and previous infection.

Proteus Mirabilis

Proteus mirabilis causes nosocomial pneumonia. It responds to third-generation cephalosporins and aminoglycosides.

Atypical Organisms

Legionella Species

Legionnaire disease was first recognized among legionnaires attending a convention in a Philadelphia hotel. Although more than 30 species of *Legionella* have been identified, most infections are caused by *L pneumophila*. This **atypical organism** colonizes domestic water and wet cooling systems, which have been implicated as sources in outbreaks. Infections by the *Legionella* species presents as Pontiac fever or pneumonia. Pontiac fever is a transient, self-limiting, influenza-like illness. *Legionella* species can cause both community- and hospital-acquired pneumonia. Clinical symptoms include cough, fever, dyspnea, confusion, abdominal pain, and diarrhea. Nonpulmonary complications include pericarditis/myocarditis, encephalomyelitis, Guillain-Barré syndrome, rhabdomyolysis, acute renal failure, paralytic ileus, and pancreatitis. Quinolones and macrolides are used to treat legionellosis. Rifampin is added to erythromycin to treat severe legionellosis.

Mycoplasma Pneumoniae

Mycoplasma pneumoniae is acquired by inhalation of respiratory droplets. It causes infection in closed populations such as those in military recruit camps and boarding schools. Epidemics of *Mycoplasma* pneumonia occur in 4-year cycles. Symptoms include fever, malaise, headache, and cough. Extrapulmonary manifestations can involve any organ. Myringitis is associated with *Mycoplasma* infection. Elevated cold hemagglutinins are seen in *Mycoplasma* infection but are nonspecific. The treatment includes fluoroquinolones, doxycyclines, and macrolides.

Chlamydophila Psittaci

Psittacosis (caused by *Chlamydophila psittaci*) occurs in people who have contact with birds and bird products. Symptoms include fever, cough, dyspnea, headache, and myalgia. Extrapulmonary manifestations are common and involve the skin, blood, kidney, liver, central nervous system, and heart. The treatment of choice is doxycycline.

Chlamydophila Pneumoniae

Outbreaks of *C pneumoniae* infection have occurred in schools, military institutions, and within families. The clinical manifestations include fever, cough, and pharyngitis. Extrapulmonary manifestations of *C pneumoniae* include arthritis, meningoencephalitis, myocarditis, endocarditis, coronary artery disease, and Guillain-Barré syndrome. Treatment includes fluoroquinolones, doxycycline, and macrolides.

Coxiella Burnetii

Cattle are the reservoir for *Coxiella burnetii*, which causes Q fever. The clinical manifestations include fever, chills, cough, fatigue, myalgia, and diarrhea. The nonpulmonary manifestations include endocarditis, hepatitis, meningoencephalitis, and osteomyelitis. Tetracyclines and fluoroquinolones are used for treatment.

Anaerobic Bacterial Infection

The major anaerobic pathogens implicated in pneumonia are *Peptostreptococcus* species, *Bacteroides melaninogenicus, Fusobacterium necrophorum, Bacteroides asaccharolyticus, Porphyromonas endodontalis*, and *Porphyromonas gingivalis*.[8] Aspiration of oropharyngeal secretions, which contain large numbers of anaerobic bacteria, is the major mechanism of anaerobic lung infection. **Anaerobic bacterial pneumonia** caused by hematogenous spread from septic phlebitis and contiguous spreads from subdiaphragmatic abscess is less common. Predisposing factors for anaerobic lung infections include decreased level of consciousness, impaired swallowing, and gastrointestinal dysfunction. Anaerobic pneumonia is usually multimicrobial.

Patients with anaerobic pneumonia may have poor dental hygiene and longer duration of symptoms compared with those with pneumococcal pneumonia. Radiographically, the posterior segment of the right upper lobe and the superior segment of the right lower lobe are commonly involved. The diagnosis of anaerobic lung infection is made by positive culture of a transtracheal aspirate or empyema. Unless promptly treated, anaerobic pneumonia can lead to necrotizing pneumonia, lung abscess, and empyema.

Clindamycin is the drug of choice to treat anaerobic pneumonia. Amoxicillin-clavulanate, ticarcillin-clavulanate, ampicillin-sulbactam, imipenem, meropenem, and a metronidazole-penicillin combination are other alternatives.

Viral Causes of Pneumonia

Viruses usually cause trivial disease limited to the upper respiratory tract. **Viral pneumonias** are uncommon but often severe. The major viruses causing pneumonia include influenza, parainfluenza, respiratory syncytial virus (RSV), cytomegalovirus (CMV), adenovirus, measles, varicella zoster, herpes simplex, Epstein-Barr, and hantavirus.

Influenza Virus

Influenza infection is characterized by yearly outbreaks, usually in the winter, and less frequent, irregular cycles of pandemics. Attack rates for influenza are highest in young children. Hospital admission and mortality rates are highest in the elderly, especially in those with underlying chronic medical conditions. Secondary bacterial pneumonia, usually caused by *S aureus* and *S pneumoniae*, is a severe complication of influenza infection. Treatment of influenza infection is usually symptomatic, with rest and adequate fluid intake being prescribed. The antiviral drugs amantadine and rimantadine are used in selected cases. Annual influenza vaccination is used as prophylaxis against influenza infection. The influenza vaccines are made annually based on surveillance of strains that are prevalent in the community. The current inactivated influenza vaccines are highly purified and associated with few side effects. The vaccine is contraindicated in people who have an allergy to hen's eggs.

> **AGE-SPECIFIC ANGLE**
>
> Influenza rates are highest in young children. Hospital admission and mortality rates are highest among the elderly.

Other Viruses

Parainfluenza viruses rarely cause pneumonia in adults. Treatment is similar to that for influenza. No vaccination is available against parainfluenza infection.

RSV is more frequent in children. Outbreaks of RSV peak in the winter months. Clinical features are similar to influenza. Aerosolized ribavirin may be used as part of the treatment.

> **AGE-SPECIFIC ANGLE**
>
> RSV infection is frequent in children, particularly in the winter months.

CMV rarely causes a problem in an immunocompetent host. However, it causes severe disease with high mortality in immunocompromised patients. The risk of primary CMV infection is high when a CMV seronegative, immunocompromised patient receives blood products or tissue from a seropositive donor. The clinical presentations include fever, dry cough, and tachypnea with hypoxemia. Radiographic abnormalities include diffuse interstitial infiltrates. Most of the patients who have positive CMV culture in respiratory secretions do not have histologic evidence of CMV pneumonia. Ganciclovir is used to treat CMV pneumonitis. Acyclovir and ganciclovir are used as prophylaxis against CMV.

Adenoviruses can cause severe illness, especially in children. There is no effective antiviral agent that can be used against adenoviruses.

Patients with measles pneumonia usually have the classic measles rash. Measles pneumonia is characterized by prolonged fever, increased cough, and progressive respiratory failure requiring mechanical ventilation. Measles in pregnant women is associated with premature labor and spontaneous abortion. Intravenous ribavirin has been used to treat measles.

Varicella zoster pneumonia is more common in immunocompromised patients. The patient presents with typical chickenpox rash followed by dry cough, dyspnea, and pleuritic chest pain. The chest radiograph usually shows diffuse nodular or reticular densities. Acyclovir is used to treat varicella zoster pneumonia. Vidarabine and foscarnet are alternatives.

Most cases of herpes simplex pneumonia occur in patients with severe immunosuppression, burns, or ARDS. Stomatitis, genital infection, ocular infection, and encephalitis are the main manifestations of herpes simplex infection. The presence of herpes simplex virus in respiratory secretions does not confirm the diagnosis of pneumonia. Histologic proof of parenchymal involvement on lung biopsy is required to confirm the diagnosis of herpes simplex pneumonia. Herpes simplex bronchitis has been associated with fever, wheezing, cough, and bronchospasm. Acyclovir, foscarnet, and vidarabine are used for treatment of herpes simplex pneumonia.

Hantavirus causes influenza-like illness with fever and myalgia, followed by dyspnea, hypoxemia, pulmonary edema, shock, and death. The major reservoir for the virus is the deer mouse. It was initially reported in the Four Corners region of Arizona, Colorado, New Mexico, and Utah.[9] There is no effective therapy to treat this virus.

Mycobacterial Causes of Pneumonia

In addition to *Mycobacterium tuberculosis*, about 19 other nontuberculous mycobacteria can cause human disease. AFB smears and mycobacterial cultures are used in the diagnosis of **mycobacterial pneumonia**. Once mycobacteria are isolated, *M tuberculosis*, *M avium-intracellulare* complex, *M gordonae*, and *M kansasii* can be identified with nucleic acid probes.

Tuberculosis

The World Health Organization (WHO) has estimated that nearly 1 billion people worldwide will be newly infected, 200 million will become ill, and 35 million will die from **tuberculosis** between the years 2000 and 2020. In the United States, the number of cases of tuberculosis has increased each year since 1985; in the preceding 30 years, a 6% annual fall in the number of cases was reported. HIV infection, homelessness, drug abuse, overcrowding, and emigration are responsible for the current rise.

Tuberculous infections are transmitted by inhalation of organisms from infected, coughing individuals. In countries with a high prevalence of tuberculosis, primary tuberculosis occurs in childhood. When infection develops, the affected persons may have malaise and fever or exhibit no symptoms at all. In most children with primary tuberculosis, the primary complex heals, and calcification of the affected lymph node and the associated primary lesion occurs. In some patients, the primary infection can progress and cause cough productive of tubercle bacilli in sputum and, in some cases, pleural effusion. Lymphatic and hematogenous spread to other organs also can be seen. Postprimary pulmonary tuberculosis usually arises from reactivation of a previously dormant primary infection or sometimes as a result of a new exogenous infection. Symptoms include malaise, anorexia, fever, night sweats, weight loss, productive cough, and hemoptysis.

AFB smears and mycobacterial cultures are performed on expectorated and induced sputum, BAL, and lung tissues to diagnose pulmonary tuberculosis. The tuberculin skin test with purified protein derivative (PPD) is used to determine an individual's exposure to mycobacterial infection, including past bacille Calmette-Guérin (BCG) vaccination. A positive test is defined as induration of 10 mm or more in diameter in high-risk individuals without HIV infection, and 5 mm in those with HIV infection. However, the test can be falsely negative in overwhelming infections, sarcoidosis, lymphoma, malignancy, and treatment with immunosuppressive drugs and corticosteroids. There are also problems with its administration as well as interpretation in individuals who have received BCG vaccination or have had nontuberculous mycobacterial infection. Interferon-gamma release assays from serum provide an additional tool to identify latent tuberculous infection in such circumstances.

Primary pulmonary tuberculosis can involve any lobe and has no typical radiologic features. More advanced tuberculosis usually involves the upper lobes (**Figure 38–3**) and the superior segments of the lower lobes with cavitation. Long-standing disease may cause fibrosis.

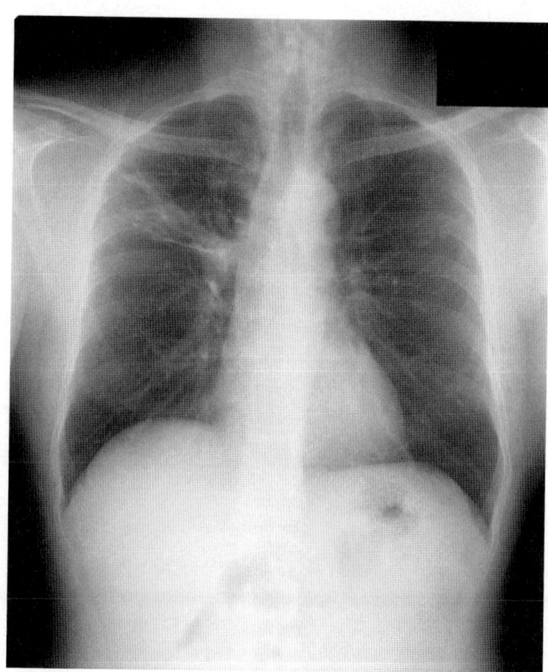

FIGURE 38–3 Posteroanterior chest radiograph of a patient with active tuberculosis pneumonia showing right upper lobe consolidation and volume loss.

Treatment of tuberculosis should include at least 6 months of isoniazid and rifampin and 2 months of pyrazinamide. In areas where the incidence of isoniazid resistance is 4% or greater, ethambutol should be added. Directly observed therapy is recommended.

BCG vaccination and isoniazid are used to prevent tuberculosis. BCG may be beneficial in healthcare workers at risk and in tuberculin-negative adults and infants from countries where tuberculosis is common.

Nontuberculous Mycobacteria

The most commonly isolated nontuberculous mycobacteria (NTM) are *M avium-intracellulare* complex, *M gordonae*, and *M kansasii*. NTM are widespread worldwide and are found in soil and water. NTM are often isolated in the absence of clinical disease. The mode of transmission of NTM infection is not clear. Many cases of pulmonary disease caused by NTM occur in smokers with COPD, silicosis, malignancy, cystic fibrosis, HIV infection, and other immunocompromised conditions. The isolation of NTM without evidence of tissue involvement by biopsy does not differentiate between colonization and disease. The diagnosis of NTM pneumonia is even more difficult in immunocompromised patients because the classic histologic response may not occur. To overcome these diagnostic difficulties, the American Thoracic Society has published diagnostic criteria of NTM lung disease for patients with clinical and radiologic features compatible with mycobacterial disease (**Box 38–4**).[10]

Chronic pulmonary disease is the most common localized manifestation of NTM infection. *M avium-intracellulare* complex, followed by *M kansasii*, is the most frequent NTM causing lung disease in the United States. Symptoms at presentation include chronic cough, sputum production, fatigue, malaise, dyspnea, fever,

BOX 38–4

American Thoracic Society Diagnostic Criteria for Pulmonary Disease Caused by Nontuberculous Mycobacteria

Clinical (both required)

1. Pulmonary symptoms, nodular or cavitary opacities on chest radiograph, or a high-resolution computed tomography scan that shows multifocal bronchiectasis with multiple small nodules

and

2. Appropriate exclusion of other diagnoses

Microbiologic

1. Positive culture results from at least two separate expectorated sputum samples. If the results from (1) are nondiagnostic, consider repeat sputum AFB smears and cultures

or

2. Positive culture result from at least one bronchial wash or lavage

or

3. Transbronchial or other lung biopsy with mycobacterial histopathologic features (granulomatous inflammation or AFB) and positive culture for NTM or biopsy showing mycobacterial histopathologic features (granulomatous inflammation or AFB) and one or more sputum or bronchial washings that are culture positive for NTM
4. Expert consultation should be obtained when NTM are recovered that are either infrequently encountered or that usually represent environmental contamination
5. Patients who are suspected of having NTM lung disease but do not meet the diagnostic criteria should be followed until the diagnosis is firmly established or excluded
6. Making the diagnosis of NTM lung disease does not, per se, necessitate the institution of therapy, which is a decision based on potential risks and benefits of therapy for individual patients

AFB, acid-fast bacillus; NTM, nontuberculous mycobacteria.

hemoptysis, and weight loss. Radiographic features of NTM pneumonia are highly variable and range from upper lobe apical opacities with cavitation to nonspecific lower lobe infiltrates and nodules. High-resolution computed tomography of the chest may show bronchiectasis in patients with *M avium-intracellulare* complex pneumonia. Skin testing is of limited use in the diagnosis of NTM pneumonia.

In the appropriate clinical setting, specific therapy with isoniazid, rifampin, and ethambutol for 18 months is recommended for pulmonary disease caused by *M kansasii*. Clarithromycin, ethambutol, and rifabutin for 18 to 20 months are recommended for the treatment of *M avium-intracellulare* lung disease. Rifabutin combined with azithromycin is used for prophylaxis against *M avium-intracellulare* complex.

Fungal Respiratory Infections

Histoplasmosis

The major endemic areas of histoplasmosis are in North and South America, especially in the Ohio and Mississippi River valleys of the United States. Cutting through logs contaminated with avian excrement, doing construction work, and being exposed to chicken coops or other bird roosts predispose people to contracting histoplasmosis. The majority of **fungal respiratory infections** resulting from exposure to *Histoplasma capsulatum* are asymptomatic. Symptoms develop in individuals exposed to a large inoculum of the organism or in immunocompromised persons. The manifestations of acute pulmonary histoplasmosis include fever, headache, malaise, and nonproductive cough. An intense inflammatory response during an acute pulmonary histoplasmosis infection can cause mediastinal granulomatosis and fibrosis leading to life-threatening complications such as superior vena cava syndrome, esophageal compression, constrictive pericarditis, and lung collapse. Healed pulmonary foci of histoplasmosis can leave calcified coin lesions. Individuals with COPD are at risk for chronic pulmonary histoplasmosis, which is associated with extensive pulmonary infiltrates, cavitation, and volume loss. Disseminated histoplasmosis is life threatening and is seen in immunocompromised patients.

H capsulatum can be seen in blood smears, sputum, cerebrospinal fluid, bone marrow, and lung tissue. Fungal cultures of sputum, bronchial washings, and lung tissues are also used for the diagnosis of histoplasmosis. In disseminated histoplasmosis, urine and sputum *Histoplasma* polysaccharide antigen may be positive.

No specific treatment is needed for asymptomatic or mildly symptomatic acute pulmonary histoplasmosis. In patients with persistent or progressive acute pulmonary histoplasmosis, itraconazole can be used. In severe cases, amphotericin B is needed. Amphotericin B is also recommended for chronic pulmonary and disseminated histoplasmosis.

Blastomycosis

Blastomycosis is endemic in the southern and upper midwestern United States. The presence of both decaying organic debris and high humidity favors the growth of *Blastomyces dermatitidis*. Blastomycosis is acquired sexually or through inhalation.

Acute blastomycosis manifests as pneumonia with fever, chills, myalgia, and productive cough. Chronic blastomycosis manifests with fever, weight loss, cough productive of purulent sputum, and hemoptysis. Chronic blastomycosis can involve the skin, bones, joints, and central nervous system. The diagnosis is made by observation of the organism or by obtaining a positive culture from sputum, bronchial lavage, pleural fluid, skin lesion, cerebrospinal fluid, or urine. Blastomycosis is treated with itraconazole or amphotericin B.

Coccidioidomycosis

Coccidioides immitis lives in soil with arid and semiarid climates. It is endemic in the southwestern United States and some countries of South America. Coccidioidomycosis peaks in the summer and late autumn. In 1994, there was an epidemic of coccidioidomycosis in the Los Angeles area among persons who were exposed to dust clouds after the earthquake.

Infection is generally initiated by inhalation of the organisms. Primary coccidioidomycosis is asymptomatic in the majority of cases. Clinical features include fever, malaise, anorexia, myalgia, cough, hemoptysis, and chest pain. An erythematous, macular rash is seen initially. The usual radiologic manifestations of primary coccidioidomycosis are patchy pulmonary infiltrates. Resolution of the infiltrates is followed by the development of a pulmonary nodule, which may cavitate. Miliary pulmonary infiltrates are seen in disseminated coccidioidomycosis. A minority of the patients with primary coccidioidomycosis may develop chronic, progressive coccidioidomycosis, characterized by apical fibronodular infiltrates. Hematogenous dissemination of coccidioidomycosis is more common in African Americans and Filipinos than in whites and may involve the skin, bones, and meninges. Smear and fungal culture of sputum, bronchial washings, and lung tissues and complement fixation and immunodiffusion serology are used to diagnose coccidioidomycosis.

Primary pulmonary coccidioidomycosis is usually self-limited and does not require antifungal therapy. However, in cases of persistent and progressive symptoms and disseminated disease and in individuals at high risk for dissemination, such as African Americans, Filipinos, immunosuppressed patients, and women in late pregnancy, antifungal therapy is indicated. Amphotericin B is the treatment of choice. Amphotericin B is also effective in chronic and disseminated coccidioidomycosis, although the disease relapses when treatment is stopped. Cavitary pulmonary lesions do not respond to antifungal therapy and may require surgical intervention.

Cryptococcosis

Cryptococcus neoformans has worldwide distribution. The organism is often found in areas contaminated with avian droppings. Infection occurs when aerosolized *Cryptococcus* organisms are inhaled. Most infections are asymptomatic. Cryptococcal disease can occur in normal or immunocompromised persons. Normal persons usually develop self-limited pneumonia without extrapulmonary manifestation, although cryptococcal meningitis can occur in some. Disseminated cryptococcosis occurs more often in patients with impaired cellular immunity, such as those with HIV infection; systemic, prolonged corticosteroid use; certain hematologic malignancies; and organ transplantation. The clinical manifestations of pulmonary cryptococcosis include dry cough, dyspnea, and chest pain. Although meningitis is the most common form of extrapulmonary cryptococcosis, skin, bones, and any other organ also can be involved. The diagnosis is made by direct visualization or culturing of the organism from sputum, bronchial washings, and lung tissue. The cryptococcal antigen test is useful for the diagnosis of cryptococcal meningitis but not respiratory tract infection. Patients with severe cryptococcal pneumonia, extrapulmonary disease, and immunosuppression need treatment with amphotericin B, with or without flucytosine.

Aspergillosis

Aspergillus molds are ubiquitous, being found in soil, dust, and water. The most common *Aspergillus* species causing human disease is *Aspergillus fumigatus*. The organism is transmitted by inhalation from the environment, especially during hospital construction alterations. Qualitative and quantitative neutrophil defects predispose a person to invasive aspergillosis.

The pulmonary manifestations of *Aspergillus* infection include hypersensitivity-type reaction, noninvasive infection, and invasive infection.[11] The hypersensitivity-type reactions include asthma, extrinsic allergic alveolitis, and allergic bronchopulmonary aspergillosis. Noninvasive infection can present as aspergilloma, and invasive infection as chronic necrotizing aspergillosis, acute invasive aspergillosis, and acute tracheobronchitis. The hypersensitivity-type manifestations are treated with systemic corticosteroids. Aspergilloma usually develops in a preexisting cavity, and the infected person may be asymptomatic or present with cough and hemoptysis. Aspergillomas are usually managed conservatively but may require surgery if recurrent or life-threatening symptoms occur. Amphotericin B, voriconazole, and caspofungin are used to treat invasive *Aspergillus* pulmonary infection.

Candidiasis

Candida species are found in soil and food and colonize the gastrointestinal tract, skin, and hospital environment. *Candida* species play a major role in nosocomial infections, particularly in the ICU and in patients with neutropenia. *Candida albicans* is the most common species causing human disease. The manifestations of *Candida* respiratory infections include bronchitis, laryngitis, epiglottitis, mycetoma, lung abscess, and pneumonia. *C albicans* is a common cause of pharyngeal infection in persons using inhaled corticosteroids. Because *Candida* organisms colonize the respiratory tract, the diagnosis of *Candida* pneumonia requires lung biopsy demonstrating tissue invasion. Amphotericin B is the treatment of choice. Amphotericin B, fluconazole, and caspofungin are used for treatment.

Actinomycosis and Nocardiosis

Actinomycosis

Actinomyces species are normally present in the mouth and have a tendency to form filaments as a result of failure to separate with growth. Actinomycosis affects men more often than women. *Actinomyces israelii* is the most commonly implicated species. After dental surgery, aspiration, or penetrating trauma, actinomycosis can involve the thoracic cage, bronchi, mediastinum, lungs, or pleura. Initial clinical features include cough, fever, hemoptysis, chest pain, weight loss, or malaise. Chest radiograph may reveal infiltrates, cavitation, lung abscess, mass lesions, or chest wall involvement. Penicillin is the drug of choice in the treatment of actinomycosis. Alternative antimicrobials include first-generation cephalosporins, imipenem, clindamycin, erythromycin, chloramphenicol, tetracycline, trimethoprim-sulfamethoxazole, or ciprofloxacin. Surgical intervention is required in patients who fail to respond to medical therapy. Hyperbaric oxygen has been used as an adjunctive therapy.

RESPIRATORY RECAP

Causes of Pneumonia

- Gram-positive bacteria: *Streptococcus pneumoniae*, *Staphylococcus aureus*
- Gram-negative bacteria: *Haemophilus influenzae*, *Moraxella catarrhalis*, *Pseudomonas aeruginosa*, *Klebsiella* species, *Escherichia coli*, *Enterobacter* species, *Acinetobacter* species, *Proteus mirabilis*
- Atypical bacteria: *Legionella pneumophila*, *Mycoplasma pneumoniae*, *Chlamydia psittaci*, *Chlamydophila pneumoniae*, *Coxiella burnetii*
- Anaerobic bacteria
- Viruses: influenza, parainfluenza, respiratory syncytial virus, cytomegalovirus, adenovirus, measles, varicella zoster, herpes simplex, hantavirus
- Mycobacteria: *Mycobacterium tuberculosis*, *M avium-intracellulare* complex, *M gordonae*, *M kansasii*
- Fungus: histoplasmosis, blastomycosis, coccidioidomycosis, cryptococcosis, aspergillosis, candidiasis

Nocardiosis

Nocardia species are ubiquitous in soil. *Nocardia asteroides* is the most common *Nocardia* species causing human disease. Nocardial infection is acquired through inhalation. Pulmonary nocardiosis occurs in patients with immunosuppression, chronic pulmonary disease, steroid use, alcoholism, alveolar proteinosis, and autoimmune diseases. Patients with pulmonary nocardiosis present with productive cough over several weeks' duration associated with fatigue, weight loss, fever, dyspnea, and chest pain. Extrapulmonary involvement can include the skin and central nervous system. The radiologic abnormalities include infiltrates, necrotizing pneumonia, cavitation, pulmonary nodules, abscesses, pleural effusion, and hilar and mediastinal lymphadenopathy. The diagnosis of pulmonary nocardiosis can be made from sputum, BAL, and transbronchial and open lung biopsies. Trimethoprim-sulfamethoxazole is the drug of choice used to treat nocardiosis. In addition to antimicrobials, surgical resection and drainage may be necessary for abscess and empyema.

Community-Acquired Pneumonia

The rate of CAP is estimated to be 28.4 per 1000 person-years in adults aged 65 years or older in the United States.[12] Risk factors for CAP include smoking, age, male gender, COPD, asthma, diabetes mellitus, congestive heart failure, lung cancer, dementia, stroke, corticosteroid therapy, immunosuppressive medications, home oxygen therapy, previous hospitalization for pneumonia, and the number of outpatient visits. The peak rates of CAP occur during the winter, coinciding with periods of influenza viral circulation.

AGE-SPECIFIC ANGLE

In the very young and the very old, the incidence of CAP is highest in the winter months.

Diagnostic Evaluation

CAP is defined by the development of a new infiltrate on chest radiograph associated with signs and symptoms suggestive of infection (refer to Box 38–1). Physical findings of rales and bronchial breath sounds have lower sensitivity and specificity than chest radiographs for the diagnosis of CAP and may be absent or altered in the elderly.[3] A chest radiograph should be routinely performed in patients with suspected pneumonia not only to help in establishing the diagnosis, excluding alternative diagnoses, and suggesting the etiologic agent, but also because of its prognostic value and identification of complications.[3] Rarely, when the chest radiograph is negative, computed tomography (CT) of the chest may reveal infiltrates.

The IDSA/ATS consensus guidelines recommend investigating patients with CAP for specific pathogens that would significantly alter empirical management decisions.[3] The spectrum of antibiotic therapy for an individual patient can be altered on the basis of diagnostic testing. Microbiologic evaluation is highly important in regions with unusual pathogens or antibiotic resistance. Some etiologic diagnoses, such as severe acute respiratory syndrome (SARS), influenza, and Legionnaire disease, have important epidemiologic implications. Moreover, trends in antibiotic resistance are more difficult to track and empirical antibiotic recommendations are less likely to be accurate without the accumulated information available from culture results.

Routine diagnostic tests to identify an etiologic diagnosis are optional for outpatients with CAP.[3] Rapid diagnostic tests may be indicated when the diagnosis is uncertain and when distinguishing influenza A from influenza B is important for therapeutic decisions. Microbiologic evaluation is needed for suspected SARS and avian (H5N1) influenza, disease caused by agents of bioterrorism, *Legionella* infection, community-acquired MRSA infection, *M tuberculosis* infection, or endemic fungal infection. Attempts to establish an etiologic diagnosis are also appropriate in selected cases associated with outbreaks, specific risk factors, or atypical presentations.

Blood cultures yield positive results for a probable pathogen in 5% to 14% of patients hospitalized with CAP.[3] The most common blood culture isolate is *S pneumoniae.* The positive yield of blood culture is lower in patients who have received antibiotics and higher in those with severe CAP. The yield of sputum bacterial cultures is influenced by the quality of collection and processing. The yield of sputum for *S pneumonia* is 40% to 50% in patients with bacteremic pneumococcal pneumonia. In patients who have received no antibiotics, the sputum Gram stain and culture results have higher yield. The yield of cultures is substantially higher with endotracheal aspirates, nonbronchoscopic BAL, bronchoscopic sampling, or transthoracic needle aspirates.[3] However, specimens obtained after initiation of antibiotic therapy are unreliable and must be interpreted carefully. Interpretation is improved with quantitative cultures of sputum, tracheal aspirations, and bronchoscopic aspirations. Many of the pathogens causing severe CAP are unaffected by a single dose of antibiotics, unlike *S pneumoniae.* Failure to detect *S aureus* or gram-negative bacilli in good-quality specimens is strong evidence against the presence of these pathogens. Sputum culture in patients with suspected Legionnaire disease improves the likelihood that an environmental source of *Legionella* can be identified.[3]

Diagnostic thoracentesis should be performed and the fluid sent for Gram stain and aerobic and anaerobic bacterial culturing if there is pleural effusion with height more than 5 cm on a lateral upright chest radiograph.[3] Although the yield with pleural fluid cultures is low, it will guide antibiotic choice and the need for drainage.

Urinary antigen tests for detection of *S pneumoniae* and *L pneumophila* serogroup 1 improve the diagnostic yield.[3] The pneumococcal antigen tests are rapid (taking about 15 minutes) and are able to detect pneumococcal pneumonia even after antibiotic therapy has been started. They have a sensitivity of 50% to 80% and a specificity of greater than 90%. False-positive results have been seen in children with chronic respiratory diseases who are colonized with *S pneumoniae* and in patients with an episode of CAP within the previous 3 months, but not in adult colonized patients with COPD.[3] For *Legionella*, the available urinary antigen assays detect only *L pneumophila* serogroup 1, which accounts for 80% to 95% of community-acquired Legionnaire disease. The assays have a sensitivity of 70% to 90% and a specificity of nearly 99% for detection of *L pneumophila* serogroup 1. The urine is positive for antigen on day 1 of illness and continues to be positive for weeks.

Rapid antigen detection tests for influenza provide an etiologic diagnosis within 15 to 30 minutes and lead to consideration of antiviral therapy.[3] Most tests show a sensitivity of 50% to 70% in adults and a specificity approaching 100%. Direct fluorescent antibody tests are available for influenza and RSV and require about 2 hours. The sensitivity of the DFA tests is 85% to 95% for influenza and 20% to 30% for RSV in adults.

The standard for diagnosis of infection with most atypical pathogens, including *Chlamydophila pneumoniae, Mycoplasma pneumoniae,* and *Legionella* species other than *L pneumophila*, relies on acute- and convalescent-phase serologic testing.[3] However, this is of limited clinical value because a single acute-phase titer is unreliable and the convalescent-phase test results will not be available until antibiotic therapy is completed. There are several PCR assays that detect respiratory pathogens, including all serotypes of *L pneumophila*. However, there are no good clinical trials and experience to define their role in CAP.

Etiology

Although a myriad of pathogens may cause CAP, only a few of them are responsible for most cases (**Table 38–2**).[3] *S pneumoniae* is the most frequently isolated pathogen. Age younger than 2 years or older than 65 years, β-lactam therapy within the previous 3 months, alcoholism, medical comorbidities, immunosuppressive illness or therapy, and exposure to a child in a day-care center are risk factors for β-lactam-resistant *S pneumoniae*. *Haemophilus influenzae* and *Moraxella catarrhalis* are common causes of CAP in patients with bronchopulmonary disease. CAP due to *S aureus*, at times methicillin resistant, occurs more frequently during an influenza outbreak.[13] Severe underlying bronchopulmonary disease, alcoholism, and frequent antibiotic therapy are risks for infection with Enterobacteriaceae and *P aeruginosa*.[3] *Streptococcus pyogenes, Neisseria meningitidis, Pasteurella multocida,* and *H influenzae* type b are less common causes of CAP.

The atypical organisms causing CAP, including *M pneumoniae, C pneumoniae, Legionella* species, and respiratory viruses, are not detectable on Gram stain and do not grow on standard bacteriologic media. With the

TABLE 38–2 Common Pathogens Causing Community-Acquired Pneumonia

Patient Type	Pathogen
Outpatient	*Streptococcus pneumoniae* *Mycoplasma pneumoniae* *Haemophilus influenzae* *Chlamydophila pneumoniae* Respiratory viruses
Non-ICU inpatient	*Streptococcus pneumoniae* *Mycoplasma pneumoniae* *Chlamydophila pneumoniae* *Haemophilus influenzae* *Legionella species* Respiratory viruses
ICU inpatient	*Streptococcus pneumoniae* *Staphylococcus aureus* *Legionella species* Gram-negative bacilli *Haemophilus influenzae*

ICU, intensive care unit.

Data from Mandell LA, Wunderink RG, Anzueto A, et al. Infectious Diseases Society of America/American Thoracic Society consensus guidelines on the management of community-acquired pneumonia in adults. *Clin Infect Dis*. 2007;44(suppl 2):S27–S72.

exception of *Legionella* species, these microorganisms are common causes of pneumonia, especially among outpatients. A study has shown respiratory viruses to be the second most common cause of CAP, with influenza being the most predominant.[14] Other common viral causes are RSV, adenovirus, and parainfluenza virus.

Of those who contract CAP, 80% can be treated as outpatients. The most significant pathogens in this setting are *S pneumoniae, H influenzae,* and influenza A virus. The incidence of *M pneumoniae* may vary according to the rapidity of its reproductive cycle and the age of the exposed population.

RESPIRATORY RECAP

Community-Acquired Pneumonia

- » Most individuals can be treated as outpatients.
- » CAP can be classified as typical and atypical.
- » Antibiotic therapy aimed against likely pathogens should be started promptly.
- » The decision to hospitalize is based on the presence of risk factors.
- » Mortality is less than 15%.

Approximately 20% to 50% of patients with CAP require hospitalization. *S pneumoniae* is the most common pathogen, followed by *H influenzae* and *M pneumoniae*. The most important difference between outpatient and hospital-treated CAP is the higher incidence of *L pneumophila* in the hospital-treated group. However, there are regional and annual variations in the incidence of *L pneumophila* pneumonia. Mixed infections account for 10% to 20% of cases of CAP. Admission to an ICU is required for 10% of patients hospitalized for CAP. In these critically ill patients, *S pneumoniae* is the most common pathogen, followed by *L pneumophila*.

The etiology of CAP is modified by age, coexisting illnesses, and geographic, seasonal, and individual factors. Elderly patients appear to suffer from a more severe course of infection. Patients with COPD are often colonized with *S pneumoniae* and *H influenzae.* Patients who abuse alcohol suffer more often from *S pneumoniae* and *K pneumoniae* infections and aspiration pneumonia. Patients with cystic fibrosis and bronchiectasis develop pneumonia caused by *P aeruginosa, S aureus,* and *H influenzae.* Severe neurologic impairment predisposes a person to aspiration pneumonia. In the developing countries, *M tuberculosis* is very common. Travel to certain endemic regions can lead to pneumonia caused by *Histoplasma capsulatum, Coccidioides immitis,* and *Blastomyces dermatitidis.* The incidence of pneumonia rises in the winter, coinciding with peaks of pneumococcal and influenza virus pneumonia. *Legionella* pneumonia is more common in the summer and autumn. *M pneumoniae* has cyclic epidemics every 3 to 4 years. Contact with avian species is associated with *C psittaci.* Domestic animals are the main source of *C burnetii.* Injection drug users are at increased risk for pneumococcal and staphylococcal pneumonia.

AGE-SPECIFIC ANGLE

Elderly patients suffer a more severe course of CAP.

Classically, the epidemiologic, clinical, and radiographic characteristics of each case have been considered to give clues for the initial etiologic assessment. Based on these characteristics, pneumonias have been classified as "typical" and "atypical." However, the usefulness of this classification of CAP has been questioned because no convincing association has been found between individual symptoms, physical findings or laboratory values, and specific etiologies.

Typical pneumonias are characterized by abrupt onset of chills, high fever, pleuritic chest pain, and cough productive of rusty or purulent sputum. Physical signs of consolidation such as bronchial breath sounds and inspiratory crackles are present. Lobar or segmental consolidation is seen on the chest radiograph. Leukocytosis is present. *S pneumoniae* is the most common cause of typical pneumonia, followed by *H influenzae,* Enterobacteriaceae, and *S aureus.* Chronic debilitating diseases such as diabetes mellitus, COPD, hepatic cirrhosis, and alcoholism increase the risk of having nonpneumococcal etiologies.

Atypical pneumonia is more common in the young. It is characterized by a flulike disease with prodromal symptoms, dry cough, myalgia, malaise, rhinorrhea, and moderate fever. Chills are rare. The white blood cell count is usually normal. Chest radiograph shows diffuse infiltrate or a focal peribronchial pattern. Usual pathogens include *M pneumoniae, C psittaci, C burnetii, C pneumoniae,* and respiratory viruses.

AGE-SPECIFIC ANGLE

Atypical pneumonia is more common in younger patients.

BOX 38–5

The CURB-65 Criteria

- Confusion
- Blood urea nitrogen (BUN) ≥ 20 mg/dL
- Respiratory rate ≥ 30 breaths/min
- Systolic blood pressure < 90 mm Hg or diastolic ≤ 60 mm Hg
- Age ≥ 65 years

Data from Lim WS, van der Eerden MM, Laing R, et al. Defining community acquired pneumonia severity on presentation to hospital: an international derivation and validation study. *Thorax.* 2003;58:377–382.

Initial Management

When evaluating patients with CAP, clinicians have to make decisions about antibiotic therapy and site of care. The IDSA/ATS consensus recommends implementing guidelines to improve process-of-care variations and relevant clinical outcomes.[3] The guidelines should be modified according to the local antibiotic resistance patterns, drug availability, and variations in healthcare systems. Protocols based on evidence-based guidelines have been associated with decrease in the time to first antibiotic dose, number of unnecessary hospital admissions, length of hospital stay, duration of hospitalization, and mortality.[3]

Based on the initial assessment of severity, the clinician has to determine the site of care for patients with CAP: outpatient, hospitalization in a medical ward, or admission to an ICU.[3] Severity-of-illness scores, such as the CURB-65 criteria, or prognostic models, such as the Pneumonia Severity Index (PSI), can be used to identify patients with CAP who may be candidates for outpatient treatment.[3,15,16] The CURB-65 scoring system (**Box 38–5**) is based on five variables associated with increased mortality in CAP.[16] In a study by Lim et al., the 30-day mortality was 0.7% when none of these prognostic markers was present and rose to 57% with the presence of five markers.[16] Patients with a CURB-65 score of 0 to 1 may be treated as outpatients, those with a score of 2 may be admitted to the wards, and patients with a score of 3 or higher may require ICU care.

The PSI is based on 20 variables independently associated with mortality (**Box 38–6**).[15] The PSI assigns points for each of the prognostic variables and stratifies patients into five mortality risk classes based on the total sum of the points. In a study by Fine et al., there were good correlations between clinical outcome measures and PSI risk classes (**Table 38–3**).[15] On the basis of associated mortality rates, it has been suggested that risk class I

BOX 38–6

The Pneumonia Severity Index (PSI) Criteria

Male gender
Age greater than 50 years
Nursing home residence
Presence of coexisting illnesses
- Neoplastic disease
- Congestive heart failure
- Cerebrovascular disease
- Renal disease
- Liver disease

Physical examination findings
- Altered mental status
- Pulse > 125 per minute
- Respiratory rate > 30 per minute
- Systolic blood pressure < 90 mm Hg
- Temperature < 35° C or > 40° C

Laboratory or radiographic findings
- Blood urea nitrogen > 30 mg/dL
- Glucose > 250 mg/dL
- Hematocrit < 30%
- Sodium < 130 mmol/L
- Arterial oxygen tension < 60 mm Hg
- Arterial pH < 7.35

Presence of pleural effusion

Modified from Chastre J, Fagon JY. Ventilator-associated pneumonia. *Am J Respir Crit Care Med.* 2002;165:867–903.

and II patients should be treated as outpatients, risk class III patients should be treated in an observation unit or with a short hospitalization, and risk class IV and V patients should be treated as inpatients.[3,15]

The use of objective criteria can play an important role in decision support about the site of care of patients with CAP. The inclusion of 20 different variables in the PSI limits its utilization in busy emergency department or outpatient settings unless they have the needed human or computerized decision support resources.[3] Compared with the PSI, the CURB-65 criteria consist of only five variables that are easily remembered. However, CURB-65 has not been as extensively studied as the PSI. The IDSA/ATS committee preferred use of the CURB-65 system to measure illness severity because of its simplicity and design.[3]

The indications for ICU admission of patients with CAP vary based on patient characteristics, physicians, hospitals, and different healthcare systems. The IDSA/ATS guidelines recommend ICU admission of patients who meet any one of the major or three of the minor criteria for severe CAP (refer to Box 38–2).[3] When

TABLE 38–3 Clinical Outcome of Patients with Community-Acquired Pneumonia According to the Pneumonia Severity Index Risk Class

Risk Class	Mortality (%)	ICU Admission (%)	Hospital Length of Stay (median, days)
I	0.1	4.3	5.0
II	0.6	4.3	6.0
III	0.9	5.9	7.0
IV	9.3	11.4	9.0
V	27.0	17.3	11.0

ICU, intensive care unit.

Data from Fine MJ, Auble TE, Yealy DM, et al. A prediction rule to identify low-risk patients with community-acquired pneumonia. *N Engl J Med.* 1997;336:243–250.

determining the site of care of patients with CAP, decision support tools should always be supplemented with clinicians' determination of subjective factors, including the patient's ability to safely and reliably take oral medication and the availability of outpatient support resources.

Antibiotic Therapy

Appropriate antimicrobial therapy is the mainstay of treatment for CAP, and the selection depends on the causative pathogen and susceptibility. Antimicrobial therapy should be started as soon as possible because delay is associated with poor outcome. Although pneumonia may be caused by a wide variety of pathogens, the initial treatment is mostly empiric, aimed at the most likely pathogens, taking into consideration local susceptibility patterns and specific risk factors.[3] For previously healthy patients with no antibiotic exposure within 3 months preceding the CAP, a macrolide or doxycycline is adequate. For patients with comorbidities or antibiotic exposure within 3 months, a respiratory fluoroquinolone or a β-lactam plus a macrolide is recommended. For patients admitted to the ICU, a β-lactam (cefotaxime, ceftriaxone, or ampicillin-sulbactam) plus azithromycin or a respiratory fluoroquinolone plus azithromycin are appropriate. In patients suspected of having anaerobic aspiration pneumonia, clindamycin or a β-lactam/β-lactamase inhibitor should be used.

If pseudomonas is a consideration, an antipneumococcal, antipseudomonal β-lactam (piperacillin-tazobactam, cefepime, imipenem, or meropenem) plus ciprofloxacin or levofloxacin or an antipneumococcal, antipseudomonal β-lactam plus aminoglycoside and azithromycin or an antipneumococcal, antipseudomonal β-lactam plus aminoglycoside and antipneumococcal fluoroquinolone should be administered. In patients with penicillin allergy, aztreonam should be substituted for the β-lactam. For suspected MRSA, add vancomycin or linezolid. Once the etiology of CAP has been identified on the basis of reliable microbiologic methods, antimicrobial therapy should be directed at that pathogen. Treatment with oseltamivir or zanamivir within 48 hours of symptom onset is recommended for influenza A.

Patients should be switched from intravenous to oral therapy when they are hemodynamically stable and are improving clinically, are able to ingest medications, and have a normally functioning gastrointestinal tract, and should be discharged from the hospital if they have no other active medical problems and have a safe environment for continued care.[3] Patients with CAP should be treated for a minimum of 5 days. They should be afebrile for 48 to 72 hours and should have no more than one CAP-associated sign of clinical instability before therapy is discontinued.

Management of Nonresponding Community-Acquired Pneumonia

Approximately 6% to 15% of hospitalized patients with CAP fail to respond to the initial antibiotic therapy and have a higher associated mortality rate compared with responders.[3] Unacceptable response manifests as clinical deterioration or nonresponse. The clinical deterioration may result in acute respiratory failure requiring ventilator support or in septic shock, usually within the first 72 hours of hospital admission. Development of respiratory failure or hypotension more than 72 hours after initial treatment is often related to intercurrent complications, deterioration in underlying disease, or development of nosocomial superinfection. The absence of or delay in achieving clinical stability is associated with older age; underlying COPD or liver disease; the presence of pleural effusion, cavitation, and multilobar infiltrates on chest radiograph; leukopenia; *Legionella* and gram-negative pneumonia; discordant antibiotic therapy; not using a fluoroquinolone; and higher PSI scores. When there is clinical deterioration or nonresponse despite therapy, clinicians should consider other diagnoses, such as pulmonary embolism, congestive heart failure, bronchiolitis obliterans with organizing pneumonia, ARDS, vasculitis and drug fever.

The median time for patients with CAP to achieve clinical stability is 3 days. Antibiotic changes during the first 72 hours should be considered only for patients with deterioration or in whom new culture data or epidemiologic clues suggest alternative etiologies.[3] Patients with CAP not responding to antibiotics may require transfer to a higher level of care, further diagnostic testing, and escalation or change in antibiotic treatment. Repeat blood cultures, urinary antigen tests for *S pneumoniae* and *L pneumophila*, and looking for other sources of infection may be helpful. Chest CT, thoracentesis, and bronchoscopy are valuable for selected patients with nonresponse. Empyema complicates about 0.7% of CAP cases and requires tube thoracostomy. The presence of risk factors for potentially untreated microorganisms may warrant temporary empiric broadening of the antibiotic regimen until results of diagnostic tests are available.

Prevention

For preventing CAP and decreasing the morbidity and mortality associated with it, pneumococcal polysaccharide vaccine and inactivated influenza vaccine are recommended for all older adults and for younger persons with medical conditions that place them at high risk for morbidity and mortality.[3] Because smokers are at high risk for pneumococcal bacteremia, they should be vaccinated both for pneumococcus and influenza. The annual live attenuated influenza vaccine is recommended for healthy persons 5 to 49 years of age, including healthcare workers and household contacts of high-risk persons. Chemoprophylaxis with oseltamivir and zanamivir can be used as an adjunct to vaccination for prevention and control of influenza. Because developing an adequate immune response to the inactivated influenza vaccine takes about 2 weeks in adults, chemoprophylaxis may be useful during this period for those with household exposure to influenza, those who live or work in institutions with an influenza outbreak, or those who are at high risk for influenza complications in the setting of a community outbreak.[3] Chemoprophylaxis also may be useful for persons with contraindications to influenza vaccine or as an adjunct to vaccination for those who may not respond well to influenza vaccine.

Prognosis

The overall mortality rate of CAP was reported to be 13.7%, ranging from 5.1% for hospitalized and ambulatory patients to 36.5% for ICU patients, in a meta-analysis published in 1996.[17] A more recent population-based study has shown the 30-day mortality rate of CAP to be 3.6% among the elderly.[12] The hospital mortality of patients with CAP admitted to the ICU may approach 50%.[18] Many factors influence the prognosis of CAP. Old age, coexisting illnesses, alcoholism, delay in antimicrobial therapy, and inappropriate initial antimicrobial therapy increase mortality. Tachypnea, hypotension, tachycardia, lack of fever, confusion, low arterial oxygen tension, leukopenia, low serum albumin levels, increased blood urea nitrogen levels, increased serum lactate dehydrogenase levels, multiple lobe infection, bacteremia, certain pathogens, and overall disease severity measured by the Acute Physiology and Chronic Health Evaluation (APACHE) prognostic system are indicators of poor outcome. Disease progression leading to requirement of mechanical ventilation, development of septic shock, ARDS, renal failure, secondary gram-negative colonization, and radiographic spread of the pneumonia are also associated with poor outcome.

Healthcare-Associated Pneumonia and Hospital-Acquired Pneumonia

HAP is usually caused by bacteria and is the second most common nosocomial infection in the United States.[4] The presence of HAP increases hospital stay by an average of 7 to 9 days and cost by more than $40,000 per patient. A 2007 study of 28 hospitals from the southeastern region of the United States showed the weight-adjusted mean cost estimate to be $25,072 per episode of VAP.[19] HAP occurs at a rate of 5 to 10 cases per 1000 hospital admissions, with the incidence increasing by 6- to 20-fold in mechanically ventilated patients. HAP accounts for up to 25% of all ICU infections and for more than 50% of the antibiotics prescribed.[4] The crude mortality rate for HAP may be as high as 30% to 70%. However, many of the critically ill patients with HAP die of their underlying disease rather than pneumonia; thus, its attributable mortality rate has not been clearly defined.

Epidemiology

There are very few studies on HAP in non-ICU patients and on HCAP. In a multicenter prospective study from Spain, the incidence of HAP in non-ICU patients was 3 per 1000 hospital admissions.[20] Risk factors for HAP were hospitalization in a medical ward, severe underlying disease, and longer hospital stay. The onset of HAP occurred an average of 15 days after hospital admission. The pathogens were established in 36% of cases and included *Streptococcus pneumoniae*, *Legionella pneumophila*, *Aspergillus* species, *Pseudomonas aeruginosa*, and Enterobacteriaceae. Bacteremia occurred in 9.3%. Complications developed in 52.1%, including respiratory failure in 34.5%, pleural effusion in 20.6%, septic shock in 9.6%, renal failure in 4.8%, and empyema in 2.4%. The overall hospital mortality rate of patients with non-ICU HAP was 26%, 13.9% of which was attributable to the pneumonia. For patients who did not receive appropriate antibiotic therapy, the crude and attributable mortality rates were 75% and 50%, respectively. Most of the patients in this Spanish study did not have oropharyngeal manipulations that would have led to aspiration of pathogens commonly implicated in VAP. Most of the patients with *L pneumophila* and *Aspergillus* species were immunosuppressed.

In a retrospective study based on an inpatient database from 59 hospitals in the United States, Kollef et al. described the microbiology and outcome of 4543 patients with microbiologically documented VAP, HAP, HCAP, and CAP.[2] They used mutually exclusive definitions for each pneumonia category. First, patients who received mechanical ventilation for at least 24 hours and had a first positive bacterial respiratory culture result after the start of ventilation were classified into the VAP group. Second, patients with a first positive bacterial respiratory culture result more than 2 days after hospital admission who did not meet the VAP definition were classified into the HAP group. Third, patients with a first positive bacterial respiratory culture result within 2 days of hospital admission who had been transferred from another healthcare facility, had been receiving long-term hemodialysis, or had had a prior hospitalization within 30 days were classified into the HCAP group. All remaining patients constituted the CAP group. The analyses were limited to the first 5 days of hospital admission. HCAP accounted for 21.7% of the pneumonias in this study (**Table 38–4**). MRSA and *Pseudomonas* species were each identified in more than 10% patients with HCAP, HAP, and VAP. HCAP and HAP were associated with mortality rates of 19.8% and 18.8%, respectively.

A study based on prospectively collected hospital-wide surveillance data has shown that patients with HAP have a similar frequency of MRSA but a lower rate of *P aeruginosa* pneumonia compared with patients with VAP.[21] The evidence for *Legionella pneumophila* as a cause of HAP is variable, but is increased in immunocompromised patients, such as organ transplant recipients or patients with HIV disease, as well as those with diabetes mellitus, underlying lung disease, or end-stage renal disease.[4] HAP due to *Legionella* species is more common in hospitals where the organism is present in the water supply or where there is ongoing construction.

Ventilator-Associated Pneumonia

Epidemiology

Critically ill patients spend about 40% of their ICU days on mechanical ventilators.[22] The National Healthcare Safety Network (NHSN) reported an overall VAP incidence rate of 4.2 per 1000 ventilator days in the United States, ranging between 2.8 in coronary care units to 12.3 in burn ICUs.[22] Multicenter studies in the Netherlands, Turkey, and Japan have reported incidence rates of 25, 26.5, and 12.6 per 1000 ventilator days, respectively.[23–25] In developing countries, the rate of VAP ranges between 10.0 and 52.7 per 1000 ventilator days, with a mean of 24.1.[26,27] Although the cumulative risk of VAP increases over time, the daily hazard rate decreases after day 5 of mechanical ventilation.[28]

Pathogenesis

VAP occurs when the balance between host defenses and microbial propensity for colonization and invasion shifts in favor of the pathogens.[4] Sources of infection include healthcare devices, the environment, and the patient. The severity of the patient's underlying disease, prior surgery, exposure to antibiotics and other medications, and exposure to invasive respiratory devices and equipment are important in the pathogenesis of HAP and VAP. VAP requires the colonization of the upper aerodigestive tract and entry of microbial pathogens into the lower respiratory tract, which can then overwhelm the host's

TABLE 38-4 Characteristics of 4543 Hospitalized Patients with Pneumonia

Characteristics	CAP	HCAP	HAP	VAP
Number (percentage)	2221 (48.9%)	988 (21.7%)	835 (18.4%)	499 (11.0%)
Male (%)	57.5	58.7	57.5	61.3
White race (%)	76.6	78.1	77.3	71.7
Median age, IQR (years)	73 (60–80)	77 (66–83)	76 (64–82)	65 (50–77)
Admitted from SNF (%)	NA	49.6	10.3	9.4
Gram-positive pathogens (%)				
S aureus (MRSA)	25.5 (8.9)	46.7 (26.5)	47.1 (22.9)	42.5 (14.6)
Streptococcus nongroup	13.4	7.8	13.9	7.0
S pneumoniae	16.6	5.5	3.1	5.8
Other gram-positive pathogens	7.1	7.7	8.1	8.6
Gram-negative pathogens (%)				
Pseudomonas spp	17.1	25.3	18.4	21.2
Haemophilus spp	16.6	5.8	5.6	12.2
Klebsiella spp	9.5	7.6	7.1	8.4
Escherichia spp	4.8	5.2	4.7	6.4
Enterobacter spp	2.9	3.5	4.3	5.6
Acinetobacter spp	1.6	2.6	2.0	3.0
Other gram-negative pathogens	4.1	9.5	3.7	6.2
Mean ± SD hospital LOS (days)	7.5 ± 7.2	8.8 ± 7.8	15.2 ± 13.6	23.0 ± 20.3
Mortality (%)	10.0	19.8	18.8	29.3

CAP, community-acquired pneumonia; HCAP, healthcare-associated pneumonia; HAP, hospital-acquired pneumonia; VAP, ventilator-associated pneumonia; IQR, interquartile range; SNF, skilled nursing facility; NA, not applicable; MRSA, methicillin-resistant *Staphulococus aureus*; SD, standard deviation; LOS, length of stay.

Data from Kollef MH, Shorr A, Tabak YP, et al. Epidemiology and outcomes of health-care-associated pneumonia: results from a large US database of culture-positive pneumonia. *Chest.* 2005;128:3854–3862.

mechanical (ciliated epithelium and mucus), humoral (antibody and complement), and cellular (polymorphonuclear leukocytes, macrophages, and lymphocytes and their respective cytokines) defenses to establish infection. Aspiration of oropharyngeal pathogens and leakage of bacteria around the endotracheal tube cuff are the primary routes of bacterial entry into the trachea. Hematogenous spread and inhalation of pathogens from contaminated aerosols are less common. Infected biofilm in the endotracheal tube, with subsequent embolization to distal airways, may also be important in the pathogenesis of VAP.

Risk Factors

There are several risk factors, modifiable and nonmodifiable, for the development of VAP. Some of these risk factors are patient related and others treatment related. Intubation and mechanical ventilation increase the risk of pneumonia 6- to 21-fold. Nasal intubation, reintubation, use of sedative and paralytic agents that depress cough and other host-protective mechanisms, endotracheal cuff pressure lower than 20 cm H_2O, supine body position, enteral feeding, hyperglycemia, and blood transfusion increase the risk of VAP. Inadequate staffing may also predispose to VAP.[4,29]

Morbidity and Mortality

The development of VAP is associated with increased morbidity and mortality. VAP prolongs the length of ICU stay by about 4 days and has an attributable mortality rate of 20% to 30%.[4,27,28] In a study from developing countries, the crude mortality rate of VAP was 44.9%.[27] However, some studies have failed to identify any attributable mortality, suggesting that the severity of underlying medical conditions may have more prognostic importance. Increased mortality rates are associated with bacteremia, especially with *Pseudomonas aeruginosa* or *Acinetobacter* species, medical rather than surgical illness, and treatment with ineffective antibiotic therapy.[4]

Diagnostic Strategies and Approaches

Diagnostic testing is required to determine whether a patient has VAP and to determine the etiologic pathogens and guide antibiotic therapy. The diagnosis of VAP is suspected when an endotracheally intubated patient develops a new or progressive radiographic infiltrate

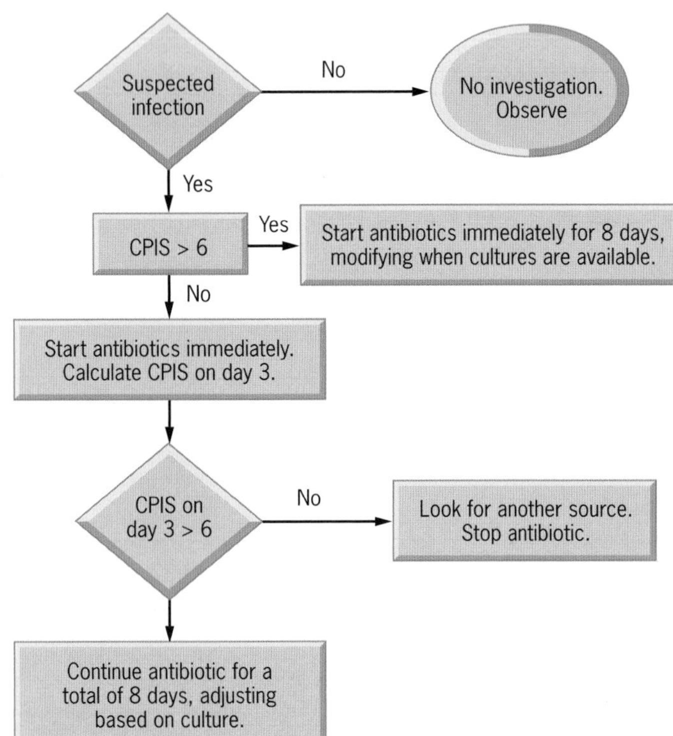

FIGURE 38–4 Approach to ventilator-associated pneumonia based on clinical pulmonary infection score.

with clinical findings (refer to Box 38-1) suggesting infection. Clinical findings of respiratory infection without lung infiltrate suggest tracheobronchitis. For patients with ARDS, VAP should be suspected even when only one of the clinical criteria is present or when unexplained hemodynamic instability or deterioration of blood gas values develops.[4]

The etiologic diagnosis of VAP usually requires a lower respiratory tract culture, but rarely may be made from blood or pleural fluid cultures. A lower respiratory tract culture needs to be collected from all patients before antibiotic therapy, but collection of cultures should not delay the initiation of therapy in critically ill patients.[4] Respiratory tract cultures can include endotracheal aspirates, BAL, or PSB specimens. Because colonization of the trachea precedes the development of VAP, a positive culture cannot always distinguish a pathogen from a colonizing organism. However, a sterile culture from the lower respiratory tract in the absence of a recent change in antibiotic therapy is strong evidence that pneumonia is not present. In addition, the absence of multidrug-resistant (MDR) microorganisms from a lower respiratory tract specimen in intubated patients in the absence of a change in antibiotics within the last 72 hours is strong evidence that they are not the causative pathogens.

Either semiquantitative or quantitative culture data can be used for the management of patients with VAP. Quantitative cultures increase the specificity of the diagnosis of VAP without deleterious consequences, and the specific quantitative technique should be chosen on the basis of local expertise and experience. Patients with suspected VAP should have blood cultures and a diagnostic thoracentesis to exclude complicating empyemas or parapneumonic effusions, if large pleural effusions are present or if the patients appear toxic.

The IDSA/ATS guidelines have incorporated clinical and bacteriologic strategies for the management of VAP.[4] Both strategies emphasize prompt empiric therapy for all patients suspected of having VAP (**Figure 38–4** and **Figure 38–5**). The presence of a new or progressive radiographic infiltrate plus at least two of three clinical features represents the most accurate clinical criteria for starting empiric antibiotic therapy.

Clinical Strategy

When the clinical approach is used, the presence of VAP is defined by new or progressive radiographic infiltrate plus at least two of the three clinical criteria (refer to Box 38–1). The etiologic cause of pneumonia is defined by semiquantitative cultures of endotracheal aspirates, with the growth reported as light, moderate, or heavy. In general, it is rare that a tracheal aspirate culture does not contain the pathogens found in invasive quantitative cultures. Absence of bacteria or inflammatory cells in a patient without a recent (within 72 hours) change in antibiotics has a strong negative predictive value. The initial antibiotic therapy is modified on the basis of the clinical response on days 2 and 3 and the findings of semiquantitative cultures of lower respiratory tract secretions. The clinical approach often leads to more antibiotic therapy than when therapy decisions are based on the findings of invasive (bronchoscopic) lower respiratory tract samples.

The clinical pulmonary infection score (CPIS) was developed to improve the specificity of clinical diagnosis (**Box 38–7**).[30,31] In a randomized clinical trial of patients with suspected pneumonia and a CPIS of 6 or lower, discontinuing antibiotic on day 3 if the CPIS remained at 6 or below was associated with lower antimicrobial therapy costs, antimicrobial resistance, and superinfection.[31] An antibiotic discontinuation policy based on identification of noninfectious etiology or resolution of signs and symptoms suggesting active infection has also been shown to decrease the duration of antibiotic therapy.[32]

Bacteriologic Strategy

The bacteriologic strategy uses quantitative cultures of lower respiratory secretions (endotracheal aspirate, BAL, or PSB specimens collected with or without a bronchoscope). Quantitative culture can be performed using the serial dilution or the calibrated loop technique. Although considered to be the gold standard method for quantitative culture, the serial dilution technique is cumbersome and labor intensive. When applied to lower respiratory tract samples obtained by bronchoscopy, the calibrated loop technique has similar accuracy to that of serial dilution for the diagnosis of VAP and is less cumbersome and time consuming.[33] Endotracheal aspiration is simpler and less costly than the bronchoscopic techniques. However, it usually identifies multiple organisms, including nonpathogens.

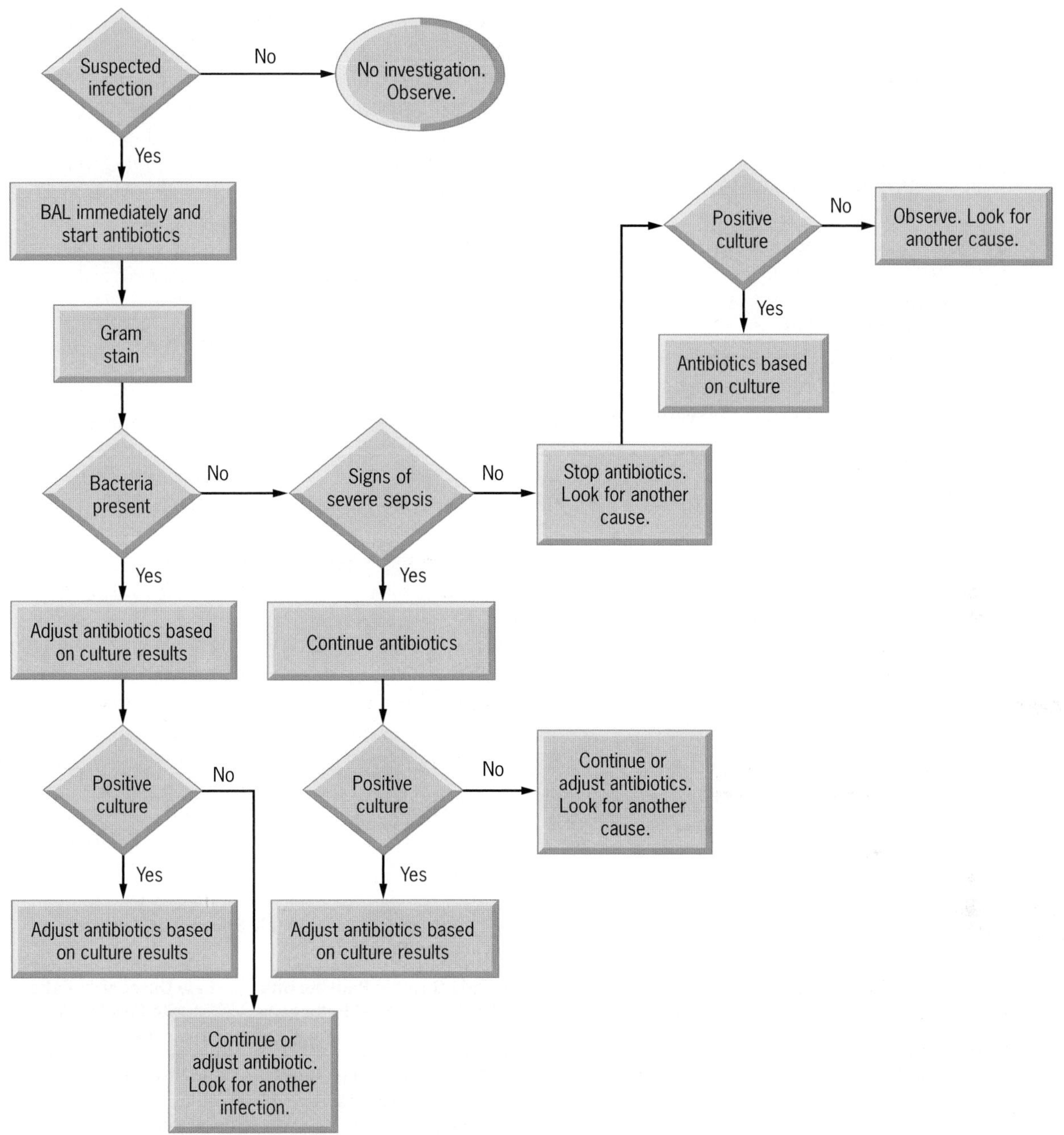

FIGURE 38–5 Approach to ventilator-associated pneumonia based on bronchoscopic findings.

Concern about upper airway colonization has led to bronchoscopic and nonbronchoscopic sampling of the distal airways in patients with suspected VAP. The advantages of the nonbronchoscopic approaches include patient safety, low cost, the ability to pass the catheters through small tracheal tubes, and no need for bronchoscopy. Nonbronchoscopic BAL and PSB can be performed by trained respiratory therapists.

Fiberoptic bronchoscopy provides the ability to sample the lung at the site of infection and minimizes contamination with upper airway microbial flora. However, it is far from perfect. When performing bronchoscopy for VAP, the standardized methodology outlined in the Memphis 1992 International Consensus report should be followed.[34] Bronchoscopic BAL for VAP requires instilling a total of at least 120 mL of saline in three to six aliquots. The bronchoscopic specimen should be processed within 30 minutes of collection to prevent loss of pathogen viability and overgrowth of contaminants. Bronchoscopic BAL is more sensitive and less specific than PSB. Although uncommon, complications of bronchoscopy include cardiac dysrhythmias, hypoxemia, bronchospasm, and infection.[35]

When using quantitative cultures, growth above a threshold concentration is required to diagnose VAP (**Box 38–8**). The bacteriologic approach has been associated with fewer and narrower-spectrum antibiotic use, and improved patient outcome.[36,37] The major concern with the bacteriologic approach is a false-negative

BOX 38–7

The Clinical Pulmonary Infection Score (CPIS)

1. Temperature in °C
   - 36.5 − 38.4 = 0
   - 38.5 − 38.9 = 1
   - ≥39 or ≤36 = 2
2. White blood cell count per liter
   - $4 \times 10^9 - 11 \times 10^9 = 0$
   - $<4 \times 10^9$ or $>11 \times 10^9 = 1$ + band form $\geq 0.5 \times 10^9 = 1$
3. Tracheal secretions
   - Absence of tracheal secretions = 0
   - Presence of nonpurulent tracheal secretions = 1
   - Presence of purulent tracheal secretions = 2
4. Oxygenation, PaO_2/FIO_2, mm Hg
   - >240 or ARDS = 0
   - ≤240 and no evidence of ARDS = 2
5. Chest radiograph
   - No infiltrate = 0
   - Diffuse or patchy infiltrate = 1
   - Localized infiltrate = 2
6. Progression of pulmonary infiltrate
   - No radiographic progression = 0
   - Radiographic progression (after exclusion of CHF and ARDS) = 2

ARDS, acute respiratory distress syndrome; CHF, congestive heart failure.

Modified from Pugin J, Auckenthaler R, Mili N, et al. Diagnosis of ventilator-associated pneumonia by bacteriologic analysis of bronchoscopic and nonbronchoscopic "blind" bronchoalveolar lavage fluid. *Am Rev Respir Dis.* 1991;143:1121–1129.

BOX 38–8

Thresholds for the Diagnosis of Ventilator-Associated Pneumonia

Endotracheal aspirates
   ≥10^5–10^6 CFU/mL
Bronchoalveolar lavage
   ≥10^4 CFU/mL
Protected specimen brush
   ≥10^3 CFU/mL

CFU, colony forming unit.

TABLE 38–5 Most Likely Etiology of Ventilator-Associated Pneumonia

Early Onset in Patients with No Risk for MDR Pathogens	Late Onset or in Patients with Risk for MDR Pathogens
Streptococcus pneumoniae	Methicillin-resistant *Staphylococcus aureus*
Haemphilus influenzae	*Pseudomonas aeruginosa*
Methicillin-sensitive *Staphylococcus aureus*	*Klebsiella pneumoniae* (ESBL producing)
Antibiotic-sensitive enteric gram-negative bacilli	*Acinetobacter spp*
Escherichia coli	Early-onset pathogens
Klebsiella pneumonia	
Enterobacter spp	
Proteus spp	
Serratia narscescens	

MDR, multidrug resistant; ESBL, extended-spectrum β-lactamase.

culture, especially in patients with a recent start or change of antibiotic therapy.

Etiology

Time of onset of pneumonia is an important epidemiologic variable and risk factor for specific pathogens and outcome in patients with HAP and VAP. Early-onset HAP and VAP, defined as occurring within the first 4 days of hospitalization, usually carry a better prognosis and are more likely to be caused by antibiotic-sensitive bacteria (**Table 38–5**).[4] Late-onset HAP and VAP (occurring after 5 days or more) are more likely to be caused by MDR pathogens and are associated with increased mortality and morbidity. However, patients with early-onset HAP who have received prior antibiotics or who have had prior hospitalization within the past 90 days are at greater risk for colonization and infection with MDR pathogens. *Pseudomonas aeruginosa* and *Staphylococcus aureus* are the two most common organisms causing VAP.[35] Most of the *S aureus* strains causing VAP are MRSA. Although oropharyngeal commensals (viridans group streptococci, coagulase-negative staphylococci, *Neisseria* species, and *Corynebacterium* species) are usually colonizers, they can cause VAP in some patients. Polymicrobial infections are especially high in patients with ARDS. Anaerobic organisms may cause HAP following aspiration in nonintubated patients, but they are rare in patients with VAP. Viruses and fungi are uncommon causes of VAP in immunocompetent patients.

Treatment

The IDSA/ATS guidelines recommend similar initial empiric antibacterial treatment for HCAP, HAP, and VAP.[4] The guidelines emphasize appropriate antibiotic therapy, while avoiding excessive antibiotics by de-escalation of initial antibiotic therapy based on microbiologic cultures and the clinical response, and shortening the duration of therapy to the minimum effective period.[4] Because several studies have shown that delay of appropriate antibiotic therapy is associated with increased mortality, empiric antibiotic therapy should be administered as soon as VAP is suspected. Patients with early-onset VAP with no risk factors for MDR pathogens should be started empirically on limited-spectrum antibiotic therapy, whereas those with late-onset VAP and those with early-onset VAP and risk factors for MDR pathogens should receive broad-spectrum antibiotics (**Box 38–9**).[4] The initial empiric antibiotics should be modified based on knowledge of the predominant pathogens in any specific clinical setting and the local patterns of antibiotic susceptibility. Moreover, once the results of respiratory tract and blood cultures become available, therapy should be narrowed (i.e., de-escalation). An empiric therapy regimen should include agents from a different antibiotic class than the patient has recently received.

Colistin may be considered as therapy for patients with VAP due to MDR *Acinetobacter* species and *P aeruginosa*.[38] Local instillation or aerosolization enhances antibiotic penetration to the lower respiratory tract. Aminoglycosides and polymyxin B are the two antibiotics that have been widely used in aerosolized forms. Although aerosolized antibiotics may play a role in treating organisms that are resistant to systemic therapy, the available data supporting their use are scarce.[39]

Duration of Antibiotic Treatment

A shorter duration of antibiotic therapy (7 to 8 days) is recommended for patients with uncomplicated HAP, VAP, or HCAP who have received initially appropriate therapy and have had a good clinical response, with no evidence of infection with nonfermenting gram-negative bacilli.[4,36] Such short-duration therapy may be associated with relapse if the etiologic agent is *P aeruginosa* or *Acinetobacter* species. Customization of the duration of antibiotic therapy based on the responses in symptoms and signs of pneumonia can shorten the duration of treatment without any adverse effect.[32]

BOX 38–9

Empiric Antibiotic Treatment for Ventilator-Associated Pneumonia

Early Onset and No Risk for MDR

Ceftriaxone *or*
Levofloxacin or moxifloxacin or ciprofloxacin *or*
ampicillin/sulbactam *or*
Ertapenem

Late Onset or High Risk for MDR

Antipseudomonal cephalosporin (cefepime or ceftazidime) *or* antipseudomonal carbapenem (imipenem or meropenem) *or* β-lactam/β-lactamase inhibitor (piperacillin-tazobactam) *and*
Antipseudomonal fluoroquinolone (ciprofloxacin, levofloxacin) or aminoglycoside (amikacin, gentamicin, or tobramycin) *and*
Linezolid or vancomycin

MDR, multidrug resistance.

Antibiotic Heterogeneity and Antibiotic Cycling

Antibiotic cycling or rotation has been advocated as a potential strategy for reducing the emergence of antimicrobial resistance. Antibiotic restriction can limit epidemics of infection with specific resistant pathogens. Heterogeneity of antibiotic prescriptions, including formal antibiotic cycling, may be able to reduce the overall frequency of antibiotic resistance. However, the long-term impact of this practice is unknown.[4]

Reasons for Deterioration or Nonresolution

Clinical improvement of VAP usually becomes apparent after the first 48 to 72 hours of therapy; therefore, the selected antimicrobial regimen should not be changed during this time unless progressive deterioration is noted or initial microbiologic studies so dictate.[4] There are several possible causes for rapid deterioration or failure to improve. Inaccurate diagnosis or host, bacterial, and therapeutic (antibiotic) factors may be responsible. Atelectasis, ARDS, pulmonary hemorrhage, congestive heart failure, pulmonary embolus with infarction, lung contusion, and chemical pneumonitis may mimic infectious pneumonia. Host factors that compromise the patient's response to infection may delay or prevent resolution of pneumonia. Bacterial resistance to the administered antibiotics and recurrent infection may cause nonresponse to therapy. Some patients with VAP can have other sources of infection or fever, including sinusitis, vascular catheter-related infection, pseudomembranous enterocolitis, or urinary tract infections. Complications of VAP, such as empyema and abscesses, can also lead to failure.

> **RESPIRATORY RECAP**
>
> **Ventilator-Associated Pneumonia**
>
> » The incidence rate of VAP ranges between 2.8 in coronary care units to 12.3 in burn ICUs.
>
> » VAP requires the colonization of the upper aerodigestive tract and entry of microbial pathogens into the lower respiratory tract.
>
> » There are modifiable and nonmodifiable risk factors for the development of VAP.
>
> » VAP is associated with increased morbidity and mortality.
>
> » When the clinical approach is used, the presence of VAP is defined by new or progressive radiographic infiltrates plus at least two of three clinical criteria.
>
> » The bacteriologic strategy uses quantitative cultures of lower respiratory secretions.
>
> » Time of onset of pneumonia is an important epidemiologic variable and risk factor for specific pathogens and outcome in patients with HAP and VAP.
>
> » Guidelines for the management of HAP, VAP, and HCAP emphasize appropriate antibiotic therapy, de-escalation of initial antibiotic therapy, and shortening the duration of therapy to the minimum effective period.
>
> » The endotracheal tube is the main risk factor for VAP; prevention should focus on minimizing aspiration of secretions.

Prevention

The development of VAP requires the colonization of the upper airways by microbial pathogens followed by their entry to the lower respiratory tract. The endotracheal tube is the main risk factor for VAP because it allows leakage of oropharyngeal secretions around the cuff and also acts as a nidus for the growth of intraluminal biofilm. Prevention of VAP should rely on a multidisciplinary and evidence-based approach. Responding to the campaign initiated by the Institute for Healthcare Improvement (IHI), many medical centers have adopted the VAP bundle, with five components aimed at improving the care of the critically ill, including reducing the incidence of pneumonia (**Box 38–10**).[40] The CDC and other authors have published comprehensive guidelines for the prevention of healthcare-associated pneumonia (**Box 38–11**).[41–43] Education and adequacy of ICU staffing are important components of VAP prevention. Staff education should aim at infection control with microbiologic surveillance data feedback. Because the hospital environment and devices may be the source of pathogens, sterilization or disinfection and maintenance of equipment and devices should be performed routinely. Unnecessary manipulation and change of ventilatory circuits should be avoided. However, contaminated condensate should be carefully emptied from ventilator circuits, and condensate should be prevented from entering either the endotracheal tube or inline medication nebulizers. Because endotracheal intubation and invasive mechanical ventilation are the main risk factors for VAP, every attempt should be made to avoid intubation and shorten the duration of invasive mechanical ventilation. Use of noninvasive positive pressure ventilation, implementation of practice protocols aimed at limiting the administration of sedation, and acceleration of weaning from mechanical ventilation help to achieve these objectives.

> **BOX 38–10**
>
> **Ventilator Bundle**
>
> Elevation of the head of the bed to between 30 and 45 degrees
>
> Daily sedation vacation
>
> Daily assessment of readiness for extubation
>
> Peptic ulcer disease prophylaxis
>
> Deep vein thrombosis prophylaxis

In patients receiving invasive mechanical ventilation, prevention should focus on minimizing aspiration of secretions. A comprehensive oral hygiene program reduces the colonization of the upper aerodigestive tract by virulent pathogens and prevents VAP.[44] Because supine patient positioning facilitates aspiration, semirecumbent positioning (30 to 45 degrees) is recommended, especially when receiving enteral feeding. Although semirecumbent positioning should be an easy target, it has not been easy to achieve even in clinical trials.[45] The endotracheal tube cuff pressure should be maintained at greater than 20 cm H_2O to prevent leakage of bacterial pathogens around the cuff into the lower respiratory tract. Randomized clinical trials have shown that endotracheal tubes with separate dorsal lumens, which allow continuous aspiration of the subglottic secretions, reduce the incidence of VAP.[46–49] However, none of these studies has shown benefit in mortality rate, length of ICU stay, or duration of mechanical ventilation. Similarly, silver-coated endotracheal tubes have been shown to reduce the incidence of VAP in a recently completed multicenter clinical trial, without improving other clinically important outcome measures.[50]

Modulation of colonization using local antiseptics and systemic antibiotics has the potential to prevent VAP. A meta-analysis of seven randomized clinical trials has shown that topical chlorhexidine reduces the incidence of VAP, with its most marked effect seen in cardiac surgery patients.[51] Selective decontamination of the digestive tract (SDD) combines oropharyngeal decontamination with gastric decontamination and systemic antibiotic administration. However, concern regarding its potential risk of promoting more widespread antibiotic resistance has limited the widespread use of SDD and its inclusion in practice guidelines.[4,43]

Randomized trials, using different doses and various study populations, have provided controversial results on the benefits of specific stress ulcer bleeding prophylaxis agents in relation to the increased risk of VAP.[4] If stress ulcer prophylaxis is indicated, the risks and benefits of each regimen should be weighed before prescribing either H_2 blockers or sucralfate.

BOX 38–11

Strategies for the Prevention of Ventilator-Associated Pneumonia

General Measures

Staff education and involvement in infection control

Adequate staffing of the intensive care unit

Preventing Colonization

Sterilization or disinfection and maintenance of equipment and devices

Standard precautions:

- Hand hygiene
- Gloving and wearing gowns when appropriate
- Tracheostomy care under aseptic conditions

Silver-coated endotracheal tube

Preventing aspiration-contaminated materials:

- Using noninvasive ventilation if possible
- Shortening duration of invasive mechanical ventilation
- Avoiding unnecessary patient transports
- Avoiding gastric overdistension
- Avoiding repeat endotracheal intubation
- Using orotracheal instead of nasotracheal intubation
- Performing continuous or frequent intermittent subglottic suctioning
- Clearing secretions above the endotracheal cuff before deflating it
- Elevating the angle of the bed at 30 to 45 degrees
- Appropriate positioning of feeding tubes

Oropharyngeal cleaning and decontamination

- Selective decontamination of the digestive tract

Pneumonia in Immunocompromised Patients Without HIV Infection

Infectious pulmonary complications are common in immunocompromised patients.[52,53] The progress in the treatment of malignancies, connective tissue diseases, and organ transplantation has led to an increased number of patients with immunologic defects. The type of immunologic defect determines the type of pneumonia that develops in these patients. Neutropenia and impaired granulocyte function compromise resistance to bacterial and fungal infections. Qualitative and quantitative defects of T lymphocyte function facilitate the development of viral, fungal (including *P jiroveci*), mycobacterial, and other intracellular microorganisms. B lymphocyte dysfunction with impaired antibody formation increases patients' vulnerability to pneumonia by encapsulated bacteria.

Clinical and Radiographic Findings

The patient's history, including previous radiation therapy, medications, CMV status (of a transplant recipient or donor), previous antibiotics, and prophylactic treatment may suggest the type of pulmonary complications that develop in the immunocompromised patient. The time and acuteness of onset also help in the differential diagnosis. In bone marrow transplant patients, bacterial and *Candida* pneumonia are often observed within 30 days of transplant, whereas CMV and *Aspergillus* species infections occur within 30 to 100 days. Acute onset is seen in bacterial or viral (influenza, adenovirus, RSV) infections, whereas subacute pneumonia occurring within 1 or 2 weeks is seen in CMV, aspergillosis, and mucormycosis. Nocardiosis and tuberculosis have chronic or insidious onset. PCP in non-HIV-infected immunocompromised patients has an acute onset.

Patients usually present with dyspnea, cough, and fever. Skin lesions are seen in mucormycosis, meningitis in cryptococcal and CMV infection, chorioretinitis in CMV, and choroidal lesions in *Candida* infections.

CMV and PCP produce diffuse reticulonodular patterns on chest radiograph, whereas extensive airspace consolidation is seen in bacterial pneumonia, pulmonary edema, and hemorrhage.[54,55] Focal infiltrates suggest bacterial or fungal pneumonia. Nodular or cavitating lesions are observed in nocardiosis, mycobacteriosis, or bacterial abscess. Infiltrates secondary to radiation pneumonitis are limited to the field of radiation. Air crescent sign is suggestive of invasive aspergillosis. Pleural effusions are rare in CMV and PCP. Mediastinal adenopathy is infrequent in PCP and more common in mycobacteriosis and nocardiosis.

Diagnostic Procedures

Diagnostic procedures should be able to give rapid and specific diagnoses. Blood culture helps identify dissemination of infection. Antibody detection for *Legionella* and *Aspergillus* species has low sensitivity and delayed results. CMV viremia, viruria, and antibody titers are useful markers of active infection but nonspecific for pneumonia. Detection of cryptococcal and *Aspergillus* antigens is highly specific but not sensitive.

Expectorated and induced sputum have low yield for PCP, mycobacteria, and *Legionella* species in non-HIV-infected immunocompromised patients. *Aspergillus*, *Cryptococcus*, and *Nocardia* species are usually considered to be colonizing agents, except in severely immunocompromised patients. Transthoracic percutaneous needle aspiration is not routinely performed because of its potential complications.

BAL is diagnostic of *P jiroveci*, *Toxoplasma gondii*, *Legionella* species, *M tuberculosis*, influenza, *Mycoplasma* species, and RSV infections. Detection of herpes simplex and CMV in BAL fluid is not an accurate indicator of pneumonia unless there is cytologic or histologic evidence of infection. The presence of fungi, bacteria, and NTM needs to be correlated with the clinical and radiographic findings. BAL can establish definite diagnosis in 33% to 66% of immunocompromised patients. Application of PCR to BAL fluid increases the sensitivity and is rapid in the detection of CMV, PCP, and mycobacterial pulmonary infection. Transbronchial lung biopsy is used in the diagnosis of CMV, *Aspergillus* species, rejection, and noninfectious etiologies. At times, open lung or thoracoscopic lung biopsies may be needed.

Causes of Pneumonia

Immunocompromised patients are vulnerable to infections caused by bacteria, mycobacteria, fungi, and viruses. Encapsulated organisms such as *S pneumoniae* are common causes of pneumonia in patients with B lymphocyte deficit such as multiple myeloma. Gram-negative organisms such as *P aeruginosa* are common causes of pneumonia in neutropenic patients.

Fungal infections are common, especially in hematologic malignancies. Prolonged neutropenia, long duration of steroid therapy, broad-spectrum antibiotic therapy, and central venous catheters are risk factors for the development of fungal infections. *Candida* pneumonia is the most common fungal pneumonia in the immunocompromised host. *Aspergillus* species cause extensive pneumonia with diffuse pulmonary hemorrhage. Pneumonias caused by *Mucor* and *Cryptococcus* species are reported occasionally. *Histoplasma* pneumonia, coccidioidomycosis, and blastomycosis should be considered in endemic areas.

> **RESPIRATORY RECAP**
>
> **Pneumonia in Immunocompromised Patients**
>
> » Pulmonary infections are common in these patients.
> » Bronchoalveolar lavage is often diagnostic.
> » Infections are caused by bacteria, mycobacteria, fungi, and viruses.
> » Noninfectious causes account for about 25% of infiltrates.

CMV infection is the most common opportunistic infection after organ transplantation and is associated with poor prognosis. In the preprophylaxis era, CMV reactivation in seropositive patients was 80% in bone marrow transplant patients, and CMV pneumonitis was diagnosed in 10% to 35% of cases, with a mortality rate of 50%. In lung transplant patients, CMV pneumonitis is reported in 16% to 58% of cases and is the most significant risk factor for early death and rejection. Herpes simplex viral pneumonitis occurs less often, and it is often associated with intraoral mucosal lesions.

Mycobacterial infections are rare in immunocompromised patients without HIV infection. PCP is a common opportunistic infection in immunocompromised patients. It also occurs in patients receiving methotrexate and systemic corticosteroids. However, its incidence has been decreasing since prophylaxis was started.

Noninfectious causes are responsible for about 25% of infiltrates in the immunocompromised patient. These causes include cytotoxic drugs, radiation, pulmonary edema, and progression of underlying disease such as carcinomatous lymphangitis or tumor, alveolar hemorrhage, lung involvement resulting from connective tissue disease, graft-versus-host disease, or bronchiolitis obliterans with organizing pneumonia (BOOP).

Therapeutic Considerations

Antimicrobial therapy is usually needed during the wait for results of diagnostic procedures. For bacterial pneumonia, a combination of antibiotics effective in the treatment of *P aeruginosa* and *S aureus* infections is usually necessary. Trimethoprim-sulfamethoxazole is used for PCP. When CMV pneumonitis is present, ganciclovir or foscarnet is used. Amphotericin B is used for invasive aspergillosis. In patients able to tolerate invasive procedures, bronchoscopy is needed when pulmonary infiltrates progress despite empiric treatment or when the diagnosis is uncertain.

Prophylaxis

Oral fluoroquinolones have been used to reduce the frequency of bacterial infection with gram-negative organisms in neutropenic patients. Acyclovir and ganciclovir have been used for CMV, and trimethoprim-sulfamethoxazole has been used for PCP.

Pneumonia in Patients with HIV Infection

The World Health Organization estimated that 33.2 million people were living with HIV/AIDS worldwide in 2007, of whom 2.5 million were newly infected, and 2.1 million died of AIDS. At the end of 2003, an estimated 1,039,000 to 1,185,000 persons in the United States were living with HIV/AIDS. Infectious lung diseases are seen in 60% to 80% of patients with HIV infection. Despite the development of effective antiretroviral therapy, the lungs remain the most common site of infection in these patients. The most common pathogens causing pneumonia in patients with HIV/AIDS are bacteria, tuberculosis, and *Pneumocystic jiroveci* (**Box 38–12**).[56] The type of pneumonia that develops in these patients depends on the geographic location, CD4 count, history of prior infection, HIV exposure category, and the virulence of the infecting organism. Pneumonias caused by bacteria, tuberculosis, influenza, and endemic mycoses are seen even with normal CD4 count. PCP occurs more often when the CD4 count drops below 200/μL.

BOX 38–12

Major Causes of Pneumonia in Patients with HIV Infection

Bacterial
- *Streptococcus pneumoniae*
- *Haemophilus influenzae*
- *Staphylococcus aureus*
- *Pseudomonas aeruginosa*

Mycobacterial
- *Mycobacterium tuberculosis*
- *Mycobacterium avium-intracellulare* complex

Fungal
- *Pneumocystis jiroveci*
- *Candida* species
- *Aspergillus* species

Viral
- Cytomegalovirus
- Herpes simplex virus

HIV, human immunodeficiency virus.

Expectorated or induced sputum, nonbronchoscopic catheter lavage, and specimens obtained by bronchoscopy and open lung biopsy are used for diagnosis. BAL has an overall sensitivity of greater than 85% in the diagnosis of pulmonary disorders in patients with HIV infection. Transbronchial lung biopsy has an additive yield to BAL, especially in patients with non-PCP pulmonary complications. Bronchoscopic brush biopsy is not used in patients with HIV infection because of its low additive yield. Open lung biopsy is rarely needed when bronchoscopy is nondiagnostic or transbronchial biopsy cannot be performed because of a bleeding disorder or positive pressure ventilation.

The differential diagnosis of pulmonary infiltrates in patients with HIV infection should include noninfectious causes such as nonspecific interstitial pneumonitis, lymphoid interstitial pneumonitis, Kaposi sarcoma, and non-Hodgkin lymphoma. The application of primary prophylaxis and antiretroviral therapy has led to a decline in PCP and tuberculous infection in developed countries.

Causes of Pneumonia

Bacterial pneumonia is the most common pneumonia in HIV-infected patients in the United States, whereas tuberculosis dominates globally.[56,57] Bacterial pneumonia is more common and is more likely to be bacteremic in patients with HIV compared with those without HIV infection. Low CD4 count and injection drug use are risk factors for bacterial pneumonia, whereas PCP prophylaxis with trimethoprim-sulfamethoxazole is protective. The most common organisms causing bacterial pneumonia are *S pneumoniae* and *H influenzae*. Infection with *P aeruginosa* is being reported more often, especially in patients with low CD4 and leukocyte count. Some patients develop recurrent bronchitis and sinusitis. Legionnaire disease is rare in patients with HIV infection. *Nocardia asteroides* and *Rhodococcus equi* can cause pneumonia in these patients. Pneumococcal vaccination is recommended for patients with HIV infection.

Despite its decline, PCP remains the most common AIDS-defining condition in the United States and other developed countries, especially in patients who do not know they have HIV infection and those who are not receiving antiretroviral therapy and PCP prophylaxis. The occurrence of PCP varies according to region, CD4 count, nutritional status, and risk factors for HIV infection. Patients with HIV infection and PCP usually present with fever, dyspnea, and nonproductive cough of several weeks' duration. The chest radiograph often reveals diffuse, bilateral interstitial infiltrates (**Figure 38–6**). Arterial blood gas measurements are used to determine the severity of infection and guide management. Hypoxemia with wide alveolar-arterial oxygen tension gradient and elevated serum lactate

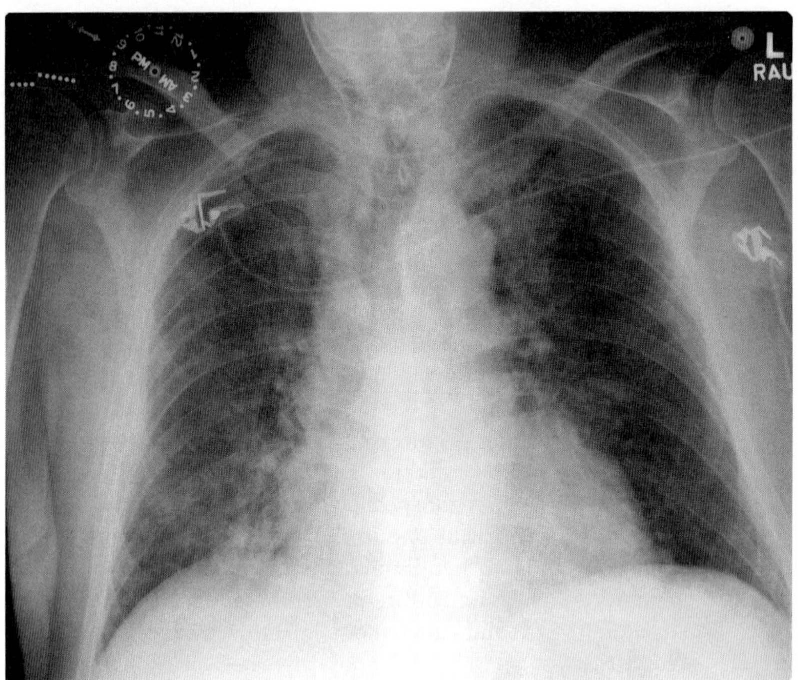

FIGURE 38–6 Portable anteroposterior chest radiograph of a patient with AIDS and *Pneumocystis* pneumonia showing bilateral diffuse infiltrates.

dehydrogenase levels are seen in patients with PCP. Because *P jiroveci* cannot be cultured in vitro, the diagnosis requires direct visualization of the cyst in special stains of respiratory specimens or lung tissue or PCR. Induced sputum has an 80% yield in the diagnosis of PCP in some centers. BAL has high sensitivity in the diagnosis of PCP. In patients with endotracheal tubes, PCP can be diagnosed by instilling 60 mL of saline in 10-mL aliquots and collecting a specimen 30 seconds after each aliquot.

Trimethoprim-sulfamethoxazole and intravenous pentamidine are the primary medications used to treat PCP. Corticosteroids are used as adjunctive therapy for AIDS patients with PCP. PCP prophylaxis should be given to all patients with HIV infection who have a history of PCP, CD4 count less than 200/μL, oral thrush, or unexplained fever. Trimethoprim-sulfamethoxazole and inhaled pentamidine have been widely used for prophylaxis against PCP.

HIV infection has a major impact on the epidemiology of tuberculosis. In the United States, 52,100 excess cases of tuberculosis were reported during the period from 1985 to 1992. At least 50% of these excess cases could be attributed to HIV infection. Among patients exposed to *M tuberculosis*, those with HIV infection have a higher probability of progressing to clinical tuberculosis than those without HIV infection. Pulmonary tuberculosis can occur at any stage during HIV infection. Chest radiographic manifestations of tuberculous pneumonia in patients with HIV infection are very variable. Even a normal chest radiograph does not exclude tuberculosis.

In patients with advanced HIV disease, hilar and mediastinal lymphadenopathy and lower lung field infiltrates are common, and cavitation is less common. Because of their anergy, these patients are considered to have a positive tuberculosis skin test when induration is 5 mm. T cell–based interferon-γ release assays are replacing the tuberculin skin test for the diagnosis of latent tuberculosis in developed countries.[57]

Expectorated and induced sputum are used for the diagnosis of pulmonary tuberculosis. BAL, transbronchial lung biopsy, and postbronchoscopy sputum analysis are used to make the diagnosis when sputum smears are negative or when patients are unable to produce sputum. The isolation of *M avium-intracellulare* complex does not correlate with pulmonary disease because it may represent colonization. Histologic evidence of tissue invasion is needed for the diagnosis of *M avium-intracellulare* complex pneumonia. Both tuberculosis and *M avium-intracellulare* complex pneumonia can present as endobronchial lesions. Stool, urine, and blood specimens should be sent for mycobacterial culture because the incidence of extrapulmonary involvement is high, especially in advanced HIV infection. Because tuberculosis is more commonly smear positive, communicable, and treatable, antituberculosis medications should be initiated when microscopy reveals AFB or caseating granulomas.

Patients with HIV infection have good response to standard antituberculosis treatment. Standard antituberculosis therapy includes 9 months of isoniazid and rifampin and 2 months of pyrazinamide. In areas where the incidence of isoniazid resistance is 4% or more, ethambutol or streptomycin is added to this regimen. Because of uncertainty about patients' adherence to therapy, direct observed therapy is preferred. One year of isoniazid is used as prophylaxis in patients with latent tuberculous infection and in those exposed to potentially infectious cases of tuberculosis. Although the WHO recommends BCG vaccination for children with HIV infection, it is not used in the United States for fear of disseminating BCG infection.

RESPIRATORY RECAP

Pneumonia in Patients with HIV

- » PCP occurs more frequently when the CD4 count is less than 200/μL.
- » Bronchoalveolar lavage is often diagnostic.
- » PCP is a common cause of mortality.
- » HIV infection has a major impact on the epidemiology of tuberculosis.

Candida and *Aspergillus* pneumonia are uncommon in patients with HIV. Because the respiratory tract may be colonized with these organisms, a positive culture from a respiratory tract specimen is not sufficient. Histologic evidence from lung tissue is needed for the diagnosis of *Candida* and *Aspergillus* pneumonia. *Aspergillus* pneumonia is usually part of disseminated infection and occurs in patients with advanced HIV infection and additional risk factors, such as neutropenia and steroid use.

In patients with HIV infection, pulmonary cryptococcosis is almost always part of a disseminated cryptococcal infection. Pulmonary histoplasmosis, coccidioidomycosis, and blastomycosis are seen in patients with HIV infection who have lived in or traveled to endemic areas. Although these endemic mycoses can develop during any stage of HIV infection, dissemination becomes more common when the CD4 count becomes low. Amphotericin B remains the antifungal therapy of choice.

Although CMV can be cultured from the BAL of many patients with HIV infection, it has not been found to be an important pathogen causing pneumonia in these patients. The clinical manifestations of CMV pneumonia are similar to those of PCP. Histologic evidence from lung tissue is needed for the diagnosis of CMV pneumonia. However, the detection of CMV in BAL may predict an increased risk of developing CMV-associated disease in other organs. Ganciclovir is used to treat CMV pneumonia. Although rare, herpes simplex virus can cause pneumonia in patients with HIV infection. Acyclovir is used to treat herpes simplex virus pneumonia.

Pneumonia in Children

Childhood pneumonia is the leading single cause of mortality in children younger than 5 years.[58] The incidence in this age group is estimated to be 0.29 and 0.05 episodes per child-year in developing and developed countries, respectively. This translates into about 156 million new episodes each year worldwide, of which 151 million episodes are in the developing world. Of all childhood CAP cases, 7% to 13% are severe enough to be life threatening and require hospitalization.

> **RESPIRATORY RECAP**
>
> **Pneumonia in Children**
>
> » Respiratory infections in children often affect the upper respiratory tract and are self-limiting.
>
> » No pathogen is identified in about 50% of cases of pneumonia in children.
>
> » The differential diagnosis includes asthma, bronchiolitis, bronchitis, bronchiectasis, foreign body aspiration, pulmonary sequestration, and atelectasis.
>
> » Most children recover fully.

The patterns of respiratory infection in children and the causative pathogens are different from those in adults. Compared with adults, children have smaller airways, more compliant thoracic cages, less efficient respiratory muscles, and underdeveloped immunologic systems that affect their response to respiratory infection. The leading risk factors contributing to pneumonia in children are male sex, lack of exclusive breastfeeding, malnutrition, indoor air pollution, passive smoking, low birth weight, premature birth, congenital respiratory diseases such as tracheoesophageal fistula and lobar sequestration, cystic fibrosis, bronchopulmonary dysplasia, congenital heart disease, neurologic impairment, a compromised immune system, crowding, and lack of measles immunization. Pneumonia is responsible for about 19% of all deaths in children younger than 5 years, of which more than 70% take place in sub-Saharan Africa and southeast Asia. Mortality is low in the developed countries.

The age of a child influences the type, frequency, and severity of the respiratory infection.[59] Viral bronchiolitis is seen in infants aged between 4 weeks and 8 months; epiglottitis is uncommon in the first year of life and peaks in incidence in the third year. Most deaths caused by respiratory infections occur in infancy.

The incidence, etiology, and optimal management of pneumonia in children have not been well defined because of the lack of a practical definition of pneumonia, the wide spectrum of microorganisms causing pneumonia in the different age groups, and the difficulties in identification of the causative pathogens. Many cases of CAP may not be diagnosed if the child is not seriously ill and chest radiographs are not performed. The incidence of pneumonia peaks at 40 episodes per 1000 children per year in children between 6 months and 5 years of age, and it falls to 11 episodes per 1000 children per year in children older than 9 years. Pneumonia is more common in the winter months.

Box 38–13 lists the common pathogens causing pneumonia in children. The most common are *Streptococcus pneumoniae* and *Haemophilus influenzae* type b,

> **BOX 38–13**
>
> **Pathogens Causing Pneumonia in Children According to Age**
>
> **Neonate**
>
> Group B streptococci
> *Escherichia coli*
> *Staphylococcus aureus*
> *Chlamydia trachomatis*
>
> **1 Month to 2 Years**
>
> Respiratory syncytial virus
> Parainfluenza viruses
> Influenza viruses
> *Streptococcus pneumoniae*
> *Haemophilus influenzae*
>
> **2 to 12 Years**
>
> *Streptococcus pneumoniae*
> *Mycoplasma pneumoniae*
> *Chlamydia pneumoniae*

followed by *Staphylococcus aureus* and *Klebsiella pneumoniae*. Both *S pneumoniae* and *H influenzae* type b infections can be prevented by immunization. Viruses alone account for 14% to 35% of cases and are more commonly identified in children younger than 5 years.[59] In children older than 5 years, *Mycoplasma pneumoniae* and *Chlamydophila pneumoniae* infections are more common. RSV is the most common viral pathogen responsible for pneumonia in children younger than 5 years, and it frequently represents an extension of bronchiolitis.

Diagnosing pneumonia in a child is more difficult than in an adult. The typical features of pneumonia, such as bronchial breathing, dull percussion note, and pleuritic pain, are uncommon in children. Bacterial pneumonia should be suspected in children aged 3 years or younger if they have fever higher than 38.5° C together with chest wall recession and a respiratory rate above 50 breaths/min.[59] For older children, difficulty in breathing is more helpful than clinical signs. The absence of the symptom cluster of respiratory distress, tachypnea, crackles, and decreased breath sounds excludes pneumonia.[60] *C trachomatis* infection causes afebrile pneumonia with dry cough in the first 2 months of life. Wheezing is more common in viral and *Mycoplasma* infection. However, it is difficult to determine the causative pathogen based on clinical findings. Cyanosis may not be detected in children with dark skin and anemia, and it is often a late sign of severe disease. The clinical presentation of pneumonia in older children and teenagers is similar to that in adults. Leukopenia can be seen in viral and severe bacterial infections.

Despite extensive investigation, no pathogen is identified in 20% to 60% of pneumonia cases in children.[59] Most children cannot expectorate sputum, and even if they do, the sputum is contaminated with upper airway commensals. Blood cultures should be performed if bacterial pneumonia is suspected.[59] Blood cultures are positive in 40% of neonates and 10% to 20% of older children with bacterial pneumonia. The detection of pneumococcal and *H influenzae* type b antigen in serum or urine is more sensitive than blood culture in childhood pneumonia. However, it is associated with high false-positive and false-negative rates. Nasopharyngeal aspirates from children younger than 18 months should be sent for viral antigen detection with or without viral culture. When significant pleural effusion is present, diagnostic thoracentesis should be performed.

There is a paucity of guidelines addressing the management of pneumonia in children.[59,61] A child with pneumonia who responds to treatment as an outpatient does not need further investigation. The British Thoracic Society guidelines have outlined criteria for hospital admission of children with pneumonia (**Box 38–14**). Oximetry should be performed in every child admitted with pneumonia.[59] Oximetry correlates with clinical outcome and length of hospital stay.

BOX 38–14

The British Thoracic Society Criteria for Hospital Admission of Children with Pneumonia

For Infants

- Oxygen saturation ≤ 92% or cyanosis
- Respiratory rate > 70 breaths/min
- Difficulty in breathing
- Intermittent apnea or grunting
- Not feeding
- Family not able to provide appropriate observation or supervision

For Older Children

- Oxygen saturation ≤ 92% or cyanosis
- Respiratory rate > 50 breaths/min
- Difficulty in breathing
- Grunting
- Signs of dehydration
- Family not able to provide appropriate observation or supervision

Modified from British Thoracic Society guidelines for the management of community acquired pneumonia in childhood. *Thorax*. 2002;57(suppl 1):1–24.

The differential diagnosis of pneumonia in children should include asthma, bronchiolitis, acute bronchitis, acute exacerbation of bronchiectasis, aspiration of a foreign body, pulmonary sequestration, and atelectasis. Children with recurrent or persistent cough productive of purulent sputum should be evaluated for the presence of cystic fibrosis, bronchial obstruction, ciliary abnormalities, congenital abnormalities of the lung (e.g., lobar sequestration, lung cysts, bronchial stenosis, cystadenomatoid malformation), esophageal atresia, tracheoesophageal fistula, and immunodeficiency disorders.

There is a paucity of well-conducted, randomized controlled trials comparing the efficacy of different antibiotics and their impact on the outcome of pneumonia in children. The choice of antibiotic depends on the child's age and knowledge of the likely pathogen in that age group. Oral antibiotics are adequate for most mild to moderately severe pneumonias. Parenteral antibiotics are needed for neonates and other children with severe pneumonia. In neonates, the antibiotic regimen should cover group B streptococcus and gram-negative organisms. A macrolide should be added to cover *C trachomatis* in certain areas. There is no specific treatment for viral pneumonia. Antibiotic usage for nonbacterial infections should be discouraged because it may lead to the development of resistance. Some children with RSV pneumonia respond to aerosolized ribavirin therapy.

Children requiring hospitalization should receive a second- or third-generation cephalosporin, with or without a macrolide depending on their ages. For children with pneumonia after viral infection, antistaphylococcal coverage should be included. In places where the incidence of penicillin-resistant *S pneumoniae* infection is high, vancomycin should be considered. Supplemental oxygen, intravenous or nasogastric fluids, postural drainage, and percussion may be needed.

Most children with pneumonia recover fully. It takes longer for radiologic recovery than clinical recovery. Severe *Mycoplasma* infection and adenoviral pneumonia can lead to permanent lung damage such as persistent collapse, bronchiolitis obliterans, bronchiectasis, and Swyer-James syndrome, which is characterized by a small hyperlucent lobe with impaired perfusion and ventilation.

Children with HIV infection present most often with respiratory illnesses. PCP is the most common infection in these children. Other causes of pneumonia include CMV, RSV, adenovirus, influenza, parainfluenza, herpes simplex, varicella zoster, encapsulated bacteria, gram-negative bacteria, mycobacteria, and fungi.

CASE STUDIES

Case 1. Community-Acquired Pneumonia

A 44-year-old African American man was admitted to the hospital because of productive cough. The patient has a history of alcohol abuse and 20 pack-a-day years of smoking. He had been in good health until 3 days before admission, when he developed a cough productive of yellow sputum. The cough was associated with fever and chills. He also had dyspnea with minimal exertion. He denied weight loss, night sweats, and previous exposure to tuberculosis. He had no visit to a physician in the previous 30 years.

On presentation to the hospital, he was in mild respiratory distress with a temperature of 102.1° F, a respiratory rate of 34 breaths/min, a blood pressure of 125/79 mm Hg, and a pulse rate of 125 beats/min. On physical examination, crackles were heard on auscultation, and dullness was present on percussion of the right lower chest. Oxygen saturation was 93% breathing room air. The serum electrolyte values, hematocrit, and platelet count were normal. His white blood cell count was 16,000 per mm^3, with 20% bands, 70% neutrophils, and 10% lymphocytes. Serum protein was 7 g/dL, and lactate dehydrogenase (LDH) was 210 U/L. A radiograph of the chest showed right pleural effusion and alveolar infiltrate involving the right middle and lower lobes.

After blood and expectorated sputum were obtained for Gram stain and culture, antibiotic therapy with intravenous erythromycin and ceftriaxone was initiated. Diagnostic thoracentesis was performed. Pleural fluid analysis showed a white blood cell count of 1000 per mm^3, with 95% neutrophils and 5% monocytes; protein 5 g/dL, LDH 198 U/L, and pH 7.37. The Gram stain and culture of the pleural fluid showed no organisms. The sputum and blood culture grew *Streptococcus pneumoniae* sensitive to penicillin.

On the second hospital day, the patient's symptoms improved and he became afebrile. On the third hospital day, the ceftriaxone and erythromycin were discontinued, and intravenous penicillin was initiated. The patient's condition continued to improve, and the intravenous penicillin was changed to oral penicillin on the fourth hospital day. He was discharged home on the fifth hospital day on oral penicillin, with a follow-up appointment to an outpatient clinic in one week.

Case 2. Pneumonia in an Immunocompromised Patient

A 26-year-old white woman was admitted to the hospital for dyspnea. The patient had a remote history of unprotected sex and injection drug use. She had weight loss of 25 pounds over a 3-month period, cough for 5 weeks, and night sweats and fever for 1 week. Her cough had been dry for the first 4 weeks, but productive of brown sputum for the last 7 days. She had dyspnea for 7 days that worsened on the day of admission. She denied exposure to tuberculosis.

On presentation to the hospital, the patient was in moderate respiratory distress with a temperature of 101.2° F, a respiratory rate of 39 breaths/min, a blood pressure of 90/55 mm Hg, and a pulse rate of 145 beats/min. Diffuse crackles were heard on auscultation of the chest. Oxygen saturation was 82% breathing room air. The serum electrolyte values were normal. The hematocrit was 23%, the platelet count was 85,000 per mm^3, and the white blood cell count was 5000 per mm^3, with 10% bands, 80% neutrophils, and 10% lymphocytes. Serum protein was 6 g/dL, and lactate dehydrogenase was 900 U/L. A radiograph of the chest showed diffuse interstitial infiltrate, with denser consolidation of the right upper lobe. Blood culture was obtained. Sputum was induced with 3% saline by use of an ultrasonic nebulizer for Gram stain, routine culture, and sensitivity; AFB stain and mycobacterial culture; and *Pneumocystis jiroveci* stains.

Intravenous trimethoprim-sulfamethoxazole and oral prednisone were administered for treatment of suspected *P jiroveci* pneumonia. On the second hospital day, her condition deteriorated, and she was transferred to the medical ICU. Her Pao_2 was 65 mm Hg breathing 100% O_2. She underwent endotracheal intubation and mechanical ventilation for hypoxemic respiratory failure. The induced sputum monoclonal antibody stain was positive for *P jiroveci*. Both the ELISA and Western blot were positive for HIV. Her CD4 count was 10/μL.

Because of failure to improve, bronchoscopy was performed on her fifth hospital day. The AFB stain of the bronchoalveolar lavage was positive, and the PCR was consistent with *Mycobacterium tuberculosis*, later confirmed with the culture result. Treatment with four antituberculosis drugs was initiated. The patient's condition gradually improved over the next 3 weeks. However, her condition deteriorated during the fourth week of her hospital stay. Repeat bronchoscopy was performed. The quantitative culture of the BAL showed 2.3 × 10^6/mL of methicillin-resistant *Staphylococcus aureus*. Her blood culture also grew methicillin-resistant *S aureus*. She died of multiple organ failure secondary to septic shock on her 35th day of hospital stay.

KEY POINTS

- Pneumonia is the inflammation and consolidation of lung tissue caused by infectious agents.
- Community-acquired pneumonia (CAP) occurs outside the hospital.
- Hospital-acquired pneumonia (HAP) and ventilator-associated pneumonia (VAP) are acquired in the hospital.
- Noninvasive and invasive procedures are used to diagnose pneumonia.
- Organisms causing pneumonia include gram-positive bacteria, gram-negative bacteria, atypical organisms, anaerobic bacteria, viruses, mycobacteria, fungi, actinomycosis, and nocardiosis.
- Most patients with CAP can be treated as outpatients.
- Pneumonia is the second most common nosocomial infection and has a high mortality rate.
- VAP is associated with increased morbidity and mortality.
- Guidelines for the management of HAP, VAP, and healthcare-associated pneumonia emphasize appropriate antibiotic therapy, de-escalation of initial antibiotic therapy, and shortening the duration of therapy to the minimum effective period.
- The endotracheal tube is the main risk factor for VAP; prevention should focus on minimizing aspiration of secretions.
- Pulmonary infections are common in immunocompromised patients, and bronchoalveolar lavage is often diagnostic.
- PCP is a common cause of mortality in patients with HIV; tuberculosis is also common in these patients.
- Children usually recover fully from pneumonia, and no pathogen is identified in about half of all cases.

REFERENCES

1. Kozak LJ, DeFraces CJ, Hall MJ. *National Hospital Discharge Survey: 2004 Annual Summary with Detailed Diagnosis and Procedure Data.* Washington, DC: National Center for Health Statistics; 2006. Vital Health Statistics 13.
2. Kollef MH, Shorr A, Tabak YP, Gupta V, Liu LZ, Johannes RS. Epidemiology and outcomes of health-care-associated pneumonia: results from a large US database of culture-positive pneumonia. *Chest.* 2005;128:3854–3862.
3. Mandell LA, Wunderink RG, Anzueto A, et al. Infectious Diseases Society of America/American Thoracic Society consensus guidelines on the management of community-acquired pneumonia in adults. *Clin Infect Dis.* 2007;44(suppl 2):S27–S72.
4. Guidelines for the management of adults with hospital-acquired, ventilator-associated, and healthcare-associated pneumonia. *Am J Respir Crit Care Med.* 2005;171:388–416.
5. Pingleton SK, Fagon JY, Leeper KV Jr. Patient selection for clinical investigation of ventilator-associated pneumonia. Criteria for evaluating diagnostic techniques. *Chest.* 1992;102:553S–556S.
6. Jennings LC, Anderson TP, Beynon KA, et al. Incidence and characteristics of viral community-acquired pneumonia in adults. *Thorax.* 2008;63:42–48.
7. Meduri GU, Mauldin GL, Wunderink RG, et al. Causes of fever and pulmonary densities in patients with clinical manifestations of ventilator-associated pneumonia. *Chest.* 1994;106:221–235.
8. Bartlett JG. Anaerobic bacterial infections of the lung. *Chest.* 1987;91:901–909.
9. Duchin JS, Koster FT, Peters CJ, et al. Hantavirus pulmonary syndrome: a clinical description of 17 patients with a newly recognized disease. The Hantavirus Study Group. *N Engl J Med.* 1994;330:949–955.
10. Griffith DE, Aksamit T, Brown-Elliott BA, et al. An official ATS/IDSA statement: diagnosis, treatment, and prevention of nontuberculous mycobacterial diseases. *Am J Respir Crit Care Med.* 2007;175:367–416.
11. Sharma OP, Chwogule R. Many faces of pulmonary aspergillosis. *Eur Respir J.* 1998;12:705–715.
12. Jackson ML, Neuzil KM, Thompson WW, et al. The burden of community-acquired pneumonia in seniors: results of a population-based study. *Clin Infect Dis.* 2004;39:1642–1650.
13. Centers for Disease Control and Prevention. Severe methicillin-resistant *Staphylococcus aureus* community-acquired pneumonia associated with influenza—Louisiana and Georgia, December 2006–January 2007. *MMWR.* 2007;56:325–329.
14. Angeles MM, Camps M, Pumarola T, et al. The role of viruses in the aetiology of community-acquired pneumonia in adults. *Antivir Ther.* 2006;11:351–359.
15. Fine MJ, Auble TE, Yealy DM, et al. A prediction rule to identify low-risk patients with community-acquired pneumonia. *N Engl J Med.* 1997;336:243–250.
16. Lim WS, van der Eerden MM, Laing R, et al. Defining community acquired pneumonia severity on presentation to hospital: an international derivation and validation study. *Thorax.* 2003;58:377–382.
17. Fine MJ, Smith MA, Carson CA, et al. Prognosis and outcomes of patients with community-acquired pneumonia. A meta-analysis. *JAMA.* 1996;275:134–141.
18. Woodhead M, Welch CA, Harrison DA, Bellingan G, Ayres JG. Community-acquired pneumonia on the intensive care unit: secondary analysis of 17,869 cases in the ICNARC Case Mix Programme Database. *Crit Care.* 2006;10(suppl 2):S1.
19. Anderson DJ, Kirkland KB, Kaye KS, et al. Underresourced hospital infection control and prevention programs: penny wise, pound foolish? *Infect Control Hosp Epidemiol.* 2007;28:767–773.
20. Sopena N, Sabria M. Multicenter study of hospital-acquired pneumonia in non-ICU patients. *Chest.* 2005;127:213–219.
21. Weber DJ, Rutala WA, Sickbert-Bennett EE, Samsa GP, Brown V, Niederman MS. Microbiology of ventilator-associated pneumonia compared with that of hospital-acquired pneumonia. *Infect Control Hosp Epidemiol.* 2007;28:825–831.
22. Edwards JR, Peterson KD, Andrus ML, et al. National Healthcare Safety Network (NHSN) report, data summary for 2006, issued June 2007. *Am J Infect Control.* 2007;35:290–301.
23. Leblebicioglu H, Rosenthal VD, Arikan OA, et al. Device-associated hospital-acquired infection rates in Turkish intensive care

units. Findings of the International Nosocomial Infection Control Consortium (INICC). *J Hosp Infect.* 2007;65:251–257.

24. Suka M, Yoshida K, Uno H, Takezawa J. Incidence and outcomes of ventilator-associated pneumonia in Japanese intensive care units: the Japanese nosocomial infection surveillance system. *Infect Control Hosp Epidemiol.* 2007;28:307–313.
25. van der Kooi TI, de Boer AS, Mannien J, et al. Incidence and risk factors of device-associated infections and associated mortality at the intensive care in the Dutch surveillance system. *Intensive Care Med.* 2007;33:271–278.
26. Jaimes F, De La RG, Gomez E, Munera P, Ramirez J, Castrillon S. Incidence and risk factors for ventilator-associated pneumonia in a developing country: where is the difference? *Respir Med.* 2007;101:762–767.
27. Rosenthal VD, Maki DG, Salomao R, et al. Device-associated nosocomial infections in 55 intensive care units of 8 developing countries. *Ann Intern Med.* 2006;145:582–591.
28. Cook DJ, Walter SD, Cook RJ, et al. Incidence of and risk factors for ventilator-associated pneumonia in critically ill patients. *Ann Intern Med.* 1998;129:433–440.
29. Hugonnet S, Uckay I, Pittet D. Staffing level: a determinant of late-onset ventilator-associated pneumonia. *Crit Care.* 2007;11:R80.
30. Pugin J, Auckenthaler R, Mili N, Janssens JP, Lew PD, Suter PM. Diagnosis of ventilator-associated pneumonia by bacteriologic analysis of bronchoscopic and nonbronchoscopic "blind" bronchoalveolar lavage fluid. *Am Rev Respir Dis.* 1991;143:1121–1129.
31. Singh N, Rogers P, Atwood CW, Wagener MM, Yu VL. Short-course empiric antibiotic therapy for patients with pulmonary infiltrates in the intensive care unit. A proposed solution for indiscriminate antibiotic prescription. *Am J Respir Crit Care Med.* 2000;162:505–511.
32. Micek ST, Ward S, Fraser VJ, Kollef MH. A randomized controlled trial of an antibiotic discontinuation policy for clinically suspected ventilator-associated pneumonia. *Chest.* 2004;125:1791–1799.
33. Afessa B, Hubmayr RD, Vetter EA, et al. Bronchoscopy in ventilator-associated pneumonia: agreement of calibrated loop and serial dilution. *Am J Respir Crit Care Med.* 2006;173:1229–1232.
34. Meduri GU, Chastre J. The standardization of bronchoscopic techniques for ventilator- associated pneumonia. *Chest.* 1992;102:557S–564S.
35. Chastre J, Fagon JY. Ventilator-associated pneumonia. *Am J Respir Crit Care Med.* 2002;165:867–903.
36. Chastre J, Wolff M, Fagon JY, et al. Comparison of 8 vs 15 days of antibiotic therapy for ventilator-associated pneumonia in adults: a randomized trial. *JAMA.* 2003;290:2588–2598.
37. Fagon JY, Chastre J, Wolff M, et al. Invasive and noninvasive strategies for management of suspected ventilator-associated pneumonia. A randomized trial. *Ann Intern Med.* 2000;132:621–630.
38. Kallel H, Hergafi L, Bahloul M, et al. Safety and efficacy of colistin compared with imipenem in the treatment of ventilator-associated pneumonia: a matched case-control study. *Intensive Care Med.* 2007;33:1162–1167.
39. Wood GC, Swanson JM. Aerosolised antibacterials for the prevention and treatment of hospital-acquired pneumonia. *Drugs.* 2007;67:903–914.
40. Berwick DM, Calkins DR, McCannon CJ, Hackbarth AD. The 100,000 Lives campaign: setting a goal and a deadline for improving health care quality. *JAMA.* 2006;295:324–327.
41. Craven DE. Preventing ventilator-associated pneumonia in adults: sowing seeds of change. *Chest.* 2006;130:251–260.
42. Kollef MH. Prevention of hospital-associated pneumonia and ventilator-associated pneumonia. *Crit Care Med.* 2004;32:1396–1405.
43. Tablan OC, Anderson LJ, Besser R, Bridges C, Hajjeh R. Guidelines for preventing health-care-associated pneumonia, 2003: recommendations of CDC and the Healthcare Infection Control Practices Advisory Committee. *MMWR Recomm Rep.* 2004;53:1–36.
44. Mori H, Hirasawa H, Oda S, Shiga H, Matsuda K, Nakamura M. Oral care reduces incidence of ventilator-associated pneumonia in ICU populations. *Intensive Care Med.* 2006;32:230–236.
45. van Nieuwenhoven CA, Vandenbroucke-Grauls C, van Tiel FH, et al. Feasibility and effects of the semirecumbent position to prevent ventilator-associated pneumonia: a randomized study. *Crit Care Med.* 2006;34:396–402.
46. Kollef MH, Skubas NJ, Sundt TM. A randomized clinical trial of continuous aspiration of subglottic secretions in cardiac surgery patients. *Chest.* 1999;116:1339–1346.
47. Mahul P, Auboyer C, Jospe R, et al. Prevention of nosocomial pneumonia in intubated patients: respective role of mechanical subglottic secretions drainage and stress ulcer prophylaxis. *Intensive Care Med.* 1992;18:20–25.
48. Smulders K, van der Hoeven H, Weers-Pothoff I, Vandenbroucke-Grauls C. A randomized clinical trial of intermittent subglottic secretion drainage in patients receiving mechanical ventilation. *Chest.* 2002;121:858–862.
49. Valles J, Artigas A, Rello J, et al. Continuous aspiration of subglottic secretions in preventing ventilator-associated pneumonia. *Ann Intern Med.* 1995;122:179–186.
50. Kollef MH, Afessa B, Anzueto A, et al. Silver-coated endotracheal tubes and incidence of ventilator-associated pneumonia: the NASCENT randomized trial. *JAMA.* 2008;300:805–813.
51. Chlebicki MP, Safdar N. Topical chlorhexidine for prevention of ventilator-associated pneumonia: a meta-analysis. *Crit Care Med.* 2007;35:595–602.
52. Rosenow EC III, Wilson WR, Cockerill FR III. Pulmonary disease in the immunocompromised host. 1. *Mayo Clin Proc.* 1985;60:473–487.
53. Wilson WR, Cockerill FR III, Rosenow EC III. Pulmonary disease in the immunocompromised host. 2. *Mayo Clin Proc.* 1985;60:610–631.
54. Conces DJ Jr. Pulmonary infections in immunocompromised patients who do not have acquired immunodeficiency syndrome: a systematic approach. *J Thorac Imaging.* 1998;13:234–246.
55. Waite S, Jeudy J, White CS. Acute lung infections in normal and immunocompromised hosts. *Radiol Clin North Am.* 2006;44:295–315.
56. Rosen MJ. Pulmonary complications of HIV infection. *Respirology.* 2008;13:181–190.
57. Davis JL, Fei M, Huang L. Respiratory infection complicating HIV infection. *Curr Opin Infect Dis.* 2008;21:184–190.
58. Rudan I, Boschi-Pinto C, Biloglav Z, Mulholland K, Campbell H. Epidemiology and etiology of childhood pneumonia. *Bull World Health Organ.* 2008;86:408–416.
59. British Thoracic Society guidelines for the management of community acquired pneumonia in childhood. *Thorax.* 2002;57(suppl 1): 1–24.
60. Murphy TF, Henderson FW, Clyde WA Jr, et al. Pneumonia: an eleven-year study in a pediatric practice. *Am J Epidemiol.* 1981;113:12–21.
61. Jadavji T, Law B, Lebel MH, et al. A practical guide for the diagnosis and treatment of pediatric pneumonia. *CMAJ.* 1997;156:S703–S711.

CHAPTER 39

Cystic Fibrosis

Teresa A. Volsko
Catherine O'Malley
Scott H. Donaldson
James R. Yankaskas
Bruce K. Rubin

OUTLINE

History
Pathogenesis
Diagnosis
Extrapulmonary Manifestations
Respiratory Manifestations
Major Respiratory Complications
Standard Therapy of Lung Disease

OBJECTIVES

1. Describe the inheritance pattern of cystic fibrosis.
2. Describe the pathogenesis of cystic fibrosis.
3. List the diagnostic criteria for cystic fibrosis.
4. Describe the numerous extrapulmonary manifestations of cystic fibrosis.
5. Describe typical respiratory manifestations of cystic fibrosis.
6. Discuss the approach to common life-threatening respiratory complications of cystic fibrosis.
7. Describe the principles of preventive care for cystic fibrosis.
8. Outline an approach to the management of an acute exacerbation of cystic fibrosis lung disease.
9. Describe the role that lung transplantation plays in the management of cystic fibrosis.

KEY TERMS

bronchial artery embolization (BAE)
cepacia syndrome
cystic fibrosis (CF)
cystic fibrosis–related diabetes (CFRD)
cystic fibrosis transmembrane conductance regulator (CFTR)
distal intestinal obstruction syndrome (DIOS)
lung transplantation
meconium ileus
steatorrhea
sweat testing

INTRODUCTION

Cystic fibrosis (CF) is an autosomal recessive genetic disorder, passed from parents to their children. Each parent must be a carrier of the gene defect if the children are to be affected. Because the parents are carriers, they are not affected by the disease. However, each child has a 25% chance of inheriting CF. Children that do not inherit the disease may be carriers of the altered gene or have a normal genetic pattern. This chapter addresses the care of a patient with cystic fibrosis.

History

Cystic fibrosis (CF) was first described as a distinct disease entity in the late 1930s independently by Dorothy H. Andersen and Guido Fanconi. Fanconi described the connection between bronchiectasis, malabsorption, and pancreatic changes associated with CF.[1] Andersen and described *cystic fibrosis of the pancreas* as a distinct disease entity in 1938.[2] Andersen conducted an extensive pathology study, describing affected infants who presented with intestinal obstruction or malnutrition as a consequence of malabsorption.[3] In those days, the diagnosis was based on the patient's clinical presentation, and effective treatment was unavailable. Children with CF usually died in the first year of life. Postmortem studies revealed obstruction of pancreatic ducts and the gut with abnormally tenacious mucus, prompting the term *mucoviscidosis*.[3]

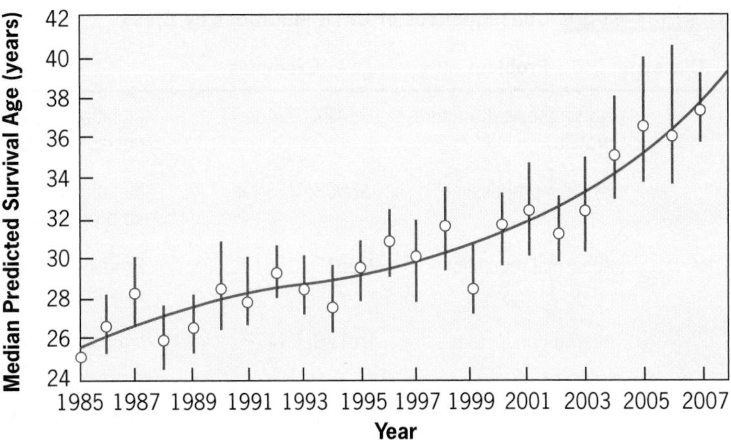

FIGURE 39–1 The median predicted survival age by life table analysis was 37 years for 2007. This represents the age to which half of the current cystic fibrosis (CF) registry population would be expected to survive, given the ages of the CF patients in the registry and the age distribution of the deaths in 2007. Ninety-five percent confidence bounds for the survival estimates are shown, indicating that the 2007 median predicted survival was between 36 years and 39 years. From Marshall PC, Penland CM, Hazle L, et al. Cystic Fibrosis Foundation: achieving the mission. *Respir Care.* 2009;54:788–795. Reprinted with permission. Created with data from Cystic Fibrosis Foundation. *Patient Registry Annual Data Report for 2007*. Bethesda, MD: Cystic Fibrosis Foundation; 2008.

In the 1950s, di Sant'Agnese and colleagues investigated cases of severe dehydration in children with CF during a summer heat wave in New York City and recognized that excessive salt loss occurred through sweat.[4] This observation led to the development of the use of pilocarpine by iontophoresis to stimulate the sweat glands and induce localized sweating.[5] The pilocarpine iontophoresis sweat test, described by Gibson and Cooke in 1959, remains a standard diagnostic test for CF. In 1989 the gene responsible for CF was cloned and its protein product was named the **cystic fibrosis transmembrane conductance regulator (CFTR)**.[6]

Today CF is recognized as the most common life-shortening genetic disease in the white population. In North America one in 29 whites carries a mutant CFTR allele, and one in 3300 live births is affected with CF. Other ethnic populations have lower mutation carrier rates, and thus lower incidences of CF disease. The Hispanic birth incidence is 1 in 9500; for Native Americans it is 1 in 11,200; African Americans, 1 in 15,300; and in the U.S. Asian population, 1 in 32,100 live births. Survival now commonly extends into adulthood, with a median survival of more than 37 years (**Figure 39–1**).[7] More than 21,000 patients with CF have been identified in the United States, and 45% are older than 18 years. This chapter describes the pathogenesis, diagnosis, and clinical manifestations of CF. Although CF is a multisystem disease, the management of acute and chronic respiratory complications is emphasized.

Pathogenesis

Genetics of Cystic Fibrosis

CF is a monogenetic classic Mendelian disorder that is inherited in an autosomal recessive pattern. Persons who carry a single mutated CFTR gene along with a normal CFTR allele are termed *carriers* and have few or no symptoms attributable to CF. Each offspring conceived from two CF carriers therefore has a one in four chance of being affected with CF, and a two in four chance of being a CF carrier.

The CFTR gene belongs to a family of membrane ATP-binding cassette (ABC) proteins that serve as molecular pumps. CFTR is a cAMP-regulated chloride channel in epithelial tissues. Since the discovery of the CFTR gene in 1989, more than 1700 individual mutations have been identified,[8] although the most common mutation (ΔF508) accounts for 66% of CF alleles reported worldwide, and thus about half of all persons with CF are homozygous for this mutation.[9] The exact prevalence of individual mutations also varies according to the ethnic group being studied, with the ΔF508 mutation being less common among nonwhite populations.

Mutations in the CFTR gene have been categorized into five groups reflecting the mechanism for loss of CFTR function (**Table 39–1**). Class I mutations result in the loss of protein production and thus absence of full-length CFTR. Class II mutations result in abnormal protein processing between the cell nucleus and plasma membrane. This class of mutations includes the common ΔF508 mutation, in which improper protein glycosylation and folding prevents normal transport to the apical cell membrane. Most of this abnormal protein is degraded in the endoplasmic reticulum. Class III mutations in the CFTR gene affect the regulation or activation or both of the CFTR chloride channel, although the channel itself successfully reaches the plasma membrane. These mutations tend to produce milder disease. Class IV mutations also reach the plasma membrane but affect the

TABLE 39–1 Consequences of CFTR Mutations by Class

Class	Problem	Examples	Features
I	No synthesis of mature protein	G542X; 394delTT	Mutations cause premature stop codons (e.g., frameshift, nonsense) or unstable mRNA.
II	Block in processing	ΔF508; N1303K	Mutations cause improper intracellular processing (folding, glycosylation), so protein may not reach plasma membrane.
III	Abnormal regulation	G551D; G551S	Protein reaches plasma membrane but is not activated properly; mutation may be mild or severe.
IV	Altered conductance	R117H; R347P	Ion conductance of the channel is altered. Partially functioning channel is often associated with pancreatic sufficiency.
V	Reduced synthesis	3489+10kbC >7T	Altered mRNA splicing sites result in reduced synthesis of normal protein; low levels of preserved synthesis often confer a milder phenotype.

RESPIRATORY RECAP

Genetics of Cystic Fibrosis

- » CF is inherited in an autosomal recessive pattern.
- » CFTR is the gene responsible for CF.
- » It is difficult to predict phenotype from CFTR mutation because of modifier genes and gene–environment interactions.

conductance of chloride through the channel pore. Class V CFTR mutations decrease the abundance of mature CFTR mRNA and protein levels and may include mutations in gene promoters or regions that influence mRNA splicing. These mutations may permit the production of adequate CFTR levels to confer a less severe disease phenotype.[10]

Predicting an individual patient's clinical phenotype has been difficult based on the specific CFTR mutations present. Some genotype–phenotype correlation has been noted, principally among a group of mutations associated with pancreatic exocrine sufficiency, milder lung disease, and borderline or even normal sweat chloride values.[10,11] In addition, certain mutations have been found in men who present solely with infertility resulting from the congenital bilateral absence of the vas deferens (CBAVD), often without other symptoms of CF disease.[12,13] The manifestations of CF in an individual depend on other genetic factors (i.e., modifier genes) and environmental factors.

CFTR Functions and Host Defense

CFTR is a chloride channel expressed in the apical membrane of epithelial cells lining the lung, pancreas, gut, sweat duct, and reproductive tract. As its name implies, however, CFTR regulates several other ion conductance pathways,[14] including sodium channels,[15–18] chloride channels other than CFTR,[19–21] and potassium channels.[22] The loss of a normally functioning CFTR therefore can have a profound impact on epithelial ion transport. In the lung, the absence of CFTR causes increased sodium absorption from the airway lumen[23,24] and a diminished capacity to secrete chloride ions via CFTR. This combination alters the local milieu, and adequate defense against invading microbes is lost.

One hypothesis for the mechanism underlying this defect rests on data showing that increased isotonic volume absorption from the airway lumen (driven by sodium hyperabsorption) depletes the periciliary liquid layer. Periciliary liquid depletion results in disruption of rotational mucus transport in vitro and is predicted to impair both ciliary and cough clearance of airway secretions in vivo.[25] Reduced airway clearance and retention of mucous plaques will in turn cause airway obstruction and allow the establishment of bacterial infection. However, mucociliary clearance is preserved in the nose of persons with CF. The middle ear and eustachian tube are also cleared by mucociliary clearance, but persons with CF do not usually develop chronic or persistent otitis media. Furthermore, persons with primary ciliary dyskinesia (PCD) have congenital absence of mucociliary transport but much milder lung disease than persons with CF. Despite absent ciliary function, cough clearance is not compromised in patients with PCD.[26]

A second hypothesis proposes that NaCl concentrations in airway surface liquid (ASL) are normally low (<50 mM NaCl) but are high in CF (>100 mM) because of the inability to absorb chloride through CFTR. Elevated NaCl concentrations in ASL may inhibit the antimicrobial effects of defensins, which are small, salt-sensitive peptides produced by airway epithelia.[27] Challenges to this hypothesis are the scarcity of defensins in ASL relative to other salt-insensitive antimicrobial molecules (e.g., lactoferrin, lysozyme)[28] and the absence of a physiologic mechanism for the generation of hypotonic fluids across the water-permeable airway epithelium.

Because CFTR expression in the lung is greatest within submucosal glands lining proximal conducting airways,[29] perhaps an alteration in glandular secretion resulting from absent CFTR is a cause of altered airway defense in CF. Indeed, CFTR is involved in generating airway surface liquid via submucosal glands in proximal airways.[30] A third hypothesis relating CFTR function

BOX 39–1

Diagnostic Criteria for Cystic Fibrosis

Phenotypic Feature

Chronic sinopulmonary disease

- Persistent infection with typical cystic fibrosis pathogens (e.g., *Staphylococcus aureus, Pseudomonas aeruginosa, Burkholderia cepacia*, atypical *Mycobacteria*)
- Chronic cough, especially with sputum expectoration
- Persistent chest radiographic abnormality (e.g., bronchiectasis, hyperinflation, atelectasis)
- Airway obstruction pattern on pulmonary function testing
- Nasal polyps and chronic sinus (but not middle ear) involvement
- Digital clubbing

Gastrointestinal or nutritional abnormality

- *Intestinal*: meconium ileus, rectal prolapse, distal intestinal obstruction syndrome
- *Pancreatic*: pancreatic insufficiency, recurrent pancreatitis (in older children and adults)
- *Hepatic*: focal biliary cirrhosis
- *Nutritional*: malnutrition, hypoproteinemia, fat-soluble vitamin deficiency

Salt loss syndrome

- Acute salt depletion, especially with water loss, such as during exercise in heat
- Chronic metabolic alkalosis

Male urogenital abnormality

- Obstructive azoospermia resulting from congenital bilateral absence of the vas deferens (CBAVD)

CFTR Abnormality

Sweat chloride test

- Result > 60 mmol/L on two occasions (minimum 75 mg of sweat collected during 30 minutes) without other causes for high sweat chloride (e.g., anorexia nervosa, atopic dermatitis)

CFTR mutational analysis

- Two identified mutant CFTR alleles

Nasal potential difference (PD) testing

- Higher basal PD
- Greater amiloride-sensitive PD
- Absent or minimal change in PD after isoproterenol in chloride free perfusion solution

The combination of one or more phenotypic abnormalities (or cystic fibrosis in a sibling, or a positive newborn screening test) with evidence of a CFTR abnormality constitutes a cystic fibrosis diagnosis. CFTR, cystic fibrosis transmembrane conductance regulator.

and host defenses therefore emphasizes that deficient secretion of fluid containing sodium chloride or sodium bicarbonate from submucosal glands or serous cells lining small airways may lead to a volume-depleted ASL layer, an ASL layer with an altered composition, or both.

Other hypotheses relating to the pathogenesis of CF lung disease exist. It has been proposed that because there is less intact mucin (mucus) in the CF airway, this may leave the airway more vulnerable to chronic bacterial infection and to the development of bacterial biofilms by organisms in the airway.[31] In addition to hypotheses describing differences in airway mucins,[32–34] others relate to the CF immune response.[35–39] These do not tightly link CFTR function with the resulting disease process and in some cases rest on observations that may be secondary to infection. Most therapies focus on airway clearance and fighting chronic bacterial infection and on modulating the hyperimmune and inflammatory response in the airway.

Diagnosis

The diagnosis of CF is based on the combination of one or more typical phenotypic features and evidence of CFTR malfunction (**Box 39–1**).[40,41] Knowledge of the broad range of clinical features that may be present in CF and appropriate access to specialized diagnostic testing are essential for an accurate diagnosis. Among the clinical features assessed are the presence of obstructive lung disease leading to bronchiectasis and infection with typical pathogens, chronic sinus disease with or without nasal polyposis, exocrine pancreatic insufficiency or recurrent pancreatitis, intestinal obstruction either at birth (meconium ileus) or later in life (distal intestinal obstruction syndrome, formerly called meconium ileus equivalent), rectal prolapse, chronic liver disease, nutritional deficiencies including protein/caloric malnutrition and complications of fat-soluble vitamin deficiency, electrolyte abnormalities such as acute salt depletion or chronic metabolic alkalosis, absence of the vas deferens resulting in obstructive azoospermia in males, and digital clubbing. A family history of CF should also be sought in support of a clinical CF diagnosis.

RESPIRATORY RECAP

Diagnosis of Cystic Fibrosis

- » Clinical features consistent with the disease
- » Family history
- » Sweat testing
- » Mutational analysis to identify CF alleles
- » Nasal epithelial potential difference measurements in response to specific pharmacologic agents

Evidence of CFTR dysfunction is typically provided by **sweat testing** with a chloride concentration of more than 60 mmol/L on two or more occasions. Values greater than 40 mmol/L are considered borderline and are more suggestive of CF in infants. Values between 60 and 80 mmol/L can also be seen in individuals with diseases other than CF. Laboratory errors are common with this technique, and even a small amount of water vapor loss from the collected sweat can concentrate ions and cause a false-positive test result. Thus, all positive and borderline tests should be repeated at a Cystic Fibrosis Foundation–accredited center.

A complementary approach to sweat testing is the use of CFTR mutational analysis to identify CF alleles. The identification of two disease-causing CFTR mutations is highly specific for the diagnosis of CF, but this approach lacks sensitivity. CFTR mutational analysis usually screens for 32 to 70 common mutations and detects up to 95% of CF alleles. The use of mutation panels customized for a given ethnic group or clinical situation (e.g., African American, pancreatic sufficient) may increase the likelihood of the identification of CF alleles. No commercially available screening panel can rule out the diagnosis of CF, however, because none test for all the known mutations capable of causing CF. Also, many mutations may have no functional consequences.

When sweat testing and CFTR mutational analysis are inconclusive, the measurement of nasal epithelial potential difference (PD) in response to various pharmacologic agents can be useful.[42,43] However, this test is only available at a few specialized research centers.

Extrapulmonary Manifestations

Upper Respiratory Tract

Nearly all patients with CF have radiographic opacification of the paranasal sinuses,[44] and a large fraction report symptoms attributable to either nasal obstruction or chronic sinusitis.[45] Symptomatic nasal polyps are particularly common toward the end of the first and during the second decade of life and occur in about 20% to 48% of all patients with CF.[46] This variation in prevalence may be attributed to differences in diagnostic method used. Manifestations include severe nasal airflow obstruction, rhinorrhea, and occasionally, widening of the bridge of the nose. Severity of lung disease is reportedly less among children with CF presenting with recurrent nasal polyps and has been attributed to a proliferative airway repair mechanism.[47] Despite the universal presence of radiographic abnormalities, symptoms attributable to sinusitis occur in fewer than 10% of children[48] and approximately 24% of adults.[49,50] The kind of bacteria isolated in CF sinus disease varies with age and may be similar to those cultured from the lower respiratory tract. *Staphylococcus aureus* and *Haemophilus influenza* are commonly found in younger children, whereas *Pseudomonas aeruginosa* appears more frequently at a later age. Unfortunately, recurrence of polyps and sinus symptoms is extremely common after surgical interventions. Thus, patients must be carefully selected when a surgical intervention for nasal or sinus disease is considered.

Exocrine and Endocrine Pancreas

Exocrine pancreatic insufficiency is present from birth in most patients with CF.[51] Enzyme deficiency results in fat and protein maldigestion, producing **steatorrhea**. Uncorrected malabsorption results in failure to gain weight and ultimately a failure of linear growth. Exocrine pancreatic insufficiency and malnutrition are managed with oral pancreatic enzyme supplementation and dietary supplements. Impaired absorption of fat-soluble vitamins (A, D, E, and K) occasionally produces symptoms of vitamin deficiency, which can be prevented with adequate supplementation. Symptoms of pancreatitis are encountered in fewer than 1% of identified adolescent and adult CF patients and are limited to those who have retained some exocrine pancreatic function.[52] However, recurrent non-ethanol-induced pancreatitis has been associated with mutations in CFTR and may be the presenting symptom in adults with CF.[53,54]

AGE-SPECIFIC ANGLE

Exocrine pancreatic insufficiency is present from birth in most patients with CF. Approximately 18% of newborns with CF have meconium ileus, and these babies uniformly have pancreatic insufficiency.

Although the exocrine pancreas is frequently affected from birth, the gradual loss of insulin production from the endocrine pancreas occurs slowly over time in patients with CF. In the United States, the overall incidence of **cystic fibrosis–related diabetes (CFRD)** or glucose intolerance is reported to be 15% to 30% of adult patients requiring chronic insulin therapy.[55] Because of the insidious onset of CFRD, screening is suggested for individuals aged 14 years and older. Measurements of 2-hour plasma glucose values obtained during an oral glucose tolerance test are a more reliable screening tool than random plasma glucose or glycosylated hemoglobin A1c measurement, performed alone or in combination.[56] Manifestations of CFRD may include failure to gain or maintain weight despite nutritional intervention, poor growth, or an unexplained chronic decline in pulmonary function.[57]

Insulin is the preferred hypoglycemic agent in CFRD, because limited islet cell reserve exists in most cases. Other facets of CFRD management, however, differ substantially from that of either type 1 or 2 diabetes mellitus. Because all CF patients require a high energy intake and generally malabsorb fat even with appropriate pancreatic enzyme supplementation, a high-calorie diet consisting of 40% fat is recommended. Caloric restriction never should be used to aid management of blood glucose in CF except in the rare pancreatic-sufficient and obese patent with CF with chronic type 2 diabetes. Insulin dosage is instead matched to the calorie and carbohydrate intake, and the presence of intercurrent infections is factored in as needed.[58] Patients also are at risk for the usual microvascular complications of diabetes;[55] therefore, similar glucose targets are used as with type 1 and type 2 diabetes mellitus. Equally important, however, is the maintenance of optimal nutrition and growth, the avoidance of severe hypoglycemia, and the need to fit this additional treatment burden within the patient's CF regimen.

Gastrointestinal Tract

Meconium ileus occurs in about 18% of newborns with CF, and true meconium ileus (as opposed to the meconium plugs commonly seen in very premature infants) is nearly diagnostic for CF.[59] A barium enema usually demonstrates a small colon, and a site of ileal obstruction may be identified. Intestinal obstruction can also be diagnosed by fetal ultrasound toward the end of pregnancy.

Later in life, intestinal obstruction may be caused by the **distal intestinal obstruction syndrome (DIOS)**. This occurs in approximately 20% of patients and usually presents with constipation, right lower quadrant abdominal pain, anorexia, nausea, vomiting, and sometimes fever.[57,60,61] As with meconium ileus, obstruction usually occurs in the terminal ileum and is associated with copious, incompletely digested intestinal contents. DIOS has been associated with poor adherence to taking pancreatic enzyme therapy and with dietary indiscretions.

> **RESPIRATORY RECAP**
>
> **Extrapulmonary Manifestations of Cystic Fibrosis**
>
> » Upper airway
> » Exocrine and endocrine pancreas
> » Gastrointestinal tract
> » Hepatobiliary system
> » Reproductive tract
> » Sweat glands

Other causes of abdominal pain include simple constipation, intussusception, intestinal adhesions from previous abdominal surgery (including for meconium ileus), or chronic appendicitis that has been partially suppressed by antibiotic therapy. Rectal prolapse occurs in up to 20% of children but is an infrequent event for adults with CF.[62] Excessive pancreatic enzyme dosages have been associated with the occurrence of fibrosing colonopathy, especially in those patients taking 6000 units or more of lipase per kilogram per meal.[63–65] Pancreatic enzyme dosages of 2500 units or less of lipase per kilogram per meal are recommended to avoid this complication. Gastroesophageal reflux disease is common and should be recognized and treated because this process may exacerbate lung disease, just as lung disease and chronic cough can worsen gastroesophageal reflux.[66–68]

Hepatobiliary System

Focal biliary cirrhosis is characteristic of CF but produces symptoms in fewer than 5% of CF patients and is the cause of death in about 2%.[69,70] Unlike many complications of CF, hepatic disease has a peak incidence during adolescence and a decreased prevalence in patients older than 20 years.[71] Hepatic abnormalities can present as hepatosplenomegaly or as a persistent elevation of hepatic enzymes (particularly alkaline phosphatase). Rarely, patients may present with esophageal varices and hemorrhage resulting from portal hypertension. Fatty liver is also common and may improve with adequate nutrition. Dysfunctional gallbladders[72] or gallstones[73] are present in 10% to 30% of patients.

Reproductive Tract

More than 98% of male patients with CF have azoospermia resulting from obstruction of the vas deferens.[74] In fact, absence of a palpable vas deferens is a useful clue to the diagnosis of CF during the evaluation of a male patient with otherwise unexplained lung disease or other manifestation of CF. Semen analysis may be required to identify the very rare man with CF who is fertile. The volume of ejaculate is usually one-third to one-half of normal, void of spermatozoa, and has a number of chemical abnormalities of seminal fluid that reflect the absence of secretions from the seminal vesicles.[75] Because spermatozoa do develop in the testis of patients with CF, despite being absent in the ejaculate, epididymal sperm microaspiration coupled with intracytoplasmic oocyte injection may allow successful conception.[76]

Although male infertility is nearly universal, female infertility is only about 20%.[74] Some women with CF are anovulatory because of chronic lung disease and malnutrition. In addition, mucus in the cervical os has abnormal electrolyte concentration and can present an obstacle to conception by impeding normal sperm migration.[77] Nevertheless, hundreds of pregnancies in women with CF have been reported. A longitudinal study of 325 pregnant women with CF reported 258 live births (79%) and 67 therapeutic abortions. Pregnancy in women with CF did not have a negative effect on pulmonary status or mortality over 2 years.[78] However, women with CF must consider their own health and expected life span in the context of family planning.

Sweat Glands

Sweat chloride is elevated in most CF patients because of reduced NaCl reabsorption in the sweat duct.[79] This abnormality forms the basis for the diagnostic sweat

AGE-SPECIFIC ANGLE

Young children with CF are most at risk for episodes of salt loss, especially in hot, arid climates and in the setting of concomitant salt/volume loss.

chloride test and may predispose patients to salt depletion. Young children are most at risk for episodes of salt loss, especially in hot, arid climates and in the setting of concomitant salt/volume loss resulting from vomiting, diarrhea, or exercise. These children present with lethargy, anorexia, and hypochloremic alkalosis. Presentation with hypochloremic alkalosis is rare in older children and adults.[79] Salt restriction is never indicated in CF, and increased salt intake should be encouraged when environmental or clinical circumstances place a patient at increased risk for salt depletion.

Respiratory Manifestations

Symptoms

Newborns with CF appear to have normal lung function, implying normal intrauterine lung development. Clinical symptoms or evidence of increased airways resistance and gas trapping often develop very early in life, although they may not be apparent until adulthood in a minority of patients. Respiratory symptoms typically include a cough that becomes persistent and productive of purulent sputum over time. Periods of clinical stability are inevitably interrupted by typical exacerbations, characterized by increased cough, sputum, fatigue, anorexia, weight loss, and decreased lung function. These exacerbations require more intensive therapy, with the goal of alleviating symptoms and restoring lost lung function through the use of antibiotics and airway clearance maneuvers. Over time exacerbations become more frequent, respond less well to interventions, and eventually result in respiratory failure.

RESPIRATORY RECAP

Respiratory Manifestations of Cystic Fibrosis

- » Clinical symptoms: cough, sputum, fatigue, anorexia, and weight loss are characteristic of an exacerbation of lung disease
- » Chest radiograph: hyperinflation, progressing to bronchiectasis that is more prominent in the upper lobes
- » Pulmonary function: airflow obstruction
- » Respiratory microbiology: airways become persistently infected with gram-negative pathogens such as *P aeruginosa* and resistant *S aureus*

Chest Radiography

Chest radiographs in CF often are normal early in the course of disease. Hyperinflation may be the first radiographic finding in children, followed by increased interstitial markings. These increased interstitial markings progress to the typical findings of cystic bronchiectasis, which is usually most pronounced in the upper lobes. The right upper lobe is more frequently and severely affected than the left for unclear reasons. Despite high densities of bacteria in airways, findings of an alveolar filling process typical of bacterial pneumonia are not generally seen even during periods of acute illness. Segmental or subsegmental atelectasis and lobar collapse are common radiographic findings related to airway obstruction and retained secretions. Although the chest radiograph demonstrates the chronic progression of lung destruction and is useful for the detection of important complications such as lobar collapse and pneumothorax, there can be little correlation between the radiograph and acute clinical changes later in the course of disease.

High-resolution computed tomography (CT) scans of the chest may be useful to detect bronchiectasis and other early pathologic changes that are not visible on routine chest radiographs, especially during the evaluation of a patient with chronic cough and sputum production who is not otherwise known to have bronchiectasis.[80] Chest CT also may be useful in the CF patient with persistent nontuberculous mycobacteria (NTM) infection, because the presence of multiple, small parenchymal nodules (so-called tree-in-bud nodules) predominating in the middle and lower lobes and patchy airspace disease are evidence of true NTM infection.[81,82]

Pulmonary Function

Pulmonary function testing is a reliable method used to evaluate the severity of CF lung disease and is an objective means to determine when a patient's clinical status has deteriorated and requires more intensive therapy. The first abnormality detected is obstruction of small airways, as indicated by reduced flow at low lung volumes (e.g., $FEF_{25-75\%}$) and gas trapping with an increase in the ratio of residual volume to total lung capacity (RV/TLC).[83] Later in the course of disease, pulmonary function tests demonstrate progressive reduction in FEV_1, followed by decreased functional vital capacity (FVC). The FEV_1 is the accepted indicator of disability and is somewhat predictive of length of survival.[84] An FEV_1 of about 30% of predicted often is used as an indication to initiate lung transplant evaluation, although other factors also should be considered.[85]

Well before spirometric abnormalities appear, bronchiectatic changes and airways obstruction may be evident. This is especially true in young children, and such changes are often detected by CT scans. Novel physiologic tests such as the lung clearance index (LCI) display superior sensitivity in the mild stages of CF and are easier for younger patients.[86] LCI is measured by performing an inert gas washout using a low concentration of an inert gas, generally sulfur hexafluoride (SF_6). In the future this technique may become a standard means for evaluating the severity of early CF lung disease.

As airway obstruction worsens, hypoxemia develops due to ventilation-perfusion mismatching. Even when oxygenation is adequate at rest, the clinician should be aware that hypoxemia may occur during sleep or with exercise in the setting of moderate to severe lung disease and should screen for it with exercise and sleep oximetry recordings.[87,88] Although significant hypoxemia tends to occur in patients with more advanced lung disease, pulmonary function test results can be a poor predictor of the need for oxygen therapy.[86] Supplemental oxygen may improve exercise performance in patients found to desaturate during exercise[89,90] and is generally effective in delaying the progression of pulmonary hypertension and cor pulmonale.[91]

Severe airway disease causes retention of carbon dioxide due to an increased dead space to tidal volume ratio (VD/VT), which in turn may worsen hypoxemia. Carbon dioxide retention usually does not occur until severe airway obstruction is present. Along with resting hypoxemia, it is a predictor of end-stage lung disease and decreased survival.[92]

Respiratory Microbiology

The respiratory tract of newborns is likely sterile but often becomes infected with pathogens early in life.[93] The CF lung is infected with distinctive bacterial organisms. Once chronic infection is established, it is rarely eradicated and consists of characteristic age-related bacteria (**Figure 39–2**). *Staphylococcus aureus* and *Haemophilus influenzae* are often the first organisms detected, although *H influenzae* rarely persists beyond childhood.[94] *S aureus* may not persist after its initial isolation during childhood or may be isolated for the first time during the adult years. The prevalence of *S aureus* is nearly 50% in newly diagnosed children, peaks at just over 55% in children aged 6 to 10 years, and then gradually decreases to 33% in patients older than 35 years. *S aureus* resistant to available β-lactam antibiotics is referred to as methicillin-resistant *S aureus* (MRSA). MRSA strains are becoming increasingly more prevalent in persons with CF. In 2008, the mean MRSA infection rate at CF centers was reported to be 22.6%, an increase from 7% in 2001.[7] Infection with MRSA is associated with more rapid decline in pulmonary function and with more frequent exacerbations than infection with *Pseudomonas*.[95]

For unclear reasons, the airways of CF patients have a propensity to become persistently infected with otherwise uncommon gram-negative pathogens. These form bacterial biofilms in the airway, making eradication particularly difficult. Among these, *Pseudomonas aeruginosa* is the most common, with the prevalence ranging from approximately 25% during the first year of life to nearly 80% in adulthood.[7] With the progression of lung disease, *P aeruginosa* is often the only organism recovered from sputum and may be present in several types of colonies, often with different antibiotic sensitivity patterns. The recovery of *P aeruginosa*, particularly the mucoid and biofilm form, from the lower respiratory tract of a child or young adult with chronic lung symptoms is highly suggestive of CF. Infection with *P aeruginosa* is a negative predictor of lung function and survival,[96] making avoidance of initial infection desirable. As a result, many clinics segregate infected patients from those who have never grown *P aeruginosa* in sputum cultures.[97] Along similar lines of reasoning, the feasibility and efficacy of the eradication of *Pseudomonas* on its initial isolation is being investigated. The Early *Pseudomonas* Infection Control (EPIC) large multicenter trials, for example, are currently under way to examine treatment strategies for early *Pseudomonas* infections in the airways of young children with CF.[98,99]

AGE-SPECIFIC ANGLE

The respiratory tract of a child with CF often becomes infected with bacteria early in life.

Burkholderia cepacia complex is highly transmissible among patients with CF and is difficult to treat because it is often resistant to antimicrobial drugs. *B cepacia* complex now includes 10 named bacterial species, with the overall prevalence of *B cepacia* complex in the United States being 2.8%.[7,100] The two most common species in

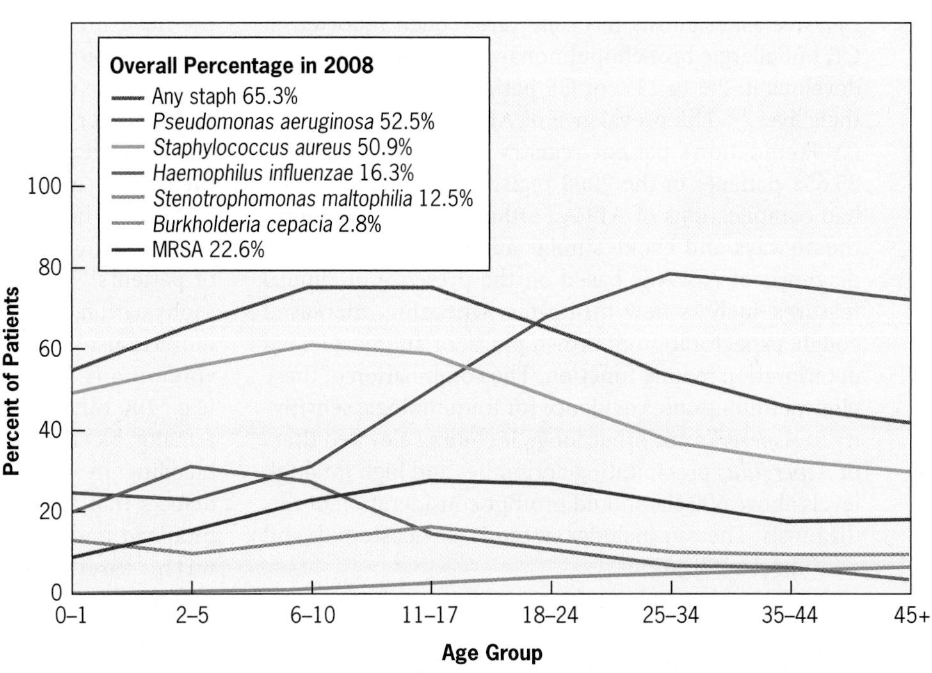

FIGURE 39–2 The prevalence of common bacterial organisms in different age groups. Reprinted from Cystic Fibrosis Foundation. *Patient Registry Annual Data Report for 2008*. Bethesda, MD: Cystic Fibrosis Foundation; 2009.

patients with CF are *B cenocepacia* and *B multivorans*, accounting for approximately 45% and 40% of infections, respectively.[99] A subset of patients will manifest the **cepacia syndrome**,[101] a rapid clinical decline with fever and sepsis after initial infection, although the precise pathogen and host factors that trigger this dramatic and often fatal decompensation are unknown. It may be that the *B cenocepacia* strain, for example, is more virulent and transmissible than the other strains.[102,103] Because strong evidence exists that person-to-person spread of *B cepacia* complex occurs, particularly with highly transmissible strains expressing the cable pilus,[104,105] stringent infection control measures are now advocated wherever CF care is provided.[106,107] Infection prevention and control measures, such as segregating infected patients, a strong emphasis on hand hygiene, and contact isolation, can help decrease the spread of this pathogen.[108]

Other gram-negative rods that may cause lung infection in CF include emerging pathogens, such as *Achromobacter xylosoxidans* and *Stenotrophomonas maltophilia*.[92] The prevalence of these bacterial species in patients in CF centers in the United States is approximately 6% for *A xylosoxidans* and 12.5% for *S maltophilia*. The impact these infections have on the progression of disease in CF is unclear. There is little evidence of cross infection, and the source of infection may be the environment.[109–111] Because these organisms are often multidrug resistant, infection prevention and control measures are usually used.

Fungi and molds are frequently cultured from the respiratory secretions of CF patients. *Aspergillus* species was reported in sputum cultures from 10.4% of children and 18.8% of adults in the 2008 CF Foundation Patient Registry,[7] although the prevalence is probably higher. Invasive aspergillosis has only rarely been reported in CF, but allergic bronchopulmonary aspergillosis (ABPA) develops in 2% to 11% of CF patients at some point in their lives.[112] The prevalence of ABPA is tracked by the CF Foundation's patient registry. Data gathered from 25,651 patients in the 2008 registry report found 4.7% had complications of ABPA.[7] Other fungi may colonize the airways and evoke similar allergic responses. The diagnosis of ABPA is based on the presence of clinical features such as new infiltrates, wheezing, increased cough, expectoration of brown plugs, or an unexplained deterioration in lung function. The combination of these clinical findings plus evidence for immunologic sensitivity to *Aspergillus* or other fungi, including elevated titers of *Aspergillus* precipitating antibodies and high total IgE levels above 500 IU, should prompt consideration of this diagnosis. Therapy includes systemic corticosteroids and antifungal medications.

Isolation of nontuberculous mycobacteria from appropriately processed[113] CF sputum is relatively common and may occur in as many as 20% of adult CF patients.[114] Preliminary data from a multicenter study suggest an overall prevalence of about 13%, with *Mycobacterium avium* complex being most common; however, there is a significant prevalence of both *M abscessus* and *M fortuitum*. *M abscessus* is thought to be more virulent and to cause more severe and invasive disease.[115–118] Patients with high mycobacterial burdens and symptoms refractory to treatment of typical bacteria may benefit from antimycobacterial therapy.

Major Respiratory Complications

Hemoptysis, pneumothorax, and respiratory failure are major pulmonary complications that tend to occur in association with more severe lung disease. In the adult CF population, major hemoptysis and pneumothorax each occurs in about 1% of patients annually. Most patients who suffer massive hemoptysis or pneumothorax can be treated successfully. Respiratory failure, as the result of progressive airway obstruction and destruction, is nearly universal and the cause of death in 94% of CF patients. Although improved therapies have delayed the development of respiratory failure, at this time respiratory failure can only be treated by **lung transplantation**.

Hemoptysis

Hemoptysis in CF may range from minor blood streaking of the sputum, requiring little intervention, to massive bleeding (more than 240 mL in 24 hours). Minor hemoptysis is common and usually self-limited, although it may indicate an exacerbation of lung disease. Massive hemoptysis in CF almost invariably comes from the bronchial artery circulation, which is at systemic arterial pressure. The new occurrence of any amount of bleeding may signal the presence of an increased infectious or inflammatory burden and the need for intensified treatment. The approach to a minor amount of hemoptysis therefore is to determine whether the patient requires treatment with antibiotics and whether medications (e.g., NSAIDs, aspirin, penicillin) or vitamin K deficiency may be contributing to the new onset of bleeding.

Massive hemoptysis (more than 240 mL in 24 hours) from bronchiectatic airways occurs in approximately 5% of patients[119] and may lead to airway obstruction and asphyxiation. Hypotension, anemia, and chemical pneumonitis also may result from massive hemoptysis. Less voluminous hemoptysis that persists for several days (e.g., 100 mL/day for 3 days) also should be considered a major bleeding event, because it may herald massive bleeding. In addition to the correction of any hemostatic defects that are present, these patients should be hospitalized and treated with antibiotics based on recent sputum culture results. Cough suppression and bed rest may be used during the acute

RESPIRATORY RECAP

Complications of Cystic Fibrosis

» Hemoptysis
» Pneumothorax
» Respiratory failure

presentation to lessen the likelihood of further bleeding but should not be continued for prolonged periods in patients with advanced lung disease who are likely to suffer from inadequate airway clearance.

When bleeding is rapid, positioning the patient with the bleeding lung in a dependent position may help prevent soiling of the nonbleeding lung. Endotracheal intubation may be required if the patient is unable to maintain a patent airway. A large orotracheal tube, which can be advanced into the main bronchus serving the nonbleeding lung, is preferable to double-lumen tubes because the small lumens of these latter devices limit airway suctioning. Attempts to localize the site of bleeding with chest radiography, CT scanning, and bronchoscopy may help direct invasive therapies aimed at the control of bleeding but often are not diagnostic and may delay therapy.

With massive bleeding, **bronchial artery embolization (BAE)** is the therapy of choice and is usually directed at tortuous and hypertrophied bronchial arteries.[120] Nonbronchial systemic collateral vessels are also frequently involved, especially in cases of recurrent hemoptysis after BAE.[121] The use of nonionic contrast material and of embolizing particles large enough to prevent distal tissue ischemia, and the avoidance of sclerosant agents have made BAE relatively safe and successful in experienced hands. Rebleeding after BAE is not uncommon and may require further attempts at BAE to achieve a successful outcome.[122] Studies have demonstrated a higher risk for rate of decline in lung function, need for lung transplantation, and death among adults with CF treated with BAE for hemoptysis.[123] Surgical resection is occasionally required for bleeding refractory to repeated attempts at BAE in patients with adequate pulmonary reserve.

Pneumothorax

The presence of subpleural air cysts is likely responsible for the increased incidence of spontaneous pneumothorax in CF. The incidence of pneumothorax is approximately 1% per year overall, but it increases with age. Pneumothorax occurs in 16% to 20% of adult patients at some time.[124] Most patients complain of a sudden increase in dyspnea or chest discomfort, although others are asymptomatic. The presence of a newly detected pneumothorax usually mandates hospitalization, whether or not chest tube insertion is planned at the outset. Asymptomatic pneumothoraces that occupy less than 20% of the hemithorax may be observed with follow-up radiographs and clinical monitoring to assess progression.

Larger pneumothoraces and those leading to symptoms should be treated with tube thoracostomy. Chest tubes may be removed once the pneumothorax has resolved and the air leak stopped. Additional tubes may be required when significant air collections persist after the initial tube placement. Chest tubes to evacuate air should generally be placed to water-seal rather than to suction because the negative pressure may inhibit the air leak from sealing. Further interventions may be necessary when a persistent air leak results in recurrent or persistent pneumothorax. Talc pleurodesis has been used to cause an inflammatory reaction that leads to obliteration of the pleural space. Although in the past pleurodesis was a relative contraindication for eventual lung transplantation, this is no longer considered to be true. A surgical approach, with either a small transaxillary thoracotomy or a thoracoscopic procedure, is usually used. Stapling across ruptured pleural blebs and pleural abrasion can be performed with a relatively low rate of recurrence.[122,125]

Respiratory Failure

Hypoxemic and hypercapnic respiratory failure occurs in the late stages of CF and accounts for most deaths. Treatment of hypoxemia may improve both the quality and duration of life while delaying the development of cor pulmonale.[126,127] As infection and inflammation progress, airway obstruction and parenchymal destruction worsen, causing ventilation-perfusion mismatch and hypoxemia. Other mechanisms also may contribute to hypoxemia, including an increased partial pressure of carbon dioxide, intrapulmonary shunt, reduced mixed venous saturation resulting from increased oxygen consumption, malnutrition, and weakness.

The use of noninvasive ventilation (NIV) may be effective alone or with long-term oxygen therapy. NIV can improve nocturnal ventilation, oxygenation, and sleep quality.[128] Treatment of hypoxemic respiratory failure is first aimed at correcting all reversible processes. This includes optimization of the treatment of airway infection, clearance of retained secretions, improving nutrition, and treating other complications that may be present. Supplemental oxygen by nasal cannula should be prescribed with the goal of maintaining a Spo_2 of 90% or above. Even when daytime oxygen saturation is adequate, hypoxemia during sleep or exercise may occur and should be assessed, especially in the setting of severe lung disease ($FEV_1 \leq 30\%$ of predicted), low resting oxygen saturation ($\leq 92\%$) or when signs of cor pulmonale are present. Because spirometry poorly predicts the occurrence of exercise- or sleep-induced hypoxemia, a low threshold for screening should exist.[86] This approach to the treatment of hypoxemic respiratory failure in CF can improve exercise capacity,[87,88] delay the development of cor pulmonale, and improve survival.[89,126]

Hypercapnic respiratory failure is the result of alveolar hypoventilation, primarily from airway obstruction and increased dead space ventilation. In addition, respiratory muscle weakness in association with muscle fatigue and malnutrition may be an important contributor. Acidosis that develops gradually from hypercapnia usually is compensated by renal mechanisms, such that an adequate acid–base balance is maintained. However, acute elevations in the P_{CO_2} will lead to acidosis and an impaired sensorium. Although hypercarbia is often the result of slowly progressive lung disease, a search for treatable causes of respiratory failure should be performed. Ventilatory assistance can be provided by NIV or with endotracheal intubation. The decision to use assisted ventilation with intubation should be based on the baseline severity of lung disease, presence of a reversible precipitating process, and whether the patient has been accepted for lung transplantation.[129,130]

In the setting of an acute, reversible process such as pneumothorax, severe hemoptysis, or suboptimal treatment of the underlying CF lung disease, assisted ventilation may buy time needed to treat the acute, superimposed process. Once the decision to ventilate a patient has been made, airway clearance, suctioning, and antibiotics should all be used. Therapy for muscle weakness with nutrition and exercise (including ambulation with assisted ventilation) should be started. Successful liberation from mechanical ventilation depends primarily on the extent of the underlying lung disease rather than the severity of the acute respiratory event. In the patient awaiting lung transplantation who has accrued enough seniority to make organ availability a possibility within days or weeks, a trial of mechanical ventilation and intensive therapy may be reasonable, with the understanding that prolonged support may not be possible. This period of support may provide a bridge to successful transplantation or may allow the patient and family to address end-of-life issues with greater control.

Patients with irreversible respiratory insufficiency are unlikely to benefit from invasive mechanical ventilation without the possibility of imminent lung transplantation. The debilitating nature of advanced lung disease makes the probability of liberation from mechanical support very low. NIV may relieve acute dyspnea and other symptoms of hypoventilation such as morning headaches, exertional dyspnea, and daytime lethargy.[131,132] NIV may also be useful as a bridge to transplantation for patients with decompensated respiratory failure.[131] In a small sample of selected CF patients with severe airflow limitation and chronic respiratory failure, the use of nocturnal NIV was well tolerated and reduced complaints of daytime respiratory muscle fatigue, and dyspnea, with no concomitant improvement in lung function.[133] Studies examining the use of NIV in CF have yielded mixed results in terms of improved quality of life, daytime gas exchange, respiratory muscle function, and quality of sleep. As with conventional mechanical ventilation, NIV may help sustain patients with respiratory failure who are waiting for lung transplantation.[118] Because of these mixed results, NIV use should be individualized and closely monitored. Polysomnography should be used to document the degree of gas exchange deterioration during sleep and the frequency of respiratory disturbances and to titrate airway pressures.

Standard Therapy of Lung Disease

Treatment of CF lung disease can be categorized as therapies used to prevent deterioration of lung function and those used to treat acute exacerbations. Although therapies are being developed that are aimed at the correction of either the gene defect or the ion transport abnormalities that characterize CF epithelia, currently available therapies either promote the physical removal of airway secretions or reduce airway infection and inflammation. Several types of therapy are often combined to provide optimal care for patients. When multiple expensive and labor-intensive treatment modalities are prescribed, careful attention should be paid to appropriate use and adherence (**Table 39–2**).

Although not addressed in detail here, nutritional support to achieve and maintain ideal body weight and treatment of complications such as CF-related diabetes are integral parts of the multidisciplinary care of patients and may directly affect the severity of lung disease and survival. The development of specialized CF care centers where expertise from multiple disciplines is applied

TABLE 39–2 Airway Clearance and Medications

Agent	Rationale
Dornase alfa	Decreases secretion viscosity by degrading DNA polymers
Bronchodilator (β-adrenergic agonist)	May aid airway clearance; protects against bronchospasm induced by expectorants and/or antibiotics
Hypertonic saline or mannitol	May improve airway surface fluid hydration, increase mucin secretion, and increase effective coughing
Airway clearance maneuvers and devices	Methods should be individualized to the patient and used more frequently when the patient is acutely sick
Antibiotic (TOBI, colistin)	Deposition may be enhanced after airway clearance

in an integrated fashion has greatly improved survival. **Box 39–2** lists typical respiratory therapist roles in the management of patients with CF.

Maintenance Therapy

CF airway secretions are difficult to clear because of their lower viscosity and higher tenacity. This is probably caused by inflammation and the presence of DNA/F-actin copolymers in sputum. If left untreated, retained phlegm leads to progressive airway obstruction and serves as a nidus for ongoing infection and inflammation. In an attempt to treat the progression of infection, inflammation, and lung destruction, airway clearance techniques have been developed to promote the expectoration of airway secretions. These techniques continue to be a cornerstone of CF therapy (**Table 39–3**).

Several means of airway clearance are available to patients with CF, with little other than systematic, individual trials to guide the clinician to the best choice for a given patient. Chest physical therapy (CPT) by hand clapping, the traditional means used to clear secretions, is usually effective, although this form of therapy is considered time and labor intensive, and adherence is poor. CPT has been shown to improve mucus clearance and pulmonary function in otherwise stable patients.[134] This method requires a caregiver capable of performing the therapy correctly. There are no data showing that postural drainage increases the effectiveness of CPT, but it does increase the risk of gastroesophageal reflux.

Alternative airway clearance therapies include breathing techniques such as autogenic drainage (AD) and the active cycle of breathing (ACB), handheld devices such as positive expiratory pressure (PEP)[135] and oscillatory PEP (OPEP),[136] and mechanical devices that deliver high-frequency chest wall compression (HFCWC).[137] These offer alternatives to traditional CPT and can be effectively self-administered, allowing for more independence. Also, the treatment times are typically less than that required for CPT. Because no single method has been shown to be consistently superior and great variability

BOX 39–2

Respiratory Therapist Roles in Cystic Fibrosis Management

- Monitoring of oxygen therapy (e.g., rest, nocturnal, exercise)
- Administering aerosol therapies
- Providing assisted ventilation (via mask or endotracheal tube)
- Performing airway clearance maneuvers
- Performing spirometry and other pulmonary function testing
- Evaluating exercise tolerance
- Educating patients
  - Proper use of inhaled medications
  - Instruction on airway clearance techniques
  - Respiratory equipment care and maintenance

TABLE 39–3 Airway Clearance Techniques

Technique	Description	Performed Independently?
Percussion, vibration	Hand percussion, shaking, and/or vibration is applied over individual lung segments. Mechanical percussors provide limited patient autonomy and may decrease fatigue in the caregiver. There is no proven benefit to adding postural drainage. Adherence is poor.	No
Active cycle of breathing (ACB)	Technique alternates (1) gentle breathing with the lower chest, (2) deep breathing with emphasis on inspiration, and (3) forced exhalation technique (FET) using the abdominal muscles and an open mouth/glottis (huff). ACB may be combined with posture positions.	Yes
Autogenic drainage	Technique alternates (1) breathing at low lung volumes to loosen peripheral secretions, (2) breathing at low to mid lung volumes to collect mucus from central airways, and (3) mucus evacuation by breathing at mid to high lung volumes. It is performed in the sitting position and requires significant teaching.	Yes
Positive expiratory pressure (PEP)	Pressure (10–20 cm H_2O) is applied via an expiratory resistor attached to a mask or mouthpiece. Tidal breathing with slightly active exhalation is used. Forced expirations and cough follow PEP to evacuate mucus. Nebulized medications may be delivered in conjunction with PEP device.	Yes
Oscillatory PEP (OPEP)	A handheld device delivers airflow oscillations in addition to positive expiratory pressure. It is essential to achieve sufficient airflow and pressure through the device, and patients with very severe lung disease may not be able to perform this technique. Technique is tiring and adherence is poor. Some devices allow nebulized medications to be delivered in conjunction with OPEP therapy.	Yes
High-frequency chest wall compression	An inflatable vest linked to a compressed air delivery system provides air pulses at various frequencies. Therapy is given over 20 to 30 minutes, with the patient sitting in an upright position.	Yes

exists between patients, several of these methods should be tried until the patient identifies those that he or she is willing and able to use.

To achieve good patient outcomes, it is essential for the respiratory therapist to understand the operation and limitations of the airway clearance devices available for use.[138] The patient's age, ability to cooperate and to properly perform the therapy, level of motivation, and degree of pulmonary impairment must be taken into consideration. The use of airway clearance protocols helps match therapeutic goals to clinical needs and guides selection and sequencing of therapy.

RESPIRATORY RECAP

Maintenance Therapy for Cystic Fibrosis

- » Airway clearance techniques
- » Aerosolized dornase alfa
- » Other mucus-modifying agents
- » Antibiotics
- » Anti-inflammatory medications

Patient and family education should include how to perform the therapy as well as how to use and clean the equipment.[139,140] Effective strategies for integrating multiple lengthy therapy sessions into the patient's daily schedule should also be reviewed.[141] Patient acceptance of a technique is crucial if adherence is to be expected.

Exercise has been shown to enhance an airway clearance regimen and assist secretion removal. Beneficial effects on health and well-being have been well documented.[142] The need for supplemental oxygen during exercise should be assessed periodically in those patients with severe airway obstruction.

Another strategy used to aid secretion removal is to modify the transportability of phlegm. Because DNA is the major polymer in CF secretions, human recombinant DNase I (dornase alfa; Pulmozyme) was developed and approved for use in CF in 1994.[143] In a well-controlled 6-month study, once-daily use of dornase improved FEV_1 by 6% above baseline and decreased the frequency of respiratory exacerbations by 28%. The response to dornase is variable, with some patients showing clear benefit and others showing no change or actually worsening. Therefore, individualized use and careful monitoring of the response are warranted. Because most patients who benefit show a response within 1 to 3 months of starting the drug, a therapeutic trial should be considered for up to 3 months while the patient is monitored for improvement in lung function and clinical symptoms. The efficacy of dornase over longer time periods is unknown.

The DNA polymer network copolymerizes with filamentous actin (F-actin) from effete airway and inflammatory cell walls.[144] This increases the rigidity of these polymers. F-actin depolymerizing agents such as thymosin beta 4 have been shown to be both effective as mucolytics and synergistic with dornase alfa in vitro, but these have not been studied in patients with CF.[145]

Several mucolytics have been used in CF, although none has been shown to improve lung function or other clinical outcomes. Among these agents, *N*-acetylcysteine (Mucomyst) is perhaps the most commonly used. This agent reduces disulfide bonds in mucins, thus making them less viscous. Unfortunately, this agent may increase epithelial inflammation. Although irritation can induce coughing, aerosol *N*-acetylcysteine has not been shown to be beneficial for persons with CF. Other mucolytic agents also have been used but have not been shown to have benefit for CF.

Hypertonic saline has been used to promote hydration of periciliary fluid, induce coughing, and induce mucus secretion. Studies examining the acute effect of hypertonic NaCl (3% to 12%) on mucociliary clearance[146–148] and studies of lung function[149] suggest benefit.[150] Some CF patients with coexistent asthma may not tolerate hypertonic solutions because of bronchospasm.[151] Similarly, inhaled dry powder mannitol has been shown to improve the biophysical and transport properties of CF sputum, and clinical trials are now in progress.[152]

Because chronic airway infection causes progression of CF lung disease, oral and inhaled antibiotics are important parts of a standard CF care regimen. In general, oral antibiotics are used episodically, when new respiratory symptoms develop or a minor decline in lung function is detected. Scheduled cycles of oral antibiotics also may be used prophylactically in the patient having frequent exacerbations. Continuous use of an oral antibiotic designed to suppress infection with *S aureus* has been a common practice, especially in Europe. Long-term use of ciprofloxacin, the primary oral agent with good activity against *P aeruginosa*, should be avoided because of the rapid emergence of resistance after 3 to 4 weeks of use.

Because of the limited number of oral antibiotics available to treat *P aeruginosa*, inhaled aminoglycosides have been used. This route of administration has the benefit of achieving high drug levels in proximal airway secretions, with minimal systemic levels or toxicity. High drug concentrations in secretions may be particularly helpful in the treatment of organisms that are resistant to antibiotic concentrations that may be achieved via the intravenous route. However, there is a natural concentration gradient of antibiotic in the airway; thus, distal secretions are exposed to progressively lower concentrations, inevitably leading to the development of antimicrobial resistance.

The best data for inhaled antibiotic efficacy exist for high-dose tobramycin. A preservative-free, concentrated preparation of tobramycin solution for inhalation (TOBI, Novartis) 300 mg twice a day taken during alternate months improves lung function and lessens the relative risk of hospitalization or treatment with intravenous antibiotics.[153] An alternative to inhaled tobramycin is colistin (75 to 150 mg, twice a day), which has good in vitro activity against *P aeruginosa* but has been less well studied in clinical trials.[154]

An alternative approach embraced by the Danish CF Centre stresses measures aimed at delaying the acquisition of *P aeruginosa* and aggressive antibiotic treatment once this organism is cultured from sputum. These measures include the segregation of patients by microbiologic status and attempts to eradicate pseudomonads when initially cultured in a patient.[94] Scheduled courses of intravenous antibiotics are also employed every 3 months for patients who are chronically infected with *Pseudomonas*. This center claims that there is improved survival using this approach compared with historical controls.[155] Significant concerns include the earlier development of bacterial antibiotic resistance, the lack of proven efficacy by controlled trials, the enormous healthcare resources involved, and the personal impact this approach has on patients.

Bronchodilators, especially those delivered via the inhaled route, are commonly prescribed in CF. Approximately one quarter of patients have bronchial hyperreactivity.[156–159] In these patients, bronchodilators may improve respiratory symptoms and airway secretion clearance. Whether these agents provide long-term benefit in CF is unknown. In general, inhaled β-adrenergic agents are used in patients with documented reversibility on spirometry or in those who receive symptomatic benefit. Inhaled anticholinergic agents, especially ipratropium bromide, may also have a role in CF.[160] Oral preparations, including theophylline, are not routinely used, have not been shown to be beneficial, and must be monitored carefully because of pharmacokinetic variability.

There is a clear rationale for using anti-inflammatory agents to decrease neutrophilic inflammation and the harmful effects of neutrophil products. Initial studies designed to test this approach used high doses of corticosteroids. Although patients receiving 1 to 2 mg/kg of prednisolone on alternate days had a slowed decline in lung function (ΔFEV_1 of –2% versus –6% in placebo group, at 48 months), there were unacceptable side effects.[161–163] Glucose metabolism abnormalities and delayed linear growth limit chronic therapy with oral corticosteroids. The risk–benefit ratio may favor their use in patients with ABPA. Inhaled steroids also have been studied in CF, but studies clearly suggest that with the exception of patients who have concomitant asthma, there are few if any benefits and some possible risks.[164]

An alternative means to decrease neutrophilic inflammation is high-dose ibuprofen. In a 4-year study, young patients (5 to 13 years) with mild lung disease ($FEV_1 \geq$ 60% of predicted) benefited from twice-daily ibuprofen at doses sufficient to achieve peak blood levels of 50 to 100 mg/L. In those who complied with therapy, the annual rate of change in FEV_1 was –1.5%, versus –3.5% in the placebo group. Nutritional status and radiographic indices of disease activity also were improved in the treated group, and few side effects were encountered.[165]

Low-dose macrolide antibiotics (clarithromycin and azithromycin) are effective as immunomodulatory medications and can decrease neutrophil-dominated airway inflammation and improve pulmonary function in patients with CF.[166] A large multicenter study demonstrated significant lung function improvement and fewer intravenous antibiotic courses in subjects with CF on azithromycin.[167] A meta-analysis of four studies with 296 participants concluded that there is a small but significant treatment effect for azithromycin in improving pulmonary function in persons with CF.[168]

Exacerbations

The course of CF lung disease is punctuated by periodic episodes of increased airway infection and inflammation with worsened lung function. These exacerbation episodes occur more frequently and become more difficult to treat as lung disease progresses and bacterial resistance develops. When exacerbations inevitably occur, an aggressive approach should be taken to reclaim lost lung function and to prevent early relapse with its associated risks.

Access to a CF center for early detection and treatment of an exacerbation is critically important. It has been reported that children with better lung function actually had *more* office sick visits, which implies that they were able to be treated promptly for pulmonary problems.[169] Typical features of an infectious exacerbation of CF lung disease include an increase in the frequency of cough and amount of sputum, diminished appetite, weight loss, fatigue, and a decrease in the FEV_1. Fever is not common, and high fever should prompt the search for other etiologies, including infection with *B cepacia* complex or atypical organisms (e.g., respiratory viruses, mycobacteria) or indwelling catheter infection. Leukocytosis is typically mild to moderate, and chest radiographs usually show little or no acute change.

During the initiation of therapy for a CF exacerbation, consideration of potential precipitating causes should include the presence of environmental allergens or irritants, inadequate airway clearance measures, allergic bronchopulmonary aspergillosis, and therapeutic medicine nonadherence. The adequacy of airway clearance at home, the severity of the exacerbation, the baseline severity of lung disease, and the complexity of the treatment regimen being instituted should be weighed during consideration of whether home therapy with intravenous antibiotics may be an option. In either environment, airway clearance maneuvers should be intensified, preferably to include airway clearance therapy at least four times daily to clear the airways. Antibiotics should be selected based on recent, pretreatment culture and sensitivity testing whenever possible. Every isolated organism is targeted when feasible, although patients often improve even when only selected organisms are targeted. *P aeruginosa*, *B cepacia* complex, and other typical gram-negative organisms (e.g., *S maltophilia*, *A xylosoxidans*) should be treated with two antibiotics from different drug classes. When both a gram-negative organism and

S aureus are cultured, antistaphylococcal therapy must be added. The duration of therapy is typically around 2 or 3 weeks but may be longer when the clinical response is slow. Pulmonary function testing near the end of a planned antibiotic course may be useful as an objective measure of the adequacy of therapy. Although some further improvement in lung function may occur even after completion of the antibiotic course, the return of lung function to preexacerbation levels is reassuring.

Lung Transplantation

Lung transplantation has become an accepted therapy for end-stage CF lung disease. The relative paucity of donor organs and subsequent long waiting times before organ availability mandate that patients be referred to transplant centers on a timely basis. With waiting times exceeding 2 years at some centers, close attention should be paid to clinical and testing results that predict a 2-year survival probability of 50%. These predictors include an FEV_1 of less than 30% of predicted, the rate of decline in lung function, and hypercapnia ($P_{CO_2} \geq 45$ mm Hg). The presence of an accelerated clinical decline, characterized by more frequent exacerbations that respond incompletely to aggressive therapy, recurrent pneumothoraces, massive hemoptysis, or panresistant organisms, should prompt consideration for earlier referral.[80–83,170] Optimal transplant candidates should not have significant nonpulmonary organ dysfunction (e.g., kidney, liver, heart), should be motivated and adherent with therapy, and should have adequate psychosocial support.

The surgical approach now preferred is sequential, bilateral transplantation rather than heart–lung transplantation. Alternatively, when a patient is not likely to survive until a cadaveric transplant can be performed, living donor lobar transplantation can be performed when healthy donors of sufficient size and correct blood type are available.[171] In either case, survival after transplantation appears no different in CF than in transplantation for other indications. The 5-year survival rate is approximately 48% and is limited primarily by opportunistic infections and chronic graft rejection, manifesting as bronchiolitis obliterans.[172]

KEY POINTS

- Cystic fibrosis is a prevalent inherited disorder that causes significant morbidity and premature mortality in those who suffer from it.
- Cystic fibrosis is the most common lethal genetic disease affecting the white population; it is autosomal recessive.
- Mutations in the CFTR gene result in several ion transport abnormalities, which in turn impair cough clearance and lung defense.
- Chronic infection and inflammation lead to progressive lung damage and respiratory failure in most patients.
- Improvements in care, including better antibiotics and nutritional support, have greatly extended survival.
- Cystic fibrosis is a multiorgan disease, with a broad spectrum of clinical manifestations.
- The combination of a typical CF clinical manifestation with evidence for abnormal CFTR is required for the diagnosis of cystic fibrosis.
- Preventive care is the cornerstone of effective CF management.
- Close monitoring of lung function, therapies aimed at airway clearance and minimization of infection, and nutritional support are necessary elements in CF care.
- Lung transplantation is an appropriate therapy for patients with severe CF lung disease. Evaluation for transplant in appropriate candidates should occur before the local waiting time for donor availability exceeds the anticipated survival time.

REFERENCES

1. Lobitz S, Velleuer E. Guido Fanconi (1892–1979): a jack of all trades. *Nat Rev Cancer.* 2006;6:893–898.
2. Andersen DH. Cystic fibrosis of the pancreas and its relation to celiac disease: a clinical and pathologic study. *Am J Dis Child.* 1938;56:344–399.
3. Farber S. Some organic digestive disturbances in early life. *J Mich Med Sci.* 1945;44:587–594.
4. di Sant'Agnese PA, Darling RC, Perera GA, et al. Abnormal electrolyte composition of sweat in cystic fibrosis of the pancreas. *Pediatrics.* 1953;12:549–563.
5. Gibson LE, Cooke RE. A test for concentration of electrolytes in sweat in cystic fibrosis on the pancreas utilizing pilocarpine by iontophoresis. *Pediatrics.* 1959;23:545–549.
6. Riordan JR, Rommens JM, Kerem B-T, et al. Identification of the cystic fibrosis gene: cloning and characterization of complementary DNA. *Science.* 1989;245:1066–1073.
7. Cystic Fibrosis Foundation. *Patient Registry Annual Data Report for 2008.* Bethesda, MD: Cystic Fibrosis Foundation; 2009.
8. Cystic Fibrosis Mutation Database. Statistics. Available at: http://www.genet.sickkids.on.ca/cftr/StatisticsPage.html.
9. Population variation of common cystic fibrosis mutations. The Cystic Fibrosis Genetic Analysis Consortium. *Hum Mutat.* 1994;4:167–177.
10. Zielenski J, Tsui LC. Cystic fibrosis: genotypic and phenotypic variations. *Annu Rev Genet.* 1995;29:777–807.
11. The Cystic Fibrosis Genotype-Phenotype Consortium. Correlation between genotype and phenotype in patients with cystic fibrosis. *N Engl J Med.* 1993;329:1308–1313.
12. Chillon M, Casals T, Mercier B, et al. Mutations in the cystic fibrosis gene in patients with congenital absence of the vas deferens. *N Engl J Med.* 1995;332:1475–1480.
13. Dork T, Dworniczak B, Aulehla-Scholz C, et al. Distinct spectrum of CFTR gene mutations in congenital absence of vas deferens. *Hum Genet.* 1997;100:365–377.
14. Greger R, Mall M, Bleich M, et al. Regulation of epithelial ion channels by the cystic fibrosis transmembrane conductance regulator. *J Mol Med.* 1996;74:527–534.
15. Stutts MJ, Rossier BC, Boucher RC. Cystic fibrosis transmembrane conductance regulator inverts protein kinase: a mediated regulation of epithelial sodium channel single channel kinetics. *J Biol Chem.* 1997;272:14037–14040.

16. Stutts MJ, Canessa CM, Olsen JC, et al. CFTR as a cAMP-dependent regulator of sodium channels. *Science.* 1995;269:847–850.
17. Mall M, Bleich M, Greger R, et al. The amiloride-inhibitable Na^+ conductance is reduced by the cystic fibrosis transmembrane conductance regulator in normal but not in cystic fibrosis airways. *J Clin Invest.* 1998;102:15–21.
18. Mall M, Bleich M, Kuehr J, et al. CFTR-mediated inhibition of epithelial Na^+ conductance in human colon is defective in cystic fibrosis. *Am J Physiol.* 1999;277:G709–G716.
19. Gabriel SE, Clarke LL, Boucher RC, et al. CFTR and outward rectifying chloride channels are distinct proteins with a regulatory relationship. *Nature.* 1993;363:263–268.
20. Egan M, Flotte T, Afione S, et al. Defective regulation of outwardly rectifying Cl^- channels by protein kinase A corrected by insertion of CFTR. *Nature.* 1992;358:581–584.
21. Kunzelmann K, Mall M, Briel M, et al. The cystic fibrosis transmembrane conductance regulator attenuates the endogenous Ca^{2+} activated Cl^- conductance of *Xenopus* oocytes. *Pflugers Arch.* 1997;435:178–181.
22. McNicholas CM, Guggino WB, Schwiebert EM, et al. Sensitivity of a renal K^+ channel (ROMK2) to the inhibitory sulfonylurea compound glibenclamide is enhanced by coexpression with the ATP-binding cassette transporter cystic fibrosis transmembrane regulator. *Proc Natl Acad Sci USA.* 1996;93:8083–8088.
23. Boucher RC, Stutts MJ, Knowles MR, et al. Na^+ transport in cystic fibrosis respiratory epithelia: abnormal basal rate and response to adenylate cyclase activation. *J Clin Invest.* 1986;78:1245–1252.
24. Cotton CU, Stutts MJ, Knowles MR, et al. Abnormal apical cell membrane in cystic fibrosis respiratory epithelium. An in vitro electrophysiologic analysis. *J Clin Invest.* 1987;79:80–85.
25. Matsui H, Grubb BR, Tartan R, et al. Evidence for periciliary liquid layer depletion, not abnormal ion composition, in the pathogenesis of cystic fibrosis airways disease. *Cell.* 1998;95:1005–1015.
26. Lindström M, Falk R, Hjelte L, et al. Long-term clearance from small airways in subjects with ciliary dysfunction. *Respir Res.* 2006;7:79.
27. Smith JJ, Travis SM, Greenberg EP, et al. Cystic fibrosis airway epithelia fail to kill bacteria because of abnormal airway surface fluid. *Cell.* 1996;85:229–236.
28. Travis SM, Conway BA, Zabner J, et al. Activity of abundant antimicrobials of the human airway. *Am J Respir Cell Mol Biol.* 1999;20:872–879.
29. Engelhardt JF, Yankaskas JR, Ernst SA, et al. Submucosal glands are the predominant site of CFTR expression in the human bronchus. *Nat Genet.* 1992;2:240–248.
30. Ballard ST, Trout L, Bebok Z, et al. CFTR involvement in chloride, bicarbonate, and liquid secretion by airway submucosal glands. *Am J Physiol.* 1999;277:L694–L699.
31. Henke MO, Renner A, Huber RM, et al. MUC5AC and MUC5B mucins are decreased in cystic fibrosis airway secretions. *Am J Respir Cell Mol Biol.* 2004;31:86–91.
32. Davril M, Degroote S, Humbert P, et al. The sialylation of bronchial mucins secreted by patients suffering from cystic fibrosis or from chronic bronchitis is related to the severity of airway infection. *Glycobiology.* 1999;9:311–321.
33. Wesley A, Forstner J, Qureshi R, et al. Human intestinal mucin in cystic fibrosis. *Pediatr Res.* 1983;17:65–69.
34. Cheng PW, Boat TF, Cranfill K, et al. Increased sulfation of glycoconjugates by cultured nasal epithelial cells from patients with cystic fibrosis. *J Clin Invest.* 1989;84:68–12.
35. Bonfield TL, Konstan MW, Berger M. Altered respiratory epithelial cell cytokine production in cystic fibrosis. *J Allergy Clin Immunol.* 1999;104:72–78.
36. Bonfield TL, Konstan MW, Burfeind P, et al. Normal bronchial epithelial cells constitutively produce the anti-inflammatory cytokine interleukin-10, which is downregulated in cystic fibrosis. *Am J Respir Cell Mol Biol.* 1995;13:257–261.
37. Bonfield TL, Panuska JR, Konstan MW, et al. Inflammatory cytokines in cystic fibrosis lungs. *Am J Respir Crit Care Med.* 1995;152:2111–2118.
38. Muhlebach MS, Stewart PW, Leigh MW, et al. Quantitation of inflammatory responses to bacteria in young cystic fibrosis and control patients. *Am J Respir Crit Care Med.* 1999;160:186–191.
39. Noah TL, Black HR, Cheng PW, et al. Nasal and bronchoalveolar lavage fluid cytokines in early cystic fibrosis. *J Infect Dis.* 1997;175:638–647.
40. Stern RC. The diagnosis of cystic fibrosis. *N Engl J Med.* 1997;336:487–491.
41. Farrell PM, Rosenstein BJ, White TB, et al. Guidelines for the diagnosis of cystic fibrosis in newborns through older adults: Cystic Fibrosis Foundation consensus report. *J Pediatr.* 2008;153:S4–S14.
42. Knowles M, Gatzy J, Boucher R. Increased bioelectric potential difference across respiratory epithelia in cystic fibrosis. *N Engl J Med.* 1981;305:1489–1495.
43. Knowles MR, Paradiso AM, Boucher RC. In vivo nasal potential difference: techniques and protocols for assessing efficacy of gene transfer in cystic fibrosis. *Hum Gene Ther.* 1995;6:445–455.
44. Gharib R, Allen RP, Joos HA, et al. Paranasal sinuses in cystic fibrosis: incidence of roentgen abnormalities. *Am J Dis Child.* 1964;108:499–502.
45. Stern RC, Jones K. Nasal and sinus disease. In: Yankaskas JR, Knowles MR, eds. *Cystic Fibrosis in Adults.* Philadelphia: Lippincott-Raven; 1999:221–231.
46. Gysin C, Alothman GA, Papsin BC. Sinonasal disease in cystic fibrosis: clinical characteristics, diagnosis and management. *Pediatr Pulmonol.* 2000;30:481–489.
47. Robertson JM, Friedman EM, Rubin BK. Nasal and sinus disease in cystic fibrosis. *Paediatr Respir Rev.* 2008;9:213–219.
48. King VV. Upper respiratory disease, sinusitis and polyposis. *Clin Rev Allergy.* 1991;9:143–157.
49. Jaffe BF, Strome M, Khaw KT, et al. Nasal polypectomy and sinus surgery for cystic fibrosis—a 10 year review. *Otolaryngol Clin North Am.* 1977;10:81–90.
50. Shwachman H, Kowalski M, Khaw KT. Cystic fibrosis: a new outlook. 70 patients above 25 years of age. *Medicine (Baltimore).* 1977;56:129–149.
51. Durie PR, Forstner GG. The exocrine pancreas. In: Yankaskas JR, Knowles MR, eds. *Cystic Fibrosis in Adults.* Philadelphia: Lippincott-Raven; 1999:261–287.
52. Shwachman H, Lebenthal E, Khaw KT. Recurrent acute pancreatitis in patients with cystic fibrosis with normal pancreatic enzymes. *Pediatrics.* 1975;55:86–95.
53. Cohn JA, Friedman KJ, Noone PG, et al. Relation between mutations of the cystic fibrosis gene and idiopathic pancreatitis. *N Engl J Med.* 1998;339:653–658.
54. Sharer N, Schwarz M, Malone G, et al. Mutations of the cystic fibrosis gene in patients with chronic pancreatitis. *N Engl J Med.* 1998;339:645–652.
55. Alves Cde A, Aquias RA, Alves AC, Santana MA. Diabetes mellitus in patients with cystic fibrosis. *J Bras Pneumol.* 2007;33:213–221.
56. Lanng S. Glucose intolerance in cystic fibrosis patients. *Paediatr Respir Rev.* 2001;2:253–259.
57. Marshall BC, Butler SM, Stoddard M, et al. Epidemiology of cystic fibrosis-related diabetes. *J Pediatr.* 2005;146:681–687.
58. Fischmann D, Nookala VK. Cystic fibrosis-related diabetes mellitus: etiology, evaluation and management. *Endoc Pract.* 2008;14:1169–1179.
59. di Sant'Agnese PA, Hubbard VS. The gastrointestinal tract. In: Taussig LM, ed. *Cystic Fibrosis.* New York: Thieme-Stratton; 1984:212–229.

60. di Sant'Agnese PA, Davis PB. Cystic fibrosis in adults. 75 cases and a review of 232 cases in the literature. *Am J Med.* 1979;66:121–132.
61. Gaskin KJ. Intestines. In: Yankaskas JR, Knowles MR, eds. *Cystic Fibrosis in Adults.* Philadelphia: Lippincott-Raven; 1999:325–342.
62. Robertson MB, Choe KA, Joseph PM. Review of the abdominal manifestations of cystic fibrosis in the adult patient. *Radiographics.* 2006;26:679–690.
63. Borowitz DS, Grand RJ, Durie PR. Use of pancreatic enzyme supplements for patients with cystic fibrosis in the context of fibrosing colonopathy. Consensus Committee. *J Pediatr.* 1995;127:681–684.
64. Fitzsimmons SC, Burkhart GA, Borowitz D, et al. High-dose pancreatic-enzyme supplements and fibrosing colonopathy in children with cystic fibrosis. *N Engl J Med.* 1997;336:1283–1289.
65. Stevens JC, Maguiness KM, Hollingsworth J, et al. Pancreatic enzyme supplementation in cystic fibrosis patients before and after fibrosing colonopathy. *J Pediatr Gastroenterol Nutr.* 1998;26:80–84.
66. Ledson MJ, Tran J, Walshaw MJ. Prevalence and mechanisms of gastro-esophageal reflux in adult cystic fibrosis patients. *J R Soc Med.* 1998;91:7–9.
67. Malfroot A, Dab I. New insights on gastro-oesophageal reflux in cystic fibrosis by longitudinal follow up. *Arch Dis Child.* 1991;66:1339–1345.
68. Stringer DA, Sprigg A, Juodis E, et al. The association of cystic fibrosis, gastroesophageal reflux, and reduced pulmonary function. *Can Assoc Radiol J.* 1988;39:100–102.
69. Colombo C, Crosignani A, Battezzati PM. Liver involvement in cystic fibrosis. *J Hepatol.* 1999;31:946–954.
70. Colombo C, Crosignani A, Melzi ML, et al. Hepatobiliary system. In: Yankaskas JR, Knowles MR, eds. *Cystic Fibrosis in Adults.* Philadelphia: Lippincott-Raven; 1999:309–324.
71. Scott-Jupp R, Lama M, Tanner MS. Prevalence of liver disease in cystic fibrosis. *Arch Dis Child.* 1991;66:698–701.
72. Jebbink MC, Heijerman HG, Masclee AA, et al. Gallbladder disease in cystic fibrosis. *Neth J Med.* 1992;41:123–126.
73. King L, Scurr E, Murugan N, et al. Hepatobiliary and pancreatic manifestations of CF: MR imaging appearances. *Radiographics.* 2000;20:767–777.
74. Lyon A, Bilton D. Fertility issues in cystic fibrosis. *Paediatr Respir Rev.* 2002;3:236–240.
75. Flume PA, Yankaskas JR. Reproductive issues. In: Yankaskas JR, Knowles MR, eds. *Cystic Fibrosis in Adults.* Philadelphia: Lippincott-Raven; 1999:449–464.
76. Silber SJ. The use of epididymal sperm for the treatment of male infertility. *Baillieres Clin Obstet Gynaecol.* 1997;11:739–752.
77. Kopito LE, Kosasky HJ, Shwachman H. Water and electrolytes in cervical mucus from patients with cystic fibrosis. *Fertil Steril.* 1973;24:512–516.
78. Fiel SB, Fitzsimmons S. Pregnancy in patients with cystic fibrosis. *Pediatr Pulmonol.* 1997;16(suppl):111–112.
79. Nussbaum E, Boat TF, Wood RE, et al. Cystic fibrosis with acute hypoelectrolytemia and metabolic alkalosis in infancy. *Am J Dis Child.* 1979;133:965–966.
80. Linnane B, Robinson P, Ranganathan S, Stick S, Murray C. Role of high-resolution computed tomography in the detection of early cystic fibrosis lung disease. *Paediatr Respir Rev.* 2008;9:168–174.
81. Moore EH. Atypical mycobacterial infection in the lung: CT appearance. *Radiology.* 1993;187:777–782.
82. Hartman TE, Swensen SJ, Williams DE. *Mycobacterium avium-intracellulare* complex: evaluation with CT. *Radiology.* 1993;187:23–26.
83. Wagener JS, Headley AA. Cystic fibrosis: current trends in respiratory care. *Respir Care.* 2003;48:234–245.
84. Konstan MW, Morgan WJ, Butler SM, et al. Scientific Advisory Group and the Investigators and Coordinators of the Epidemiologic Study of Cystic Fibrosis: risk factors for rate of decline in forced expiratory volume in one second in children and adolescents with cystic fibrosis. *J Pediatr.* 2007;151:134–139.
85. Boehler A. Update on cystic fibrosis: selected aspects related to lung transplantation. *Swiss Med Wkly.* 2003;133:111–117.
86. Davies JC, Cunningham S, Alton EW, Innes JA. Lung clearance index in CF: a sensitive marker of lung disease severity. *Thorax.* 2008;63:96–97.
87. Ballard RD, Sutarik JM, Clover CW, et al. Effects of non-REM sleep on ventilation and respiratory mechanics in adults with cystic fibrosis. *Am J Respir Crit Care Med.* 1996;153:266–271.
88. Bradley S, Solin P, Wilson J, et al. Hypoxemia and hypercapnia during exercise and sleep in patients with cystic fibrosis. *Chest.* 1999;116:647–654.
89. Marcus CL, Bader D, Stabile MW, et al. Supplemental oxygen and exercise performance in patients with cystic fibrosis with severe pulmonary disease. *Chest.* 1992;101:52–57.
90. Nixon PA, Orenstein DM, Curtis SE, et al. Oxygen supplementation during exercise in cystic fibrosis. *Am Rev Respir Dis.* 1990;142:807–811.
91. Fraser KL, Tullis DE, Sasson Z, et al. Pulmonary hypertension and cardiac function in adult cystic fibrosis: role of hypoxemia. *Chest.* 1999;115:1321–1328.
92. Kerem E, Reisman J, Corey M, et al. Prediction of mortality in patients with cystic fibrosis. *N Engl J Med.* 1992;326:1187–1191.
93. Khan TZ, Wagener JS, Bost T, et al. Early pulmonary inflammation in infants with cystic fibrosis. *Am J Respir Crit Care Med.* 1995;151:1075–1082.
94. Gilligan PH. Microbiology of cystic fibrosis lung disease. In: Yankaskas JR, Knowles MR, eds. *Cystic Fibrosis in Adults.* Philadelphia: Lippincott-Raven; 1999:93–114.
95. Dasenbrook EC, Merlo CA, Diener-West M, et al. Persistent methicillin-resistant *Staphylococcus aureus* and rate of FEV_1 decline in cystic fibrosis. *Am J Respir Crit Care Med.* 2008;178:814–821.
96. Saiman L, Siegel J. Infection control in cystic fibrosis. *Clin Microbiol Rev.* 2004;17:57–71.
97. Frederiksen B, Koch C, Hoiby N. Changing epidemiology of *Pseudomonas aeruginosa* infection in Danish cystic fibrosis patients (1974–1995). *Pediatr Pulmonol.* 1999;28:159–166.
98. Pressler T, Frederiksen B, Skov M, et al. Early rise of anti-*Pseudomonas* antibodies and a mucoid phenotype of *Pseudomonas aeruginosa* are risk factors for development of chronic infection—a case control study. *J Cyst Fibros.* 2006;5:9–15.
99. Li Z, Kosorok MR, Farrell PM, et al. Longitudinal development of mucoid *Pseudomonas aeruginosa* infection and lung disease progression in children with cystic fibrosis. *JAMA.* 2005;293:581–588.
100. LiPuma JJ. Update on the *Burkholderia* nomenclature and resistance. *Clin Microbiol Newsletter.* 2007;29(9):65–69.
101. Lewin LO, Byard PJ, Davis PB. Effect of *Pseudomonas cepacia* colonization on survival and pulmonary function of cystic fibrosis patients. *J Clin Epidemiol.* 1990;43:125–131.
102. Aris R, Routh J, LiPuma J, et al. *Burkholderia cepacia* complex in cystic fibrosis patients after lung transplantation: survival linked to genomovar type. *Am J Respir Crit Care Med.* 2001;164:2102–2106.
103. Mahenthiralingam E, Vandamme P, Campbell M, et al. Infection with *Burkholderia cepacia* complex genomovars in patients with cystic fibrosis: virulent transmissible strains of genomovar III can replace *Burkholderia multivorans. Clin Infect Dis.* 2001;33:1469–1471.
104. Holmes A, Nolan R, Taylor R, et al. An epidemic of *Burkholderia cepacia* transmitted between patients with and without cystic fibrosis. *J Infect Dis.* 1999;179:1197–1205.

105. Sun L, Jiang RZ, Steinbach S, et al. The emergence of a highly transmissible lineage of cbl+ *Pseudomonas (Burkholderia) cepacia* causing CF centre epidemics in North America and Britain. *Nat Med.* 1995;1:661–666.
106. Goldstein R, Sun L, Jiang RZ, et al. Structurally variant classes of pilus appendage fibers coexpressed from *Burkholderia (Pseudomonas) cepacia. J Bacteriol.* 1995;177:1039–1052.
107. LiPuma JJ, Dasen SE, Nielson DW, et al. Person-to-person transmission of *Pseudomonas cepacia* between patients with cystic fibrosis. *Lancet.* 1990;336:1094–1096.
108. Saiman L, Siegel J. Infection control in cystic fibrosis. *Clin Microbiol Rev.* 2004;17:57–71.
109. Krzewinski JW, Nguyen CD, Foster JM, Burns JL. Use of random amplified polymorphic DNA polymerase chain reaction to determine the epidemiology of *Stenotrophomonas maltophilia* and *Achromobacter (Alcaligenes) xylosoxidans* from patients with cystic fibrosis. *J Clin Microbiol.* 2001;39:3597–3602.
110. Valdezate S, Vindel A, Maiz L, et al. Persistence and variability of *Stenotrophomonas maltophilia* in cystic fibrosis patients, Madrid, 1991–1998. *Emerg Infect Dis.* 2001;7:113–121.
111. Davies JC, Rubin BK. Emerging and unusual gram-negative infections in cystic fibrosis. *Semin Respir Crit Care Med.* 2007;28:312–321.
112. Knutsen A, Slavin RG. Allergic bronchopulmonary mycosis complicating cystic fibrosis. *Semin Respir Infect.* 1992;7:179–192.
113. Whittier S, Hopfer RL, Knowles MR, et al. Improved recovery of mycobacteria from respiratory secretions of patients with cystic fibrosis. *J Clin Microbiol.* 1993;31:861–864.
114. Kilby JM, Gilligan PH, Yankaskas JR, et al. Nontuberculous mycobacteria in adult patients with cystic fibrosis. *Chest.* 1992;102:70–75.
115. Oliver KN. Nontuberculosis mycobacteria. I: multicenter prevalence study in cystic fibrosis. *Am J Respir Crit Care Med.* 2003;167:828–834.
116. Cullen AR, Cannon CL, Mark EJ, Colin AA. *Mycobacterium abscessus* infection in cystic fibrosis. *Am J Respir Crit Care Med.* 2000;161:641–645.
117. Esther CR Jr. *Mycobacterium abscessus* infection in young children with cystic fibrosis. *Pediatr Pulmonol.* 2005;40:39–44.
118. Griffith DE, Girard WM, Wallace RJ. Clinical features of pulmonary disease caused by rapidly growing mycobacteria: an analysis of 154 patients. *Am Rev Respir Dis.* 1993;147:1271–1278.
119. Stern RC, Wood RE, Boat TF, et al. Treatment and prognosis of massive hemoptysis in cystic fibrosis. *Am Rev Respir Dis.* 1978;117:825–828.
120. Yoon W, Kim JK, Kim YH, et al. Bronchial and nonbronchial systemic artery embolization for life-threatening hemoptysis: a comprehensive review. *Radiographics.* 2002;22:1395–1409.
121. Brinson GM, Noone PG, Mauro MA, et al. Bronchial artery embolization for the treatment of hemoptysis in patients with cystic fibrosis. *Am J Respir Crit Care Med.* 1998;157:1951–1958.
122. Barben JU, Ditchfield M, Carlin JB, et al. Major haemoptysis in children with cystic fibrosis: a 20 year retrospective study. *J Cyst Fibros.* 2003;2:105–111.
123. Vidal V, Therasse E, Berthiaume Y, et al. Bronchial artery embolization in adults with cystic fibrosis: impact on the clinical course and survival. *J Vasc Interv Radiol.* 2006;17:953–958.
124. Schidlow DV, Taussig LM, Knowles MR. Cystic Fibrosis Foundation consensus conference report on pulmonary complications of cystic fibrosis. *Pediatr Pulmonol.* 1993;15:187–198.
125. Yankaskas JR, Egan TM, Mauro MA. Major complications. In: Yankaskas JR, Knowles MR, eds. *Cystic Fibrosis in Adults.* Philadelphia: Lippincott-Raven; 1999:175–193.
126. Nocturnal Oxygen Therapy Trial Group. Continuous or nocturnal oxygen therapy in hypoxemic chronic obstructive lung disease: a clinical trial. *Ann Intern Med.* 1980;93:391–398.
127. Spier S, Rivlin J, Hughes D, et al. The effect of oxygen on sleep, blood gases, and ventilation in cystic fibrosis. *Am Rev Respir Dis.* 1984;129:712–718.
128. Wedzicha JA, Muir JF. Noninvasive ventilation in chronic obstructive pulmonary disease, bronchiectasis and cystic fibrosis. *Eur Respir J.* 2002;20(3):777–784.
129. Vedam H, Moriarty C, Torzillo PJ, et al. Improved outcomes of patients with cystic fibrosis admitted to the intensive care unit. *J Cyst Fibros.* 2004;3:8–14.
130. Sood S, Paradowski LJ, Yankaskas JR. Outcomes of ICU care in adults with cystic fibrosis. *Am J Respir Crit Care Med.* 2001;163:335–338.
131. Young AC, Wilson JW, Kotsimbos TC, Naughton MT. Randomised placebo controlled trial of non-invasive ventilation for hypercapnia in cystic fibrosis. *Thorax.* 2008;63:72–77.
132. Holland AE, Denehy L, Ntoumenopoulos G, et al. Non-invasive ventilation assists chest physiotherapy in adults with acute exacerbations of cystic fibrosis. *Thorax.* 2003;58:880–884.
133. Granton JT, Shapire C, Keston S. Noninvasive respiratory support in advanced lung disease from cystic fibrosis. *Respir Care.* 2002;47:675–681.
134. van der Schans CP. Conventional chest physical therapy for obstructive lung disease. *Respir Care.* 2007;52:1198–1209.
135. Myers TR. Positive expiratory pressure and oscillatory positive expiratory pressure therapies. *Respir Care.* 2007;52:1308–1327.
136. Volsko TA, DiFiore J, Chatburn RL. Performance comparison of two oscillating positive expiratory pressure devices: Acapella vs Flutter. *Respir Care.* 2003;48:124–130.
137. Chatburn RL. High frequency assisted airway clearance. *Respir Care.* 2007;52:1224–1237.
138. Volsko TA. The value of conducting laboratory investigations on airway clearance devices. *Respir Care.* 2008;53:311–313.
139. Lester ML, Flume PA, Gray SL, et al. Nebulizer use and maintenance by cystic fibrosis patients: a survey study. *Respir Care.* 2004;49:1504–1508.
140. Homnick DN. Making airway clearance successful. *Paediatr Respir Rev.* 2007;8:40–45.
141. Havermans T, De Boeck K. Cystic fibrosis: a balancing act? *J Cyst Fibros.* 2007;6:161–162.
142. Fereday J, MacDougall C, Spizzo M, et al. "There's nothing I can't do—I just put my mind to anything and I can do it": a qualitative analysis of how children with chronic disease and their parents account for and manage physical activity. *BMC Pediatr.* 2009;9:1–16.
143. Fuchs HJ, Borowitz DS, Christiansen DH, et al. Effect of aerosolized recombinant human DNase on exacerbations of respiratory symptoms and on pulmonary function in patients with cystic fibrosis. The Pulmozyme Study Group. *N Engl J Med.* 1994;331:637–642.
144. Voynow JA, Rubin BK. Mucus, mucins, and sputum. *Chest.* 2009;135:505–512.
145. Kater A, Henke MO, Rubin BK. The role of DNA and actin polymers on the polymer structure and rheology of cystic fibrosis sputum and depolymerization by gelsolin or thymosin beta 4. *Ann N Y Acad Sci.* 2007;1112:140–153.
146. Robinson M, Hemming AL, Regnis JA, et al. Effect of increasing doses of hypertonic saline on mucociliary clearance in patients with cystic fibrosis. *Thorax.* 1997;52:900–903.
147. Robinson M, Regnis JA, Bailey DL, et al. Effect of hypertonic saline, amiloride, and cough on mucociliary clearance in patients with cystic fibrosis. *Am J Respir Crit Care Med.* 1996;153:1503–1509.
148. Daviskas E, Anderson SD, Gonda I, et al. Inhalation of hypertonic saline aerosol enhances mucociliary clearance in asthmatic and healthy subjects. *Eur Respir J.* 1996;9:725–732.

149. Eng PA, Morton J, Douglass JA, et al. Short-term efficacy of ultrasonically nebulized hypertonic saline in cystic fibrosis. *Pediatr Pulmonol.* 1996;21:77–83.
150. Wark P, McDonald VM. Nebulised hypertonic saline for cystic fibrosis. *Cochrane Database Syst Rev.* 2009;(2):CD001506.
151. Rodwell LT, Anderson SD. Airway responsiveness to hyperosmolar saline challenge in cystic fibrosis: a pilot study. *Pediatr Pulmonol.* 1996;21:282–289.
152. Daviskas E, Anderson SD, Jaques A, Charlton B. Inhaled mannitol improves the hydration and surface properties of sputum in patients with cystic fibrosis. *Chest.* 2009 (in press). doi: 10.1378/chest.09-2017.
153. Ramsey BW, Pepe MS, Quan JM, et al. Intermittent administration of inhaled tobramycin in patients with cystic fibrosis. Cystic Fibrosis Inhaled Tobramycin Study Group. *N Engl J Med.* 1999;340:23–30.
154. Jensen T, Pedersen SS, Game S, et al. Colistin inhalation therapy in cystic fibrosis patients with chronic *Pseudomonas aeruginosa* lung infection. *J Antimicrob Chemother.* 1987;19:831–838.
155. Frederiksen B, Lanng S, Koch C, et al. Improved survival in the Danish center-treated cystic fibrosis patients: results of aggressive treatment. *Pediatr Pulmonol.* 1996;21:153–158.
156. Hordvik NL, Konig P, Morris D, et al. A longitudinal study of bronchodilator responsiveness in cystic fibrosis. *Am Rev Respir Dis.* 1985;131:889–893.
157. Hordvik NL, Sammut PH, Judy CG, et al. Effects of standard and high doses of salmeterol on lung function of hospitalized patients with cystic fibrosis. *Pediatr Pulmonol.* 1999;27:43–53.
158. Hordvik NL, Sammut PH, Judy CG, et al. The effects of albuterol on the lung function of hospitalized patients with cystic fibrosis. *Am J Respir Crit Care Med.* 1996;154:156–160.
159. Konig P, Poehler J, Barbero GJ. A placebo-controlled, double-blind trial of the long-term effects of albuterol administration in patients with cystic fibrosis. *Pediatr Pulmonol.* 1998;25:32–36.
160. Sanchez I, De Koster J, Holbrow J, et al. The effect of high doses of inhaled salbutamol and ipratropium bromide in patients with stable cystic fibrosis. *Chest.* 1993;104:842–846.
161. Auerbach HS, Williams M, Kitkpatrick JA, et al. Alternate-day prednisone reduces morbidity and improves pulmonary function in cystic fibrosis. *Lancet.* 1985;2:686–688.
162. Eigen H, Rosenstein BJ, Fitzsimmons S, et al. A multicenter study of alternate-day prednisone therapy in patients with cystic fibrosis. Cystic Fibrosis Foundation Prednisone Trial Group. *J Pediatr.* 1995;126:515–523.
163. Rosenstein BJ, Eigen H. Risks of alternate-day prednisone in patients with cystic fibrosis. *Pediatrics.* 1991;87:245–246.
164. Balfour-Lynn IM, Welch K. Inhaled corticosteroids for cystic fibrosis. *Cochrane Database Syst Rev.* 2009;(1):CD001915.
165. Konstan MW, Byard PJ, Hoppel CL, et al. Effect of high-dose ibuprofen in patients with cystic fibrosis. *N Engl J Med.* 1995;332:848–854.
166. López-Boado YS, Rubin BK. Macrolides as immunomodulatory medications for the therapy of chronic lung diseases. *Curr Opin Pharmacol.* 2008;8:286–291.
167. Saiman LB, Marshall C, Mayer-Hamblett N, et al. for the Macrolide Study Group. Azithromycin in patients with cystic fibrosis chronically infected with *Pseudomonas aeruginosa*: a randomized controlled trial. *JAMA.* 2003;290:1749–1756.
168. Southern KW, Barker PM, Solis A. Macrolide antibiotics for cystic fibrosis. *Cochrane Database Syst Rev.* 2004;CD002203.
169. Padman R, McColley SA, Miller DP, et al. Infant care patterns at epidemiologic study of cystic fibrosis sites that achieve superior childhood lung function. *Pediatrics.* 2007;199:531–537.
170. Rosenblatt RL. Lung transplantation in cystic fibrosis. *Respir Care.* 2009:54:777–787.
171. Cohen RG, Barr ML, Schenkel FA, et al. Living-related donor lobectomy for bilateral lobar transplantation in patients with cystic fibrosis. *Ann Thorac Surg.* 1994;57:1423–1427.
172. Yankaskas JR, Mallory GB Jr. Lung transplantation in cystic fibrosis: consensus conference statement. *Chest.* 1998;113:217–226.

CHAPTER 40

Acute Lung Injury and the Acute Respiratory Distress Syndrome

Michael A. Gentile
Christopher E. Cox

OUTLINE

Definition
Incidence
Etiology
Clinical Manifestations
Pathobiology
The National Institutes of Health ARDS Network
Management
Outcomes

OBJECTIVES

1. Define acute lung injury (ALI) and acute respiratory distress syndrome (ARDS).
2. List common risk factors for ALI and ARDS.
3. Recognize the clinical, radiographic, and pathophysiologic features of ALI and ARDS.
4. Describe the pathobiology of ALI and ARDS.
5. Discuss the experimental and proven therapeutic interventions for ALI and ARDS, including pharmacologic and mechanical therapies.
6. Describe how ALI and ARDS affect long-term physical functioning and quality of life.

KEY TERMS

acute lung injury (ALI)
acute respiratory distress syndrome (ARDS)
ARDS Network (ARDSnet)
lung injury score
mechanical ventilation
oxygenation index (OI)
PaO_2/FIO_2 ratio
plateau pressure
positive end-expiratory pressure (PEEP)
primary ARDS
prone position
secondary ARDS

INTRODUCTION

Acute lung injury (ALI) and the **acute respiratory distress syndrome (ARDS)** are a spectrum of critical illnesses characterized by diffuse damage to the alveolocapillary lung structures with hypoxemia and noncardiogenic pulmonary edema. ARDS is a worldwide public health issue with significant morbidity and mortality that affects both medical and surgical patients. Respiratory therapists play an essential role in the early recognition of ALI and ARDS and contribute to the multidisciplinary team approach required to manage these life-threatening conditions. Having a solid understanding of the epidemiology, diagnosis, and management of ALI and ARDS is essential in the care of these critically ill patients.

Definition

The first clinical description of ARDS was in 1967, when Ashbaugh et al.[1] identified 12 patients with trauma, aspiration, and pulmonary infection who presented with acute dyspnea, hypoxia, diffuse pulmonary infiltrates, and decreased pulmonary compliance. This was initially termed "adult" respiratory distress syndrome to distinguish it from neonatal acute respiratory failure that had similar physiologic derangements but was due to immature lungs with inadequate surfactant production.[2] Later, the name was changed to "acute" respiratory distress syndrome as it became apparent that diffuse lung injury from a variety of causes could affect both adult and pediatric populations.

In 1994, the American–European Consensus Conference (AECC) recommended the definition for use in the identification of patients with ARDS as "an acute clinical illness characterized by the development of bilateral pulmonary infiltrates on chest radiograph and severe hypoxemia with a $Pa{O_2}/F{IO_2}$ ratio of less than 200 mm Hg in the absence of congestive heart failure."[3] The AECC also recognized a less severe form of ARDS, termed acute lung injury (ALI), with similar clinical findings but with a qualifying $Pa{O_2}/F{IO_2}$ of less than 300 (**Table 40–1**). These definitions continue to be used today in the identification of patients at risk for ALI and ARDS.

The effort to standardize the definition of ALI and ARDS is important to facilitate communication among clinicians and to accurately describe populations in clinical trials. Unfortunately, this broad and simplistic AECC definition does not take into account important physiologic factors affecting $Pa{O_2}/F{IO_2}$ (i.e., positive airway pressure and $F{IO_2}$ levels), and it ignores both etiologic and host factors that likely affect the biochemical, cellular, and genetic pattern of the illness. This can lead to inclusion of a wide variety of different clinical phenotypes in clinical studies, which can make interpretation and generalizability of trial results difficult.

From a physiologic perspective, one approach to a more accurate characterization of lung injury is the **lung injury score** developed by Murray.[4] It incorporates the level of **positive end-expiratory pressure (PEEP)**, the **$Pa{O_2}/F{IO_2}$ ratio**, a chest radiograph score, and lung compliance into a summary score that can be used to describe the severity of lung injury and to follow the course of the disease.

Another method used to quantify physiologic abnormalities in ARDS is to calculate the **oxygenation index (OI)**:

$$OI = [(\bar{P}aw \times F{IO_2})/Pa{O_2})] \times 100$$

where $\bar{P}aw$ is mean airway pressure. The OI incorporates $F{IO_2}$ and $\bar{P}aw$.[5,6] The OI has also been suggested as a severity score for use of methods such as high-frequency oscillatory ventilation (HFOV) and extracorporeal life support (ECLS).[5,6]

In the future, there will likely be newer methods to better characterize ARDS. For example, cytokine profiles, inflammatory cellular responses, genetic expression patterns, comorbidities, and accompanying organ injuries all have the potential to be used to characterize the various clinical phenotypes of ARDS.

Incidence

Efforts to determine the prevalence of ARDS have resulted in widely varying estimates. An initial report by the National Institutes of Health in 1972 estimated 75 cases of ARDS per 100,000 population (approximately 150,000 cases of ARDS per year) in the United States.[7] Other studies have often found lower estimates, ranging from 3 to 13.5 cases per 100,000 population.[8–10] The most recent study suggested a range of 79 to 86 per 100,000 person-years.[11] Approximately 10% to 15% of patients admitted to the intensive care unit (ICU) meet the AECC diagnostic criteria for ALI or ARDS.[12]

Etiology

Multiple clinical conditions have been associated with the development of ALI and ARDS (**Box 40–1**).[13] Risk factors can be described as those that cause direct injury to the lungs (such as pneumonia, aspiration of gastric contents, inhalation of toxic gases, or pulmonary contusion)—so-called **primary ARDS**—and those that cause indirect injury to the lung (such as sepsis and multiple trauma)—so-called **secondary ARDS**. Indeed, in the

TABLE 40–1 American–European Consensus Conference Definition of ALI and ARDS

Condition	$Pa{O_2}/F{IO_2}$ Ratio	Chest Radiograph	PAWP
ALI	≤300 mm Hg regardless of PEEP	Bilateral infiltrates	≤18 mm Hg or no clinical evidence of left atrial hypertension
ARDS	≤200 mm Hg regardless of PEEP	Bilateral infiltrates	≤18 mm Hg or no clinical evidence of left atrial hypertension

ALI, acute lung injury; ARDS, acute respiratory distress syndrome; PAWP, pulmonary artery wedge pressure; PEEP, positive end-expiratory pressure.

Reprinted with permission of the American Thoracic Society. Copyright © American Thoracic Society. From Bernard GR, Artigas A, Brigham KL, et al. The American–European Consensus Conference on ARDS: definitions, mechanisms, relevant outcomes, and clinical trial coordination. *Am J Respir Crit Care Med.* 1994;149:818–824. Official Journal of the American Thoracic Society; Diane Gern, Publisher.

BOX 40-1

Clinical Disorders Associated with ALI and ARDS

Direct Lung Injury (Primary Lung Injury)

Common causes
- Pneumonia
- Aspiration of gastric contents

Less common causes
- Pulmonary contusion
- Fat emboli
- Near-drowning
- Inhalation injury
- Reperfusion pulmonary edema after cardiopulmonary bypass

Indirect Lung Injury (Secondary Lung Injury)

Common causes
- Sepsis
- Trauma with shock and blood product transfusion

Less common causes
- Drug overdose
- Cardiopulmonary bypass
- Acute pancreatitis
- Transfusion of blood products

From Ware LB, Matthay MA. The acute respiratory distress syndrome. *N Engl J Med.* 2000;342:18:1334–1348.

case of indirect injury, ARDS is thought to be the result of systemic inflammation, which results in the release of proinflammatory mediators and neutrophil migration to the alveoli. Overall, patients with sepsis are those at the highest risk to develop ALI and ARDS, with a 40% incidence.[14] Secondary risk factors such as low serum pH, chronic lung disease, and chronic alcohol abuse have been associated with an increased risk for ALI and ARDS.[15] If patients with ARDS from a direct lung injury subsequently develop sepsis or shock, they can develop an indirect lung injury as well. Thus, the distinction between direct and indirect injury often is blurred.

Defining risk factors can help predict the onset of ALI and ARDS. Among those patients with a risk factor of sepsis, trauma, or aspiration, approximately 50% of patients who developed ALI and ARDS did so within 24 hours of meeting risk criteria.[15–17] Of the nearly 85% of those who ultimately develop ALI or ARDS, risk of occurrence is highest within the first 72 hours.[15–17] Clearly identified risk factors for ALI or ARDS can assist in the management of

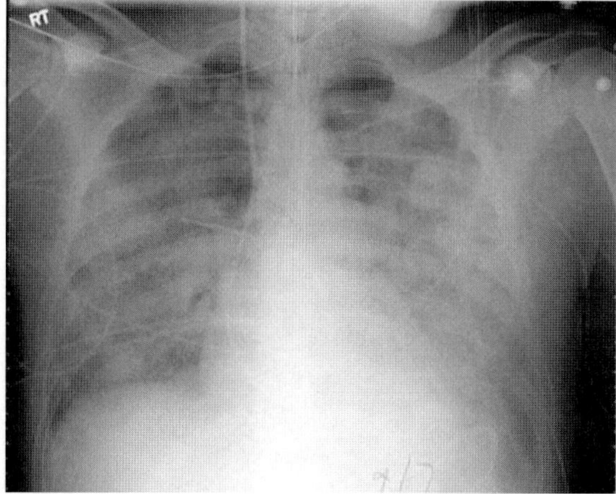

FIGURE 40–1 Anteroposterior supine radiograph of a patient with acute respiratory distress syndrome.

these patients in a timely fashion, with the goal of early detection, supportive management, and effective multidisciplinary care to optimize clinical outcomes.

Clinical Manifestations

Most patients with ALI or ARDS are symptomatic with progressive dyspnea and acutely abnormal oxygenation. Profound hypoxemia (e.g., a Pa_{O_2} of 60 mm Hg or an F_{IO_2} of 0.50) is primarily the result of shunt caused by atelectasis and alveolar flooding. In addition, disturbance of the normally protective mechanism of hypoxic pulmonary vasoconstriction contributes to shunt and hypoxemia. Patients in the first few days of ALI or ARDS experience a decrease in lung compliance, partly because of alveolar and interstitial edema, but also due to surfactant function impairment. Decreased compliance and hypoxemia together lead to rapid, shallow breathing with increased minute ventilation and an increased work of breathing. This usually culminates in the need for mechanical ventilatory support.

Chest radiographic findings show bilateral opacities reflecting inflammatory exudates and noncardiogenic pulmonary edema (**Figure 40–1**). The opacities may be confluent, patchy, or asymmetric and can be complicated by pleural effusions and heart failure. Because ALI and ARDS can represent a myriad of disease processes, the chest radiograph may also range from mild edema to profound whiteout, both extremes meeting the radiographic criteria for a diagnosis of ALI or ARDS. Subsequent chest radiographs in patients with persistent ARDS may reveal evidence of barotrauma such as pneumothoraces, pneumomediastinum, or pneumatoceles.[18]

Despite the appearance of diffuse infiltrates on the frontal chest radiograph, ARDS is not a homogeneous process. Although not commonly obtained for the diagnosis of ALI or ARDS, computed tomography (CT) of the chest demonstrates the heterogeneity of this disease (**Figure 40–2**).[19,20] More dependent portions of the lungs often demonstrate greater atelectasis than the more

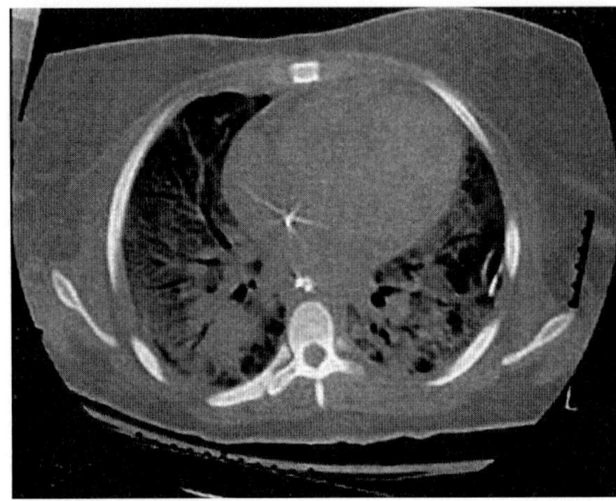

FIGURE 40–2 Computed tomography (CT) of the chest of a patient with acute respiratory distress syndrome.

nondependent areas. This helps explain the different effects of positive airway pressure seen in these different regions of the lung.[20,21]

In patients for whom this disease process continues longer than 3 to 7 days, the clinical characteristics often change. Profound hypoxemia may subside, but poor compliance often continues, in part because of fibrosis. Rather than intrapulmonary shunting, the problem at this phase, known as the fibroproliferative phase of ARDS, is increasing dead space (high-$\dot{V}/\dot{Q}$ regions) resulting in increasing minute ventilation requirements. Dead space in excess of 70% may occur and has been associated with high mortality.[22] The increased dead space as well as obstruction and destruction of pulmonary capillaries from microthrombi is attributed to fibrosis. These effects can lead to pulmonary hypertension and, in some cases, to right heart dysfunction.[23]

Pathobiology

The increased alveolar permeability in ALI and ARDS causes hypoxemia. Pathologically, ALI and ARDS are characterized by acute alveolar inflammation, neutrophil activation, surfactant deficiencies, damage to the alveolocapillary membrane (increased permeability, neutrophil and bacterial migration), and development of proteinaceous pulmonary edema and alveolar collapse.[17]

Destruction of the type I alveolar epithelial cells leads to detachment from their underlying basement membrane. This results in impairment of the normal anatomic barrier, which leads to increased permeability and resultant influx of protein-rich edema fluid into the interstitium and alveolar space (**Figure 40–3**). This denuded basement membrane becomes covered with a layer of fibrin, known as the hyaline membrane. These findings are described pathologically as diffuse alveolar damage. In patients with persistent lung injury (3 to 7 days after initial lung injury), the disease process progresses to a stage at which the basement membrane is replaced with a more fibrotic material enhanced by proliferation of alveolar type II cells. This fibrosis, in addition to contributing to the poor compliance of the lung, can contribute to loss of the alveolocapillary interface. Additional destruction of the pulmonary vasculature caused by fibrosis and thrombosis can lead to pulmonary hypertension.[24,25]

Although no clinically available systemic marker exists that correlates with lung injury, the study of alveolar fluid in patients with ALI and ARDS has been important in learning about the inflammatory response in the lungs of these patients. Comparison of the protein concentration in pulmonary edema fluid to the protein concentration in plasma soon after initiation of mechanical ventilation for respiratory failure has shown a consistently higher ratio in patients with permeability pulmonary edema (ALI and ARDS) than in patients with hydrostatic pulmonary edema (left heart failure).[26]

Bronchoalveolar lavage (BAL) is safe in this patient population and has been used to identify cells or inflammatory mediators that are consistent with ALI and ARDS or to predict which patients have a worse prognosis.[27] Although no one marker has proven to be both sensitive and specific, BAL results have provided a better understanding of the inflammation occurring in the alveolar space.[28–30] Analysis of BAL fluid in patients with early ARDS reveals a high percentage of neutrophils, usually present in only trace amounts in a normal lung lavage. As lung injury progresses, neutrophils tend to be replaced with alveolar macrophages and lymphocytes. However, there is a higher mortality in patients with persistence of alveolar neutrophils, due to their destructive nature and release of cellular debris.[31,32]

The National Institutes of Health ARDS Network

In 1994, the National Heart, Lung and Blood Institute of the National Institutes of Health (NIH) developed a clinical network to perform multicenter clinical trials of treatments for ALI and ARDS.[33] This group, the **ARDS Network (ARDSnet)**, is a clinical research network that consists of 40 hospitals, organized into 12 clinical sites, and a coordinating center. The ARDSnet was established to accelerate the development of successful management strategies for ALI and ARDS. The goal of the ARDSnet is to test promising agents, devices, and management strategies to improve the care of patients with ALI and ARDS.

Management

Management of patients with ALI and ARDS involves a multidisciplinary approach. Treatment of the underlying and causative pathophysiology is paramount. This includes hemodynamic management, appropriate use of antibiotics, and surgical intervention when required. These actions are used in conjunction with supportive care involving lung-protective mechanical ventilation strategies and prevention of nosocomial infection.

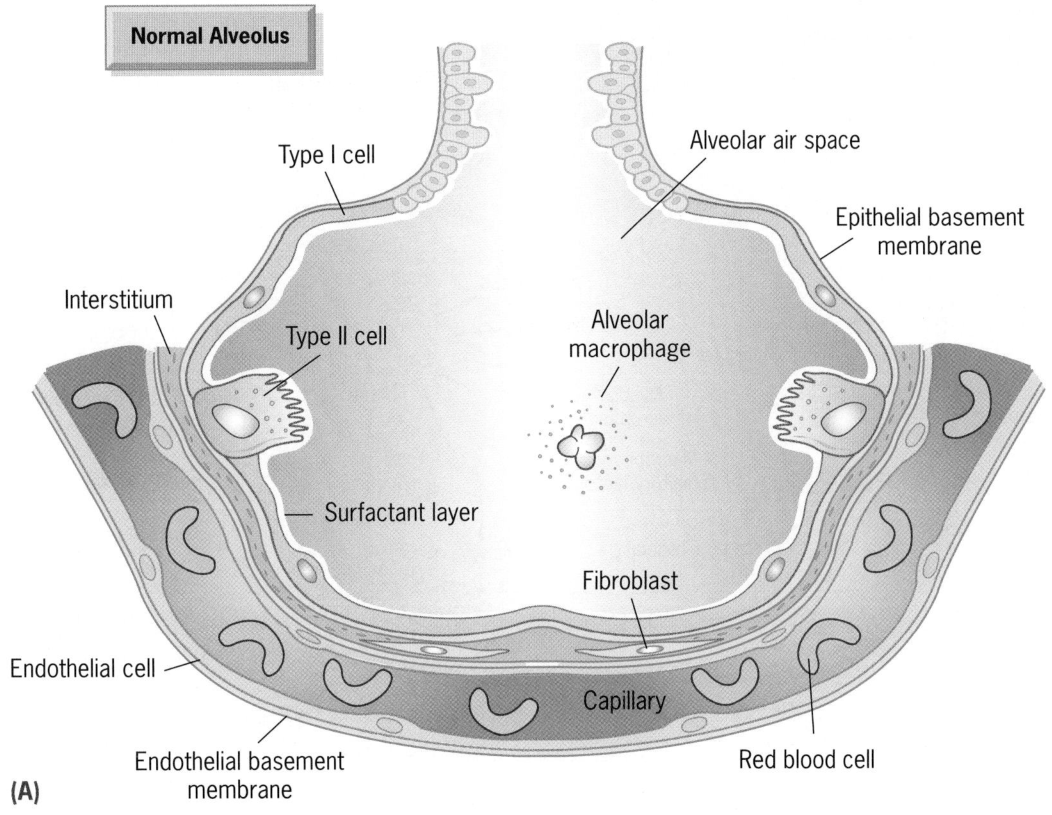

FIGURE 40–3 (**A**) Normal alveolus. (*continues*)

Positive Pressure Ventilation

Patients with ALI and ARDS present in either respiratory distress or respiratory failure (i.e., patients with symptomatic but not life-threatening physiology vs. patients with life-threatening physiology). For respiratory distress, dyspnea and hypoxemia should be treated with high-flow oxygen and preparations made for escalation of care, including endotracheal intubation. Because the course of ALI and ARDS may include hemodynamic instability, sedation, and multisystem organ failure, most patients are not candidates for noninvasive ventilation (NIV). Endotracheal intubation should be performed electively ahead of the patient progressing to full respiratory failure.

Mechanical ventilation is usually required due to the severity of hypoxemia and can be life saving for patients with ALI and ARDS. The goal of mechanical ventilation for these patients is support of gas exchange without inducing further injury to the lungs. Because of the heterogeneity of the lungs of patients with ALI and ARDS, mechanical ventilation strategies include alveolar recruitment while avoiding overdistention of normal lung units. Prolonged exposure to large tidal volume (V_T), high alveolar pressures, and high F_{IO_2} can cause destruction of the lung epithelium (both physically and by free radical formation) and release of inflammatory mediators.

High pressure can overdistend alveoli and contribute to a cascade of lung and systemic inflammatory responses that can worsen the underlying lung injury (ventilator-induced lung injury, or VILI). VILI can manifest as air leak (barotrauma), diffuse alveolar damage by overinflation (volutrauma), or shear stress when collapsed lung units repeatedly open and close (atelectrauma). *Biotrauma* refers to the migration of bacteria, neutrophils, and proinflammatory mediators from the lungs through the porous alveolocapillary membrane with eventual effects on distal organs. Growing appreciation for VILI has placed an emphasis on avoiding alveolar overdistention and cyclic alveolar collapse and reexpansion.

In the past, V_T was commonly set at 10 to 15 mL/kg of body weight to normalize gas exchange. What has been termed *lung-protective ventilation* reduces the V_T to near-normal ranges (4 to 8 mL/kg ideal body weight), thus decreasing the injurious alveolar stretch and subsequent release of inflammatory mediators. The use of a lung-protective ventilation strategy has been shown to reduce mortality and should be employed in all patients with ALI and ARDS.[34–40]

The best evidence supporting lung-protective ventilation comes from the ARDSnet study of higher versus lower V_T.[40] In this study, 861 patients were randomized to a V_T of 6 mL/kg (lung protective) or 12 mL/kg

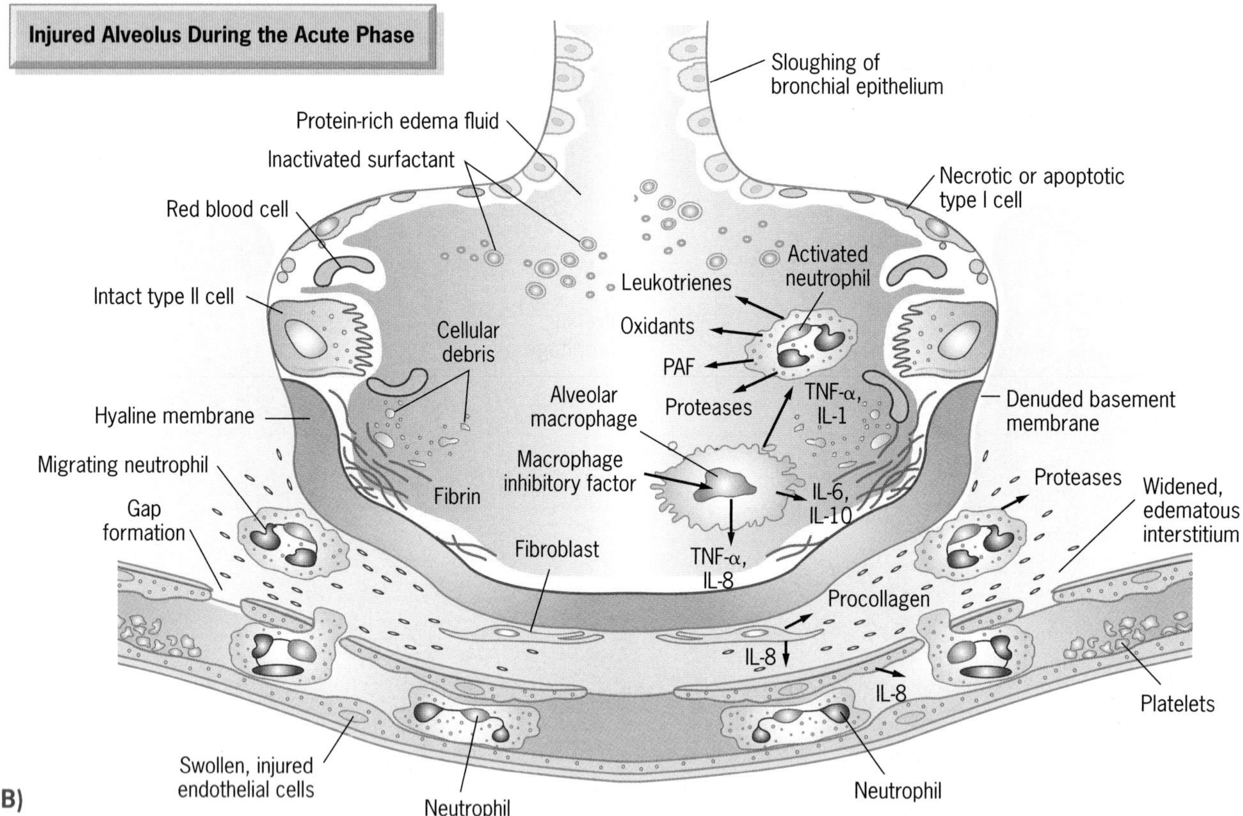

FIGURE 40–3 Continued. (**B**) The injured alveolus in the acute phase of the acute respiratory distress syndrome. Neutrophils are shown adhering to the injured capillary endothelium and marginating through the interstitium into the airspace, which is filled with protein-rich edema fluid. In the airspace, an alveolar macrophage is secreting cytokines, interleukins 1, 6, 8, and 10 (IL-1, IL-6, IL-8, and IL-10), and tumor necrosis factor α (TNF-α), which act locally to stimulate chemotaxis and activate neutrophils. Macrophages also secrete other cytokines, including IL-1, IL-6, and IL-10. Interleukin-1 can also stimulate the production of extracellular matrix by fibroblasts. Neutrophils can release oxidants, proteases, leukotrienes, and other proinflammatory molecules, such as platelet-activating factor (PAF). A number of anti-inflammatory mediators are also present in the alveolar milieu, including interleukin-1 receptor antagonist, soluble tumor necrosis factor receptor, autoantibodies against interleukin-8, and cytokines such as IL-10 and IL-11 (not shown). The influx of protein-rich edema fluid into the alveolus has led to the inactivation of surfactant. Adapted from Ware LB, Matthay MA. The acute respiratory distress syndrome. *N Engl J Med.* 2000;432:18:1334–1348.

(traditional), based on ideal body weight. **Plateau pressure** was limited to 30 cm H_2O in the lung-protective group and 50 cm H_2O in the traditional group. A significant mortality difference was noted: 31% in the lung-protective group compared with 40% in the traditional group. In addition, levels of plasma interleukin-6, an important inflammatory cytokine, were noted to be lower in the lung-protective group. These data support the hypothesis that alveolar stretch can propagate systemic inflammation and can subsequently lead to multiple organ dysfunction and death.[40]

Raising F_{IO_2} improves Pa_{O_2} in low-$\dot{V}/\dot{Q}$ units but has little effect on Pa_{O_2} in the presence of shunt. High F_{IO_2} can cause lung damage through free radical formation (oxygen toxicity). Thus, efforts should be made to minimize FiO_2 exposure.[41,42] PEEP improves oxygenation by maintaining alveolar recruitment and thereby reducing shunt. Increased alveolar recruitment with PEEP also improves lung compliance and likely reduces VILI from shear forces that result when alveoli repetitively open and close.[21,34] However, PEEP has some potential negative effects as well. By increasing intrathoracic pressure, it can decrease venous return and cardiac output. Additionally, PEEP can result in overdistention of open alveoli, VILI, and barotrauma.[43] The overdistention also can increase resistance to blood flow to ventilated areas, resulting in an increase in dead space.

Investigators have proposed various mechanical (e.g., pressure–volume curve) or radiographic (e.g., CT) approaches to optimize PEEP and F_{IO_2} settings. These approaches are cumbersome and impractical for routine use. Thus, balancing PEEP and F_{IO_2} to provide adequate gas exchange (e.g., Pa_{O_2} of 55 to 80 mm Hg) is often empiric. PEEP–F_{IO_2} tables were developed to assist clinicians in selecting the appropriate combinations of PEEP and F_{IO_2}. Attention to blood pressure, plateau pressure, and cardiac output (directly or by assessment of end-organ perfusion) is also important. Large multicenter randomized trials have evaluated higher versus moderate PEEP levels and have failed to show superiority of higher PEEP levels.[44–46] A meta-analysis of these studies confirmed that although a trend favored higher PEEP, the pooled results did not reach statistical significance.[47] The results of a subsequent meta-analysis suggest that higher levels of PEEP should be used with ARDS, whereas modest levels of PEEP should be used with ALI.[48] PEEP should not be abruptly discontinued. Even a brief reduction in PEEP may be associated with alveolar derecruitment, rapid arterial oxygen desaturation, and possibly pulmonary hypertension. This is particularly important during endotracheal suctioning.

High-frequency oscillatory ventilation (HFOV) delivers small VT, increased $\bar{P}aw$, and frequencies of 1 to 15 Hz (1 Hz = 60 breaths/min). Oxygenation is related to $\bar{P}aw$, facilitating the maintenance of end-expiratory lung volume, which may minimize VILI.[49] An observational study of adult patients with severe ARDS failing conventional ventilation reported a decrease in OI after starting HFOV.[50] There was no significant decrease in cardiac output despite significant increases in $\bar{P}aw$. The overall survival rate was 47%, and the number of days on conventional ventilation before initiating HFOV was associated with mortality. Another study reported that early institution of HFOV was a significant factor for improved mortality.[51] In a randomized controlled trial in adults with ARDS, found that 30-day mortality was 37% in the HFOV group and 52% in the conventional ventilation group, but this difference did not reach statistical significance.[52] Moreover, higher-than-recommended VT were used in the conventional ventilation group. The use of HFOV in the care of patients with ARDS is controversial.[53]

Extracorporeal Life Support

Despite maximal supportive care with mechanical ventilation, some patients with ARDS experience severe refractory hypoxemia. Extracorporeal life support (ECLS) uses venoarterial and venovenous approaches to remove CO_2 and add O_2 to blood. Venoarterial systems can provide complete cardiopulmonary bypass, whereas the simpler venovenous systems provide only partial support. Extracorporeal techniques provide adequate gas exchange with a lower inspired FIO_2 and reduced ventilation pressures. Complications include clot formation in the circuit, bleeding due to systemic anticoagulation, and technical failure. These complications are more common with venoarterial ECLS. Several studies have reported benefit with the use of ECLS in patients with ARDS and severe respiratory failure.[54,55] One study[55] reported improvement in survival without severe disability at 6 months in patients transferred to a specialist center for consideration of ECLS treatment compared with continued conventional ventilation. However, aspects of the design of this study have been criticized, and the role of ECLS in severe ARDS remains unclear.

Pharmacologic Agents

Given the inflammatory response in ALI and ARDS, the use of corticosteroids seems reasonable, given that they are potent inhibitors of inflammation. However, an appropriate balance of proinflammatory and anti-inflammatory mediators must be maintained.[56] Corticosteroids used early in the course of ARDS have not proven beneficial.[57–59] Small studies have not convincingly proven the benefit of steroids in the late, fibroproliferative phase of ARDS. One of these demonstrated an improvement in lung injury score and mortality, but the small sample size and crossover design of the trial warrant further confirmation.[59] A randomized controlled trial sponsored by the ARDSnet addressed the potential benefits of corticosteroids in late-stage ARDS.[60] Patients with ALI or ARDS of at least 7 days' duration were randomized to either intravenous methylprednisolone or placebo in a double-blind fashion. At 60 days, the hospital mortality rate was the same in each group. These results do not support the routine use of methylprednisolone for persistent ARDS despite the improvement in cardiopulmonary physiology.

Other anti-inflammatory agents such as ibuprofen, ketoconazole, and lisophylline have been shown to be ineffective in large randomized trials.[61,62] Some trials have investigated treatment with surfactant therapy.[63,64] Several different surfactant replacement products and delivery devices have been evaluated, but studies to date have not reported an improvement in survival.

Interventions with vitamin E or *N*-acetylcysteine have been pursued with varying results.[65–67] In a randomized controlled study comparing standard enteral feeding to a formula replete with antioxidants, fish oil, and borage oil (immunonutrition), the investigators reported less alveolar inflammation, shorter time on the ventilator and in the ICU, and fewer organ failures in patients receiving the intervention.[68] However, it remains to be determined whether this improves survival.

Inhaled nitric oxide (iNO) can decrease pulmonary artery pressure, improve right ventricular function, and improve ventilation-perfusion matching, leading to improved oxygenation.[69–71] Despite these potential advantages, randomized controlled trials of iNO in patients with ALI and ARDS did not have an effect on mortality or any other meaningful outcomes.[72,73] Its routine use is discouraged, especially given the significant expense associated with iNO. Other inhaled vasodilators, such as prostacyclin, are also used in patients with ARDS, but the effect of these agents on patient outcome is unknown.[74]

Patient Position

Changes in body position may improve oxygenation, particularly in patients with very asymmetric disease where the lateral decubitus position may improve ventilation-perfusion matching. The use of the **prone position** is based on restoration of ventilation to dorsal areas of the lung that are collapsed in the supine position. Physiologic data suggest that gas exchange is improved in the prone position,[75] presumably because it improves shunt.[76–78] Clinical improvement appears best in the early, exudative phase of ARDS. Although benefit may be seen in trauma patients with ARDS, the potential for complications is higher.[79] Prone positioning should be performed in a facility that is familiar with the procedure and that has the resources to safely perform the maneuver. Complications include removal of tubes and lines, pressure necroses, and ocular injury. Although the prone position results in improvement in oxygenation, it has not been shown to affect mortality or other meaningful outcomes.[80] Routine use of prone positioning is not recommended, but it may be considered in the setting of severe refractory hypoxemia.

Fluid Management

Because the pathophysiology of ALI and ARDS is characterized by lung edema formation, there has been longstanding interest in how best to manage fluids in these patients. On one hand, dry lungs would be expected to have better gas exchange and mechanical function. But on the other hand, fluid restriction and diuresis in a dry strategy may compromise cardiac output and oxygen delivery. An ARDSnet study showed that a strategy of even fluid balance led to shorter ventilator duration compared with a traditional strategy that usually results in 1 liter or more positive fluid balance per day. Importantly, this conservative fluid strategy did not increase the incidence of shock or renal failure.[81]

Outcomes

Mortality rates declined from a range of 60% to 70% in the early 1980s to 30% to 40% in the mid-1990s.[82,83] A 2009 examination of 18,900 patients from 89 published clinical trials reported a mortality of 44.3%, with 44% in observation studies and 36.2% in randomized controlled trials.[84] Another study evaluating the effect of age on survival reported advanced age as an independent risk factor for increased mortality in patients with ARDS.[85]

Approximately one-third of the mortality occurs within the first 72 hours after onset. The cause of death in these patients is usually related to their underlying risk, such as sepsis or trauma. Only a minority (15%) of patients die from respiratory failure. The majority of ARDS mortality is in the setting of sepsis or multisystem organ failure.[86,87]

Assessments of pulmonary function, neuropsychiatric testing, and quality of life are important markers of outcome. Pulmonary function tests performed within 2 weeks of extubation have shown substantial restrictive impairments.[86] Pulmonary function improved at 3 months, and further improvement was seen at 6 months. Little additional improvement was noted after that time, and no further gains were noted at 1 year. Most pulmonary function tests returned to normal at 1 year or had mild to moderate restriction, with an abnormal diffusing capacity being most common. This abnormal diffusing capacity is consistent with the known vascular destruction that occurs as part of the acute process of ARDS. Whereas many patients require oxygen at the time of hospital discharge, a persistent gas exchange abnormality at 1 year is uncommon, except for oxygen desaturation occasionally seen with exercise. Ultimate lung function is most consistently associated with the severity of the original lung injury and with duration of mechanical ventilation.

The impact of ARDS on quality of life was assessed by comparison of these patients with non-ARDS patients with similar levels of critical illness.[87] ARDS survivors were noted to have lower health-related quality of life scores. Decrements in perceived quality of life may persist for over a year. When tested at the 1-year interval, one-third of the patients had generalized cognitive decline, and 75% had at least one impairment in memory, attention, concentration, or mental processing speed.[88]

Although the outcome measures of pulmonary function, quality of life, and cognitive functioning are not as clearly defined or as readily attainable as mortality rates, they do represent a significant impact on the lives of the survivors.[89] Better understanding of these deficits will allow future research efforts to focus on these issues and will direct appropriate resources toward the care of these patients.

KEY POINTS

- Current practice uses the AECC criteria for ALI and ARDS.
- Because of differences in definitions and study design, no clear national or worldwide incidence of ARDS can be estimated at this time.
- The most common risk factors for ARDS are sepsis, aspiration of gastric contents, transfusions, and severe trauma.
- More than half of patients who develop ARDS do so within 24 hours of the risk onset.
- ARDS is a heterogeneous disease and is characterized by alveolar inflammation and increased permeability of the alveolocapillary membrane.
- There are no proven effective drug therapies for ARDS.
- The most important therapeutic advance for treatment of ARDS has been the identification of lung-protective ventilatory strategies.
- Use a tidal volume of 6 mL/kg ideal body weight and a plateau pressure of less than 30 cm H_2O.
- Use PEEP to maintain alveolar recruitment.
- Mortality for ARDS patients has decreased from nearly 70% in the 1980s to approximately 40% by 2009.
- ARDS survivors have mild to moderate pulmonary restriction and decreased diffusing capacity at 1 year.
- Decrements in quality of life and cognitive function also are noted in ARDS survivors.

REFERENCES

1. Ashbaugh DG, Bigelow DB, Petty TL, et al. Acute respiratory distress in adults. *Lancet.* 1967;12:319–323.
2. Petty TL, Ashbaugh DG. The adult respiratory distress syndrome; clinical features, factors influencing prognosis and principles of management. *Chest.* 1971;233–239.
3. Bernard GR, Artigas A, Brigham KL, et al. The American–European consensus conference on ARDS: definitions, mechanisms, relevant outcomes, and clinical trial coordination. *Am J Respir Crit Care Med.* 1994;149:818–824.
4. Murray JF, Matthay MA, Luce JM, et al. An expanded definition of the adult respiratory distress syndrome. *Am Rev Resp Dis.* 1988;138:720.
5. Mehta S, Granton J, MacDonald RJ, et al. High-frequency oscillatory ventilation in adults. *Chest.* 2004;126:518–527.
6. Monchi M, Bellenfant F, Cariou A, et al. Early predictive factors of survival in the acute respiratory distress syndrome. A multivariate analysis. *Am J Respir Crit Care Med.* 1998;158:1076–1081.
7. National Heart and Lung Institutes. *Task Force Report on Problems, Research Approaches, Needs.* Washington, DC: U.S. Government Printing Office; 1972:167–180.
8. Villar J, Slutsky AS. The incidence of the adult respiratory distress syndrome. *Am Rev Respir Dis.* 1989;140:814–816.
9. Lewandowski K, Metz J, Deutschmann C, et al. Incidence, severity, and mortality of acute respiratory failure in Berlin, Germany. *Am J Respir Crit Care Med.* 1995;151:1121–1125.
10. Thomsen GE, Morris AH. Incidence of the adult respiratory distress syndrome in the state of Utah. *Am J Respir Crit Care Med.* 1995;152:965–971.
11. Rubenfeld GD, Caldwell E, Peabody E, et al. Incidence and outcomes of acute lung injury. *N Engl J Med.* 2005;353:1685–1693.
12. Frutos-Vivar F, Nin N, Estaban A. Epidemiology of acute lung injury and acute respiratory distress syndrome. *Curr Opin Crit Care.* 2004;10:1–6.
13. Ware LB, Matthay MA. The acute respiratory distress syndrome. *N Engl J Med.* 2000;432:1334–1348.
14. Hudson LD, Milberg JA, Anardi D, et al. Clinical risks for development of the acute respiratory distress syndrome. *Am J Respir Crit Care Med.* 1995;151:293–301.
15. Doyle RL, Szaflarski N, Modin GW, et al. Identification of patients with acute lung injury. Predictors of mortality. *Am J Respir Crit Care Med.* 1995;152:1818–1824.
16. Hudson LD, Steinberg KP. Epidemiology of acute lung injury and ARDS. *Chest.* 1999;116:74S–82S.
17. Piantadosi CA, Schwartz DA. The acute respiratory distress syndrome. *Ann Intern Med.* 2004;141:460–471.
18. Steinberg KP. Diffuse pulmonary infiltrates and acute respiratory distress syndrome. In: Root RK, ed. *Clinical Infectious Diseases: A Practical Approach.* New York: Oxford University Press; 1999:557–564.
19. Gattinoni L, Caironi P, Valenza F, et al. The role of CT-scan studies for the diagnosis and therapy of acute respiratory distress syndrome. *Clin Chest Med.* 2006;27:559–570.
20. Gattinoni L, Caironi P, Cressoni M, et al. Lung recruitment in patients with the acute respiratory distress syndrome. *N Engl J Med.* 2006;354:1775–1786.
21. Gattinoni L, Pelosi P, Crotti S, et al. Effects of positive end-expiratory pressure on regional distribution of tidal volume and recruitment in adult respiratory distress syndrome. *Am J Respir Crit Care Med.* 1995;151:1807–1814.
22. Nuckton TJ, Alonso JA, Kallet RH, et al. Pulmonary dead-space fraction as a risk factor for death in the acute respiratory distress syndrome. *N Engl J Med.* 2002;346:1281–1286.
23. Brower RG, Ware LB, Berthiaume Y, et al. Treatment of ARDS. *Chest.* 2001;120:1347–1367.
24. Artigas A, Bernard GR, Carlet J, et al. The American–European Consensus Conference on ARDS. Part 2. Ventilatory, pharmacologic, supportive therapy, study design strategies, and issues related to recovery and remodeling. *Am J Respir Crit Care Med.* 1998;157:1332–1347.
25. Idell S. Endothelium and disordered fibrin turnover in the injured lung: newly recognized pathways. *Crit Care Med.* 2002;30:S274–S280.
26. Matthay MA, Wiener-Kronish JP. Intact epithelial barrier function is critical for the resolution of alveolar edema in humans. *Am Rev Respir Dis.* 1990;142:1250–1257.
27. Steinberg KP, Mitchell DR, Maunder RJ, et al. Safety of bronchoalveolar lavage in patients with adult respiratory distress syndrome. *Am Rev Respir Dis.* 1993;148:556–561.
28. Pugin J, Verghese G, Widmer M, et al. The alveolar space is the site of intense inflammatory and profibrotic reactions in the early phase of acute respiratory distress syndrome. *Crit Care Med.* 1999;27:237–238.
29. Goodman RB, Strieter RM, Martin DP, et al. Inflammatory cytokines in patients with persistence of the acute respiratory distress syndrome. *Am J Respir Crit Care Med.* 1996;154:601–611.
30. Martin TR. Lung cytokines and ARDS. *Chest.* 1999;116:2S–8S.
31. Steinberg KP, Milberg JA, Martin TR, et al. Evolution of bronchoalveolar cell populations in the adult respiratory distress syndrome. *Am J Respir Crit Care Med.* 1994;150:113–122.
32. Meduri GU, Headley S, Kohler G, et al. Persistent elevation of inflammatory cytokines predicts a poor outcome in ARDS. Plasma IL-1 and IL-6 levels are consistent and efficient predictors of outcome over time. *Chest.* 1995;107:1062–1073.
33. Kallet RH. What is the legacy of the National Institutes of Health Acute Respiratory Distress Syndrome Network? *Respir Care.* 2009;54:912–924.
34. Webb HH, Tierney DF. Experimental pulmonary edema due to intermittent positive pressure ventilation with high inflation pressures: protection by positive end-expiratory pressure. *Am Rev Respir Dis.* 1974;110:556–565.
35. Dreyfuss D, Saumon G. Role of tidal volume, FRC, and end-inspiratory volume in the development of pulmonary edema following mechanical ventilation. *Am Rev Respir Dis.* 1993;148:1194–1203.
36. Brochard L, Roudot-Thoraval F, Roupie E, et al. Tidal volume reduction for prevention of ventilator-induced lung injury in acute respiratory distress syndrome. The Multicenter Trial Group on Tidal Volume Reduction in ARDS. *Am J Respir Crit Care Med.* 1998;158:1831–1838.
37. Stewart TE, Meade MO, Cook DJ, et al. Evaluation of a ventilation strategy to prevent barotrauma in patients at high risk for acute respiratory distress syndrome. *N Engl J Med.* 1998;338:355–361.
38. Amato MB, Barbas CS, Medeiros DM, et al. Effect of a protective-ventilation strategy on mortality in the acute respiratory distress syndrome. *N Engl J Med.* 1998;338:347–354.
39. Ranieri VM, Suter PM, Tortorella C, et al. Effect of mechanical ventilation on inflammatory mediators in patients with acute respiratory distress syndrome: a randomized controlled trial. *JAMA.* 1999;282:54–61.
40. The Acute Respiratory Distress Syndrome Network. Ventilation with lower tidal volumes as compared with traditional tidal volumes for acute lung injury and the acute respiratory distress syndrome. *N Engl J Med.* 2000;342:1301–1318.
41. Singer MM, Wright F, Stanley LK, et al. Oxygen toxicity in man. A prospective study in patients after open-heart surgery. *N Engl J Med.* 1970;283:1473.
42. Frank L, Roberts RJ. Endotoxin protection against oxygen-induced acute and chronic lung injury. *J Appl Physiol.* 1979;47:577–581.
43. Rouby JJ, Lu Q, Goldstein I. Selecting the right level of positive end expiratory pressure in patients with acute respiratory distress syndrome. *Am J Respir Crit Care Med.* 2002;165:1182–1186.
44. Brower RG, Lanken PN, MacIntyre N, et al. Higher versus lower positive end-expiratory pressures in patients with the acute respiratory distress syndrome. *N Engl J Med.* 2004;351:327–336.
45. Meade MO, Cook DJ, Guyatt GH, et al. Ventilation strategy using low tidal volumes, recruitment maneuvers, and high positive

end-expiratory pressure for acute lung injury and acute respiratory distress syndrome: a randomized controlled trial. *JAMA.* 2008;299:637–645.
46. Mercat A, Richard JC, Vielle B, et al. Positive end-expiratory pressure setting in adults with acute lung injury and acute respiratory distress syndrome: a randomized controlled trial. *JAMA.* 2008;299:646–655.
47. Oba Y, Thameem DM, Zaza T. High levels of PEEP may improve survival in acute respiratory distress syndrome: a meta analysis. *Respir Med.* 2009;103:1174–1181.
48. Briel M, Meade M, Mercat A, Brower RG, et al. Higher vs lower positive end-expiratory pressure in patients with acute lung injury and acute respiratory distress syndrome: systematic review and meta-analysis. *JAMA.* 2010;303:865–873.
49. Pillow JJ. High-frequency oscillatory ventilation: mechanisms of gas exchange and lung mechanics. *Crit Care Med.* 2005;33:S135–141.
50. Fort P, Farmer C, Westerman J, et al. High frequency oscillatory ventilation for adult respiratory distress syndrome—a pilot study. *Crit Care Med.* 1997;25:937–947.
51. Mehta S, Lapinsky SE, Hallett DC, et al. Prospective trial of high-frequency oscillation in adults with acute respiratory distress syndrome. *Crit Care Med.* 2001;29:1360–1369.
52. Derdak S, Mehta S, Stewart TE, et al. Multicenter Oscillatory Ventilation for Acute Respiratory Distress Syndrome Trial (MOAT) study investigators: high-frequency oscillatory ventilation for acute respiratory distress syndrome in adults. *Am J Respir Crit Care Med.* 2002;166:801–808.
53. Fessler HE, Hess DR. Respiratory controversies in the critical care setting. Does high-frequency ventilation offer benefits over conventional ventilation in adult patients with acute respiratory distress syndrome? *Respir Care.* 2007;52:595–608.
54. The Australia and New Zealand Extracorporeal Membrane Oxygenation Influenza Investigators. Extracorporeal membrane oxygenation for 2009 influenza (H1N1) acute respiratory distress syndrome. *JAMA.* 2009;302:1535–1545.
55. Peek GJ, Mugford M, Tiruvoipati R, et al. Efficacy and economic assessment of conventional ventilatory support versus extracorporeal membrane oxygenation for severe adult respiratory failure (CESAR): a multicentre randomised controlled trial. *Lancet.* 2009;374:1351–1363.
56. Martin TR. Cytokines and the acute respiratory distress syndrome (ARDS): a question of balance. *Nature Med.* 1997;3:272–273.
57. Lefering R, Neugebauer EA. Steroid controversy in sepsis and septic shock: a meta-analysis. *Crit Care Med.* 1995;23:1294–1303.
58. Cronin L, Cook DJ, Carlet J, et al. Corticosteroid treatment for sepsis: a critical appraisal and meta-analysis of the literature. *Crit Care Med.* 1995;23:1430–1439.
59. Meduri GU, Headley AS, Golden E, et al. Effect of prolonged methylprednisolone therapy in unresolving acute respiratory distress syndrome: a randomized controlled trial. *JAMA.* 1998;280:159–165.
60. Steinberg KP, Hudson LD, Goodman RB, et al. Efficacy and safety of corticosteroids for persistent acute respiratory distress syndrome. *N Engl J Med.* 2006;354:1671–1684.
61. The Acute Respiratory Distress Syndrome Network. Ketoconazole for early treatment of acute lung injury and acute respiratory distress syndrome: a randomized controlled trial. The ARDS Network. *JAMA.* 2000;283:1995–2002.
62. Bernard GR, Wheeler AP, Russell JA, et al. The effects of ibuprofen on the physiology and survival of patients with sepsis. The Ibuprofen in Sepsis Study Group. *N Engl J Med.* 1997;336:912–918.
63. Weg JG, Balk RA, Tharratt RS, et al. Safety and potential efficacy of an aerosolized surfactant in human sepsis-induced adult respiratory distress syndrome. *JAMA.* 1994;272:1433–1438.
64. Gregory TJ, Steinberg KP, Spragg R, et al. Bovine surfactant therapy for patients with acute respiratory distress syndrome. *Am J Respir Crit Care Med.* 1997;155:1309–1315.
65. Domenighetti G, Suter PM, Schaller MD, et al. Treatment with *N*-acetylcysteine during acute respiratory distress syndrome: a randomized, double-blind, placebo-controlled clinical study. *J Crit Care.* 1997;12:177–182.
66. Jepsen S, Herlevsen P, Knudsen P, et al. Antioxidant treatment with *N*-acetylcysteine during adult respiratory distress syndrome: a prospective, randomized, placebo controlled study. *Crit Care Med.* 1992;20:918–923.
67. Suter PM, Domenighetti G, Schaller MD, et al. *N*-acetylcysteine enhances recovery from acute lung injury in man. *Chest.* 1994;105:190–194.
68. Gadek, JE, DeMichele SJ, Karlstad MD, et al. Effect of enteral feeding with eicosapentaenoic acid, gamma-linoleic acid, and antioxidants in patients with acute respiratory distress syndrome. Enteral Nutrition in ARDS Study Group. *Crit Care Med.* 1999;27:1409–1420.
69. Rossaint R, Falke KJ, Lopez F, et al. Inhaled nitric oxide for the adult respiratory distress syndrome. *N Engl J Med.* 1993;328:399–405.
70. Frostell CG, Blomqvist H, Hedenstierna G, et al. Inhaled nitric oxide selectively reverses human hypoxic pulmonary vasoconstriction without causing systemic vasodilation. *Anesthesiology.* 1993;78:427–435.
71. Gerlach H, Rossaint R, Pappert D, et al. Time-course and dose-response of nitric oxide inhalation for systemic oxygenation and pulmonary hypertension in patients with adult respiratory distress syndrome. *Eur J Clin Invest.* 1993;23:499–502.
72. Dellinger RP, Zimmerman JL, Taylor RW, et al. Effects of inhaled nitric oxide in patients with acute respiratory distress syndrome: results of a randomized phase II trial. Inhaled Nitric Oxide in ARDS Study Group. *Crit Care Med.* 1998;26:15–23.
73. Michael JR, Barton RG, Saffle JR, et al. Inhaled nitric oxide versus conventional therapy: effect on oxygenation in ARDS. *Am J Respir Crit Care Med.* 1998;157:1372–1380.
74. Siobal MS, Hess DR. Are inhaled vasodilators useful in acute lung injury and acute respiratory distress syndrome? *Respir Care.* 2010;55:144–161.
75. Albert RK, Hubmayr RD. The prone position eliminates compression of the lungs by the heart. *Am J Respir Crit Care Med.* 2000;161:1660–1665.
76. Lamm WJE, Graham MM, Albert RK. Mechanism by which the prone position improves oxygenation in acute lung injury. *Am J Respir Crit Care Med.* 1994;150:184–193.
77. Nakos G, Tsangaris I, Kostanti E, et al. Effect of the prone position on patients with hydrostatic pulmonary edema compared with patients with acute respiratory distress syndrome and pulmonary fibrosis. *Am J Respir Crit Care Med.* 2000;161:360–368.
78. Jolliet P, Bulpa P, Chevrolet J. Effects of the prone position on gas exchange and hemodynamics in severe acute respiratory distress syndrome. *Crit Care Med.* 1998;26:1977–1985.
79. Offner PJ, Haenel JB, Moore EE, et al. Complications of prone ventilation in patients with multisystem trauma with fulminant acute respiratory distress syndrome. *J Trauma.* 2000;48:224–228.
80. Sud S, Sud M, Friedrich JO, et al. Effect of mechanical ventilation in the prone position on clinical outcomes in patients with acute hypoxemic respiratory failure: a systematic review and meta-analysis. *CMAJ.* 2008;178:1153–1161.
81. Wheeler AP, Bernard GR, Thompson BT, et al. Pulmonary-artery versus central venous catheter to guide treatment of acute lung injury. *N Engl J Med.* 2006;354:2213–2224.
82. Montgomery AB, Stager MA, Carrico CJ, et al. Causes of mortality in patients with the adult respiratory distress syndrome. *Am Rev Respir Dis.* 1985;132:485–489.
83. Milberg JA, Davis DR, Steinberg KP, et al. Improved survival of patients with acute respiratory distress syndrome (ARDS): 1983–1993. *JAMA.* 1995;273:306–309.
84. Phua J, Badia JR, Adhikari KJ, et al. Has mortality from acute respiratory distress syndrome decreased over time? *Am J Respir Crit Care Med.* 2009;179:220–227.

85. Sprenkle MD, Caldwell ES, Rubenfeld GD, et al. Mortality following acute respiratory distress syndrome (ARDS) among the elderly. *Am J Respir Crit Care Med*. 1999;159:A717.
86. McHugh LG, Milberg JA, Whitcomb ME, et al. Recovery of function in survivors of the acute respiratory distress syndrome. *Am J Respir Crit Care Med*. 1994;150:90–94.
87. Herridge MS, Cheung AM, Tansey CM, et al. One-year outcomes in survivors of the acute respiratory distress syndrome. *N Engl J Med*. 2003;348:683–693.
88. Hopkins RO, Weaver LK, Pope D, et al. Neuropsychological sequelae and impaired health status in survivors of severe acute respiratory distress syndrome. *Am J Respir Crit Care Med*. 1999;160:50–56.
89. Cox CE, Docherty SL, Brandon DH, et al. Surviving critical illness: acute respiratory distress syndrome as experienced by patients and their caregivers. *Crit Care Med*. 2009;37:2702–2708.

CHAPTER 41

Postoperative Respiratory Care

Mark Simmons
Priscilla Simmons

OUTLINE

OBJECTIVES

1. List the steps in preoperative assessment and management.
2. Identify factors that increase the risk of postoperative pulmonary complications.
3. List the studies commonly performed during preoperative testing.
4. Identify the intraoperative factors that contribute to postoperative pulmonary complications.
5. Describe the common assessment and management practices employed to combat postoperative respiratory failure.
6. Discuss the etiology, risk factors, clinical manifestations, diagnostic findings, and management of postoperative atelectasis.
7. Discuss the etiology, risk factors, clinical manifestations, diagnostic findings, and management of postoperative thromboembolic disease and pulmonary embolism.
8. Discuss the etiology, risk factors, clinical manifestations, diagnostic findings, and management of postoperative pneumonia.

KEY TERMS

atelectasis
deep vein thrombosis (DVT)
enteral tube feeding (ETF)
heparin
impedance plethysmography
myocardial ischemia
partial thromboplastin time (PTT)
patient-controlled analgesia (PCA)
pneumonia
pulmonary embolism (PE)
thrombolytic
tissue plasminogen activator (TPA)
total parenteral nutrition (TPN)

INTRODUCTION

Despite advances in the care of surgical patients, pulmonary complications are the leading cause of postoperative morbidity and death. Most patients having thoracic or upper abdominal surgery will have a decrease in pulmonary function after surgery as a result of decreased lung volumes, diaphragmatic dysfunction, and gas exchange abnormalities. In addition, anesthesia may depress the postoperative respiratory drive. Inhibition of cough and impaired airway clearance can contribute to risk of infection. However, many of these patients compensate for any decrease in pulmonary function with their pulmonary reserves. Postoperative pulmonary complications occur in approximately 7% of patients with normal preoperative lung function, and respiratory failure is rare without preexisting cardiopulmonary or neuromuscular disorders. With increased risk factors, however, pulmonary complications have been reported to be as high as 70%.[1] This chapter addresses some of the preoperative, intraoperative, and postoperative factors that increase the risk of postoperative pulmonary complications and respiratory failure. Also included is management of the postoperative patient to prevent postoperative respiratory failure.

Preoperative Assessment and Management

The goal of preoperative evaluation is to identify patients who are at risk for intraoperative or postoperative complications. If a patient at risk is identified, the next step is to determine how complications can be prevented. In some cases this may mean postponement of surgery or a change in the anesthesia or surgical plan. Other interventions include modification of risk factors such as smoking. The use of pulmonary medications and deep breathing exercises also may be appropriate for the prevention of postoperative complications.

> **RESPIRATORY RECAP**
>
> **Key Considerations in Preoperative Assessment and Management**
>
> » History and physical exam
> » Detailed planning of surgery and postsurgical care and complications
> » Patient education

An important first step in preoperative management is obtaining a patient history. A careful history may identify conditions that could increase the risk of postoperative pulmonary complications and note indications for preoperative screening tests. Detailed preoperative planning of the surgery is necessary, including considerations for postoperative care and complications to avoid.

Preoperative patient education is important. The patient should be informed of the type of surgery planned, the pain intensity expected postoperatively, and the type of respiratory therapy that may be required after surgery. Clearly, preoperative instruction about planned postoperative respiratory care procedures is important for effectiveness following surgery.[2,3] When patients are educated about postoperative expectations, they may require less analgesia in the postoperative period.

Multiple factors have been identified as risk factors for postoperative complications (**Box 41–1**).[2,4–9] Many of these are discussed in the following subsections.

> **BOX 41–1**
>
> **Patient Factors Increasing the Risk of Postoperative Pulmonary Complications**
>
> Age greater than 50 years
> Smoking history
> Preexisting pulmonary disease
> Obesity
> Obstructive sleep apnea
> Upper respiratory tract infection
> Heart failure
> Nutritional status

Age

Age is an independent morbidity and mortality risk factor for many diseases. When compared with patients younger than 50 years, aged patients had the following odds ratios for increased chance of postoperative pulmonary complications: 50 to 59 years, 1.5; 60 to 69 years, 2.28; 70 to 79 years, 3.9; and 80 years or older, 5.63.[2] Postoperative complications occur in half of patients older than 70 years. In the elderly, calcium channel blockers can affect mental function. Narcotics and sedatives can further compromise postoperative ventilatory function, leading to respiratory failure. Cardiopulmonary, hepatic, renal, and nervous system reserves are reduced in the elderly, which increases their susceptibility to decompensation.[10] Older people (older than 75 years) also have an augmented inflammatory response. These factors result in increased postoperative mortality rates.

> **AGE-SPECIFIC ANGLE**
>
> The elderly are at increased risk for postoperative respiratory complications.

Box 41–2 lists pulmonary changes seen in the elderly patient. Because of these changes, the use of supplemental oxygen is recommended after any operative procedure in the elderly. The increased work of breathing that accompanies increased age compromises capacity to meet the additional workload demand following surgery and may contribute to postoperative respiratory failure.

The elderly also have a decreased cardiac stress response and an increased association with coronary artery disease, placing them at high risk for cardiac

> **BOX 41–2**
>
> **Changes in the Pulmonary and Thoracic Systems of Elderly Individuals**
>
> Increased chest wall rigidity
> Increased expenditure of energy to move chest wall
> Decreased respiratory muscle strength (by 20% at age 70 years)
> Decreased functional surface area for gas exchange (by 15% at age 70 years)
> Increased $\dot{V}/\dot{Q}$ mismatch and decreased Pa_{O_2}
> Diminished response to hypoxemia and hypercapnia
> Decreased vital capacity
> Increased closing volume

AGE-SPECIFIC ANGLE

Operative factors affecting cardiovascular function have a greater effect on the elderly.

complications. Factors influencing cardiovascular function (e.g., hypotension, fluid volume, positive pressure ventilation) can have greater effects on the elderly than they do on the young.[10] Each of these factors increases the probability of pulmonary complications after surgery in the elderly.

Smoking History

A 20-pack-year or greater smoking history results in a higher incidence of postoperative complications when compared with a lower pack-year history. Smoking cessation has been shown to be beneficial in decreasing pulmonary complications of general anesthesia and surgery. Smoking cessation for 4 to 8 weeks prior to surgery yielded a significant decrease in pulmonary complications compared with those who continued to smoke.[4,11–14] Persons who had stopped smoking for more than 6 months had complication rates similar to those who never smoked. Heavy smokers have a higher rate of pulmonary complications than light smokers and may benefit from refraining from smoking for even 1 day before surgery. This allows carboxyhemoglobin levels to decrease and improves oxygen-carrying capacity.

Preexisting Lung Disease

Patients with asthma and chronic obstructive pulmonary disease (COPD) are at increased risk for postoperative complications. Chronic lung disease has been identified as the most significant factor for increased risk of postoperative pulmonary complications, including respiratory failure. Patients with COPD have an increase in postoperative complications ranging from 26% to 78%, and patients with symptomatic asthma also have an increased risk of morbidity from anesthesia. Surgery on these patients should occur when they are symptom free or when their symptoms are well controlled. There is no increased postoperative risk for patients with well-controlled asthma.[2–4]

Increased residual volume, decreased forced expiratory volume in the first second of exhalation (FEV_1), decreased diffusing capacity of the lung for carbon dioxide (D_{LCO}), and excessive sputum production are predictive for postoperative pulmonary complications.[15] Preoperative dyspnea also has been shown to correlate with increased postoperative complications. The use of antibiotics, bronchodilators, and steroids can reduce the risk of postoperative complications in high-risk patients. Antibiotics should be reserved for patients with evidence of infected sputum.[16] It seems reasonable, in these patients, to use a course of preoperative antibiotic therapy to eliminate the infection and delay surgery until the infection has resolved. This may reduce the risk of postoperative pneumonia.

Patients with pulmonary disease and hypoxemia are at increased risk for **myocardial ischemia** and cardiac complications.[17] Pulmonary complications are also among the most common encountered in patients with cardiac compromise. Patients with cardiopulmonary disease who undergo elective surgery should have their lung function optimized, be free of pulmonary infections, and have their heart failure controlled.

Obesity

Surgical mortality is not increased in obese patients, but morbidly obese patients are at increased risk for complications such as reduced lung volumes, atelectasis, ventilation-perfusion ($\dot{V}/\dot{Q}$) mismatch, and persistent hypoxemia. Comorbid conditions such as diabetes, asthma, and heart conditions commonly exist in the obese patient. However, obesity has not consistently been shown to be a risk factor for postoperative complications.[2,4] The discrepancy among reports may be due to inadequate distinguishing of obesity itself from comorbid conditions. Although obesity alone is not currently identified to be a significant risk factor for postoperative pulmonary complications, delaying surgery in morbidly obese patients may be appropriate until some weight loss can be achieved.

Morbidly obese patients undergo surgery for many, often nonelective, reasons. Bariatrics is the branch of medicine that deals with the prevention, control, and treatment of obesity. Bariatric surgery should be considered an elective procedure. Although weight-related comorbidities (diabetes and hypertension) are more prevalent in bariatric patients, they do not appear to increase surgical risk if they are managed preoperatively.[18,19] Obstructive sleep apnea (OSA) is also common in bariatric patients, but little evidence links OSA with perioperative complications.[20] It is reasonable to recommend the continuation of postoperative continuous positive airway pressure (CPAP) in these patients who use CPAP for sleep. Postoperative treatment for bariatric patients includes a head-up body position to improve lung volumes and decrease atelectasis and shunting. Although mortality rates are low immediately following bariatric surgery, one of the leading causes of death is pulmonary embolus.[21] Prophylactic use of lower extremity compression devices, low-dose heparin therapy, and early ambulation should be considered. The placement of a vena caval filter is recommended in patients who have a history of a hypercoagulable condition.[20]

General Health Status

Coronary artery disease is common in the surgical population, with up to 50% of postoperative deaths resulting from cardiac events. Most of these events are ischemic. Catecholamine release during surgery can predispose the patient to arrhythmias and possible coronary artery plaque rupture. Recent data indicate that use of beta blockers during the perioperative period can decrease ischemia and the incidence of myocardial infarction.[22] Heart failure has been shown to be a significant risk factor for postoperative pulmonary complications.[2] Stable heart function and careful management are required for patients undergoing surgery.

There is little information in the literature regarding pulmonary complications in patients with recent upper airway infections. It may be prudent to defer elective surgery in this patient population until the infection has resolved.

Little evidence addresses the risk of postoperative pulmonary complications in patients with OSA. However, OSA has the potential of increasing pulmonary complications.[23] It is prudent for patients with known OSA to use CPAP during sleep in the postoperative period.

Nutritional Status

Serum albumin levels less than 3.6 g/dL place the patient at risk for postoperative complications. Patients with a serum albumin value less than 2.5 g/dL or those with more than 10% weight loss should have nutritional repletion for 7 to 10 days before surgery. If diet alone cannot correct the problem, nutritional support may be indicated. Preoperative **total parenteral nutrition (TPN)** (i.e., intravenous administration) for malnourished patients is only indicated in selected patients. In general, postoperative administration of TPN has had dismal results. On the other hand, **enteral tube feeding (ETF)** (i.e., gastrointestinal administration) is well tolerated as long as the patient has adequate gastric motility and emptying. ETF improves postoperative morbidity and mortality better than TPN when used for preoperative nutritional support.[24–26]

Poor nutritional status in critically ill patients undergoing major surgery is associated with reduced systemic immunity and an exaggerated stress response. Weight loss (more than 10% from baseline), low ideal body weight (less than 85%), hypoalbuminemia, and protein-calorie malnutrition are all predictors of increased postoperative complications such as infection, organ system failure, delayed wound healing, and delayed functional recovery. Patients with at least one of these abnormalities have a significant increase in incidence of overall surgical complications, major complications, and increased length of stay compared with patients who have all normal markers. Severely malnourished patients have a high risk of postoperative complications.

Preoperative Testing

Millions of surgical operations and procedures are performed in the United States each year, with estimated billions of dollars being spent on preoperative laboratory and diagnostic studies. In general, these studies should be performed for specific clinical indications and not as a routine preoperative screen unless they will influence patient treatment and outcome. Little evidence supports routine screening of healthy patients with electrocardiograms (ECGs), chest radiographs, pulmonary function tests (PFTs), echocardiograms, or blood chemistry panels.[3,4,27,28] A complete history and physical, however, are a very important part of the preoperative assessment. It is during this time that significant risk factors should be identified. Following the history and physical, the appropriate screening tests can be determined.

RESPIRATORY RECAP

Preoperative Laboratory and Diagnostic Studies

- » Electrocardiogram
- » Chest radiograph
- » Arterial blood gas measurements
- » Pulmonary function testing

Electrocardiogram

A preoperative ECG is important for the patient with a history of circulatory and cardiac problems.[27] An ECG should not be performed as a routine preoperative screen or based on patient age alone. **Box 41–3** lists clinical indications for preoperative ECG. Exercise testing along with ECG monitoring is being done more frequently prior to surgery, especially in older patients. However, no data support its routine use in evaluation of patients prior to general surgery.

Chest Radiograph

Chest radiographs are not recommended as part of a routine protocol in healthy patients. Chest radiographs should be individualized and based on clinical indications.[27] Chest radiographs are indicated in patients with acute, progressive, or chronic cardiopulmonary disease and in patients at high risk for developing postoperative pulmonary complications. Abnormal chest radiographs are more frequent in older patients. It is reasonable to perform chest radiography on patients older than

BOX 41–3

Clinical Indications for Preoperative Electrocardiogram

Hypertension
Congestive heart failure
Diabetes
Chest pain
Dizziness
Syncope
Cerebral and peripheral vascular disease
Shortness of breath
Palpitations
Ankle edema
Abnormal valvular murmurs

50 years who are undergoing high-risk surgical procedures. **Box 41–4** lists indications for preoperative chest radiographs.

Arterial Blood Gas Measurements

Arterial blood gas measurements are not recommended as a general preoperative screening test,[27] but are indicated in patients with new or changing lung disease and in patients at high risk for lung disease. Patients with an increased $Paco_2$ have an increased incidence of postoperative pulmonary complications. A chronically elevated $Paco_2$ greater than 45 mm Hg predicts a high risk for pulmonary complications or death. A Pao_2 below 50 mm Hg may be a relative contraindication to surgery.

Pulmonary Function Tests

All patients who are candidates for lung resection should have pulmonary function testing. However, pulmonary function testing as a general preoperative screen for the presence of pulmonary disease in patients without a suggestive clinical history is not indicated and should not be done to predict postoperative pulmonary complications.[29] For abdominal and cardiac surgery, the predictive value of spirometry and determination of lung volumes is unproven. Spirometry should be obtained before the initiation of general anesthesia if the patient's respiratory symptoms have changed. Spirometry is indicated in patients with severe pulmonary dysfunction to assess whether pulmonary rehabilitation is indicated to improve the pulmonary condition prior to surgery.[8] Pulmonary function testing is also recommended in patients with neuromuscular disease, chest wall and spinal deformities, and morbid obesity. In patients with COPD, pulmonary function testing may help to assess the probability of early extubation.

BOX 41–4

Indications for Preoperative Chest Radiograph

- Pneumonia
- Pulmonary edema
- Atelectasis
- Aortic aneurysm
- Mediastinal or pulmonary masses
- Tracheal deviation
- Cardiomegaly
- Pulmonary hypertension
- Chronic obstructive pulmonary disease
- Pulmonary embolism
- Dextrocardia

Intraoperative Risk Factors

Several intraoperative factors contribute to postoperative pulmonary complications. These include surgical incision site, duration of surgery, type of anesthesia used during surgery, monitoring, and fluid management.

Surgical Incision Site

Surgical incision site is the most important factor in predicting the overall risk of postoperative pulmonary complications. Thoracic and upper abdominal incisions have been shown to have the most negative effects on pulmonary function and carry the highest rate of postoperative pulmonary complications. In general, the closer the incision is to the diaphragm, the greater the risk of pulmonary complications. Compared with lower abdominal surgeries, upper abdominal procedures double the risk.[30,31] Upper abdominal and thoracic surgeries carry a 20% to 70% pulmonary complication rate, compared with a 4% pulmonary complication rate after urologic and orthopedic surgery. The use of muscle-sparing thoracotomy may improve postoperative muscle strength and lung function.[8] Aortic surgery, head and neck surgery, neurosurgery, and abdominal aortic aneurysm surgery are also listed as high-risk procedures.[28,32,33]

RESPIRATORY RECAP

Intraoperative Factors Contributing to Postoperative Pulmonary Complications

» Surgical incision site
» Duration of surgery
» Type of anesthesia
» Monitoring during anesthesia
» Intraoperative fluid management

Duration of Surgery

Reduced lung volume is a major factor contributing to postoperative pulmonary complications following surgery. Vital capacity can be reduced by 50% to 60% and remain decreased for up to a week. Supine positioning decreases the functional residual capacity (FRC) by 10% to 15%. General anesthesia can further decrease the FRC up to 30%. Postoperative complications double if surgery lasts longer than 3 hours.[4,31]

Type of Anesthesia

Although there are conflicting data, it appears that patients who receive only general anesthesia are at higher risk for pulmonary complications than those who receive epidural or spinal anesthesia, with or without general anesthesia. Patients receiving epidural or spinal anesthesia had a 39% reduction in the risk of pneumonia and a 59% reduction in the risk of respiratory depression.[34] Long-acting neuromuscular blockers, such as pancuronium, lead to a higher incidence of pulmonary complications than shorter-acting agents.

Monitoring

Intraoperative monitoring may decrease anesthetic risks for cardiopulmonary compromise, thus reducing postoperative complications. Although the evidence is scant, most clinicians agree that the addition of physiologic monitoring intraoperatively, especially pulse oximetry and capnography, has improved postoperative outcomes.

Fluid Management

Proper fluid management is important for maintaining renal function, ensuring gastrointestinal integrity, and maintaining oxygen delivery. Blood loss and lack of fluids can lead to hypotension, poor organ perfusion, and insufficient oxygen delivery. Intraoperative blood loss greater than 1200 mL also has been associated with increased pulmonary complications. Excessive fluids may lead to edema, congestive heart failure, and hypertension.[35] Massive volume resuscitation can result in abdominal compartment syndrome, in which the increased intra-abdominal pressure results in increased work of breathing and decreased renal blood flow.

Postoperative Respiratory Failure: Assessment and Management

Postoperative pulmonary complications are common and contribute to postoperative morbidity and mortality. Common postoperative complications include atelectasis, infection, respiratory failure, exacerbation of underlying chronic lung disease, and bronchospasm. The goal is to prevent these complications. Postoperative respiratory management includes pain control, mobilization, deep breathing, airway clearance, ventilator liberation, nutritional support, and oxygen therapy.[16,36]

RESPIRATORY RECAP

Components of Postoperative Management

- » Pain control
- » Mobilization
- » Lung expansion therapy
- » Airway clearance
- » Ventilator liberation
- » Nutritional support
- » Oxygen therapy

Hypoxemia

Mild hypoxemia is treated with low concentrations of oxygen, most commonly by nasal cannula. Severe cases of hypoxemia require more aggressive therapy with the use of CPAP or mechanical ventilation with positive end-expiratory pressure (PEEP). Atelectasis is a major contributor to postoperative hypoxemia, and lung volume expansion therapies such as incentive spirometry, intermittent positive pressure breathing (IPPB), positive expiratory pressure (PEP), or CPAP may be required.[37]

Hypercapnia

If the central respiratory drive is blunted, an increased Pa_{CO_2} will occur. The use of anesthetics and analgesics during and after surgery is the major cause of short-term acute respiratory failure following surgery. Once sedation has been terminated and the drug is metabolized or excreted, most postoperative patients can ventilate appropriately if pain control measures are used. Treatment is aimed at the underlying etiology. Mechanical ventilation can be maintained until the cause of respiratory failure is reversed. The use of respiratory stimulants is controversial and is not recommended.

Motor neuron disorders, respiratory muscle weakness, chest wall abnormalities, and diaphragmatic or abdominal conditions also can result in hypercapnia. Postoperative respiratory failure resulting from ventilatory pump dysfunction is uncommon except with preexisting preoperative factors. Diaphragmatic paralysis can occur after some surgeries and may contribute to respiratory failure. Muscle weakness may result from drugs used intraoperatively or during the postoperative period. Pain can also be a factor preventing the normal use of the ventilatory bellows. Treatment is directed toward the underlying disorder, and mechanical ventilation can be used for supportive care.

Nutrition

The integrity of the gut affects immune defenses, organ function, and whether the stress response is provoked or attenuated. If a patient is unable to eat, initiation of ETF may be desirable. Generally ETF is well tolerated and improves postoperative morbidity and mortality better than parenteral nutrition.[24,25] **Box 41–5** lists the positive aspects of ETF. When compared with control subjects who received no feedings, nutritional intervention in the perioperative period has shown a benefit of reduced postoperative morbidity. A group of trauma patients receiving ETF for 5 to 7 days had a lower rate of sepsis compared with a group receiving intravenous fluid

BOX 41–5

Advantages of Enteral Tube Feedings Compared with Total Parenteral Nutrition in the Postoperative Patient

- Increased integrity of gastrointestinal system
- Improved immune defenses
- Improved organ function
- Attenuated immune response
- Decreased nosocomial infections
- Improved return of cognitive function
- Decreased mortality
- Less expensive
- Decreased septic complications

administration. Patients with liver transplantation had a lower viral infection rate with administration of ETF.[26] It should be noted, however, that the routine use of a nasogastric tube following surgery increases the risk of aspiration pneumonia and atelectasis. Nasogastric tubes should be used only when indicated.

Pain Management

The use of analgesics (pain medications) is essential after surgery, particularly following thoracic and abdominal surgery. Effective pain control will encourage early ambulation and deep breathing. Ineffective pain management may lead to serious pulmonary complications. Analgesia can be delivered orally, parenterally, or via epidural catheters. For epidural catheterization, the tip of a needle is positioned within the epidural space in the spinal column.[38,39] Once positioned, a thin catheter is threaded through the needle, and the needle is removed. The catheter is secured to the patient and is used to administer intermittent or continuous analgesia.

Patient-controlled analgesia (PCA) is a popular method of pain control. PCA allows the patient to titrate the amount of analgesic he or she receives by simply pressing a button. There is a limit set on the delivering device, which prevents the patient from overdosing on the drug. PCA can be used with IV or epidural analgesic administration. The benefits of PCA include active involvement of the patient, lesser amounts of drug usage, more rapid analgesic action, and better pain control with minimal side effects.[36,40]

Patient Temperature

Postoperative hypothermia causes vasoconstriction and may decrease tissue perfusion, resulting in metabolic acidosis. If shivering is present, it will increase oxygen consumption and carbon dioxide production. This may increase the risk of myocardial ischemia and hypercapnic ventilatory failure.

Muscle Strength

Postoperative sedation may lead to respiratory depression as a result of muscle weakness. The diaphragm is the last muscle to become paralyzed and the first to recover from neuromuscular blockade. A 5-second head-lift or leg-lift evaluation may be a good indicator of a patient's ability to maintain an adequate airway. If previously sedated patients who are alert and following commands can lift their extremities for 5 seconds, the diaphragm should be functional and they should be able to protect their airway. The 5-second lift test has correlated well with the maximal inspiratory pressure, which checks respiratory muscle strength.[41]

Lung Expansion

Pulmonary complications are the most common form of postoperative morbidity experienced by patients who undergo general surgical abdominal and thoracic procedures. The high incidence of pulmonary complications in the postoperative period is likely due to pain and the inability to take deep breaths because of decreased diaphragmatic function, chest wall dysfunction, and alterations in mechanics. Some studies have shown that forced vital capacity and peak flow can be decreased by as much as 50%. Functional residual capacity may be decreased by as much as 10% to 15% in lower abdominal surgery, 30% in upper abdominal surgery, and 35% in thoracic surgery in the postoperative period and may not return to normal for 3 to 6 days. Transdiaphragmatic pressure has been shown to decrease by as much as 70% in abdominal surgery, and normal function may not return for 1 week. In some cases, adequate pain management does not reduce this impairment, which seems to occur from diaphragm dysfunction itself.

Another important element in the etiology of postoperative respiratory complications is the lung volume at which airway closure occurs. Factors that increase closing volumes include increased age, tobacco use, fluid overload, bronchospasm, and airway secretions.[8] With a decreased FRC or increased closing volume, the lungs are predisposed to airway closure and atelectasis, leading to $\dot{V}/\dot{Q}$ mismatch, hypoxemia, retained secretions, and respiratory failure. Deep breathing exercises and pulmonary hygiene are important postoperative considerations for impending pulmonary complications. Several techniques for lung expansion are available, including IPPB, incentive spirometry, PEP breathing, deep breathing and coughing, CPAP, and others. Pulmonary complications, specifically atelectasis, pneumonia, and pulmonary embolism, represent the leading causes of postoperative morbidity and mortality.

Atelectasis

Etiology and Risk Factors

Atelectasis is the collapse of previously expanded lung tissue. Collapse may be minimal and diffuse. It may be difficult to see on chest radiographs (microatelectasis); or, it may involve whole segments, lobes, or a lung and be easily seen on chest radiographs. Atelectasis is one of the most common noninfectious pulmonary complications after surgery. Studies have reported that 20% to 25% of lung tissue in the basal lung areas collapses after induction with general anesthesia. Furthermore, the use of high concentrations of oxygen (more than 40%) contributes to the collapse. Atelectasis is reported in a wide range of patients (6% to 75%) having abdominal or thoracic surgery. The incidence of clinically significant atelectasis after abdominal surgery is 15% to 20%, with the left lower lobe being the most common area for atelectasis.[42]

Atelectasis may be caused by many factors, including small, monotonous tidal volumes and inadequate lung distending forces, airway obstruction with gas absorption, and reduction in surfactant levels. These conditions are likely in postoperative patients who are sedated, have significant pain, and often have poor clearance of airway secretions. Any condition that interferes with the generation of negative pleural pressure predisposes to atelectasis. Examples include weak inspiratory muscles because of sedation, advanced age, obesity, chest wall deformities, pulmonary fibrosis, abdominal and thoracic surgery, and pain.

Retained secretions may be the common factor in the development of postoperative atelectasis when the patient has an inadequate cough. Furthermore, anesthetics and a lack of humidity can diminish airway mucus transport during the intraoperative period. Surfactant levels may also be decreased in the lungs of postoperative patients as a result of the anesthetic, high concentrations of oxygen, and the absence of deep breathing. Intraoperative aspiration may also contribute to airway compromise.

AGE-SPECIFIC ANGLE

Elderly patients are at greater risk for atelectasis.

Clinical Manifestations and Diagnostic Findings

Some of the signs and symptoms of atelectasis include fine late inspiratory crackles, bronchial-type breath sounds, diminished breath sounds, increased breathing frequency and dyspnea, increased heart rate, and hypoxemia. The significance of each of these findings depends on the degree of atelectasis present. Atelectasis also can lead to respiratory failure and pneumonia. The presence of a fever in a patient with atelectasis is most often associated with infection resulting from retained secretions. Although contrary to common teaching, atelectasis without infection does not result in fever.[42]

Atelectasis is one of the most commonly encountered abnormalities on chest radiographs. At times it may be overlooked and at other times may be confused with other intrathoracic pathology such as **pneumonia**. Some of the radiographic signs of atelectasis include localized increase in density or opacity, air bronchograms, displacement of lobar fissures, elevation of the diaphragm, mediastinal shift, hilar displacement, regional change in rib spacing, hyperinflation of surrounding lung, and generalized volume reduction.

Pulmonary function tests reveal a decreased FRC, a decreased vital capacity (VC), and decreased compliance. An arterial blood sample often shows an uncompensated respiratory alkalosis with hypoxemia. The hypoxemia is a result of $\dot{V}/\dot{Q}$ mismatch and areas of right-to-left shunt. General anesthesia inhibits hypoxic pulmonary vasoconstriction, which further contributes to $\dot{V}/\dot{Q}$ mismatch and increased work of breathing.

RESPIRATORY RECAP

Signs and Symptoms of Postoperative Atelectasis

- » Inspiratory crackles
- » Bronchial breath sounds
- » Diminished breath sounds
- » Tachypnea
- » Dyspnea
- » Tachycardia
- » Hypoxemia

Management

Treatment for atelectasis depends on the severity and etiology of the problem. Preventive treatment is best. Preoperative patient education and training, when the patient is alert, responsive to instruction, and without pain, may play a significant role in preventing postoperative complications. Smoking cessation at least 8 weeks before surgery has also been shown to improve postoperative outcomes.

With minimal postoperative atelectasis, no special intervention is needed. Spontaneous coughing, deep breathing, and mobilization (walking) should be sufficient to reverse any pulmonary impairment. In moderate cases, incentive spirometry, IPPB, PEP therapy, and CPAP can be used to help prevent or reverse atelectasis.[37] Chest physiotherapy (CPT) and the use of bronchodilators may improve bronchial hygiene and aid in removal of secretions in some patients, but these are usually not indicated in this patient population. Deep breathing and coughing are as effective as other modes of therapy for the treatment of atelectasis; no individual approach to lung inflation therapy is significantly superior to another. Although these treatments are similar in their ability to prevent pulmonary complications, each has been shown to be better than no treatment at all. Some studies have demonstrated PEP and CPAP therapy to be more effective than deep breathing or incentive spirometry.[43]

Low-risk surgical patients probably do not need respiratory therapy, but even with therapy, an estimated 25% of high-risk patients will suffer from postoperative pulmonary complications. Short-term oxygen therapy is often indicated. In rare severe cases, mechanical ventilation with PEEP and high oxygen levels may be indicated to reinflate collapsed areas and support oxygenation until the patient has improved. Therapeutic fiberoptic bronchoscopy may be indicated to remove mucus plugs if they are the cause of airway obstruction and atelectasis.

RESPIRATORY RECAP

Management of Postoperative Atelectasis

- » Prevention
- » Patient education
- » Smoking cessation
- » Spontaneous coughing
- » Deep breathing exercises
- » Incentive spirometry
- » Intermittent positive pressure breathing (IPPB)
- » Mobilization
- » Positive expiratory pressure (PEP)
- » Airway clearance therapy
- » CPAP therapy
- » Oxygen therapy
- » Mechanical ventilation

Pulmonary Emboli and Pulmonary Thromboembolic Disease

Etiology and Risk Factors

The most common cause of **pulmonary embolism (PE)** is venous thromboembolism. Blood clots formed in the leg veins travel to the lungs, where they obstruct pulmonary vessels. Blood clotting in the legs and pelvis, **deep vein thrombosis (DVT)**, occurs as a result of venostasis in surgical patients and from other causes of immobility. It may also occur due to damage to the endothelial wall of the blood vessels and hypercoagulability states. Risk factors associated with DVT include age greater than 70 years, obesity, congestive heart failure, presence of malignancies, burns, use of estrogen-containing drugs, and postoperative states.

Clinical Manifestations and Diagnostic Findings

Signs and symptoms of acute PE include abrupt onset of cough, pleuritic chest pain, anxiety, and tachycardia. Tachypnea and dyspnea are the most common findings present, even in patients without hypoxemia. Lung auscultation may reveal wheezing or crackles. Hemoptysis may occasionally occur. The lower extremities may reveal some tenderness or swelling associated with DVT, but PE often occurs as the first sign of DVT.

The severity of symptoms and degree of compromise depend on the magnitude of occlusion of the pulmonary vessels and the amount of preexisting cardiopulmonary disease. As a result of venous occlusion, hypoxemia usually occurs. This is due to $\dot{V}/\dot{Q}$ mismatch, bronchoconstriction, decreased surfactant production, atelectasis, and shunting. In healthy patients, right-sided heart dysfunction does not usually occur unless occlusion of 50% or more (massive occlusion) of the pulmonary vasculature occurs. In patients with cardiopulmonary disease, hemodynamic collapse can occur with less than massive occlusion. Although pulmonary occlusion can be extensive, pulmonary infarction is uncommon because the lung receives oxygen from three sources: pulmonary circulation, bronchial circulation, and the alveolar gas.

PE can occur with few symptoms, or it may be mistaken for other diseases or coexist with them. PE is commonly mistaken for pneumonia. The diagnosis of PE includes clinical suspicion, physical exam, chest radiograph, ECG, and arterial blood gas measurements. Chest radiographs may be normal, or an infiltrate may be present. Radiographs are often not specific enough to be of great help. In some cases a wedge-shaped density called a Westermark sign may be present. The ECG may have nonspecific alterations. Arterial blood gas values often show a respiratory alkalosis and hypoxemia.

> **RESPIRATORY RECAP**
>
> **Signs and Symptoms of Postoperative Pulmonary Embolism**
>
> » Abrupt onset of cough
> » Pleuritic chest pain
> » Anxiety
> » Tachycardia
> » Hypoxemia

Noninvasive studies used to diagnose DVT include **impedance plethysmography** and Doppler ultrasound. Invasive contrast venography is the gold standard in the diagnosis of DVT. The hazard associated with venography is mobilization of the clot. To diagnosis PE, the $\dot{V}/\dot{Q}$ scan is used to evaluate perfusion defects combined with areas of normal ventilation. The pulmonary angiogram, although considered the gold standard to determine the presence of PE, is invasive and carries with it a higher risk of complications than the $\dot{V}/\dot{Q}$ scan. Because of the increased risk of complications, pulmonary angiography is often used as a last resort. Because of its widespread availability, spiral (helical) CT scanning with intravenous contrast is now being used to help diagnose suspected PE.

Management

Prophylaxis of PE involves prevention of DVT, including compression wraps (stockings) or pneumatic boots with intermittent inflation and early ambulation and leg exercises. Anticoagulation therapy is also indicated. Anticoagulation therapy with **heparin** is considered therapeutic if the clotting time or **partial thromboplastin time (PTT)** is 2 to 2.5 times the control. If venous thrombosis is present, heparin will prevent further clot formation but will not dissolve clots already present. Warfarin is another anticoagulant used by patients who are at risk for thromboembolism. These at-risk conditions include atrial fibrillation, presence of prosthetic heart valves, and previous thromboembolism.[44,45] Although bleeding from the surgical site is a risk when using anticoagulants, withholding or reducing anticoagulants may increase the risk of thromboembolism, including stroke. Several factors influence the risk the bleeding in patients using anticoagulants. These include patient age, disease presence, type of surgery, other drug use such as aspirin or antiplatelet agents, and the degree of anticoagulation as determined by the international normalized ratio (INR). The INR is used to determine the degree of anticoagulation in patients who are on oral (warfarin) anticoagulation therapy. Once the INR is below 2.0, surgery can be preformed with relative safety. The INR is normally kept between 2.0 and 3.0 for optimal therapeutic levels.[46,47]

> **RESPIRATORY RECAP**
>
> **Management of Postoperative Pulmonary Embolism**
>
> » Prophylaxis/prevention of DVT
> » Anticoagulation therapy
> » Thrombolytic therapy
> » Insertion of IVC filters
> » Surgery

If clots are already present, **thrombolytic** therapy will help dissolve clots. Common thrombolytics include streptokinase, urokinase, and **tissue plasminogen activator**

(TPA). The use of thrombolytic therapy must be balanced against the risk of bleeding in postoperative patients. An inferior vena caval (IVC) filter (Greenfield or bird's nest filter) can be inserted to prevent clots originating in the lower extremities from reaching the lungs. These implanted filters intercept clots, thus preventing PE. Surgical removal of the embolus may rarely be attempted. Supportive therapy includes supplemental oxygen and, in severe cases of acute respiratory failure, mechanical ventilation with PEEP and high oxygen levels.

Pneumonia

Etiology and Risk Factors

Hospital-acquired pneumonia (HAP), ventilator-associated pneumonia (VAP), and healthcare-associated pneumonia (HCAP) are important causes of morbidity and mortality in the healthcare setting. Nosocomial pneumonia (hospital acquired after more than 48 hours following admission) accounts for 15% of all hospital-acquired infections, with half occurring in surgical patients. Postoperative pneumonia has been reported to occur in 18% of patients undergoing elective upper or lower abdominal and thoracic surgery. Pneumonia carries the highest mortality rate from hospital-acquired infections. It is the most common cause of death among surgical patients, with a reported mortality rate of 20% to 50% and up to 90% mortality in patients with acute respiratory distress syndrome.

RESPIRATORY RECAP

Signs and Symptoms of Postoperative Pneumonia

- » Fever
- » Shaking chills
- » Cough
- » Hemoptysis
- » Tachypnea
- » Dullness to percussion
- » Crackles
- » Purulent sputum
- » Pleuritic chest pain

Risk factors for development of pneumonia include immunosuppression, malnutrition, COPD, and age greater than 65 years. Additional risk factors for development of nosocomial pneumonia include major thoracic and upper abdominal surgery, greater than 1,200 mL blood loss during surgery, altered protective effects of the glottic area, ineffective cough, inhibition of ciliary motion, and impaired consciousness leading to increased chance of aspiration. Postoperative patients are at high risk especially when they are intubated, have a nasogastric tube in place, have had general anesthesia, have swallowing difficulties, or have regurgitation of gastric contents.

Clinical Manifestations and Diagnostic Findings

Signs and symptoms of pneumonia include fever, shaking chills, cough, hemoptysis, tachypnea, dullness to percussion, crackles, purulent sputum production, and pleuritic chest pain. However, some of the usual clinical manifestations are often unclear and may be overshadowed by an underlying illness when pneumonia develops while a patient is in the hospital. When a bacterial pneumonia is present, laboratory data include increased white blood cell count (leukocytes), increased granulocytes (neutrophilia), and an increased percentage of immature neutrophils (referred to as a shift to the left). Arterial blood gas measurements show hypoxemia with respiratory alkalosis. Chest radiographs vary according to the type of pneumonia present. Lobar pneumonia presents as a homogenous infiltrate with air bronchograms. Nonhomogeneous, patchy, nonlobar densities occur with bronchopneumonia. A diffuse bilateral reticular density often indicates a viral infection.

Management

Prevention is the best course of action. Proper hand hygiene is essential. Deep breathing maneuvers and coughing are indicated for secretion removal. Bronchodilator therapy and airway clearance therapies are usually not indicated for consolidative pneumonia. Administration of antibiotics is the most important therapy. If isolation of the causative agent is possible, culture and sensitivity tests should direct proper antimicrobial use. If the agent cannot be isolated, initial general antimicrobial therapy (empiric therapy) includes the following drug options: extended-spectrum penicillins (ampicillin/sulbactam), cephalosporins (ceftriaxone, cefotaxime, cefepime), the fluoroquinolones (levofloxacin, moxifloxacin, ciprofloxacin), a β-lactam (ertapenem), and aminoglycosides (tobramycin, vancomycin) or an oxazolidinone (linezolid). The actual drug regimen will vary depending on suspected microbial infection and other complicating patient factors and can be modified based on knowledge of local pathogens and their susceptibility to antibiotics.[48] Oxygen is often needed for hypoxemia. In severe cases, mechanical ventilation with PEEP may be indicated.

RESPIRATORY RECAP

Management of Postoperative Pneumonia

- » Antibiotics
- » Oxygen
- » Mechanical ventilation with PEEP

Mechanical Ventilation

Postoperative mechanical ventilation is occasionally required, most commonly due to the residual respiratory depressant effects of anesthesia. This often involves several hours of ventilatory support in the postanesthesia care unit, after which the patient is extubated. After cardiac surgery, the patient is mechanically ventilated in the intensive care unit for several hours, after which fast-track ventilator discontinuation protocols are used to rapidly liberate the patient from the ventilator. After neurosurgery, mechanical ventilation may be needed because of respiratory depression and to assist with the control of intracranial pressure. After thoracic surgery, mechanical ventilation is often required because of the extent of surgical trauma to the thorax.

The principles of mechanical ventilation are similar for the postoperative patient as for other patients requiring this therapy. Appropriate ventilatory support is provided, with attention to the prevention of iatrogenic injuries such as overdistention, auto-PEEP, and hemodynamic compromise. Some postoperative patients (e.g., after neurosurgery) may have relatively normal lungs and chest wall. Others may have relatively normal lung function, but surgical chest wall trauma (e.g., after cardiac surgery). Thoracic surgery patients may be difficult to manage because they have surgical chest wall trauma, lung resection with risk of pneumothorax, and underlying lung disease such as COPD.

Mechanical ventilation places a patient at high risk for development of pneumonia. VAP occurs in 9% to 27% of mechanically ventilated patients, and mortality rates vary from 27% to 50%. A set of procedures used to prevent VAP is included in what is known as a *ventilator bundle*. The ventilator bundle for prevention of VAP includes elevating the head of the bed by at least 30 degrees, providing sedation vacations for assessment of extubation potential, peptic ulcer prophylaxis, oral care to decrease microbial flora, and DVT prophylaxis. Other procedures that may help decrease VAP include use of protective covers for suction and resuscitation equipment, decontamination of the stomach, use of silver-coated endotracheal tubes,[49] and continuous subglottic suction with specially designed endotracheal tubes. Some of these techniques and devices need more study before their effectiveness in reducing VAP is known. The goal is to prevent VAP and thereby reduce medical costs, patient morbidity, and mortality.

KEY POINTS

- An important first step in preoperative management is obtaining a patient history.
- Age, smoking history, preexisting lung disease, and poor nutritional status are risk factors for postoperative respiratory complications.
- Little evidence exists that routine screening of healthy patients with ECGs, chest radiographs, PFTs, echocardiograms, or blood chemistry panels significantly alters outcomes.
- Intraoperative factors that affect postoperative pulmonary complications include surgical incision site, duration of surgery, type of anesthesia, monitoring during anesthesia, and intraoperative fluid management.
- Postoperative respiratory management includes pain control, early mobilization, deep breathing, airway clearance therapy, early ventilator liberation, early feeding, and oxygen therapy, as indicated.
- Atelectasis, pulmonary embolism, and pneumonia are common postoperative problems.

REFERENCES

1. Fisher BW, Majumdar SR, McAlister FA. Predicting pulmonary complications after nonthoracic surgery: a systematic review of blinded studies. *Am J Med.* 2002;112:219.
2. Smetana GW, Lawrence VA, Cornell JE. Preoperative pulmonary risk stratification for noncardiothoracic surgery: systematic review for the American College of Physicians. *Ann Intern Med.* 2006;144:581.
3. Smetana GW. Preoperative pulmonary evaluation. *N Engl J Med.* 1999;340:937.
4. McAlister FA, Khan NA, Straus SE, et al. Accuracy of the preoperative assessment in predicting pulmonary risk after nonthoracic surgery. *Am J Respir Crit Care Med.* 2003;167:741.
5. Bapoje SR, Whitcker JF, Schulz T, et al. Preoperative evaluation of the patient with pulmonary disease. *Chest.* 2007;13:1637–1645.
6. Sigworth S. Preoperative evaluation of hospitalized patients. *Mt Sinai J Med.* 2008;75:442–448.
7. Kanat F, Golcuk A, Teke T, Golcuk M. Risk factors for postoperative pulmonary complications in upper abdominal surgery. *ANZ J Surg.* 2007;77:135–141.
8. Ferguson MK. Preoperative assessment of pulmonary risk. *Chest.* 1999;115:58S–63S.
9. McAlister F, Beertsch K, Man J, et al. Incidence of and risk factors for pulmonary complications after nonthoracic surgery. *Am J Respir Crit Care Med.* 2005;171:514.
10. Oskuig RM. Special problems in the elderly. *Chest.* 1999; 115:158S–164S.
11. Lindstrom D, Sadr AO, Wladis A, et al. Effects of a perioperative smoking cessation intervention on postoperative complications: a randomized trial. *Ann Surg.* 2008;5:739–745.
12. Theadom A, Cropley M. Effects of preoperative smoking cessation on the incidence and risk of intraoperative and postoperative complications in adult smokers: a systematic review. *Tob Control.* 2006;5:352–358.
13. Moller A, Tonnesen H. Risk reduction: perioperative smoking intervention. *Best Pract Res Clin Anaesthesiol.* 2006;2:237–248.
14. Warner D. Preoperative smoking cessation: the role of the primary care provider. *Mayo Clin Proc.* 2005;80:252.
15. Mitchell CK, Smoger SH, Pfeifer MP, et al. Multivariate analysis of factors associated with pulmonary complications following general elective surgery. *Arch Surg.* 1998;133:194–198.
16. Lawrence V, Cornell J, Smetana G. Strategies to reduce postoperative pulmonary complications after noncardiothoracic surgery: systematic review for the American College of Physicians. *Ann Intern Med.* 2006;144:596–608.
17. Belzberg H, Rivkind AI. Preoperative cardiac preparation. *Chest.* 1999;115:82S–95S.
18. Reiss KP, Baker MT, Lambert PJ, et al. Effect of preoperative weight loss on laparoscopic gastric bypass outcomes. *Surg Obes Related Dis.* 2008;4:704–708.
19. Ramaswamy A, Gonzalez R, Smith CD. Extensive preoperative testing is not necessary in morbidly obese patients undergoing gastric bypass. *J Gastrointest Surg.* 2004;2:159–164.
20. McGlinch BP, Que FG, Nelson JL, et al. Perioperative care of patients undergoing bariatric surgery. *Mayo Clin Proc.* 2006;81(10 suppl):S25–S33.

21. Meelinek J, Livingston E, Cortina G, Fishbein MC. Autopsy findings following gastric bypass surgery for morbid obesity. *Arch Pathol Lab Med.* 2002;126:1091.
22. Hollenberg SM. Preoperative cardiac risk assessment. *Chest.* 1999;115:51S–57S.
23. Gupta RM, Parvizi J, Hanssen AD, Gay PC. Postoperative complications in patients with obstructive sleep apnea syndrome undergoing hip or knee replacement: a case-control study. *Mayo Clin Proc.* 2001;76:897.
24. Stack JA, Babineau TJ, Bristrian BR. Assessment of nutritional status in clinical practice. *Gastroenterologist.* 1996;4:8S–15S.
25. Kudsk KA, Tolley EA, DeWitt RC, et al. Preoperative albumin and surgical site identify surgical risk for major postoperative complications. *JPEN.* 2003;1:1–9.
26. Hasse JM, Blue LS, Liepa GU, et al. Early enteral nutrition support in patients undergoing liver transplantation. *J Parenter Enteral Nutr.* 1995;19:437–443.
27. Fischer SP. Cost-effective preoperative evaluation and testing. *Chest.* 1999;115:96S–110S.
28. Smetana GW, Macpherson DS. The case against routine preoperative laboratory testing. *Med Clin North Am.* 2003; 87:7.
29. Qaseem A, Snow V, Fitterman N, et al. Risk assessment for and strategies to reduce perioperative pulmonary complications for patients undergoing noncardiothoracic surgery: a guideline from the American College of Physicians. *Ann Intern Med.* 2006;144:575.
30. Moller AM, Maaloe R, Pedersen T. Postoperative intensive care admittance: the role of tobacco smoking. *Acta Anaesthesiol Scand.* 2001;45:345.
31. Brooks-Brunn JA. Predictors of postoperative complications following abdominal surgery. *Chest.* 1997;111:564.
32. Arozullah AM, Daley J, Henderson WG, Khuri SF. Multifactorial risk index for predicting postoperative respiratory failure in men after major noncardiac surgery. The National Veterans Administration Surgical Quality Improvement Program. *Ann Surg.* 2000;232:242.
33. Arozullah AM, Khuri SF, Henderson WG, Daley J. Development and validation of a multifactorial risk index for predicting postoperative pneumonia after major noncardiac surgery. *Ann Intern Med.* 2001;135:847.
34. Rodgers A, Walker N, Schug S, et al. Reduction of postoperative mortality and morbidity with epidural or spinal anesthesia: results from overview of randomized trials. *BMJ.* 2000;321:1493.
35. Rosenthal MH. Intraoperative fluid management—what and how much? *Chest.* 1999;115:130S–137S.
36. Peeters-Asdourian C, Gupta S. Choices in pain management following thoracotomy. *Chest.* 1999;115:122S–124S.
37. Squadrone V, Coha M, Cerutti E, et al. Continuous positive airway pressure for treatment of postoperative hypoxemia: a randomized trial. *JAMA.* 2005;293:589–595.
38. Howell CJ, Dean T, Lucking L, et al. Randomized study of long term outcome after epidural versus non-epidural analgesia during labour. *BMJ.* 2002;325:357.
39. Sitsen E, van Poorten F, van Alphen W, et al. Postoperative epidural analgesia after total knee arthroplasty with sufentanil 1 microg/ml combined with ropivacaine 0.2%, ropivacaine 0.125%, or levobupivacaine 0.125%: a randomized, double-blinded comparison. *Reg Anesth Pain Med.* 2007;6:475–480.
40. Ballantyne J, Kupelnick B, McPeek B, Lau J. Does the evidence support the use of spinal and epidural anesthesia for surgery? *J Clin Anesth.* 2005;5:382–391.
41. Pavlin EG, Holle RH, Schoene RB. Recovery of airway protection compared with ventilation in humans after paralysis with curare. *Anesthesiology.* 1996;70:381–385.
42. Platell C, Hall JC. Atelectasis after abdominal surgery. *J Am Coll Surg.* 1997;185:584–592.
43. Ferreyra G, Baussano I, Squadrone V, et al. Continuous positive airway pressure for treatment of respiratory complications following abdominal surgery: a systematic review and meta-analysis. *Ann Surg.* 2008;247(4):617–626.
44. Dunn A, Turpie A. Perioperative management of patients receiving oral anticoagulants: a systematic review. *Arch Intern Med.* 2003;163:901.
45. Douketis J, Berger P, Dunn A, et al. The perioperative management of antithrombotic therapy: American College of Physicians evidence-based clinical practice guidelines (8th edition). *Chest.* 2008;133:299S.
46. Torn M, Rosendaal F. Oral anticoagulation in surgical procedures: risks and recommendations. *Br J Haematol.* 2003;123:676.
47. Kovich O, Otley C. Thrombotic complications related to discontinuation of warfarin and aspirin therapy perioperatively for cutaneous operation. *J Am Acad Dermatol.* 2003;48:233.
48. Guidelines for the management of adults with hospital-acquired, ventilator-associated, and health-care associated pneumonia. *Am J Respir Care Med.* 2005;171:388–416.
49. Relelo J, Kollef M, Diaz E, et al. Reduced burden of bacterial airway colonization with a novel silver-coated endotracheal tube in a randomized multiple-center feasibility study. *Crit Care Med.* 2006;34:2766.

CHAPTER 42

Cardiac Failure

William S. Stigler
Benjamin D. Medoff

OUTLINE

OBJECTIVES

1. Discuss the epidemiology and etiology of cardiac failure.
2. Describe the physiology of normal cardiac function, the pathophysiology of abnormal cardiac function, and the pathophysiology of pulmonary edema.
3. Describe the determinants of ventricular function.
4. List the symptoms and signs of cardiac failure.
5. Discuss the basic ways in which the heart and lungs interact.
6. Discuss the common causes and treatment of cardiac failure.
7. Discuss the treatment of chronic and acute cardiac failure.
8. Discuss issues related to noninvasive and invasive ventilation of patients with cardiac failure.

KEY TERMS

afterload
cardiac failure
cardiac output ($\dot{Q}c$)
cardiomyocytes
cardiomyopathy
contractility
coronary angiography
coronary artery bypass surgery
diastole
diastolic dysfunction
echocardiography
hepatojugular reflux
intra-aortic balloon pump (IABP)
oncotic pressure
orthopnea
percutaneous coronary intervention (PCI)
preload
pulmonary edema
pulmonary vascular resistance (PVR)
Starling's law of cardiac function
stroke volume
systole
systolic dysfunction
venous return
ventricular interdependence

INTRODUCTION

Cardiac failure is the final common pathway of almost all forms of heart disease. The high prevalence of heart disease has made cardiac failure one of the most common problems encountered in hospitalized patients. Cardiac failure results in a broad range of symptoms and presentations and, in extreme cases, respiratory failure requiring mechanical ventilation. Mechanical ventilation of these patients can be challenging because of the complexity of the cardiopulmonary interactions and concomitant cardiac problems such as myocardial ischemia. Proper care of the ventilated patient with cardiac failure requires knowledge of the clinical manifestations and an understanding of the basic pathophysiology.

Definition

Cardiac failure is defined by the American College of Cardiology and American Heart Association as a complex clinical syndrome that can result from any structural or functional cardiac disorder that impairs the ventricle from filling with or ejecting blood. The cardinal manifestations of cardiac failure are dyspnea and fatigue, which may limit exercise tolerance, and fluid retention, which may lead to pulmonary congestion and peripheral edema.[1] Because cardiac failure is a complex syndrome, others define it in various ways, including an inability for cardiac function to meet the body's metabolic demands without increasing filling pressures.

Epidemiology

Cardiac failure is a common cause of morbidity and mortality in the United States and worldwide, accounting for 12 to 15 million office visits and 6.5 million hospital days each year. In recent years, the number of hospitalizations with cardiac failure has increased substantially. Cardiac failure is linked closely with cardiovascular diseases such as coronary artery disease, hypertension, and diabetes.

Incidence

The incidence of cardiac failure is estimated to be 3 to 10 persons per 1000 population each year. Cardiac failure disproportionally affects the elderly; the incidence rate is 10 persons per 1000 population after age 65 years, and the rate continues to increase after age 65 years. Despite improved therapeutic interventions for many of the underlying diseases leading to cardiac failure, the incidence has not declined over the last two decades.

Mortality

Clearly establishing mortality due to cardiac failure is difficult because the syndrome is a manifestation of myriad underlying processes. However, cardiac failure is an associated cause in 1 in 8 deaths; 52.3 per 1000 deaths are attributable entirely to cardiac failure. Data from the Framingham Heart Study cohort demonstrate that 80% of men and 70% of women younger than 65 years with cardiac failure will die within 8 years. The mortality of cardiac failure approaches that observed in cancer and acquired immunodeficiency syndrome (AIDS), with 1-year and 5-year mortality rates of 22% and 42%, respectively.[2]

Etiology

Cardiac failure results from a large number of primary cardiac diseases as well as systemic diseases. The most common etiologies include coronary artery disease (CAD), hypertension, alcohol, and idiopathic dilated **cardiomyopathy**. **Box 42–1** lists many of the possible etiologies of cardiac failure.

Cardiac Physiology

The heart is a mechanical pump that circulates blood through the pulmonary and systemic circulations. The intact performance of the heart requires a complex series of events that coordinates excitation at the individual myocyte to contraction of the heart muscle itself. To generate an adequate cardiac output, the heart must contract and pump blood out (systolic function) and also relax and refill the chambers with blood (diastolic function). Overall cardiac function is regulated by numerous neurohumoral and mechanical factors that can be manipulated with various pharmacologic agents.

Cellular Biology and Biochemistry of Cardiac Function

The heart is composed of cardiac muscle cells (**cardiomyocytes**) organized into linear series called *myofibers*. The myocytes contain the sarcomere, the basic contractile apparatus of the heart, as well as numerous mitochondria for energy production. In addition, the heart has specialized myocytes that initiate and propagate the action potential that causes contraction of the muscle cells.

The smallest unit of muscle that contracts is the sarcomere. Contraction of the myocyte is initiated by cell membrane depolarization. The conducting cells of the heart initiate the action potential that propagates to the muscle cells. When stimulated, myocytes release calcium; the calcium interacts with actin and myosin, the proteins forming the sarcomere, stimulating shortening and therefore contraction of the cells. Through an active process, calcium is again stored in the cell, allowing for relaxation. Both the contraction and the relaxation of the myocyte are energy-dependent functions.[3]

Cardiac Pump Function

The heart rhythmically contracts and continually empties and fills with blood, thus propelling blood through the circulation. The cardiac cycle consists of a period of contraction (**systole**), during which the heart pumps blood into the pulmonary and systemic circulation, followed by a relaxation period (**diastole**), during which venous blood returns to the heart. With each cardiac cycle, a volume of blood is ejected, termed the **stroke volume** of the heart. The product of the stroke volume and heart rate (in beats per minute) gives the **cardiac output ($\dot{Q}c$)**, expressed as L/min.

After the blood is ejected, the heart quickly fills with blood from the venous circulation, termed **venous return**. In the steady state the venous return must equal the $\dot{Q}c$. The concept of matched venous return and $\dot{Q}c$ is important in the determination of overall function, because processes that affect the venous return must then affect $\dot{Q}c$, and vice versa.

BOX 42-1

Diagnoses Associated with Cardiac Failure

- Acute ischemia
- Dilated cardiomyopathy
  - Chronic ischemic disease
  - Idiopathic
  - Tachycardia induced
  - Myocarditis (e.g., viral, giant cell)
  - Chagas disease
  - Toxin or drug mediated (e.g., Adriamycin, cobalt)
  - Sarcoidosis
  - Hemochromatosis
  - Thyroid disease
  - Heredity
- Restrictive cardiomyopathy
  - Hypertrophic cardiomyopathy
  - Infiltrative disorders (amyloid, malignancy)
  - Idiopathic
- Valvular or mechanical disease
  - Aortic stenosis
  - Aortic insufficiency (acute and chronic)
  - Mitral stenosis
  - Mitral regurgitation (acute and chronic)
  - Ventricular septal defect (acute and chronic)
  - Free wall rupture
- Arrhythmia
  - Tachycardia
  - Bradycardia
- Pericardial disease
  - Constrictive pericarditis
  - Constrictive/effusive pericarditis
  - Pericardial tamponade
- Right heart failure
  - Valvular (pulmonary stenosis/insufficiency, tricuspid regurgitation)
  - Eisenmenger syndrome (e.g., atrial septal defect)
  - Pulmonary hypertension (e.g., pulmonary embolism, primary)
- High-output failure
  - Arteriovenous shunting
  - Paget disease
  - Thyroid disease
  - Beriberi
- Miscellaneous
  - Vasculitis (e.g., Churg-Strauss, Wegener)
  - Carcinoid
  - Scleroderma
  - Eosinophilic cardiomyopathy (Löffler endocarditis)

Additionally, the left ventricle (LV) and the right ventricle (RV) interact with one another through a complex interplay termed **ventricular interdependence**. This concept introduces greater complexity because an understanding of LV function must take into account changes in RV dimensions and function. These aspects of the RV vary with alterations of venous return, pulmonary vascular resistance, and intrathoracic pressure changes.[4]

Determinants of Ventricular Function

Preload

Mechanical factors affect myocyte and myocardial contraction. **Starling's law of cardiac function** states that the longer the initial sarcomere length, the greater the force generated with contraction. The degree of precontraction stretch of the sarcomere is termed the **preload**. In general, $\dot{Q}c$ increases as preload increases, a function known as the Frank-Starling relationship. However, as preload continues to increase, the $\dot{Q}c$ eventually reaches a plateau and can decline if too great of a load is placed on the cardiac myocyte. The preload of the ventricle may be approximated by the ventricular end-diastolic volume (EDV) (**Figure 42–1**). Unfortunately, this is a difficult variable to measure clinically, and the end-diastolic pressure (EDP) is often used as a surrogate. The ventricular diastolic filling pressure also represents a back pressure limiting venous return (**Figure 42–2**). The relationship between preload and $\dot{Q}c$ requires consideration of both intrinsic ventricular function and venous return (**Figure 42–3**).

Afterload

The load that opposes myocardial shortening is called the **afterload**. There is an inverse relationship between the force generated by the cardiac muscle against a load and the degree and velocity of muscle shortening. As the afterload is increased at any fixed degree of contractility,

RESPIRATORY RECAP

Determinants of Ventricular Function

- » Preload
- » Afterload
- » Contractility

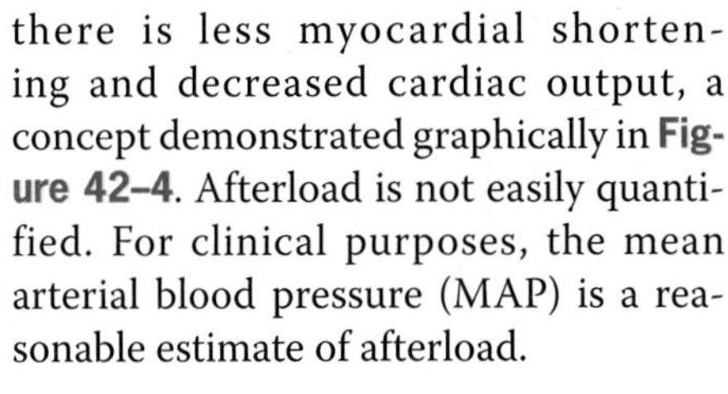

there is less myocardial shortening and decreased cardiac output, a concept demonstrated graphically in **Figure 42–4**. Afterload is not easily quantified. For clinical purposes, the mean arterial blood pressure (MAP) is a reasonable estimate of afterload.

Contractility

Contractility defines the intrinsic strength of contraction independent of preload and afterload. The myocardium can alter contractility in many ways. In general, measures that increase the concentration or availability of cellular calcium ions increase the contractility. The effect of changes in contractility can be demonstrated graphically as a change in the relationship between stroke volume and preload or afterload (**Figure 42–5**). An increase in contractility improves

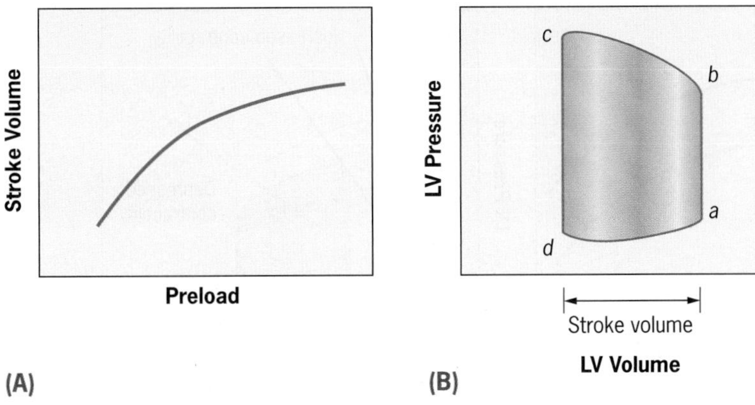

FIGURE 42–1 (**A**) Relationship between preload and stroke volume. (**B**) The pressure–volume loop. For a single cardiac cycle, left ventricular (LV) pressure is plotted against LV volume. Point *a* represents end-diastole and the start of isovolemic contraction. Ventricular pressure increases without a change in volume until ejection starts at point *b*, which represents the opening of the aortic valve. During ejection, ventricular volume decreases. Point *c* represents end-systole and the start of isovolumic relaxation. The aortic valve closes near end-systole. Ventricular pressure continues to fall until ventricular filling starts with the opening of the mitral valve at point *d*. Ventricular pressure increases very slightly during diastolic filling. Modified from Wanneburg T, Little WC. Regulation of cardiac output. In: Brown DL, ed. *Cardiac Intensive Care*. WB Saunders; 1998.

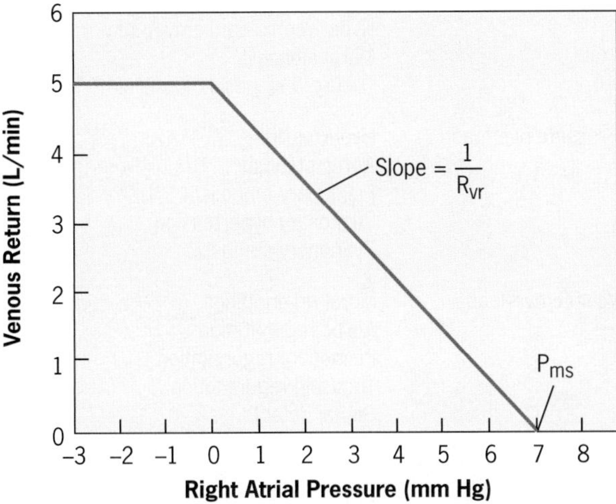

FIGURE 42–2 Normal venous return curve. Relationship between right atrial pressure and the venous return. R_{vr}, resistance to venous return; P_{ms}, mean systemic pressure. Modified from Brienza N, et al. Peripheral control of venous return in critical illness: role of the splanchnic vascular compartment. In: Dantzker DR, Scharf SM, eds. *Cardiopulmonary Critical Care*. 3rd ed. WB Saunders; 1998.

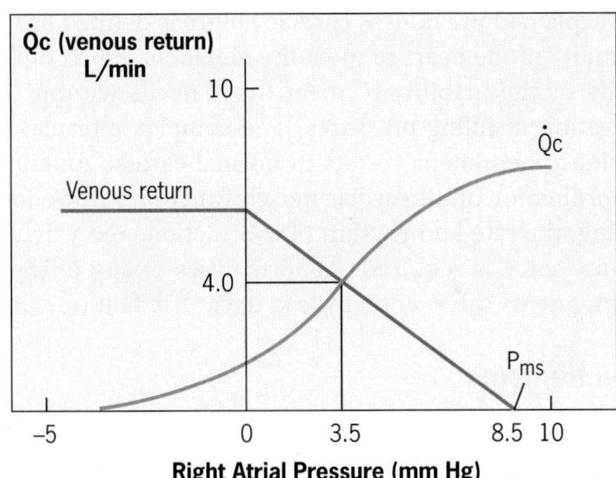

FIGURE 42–3 Venous return and cardiac output as a function of right atrial pressure. The intersection of the two curves represents the steady-state cardiac output of the heart under the given loading conditions. With kind permission from Springer Science+Business Media. *Can J Anesth*. The role of the vasculature in venous return and cardiac output: historical and graphical approach. 1997;44:849–867. Jacobsohn E, Chorn R, O'Connor M.

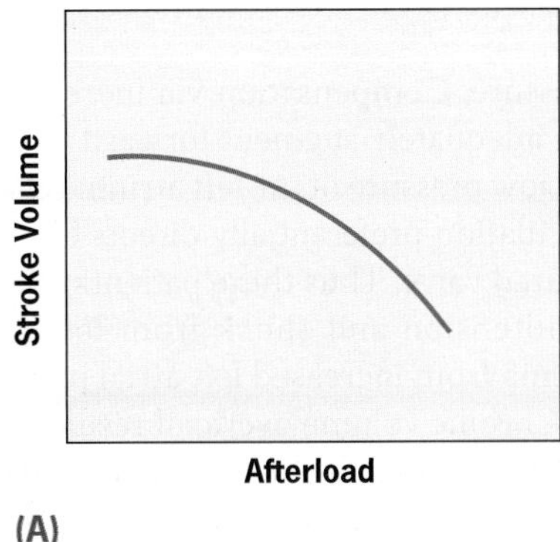

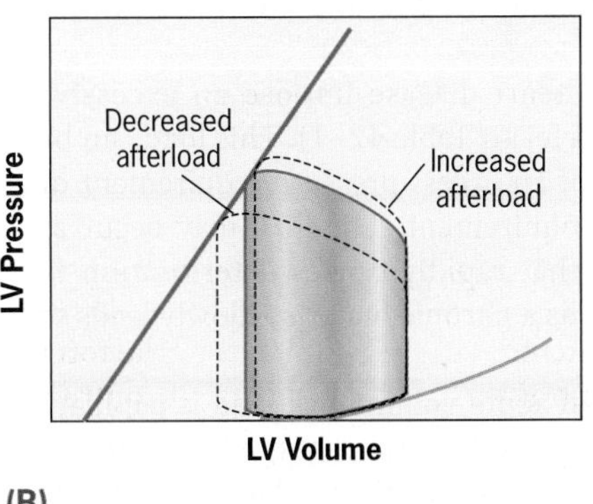

FIGURE 42–4 (**A**) Effects of afterload on stroke volume. (**B**) Effects of afterload on the pressure–volume curve of the left ventricle (LV). Modified from Wanneburg T, Little WC. Regulation of cardiac output. In: Brown DL, ed. *Cardiac Intensive Care*. WB Saunders; 1998:55–62.

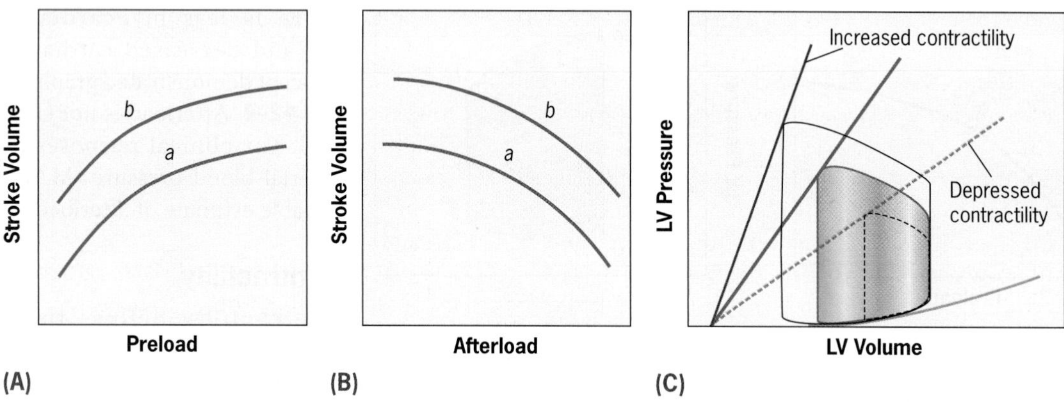

FIGURE 42–5 (**A**) Effects of changes in contractility on stroke volume as shown as a function of preload. For curve b, the contractility is greater than curve a. (**B**) Effects of changes in contractility as a function of afterload. (**C**) Effects of changes of contractility on the pressure–volume curve. LV, left ventricle. Modified from Wanneburg T, Little WC. Regulation of cardiac output. In: Brown DL, ed. *Cardiac Intensive Care*. WB Saunders; 1998.

the relative cardiac performance for a given preload and afterload. Similarly, decrements in contractility will alter this relationship in a negative fashion.

Pathophysiology of Cardiac Failure

As explained previously, cardiac failure is defined as the inability of the heart to meet the metabolic needs of the body or the inability to meet those needs without an elevation in filling pressures. The complex interplay of various phenomena results in normal cardiac function. Coordination of the cardiac muscle function with venous filling, the rate and rhythm of contraction, and valvular competence is required. Abnormalities of any of these components can eventually lead to cardiac failure.

Mechanisms

Impairment of contractile function includes primary muscle disorders such as myocardial infarction and rhythm disorders. **Table 42–1** lists common cardiac disorders that can lead to heart failure via this pathway. In these disorders, the primary problem is the inability of the heart to pump because of either direct impairment in the force of contraction or in the frequency of contractions (as in arrhythmias). This form of heart failure is often called **systolic dysfunction** and can be represented graphically as a shift in the Starling curve downward (**Figure 42–6**).

Many forms of heart disease impose an excessive load on the heart (refer to Table 42–1). This load can be either in the form of an excess pressure requirement or an excess volume requirement. The load may occur as an acute overload that rapidly causes deterioration in cardiac function or as a chronic load that slowly leads to cardiac failure.

An example of an acute volume overload is papillary muscle rupture and acute mitral regurgitation. In this situation, the heart suddenly ejects a large amount of blood from the left ventricle through the mitral valve into the left atrium during systole, thus reducing the forward $\dot{Q}c$ to the systemic circulation and increasing left atrial pressure. Compensation via increased contractility may not adequately augment forward stroke volume because the low pressure of the left atrium relative to the systemic circulation preferentially directs blood flow through the injured valve. Thus these patients will often present with hypotension and shock from low $\dot{Q}c$ and pulmonary edema from increased left atrial pressure.

Chronic volume overload results from disorders such as progressive aortic or mitral valve regurgitation, in which initially a small portion of the stroke volume is regurgitated into the ventricle. The result is a decrease in the true forward $\dot{Q}c$ at a given LVEDV. Under such conditions the slow progression of the degree of regurgitation

TABLE 42–1 Pathophysiology of Cardiac Failure with Clinical Examples

Pathophysiology	Clinical Examples
Restricted filling	Restrictive cardiomyopathy Constrictive pericarditis Tamponade Hypertrophic cardiomyopathy Mitral stenosis Tricuspid stenosis
Pressure overload	Hypertension Aortic stenosis Pulmonary embolism Pulmonary hypertension Pulmonary stenosis
Volume overload	Mitral regurgitation Aortic regurgitation Pulmonary regurgitation Tricuspid regurgitation Septal defects
Contractile impairment	Ischemia (chronic or acute) Dilated cardiomyopathy Myocarditis
Arrhythmia	Tachycardia Bradycardia

From Timmis AD, Nathan AW. *Essentials of Cardiology*. Oxford: Blackwell Scientific; 1993.

allows the heart to compensate with slow dilation and an increase in mass, which helps to normalize wall stress and preserve the forward stroke volume (**Figure 42–7**), although this leads to a chronic increase in LVEDV and LV wall thickness.

In acute pressure overload, a high afterload reduces the forward output of the heart. Because of the acute nature of the overload, the compensatory mechanisms of the heart (increased LVEDV and increased contractility) may be inadequate to augment forward flow, leading to elevated filling pressures with pulmonary edema. Acute pressure overload is typified by hypertensive emergency, a process in which there is a sudden and severe increase in systemic blood pressure. **Figure 42–8** illustrates the relationship between $\dot{Q}c$ and arterial pressure.

Chronic pressure overload, as exemplified by chronic hypertension and aortic stenosis, results in a sustained increase in afterload and ventricular wall stress. Over time the cardiomyocytes will adapt to this stress by hypertrophy, and clinically this adaptation can result in thickened ventricular walls. A pressure overload such as aortic stenosis can be demonstrated graphically as shown in **Figure 42–9**.

As the increased load continues, adaptive mechanisms will eventually fail to compensate and the signs of cardiac failure will become evident. The end result is systolic dysfunction. This process differs from the previously described mechanism because the original cause of the dysfunction is not a primary disorder of the contractile apparatus but, ultimately, is caused by exhausted compensation.

Alteration of ventricular filling may accompany a number of different cardiac disorders (refer to Table 42–1). The disorders range from myocardial valvular disease to pericardial disease. In these disorders, the abnormally high filling pressures are required to achieve the preload necessary to deliver an adequate stroke volume.[3]

The failure of the cardiac muscle to relax normally is often called **diastolic dysfunction** or heart failure with preserved ejection fraction (HFpEF) and represents a common and significant cause of cardiac failure. HFpEF results in elevated filling pressures and

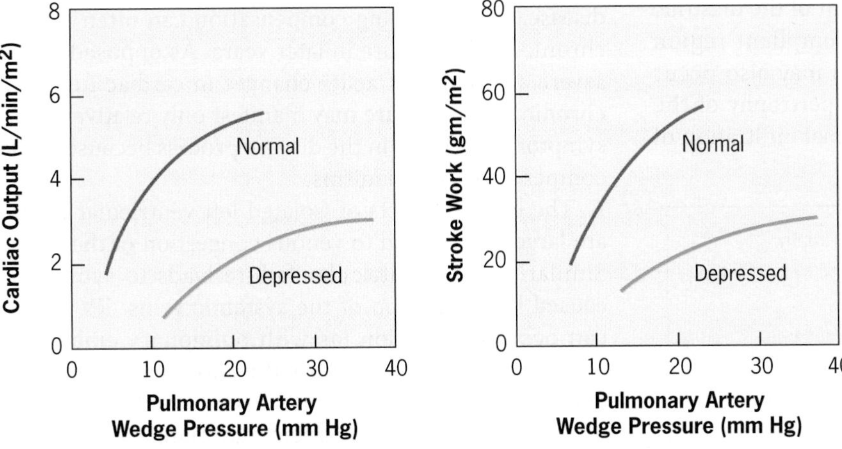

FIGURE 42–6 The effect of a decrease in contractility on the Starling relationship. This article was published in Little WC, Braunwald E. Assessment of cardiac function. In: Braunwald E, ed. *Heart Disease: A Textbook of Cardiovascular Medicine*. 5th ed. Copyright Elsevier (WB Saunders) 1997.

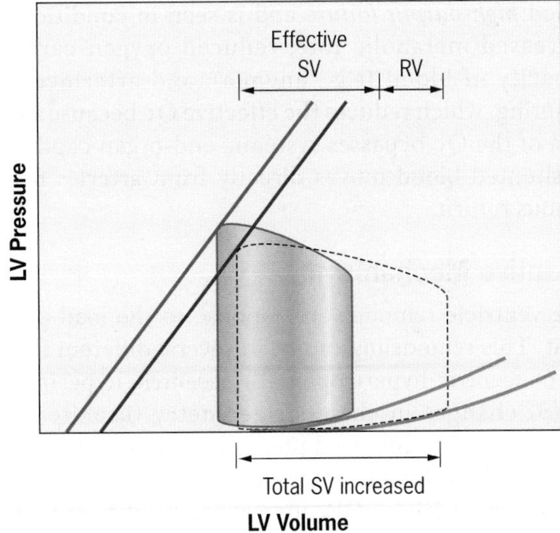

FIGURE 42–7 The effect of a chronic volume overload on the pressure–volume curve of the left ventricle (LV). RV, regurgitant volume; SV, stroke volume. Modified from Wannenburg T, Little WC. Regulation of cardiac output. In: Brown DL, ed. *Cardiac Intensive Care*. WB Saunders; 1998.

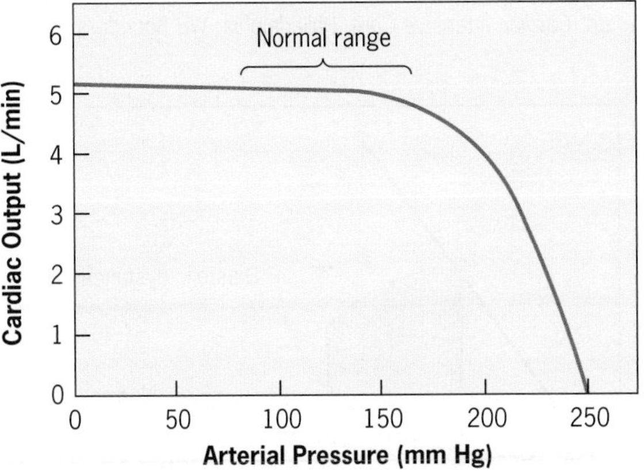

FIGURE 42–8 Constancy of cardiac output up to a pressure level of 160 mm Hg. Only when the arterial pressure rises above the normal operating pressure range does the pressure load cause the cardiac output to fall. This article was published in Guyton AC, Hall JE. *Textbook of Medical Physiology*. 10th ed. Copyright Elsevier (WB Saunders) 2000.

> **RESPIRATORY RECAP**
>
> **Mechanisms of Cardiac Failure**
>
> » Primary impaired myocardial contractile function
> » Excessive ventricular load (pressure or volume)
> » Restricted ventricular filling
>
> *Note:* These mechanisms of cardiac failure are not mutually exclusive, and many forms of heart disease show components of all three pathways.

symptoms of pulmonary and systemic congestion despite normal systolic function. HFpEF is caused by processes that affect the active (energy-dependent) and passive (compliance) relaxation of the ventricle.[5,6] Many conditions cause diastolic dysfunction. As previously noted, early in diastole the ventricular relaxation is an energy-requiring process, so cardiac ischemia is a common cause of both diastolic and systolic dysfunction. Volume overload can cause relative diastolic dysfunction by increasing the LVEDV, thus increasing the LV filling pressures because of a shift of the diastolic pressure–volume curve into a less compliant region (**Figure 42–10**). Diastolic dysfunction may also occur with an increase in afterload. With hypertrophy of the myocardium or in conditions of abnormal infiltration of the myocardium, the ventricles are less compliant, and the diastolic pressure volume curve will shift upward (refer to Figure 42–10). Extrinsic compression of the heart does not affect the intrinsic relaxation of the myocardium but reduces the distensibility of the heart and thus displaces the pressure–volume curve upward.

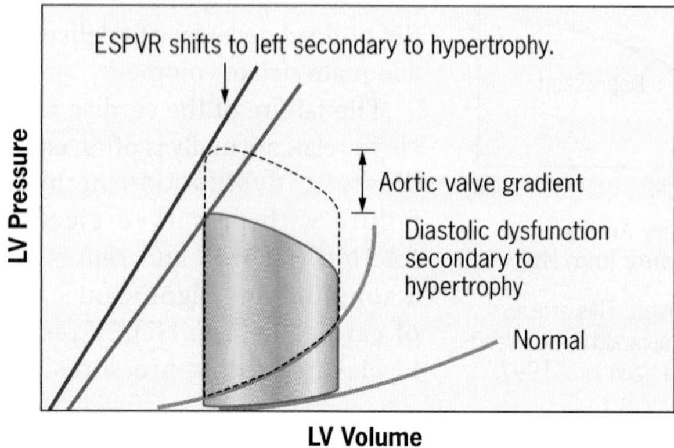

FIGURE 42–9 The effect of a chronic pressure overload (aortic stenosis) on the pressure–volume curve of the left ventricle (LV). ESPVR, end-systolic pressure–volume relationship. Modified from Wannenburg T, Little WC. Regulation of cardiac output. In: Brown DL, ed. *Cardiac Intensive Care*. Philadelphia: WB Saunders; 1998.

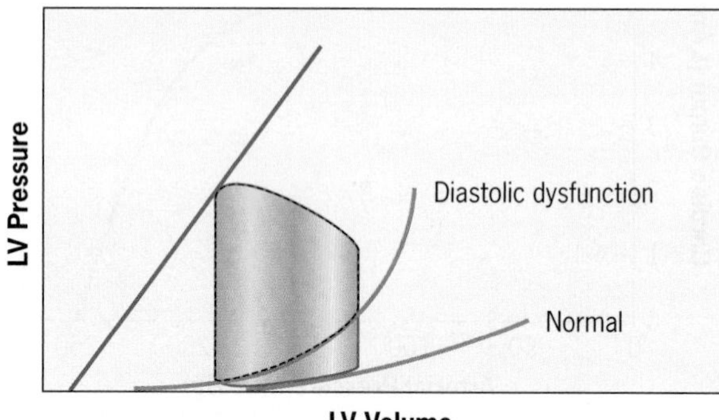

FIGURE 42–10 Diastolic dysfunction leads to an elevation of the diastolic pressure–volume curve of the left ventricle (LV). Modified from Wannenburg T, Little WC. Regulation of cardiac output. In: Brown DL, ed. *Cardiac Intensive Care*. Philadelphia: WB Saunders; 1998.

Classification

The temporal course of cardiac failure is an important etiologic consideration. Myocardial infarction, myocarditis, and pulmonary emboli may cause acute cardiac failure. An acute, severe change in cardiac function can cause pulmonary edema and shock resulting from the inability of the heart to adapt rapidly to loss of myocardium or a dramatic increase in load. Chronic cardiac failure is seen in conditions such as coronary artery disease, hypertensive heart disease, and chronic valvular disease. Long-standing compensation can often lead to chronic cardiac failure in later years. As opposed to the severe symptoms of acute changes in cardiac function, chronic cardiac failure may manifest only relatively mild symptoms until late in the disease process because of the compensatory mechanisms.

The clinical effects of isolated left ventricular failure are largely attributed to venous congestion of the lungs. Similarly, right ventricular failure leads to symptoms caused by congestion of the systemic veins. RV failure can occur in isolation (as with pulmonary embolism) or concurrent with LV failure (biventricular failure). RV failure most commonly results from LV failure. In cases of biventricular failure a patient may manifest symptoms of predominantly right or left ventricular failure, or both.

Most forms of cardiac failure are characterized by a reduction in the $\dot{Q}c$ either at rest or with exercise. In certain uncommon conditions, the tissue demand for oxygen cannot be met despite a high $\dot{Q}c$. This is called *high-output failure* and is seen in conditions of increased metabolic rate, reduced oxygen-carrying capacity of blood (e.g., anemia), and arteriovenous shunting, which reduces the effective $\dot{Q}c$ because a portion of the $\dot{Q}c$ bypasses systemic end-organ capillaries as shunted blood moves directly from arteries to the venous return.

Adaptive Mechanisms

The ventricle remodels in response to the load placed on it. This remodeling can be in several different forms: (1) concentric hypertrophy, (2) eccentric hypertrophy, or (3) changes in chamber geometry (usually more sphere-like). A prolonged pressure load on the myocardium leads to fundamental changes in cardiac muscle. In experimental models, increased systolic wall stress upregulates growth factors that increase the number of mitochondria and increase myofibril mass. The new myofibrils are usually laid down in parallel, leading to myocyte hypertrophy and, ultimately, to a concentrically thicker ventricle. Physiologically, a thicker ventricle serves to normalize increased wall stress. Wall stress can be calculated by the law of Laplace:

Wall stress = (Pressure × Radius)/(2 × Wall thickness)

Thus, the pressure the ventricle contracts against is directly proportional to wall stress. As the ventricle increases its thickness, wall stress decreases, which in turn improves cardiac performance to a point. However, this improved performance is at the price of increased oxygen demand and possible diastolic dysfunction.

The dilated ventricle has increased diastolic wall stress caused by increased diastolic volume (due to an increased radius). In an effort to accommodate the increased volume, myocytes increase the number of sarcomeres in series, thus increasing the radius and length of the ventricle. As the chamber radius increases, so does systolic wall stress, and the ventricle is therefore stimulated to increase in thickness. Thus, volume overload induces ventricular dilation and hypertrophy to compensate for the increased diastolic wall stress. This adaptation initially allows compensation for increased diastolic load at normalized wall stress.

The ventricle changes in shape in response to the specific, chronic load placed on it in order to optimize function. Chronic pressure loads induce thickened ventricles with small cavities, whereas chronic volume loads cause dilation of the ventricle. These ventricular shape changes have effects on both systolic and diastolic performance, as well as on oxygen use. These adaptive compensatory changes may become ineffective if the heart thickens or dilates excessively, and cardiac failure may ensue.[3]

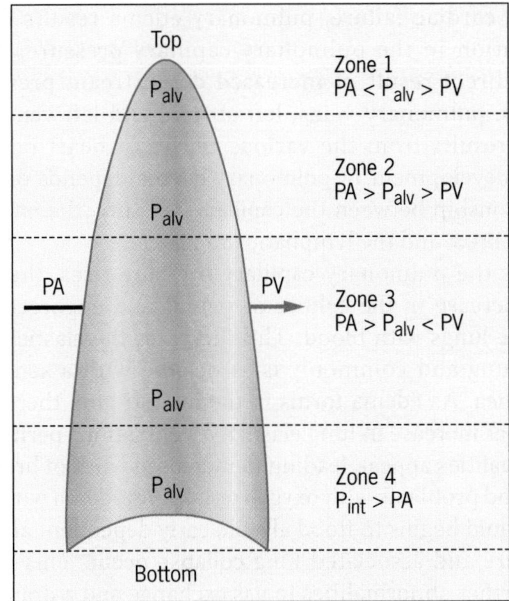

FIGURE 42–11 The four perfusion zones of the lung. The heights of the thick black lines represent pulmonary arterial (PA) and pulmonary venous (PV) pressures. P_{alv}, alveolar pressure; P_{int}, interstitial pressure. Modified from Gaine SP, et al. Pathophysiology of the pulmonary vascular bed. In: Dantzker DR. Scharf SM, eds. *Cardiopulmonary Critical Care*. 3rd ed. WB Saunders; 1998.

Pathophysiology of Pulmonary Edema

Pulmonary edema is the accumulation of excess fluid in the interstitial and alveolar spaces in the lung. The large capillary network of the pulmonary circulation has extensive interaction with the air-filled alveoli. The interstitium between the capillary endothelial cells and the alveolar epithelial cells is quite thin and made up of a basement membrane, connective tissue, and cellular elements. Normally a continuous flux of fluid and proteins is transported between the pulmonary circulation and the lung interstitium, with a net flow from the capillaries into the interstitial tissue. Excess fluid is removed from the interstitium by the lymphatic system. Pulmonary edema develops when there is an increase in the flux of fluid going into the lung interstitium that overwhelms the lymphatic drainage. Normally the lymphatic drainage actively takes up interstitial fluid and removes it from the interstitial space at about 20 mL/hour. With chronic pulmonary edema, the pulmonary lymphatics hypertrophy and increased amounts of fluid can be removed (up to 200 mL/hour).

Pulmonary edema can result from any of a number of causes that create an increased influx of fluid to the interstitium. These mechanisms include increased pulmonary capillary pressure as in cardiac failure, decreased blood oncotic pressure, and increased capillary permeability. Increased fluid flux into the interstitium eventually overwhelms the lymphatic drainage, and fluid initially collects in the most compliant regions of the interstitium around vessels and airways. With increased accumulation, fluid begins to collect in the alveolocapillary membrane and eventually floods the alveoli.

> **RESPIRATORY RECAP**
>
> **Mechanisms of Pulmonary Edema**
>
> » Increased pulmonary capillary pressure as in cardiac failure
> » Decreased blood oncotic pressure
> » Increased capillary permeability

Gravity directs the majority of lung blood flow toward the most dependent regions of the lung. Pulmonary perfusion pressure and pulmonary venous pressure increase from the apex to the base in the upright lung (**Figure 42–11**). Thus, edema is most likely to form in the dependent regions (West zone III). As interstitial pressure increases, the lumen of the pulmonary vessels may be compressed in the dependent regions, leading to a decrease in their perfusion (West zone IV) and redistribution of the blood flow into the nondependent regions. This is the cause of the increased apical vascular markings commonly seen on chest radiographs of patients with pulmonary edema.

In cardiac failure, pulmonary edema results from elevation in the pulmonary capillary pressure. This is a direct result of increased downstream pressure in the pulmonary veins, left atrium, and left ventricle that results from the various causes of heart failure. The development of pulmonary edema depends on the relationship between the capillary pressure, the **oncotic pressures**, and the lymphatic drainage.

As the pulmonary capillary pressure rises, there is an increase in the caliber of vessels and engorgement of the lungs with blood. This increases the elasticity of the lung and commonly is associated with a sense of dyspnea. As edema forms in the interstitium, there is a further increase in lung elasticity. Ventilation–perfusion inequalities appear, leading to increased work of breathing and problems with oxygen uptake. As edema worsens and fluid begins to flood alveoli, early dependent airway closure and associated lung collapse occur. This leads to further abnormalities in gas exchange and a dramatic increase in elasticity and work of breathing. In addition, engorged blood vessels may reduce the caliber of small airways and increase airways resistance. This can then cause a decreased vital capacity and air trapping. Often the airway edema predisposes patients to bronchospasm, and they may develop wheezing, sometimes called cardiac asthma. Gas exchange abnormalities may be quite severe, with hypoxia followed by hypercapnia as the patient begins to fatigue. In acute severe pulmonary edema, the patient may rapidly progress to respiratory failure. Rapid diagnosis and application of therapy can be life saving and often can avoid the use of mechanical ventilation.

Heart–Lung Interactions

The heart and lungs are pressure-driven systems that share the primary responsibility for oxygen uptake and delivery to the body. They also share a common space (the thorax) and thus are linked anatomically. The heart and lung interactions based on these physiologic links often have profound consequences in critical illness. With each breath the lungs and thorax change, both in volume and in intrathoracic pressure. These fluctuations can affect cardiac function by inducing changes in the heart rate, preload, afterload, venous return, and contractility of the heart. The heart–lung interactions in cardiac failure can be especially challenging because the heart is less likely to tolerate fluctuations in these physiologic variables. A basic understanding of these interactions is important in the guidance of therapy such as mechanical ventilation.

Changes in Intrathoracic Pressure

The changes in pleural pressure with ventilation affect the pressures at the heart's surface. The cardiac surface pressure will affect cardiac filling pressures based on the compliance of the myocardium. In addition, cardiac filling volume is dependent on the transmural pressure, or the distending stress across the wall of the cardiac chamber. Thus, the pleural pressure swings during respiration can affect preload and afterload of the heart. For example, a decrease in pleural pressure during inspiration will be transmitted to the surface of the heart. During inspiration, the right atrial pressure falls relative to the systemic extrathoracic venous circulation, and venous filling of the right atrium is enhanced. This leads to an increase in venous return and right atrial volume during inspiration. Similarly, assuming a constant arterial pressure, a decrease in the pleural pressure that also lowers cardiac surface pressure will increase afterload by increasing the LV transmural pressure. An increase in intrathoracic pressure can decrease afterload by a similar mechanism. Normally these are small changes, but if there are large swings in the pleural pressure (as with respiratory distress) or if cardiac function is reduced, the effects can be more significant. The cardiac surface pressure also depends on the pericardial compliance and pressure, which is sensitive to changes in the volume of the cardiac chambers. Thus, the change in cardiac surface pressure with a change in pleural pressure can be quite variable.

RESPIRATORY RECAP

Heart–Lung Interactions

- » Intrathoracic pressure changes
- » Lung volume changes
- » Pulmonary vascular resistance
- » Mechanical effects of lung expansion
- » Abdominal pressure changes
- » Ventricular interdependence

Changes in Lung Volume

Changes in lung volume can influence cardiovascular performance by a number of different mechanisms. These mechanisms include changes in autonomic tone, changes in **pulmonary vascular resistance (PVR)**, direct mechanical compression of the cardiac fossa, increases in intra-abdominal pressure, and ventricular interdependence. Such effects are manifest with every breath and can become quite significant during periods of sustained inflation as with mechanical ventilation and high positive end-expiratory pressure (PEEP).

Changes in Pulmonary Vascular Resistance

The major determinants of pulmonary blood flow are RV systolic performance and the PVR. The PVR is highly dependent on the volume of the lungs. As alveoli expand, the vessels surrounding them are compressed, thus increasing the resistance to flow. Vessels outside of the alveoli are pulled open during lung inflation by radial traction, which decreases vascular resistance. The net effect of the opposing changes is that PVR is lowest at the functional residual capacity (FRC) of the lungs. Decreases or increases in resting lung volume

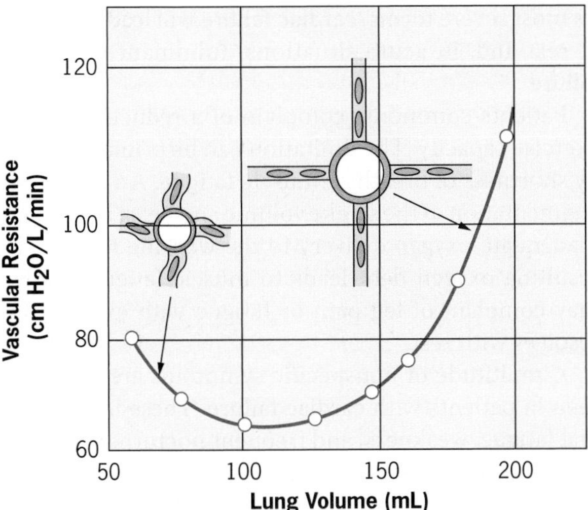

FIGURE 42–12 Effect of lung volume on the pulmonary vascular resistance. The effect of lung volume on the caliber of extra-alveolar vessels also is shown. Modified from West JB. *Respiratory Physiology*. Lippincott Williams & Wilkins; 1990.

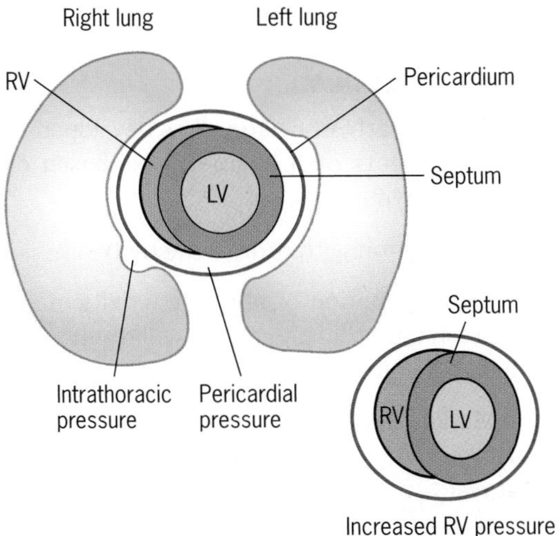

FIGURE 42–13 The anatomic relationship between the heart and lungs. RV, right ventricle; LV, left ventricle. This article was published in Scharf SM. Mechanical cardiopulmonary interactions in critical care. In: Dantzker DR. Scharf SM, eds. *Cardiopulmonary Critical Care*. 3rd ed. Copyright Elsevier (WB Saunders) 1998.

cause an increase in the PVR (**Figure 42–12**). An increase in PVR increases RV afterload and thus may decrease cardiac performance. In cardiac failure, alveolar edema may cause alveolar collapse and an increase in PVR. The use of PEEP may restore resting lung volume to the normal FRC and decrease PVR. If applied in excess, PEEP can increase lung volume above FRC and increase the PVR.[7,8]

Mechanical Effects of Lung Expansion

As the lungs expand, they can affect the heart by physically pushing against the cardiac fossa (**Figure 42–13**). This will increase the pressure surrounding the heart and can affect filling of the ventricles. The

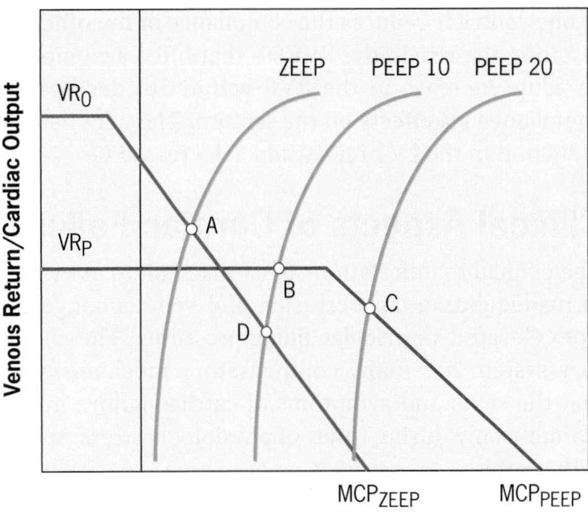

FIGURE 42–14 Effects of positive end-expiratory pressure (PEEP) on the determinants of venous return. VR_0, venous return curve with zero PEEP (ZEEP); VR_P, venous return with PEEP; MCP, mean circulatory pressure. This article was published in Scharf SM. Mechanical cardiopulmonary interactions in critical care. In: Dantzker DR. Scharf SM, eds. *Cardiopulmonary Critical Care*. 3rd ed. Copyright Elsevier (WB Saunders) 1998.

effect is independent of the pleural pressure change and dependent on lung volume. In patients with hyperinflation (as with chronic obstructive pulmonary disease [COPD]), the lungs can exert a fair amount of pressure around the heart and adversely affect ventricular filling.

Abdominal Pressure Changes

The descent of the diaphragm with respiration compresses the abdominal compartment and increases abdominal pressure. This increases the abdominal vascular pressures and increases the driving pressure for venous return. If the patient is receiving positive pressure ventilation, the increase in abdominal pressure may partially compensate for the increase in right atrial pressure induced by the positive pressure. Thus, the application of PEEP can have complicated effects on the venous return depending on the change in abdominal pressure and previous filling pressure of the ventricle (**Figure 42–14**).

Ventricular Interdependence

Although not a true heart–lung interaction, ventricular interdependence is often discussed in this setting. Changes in the volume and performance of one ventricle will affect the other ventricle through two general mechanisms. The filling of the LV depends on the output of the RV. Thus, a reduction in RV performance will reduce LV output by reducing LV preload. This is often called the *series interaction*. In addition, the ventricles are both surrounded by the relatively nondistensible sac called the pericardium, and both ventricles share a common intraventricular septum. This anatomic coupling results in parallel interactions in which an increase in the volume of one ventricle reduces the compliance of the other. For instance, the rise in the RVEDV that often accompanies an acute increase in the PVR will act to decrease LV compliance via effects on the septum. The net effect is a reduction in the LV preload and a decreased $\dot{Q}c$.

Clinical Aspects of Cardiac Failure

The clinical manifestations of cardiac failure are related to inadequate organ perfusion and venous congestion from elevated ventricular filling pressures. The circulatory system has many compensatory mechanisms, so that the signs and symptoms of cardiac failure may be manifest only during times of physiologic stress, such as with exercise.

Symptoms

The increased pulmonary capillary pressure and resulting interstitial edema seen in cardiac failure commonly lead to difficulty in breathing or an increased awareness of breathing. Most of the dyspnea can be attributed to an increased work of breathing resulting from decreased pulmonary function and increased ventilatory drive. Pulmonary edema increases lung elastance and can increase airways resistance, thus increasing the pressure changes needed to move air in and out of the lungs. Ventilation and perfusion abnormalities lead to hypoxemia and hypercapnia, which increase the drive to breathe. With extreme decreases in $\dot{Q}c$, respiratory muscle fatigue can develop as a result of poor oxygen delivery to the respiratory muscles and further exacerbate the patient's dyspnea. Thus, dyspnea may be caused by either pulmonary congestion or a low-output state.

The breathlessness of cardiac failure can manifest in many different ways. Most commonly the patient with cardiac failure has dyspnea on exertion. This symptom can be a slowly progressive process, so it is important to ascertain the changes in the patient's exercise tolerance over time. As cardiac failure progresses, the patient may develop breathlessness when recumbent (**orthopnea**). This symptom likely results from decreased pooling of blood in the lower extremities in the supine position. This displaces blood into the central circulation, increases filling pressures, and increases interstitial edema. The patient may report a change in the number of pillows required to sleep or, in severe cases, the need to sleep in a chair. Breathlessness can occur suddenly during sleep, so-called paroxysmal nocturnal dyspnea (PND). Patients will relate terrifying episodes of air hunger during the night requiring them to sit upright. PND may result from sudden bronchospasm related to airway edema. Often the symptoms resolve once the patient is upright for a period of time. Finally, in its most severe forms, cardiac failure will lead to dyspnea at rest and, in acute situations, fulminant respiratory failure.

> **RESPIRATORY RECAP**
>
> **Symptoms of Cardiac Failure**
> - Dyspnea
> - Reduced exercise capacity
> - General fatigue, weakness, nocturia
> - Peripheral edema

Patients commonly complain of a reduction in their exercise capacity. The limitation can be primarily caused by shortness of breath or muscle fatigue. An insufficient augmentation of the stroke volume and heart rate leads to inadequate oxygen delivery to the working muscle. The resulting oxygen debt leads to muscle fatigue. Patients may complain of leg pain or fatigue with exertion that resolves with rest.

A multitude of nonspecific symptoms are commonly seen in patients with cardiac failure. These include general fatigue, weakness, and frequent nocturnal urination. Occurrences of mental status changes or confusion are signs of a drastically reduced $\dot{Q}c$. Patients with right heart failure, either isolated or resulting from left heart failure, will commonly complain of peripheral edema. The legs are involved most commonly. Dyspnea is not a prominent feature of right heart failure and is usually seen only with severe RV dysfunction.

Functional Classification

The New York Heart Association has developed a classification of patients with heart disease based on the severity of their symptoms.[9]

Class I: No limitation with ordinary activity

Class II: Slight limitation of physical activity; no symptoms at rest, but ordinary activity will result in fatigue, dyspnea, palpitation, or angina

Class III: Marked limitation of physical activity; less than ordinary activity results in symptoms, but comfortable at rest

Class IV: Inability to carry on any physical activity without discomfort; symptoms present at rest

Physical Examination

The physical signs of cardiac failure are often nonspecific, and many findings may be absent in patients, even with severe chronic heart failure. In the correct clinical setting, signs of elevated cardiac filling pressures can be diagnostic of cardiac failure. The following physical signs are suggestive of cardiac failure.

Fluid retention and elevated right filling pressures can lead to the extravasation of fluid into the extravascular space, which is usually seen in the legs or back. Commonly the edema is symmetrical and manifests over several days. An enlarged and/or pulsatile liver can result from elevated filling pressures and tricuspid regurgitation. Ascites can be seen in severe cases. In a recumbent patient with the head of bed at 45 degrees, the upper excursion of the pulsations in the internal jugular vein are normally not more than 3 cm above the sternal angle. With elevated right ventricular filling pressures, the level will be elevated. Some patients will have a normal jugular venous pressure (JVP) but will elevate the JVP inappropriately when the abdomen is compressed over the liver. This sign is called **hepatojugular reflux** and, if present and sustained, suggests altered RV compliance or RV failure or both.

The transudation of fluid into the pulmonary parenchyma leads to airway and alveolar collapse. The expansion of these regions with inspiration leads to characteristic wet crackles, best heard in the dependent regions. The presence of airway edema with bronchospasm will create high-pitched wheezes similar to those in patients with asthma. Crackles and wheezes together in a patient with sudden-onset shortness of breath are highly suggestive of pulmonary edema. Cheyne-Stokes respirations are occasionally seen in cardiac failure. This characteristic pattern of alternating hyperpneas and apneas results from a slow circulation time between the lungs and brain. Patients are often unaware of the breathing pattern, and it may manifest only during sleep.

RESPIRATORY RECAP

Physical Examination in Cardiac Failure

- Peripheral edema
- Congestive hepatomegaly
- Elevated jugular venous pressure
- Pulmonary auscultation: dependent lung crackles and wheezes
- Cheyne-Stokes breathing pattern
- Abnormal cardiac palpation
- Cardiac auscultation: S_3, S_4, murmurs

The contraction of the heart can normally be felt as a small impulse on the chest below the left nipple. With enlargement of the left ventricle, this point of maximal impulse will be displaced inferiorly and laterally on the chest. The impulse may become quite enlarged and diffuse with severe LV dilation. With hypertrophy of the left ventricle, the impulse may feel stronger and more sustained. The right ventricular impulse is not usually felt, but with RV strain or dilation, a lift may be felt just to the left of the sternum. This parasternal lift is suggestive of RV enlargement or failure. With pulmonary hypertension, a tap may be felt over the left base of the heart, a sign known as a pulmonary artery (PA) tap. Finally, severe murmurs can occasionally be palpated as thrills over the precordium.

The presence of a third heart sound (S_3) after the closure of the aortic and pulmonary valves is suggestive of cardiac failure. The sound likely represents the deceleration of blood in the right or left ventricle during early diastole. A fourth heart sound (S_4) occurring in late diastole is found in patients with thick noncompliant ventricles and likely results from vibrations during atrial contraction. Other cardiac sounds, such as murmurs, which result from turbulent flow, can result from stenosis or regurgitation of any of the four valves. The presence of murmurs can provide clues to the etiology of cardiac failure.

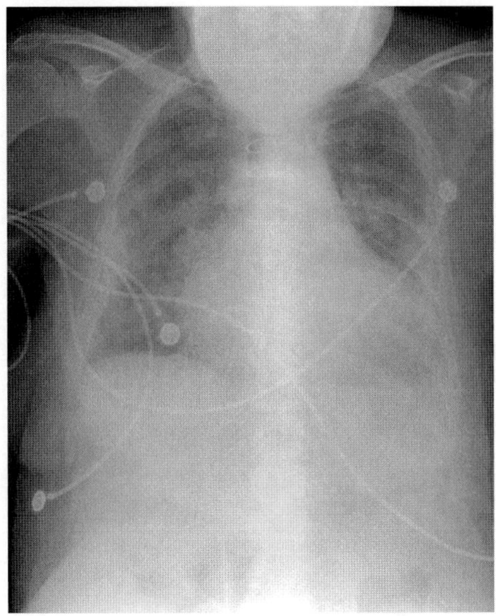

FIGURE 42–15 Anteroposterior chest radiograph of a patient with cardiac failure.

Radiography

The chest radiograph (**Figure 42–15**) provides a relatively inexpensive and easy way to assess the lung fields and the size of the heart. Pulmonary edema is often evident on a chest radiograph as basilar infiltrates with pulmonary vascular redistribution. The infiltrates range from subtle interstitial markings to frank alveolar exudates. As blood flow is redistributed to the nondependent vessels, the upper lobe vasculature appears plump and indistinct. Bilateral pleural effusions and enlargement of the cardiac silhouette also are commonly seen. In chronic cardiac failure, the chest radiograph may be quite unremarkable apart from cardiomegaly. In addition, radiographic changes may lag behind clinical changes. Nevertheless, the chest radiograph remains a cornerstone for the diagnosis and follow-up of cardiac failure.

Measurement and Monitoring of Cardiac Function

Electrocardiography

The electrocardiogram (ECG) records the electrical impulses propagated in the heart (**Figure 42–16**). The impulses are recorded in two planes and at 12 different positions (leads). By examining the resulting complexes, one can determine the heart rate, the rhythm, and whether there are any abnormalities in conduction or repolarization. In addition, the patterns on the ECG may be diagnostic of certain cardiac disorders. Most notably, the syndrome of cardiac ischemia or infarction can be diagnosed by certain abnormalities on the electrocardiogram.

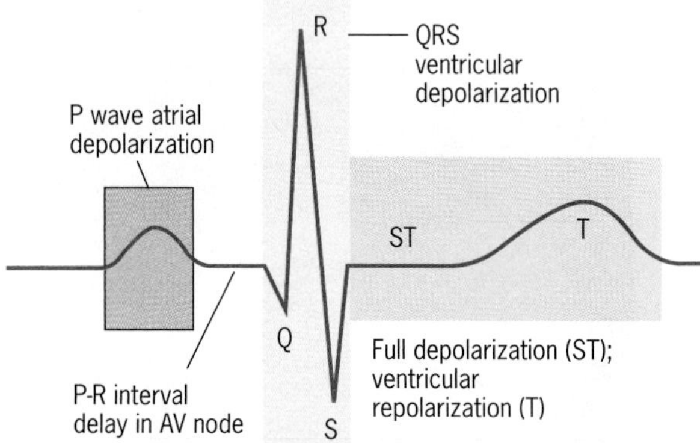

FIGURE 42–16 Normal electrocardiogram waveform. AV, arteriovenous.

Echocardiography

Echocardiography is a noninvasive form of cardiac imaging used extensively to diagnose a variety of valvular and myocardial diseases. The images provide a wealth of information about cardiac pump function as well as valvular and pericardial disease. Many forms of cardiac disease can be definitively diagnosed with echocardiography. Injection of small air bubbles into a vein provides contrast within the cardiac chambers. Crossover of bubbles into the left-sided chambers allows identification of intracardiac and intrapulmonary shunts.

Exercise Stress Test

The exercise stress test is used to diagnose cardiac ischemia resulting from CAD as a cause of chest pain or cardiac dysfunction. The patient is exercised on a treadmill with electrocardiographic and blood pressure monitoring. ECG changes indicative of ischemia are a reasonably reliable method used to detect CAD.

Radionucleotide Imaging

The sensitivity and specificity of exercise ECG stress testing can be increased by imaging of myocardial perfusion with a radioisotope. The isotope is injected during peak exercise, and the heart is imaged with a gamma camera. The heart is then reimaged at rest and compared with the exercise images. Alternatively, images can be taken during infusion of a chemical agent, such as dobutamine or adenosine, which induces ischemia or changes in myocardial perfusion. Areas of myocardium that have altered perfusion caused by ischemia or infarction will not take up the isotope. At rest those areas that were ischemic during exercise (or chemical infusion) now perfuse and take up isotope.

> **RESPIRATORY RECAP**
>
> **Measurement and Monitoring of Cardiac Function**
>
> » Electrocardiogram
> » Echocardiogram
> » Exercise stress test
> » Radionucleotide imaging
> » Coronary angiography
> » CT angiography
> » Hemodynamic monitoring

Coronary Angiography

Direct imaging of the coronary arteries is possible by cardiac catheterization (**coronary angiography**). This technique is used to assess the extent and severity of CAD as a cause for chest pain or cardiac dysfunction. Special catheters are inserted into the aorta and into the origins of the right and left coronary arteries. Contrast dye is injected as radiographic images are obtained. The information obtained can identify atherosclerotic lesions as well as coronary anomalies, areas of spasm, and acute thrombi. Contrast dye also can be injected into the left ventricle and, with subsequent imaging, the cardiac pump function (ejection fraction) can be assessed. In addition, valvular disease can be diagnosed and quantified by imaging and direct pressure measurements.

Computed Tomographic Angiography

Computed tomographic (CT) angiography is an emerging imaging technique for assessment of risk of coronary artery disease. Use of CT imaging in cardiac disease includes both assessment of coronary calcium and CT angiography for evaluation of obstructing lesions in the coronary vessels. The exact use of CT angiography continues to evolve as the technology allows for higher-resolution visualization of the coronary anatomy.[10]

Hemodynamic Monitoring

Direct measurements of the intracardiac and pulmonary vascular pressures are possible through the use of the pulmonary artery catheter. This catheter is equipped with a balloon on the tip that allows it to float from a central vein (internal jugular, subclavian, or femoral) into the right atrium, right ventricle, pulmonary artery, and then into a pulmonary artery occlusion position (often called the wedge pressure). A column of fluid within the catheter allows pressure fluctuations to be transmitted to a transducer and then displayed graphically for analysis. **Figure 42–17** shows a normal set of tracings.

The pulmonary artery occlusion technique creates a static column of blood in a section of the pulmonary vasculature. The measured pressure is a pulmonary venous pressure, which closely approximates left atrial pressure. The mean left atrial pressure also estimates the pressure in the pulmonary capillary circulation. If elevated, fluid may move from the capillaries into the pulmonary interstitium, thereby creating pulmonary edema. These catheters also have the ability to perform measurements of the $\dot{Q}c$ using the thermodilution technique.

Determination of the filling pressures and $\dot{Q}c$ can provide a wealth of information in the setting of pulmonary edema or hypotension. In the case of pulmonary

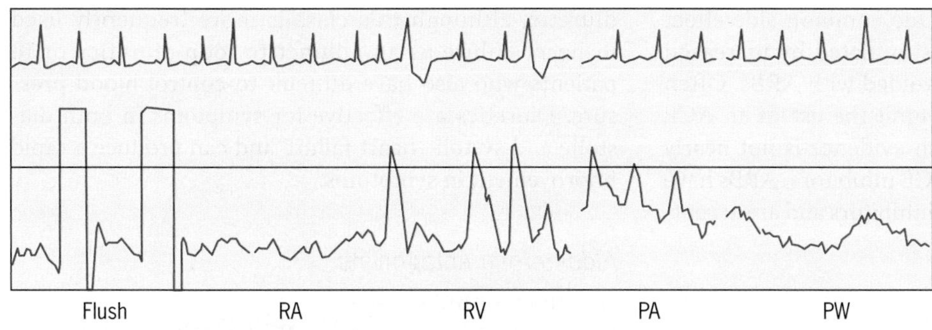

FIGURE 42–17 Normal tracing from a pulmonary artery catheter as it is advanced from the right atrium (RA), right ventricle (RV), pulmonary artery (PA), and into the occlusion or "wedge" (PW). Modified from Leatherman JW, Marini JJ. Pulmonary artery catheterization: interpretation of pressure recordings. In: Tobin MJ, ed. Principles and Practice of Intensive Care Monitoring. New York: McGraw-Hill; 1998.

edema, an elevated pulmonary artery occlusion pressure suggests a cardiac cause for the edema, whereas a low occlusion pressure suggests a capillary leak syndrome (as with acute respiratory distress syndrome [ARDS]). In the setting of hypotension, a low $\dot{Q}c$ with high filling pressures is suggestive of cardiogenic failure or cardiogenic shock.

Treatment Guidelines for Chronic Cardiac Failure

The initial approach to the patient with cardiac failure is to identify the underlying cause and, if possible, treat or remove it. Unfortunately, in the majority of cases of cardiac failure, the underlying cause cannot be easily reversed, so treatment of symptoms is a major goal of therapy. The management of cardiac failure is, however, no longer confined to symptom relief. Treatment to prevent or delay progression of disease and LV remodeling is now the primary focus of many interventions.

The goals of therapy are twofold. The first goal is symptom control and improvement in quality of life. Relieving circulatory congestion and increasing oxygen delivery are the major mechanisms employed to improve symptoms. The second goal is to prevent or delay the progression of the cardiac dysfunction and to prevent the complications that increase mortality. The following discussion is a brief overview of general treatment measures.

Nonpharmacotherapy

In general, lifestyle modification should consist of attempts to optimize diet and exercise, patient education regarding their disease, and avoidance of items that might exacerbate heart failure. In most patients, a modest sodium restriction can be helpful in preventing volume expansion that can lead to pulmonary edema and peripheral edema. Additionally, patients should be taught to weigh themselves frequently because even minor changes in weight can precede obvious clinical signs of volume overload and deterioration of cardiac failure. Although there is no proven benefit of exercise, experts generally recommend physical activity to prevent physical deconditioning. Patients are instructed to avoid toxins and medications that can either worsen their underlying cardiac disease or exacerbate the symptoms of cardiac failure. For example, alcohol should be avoided, especially when the etiology of the cardiac failure is a nonischemic alcohol-induced cardiomyopathy, because patients can have some recovery of function with cessation. Smoking cessation is also a priority given the association of smoking with cardiovascular disease. Obesity has been linked to many cardiac risk factors, including hypertension and diabetes, and patients should be encouraged to lose weight via lifestyle changes such as diet and exercise. Bariatric surgery can be considered in the morbidly obese with significant comorbidities. Aggressive treatment of other cardiovascular comorbidities is also important.

Pharmacotherapy

The treatment of chronic cardiac failure has progressed greatly in the last several decades. Treatment is directed not only at symptom control but also at long-term reductions in morbidity and mortality. Many treatments have been shown to delay or prevent progression of cardiac dysfunction and improve mortality. Thus, even asymptomatic patients with LV dysfunction require thorough evaluation and aggressive treatment.

Angiotensin-Converting Enzyme Inhibitors and Angiotensin Receptor Blockers

Angiotensin-converting enzyme inhibitors, also called ACE inhibitors, have become the mainstay of treatment for chronic cardiac failure. They are one of the most well-studied classes of agents for heart failure and have multiple proposed benefits. Hemodynamic effects include vasodilation leading to a reduction in afterload and an increase in $\dot{Q}c$. ACE inhibitors are also believed to have beneficial effects on cardiac remodeling, thereby helping to prevent decompensation related to the adaptive mechanisms described previously. Overall, data support the claim that this class of medications improves symptoms and reduces hospital admissions and death. Unless a patient with reduced systolic function has a contraindication or experiences a severe adverse effect, he or she should be prescribed an ACE inhibitor.

Although ACE inhibitors are now a first-line therapy in cardiac failure, angiotensin receptor blockers (ARBs) are considered a reasonable alternative in patients unable to tolerate an ACE inhibitor. One common side effect of ACE inhibitors is a cough stimulated by increased bradykinin; this effect can be avoided with ARBs. Often the cough is severe enough to limit the use of an ACE inhibitor. Although the research evidence is not nearly as extensive as that regarding ACE inhibitors, ARBs have proven benefits similar to ACE inhibitors and are acceptable second-line agents.

β-Blockers

β-blockers have been used to treat heart failure caused by cardiac ischemia and diastolic dysfunction for many years. Although they slow relaxation, clinically they control symptoms of diastolic heart failure by slowing the heart rate and providing overall more time for filling during diastole. The use of β-blockers in systolic dysfunction seems counterintuitive because of their negative inotropic effects and decrease in contractility, but is clearly effective. Initial studies in the 1970s suggested that β-blockade improved symptoms and cardiac function in patients with systolic heart failure. Smaller studies in the 1980s confirmed these results,[11,12] but β-blockade to treat cardiac failure caused by LV dysfunction did not become accepted therapy until recently. One reason for this is the lack of a mechanistic consensus on how β-blockers are beneficial in cardiac failure. β-blockers alter the sympathetic axis and affect the β-receptor signaling cascade. Because excessive, sustained neurohumoral activation is common in cardiac failure and contributes to myocyte dysfunction and deleterious chamber remodeling, blockade of this pathway actually improves cardiac function in the long term by inhibiting adverse remodeling.[13]

Because of early reports of increased bronchospasm in patients with underlying reactive airways (both asthma and COPD), there is often concern about administering β-blockers to these patients. However with the development of the more specific cardioselective β-blockers, which act preferentially on the β_1 receptor, there is little evidence to suggest an increased risk of exacerbating asthma or COPD with this class of β-blocker. A large meta-analysis concluded that cardioselective β-blockers do not produce significant adverse effects in patients with mild to moderate reactive airways.[14]

Diuretics

Diuretics are a class of drugs that prevent sodium reabsorption in the kidney and promote sodium loss in the urine. This effect increases salt and water excretion and in heart failure helps reduce circulatory congestion. The physiologic effect of reduced circulating volume is a reduction in filling pressures and thus less transudation of fluid from the systemic and pulmonary circulation. There are several classes of diuretics, but the one most commonly used for cardiac failure is the loop diuretic. Commonly used loop diuretics are furosemide and torsemide. Another frequently used class is the thiazide diuretic, although this class is more frequently used in heart failure as an adjunct to loop diuretics or in patients who also have difficult-to-control blood pressure. Diuretics are effective for symptoms in both diastolic and systolic heart failure and can produce a rapid improvement in symptoms.

Aldosterone Antagonists

> **RESPIRATORY RECAP**
>
> **Pharmacotherapy for Cardiac Failure**
>
> » ACE inhibitors
> » β-blockers
> » Diuretics
> » Aldosterone antagonists
> » Hydralazine and nitrates
> » Digoxin

In select populations, the addition of an aldosterone antagonist such as spironolactone can be considered. Aldosterone antagonists work in the same pathway as ACE inhibitors, thereby having the similar hemodynamic effect of decreasing afterload. They also have a weak diuretic effect. This class of medications has proven beneficial in carefully selected patients with severe heart failure symptoms and LV dysfunction following myocardial infarction. Patients must be monitored closely, however, for development of potentially life-threatening hyperkalemia, and use of aldosterone antagonists should be avoided in the setting of renal dysfunction.

Hydralazine and Nitrates

Hydralazine is an effective vasodilator that when combined with isosorbide dinitrate has been shown to modestly improve survival in patients with cardiac failure. Hydralazine is primarily an arterial vasodilator whose mechanism of action is unclear. Nitrates such as isosorbide dinitrate work by releasing nitric oxide and work as venodilators at low doses as well as arterial vasodilators at higher doses. The venodilation effect acts to decrease preload, thereby improving $\dot{Q}c$. The combination of hydralazine and nitrates should be considered in patients who cannot tolerate either ACE inhibitors or ARBs. A frequent indication is in the patient who develops hypotension and renal failure during treatment with an ACE inhibitor.

Digoxin

Derived from the leaves of the digitalis plant, digoxin is one of the oldest medications in use. This cardiac glycoside is a potent inhibitor of sodium and potassium exchange across the cardiac cell membranes. The excess sodium available within the cell increases calcium flux into the cell. The increased availability of cytosolic calcium increases the velocity and force of muscle shortening. Digoxin thus has a positive inotropic effect. Digoxin also increases the sensitivity of the baroreceptors, leading to a decrease in the sympathetic activation seen in cardiac failure.

The benefit of digoxin therapy is counterbalanced by the risk for toxicity. Increased serum levels of digoxin are associated with mental status changes, arrhythmias, and sinus arrest. Moreover, the drug has numerous interactions with other medications and has a reduced clearance in patients with renal failure. Studies of digoxin therapy in patients with systolic dysfunction have failed to show a mortality benefit, although digoxin did reduce symptoms and hospitalizations. In patients who have failed to respond appropriately to other treatment modalities, digoxin can be a useful adjunct therapy.[15]

Percutaneous Coronary Intervention

Percutaneous coronary intervention (PCI) consists primarily of either balloon angioplasty or placement of stents in occluded or stenotic coronary arteries. In conjunction with coronary angioplasty, in which contrast dye is used to evaluate the coronary circulation, PCI can be used to improve flow through affected arteries. The clearest indication for PCI is in the setting of acute coronary syndrome (described later in this chapter); however, there can be a role in cardiac failure if there is evidence of viable myocardium on radionucleotide imaging or in acute decompensated heart failure. Patients with a new diagnosis of cardiac failure generally should undergo coronary angiography to assess for evidence of ischemic disease and consideration of intervention to improve functional ability.[16–18]

Surgical Treatments

Coronary Revascularization

Coronary revascularization with **coronary artery bypass surgery** can improve myocardial function by reducing ischemia. In some cases so-called hibernating myocardium (myocardium rendered hypocontractile because of chronic hypoperfusion) can return to normal contractile function after restoration of normal blood flow. Other surgical procedures considered for patients with cardiac failure include valvular repairs or replacements and limited septal myomectomies for patients with hypertrophic obstructive cardiomyopathy.

Heart Transplantation

Advances in the techniques of heart transplantation and immunosuppression have improved survival. Patients who undergo transplantation experience a near-normal quality of life but remain at risk for rejection, increased rates of infection, and a unique coronary vasculopathy that leads to severe CAD. The major limitation in cardiac transplantation is organ availability.

Treatment Guidelines for Acute Cardiac Failure

Acute cardiac failure is notable for an acute deterioration of symptoms usually characterized by pulmonary congestion, and often constitutes a medical emergency. Etiologies of acute cardiac failure are discussed in previous sections, but in general terms common precipitants in patients with preexisting cardiac dysfunction include nonadherence to therapy or diet recommendations, hypertensive crisis, and cardiac ischemia. As opposed to the extensive data supporting many of the therapies in chronic cardiac failure, therapy for acute cardiac failure is largely empiric but focuses on similar pathophysiologic variables, including alteration of preload, afterload, and contractility. Because acute cardiac failure can result in fulminant respiratory failure, patients often require support with positive pressure ventilation, both intubation and noninvasive ventilation.[15]

Pharmacologic Therapy

In the patient with acute severe pulmonary edema and volume overload, intravenous dosing of a loop diuretic may be necessary for rapid treatment of symptoms. Bolus dosing is usually effective; however, continuous drips may be more effective and have been associated with fewer side effects. If loop diuretics alone are not effective, then the addition of a thiazide diuretic may be useful. In patients who experience restlessness, anxiety, chest pain, and severe dyspnea, morphine can relieve some of these symptoms in addition to causing mild vasodilation and reduction of preload. For patients who are not hypotensive, vasodilators can be beneficial in acute cardiac failure because they decrease both afterload and preload. Frequently, IV nitrates are used. Nitroglycerin is primarily a venodilator and can affect preload, whereas nitroprusside can reduce both preload and afterload.

Tailored Therapy

In patients with severely decompensated heart failure, aggressive intravenous therapy with diuretics and vasodilators can be administered with concurrent hemodynamic monitoring. A pulmonary arterial catheter can provide important information regarding serial determination of filling pressures and allow optimal titration of vasodilators and volume status. Occasionally, intravenous inotropes such as dobutamine or milrinone are needed to augment the cardiac output and help optimize hemodynamics. Tailored therapy remains a useful intervention in patients with severe cardiac failure.

> **RESPIRATORY RECAP**
>
> **Treatments for Acute Cardiac Failure**
>
> » Pharmacologic therapy
> » Tailored therapy
> » Intra-aortic balloon pump

Intra-aortic Balloon Pump

The **intra-aortic balloon pump (IABP)** uses the principle of counterpulsation to support the failing heart. The catheter-based balloon is inserted into the descending aorta just below the aortic arch. The balloon is then inflated during diastole, causing increased coronary blood flow, and deflated during systole, causing decreased afterload. An IABP is especially effective in cardiogenic shock caused by myocardial ischemia because it decreases myocardial oxygen demand while increasing coronary perfusion. IABPs can be inserted safely in emergency situations and often can bridge a critically ill patient to corrective surgery.

Acute Myocardial Infarction

Acute myocardial infarction occurs when there is partial or complete occlusion of the coronary circulation. Infarction occurs most commonly when there is rupture of a plaque in one of the coronary arteries, resulting in thrombosis and obstruction of blood flow to the tissue it supplies. The end result of absent or reduced blood flow is tissue hypoxia and cell death unless blood flow is improved quickly. Acute coronary syndrome can manifest itself clinically in a variety of ways; however, the most common complaints are severe chest pain radiating to the left arm and jaw, dyspnea, nausea, and a sense of impending doom. Often the patient will appear uncomfortable and diaphoretic. The diagnosis can be confirmed by ECG and measurement of serum cardiac biomarkers such as troponin.

There are many subclassifications of acute coronary syndromes, but the most urgent is the ST-elevation myocardial infarction (STEMI), which warrants prompt intervention to prevent irreversible damage to the myocardium. Initial treatment involves the administration of aspirin and other anticoagulants such as heparin and clopidogrel to help prevent platelet adhesion and thrombosis; nitroglycerin to assist with coronary vasodilation; supplemental oxygen to alleviate tissue hypoxia; and often morphine if the patient has persistent chest pain. In centers where cardiac catheterization is available or can be obtained within 90 minutes, the patient should undergo PCI with angioplasty or placement of a stent to obtain revascularization of the affected artery. If PCI is unavailable, then medical thrombolysis can be attempted.[19]

Ventilatory Support of the Patient with Cardiac Failure

Pulmonary edema is associated with increased lung elastance, increased airway resistance, and lung collapse. Thus, pulmonary edema from any cause leads to increased work of breathing and hypoxemia. The large negative intrathoracic pressure swings may increase afterload for the strained left ventricle. Hypoxic pulmonary vasoconstriction will increase afterload of the right ventricle. In severe cases the patient may not be able to maintain adequate ventilation and oxygen delivery. This can then further exacerbate myocardial dysfunction because of cellular hypoxia and acidosis, especially when the heart failure is caused by cardiac ischemia. The increased work of the respiratory muscles also may steal oxygen from the working myocardium. Thus, combined cardiac failure and respiratory distress begets more cardiac failure.

If the cycle of respiratory failure can be temporarily interrupted, therapy aimed at treating the cardiac abnormalities can be used and the process can be reversed. Positive pressure ventilation is an ideal mechanism used to stabilize the acutely decompensated patient. Positive pressure ventilation improves oxygenation by recruiting collapsed lung and decreases the work of breathing by unloading the respiratory muscles. In addition, positive intrathoracic pressure may improve forward $\dot{Q}c$. Chronic therapy with noninvasive positive pressure ventilators may have a role in selected patients with sleep-disordered breathing and heart failure.

Noninvasive Ventilation

In the past, many patients with respiratory failure caused by cardiac failure were intubated for mechanical ventilation. However, experience with noninvasive ventilation (NIV) by face mask has provided encouraging results. In some cases the patient can be stabilized and endotracheal intubation can be prevented by the use of mask continuous positive airway pressure (CPAP) at 5 to 10 cm H_2O. Inspiratory pressure also can be applied to further unload the respiratory muscles. A systematic review of the use of NIV as compared with conventional medical therapy for acute cardiopulmonary edema found that NIV (consisting of CPAP or bilevel NIV) outperformed medical therapy in terms of mortality, intubation rates, and physiologic parameters.[20]

In patients with active cardiac ischemia, heavy sedation and controlled mechanical ventilation through an endotracheal tube significantly reduces the work of breathing, reduces the work of the myocardium, and allows the most effective oxygen delivery to the ischemic myocardium. Patients with hemodynamic instability, arrhythmias, and a depressed mental status or some patients undergoing invasive procedures (such as cardiac catheterization) should be managed with intubation and mechanical ventilation.

Invasive Mechanical Ventilation

Intubation of the patient with cardiac failure may prove challenging because of underlying hemodynamic abnormalities. The necessary sedation for this procedure can potentially cause hypotension and arrhythmias. Thus, monitoring of the rhythm and blood pressure is essential. Very few sedating medications do not have some cardiovascular depressive actions. One exception is etomidate, which is a hypnotic agent with minimal cardiovascular depressant actions. Etomidate is the recommended induction agent for intubation of patients with cardiovascular instability. After intubation the patient will likely require continued sedation. Low doses of benzodiazepines and opiates are often sufficient.

No controlled trials on various modes of ventilation in cardiac failure have been conducted. The clinician should use the mode that provides the most effective and comfortable ventilation for the patient. Patients with mild or chronic cardiac failure and significant pulmonary edema may be managed with minimal ventilatory support and spontaneous ventilation with a mode such as pressure support. Most patients with severe cardiac failure will benefit from full ventilatory support. Pressure control or volume control ventilation can be used for cardiac failure as long as adequate ventilation and oxygenation are maintained without hyperinflation or significant lung collapse. Pressure support or pressure control may allow patients to set their own inspiratory flows and may permit less sedation by providing a comfortable form of ventilation. Tidal volume should be 8 mL/kg with an inspiratory time of 0.8 to 1.2 seconds. Plateau pressure should be monitored and kept below 30 cm H_2O. An adequate rate should be provided if heavy sedation is used. FIO_2 should be set at 1.0 and then decreased to the lowest level that maintains SpO_2 above 90%. PEEP is initially set at 5 cm H_2O and titrated as needed for oxygenation if tolerated hemodynamically.

RESPIRATORY RECAP

Mechanical Ventilation for Cardiac Failure

- » A mode should be chosen that is effective and comfortable for the patient.
- » Avoid peak alveolar pressure above 30 cm H_2O.
- » Use an initial tidal volume of 8 mL/kg.
- » Use an initial inspiratory time of 0.8 to 1.2 seconds.
- » An initial FIO_2 of 1.0 should be chosen.
- » An initial PEEP of 5 cm H_2O should be chosen.

Cardiac Effects of Mechanical Ventilation

Positive pressure ventilation has many potential effects on the cardiovascular system. The filling of the ventricles is highly dependent on the pressures surrounding the heart. Cardiac surface pressure depends on the pericardial pressure, intrathoracic pressure, and lung volume around the heart. Changes in lung volume also will affect PVR and thus RV performance. In turn, RV performance can affect LV performance via series and parallel interactions. Thus, the overall effects of the application of positive pressure ventilation in the individual patient are highly unpredictable and can be beneficial (reduced work of breathing, reduced edema, increased $\dot{Q}c$) or potentially detrimental (hypotension, hyperinflation, ischemia). Therefore, a careful titration of respiratory support during monitoring of all available aspects of cardiovascular performance (i.e., blood pressure, heart rate, filling pressures, $\dot{Q}c$, arterial blood gases, electrocardiogram) may be the optimal method of ventilation in the patient with cardiac failure.

The most effective means to increase intrathoracic positive pressure is the application of PEEP. In addition to potentially reducing afterload and preload, PEEP prevents alveolar derecruitment. Collapsed lung units increase intrapulmonary shunt, increase PVR, and induce hyperinflation in open lung units by reducing the amount of lung available to accommodate the delivered tidal volume. In addition, cyclic opening and closure of alveoli over each ventilatory cycle can be injurious. Optimal ventilatory settings should prevent derecruitment by ventilating above the closing pressures of the lung units.

In patients with dilated cardiomyopathy, PEEP has been shown to improve $\dot{Q}c$ without increasing the oxygen requirements of the LV. It is widely believed that this effect is from a reduced afterload on the LV induced by the positive intrathoracic pressure. The afterload on the heart can be estimated by the transmural pressure across the LV, and since PEEP can increase cardiac surface pressure, it will reduce afterload, assuming the arterial pressure does not increase. However, this increase in $\dot{Q}c$ is not seen in patients with normal cardiac function or normal volume status, suggesting that the mechanism of benefit may not be as simple as a reduced afterload. It is hypothesized that the increase that occurs in patients with cardiac failure when placed on positive pressure ventilation may be caused by displacement of blood from the thorax leading to reduced ventricular volumes and improved contraction due to less pericardial constraint. In addition, PEEP may be beneficial by redistributing edema to the perivascular spaces and reducing PVR by limiting lung collapse. Based on the complex effects of PEEP, a careful increase in pressure is recommended, while simultaneously monitoring oxygenation, blood pressure, the electrocardiogram, and the $\dot{Q}c$ if possible.

Discontinuing Mechanical Ventilation

Acute respiratory failure from pulmonary edema is often rapidly reversible and does not usually require prolonged mechanical ventilation. Often the patient can be extubated without a prolonged weaning of support. However, the sudden loss of positive pressure in the thorax can lead to acute edema and rapid failure in fragile patients. Ongoing cardiac ischemia is associated with failure to wean and should be corrected before ventilatory support is removed.

Chronic Noninvasive Ventilation in Sleep-Disordered Breathing

Many patients with chronic cardiac failure have sleep-disordered breathing, including Cheyne-Stokes respiration and sleep apnea. Perhaps as many as 40% to 50% of patients with cardiac failure also have obstructive sleep apnea (OSA) or Cheyne-Stokes respiration with central sleep apnea (CSR-CSA). In patients with cardiac failure, the presence of sleep-disordered breathing is associated with a poor prognosis and a higher mortality.

BOX 42–2

Effects of Obstructive Sleep Apnea on Cardiovascular Function

Negative Intrathoracic Pressure

- Increased left ventricular systolic transmural pressure (i.e., afterload)
- Reduced stroke volume and cardiac output

Hypoxemia and Hypercapnia

- Increased respiratory drive and sympathetic nervous system activity
- Pulmonary vasoconstriction and hypertension leading to increased right ventricular afterload
- Systemic vasoconstriction and hypertension
- Cardiac arrhythmias (bradycardia, heart block, ventricular and supraventricular tachycardias)

Arousal

- Increased central sympathetic nervous system activity
- Increased systemic blood pressure
- Increased heart rate

Box 42–2 lists the extensive cardiovascular effects of apneic episodes.

It is clear that these effects work in concert to increase afterload and overload the myocardium. It has been suggested that these pathophysiologic effects may contribute to the progression of cardiac failure. There is increasing evidence that treatment of these disorders with nocturnal mask CPAP is associated with marked improvements in cardiac function and the symptoms of cardiac failure.

The assessment of all patients with cardiac failure should include questions about sleep disorders and symptoms of sleep deprivation, snoring, and apneas. Any suggestion of sleep-disordered breathing should prompt a thorough evaluation with a sleep study and treatment if indicated.[21]

CASE STUDIES

Case 1. Ischemic Congestive Heart Failure

A 55-year-old man (80 kg) with a history of CAD and prior infarction presented with chest pain and shortness of breath. The patient presented with an anterior myocardial infarction (MI) 6 months ago and underwent emergent coronary angioplasty with stent placement to his left anterior descending (LAD) coronary artery. His LV function after MI was moderately impaired at an LVEF of 40%. He was managed with aspirin, β-blockers, and an ACE inhibitor. Over the last 2 weeks he has noted return of his chest pain with exertion, and on the day of presentation he had two 20-minute episodes of pain at rest. The last one was associated with some mild dyspnea. Shortly before presenting he developed severe crushing chest pain and became quite dyspneic. An ambulance was called, and he was taken to the emergency department. On presentation he was in respiratory distress, sitting upright, and sweating, with marked use of accessory muscles. His respiratory rate was 36 breaths/min, heart rate 110 beats/min, and blood pressure 150/100 mm Hg, and oxygen saturation was 91% on 15 L/min oxygen via face mask. On exam the patient appeared to have distended neck veins. His chest had diffuse crackles and wheezes throughout. Cardiac exam was notable for tachycardia and a summation gallop. An ECG showed T-wave inversions and ST depression in leads V_2 to V_6, and a chest radiograph showed moderate pulmonary edema.

The patient clearly has congestive heart failure (CHF) from myocardial ischemia. In this case, the lack of oxygen delivery to the working myocardium led to depletion in ATP and dysfunction of both contraction and relaxation of cardiac muscle. This insult resulted in elevated LV filling pressures and pulmonary edema. The patient has evidence of a marked increase in work of breathing that is likely contributing to the ischemia by increasing his oxygen delivery requirements. If the patient begins to retain carbon dioxide, the resulting acidosis may lead to further myocardial dysfunction and increase the risk of arrhythmias. Efforts to restore oxygen supply to the heart might be more successful if the patient were intubated and heavily sedated.

The therapeutic strategy is to intubate the patient and provide full mechanical ventilatory support. Pressure or volume ventilation so that the volumes are 600 mL and inspiratory time is 0.8 to 1.2 seconds with a rate of 12 to 16 breaths/min is a good starting point. The F_{IO_2} should be 1.0 to start. PEEP of 5 cm H_2O should be applied, and if the blood pressure tolerates this, a slow increase to 10 cm H_2O could be attempted. In the meantime the patient should be treated with anticoagulation (aspirin, heparin, a II/IIIa inhibitor), intravenous nitroglycerin, and diuretics. Consultation with a cardiologist for possible cardiac catheterization also should be obtained.

Case 2. Acute Aortic Valve Insufficiency

A 28-year-old man complains of fevers, chills, and shortness of breath. The patient has a history of rheumatic fever as a child but has otherwise been in good health. Three days before presentation he injected intravenous heroin with a dirty needle. The day before presentation he noted chills and sweats. On the morning of presentation he had a rapid progression of dyspnea and nausea. He felt weak when standing and finally collapsed in his home. The patient was brought to the emergency department awake but in respiratory distress. His blood pressure was 110/40 mm Hg, heart rate 120 beats/min, respiratory rate 30 breaths/min, temperature 102° F, and oxygen saturation 88% on 10 L/min oxygen by face mask. Physical exam was notable for signs of increased work of breathing and crackles on chest auscultation. His cardiac exam disclosed an elevated JVP, a hyperdynamic precordium on palpation, tachycardia, and a loud diastolic murmur at the left lower sternal border on auscultation. A summation gallop also was noted. The patient's extremities were cool and without edema. Laboratory evaluation disclosed an elevated white count; an ECG showed tachycardia with some nonspecific T-wave changes. The chest radiograph showed pulmonary edema. An urgent echocardiogram showed 4+ aortic regurgitation with LV dilation. LV systolic function appeared intact. A large vegetation was seen on one of the aortic cusps, and the other cusps appeared thickened.

This patient has acute aortic valve endocarditis, likely from a staphylococcal infection. The infection was probably acquired from his IV drug use and involved his aortic valve, which may have been damaged previously from the episode of rheumatic fever. The infection has eroded his aortic valve and produced acute aortic insufficiency. In this case the LV acutely has a large regurgitant volume load. When the aortic valve eroded, there was an acute increase in diastolic volume caused by regurgitation of blood from the aorta. This led to LV dilation and increased diastolic wall stress and elevated filling pressures. The elevated filling pressures led to pulmonary edema and dyspnea. The $\dot{Q}c$ is decreased because of the regurgitation of blood into the LV, but the heart has partially compensated by increasing its rate and augmenting its stroke volume. Unfortunately, the $\dot{Q}c$ is not adequate to meet the body's demands, and the patient is developing tissue hypoperfusion and cardiogenic shock.

Management in this case begins with stabilization of the respiratory system. Oxygen delivery and respiratory muscle unloading are required. Positive pressure ventilation also may help cardiac function by reducing the afterload and the amount of blood regurgitated into the LV. A trial of noninvasive ventilation with bilevel pressure support and PEEP may be attempted in this case. If the patient does not tolerate this intervention, he may require intubation, sedation, and ventilation with pressure support and PEEP. PEEP can be started at 5 cm H_2O and increased as tolerated to support oxygenation and reduce afterload. In the meantime, antibiotic therapy and intravenous afterload reducers (such as sodium nitroprusside) can be administered. The patient should be considered for urgent surgical replacement of the aortic valve given the severity of heart failure.

Case 3. Diastolic Dysfunction from Hypertension

An 80-year-old woman with a long history of hypertension and COPD presented with a fractured hip after a fall. She underwent surgical fixation of the fracture that evening. Postoperatively she was observed to develop atrial fibrillation with a rapid ventricular response. Shortly afterward she complained of shortness of breath. The patient was sitting upright in bed, was diaphoretic, and was in moderate respiratory distress. Blood pressure was 180/100 mm Hg, heart rate was 140 to 160 beats/min and irregular, and temperature was 101° F. Oxygen saturation was 90% on 8 L/min oxygen via nasal cannula. Physical exam disclosed slight wheezing and crackles on chest auscultation. A chest radiograph was consistent with pulmonary edema. An ECG revealed atrial fibrillation without ischemic changes. An echocardiogram disclosed a thickened and hyperkinetic LV with normal chamber dimensions and ejection fraction.

This patient has pulmonary edema from diastolic dysfunction. The cause of her pulmonary edema is multifactorial. First, the heart is thickened from long-standing hypertension and likely has baseline abnormalities in relaxation. With atrial fibrillation, the contribution to ventricular filling from the atrial contraction was lost. Normally, atrial contraction serves to increase LVEDP without a large concurrent rise in mean left atrial pressure (LAP). Loss of atrial contraction causes a rise in the mean LAP and can contribute to pulmonary edema. The rapid ventricular rate that results from atrial fibrillation also may impede diastolic function by limiting the diastolic interval available for filling.

In this case, therapy should be directed at restoration of a normal sinus rhythm. The respiratory status is reasonably stable at present and can be managed with supplemental oxygen alone. The quickest and easiest method to restore a normal sinus rhythm is synchronized electric cardioversion. If this is unsuccessful or the patient reverts to atrial fibrillation, an antiarrhythmic drug may help convert and stabilize the rhythm. If attempts at cardioversion fail, the patient may be rate controlled with a variety of agents. The calcium channel blockers diltiazem or verapamil are effective at rate control. Both can be given by continuous intravenous infusion. β-blockers also can be used and are ideal after myocardial infarction. The antiarrhythmic amiodarone can slow the heart rate and may help cardiovert the patient back into normal sinus rhythm. Further supportive therapy with nitroglycerin and diuretics also may be used in this situation. Effective pain control, treatment of bronchospasm (with a nonabsorbed anticholinergic, such as ipratropium, that will not stimulate the heart), and reduction of fever are important methods to reduce the cardiac stimulation from catecholamine release.

Case 4. Chronic Congestive Heart Failure from Cardiomyopathy of Coronary Artery Disease

A 55-year-old man with a history of CHF and multiple myocardial infarctions presented with slowly progressive fatigue and shortness of breath over the last week. The patient had his first MI at age 45 years. He initially did well with medical management but at age 53 had a large anterior MI. His course after this MI has been notable for multiple episodes of cardiac failure. After the MI, he was found to have two-vessel coronary disease and a decreased ejection fraction at 20%. He has been managed with an ACE inhibitor and diuretics while he awaits cardiac transplantation. About 3 months ago he was started on carvedilol. The patient was traveling in Italy the last 3 weeks and admits to noncompliance with his low-salt diet. He also ran out of his lisinopril 10 days ago. About 1 week ago he noted some increased dyspnea with exertion and fatigue. The last 3 days he has been sleeping on three to four pillows instead of his usual two, and last night he woke up twice very short of breath. He denies any chest pain but has had some pedal edema.

On exam he was in mild respiratory distress and had a periodic breathing pattern, especially when distracted or resting. Blood pressure was 110/70 mm Hg, heart rate 75 beats/min, and oxygen saturation 95% on 2 L/min nasal cannula. Auscultation of his chest was notable only for a few mild crackles at the bases. His neck veins were elevated to his jaw, there was a large displaced LV apical impulse, and on auscultation a loud S_3 was noted. His legs had 2+ to 3+ pitting edema. Laboratory evaluation was unremarkable, and an ECG showed his usual left bundle branch pattern. A chest radiograph showed cardiomegaly and small bilateral effusions. No pulmonary edema was noted. He was transferred to the critical care unit and while sleeping was noted to desaturate during periods of apnea.

This patient has decompensated cardiac failure from medical and dietary noncompliance. Although conservative therapy with diuretics and restarting of his ACE inhibitor may work, an attempt at tailored therapy may provide better long-term results. In this patient a pulmonary artery catheter could be placed to guide therapy. Intravenous diuretics and vasodilators could be used to obtain the lowest filling pressures that provide an adequate $\dot{Q}c$. If needed, an inotrope such as dobutamine could be added. Once hemodynamics are optimized, oral therapy would begin. The presence of periodic breathing is the result of his cardiac failure. An attempt to treat this with noninvasive positive pressure ventilation may help his left ventricular function and overall well-being.

Case 5. Coronary Bypass Surgery

A 68-year-old man with a history of angina underwent coronary bypass surgery for three-vessel disease. When coming off the pump, he experienced hypotension that required high doses of a norepinephrine infusion to stabilize his blood pressure. The patient remained intubated and sedated and was transported to the intensive care unit. He was ventilated with volume ventilation at 8 mL/kg, PEEP 5 cm H_2O, F_{IO_2} of 1.0, and a rate of 12/min. With this he was hypoxemic with a blood gas of pH 7.46, Pa_{CO_2} of 34 mm Hg, and Pa_{O_2} of 50 mm Hg. The pulmonary artery catheter disclosed a right atrial pressure of 14 mm Hg, an RV pressure of 45/14 mm Hg, a pulmonary artery pressure (PAP) of 45/20 mm Hg, and a pulmonary artery occlusion pressure (PAOP) of 8 mm Hg. The $\dot{Q}c$ was normal at 3.8 L/min. A chest radiograph and an ECG were within normal limits. An emergent echocardiogram was notable for a hypocontractile RV with preserved LV function. A patent foramen ovale with right-to-left shunting was noted when air contrast was injected.

This patient has shock from isolated RV dysfunction after cardiopulmonary bypass during cardiac surgery. RV dysfunction after bypass is a well-described complication of cardiac surgery. Several possible etiologies for this dysfunction include air emboli, RV infarction, and stunned myocardium. Air embolism can be fatal and requires prompt treatment with removal of the air or hyperbaric oxygen therapy. The other forms of RV dysfunction after cardiac surgery can reverse if given enough time. The goal is to support the patient with vasoactive drugs until the RV function returns.

In this case the situation is complicated by an intracardiac shunt. The foramen ovale is a hole that exists in utero between the atria. It closes after birth and in most people is fused. A significant portion of the population has a nonfused foramen ovale that remains closed because the left-sided atrial pressure is greater than the right-sided atrial pressure. In this patient, when the pressure increased in the right atrium in association with the decreased compliance of the RV, the foramen ovale opened and shunted blood from the right atrium to the left atrium. This shunted blood is the cause of the refractory hypoxemia.

This patient was stabilized hemodynamically with norepinephrine. The challenge is to reduce the shunt. Increasing PEEP, which generally improves oxygenation in patients with lung disease, may actually be detrimental in this case because it can increase pulmonary vascular resistance and thus increase the fraction of right-to-left shunted blood. Intravenous vasodilators such as nitroprusside and nitroglycerin can lower the PVR but also can lower systemic blood pressure. In addition, these agents will reduce hypoxic vasoconstriction and may potentially worsen hypoxemia. Inhaled nitric oxide is a potent vasodilator with a short half-life. When inhaled, it selectively dilates the pulmonary arteries and improves ventilation-perfusion matching by preferentially dilating the vasculature of ventilated lung units. In this case, a trial of inhaled nitric oxide reduced the shunt and improved RV function by reducing PVR.

KEY POINTS

- Cardiac failure is a common occurrence in hospitalized patients and often causes respiratory failure.
- Although there are numerous causes for cardiac failure, it ultimately results from an abnormality of contraction, excessive load, and/or restricted filling.
- Symptoms vary from patient to patient but usually manifest with fatigue and dyspnea on exertion. Often the symptoms occur late in the disease process.
- Treatment for cardiac failure requires a knowledge of its complex pathophysiology.
- The majority of treatments for cardiac failure stabilize the disease and do not reverse the process.
- ACE inhibitors, β-blockers, and diuretics remain the mainstay of therapy in patients with cardiac failure.
- Mechanical ventilation for patients with respiratory failure can be very effective in reversing the abnormalities resulting from pulmonary edema.
- The interactions of the lungs and heart are complex in patients with heart failure, and the use of positive pressure ventilation can often lead to unpredictable results if not used carefully.

REFERENCES

1. Hunt SA, et al. ACC/AHA 2005 guideline update for the diagnosis and management of chronic heart failure in the adult: a report of the American College of Cardiology/American Heart Association Task Force on Practice Guidelines. *Circulation.* 2005;112:e154–e235.
2. Lloyd-Jones D, et al. Heart disease and stroke statistics 2009 update. A report from the American Heart Association Statistics Committee and Stroke Statistics subcommittee. *Circulation.* 2009;119:e21–e181.
3. Opie LA. *The Heart: Physiology from Cell to Circulation.* Philadelphia: Lippincott Wilkins & Williams; 1998.
4. Guyton AC, Hall JE. *Textbook of Medical Physiology.* 10th ed. Philadelphia: Saunders; 2000:96–174.
5. Ouzounian M. Diastolic heart failure: mechanisms and controversies. *Nat Clin Pract Cardiovasc Med.* 2008;5:375–386.
6. Ashrafian H. The pathophysiology of heart failure: a tale of two old paradigms revisited. *Clin Med.* 2008;8:192–197.
7. Monnet X. Cardiopulmonary interactions in patients with heart failure. *Curr Opin Crit Care.* 2007;13:6–11.
8. Pinsky MR. Cardiovascular issues in respiratory care. *Chest.* 2005;128:592S–597S.
9. New York Heart Association Criteria Committee. *Disease of the Heart and Blood Vessels: Nomenclature for Diagnosis.* Boston: Little Brown; 1964:114.
10. Miller JM, Rochitte CE, et al. Diagnostic performance of coronary angiography by 64-row CT. *N Engl J Med.* 2008;359:2324–2336.
11. Engelmeier RS, O'Connell JB, Walsh R, et al. Improvement in symptoms and exercise tolerance by metoprolol in patients with dilated cardiomyopathy: a double-blind, randomized, placebo-controlled trial. *Circulation.* 1985;72:536–546.
12. Anderson JL, Lutz JR, Gilbert EM, et al. A randomized trial of low-dose β-blockade therapy for idiopathic dilated cardiomyopathy. *Am J Cardiol.* 1985;55:471–475.
13. Krumholz HM. β-blockers for mild to moderate heart failure. *Lancet.* 1999;353:2.
14. Salpeter SR, Ormiston TM, Salpeter EE. Cardioselective β-blockers in patients with reactive airway disease: a meta-analysis. *Ann Intern Med.* 2002;137:715–725.
15. Cohen-Solal A, et al. ESC guidelines for the diagnosis and treatment of acute and chronic heart failure 2008. *Eur Heart J.* 2008;29:2388–2442.
16. Boden WE, Gupta V. Reperfusion strategies in acute ST-segment elevation myocardial infarction. *Curr Opin Cardiol.* 2008;23:613–619.
17. Flaherty JD, Davidson CJ, Faxon DP. Percutaneous coronary intervention for myocardial infarction with left ventricular dysfunction. *Am J Cardiol.* 2008;102:38G–41G.
18. 2009 focused updates: ACC/AHA guidelines for the management of patients with ST-elevation myocardial infarction (updating the 2004 guideline and 2007 focused update) and ACC/AHA/SCAI guidelines on percutaneous coronary intervention (updating the 2005 guideline and 2007 focused update). *JACC.* 2009;53:2205–2241.
19. White HD, Chew DP. Acute myocardial infarction. *Lancet.* 2008;372:570–584.
20. Vital FMR. Non-invasive positive pressure ventilation (CPAP or bilevel NPPV) for cardiogenic pulmonary edema. *Cochrane Rev.* 2009;1:1–26.
21. Naughton MT. Common sleep problems in ICU: heart failure and sleep-disordered breathing syndromes. *Crit Care Clin.* 2008;24:565–587.

CHAPTER 43

Trauma

Bryce R. H. Robinson
Richard D. Branson

OUTLINE

OBJECTIVES

1. Discuss the evaluation of a trauma patient with respect to a primary and secondary survey.
2. List the components of the ABCDE algorithm for assessing the trauma patient.
3. Describe the injuries following trauma that may require respiratory support.
4. Identify common life-threatening injuries encountered during the primary survey.
5. Describe common injuries encountered during the secondary survey.
6. Discuss the importance of pain control.
7. Describe the mechanism of head trauma and traumatic brain injury.
8. Discuss methods to monitor and treat acute traumatic brain injury.

KEY TERMS

Beck's triad
blunt trauma
cardiac tamponade
epidural hematoma
hemothorax
hypovolemic shock
penetrating trauma
pneumothorax
primary survey
pulmonary contusion
secondary survey
subarachnoid (intracerebral) hematoma
subdural hematoma

INTRODUCTION

Regardless of the mechanism or anatomic location of injury, the initial evaluation and care of the traumatically injured patient is structured by principles delineated by the advanced trauma life support (ATLS) program of the American College of Surgeons Committee on Trauma.[1] ATLS focuses on the rapid initial assessment and treatment of life-threatening injuries, reevaluation and stabilization of the traumatically injured, and principles for the transfer of these patients to a higher-level care if warranted. Trauma patients die in certain reproducible time frames. A patient without a definitive airway will die of hypoxia more rapidly than a patient with hypovolemic shock. The purpose of this chapter is to familiarize care providers with the evaluation and treatment of injuries to the chest and head.

The Primary and Secondary Surveys

The **primary survey** uses the mnemonic ABCDE for an orderly evaluation and treatment of traumatic injuries based on the rapidity of lethality. *A* stands for airway and cervical spine protection, *B* for breathing, *C* for circulation, *D* for deficits, and *E* for exposure (**Figure 43–1**). While the primary survey is occurring, care providers are simultaneously recording vital signs, starting resuscitation, drawing pertinent laboratory specimens, inserting clinically relevant urinary or gastric catheters, obtaining chest and pelvic radiographs, and performing the focused assessment by sonography for trauma (FAST) exam.

The **secondary survey** of the trauma patient is a head-to-toe physical examination that includes a thorough history using the AMPLE mnemonic. AMPLE stands for *a*llergies, current *m*edications used, *p*ast illnesses/*p*regnancy, *l*ast meal, and *e*vents/*e*nvironment related to the traumatic injury. The secondary exam is not performed until the patient is deemed stable by completion of the primary survey and this is confirmed with normal vital signs while resuscitation is under way. After the primary and secondary surveys are complete, patients are triaged for further radiographic evaluation, operative intervention, or inter- or intrahospital transfer or admission.

A: Airway
B: Breathing
C: Circulation
D: Deficits
E: Exposure

FIGURE 43–1 Primary survey.

Thoracic Trauma

Injuries to the chest can be broadly classified as having either a blunt or penetrating mechanism. Traumatic injuries are responsible for approximately 180,000 deaths and 9 million disabling injuries in the United States each year.[2] This mechanism constitutes the fourth leading cause of death for all Americans and is the leading cause of death for those aged 1 to 44 years.[3,4] Twenty-five percent of deaths from **blunt trauma** are the direct result of thoracic injury.[2] For those who survive their initial injuries, blunt thoracic injuries are responsible for 8% of traumatic hospital admissions.[5] Motor vehicle crashes (MVCs) are the dominant cause of blunt force resulting in chest injury.

Penetrating trauma is a common injury pattern endemic to urban trauma centers in the United States. Injuries from stab wounds and handguns result in low-velocity (<1500 ft/s) wounds with injured tissue centered at the trajectory of the object. High-velocity (>1500 ft/s) injuries occur with military assault weapons or hunting rifles. These injuries incur a remarkable amount of tissue damage not only by the trajectory of the missile but also by the simultaneous blast effect, which creates widespread contusion and hemorrhage. High-velocity missiles often are designed to fragment or tumble as they travel, increasing the diameter of the pathway created and resulting in multiple locations of perforation and hemorrhage. Even at the busiest of urban trauma centers, however, penetrating chest injury accounts for only 7% of trauma admissions and 16% of penetrating admissions; these injuries are almost exclusively low-velocity injuries.[6]

RESPIRATORY RECAP

Types of Thoracic Trauma

» Blunt
» Penetrating

Airway and Breathing Injuries

Airway injuries detected during the primary survey take precedence over any other injury detected initially due to the temporal nature of their lethality. Initial inspection of the airway includes observing the quality and quantity of air movement at the nose, mouth, and chest. Auscultation of air movement is carried down to the chest onto the lung fields. Inspection of the oropharynx for obstruction occurs rapidly along with the evaluation of the accessory muscles of respiration, specifically, the intercostals and supraclavicular groups.

Laryngotracheal Injuries

Laryngotracheal injuries occurring in the neck or at the thoracic outlet can directly affect the patency of the airway. These injuries occur in both blunt and penetrating mechanisms. Signs and symptoms of presentation include stridor, neck tenderness, hematomas of the neck or upper chest, and subcutaneous emphysema. The evaluation of these injuries requires the use of direct laryngoscopy as well as bronchoscopy. Establishment of a definitive airway is imperative before obstruction occurs, although improperly placed endotracheal airways can worsen an already precarious situation. If such an injury is suspected, operative evaluation and intervention is required.[7]

RESPIRATORY RECAP

Airway and Breathing Injuries

» Laryngotracheal injuries
» Dislocation of the sternoclavicular heads
» Pneumothorax

Obstruction of the airway can occur by a dislocation of the sternoclavicular heads secondary to frontal or lateral blunt impact. Palpation of the sternum with evident posterior dislocation should alert the care team to such an injury. Patients may complain of sternal pain, stridor, and dysphasia due to the direct compression of mediastinal structures. The diagnosis is often confirmed by specific angled radiographs or computed tomography (CT) or both. Closed reduction is the preferred method for correction, although operative open reduction and fixation may be necessary.[8]

Pneumothorax

One of the most common and potentially lethal injuries encountered in chest trauma is a **pneumothorax**. It is estimated that 20% of patients who present to a trauma center alive have a pneumothorax,[9] which is the presence of air in the pleural space between the lung and the posterior thoracic wall. Universal signs of pneumothorax are chest pain and respiratory distress. Subcutaneous emphysema found on exam indicates the presence of air escaping from the chest cavity into the subcutaneous tissue from a pneumothorax etiology. The classic yet subtle findings of tracheal deviation and hyperresonance on percussion are difficult and rare to detect in the noisy and busy trauma bay.

Definitive diagnosis is made by chest radiograph, although clinical signs and symptoms can delineate the diagnosis. However, the rate of missed anterior pneumothoraces on supine anteroposterior chest radiographs is estimated to be between 20% and 35%.[10] Evidence is emerging regarding the utility of detecting pneumothoraces by ultrasound as an adjunct of the FAST exam, although utility may be limited if subcutaneous emphysema is present.[11] Nonetheless, with the increasing rate of CT use for both abdominal and chest imaging, more and more pneumothoraces are being detected. The clinical relevance of these occult pneumothoraces is questionable, however.

There are three subtypes of pneumothoraces: simple, open, and tension. A simple pneumothorax is one that presents as a collection of air in the pleural space. An open pneumothorax differs in that such an injury is associated with a chest injury that allows air to enter the negatively pressured thoracic cavity. An equalization of pressure between the atmosphere and the chest then occurs. With each inspiration, air is preferentially drawn into the chest via the wound if the diameter of the wound is approximately two-thirds or more greater than that of the trachea. Initial treatment of an open pneumothorax is to place a sterile dressing to the wound with three of four sides taped to the chest. Having one side free allows air to exit the chest during exhalation but prevents air entry into the chest cavity during inspiration by a flap valve mechanism. After application of the dressing, a chest tube should be placed away from the wound site. Preferably, a 32-French or larger tube should be placed in the fourth to fifth rib interspace anterior to the midaxillary line. The chest tube is then attached to a underwater seal system, and suction may be applied to prevent air accumulation in the pleural space (**Figure 43–2**).

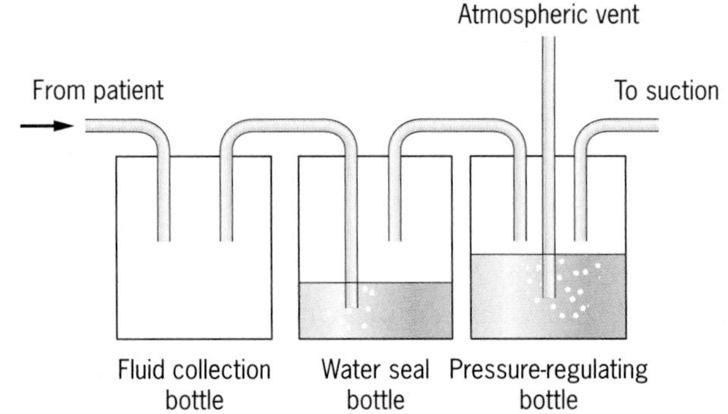

FIGURE 43–2 Schematic of underwater seal showing component parts.

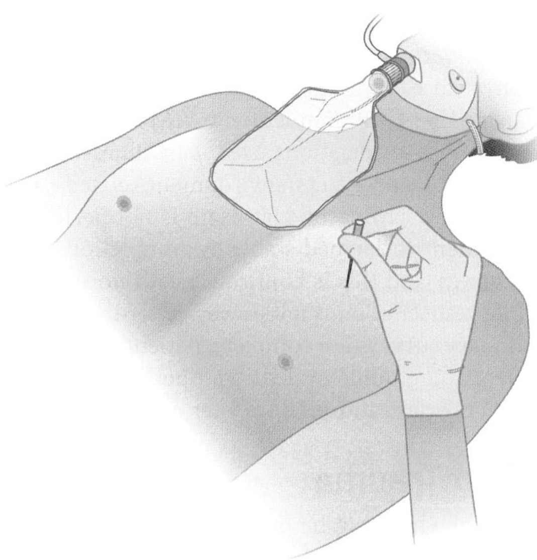

FIGURE 43–3 Chest needle for treating pneumothorax.

The most lethal of the subtypes is the tension pneumothorax. A tension pneumothorax occurs via air entering the chest from a lung or chest wall injury but being unable to escape. With enough air entering the cavity through a one-way valve system, pressure accumulates in the chest. This intrathoracic pressure can be higher than the intrinsic venous pressure required to return blood to the heart and may displace the mediastinum. As the pressure builds, less and less blood is able to enter the right heart. This increasing pressure also causes ipsilateral and even contralateral lung parenchymal collapse. Hemodynamic failure and death are imminent unless the pressure is relieved, allowing the return of cardiac preload and pulmonary ventilation and oxygenation.

The diagnosis of tension pneumothorax is made clinically and should not be delayed by waiting for diagnostic imaging. Clinical signs and symptoms include those found for simple pneumothorax, but the presence of tracheal deviation, hyperresonance, and neck vein distention may be more pronounced, although still difficult to detect. Treatment of this breathing emergency starts with immediate chest decompression. This can be accomplished by placing a 14-gauge, 4.5-cm IV catheter needle into the second intercostal space in the midclavicular line on the affected side (**Figure 43–3**). Such decompression is not without drawbacks, in that it is estimated that 30% of trauma patients have a chest wall thickness greater than 5 cm.[12] Definitive treatment often requires the placement of a chest tube.

TABLE 43-1 Estimated Blood Loss* Based on Patient's Initial Presentation†

	Class I	Class II	Class III	Class IV
Blood loss (mL)	Up to 750	750–1500	1500–2000	>2000
Blood loss (% blood volume)	Up to 15%	15–30%	30–40%	>40%
Heart rate	<100	100–120	120–140	>140
Blood pressure	Normal	Normal	Decreased	Decreased
Pulse pressure (mm Hg)	Normal or increased	Decreased	Decreased	Decreased
Respiratory rate	14–20	20–30	30–40	>35
Urine output (mL/hr)	>30	20–30	5–15	Negligible
Central nervous system/mental status	Slightly anxious	Mildly anxious	Anxious, confused	Confused, lethargic
Fluid replacement	Crystalloid	Crystalloid	Crystalloid and blood	Crystalloid and blood

*For a 70-kg male.

†The guidelines in this table are based on the 3-for-1 (3:1) rule, which derives from the empiric observation that most patients in hemorrhagic shock require as much as 300 mL of electrolyte solution for each 100 mL of blood loss. Applied blindly, these guidelines may result in excessive or inadequate fluid administration. For example, a patient with a crush injury to an extremity may have hypotension that is out of proportion to his or her blood loss and may require fluids in excess of the 3:1 guidelines. In contrast, a patient whose ongoing blood loss is being replaced by blood transfusion requires less than 3:1. The use of bolus therapy with careful monitoring of the patient's response may moderate these extremes.

From Shock. In: American College of Surgeons Committee on Trauma. *Advanced Trauma Life Support for Doctors: Student Course Manual.* 8th ed. Chicago: American College of Surgeons; 2008:55–71. Reprinted with permission.

Circulation Injuries

After the clearance of potential breathing injuries, the focus shifts to those injuries that can affect the circulatory system. The initial assessment of hemodynamically unstable patients focuses on the palpation of distal pulses in both the upper and lower extremities. The strength, rate, and rhythm of these pulses need to be evaluated. Objective measurement of vital signs needs to occur. This includes the measurement of heart rate, blood pressure, and respiratory rate. As these parameters are being assessed, a cardiac monitor and pulse oximeter should be attached to the patient. Careful interpretation of the cardiac rhythm is necessary if one suspects blunt thoracic injury, because arrhythmias may occur with such an injury pattern.

Hypovolemic Shock

The diagnosis and treatment of **hypovolemic shock** is the focus at this step in the primary survey. Tissue hypoperfusion from intravascular blood loss (hemorrhagic hypovolemic shock) is the most commonly encountered shock state of injured patients. Signs and symptoms of hemorrhagic hypovolemia include tachycardia, hypotension, and pallor of the skin. Hemorrhage is classified into four categories, using vital signs to aid in the quantification of blood loss (**Table 43–1**). Class I hemorrhage is characterized by a 70-kg patient losing up to 15% of his blood volume (<750 mL). Vital signs are often unchanged in a young, healthy—albeit injured—patient with this class of hemorrhage. Class II hemorrhage is characterized by an increase in the heart rate to more than 100 beats per minute for those who have lost 15% to 30% (750–1500 mL) of their volume. Hypotension is the hallmark of class III hemorrhage. These patients have lost 30% to 40% (1500–2000 mL) of their blood volume, affecting their ability to maintain a normal blood pressure. Class IV hemorrhage encompasses patients who have lost more than 40% of their volume (>2000 mL). These patients are in extremis, near the point of death. Those patients who have sustained a thoracic injury and present with a circulatory deficit detected on the primary survey have by definition fallen into at least class II if they exhibit signs of tachycardia, and class III if they are hypotensive.

Controversy surrounds the definition of hypotension. Traditionally, hypotension has been defined as a patient with a systolic blood pressure less than 90 mm Hg. However, little evidence supports this rigid physiologic cutoff, with emerging work demonstrating an inflection of mortality beginning at 110 mm Hg.[13]

Hemothorax

Massive **hemothorax** is the accumulation of more than 1500 mL of blood in the chest cavity. Such an injury is most commonly caused by a penetrating mechanism, although blunt trauma may be implicated. The classic physical findings of a massive hemothorax are a patient in hemorrhagic shock with decreased breaths sounds and/or dullness to percussion isolated to the affected hemithorax.

The treatment of a massive hemothorax begins with correcting the physiologic derangements associated with hemorrhagic shock. Initial crystalloid resuscitation often occurs in the prehospital environment. This resuscitation continues as the patient is cared for by the evaluating trauma team, although evidence is emerging that a balanced blood product resuscitation of fresh, frozen plasma to packed red blood cells may benefit those individuals undergoing a massive transfusion (more than 10 units of blood products in 24 hours).[14–16] Care needs to be taken regarding the amount of resuscitation a patient undergoes. Aggressive fluid resuscitation may be detrimental to the hypotensive patient with penetrating injuries before bleeding is controlled, in that such resuscitation may prevent appropriate clotting at the site of injury and may lead to increased mortality.[17]

The management of a massive hemothorax depends on the stability of the patient and the quantification of the hemothorax. In the unstable patient with clinical signs of massive hemothorax, immediate chest cavity decompression is warranted concurrently with ongoing resuscitation. In the hemodynamically stable patient, diagnostic imaging is often performed while the primary and secondary surveys are occurring. Commonly the diagnosis is made by chest radiography, although between 200 and 300 mL of blood needs to be present in the chest for it to be seen on the radiograph. Placing the patient in an upright position will cause the blood to layer in the base of thorax, thus increasing the sensitivity of the radiograph. In the acute setting, this may be the sole imaging from which the diagnosis is made and treatment initiated. This positioning may not be appropriate in those patients in whom a spinal cord injury is suspected. The presence and size of a hemothorax are much more difficult to assess with supine chest radiograph.

Adjuvant methods of imaging are of growing interest in those hemodynamic patients without signs of a massive hemothorax but with evidence of blood within the chest (simple hemothorax). CT is a highly accurate diagnostic study for the evaluation of chest structures and pathology, although it means both a dramatic increase of cost and radiation exposure as compared with chest radiography.[18] Opponents of the routine use of CT imaging contend that its high sensitivity identifies pathology that is clinically nonsignificant.[19] However, such imaging has been demonstrated to be superior over chest radiography in the evaluation of patients with suspected retained hemothorax later in the course of care.[20]

Treatment of both a massive hemothorax and simple hemothorax focuses on the complete evacuation of fluid from the chest cavity. This is first performed by placement of a chest tube into the affected side as described previously. When a massive hemothorax is present, the initial output from the chest tube is dramatic. If more than 1500 mL is immediately evacuated, it is very likely the patient will require emergent thoracotomy, thus necessitating the appropriate surgical consultation. Continued bleeding from the chest (>200 mL per hour for 2 to 4 hours) is traditionally cited as criteria for emergent thoracotomy. Even with these recommended criteria for surgical intervention, the patient's clinical signs and physiology take precedence for determining operative intervention. A patient in hemorrhagic shock, although with output less than the criteria just described, who requires ongoing resuscitation (likely with blood products) is likely experiencing ongoing blood loss and thus will require surgical intervention to control it.

Cardiac Tamponade

Cardiac tamponade is an injury that is most commonly seen after a penetrating injury, although blunt mechanisms have been reported. Cardiac tamponade is defined by the filling of the pericardial sac with blood from the heart, the great vessels, or pericardial vessels. Because the pericardial sac is a fibrous structure with a fixed volume, ever-increasing small amounts of blood that leak into it cause an increase in pressure within this closed space (**Figure 43–4**). This pressure increase directly restricts the activity of the heart and prevents adequate cardiac filling.

> **RESPIRATORY RECAP**
>
> **Circulation Injuries**
> - Hypovolemic shock
> - Hemothorax
> - Cardiac tamponade

The diagnosis of cardiac tamponade is classically described as **Beck's triad**, which consists of venous pressure elevation (jugular venous distention), a decline in arterial pressure, and muffled heart sounds. In reality, such a triad is difficult to diagnose in a busy and noisy trauma bay. Patients with tamponade present with a

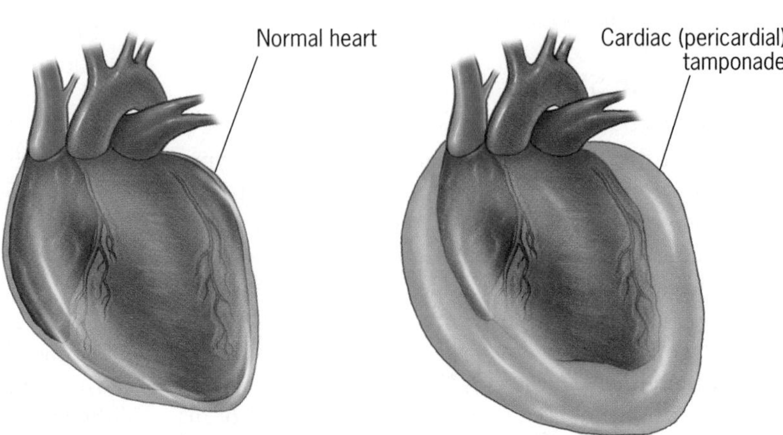

FIGURE 43–4 Cardiac tamponade.

spectrum of findings that range from a subtle decrease in blood pressure to hemodynamic collapse with cardiac arrest. A high index of suspicion is required to make a rapid diagnosis. The use of ultrasound has made the detection of pericardial fluid rapid and accurate at the bedside of these patients. The FAST exam allows clinicians to detect blood not only in the pericardial space but also in the abdomen by noninvasive means.[21] Although the precision of such a test is operator dependent, the initial accuracy rate of the FAST exam has been found to be at least 90% from the outset of the experience of the individual clinician.[22]

The treatment of cardiac tamponade begins with volume resuscitation. The goal of intravenous fluids is to increase the central venous pressure to overcome the restrictive pressure created by the accumulated pericardial blood. With an increase in cardiac output created, transient increases in the hemodynamics of the patient are expected. Evacuation of the pericardial blood is necessary for the relief of the tamponade physiology. This is best performed in the operating room by a surgical team experienced in repairing injuries to the heart. If surgical intervention is not available, pericardiocentesis using ultrasound is a means to aspirate pericardial blood. This is merely a temporizing measure in that blood may reaccumulate if the cardiac injury is not surgically repaired.

Injuries Encountered During the Secondary Survey

The secondary survey begins after the primary survey is complete and all immediate life-threatening injuries have been addressed. If the patient decompensates hemodynamically during any part of the primary or secondary survey, the clinician must start reevaluating causes using the ordered nature of the primary survey. Injuries described earlier in this chapter may not be detected until the secondary survey based on the temporal nature of their acuity. The secondary survey focuses on an in-depth physical examination of the patient from head to toe. While this exam is occurring, radiographic and laboratory data are collected by members of the team.

If the chest radiograph was not obtained during the primary survey, it should be performed at this time. The anteroposterior chest radiograph is the single most valuable diagnostic study in the evaluation of any patient with chest trauma. Findings on the chest radiograph can suggest the amount of velocity incurred during blunt impact. Multiple broken ribs—specifically, fractures of the first or second ribs—can indicate a high-velocity impact. The chest radiograph may also demonstrate findings to aid in the diagnosis of the eight lethal injuries of the chest, which are tracheobronchial injuries, pneumothorax, hemothorax, pulmonary contusion, blunt cardiac injury, aortic injury, diaphragmatic injury, and esophageal injury. Detection of these injuries during the secondary survey may be subtle as compared with those that present during the primary survey; thus, a high index of suspicion is required for detection.

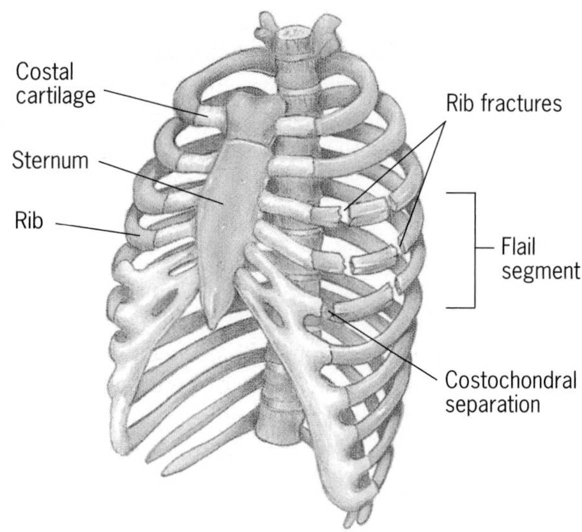

FIGURE 43–5 Flail chest.

Pulmonary Contusion

A **pulmonary contusion** is a bruise of the lung parenchyma. The initial trauma, whether direct injury from a blunt impact or contusion injury from a penetrating mechanism, causes the rupture of small blood vessels within the lung or direct injury to lung alveoli. Interstitial edema and intra-alveolar hemorrhage are the end result at the tissue level.[23]

Pulmonary contusion may occur without rib fractures, although the presence of a contusion is almost pathognomonic when a flail segment is present. A flail chest results from two or more ribs that are fractured in two or more locations, sternal fracture, or costochondral separation (**Figure 43–5**). The term *flail* refers to the paradoxical motion of the affected chest wall segment caused by the lack of structural integrity. During inspiration, the flail segment is drawn into the chest (due to negative intrapleural pressure) while the rest of the thorax expands outward. During exhalation, the opposite occurs, with the flail segment being pushed outward while the rest of the chest retracts. Because the chest wall becomes unstable during impact, the moving segment directly injures the lung parenchyma deep to the thoracic wall.

Pulmonary contusion alters the ventilation-perfusion ($\dot{V}/\dot{Q}$) match and may lead to arterial hypoxia. Patients with significant hypoxia may require intubation rapidly after injury due to the progressive nature of this disease. Pulmonary contusions often develop at 48 hours after injury, with maximal ($\dot{V}/\dot{Q}$) mismatching occurring during this period.[24] Because of the expected progressive nature of significant pulmonary contusions, elective intubation prior to respiratory failure should be considered early in the patient's management. Once the patient's airway is controlled, manipulations of mean airway pressure (e.g., positive end-expiratory pressure, inspiratory-to-expiratory ratio) should be considered to reinflate collapsed pulmonary segments and alveoli to maximize oxygenation. The treatment of contusion is entirely supportive, with resolution occurring at approximately 1 week.

Blunt Cardiac Injury

Much like pulmonary contusion is an injury that occurs to lung parenchyma, blunt cardiac injury is trauma to cardiac tissue resulting from a blunt mechanism. Blunt cardiac injury can result in bruising to the heart myocardium, coronary artery injury, chamber rupture, valvular injury, or a combination of these. Cardiac rupture is possible, although it is usually associated with a high transfer of energy such as seen with high-speed MVCs or falls from substantial height.

Patients with blunt cardiac injury present commonly with chest pain. Often these patients have multiple chest wall injuries that can confound this finding. Screening the asymptomatic patient with electrocardiograms (ECGs) and cardiac enzyme levels, the gold standard for myocardial ischemia, has little value in this injury.[25,26] Symptomatic patients are defined by the finding of hemodynamic instability and dysrhythmias on ECG. These include atrial fibrillation, premature ventricular contractions, sinus tachycardia, bundle-branch block, and ST segment changes. These patients warrant evaluation by echocardiography to determine the presence of pericardial fluid, to quantify the presence of cardiac wall motion abnormality, and to measure cardiac contractility.

Treatment of a blunt cardiac injury follows the same principles described for a penetrating cardiac injury. If pericardial fluid is demonstrated by the initial FAST exam or formal echocardiography, timely drainage of the pericardial space needs to occur, with the possibility that surgical repair of such an injury may be required. In the patient with dysrhythmias or conduction abnormalities found on ECG, supportive care needs to be provided in an intensive care environment with the possibility of concomitant cardiac pharmacology. Nonetheless, these dysrhythmias are often self-limiting, with resolution within 24 to 48 hours.

Aortic Injury

The great majority of injuries to the thoracic aorta have a penetrating mechanism of injury. Unfortunately, these injuries often have a fatal outcome. The identification of an aortic injury by a blunt mechanism often requires a great deal of insight during the secondary survey. The proximal descending aorta is the most common site for injury via a blunt mechanism because of its mobility and susceptibility to shear forces in relation to an otherwise relatively fixed structure.[27] Common types of injuries include a dissection (a tear of the innermost tissue layer of the aorta), a pseudoaneurysm (a full-thickness injury that is contained by surrounding tissue), and rupture, which often is fatal.

The presentation of patients with such an injury pattern is subtle at best in a busy trauma bay. Nonspecific clinical signs of a thoracic aorta injury include chest pain, shortness of breath, multiple rib fractures, or a sternal fracture and asymmetric upper extremity blood pressures. Traditional means of diagnosis begin with the chest radiograph. Findings may include a widened mediastinum, loss of the aortopulmonary window, depression of the left main bronchus, blunting of the aortic knob, or deviation of the esophagus or trachea. Abnormalities on chest radiography or a high clinical suspicion dictate the need for further imaging. The historical gold standard for the evaluation of the aorta has been catheter arteriography, although more centers are relying on spiral chest CT because of its speed, accuracy, and noninvasive nature.[28]

When an injury is found, the first step is expedient admission into a critical care environment. The main focus of such an admission is the control of blood pressure via beta blockade to reduce shear forces that are generated by blood flow at the area of injury.[29] Although this treatment is classic teaching for intensivists, the evidence behind such pharmacology is remote and lacks prospective validation. The traditional treatment for such injuries has been open surgical repair, whether primary or by replacement of the injured segment by an interposition graft. Endovascular techniques are rapidly becoming an alternative approach for operations that carry great inherent morbidity.[30]

Diaphragmatic Injury

Detecting injuries to the diaphragm is often very difficult. The dynamic movement of this structure makes predicting penetrating injuries based on trajectory a guess at best. Penetrating injuries to the diaphragm occur almost three times more frequently than injuries to the diaphragm due to a blunt mechanism.[31] Such penetrating injuries are extremely small, the size of the bullet or the width of a knife, and often are diagnosed and repaired intraoperatively. Blunt trauma often creates large tears secondary to a blow-out effect as force is applied to the external thorax or abdomen. These blunt lacerations are more commonly diagnosed on the left rather than the right because the liver acts to protect or obscure the right hemidiaphragm.

The utility of the screening chest radiograph has been described previously. Diaphragmatic injuries are often missed or misinterpreted as normal anatomic variations. If an injury is suspected of the left hemidiaphragm, a nasogastric tube should be placed and a repeat chest radiograph taken. With a nasogastric tube in place, the clinician has an improved ability to determine whether the stomach is within the thoracic cavity. A hemothorax may obscure clear radiographic evaluation of the left diaphragm, and thus a chest tube should be placed before further evaluation. If the diagnosis continues to be unclear, some advocate upper gastrointestinal contrast studies or CT imaging of the chest and abdomen. Unfortunately, there are few specific findings attributable to diaphragmatic injuries, which contributes to a high false-negative rate for these tests.[32]

Operative intervention may be required for the diagnosis to be made in those patients for whom there is a high suspicion of injury. The routine use of laparoscopy for the evaluation of the left hemidiaphragm for penetrating injuries has demonstrated a significant number of otherwise occult injures.[33–35] Penetrating injuries detected during laparoscopy or thoracoscopy may be repaired using minimally invasive techniques if further exploration is not required. Larger or more complex injuries may require a traditional open abdominal or thoracic approach, especially if synthetic mesh is necessary for diaphragmatic closure.

Esophageal Injury

Injuries to the thoracic esophagus are mainly due to gun shot wounds because of the central and deep location of the structure. Penetrating injuries to the esophagus are associated with other central chest injuries (heart, lungs, and great vessels) and thus are associated with a large mortality. Blunt injuries have been reported, although these are suspected to be the result of a blow-out type of mechanism due to force being placed on the chest or abdomen.

Signs and symptoms of an esophageal injury are nonspecific and are often clouded by the patient having multiple severe injuries. A delay in detection of an injury can be catastrophic because of the resultant increase in thoracic contamination, which leads to a higher risk of mediastinitis, sepsis, and death.[36] The evaluation of blunt esophageal injury should be considered in patients with injuries consistent with significant thoracic force. A chest radiograph should be obtained, although accuracy for injury is low. Findings of pneumomediastinum should alert the care team to a possible injury and prompt further evaluation. A high index of suspicion or abnormalities detected on chest radiography should direct the clinician to contrast studies of the esophagus or esophagoscopy, or both. Diagnosed injuries require expedient surgical repair with wide drainage of the contaminated pleural cavity.

Chest Wall Injury

Injuries to the chest often include injuries of the bony thorax, specifically the ribs, clavicles, sternum, and scapulas. Fracture of the upper ribs (ribs 1 and 2), scapula, or sternum requires a great deal of force and thus may give insight into the amount of energy transferred to the chest wall. Such an injury pattern may demand evaluation of the head, spine, lungs, heart, and the great vessels. Fractures of the lower ribs (ribs 10 through 12) may lead to thoracoabdominal injuries, specifically of the spleen and liver.

Although often underappreciated, the sequela from bone pain of the thorax can be dramatic. The ability of patients to participate in incentive spirometry, clear secretions, ventilate, and oxygenate is compromised by such pain. In the elderly population, the effects of simple rib fractures can be morbid, likely as a result of the impending consequences of poor pulmonary toilet.[37,38] Splinting of the chest wall may aid in local pain control, although it is contraindicated because of the negative consequences of inadequate pulmonary toilet due to chest wall immobility.

> **RESPIRATORY RECAP**
>
> **Injuries Found on Secondary Survey**
> - » Pulmonary contusion
> - » Blunt cardiac injury
> - » Aortic injury
> - » Diaphragmatic injury
> - » Esophageal injury
> - » Chest wall injury

Aggressive pain control should be a primary endpoint for this patient population regardless whether surgical fixation is warranted. The failure to provide adequate pain control has been associated with hypoventilation, retained secretions, atelectasis, pneumonia, and respiratory failure.[39] Methods of pain medication delivery include parenteral methods (intravenous and intramuscular), enteral means, epidural delivery, and local techniques, including nerve blocks, intrapleural catheters, and extrapleural catheters. These techniques can be controlled by the care team or by the patient. In the latter case, the patient dictates how much pain control is needed by pushing the button of a patient-controlled analgesia (PCA) device.[40] PCA devices prevent periods of breakthrough pain that may delay progress in pulmonary toilet, atelectasis, and cough. PCA devices can have preprogrammed lock-outs for the amount or frequency of medications delivered.

Parenteral narcotics continue to be the standard method by which clinicians treat thoracic pain. Narcotics can be delivered by all of the methods just described. The amount required for pain control is individualized to the patient and thus requires that patients be monitored and evaluated by objective pain measurement tools.[41] Traditionally, approaches focus on the use of short-acting parenteral narcotics for procedural pain or pain control while intubated, with a transition to PCA methods when the patient is able to participate in his or her care. A conversion to longer-acting enteral narcotics often occurs when a diet can be tolerated and more chronic pain medication needs are established. Regardless of whether a narcotic is provided enterally or parenterally, the side effects of confusion, respiratory depression, and cough suppression may occur. A careful balance needs to be achieved between the side effects of narcotic usage and the benefits created by pain-controlled pulmonary care.

The use of regional anesthetics can add a great deal to chest wall pain control while limiting exposure to side effects. Continuous epidural infusions of narcotic and local anesthetics have been successful in controlling chest pain and improving respiratory function. For thoracic trauma patients, it has been demonstrated that epidural delivery of anesthesia may be superior to PCA methods for the control of pain and improvement of pulmonary function.[41] The use of epidural anesthetics has demonstrated an increase in maximum inspiratory and expiratory pressures, vital capacity, and peak expiratory flow. Parenteral narcotics often cause a respiratory depression that leads to a decrease in Pao_2 and increase in $Paco_2$. Epidural analgesia prevents this problem by maintaining normal Pao_2 and $Paco_2$ levels. Epidurals are not without issues, however. Complications at the insertion site, as well as spinal cord injury, have been associated with their use. Epidural analgesia also can cause profound vasodilatory hypotension if fluid management strategies as well as epidural medication infusions are not closely monitored. The use of intercostal catheters with or without medication pumps for the administration of local anesthetic has also been reported, although placement of the catheters requires surgical expertise and the benefits it adds to epidural analgesia are unclear.[43,44]

Head Trauma

Head injuries are commonly encountered by those caring for the traumatically injured. Although most injuries are categorized as minor, it is imperative for the care team to provide timely evaluation and treatment to prevent secondary brain injury in those patients with any signs or symptoms of traumatic brain injury (TBI). Injuries can be the result of either penetrating or blunt mechanisms. Treatment of the patient with a traumatic head injury follows the same orderly steps described previously and outlined by the ATLS guidelines of the American College of Surgeons Committee on Trauma.[45] The focus of the ABCDE and later secondary survey is the identification of a treatable mass lesion, prevention of hypoxia, and the avoidance of hypotension to secure adequate cerebral perfusion pressure.

Intracranial Physiology

To understand primary brain injury and to prevent secondary injury, it is important to focus on the unique anatomy and physiology of the head. The brain is enveloped by the arachnoid mater, then by the dura mater, and finally encased by the skull. Because of the nonexpandable nature of the skull, the Monro-Kellie doctrine states that the total volume of the intracranial contents must remain constant. These contents include the brain, the cerebrospinal fluid (CSF), and venous blood. If a patient were to have an increase in intracranial blood after a traumatic injury, the resultant volume of CSF and venous blood must exit the skull or intracranial pressure (ICP) will rise (**Figure 43–6**). With both CSF and venous blood being removed by compensatory mechanisms from the intracranial space, ICP will exponentially rise if such a lesion is not externally decompressed.

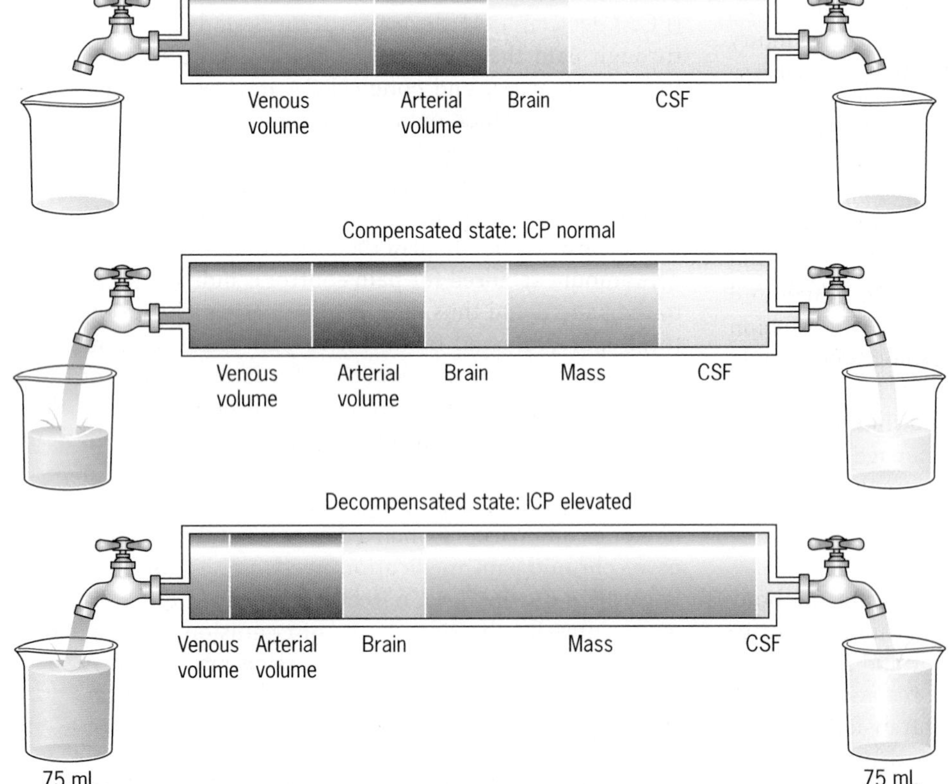

FIGURE 43–6 The Monro-Kellie doctrine. Reproduced from *Advance Trauma Life Support*. 8th ed. 2008. With permission of the American College of Surgeons.

Blood flow to the brain is directly dependent on the pressure head of the systemic blood pressure but is negated by elevated ICP. When ICP rises, a reflexive increase in mean arterial pressure (MAP) occurs to maintain the appropriate cerebral perfusion pressure (CPP). CPP is defined as the difference between MAP and ICP. The goal of medical and surgical maneuvers is to maintain CPP above 60 mm Hg. This is done by decreasing ICP or increasing MAP, or both. If a normal CPP is unobtainable, cerebral ischemia may result. Normally, the autoregulation of arterial blood flow to the brain has a dramatic ability to maintain a constant flow over a wide range of systemic pressures. In the injured brain, the auto-regulation of flow is decreased, thus making the brain more susceptible to fluctuations of MAP.

Types of Intracranial Lesions

The anatomic layer in which blood is present and whether the lesion is focal or diffusely located define traumatic intracranial lesions. Focal lesions include epidural, subdural, and subarachnoid or intracerebral hematomas. Diffuse injuries are often referred to as *diffuse axonal injuries* or *shear injuries*. Most intracranial lesions are often characterized early in the course of care by obtaining a head CT.

Epidural Hematoma

An **epidural hematoma** is a collection of blood occurring in the potential space between the dura mater and the posterior wall of the skull. These hematomas occur rarely, affecting 0.9% of those with brain injuries and 9% of those in coma.[45] The etiology of such a bleed is the injury of a blood vessel within this space. Blood that accumulates has a biconvex or lenticular shape on head CT because the clot pushes the dura mater away from the posterior wall of the skull (**Figure 43–7**). Epidural hematomas that accumulate in the temporal or temporoparietal area of the skull often are caused by an injury of the middle meningeal artery.

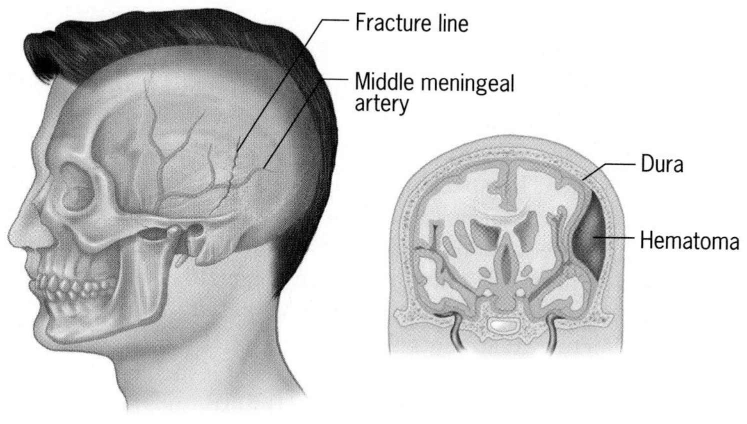

FIGURE 43–7 Epidural hematoma.

Subdural Hematoma

A **subdural hematoma** is the result of vascular injury that occurs in the space between the dura mater and the arachnoid mater. Blood that accumulates is often a result of shear injuries of bridging blood vessels originating from the cerebral cortex that travel within this potential space. Subdural hematomas are more common than epidural hematomas in that they occur in approximately 30% of severe brain injuries.[45] The underlying brain injury from a subdural hematoma is often more severe than from an epidural hematoma. On head CT, subdural hematomas have the appearance of curving to conform to the contours of the brain (**Figure 43–8**).

> **RESPIRATORY RECAP**
>
> **Types of Intracranial Lesions**
>
> » Epidural hematoma
> » Subdural hematoma
> » Subarachnoid (intracerebral) hematoma
> » Diffuse axonal injury

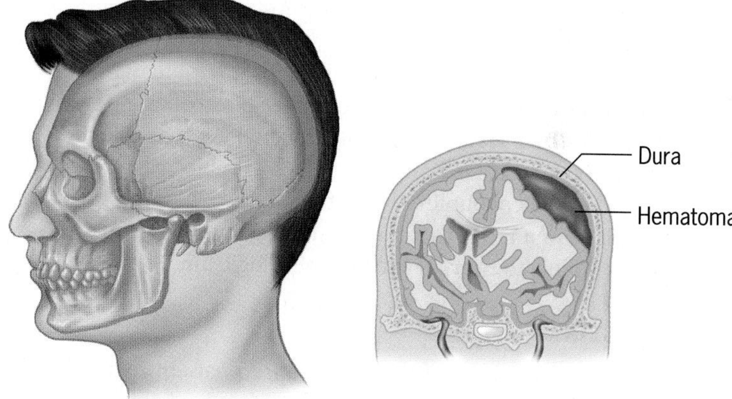

FIGURE 43–8 Subdural hematoma.

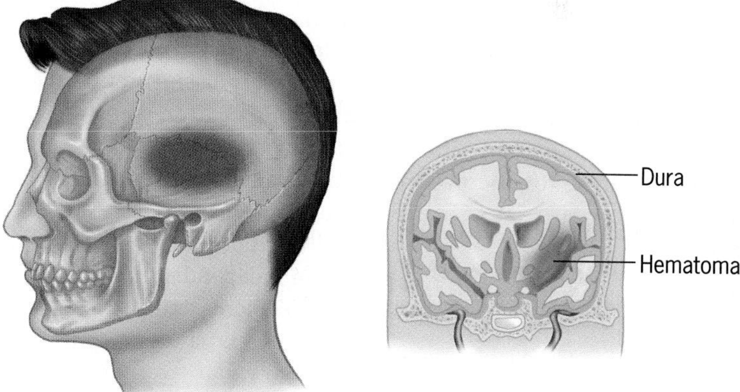

FIGURE 43–9 Subarachnoid (intracerebral) hematoma.

Subarachnoid Hematoma

Blood that accumulates under the arachnoid mater can have the diffuse appearance common with a **subarachnoid (intracerebral) hematoma** or be a discrete collection as seen with this type of hematoma (**Figure 43–9**). Traumatic subarachnoid hemorrhages have the potential to induce cerebral vasospasm, although the risk is lower than in aneurysmal subarachnoid hemorrhage.[46] Hematomas that occur within the parenchyma may occur in any region of the brain and have the ability to increase in size with time. Often, serial head CT exams are warranted to follow the mass effect of such a bleed.

Diffuse Axonal Injury

Injuries that involve discrete nerve injuries due to shearing forces present during the traumatic event are often referred to as diffuse axonal injuries. With multiple nerves being fractured, the potential for pathway injury is present. The spectrum of injury varies from mild concussive symptoms to severe traumatic brain injury. Unfortunately, axonal injury is often difficult to appreciate on head CT and may require magnetic resonance imaging (MRI) for quantification. At present, there are no effective treatments for diffuse axonal injury. The possibility for neuronal healing is present if such nerves are merely injured, not severed, and the exposure to secondary injury is limited.

Primary Survey Issues of Head Injury

The primary and secondary survey of a patient with a head injury occurs in the same organized format as it does with any other traumatically injured patient. The effects of brain injury are exacerbated by preventable secondary injury that is encountered and treated during these surveys. It is imperative that the trauma team addresses these issues rapidly to prevent further neurologic injury.

Hypoxia

The primary survey of the head-injured patient focuses on the prevention of hypoxia. Whether that involves placing a definitive airway or simply providing oxygen to the patient, such interventions need to occur quickly. Those patients who present with severe brain injury may need endotracheal intubation if they are unable to protect their airway or the care team is concerned about the evolution of hypoxia. Pulse oximetry is a useful adjunct in these patients in that a continuous measurement of the blood oxygen saturation is immediately available to all caring for the patient. Hypoxia has been reported to occur in approximately 22% of those with TBI and is an independent predictor of increased morbidity and mortality.[47,48] It appears that even short periods of hypoxia have a significant effect. In one report, an Spo_2 of 90% or less for a median duration of 12 to 20 minutes was found to be an independent predictor of death.[49]

RESPIRATORY RECAP

Primary Survey Issues of Head Injury
- » Hypoxia
- » Hyperventilation
- » Hypotension
- » Deficits

Hyperventilation

For many years, hyperventilation has been a cornerstone in the care of the patient with severe TBI. Hyperventilating the patient to a $Paco_2$ of less than 25 mm Hg has been demonstrated to rapidly reduce ICP. However, the mechanism for this reduction is cerebral vasoconstriction, with an ultimate reduction of cerebral blood flow.[50] This iatrogenic reduction in cerebral blood flow on top of the innate critical reduction of flow after injury may increase the risk of cerebral ischemia. Cohorts that received prophylactic hyperventilation showed a significantly reduced outcome at 3 and 6 months compared with those who did not receive such treatment.[51] Because of this established risk, the use of prophylactic hyperventilation is not recommended; it should only be used as a temporizing measure for the acute reduction of elevated ICP.[52]

Hypotension

The resuscitation of the TBI patient begins immediately in the prehospital setting and continues throughout the patient's evaluation and stay to defend against the deleterious effects of hypotension upon secondary brain injury. Previous work has demonstrated that a single episode of hypotension (<90 mm Hg systolic blood pressure) is associated with an increase in morbidity and a doubling of mortality.[52] The correction of hypotension by fluid resuscitation has been shown to have an impact on beneficial neurologic outcome.[53] Whether resuscitation should occur needs to take into account the CPP of the patient. A systolic blood pressure above 90 mm Hg may not be appropriate if the CPP is compromised. These patients likely would benefit from a closely monitored environment so that alterations in blood pressure can be quickly corrected.

Deficits

The *D* of the primary survey represents evaluating the patient for any neurologic deficits. For a patient who has sustained a traumatic brain injury, calculating the Glasgow Coma Scale (GCS) score is imperative. This scale is an objective clinical measurement of the severity of brain injury. The best GCS score a patient can achieve is 15, whereas the worst is 3. Brain injury is categorized as minor if the score is between 15 and 13, moderate if between 12 and 9, and severe if less than 9. When calculating the GCS score, one uses the highest score response for each of the eye, motor, and verbal components. Accurate scoring is important in that it aids in the prediction of long-term outcome from a variety of injury patterns.

Secondary Survey Issues of Head Injury

The secondary survey exam of a head-injured patient needs to include a thorough neurologic examination. Such an exam needs to be carefully documented so that all others who examine the patient have a clear understanding of the baseline exam. If changes should arise in the neurologic exam, a worsening of the neurologic injury needs to be excluded.

After the secondary survey is complete, an emergency head CT scan is the diagnostic study of choice for all those with moderate or severe brain injury. Controversy exists over the indications for head CT in those with mild brain injury.[54] Regardless, transport of the patient to the CT scanner occurs only after achieving hemodynamic stability. If a change in neurologic exam is encountered during the patient's hospital stay, a repeat head CT is likely indicated.

Treatment of Head Injuries

Medical therapy for the treatment of intracranial injuries focuses on the pharmacologic treatment of elevated ICP. Hyperosmolar agents are the backbone of such therapy. These include mannitol and hypertonic saline. Mannitol acts to lower ICP by creating an osmotic shift of water out of the brain into the intravascular space. Although effective for acutely decreasing ICP, mannitol is a potent diuretic that may exacerbate hypotension. Because of this side effect, the recommended use of mannitol is limited to when signs of transtentorial herniation or progressive neurologic deterioration are present.[55] The use of hypertonic saline to induce an osmotic mobilization similar to mannitol is gaining interest. The use of hypertonic saline as both a bolus agent for treatment of acute ICP and as a continuous infusion for prolonged treatment has been reported, but its long-term efficacy is still unclear.[55]

The surgical treatment of traumatic brain injuries focuses on the rapid decrease of ICP either by open evacuation of the hematoma or by removal of CSF via intraventricular drains. Both of these methods require the expertise of a neurosurgeon in the setting of emergency care. Evidence is emerging that the measurement of brain tissue oxygen levels by an intracranial catheter with the intended goal of manipulating oxygen delivery may have a beneficial effect.[56,57] Nonetheless, placement of these catheters requires neurosurgical support, with values being interpreted by an experienced critical care team.

KEY POINTS

- The mnemonic ABCDE provides for an orderly evaluation and treatment of traumatic injuries.
- The secondary survey of the trauma patient is a head-to-toe physical examination.
- Injuries to the chest can be broadly classified as having either a blunt or penetrating mechanism.
- Traumatic airway and breathing injuries include laryngotracheal injuries, dislocation of the sternoclavicular heads, and pneumothorax.
- There are three subtypes of pneumothoraces: simple, open, and tension.
- Hemorrhage is classified into four categories, using vital signs to aid in the quantification of blood loss.
- Massive hemothorax is accumulation of more than 1500 mL of blood in the chest cavity.
- Treatment of both a massive hemothorax and simple hemothorax focuses on the complete evacuation of fluid from the chest cavity.
- Cardiac tamponade is defined as the filling of the pericardial sac with blood from the heart, the great vessels, or pericardial vessels.
- Lethal injuries of the chest include tracheobronchial injuries, pneumothorax, hemothorax, pulmonary contusion, blunt cardiac injury, aortic injury, diaphragmatic injury, and esophageal injury.
- A flail chest results from two or more ribs that are fractured in two or more locations, sternal fracture, or costochondral separation.
- Pulmonary contusions often develop at 48 hours after injury, with maximal ventilation-perfusion mismatching occurring during this period.
- Although often underappreciated, the sequela from bone pain of the thorax can be dramatic.
- Traumatic brain injuries can cause epidural hematoma, subdural hematoma, subarachnoid hemorrhage, or diffuse axonal injury.
- Prophylactic hyperventilation is not recommended and should only be used as a temporizing measure for the acute reduction of elevated ICP.
- The correction of hypotension by fluid resuscitation improves neurologic outcome.
- Medical therapy for the treatment of intracranial injuries focuses on pharmacologic treatment of elevated ICP.
- Surgical treatment of traumatic brain injuries focuses on the rapid decrease of ICP.

REFERENCES

1. American College of Surgeons Committee on Trauma. *Advanced Trauma Life Support for Doctors: Student Manual.* 8th ed. Chicago: American College of Surgeons; 2008.
2. Calhoon JH, Trinkle JK. Pathophysiology of chest trauma. *Chest Surg Clin North Am.* 1997;7:199–211.
3. Centers for Disease Control and Prevention. Injury prevention and control: data and statistics (WISQARS). Available at: http://www.cdc.gov/ncipc/wisqars/default.htm.
4. MacKenzie EJ, Fowler CJ. Epidemiology. In: Moore EE, Feliciano DV, Mattox KL, eds. *Trauma.* New York: McGraw-Hill; 2004:21–39.
5. Peterson RJ, Tepas JJ, Edwards FH, et al. Pediatric and adult thoracic trauma: age-related impact on presentation and outcome. *Ann Thorac Surg.* 1994;58:14–18.
6. Demetriades D, Velmahos GD. Penetrating injuries of the chest: indications for operation. *Scand J Surg.* 2002;91:41–45.
7. Mathisen DJ, Grillo H. Laryngotracheal trauma. *Ann Thoracic Surg.* 1987;43:254–262.

8. Meyer FN. Upper extremity and hand injuries. In: Moore EE, Feliciano DV, Mattox KL, eds. *Trauma*. New York: McGraw-Hill; 2004:901–937.
9. Di Bartolomeo S, Sanson G, Nardi G, et al. A population based study on pneumothorax in severely traumatized patients. *J Trauma*. 2001;51:677–682.
10. Livingston DH, Hauser CJ. Trauma to the chest wall and lung. In: Moore EE, Feliciano DV, Mattox KL, eds. *Trauma*. New York: McGraw-Hill; 2004:507–538.
11. Dulchavsky SA, Schwarz KL, Kirkpatrick AW, et al. Prospective evaluation of thoracic ultrasound in the detection of pneumothorax. *J Trauma*. 2001;50:201–205.
12. Marinaro JL, Kenny CV, Smith SR, et al. Needle thoracostomy in trauma patients: what catheter length is adequate? *Acad Emerg Med*. 2003;10:495.
13. Eastridge BJ, Salinas J, McManus JG, et al. Hypotension begins at 110 mm Hg: redefining "hypotension" with data. *J Trauma*. 2007;63:291–299.
14. Borgman MA, Spinella PC, Perkins JG, et al. The ratio of blood products transfused affects mortality in patients receiving massive transfusions at a combat support hospital. *J Trauma*. 2007;63:805–813.
15. Holcomb JB, Jenkins D, Rhee P, et al. Damage control resuscitation: directly addressing the early coagulopathy of trauma. *J Trauma*. 2007;62:307–310.
16. Sperry JL, Ochoa JB, Gunn SR, et al. An FFP:PRBC transfusion ratio of ≥1:1.5 is associated with a lower risk of mortality after massive transfusion. *J Trauma*. 2008;65:986–993.
17. Bickell WH, Wall MJ, Pepe PE, et al. Immediate versus delayed fluid resuscitation for hypotensive patients with penetrating torso injuries. *N Engl J Med*. 1994;331:1105–1109.
18. Stafford RE, Linn J, Washington L. Incidence and management of occult hemothoraces. *Am J Surg*. 2006;192:722–726.
19. Kwon A, Sorrells DL, Kurkchubasche AG, et al. Isolated computed tomography diagnosis of pulmonary contusion does not correlate with increased morbidity. *J Pediatr Surg*. 2006;41:78–82.
20. Velmahos GC, Demetriades D, Chan L, et al. Predicting the need for thoracoscopic evacuation of residual hemothorax: chest radiograph is insufficient. *J Trauma*. 1999;46:65–70.
21. Rozycki GS, Feliciano DV, Schmidt JA, et al. The role of ultrasound in patients with possible penetrating cardiac wounds: a prospective multicenter study. *J Trauma*. 1999;46:542–551.
22. McCarter FD, Luchette FA, Molloy M, et al. Institutional and individual learning curves for focused abdominal ultrasound for trauma: cumulative sum analysis. *Ann Surg*. 2000;231:689–700.
23. Fulton RL, Peters ET. Compositional and histologic effects of fluid therapy following pulmonary contusion. *J Trauma*. 1974;14:783–790.
24. Fulton RL, Peters ET. The progressive nature of pulmonary contusion. *Surgery*. 1979;67:499–506.
25. Weiss RL, Brier JA, O'Conner W, et al. The usefulness of transesophageal echocardiography in diagnosing cardiac contusions. *Chest*. 1996;109:73–77.
26. Bertinchant JP, Polge A, Mohty D, et al. Evaluation of incidence, clinical significance, and prognostic value of circulating cardiac troponin I and T elevation in hemodynamically stable patients with suspected myocardial contusions after blunt chest trauma. *J Trauma*. 2000;48:924–931.
27. Williams JS, Graff JA, Uku JM, et al. Aortic injury in vehicular trauma. *Ann Thorac Surg*. 1994;57:727–730.
28. Demetriades D, Velmahos GC, Scalea TM, et al. Diagnosis and treatment of blunt thoracic aortic injuries: changing perspectives. *J Trauma*. 2008;64:1415–1418.
29. Wheat MW, Palmer RF, Bartley TD, et al. Treatment of dissecting aneurysm of the aorta without surgery. *J Thorac Cardiovasc Surg*. 1965;50:364–373.
30. Lee JT, White RA. Current status of thoracic aorta endograft repair. *Surg Clin North Am*. 2004;84:1295–1318.
31. Demetriades D, Murray JA. Traumatic diaphragmatic hernias. In: Fitzgibbons RJ, Greenburg AG, eds. *Nyhus and Condon's Hernia*. Philadelphia: Lippincott Williams & Wilkins; 2002:503–511.
32. Chen JC, Wilson SE. Diaphragmatic injuries: recognition and management in sixty-two patients. *Am Surg*. 1991;57:810–815.
33. Friese RS, Coln CE, Gentilello LM. Laparoscopy is sufficient to exclude occult diaphragm injury after penetrating abdominal trauma. *J Trauma*. 2005;58:789–92.
34. Powell BS, Magnotti LJ, Schroeppel TJ, et al. Diagnostic laparoscopy for the evaluation of occult diaphragmatic injury following penetrating thoracoabdominal trauma. *Injury*. 2008;39:530–534.
35. Scharff JR, Naunheim KS. Traumatic diaphragmatic injuries. *Thorac Surg Clin*. 2007;17:81–85.
36. Abbas G, Schuchert MJ, Pettiford BL, et al. Contemporaneous management of esophageal perforation. *Surgery*. 2009;146:749–755.
37. Bulger EM, Arneson MA, Mock CN, et al. Rib fractures in the elderly. *J Trauma*. 2000;48:1040–1046.
38. Bergeron E, Lavoie A, Clas D, et al. Elderly trauma patients with rib fractures are at greater risk of death and pneumonia. *J Trauma*. 2003;54:478–485.
39. Desai P. Pain management and pulmonary dysfunction. *Crit Care Clin*. 1999;15:151–166.
40. White PE. Use of patient-controlled analgesia for management of acute pain. *JAMA*. 1988;259:243–247.
41. Sessler CN, Grap MJ, Ramsay MA. Evaluating and monitoring analgesia and sedation in the intensive care unit. *Crit Care*. 2008;12(suppl 3):S2.
42. Moon MR, Luchette FA, Gibson SW, et al. Prospective, randomized comparison of epidural versus parenteral opioid analgesia in thoracic trauma. *Ann Surg*. 1999;229:684–691.
43. Haenel JB, Moore FA, Moore EE, et al. Extrapleural bupivacaine for amelioration of multiple rib fracture pain. *J Trauma*. 1995;38:22–27.
44. Allen MS, Halgren L, Nichols FC III, et al. A randomized controlled trial of bupivacaine through intracostal catheters for pain management after thoracotomy. *Ann Thorac Surg*. 2009;88:903–910.
45. Fildes J. Head trauma. In: American College of Surgeons Committee on Trauma. *Advanced Trauma Life Support for Doctors: Student Manual*. 8th ed. Chicago: American College of Surgeons; 2008:131–151.
46. Martin NA, Doberstein C, Zane C, et al. Posttraumatic cerebral arterial spasm: transcranial doppler ultrasound, cerebral blood flow, and angiographic findings. *J Neurosurg*. 1992;77:575–583.
47. Chestnut RM, Marshall LF, Klauber MR, et al. The role of secondary brain injury in determining outcome from severe head injury. *J Trauma*. 1993;34:216–222.
48. Murray GD, Butcher I, McHugh GS, et al. Multivariable prognostic analysis in traumatic brain injury: result from the IMPACT study. *J Neurotrauma*. 2007;24:329–337.
49. Jones PA, Andrews PJD, Midgely S, et al. Measuring the burden of secondary insults in head injured patients during intensive care. *J Neurosurg Anesthesiol*. 1994;6:4–14.
50. Raichle ME, Plum F. Hyperventilation and cerebral blood flow. *Stroke*. 1972;3:566–575.
51. Muizelaar JP, Marmarou A, Ward JD, et al. Adverse effects of prolonged hyperventilation in patients with severe head injury: a randomized clinical trial. *J Neurosurg*. 1991;75:731–739.

52. Bratton SL, Chestnut RM, Ghajar J, et al. Guidelines for the management of severe traumatic brain injury. XIV. Hyperventilation. *J Neurotrauma*. 2007;24(suppl 1):S87–S90.
53. Vassar MJ, Fischer RP, O'Brian PE, et al. A multicenter trial for resuscitation of injured patients with 7.5% sodium chloride. The effect of added dextran 70. The Multicenter Group for the Study of Hypertonic Saline in Trauma Patients. *Arch Surg.* 1993;128:1003–1011.
54. Stiell IG, Wells GA, Vandemheen K, et al. The Canadian CT head rule for patients with minor head injury. *Lancet.* 2001;357:1391–1396.
55. Bratton SL, Chestnut RM, Ghajar J, et al. Guidelines for the management of severe traumatic brain injury. II. Hyperosmolar therapy. *J Neurotrauma*. 2007;24(suppl 1):S14–S20.
56. Stiefel MF, Spiotta A, Gracias VH, et al. Reduced mortality rate in patients with severe traumatic brain injury treated with brain tissue oxygen monitoring. *J Neurosurg.* 2005;103:805–811.
57. Narotam PK, Morrison JF, Nathoo N. Brain tissue oxygen monitoring in traumatic brain injury and major trauma: outcome analysis of a brain tissue oxygen-directed therapy. *J Neurosurg.* 2009;111:672–682.

CHAPTER 44

Burn and Inhalation Injury

Robert L. Sheridan
Daniel F. Fisher

OUTLINE

OBJECTIVES

1. Describe the four phases of burn management.
2. Use the Lund-Browder chart to evaluate the extent of a burn injury.
3. Compare first-, second-, third-, and fourth-degree burns.
4. Discuss issues related to fluid resuscitation of patients with a burn injury.
5. Describe the effect of circumferential burn wounds of the torso on ventilatory function.
6. Discuss issues related to cutaneous heat and water loss in patients with a burn injury.
7. Discuss the physiology of inhalation injury.
8. Describe the diagnosis of inhalation injury.
9. List five predictable events in patients with inhalation injury.
10. Describe the management of upper airway obstruction, bronchospasm, small airway obstruction, pulmonary infection, and respiratory failure in patients with an inhalation injury.
11. Describe the treatment of patients with carboxyhemoglobinemia.

KEY TERMS

carboxyhemoglobin (HbCO)
CO-oximetry
eschar
escharotomy
fluid resuscitation
hyperbaric oxygen therapy
inhalation injury
total body surface area (TBSA)

INTRODUCTION

The term *burn* refers to the denaturing and destruction of tissue proteins and bone caused by thermal, electrical, or chemical injury. A major burn is defined as covering 25% or more of **total body surface area (TBSA)**.[1] The quality of life and the outcome for major burn patients has improved dramatically over the past 20 years.[2–4] This change began with a realization that the natural history of burns can be changed by prompt surgery; the early removal of **eschar** and immediate biologic closure of the resulting open wounds prevents the otherwise inevitable development of burn wound sepsis. However, to support a patient with a serious burn injury and associated respiratory failure through the physiologic trial of staged wound closure is not a simple undertaking. Patients who experience a major burn injury do better when cared for at a specialty burn center staffed with experienced personnel.[5]

Burn Injury

Phases of Burn Care

Patients with large burns typically have a deep, painful wound and are at risk for sepsis and progressive multiorgan dysfunction. Immediate clinical needs must be met, but an organized, overall plan of care must also be created. The initial evaluation of the burn patient should follow the recommendations established by the advanced trauma life support (ATLS) guidelines.[2,6–8] Burn injuries may distract the caregiver from other injuries; therefore, careful attention needs to be paid to ensure that a complete examination is performed. The patient must be screened for other injuries and comorbid conditions.[1,2,6] This organized plan of care has four phases (**Table 44–1**).[9]

The first phase, the initial evaluation and resuscitation, extends from day 1 through day 3. Providing adequate **fluid resuscitation** for the treatment of the resulting burn shock has been recognized as the most important factor in treating patients with burn injury.[10–12] Burn shock is the major cause of morbidity and mortality in the burn patient.

The second phase, initial wound excision and biologic closure, extends from day 1 through day 7. During this phase, the surgery is performed that changes the natural history of the injury. Typically, this period involves a series of staged operations to excise and debride the wound and place temporary covering over the denuded areas.

The third phase, definitive wound closure, lasts from day 7 through week 6. It involves replacement of temporary wound covers with definitive cover, as well as closure and acute reconstruction of burns that have a small surface area but are highly complex, such as wounds on the face and hands.

The final stage involves rehabilitation, reconstruction, and reintegration. Although this final stage actually begins during the resuscitation period, it becomes very time consuming and involved toward the end of the acute hospital stay.

Physiology of Burn Injury

An extensive cutaneous burn wound has a profound influence on pulmonary function, and accurate evaluation of the wound is important. This task can prove to be difficult even for an experienced burn surgeon because a burn wound is a dynamic injury and will alter based on both extrinsic and intrinsic factors, such as amount of resultant edema, release of inflammatory mediators, and initial treatment of the wound.[1,13]

Burns should be evaluated for extent, depth, and circumferential components (**Box 44–1**). Initially, it is critical to have a good estimate of total body surface area involvement to determine the course and aggressiveness of the resuscitative efforts. The extent of the burn injury is best estimated with a Lund-Browder chart, which accounts for variance in body proportions with growth (**Figure 44–1**). An alternative in adults is the Wallace rule of nines, which divides the body into sections representing 9% of body surface area. This is a rapid method of estimating burn surface area, but the rule of nines has a tendency to overestimate the extent of the burn, which can lead to excessive fluid resuscitation.[2,10,14,15] Another surface area estimation technique uses the palmar surface of the patient's hand (without fingers), which represents approximately 1% of the body surface area.

It is vital to have an accurate assessment of the burn area and severity for the needs of fluid resuscitation. Having an understanding of the limitations of each of these methods also will affect the resuscitation efforts. The wide variation of burn size estimates from any of these techniques has been a driving force for developing several computer models to aid the surgeon in obtaining a more accurate and reproducible measurement of body surface area involvement.[16,17] When using the computer models, a digital image is taken of the patient, and the burn area is calculated using either two-or three-dimensional graphics, or the areas affected are drawn on a representation of the patient's body type (**Figure 44–2**). The benefits of these estimation methods are

TABLE 44–1 Four Phases of Burn Care

Phase	Timing	Treatment Objectives
Initial evaluation and resuscitation	First 72 hours	To achieve accurate fluid resuscitation and perform a thorough evaluation
Initial wound excision and biologic closure	Days 1 through 7	To identify and remove all full-thickness wounds and obtain biologic closure
Definitive wound closure	Day 7 through week 6	To replace temporary covers with definitive ones and close small, complex wounds
Rehabilitation, reconstruction, and reintegration	Entire hospitalization	Initially to maintain range of motion and reduce edema; subsequently to strengthen and prepare patients for return to community

BOX 44–1

Evaluation of the Burn Wound

Extent

Lund-Browder chart: An age-specific chart that accounts for changes in body proportions. This is the preferred method used to determine the extent of a burn injury.

Wallace rule of nines: A rough method of estimation that assumes adult body proportions. The head and neck are roughly 9%; the anterior and posterior chest are 9% each; the anterior and posterior abdomen (including buttocks) are 9% each; each upper extremity is 9%; each thigh is 9%; each leg and foot is 9%; and the genitals are 1%.

Palmar surface of the hand: The palmar surface of a person's hand (without the fingers) is approximately 1% of the body surface over all age groups.

Depth

First degree: Red, dry, painful wounds that often are deeper than they appear; sloughing occurs the next day.

Second degree: Red, wet, very painful wounds. Their depth, ability to heal, and propensity to form hypertrophic scars vary immensely.

Third degree: Leathery, dry, insensate, waxy wounds that do not heal.

Fourth degree: Wounds that involve underlying subcutaneous tissue, tendon, or bone.

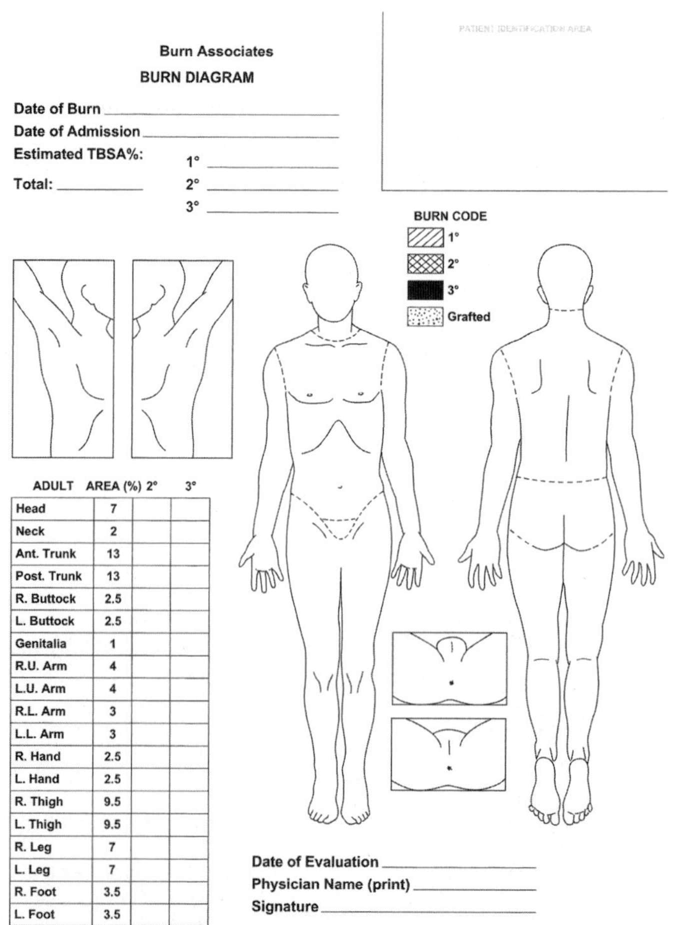

PATIENT IDENTIFICATION AREA

Burn Associates
BURN DIAGRAM

Date of Burn ____________
Date of Admission ____________
Estimated TBSA%: 1° ________ 2° ________ 3° ________
Total: ________

BURN CODE
1°
2°
3°
Grafted

ADULT	AREA (%)	2°	3°
Head	7		
Neck	2		
Ant. Trunk	13		
Post. Trunk	13		
R. Buttock	2.5		
L. Buttock	2.5		
Genitalia	1		
R.U. Arm	4		
L.U. Arm	4		
R.L. Arm	3		
L.L. Arm	3		
R. Hand	2.5		
L. Hand	2.5		
R. Thigh	9.5		
L. Thigh	9.5		
R. Leg	7		
L. Leg	7		
R. Foot	3.5		
L. Foot	3.5		

Date of Evaluation ____________
Physician Name (print) ____________
Signature ____________

FIGURE 44–1 Lund-Browder chart for estimating body surface area involvement.

that the computed TBSA involvement is reproducible and can be obtained quickly even by clinicians who may have limited burn experience, and the injury maps can be sent along with the patient when he or she is transferred to a regional burn center. The initial injury is also better documented for evaluation by the burn surgeon. A more direct need for having accurate burn maps is for determining the fluid requirements for the patient based on the severity of the injury. Inaccurate estimates can lead to improper fluid resuscitation. Providing too little fluid during the initial resuscitation can lead to organ system failure. Too much fluid will contribute to systemic edema, which decreases peripheral circulation, leading to collateral tissue injury.[14,15]

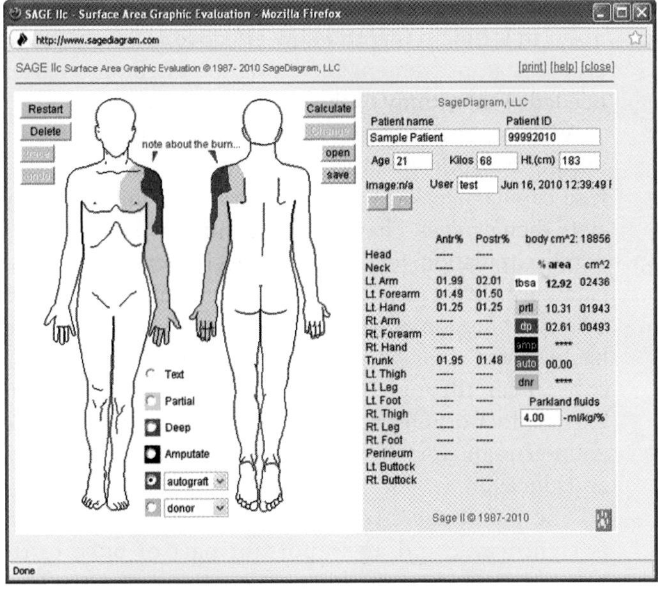

FIGURE 44–2 Surface Area Graphic Evaluation (SAGE II) screen: digital burn diagram.

Burns are classified as first, second, third, or fourth degree (**Figure 44–3**). In addition, they are classified by the depth of the injury, ranging from superficial to full-thickness and finally to deep dermal.[18] It can be difficult for even an experienced examiner to accurately determine the depth of a burn early on. As a general rule, depth usually is underestimated on the initial examination.[13,18,19]

An understanding of the physiologic aberrations that occur with serious burns allows clinicians to provide respiratory care in the burn unit. Successfully resuscitated burn patients manifest a sequence of predictable physiologic changes (**Table 44–2**). These changes can be anticipated, which aids in patient management.

Individuals who suffer serious burns experience diffuse capillary leakage, which is in direct response to wound-released mediators.[9,20,21] The result is

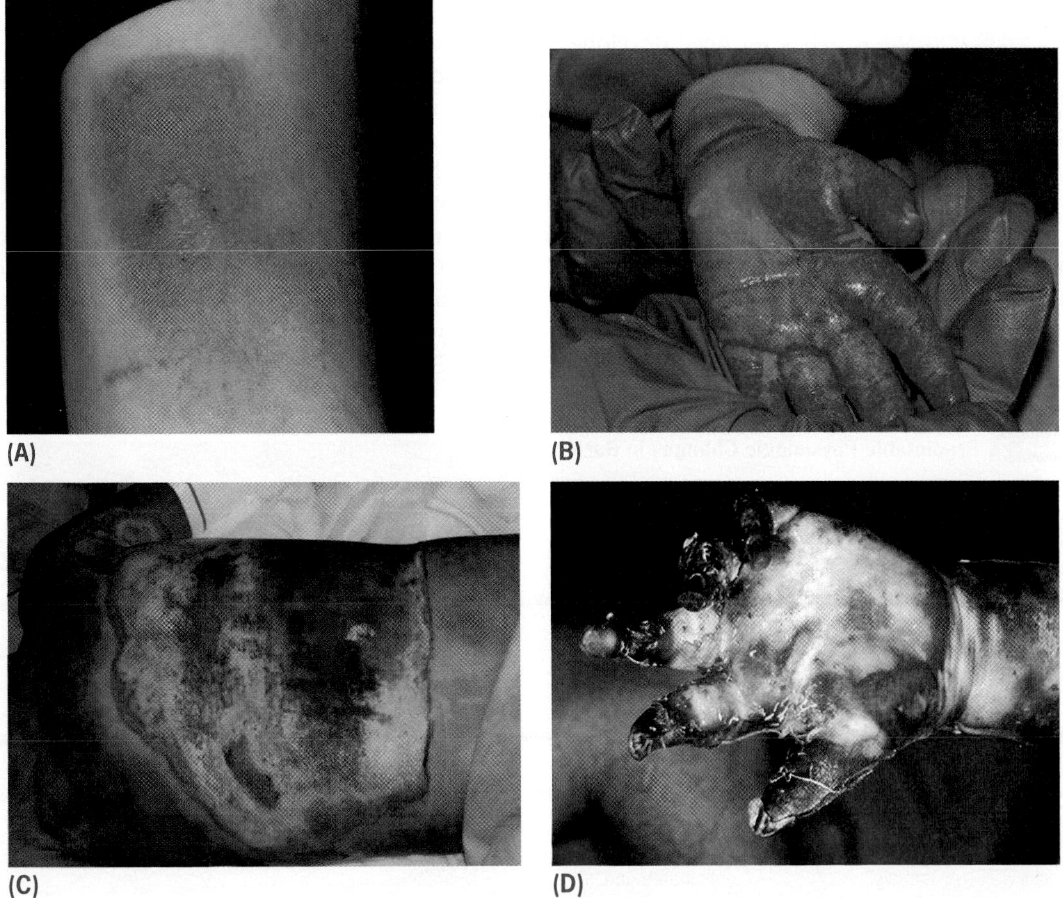

FIGURE 44–3 Various degrees of burn severity. (**A**) First degree. (**B**) Second degree. (**C**) Third degree. (**D**) Fourth degree.

extravasation of fluids, electrolytes, and moderate-sized colloid molecules, which explains the enormous fluid resuscitation requirements of burn patients. A number of formulas have been developed that attempt to predict resuscitation volume requirements based on body weight or surface area and burn size.[1,11,12,14,16,18,22] These formulas all depend on the accurate estimation of body surface area's involvement. It has been shown that even with these formulas, excessive fluid can be delivered to the patient in a phenomenon referred to as fluid creep, which refers to delivery of more than predicted volumes of fluid during resuscitation.[13,15] This does not suggest that the fluid resuscitation formulas are in error, but rather reminds the clinician to be aware that the resulting edema can have deleterious effects on the burn wound.

A number of variables affect resuscitation requirements, in-cluding delay in initiation of resuscitation, inhalation injury, and the depth and vapor transmission characteristics of the wound itself. No two injuries are exactly alike, and no formula has yet been developed that can predict with acceptable accuracy the volume requirements in all patients.[13,14] For these reasons, a resuscitation formula can only help determine the initial volume infusion rate and roughly predict overall requirements. Because inaccurate volume administration is associated with substantial morbidity, it is essential that burn resuscitation be guided by hourly reevaluation of resuscitation end points.

RESPIRATORY RECAP

Diffuse Capillary Leakage

- Burn patients have a substantial need for fluid replacement for the first 24 hours after the injury.
- Fluid resuscitation: kg per percent TBSA of lactated Ringer's solution during the first 24 hours after burn.
  - Half of this amount is given during the first 8 hours.
  - The remainder is given over the next 16 hours.
- An abrupt decline in fluid requirement occurs 18 to 24 hours after injury.
- After 24 hours, tissue edema begins to subside and urine output increases as excess fluid is reabsorbed and cleared.

Circumferential or near-circumferential burn wounds of the torso require special monitoring; such wounds may interfere with ventilation as soft tissues swell beneath the inelastic eschar and may require **escharotomy** (**Figure 44–4**). The need for escharotomy must be recognized in a timely way to allow effective intervention. A dramatic improvement in ventilation is common after needed escharotomy of the chest and abdomen.

With successful resuscitation, volume requirements decline abruptly 18 to 24 hours after injury as the diffuse capillary leakage abates. A systemic inflammatory state then evolves, characterized clinically by a hyperdynamic circulation, fever, and massively increased protein catabolism. This physiologic state is thought to be caused by a combination of wound colonization, with release of bacteria and their by-products; translocation of similar substances through a compromised gastrointestinal barrier; foci of infection; and augmented release of the counter-regulatory hormones cortisol, catecholamines, and glucagon.

The metabolic stress associated with a large burn is significant, and an important part of burn critical care is support of this physiologic condition. This therapy takes the form of accurate fluid repletion, nutritional support, control of environmental temperatures, prompt removal of nonviable tissue with physiologic wound closure, support of the gastrointestinal barrier, and proper management of pain and anxiety. An additional and critical component is support of body temperature. Burn patients have extensive evaporative water and energy losses if they are maintained in the typical cool, dry air of a general hospital. Burn units and operating rooms must be engineered to maintain a high ambient temperature and relative humidity level to avoid the difficult problem of hypothermia and humidity deficit of the airway, which could result in thickened pulmonary secretions.

TABLE 44–2 Predictable Physiologic Changes in Burn Patients

Time Frame	Change	Treatment Steps
Resuscitation period (days 0 to 3)	Massive capillary leakage	Fluid resuscitation
Post-resuscitation period (day 3 to 95% definitive wound closure)	Hyperdynamic and catabolic state with high risk of infection	Early wound closure to prevent sepsis (nutritional support is essential)
Recovery period (95% definitive wound closure to 1 year after injury)	Continuing catabolic state and risk of nonwound sepsis	Nutritional support essential; complications anticipated and treated

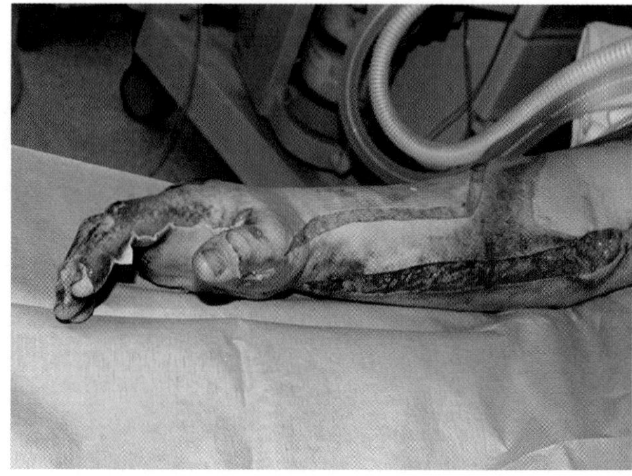

FIGURE 44–4 Escharotomy of right arm.

Inhalation Injury

Inhalation injury describes damage to the lungs by the inspiration of superheated gases (temperatures greater than 150° C), steam, or noxious products of incomplete combustion. Smoke inhalation injury has been reported to affect anywhere from 5% to 35% of hospitalized burn patients.[10,21,23,24] Early consequences of inhalation injury include increased alveolar permeability, acute pulmonary edema, and an accumulation of both pro- and anti-inflammatory cytokines that are indicators for acute lung injury (ALI) or acute respiratory distress syndrome (ARDS).[20,23] The presence of inhalation injury can adversely affect both gas exchange and hemodynamics.[25]

The severity of inhalation injury varies widely and cannot be predicted at the initial evaluation because of the poor correlation between diagnostic criteria and severity of injury, as well as the delayed onset of symptoms. Inhalational injury coupled with thermal injury has a profound effect on mortality: the mortality rate for a person who sustains an inhalation injury with a major burn doubles when compared with the mortality rate predicted based on age and burn size alone.[10]

Inhalational injuries can be divided into the following different phases based on varying pathology and treatment requirements: exudative, degenerative, proliferative, and reparative.[21]It is also important to note the sites affected by the injury: inhalation injury caused at the site as a result of inspiring noxious gases, upper airway heat injury, or lower airway chemical injury. Although there is no specific treatment for inhalation injury, supportive, lung-protective strategies exist for acute lung injury and can be used in management of the injury. Management involves providing the support required to compensate for decrements in gas exchange while the injured endobronchial and alveolar mucosae regenerate.

Smoke inhalation is the most common form of inhalation injury. The components of smoke are determined by the burning material and the availability of oxygen where the fire has taken place. The concentration of smoke inspired depends on the confines of the space where the fire is occurring as well as the duration of exposure. The larynx is one of the most affected organs in inhalation injury, thus resulting in upper airway dysfunction later in the healing process.[26]

Physiology of Inhalation Injury

An inhalation injury involves the entire respiratory system, from the upper airway to the alveoli, to a variable and unpredictable degree. Two properties of the inspired irritant gases are worthwhile in noting the site of damage during inhalation injury: water solubility and chemical reactivity. These two properties will affect where along the airway tract the damage occurs.Water-soluble gases will dissolve into the mucous layer of the upper airway. Gases and other particulates can form concentration gradients throughout the upper and lower airways.[27]

The morbidity of severe burns is increased when accompanied by smoke inhalation because of the stimulation of the inflammatory response and loss of small airway patency.[25,28] It is the presence of these inflammatory mediators that can result in ALI or ARDS evidence derived from animal models demonstrates that it is this systemic inflammatory response that triggers an increase in cell death or apoptosis.[28] The debris from the dead cells and hypersecretion of mucus glands contribute to the small airway occlusion. During the initial phase of the injury, superheated gas and liquid burn the upper airway, with resultant mucosal edema and airway obstruction presenting in later stages, which explains why the severity of an inhalational injury can be misleading during the primary evaluation of the patient.

The pathophysiology of inhalational injury with subsequent smoke inhalation can be divided into two subcategories: upper airway involvement and lower airway involvement.[21]The structures of the upper airway, tongue, and oropharynx, including the larynx, act as a heat sink and absorb a large portion of the heat energy, confining the burns to the upper airway. Smoke and the irritating gases that are inspired along with the heated air can trigger bronchospasm and result in inflammation of the lung parenchyma, releasing histamines and cytokines.[21,25] The major airways are denuded of their normal mucosal layer, which impairs the ciliary transport mechanism until resurfacing occurs.[29] The smaller airways become obstructed with sloughed endobronchial debris and accumulated secretions (**Figure 44–5**).

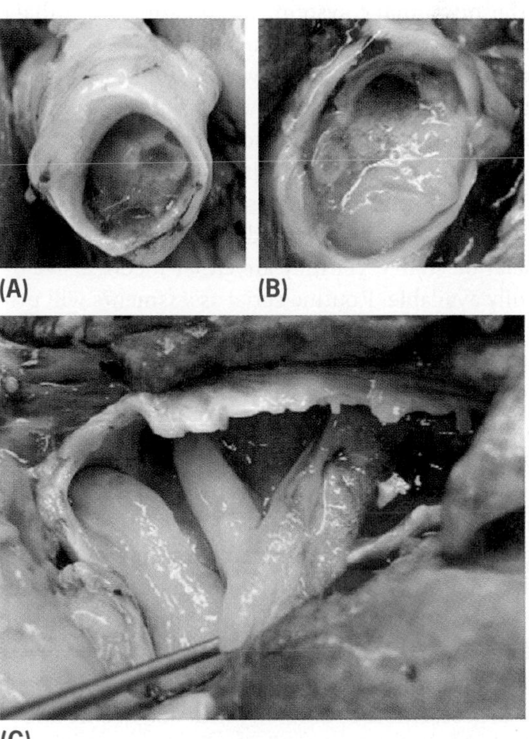

FIGURE 44–5 Macroscopic picture of airway obstructive cast 48 hours after cutaneous burn and smoke inhalation in a sheep. (**A**) Trachea. (**B**) Bronchi. (**C**) Smaller bronchi.

With the mucociliary transport system disrupted, along with the accumulation of cellular debris within the small airways, inhalation injury promotes changes in the lung that favor pneumonia.[30] Pneumonia and tracheobronchitis frequently occur in partially obstructed lung units. The alveolar epithelium is disrupted by toxic products released by the burning of synthetic products, resulting in alveolar flooding.[21,24,25,27] The clinically important sequelae include loss of airway patency secondary to mucosal edema, bronchospasm, intrapulmonary shunting from small airway occlusion, diminished compliance secondary to alveolar flooding and collapse, pneumonia secondary to loss of ciliary clearance, and respiratory failure secondary to a combination of the previously stated factors.

Diagnosis of Inhalation Injury

Numerous proposals have been made to develop a mechanism to aid in the diagnosis and severity scoring of an inhalation injury.[10,20,23,25] This has proved to be a daunting task. Diagnosing inhalation injury is difficult because of the lack of uniformity in the criteria and absence of generally accepted and applied methods for quantifying inhalation injury.[31] Some patients who have an inhalation injury will present with an initial Pao_2/Fio_2 ratio that is relatively benign. It is only after the initial resuscitation and the redistribution of fluids within the tissue that there may be a significant change in the Pao_2/Fio_2.[22]

Because the Pao_2/Fio_2 ratio can be misleading early on in the injury and may not reflect the dysfunction of the pulmonary system, the diagnosis of inhalation injury is based on the clinical presentation of the patient and the circumstances in which the burn injury was obtained.[21,23] Inhalation injury should be suspected if there is evidence of carbonaceous material surrounding the nose and mouth, if the fire was in a closed area, and if there is singed skin or nasal hairs. A limited number of tests have been proposed to aid in the diagnosis of inhalation injury, yet they are either inconclusive or not readily available. Routine serial assessments will provide similar conclusions.

Current methods of diagnosing inhalation injury include the history, physical examination, chest radiograph, bronchoscopy, the Pao_2/Fio_2 ratio, and radioisotope scanning (if available). Because there are no specific preemptive therapies for inhalation injury and because current diagnostic measures only loosely predict the degree of subsequent pulmonary dysfunction, diagnostic tests are used only for general evaluation and prognosis. The underlying difficulty with diagnosis is that, unlike with a cutaneous burn, inhalation injuries evolve over time and involve the entire respiratory system to a variable degree. Another difficulty with diagnosing and grading inhalation injury is the lack of consensus of a grading system for inhalation injury.[31] For these reasons, patients at risk for this diagnosis generally are classified as having or not having sustained inhalation injury, with no effort made to quantify the degree of injury.

Typically, the diagnosis is derived through the history of the burn, physical examination, and bronchoscopic findings. The circumstances surrounding the burn can provide to the burn surgeon clues as to whether an inhalation injury has occurred. Burns sustained in a closed space or aspiration of hot steam or liquid are pertinent points of the history. Physical findings suggesting the diagnosis include carbonaceous debris in the mouth or sputum, singed nasal hairs, and facial burns. The chest radiograph generally is normal initially, which is consistent with the evolution of these injuries over time.

In addition to bronchoscopy, invasive measures sometimes used include radioisotope scanning and determination of the serum carboxyhemoglobin level. Although logistically more complicated in young children, most clinicians use bronchoscopy as the gold standard for diagnosis of inhalation injury. Bronchoscopic findings consistent with this diagnosis include carbonaceous endobronchial debris and mucosal pallor and ulceration (**Figure 44–6**). One study has suggested that inflammatory mediators found in pulmonary secretions can be used to score the extent and severity of the inhalation injury.[20] Two of the findings of this study were surprising: early rise of a specific mediator actually was a positive sign for a positive outcome, and the severity of the injury did not correlate with the level of the cytokines.

Two types of radioisotope imaging have been used to diagnose inhalation injury: intravenous administration of technetium-99 or inhalation administration of xenon-133. Both radioisotopes are rapidly cleared by normal lungs, and asymmetric or delayed clearance is consistent with the diagnosis of inhalation injury. Although physiologically sound, xenon and technetium scanning have not been widely used because of their logistic difficulty and expense.

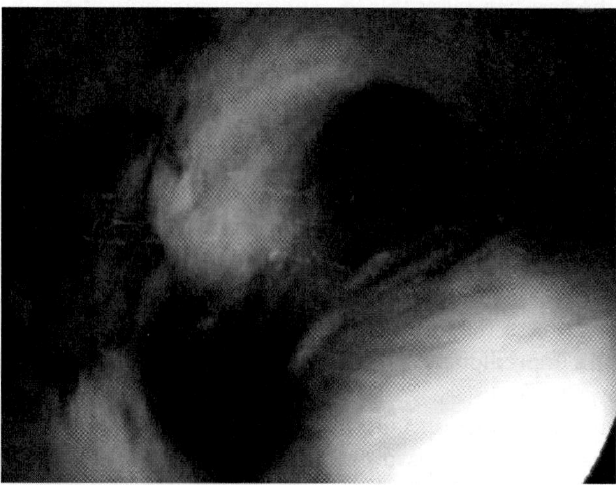

FIGURE 44–6 Bronchoscopic image of airway after sustaining inhalation injury. Note the carbonaceous buildup and inflammation of the airway wall.

In small clinical series, tracheobronchial cytologic studies and biopsy have been reported to facilitate the diagnosis of inhalation injury, but these techniques have not been widely used because of logistic difficulties and potential complications. Work continues in the area of finding biological markers for grading the severity of inhalation injury.[9,20,31]

Management of Inhalation Injury

When a diagnosis of inhalation injury is suspected or confirmed, management is supportive only. Treatment of inhalation injury can be broken down into several categories: ventilator management, pharmacologic treatment to aid pulmonary function using aerosolized medications, early tracheostomy, and using evidence-based medicine to optimize patient outcomes.[23] As noted earlier, there are no prophylactic or preemptive therapies for inhalation injury. There is no clear-cut value in using prophylactic antibiotics, and there is evidence to show that such use would promote selection of antibiotic-resistant strains colonizing the airway. Although many patients demonstrate reactive bronchospasm and benefit from early institution of nebulized β-agonists, steroids are infrequently required to treat acute bronchospasm. The practice of nebulizing heparin alone or along with *N*-acetylcysteine has been studied as a means to prevent or lessen the effects of small airway obstruction resulting from the sloughing of epithelial cells, excessive mucus production, and the formation of fibrin casts in a sheep model.[32,33] This practice has been undertaken by several burn centers, but the supporting evidence is mainly anecdotal.[23,24,32,33] However, it is extremely important to maintain high relative humidity within the ventilator circuit to prevent a humidity deficit of the airways that results in the desiccation of the secretions of the distal airways. Providing good pulmonary hygiene is also crucial.[34] There is no known benefit from prophylactic administration of antibiotics in these patients, and cavalier use of these drugs may select for resistant species.

> **RESPIRATORY RECAP**
>
> **Management of Inhalation Injury**
>
> » Upper airway obstruction should be bypassed with endotracheal intubation or a tracheostomy; careful attention must be given to the endotracheal tube's position and patency.
>
> » Bronchospasm should be treated with inhaled bronchodilators.
>
> » Adequate humidification of the airway needs to be provided to lessen the chances of secretion desiccation.
>
> » Pulmonary infection should be managed with a focus on organisms identified by sputum culture.
>
> » Respiratory failure is managed with positive end-expiratory pressure and low tidal volumes to avoid alveolar overdistension and subsequent ventilator-induced lung injury.

Lung-protective strategies should be used in the ventilator management of these patients. The use of a low-tidal-volume (VT) approach similar to the National Heart, Lung and Blood Institute's ARDSnet protocol is an acceptable method of managing these patients because it keeps ventilating pressures down, which would otherwise add to the already sustained lung injury.[35] Other practices to consider are permissive hypercapnia and prone positioning.[35,36]

In patients with inhalation injury, five predictable events occur that have important clinical implications and require intervention: acute upper airway obstruction, bronchospasm, small airway obstruction, infection, and respiratory failure.

Acute Upper Airway Obstruction

During inhalation injury, airway obstruction caused by mucosal edema evolves over time (usually within the first 4 to 24 hours after injury) and ideally is anticipated and managed with intubation.[24] Early intubation should be considered in the patient with suspected inhalation injury. In general, most intubation attempts of these often-difficult airways can be approached in a studied manner if the impending obstruction is anticipated. After resuscitation has occurred, edema of the upper airway can change the anatomic structures from a relatively easy intubation to a difficult airway requiring a well-experienced anesthesiologist or even a surgical airway. Failure to recognize impending airway obstruction can result in serious morbidity and even mortality in burn patients. Clinicians should be alert in cases involving hot liquid aspiration, which can lead to sudden loss of airway patency early[9] and to the late occurrence of the sequelae of upper airway burns.[10,23,27,37] The critical importance of initial airway evaluation and proper control cannot be overemphasized, and this need continues throughout the period of intubation.

Oral endotracheal tubes are often used because they are easy to place and are subjectively more comfortable for the patient than nasal endotracheal tubes. Tubes should be secured in a manner that allows room for stabilization and easy adjustment as facial edema changes, but not for gross movement of the airway that might risk unintended extubation. Because the lips are not reliable landmarks, placement of the endotracheal tube must be monitored by notation of the centimeter mark at the incisor or gum. It is useful if this information is posted near the head of the bed for quick reference during routine and emergency airway care.

The security of the endotracheal tube should be verified regularly, because reintubation after accidental extubation can be incredibly difficult in burn patients, who commonly have significant facial and oropharyngeal edema. Clinicians who care for these patients should be equipped to deal with sudden airway emergencies and have the appropriate equipment on hand for managing a difficult, unstable airway. Maintenance of endotracheal tubes in burn patients is complicated by shifts in extravascular volume. The method used to secure the tube should facilitate simple loosening and tightening as needed. When facial burns are present, adhesive tape is seldom useful. Cloth ties can be effectively used to secure tubes.

Another aspect of good airway care should be maintaining adequate cuff pressure in the cuff of the airway to prevent or at least minimize leakage and aspiration of trapped material from the oropharynx into the lungs. Maintaining the head of the patient's bed, if physiologically possible, at a 30-degree supine angle will also help minimize silent aspiration and potential ventilator-associated pneumonia (VAP).[34] By following these easy interventions, the incidence of nosocomial pneumonia can be decreased, and this is a population where pulmonary involvement can double the morbidity of the underlying injury.[34]

The proper indication and optimum timing for tracheostomy in the burn patient remains the subject of wide debate. However, the consensus is that adult burn patients in whom protracted intubation is expected are proper candidates, ideally after anterior neck burns have been addressed.

Bronchospasm

Intense bronchospasm from aerosolized irritants is common during the first 24 to 48 hours after injury, especially in young children. This condition is well managed with inhaled β-agonists in most patients, although some require low-dose epinephrine infusions or parenteral or inhaled steroids. Another option would be the use of heliox if the patient's oxygen requirements were minimal. Use of continuous nebulization of high-dose β-agonists is another option.

Ventilatory strategies should be designed to minimize auto-PEEP (positive end-expiratory pressure) in this setting, much as would be done to ventilate a patient with status asthmaticus. Techniques used to minimize auto-PEEP, such as using short inspiratory times and high inspiratory flow rates, as well as attempting to match the auto-PEEP with applied PEEP, often may be necessary, but if air trapping is severe, some degree of carbon dioxide retention is acceptable. Most current-generation critical care ventilators are equipped with graphic displays, and understanding how to interpret these waveforms can aid the practitioner during the treatment of auto-PEEP or demonstrate airway occlusion. Routine monitoring of both the plateau airway pressure (Pplat) and mean airway pressure should be done to assess the patient's gas exchange and transport status.[35]

> **AGE-SPECIFIC ANGLE**
>
> Intense bronchospasm caused by aerosolized irritants is a particular problem in children because of their overall smaller airways.

Small Airway Obstruction

During the first 24 hours after inhalation injury, airway obstruction is essentially limited to the bronchial airways. Major components of this obstructive material are mucus from extensive glandular secretion, inflammatory cells, fibrin, and exfoliated epithelial cells.[24] As necrotic endobronchial debris sloughs, pulmonary hygiene often become increasingly difficult. An aggressive program of pulmonary hygiene, including suctioning and bronchoscopy is an important component of care. Along with aggressive secretion clearance techniques, it is vitally important to provide adequate humidification of inspired gases. Therapeutic bronchoscopy can greatly facilitate clearance of the airways as well as allow the clinician to evaluate the condition of the airway mucosa. Small endotracheal tubes can suddenly become occluded; staff members should be prepared to respond promptly (**Box 44–2**). Vigilant pulmonary hygiene is an essential component of the management of patients with inhalation injury. It is crucial to provide 100% relative humidity to these patients and decrease the potential for humidity deficit that might thicken pulmonary secretions and increase the chances of occluding the endotracheal tube.

The use of mucolytic agents in treating small airway obstruction has been shown not to be as effective as was once believed. The main components of bronchial and small airway casts are fibrin and cellular debris. Use of mucolytic agents has not been shown to be effective in either clinical practice or animal models.[32]

Pulmonary Infection

Pulmonary infection develops in 30% to 50% of patients with inhalation injury. Pneumonia without the presence of inhalation injury increases the mortality of burn injury up to 40%.[38] It frequently is difficult to distinguish between pneumonia and tracheobronchitis (purulent infection of the denuded tracheobronchial tree), but the difference often has little practical clinical importance. Infection typically occurs toward the end of the first postinjury week; patients with serious inhalation injuries often are seen to deteriorate at this time. A patient with newly purulent sputum, fever, and perhaps diminished gas exchange should be treated with antibiotics, which should be focused after sputum culture information has been obtained. To repeat an important point: the physiology of inhalation injury, which involves injury to endobronchial mucosa with hampered mucociliary clearance, makes good pulmonary hygiene a particularly important component of management.

Respiratory Failure

Respiratory failure is not uncommon in individuals with inhalation injury, and its management is discussed elsewhere in this book. Respiratory failure among these patients is caused as often by sepsis as by inhalation injury. As in other forms of respiratory failure, the lung volume that can be recruited with mechanical ventilation is limited, and over vigorous attempts to force high pressures into these lungs exacerbate the underlying injury. These patients do well with a pressure-limited ventilation strategy based on permissive hypercapnia

BOX 44–2

Evaluation and Initial Management of Deterioration of the Patient–Ventilator System

A sudden deterioration of the patient–ventilator unit requires immediate assessment for any of four problems: mechanical malfunction, obstruction of the artificial airway, displacement of the endotracheal tube from the trachea or into the main stem bronchus, or pneumothorax.

1. Assess the patient and observe the patient's inspiratory efforts (if any) and compare them with the cycling of the ventilator. Auscultate breath sounds:
   a. If wheezing, provide β_2-agonists.
   b. If coarse, suction the airway.
   c. If the breath sounds are unilaterally decreased, consider a main stem intubation or pneumothorax.
   d. If the breath sounds are absent bilaterally, consider an occluded artificial airway.
2. Observe the monitors.
   a. Is the patient hemodynamically stable?
   b. Check the Spo_2 and provide maximal inspired oxygen. Remember: In an emergency, oxygen buys time.
3. Check the ventilator.
   a. Determine which alarms are being triggered. Knowing this is helpful in troubleshooting mechanical problems.
   b. Check the ventilator waveforms; look at the flow–time curve to determine whether the patient is receiving adequate flow, or whether the inspiratory time is either too long or too short.
   c. Are the parameters set on the ventilator correct for the patient's needs? If the patient was initially paralyzed and is now able to move and spontaneously trigger the ventilator, it is possible that changes will need to be made.
   d. Is the ventilator functioning as expected? If not, remove the patient from the ventilator, manually ventilate, and exchange with another ventilator.
4. If unable to quickly assess and correct the problem, it may be necessary to disconnect the patient from the ventilator and provide manual breaths with a bag-valve device while troubleshooting the problem. Remember, for patients who require high levels of positive end-expiratory pressure (PEEP), alveolar derecruitment will occur if the patient is manaully ventilated without PEEP.
5. If unable to manually ventilate, the tube may be severely occluded, and extubation followed by mask ventilation may be required.
6. In the event a new airway cannot be passed into the trachea, a surgical airway (cricothyroidotomy, tracheostomy) may be required.

(**Box 44–3**). If this approach fails, innovative methods of support should be considered, such as extracorporeal membrane oxygenation or inhaled nitric oxide. Prone positioning also has been shown to improve oxygenation. In this position the posterior portions of the lungs, which are compressed by the diaphragm and heart, can be recruited through provision of a more uniform pleural pressure gradient. With adequate personnel, the patient can be quickly and safely repositioned while special attention is given to maintenance of the airway and central lines.[34]

Some centers have suggested the use of volumetric diffusive respiration in burn patients. This modality is not readily available in adults in all burn centers, nor has it shown any definitive benefit over more conventional methods of mechanical ventilation. This is essentially pressure-controlled ventilation with a superimposed subtidal oscillation that facilitates clearance of endobronchial debris. Although the initial data have been encouraging, burn patients with inhalation injury and respiratory failure can be very well managed with any mode of ventilation with which the center is comfortable, paying particular attention to volumes, airway pressures, and aggressive pulmonary hygiene.[10,21,23,38]

Ventilator discontinuation and extubation of burn patients follows the general guidelines applicable to other patients. However, this patient group has some unique aspects that must be taken into consideration (**Box 44–4**). Of particular importance is the balance of the pain medication needs of patients with large wounds and donor sites with the need for an alert sensorium for extubation. There is evidence of benefit from combined spontaneous breathing trials along with routine periodic sedation discontinuation in order to assess mental status.[39–41]

BOX 44–3

Therapeutic Responses to Progressive Respiratory Failure

Address bronchospasm with nebulized β_2-agonist agents.
Address poor chest wall compliance that occurs secondary to overlying eschar with escharotomies.
Ensure ventilator synchrony with adequate opiate and benzodiazepine infusions. Neuromuscular blockade occasionally may be required.
Reset end point of ventilation to a physiologic pH (7.2 or higher). Allow gradual onset of hypercapnia as long as the patient does not have a head injury.
Reset end point of oxygenation to an arterial saturation of at least 88%, typically associated with an arterial oxygen content of 55 mm Hg or higher.
Optimize inflating pressures.
Utilize a lung-protective, low-tidal-volume approach to ventilation. Follow ARDSnet guidelines for adjusting tidal volumes based on predicted body weight for the patient.
Keep plateau pressure (Pplat) below 30 cm H_2O.
Choose optimum positive end-expiratory pressure (PEEP).
Choose optimum mean airway pressure. Lengthen inspiratory time to a target mean airway pressure of 20 to 25 cm H_2O, as long as auto-PEEP is not detectable.
If these measures are inadequate, consider the use of innovative adjuncts, such as inhaled nitric oxide or extracorporeal support.

BOX 44–4

Important Considerations in Ventilator Discontinuation and Extubation of a Patient with a Burn Injury

Sensorium: The patient must be awake and alert enough to protect the airway.
Airway patency: Upper airway edema must be resolved to the extent that an air leak is audible around the endotracheal tube (with the cuff deflated if the tube is cuffed) at a moderate inflating pressure (20 to 30 cm H_2O).
Muscle strength: Strength must be adequate for ventilation. An indirect measure of this is a tidal volume of 6 to 10 mL/kg and a maximum inspiratory pressure (PImax) less than −20 cm H_2O.
Compliance: Combined chest wall and lung compliance must be high enough that work of spontaneous breathing is not excessive. Respiratory system compliance should be at least 50 mL/cm H_2O.
Gas exchange: The PaO_2/FIO_2 should be greater than 200 mm Hg.
Spontaneous breathing trial (SBT): The successful completion of an SBT.

Carbon Monoxide Exposure

Many patients injured in structural fires inhale carbon monoxide (CO), and many are obtunded from a combination of CO, anoxia, and hypotension. Carbon monoxide is produced from incomplete combustion, or combustion in a low-oxygen atmosphere. CO binds avidly to heme-containing enzymes, particularly hemoglobin and the cytochrome proteins, which inhibits cellular respiration.[21,42,43] The formation of **carboxyhemoglobin (HbCO)** results in an acute physiologic anemia, much like an isovolemic hemodilution. A HbCO concentration of 50% is physiologically similar to an isovolemic hemodilution to 50% of a baseline hemoglobin level. Moreover, CO causes a leftward shift of the oxyhemoglobin dissociation curve, which decreases oxygen release to the tissue. Therefore, the routine occurrence of unconsciousness at this HbCO level makes it clear that other mechanisms are involved in the pathophysiology of CO injury. It is likely that CO binding to the cytochrome system in the mitochondria, which interferes with oxygen utilization, is more toxic than CO binding to hemoglobin. Many patients with severe CO exposure also have been exposed to cyanide, which is released from burning synthetics. However, the degree of exposure rarely is such that specific treatment is required.

For unknown reasons, 5% to 25% of patients with serious CO exposure have been reported to develop delayed major neurologic sequelae.[42,43] These patients can be managed with 100% isobaric oxygen or with **hyperbaric oxygen (HBO) therapy**. The half-life of HbCO is about 5 hours breathing 21% oxygen at ambient pressure, about 74 minutes breathing 100% oxygen at ambient pressure (range 26–148 min), and less than 30 minutes breathing 100% oxygen at 3 atm. If serious exposure has occurred and is manifested by overt neurologic impairment or a high HbCO level, HBO treatment probably is reasonable if it can be safely administered. With inhalation injury, 100% oxygen should be administered until a safe HbCO level is reached.

> **RESPIRATORY RECAP**
>
> **Carboxyhemoglobinemia**
> - » Measure carboxyhemoglobin (HbCO) with CO-oximetry.
> - » Administer 100% oxygen.
> - » Consider hyperbaric oxygen therapy, particularly in patients with neurologic depression or delayed neurologic sequelae.

With inhalation injury the HbCO level should be measured with **CO-oximetry**. In the presence of HbCO, traditional pulse oximetry is unreliable and potentially misleading. Two-wavelength pulse oximetry does not measure HbCO. The pulse oximeter displays a high oxygen saturation (Spo_2) despite significant HbCO, misleading the clinician to believe that HbCO is not present. New generation multiple wavelength pulse oximeters allow noninvasive measurement of HbCO. Because HbCO does not affect gas exchange in the lungs, a patient with HbCO who is breathing 100% oxygen may have a very high Pao_2 (more than 400 mm Hg) despite a low hemoglobin oxygen saturation as measured by CO-oximetry. The high Pao_2 competes with CO for hemoglobin binding sites, resulting in eventual displacement of CO from the hemoglobin.

HBO therapy has been proposed as a means to improve the prognosis of those who suffer serious CO exposure, but its use remains controversial. On a busy burn service the question of which patient to treat in the hyperbaric chamber commonly arises. Most patients who undergo hyperbaric oxygen therapy are treated in a monoplace hyperbaric chamber (**Figure 44–7**). Treatment regimens vary, but a typical one is 2 or 3 atm for 90 minutes, with two 10-minute air breaks to reduce the incidence of oxygen toxicity seizures. Providing HBO to a patient in a monoplace chamber severely limits access to the patient during treatment, so patients in unstable condition are poor candidates. Other relative contraindications are wheezing or air trapping, which increase the risk of pneumothorax, and high fever, which increases the risk of seizures.[42]

If a patient must be mechanically ventilated during HBO therapy, adequate preparation before the chamber door is closed can prevent most complications. Before the patient is placed in the chamber, the endotracheal tube cuff must be deflated and refilled with an appropriate volume of sterile water; converting to a fluid-filled cuff prevents collapse of the cuff during the compression phase of the treatment. The airway must be well positioned and adequately stabilized because patients who inadvertently awaken during the therapy may attempt self-extubation. For the same reason, patients must be well restrained before HBO treatment regardless of their mental status. They must be evaluated for bronchospasm and aggressively treated with bronchodilators just before treatment. Suctioning of both the lower respiratory tract and the oral pharynx is helpful because this cannot be done while the patient is in the hyperbaric chamber. Prophylactic myringotomies are recommended for unconscious or intubated patients to prevent tympanic membrane rupture.

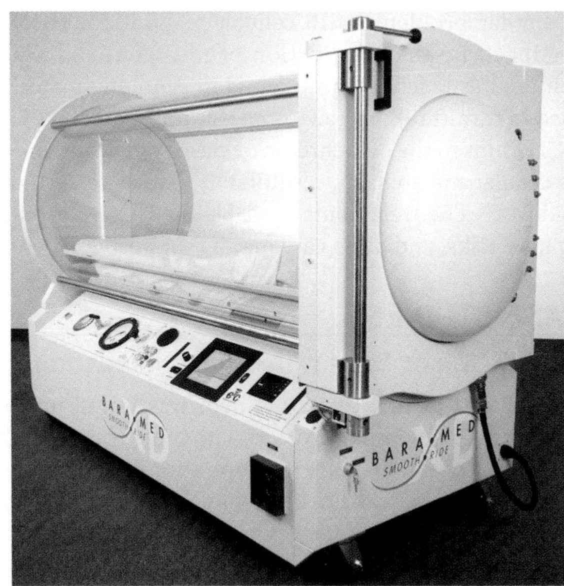

FIGURE 44–7 Monoplace hyperbaric chamber.

Ventilators used with monoplace HBO chambers are modified versions of a pressure-limited, time-cycled device. A base rate is maintained, but all spontaneous breathing efforts are unassisted. Patients who suddenly awaken during therapy and who cough or inspire vigorously can aspirate oral secretions, leading to an increase in airway pressure and a reduction in tidal volume. These same clinical signs occur with other clinical complications, such as a kinked endotracheal tube, mainstem intubation, pneumothorax, or bronchospasm. Assessment and ascertaining the cause are difficult because the clinician is isolated from the patient. It may be best, if clinically appropriate, to adequately sedate the patient and avoid spontaneous breathing during the course of treatment.

Hydrogen Cyanide Poisoning

Although carbon monoxide poisoning is the more common condition to treat with inhalation injury, hydrogen cyanide (HCN) poisoning can be present and can result in similar problems with cellular respiration. HCN is produced by the combustion of nitrogen-containing compounds (such as those found in synthetic materials used in furniture) in a low-oxygen atmosphere. Like CO, HCN binds to the cytochrome oxidase system and inhibits cellular metabolism, resulting in tissue and systemic acidosis.[21] The treatments available for HCN poisoning do have risks, and often care may be supportive.[21]

CASE STUDIES

Case 1. Minor Burn with Smoke Inhalation

A 5-foot 10-inch, 47-year-old man was found unconscious on a smoldering mattress with minor burns to the right arm, chest, and thigh. Respirations were shallow and erratic, pulse was 110 beats/min, blood pressure was 140/90 mm Hg, and there was no apparent cyanosis. The patient could not be aroused and was orally intubated at the scene. He was manually ventilated at an F_{IO_2} of 1.0 and transported to the emergency department.

On admission, the patient was mechanically ventilated with continuous mandatory ventilation, pressure control set at 20 cm H_2O, an inspiratory time of 1 second, a respiratory rate of 12 breaths/min, a PEEP of 5 cm H_2O, and an F_{IO_2} of 1.0. The returned tidal volume was approximately 600 mL (≈8 mL/kg predicted body weight [PBW]). A chest radiograph revealed the endotracheal tube to be 3.5 cm above the carina, with no evidence of pneumothorax or other chest trauma. The patient's pupils were sluggish but reactive. The heart rate and blood pressure remained 110 beats/min and 140/90 mm Hg, respectively. The Sp_{O_2} was 100%.

A toxicology screen was drawn. The arterial blood gas values were as follows: pH, 7.45; Pa_{CO_2}, 34 mm Hg; and Pa_{O_2}, 360 mm Hg. The HbCO level as assessed by CO-oximetry was 38%. Auscultation of the chest revealed mild diffuse bronchospasm, which resolved with administration of albuterol (six puffs via metered dose inhaler [MDI]). There was no evidence of air trapping or auto-PEEP. Because of the patient's depressed level of consciousness and elevated CO level, the decision was made to treat him with HBO.

At the HBO treatment center, the airway was restabilized, the patient's oropharynx and endotracheal tube were suctioned, and an additional four puffs of albuterol via MDI were delivered. The endotracheal cuff was deflated and refilled with the same volume of sterile water to prevent collapse of the cuff during HBO therapy. Bilateral myringotomies were performed to avoid inadvertent rupture of the ear drums. All intravenous fluids and medications were transferred to specialized infusion pumps designed to operate within the HBO chamber. The patient was connected to a specialized HBO mechanical ventilator at the following settings: V_T, 600 mL; respiratory rate, 12 breaths/min; F_{IO_2}, 1.0; and PEEP, 0 cm H_2O. The patient was placed in the HBO monochamber, and the chamber was pressurized to 3 atmospheres absolute (ATA). After approximately 15 minutes at this pressure, the V_T became erratic, and the peak inspiratory pressure increased by 15 cm H_2O. The patient became progressively more awake and attempted to remove the endotracheal tube. Initial attempts to sedate the patient failed, and anesthesia was induced with propofol. The patient was maintained with periodic boluses of propofol for the duration of the treatment, and there were no further complications.

After the HBO treatment, the patient was admitted to the burn intensive care unit (ICU), and all sedation was withdrawn. Assessment of ventilatory mechanics and level of consciousness demonstrated intact ventilatory function and responsiveness to commands. The patient was extubated and observed for 12 hours before being transferred to a non-ICU floor and subsequently discharged.

Case 2. Second- and Third-Degree Burns (70% TBSA) with Severe Inhalation Injury

A 5-foot 6-inch, 67-year-old unconscious woman was rescued from a kitchen fire with severe burns over much of her body. Assessment at the scene found significant facial burns and carbonaceous debris in the upper airway. The respiratory rate was 46 breaths/min and labored. The patient was orally intubated, manually ventilated with 100% oxygen, and transported to the emergency department.

On admission the heart rate was 135 beats/min and the blood pressure was 150/100 mm Hg. There was profound wheezing throughout all lung fields. The patient was mechanically ventilated with volume control ventilation and a V_T of 475 mL (8 mL/kg PBW), a respiratory rate of 16 breaths/min, a descending ramp flow pattern, and peak inspiratory flow adjusted to provide an inspiratory time of 1.0 second (≈50 L/min). PEEP was 5 cm H_2O,and $F_{IO_2}$was 1. The arterial blood gas values with these settings were as follows: pH 7.35, Pa_{CO_2} 66 mm Hg, and Pa_{O_2} 82 mm Hg. The CO level was 27%. Ventilator graphics indicated significant flow present at end-exhalation along with a decreased peak expiratory flow. Total PEEP was measured and found to be 17 cm H_2O (12 cm H_2O of auto-PEEP). Pplat was 31 cm H_2O. Albuterol was administered via nebulizer continuously over the next hour with little effect on the total PEEP.

The ventilator was adjusted to address the significant amount of auto-PEEP present by increasing the amount of applied PEEP to counterbalance auto-PEEP, and V_T was reduced to 415 mL (7 mL/kg PBW). The inspiratory time was kept at 1.0 second to remain in synchrony with the patient's own inspiratory timing. On reassessment the total PEEP was 6 cm H_2O. Although air trapping was reduced, the diffuse bronchospasm remained refractory to aggressive β-agonist therapy. HBO therapy was rejected because of the significant risk of barotrauma. The F_{IO_2} was titrated to maintain an Sp_{O_2} greater than or equal to 88%.

Over the next several days, the patient's arterial blood gas values deteriorated, requiring increases in applied PEEP up to 18 cm H_2O and an FIO_2 between 0.6 and 1. Air trapping continued to be a problem, and ventilator strategies were modified to include permissive hypercapnia. Bronchoscopy was performed several times to facilitate pulmonary hygiene. The bronchoscopy also revealed significant airway injury and edema.

By the fifth day of hospitalization, the patient showed signs of sepsis (increased fever and labile blood pressure) and purulent sputum. Appropriate antibiotic therapy was instituted, and the blood pressure was supported with vasopressors. Oxygenation worsened dramatically on day 6 despite various maneuvers to recruit lung volumes and increase the mean airway pressure. The blood pressure became progressively more unstable until the patient suffered cardiopulmonary arrest. Cardiopulmonary resuscitation was performed but was unsuccessful.

KEY POINTS

- Respiratory failure is a leading cause of morbidity and mortality in the burn unit.
- An organized plan of care for patients with burn injury has four phases: initial evaluation and resuscitation, initial wound excision and biologic closure, definitive wound closure, and rehabilitation.
- Burn wounds should be evaluated for extent, depth, and circumferential components.
- Adequate fluid resuscitation is vital during the first 24 hours after injury.
- Approximately 20% of burn injury patients suffer inhalation injury.
- Five predictable events occur in patients with inhalation injury: acute upper airway obstruction, bronchospasm, small airway obstruction, infection, and respiratory failure.
- All clinicians who care for burn patients should be prepared to deal with airway emergencies.
- Carboxyhemoglobin is treated with 100% oxygen or hyperbaric oxygen therapy, or both.

REFERENCES

1. Hettiaratchy S, Papin R. Initial management of a major burn: I—overview. *BMJ*. 2004;328:1555–1557.
2. Pauldine P, Gibson BR, et al. Considerations in burn critical care. *Contemp Crit Care*. 2008;6(3):1–12.
3. Namias N. Advances in burn care. *Curr Opin Crit Care*. 2007;13:405–410.
4. Meshulam-Derazon S, Nachumovsky S, et al. Prediction of morbidity and mortality on admission to a burn unit. *Plast Reconstr Surg*. 2006;118:116–120.
5. Sheridan R, Barillo D, Herndon D, et al. Burn specialty teams. *J Burn Care Rehabil*. 2005;26:170–173.
6. Allison K, Porter K. Consensus on the prehospital approach to burns patient management. *Emerg Med J*. 2004;21:112–114.
7. Pham TN, Cancio LC, Gibran NS. American Burn Association practice guidelines: burn shock resuscitation. *J Burn Care Res*. 2008;29(1):257–266.
8. Saffle JR, Davis B, et al. Recent outcomes in the treatment of burn injury in the United States: a report from the American Burn Association Patient Registry. *J Burn Care Rehabil*. 1995;16:219–232.
9. Sheridan RL. Airway management and the respiratory care of the burn patient. *Int Anesthesiol Clin*. 2000;38(3):129–145.
10. Endorf FW, Gamelli RL. Inhalation injury, pulmonary perturbations, and fluid resuscitation. *J Burn Care Res*. 2007;28:80–83.
11. Holm C, Melcer B, Hörbrand F, et al. Intrathoracic blood volume as an end point in resuscitation of the severely burned: an observational study of 24 patients. *J Trauma*. 2000;48(4):728–734.
12. Klein MB, Hayden D, et al. The association between fluid administration and outcome following major burn: a multicenter study. *Ann Surg*. 2007;245:622–628.
13. Hettiaratchy S, Papin R. Initial management of a major burn: II—assessment and resuscitation. *BMJ*. 2004;329:101–103.
14. Cartotto RC, Innes M, et al. How well does the Parkland formula estimate actual fluid resuscitation volumes? *J Burn Care Rehabil*. 2002;23:258–265.
15. Saffle JR. The phenomenon of "fluid creep" in burn resuscitation. *J Burn Care Res*. 2007;28:382–395.
16. Neuwalder JM, Sampsono C, et al. A review of computer-aided body surface area determination: SAGE II and EPRI's 3D Burn Vision. *J Burn Care Res*. 2002;23:55–59.
17. Miller SF, Finley RK, et al. Burn size estimate reliability: a study. *J Burn Care Rehabil*. 1991;12:546–559
18. Pappini R. Management of burn injuries of various depths. *BMJ*. 2004;329:158–160.
19. Benson A, Dickson WA, Boyce DE. ABC of wound healing: burns. *BMJ*. 2006:332:649–652.
20. Kurzius-Spencer M, Foster K, et al. Tracheobronchial markers of lung injury in smoke inhalation victims. *J Burn Care Res*. 2008;29:311–318.
21. Fraser JF, Mullany D, et al. Inhalational injury in patients with severe thermal burns. *Contemp Crit Care*. 2007;4(9):1–10.
22. Hammond JS, Ward CG. Transfers from emergency room to burn center: errors in burn size estimate. *J Trauma*. 1987;27(10): 1161–1165.
23. Palmieri TL. Inhalation injury: research progress and needs. *J Burn Care Res*. 2007;28(4):549–554.
24. Cox RA, Mlcak RP, et al. Upper airway mucus deposition in lung tissue of burn trauma victims. *Shock*. 2008;29(3):356–361
25. Brown D, Archer SB, et al. Inhalation injury severity scoring system: a quantitative method. *J Burn Care Rehabil*. 1996;17:552–557.
26. Valdez TA, Desai U, et al. Early laryngeal inhalation injury and its correlation with late sequelae. *Laryngoscope*. 2006;116:283–287.
27. Smith DD. Acute inhalation injury. *Clin Pulm Med*. 1999;6(4): 224–235.
28. Vertrees RA, Nasaon R, et al. Smoke/burn injury-induced respiratory failure elicits apoptosis in ovine lungs and cultured cells, ameliorated with arteriovenous CO_2 removal. *Chest*. 2004;125:1472–1482.
29. Gaissert HA, Lofgren RH, Grillo HC. Upper airway compromise after inhalation injury: complex strictures of the larynx and trachea and their management. *Ann Surgery*. 1993;218(5):672–678.
30. Edelman DA, Khan N, et al. Pneumonia after inhalational injury. *J Burn Care Res*. 2007;28:241–246.
31. Woodson LC. Diagnosis and grading of inhalation injury.*J Burn Care Res*. 2009;30(1)1–3.
32. Holt J, Saffle JR, et al. Use of inhaled heparin/*N*-acetylcysteine in inhalation injury: does it help? *J Burn Care Res*. 2008;29:192–195.
33. Enkhbaatar P, Cox RA, et al. Aerosolized anticoagulants ameliorate acute lung injury in sheep after exposure to burn and smoke inhalation. *Crit Care Med*. 2007;35:2805–2810.

34. Blamoun J, et al. Efficacy of an expanded ventilator bundle for the reduction of ventilator-associated pneumonia in the medical intensive care unit. *Am J Infect Control.* 2009;37(2):172–175.
35. Acute Respiratory Distress Syndrome Network. Ventilation with lower tidal volumes as compared with traditional tidal volumes for acute lung injury and the acute respiratory distress syndrome. *N Engl J Med.* 2000;342:1301–1308.
36. Galiatsou E, et al. Prone position augments recruitment and alveolar overdistention in acute lung injury. *Am J Respir Crit Care Med.* 2006;174:187–197.
37. Liao W, Yeh F, et al. Delayed tracheal stenosis in an inhalation burn patient. *J Trauma.* 2008;64:E37–E40.
38. Freiburg C, Igneri P, et al. Effects of differences in percent total body surface area estimation on fluid resuscitation of transferred burn patients. *J Burn Care Res.* 2007;28:42–48.
39. Sessler CN, Grap MJ, Ramsay MAE. Evaluating and monitoring analgesia and sedation in the intensive care unit. *Crit Care.* 2008;12(suppl 3):S2.
40. Nelson BJ, Weinert CR, Bury CL, et al. Intensive care unit drug use and subsequent quality of life in acute lung injury patients. *Crit Care Med.* 2000;28:3626–3630.
41. Girard TD, Kress JP, Fuchs BD, et al. Efficacy and safety of a paired sedation and ventilator weaning protocol for mechanically ventilated patients in intensive care (Awakening and Breathing Controlled trial): a randomized controlled trial. *Lancet.* 2008; 371:126–134.
42. Weaver LK, Hopkins RO, Chan KJ, et al. Hyperbaric oxygen for acute carbon monoxide poisoning. *N Engl J Med.* 2002;347:1057–1067.
43. Brown KL, Wilson RF, White MT. Carbon monoxide-induced status epilepticus in an adult. *J Burn Care Res.* 2007;28:533–536.

CHAPTER 45

Neuromuscular Dysfunction

Francis C. Cordova
John Mullarkey
Gerard J. Criner

OUTLINE

Overview
Pathophysiology of Neuromuscular Disease on Respiratory Failure
Evaluation of Respiratory Function in Patients with Neuromuscular Disease
Upper Motor Neuron Disorders
Lower Motor Neuron Disorders
Disorders of the Peripheral Nerves
Disorders of the Neuromuscular Junction
Inherited Myopathies
Acquired Inflammatory Myopathies
Treatment of Neuromuscular Dysfunction

OBJECTIVES

1. Discuss the effects of neuromuscular disease on respiratory function during wakefulness and sleep.
2. Discuss the relevance of clinical history, physical examination, and pulmonary function testing in the evaluation of respiratory function in patients with neuromuscular disease.
3. Describe neuromuscular disease associated with upper neuron lesions, lower motor neuron lesions, disorders of peripheral nerves, disorders of the neuromuscular junction, and inherited and acquired myopathies.
4. Discuss the treatment of respiratory dysfunction in patients with neuromuscular disease.
5. Describe the role of respiratory muscle training, assisted coughing, glossopharyngeal breathing, mechanical ventilatory support, and diaphragmatic pacing.

KEY TERMS

acid maltase deficiency
amyotrophic lateral sclerosis (ALS)
Becker muscular dystrophy (BMD)
botulism
Cheyne-Stokes breathing
critical illness polyneuromyopathy (CIPNM)
diaphragmatic pacing
Duchenne muscular dystrophy (DMD)
fascioscapulohumeral muscular dystrophy (FSH)
glossopharyngeal breathing
Guillain-Barré syndrome (GBS)
Lambert-Eaton syndrome (LEMS)
limb-girdle muscular dystrophy
maximum expiratory pressure (MEP or PEmax)
maximum inspiratory pressure (MIP or PImax)
mitochondrial myopathy
mouth occlusion pressure ($P_{0.1}$)
multiple sclerosis (MS)
muscular dystrophy
myasthenia gravis (MG)
myotonic dystrophy
Parkinson disease
postpoliomyelitis syndrome
sniff test
stroke
systemic lupus erythematosus (SLE)
tetraplegia
transdiaphragmatic pressure (Pdi)

INTRODUCTION

The respiratory system can be divided into two functional parts: the lungs, where gas exchange occurs, and the respiratory muscles and rib cage, which act as a vital pump to enable normal gas exchange. Neuromuscular diseases are a diverse group of neurologic disorders that range from primary muscle diseases that impair all skeletal muscle functions to conditions that selectively involve only the diaphragm. The severity of respiratory muscle dysfunction depends on the type of neuromuscular disease, the pattern of respiratory muscle involvement (inspiratory or expiratory muscle), and whether or not effective medical therapies (e.g., plasmapheresis in Guillain-Barré syndrome) are available. The respiratory pump may be impaired at the level of the central nervous system, spinal cord, peripheral nerve, neuromuscular junction, or respiratory muscles. A thorough understanding of the neuroanatomic and pathologic changes brought on by the different neuromuscular disorders is important in the diagnosis and treatment of these diseases. This chapter discusses in detail the etiology, pathophysiology, and treatment of ventilatory dysfunction in the setting of neuromuscular disease.

Overview

Although the list of diseases usually classified under the heading of neuromuscular disorders includes a heterogeneous and pathologically diverse composite of neurologic and muscular diseases (**Table 45–1**), they all commonly lead to a stereotypic clinical course of ineffective cough, recurrent pulmonary infections, and ventilatory insufficiency in advanced disease. Chronic respiratory failure, in association with pulmonary sepsis, is the most common cause of death in these patients.

Some neuromuscular disorders may remain unrecognized by both patients and physicians alike until an intercurrent illness leads to acute respiratory failure. In such cases, neuromuscular dysfunction is only suspected once patients fail to wean from mechanical ventilation. In a study involving 293 chronic ventilator-dependent patients, 17% of patients had an underlying neuromuscular disease as the major factor contributing to the development of respiratory failure.[1] Neuromuscular dysfunction frequently contributes to the need for prolonged mechanical ventilation. Overall, the incidence of neuromuscular disease resulting in prolonged mechanical ventilation has been reported to range from 10% to 25% in various ventilator rehabilitation units across the country.[1]

Pathophysiology of Neuromuscular Disease on Respiratory Function

The changes that occur in ventilation in chronic neuromuscular disorders can best be understood by studying the impact of neuromuscular disease on the respiratory system's different functional components. Neuromuscular diseases can affect the integrity of the respiratory system by affecting its closely interrelated functional parts, such as control of breathing, respiratory muscle function, lung and chest wall mechanics, and upper airway function. In general, the commonly observed changes in respiratory system found in patients with moderately advanced chronic neuromuscular dysfunction are normal or high central respiratory drive (except in certain diseases that affect the brain stem, such as poliomyelitis); a restrictive ventilatory pattern manifested as a reduction in forced vital capacity and an increase in residual volume; a reduction in respiratory muscle strength; and upper airway dysfunction, which may present as upper airway obstruction, recurrent aspiration pneumonia, and obstructive sleep apnea. All of these pathologic changes may present as subtle signs and symptoms during restful breathing, but become magnified during sleep and exercise (**Figure 45–1**).

TABLE 45–1 Levels of Pathologic Injury in Neuromuscular Diseases

Level	Disease
Upper Motor Neuron	
Cerebral	Stroke
Spinal cord	Trauma
Lower Motor Neuron	
Anterior horn cells	Poliomyelitis
	Amyotrophic lateral sclerosis
Peripheral nerves	Phrenic nerve injury
	Diabetes mellitus
	Guillain-Barré syndrome
	Critical illness polyneuropathy
Neuromuscular junction	Myasthenia gravis
	Lambert-Eaton syndrome
	Botulism
	Aminoglycosides
Muscle	Dystrophy
	Acid maltase deficiency
	Corticosteroids
	Acute intensive care myopathy

Control of Breathing

The ventilatory responses to hypoxia and hypercapnia are used to assess the response of the peripheral and central chemoreceptors to chemical stimuli. In normal individuals, the relationship between oxygen saturation and ventilation is linear, such that a fall in oxygen saturation by 1% will trigger an increase of approximately 1 L/min in minute ventilation. A much steeper linear increase in minute ventilation is seen during hypercapnic breathing test. For very 1 mm Hg rise in $Paco_2$, ventilation increases by 2.5 to 3 L/min. The normally predictable increases in ventilation that occur in response to hypoxia and hypercapnia become disturbed in some neuromuscular disorders.

Several studies have shown that patients afflicted with neuromuscular disorders exhibit hypoventilation out of proportion to the severity of the respiratory muscle weakness.[2,3] However, definite conclusions cannot be drawn from these early studies because the ventilatory response to metabolic stress is not considered a good index of central respiratory drive in the presence of respiratory muscle weakness. The blunted ventilatory responses to hypoxic and hypercapnic challenges observed in patients with chronic neuromuscular disease may be related to inability of the respiratory pump to increase the work of breathing in response to increases in respiratory drive due to respiratory muscle weakness. Alternatively, abnormal chest wall and lung mechanics, a defective afferent input from diseased respiratory muscles, upper airway involvement,[4,5] and upper motor neuron disorders[6] may all contribute to hypoventilation in selected neuromuscular disorders. A more accurate test of central respiratory drive that is independent of underlying respiratory mechanics is the **mouth occlusion pressure ($P_{0.1}$)**. $P_{0.1}$ refers to the maximum negative mouth pressure generated during the first 100 milliseconds of inspiration measured during complete airway occlusion. Because $P_{0.1}$ is obtained during early inspiration, a small

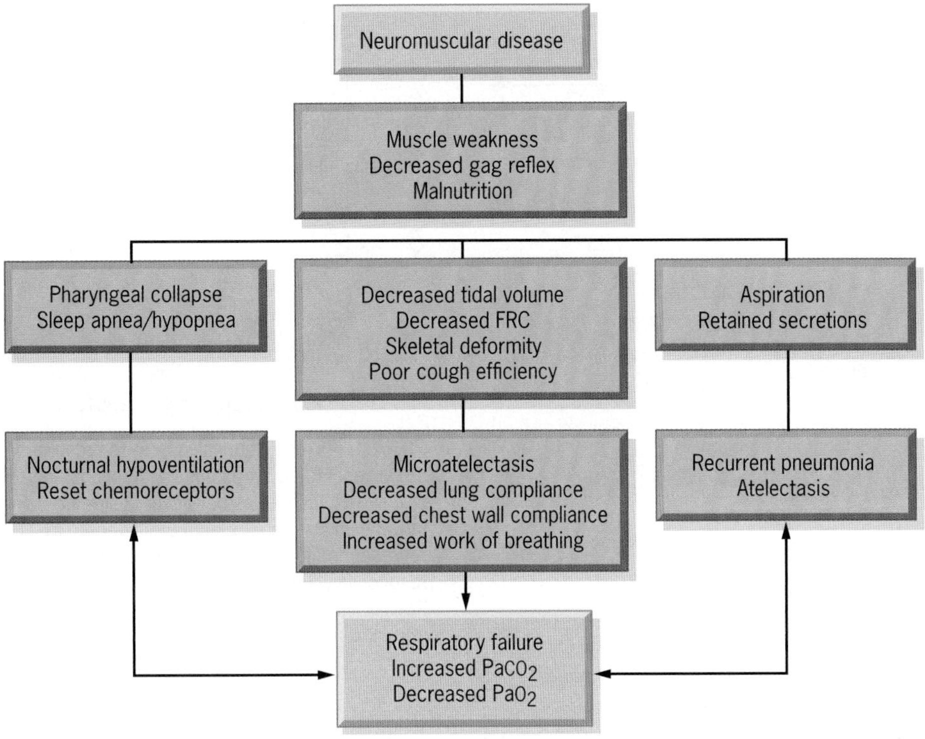

FIGURE 45–1 Pathophysiology of respiratory failure in patients with neuromuscular diseases. Reproduced from Hill NS, Braman S. 1999. Noninvasive ventilation in neuromuscular disease. In: Cherniack NS, Altose MD, Homma I, eds. *Rehabilitation of the Patient with Respiratory Disease*. New York: McGraw-Hill. (© The Mc-Graw-Hill Companies, Inc.)

fraction of total inspiratory time, it is not influenced by volitional effort. In addition, because $P_{0.1}$ requires only a fraction of maximum inspiratory muscle strength, it remains valid even in the presence of moderately severe inspiratory muscle weakness.

In contrast to studies that have used ventilation to assess central respiratory drive, $P_{0.1}$ has been found to be normal, or increased, in patients with neuromuscular diseases despite the presence of substantial muscle weakness. Indeed, several studies have shown that despite significant reductions in respiratory muscle strength, $P_{0.1}$ values in patients with Duchenne muscular dystrophy, myotonic dystrophy, and a variety of other neuromuscular diseases are one- to twofold higher than in normal controls.[7,8] One study found that partial curarization of the spontaneously breathing cat produced a marked increase in phrenic nerve discharge despite a significant decrease in minute ventilation.[9] Similar increases in $P_{0.1}$ were observed in normal human volunteers after severe muscle weakness was induced by curarization.[10] Thus, it appears that central respiratory drive, as measured by $P_{0.1}$, is usually preserved in most patients with underlying neuromuscular diseases.

> **RESPIRATORY RECAP**
>
> **Control of Breathing**
>
> » The central respiratory drive in the brain is sensitive to changes in $PaCO_2$ and PaO_2.
>
> » The mouth occlusion pressure ($P_{0.1}$) is an accurate measure of the central respiratory drive.
>
> » Respiratory drive is preserved in patients with neuromuscular disease.

Respiratory Muscle Function

The respiratory muscles consist of muscles of the upper airway, the diaphragm, chest wall, and abdomen muscles. The respiratory muscles can be further functionally divided into the inspiratory and expiratory muscles. The inspiratory muscles produce rib cage expansion and generate negative intrathoracic pressure, thereby facilitating inspiratory airflow. During rest, exhalation is passive and is driven by the lung and chest wall elastic recoil pressures. However, active contraction of the expiratory muscles occurs under conditions in which increased expiratory airflow is required, such as during coughing, exercise, and airways obstruction. **Table 45–2** lists the innervation of the different respiratory muscles and their major functions.

Patients with moderate to severe respiratory muscle weakness due to neuromuscular disease often complain of fatigue, poor sleep quality, and dyspnea, especially on exertion. However, a significant percentage of these patients may be asymptomatic despite moderate to severe weakness of the inspiratory and expiratory muscles. It has been reported that 27% of the patients with moderately advanced neuromuscular disease who had severe reduction in both the inspiratory

TABLE 45–2 Innervation of the Respiratory Muscles

Muscle Group	Nerve
Upper airway	
Palate, pharynx	Glossopharyngeal, vagus, spinal accessory
Genioglossus	Hypoglossal
Inspiratory	
Diaphragm	Phrenic
Scalenes	Cervical (C4 through C8)
Parasternal intercostals	Intercostal (T1 through T7)
Sternocleidomastoid	Spinal accessory
Lateral external intercostals	Intercostal (T1 through T12)
Expiratory	
Abdominal	Lumbar (T7 through T11)
Internal intercostals	Intercostal (T1 through T12)

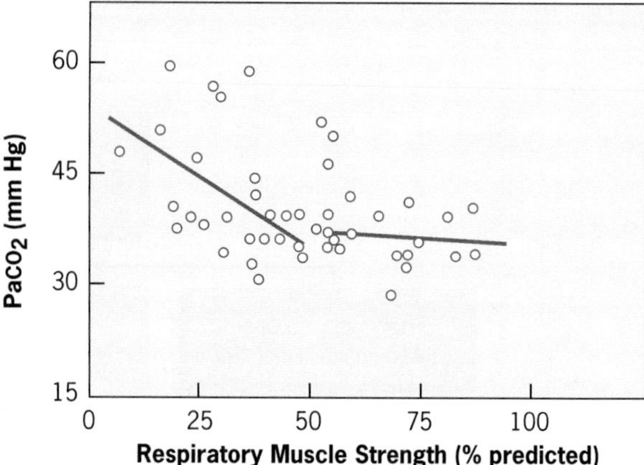

FIGURE 45–2 Relationship between respiratory muscle strength and arterial $PaCO_2$ in patients with myopathies. The data suggest that hypercapnia does not occur until the respiratory muscle strength is less than 30% of predicted. Red and blue circles represent patients with and without concomitant lung disease, respectively. Reproduced from *Thorax*, Braun NMT, Arora NS, Rochester DF, vol. 38, pages 616–623. © 1983, with permission from BMJ Publishing Group Ltd.

and expiratory muscles had no respiratory complaints.[11] Similarly, another study reported that as many as 50% of patients with severe respiratory muscle weakness due to chronic neuromuscular disease were asymptomatic.[12] It is unclear why there is such a poor correlation between the extent of respiratory muscle weakness and clinical symptoms exhibited by patients. It is possible that the presence of significant respiratory muscle weakness is masked by the inability to achieve significant exercise because of generalized muscle weakness that enforces a sedentary lifestyle. Whatever the case, a substantial number of patients may have significant neuromuscular impairment of the respiratory system that may go initially unnoticed.

> **RESPIRATORY RECAP**
>
> **Respiratory Muscle Function**
>
> » Isolated or combined inspiratory, expiratory, and bulbar weakness can be seen in neuromuscular diseases.
>
> » Respiratory muscle weakness can be present in the absence of respiratory muscle weakness.

The particular type of underlying neuromuscular disorder determines the pattern and severity of respiratory muscle weakness. Some diseases cause global respiratory muscle dysfunction, whereas others cause preferential weakness of the inspiratory or expiratory muscles. Moreover, decreases in inspiratory and expiratory muscle strength may not correlate with general muscle strength assessment.[12] Primary muscle diseases (e.g., polymyositis) may cause more significant impairment of the respiratory muscles compared with the neuropathies. The relationship between inspiratory muscle strength and the onset of ventilatory insufficiency is not linear. Once maximum inspiratory mouth pressure decreases to less than 30% of predicted, hypercapnia ensues (**Figure 45–2**).[13] The clinical course of respiratory muscle dysfunction in different neuromuscular diseases may also be varied. It can be relentlessly progressive (amyotrophic lateral sclerosis), reversible with therapy (Guillain-Barré syndrome, myasthenia gravis), or improve with time (critical care polyneuropathy).

Lung and Chest Wall Mechanics

Lung volume studies in patients with chronic respiratory muscle weakness often show a restrictive ventilatory pattern with a reduction in total lung capacity (TLC) and forced vital capacity (FVC). There is a moderate decrease in both inspiratory and expiratory reserve volumes. The decrease in FVC is mainly due to respiratory muscle weakness, and its decrease generally parallels the progression of the underlying neuromuscular disease. However, because of the sigmoidal shape of the pressure–volume curve, vital capacity is relatively well preserved until respiratory muscle weakness is well advanced (**Figure 45–3**). Indeed, the fall in FVC has been shown to be out of proportion to the reduction in inspiratory muscle strength. It has been reported that a reduction in lung compliance of 40% in 25 patients with moderate to severe neuromuscular disease.[14] Additionally, respiratory muscle weakness may also account for a lower vital capacity in these patients. The exact cause or causes of reduced lung compliance in neuromuscular disease patients remain speculative. Several proposed explanations include failed maturation of normal lung tissue in congenital neuromuscular diseases; the presence of micro- or macroatelectasis; an increased alveolar surface tension caused by breathing chronically at low tidal volumes; and an alteration in lung tissue elasticity.

Patients with neuromuscular disease have a rapid, shallow breathing pattern similar to patients with interstitial lung disease. The exact mechanism of this abnormal breathing pattern is unclear but is thought to be secondary to changes in lung and chest wall elastic

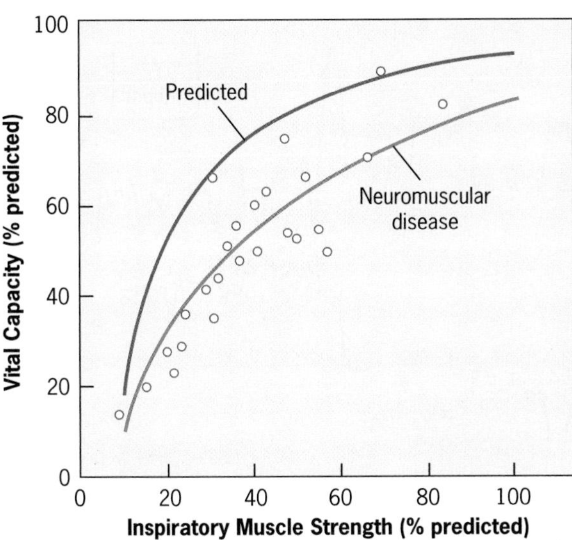

FIGURE 45–3 Relationship between inspiratory muscle strength and vital capacity. The orange line represents the regression line calculated in 25 patients with neuromuscular diseases showing the disproportionate fall in vital capacity for the given degree of inspiratory muscle weakness. The blue line represents the predicted relationship between vital capacity and inspiratory muscle strength. Reproduced from *Thorax*, De Troyer A, Borensteinm S, Cordier R, vol. 35, pages 603–610. © 1980, with permission from BMJ Publishing Group Ltd.

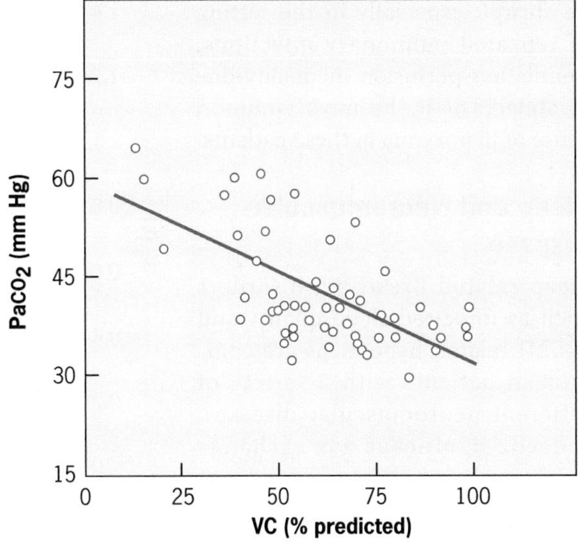

FIGURE 45–4 Relationship between vital capacity and arterial $PaCO_2$, showing that hypercapnia occurs when the vital capacity is less than 50% of predicted. Red and blue circles represent patients with and without concomitant lung disease, respectively. Reproduced from *Thorax*, Braun NMT, Arora NS, Rochester DF, vol. 38, pages 616–623. © 1983, with permission from BMJ Publishing Group Ltd.

recoil. Animal studies have demonstrated that breathing at small tidal volumes is associated with reductions in lung compliance and may lead to increased alveolar surface tension. In addition, the lower ventilatory demand induced by a sedentary lifestyle leads to lower lung mechanical stress and over time may result in a reduction in lung tissue elasticity.

Similar to the changes seen in the lungs, a significant reduction in chest wall compliance has been reported in patients with chronic neuromuscular disease.[15] The mechanisms of the reduction in chest wall compliance are unclear but may be caused by increased rib cage stiffness due to decreased distensibility of chest wall structures (i.e., tendons, ligaments, costovertebral and costosternal articulations). In patients with type 1 spinal muscular atrophy, the relative preservation of diaphragm strength in the face of marked weakness of the intercostals commonly leads to chest wall deformity characterized by sternal recession and a small bell-shaped chest.

> **RESPIRATORY RECAP**
>
> **Respiratory Mechanics**
>
> » Lung volume shows a restrictive pattern due to reduced chest wall and lung compliance.
>
> » The breathing pattern is rapid and shallow.
>
> » The decrease in FVC is relatively attenuated until the respiratory muscle weakness is severe.

Although a low vital capacity is almost always seen in moderately advanced neuromuscular disease, the changes in functional residual capacity (FRC) and residual volume (RV) are variable and depend on the type, severity, and stage of neuromuscular disease. Most studies report FRC to be unchanged or lower.[11] Similar variable findings have been reported for RV.[4] In general, patients with neuromuscular diseases have moderate reductions in TLC and FRC, with a normal RV.

Gas Exchange Abnormalities

Hypercapnia and hypoxemia are late findings in patients with neuromuscular disease. Hypercapnia with a relatively normal FVC and static maximum respiratory pressures should raise the possibility of sleep-related breathing disorders (e.g., obstructive sleep apnea, obesity hypoventilation syndrome), the presence of parenchymal lung disease such as chronic obstructive airway disease, or problems with central respiratory drive such as chronic hypoventilation syndrome or hypothyroidism. Even with normal daytime gas exchange parameters, significant hypoxemia and alveolar hypoventilation may occur during sleep, especially during rapid eye movement (REM) sleep, when the activity of the accessory muscles is diminished. In advanced neuromuscular diseases, evidence of alveolar hypoventilation on blood gas examination is likely when the FVC is less than 55% of predicted (**Figure 45–4**) or when the respiratory muscle strength (average of percent predicted inspiratory and expiratory muscle strength) is less than 30% of normal.[16,24] In addition, hypercapnia is likely if the FVC is less than 1 L. However, the onset of hypercapnia in the setting of advanced neuromuscular disease may be abrupt, especially in the setting of repeated pulmonary infections. Ventilation-perfusion inequality due to atelectasis is the most common cause of hypoxemia in these patients.

Sleep and Neuromuscular Disease

Sleep-related breathing disorders such as impaired sleep quality and (REM) related hypopneas are common in patients with a variety of different neuromuscular diseases. Indeed, significant gas exchange abnormalities may be present and even unsuspected when daytime hypoxemia and hypercapnia are absent. In addition, sleep study usually shows an increased number of awakenings, sleep fragmentation, and disorganization, along with reduced total sleep time.

Several physiologic changes occur in the respiratory system during sleep, especially during REM sleep. Alveolar hypoventilation, causing a 2 to 3 mm Hg rise in Pa_{CO_2}, occurs during sleep in normal individuals. An inhibition of accessory inspiratory muscle activity during REM sleep may lead to a significant reduction in alveolar ventilation in patients with underlying diaphragm weakness.

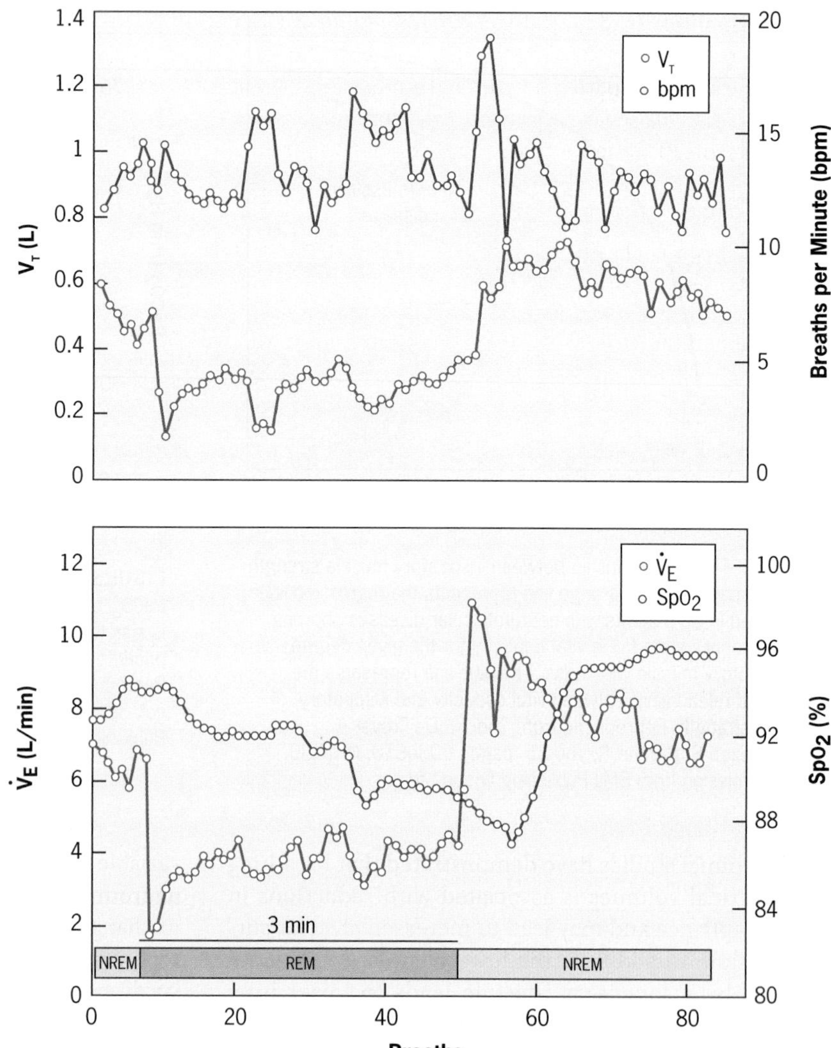

FIGURE 45–5 Both panels show the decrease in tidal volume (V_T) and minute ventilation ($\dot{V}_E$) with no change in respiratory rate during transition from nonrapid eye movement (NREM) sleep to rapid eye movement (REM) sleep. Hypoventilation due to decrease in V_T during REM sleep appears to be the main reason leading to nocturnal oxygen desaturation in patients with limited pulmonary reserve. Modified from Becker H, et al. Breathing during sleep in patients with nocturnal desaturation. *Am J Respir Crit Care Med.* 1999;159:112–118.

Hypoventilation during sleep is the major cause of sleep-related oxygen desaturation. In a study of 26 patients with chronic respiratory failure and nocturnal oxygen desaturation (patients with chronic airways obstruction, obesity hypoventilation, neuromuscular disease), minute ventilation decreased by 21% during non-REM sleep and by 39% during REM sleep compared with wakefulness (**Figure 45–5**).[17] The decrease in minute ventilation was mainly due to a decrease in tidal volume and was found to be independent of the underlying lung disease. Phasic REM sleep–induced changes in breathing pattern superimposed on the rapid, shallow breathing pattern commonly observed in neuromuscular patients will lead to further increases in dead space ventilation, resulting in more profound degrees of hypoxemia and hypercapnia. In addition to these sleep-induced breathing abnormalities, weakness of the pharyngeal muscles in certain neuromuscular diseases may predispose patients to obstructive sleep apnea and hypopnea due to loss of upper airway tone, especially during REM sleep.

If nocturnal hypoventilation is severe and remains clinically unrecognized, daytime hypercapnia and hypoxemia may ensue even in the absence of severe respiratory muscle dysfunction. Nocturnal gas exchange abnormalities usually precede abnormalities in daytime arterial blood gas results.[18–20] Indeed, most patients with normal nocturnal gas exchange are unlikely to have abnormal daytime values.

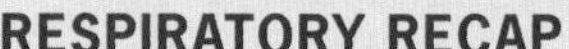

RESPIRATORY RECAP

Gas Exchange Abnormalities

- » Daytime hypercapnia is likely when FVC is less than 55% or respiratory muscle weakness is less than 30%.
- » Hypercapnia is a late sign of respiratory muscle weakness.

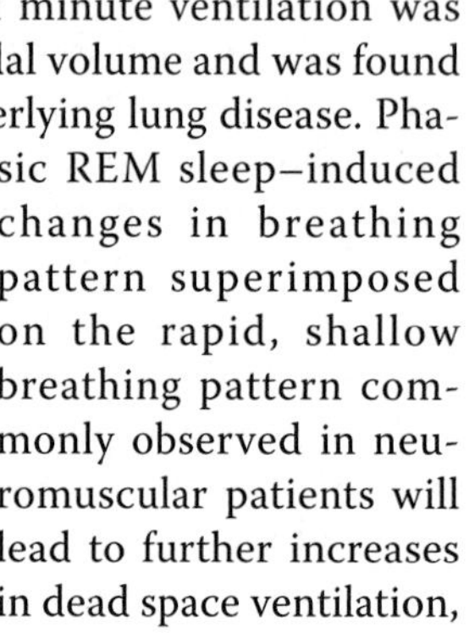

Abnormalities in daytime gas exchange and certain parameters of respiratory mechanics are useful in predicting the subset of patients with neuromuscular disease who are at risk for severe nocturnal oxygen desaturation. In a study of 20 patients with a variety of moderately advanced neuromuscular diseases, it was found that the degree of REM-related oxygen desaturation is directly related to the severity of daytime hypercapnia and hypoxemia.[18] Absolute values for vital capacity, as well as the decrement in vital capacity measured in the supine compared with the seated position, also correlate with the nadir in oxygen saturation measured during REM sleep. The mean decrease in vital capacity measured in the seated compared with supine posture was 21%. In patients with primary myopathies, FVC less than 60% is associated with the development of REM-associated hypopneas. Nocturnal hypopneas occur during REM and non-REM sleep once the vital capacity is less than 40% and the **maximum inspiratory pressure (MIP or Pımax)** is greater than −30 cm H_2O.[19] **Figure 45–6** shows the evolution of respiratory failure in patients with neuromuscular disease.

> **RESPIRATORY RECAP**
>
> **Sleep-Disordered Breathing**
>
> » Nocturnal hypoventilation is common and may herald the onset of daytime hypercapnia.
>
> » FVC less than 40% and maximum inspiratory pressure less than 30 cm H_2O predict REM- and non-REM-associated hypoventilation.

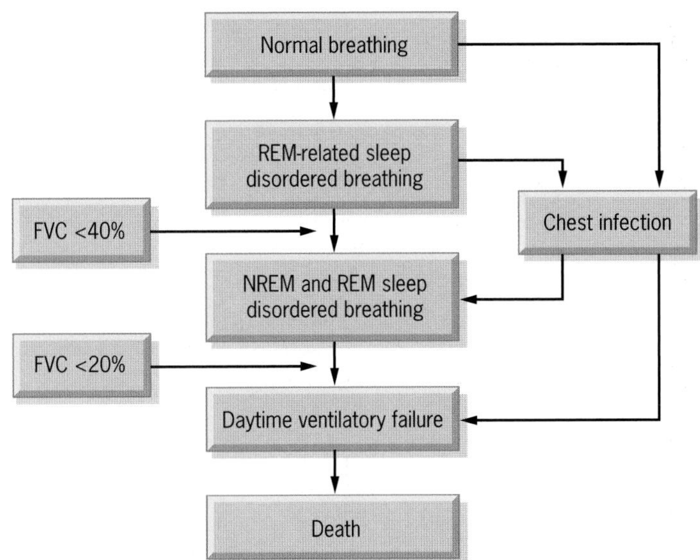

FIGURE 45–6 Respiratory insufficiency in patients with neuromuscular disease is manifested initially as sleep-related breathing disorder during REM sleep and later in NREM sleep. Chronic hypercapnic respiratory failure ensues once forced vital capacity is less than 20% of predicted or in the presence of chest infection. From Simonds AK. Recent advances in respiratory care for neuromuscular disease. *Chest.* 2006;130:1882. Reprinted with permission.

Upper Airway Function

Some neuromuscular diseases involve the bulbar muscles and therefore impair upper airway function. Upper airway dysfunction is commonly manifested by repeated pulmonary aspiration, stridor, obstructive sleep apnea, and hypopnea. In patients with chronic neuromuscular disorders, upper airway dysfunction is more common in those who exhibit respiratory muscle weakness than those patients without such weakness.

The flow–volume loop is a useful screening tool to detect significant upper airway dysfunction. Indeed, an abnormal flow–volume loop has a high sensitivity and specificity in predicting bulbar and upper airway involvement in patients with neuromuscular dysfunction.[5] **Figure 45–7** shows a typical flow–volume loop in a patient with motor neuron disease with bulbar involvement. Sawtoothing of the flow contour can occur in patients with Parkinson disease.[4] In addition, variable extrathoracic obstruction that reverses with drug therapy has been described in patients with myasthenia gravis.[21] Certain features of the flow–volume contour have been shown to correlate with reduced maximum static inspiratory and expiratory mouth pressures: a reduced peak expiratory flow, decreased slope of the ascending limb of the maximum expiratory curve, a drop-off of the

> **RESPIRATORY RECAP**
>
> **Upper Airway Muscles**
>
> » Weakness of the bulbar muscles leads to recurrent aspiration, pneumonia, and upper airway obstruction.
>
> » The flow–volume loop is useful in detecting upper airway obstruction.

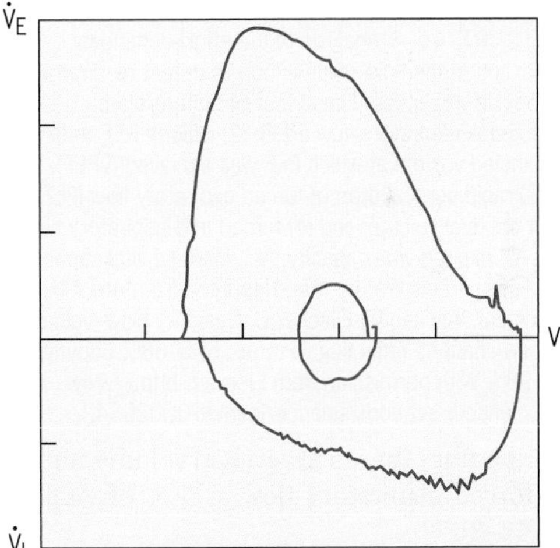

FIGURE 45–7 An example of a flow–volume loop in a patient with motor neuron disease, showing inspiratory flow limitation suggestive of partial upper airway obstruction. Modified from Vincken W, Ellecker G, Cosio M. Detection of upper airway muscle involvement in neuromuscular disorders using flow-volume loop. *Chest.* 1986;90:52–54.

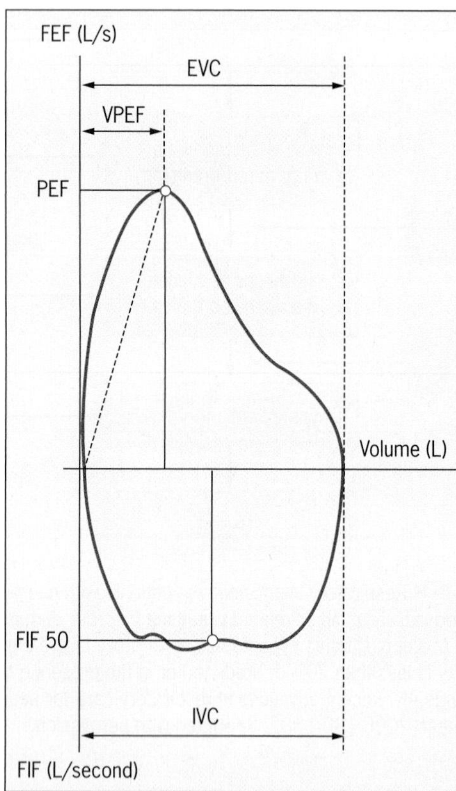

FIGURE 45–8 Analysis of the effort-dependent portion of the flow–volume loop to detect respiratory muscle weakness. These four parameters are (1) peak expiratory flow (PEF); (2) ratio of PEF to the exhaled volume at which PEF was achieved (VPEF); (3) rapid vertical drop of forced expiratory flow (FEF) at residual volume; and (4) forced mid-inspiratory flow. EVC, expired vital capacity; IVC, inspired vital capacity; FIF, forced inspiratory flow. Reprinted from *Am J Med*, vol. 83, Vincken W, Ellecker G, Casio M. Flow–volume loop changes reflecting . . . , pp. 673–680, copyright 1987. With permission from Elsevier. http://www.sciencedirect.com/science/journal/00029343.

forced expiratory flow near residual volume, and a reduction in forced inspiratory flow at 50% of vital capacity (**Figure 45–8**).[5,22]

Evaluation of Respiratory Function in Patients with Neuromuscular Disease

Clinical History

The diagnosis of the etiology of muscle weakness may not be readily made on initial clinical evaluation because of the overlapping syndromes among the different neuromuscular diseases. The predominant signs and symptoms of a particular neuromuscular disease depend on the patient's age at the presentation of the clinical symptoms; the acuity, severity, and clinical course of the disease; and the pattern of neuromuscular weakness. Diseases that predominantly affect the pump function of the respiratory system will present as dyspnea, weak cough, and recurrent respiratory tract infections, whereas diseases that primarily affect the limb muscles will present as impaired patient mobility early in the disease evolution. Once respiratory muscles are affected in advanced neuromuscular disease, respiratory failure may occur abruptly due to an intercurrent illness or slowly over months and years, culminating in chronic hypercapnic respiratory failure. However, in some neuromuscular diseases, a typical presentation will help with the correct diagnosis. For example, an acute ascending paralysis of the lower extremities suggests Guillain-Barré syndrome, waxing and waning of neurologic symptoms is commonly seen in multiple sclerosis, and skeletal muscle weakness with repetitive action of a particular muscle group is highly suspicious of myasthenia gravis unless proven otherwise.

In the majority of the neuromuscular diseases, respiratory muscle weakness usually occurs insidiously and is typically associated with weakness of other skeletal muscle groups. However, up to 50% of patients with significant respiratory muscle weakness may be asymptomatic until they present with overt respiratory failure.[2] Thus, it is no surprise that acute respiratory failure has been reported as the initial presentation in patients with motor neuron disease, myasthenia gravis, and adult-onset acid maltase deficiency, and has also been reported with mitochondrial myopathy. In clinical practice, pulmonary physicians and respiratory therapists are involved in the care of these patients when these patients develop either acute respiratory failure or acute or chronic hypercapnic respiratory failure.

In patients who develop acute respiratory failure, the nature of the neuromuscular disease is often not clinically apparent, and the clinical history is often dominated by the symptoms of the precipitating illness that led to respiratory failure. These patients often require early intubation and mechanical ventilation and appropriate treatment of the precipitating intercurrent illness. In most cases, respiratory muscle weakness due to a neuromuscular disease comes to light only after the patient has failed multiple weaning trials.

> **RESPIRATORY RECAP**
>
> **Acute Respiratory Failure in Neuromuscular Disease**
>
> » Weak cough, inability to clear oral secretions, and failure to wean from mechanical ventilation should prompt neuromuscular disease workup.

In patients who have chronic stable neuromuscular diseases, such as amyotrophic lateral sclerosis (ALS) or congenital myopathies, progressive respiratory muscle weakness occurs over months and years, eventually leading to chronic progressive hypercapnic respiratory failure. The challenge to both respiratory physicians and therapists is to detect early signs of respiratory muscle weakness before the onset of fulminant respiratory failure and to prevent complications such as aspiration, recurrent respiratory tract infections, and cor pulmonale as well as to preserve remaining lung function. Some studies have shown that early institution of noninvasive positive pressure ventilation may attenuate the decline in respiratory muscle function in certain diseases.[23] The common symptoms of respiratory muscle weakness are dyspnea (especially with activity), inability to clear secretions, and weak cough; frequent respiratory tract infections and choking episodes are often elicited several months before these patients seek medical attention. The presence of chronic headache, lethargy, and somnolence suggests significant daytime and nocturnal hypercapnia. As previously discussed, nocturnal hypercapnia usually heralds the onset of chronic respiratory failure.

Physical Examination

A thorough physical examination and a detailed neurologic assessment may reveal a previously undiagnosed neuromuscular disorder. This is particularly true in patients who have mild respiratory muscle weakness but develop acute respiratory failure due to increased ventilatory demand from an acute illness such as an infection. In patients with early or mild neuromuscular weakness, respiratory muscle weakness may not be detected on routine physical examination. Limb muscle weakness is often only recognized after the patient fails multiple weaning attempts. Nevertheless, certain physical examination findings indicate significant respiratory muscle weakness. Tachypnea at rest is very common with the onset of respiratory muscle weakness. As the respiratory muscle weakness progresses, the increase in respiratory rate may be followed by signs of high respiratory workload such as nasal flaring, recruitment of the accessory muscles, and intercostal as well as subcostal retractions. Further progressive weakness of the respiratory muscles will eventually lead to paradoxical inward motion of the rib cage and outward displacement of the abdomen during inspiration. Abnormal paradoxical motion of the rib cage and abdomen may indicate either impending respiratory failure or diaphragm weakness. Indeed, paradoxical inward movement of the abdomen on inspiration that worsens with recumbent position is typically seen in diaphragm weakness.

> **RESPIRATORY RECAP**
>
> **Signs of Respiratory Muscle Weakness**
>
> » Subcostal retraction is a sign of diaphragm weakness and heralds impending respiratory failure.
>
> » Tachypnea and use of the respiratory accessory muscles at rest are signs of respiratory muscle weakness.

Arterial Blood Gas Measurements

Abnormalities in arterial blood gas values occur late in patients with severe respiratory muscle weakness and should not be relied on before ventilatory support is initiated. Hypoxemia is commonly the result of microatelectasis due to ineffective cough and retained secretions causing ventilation-perfusion mismatch or intrapulmonary shunting. More important, alveolar hypoventilation due to respiratory muscle weakness or decreased central respiratory drive may also contribute significantly to hypoxemia. Hypoxemia due mainly to alveolar hypoventilation may be detected by a normal alveolar–arterial oxygen gradient. Pulse oximetry, which is a measure of arterial oxyhemoglobin saturation, is useful in detecting hypoxemia but is an insensitive indicator of hypoventilation.

> **RESPIRATORY RECAP**
>
> **Gas Exchange**
>
> » Hypoxemia is caused by retained secretions and atelectasis.
>
> » Hypercarbia is caused by alveolar hypoventilation.

Hypercarbia is a late finding in severe respiratory muscle weakness. In fact, hypercarbia does not occur until the respiratory muscle strength is less than 50% of predicted. Careful analysis of the pH and bicarbonate level is helpful in detecting the presence of acute or chronic hypercapnic respiratory failure. Sleep-induced breathing disturbances may also lead to hypercarbia, as previously discussed, and should be carefully studied in susceptible patients.

Pulmonary Function Tests

Spirometry and lung volume studies are helpful in the initial evaluation as well as in the follow-up of patients with neuromuscular disease. In general, spirometry produces a restrictive pattern characterized by a reduction in FVC and a normal ratio of forced expiratory volume in 1 second to forced vital capacity (FEV_1/FVC). Moreover, there is a decrease in effort-dependent expiratory flow, such as peak expiratory airflow measurement, whereas FEV_1 and measurement of midexpiratory flow rates ($FEF_{25-75\%}$ or FEF_{50}) are often greater than normal predicted values in these patients because of decreased lung compliance resulting in increased lung elastic recoil. Lung volume studies demonstrate a low total lung capacity but a high residual volume due to expiratory muscle weakness. The diffusion capacity is usually normal.

Serial measurement of FVC is helpful in following the progression of respiratory muscle weakness in patients with chronic neuromuscular disease and in the timing of institution of noninvasive positive pressure ventilation. In patients with rapidly progressive respiratory muscle weakness such as seen in Guillain-Barré syndrome, daily measurement of FVC (<10 mL/kg or <1 L) helps in decisions regarding elective airway intubation and mechanical ventilation. Alternatively, FVC can be used as one of the criteria for the initiation of weaning trials and liberation from mechanical ventilation.

Upper airway dysfunction, commonly seen in chronic neuromuscular diseases, may be detected easily by

RESPIRATORY RECAP

Spirometry

» FVC is the most important indicator of disease progression and need for ventilator support.

analyzing the flow–volume loop. For example, an inspiratory plateau of the flow waveform is indicative of extrathoracic upper airway obstruction. In patients with Parkinson disease, instability of the upper airway muscles is reflected in sawtoothing of the contour of the flow–volume loop. An abnormal flow–volume loop in patients with neuromuscular disease is both highly sensitive and specific for predicting bulbar dysfunction in these patients.[5]

Radiographic Assessment

In patients with inspiratory muscle weakness, lung volume appears small on chest radiograph because of an elevated bilateral hemidiaphragm. This radiographic picture can be easily dismissed as a poor inspiratory film. The presence of bilateral basal bandlike atelectasis is suggestive of chronic loss of lung volume due to weak respiratory muscles. Unilateral hemidiaphragm paralysis can be easily recognized on routine chest radiograph as an elevated hemidiaphragm on the one side. The elevation of a hemidiaphragm due to paralysis can be confirmed by performing a **sniff test** under fluoroscopy, which may demonstrate a paradoxical upward movement of the affected hemidiaphragm during a rapid sniff maneuver.

RESPIRATORY RECAP

Chest Radiography

» Chest radiograph typically shows small lung volume and basilar atelectasis.

Assessment of Respiratory Muscle Function

Maximum Mouth Pressures

Maximum static respiratory pressures, measured at the airway opening during a voluntary contraction against an occluded airway, are the most sensitive tests to assess respiratory muscle dysfunction in patients with moderately advanced neuromuscular disease even in the absence of symptoms and normal ventilatory function.[11] The extent of respiratory muscle weakness can be quantified by measuring PImax and **maximum expiratory pressure** (MEP or PEmax) that can be generated by the respiratory muscles. Measurement of static mouth pressures is affected by lung volume. PImax is greatest when measured near residual volume, when the inspiratory muscles are at their optimum precontraction operating length. In contrast, PEmax is greatest when measured near total lung capacity, when the inward recoil of the respiratory system and the ability of the expiratory muscles to generate force are greatest. **Table 45–3** shows normal values for maximum static inspiratory and expiratory muscle strength in adults. Reported values vary widely in different studies and may be due to differences in the techniques used or to repeated measurements inducing a learning effect.

In chronic neuromuscular disease, PImax and PEmax are frequently decreased and range from 37% to 52% of normal.[7,16] In one study of 16 patients with a variety of chronic neuromuscular diseases, the mean static inspiratory pressure measured with an esophageal balloon was 43% of predicted.[15,24] In patients with proximal myopathies, hypercapnic respiratory failure was likely when the average PImax and PEmax values were less than 30% of predicted or vital capacity was less than 55% of predicted.[24] A reduction in PImax and PEmax may also be seen in patients with only mild generalized nonrespiratory muscle weakness. In a study of 30 patients with stable chronic neuromuscular weakness, up to 30% of patients with relatively preserved general muscle strength had unsuspected severe respiratory muscle weakness (less than 50% predicted).[22] Measurement of PImax and PEmax should be routine in the assessment of respiratory status in patients with neuromuscular disease regardless of the severity of the underlying neurologic disease or absence of respiratory symptoms.

TABLE 45–3 Selected Normal Maximum Static Airway Pressure Values in Adults

Study	Sex	PImax (cm H_2O)	PEmax (cm H_2O)
Black LF, Hyatt RE. Maximal static respiratory pressures in generalized neuromuscular disease. *Am Rev Respir Dis.* 1971;103:641–649.	Male Female	124±22 87±16	233±42 152±27
Braun NMT, Arora NS, Rochester DF. Respiratory muscle and pulmonary function in polymyosities and other proximal myopathies. *Thorax.* 1983;38:616–623.	Male Female	127±28 91±25	216±41 138±39
Vincken W, Ghezzo H, Cosio MG. Maximal static respiratory pressures in adults: normal values and their relationship to determinants of respiratory function. *Bull Eur Physiopathol Respir.* 1987;23(5):435–439.	Male Female	105±25 71±23	140±38 89±24

PImax, maximum inspiratory pressure; PEmax, maximum expiratory pressure.

FVC is also a useful index of global respiratory muscle function. Moreover, it is easy to measure and can be done serially at the bedside to predict impending respiratory failure and the need for ventilatory support. Ventilatory support is often required once FVC is less than 10 to 15 mL/kg or the PImax is greater than –20 to –25 cm H_2O. Mechanical ventilation may be required in select patients above these threshold values in the presence of additional respiratory loads such as occur with pneumonia, atelectasis, or inability to clear secretions. Although measurements of PImax, PEmax, or FVC are useful in quantifying global respiratory muscle strength, they do not distinguish selective weakness of certain respiratory muscle groups.

Maximum Voluntary Ventilation

Maximum voluntary ventilation (MVV) is a commonly performed maneuver in which the subject is asked to breathe in and out as deeply and as fast as he or she can in 15 to 30 seconds. It is a reflection of the global integrity of the respiratory system as a whole. Thus, MVV decreases with loss of coordination of the respiratory muscles, deformity of the thoracic bellow, neurologic diseases, deconditioning, and ventilatory defects. The MVV is a useful test to assess respiratory muscle endurance. However, the MVV maneuver is dangerous in patients with myasthenia gravis because it may precipitate acute respiratory failure.

Transdiaphragmatic Pressure Measurement

In contrast to maximum static pressures, which measure global respiratory function, **transdiaphragmatic pressure (Pdi)** specifically measures diaphragm strength. Although transdiaphragmatic pressure measurement is invasive and is not readily available in clinical practice, it may be useful in certain clinical conditions such as phrenic nerve paralysis following cardiac surgery, or in cases of idiopathic diaphragm paralysis.

Measurement of diaphragm strength is made by measuring esophageal (Pes) and gastric (Pga) pressures via balloon-tipped catheters placed in the mid-esophagus and in the stomach, respectively. Pdi is then calculated as Pga minus Pes. Several maneuvers with varying degree of difficulty have been used during the measurement of Pdi to obtain maximal voluntary activation of the diaphragm. Pdi obtained during a maximal sniff maneuver (Pdi_{sniff}) is the easiest to perform, whereas Pdi_{max} obtained via a Mueller maneuver combined with active expulsion appears to be the most reproducible and maximal maneuver to measure transdiaphragmatic pressure.[4] Transdiaphragmatic pressure measurement is limited by the need for esophageal and gastric balloon placement, and there is a large variation in measured values (as high as 40%) even in normal individuals. The wide intrasubject variability of Pdi is due to submaximal efforts or activation of the intercostal and accessory muscles, which results in falsely low Pdi values. Direct stimulation of the phrenic nerve, by consistently obtaining maximal stimulation of the diaphragm, avoids variability in measured Pdi when only volitional effort is used.

The phrenic nerve is easily stimulated in the neck as it traverses the posterior border of the sternocleidomastoid muscle at the level of the cricoid cartilage. Phrenic nerve stimulation may be performed with either a transcutaneous electrode or a magnetic coil.[25] Care should be taken to ensure supramaximal stimulation as indicated by maximum diaphragm muscle action potential.

> **RESPIRATORY RECAP**
>
> **Assessment of Respiratory Muscle Function**
>
> » Maximum inspiratory and expiratory pressures, maximum voluntary ventilation, and FVC should be assessed.
>
> » Transdiaphragmatic pressures measure diaphragm muscle strength.
>
> » Serial FVC, PImax, and PEmax measurements are useful in predicting impending respiratory failure.

A single, unfused twitch contraction of the diaphragm following electrophrenic stimulation is known as Pdi_{twitch}. Pdi_{twitch} is not widely used clinically because of the invasiveness of the procedure and the large coefficient of variation reported in some studies measuring Pdi during volitional efforts. In a study involving 10 patients with diaphragm weakness and 20 normal subjects as controls, there was a large overlap in Pdi_{twitch} between patients with diaphragm weakness (3–27 cm H_2O) and control subjects (9–33 cm H_2O).[26] The Pdi_{twitch} was only consistently decreased when diaphragm weakness was severe. The appropriate role of electrophrenic stimulation in the assessment of respiratory muscle weakness is unclear; currently, it is considered a research tool until further information becomes available.

Upper Motor Neuron Disorders

Stroke

Stroke following an embolic or thrombotic vascular event is one of the major causes of morbidity and mortality in developed countries. Due to the neuroanatomic and functional organization of the brain, different stroke syndromes have a predictable effect on the respiratory system that can be clinically recognized. For example, an acute hemispheric stroke may lead to loss of upper airway function and Cheyne-Stokes breathing, whereas a small stroke in the dorsolateral area of the medulla will lead to sudden death due to respiratory arrest. The pulmonary consequences of the different stroke syndromes include loss of upper airway function, abnormal breathing patterns, decreased diaphragmatic excursion, and loss of automatic or voluntary control of breathing.

> **RESPIRATORY RECAP**
>
> **Stroke**
>
> » Cheyne-Stokes breathing is seen in cortical stroke.
>
> » Swallowing incoordination due to upper airway dysfunction is common.

Upper airway dysfunction resulting in swallowing dyscoordination is a common finding following stroke. This frequently leads to aspiration of oropharyngeal contents, resulting in aspiration pneumonia. Different abnormal breathing patterns may be observed following an acute hemispheric stroke or in rostrocaudal loss of brain stem function, as in brain herniation due to elevated intracerebral pressure. Hemispheric stroke often results in **Cheyne-Stokes breathing**, which is a breathing pattern characteristically described as cyclical hyperpnea and hypopnea often terminating in apnea. Cheyne-Stokes breathing is thought to be due to increased responsiveness to carbon dioxide as a result of interruption of normal cortical inhibition. Brain stem stroke located in the midbrain may lead to central neurogenic hyperventilation, whereas apneustic and ataxic breathing may be seen following injury to the pontomedullary area of the brain stem. After an acute hemispheric stroke, voluntary contraction of the respiratory muscles is reduced on the side of hemiparesis as shown by electromyographic (EMG) activity of the diaphragm and intercostal muscles.

Respiration is under both voluntary and automatic control. The loss of automatic control of respiration (Ondine's curse) occurs following injury to the descending reticulospinal tract in the pons or the nucleus of the vagus, ambiguus, and para-ambiguus. The most common stroke syndrome associated with Ondine's curse is unilateral lateromedullary infarction.[27] A midpontine lesion, which results in the locked-in syndrome, may lead to a loss in the voluntary control of breathing.

Spinal Cord Injury

The degree of respiratory impairment and the need for chronic ventilator support depend on the level and extent of the spinal cord injury. Following traumatic injury to the spinal cord, paresis or paralysis can be easily elicited at or below the level of spinal injury. High cervical cord injury above the origin of the phrenic nerve (C1 through C3) leads to paralysis of all the major respiratory muscles except the accessory and bulbar muscles. All patients with high cervical injury invariably require chronic ventilator support. Injury at the level of the phrenic nerve roots (C3 through C5) results in weakness or total paralysis of the diaphragm, requiring continuous ventilatory support. Lower cervical cord injury below the origin of the phrenic nerve (C5 through C6) causes paralysis of the intercostal and abdominal muscles, but because diaphragm function remains intact, the need for long-term ventilator support is obviated. However, these patients often require ventilatory support in the acute setting. Thus, the requirement for chronic ventilatory support depends on the level of spinal injury, the ability of the accessory muscles to support ventilation, and the response to strengthening deconditioned muscles.

> **RESPIRATORY RECAP**
>
> **Spinal Cord Injury**
>
> » High cervical injury or injury of the phrenic nerve roots (C3 through C5) requires chronic respiratory support.
>
> » Low cervical injury leads to ineffective cough and atelectasis.

The effect of the level of spinal cord injury on the mechanical properties of the respiratory system is the same as previously described in patients with chronic neuromuscular disease. Among the changes that may be seen on the respiratory system are a reduction in inspiratory muscle strength to 60% of predicted; a 20% to 30% reduction in both lung and chest wall compliance; and a 50% to 80% reduction in predicted vital capacity, with total lung capacity also moderately reduced.[28] The reduction in lung and chest wall compliance can be observed as early as the first week of injury and usually reaches its nadir by the first month after injury.[28] The reduction in lung compliance may be partly explained by the presence of small lung volumes due to airway closure and atelectasis. On the other hand, the reduction in chest wall compliance is thought to be due to stiffness and ankylosis of the rib cage due to a rapid, shallow breathing pattern and limited chest wall excursion.

In patients with **tetraplegia**, there is a paradoxical increase in FVC measured in the supine compared with the seated position that occurs without a significant increase in total lung capacity. The increase in FVC observed during the supine position is due to cephalad displacement of the end-expiratory position of the diaphragm as a result of gravitational effects on the abdominal visceral organs. The overall effect of these changes is to enable the diaphragm to operate on an optimal portion of its length–tension curve. Alternatively, the increase in FVC in the supine position may be due to a decrease in residual volume since total lung capacity is slightly decreased or unchanged. It has been shown that RV decreases in the supine position by 30% to 38% of seated values in both tetraplegics and paraplegics.[29] They showed that the decrease in RV was due to paralysis of the abdominal muscles and the effect of gravity on the abdominal contents. They further showed that the decrease in RV was not related to an abnormal increase in intrathoracic blood volume as a result of gravitationally induced fluid shifts.

> **RESPIRATORY RECAP**
>
> **Tetraplegia**
>
> » FVC increases in the supine position in patients with tetraplegia because the diaphragm is at its optimal operating length.
>
> » In low cervical injury, training of the clavicular portion of the pectoralis major muscle may improve cough in some patients.

In tetraplegic patients with relatively intact diaphragm function, paradoxical inward motion of the upper rib cage during inspiration occurs due to parasternal and scalene muscle weakness. This abnormal pattern of breathing is even more marked in the supine position than when the subject is seated. In high tetraplegic patients (above C3 through C5), short periods of spontaneous respiration are possible because of contraction of the sternocleidomastoid and trapezius muscles. Analysis of rib cage motion in these patients shows an increase in upper rib cage diameter due to the action of the neck accessory muscles in pulling the sternum cranially and expanding the upper rib cage.

It was previously believed that all of the expiratory muscles were paralyzed in low cervical cord injury. As a result, both cough and other expiratory maneuvers would be passive and solely rely on chest wall elastic recoil. An ineffective cough leads to mucus retention, atelectasis, and pneumonia.[30] Indeed, pneumonia is still the leading cause of death in this subset of neurologically impaired patients.[31] EMG activity of the clavicular portion of the pectoralis major is present during voluntary expiration and cough in patients with traumatic low cervical cord injury.[32] Contraction of the clavicular portion of the pectoralis major decreases upper rib cage diameter during cough and could decrease expiratory reserve volume by 60% with the shoulders maintained in abduction. These findings suggest that an active cough can be generated by the clavicular portion of the pectoralis muscles in some tetraplegic patients. The authors concluded that abdominal binding with nonelastic straps to minimize dissipation of intrathoracic forces and training of the clavicular portion of the pectoralis muscle could further improve the effectiveness of cough in tetraplegic patients. Furthermore, 6 weeks of isometric training of the pectoralis muscle increases maximum pectoralis muscle isometric strength and thereby improves cough effectiveness.[33]

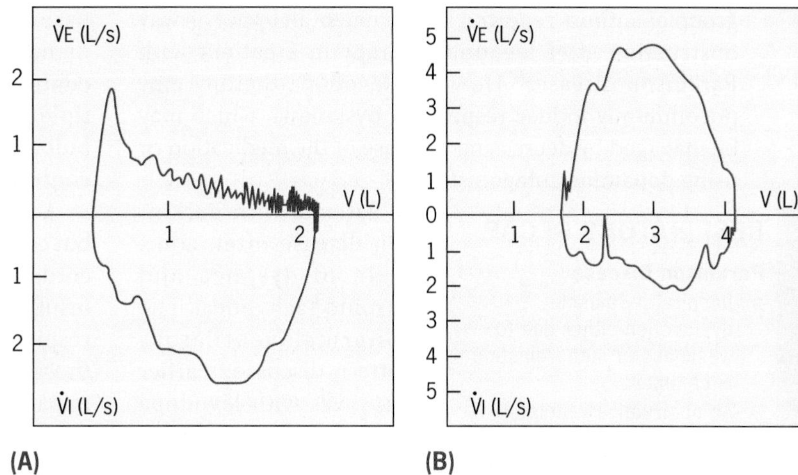

FIGURE 45-9 Two types of abnormal flow–volume loop in patients with extrapyramidal disorders. **(A)** Type A flow–volume loop is characterized by respiratory flutter, a regular consecutive flow deceleration and acceleration representing alternating abduction and adduction of the glottic opening. **(B)** Type B flow–volume loop is characterized by grossly abnormal pattern with abrupt changes in flow indicating intermittent upper airway obstruction due to irregular jerky movements of the glottic structures. V̇E, expiratory flow; V̇I, inspiratory flow. Adapted from Vincken WG, et al. Involvement of upper airway muscles in extrapyramidal disorders: a cause of airflow limitation. *N Engl J Med.* 1984;311:438–442.

Parkinson Disease

Parkinson disease was first described by James Parkinson in 1817 as a symptom complex of cogwheel rigidity, resting tremors, bradykinesia, shuffling gait, and postural instability. The disease affects about 1% of the population older than 50 years and has a disease prevalence of 200 cases per 100,000 individuals. Parkinsonism may be categorized as primary (i.e., idiopathic) or secondary due a variety of causes such as viral encephalitis and drugs. However, the pathologic findings in primary and secondary parkinsonism are the same and are characterized by the degeneration of pigmented neurons in the substantia nigra, resulting in disruptions of dopaminergic neural pathways.

Ventilatory failure, upper airway obstruction, and aspiration can complicate the clinical course of patients with Parkinson disease. In fact, respiratory infection is the most common cause of death in these patients. Both obstructive and restrictive ventilatory patterns have been noted on pulmonary function testing, with about one-third of patients with Parkinson disease having an obstructive ventilatory defect. Both peak inspiratory and expiratory flows are reduced, which may be related to upper airway dysfunction. A concomitant restrictive ventilatory defect appears to be due to weakness and stiffness of the respiratory muscles.

Respiratory muscle dysfunction is common in patients with Parkinson disease.[34] This is usually manifested as either a decrease in respiratory muscle strength or poor coordination, especially when performing repetitive ventilatory tasks similar to what is observed in the limb muscles. Both maximum static inspiratory and expiratory pressures are reduced in Parkinson disease.[4] Poor muscle control, as manifested by difficulty in performing repetitive inspiratory resistive efforts, may be seen even in patients with normal pulmonary function results and respiratory muscle strength. In addition, the performance of this maneuver was associated with a higher oxygen cost of breathing and reduced efficiency of breathing.[35]

Upper airway muscle dysfunction is most likely the cause of the obstructive ventilatory pattern in patients with extrapyramidal disorders.[4] Of 27 patients, 24 showed either regular (type A) or irregular (type B) flow oscillations on both the inspiratory and expiratory flow–volume loops (**Figure 45-9**). Oscillations on the flow–volume loop were due to upper airway muscle dyskinesia, which was confirmed by direct endoscopic evaluation. Some patients showed frank intermittent airway closure that caused signs and symptoms of upper airway obstruction. A reduction in FEV_1 should alert the clinician to the possibility of upper airway muscle dysfunction in patients with parkinsonism. The same group of authors reported improvement in upper airway obstruction after levodopa therapy in a patient with Parkinson disease.[36] However, levodopa therapy may uncommonly induce respiratory dyskinesia, which may be managed by decreasing the dose of the medication or using dopamine antagonists.

RESPIRATORY RECAP

Parkinson Disease

- » Respiratory muscle dysfunction either due to weakness or incoordination is common.
- » An obstructive ventilatory pattern is often caused by upper airway dysfunction.

Patients with Parkinson disease often complain of dyspnea and chronic tachypnea. The abnormal ventilatory pattern discussed earlier improves with levodopa treatment[35] and returns to baseline once therapy is stopped. A modest improvement in FEV_1, FVC, and peak expiratory flow rate has been reported after 1 week of levodopa therapy in 9 of 10 patients with Parkinson disease.[37] Four patients continued to have small, sustained improvements in expiratory flow after 2 weeks of therapy. Patients who did not respond to levodopa therapy did not show an improvement in ventilatory function.

Medications commonly used in the treatment of Parkinson disease can cause pulmonary complications. Levodopa has been reported to cause dyspnea and respiratory distress, presumably due to respiratory muscle dyskinesia. Ergot derivatives such as bromocriptine can cause pleural effusion, pleural thickening, or pulmonary infiltrates.

Multiple Sclerosis

Multiple sclerosis (MS) is a demyelinating disease of the central nervous system clinically characterized by repeated remissions and exacerbations of symptoms. Multiple sclerosis is the most common neurologic disease affecting young adults, with an estimated 350,000 to 400,00 cases in the United States. The exact etiology of the disease remains elusive, although epidemiologic evidence points to both genetic and environmental factors. Classic clinical symptoms include paresthesias, motor weakness, diplopia, blurred vision, bladder incontinence, and ataxia. Symptoms are typically aggravated by an increase in temperature, which causes conduction block in partially demyelinated fibers. The disease may demonstrate remissions and relapses or follow a chronic progressive course. Pathologically, lesions or plaques have a predilection to involve the periventricular white matter of the cerebral hemisphere, the optic nerve, brain stem, and the cervical spinal cord. Because multiple sclerosis can cause focal lesions anywhere in the central nervous system, different patterns of respiratory impairment can occur. Involvement of the respiratory centers in the medulla can affect either the voluntary or automatic breathing (Ondine's curse) and produce apneustic breathing, paroxysmal hyperventilation, obstructive sleep apnea, or neurogenic pulmonary edema.[38] The three most common patterns of respiratory involvement in multiple sclerosis include respiratory muscle weakness, bulbar dysfunction, and abnormalities in respiratory control.[39]

Acute respiratory failure is rarely encountered in MS, but can occur due to severe demyelination of the cervical cord.[40] Diaphragmatic paralysis resulting in respiratory insufficiency has also been reported.[41] More commonly respiratory failure presents insidiously, affecting only those with advanced MS. Even with severe disability and impaired respiratory muscle function, patients with multiple sclerosis seldom complain of dyspnea. The paucity of respiratory complaints may be due to restricted motor activities and greater expiratory than inspiratory muscle weakness. Clinical signs that may be helpful in predicting respiratory muscle involvement are a weak cough and the inability to clear secretions, a limited ability to count on a single exhalation, and the presence of upper extremity weakness.

RESPIRATORY RECAP

Multiple Sclerosis

- » Demyelination of the central nervous system can affect the respiratory center in the medulla and nerve innervation to the bulbar and respiratory muscles.
- » Pulmonary impairment depends on the severity of the disease and the functional capacity of the patient.

Expiratory muscles appear to be more frequently involved than the inspiratory muscles in MS patients. Analysis of pulmonary function tests in 25 patients with varying severity of multiple sclerosis showed that FVC, MMV, and PEmax are normal in ambulatory MS patients but were severely reduced (39%, 32%, and 36%, respectively) in bedridden patients.[42] Pulmonary dysfunction depends to a large extent on the severity of the disease and the functional capacity of the patient. Those patients who were wheelchair-bound with upper extremity involvement also showed moderate reductions in FVC, MVV, and PEmax. In addition, patients who were quadriplegic and who exhibited prominent bulbar muscle involvement were at high risk for acute respiratory failure.

Close respiratory monitoring is required in these patients. Arterial blood gas results are frequently normal even with abnormal respiratory muscle function. Advanced multiple sclerosis is frequently complicated by aspiration, atelectasis, and pneumonia.

Treatment of multiple sclerosis includes adrenocorticotropic hormone (ACTH), high-dose corticosteroids, immunosuppressive agents such as cyclophosphamide and azathioprine, intravenous immunoglobulin therapy, and plasmapheresis. ACTH and prednisone have been shown to hasten the resolution of clinical symptoms in controlled studies.[43] Methylprednisolone 1 g daily for 5 days with or without prednisone taper may be helpful in MS patients with severe respiratory complications. Plasmapheresis has been shown to improve clinical symptoms in patients with severe acute exacerbation and in the relapsing/remitting variety of MS with acute exacerbation.[44] A beneficial effect of intravenous immunoglobulin has been reported in patients with quadriplegia and respiratory failure following an attack of MS.

Both positive and negative noninvasive pressure ventilation have been successfully used in MS patients with intact bulbar function.[45,46] In the presence of bulbar dysfunction and respiratory failure, tracheotomy and positive pressure ventilation are usually required.

Lower Motor Neuron Disorders

Amyotrophic Lateral Sclerosis

Amyotrophic lateral sclerosis (ALS) is a progressive neurodegenerative disorder of both upper and lower motor neurons leading to a loss of skeletal muscle strength, including the respiratory muscles. The incidence of ALS is 1 to 2 cases per 100,000 people. Males are more commonly affected than females, with a ratio of 2:1 involvement. The majority of ALS cases are sporadic (classic ALS), but 5% to 10% of cases are due to an autosomal dominant inheritance (familial ALS). Death is usually due to progressive respiratory failure and repeated respiratory infections. Approximately 80% of ALS patients die within 5 years of initial diagnosis.

The exact etiology of ALS is unknown. A genetic mutation encoding copper-zinc superoxide dismutase, a free oxygen radical scavenger, has been identified in 10% to 15% of familial ALS patients, thus suggesting a susceptibility of the neurons to oxidative stress. Evidence suggests that the motor neurons are susceptible to glutamate-induced neurotoxicity. Glutamate is the principal excitatory brain neurotransmitter. A decreased uptake of glutamate may lead to overstimulation of the glutamate receptors, leading to an increase in intracellular calcium, which then triggers proteolytic enzymes, causing cell membrane injury.

The usual clinical presentation in two-thirds of ALS patients is progressive weakness of the distal extremities, although early involvement of the bulbar muscles occurs in 25% of cases. Acute respiratory failure[16,47] and nocturnal hypoventilation[48] have been described as initial presentations of ALS. Early involvement of the phrenic nerve neurons within the cervical cord is implicated in this type of presentation.

Although respiratory muscle impairment is usually only evident in advanced stages of the disease, abnormalities in pulmonary function tests are apparent even in patients with mild weakness of the extremities. Serial lung function studies in ALS patients who die show progressive reductions in FVC and MVV, as well as progressive increases in RV compared with patients who survive.[6] Both PImax and PEmax are reduced to 34% and 47% of predicted, respectively.[6,49] In ALS patients who are dyspneic but with relatively preserved pulmonary function tests, PImax and PEmax are frequently abnormal.[49] PImax greater than −60 cm H_2O is 100% sensitive for predicting survival of less than 18 months. However, FVC is the most specific test for predicting survival.

Flow–volume curve shape may identify a subset of patients with greater expiratory muscle weakness. In patients with severe weakness of the expiratory muscles, the flow–volume loop will show a concavity of the maximal expiratory curve, with a sharp drop-off in flow at lower lung volumes. This group of ALS patients exhibits lowers maximal expiratory pressures, smaller vital capacities, and higher residual volumes compared with patients with more normal flow–volume loop contours.[50] Upper airway dysfunction may be detected by oscillations of the flow–volume loop or by direct laryngoscopy. As the disease advances, FVC is reduced and RV is elevated; however, in contrast to other chronic neuromuscular diseases, TLC and FRC are relatively well preserved. These changes are due to earlier involvement of the abdominal muscles with preservation of intercostal and diaphragm function. Weakness of the abdominal muscles causes a reduction in PEmax and an increase in RV. In addition, spasticity of the intercostal muscles may attenuate the stiffness of the chest wall, thus preserving lung volumes. However, expiratory muscle weakness is often associated with inspiratory muscle weakness.[50] Adequate oxygenation is usually well maintained even with severe deterioration in spirometry. Arterial blood gas monitoring is not useful in early disease. Spirometry, however, is still important in the initial evaluation of patients with ALS because impairment in ventilatory function is frequently underestimated, even by experienced examiners.

> **RESPIRATORY RECAP**
>
> **Amyotrophic Lateral Sclerosis**
>
> » Progressive weakness of the distal extremities is the most common presentation, but bulbar muscle weakness occurs in one-fourth of patients.
>
> » Serial FVC values and measurements of respiratory muscle strength are useful guides as to when to initiate noninvasive ventilation (NIV).
>
> » NIV improves gas exchange and quality of life and decreases mortality.

The comprehensive management of ALS patients should include measures to alleviate symptoms, and specific drug therapy to alter the progressive clinical course. Riluzole, an antiglutamate drug, is approved by the U.S. Food and Drug Administration (FDA) for the treatment of ALS. Riluzole is the only treatment that has been shown to prolong survival in ALS.[51] It should be given to patients once a diagnosis of ALS is made. Other antiglutamate drugs (such as gabapentin) or neurotrophic factors (such as insulin-like growth factors or glial-derived neurotrophic factor) are currently under investigation.

Despite optimal medical therapy, disease progression invariably occurs, resulting in respiratory insufficiency that requires some form of ventilatory assistance. The onset of respiratory failure often signals a rapid decline in global as well as functional status. The need for mechanical ventilation should be discussed with the patient and family early on to prevent rapid decline in lung function. In a survey of ALS patients, the majority of patients considered mechanical ventilation during the early phase of their disease but eventually declined artificial ventilation as the disease progressed.[52]

In ALS patients who develop respiratory symptoms or have moderate or rapid reductions in lung function, noninvasive forms of ventilation (NIV) should be considered. In patients who can tolerate nasal noninvasive pressure ventilation, the risk of death is decreased by a factor of 3.1.[23] In a study involving 122 patients with ALS who were offered NIV once they developed dyspnea or an FVC less than 50% predicted or a fall of more than 15% in FVC in 3 months' follow-up.[53] Those patients who used NIV more than 4 hours per day not only showed a slower decline in lung function but also decreased mortality.

A randomized, controlled trial assessed the effect of noninvasive mechanical ventilation versus standard care on survival and quality of life in a cohort of patients with ALS. Patients were clinically followed every 2 months and were randomly assigned to noninvasive ventilation or standard care when they developed orthopnea with a PImax of greater than 60% or the presence of hypercarbia. NIV improved survival and improved the quality of life in patients with no bulbar or with moderate bulbar symptoms compared to the best supportive care.[51] In patients with severe bulbar symptoms, NIV improved only the quality of life. In the intensive care unit (ICU) setting, NIV should be tried first in ALS patients who experience acute or chronic respiratory insufficiency, especially in the absence of significant bulbar symptoms. Patients with significant bulbar symptoms usually cannot tolerate NIV because of difficulty handling oral secretions. Some patients with acute respiratory decompensation may have a partial improvement in respiratory muscle strength after a period of ventilatory assistance.

Aminophylline has also been reported to improve respiratory muscle strength in ALS patients. One study reported theophylline significantly increased respiratory muscle strength after resistive breathing.[54] The negative inspiratory pressure, forced vital capacity, and peak inspiratory flow increased by 28%, 10%, and 12%, respectively, in that study.

Poliomyelitis and Postpoliomyelitis Muscular Dystrophy

Poliomyelitis was the most common cause of respiratory failure in the early part of the 20th century, before the advent of the widespread use of the oral polio vaccine. Acute poliomyelitis is now rare in the United States, and recent cases of poliomyelitis are due to exposure to oral polio vaccine and unimmunized individuals. Although most cases of acute polio infections are nonparalytic, as many as 25% of cases are the paralytic form of poliomyelitis that leads to respiratory muscle weakness requiring assisted ventilation. In most cases, respiratory muscle function improves after the acute episode so that assisted ventilation is no longer required. However, progressive muscle weakness may occur years later.

Postpoliomyelitis syndrome is recognized as a progressive muscle weakness occurring on average 29 years after recovery from an acute episode of poliomyelitis. Approximately 20% to 60% of poliomyelitis survivors will develop postpoliomyelitis syndrome, with a mean age of onset of 51 years. These patients may complain of dyspnea, exercise intolerance, sleep-related symptoms such as daytime hypersomnolence and morning headaches, and muscle weakness. Muscles that were previously involved are primarily involved in this syndrome, although other muscle groups may also be affected due to previous subclinical involvement.[55]

Several theories have been proposed to explain the pathogenesis of postpoliomyelitis syndrome, including susceptibility to aging of reinnervated motor units,[56] chronic compensatory overuse of damaged muscle fiber,[57] and immune-mediated attack on the abnormal motor units, but the basic pathophysiology appear to be denervation and aberrant reinnervation of motor units.[55]

RESPIRATORY RECAP

Postpoliomyelitis Syndrome

- Respiratory muscle weakness recurs about 30 years after recovery from acute poliomyelitis.
- Sleep-disordered breathing, both obstructive and central, is common.
- NIV is effective in the reversal of sleep-associated breathing dysfunction.

Postpoliomyelitis syndrome often presents insidiously as chronic respiratory failure secondary to respiratory muscle weakness. Serial monitoring of FEV_1, FVC, PImax, and PEmax may be helpful in predicting which subset of patients with a prior history of polio develop chronic respiratory failure.[58] The average yearly decline in FVC has been estimated at 18.6 mL/year, or 1.9%. Once the VC is less than 1 L, assisted ventilation is often required.[59] NIV is effective in reversing chronic hypoventilation and its associated symptoms.[59,60] Nocturnal NIV may also improve respiratory muscle strength and exercise capacity.[60]

Sleep-related breathing disorders are common in patients with postpoliomyelitis syndrome,[55,61–63] even in patients who are already on nocturnal ventilatory support.[61] Hypersomnolence was the most common presenting symptom in one review, present in 32 of 35 postpoliomyelitis patients.[62] The most frequently identified sleep-related breathing disorders were obstructive sleep apnea (19 of 35), hypoventilation (7 of 35), and mixed apnea and hypopnea (9 of 35). Patients with bulbar dysfunction have a greater frequency of sleep apnea compared with those with intact bulbar muscle function. Detailed questioning concerning sleep-related symptoms during initial evaluation helps select those patients with postpoliomyelitis syndrome who may benefit from a formal sleep study evaluation. Even patients who are already on nocturnal assisted ventilation may benefit from a sleep study, especially if they have daytime hypersomnolence, fatigue, and morning headache.

Postpoliomyelitis syndrome may also present as recurrent aspiration due to upper airway muscle weakness, and vocal cord paralysis.[64] Asymmetric involvement of the thoracic muscles may lead to kyphoscoliosis and may further compromise respiratory muscle function. Central hypoventilation due to involvement of the brain stem's respiratory center has also been reported.[65]

Disorders of the Peripheral Nerves

Phrenic Nerve Injury

Unilateral or bilateral diaphragm paralysis can occur following phrenic nerve injury. Phrenic nerve injury may be seen following cardiac surgery, trauma, mediastinal tumors, pleural space infection, or forceful neck manipulation.[66] Phrenic nerve injury during cardiac surgery is due either to cold exposure[67] or mechanical stretching of the nerve during surgery.[68] Diaphragm paralysis may also be seen with motor neuron disease, myelopathies, neuropathies, and myopathies. However, the majority of cases of diaphragm weakness are idiopathic.

Dyspnea is the main complaint of patients with bilateral diaphragm weakness, especially when lying down. Cranial displacement of the diaphragm by the abdominal visceral contents in the supine position can further impair the pump function of an already weakened diaphragm. Thus, unexplained severe orthopnea and thoracoabdominal paradoxical breathing especially in the supine position are clinical clues to the presence of diaphragm dysfunction. Unilateral diaphragm weakness is usually well tolerated by patients even when the FVC and TLC are mildly reduced.

Bilateral diaphragm paralysis usually is identified as a restrictive ventilatory defect on pulmonary function testing. The vital capacity is typically reduced to less than 50% of predicted in the erect posture. The chest radiograph typically shows either a unilateral or bilateral elevated hemidiaphragm, depending on the location of the phrenic nerve injury. However, both parenchymal and pleural diseases such as atelectasis, pulmonary fibrosis, or subpulmonic fluid collections may mimic the radiographic picture of diaphragm paralysis, making the diagnosis difficult and frequently even delayed.[69]

Fluoroscopy can confirm diaphragmatic weakness or paralysis. The diaphragm is viewed under fluoroscopy while the patient performs a sniff maneuver (sniff test). The rapid increase in intrapleural pressure during the sniff maneuver will cause a paradoxical cephalad movement of the weak hemidiaphragm. Fluoroscopy is not useful in bilateral diaphragm weakness because both hemidiaphragms may descend normally during a sniff maneuver despite profound weakness due to sudden relaxation of the abdominal muscles. The sniff test should be interpreted with caution because paradoxical movement can be seen in up to 6% of normal individuals. The paradoxical movement should be at least 2 cm to increase the specificity of the test.

Ultrasound examination of the diaphragm has been reported to be useful in assessing diaphragm contractile function.[70] This technique has the advantage of being rapid, easy to use, noninvasive, and without radiation exposure. The utility of this technique to assess diaphragm function in a variety of clinical scenarios is unclear at the present time and needs further study.

RESPIRATORY RECAP

Phrenic Nerve Injury

- » Injury can lead to unilateral or bilateral diaphragm paralysis.
- » Severe orthopnea and abdominal rib cage paradox are clues to the diagnosis.
- » Chest radiograph shows elevated hemidiaphragm (unilateral) or small lung volume (bilateral).
- » Fluoroscopy (sniff test) or ultrasound of the diaphragm are useful tests for diagnosis of diaphragm paralysis.

In patients with mild diaphragm weakness, both pulmonary function tests and radiographic examinations may be reported as normal. In this case, measurement of transdiaphragmatic pressure (Pdi), with all of the limitations discussed earlier in mind (i.e., intersubject variability, invasive procedure, and the need for full patient cooperation), is useful in the diagnosis and quantification of diaphragm weakness.[70] Total diaphragm paralysis is diagnosed when there is no pressure difference across the two sides of the diaphragm (Pdi = 0) during forceful inspiratory maneuvers against an occluded airway.

Sleep may worsen ventilatory failure in patients with bilateral diaphragm paralysis because of a loss of respiratory accessory muscle activity during REM sleep. However, significant nocturnal hypoventilation or daytime hypercapnia was not present in six patients with isolated bilateral diaphragm paralysis.[71]

Recovery from diaphragm weakness depends on the etiology. In phrenic injury after cardiac surgery, 80% of patients will recover nerve function in 6 months, and 90% will recover in 1 year.[72]

Guillain-Barré Syndrome

Guillain-Barré syndrome (GBS) is an acute idiopathic polyneuritis that usually presents as an ascending symmetric paralysis of the lower extremities associated with absent tendon reflexes and autonomic dysfunction. The degree of motor weakness is variable, ranging from mild paresis to complete paralysis. Maximum weakness of the lower extremities occurs within 2 weeks in 50% of cases and in 4 weeks in 80%. Facial (60%), ocular (15%), and oropharyngeal (50%) muscles may be involved. The objective findings of sensory loss are variable, occurring in 40% to 70% of patients. Varying degrees of autonomic dysfunction, such as cardiac arrhythmia, blood pressure lability, gastrointestinal dysfunction, pupillary dysfunction, sweating abnormalities, and urinary retention, can occur in as many as 65% of patients, as reported in one series. Involvement of the bulbar and respiratory muscles may lead to swallowing dysfunction, increased risk of aspiration, and respiratory failure.

Diagnostic criteria for GBS have been reported.[73] Other variants of GBS (e.g., with asymmetric involvement of the extremities, presence of ataxia, or absence of paresthesia) have also been described. In over 70% of cases, the syndrome is preceded by a history of a recent viral or bacterial infection. The diagnosis of GBS is confirmed by abnormal cerebrospinal fluid (CSF) and nerve conduction studies. The CSF examination characteristically shows an increased protein content with a paucity of cells, commonly referred to as albuminocytologic dissociation. Nerve conduction study typically shows multifocal demyelination.

Although the exact etiology of GBS is unknown, several risk factors have been identified that may precipitate the disease. These risk factors include viral illnesses (e.g., cytomegalovirus, Epstein-Barr virus), *Mycoplasma pneumoniae* infection, influenza vaccination, recent surgery, and malignancy (lymphoma). A strong association between antecedent *Campylobacter jejuni* infection and GBS has also been found. The current concept suggests that GBS is a self-limited, reactive autoimmune disease in which an aberrant immune response is directed against bacterial lipopolysaccharides that share similar epitopes with the myelin sheath or Schwann cell basement membrane.

RESPIRATORY RECAP

Guillain-Barré Syndrome

» Ascending symmetric paralysis of the lower extremities is a common presentation.
» Acute respiratory failure is a serious complication in one-third of patients.
» Bulbar muscle weakness increases the risk of aspiration and may warrant early intubation.
» Indications for ventilatory support include an FVC less than 12 mL/kg, respiratory distress, inability to handle oral secretions, hypoxemia, and hypercarbia.
» Autonomic dysfunction is common and can cause hemodynamic instability.

Respiratory failure requiring assisted ventilation occurs in 15% to 30% of cases.[74] Once respiratory muscle dysfunction is evident and requires ICU care, up to 62% of patients will require ventilatory assistance. The average duration of mechanical ventilation in two large series was 50 to 55 days.[74,75] Most patients will require tracheostomy because of the need for prolonged mechanical ventilation and to facilitate pulmonary hygiene. Ropper suggested that tracheostomy be delayed up to 10 days to avoid the procedure in patients who rapidly improve.[75]

A severe reduction in maximum transdiaphragmatic pressures has been documented during acute ventilatory failure and during recovery from the illness.[76] Among the pulmonary function tests, serial vital capacity measurement is the most useful test in predicting the need for mechanical ventilation. Several studies have shown that a VC of 12 to 15 mL/kg is a sign of imminent respiratory failure.[74,75,77,78] In patients who developed respiratory failure as a result of Guillain-Barré syndrome, the VC measured serially decreased from a mean of 2.5 L to 0.9 L within 2 weeks. In a study of 81 GBS patients who required mechanical ventilation, the average FVC at the time of intubation was 33±11%. Other indications for intubation and ventilatory support include respiratory distress, inability to handle oral secretions, hypoxemia ($Pa{O_2}$ less than 70 mm Hg on room air, or alveolar–arterial O_2 difference of more than 300 mm Hg with $F{IO_2}$ of 1.0), and hypercapnia. Other predictors of the need for mechanical ventilation include time between onset of disease and hospital admission of less than 7 days, inability to lift the head, presence of bulbar dysfunction, and the presence of anti-GQ1b antibodies.

Neurophysiologic testing is helpful in predicting the need for mechanical ventilation.[76] Of the 154 patients included in this study, patients with the demyelinating form of GBS required mechanical ventilation more often than patients with axonal or equivocal findings on electrophysiology. The risk of acute respiratory failure was only 2.5% if the proximal/distal compound muscular amplitude potential ratio was greater than 55% and FVC was greater than 80%. It is prudent to initiate early intubation and assisted ventilation to avoid complications that may arise from emergent intubation.[76] Arterial blood gas analysis is used to ensure adequate oxygenation and ventilation. Hypercapnia is a late sign of ventilatory failure. The average $Pa{CO_2}$ at the time of intubation when VC is less than 12 mL/kg was 43 mm Hg in two large series of GBS patients.[75]

Upper airway dysfunction due to bulbar involvement may occur in GBS. This may lead to inability to swallow oral secretions, increasing the risk of aspiration. The presence of nasal voice, abnormal gag reflex, dysarthria, and poor mobility of pharyngeal muscles suggests significant bulbar muscle dysfunction. The swallowing mechanism can be roughly assessed at the bedside by asking the patient to drink sips of water and observing for coughing spells. Once significant bulbar dysfunction is observed, early intubation may be necessary to protect the airway even if respiratory muscle strength is still adequate. A study suggested that delaying intubation may increase the risk of early-onset pneumonia.[76]

Autonomic dysfunction can occur in 65% of patients with GBS. Common manifestations of autonomic dysfunction include labile blood pressure, sinus tachycardia, excessive sweating, urinary retention, and ileus. Autonomic dysfunction is commonly prevalent in patients who require mechanical ventilation and during the progressive and plateau phases of the illness. Particular care should be observed during endotracheal suctioning because it can precipitate tachyarrhythmias and bradyarrhythmias and even asystole from vagal stimulation. Moreover, patients may be overly sensitive to vasoactive medications. Management of severe ileus includes bowel rest and therapeutic trials with erythromycin or neostigmine. The use of pro-motility agents is contraindicated in patients with dysautonomia.

Aggressive pulmonary toilet is indicated to prevent as well as treat atelectasis. Atelectasis may require repeated bronchoscopy and may decrease the incidence of nosocomial pneumonia.[74] Subcutaneous heparin is preferred for deep venous thrombosis prophylaxis compared with pneumatic boots to avoid prolonged foot drop due to compression of the peroneal nerve. Corticosteroids are not beneficial and may be harmful. Weaning may be started once VC exceeds 8 to 10 mL/kg, adequate oxygenation can be achieved with an F_{IO_2} of 0.4 or less, and patients are able to double their minute ventilation.

Immune modulation using either plasma exchange or intravenous immunoglobulin infusion is the mainstay of therapy in GBS. The maximum inspiratory force at the time of successful weaning is more negative than 40 cm H_2O. In two multicenter trials, plasmapheresis (250 mL/kg every 2 days for a total of five treatments) using either albumin or fresh frozen plasma as replacement fluid showed short-term benefits in early motor recovery and ambulation, reduced the number of patients who required assisted ventilation, and shortened the duration of mechanical ventilation.[79–81] Immunotherapy should be started within 2 weeks of onset of symptoms or as early as possible. However, in patients with rapidly deteriorating clinical symptoms, plasmapheresis may still offer some benefit even if the duration of the disease is more than 3 weeks.[75] Intravenous immunoglobulin (IVIG) given within 2 weeks of the onset of GBS may be as effective as plasma exchange therapy.[80] In approximately 10% of patients, relapse of neurologic symptoms may follow plasma exchange treatment due to antibody rebound. In such circumstances, additional plasma exchange treatment or IVIG treatment is helpful.

Because IVIG is easier to administer, it is preferred over plasma exchange unless there are specific contraindications to its use, such as low serum immunoglobulin A, presence of uncontrolled hypertension, and a hyperosmolar state. There is no additional benefit conferred by sequential treatment consisting initially of plasmapheresis followed by IVIG when compared with either treatment alone. Corticosteroids alone confer no therapeutic benefit and may slow recovery in GBS; their use is not recommended.[82] The combination of IVIG and intravenous methylprednisolone may hasten recovery, but there has been no documented beneficial effect on long-term outcome.[82,83]

With the advent of modern ICU care, mortality from Guillain-Barré syndrome dropped from 15% in the 1970s to between 3% and 4% in the 1980s. Common complications are pneumonia, recurrent aspiration, and pulmonary thromboembolic disease. Prognosis for recovery is generally good, but only 15% of patients will have no neurologic residuals. Factors associated with poor prognosis are older age, lower mean compound muscle action potential amplitudes during distal stimulation (less than 20% of normal), need for ventilatory support, and rapid progression to severe weakness in less than 1 week.

Critical Illness Polyneuropathy and Neuromyopathy

Critical illness polyneuromyopathy (CIPNM), presenting as flaccid paralysis of both upper and lower extremities, is a common sequela of severe sepsis and multisystem organ failure in both surgical and medical intensive care units. The incidence of CIPNM depends on the severity of illness, the diagnostic criteria used, and the timing of examination from the onset of the critical illness. In prospective studies, 25% to 63% of patients who required mechanical ventilation for at least 7 days developed CIPNM.[84] Patients with sepsis and sepsis syndrome have the highest incidence of CIPNM, approaching 70% to 100%. Axonal polyneuropathy was initially thought to be the main pathologic change in ICU-acquired weakness. However, EMG and muscle biopsy studies showed that acute myopathy coexists with polyneuropathy, and in fact often exists as a separate clinical entity. Four categories of the syndrome are recognized (**Table 45–4**). In a prospective study of 30 patients with critical illness polyneuropathy, biopsy of the quadriceps femoral muscle showed neuropathic changes in 37%, myopathy in 40%, and both neuropathic and myopathic changes in 23% of patients. Muscle necrosis was also present in 30% of the muscle biopsy specimens.[85]

Several risk factors, other than severe sepsis and multisystem organ failure, have been identified in the

TABLE 45–4 Acute Weakness Syndrome in the Intensive Care Unit

Myopathy	Acute necrotizing myopathy Disuse atrophy
Neuromuscular junction abnormalities	Myasthenia-like syndrome Prolonged neuromuscular blockade
Neuropathy	Critical illness polyneuropathy Acute motor neuropathy
Polyneuromyopathy	Combination of neuropathy and myopathy

development of CIPNM. These include prolonged use of corticosteroids and neuromuscular blocking agents, persistent hyperglycemia, hyperosmolality, immobility, use of aminoglycosides, and prolonged mechanical ventilation.[86] Global measures of the severity of critical illness, such as the Acute Physiology, Age, and Chronic Health Evaluation (APACHE) III and the Sequential Organ Failure Assessment Score (SOFA) are also important predictors of the occurrence of CIPNM. Aggressive control of stress-induced hyperglycemia has been reported to decrease the incidence of CIPNM in both surgical and medical ICUs.[88–89] In a prospective, randomized, controlled trial, intensive insulin therapy to maintain normoglycemia (blood glucose levels between 80 and 110 mg/dL) decreased the incidence of critical illness polyneuropathy by 44% compared with conventional insulin therapy (blood glucose level between 180 and 200 mg/dL). The risk of CIPNM was significantly correlated with the mean blood glucose level. In patients who required mechanical ventilatory support for more than 7 days, intensive insulin therapy decreased the duration of mechanical ventilation with an absolute risk reduction of −11.6%. In addition, CIPNM resolved faster in the intensive insulin treatment group compared with the control group, which partially explained the decreased duration of mechanical ventilation.[90] In multivariate analysis, independent predictors of the development of polyneuropathy include conventional insulin treatment and vasopressor support of more than 3 days.

RESPIRATORY RECAP

Critical Illness Polyneuromyopathy

- » Critical illness polyneuromyopathy is the most common cause of weakness in the ICU.
- » Acute ICU myopathy is the most common CIPNM.
- » CIPNM is a common cause of failure to wean from ventilatory support in patients with severe sepsis and multisystem organ failure.
- » Quadriparesis in an awake ICU patient following severe sepsis is the usual presentation.
- » Control of hyperglycemia can decrease the incidence of CIPNM.

The pathogenesis of CIPNM is not well understood. An exaggerated immune response to severe injury is thought to be the main pathogenic pathway leading to nerve and muscle injury. Both systemic and local inflammatory response mediated by tumor necrosis factor alpha and interleukins 1 and 12 and the recruitment of T helper 1 cells, monocytes, macrophages, and neutrophils lead to endothelial cell injury, increased microvascular permeability, and endoneurial edema resulting in decreased blood flow to the nerve and muscle tissue. The end result of this injury is primary axonal degeneration of the sensory and motor fibers and muscle atrophy with loss of contractile proteins and membrane inexcitability. In animal models, sepsis triggers enhanced muscle protein proteolysis through the ubiquitin-proteosome and calpain system, causing myofibrillar degradation and disruption of the sarcomere. Moreover, animal models of critical illness myopathy reveal altered membrane expression and function of the sodium channels. It has been suggested that critical illness myopathy is not only due to selective myosin loss but also due to muscle fiber membrane electrical inexcitability caused by defective sodium channel regulation.[91]

The syndrome is often suspected initially because of failure to wean from mechanical ventilation as patients recover from their life-threatening illnesses or the presence of new symmetric weakness of both upper and lower extremities. About one-third of these patients have difficulty weaning from the ventilator, and 70% have evidence of peripheral neuropathy.[92] The muscle weakness is most prominent in the lower extremities and is accompanied by muscle wasting and reduced or absent tendon reflexes. Facial muscle weakness, presence of asymmetric weakness of the limbs, or pyramidal signs should prompt further workup to rule out other neurologic causes of weakness. Assessment of peripheral muscle strength can sometimes be difficult in uncooperative patients because of the use of sedative-hypnotic agents or the presence of either delirium or metabolic encephalopathy. Nevertheless, if motor strength assessment is possible, a standardized muscle examination can be used to assess the degree of weakness in individual muscle groups.

The diagnosis of critical care polyneuropathy is supported by nerve conduction and EMG (ENMG) studies, which typically show the presence of axonal polyneuropathy with or without the presence of concomitant myopathy. In axonal polyneuropathy, ENMG testing shows a reduction in the amplitude of the compound action potential with normal conduction velocity on motor nerve stimulation, and spontaneous electrical activity on muscle needle recording. This ENMG pattern can be seen in 70% to 100% of ICU patients with severe sepsis and after 5 to 7 days of mechanical ventilation. A myopathic pattern on ENMG is suggested by the presence of a prolonged compound muscle action potential and a short duration and low amplitude of motor unit potentials on voluntary activation. Creatine phosphokinase (CPK) levels are either normal or slightly elevated in CIPNM. Muscle and nerve biopsy can be used to confirm the diagnosis but are not routinely indicated. Muscle biopsy usually shows type II fiber atrophy and occasionally type I atrophy and muscle necrosis. Immunohistochemistry and electron microscopy show a loss of myosin thick filaments. In the right clinical setting, extensive neurologic testing or biopsy of the nerve or muscle is not required to make a confident diagnosis of CIPNM.

The differential diagnosis of muscle weakness in the ICU setting encompasses multiple central nervous system pathologies, including head and spinal cord injury. In acute spinal injury, spinal shock may cause quadriparesis and areflexia mimicking polyneuropathy. Muscle weakness associated with ptosis and bulbar weakness suggests a neuromuscular junction disease such as myasthenia gravis. Axonal variants of Guillain-Barré syndrome are distinguished by the presence of weakness before admission to the ICU, a preceding history of *Campylobacter jejuni* infection, and positive serologic test for anti-GM1 or anti-GD1a antibodies. Prolonged use of neuromuscular blocking agents, especially in the presence of hepatic and renal failure, can lead to persistent neuromuscular blockade due to delayed clearance of the drugs.

Because there is no specific treatment for CIPNM, avoidance of recognized risk factors is important in decreasing the incidence and morbidity and mortality associated with this disease process. Preventive measures include tight blood glucose control, avoidance or minimization of corticosteroids and/or neuromuscular blocking agents, early mobilization and physical therapy, and the institution of a daily interruption of sedation to avoid sedation-related immobilization.

For those patients who survive the acute phase of their injury, CIPNM prolongs the ICU and hospital length of stay, prolongs the duration of mechanical ventilation, and increases mortality. Critical illness neuromyopathy is a predictor of prolonged weaning.[93,94] Clinical recovery of nerve function is often prolonged and is usually associated with residual weakness that causes persistent functional impairment. In a cohort of 100 patients with acute respiratory distress syndrome followed for 1 year, muscle wasting and weakness were the most significant extrapulmonary complications that contributed to persistent functional impairment.[95] The detrimental effect of CIPNM on long-term outcome is best shown by a composite review of 36 studies involving 263 patients. Complete functional recovery occurred in 68% of patients; however, persistent neurologic deficits in the form of absent or reduced deep tendon reflexes, glove and stocking sensory loss, muscle atrophy, painful hyperesthesia, and persistent severe disability due to quadriparesis, quadriplegia, or paraplegia occurred in 28% of patients.[96]

Disorders of the Neuromuscular Junction

Myasthenia Gravis

Myasthenia gravis (MG) is an autoimmune disorder characterized by impaired transmission of neural impulses across the neuromuscular junction due to the destruction of the postsynaptic acetylcholine receptors. It is the most common neuromuscular transmission disorder, with an estimated incidence of 10 to 20 cases per million people and a prevalence of 100 to 200 cases per million. Younger women of childbearing age are affected twice as frequently as men. Thymic tumors are seen in 10% of cases, mostly in older men.

The typical presentation of the myasthenic patient is fluctuating weakness of the involved voluntary muscles that improves with rest or with the administration of anticholinesterase agents (positive Tensilon test) or both. Ocular, facial, and neck muscles are commonly involved. In the generalized form of the disease, variable involvement of bulbar, limb, and respiratory muscles also occurs. Bulbar muscle weakness such as dysarthria, dysphagia, and fatigable chewing is the initial presenting symptom in 15% of cases. Approximately 50% to 60% of patients with the ocular form of the disease progress to generalized weakness involving the oropharyngeal muscles, diaphragm, and other respiratory muscles and limbs within the first 2 years of the onset of symptoms. Respiratory muscle weakness is seen in one-third of patients and may occur in the absence of peripheral muscle weakness. On physical examination, fatigability of the involved muscles can be elicited by asking the patient to do repetitive or sustained muscle activity such as looking upward for several minutes to elicit lid or ocular muscle weakness.

The Tensilon test is a simple test that can be done at the bedside to confirm the diagnosis of myasthenia gravis. Tensilon (edrophonium), a short-acting inhibitor of acetylcholinesterase, can be given intravenously to elicit a transient improvement in muscle weakness. A positive Tensilon test highly suggests myasthenia gravis, but a positive test has also been reported in patients with Lambert-Eaton syndrome, botulism, and ALS. In patients with moderately generalized myasthenia gravis, pulmonary function testing reveals a mild reduction in FVC and a moderate reduction in both inspiratory and expiratory strength, indicating respiratory muscle weakness.

A serologic test may also be used to support the diagnosis of myasthenia gravis. Antibodies to acetylcholine receptors are seen in 80% of patients with generalized myasthenia and 60% of those with ocular myasthenia. The concentration of the acetylcholine receptor antibodies does not correlate with the severity of disease. Acetylcholine receptor antibodies have been found in Lambert-Eaton syndrome and in systemic lupus erythematosus. Studies showed that the presence of anti–muscle specific kinase (MuSK) antibodies identifies a subgroup of patients with myasthenia gravis who have a higher incidence of bulbar weakness (100% vs. 58%) and respiratory failure (46% vs. 7%) compared with seronegative patients.[97–99] Greater involvement of the respiratory muscles was also reported in patients who tested positive for anti-MuSK.

Electrodiagnostic study is nonspecific for MG but characteristically shows a 10% to 15% decrease in amplitude of the action potential during slow repetitive stimulation in 77% of myasthenic patients. Single-fiber EMG is abnormal in 92% of the patients and is thought to be the most sensitive test, even in patients with a negative serum antibody against acetylcholine receptor or a normal repetitive nerve stimulation test.

Respiratory muscle weakness can occur in the absence of peripheral muscle weakness.[100,101] However, respiratory muscle weakness in MG typically occurs late in the disease process. In patients with moderately generalized MG, performance of pulmonary function tests before the administration of Mestinon reveals mild reduction in FVC and moderate reduction in both maximum static inspiratory (46% of predicted) and expiratory pressures (48% of predicted). There is no evidence of restrictive or obstructive lung disease. Like other chronic neuromuscular diseases, the breathing pattern of patients with MG is rapid and shallow. After Mestinon treatment, FVC, FEV_1, PImax, and PEmax show significant improvement, although respiratory muscle strength does not completely normalize. Arterial blood gas examination is unreliable in predicting the severity of respiratory muscle weakness.

Acute respiratory failure usually occurs in the setting of either myasthenic or cholinergic crisis, or as the initial presentation of the disease. *Myasthenic crisis* refers to an exacerbation of myasthenia gravis leading to respiratory failure that necessitates the use of mechanical ventilation. This is usually precipitated by discontinuation or decrease in the dosage of anticholinergic medications, surgery (thymectomy), administration of neuromuscular blocking medications (e.g., aminoglycosides, curare-like drugs), or emotional crisis.

RESPIRATORY RECAP

Myasthenia Gravis

- » Myasthenia gravis (MG) is an autoimmune disease presenting as fluctuating weakness of ocular, facial, and neck muscles. The muscle weakness improves with anticholinesterase agents.
- » In generalized MG, respiratory muscle weakness can lead to acute respiratory failure.
- » Both myasthenic crises and cholinergic (due to excess of anticholinesterase medications) crises can lead to acute respiratory failure.
- » Surgery can precipitate postoperative respiratory failure.
- » Noninvasive ventilation can be helpful in the management of respiratory failure.

Myasthenic crisis can be confirmed by performing Tensilon testing that results in an improvement in muscle strength. Approximately 15% to 20% of patients with myasthenia gravis will experience myasthenic crises, often in the first year of illness. Thymomas are associated with a more fulminant course of MG and are present in one-third of patients who experience myasthenic crises. The initiation of corticosteroid therapy can paradoxically cause a transient increase in muscle weakness during the first and second week of therapy, especially in patients with severe bulbar symptoms and generalized myasthenia gravis.

Cholinergic crisis refers to the worsening of motor weakness due to an excess of anticholinesterase medications, which causes depolarizing blockade at the myoneural junction. This can be diagnosed and differentiated from myasthenic crisis by the presence of muscarinic symptoms such as hypersalivation, sweating, an increase in bronchial secretions, nausea and vomiting, and diarrhea. In addition, these symptoms may worsen with Tensilon testing. Nicotinic symptoms such as fasciculations and cramps are rare. A brittle crisis occurs when the disease is difficult to treat and the patient alternates between myasthenic and cholinergic crises.

Surgery after thymectomy can precipitate acute respiratory failure. In a series of 22 patients, the mean duration of mechanical ventilation was 8 days, with 6 patients (32%) requiring tracheostomy for prolonged mechanical ventilation.[102] Postoperative care of these patients is important because respiratory failure usually occurs within 24 hours of surgery in more than 50% of patients. Serial measurements of VC, PImax, and PEmax are helpful in detecting the onset of respiratory failure. It is important to remember that the dosing schedule of anticholinesterase medications will affect the measurement of respiratory parameters. The maximum improvement in respiratory muscle strength occurs about 2 hours after the drug is given, and slowly declines before the next dose is given. Consequently, VC, PImax, and PEmax should be measured 30 minutes before the next dose of anticholinesterase agents. No single respiratory parameter reliably predicts the need for mechanical ventilation. However, once VC is less than 15 mL/kg, PImax is greater than –30 cm H_2O, and PEmax is less than 30 cm H_2O, assisted ventilation should be considered.

Other clinical signs of impending acute respiratory failure include signs of upper airway obstruction due to vocal cord paralysis or inability to handle secretions due to severe bulbar involvement. Flow–volume loop analysis may show variable extrathoracic airway obstruction with the characteristic inspiratory plateau in cases of upper airway obstruction. Bilateral basal atelectasis on chest radiograph signifies poor clearance of airway secretions due to a weak cough and is often accompanied by a rapid, shallow breathing pattern. Hypercapnia is a late sign of respiratory muscle fatigue.

Several clinical parameters have been proposed as predictors of postoperative respiratory failure after thymectomy.[103,104] Severity of disease (Osserman groups 3 and 4), especially with the presence of bulbar symptoms and low VC, appears to be the most important factor in predicting postoperative respiratory failure. In a series of 14 of 122 patients who developed respiratory failure following transsternal thymectomy, independent predictors of postoperative myasthenic crises causing acute respiratory failure included preoperative bulbar symptoms, higher serum levels of acetylcholine receptor antibodies (>100 nmol/L), and intraoperative blood loss.[103–107]

Sleep-related breathing disturbances may occur in patients with myasthenia gravis. Abnormal sleep study results in MG patients usually reveal mixed central apneas and hypopneas. Patients should be asked about sleep-related symptoms such as daytime hypersomnolence, nocturnal and early morning awakening, and morning headaches. Older patients with moderate obesity and daytime alveolar hypoventilation and restrictive lung defect should undergo sleep study to screen for sleep apnea and nocturnal hypoventilation. The incidence of sleep apnea is higher in patients with a longer duration of MG.

Treatment of MG includes anticholinesterase agents, high-dose corticosteroids, and plasmapheresis in patients who are refractory to steroids and immunosuppressive therapy. Anticholinesterase agents are the first line of treatment. Most patients will improve significantly with this treatment, but only a few patients will regain normal function. Remission can be induced in up to 80% of patients with corticosteroids. However, initiation of corticosteroid therapy may cause temporary worsening of muscle weakness, usually on the 6th to 10th day of therapy. Close observation for signs of respiratory insufficiency is advisable. Other immunosuppressive agents (e.g., azathioprine, cyclosporine) are also useful in MG either alone or in combination with steroids.

Thymectomy has been shown, in retrospective study, to improve survival and clinical symptoms even in the absence of thymoma in patients with myasthenia gravis compared with patients who were treated medically.[108] In patients who are younger than 55 years, thymectomy is recommended to prevent malignant transformation of the thymoma. Up to 80% of patients with no thymoma will improve clinically following thymectomy, but the response may be delayed. Because there are no randomized controlled studies documenting the benefit of thymectomy in myasthenia gravis, and given the presence of confounding variables such as age, gender, and severity of myasthenia gravis, the American Academy of Neurology recommends thymectomy in patients with nonthymomatous autoimmune myasthenia gravis only as an option to increase the probability of remission or improvement.[108]

In patients with myasthenic crisis, plasmapheresis and IVIG are effective short-term treatments and help to prepare the symptomatic myasthenia patient for surgery.[109] Improvement in muscle strength is usually apparent in 2 to 3 days, but the improvement does not continue beyond several weeks unless immunosuppressant agents are administered concurrently. Intravenous immunoglobulin given at 1.2 to 2 g/kg over 2 to 5 days has been shown to result in a clinical response comparable with plasmapheresis. However, in a retrospective multicenter study of patients with myasthenic crises, plasmapheresis increased the ability to extubate the patient and improved the patient's functional status at 2 weeks.[109]

Immunosuppressant medications are not appropriate therapy in myasthenic crises because a therapeutic response is often delayed for weeks to months. Corticosteroids have been used in patients who were refractory to plasmapheresis or IVIG; however, steroids may cause a transient worsening of muscle weakness. Corticosteroids and cholinesterase inhibitors are best started several days after a clinical response to plasmapheresis is observed in order to avoid weakness due to corticosteroids and to avoid cholinergic crises.

Acute respiratory failure in patients with myasthenia gravis is usually treated with invasive mechanical ventilation. Noninvasive mechanical ventilation is an alternative ventilatory strategy in patients with severe myasthenic crises with early respiratory failure even in the presence of bulbar symptoms. In a retrospective study of 60 episodes of acute respiratory failure in 52 patients, NIV and invasive mechanical ventilation were the initial method of ventilatory support in 24 and 36 episodes of acute respiratory failure, respectively.[106] In the NIV group, 14 patients (58%) were successfully treated with NIV alone; 10 (52%) eventually required invasive mechanical ventilation. The use of NIV avoids the need for airway intubation, decreases the duration of mechanical ventilation, and decreases both ICU and hospital length of stay. The only predictor of failure of NIV to initially treat respiratory failure in MG was a $Paco_2$ of more than 45 mm Hg. Thus, NIV should be used early in acute respiratory failure, before the onset of hypercapnia. In patients who required invasive ventilatory support, aggressive respiratory management including the use of sighs, positive end-expiratory pressure, frequent suctioning, chest physiotherapy, turning in bed, and the use of antibiotics decreased the prevalence of both atelectasis and bronchopneumonia.

Spontaneous breathing trials can be initiated once an improvement in respiratory status is documented. This includes a PImax less than −20 cm H_2O, PEmax greater than 40 cm H_2O, and FVC greater than 10 mL/kg. In a retrospective study of 46 episodes of acute respiratory failure due to myasthenia gravis, extubation failure (defined as the need for reintubation or tracheostomy, or death while on the ventilator) occurred in 44% of cases. Risk factors associated with extubation failures included male sex, history of previous myasthenic crises, atelectasis, and more than 10 days of mechanical ventilation. The FVC, PImax, and PEmax were lower in patients who failed extubation but were not statistically different compared with patients who were successfully extubated. Those patients who had lower pH, lower FVC, the presence of atelectasis, and the need for NIV support had a higher risk for reintubation.[107] These data suggest that other factors, such as respiratory muscle fatigue, the presence of bulbar weakness, and the inability to handle upper airway secretions, are not measured by standard weaning parameters and should be considered before attempting extubation.

Lambert-Eaton Syndrome

Lambert-Eaton syndrome (LEMS) is a rare myasthenic-like disorder resulting from a impaired release of acetylcholine from presynaptic terminals. Antibodies against the voltage-gated calcium channel, a large transmembrane protein, interfere with normal calcium flux necessary for the release of acetylcholine into the neuromuscular synapse.[110] The disease is commonly associated with small cell carcinoma of the lung but has also been reported in patients with Hodgkin lymphoma, atypical carcinoid, and malignant thymoma. The prevalence of LEMS in patients with small cell lung cancer is estimated to be 3%.[111] The syndrome can occur throughout the course of the disease but can also serve as a marker of undiagnosed malignancy. In patients without malignancy, LEMS has been associated with autoimmune disorders such as type 1 diabetes mellitus and autoimmune thyroid disorders.

Unlike in myasthenia gravis, limb and girdle muscles are predominantly involved more than ocular and bulbar muscles. Although respiratory failure is infrequent, respiratory muscle weakness is often detected on pulmonary function tests. Acute respiratory failure has been reported as the initial manifestation of LEMS and should be considered as a differential diagnosis in patients with neuromuscular weakness.[112] The diagnosis of LEMS is confirmed by the presence of antibodies against the voltage-gated calcium channel and electrodiagnostic studies.

Botulism

Botulism is a rare disorder caused by toxin produced by *Clostridium botulinum*. Toxin may be ingested via improperly cooked food, wound contamination by the organisms, or absorption of the toxin from the gastrointestinal tract, particularly in infants. There are eight types of toxins, although human disease is caused by types A, B, or E. Botulinum toxin binds with the calcium channel in the presynaptic terminals, impairing neuromuscular transmission of acetylcholine. Gastrointestinal symptoms predominate early in the course of the disease, followed by neurologic impairment including descending paralysis of the neck, trunk, and limb muscles. Weakness of the respiratory muscles requiring ventilatory support is frequent, especially with botulinum type A toxins. Spirometry usually reveals a restrictive ventilatory defect. Recovery from respiratory muscle weakness may take months, requiring prolonged ventilatory support. The average duration of ventilatory support for type A poisoning is 58 days, in contrast to 26 days in type B botulism.[113] Exertional dyspnea and poor exercise tolerance may persist even with normal lung functions.

Inherited Myopathies

Muscular dystrophies refer to a heterogeneous group of progressive, hereditary degenerative skeletal muscle diseases. The respiratory muscles, like any skeletal muscles, become progressively weaker, eventually culminating in respiratory failure and death. In fact, respiratory complications are the most common cause of death in these diseases.

Duchenne and Becker Muscular Dystrophies

Both **Duchenne muscular dystrophy (DMD)** and **Becker muscular dystrophy (BMD)** are progressive myopathies inherited as X-linked recessive traits. Duchenne muscular dystrophy is the most common muscular dystrophy, with an incidence of approximately 1 in 3300 male births and a prevalence rate of 3 per 100,000. Becker muscular dystrophy is less common than DMD and usually has a milder clinical course. Both diseases are caused by mutation of the gene for skeletal protein dystrophin. Dystrophin gene mutations are caused by gene deletions in 65% of patients with DMD, and 85% of patients with BMD. The dystrophin protein is thought to stabilize the membrane-bound dystrophin-associated glycoprotein complex and prevent it from degradation. The loss of this associated protein as a result of dystrophin deficiency leads to the degenerative changes that are found in muscular dystrophy.

> **RESPIRATORY RECAP**
>
> **Duchenne Muscular Dystrophy**
>
> - DMD is a sex-linked recessive disorder associated with progressive myopathy, culminating in respiratory failure. Becker muscular dystrophy is a milder form of the disease.
> - The progression of muscle weakness can be followed by measuring serial vital capacity and maximum mouth pressures.
> - Cardiomyopathy is common and can precipitate respiratory failure.
> - Development of kyphoscoliosis can contribute to ventilatory pump failure.
> - NIV can be used initially, but many patients ultimately require tracheotomy.
> - Corticosteroid therapy may improve muscle strength and functional capacity for a few years.

Patients are usually symptomatic early in life, usually at 2 to 3 years of age. Early presenting symptoms are gait disturbances and delayed motor development. Transient improvement may be seen between 3 and 6 years of age (honeymoon period) in DMD, followed by relentless deterioration and becoming wheelchair bound by age 13 years. In contrast, patients with BMD have a milder clinical course and usually do not become wheelchair bound until age 16 years or older. Physical examinations show limb-girdle muscle weakness and pseudohypertrophy of the calf muscles. Muscle weakness is symmetric and selectively affects the proximal and lower limb muscles first before the distal and upper extremity muscle groups. When trying to stand from the floor, affected children often use hand support to push themselves to an upright position (Gower sign). Leg pain is a prominent symptom early in the disease.

Cardiomyopathy is common and becomes clinically significant during the teenage years. In a certain variant of muscular dystrophy called X-linked dilated cardiomyopathy, heart failure occurs early on because the heart muscle is primarily involved. Cognitive impairment in areas of working memory and executive function has been reported. Intestinal hypomotility, presenting as pseudo-obstruction, is a recognized complication in DMD. This gastrointestinal manifestation is thought to be due to smooth muscle degeneration.

The diagnosis is based on myopathic symptoms and signs, a markedly increased in creatine kinase values, myopathic changes on EMG, and muscle biopsy. A positive family history also is helpful in supporting the diagnosis. The diagnosis is confirmed by a mutation of the dystrophin gene in DNA from peripheral leukocytes or by the absence of or an abnormal dystrophin gene in muscle biopsy. Despite modern respiratory care and better understanding of the abnormal pulmonary mechanics of this disease, survival after the age of 25 is rare. The most common cause of death is progressive respiratory insufficiency and heart failure due to cardiomyopathy.

In Becker muscular dystrophy, the onset of the disease is usually between the ages of 5 and 15 years and in some instances in the third to fourth decade of life. The pattern of muscle weakness is similar to DMD but milder. Cardiac and cognitive impairment are usually uncommon. Gastrointestinal involvement is usually absent. The patients usually remain ambulatory beyond 16 years and into early adulthood and live beyond the age of 30 years. Death as a result of respiratory failure and cardiomyopathy usually occurs between 30 and 60 years of age.

Pulmonary symptoms are often minimal early on despite significant weakness of the respiratory muscles. Serial pulmonary function tests and a few select ancillary procedures such as chest radiography and polysomnography can detect the severity of respiratory muscle weakness and the onset of secondary complications such as scoliosis, abnormal chest wall mechanics, atelectasis due to ineffective cough, and sleep-related breathing disorders. Measurements of FVC, PEmax, and PImax, when done correctly and in serial fashion, are simple and reproducible tests that are useful in the assessment of respiratory muscle strength. It is important to remember, however, that VC increases with growth during the first decade before it plateaus and progressively decreases and thus may mask early respiratory muscle dysfunction. After age 12 years, VC decreases by about 5% to 6% per year. Maximum inspiratory force is a more useful value during the formative years because it declines gradually despite body growth. Once the initial screening tests show respiratory muscle dysfunction, a more complete battery of pulmonary tests may be needed to further define respiratory muscle endurance, the extent of expiratory muscle weakness, selective weakness of specific respiratory muscle groups, and abnormalities in lung and chest wall mechanics. Once the FVC falls below 1 L, the median survival is 3.1 years, and the 5-year survival is only 8%.[114] An FEV_1 of less than 40% is a sensitive predictor of sleep hypoventilation. Daytime hypercapnia occurs once FEV_1 is less than 20%.[115] Kyphoscoliosis is common and may contribute to a restrictive ventilatory defect.

Maximum voluntary ventilation is useful in detecting respiratory muscle fatigue, but should be avoided in severely weakened patients. Measurement of PEmax is important because involvement of the expiratory muscles (PEmax < 60 cm H_2O) will lead to ineffective cough and inability to handle airway secretions. Because maximum inspiratory pressure measures global inspiratory muscle strength, predominant involvement of the diaphragm muscle may be missed unless transdiaphragmatic pressure is measured using a balloon catheter in the esophagus and the stomach as described previously. This procedure, however, is invasive, and many patients may not be able to tolerate it. Alternatively, weakness of the diaphragm can be inferred noninvasively by a greater than 25% decrement in VC from the seated to supine position and by fluoroscopic visualization of diaphragmatic excursion (sniff test). These noninvasive tests, however, are not sensitive enough, especially in mild diaphragm weakness.

Although respiratory muscle weakness is progressive, hypercapnia is uncommon in the absence of complicating pulmonary infections. The maintenance of alveolar ventilation in early disease suggests that patients with Duchenne muscular dystrophy have intact diaphragm function until late in the course of the disease. Once hypercapnia sets in, the course is rapidly progressive and prognosis is poor. Mean duration of survival after onset of hypercapnia is about 10 months.[116] Hypoxemia due to ventilation-perfusion inequality is common in moderate to severe disease.

Because ventilation is primarily accomplished by the diaphragm in patients with muscular dystrophy, nocturnal hypoventilation may occur especially during REM sleep, when activity of the chest wall and neck muscles is diminished. Indeed REM-induced hypoventilation has been documented even in patients with normal daytime gas exchange.[117] Sleep-related hypoxemia may contribute to respiratory insufficiency and to the development of cor pulmonale. Hypoxemia is worst during REM sleep when the contribution of the accessory muscles is abolished. Supplemental oxygen may prolong the episode of hypopnea and apnea but does not appear to be clinically significant.[118] NIV has been used successfully in patients with sleep-disordered breathing and DMD.[117–119] In a study of 10 patients with DMD who had pronounced nocturnal oxygen desaturation but normal daytime blood gas values, nocturnal NIV was successfully used to prevent nocturnal oxygen desaturation. Moreover, the progressive decline in lung function appeared to be attenuated with NIV for up to 2 years in follow-up.[117]

Corticosteroids have been shown to improve muscle strength and increase the number of years of effective ambulation as well as preventing decline in VC and PImax.[120] In a randomized, double-blind study, prednisone given at a dose of either 0.75 mg/kg per day or

1.5 mg/kg per day resulted in increased muscle strength and reduced the rate of decline of muscle weakness.[120] Improvement can usually be seen within 10 days of therapy and requires at least 0.75 mg/kg per day of prednisone. Maximal improvement is usually seen at 3 months and is sustained for about 3 years. Side effects associated with prednisone (weight gain, hypertension, behavioral changes, growth retardation, and cataracts) usually necessitate dose reduction of prednisone to 0.35 mg/kg per day.[121]

A synthetic derivative of prednisone, deflazacort, is used in Europe but is currently not available in the United States. Deflazacort may have fewer side effects compared with prednisone, especially regarding weight gain. Clinical studies showed that both deflazacort and prednisone are equally effective in slowing the decline of muscle strength and improving muscle strength and functional performance.[122] A meta-analysis of 15 studies showed that deflazacort improves strength and motor function, but its benefits over prednisone remain unclear.[123] Oxandrolone, a synthetic anabolic steroid, has also been shown to have a beneficial effect comparable with prednisone. In a large randomized controlled trial, oxandrolone significantly improved the mean change in quantitative muscle strength but not the average manual muscle strength when compared with placebo.[124]

Other treatment options that are being actively investigated include gene and stem cell therapy, aminoglycosides, creatine monohydrate, and cyclosporine. The gene mutation known as a stop codon is present in up to 15% of patients with DMD.[125] Aminoglycosides have been shown to suppress the stop codons by causing misreading of RNA, allowing insertion of different amino acids at the site of the stop codon. In the mdx mouse, treatment with gentamicin resulted in dystrophin expression at 10% to 20% of that detected in normal muscle.[125]

Ambulation should be maintained and encouraged as long as possible to retard the development of scoliosis. Surgical correction of severe scoliosis may be helpful in partially correcting the restrictive ventilatory defect, although studies show no significant improvement in respiratory function in patients who undergo spinal fusion surgery. **Table 45–5** presents guidelines for perioperative management of patients with DMD. NIV and assisted coughing techniques should be initiated before the contemplated procedure if the FVC is less than 50% and the peak cough flow less than 270 L/min.[126] Potential cardiac and gastrointestinal complications should be anticipated and treated appropriately. General physiotherapy is important in preventing contractures.

Patients with chronic neuromuscular disease are at risk for respiratory muscle fatigue because weakened respiratory muscles are working against a high elastic load to maintain the same degree of alveolar ventilation. However, the effect of respiratory muscle training is variable, with some studies reporting substantial improvement whereas other studies show minimal or no significant improvement in respiratory muscle performance.[127–129] Certainly, vigorous respiratory training could be hazardous in patients with advanced disease because it may increase the ventilatory burden on already weakened respiratory muscles. It has been reported that patients with DMD may have defective nitric oxide release during exercise, potentially causing more muscle injury during exercise.[130,131] Thus, respiratory muscle strength training is currently not recommended.[132]

Proper nutrition is important in the maintenance of respiratory muscle function; VC declines as nutritional status deteriorates. In addition, PEmax and PImax correlate with body mass in both normal and malnourished persons. High-protein, low-calorie diets aiming to achieve ideal weight may be beneficial.

TABLE 45-5 Guidelines for Perioperative Management of Patients with Duchenne Muscular Dystrophy

Before Procedure	During Procedure	After Procedure
Consult anesthesiology, pulmonary, cardiology	Succinylcholine should be avoided	Consider extubation to NIV
Measure preoperative FVC, PImax, PEmax, PCF, SpO_2; FVC <50%: consider NIV; PCF < 270 L/min: consider manual and MIE training	Options for respiratory support include endotracheal intubation, laryngeal mask airway, and NIV	Use supplemental oxygen cautiously Monitor SpO_2 and end-tidal CO_2 Look for hypoventilation, atelectasis, airway secretions
Optimize nutritional status	Consider assisted ventilation if FVC < 50%, especially if < 30%	Use manually assisted cough and MIE if PEmax is < 60 cm H_2O or PCF < 270 L/min
Discuss resuscitation parameters and advance directives, if applicable	Monitor SpO_2 or end-tidal carbon dioxide intraoperatively	Adequate pain control; if sedation and hypoventilation occur, delay extubation for 24 to 48 hours or use NIV Treat constipation and consider prokinetic agents Initiate nutritional support if extubation delayed for more than 24 to 46 hours

NIV, noninvasive ventilation; FVC, forced vital capacity; PImax, maximum inspiratory pressure; PEmax, maximum expiratory pressure; PCF, peak cough flow; SpO_2, oxygen saturation measured by pulse oximetry; MIE, maximum inspiratory effort.

Nocturnal NIV in patients with DMD has been reported to improve survival and quality of sleep, decrease daytime sleepiness, improve well-being and independence, improve gas exchange, and attenuate the rate of decline of lung function compared with non-ventilated control patients.[133–138] Assisted ventilation is required once signs of respiratory insufficiency or symptoms of sleep-related breathing disorders are present. Once VC falls to between 300 to 950 mL, or less than 50% of predicted, assisted ventilation is often required. Chronic hypercapnic respiratory failure usually develops when the VC is between 500 and 700 mL. Intermittent nasal positive pressure ventilation has been shown to prolong survival and attenuate the decline in VC and MVV in a small controlled study involving patients with advanced DMD. Successful long-term assisted ventilation has been reported in DMD.[136] Intermittent noninvasive ventilation may be used initially for chronic alveolar ventilation, but all patients eventually require positive pressure ventilation via a tracheostomy as the disease advances. Tracheostomy is eventually needed to provide access to the airway secretions in patients who are too weak to cough.

Myotonic Dystrophy

Myotonic dystrophy type 1 (MD type 1) is the most common form of hereditary muscular dystrophy in adults, with an estimated incidence of 1 in 8000. The myotonic dystrophy gene, which is transmitted in an autosomal dominant pattern, is located on the long arm of chromosome 19. The genetic defect in myotonic dystrophy is thought to be due to an amplified trinucleotide CTG repeat that encodes a serine–threonine protein kinase. In normal individuals, the two alleles contain between 5 to 50 copies of the CTG repeat. In patients with MD type 1, there are 50 to 80 copies of the CTG repeat in mildly affected or asymptomatic patients; symptomatic subjects have between 80 and 2000 or more copies. A subset of patients with myotonia and proximal muscle weakness without CTG repeat expansion on chromosome 9 is known; this condition is called myotonic dystrophy type 2, or proximal myotonic myopathy.[139]

Symptoms usually present during adolescence and early adulthood, although the syndrome may be recognized as early as infancy. The cardinal symptoms of myotonic dystrophy are myotonia (delayed relaxation after contraction), weakness and wasting affecting facial muscles and distal limb muscles, frontal balding in males, cataract, cardiomyopathy with conduction block, multiple endocrinopathies (e.g., hyperinsulinism, diabetes, adrenal insufficiency, infertility), hypersomnia, low intelligence, and dementia.

Chronic respiratory failure is common in myotonic dystrophy even in the presence of only mild limb muscle weakness.[97] This is due to the presence of several factors other than respiratory muscle weakness, such as increased respiratory elastance, low central ventilatory drive, and sleep-related breathing disorder, which act in concert to impair lung function. Moreover, myotonia of the respiratory muscles can contribute to an increased work of breathing by increasing the impedance to breathing. Weakness of the expiratory muscles is much more severe compared with the inspiratory muscles in these patients. However, weakness of the inspiratory muscles becomes severe once proximal muscle weakness becomes apparent, heralding the onset of alveolar hypoventilation.

Early studies showed a high incidence of hypercapnia and blunted ventilatory response to CO_2, suggesting abnormal central respiratory drive. However, subsequent studies have shown that these patients have either a normal or high central ventilatory drive. The abnormal ventilatory response to both hypoxia and hypercarbia has been attributed to respiratory muscle weakness and fatigue. In addition, these patients also may have a chaotic breathing pattern due to impaired afferent input from the respiratory muscles. Daytime hypersomnolence, possibly due to a low central ventilatory drive or sleep apnea, may contribute to the high prevalence of chronic hypercapnia in these patients.[97]

Patients with myotonic dystrophy are particularly susceptible to general anesthesia and respiratory depressants. Avoidance of general anesthesia and muscle relaxants is recommended. If surgery is required, postoperative respiratory monitoring is required. The presence of pharyngeal and laryngeal dysfunction manifesting as nasal speech increases the risks of aspiration. Sleep-related breathing disorders, both central and obstructive sleep apnea, are common in myotonic dystrophy. Nocturnal nasal positive pressure ventilation should be tried once hypercapnia (P_{CO_2} greater than 50 mm Hg) and hypoxemia ($Sp_{O_2} < 85\%$) occur.

Acid Maltase Deficiency

Enzymatic defects in the metabolism of carbohydrates (glycogen) lead to an abnormal accumulation of glycogen in the liver, kidney, and cardiac and skeletal muscles. **Acid maltase deficiency** (Pompe disease) is a type II glycogen storage disease that arises because of a deficiency of the lysosomal enzyme responsible for the hydrolysis of both the alpha 1-4 and alpha 1-6 linkages of the glycogen. It is a rare (1 in 40,000 births), inherited, and often fatal disorder that disables the heart and muscles. The disease presents in three clinical forms: infantile, childhood, and adult form. In adult-onset disease, the age of onset is usually after age 20 years. The syndrome typically presents with truncal and proximal limb weakness. Respiratory muscle weakness invariably leads to respiratory failure and REM-associated breathing disturbances.

Severe weakness of the diaphragm, out of proportion to limb muscle weakness, may be the predominant clinical manifestation of the disease, which results in respiratory failure. These patients are often misdiagnosed because of the presence of nonspecific symptoms of fatigue, hypersomnolence, morning headaches, and orthopnea. The diagnosis of diaphragm weakness is suspected when paradoxical motion of the abdomen on inspiration is evident, leading to additional neurologic evaluation.[98] Autopsy studies have shown predominant involvement of the proximal respiratory muscles, reflecting predominance of type 1 muscle fibers, which are less efficient in the synthesis and storage of glycogen compared with type 2 muscle fibers. Diagnostic studies reveal elevated serum muscle enzyme levels, myopathic changes on EMG, and vacuoles with glycogen content on muscle biopsy. The diagnosis is confirmed by reduced acid maltase content in muscle and urine assays. Inspiratory muscle training and a high-protein diet may be beneficial.[99,140] Enzyme replacement therapy (alglucosidase alfa) has been shown to decrease heart size, maintain normal heart function, improve muscle function, tone, and strength, and reduce glycogen accumulation.

Fascioscapulohumeral Muscular Dystrophy

Fascioscapulohumeral muscular dystrophy (FSH) is an autosomal dominant dystrophy that affects primarily the face and the proximal portion of the upper extremities. The defective gene has been localized to chromosome 4q35. In normal subjects, the number of D4Z4 repeats in chromosome 4q35 ranges from 11 to more than 100. In contrast, most patients with FSH have 1 to 10 residual repeat units within the subtelomere of chromosome 4q. This forms the basis of the genetic testing, which is positive in 95% to 98% of patients with typical FSH. It has been hypothesized that deletion of D4Z4 repeat units in chromosome 4q35 leads to overexpression of one or more disease genes. In the infantile form of FSH, the disease usually manifests very early in life and is rapidly progressive; patients are usually confined to wheelchairs by the age of 9 to 10 years. In contrast, the classic form of FSH is slowly progressive, with long periods of disease inactivity. The disease usually affects young adults between the second and third decade of life. The initial manifestations of the disease usually are difficulty in raising the arms above the head and winging of the scapula. Facial weakness is manifested by the inability to close the eyes, purse the lips, and to whistle. In 20% of patients with FSH, the disease also affects pelvic girdle and trunk muscles, which may impair respiratory function. Spirometry often shows decreased FVC, but facial weakness makes the test unreliable due to poor lip seal.

Limb-Girdle Muscular Dystrophy

Limb-girdle muscular dystrophy is a heterogeneous group of muscle dystrophies that are mainly characterized by weakness of the shoulder and pelvic girdles with sparing of the distal, facial, and extraocular muscles. The mode of inheritance is variable, but the recessive forms are the most common. Similar to other congenital myopathies, symptoms usually become evident during childhood or early adult life. Late-onset disease usually has a benign course. Creatine kinase is usually moderately elevated. EMG shows myopathic changes. Muscle biopsy reveals dystrophic changes with degeneration and regeneration of the muscle fibers, fiber splitting, internal nuclei, fibrosis, and moth-eaten and whorled fibers. Hypercapnic respiratory failure is uncommon even with moderate respiratory muscle weakness. However, bilateral paresis of the diaphragm may lead to ventilatory failure. Cardiac involvement is rare.

Mitochondrial Myopathy

Mitochondrial myopathy, one of the manifestations of hereditary mitochondrial disorders, occurs due to a point mutation in mitochondrial DNA (gene mutation at 3250). This group of mitochondrial disorders can also affect other organ systems, particularly the brain. Mitochondrial disorders that manifest polymyopathy as part of the syndrome include myoneural-gastrointestinal encephalopathy; myoclonic epilepsy with ragged red fibers (MERRF); and mitochondrial encephalomyopathy, lactic acidosis, and stroke (MELAS). The disease may present initially in childhood, but onset during adulthood has also been described. The usual clinical manifestations are symmetric proximal muscle weakness that occurs in isolation or in association with central nervous system dysfunction and metabolic derangements. Acute respiratory failure as the initial presentation of the disorder has also been reported.[141] Muscle biopsy is often required to confirm the diagnosis. Modified trichome stains show marked enlargement of the mitochondria with a reddish tinge, the so-called ragged red fibers. No specific treatment is available. The use of sedative drugs should be avoided.

Acquired Inflammatory Myopathies

Systemic Lupus Erythematosus

Systemic lupus erythematosus (SLE) is an autoimmune disease that can affect almost all organ systems. The pulmonary complications of SLE can be classified as (1) pleuritis and pleural effusions, (2) acute lupus pneumonitis, (3) interstitial lung disease, and (4) respiratory muscle weakness.

Respiratory muscle weakness and diaphragm muscle dysfunction may occur without significant limb weakness. It is estimated that up to 25% of patients with SLE have significant diaphragm weakness even in the absence of generalized myopathy. The diaphragm weakness can be apparent on the chest radiograph, which shows bilateral diaphragm elevation, called by Hoffbrand and Beck the "shrinking lung syndrome."[142]

Steroid Myopathy

Unlike the acute myopathy encountered in the ICU setting, steroid myopathy results from the prolonged use of corticosteroids (as short as 2 weeks of therapy). Myopathy can occur with any glucocorticosteroid preparation but is unusual in patients treated with less than 10 mg/day of prednisone or its equivalent. Myopathy induced by glucocorticoids is largely due to their direct catabolic effects and interference with insulin-like growth factor-1 signaling, which leads to increased myocyte apoptosis. It usually manifests subacutely as proximal limb and girdle muscle weakness. Thus, affected patients have difficulty combing their hair, reaching overhead for an object, and climbing stairs. Muscle enzyme levels are usually normal. EMG is either normal or reveals only slight myopathic changes. Muscle biopsy usually shows loss of type IIa muscle fibers with no evidence of inflammation or fiber necrosis. There is a poor correlation between the total dose of steroids given and the severity of muscle weakness. A gradual improvement in muscle strength is usually observed with discontinuation or significant reduction in corticosteroid dosage.

Treatment of Neuromuscular Dysfunction

Specific medical therapies for each of the neuromuscular disorders have been discussed previously. The proper care of these complicated patients often requires a multidisciplinary team of healthcare workers consisting of pulmonary specialists, respiratory therapists, pulmonary trained nurses, physiatrists, physical therapists, nutritionists, social workers, and clinical psychologists. Depending on the acuity of care required in an individual case, patients can be initially treated in an ICU setting until the resolution of their acute illness and then transferred to a respiratory rehabilitation unit specializing in the care of these patients. Frequent family interaction with the healthcare team is beneficial to facilitate the transition of care from the hospital to home. It is helpful to admit patients with stable chronic respiratory failure to a noninvasive respiratory rehabilitation unit for a few days to familiarize them with the different types of noninvasive ventilator support available in a relaxed and supportive environment.

> **RESPIRATORY RECAP**
>
> **Treatment of Neuromuscular Dysfunction**
>
> » Respiratory muscle training may be helpful.
> » Assisted coughing techniques are useful in clearance of airway secretions.
> » Glossopharyngeal breathing (frog breathing) allows short periods of spontaneous ventilation in ventilator-dependent patients.
> » Noninvasive ventilation includes positive and negative pressure devices, rocking beds, and pneumobelts.
> » Diaphragmatic pacing is an option in ventilator dependent patients with high cervical cord injury.

The goals of therapy in the treatment of patients with chronic neuromuscular diseases are similar to those for other groups of patients with chronic lung disease: to maintain lung function and to restore independent and functional lifestyle for as long as possible. Clearly, some patients with advanced disease will not be able to achieve these goals. Nevertheless, a rapid decline in lung function may be avoided by following judicious pulmonary rehabilitation techniques such as the use of respiratory aid devices to facilitate clearance of airway secretions, early use of noninvasive ventilation to augment alveolar ventilation, especially during periods of acute decline, and the timely treatment of respiratory infections with appropriate antibiotics. Maintenance of proper nutrition is of utmost importance. Both obesity and undernutrition can further contribute to respiratory muscle dysfunction. The decreased chest wall compliance observed in obese patients will lead to an increased work of breathing and may induce respiratory muscle fatigue in already weakened respiratory muscles. On the other hand, undernutrition has also been shown to decrease respiratory muscle strength in a variety of chronic lung diseases.

Respiratory Muscle Training

Respiratory muscle training improves strength and ventilatory endurance in normal subjects and in patients with pulmonary diseases. The clinical benefits of regular exercise training aim specifically toward increasing ventilatory capacity and facilitating the clearance of airway secretions in patients with chronic neuromuscular diseases. Uncontrolled studies performed in patients with muscular dystrophy have shown that inspiratory muscle training may improve respiratory muscle endurance and strength.[99,143] In a prospective, controlled trial of 19 patients with DMD, 9 patients who received respiratory muscle training 30 minutes a day, 5 days a week, for 2 months showed no significant improvements in VC or in PImax and PEmax values at the end of the 2-month training period compared with baseline; however, both increased inspiratory and expiratory times during loaded breathing suggested an improvement in respiratory muscle endurance.[144] In contrast, studies looking at the effect of inspiratory resistive training in tetraplegic patients showed an improvement in inspiratory muscle strength and endurance after 6 to 16 weeks of exercise.[145,146] Furthermore, 6 weeks of pectoralis muscle isometric training significantly increased expiratory reserve volume in C6 through C8 tetraplegic patients.[33] The increase in expiratory reserve volume in these patients may have improved effective cough and diminished the incidence of lower respiratory tract infections.

Concerns have been raised about the potential detrimental effects of respiratory muscle training in patients with advanced neuromuscular weakness. Breathing through resistive loads may potentially lead to muscle fiber damage and fatigue already weakened respiratory muscles. Moreover, no study has correlated any improvement in respiratory mechanics with an improvement in

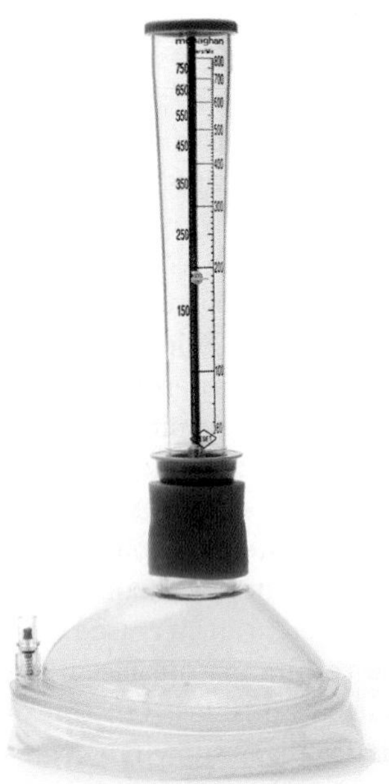

FIGURE 45–10 Peak cough flow meter with an air-cushion face mask.

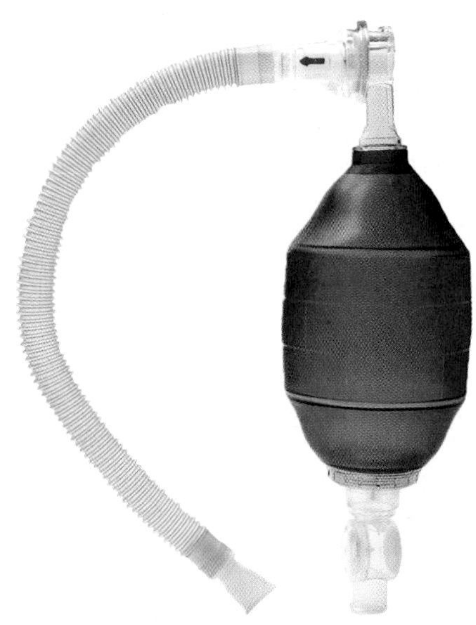

FIGURE 45–11 Resuscitator bag, one-way valve, flexible tube, and mouthpiece for manual hyperinflation.

clinical outcome. Thus, the beneficial effect of respiratory muscle training remains unresolved.

Assisted Coughing

Effective mucus clearance depends on the mucociliary escalator and cough. Cough is usually the limiting function in patients with a neuromuscular dysfunction. This may result from ineffectiveness in phase 1, phase 2, or both phases, depending on the pathology. A weakness of inspiratory muscles such as the diaphragm will limit inspiratory volume. A weakness in abdominal muscles will limit the effect of compressing gas in the lungs. When the peak cough flow is less than 160 L/min (**Figure 45–10**), the patient needs assistance in clearing secretions. Modalities that assist the patient with an ineffective cough include hyperinflation, quad cough, insufflator/exsufflator cough assist, and mechanical aspiration.

Spontaneous cough efforts can be improved in patients with weak inspiratory muscle strength using manual or mechanical insufflation. Manual hyperinflation can be administered using a resuscitator bag with a one-way valve and mouthpiece (**Figure 45–11**). A series of breath-stacking maneuvers is applied until the lungs are maximally insufflated. Mechanical insufflation can also be administered mechanically using volume control ventilation with a mouthpiece. The stored elastic recoil energy of the lungs may produce a peak cough flow sufficient to clear secretions.

The cough assist (insufflator/exsufflator) inflates the lungs with a positive pressure and then produces a negative pressure to create a peak cough flow great enough to clear secretions. Positive and negative pressures between 10 and 60 cm H_2O are selected according to patient tolerance and the effectiveness of the treatments. Inhalation and exhalation times of 1 to 3 seconds and a pause of 0 to 5 seconds may be selected. The ability of the patient to tolerate the settings and the effectiveness of the therapy will dictate the best settings. Most patients will need an oronasal mask as the patient interface if they cannot tighten their lips on a mouthpiece. If a mouthpiece is used, a nose clip will also be necessary. The cough assist can also be attached to a tracheostomy tube.

The quad cough is used to strengthen the patient's cough efforts. The clinician places the thumb of each hand below the xiphoid process, with all fingers placed below the ribs. The patient takes a deep inhalation and coughs on exhalation. The clinician pushes in and up as the patient coughs. Quad cough can be combined with hyperinflation or the cough assist (insufflator/exsufflator).

If the patient has excessive airway secretions, airway clearance therapies such as postural drainage, high-frequency chest wall compression, positive expiratory pressure (PEP), and oscillatory PEP can be used. However, the effectiveness of these therapies is often limited for patients with neuromuscular dysfunction. Inhaled bronchodilators have limited value in patients with neuromuscular disease unless the patient also has pulmonary disease such as asthma. Tracheal suction is useful in some patients with a tracheostomy tube, but nasotracheal suction is not usually indicated. In patients with bulbar disease and poor swallowing function, oral suction is helpful.

Glossopharyngeal Assistance

Glossopharyngeal breathing, also known as frog breathing, is a technique involving the use of oropharyngeal muscles to inject air into the trachea and thus augment

TABLE 45–6 Indications for Mechanical Ventilation in Patients with Neuromuscular Disorders

Acute respiratory failure	Severe dyspnea Marked accessory muscle use Inability to handle secretions Unstable hemodynamic status Hypoxemia refractory to supplemental O_2 Acute respiratory acidosis
Chronic respiratory failure	
Nocturnal hypoventilation	Morning headache Lethargy Nightmares Enuresis
Nocturnal oxygen desaturation	$SpO_2 < 88\%$ despite supplemental O_2
Cor pulmonale	Due to hypoventilation with $PaCO_2 > 45$ mm Hg, pH < 7.32

TABLE 45–7 Comparisons of Clinical Factors Favoring Invasive Versus Noninvasive Mechanical Ventilation in Patients with Neuromuscular Disease

Invasive Ventilation (Endotracheal Intubation)	Noninvasive Ventilation
Copious secretions Poor airway control Inability to tolerate or failure of noninvasive ventilation Impaired cognition Unstable hemodynamics	Awake, cooperative patient Good airway control Minimal secretions Hemodynamic stability

ventilation to provide short periods of spontaneous ventilation, improve effective cough, and increase the volume of the voice. With this technique, the patient gulps in air by lowering and raising the tongue against the palate in a pistonlike fashion, thereby injecting air into the trachea. With practice, patients may be able to gulp in 50 to 150 mL of air every half second. With six to eight successive gulps, a tidal volume of approximately 500 to 600 mL may be achieved and sustained for several hours, thus liberating the patient from ventilatory support. Although some patients have difficulty in learning and mastering the technique, patients with spinal cord injuries, postpolio syndrome, and other neuromuscular diseases have successfully used this technique.

Mechanical Ventilation

Although ventilatory insufficiency leading to chronic respiratory failure is a common sequela of progressive neuromuscular diseases, acute respiratory failure is commonly seen after aspiration pneumonia, lower respiratory tract infections, or other acute illnesses that place an additional burden on already compromised ventilatory reserve. Pneumonia is the most common cause of increased morbidity and mortality in patients with advanced chronic neuromuscular disease. Once impending respiratory failure is recognized, mechanical ventilation should be used early to support spontaneous breathing until the acute precipitating event is identified and treated. **Table 45–6** lists the indications for mechanical ventilation.

In patients who present with severe dyspnea, acute hypercapnia with respiratory acidosis, moderate to severe hypoxemia, and hemodynamic instability, translaryngeal intubation and mechanical ventilation is often necessary and is preferred over noninvasive mechanical ventilation. In some clinical situations, NIV may be used to augment minute ventilation in patients who present with acute hypercapnic respiratory failure who remain alert and cooperative, with intact upper airway function and minimal airway secretions. **Table 45–7** compares invasive ventilation and NIV.

In patients who present with chronic respiratory failure or acute or chronic respiratory failure due to progression of their underlying neuromuscular disorder, NIV has been effective in reversing hypercapnia and hypoxemia and is the treatment of choice because of patient comfort, effectiveness, and portability. Moreover, NIV has been shown to decrease the incidence of pneumonia and reduce hospitalization rates in a survey of 654 patients with neuromuscular diseases with up to 20 years of follow-up.[147] In this group of patients, the manifestation of chronic respiratory insufficiency may be subtle, with the onset of dyspnea occurring gradually over days to weeks. Common complaints include lethargy, fatigue, daytime sleepiness, morning headache, and occasionally nightmares and enuresis. These patients often have nocturnal hypercapnia with normal arterial gas values during daytime. Nocturnal oximetry or polysomnogram may be indicated to detect the presence of nocturnal oxygen desaturation and hypercapnia, which may contribute to daytime symptoms. The presence of nocturnal hypoventilation usually leads to chronic hypercapnia and progressive symptoms of respiratory failure within 2 years. In a randomized controlled trial of 26 patients with nocturnal hypercapnia and daytime normocapnia, nocturnal NIV decreased the severity of hypercapnia and improved arterial oxygen saturation. In patients who were randomized to the control group, 9 of 10 required NIV for daytime hypercapnia after a mean follow-up of 8.3 months.[134]

Noninvasive mechanical ventilation can be divided into noninvasive positive pressure ventilation and noninvasive negative pressure ventilation. **Table 45–8** lists the benefits and limitations of both forms of NIV. Noninvasive positive pressure ventilation is preferred over negative pressure ventilation because of ease of use, portability, and maintenance of upper airway patency during sleep. In addition, noninvasive positive pressure provides

TABLE 45–8 Advantages and Disadvantages of Positive and Negative Pressure Ventilation Used in Patients with Neuromuscular Disease

Type	Advantages	Disadvantages
Negative pressure ventilators (tank, pulmowrap, cuirass)	Dependable Airway cannulation not required Minimal hemodynamic effect Maintenance of speech	Cumbersome Predispose to obstructive apnea Limit nursing care Controlled ventilation
Positive pressure by mask or mouthpiece	Avoids upper airway obstruction Pressure preset, compensates leak Patient-initiated machine breaths	Aerophagia Pressure sores Leaks Problems with interface

better maintenance of alveolar ventilation and airway stability during sleep. Different types of masks may be used (e.g., nasal, oronasal, full face mask) depending on patient comfort and preference. In patients with significant mouth air leaks, the use of a chin strap or changing to an oronasal or total face mask will often solve the problem.[148–151] In chronic NIV use, facial ulcers may rarely develop due to contact pressure from a particular mask interface. In this situation, using two different mask interfaces and rotating their use may promote healing of the facial ulcers and prevent recurrence. Alternatively, mouthpiece interfaces—either a generic mouthpiece with a plastic lip seal or one custom fitted by orthodontics—have been used to administer continuous ventilatory support in some patients.[152]

A wide variety of positive pressure ventilators may be used to deliver NIV. In the intensive care setting, use of a standard ICU ventilator allows either continuous mandatory ventilation or pressure support mode. Some features that are available in standard ventilators that are useful in the acute care setting are the ability to monitor respiratory pattern and to supply supplemental oxygen. In patients with stable chronic respiratory failure, portable bilevel ventilators are widely used.

The initial ventilator settings should be low and slowly increased to achieve an increase in tidal volume of 30% to 50% and/or a decrease in $Paco_2$ of 5 to 10 mm Hg. The expiratory airway pressure during present bilevel ventilation is usually set at 4 cm H_2O or greater to minimize rebreathing, increase functional residual capacity, or counterbalance auto-PEEP. Supplemental oxygen can be titrated into the circuit of the bilevel ventilator.

The duration of ventilatory assistance depends on the severity of respiratory failure and patient tolerance. In the acute setting, ventilatory assistance of 20 hours or more may be needed. In the chronic setting, patients use NIV during the daytime for a few hours followed by nocturnal use of 6 to 8 hours once they become accustomed to the NIV settings. A Cochrane review that included eight randomized or quasi-randomized controlled studies on the efficacy of nocturnal mechanical ventilation for chronic hypoventilation in patients with neuromuscular and chest wall disorders concluded that NIV resulted in short-term improvement of symptoms of chronic hypoventilation, daytime hypercapnia, and nocturnal mean oxygen saturation compared with no ventilation. In three studies in which 1-year mortality rate was reported, the estimated risk of death following nocturnal ventilation was significantly reduced. The survival advantage of NIV was shown only in patients with ALS.[133]

Negative pressure ventilators intermittently apply subatmospheric pressures to the thorax and abdomen to increase transpulmonary pressure and inflate the lungs. The efficacy of negative pressure ventilation is determined by thoracic and abdominal compliance and the surface area over which the negative pressure is applied. Tank ventilators are the most efficient form of negative pressure ventilation because of the amount of body surface area covered compared with cuirass ventilators, which cover only the upper torso. Tank ventilators are reliable, but they are seldom used today because they are large, cumbersome, have the potential to induce claustrophobia, and interfere with nursing care. Chest cuirass ventilators are more portable than tank ventilators but must be used in the recumbent position to be effective. A limitation to all forms of negative pressure ventilators is that they may induce obstructive sleep apnea due to upper airway collapse during a mechanically delivered breath.

In patients with mild to moderate ventilatory failure, rocking beds and pneumobelts may be used, depending on patient preference, comfort, and the amount of ventilatory support required by the individual patient. These devices act as abdominal displacement devices that augment diaphragmatic motion by displacing abdominal viscera against gravity. The rocking bed consists of a mattress on a motorized platform that rocks in an arc of 40 degrees with the patient recumbent. As the bed moves with the head dependent, gravity induces the abdominal contents and diaphragm to move cranially, assisting exhalation. In the next cycle, as the bed tilts upward, gravity acts to move the diaphragm and abdominal contents in a caudad direction, assisting inspiration. The bed rocks between 12 to 24 times per minute and may be adjusted to optimize patient comfort so as to achieve the desired minute ventilation. The pneumobelt is an inflatable bladder that is worn over the anterior abdomen and is connected to a positive ventilator that intermittently inflates it. With the patient seated upright, bladder inflation increases intra-abdominal pressure, forcing the diaphragm cephalad and thereby inducing active exhalation. When the bladder deflates, gravity moves the abdominal contents and diaphragm caudally, thereby facilitating passive inspiration.

Both devices are limited by their constraint on patients and posture and the amount of ventilatory assistance they provide. The rocking bed is bulky and stationary. Similarly, the pneumobelt requires that the patient use it in the upright posture, and some patients complain of pain and discomfort when high bladder inflation pressures are required to sufficiently augment ventilation.

With the increasing popularity of NIV, several studies have showed impressive improvements in daytime gas exchange even though NIV was given only at night or intermittently throughout the 24-hour period. At the end of 3 months of NIV, the Pa_{O_2} increased by approximately 15 mm Hg while Pa_{CO_2} decreased by approximately 14 mm Hg.[133,134,150,152] Moreover, these patients had a significant improvement in their symptoms and functional capacity. The exact mechanisms responsible for the improvement of daytime gas exchange in patients with neuromuscular diseases using chronic intermittent noninvasive ventilation are unknown. Some of the proposed mechanisms are that (1) intermittent ventilatory assistance rests already fatigued respiratory muscles; (2) the Pa_{CO_2} central threshold is reset by preventing nocturnal alveolar hypoventilation; (3) ventilation-perfusion matching is improved; and that (4) the higher lung volume achieved during assisted ventilation improves lung and chest wall compliance, which decreases the work of breathing.

Diaphragmatic Pacing

Diaphragmatic pacing consists of a radio frequency transmitter and an antenna that discharges signals to a receiver to transmit electrical impulses to an electrode placed over the phrenic nerve or directly on the diaphragm in some cases. Both the electrodes and receiver are surgically implanted. Electrode implantation around the phrenic nerves can be divided via a cervical and thoracic approach; however, the thoracic approach is preferred to ensure stimulation of all phrenic nerve roots while avoiding the brachial plexus. The subcutaneous receiver is usually placed in the lower anterolateral rib cage to allow it to be superficial, but placed in an area where soft tissue movement is limited.

The group of patients who appear to benefit most from this technology are ventilator-dependent patients following high cervical cord injury. The central nervous system injury must be above the second or third cervical level, above the origin of the phrenic nerve root. Approximately one-third of patients with this type of injury may be suitable for this type of treatment. Potential candidates for diaphragmatic pacing include patients with complete upper cervical injuries leading to apnea, those with some types of central sleep apnea such as congenital central alveolar hypoventilation syndrome, and those with brain stem tumors or infarction. In addition, candidates should have normal cognitive function, complete respiratory muscle paralysis without recovery for 3 months, and viable phrenic nerves. Contraindications to diaphragmatic pacing include failure of the diaphragm to contract with percutaneous stimulation of the phrenic nerves, coma, and severe primary pulmonary disease. A period of diaphragm conditioning is necessary in patients who have had no diaphragm function for more than 6 months. Successful implantation and conditioning of the diaphragm allows the patients to be independent from ventilator support for prolonged periods of time and enables them to regain speech and olfaction.[153]

In retrospective studies of patients with ventilatory failure due to high spinal cord injury, brain stem injury, and congenital central alveolar hypoventilation, long-term diaphragm pacing full time was well tolerated in carefully selected patients.[153–155] In a study of 50 adult patients with high spinal cord injuries, direct diaphragm stimulation by a device inserted via laparoscopic technique was successful in liberating the patients from the ventilator for at least 4 hours each day in 96% of cases. For patients with ALS, diaphragmatic pacing delayed the need for mechanical ventilation for up to 2 years.[156] The widespread use of diaphragmatic pacing is limited by its high cost, the potential for sudden failure of the hardware, the development of upper airway obstruction, and the induction of diaphragm fatigue.

KEY POINTS

- Neuromuscular diseases impair the pump function of the respiratory muscles, leading to chronic respiratory failure or failure to wean from mechanical ventilation.
- Severe respiratory muscle weakness may occur in the absence of clinical symptoms.
- Measurements of static respiratory muscle strength and vital capacity help predict impending respiratory failure.
- Sleep-related breathing disorders and nocturnal oxygen desaturation may occur and often precede changes in daytime gas exchange abnormalities.
- A strong clinical suspicion is often required for the proper diagnosis and treatment of neuromuscular diseases.
- Upper motor neuron lesions include stroke, spinal cord injury, Parkinson disease, and multiple sclerosis.
- Lower motor neuron lesions include amyotrophic lateral sclerosis, poliomyelitis, and postpoliomyelitis muscular dystrophy.
- Disorders of peripheral nerves include phrenic nerve injury, Guillain-Barré syndrome, and critical illness polyneuropathy.

- Disorders of the neuromuscular junction include myasthenia gravis, Lambert-Eaton syndrome, and botulism.
- Inherited myopathies include Duchenne muscular dystrophy, Becker muscular dystrophy, myotonic dystrophy, acid maltase deficiency, fascioscapulohumeral muscular dystrophy, limb-girdle muscular dystrophy, and mitochondrial myopathy.
- Acquired inflammatory myopathies include systemic lupus erythematosus, acute ICU steroid myopathy, and chronic steroid myopathy.
- NIV is the preferred mode of ventilatory assistance in patients with respiratory insufficiency who have intact bulbar function.

REFERENCES

1. Votto J, Brancifort J, Scalise P, Wollschlager C, Zwillich CW. COPD and other diseases in chronically ventilated patients in a prolonged respiratory care unit. *Chest.* 1998;113:86–90.
2. Johnson DC, Kazemi H. Central control of ventilation in neuromuscular disease. *Clin Chest Med.* 1994;15(4):607–617.
3. Spinelli A, Marconi G, Gorini M, Pizzi A, Scano G. Control of breathing in patients with myasthenia gravis. *Am Rev Respir Dis.* 1992;145:1359–1366.
4. Vincken WG, Gauthier SG, Dollfuss RE, Hanson RE, Darauay CM, Cosio MG. Involvement of upper airway muscles in extrapyramidal disorders: a cause of airflow limitation. *N Engl J Med.* 1984;311:438–442.
5. Vincken W, Ellecker G, Cosio M. Detection of upper airway muscle involvement in neuromuscular disorders using flow-volume loop. *Chest.* 1986;90:52–57.
6. Mier-Jedrzejowicz A, Green M. Respiratory muscle weakness associated with cerebellar atrophy. *Am Rev Respir Dis.* 1988;137:673–677.
7. Baydur A. Respiratory muscle strength and control of ventilation in patients with neuromuscular disease. *Chest.* 1991;99:330–338.
8. Begin R, Bureau MA, Lupien L, et al. Control of breathing in Duchenne's muscular dystrophy. *Am J Med.* 1980;69:227–234.
9. Paton W, Aaimia E. The action of tubocurarine and of decamethonium on respiratory and other muscles in the cat. *J Physiol.* 1951;112:311–331.
10. Holle R, Shoene R, Pavlin E. Effect of respiratory muscle weakness in $P_{0.01}$ induced by partial curarization. *J Appl Physiol.* 1984;57:1150–1157.
11. Demedts M, Beckers J, Rochette F, Bulcke J. Pulmonary function in moderate neuromuscular disease without respiratory complaints. *Eur J Respir Dis.* 1982;63:62–67.
12. Vincken W, Elleker MG, Cosio M. Determinants of respiratory muscle weakness in stable neuromuscular disorders. *Am J Med.* 1987;82:53–58.
13. Toussaint M, Steens M, Soudon P. Lung function accurately predicts hypercapnia in patients with Duchenne muscular dystrophy. *Chest.* 2007;131:368–375.
14. De Troyer A, Borenstein S, Cordier R. Analysis of lung volume restriction in patients with respiratory muscle weakness. *Thorax.* 1980;35:603–610.
15. Estenne M, Heilporn A, Delhez L, Yernault J, De Troyer A. Chest wall stiffness in patients with chronic respiratory muscle weakness. *Am Rev Respir Dis.* 1983;128:1002–1007.
16. Gibson GJ, Pride NB, Newsom D, Loh LC. Pulmonary mechanics in patients with respiratory muscle weakness. *Am Rev Respir Dis.* 1977;115:389–395.
17. Becker H, Piper A, Flynn W, et al. Breathing during sleep in patients with nocturnal desaturation. *Am J Respir Crit Care Med.* 1999;159:112–118.
18. Bye PTP, Ellis ER, Issa FG, Donnelly PM, Sullivan CE. Respiratory failure and sleep in neuromuscular disease. *Thorax.* 1990;45:241–247.
19. Ragette R, Mellies U, Schwake C, et al. Patterns and predictors of sleep disordered breathing in primary myopathies. *Thorax.* 2002;57:724–728.
20. Goldstein R, Molotiu N, Skrastins R, et al. Reversal of sleep-induced hypoventilation and chronic respiratory failure by nocturnal negative pressure ventilation in patients with restrictive ventilatory impairment. *Am Rev Respir Dis.* 1987;135:1049–1055.
21. Schmidt-Nowara W, Marder E, Feil P. Respiratory failure in myasthenia gravis due to vocal cord paralysis. *Arch Neurol.* 1984;41:567.
22. Vincken W, Elleker MG, Cosio MG. Flow-volume loop changes reflecting respiratory muscle weakness in chronic neuromuscular changes. *Am J Med.* 1987;83:673–680.
23. Aboussouan L, Khan S, Meeker D, et al. Effect of noninvasive positive pressure ventilation on survival in amyotrophic lateral sclerosis. *Ann Intern Med.* 1997;6:450–453.
24. Braun NMT, Arora NS, Rochester DF. Respiratory muscle and pulmonary function in polymyosities and other proximal myopathies. *Thorax.* 1983;38:616–623.
25. Laporta D, Grassino A. Assessment of transdiaphragmatic pressure in humans. *J Appl Physiol.* 1996;58:1469–1476.
26. Mier A, Brophy C, Moxham J, Green M. Twitch pressures in the assessment of diaphragm weakness. *Thorax.* 1989;44:990–996.
27. Vingerhoets F, Bogousslavsky J. Respiratory dysfunction in stroke. *Clin Chest Med.* 1994;15(4):729–737.
28. Scanlon PD, Loring SH, Pichurko BM, et al. Respiratory mechanics in acute quadriplegia. *Am Rev Respir Dis.* 1989;139:615–620.
29. Estenne M, De Troyer A. Mechanism of the postural dependence of vital capacity in tetraplegic subjects. *Am Rev Respir Dis.* 1987;135:367–371.
30. Fishburn MJ, Marino RJ, Ditunno JF. Atelectasis and pneumonia in acute spinal cord injury. *Arch Phys Med Rehabil.* 1990;71:197–200.
31. De Vivo MJ, Kartus PL, Stover SL, Rutt RD, Fine PR. Cause of death for patients with spinal cord injuries. *Arch Intern Med.* 1989;149:1761–1766.
32. De Troyer A, Estenne M, Heilporn A. Mechanism of active expiration in tetraplegic subjects. *N Engl J Med.* 1986;314:740–744.
33. Estenne M, Knoop C, Vanvaerenbergh J, Heilporn A, De Troyer A. The effect of pectoralis muscle training in tetraplegic subjects. *Am Rev Respir Dis.* 1989;139:1218–1222.
34. Bogaard JM, Hovestadt A, Meerwaldt J, Meche FGA, Stigt J. Maximal expiratory and inspiratory flow-volume curves in Parkinson's disease. *Am Rev Respir Dis.* 1989;139:610–614.
35. Estenne M, Hubert M, De Troyer A. Respiratory muscle involvement in Parkinson's disease. *N Engl J Med.* 1984;311:1516–1517.
36. Vincken WG, Darauay CM, Cosio MG. Reversibility of upper airway obstruction after levodopa therapy in Parkinson's disease. *Chest.* 1989;96:210–212.
37. Mehta AD, Wright WB, Kirby BJ. Ventilatory function in Parkinson's disease. *BMJ.* 1978;1:1456–1457.
38. Carter JL, Noseworthy JH. Ventilatory dysfunction in multiple sclerosis. *Clin Chest Med.* 1994;15:693–703.
39. Howard RS, Wiles CM, Hirsch NP. Respiratory involvement in multiple sclerosis. *Brain.* 1992;115:479
40. Kuwahira I, Kondo T, Ohta Y, et al. Acute respiratory failure in multiple sclerosis. *Chest.* 1990;97:246
41. Balbierz J, Ellenberg M, Honet J. Complete hemidiaphragmatic paralysis in a patient with multiple sclerosis. *Am J Phys Med Rehabil.* 1988;67:161
42. Smeltzer S, Utell M, Rudick R, et al. Respiratory function in multiple sclerosis. *Arch Neurol.* 1988;45:1245.

43. Carter JL, Rodriquez M. Immunosuppressive treatment of multiple sclerosis. *Mayo Clin Proc.* 1984;64:664.
44. Weiner HL, Dau PC, Khatri BO, et al. Double-blind study of true vs. sham plasma exchange in patients treated with immunosuppression for acute attacks of multiple sclerosis. *Neurology.* 1989;39:1143–1149.
45. Bach J, Alba A, Saporito L. Intermittent positive pressure ventilation via the mouth as an alternative to tracheostomy for 257 ventilator users. *Chest.* 1993;103:174–182.
46. Splaingard M, Frates R, Jefferson L, et al. Home negative pressure ventilation: report of 20 years of experience in patients with neuromuscular disease. *Arch Phys Med Rehabil.* 1985;66:239–243.
47. Fromm GB, Wisdom PJ, Block AJ. Amyotrophic lateral sclerosis presenting with respiratory failure. *Chest.* 1977;71:612–614.
48. Carre PC, Didier AP, Tiberge YM, Arbus LJ, Leophonte PJ. Amyotrophic lateral sclerosis presenting with sleep hypopnea syndrome. *Chest.* 1988;93:1309–1312.
49. Black LF, Hyatt RE. Maximal static respiratory pressures in generalized neuromuscular disease. *Am Rev Respir Dis.* 1971;103:641–649.
50. Kreitzer SM, Saunders NA, Tyler HR, Ingram RH. Respiratory muscle function in amytrophic lateral sclerosis. *Am Rev Respir Dis.* 1978;117:437–447.
51. Bourke SC, Tomlinson M, Williams TL, Bullock RE, Shaw PJ, Gibson GJ. Effects of non-invasive ventilation on survival and quality of life in patients with amyothrophic lateral sclerosis: a randomized controlled trial. *Lancet Neuro.* 2006;5;140–147.
52. Silverstein M, Stocking C, Antel J. Amyotrophic lateral sclerosis and life-sustaining therapy: patients' desires for information, participation in decision making, and life-sustaining therapy. *Mayo Clin Proc.* 1991;66:906–913.
53. Kleopa K, Sherman M, Neal B, Neal B, Heiman-Patterson T. Bipap improves survival and rate of pulmonary function decline in patients with ALS. *J Neuro Sci.* 1999;164:82–88.
54. Schiffman PL, Belsh JM. Effect of inspiratory resistance and theophylline on respiratory muscle strength in patients with amyotrophic lateral sclerosis. *Am Rev Respir Dis.* 1989;139:1418–1423.
55. Dalakas MC, Elder G, Hallett M, et al. A long term follow-up study of patients with post-poliomyelitis neuromuscular symptoms. *N Engl J Med.* 1986;314:959–963.
56. Cashman N, Maselli R, Wollman R, Roos R, Simon R, Antel J. Late denervation in patients with antecedent paralytic poliomyelitis. *N Engl J Med.* 1981;317:7–12.
57. Perry J, Barnes G, Gronley J. The postpolio syndrome: an overuse phenomenon. *Clin Orthop Related Res.* 1988;223:145–162.
58. Deans E, Ross J, Road JD, Courtenay L, Madill KJ. Pulmonary function in individuals with a history of poliomyelitis. *Chest.* 1991;100:118–123.
59. Bach JR, Alba AS, Bohatiuk G, Saporito L, Lee M. Mouth intermittent positive pressure ventilation in the management of postpolio respiratory insufficiency. *Chest.* 1987;91:859–864.
60. Curran FJ, Colbert AP. Ventilator management in Duchenne muscular dystrophy and post-myelitis syndrome: a twelve years' experience. *Arch Phys Med Rehabil.* 1989;70:180–185.
61. Hill R, Robbins AW, Messing R, Arora NS. Sleep apnea syndrome after poliomyelitis. *Am Rev Respir Dis.* 1983;127:129–131.
62. Dean A, Graham B, Dalakas M, Sato S. Sleep apnea in patients with postpolio syndrome. *Ann Neurol.* 1998;43:661–664.
63. Hsu A, Staats B. "Postpolio" sequelae and sleep-related disordered breathing. *Mayo Clin Proc.* 1998;73(3):216–224.
64. Canon S, Ritter FN. Vocal cord paralysis after post-myelitis syndrome. *Laryngoscope.* 1987;97:981–983.
65. Solliday N, Gaensler E, Schwaber J, Parker T. Impaired central chemoreceptor function and chronic hypoventilation many years following poliomyelitis. *Respiration.* 1974;31:177–192.
66. Pandit A, Kalra S, Woolcock A. An unusual cause of bilateral diaphragm paralysis. *Thorax.* 1992;47:201.
67. Large B, Heywood LJ, Flower CD, Cory-Pearce R, Wallwork J, English TAH. Incidence and aetiology of a raised hemidiaphragm after cardiopulmonary bypass. *Thorax.* 1985;40:444–447.
68. Markand ON, Moorthy SS, Mahomed Y, King RD, Brown JW. Postoperative phrenic nerve palsy in patients with open-heart surgery. *Thorax.* 1985;35:603–610.
69. Chan CK, Loke J, Virgulto JA, Mohsenin V, Ferranti R, Lammertse T. Bilateral diaphragmatic paralysis: clinical spectrum, prognosis, and diagnostic approach. *Arch Phys Med Rehabil.* 1988;69:976–979.
70. Mier-Jedrzejowicz A, Brophy C, Moxham J, Green M. Assessment of diaphragm weakness. *Am Rev Respir Dis.* 1988;137: 877–883.
71. Laroche CM, Carroll N, Moxham J, Green M. Clinical significance of severe isolated diaphragm weakness. *Am Rev Respir Dis.* 1988;138:862–866.
72. DeVita MA, Robinson LR, Rehder J, Hattler B, Cohen C. Incidence and natural history of phrenic nerve neuropathy occurring during open heart surgery. *Chest.* 1993;103:850–856.
73. Asbury A, Cornblath D. Assessment of current diagnostic criteria for Guillain-Barré syndrome. *Ann Neurol.* 1990;27(suppl):S21–S24.
74. Gracey DR, McMihan JC, Divertie MB, Howard FM. Respiratory failure in Guillain-Barré syndrome. *Mayo Clin Proc.* 1982;57:742–746.
75. Ropper AH. The Guillain-Barré syndrome. *N Engl J Med.* 1992;326(6):1130–1136.
76. Orlikowski D, Sharshar T, Porcher R, Annane D, Raphael JC, Clair B. Prognosis and risk factors of early onset pneumonia in ventilated patients with Guillain-Barré syndrome. *Intensive Care Med.* 2006;32:1962–1969.
77. Borel CO, Tilford C, Nichols DG, Hanley DF, Traystman RJ. Diaphragmatic performance during recovery from acute ventilatory failure in Guillain-Barré syndrome and myasthenia gravis. *Chest.* 1991;99:444–451.
78. Chevrolet J, Deleamont P. Repeated vital capacity measurements as predictive parameters for mechanical ventilation need and weaning success in the Guillain-Barré syndrome. *Am Rev Respir Dis.* 1991;144:814–818.
79. Guillain-Barré Syndrome Study Group. Plasmapheresis and acute Guillain-Barré syndrome. *Neurology.* 1985;35:1096–1104.
80. French Cooperative Group on Plasma Exchange in Guillain-Barré Syndrome. Efficiency of plasma exchange in Guillain-Barré syndrome: role of replacement fluids. *Ann Neurol.* 1987;22:753–761.
81. van der Meche FGA, Schmitz PIM, The Dutch Guillain-Barré Study Group. A randomized trial comparing intravenous immune globulin and plasma exchange in Guillain-Barré syndrome. *N Engl J Med.* 1992;326:1123–1129.
82. Hughes RAC, Swan AC, van Koningsveld R, van Doorn P. Corticosteroids for Guillain-Barré syndrome. *Cochrane Database Syst Rev.* 2007;(4):16625544.
83. Hughes RAC, Swan AV, Raphael JC, Annane D, Koningsveld RV, van Dorn PA. Immunotherapy for Guillain-Barré syndrome: a systematic review. *Brain.* 2007;130:2245–3357.
84. Leijten F, De Weerd A, Poortvliet D, De Ridder V, Ulrich C, Harink-De Weerd J. Critical illness polyneuropathy in multiple organ dysfunction syndrome and weaning from the ventilator. *Intensive Care Med.* 1996;22:856–861.
85. De Letter MA, van Doorn PA, Savelkoul HF, at al. Critical illness polyneuropathy and myopathy (CIPNM): evidence for local immune activation by cytokine-expression in the muscle tissue. *J Neuroimmunol.* 2000;106:206–213.
86. Bednarik J, Vondracek P, Dusek L, Moravcova E, Cundrle I. Risk factors for critical illness polyneuropathy. *J Neurol.* 2005;252:343–351.

87. Van den Berghe G, Schoonheydt K, Becx P, et al. Insulin therapy protects the central and peripheral nervous system of intensive care patients. *Neurology*. 2005;64:1348–1353.
88. Van den Berghe G, Wouters P, Weekers F, et al. Intensive insulin therapy in the critically ill patient. *N Engl J Med*. 2001;345:1359–1367.
89. Van de Berghe G, Wilmer A, Hermans G, et al. Intensive insulin therapy in the medical ICU. *N Engl J Med*. 2006;354:449–461.
90. Hermans G, Wilmer A, Meerseman W, et al. Impact of intensive insulin therapy on neuromuscular complication and ventilator dependency in the medical intensive care unit. *Am J Respir Crit Care Med*. 2007;175:480–489.
91. Allen DC, Arunnachalam R, Mills KR. Critical illness myopathy: further evidence from muscle-fiber excitability studies of an acquired channelopathy. *Muscle Nerve*. 2008;37:14–22.
92. Witt N, Zochodne D, Bolton C. Peripheral nerve function in sepsis and multiple organ failure. *Chest*. 1991;199:176–184.
93. Garnacho-Montero J, Amaya-Villar R, Garcia-Garmendia JL, et al. Effect of critical illness polyneuropathy on the withdrawal from mechanical ventilation and the length of stay in septic patients. *Crit Care Med*. 2005;33:349–354.
94. De Jonghe B, Bastuji-Garin S, Sharshar T, et al. Does ICU acquired paresis lengthen weaning from mechanical ventilation? *Intensive Care Med*. 2004;30:1117–1121.
95. Herridge, MS, Cheung AM, Tansey CM, Matte-Martyn A, et al. One-year outcomes in survivors of the acute respiratory distress syndrome. *N Engl J Med*. 2003;348:683–693.
96. Latronico N, Peli E, Botteri M. Critical illness myopathy and neuropathy. *Curr Opin Crit Care*. 2005;11:126–132.
97. Begin P, Mathieu J, Almirall J, Grassino A. Relationship between chronic hypercapnia and inspiratory-muscle weakness in myotonic dystrophy. *Am J Respir Crit Care Med*. 1997;156:133–139.
98. Sivak E, Ahmad M, Hanson M, Mitsumoto H. Respiratory insufficiency in adult-onset acid maltase deficiency. *South Med J*. 1987;80(2):205–208.
99. Martin R, Sufit R, Ringel S, et al. Respiratory muscle improvement by muscle training in adult-onset acid maltase deficiency. *Muscle Nerve*. 1983;6:201–203.
100. Sanders DB, El Salem K, Massey JM, et al. Clinical aspects of MuSK antibody positive seronegative MG. *Neurology*. 2003;60:1978–1980.
101. Dushay KM, Zibrak JD, Jensen WA. Myasthenia gravis presenting as isolated respiratory failure. *Chest*. 1990;97:232–234.
102. Gracey DR, Divertie MB, Howard FM Jr. Mechanical ventilation for respiratory failure in myasthenia gravis. *Mayo Clin Proc*. 983;58:597–602.
103. Watanabe A, Watanabe T, Obama T, et al. Prognostic factors for myasthenic crises after transsternal thymectomy in patients with myasthenia gravis. *J Thorac Cardiovasc Surg*. 2004;127:868–876.
104. Juel VC. Myasthenia gravis: management of myasthenic crises and perioperative care. *Semin Neurol*. 2004;24:75–81.
105. Varelas PN, Chua HC, Natterman J, Barmadia L, et al. Ventilatory care in myasthenia gravis crisis: assessing the baseline adverse event rate. *Crit Care Med*. 2002;30:2663–2668.
106. Seneviratne J, Mandrekar J, Wijdicks EFM, Rabinstein AA. Noninvasive ventilation in myasthenic crisis. *Arch Neurol*. 2008;65(1):54–58.
107. Seneviratne J, Mandrekar J, Wijdicks FM, Rabinstein AA. Predictors of extubation in myasthenic crisis. *Arch Neurol*. 2008;65(7):929–933.
108. Gronseth GS, Barohn RJ. Practice parameter: thymectomy for autoimmune myasthenia gravis (an evidence-based review). Report of the quality standards subcommittee of the American Academy of Neurology. *Neurology*. 2000;55:7–15.
109. Qureshi AI, Choudhry MA, Akbar MS, et al. Plasma exchange versus intravenous immunoglobulin treatment in myasthenic crises. *Neurology*. 1999;52:629–632.
110. Lang B, Pinto A, Giovanini F, et al. Pathogenic autoantibodies in the Lambert-Eaton myasthenic syndrome. *Ann N Y Acad Sci*. 2003;998:187.
111. Elrington GM, Murray NM, Spiro SG, Newsom-Davis J. Neurological paraneoplastic syndromes in patients with small cell lung cancer. A prospective survey of 150 patients. *J Neurol Neurosurg Psychiatry*. 1991;54:764.
112. Nicolle MW, Stewart DJ, Remtulla H, et al. Lambert-Eaton myasthenic syndrome presenting with severe respiratory failure. *Muscle Nerve*. 1996;19:1328.
113. Hughes JM, Blumenthal JR, Merson MH, et al. Clinical features of type A and type B food-borne botulism. *Ann Intern Med*. 1981;95:442–445.
114. Phillips MF, Quinlivan RC, Edwards RH, Calverley PM. Changes in spirometry over time as prognostic marker in patients with Duchenne muscular dystrophy. *Am J Respir Crit Care Med*. 2001;164:2191–2194.
115. Hukins CA, Hillman DR. Daytime predictors of sleep hypoventilation in Duchenne muscular dystrophy. *Am J Respir Crit Care Med*. 2000;161:166–170.
116. Vianello A, Bevilacqua M, Salvador V, Cardaioli C, Vincenti E. Long-term nasal intermittent positive pressure ventilation in advanced Duchenne's muscular dystrophy. *Chest*. 1994;105:445–449.
117. Fanfulla F, Berardinelli A, Gaultieri G, Zoia M. The efficacy of noninvasive mechanical ventilation on nocturnal hypoxemia in Duchenne's muscular dystrophy. *Monaldi Arch Chest*. 1998;53:9–13.
118. Guilleminault C, Philip P, Robinson A. Sleep and neuromuscular disease: bilevel positive airway pressure by nasal mask as a treatment for sleep disordered breathing in patients with neuromuscular disease. *J Neurol Neurosurg Psychiatry*. 1998;65:225–232.
119. Smith PEM, Calverley PMA, Edwards RHT, Evans GA, Campbell EJM. Practical problems in the respiratory care of patients with muscular dystrophy. *N Engl J Med*. 1987;316:1197–1205.
120. Mendell JR, Moxley RT, Griggs RC, et al. Randomized, double-blind six months trial of prednisone in Duchenne's muscular dystrophy. *N Engl J Med*. 1989;320:1592–1597.
121. Backman E, Henriksson KG. Low-dose prednisolone treatment in Duchenne and Becker muscular dystrophy. *Neuromuscul Disord*. 1995;5:233–241.
122. Bonifati MD, Ruzza G, Bonometto P, et al. A multicenter, double-blind, randomized trial of deflazacort versus prednisone in Duchenne muscular dystrophy. *Muscle Nerve*. 2000;23:1344–1347.
123. Campbell C, Jacob P. Deflazacort for the treatment of Duchenne dystrophy: a systematic review. *BMC Neurol*. 2003;3:7.
124. Fenichel GM, Florence JM, Pestronk A, et al. A randomized efficacy and safety trial of oxandrolone in the treatment of Duchenne dystrophy. *Neurology*. 2001;56:1075–1079.
125. Barton-Davis ER, Cordier L, Shoturma DI, et al. Aminoglycoside antibiotics restore dystrophin function to skeletal muscles of mdx mice. *J Clin Invest*. 1999;104:375–381.
126. Birnkrant DJ, Panitch HB, Benditt JO, et al. American College of Chest Physicians statement on the respiratory and related management of patients with Duchenne muscular dystrophy undergoing anesthesia and sedation. *Chest*. 2007;132:1977–1986.
127. Wanke T, Toifl K, Merkle M, Formanek D, Lahrmann H, Zwick H. Inspiratory muscle training in patients with Duchenne muscular dystrophy. *Chest*. 1994;105:475–482.
128. Gozal D, Thiriet P. Respiratory muscle training in neuromuscular disease: long-term effects on strength and load perception. *Med Sci Sports Exerc*. 1999;31:1522–1527.
129. Smith PE, Coakley JH, Edwards RH. Respiratory muscle training in Duchenne muscular dystrophy. *Muscle Nerve*. 1988;11:784–785.
130. Stamler J, Meisser G. Physiology of nitric oxide in skeletal muscle. *Physiol Rev*. 2001;81:209–237.
131. Sander M, Chavoshan B, Harris S, et al. Functional muscle ischemia in neuronal nitric oxide synthase-deficient skeletal muscle of children with Duchenne muscle dystrophy. *Proc Natl Acad Sci USA*. 2000;97:13818–13823.

132. ATS Consensus Statement. Respiratory care of patients with Duchenne muscular dystrophy. *Am J Respir Crit Care Med.* 2004;170:456–465.
133. Annane D, Orlikowski D, Chevret S, Chevrolet JC, Raphael JC. Nocturnal mechanical ventilation for chronic hypoventilation in patients with neuromuscular and chest wall disorders. *Cochrane Database Syst Rev.* 2007;(4):CD001941.
134. Ward S, Chatwin M, Heather S, Simonds AK. Randomized controlled trial of non-invasive ventilation (NIV) for nocturnal hypoventilation in neuromuscular and chest wall disease patients with daytime normocapnia. *Thorax.* 2005;60:1019–1024.
135. Simonds AK, Muntoni F, Heather S, Fielding S. Impact of nasal ventilation on survival in hypercapnic Duchenne muscular dystrophy. *Thorax.* 1998;53:949–952.
136. Baydur A, Layne E, Aral H, et al. Long term non-invasive ventilation in the community for patients with musculoskeletal disorders: 46 years of experience and review. *Thorax.* 2000;55:4–11.
137. Barbe F, Quera-Salva MA, de Lattre J, Gajdos P, Agusti AG. Long-term effects of nasal intermittent positive-pressure ventilation on pulmonary function and sleep architecture in patients with neuromuscular diseases. *Chest.* 1996;110:1179–1183.
138. Simonds AK. Recent advances in respiratory care for neuromuscular disease. *Chest.* 2006;130:1879–1886.
139. Thornton Ca, Griggs RC, Moxley RT 3rd. Myotonic dystrophy with no trinucleotide repeat expansion. *Ann Neurol.* 1994;35:269–272.
140. Margolis ML, Hill AR. Acid maltase deficiency in an adult: evidence for improvement in respiratory function with high-protein dietary therapy. *Am Rev Respir Dis.* 1986;134:328–331.
141. Lynn DJ, Woda RP, Mendell JR. Respiratory dysfunction in muscular dystrophy and other myopathies. *Clin Chest Med.* 1994;15(4):661–674.
142. Hoffbrand B, Beck E. "Unexplained" dypnea and shrinking lungs in systemic lupus erythematosus. *Br Med J.* 1965;1:1273–1277.
143. DiMarco A, Kelling J, DiMarco M, et al. The effects of inspiratory resistive training on respiratory muscle function in patients with muscular dystrophy. *Muscle Nerve.* 1985;8:284–290.
144. Martin A, Stern L, Yeates J, Lepp D, Little J. Respiratory muscle training in Duchenne dystrophy. *Med Child Neurol.* 1986;8:284–290.
145. Gross D, Ladd H, Riley E, Macklem P, Grassino A. The effect of training on strength and endurance of the diaphragm in quadriplegia. *Am J Med.* 1980;68:27–35.
146. Huldtgren A, Fugl-Myers A, Jonasson E, Bake B. Ventilatory dysfunction and respiratory rehabilitation in post-traumatic quadriplegia. *Eur J Respir Dis.* 1980;61:347–356.
147. Bach JR, Rajaraman R, Ballanger F, et al. Neuromuscular ventilatory insufficiency: effect of home mechanical ventilator use vs oxygen therapy on pneumonia and hospitalization rates. *Am J Phys Med Rehabil.* 1998;77:8–19.
148. Criner G, Travaline J, Brennan K, Kreimer D. Efficacy of a new full face mask for noninvasive positive pressure ventilation. *Chest.* 1994;106:1109–1115.
149. Roy B, Cordova F, Travaline J, et al. Full face mask for noninvasive positive pressure ventilation in patients with acute respiratory failure. *J Am Osteopath Assoc.* 2007;107:148–156.
150. Gay P, Patel A, Viggiano R, et al. Nocturnal nasal ventilation for treatment of patients with hypercapneic respiratory failure. *Mayo Clin Proc.* 1991;144:1234–1239.
151. Heckmatt J, Loh L, Dubowitz V. Nighttime nasal ventilation in neuromuscular disease. *Lancet.* 1990;335:579–581.
152. Bach J, Alba A, Saporito L. Intermittent positive pressure ventilation via the mouth as an alternative to tracheostomy for 257 ventilator users. *Chest.* 1993;103:174–182.
153. Elefteriades JA, Hogan JF, Handler A, Loke JS. Long-term follow-up of bilateral pacing of the diaphragm in quadriplegia. *N Engl J Med.* 1992;326:1433.
154. Elefteriades JA, Quin JA, Hogan JF, et al. Long term follow-up of pacing of the conditioned diaphragm in quadriplegia. *Pacing Clin Electrophysiol.* 2002;25:897.
155. Garrido-Garcia H, Mazaira Alvarez J, Martin Escribano P, et al. Treatment of chronic ventilatory failure using a diaphragmatic pacemaker. *Spinal Cord.* 1998;36:310.
156. Onders RP, Elmo M, Khansarinia S, et al. Complete worldwide operative experience in laparoscopic diaphragm pacing: results and differences in spinal cord injured patients and amyotrophic lateral sclerosis patients. *Surg Endosc.* 2009;23:1433–1440.

CHAPTER 46

Obstructive Sleep Apnea

Bashir A. Chaudhary
Arthur Taft
Shelley C. Mishoe

OUTLINE

Descriptions and Common Terms
Obstructive Sleep Apnea
Complications of Obstructive Sleep Apnea
Diagnosis of Obstructive Sleep Apnea
Treatment of Obstructive Sleep Apnea
Mortality Associated with Obstructive Sleep Apnea

OBJECTIVES

1. Define obstructive sleep apnea.
2. Compare obstructive sleep apnea, central sleep apnea, and mixed apnea.
3. Discuss the prevalence and pathogenesis of obstructive sleep apnea.
4. Describe the clinical features of obstructive sleep apnea.
5. Describe the effects of obstructive sleep apnea on the central nervous system, cardiovascular system, pulmonary system, endocrine system, renal system, gastrointestinal tract, eyes, psychiatric function, and sexual dysfunction.
6. Describe the role of the following in the treatment of obstructive sleep apnea: weight loss, posture, continuous positive airway pressure, oral appliances, surgery, pharmacologic therapy, and mechanical devices.
7. Compare the advantages and disadvantages of various treatment strategies for obstructive sleep apnea.

KEY TERMS

apnea
arousals
central apnea
complex sleep apnea syndrome
continuous positive airway pressure (CPAP)
hypersomnolence
hypopnea
mixed apnea
obstructive apnea
oral appliance
polysomnography
sleep apnea
uvulopalatopharyngoplasty (UPPP)

INTRODUCTION

This chapter defines obstructive sleep apnea, from its prevalence and pathogenesis to its affect on the different systems of the body. Sleep apnea is a chronic disorder. Obstructive apnea is characterized by continued chest and abdominal efforts to breath during periods of airflow cessation. This chapter concludes with a discussion of the advantages and disadvantages of various treatment strategies and how treatment can prolong a patient's life.

Descriptions and Common Terms

Symptoms suggestive of sleep apnea were well described in Charles Dickens's novel *The Pickwick Papers*. In 1906, William Osler in his book *The Principles and Practice of Medicine* referred to obese patients with uncontrollable sleepiness as *Pickwickians*, "like the fat boy Joe in *Pickwick Papers*." The recognition of episodic cessation of breathing during sleep in drowsy patients heralded the modern era of sleep medicine. **Sleep apnea** is a chronic disorder characterized by daytime **hypersomnolence**, snoring, disrupted sleep, hypoxemia, and repeated episodes of **hypopnea** or **apnea**, or both, during sleep.[1] **Table 46–1** lists some of the common terms used for describing sleep-related breathing problems.

During the past 30 years, a large amount of literature has been published about various aspects of sleep apnea. Two longitudinal studies have provided a wealth of information about the long-term effects of sleep apnea. The Wisconsin Sleep Cohort Study is an epidemiologic study of sleep apnea and other sleep problems, based on a random sample of 1522 Wisconsin state employees, that began in 1989.[2] In 1994 the National Heart, Lung and Blood Institute initiated the Sleep Heart Health Study as a multicenter prospective cohort study to assess the contribution of sleep apnea to hypertension and cardiovascular disease.[3]

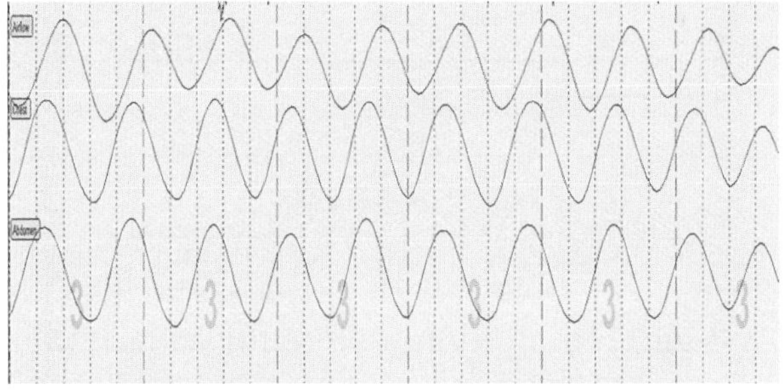

FIGURE 46–1 Normal breathing pattern. Upper tracing: airflow. Middle tracing: chest movements. Lower tracing: abdominal movements.

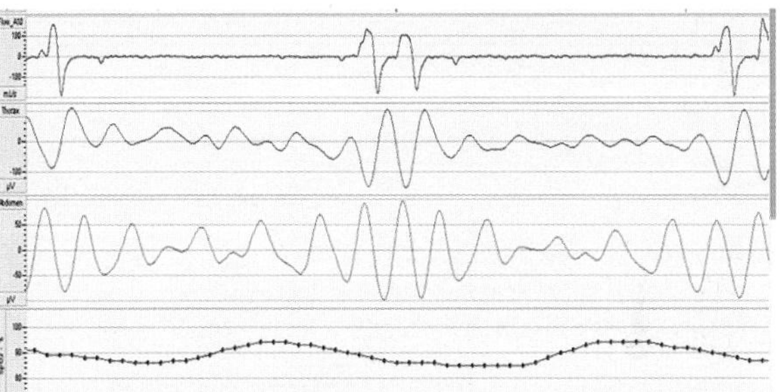

FIGURE 46–2 Obstructive apnea. First tracing: airflow. Second tracing: chest movements. Third tracing: abdominal movement. Fourth tracing: oxygen saturation.

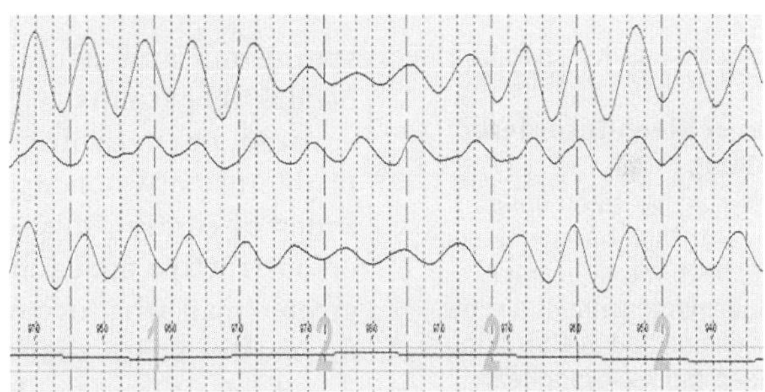

FIGURE 46–3 Hypopnea. First tracing: airflow. Second tracing: chest movements. Third tracing: abdominal movements. Fourth tracing: oxygen saturation.

Types of Sleep-Disordered Breathing

Three types of sleep apnea are recognized: obstructive apnea, central apnea, and mixed apnea.[1] During normal sleep, chest and abdominal movements are in synchrony and airflow is normal (**Figure 46–1**). **Obstructive apnea** is characterized by continued chest and abdominal efforts to breath during periods of airflow cessation (**Figure 46–2**). Sometimes the obstruction is not complete and airflow does not cease, but diminishes to 50% or less of average. These episodes are known as hypopneas (**Figure 46–3**). **Central apnea** is characterized by cessation of both the effort to breathe and airflow (**Figure 46–4**). **Mixed apnea** has characteristics of both types of apnea: central in the beginning and obstructive at the end (**Figure 46–5**). Mixed apnea often is combined with obstructive apnea, since the pathogenesis and clinical manifestations are similar. The usual description of sleep apnea refers to patients with obstructive sleep apnea (OSA).

Central sleep apnea is an uncommon disorder that causes mild sleep-related

TABLE 46–1 Definitions for Describing Sleep-Related Breathing Problems

Term	Definition
Apnea	Cessation of airflow for at least 10 seconds
Obstructive apnea	Continuation of chest and abdominal effort during apnea
Central apnea	Cessation of both airflow and the respiratory effort
Mixed apnea	Both central and obstructive apnea characteristics
Hypopnea	Reduction of airflow by 30% with oxygen desaturation of at least 4%
Apnea index	Number of apneas per hour of sleep
Hypopnea index	Number of hypopneas per hour of sleep
Apnea-hypopnea index (AHI)	Number of apneas and hypopneas per hour of sleep
Respiratory disturbance index	Apneas, hypopneas, and respiratory arousals per hour of sleep
RERA index	Number of respiratory effort–related arousals per hour of sleep

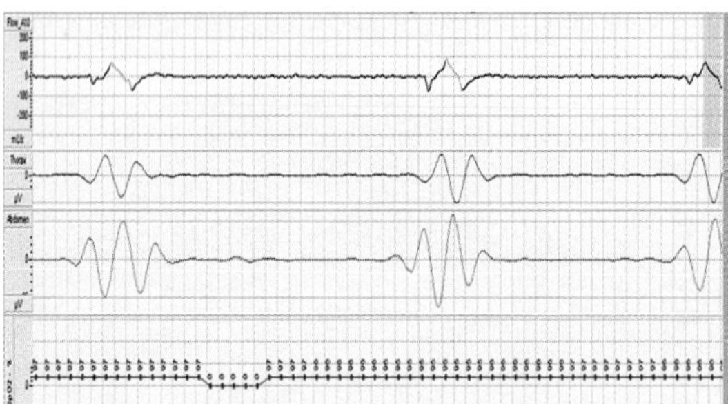

FIGURE 46–4 Central sleep apneas. First tracing: airflow. Second tracing: chest movements. Third tracing: abdominal movement. Fourth tracing: oxygen saturation.

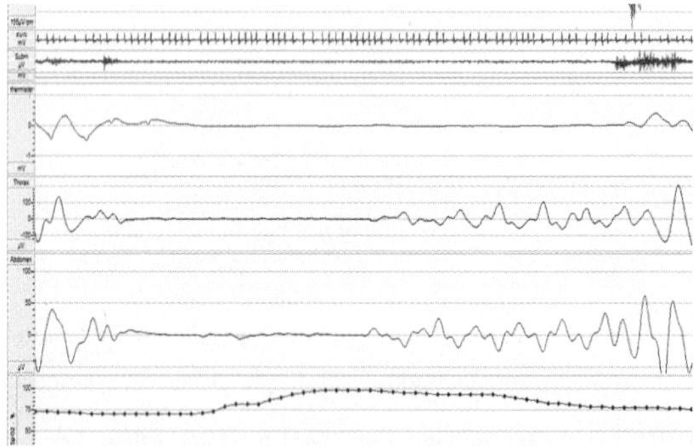

FIGURE 46–5 Mixed apneas. First tracing: airflow. Second tracing: chest movements. Third tracing: abdominal movements. Fourth tracing: oxygen saturation.

> **RESPIRATORY RECAP**
>
> **Types of Sleep-Disordered Breathing**
>
> » *Obstructive sleep apnea*: greater than normal episodes of chest and abdominal movements without airflow or diminished airflow during sleep (apnea-hypopnea index [AHI] > 5), causing pathophysiologic changes while awake.
>
> » *Central sleep apnea*: episodes of cessation of airflow and chest/abdominal movements during sleep, greater than expected (AHI > 5).
>
> » *Mixed sleep apnea*: episodes of both types of apnea, central in the beginning and obstructive at the end.
>
> » *Complex sleep apnea*: central sleep apnea as a result of treating OSA.
>
> » *Upper airway resistance breathing*: a milder sleep disorder with episodes of apnea and hypopnea greater than normal, but less than with OSA.

symptoms and usually occurs in patients with cardiac or neurologic problems.[4,5] When episodes of central, mixed, or obstructive apnea are greater than what occurs normally, sleep-disordered breathing may be diagnosed by **polysomnography**. Patients have clinical symptoms similar to OSA. Some patients who are treated for OSA develop central apneas during therapy, referred to as **complex sleep apnea syndrome**.

Initially, the presence of 30 apneas during a 6- to 8-hour polysomnogram and/or an apnea index of 5 were used to define sleep apnea.[1] The apnea index is the frequency of apneas per hour of sleep. With the recognition that hypopnea can produce clinical symptoms similar to those of apneas, a combination of apnea and hypopnea was suggested as the definition of sleep hypopnea.[6] Currently, sleep apnea is diagnosed when the apnea-hypopnea index (AHI, defined as the number of apneas plus hypopneas per hour) is 5 or more.[2] The severity of sleep apnea is considered mild if the AHI is 5 or higher, moderate if the AHI is 15 or higher, and severe if the AHI is 30 or higher.[7]

The presence of daytime hypercapnia and hypoxemia defines hypercapnic and hypoxemic respiratory failure. Sleepy obese patients with respiratory failure were diagnosed as having Pickwickian syndrome before it was known that the underlying cause for their symptoms was the sleep-disordered breathing.

A milder sleep-related breathing problem is upper airway resistance syndrome (UARS). In UARS, the sleep study does not show apneas, but there is an increase in the number of **arousals** related to increased respiratory effort. The arousals are identified by an electroencephalogram (EEG) pattern similar to awakening, but lasting less than 15 seconds. These are called *respiratory effort–related arousals* (RERAs). These patients have upper airway narrowing but are able to maintain airflow in the normal range with increased respiratory effort. The increased effort required to keep breathing in the normal range results in repeated nocturnal arousals.[8] Consequently, the symptoms are similar to OSA.

Prevalence

Sleep apnea is a very common disorder. The Wisconsin Sleep Cohort Study has provided valuable information about risk factors and the prevalence of sleep apnea in a community population.[2,9] Using the criteria of an AHI of more than 5 and the presence of daytime sleepiness revealed a prevalence of 2% in women and 4% in men. The prevalence is about 17% (24% in men and 9% in women) if sleep apnea is defined by solely an AHI of more than 5. It is estimated that about 6% of the general population has moderate sleep apnea (defined as an AHI of 15 or above). The prevalence of sleep apnea increases with age and obesity. People older than 65 years are about three times more likely to have sleep apnea compared with middle-aged persons.

Most patients clinically diagnosed to have sleep apnea are obese. There is progressive increase in the prevalence of sleep apnea with increasing severity of obesity. A person with a body mass index (BMI) of 30 has more than a 30% chance of having sleep apnea. A BMI of 40 increases the chance of having sleep apnea to 50%.[10] Neck circumference is a better predictor for the presence of sleep apnea than BMI. A neck circumference of 16 inches in women and 17 inches in men suggests the high likelihood of sleep apnea, requiring further testing to confirm it.

About one-third of patients with hypertension have sleep apnea. The prevalence is more than 50% in patients

TABLE 46–2 Common Risk Factors Associated with Sleep Apnea

Obesity	Most patients are obese (body mass index >30 kg/m^2)
Age	Progressive increase in incidence with age
Gender	Twice as common in men
Snoring	Almost all sleep apnea patients snore
Sleepiness	Very common in sleep apnea
Alcohol use	Increases the number of apneas
Hypertension	Three times more common in hypertensive patients
Congestive heart failure (CHF)	Over half of CHF patients have sleep apnea
Stroke	Over two-thirds of acute stroke patients have sleep apnea
Hypothyroidism, acromegaly	High incidence of sleep apnea
Medications	Sedatives and narcotics increase the number of apneas
Upper airway abnormalities	Higher incidence in persons with upper airway narrowing
Family history	Two to four times higher risk among family members regardless of other factors such as obesity, age, or gender

RESPIRATORY RECAP

Prevalence of Sleep Apnea

» People older than 65 years are three times more likely to develop sleep apnea syndrome than middle-aged persons.

» The risk of sleep apnea is two to four times higher among family members of sleep apnea patients regardless of age, weight, or gender.

with hypothyroidism and acromegaly. Persons with anatomic upper airway abnormalities have a high prevalence of the disease.[11]

The prevalence of sleep apnea in many Asian populations is similar to that in the United States, even though obesity is uncommon among Asians.[12] This may be related to craniofacial characteristics of Asian populations.

There is a two to four time higher risk of sleep apnea among the family members of sleep apnea patients, independent of the effects of obesity, gender, and age. The risk of sleep apnea increases with the number of affected family members. **Table 46–2** shows some of the common risk factors for the presence of sleep apnea.

Obstructive Sleep Apnea

Pathogenesis

Hypopnea and apnea result from the narrowing and occlusion of the upper airway.[13,14] The upper airway from the back of the nasal septum to the epiglottis has minimal bony support and can collapse easily. Normally this region is maintained open by a balance of the forces that tend to dilate and the forces that tend to narrow this area. Forces that tend to dilate this area include the tonic and phasic activity of the genioglossus (tongue) and upper airway muscles. The tonic activity is present throughout the respiratory cycle, and the phasic activity is present during inspiration. Conversely, inspiration creates negative pressure inside the airway. The negative pressure inside a collapsible tube can reduce the size of the tube. Increased inspiratory effort opens the intrathoracic airway but reduces the luminal area of the upper airway. This effect is similar to sucking though a collapsible straw. The harder one sucks at the straw, the narrower the lumen of the straw becomes. Airflow linearly decreases as the pressure in the upper airway becomes negative. When the negative pressure exceeds a critical pressure (e.g., −10 cm H_2O in normal persons), airway occlusion occurs.[15]

During sleep, as the tone of the pharyngeal dilator muscles decreases, the soft palate and the tongue move backward, causing narrowing of the oropharynx. Maximum narrowing occurs during rapid eye movement (REM) sleep, when the muscle tone is further reduced, and also in the supine posture, where gravity has the greatest effect. Thus, occasional apnea and hypopnea can occur during REM sleep and in supine posture, even in normal individuals. The site of occlusion is variable and may occur at multiple sites, but most commonly occurs at the velopharynx and in the retroglossal area. The velopharynx consists of the velum (soft palate), the lateral pharyngeal walls (side walls of the throat and the posterior pharyngeal wall), and the back wall of the throat. The velum rests against the back of the tongue during normal nasal breathing. During inhalation, air can flow through the nose and pharynx to the lungs without obstruction. Velopharyngeal closure occurs during speech, swallowing, gagging, vomiting, sucking, blowing, and whistling. Velopharyngeal closure during sleep is a major contributing cause of obstructive sleep apnea.

RESPIRATORY RECAP

Pathogenesis of Obstructive Sleep Apnea

» The pathogenesis of OSA syndrome is related to upper airway anatomy characteristics, pharyngeal tone during sleep, airway pressure changes during inspiration, and inspiratory efforts associated with airway narrowing or occlusion.

Four interdependent factors that play a role in upper airway occlusion during sleep are narrowing of the pharyngeal cavity, decreased activity of the pharyngeal dilator muscles, increased respiratory effort (i.e., more negative intraluminal pressure), and increased compliance (collapsibility) of the pharyngeal airway. Fat deposition in the neck and tongue causes narrowing of the upper airway and enlargement of the tongue. Many abnormalities that can cause narrowing of the upper airway have been identified (**Table 46–3**). Alcohol and sedatives reduce upper airway muscle activity, predisposing patients to apnea.[16] These substances result in narrowing of the airway from the decreased muscle tone. This leads to reduced airflow, causing an increased respiratory effort to try to restore the airflow. However, narrowing above the site of occlusion (i.e., upstream resistance) causes more negative intraluminal pressure, leading to even more narrowing. Thus, a vicious cycle occurs in which the harder the patient tries to breathe, the more the airways become obstructed. Deposition of fat makes the upper airway more compliant; that is, a small increase in negative pressure can pull the upper airway muscles together. Thus, in obese patients with sleep apnea, occlusion occurs with less negative pressure and, at times, even with positive airway pressure.[15]

Clinical Features

Apneas cause hypoxemia and hypercapnia, which are terminated by arousals. Most of the clinical manifestations of sleep apnea result from repeated arousals and hypoxemia. Snoring, daytime hypersomnolence, and disturbed sleep are the usual reasons patients seek medical attention. Many times, patients are unaware of their problems and are brought for evaluation because their spouses are bothered by the snoring and disturbed sleep. **Box 46–1** lists the usual symptoms associated with OSA. A wide spectrum of clinical manifestations exists, ranging from mild nocturnal snoring and daytime tiredness to acute or chronic hypoxemic and hypercapnic respiratory failure (**Table 46–4**).

Snoring is the most common symptom among patients with OSA. It is usually loud enough to be heard from outside the room. The loudness of snoring is a predictor of the severity of sleep apnea. The snoring may be continuous, but usually it has an intermittent pattern. Snoring is caused by the oscillation of pharyngeal soft tissues. Snoring is common in the general population, and it is estimated that about 48% of men and 34% of women snore habitually.[17] Snoring is present in almost all patients seen in sleep clinics. Occasionally a patient with sleep apnea may deny snoring, but either he or she is sleeping alone or the denial is not corroborated by the bed partner. The snoring is often described as being similar to the noise coming from a freight train. Loud snoring disturbs the bed partner's sleep and frequently leads to sleeping in separate beds or rooms.

TABLE 46–3 Common Upper Airway Abnormalities Associated with Obstructive Sleep Apnea

Nose	Enlarged turbinates, deviated septum, polyps, nasal valve dysfunction
Nasopharynx	Enlarged adenoids, tumors, pharyngeal flap
Oropharynx	Enlargement of uvula and soft palate, tonsillar hypertrophy, tumor, macroglossia
Larynx	Vocal cord paralysis, epiglottic edema
Jaw	Micrognathia, retrognathia

BOX 46–1

Symptoms of Sleep Apnea

Daytime Symptoms
- Sleepiness
- Nonrefreshing sleep
- Morning headaches
- Intellectual dysfunction
- Personality changes

Nighttime Symptoms
- Snoring
- Apneic, choking, gasping awakenings
- Restless sleep
- Nocturia
- Dry mouth
- Drooling
- Diaphoresis
- Erectile dysfunction

TABLE 46–4 Clinical Spectrum of Sleep Apnea

	Snoring	Arousals	Somnolence	Hypoxemia	Hypercarbia
Normal	–	–	–	–	–
Snorers	+	+–	–	–	–
UARS*	++	+	+–	–	–
Mild sleep apnea	+++	++	+	+–	–
Moderate sleep apnea	++++	+++	++	+	–
Severe sleep apnea	++++	++++	+++	+++	+–
Sleep apnea with respiratory failure	++++	++++	++++	++++	+

*UARS, upper airway resistance syndrome.

Hypersomnolence during the daytime is one of the main reasons for seeking evaluation. Falling asleep during periods of relative inactivity, such as watching television, driving, and attending meetings, is common. In advanced cases, the patient may fall asleep even when engaged in an activity (e.g., talking, walking, eating). Many patients seen in sleep clinics complain of daytime tiredness and general decreased performance. However, in sleep studies performed in the general population, regardless of the presence of symptoms, sleepiness is present in only about 50% of the subjects who are diagnosed to have sleep apnea.[18] Sleepiness is also uncommon in sleep apnea patients with congestive heart failure.[19] Some patients complain of daytime tiredness instead of sleepiness. "I am tired of being tired" is a common complaint. Both repeated nocturnal awakenings (i.e., sleep fragmentation) and hypoxemia have been implicated as the cause of daytime somnolence, but sleep fragmentation appears to be the main determinant.[20]

Sleepiness is usually assessed by the Epworth Sleepiness Scale (ESS), in which the patient is asked to rate the likelihood of falling asleep from 0 (no chance of dozing off) to 3 (high chance of dozing off) in eight situations (sitting and reading, watching TV, sitting inactive in a public place, as a passenger in a car for an hour, lying down in the afternoon, sitting and talking to someone, sitting quietly after lunch, and in a car while stopped in traffic).[21] An ESS score of 10 or more is suggestive of significant daytime sleepiness.[20] Objective assessment of daytime sleepiness can be obtained by the Multiple Sleep Latency Test (MSLT), in which a patient is given an opportunity to nap for 20 minutes.[22] This is repeated every 2 hours four more times. The time it takes to fall asleep during these five naps is calculated. The mean sleep latency in the general population is more than 8 minutes. In patients with sleepiness, the mean sleep latency is less than 8 minutes. This test, however, is not needed for routine care of sleep apnea patients.

Other symptoms are common with OSA. The sleep pattern of patients with OSA is characterized by frequent tossing and turning. Patients wake up repeatedly from their sleep because of choking, shortness of breath, dry mouth, or for no apparent reason. Some patients' primary complaint may be the inability to have a good night sleep. Nocturnal sweating, probably related to increased breathing effort, is common. Hallucinations may occur because of awakening from REM sleep. Patients do not feel fresh when they wake up in the morning. Morning headaches, personality changes, and decreased hearing acuity are common.

Complications of Obstructive Sleep Apnea

Blood gas abnormalities, repeated arousals, and increased negative intrathoracic pressure are the main mechanisms responsible for a myriad of complications occurring in severe sleep apnea patients. Many biochemical abnormalities have been identified that may be playing a role in the pathogenesis of these complications. Hypoxemia occurs with apneic episodes and, with increasing severity of the disease, may become sustained and occur during the daytime. Hypoxemia appears to be the main determinant of most sleep apnea–related complications.

Hypoxemia causes tissue ischemia, induces pulmonary artery constriction leading to pulmonary hypertension, and causes increased sympathetic discharge (catecholamines). Long-standing pulmonary hypertension may result in right-sided heart failure, or cor pulmonale. Transient hypercapnia also occurs with apneas and can become sustained and chronic. If left untreated, this can lead to chronic respiratory failure. Repeated arousals from sleep lead to higher catecholamine release during the night. Increased respiratory effort needed to overcome upper airway narrowing causes increased negative pressure in the chest cavity. This increased negative intrathoracic pressure affects the heart in two ways. It makes it easier for blood to come back to the right side of the heart but makes it more difficult for the left heart to pump blood into the aorta. Because of the increased negative pressure around it (i.e., the heart is being pulled to the outside), the heart has to work harder (produce more positive pressure) to pump the blood out. This increased cardiac workload may lead to left-sided heart failure.

Patients with OSA have increased blood levels of C-reactive protein (CRP), a marker of inflammation.[23] An elevated CRP level causes blunting of endothelium-dependent vasodilation and correlates with increased risk of developing cardiovascular disease. Similarly, levels of fibrinogen, tumor necrosis factor-α (TNF-α), interleukin-6 (IL-6), homocysteine, and other biomarkers are increased,[24] causing increased cardiovascular disease. Leptin is a protein secreted by fat cells and is thought to be an appetite suppressant. Serum leptin levels are high in patients with OSA, suggesting there is resistance to this protein.[25] Increased leptin levels are linked to cardiovascular disease.[26] Circulating nitric oxide level is decreased with OSA, and the level improves with therapy.[27]

Almost all parts of the body are affected by the presence of sleep apnea. Complications are common and become more frequent as the severity of disease increases. Some of the common complications of OSA are discussed in the following subsections according to their effects on various systems of the body.

Central Nervous System

Cognitive dysfunction and sleepiness are common in patients with OSA. Neuropsychological measures of overall performance are moderately impaired, and cognitive abilities have an inverse correlation with oxygen desaturation and apnea. Patients may have problems related to attention, concentration, memory, and vigilance. Some patients become irritable and have difficulty with social interaction. Sleepiness at work is associated with reduced efficiency. Sleepiness in patients who operate heavy equipment or drive for work, such as long-haul truck drivers and bus drivers, may be particularly hazardous. The rate of automobile accidents in patients with sleep apnea is about three times higher than in the general population. The rate of auto accidents goes down as patients are successfully treated.[28] Most children with lack of adequate sleep resist sleepiness and are restless during the day. These patients may be labeled as having attention deficit hyperactivity disorder (ADHD). Children and adults with ADHD who snore need to be evaluated for possible sleep apnea.[29]

Cardiovascular

Sleep apnea has been implicated in many cardiovascular abnormalities.[30] Cardiac arrhythmias and both right and left ventricular dysfunction ultimately leading to congestive heart failure can occur in patients with OSA. The heart rate slows during an apneic episode and speeds up when the apnea is terminated. Nocturnal bradycardia (30 to 50 beats per minute) during apneic episodes, followed by tachycardia (90 to 120 beats per minute) at the resolution of apnea is the most common pattern of arrhythmias.[31] Other cardiac arrhythmias are seen in about 20% of patients undergoing polysomnography. These arrhythmias occur more frequently in patients with hypoxemia and include premature atrial and ventricular contractions, atrial and ventricular tachycardia, sinus pauses, and heart block. The incidence of OSA in patients with atrial fibrillation is high, and the recurrence rate of fibrillation after cardioversion remains high if the OSA remains untreated.[32] Both right and left ventricular hypertrophy and congestive cardiac failure can develop secondary to OSA. Additionally, the incidence of both central and obstructive sleep apnea is very common in patients with congestive heart failure.[33]

Hypertension occurs in about 50% of patients with sleep apnea; conversely, the prevalence of sleep apnea in the hypertensive population is estimated to be about 30%. There is a progressive increase in the prevalence of hypertension with the severity of sleep apnea, but even mild sleep apnea is associated with an increased prevalence of hypertension.[34] The prevalence of hypertension is about two to three times higher in sleepy patients compared with nonsleepy patients.[18] Almost all male patients and two-thirds of female patients with refractory hypertension (defined as continued elevation of blood pressure in spite of taking three or more antihypertensive medications) have OSA.[35] The likelihood of developing hypertension over time progressively increases with the severity of OSA. Although both hypertension and sleep apnea occur more commonly in middle-aged obese men, sleep apnea is an independent risk factor for hypertension. Successful therapy for sleep apnea may lead to improvement in hypertension.[30]

Patients with OSA have an increased incidence of angina, myocardial infarction, and congestive heart failure.[30] Like hypertension, smoking, and obesity, OSA is considered an independent risk factor for myocardial infarction. The prevalence of OSA is higher in patients with cardiovascular disorders than in the general population.

There is a strong association between sleep apnea and cerebral vascular accidents.[5] Patients with OSA are about two to three times more likely to develop stroke compared with controls. Because OSA is a risk factor for hypertension, which is one of the strongest risk factors for stroke, it is not surprising that the risk of stroke is increased. It appears, however, that the risk of stroke in patients with sleep apnea is higher even in the absence of hypertension. The prevalence of OSA in patients with stroke is very high. More than two-thirds of patients admitted with acute stroke have sleep apnea.[5]

Pulmonary

Pulmonary hypertension during apneic episodes is common. In patients with severe hypoxemia, extremely high levels of pulmonary hypertension may be observed.[36] Sustained pulmonary hypertension during the day is found in about 20% of patients with OSA, primarily in those with hypoxemia and hypercapnia during the day and severe oxygen desaturation during the night.[37] Occasionally, acute pulmonary edema may be the presenting feature of the disease in patients with severe sleep apnea.[36] A paradoxical shift of the interventricular septum can occur because of increased right ventricular pressure.[36]

Endocrine

The prevalence of type 2 diabetes is higher in patients with OSA; conversely, the prevalence of OSA is higher in patients with type 2 diabetes.[38] Although obesity is a common risk factor for both diseases, OSA is an independent risk factor for the development of insulin resistance. There is improvement in insulin resistance with **continuous positive airway pressure (CPAP)** therapy in patients with OSA and diabetes.[38]

Renal

Proteinuria is known to commonly occur in obese patients, but it appears that sleep apnea may be a stronger determinant of its frequency and severity.[39] Proteinuria may be significant enough to be in the nephrotic range and is usually reversible with adequate therapy for sleep apnea.[40] Proteinuria usually occurs in patients with severe sleep apnea and appears to be related to the degree of hypoxemia.[41,42]

Gastrointestinal Tract

Gastroesophageal reflux symptoms are present in more than 50% of patients with OSA. Patients with reflux disease have a higher prevalence of snoring and sleep apnea.

The paradoxical breathing pattern (chest and abdomen moving in opposite directions) during apneic episodes predisposes the development of reflux. Increased negative intrathoracic pressure during an apneic episode encourages the movement of gastric acid into the esophagus. At the same time, abdominal pressure is increased due to the inward movement of the abdominal muscles causing the same effect. Therapy with CPAP leads to improvement in reflux symptoms.[43]

Ophthalmic

Several associations between OSA and various eye-related problems have been suggested. Optic disk swelling, teardrop retinal hemorrhages, normotensive glaucoma, ischemic optic neuropathy, and increased intracranial pressure associated with disc edema (pseudotumor cerebri) have all been reported in patients with OSA.[44]

Psychiatric

Sleep disturbances are frequently seen in patients with depression. Depression is common in patients with sleep apnea. Patients with depression and hypertension have a high prevalence of sleep apnea. CPAP therapy results in improvement in symptoms of depression in many patients with sleep apnea and depression.[45]

Sexual

Erectile dysfunction is common in patients with severe OSA, particularly in patients with hypoxemia. CPAP therapy is associated with improvement in erectile dysfunction.[46]

Diagnosis of Obstructive Sleep Apnea

Many clinical findings, such as degree of obesity, neck circumference, snoring, nocturnal choking, hypertension, age, sleepiness during driving, and the presence of upper airway abnormalities, have been identified as predictors of the presence of OSA. A flow–volume loop usually shows the presence of upper airway obstruction or a sawtooth pattern, or both.[47] Holter monitoring can reveal characteristic arrhythmias present predominantly during sleep. None of these, however, is strong enough to obviate the need for polysomnography for a definite diagnosis.

Nocturnal pulse oximetry showing repeated episodes of oxygen desaturation is strongly suggestive of sleep apnea.[48] In many countries an oxygen desaturation of 4% is considered equivalent to an apneic episode. Instead of using the AHI, an oxygen desaturation index (ODI) is reported. In most patients with sleep apnea and hypoxemia there is high correlation between the AHI and ODI. However, hypoxemia may not be present in patients with mild sleep apnea.

Overnight polysomnography, with recording of the electroencephalogram, electro-oculogram, electromyogram, electrocardiogram, oronasal airflow, chest and abdominal movements, and oxygen saturation, remains the standard diagnostic test for sleep apnea. Polysomnography reveals the frequency, type, and duration of apnea and hypopnea; the presence of cardiac arrhythmias; and the quality and quantity of sleep. In addition, the presence of repeated arousals and episodes of nocturnal myoclonus that can produce hypersomnolence can be identified. The American Academy of Sleep Medicine has published guidelines for scoring of sleep and sleep-related breathing problems.[49]

Usually, single-night polysomnography is a sufficiently sensitive test to exclude clinically significant sleep apnea. Sometimes, however, the first polysomnogram may be falsely negative. Factors that may cause a false-negative polysomnogram include a technically poor study, an inadequate amount of sleep, reduced REM sleep, sleeping in a lateral posture, recent weight loss, or recent therapy for suspected sleep apnea.[50]

> **RESPIRATORY RECAP**
>
> **Complications of Sleep-Disordered Breathing**
>
> » Sleep-disordered breathing causes a variety of serious complications affecting the cardiac, pulmonary, psychological, sexual, endocrine, central nervous, renal, vascular, and ophthalmic systems.
>
> » Central nervous system complications manifest as cognitive, emotional, and psychological problems that often are not associated with sleep apnea syndrome without a proper diagnosis.

Treatment of Obstructive Sleep Apnea

Tracheostomy was considered the standard treatment for very sick patients with OSA during the 1970s. Currently, most patients, including those with acute or chronic respiratory failure, can be adequately treated with CPAP therapy. **Oral appliances** also are considered first-line therapy for mild sleep apnea. Surgical therapy can be used if there are significant correctable anatomic abnormalities. Other helpful strategies include weight loss, sleeping in nonsupine posture, and avoiding aggravating factors such as alcohol, smoking, sedatives, and narcotics. Treatment of diseases contributing to sleep apnea, such as hypothyroidism, can also improve sleep apnea symptoms.

Weight Loss

Fat deposition in neck and pharyngeal tissue contributes to the anatomic and physiologic narrowing of the upper airway. Weight loss is quite effective in reducing the number of apneas and improving nocturnal oxygen desaturation and the quality of sleep. Generally, for every 1% decrease in weight there is a 3% decrease in the apnea-hypopnea index.[51,52] Usually, about a 10% to 20%

weight loss is needed for a significant effect on clinical symptoms to be seen. In some patients, however, even a modest amount of weight loss may have a significant effect on the severity of sleep apnea. Regular follow-up with dietary counseling and nutritional consultation is helpful. Weight reduction surgery or medications can also be considered in patients with significant weight-related problems.

Posture

Sleeping on the back is associated with the highest number of apneas and hypopneas. Sleeping on the side improves apnea and hypopnea and, in some patients, may totally control the problem.[53] Sleeping with a tennis ball sewn in the back of the shirt or a lateral wedge pillow can help reduce time spent sleeping on the back. Most spouses are aware of this improvement and use "elbow therapy" to make sure the patient sleeps on his or her side. Sleeping with the head and upper body elevated to 30 to 60 degrees has been effective in decreasing the severity of sleep apnea.[54]

Positive Airway Pressure Therapy

Positive airway pressure (PAP) for treating OSA was first described in 1981[55] and has become the most commonly used therapy for sleep apnea.[56,57] Positive airway pressure acts as a pneumatic splint in the upper airway counteracting the negative inspiratory pressure and preventing airway collapse (**Figure 46–6**). There is progressive increase in the upper airway size with increasing positive airway pressure. It is now considered the first-line therapy for sleep apnea and can be successfully used in most patients.

PAP can be applied using many techniques. The most common method is to apply preselected constant pressure during sleep from an airflow generator (machine). Because the same pressure level is maintained during both inspiration and expiration, it is called continuous positive airway pressure (CPAP) therapy. Many patients are uncomfortable during exhalation when they breathe against the airflow, which is still coming in at the same pressure level. The normal respiratory pattern is altered during CPAP therapy, with exhalation becoming active. Most CPAP machines provide pressures ranging from 0 to 20 cm H_2O. The most commonly used CPAP pressure range for treating OSA is between 8 and 10 cm H_2O.

Bilevel machines provide two pressure levels: higher pressure during inspiration and a lower pressure during exhalation. The pressure difference is usually about 4 cm H_2O. Because of the lowered expiratory pressure during bilevel therapy, exhalation may be less uncomfortable than with CPAP. It was anticipated that the compliance would be better with bilevel machines than with CPAP. However, compliance does not seem to be better with bilevel machines.[57] Bilevel machines are most commonly used when the pressure level during expiration is high (mostly above 15 cm H_2O), to the point that the patient cannot tolerate CPAP therapy. Bilevel machines are more expensive than CPAP machines.

Auto-titrating PAP machines detect airway narrowing and progressively adjust the pressure until airflow becomes normal again. They are being used for the diagnosis and therapy of obstructive sleep apnea and to predict the pressure needed for CPAP therapy.[58] The mean pressure with auto-titrating machines is lower than with CPAP machines because the pressure goes to the maximum only when needed. Again, these machines have not been shown to improve compliance

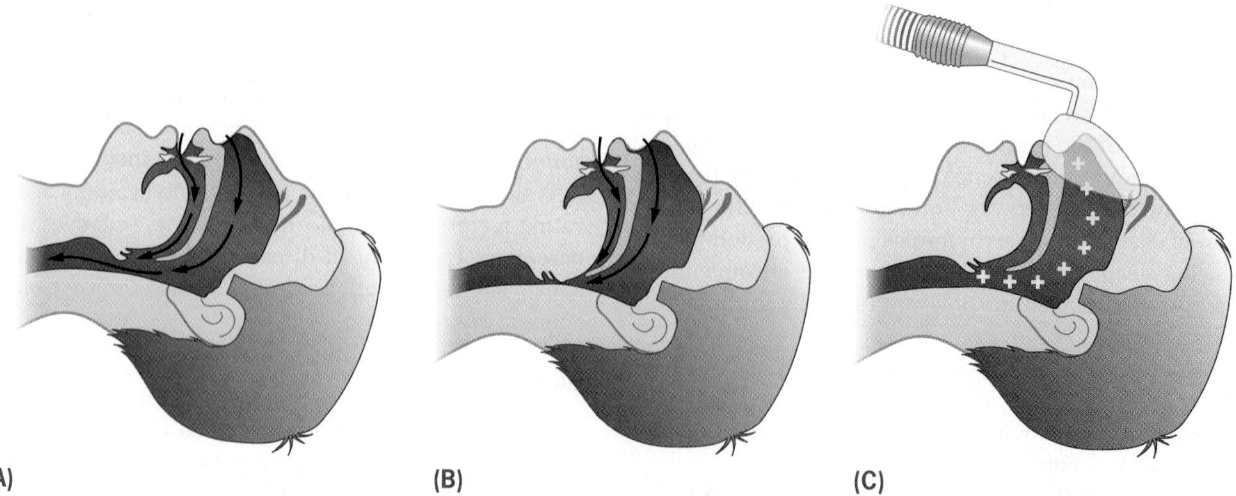

FIGURE 46–6 (**A**) Normal upper airway. (**B**) Upper airway obstruction. (**C**) Upper airway obstruction relieved with the addition of continuous positive airway pressure (CPAP) circuit for acute respiratory failure. Adapted from Branson RD. Spontaneous breathing systems: IMV and CPAP. In: Branson RD, Hess DR, Chatburn RL, eds. *Respiratory Care Equipment*. 2nd ed. JB Lippincott; 1999.

with CPAP therapy. They have the potential to decrease the need for CPAP titration studies. One drawback with auto-titrating machines is that these machines can overcompensate if there is leakage around the mask or if the mouth is open. This overcompensation can unnecessarily increase the airway pressure. This increase in pressure has the potential to cause even more air leakage and can also disturb sleep. Conversely, the patient may be undertreated because of the time delay in reaching the optimal pressure needed to correct apneas. Because one of the mechanisms in some auto-titrating machines is the detection of reduced inspiratory airflow, these machines may not be able to treat patients with central apneas. Also, they may not be able to treat patients with OSA who develop central apnea during CPAP therapy (complex sleep apnea). Auto-titrating CPAP machines are more expensive than conventional CPAP machines.

A useful feature of CPAP machines is a ramp, in which the pressure starts at a low level and gradually increases to the prescribed level. A ramp helps some patients better tolerate this therapy. The newer CPAP machines have the capability of reducing pressure (expiratory pressure relief and C-Flex modes) briefly by 1 to 4 cm H_2O at the beginning of exhalation, which may improve patient comfort and compliance.

Many different interfaces are available for CPAP. Oronasal masks are big and cover both nose and mouth. These masks are useful for patients who keep their mouth open during PAP therapy. Nasal masks are smaller and cover only the nose. Oral masks deliver air through the mouth and generally are less well tolerated than other masks. Nasal pillows or prongs are used to deliver air directly into the nose. These pillows avoid skin-contact abrasions but may cause irritation of the nares.

The immediate effect of CPAP usage is the elimination of snoring. (Spouses sleep much better and love this therapy!) Nighttime awakenings and visits to the bathroom are decreased.[59] Patients feel rested upon awakening, and the frequency of morning headaches is decreased. Daytime sleepiness and tiredness are reduced or eliminated in a significant number of patients. Improvement in sleep-related complications (driving, functioning at work) is noted. There is improvement in cognitive functions. Long-term CPAP usage is associated with improvement in most of the complications of sleep apnea.[56]

The side effects of PAP therapy are caused either by the interface or the air pressure and flow (**Table 46–5**). Newer PAP machines produce only a minimal humming noise. The main reason for noise at the face is the leakage of air because of poor fit or movement of the mask. Some patients may get entangled with the circuit. Fitting the mask too tightly can lead to skin irritation and skin abrasions at the contact site. The nasal bridge is the usual site of skin and bony erosion. Many patients complain of nasal or oral dryness, nasal congestion, sneezing, and even nosebleeds.[60] The use of heated humidity reduces symptoms in most patients.[61,62] Chin straps can help in keeping the mouth closed, thereby reducing oral dryness in patients who keep their mouth open during PAP therapy. Rhinorrhea can be helped by using intranasal ipratropium. Pressures in the lower range are well tolerated; however, at higher pressures, some patients experience hyperinflation. In such patients, the CPAP apparatus can be modified to give lower pressure during exhalation. Swallowing air (aerophagy) may be associated with CPAP use and can be reduced by using lower pressure. Pneumothorax is potentially a serious complication but occurs rarely in the usual pressure range used for sleep apnea. Pneumocephaly is also rare and is related to air leakage from the nose to cranium.

The major reason for the failure of PAP therapy is lack of adherence to the treatment plan. Most new PAP machines have the capability to provide hourly, nightly, and long-term data about when the machine is turned on and the actual usage of the machine. Because the beneficial effect of PAP therapy is directly proportional to the amount of time it is used, all-night usage should be encouraged. Arbitrarily, a patient is considered compliant if his or her PAP machine usage is a minimum of 4 hours per night on 70% of the nights under consideration.[63,64] Patient adherence during the first month predicts long-term usage. Adherence is better in patients with severe symptoms and in better-educated individuals. A higher pressure level does not reduce patient adherence, as is sometimes assumed. Patient adherence to therapy can be improved by positive reinforcement and treatment of PAP-related side effects (e.g., uncomfortable mask, oronasal dryness). Unfortunately, only about 55% of patients use CPAP therapy regularly, which is an adherence rate similar to the intake rate of oral medications for other medical diseases.

TABLE 46–5 Complications Related to Positive Airway Pressure Therapy

Cause	Complication
Machine	Noise
Circuit	Entanglement, rebreathing
Interface	Skin abrasions, claustrophobia, leaks, rebreathing
Airflow and pressure	
Nose	Dryness on nose and throat, rhinorrhea, congestion, epistaxis
Sinus	Discomfort
Eyes	Conjunctivitis
Chest	Discomfort, expiratory difficulty, hyperinflation, pneumothorax
Gastrointestinal system	Aerophagy
Central nervous system	Pneumocephalus

The Centers for Medicare and Medicaid Services has recommended AHI-based criteria for CPAP therapy. Reimbursement for CPAP is approved if the patient has an AHI of 15 or above (moderate and severe sleep apnea). Reimbursement is also approved for patients with an AHI greater than or equal to 5 and less than or equal to 14 (mild sleep apnea) who have at least one of the following: (1) symptoms of excessive daytime sleepiness; (2) impaired cognition, mood disorders, or insomnia; or (3) cardiovascular disease such as hypertension, ischemic heart disease, or history of stroke.

Oral appliances are used to enlarge the oropharynx by either advancing the mandible or keeping the tongue in a forward position.[65,66] Mandibular repositioning appliances (MRAs) cause forward and downward movement of the mandible when attached to one or both dental arches. Tongue-retaining devices (TRDs) keep the tongue in the anterior position by creating negative pressure in a plastic bulb, a flange that fits between the lips and the teeth. Oral appliances increase the airway space in both the retropalatal and retroglossal areas. Both types of devices also increase upper airway muscle tone, thereby making it easier for the airway to remain open. Previously, these appliances required dental impressions, bite registration, and fabrication by a dental laboratory. However, the newer appliances are available in prefabricated, thermolabile forms that can be molded in the office or at home.

Oral appliances are generally used in patients who present with snoring, upper airway resistance syndrome, or mild sleep apnea that does not respond to conservative therapy. These appliances can also be used in patients who have moderate or severe sleep apnea and cannot use CPAP therapy. Oral appliances are not considered the first-line therapy for severe sleep apnea.

Oral appliances are effective in reducing the severity of symptoms and various objective measures used to express the severity of sleep apnea. There is significant improvement in the intensity and frequency of snoring in most patients. Reduction in daytime sleepiness occurs in most patients. Apnea and hypopnea are improved, and the rate of improvement depends on how the improvement is defined. The success rate is about 65% if the most liberal definition of improvement (i.e., 50 % reduction in AHI) is used. The success rates are 52% and 42% if AHI reductions down to 10 or 5 are used, respectively. About one-half of patients continue to have significant apneas, and about 10% may have worsening of AHI with these appliances. The four main predictors of successful therapy with oral appliances are lower severity of OSA, lower body mass index, more severe OSA when the patient sleeps on his or her back compared with his or her side, and the amount of mandibular or tongue advancement by the appliance.[67] Improvement is least in obese patients with severe OSA, particularly those who do not have significant improvement in apneas in the nonsupine posture. The usual protrusion of mandible necessary to improve OSA varies between 5 and 10 mm. Improvement is seen in only one-third of patients if the protrusion is 50% of the maximum, but increases with more protrusion.

The compliance rate with oral appliances is high, and about three-fourths of patients use their appliance regularly. Compliance rate falls somewhat over time because of side effects and lack of efficacy. Overall compliance rates are similar to CPAP in various crossover studies.

Some oral discomfort occurs, but most patients tolerate these appliances well. Common side effects include mouth dryness, excessive salivation, tooth discomfort, occlusive change, and jaw pain. Side effects may improve with continued use. In addition, long-term use may result in a mild reduction in overbite or overjet and minor movements of teeth. In some patients bite changes persist after cessation of therapy.

Currently, oral appliances and CPAP are considered the first lines of therapy for mild sleep apnea. The patient acceptance rate is high, and many patients prefer these appliances compared with CPAP therapy. The reduction in apneas and hypopneas and oxygen desaturation is less than with CPAP therapy, but the improvement in symptoms is similar. The improvement in apneas and hypopneas is better with oral appliances than with surgical therapy.[68]

Edentulous patients are unable to use MRAs but may be able to use TRDs. Patients should have at least six teeth in each dental arch to be able to hold an MRA, and they should be able to open the mouth and protrude the mandible forward. Significant temporomandibular joint problems and severe bruxism are contraindications for oral appliance therapy.

Surgery

Tracheostomy has been very effective in eliminating apnea and reversing the consequences of apnea; however, complications commonly occur. Most patients are reluctant to have it done; consequently, tracheostomy is rarely performed for OSA. Although many surgical procedures can be undertaken to correct anatomic abnormalities and to open the upper airway (**Box 46–2**), **uvulopalatopharyngoplasty (UPPP)** remains the most common surgical procedure.[69]

Upper airway obstruction in sleep apnea usually occurs at the retropalatal and /or retroglossal area. UPPP enlarges the posterior pharynx by removing the uvula, tonsils, and excessive tissue from the lateral pharyngeal wall and pharyngopalatal arch. Following surgery, symptomatic improvement may be reported by up to 90% of patients. Objective improvement (50% reduction in apneas) occurs in about two-thirds of patients, and cure (reduction of apneas to the normal range) is seen in less than half.[70,71] Unfortunately, many patients have recurrence of symptoms of OSA after initial improvement. Some patients have worsening of apneas and hypopneas

BOX 46–2

Surgical Therapies for Sleep Apnea Syndromes

Uvulopalatopharyngoplasty (UPPP)
Genioglossal advancement
Partial glossectomy
Hyoid bone advancement
Maxillomandibular advancement
Tracheostomy
Combinations

after surgery. Many modifications of UPPP, including laser-assisted uvuloplasty (LAUP) and radio frequency ablation, have not been any more successful.

The efficacy of UPPP is highest in patients with mild to moderate sleep apnea. Patients with severe OSA and particularly those who have excessive body weight are not helped much by this procedure. The failure of UPPP is probably related to the multiplicity of causes of OSA and multiple sites of airway obstruction. Multiple modalities, including computed tomography of the upper airway, cephalometric analysis, pharyngeal pressure measurements, the Mueller maneuver, and direct visualization by nasoendoscope, have been used to predict the site of airway obstruction and the success of UPPP, but none of the techniques has been consistently beneficial.

Many other surgical procedures have been used for enlarging the upper airway. The overall success rate with additional procedures has been reported by some centers to be better than UPPP alone.[70] Correction of deviated nasal septum and resection of enlarged turbinates and nasal polyps can enlarge the nasal passage. The tongue (genioglossus muscle) is attached to the inner side of the mandible at the geniotubercle. Pulling the geniotubercle forward to attach it to the front part of the mandible (mandibular osteotomy) can put tension on the tongue, preventing it from falling back to the pharynx. Moving the lower jaw forward alone or with the upper jaw (mandibular or maxillomandibular osteotomy) can increase the space at the base of the tongue. Partial resection of the center part of the tongue (midline glossectomy) has been tried in a few patients.

Surgical procedures are associated with pain, bleeding, infection, and even deaths. Persistent side effects related to UPPP surgery occur in about half of the patients and include difficulty swallowing, globus sensation, and voice changes.[70] Because of complications and the low success rate, surgical therapy is usually considered when patients do not want to use CPAP or oral appliances. If there are significant anatomic abnormalities causing airway obstruction, such as enlarged tonsils, adenoids, or deviated nasal septum, surgical therapy may be considered as the primary therapy.

Pharmacologic Therapy

Many pharmacologic agents have been tried, but none has been consistently effective. Drugs have the potential to improve apneas by many different mechanisms. Because apneas occur more frequently during REM sleep, reduction of this sleep stage by medications may be beneficial. Most antidepressant agents significantly reduce REM sleep time. In those patients with mild sleep apnea who have the majority of their apneic episodes occurring in REM sleep, a trial of a nonsedating tricyclic antidepressant (e.g., protriptyline) or selective serotonin reuptake inhibitor (SSRI) such as fluoxetine can be undertaken to see if improvement occurs in apneas and oxygen desaturation. These antidepressants also reduce upper airway narrowing by increasing the upper airway muscle tone.[72,73] Medroxyprogesterone stimulates ventilation and was initially shown to have some beneficial effect, but subsequent studies have shown no improvement in apneas.[74] Because of the limited clinical benefit and the potential for many side effects, drug therapy is not considered as a standard therapy for OSA.

Oxygen therapy can improve nocturnal oxygen desaturation as well as the frequency of apnea.[75] A high concentration of inspired oxygen therapy may prolong apneic episodes and should be avoided. In patients who present with acute respiratory failure, oxygen therapy is used in conjunction with CPAP and diuretic therapy. Long-term oxygen therapy usually is reserved for patients who remain hypoxemic despite other forms of therapy.

Treatment of diseases that cause upper airway narrowing and apnea may be beneficial. Treatment of nasal allergies and the use of nasal steroids, decongestants, and antihistamine may improve nasal breathing in patients with rhinitis.[76] About 10% of patients with snoring and apneas can benefit from nasal vasoconstrictors. Apneas commonly occur in patients with hypothyroidism and acromegaly. Hypothyroidism causes narrowing of the upper airways and reduced ventilatory drive.[77] The possibility of hypothyroidism should be considered during evaluation of patients with sleep apnea. Drug therapy of these disorders is associated with an improvement of apneas and nocturnal oxygen desaturation. Successful therapy of these disorders may reduce the need for long-term CPAP.

RESPIRATORY RECAP

Treatment of Obstructive Sleep Apnea

- » There are many types of treatments, including mechanical, surgical, and pharmacologic approaches.
- » The mechanical approach using positive airway pressure is one of the most common and effective treatments for OSA syndrome.
- » Only about 55% of patients use the PAP device every night during sleep.

Some patients remain significantly sleepy in spite of adequate therapy of sleep apnea. The reason for the residual sleepiness is not clear. It has been suggested that it may be related to hypoxemic damage to wake-promoting regions of the brain.[78] Wakefulness-promoting medications such as modafinil may be considered in patients who continue to remain sleepy.[79] This medication improves daytime alertness; however, there is a potential risk that the patient may reduce the usage of CPAP therapy. The patient needs to be informed that this medication does not reduce apneas or apnea-related hypoxemia.

Mechanical Devices

In selected patients, nasopharyngeal tubes that can keep the upper airway open have been used successfully.[80] The control of apnea and hypopnea is less than with CPAP therapy, and the quality of sleep remains poor. Nasopharyngeal tubes are not well tolerated and have limited clinical utility.

Both external and internal dilators have been tried to treat patients with OSA.[81–83] There is improvement in snoring intensity, and some reduction in apneas, although patients continue to have oxygen desaturation and poor quality of sleep. Nasal dilators can be tried to reduce snoring but are not recommended as therapy of moderate and severe sleep apnea.

Mortality Associated with Obstructive Sleep Apnea

Many studies have shown increased cardiovascular morality in untreated sleep apnea patients, but the mortality rates have not been consistent. Morality rate variability seems to be related to multiple factors, including the severity of disease, age, obesity, hypertension, medical illnesses, and therapy. Most studies show increased mortality in moderate to severe OSA, whereas the role of mild sleep apnea is not clear. Increased mortality rates have been shown in both clinical and community populations with sleep apnea. A study of a community population (the Wisconsin Sleep Cohort) with 18 years of follow-up showed that after adjustments for age, sex, and body mass index, all-cause mortality was 3.8 times higher in patients with severe OSA compared with those with no sleep-disordered breathing.[84] In the same study, the cardiovascular mortality in severe OSA was 5.2 times compared with normal subjects. Other studies have shown annual mortality rates of 2% to 4% but have also emphasized the contribution of associated risk factors.

> **RESPIRATORY RECAP**
>
> **Mortality Associated with Obstructive Sleep Apnea**
>
> » Untreated OSA syndrome can result in serious complications and even death.
>
> » Proper diagnosis and patient adherence to required treatments is imperative. The respiratory therapist plays an important role in the diagnosis, treatment, education, and management of the patient.

Sleep apnea causes increased highway and industrial accidents.[28,85] Increased mortality may occur in the perioperative period from anesthesia and medications. Successful therapy of sleep apnea is associated with reduction in mortality. However, cardiovascular events such as angina and myocardial infarction and the death rates in patients with severe OSA who are treated with CPAP therapy are similar to controls.[86]

KEY POINTS

- Sleep apnea is common and is associated with significant complications and even death in patients who remain untreated.
- Persons who exhibit symptoms suggestive of sleep apnea should see a sleep specialist who can perform polysomnography, leading to the appropriate diagnosis and treatment.
- The most common type of sleep-disordered breathing is obstructive sleep apnea (OSA).
- Respiratory therapists should have an understanding of the basics of polysomnography and sleep-disordered breathing because they may frequently be in contact with persons who have undiagnosed sleep apnea.
- Several different treatment modalities are available to alleviate the symptoms and reverse most of the complications associated with this disease.
- Respiratory therapists have an important role in the diagnosis, treatment, and management of sleep apnea.
- Patient education is a key component of patient adherence to treatment of OSA.
- Successful therapy can significantly improve quality of life.

REFERENCES

1. Guilleminault C, Tilkian A, Dement WC. The sleep apnea syndromes. *Annu Rev Med.* 1976;27:465–484.
2. Young T, Palta M, Dempsey J, et al. The occurrence of sleep-disordered breathing among middle-aged adults. *N Engl J Med.* 1993;328:1230–1235.
3. Daniel J, Gottlieb. The Sleep Heart Health Study: a progress report. *Curr Opin Pulm Med.* 2008;14:537–542.
4. Yumino D, Bradley TD. Central sleep apnea and Cheyne-Stokes respiration. *Proc Am Thorac Soc.* 2008;5:226–236.
5. Yaggi HK, Concato J, Kernan W, et al. Obstructive sleep apnea as a risk factor for stroke and death. *N Engl J Med.* 2005;353:2034–2041.
6. Gould GA, Whyte KF, Rhind GB, et al. The sleep hypopnea syndrome. *Am Rev Respir Dis.* 1988;137:895–898.
7. Epstein LJ, Kristo D, Strollo PJ, et al. Clinical guideline for the evaluation, management and long-term care of obstructive sleep apnea in adults. *J Clin Sleep Med.* 2009;5:263–276.
8. Guilleminault C, Stoohs R, Clerk A, et al. A cause of excessive daytime sleepiness: the upper airway resistance syndrome. *Chest.* 1993;104:781–787.

9. Young T, Skatrud J, Peppard PE. Risk factors for obstructive sleep apnea in adults. *JAMA*. 2004;29:2013–2016.
10. Resta O, Foschino-Barbaro MP, Legari G, et al. Sleep related breathing disorders, loud snoring and excessive daytime sleepiness in obese subjects. *Int J Obes Relat Metab Disord*. 2001;25:669–675.
11. Strohl K, Redline S. Recognition of obstructive sleep apnea. *Am J Respir Crit Care Med*. 1996;154:279–289.
12. Lam B, Lam DC, Ip MS. Obstructive sleep apnoea in Asia. *Int J Tuberc Lung Dis*. 2007;11:2–11.
13. White DP. Pathogenesis of obstructive and central sleep apnea. *Am J Respir Crit Care Med*. 2005;172(11):1363–1370.
14. Ryan CM, Bradley TD. Pathogenesis of obstructive sleep apnea. *J Appl Physiol*. 2005;99(6):2440–2450.
15. Gleadhill IC, Schwartz AR, Schubert N, et al. Upper airway collapsibility in snorers and in patients with obstructive hypopnea and apnea. *Am Rev Respir Dis*. 1991;143:1300–1303.
16. Peppard PE, Austin D, Brown RL. Association of alcohol consumption and sleep disordered breathing in men and women. *J Clin Sleep Med*. 2007;3:265–270.
17. Ohayon MM, Guilleminault C, Priest RG, Caulet M. Snoring and breathing pauses during sleep: telephone interview survey of a United Kingdom population sample. *BMJ*. 1997;314:860–863.
18. Kapur VK, Resnick HE, Gottlieb DJ. Sleep disordered breathing and hypertension: does self reported sleepiness modify the association? *Sleep*. 2008;31:1127–1132.
19. Arzt M, Young T, Finn L, et al. Sleepiness and sleep in patients with both systolic heart failure and obstructive sleep apnea. *Arch Intern Med*. 2006;166:1716–1722.
20. Johns MW. Daytime sleepiness, snoring, and obstructive sleep apnea. The Epworth Sleepiness Scale. *Chest*. 1993;103:30–36.
21. Johns MW. A new method for measuring daytime sleepiness: the Epworth Sleepiness Scale. *Sleep*. 1991;14:540–545.
22. Littner MR, Kushida C, Wise M, et al. Practice parameters for clinical use of the multiple sleep latency test and the maintenance of wakefulness test. *Sleep*. 2005;28:113–121.
23. Lui MM, Lam JC, Mak HK, et al. C-reactive protein is associated with obstructive sleep apnea independent of visceral obesity. *Chest*. 2009;135:950–956.
24. Bravo Mde L, Serpero LD, Barcelo A, et al. Inflammatory proteins in patients with obstructive sleep apnea with and without daytime sleepiness. *Sleep Breath*. 2007;11:177–185.
25. Kapsimalis F, Varouchakis G, Manousaki A, et al. Association of sleep apnea severity and obesity with insulin resistance, C-reactive protein, and leptin levels in male patients with obstructive sleep apnea. *Lung*. 2008;186:209–217.
26. Schafer H, Pauleit D, Sudhop T, et al. Body fat distribution, serum leptin, and cardiovascular risk factors in men with obstructive sleep apnea. *Chest*. 2002;122:829–839.
27. Atkeson A, Yeh SY, Malhotra A, Jelic S. Endothelial function in obstructive sleep apnea. *Prog Cardiovasc Dis*. 2009;51:351–362.
28. Ellen RL, Marshall SC, Palayew M, et al. Systematic review of motor vehicle crash risk in persons with sleep apnea. *J Clin Sleep Med*. 2006;2:193–200.
29. Naseem S, Chaudhary B, Collop N. Attention deficit hyperactivity disorder in adults and obstructive sleep apnea. *Chest*. 2001;119:294–296.
30. Parish JM, Somers VK. Obstructive sleep apnea and cardiovascular disease. *Mayo Clin Proc*. 2004;79:1036–1047.
31. Guilleminault C, Connolly SJ, Winkle RA. Cardiac arrhythmia and conduction disturbances during sleep in 400 patients with sleep apnea syndrome. *Am J Cardiol*. 1983;52:490–494.
32. Caples SM, Somers VK. Sleep-disordered breathing and atrial fibrillation. *Prog Cardiovasc Dis*. 2009;51:411–415.
33. MacDonald M, Fang J, Pittman SD, et al. The current prevalence of sleep disordered breathing in congestive heart failure patients treated with beta-blockers. *J Clin Sleep Med*. 2008;4:38–42.
34. Nieto FJ, Young TB, Lind BK, et al. Association of sleep disordered breathing, sleep apnea and hypertension in a large community based study. Sleep Heart Health Study. *JAMA*. 2000;283:1829–1836.
35. Logan AG, Perlikowski SM, Mente A, et al. High prevalence of unrecognized sleep apnea in drug-resistant hypertension. *J Hypertens*. 2001;19:2271–2277.
36. Chaudhary BA, Nadimi M, Chaudhary TK, Speir WA. Pulmonary edema due to obstructive sleep apnea. *South Med J*. 1984;77:499–501.
37. Atwood CW Jr, McCrory D, Garcia JG, et al. Pulmonary artery hypertension and sleep disordered breathing. *Chest*. 2004;126:72s–77s.
38. Tasali, E, Mokhlesi B, Van Cauter E. Obstructive sleep apnea and type 2 diabetes: interacting epidemics. *Chest*. 2008; 133:496–506.
39. Chaudhary BA, Sklar AH, Chaudhary TK, et al. Sleep apnea, proteinuria, and nephrotic syndrome. *Sleep*. 1988;11:69–74.
40. Sklar AH, Chaudhary BA. Reversible proteinuria in obstructive sleep apnea syndrome. *Arch Intern Med*. 1988;148:87–89.
41. Chaudhary BA, Rehman O, Brown T. Proteinuria in patients with sleep apnea. *J Fam Pract*. 1995;40:139–141.
42. Faulx MD, Storfer-Isser A, Kirchner HL, et al. Obstructive sleep apnea is associated with increased urinary albumin excretion. *Sleep*. 2007;30:923–929.
43. Green BT, Broughton WA, O'Conner JB. Marked improvement in nocturnal gastroesophageal reflux in a large cohort of patients with obstructive sleep apnea treated with continuous positive airway pressure. *Ann Internal Med*. 2003;163:41–45.
44. Marcus DM, Lynn J, Miller JJ, et al. Sleep disorders: a risk factor for pseudotumor cerebri. *J Neuroophthalmol*. 2001;21:121–123.
45. Schwartz DJ, Karatinos G. For individuals with obstructive sleep apnea, institution of CPAP therapy is associated with an amelioration of symptoms of depression which is sustained long term. *J Clin Sleep Med*. 2007;3:631–635.
46. Goncalves MA, Guilleminault C, Ramos E, et al. Erectile dysfunction, obstructive sleep apnea syndrome and nasal CPAP treatment. *Sleep Med*. 2005;6:333–339.
47. Dennison FH, Taft AA, Chaudhary BA. Noise or upper airway disorder? *Respir Care*. 1993;38:202–206.
48. Zou D, Grote L, Peker Y, et al. Validation of a portable monitoring device for sleep apnea diagnosis in a population based cohort using synchronized home polysomnography. *Sleep*. 2006;29:367–374.
49. Iber C, Ancoili-Israel S, Chesson A, Quan SF, for the American Academy of Sleep Medicine. *The AASM Manual for the Scoring of Sleep and Associated Events: Rules, Terminology and Technical Specifications*. 1st ed. Westchester, IL: American Academy of Sleep Medicine; 2007.
50. Dean R, Chaudhary BA. Negative polysomnogram in patients with obstructive sleep apnea syndrome. *Chest*. 1992;101:105–108.
51. Veasey SC, Guilleminault C, Strohl KP, et al. Medical therapy for obstructive sleep apnea: a review by the Medical Therapy for Obstructive Sleep Apnea Task Force of the Standards of Practice Committee of the American Academy of Sleep Medicine. *Sleep*. 2006;29:1036–1044.
52. Young T, Peppard PE, Taheri S. Excess weight and sleep-disordered breathing. *J Appl Physiol*. 2005;99:1592–1599.
53. Chaudhary BA, Chaudhary T, Kolbeck RC, et al. Therapeutic effect of posture in sleep apnea. *South Med J*. 1986;79:1061–1063.
54. Neil AM, Angus SM, Sajklov D, McEvoy RD. Effects of sleep posture on upper airway stability in patients with obstructive sleep apnea. *Am J Respir Care Med*. 1997;155:199–204.
55. Sullivan CE, Issa FG, Berthon-Jones M, Eves L. Reversal of obstructive sleep apnea by continuous positive pressure applied through the nares. *Lancet*. 1981;1:862–865.
56. Kakkar RK, Berry RB. Positive airway pressure treatment for obstructive sleep apnea. *Chest*. 2007;132:1057–1072.

57. Kushida CA, Littner MR, Hirshkowitz M, et al. Practice parameters for the use of continuous and bilevel positive airway pressure devices to treat adult patients with sleep-related breathing disorders. *Sleep.* 2006;29:375–380.
58. Morgenthaler TI, Aurora RN, Brown T, et al. Practice parameters for the use of autotitrating continuous positive airway pressure devices for titrating pressures and treating adult patients with obstructive sleep apnea syndrome: an update for 2007. *Sleep.* 2008;31:141–147.
59. Fitzgerald MP, Mulligan M, Parthasarathy S. Nocturic frequency is related to severity of obstructive sleep apnea, improves with continuous positive airways treatment. *Am J Obstet Gynecol.* 2006;194:1399–1403.
60. Hoffstein V, Viner S, Mateika S, Conway J. Treatment of obstructive sleep apnea with nasal continuous positive airway pressure: patient compliance, perception of benefits, and side effects. *Am Rev Respir Dis.* 1992;145:841–845.
61. Neill AM, Wai HS, Bannan SP, et al. Humidified nasal continuous positive airway pressure in obstructive sleep apnoea. *Eur Respir J.* 2003;22:258–262.
62. Massie CA, Hart RW, Peralez K, Richards GN. Effects of humidification on nasal symptoms and compliance in sleep apnea patients using continuous positive airway pressure. *Chest.* 1999;116:403–408.
63. Pepin JL, Krieger J, Rodenstein D, et al. Effective compliance during the first 3 months of continuous positive airway pressure. A European prospective study of 121 patients. *Am J Respir Crit Care Med.* 1999;160:1124–1129.
64. Kribbs NB, Pack AI, Kline LR, et al. Objective measurement of patterns of nasal CPAP use by patients with obstructive sleep apnea. *Am Rev Respir Dis.* 1993;147:887–895.
65. Ferguson KA, Cartwright R, Rogers R, et al. Oral appliances for snoring and obstructive sleep apnea: a review. *Sleep.* 2006; 29;244–262.
66. Kushida CA, Morgenthaler TI, Littner MR, et al. Practice parameters for the treatment of snoring and obstructive sleep apnea with oral appliances: an update for 2005. *Sleep.* 2006;29:240–243.
67. Hoekema A, Doff MHJ, de Bont LGM, et al. Predictors of obstructive sleep apnea-hypopnea treatment outcome. *J Dent Res.* 2007;86:1181–1186.
68. Walker-Engstrom ML, Tegelberg A, Wilhelmsson B, Ringqvist I. 4-year follow-up of treatment with dental appliance or uvulopalatopharyngoplasty in patients with obstructive sleep apnea: a randomized study. *Chest.* 2002;121:739–746.
69. Fujita S, Conway W, Zorick F, Roth T. Surgical correction of anatomic abnormalities in obstructive sleep apnea syndrome: uvulopalatopharyngoplasty. *Otolaryngol Head Neck Surg.* 1981;89:923–934.
70. Franklin KA, Anttila H, Axelsson S, et al. Effects and side-effects of surgery for snoring and obstructive sleep apnea—a systematic review. *Sleep.* 2009;32:27–36.
71. Harmon JD, Chaudhary BA. Uvulopalatoplasty and obstructive sleep apnea. *South Med J.* 1986;79:197–200.
72. Smith PL, Haponik EF, Allen RP, Bleecker ER. The effects of protriptyline in sleep-disordered breathing. *Am Rev Respir Dis.* 1983;127:8–13.
73. Hanzel DA, Proia NG, Hudgel DW. Response of obstructive sleep apnea to fluoxetine and protriptyline. *Chest.* 1991;100:416–421.
74. Rajagopal KR, Abbrecht PH, Jabbari B. Effects of medroxyprogesterone acetate in obstructive sleep apnea. *Chest.* 1986;90:815–821.
75. Fletcher EC, Munafo DA. Role of nocturnal oxygen therapy in obstructive apnea: when should it be used? *Chest.* 1990;98:1497–1504.
76. Kiely JL, Nolan P, McNicholas WT. Intranasal corticosteroid therapy for obstructive sleep apnoea in patients with co-existing rhinitis. *Thorax.* 2004;59:50–55.
77. Kittle WM, Chaudhary BA. Sleep apnea and hypothyroidism. *South Med J.* 1988;81:1421–1425.
78. Zhan G, Serrano F, Fenik P, et al. NADPH oxidase mediates hypersomnolence and brain oxidative injury in a murine model of sleep apnea. *Am J Respir Crit Care Med.* 2005;172:921–929.
79. Santamaria J, Iranzo A, Ma Montserrat J, de Pablo J. Persistent sleepiness in CPAP treated obstructive sleep apnea patients: evaluation and treatment. *Sleep Med Rev.* 2007;11:195–207.
80. Karlson KH Jr, Chaudhary BA, Porubsky ES. Long-term nasopharyngeal intubation in obstructive sleep apnea. *Pediatr Pulmonol.* 1987;3:440–442.
81. Gosepath J, Amedee RG, Romantschuck S, Mann WJ. Breathe Right nasal strips and the respiratory disturbance index in sleep related breathing disorders. *Am J Rhinol.* 1999;13:385–389.
82. Schonhofer B, Franklin KA, Brunig H, et al. Effect of nasal-valve dilation on obstructive sleep apnea. *Chest.* 2000;118:587–590.
83. Ellegard E. Mechanical nasal alar dilators. *Rhinology.* 2006; 44:239–348.
84. Yong T, Finn L, Peppard PE, et al. Sleep-disordered breathing and mortality: eighteen-year follow-up of the Wisconsin Sleep Cohort. *Sleep.* 2008;31:1071–1078.
85. Ulfberg J, Carter N, Edling C. Sleep-disordered breathing and occupational accidents. *Scand J Work Environ Health.* 2000;26:237–242.
86. Marin JM, Carrizo SJ, Vicente E, Agusti AG. Long-term cardiovascular outcomes in men with obstructive sleep apnoea-hypopnoea with or without treatment with continuous positive airway pressure: an observational study. *Lancet.* 2005;365:1046–1053.

CHAPTER 47

Lung Cancer

Maha Farhat

OUTLINE

Classification
Epidemiology
Risk Factors and Etiology
Presentation
Solitary Pulmonary Nodule
Diagnosis
Workup and Staging
Treatment
Prognosis
Prevention
Future Directions
Case Studies

OBJECTIVES

1. Discuss the magnitude of the worldwide problem of bronchogenic cancer.
2. Classify the different types of lung cancer.
3. Explain the importance of cigarette smoking as a risk factor for lung cancer.
4. Describe the approach to staging of small cell and non-small-cell lung cancer.
5. List the different treatment options for lung cancer and the associated prognoses.
6. Discuss possible future advances in the screening, diagnosis, and treatment of lung cancer.

KEY TERMS

adenocarcinoma
adjuvant therapy
benign
bronchogenic carcinoma
chemotherapy
malignant
mediastinoscopy
metastasis
neoadjuvant therapy
non-small-cell lung cancer (NSCLC)
radiotherapy
small cell lung cancer (SCLC)
solitary pulmonary nodule (SPN)
squamous cell carcinoma
transbronchial needle aspiration (TBNA)
tumor suppressor gene

INTRODUCTION

Bronchogenic cancer is a common disease with major health implications. Each year, approximately 196,000 patients are diagnosed with primary carcinoma of the lung in the United States,[1] and 84% die within 5 years.[2] Lung cancer causes as many as 1 million deaths annually worldwide,[3] and it currently is the leading cause of death from cancer in adults. Although it is largely preventable, lung cancer kills more people than breast cancer, colon cancer, and prostate cancer combined. Despite extensive research, the mortality rate for lung cancer has not improved substantially over the past several decades. The U.S. cost of treatment is estimated to be $9.6 billion a year.[1] This makes lung cancer one of the most expensive cancers to treat in the country. As the frequency of smoking has decreased, the incidence of lung carcinoma in men has declined, and in the past 10 years the incidence in women has finally started to decline as well, albeit at a lower rate. This fact, in addition to new chemotherapeutic agents, recent advances in diagnostic technology, and novel treatment strategies, offers some basis for optimism. However, the persistently dismal prognosis of patients with lung cancer in developed countries and the continued rising incidence of disease among both women and men in developing countries show that this disease remains a substantial cause for concern.[1–3]

Classification

Lung tumors can be classified as primary or secondary, **benign** or **malignant**, endobronchial or parenchymal. **Box 47–1** presents the World Health Organization's histologic classification of lung and pleural tumors.

Epithelial tumors of the lung, or **bronchogenic carcinomas**, are by far the most common type of primary pulmonary tumor (other histologies constitute well under 1%). Bronchogenic carcinomas are classified as **small cell lung cancer (SCLC)** or **non-small-cell lung cancer (NSCLC)**. NSCLC includes **squamous cell carcinoma**, marked by histologic evidence of keratinization; **adenocarcinoma**, marked by glandular organization and mucus secretion; and large cell undifferentiated cancer, a diagnosis of exclusion when there is no evidence of either squamous or glandular differentiation with light microscopy. Recent advances in electron microscopy and immunohistochemistry have led to an expansion of the original classification, providing subtypes of NSCLC. These subtypes do not have a major influence on management of the disease, although some differences in presentation and pattern of spread have been noted.

RESPIRATORY RECAP

Lung Cancer Classification
- Primary or secondary
- Benign or malignant
- Endobronchial or parenchymal

Over the past 30 to 40 years, the relative incidence of adenocarcinomas has increased. Adenocarcinomas are the most common subtype of bronchogenic carcinoma and are by far the most common type in lifetime nonsmokers. They have a slightly greater propensity for early distant spread, especially to the brain,

BOX 47–1

World Health Organization's Histologic Classification of Lung and Pleural Tumors

Tumors of the Lung

Malignant Epithelial Tumors

- Squamous cell carcinoma
  - Papillary
  - Clear cell
  - Small cell
  - Basaloid
- Small cell carcinoma
  - Combined small cell carcinoma
- Adenocarcinoma
  - Adenocarcinoma, mixed subtype
  - Acinar adenocarcinoma
  - Papillary adenocarcinoma
  - Bronchoalveolar carcinoma
    - Nonmucinous
    - Mucinous
    - Mixed mucinous and nonmucinous or indeterminate
  - Solid adenocarcinoma with mucin
    - Fetal adenocarcinoma
    - Mucinous ("colloid") carcinoma
    - Mucinous cystadenocarcinoma
    - Signet ring adenocarcinoma
    - Clear cell adenocarcinoma
- Large cell carcinoma
  - Large cell neuroendocrine carcinoma
    - Combined large cell neuroendocrine carcinoma
  - Basaloid carcinoma
  - Lymphoepithelioma-like carcinoma
  - Clear cell carcinoma
  - Large cell carcinoma with rhabdoid phenotype
- Adenosquamous carcinoma
- Sarcomatoid carcinoma
  - Pleomorphic carcinoma
  - Spindle cell carcinoma
  - Giant cell carcinoma
  - Carcinosarcoma
  - Pulmonary blastoma
- Carcinoid tumor
  - Typical carcinoid
  - Atypical carcinoid
- Salivary gland tumors
  - Mucoepidermoid carcinoma
  - Adenoid cystic carcinoma
  - Epithelial-myoepithelial carcinoma
- Preinvasive lesions
  - Squamous carcinoma in situ
  - Atypical adenomatous hyperplasia
  - Diffuse idiopathic pulmonary neuroendocrine cell hyperplasia

Benign Epithelial Tumors

- Papillomas
  - Squamous cell papilloma
    - Exophytic
    - Inverted
  - Glandular papilloma
  - Mixed squamous cell and glandular papilloma
- Adenomas
  - Alveolar adenoma
  - Papillary adenoma
  - Adenomas of salivary gland type
    - Mucous gland adenoma
    - Pleomorphic adenoma
    - Others
  - Mucinous cystadenoma

RESPIRATORY RECAP

Types of Bronchogenic Carcinoma

- Small cell lung cancer
- Non-small-cell lung cancer

compared with squamous cell tumors. These tumors most often are peripheral and include bronchoalveolar carcinoma, a subtype with unique behavior. The reason for the increased risk of adenocarcinoma is unclear but may be related to changes in smoking behavior (depth of inspiration, type of filter, nitrosamine content). Squamous cell tumor incidence was superseded by that of adenocarcinoma in men in the mid-1990s. Squamous cell tumors arise from the proximal respiratory epithelium and can form large central masses, often with associated necrosis. Large cell tumors are the least common type of NSCLC. Similar to adenocarcinomas, they are most often peripheral, but they may be necrotic (more similar to squamous cell tumors).

SCLC differs from NSCLC in its cell of origin and its aggressiveness. Although tumors with mixed histology have led to the idea of a pluripotent stem cell origin for all bronchogenic cancers, small cell cancers appear to be derived from the neuroendocrine cells of the airway, the so-called enterochromaffin or amine precursor uptake and decarboxylation (APUD) cells. SCLC is highly associated with tobacco smoking, especially heavy smoking, and accounts for 15% to 25% of all bronchogenic carcinomas.[4] Overall the relative incidence of SCLC has been declining and has mirrored that of squamous cell carcinoma. The name derives from the histologic appearance of the tumors, which are seen as small, round, blue cells with hematoxylin-eosin staining. These tumor cells are about twice as big as lymphocytes and have a high

Mesenchymal Tumors
- Epithelioid hemangioendothelioma
- Angiosarcoma
- Pleuropulmonary blastoma
- Chondroma
- Congenital peribronchial myofibroblastic tumor
- Diffuse pulmonary lymphangiomatosis
- Inflammatory myofibroblastic tumor
- Lymphangioleiomyomatosis
- Synovial sarcoma
  - Monophasic
  - Biphasic
- Pulmonary artery sarcoma
- Pulmonary vein sarcoma

Lymphoproliferative Tumors
- Marginal zone B-cell lymphoma of the MALT type
- Diffuse large B-cell lymphoma
- Lymphomatoid granulomatosis
- Langerhans cell histiocytosis

Miscellaneous Tumors
- Hamartoma
- Sclerosing hemangioma
- Clear cell tumor
- Germ cell tumors
  - Teratoma, mature
  - Immature
  - Other germ cell tumors
- Intrapulmonary thymoma
- Melanoma

Metastatic Tumors

Tumors of the Pleura

Mesothelial Tumors
- Diffuse malignant mesothelioma
  - Epithelioid mesothelioma
  - Sarcomatoid mesothelioma
  - Desmoplastic mesothelioma
  - Biphasic mesothelioma
- Localized malignant mesothelioma
- Other tumors of mesothelial origin
  - Well-differentiated papillary mesothelioma
  - Adenomatoid tumor

Lymphoproliferative Disorders
- Primary effusion lymphoma
- Pyothorax-associated lymphoma

Mesenchymal Tumors
- Epithelioid hemangioendothelioma
  - Angiosarcoma
- Synovial sarcoma
  - Monophasic
  - Biphasic
- Solitary fibrous tumor
- Calcifying tumor of the pleura
- Desmoplastic round cell tumor

Adapted from Travis WD, Brambilla E, Muller-Hermelink HK, Harris CC. *Pathology and Genetics of Tumours of the Lung, Pleural, Thymus and Heart.* World Health Organization Classification of Tumours. Lyon, France: IARC Press; 2004.

mitotic rate and metastatic potential. Small cell tumors have a rapid doubling time, and early distant spread is the rule. Although small cell cancers are sensitive to chemotherapy and radiotherapy, the survival rate is dismal. This is partly because SCLC frequently presents in an advanced stage.

Epidemiology

The incidence of lung cancer in the United States in 2004 was about 73 cases per 100,000 population, amounting to a total of 196,000 new cases each year.[1] Incidence peaked in the mid-1980s in men, and around the year 2000 in women. These trends have followed the peak and decline in cigarette smoking in the United States; worldwide, however, the rate of cigarette smoking has dramatically increased in the past two decades.[5] At the current rate the worldwide incidence of lung cancer is expected to continue to increase and may reach a staggering level. Although traditionally considered a disease of men, lung cancer increasingly is seen in women, who account for 44% of new cases.[1] These gender-specific trends are largely explained by smoking behaviors. The increase in tobacco use among girls and young women makes these data a matter of particular concern.[6,7]

Risk Factors and Etiology

The major risk factor for lung cancer is cigarette smoking (**Table 47–1**). Thus, lung cancer differs from most other cancers in that it is largely preventable. The relative risk of developing lung cancer is 10 to 30 times higher for smokers than for lifelong nonsmokers. For a heavy smoker, the lifetime risk of developing lung cancer may be as high as 30% and is proportional to the total quantity and duration of cigarette use. Until recently the link between lung cancer and cigarette smoke was largely based on correlations and associations. However, a direct link was eventually demonstrated by the induction of damage to specific loci of a **tumor suppressor gene** (p53, seen in roughly 60% of lung cancers) by benzopyrene, a chemical in tobacco smoke.[5] Moreover, proto-oncogenes can produce proteins that regulate cell growth and differentiation. For example, mutations of the ras proto-oncogenes have been identified in as many as one-third of patients with NSCLC, with K-ras mutations commonly identified in adenocarcinomas in smokers.[8] Other carcinogens present in industrial pollutants can act similarly to tobacco smoke carcinogens and induce initial genetic abnormalities that lead to epithelial cell proliferation. The genetic abnormalities seen vary among different carcinoma histologies and between smokers and nonsmokers. Clearly, evidence is emerging to explain the mechanisms underlying the development of lung carcinoma and its induction by carcinogens. The genetic abnormalities thus identified hold promise in devising new methods for the early detection and therapy of lung carcinoma.[9]

RESPIRATORY RECAP

Primary Risk Factor for Lung Cancer

» The major risk factor for lung cancer is cigarette smoking.

TABLE 47–1 Relative Risk of Lung Cancer

Patient History	Risk Ratio*
Never smoked; no significant industrial contact	1
Cigarette smoker	
½ pack/day	15
½ to 1 pack/day	17
1 to 2 packs/day	42
More than 2 packs/day	64
Cigar smoker†	3
Pipe smoker†	8
Former smoker	2–10
Nonsmoking woman exposed to secondhand smoke	1.4–1.9
Asbestos worker	
Nonsmoker	5
Cigarette smoker	92
Uranium miner	
Nonsmoker	7
Cigarette smoker	38
Relatives of lung cancer patients	
Nonsmoker	4
Cigarette smoker	14

*The risk ratio is the relative risk of an individual developing lung cancer compared with the risk faced by a comparable individual without the listed exposure.

†Although cigarette smoking carries the greatest risk of lung cancer, the differences among tobacco products are small when adjusted to similar amounts of tobacco consumption.

From Murray JF, Nadel JA. *Textbook of Respiratory Medicine*. 2nd ed. Philadelphia: WB Saunders; 1994. Reprinted with permission.

Environmental tobacco smoke (ETS), also known as secondhand smoke, has important health effects as well. Although the amount of exposure is clearly less than in smokers, the onset of exposure generally occurs at a younger age. Although it varies across studies, the relative risk of lung cancer increases above that of lifelong nonsmokers in a dose-dependent fashion and is on the order of 1.2 to 1.3 times that in nonsmokers. The recognition of the significance of ETS has led to public health policies to reduce smoking and exposure in public spaces.

Risk factors unrelated to tobacco use that have also been proven to increase the risk for lung cancer development include exposure to chromium, asbestos, bischloromethyl ether, ionizing radiation, nickel, mustard gas, arsenic, radon, and polycyclic aromatic hydrocarbons (**Box 47–2**).[10–12] Risk factors may act in concert to increase the risk of lung cancer substantially—for example, smoking in a patient with asbestosis.[13] Low-level exposure to

BOX 47–2

Occupational Carcinogens for Lung Cancer

Proven Carcinogens

- Passive/environmental tobacco smoke
- Metals (e.g., arsenic, chromium, iron oxide, nickel)
- Asbestos
- Industrial (bischloromethyl ether)
- Radon gas
- Mustard gas
- Polycyclic aromatic hydrocarbons
- Ionizing radiation

Suspected Carcinogens

- Air pollution
- Acrylonitrile
- Beryllium
- Vinyl chloride
- Silica
- Wood dust
- History of tuberculosis

Data from Murray JF, Nadel JA. *Textbook of Respiratory Medicine*. 2nd ed. Philadelphia: WB Saunders; 1994; and Hanley ME, Welsh CH. *CURRENT Diagnosis and Treatment in Pulmonary Medicine*. New York: McGraw-Hill; 2003.

TABLE 47–2 Initial Symptoms of Bronchogenic Carcinoma*

Symptom	Occurrence (%)
Cough	21
Hemoptysis	21
Chest pain	16
Dyspnea	12
Extrathoracic pain	6
Anorexia and weight loss	5
Cervical mass	5
Fatigue	3
Superior vena caval obstruction	3
Hoarseness	3
Central nervous system symptoms	3
Shoulder pain	2
Clubbing of the fingers	1

*Patients were seen at University of Texas MD Anderson Cancer Center, Houston, Texas.

From Murray JF, Nadel JA. *Textbook of Respiratory Medicine*. 2nd ed. Philadelphia: WB Saunders; 1994. Reprinted with permission.

asbestos (e.g., nonoccupational exposure) without the development of asbestosis does not significantly change the risk of lung cancer.[14]

Genetic and dietary factors also may increase the risk of lung cancer.[15] First-degree relatives of patients with lung cancer have a twofold to threefold higher risk. It was initially believed that females were at increased risk of lung cancer at all levels of tobacco use, but further epidemiologic evidence has brought this hypothesis into question.[16] In addition, numerous recent studies suggest that certain benign diffuse parenchymal lung diseases (e.g., scleroderma, sarcoidosis, idiopathic pulmonary fibrosis, emphysema) may increase the relative risk of developing lung cancer.[17–22]

Infection with the human immunodeficiency virus (HIV) may influence the development and progression of lung cancer and other non-AIDS–defining malignancies. This has been particularly notable since the advent of highly active antiretroviral therapy (HAART) and the dramatic reduction in the rate of AIDS-defining illnesses, including malignancies, and the prolongation of life expectancy for patients with HIV infection. The reasons behind this increased risk are not clear, but it is postulated that the prolonged survival on HAART with only partial recovery of the immune system can account for this observation.[23,24]

Presentation

Bronchogenic cancers may be found incidentally, through active screening, or because of local or systemic symptoms.[25] Because the outcome for individuals with symptomatic lung cancer is dismal, prevention has been emphasized. Yet as it stands, screening for lung cancer is neither recommended nor widely practiced because of lack of evidence supporting its benefits. Unfortunately, roughly 90% of patients found to have lung cancer are symptomatic at presentation.

Symptoms of lung cancer are of three types: symptoms related to the primary lesion, those related to distal spread or **metastasis**, and those related to paraneoplastic phenomena. Symptoms related to the primary lesion, such as cough, are common at presentation (**Table 47–2**). Along with dyspnea and hemoptysis, cough often is thought to indicate a central tumor. Persistent pneumonic infiltrates or recurrent same-segment pneumonias should suggest an obstructing airway lesion. Similarly, a unifocal wheeze on physical examination may be a diagnostic clue to an obstructing airway lesion.

Dyspnea that occurs as a direct result of lung cancer may be caused by airway obstruction with atelectasis, postobstructive pneumonitis, lymphangitic spread of the tumor, or a compressive malignant pericardial or pleural effusion. Local invasion of the phrenic nerve or the diaphragm may contribute to dyspnea related to diaphragmatic dysfunction.

Hemoptysis is a common symptom in patients with lung cancer, to some extent reflecting concurrent chronic bronchitis. Although lung cancer is in the differential diagnosis of massive hemoptysis because in rare cases tumors may erode into hilar vessels, low-volume but recurrent hemoptysis is most characteristic of bleeding tumors. Typically a high-resolution computed tomographic (CT) scan of the chest is performed to help identify suspicious lesions, direct bronchoscopy, and define common benign etiologies such as bronchiectasis.[26]

> **RESPIRATORY RECAP**
>
> **Presentation of Lung Cancer**
> - Dyspnea
> - Hemoptysis
> - Chest pain
> - Dysphagia
> - Clubbing of the fingers
> - Endocrine syndromes
> - Neurologic syndromes
> - Signs of metastases

Substantial chest pain in lung cancer patients usually represents extension of a peripheral mass to the pleura or the chest wall. Pancoast syndrome is chest wall and spinal nerve root/sympathetic chain invasion by an apical bronchogenic tumor, the so-called superior sulcus tumor.[27] The syndrome consists of pain in the shoulder and medial scapula, an ulnar distribution of radicular pain or muscle atrophy (or both), and Horner's syndrome (unilateral ptosis, miosis, anhydrosis, and enophthalmos). Superior sulcus tumors are most commonly squamous cell carcinomas.

Local spread of proximal tumors or lymph node masses may also cause dysphagia related to esophageal compression, hoarseness related to recurrent laryngeal nerve involvement, chylothorax secondary to thoracic duct compromise, or superior vena caval (SVC) syndrome related to central venous obstruction. Although the differential diagnosis is wide, the most common cause of the SVC syndrome is intraluminal thrombosis related to extrinsic compression by bronchogenic cancer, usually SCLC. Patients with SVC syndrome have symptoms and signs of upper body venous congestion, such as headache or flushing, plethora, and a prominent upper body pattern of venous collaterals. Although controversy exists as to whether SVC syndrome is a true emergency, chemoradiotherapy in SCLC promptly resolves the syndrome.[28] Commonly these patients also require anticoagulation.

Lesions in the lung that represent the spread of a primary lung cancer consist of secondary nodules, lymphangitic spread, and tumor emboli. Tumor emboli, increasingly recognized as a syndrome, may result in subacute or acute dyspnea, disseminated intravascular coagulation, and obstructive shock. The diagnosis may be made by cytologic analysis of a wedged sample obtained by pulmonary artery (PA) catheter. This is rarely performed because of concern for the morbidity associated with PA catheter placement. Lymphangitic spread, which causes dry cough, weight loss, and progressive dyspnea, may manifest as asymmetric pulmonary edema on the chest radiograph. In the appropriate clinical context, the presence of Kerley B lines on the chest radiograph is suggestive of this diagnosis (especially if unilateral) and is highly characteristic on high-resolution CT if they are seen as thickened, beaded, intralobular septae. The diagnosis also is made with high sensitivity and specificity by transbronchial biopsy.

Spread of the tumor itself can result in a variety of manifestations, depending on the mechanism.[29] Extrathoracic symptoms may be related to hematogenous spread of the cancer itself. Common sites include the central nervous system (CNS), bone (axial more often than appendicular skeleton), liver, and adrenal glands. CNS and bone lesions are exceedingly important, because they may lead to substantial pain and disability and often are amenable to palliation, usually through radiotherapy. Liver and adrenal metastases, however, are often asymptomatic and may be suspected because of an infiltrative picture of elevated liver enzyme levels or may be found on a CT scan of the chest or abdomen.

The paraneoplastic manifestations of bronchogenic carcinoma are those that are unrelated to the mechanical effects of primary or metastatic tumor. These paraneoplastic syndromes may occur in at least 10% of lung cancer patients (**Table 47–3** and **Box 47–3**). Several specific syndromes deserve mention. Weight loss is a common feature of lung cancer and is thought to be a paraneoplastic syndrome associated with enhanced inflammatory cytokine production, which results in anorexia and hypermetabolism. The debility associated with weight loss is an important negative prognostic factor.[30,31]

Clubbing of the fingers, which is caused by an increase in subungual soft tissue with associated straightening of the nail bed (Lovibond angle), is an important, albeit nonspecific, finding in lung cancer. Other causes of clubbing include chronic pulmonary infections (bronchiectasis, lung abscess, or empyema), restrictive lung diseases (idiopathic pulmonary fibrosis, pulmonary alveolar phospholipoproteinosis), cyanotic congenital heart disease, infective endocarditis, inflammatory bowel disease, and alcoholic cirrhosis.[32] Both clubbing and the related hypertrophic pulmonary osteoarthropathy (HPO), a symmetric, painful syndrome involving the long bones, are less commonly seen in SCLC than NSCLC. Both signs may disappear with successful tumor therapy. One interesting association has been made between unilateral

TABLE 47–3 Endocrine and Hematologic Syndromes Associated with Lung Tumors

Syndrome	Tumor	Proteins/Cytokines Involved
Hypercalcemia of malignancy	Non-small cell	Parathyroid hormone–related peptide, parathormone
Hyponatremia of malignancy	Small cell Non-small cell	Antidiuretic hormone (arginine vasopressin) Atrial natriuretic peptide
Ectopic ACTH syndrome	Small cell Carcinoid	Adrenocorticotropic hormone Corticotropin-releasing hormone
Acromegaly	Carcinoid, small cell	Growth hormone–releasing hormone
Granulocytosis	Non-small cell	C-CSF, GM-CSF, IL-6
Thrombocytosis	Non-small cell, small cell	IL-6
Thromboembolism	Non-small cell, small cell	Unknown

ACTH, adrenocorticotropic hormone; C-CSF, granulocyte colony-stimulating factor; GM-CSF, granulocyte-macrophage colony-stimulating factor; IL-6, interleukin 6.

BOX 47–3

Lung Cancer Paraneoplastic Syndromes

- Cachexia (e.g., anorexia, weight loss, weakness)
- Fever
- Hypertension
- *Endocrinologic*: hypercalcemia, hyponatremia, Cushing syndrome, gynecomastia, acromegaly, hypoglycemia
- *Neurologic*: Lambert-Eaton myasthenic syndrome, peripheral neuropathy, cerebellar degeneration, limbic encephalitis, encephalomyelitis
- *Musculoskeletal*: clubbing, hypertrophic pulmonary osteoarthropathy, dermatomyositis, polymyositis
- *Hematologic*: anemia, autoimmune hemolytic anemia, leukocytosis/thrombocytosis, vasculitis, noninfectious thrombotic endocarditis, idiopathic thrombocytopenic purpura

From Hanley ME, Welsh CH. *CURRENT Diagnosis and Treatment in Pulmonary Medicine.* New York: McGraw-Hill; 2003. Reprinted with permission.

facial pain and HPO in a small number of patients with lung cancer. Both syndromes have been postulated to result from afferent vagal nerve compression from an intrathoracic tumor.

Endocrine syndromes are another relatively common feature of lung cancer, especially SCLC. The syndrome of inappropriate antidiuretic hormone secretion (SIADH, manifesting with hyponatremia) and ectopic Cushing syndrome (manifesting with weakness, glucose intolerance, and hypokalemia related to an excess of adrenocorticotropin hormone) may be found in patients with established malignancy or may be the first clue to a previously occult tumor. Hypercalcemia, seen most often with squamous cell carcinoma, presents with malaise, dehydration, and gastrointestinal and neurologic abnormalities. Differentiating paraneoplastic hypercalcemia from metastatic bone hypercalcemia that occurs secondary to osseous metastases (through identification of excess parathyroid hormone–related peptide) may be important in the determination of therapy. Hypercalcemia is a very poor prognostic factor in patients with bronchogenic carcinoma.[33]

Neurologic syndromes are recognized as devastating paraneoplastic manifestations of lung cancer. The antibody ANNA-1 (anti-Hu) is associated with SCLC and can have a variety of clinical manifestations. In addition to cerebellar ataxia and a sensory neuropathy, ANNA-1 can lead to alterations in gastric motility, manifesting with nausea, anorexia, and weight loss. Although SCLC often is localized to the chest at the time of diagnosis, the overall survival rate is still dismal. Although some authors report slower tumor growth in patients with ANNA-1, the prognosis remains poor because of associated weight loss, malnutrition, and immobility from gait ataxia.[30–33]

Solitary Pulmonary Nodule

A **solitary pulmonary nodule (SPN)**, a lesion seen on the chest radiograph, is completely surrounded by lung parenchyma, without other radiographic abnormalities such as pleural effusion or adenopathy. An arbitrary size cutoff of 3 cm distinguishes SPN from pulmonary masses, which generally are malignant. SPNs, or *coin lesions*, usually are asymptomatic and generally are found on routine radiographs. In adults, an SPN is considered malignant until proven otherwise, but a number of alternative etiologies are included in the differential diagnosis (**Box 47–4** and **Table 47–4**).[34]

Diagnostic algorithms and advances in imaging have focused on differentiation of benign lesions from malignant ones. This distinction is important because an SPN is the most curable presentation of bronchogenic carcinoma. The 5-year survival rate for resected T1N0M0 lesions ranges from 60% to 90%. In addition, nonsurgical identification of a benign lesion may eliminate the need for thoracotomy or thoracoscopy. The U.S. Veterans Administration Cooperative Armed Forces Study reported in 1975 that only one-third of resected SPNs were malignant.[35] However, a more recent study reported that the percentage of resected SPNs found to be malignant had increased.[36] The percentage ranged from 55% to 60% from 1981 to 1983 and from 90% to 100% from 1990 to 1994. This reflects the greater ability of computed tomography to identify benign lesions. The local frequency of malignant SPN depends to a large extent on the likelihood of obtaining chest radiographs in young people, the population's age distribution, the smoking prevalence, and the prevalence of infectious granulomatous disease, such as endemic fungi and tuberculosis. The differential diagnosis of an SPN also includes metastatic nodules, adenomas and other benign tumors, hamartomas, embolic phenomena, and nodules associated with rheumatologic lesions.

Historical risk factors for a malignant cause of an SPN include age over 35 years, exposure to tobacco or another known lung carcinogen, and previous malignancy (or metastatic disease). Radiographic signs of malignancy include larger size (more than 2 cm in diameter) and a spiculated border (**Figure 47–1**, **Figure 47–2**, and **Figure 47–3**). Most important, when comparison of current radiographs with previous ones shows growth of the nodule, with a volumetric doubling time of 20 to 400 days, malignancy is likely. Signs of benignity include stable lesions (i.e., no growth over a 2-year period) and calcification. Although not 100% specific, an increased calcium content of nodules correlates with benign diagnoses, and certain patterns (popcorn, laminated, diffuse, and central calcification) are very suggestive of benignity. On the other hand, peripheral eccentric calcification is thought to be compatible with a diagnosis of malignancy.

Possible approaches to clinically indeterminate nodules include serial follow-up, transthoracic or bronchoscopic

BOX 47–4

Causes of Solitary Pulmonary Nodules

Malignant Nodules

- Bronchogenic carcinoma
  - Adenocarcinoma
  - Squamous cell carcinoma
  - Small cell carcinoma
- Metastatic lesions
  - Breast
  - Head and neck
  - Melanoma
  - Colon
  - Kidney
  - Sarcoma
  - Germ cell tumor
  - Others
- Pulmonary carcinoid

Benign Nodules

- Infectious granuloma
  - Histoplasmosis
  - Coccidioidomycosis
  - Tuberculosis
  - Atypical mycobacteria
  - Cryptococcosis
  - Blastomycosis
- Other infections
  - Bacterial abscess
  - *Dirofilaria immitis*
  - *Echinococcus cyst*
  - Ascariasis
  - *Pneumocystis carinii*
  - Aspergilloma
- Benign neoplasms
  - Hamartoma
  - Lipoma
  - Fibroma
- Vascular
  - Arteriovenous malformation
  - Pulmonary varix
- Developmental
  - Bronchogenic cyst
- Inflammatory
  - Wegener granulomatosis
  - Rheumatoid nodule
- Other
  - Amyloidoma
  - Rounded atelectasis
  - Intrapulmonary lymph nodes
  - Hematoma
  - Pulmonary infarct
  - Pseudotumor (loculated fluid)
- Mucoid impaction

TABLE 47–4 Clinical and Radiologic Criteria in the Differentiation of Benign and Malignant Solitary Pulmonary Nodules

Criteria	Benign Nodule	Malignant Nodule
Clinical		
Age	Under 35 years of age; exception is hamartoma	Over 35 years of age
Symptoms	Absent	Present
Past history and functional inquiry	Geographic area with high incidence of granulomata; exposure to tuberculosis; nonsmoker	Diagnosis of primary lesion elsewhere; smoker; exposure to carcinogens
Radiographic		
Size	Small (<5 mm diameter are 1% malignant)	Large (>2 cm diameter are 80% malignant)
Location	No predilection except for tuberculosis (upper lobes)	Predominantly upper lobes except for lung metastases
Contour	Margins smooth	Margins spiculated
Calcification	Almost pathognomonic of a benign lesion if laminated, diffuse, or central	Rare, may be eccentric (engulfed granuloma)
Satellite lesions	More common	Less common
Serial studies showing no change over 2 years	Almost diagnostic of benign lesion	Most unlikely (one exception is small nodules of bronchoalveolar carcinoma)
Doubling time	<30 or >490 days	Between these extremes
Computed Tomography		
Calcification	Diffuse or central	Absent or eccentric
Fat	Virtually diagnostic of hamartoma	Absent
Bubblelike lucencies	Uncommon	Common in adenocarcinomas
Enhancement with intravenous contrast material	<15 hounsfield units (HU)	>25 HU

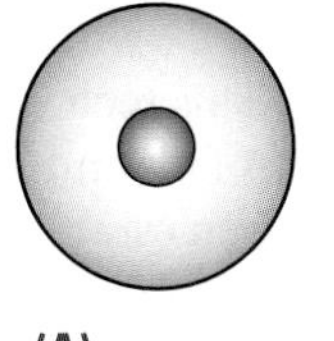
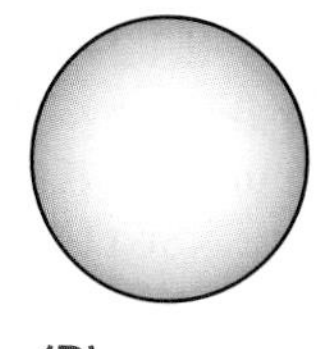
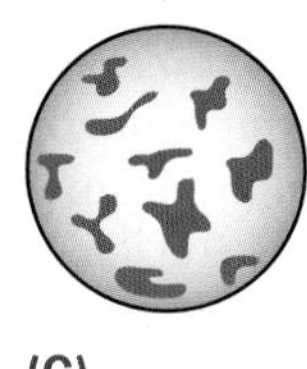
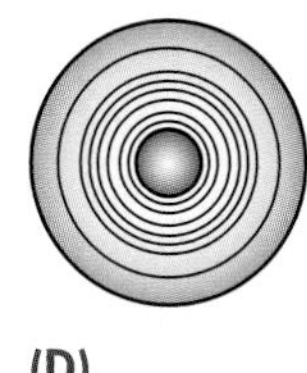

FIGURE 47–1 Patterns of benign calcification. Schematic representation of different patterns of benign calcification. **(A)** Target. **(B)** Diffuse. **(C)** Popcorn. **(D)** Lamellated calcification. Redrawn with permission from Stark P. Computed and positron emission tomographic scanning of pulmonary nodules. In: *UpToDate*, Basow DS, ed. UpToDate, Waltham, MA 2010. Copyright © 2010 UpToDate, Inc. For more information visit www.uptodate.com.

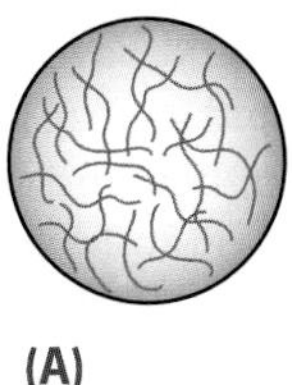
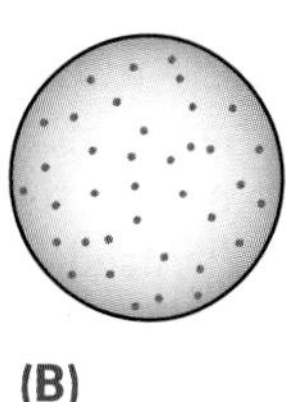
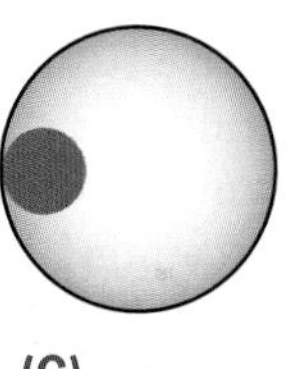
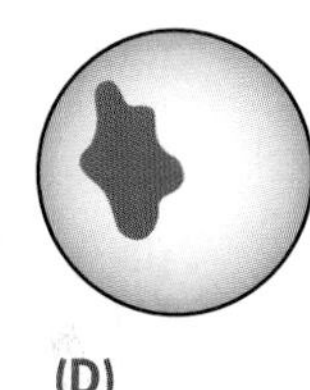

FIGURE 47–2 Patterns of malignant calcification. Schematic representation of different patterns of malignant calcification. **(A)** Reticular. **(B)** Psammomatous (punctate). **(C)** Eccentric. **(D)** Amorphous calcification. Redrawn with permission from Stark P. Computed and positron emission tomographic scanning of pulmonary nodules. In: *UpToDate*, Basow DS, ed. UpToDate, Waltham, MA 2010. Copyright © 2010 UpToDate, Inc. For more information visit www.uptodate.com.

lung biopsy, contrast CT scanning, and positron emission tomography (PET) scanning. The choice of approach depends on the pretest probability of a diagnosis of malignancy, local practice patterns, and the patient's values (i.e., the individual's comfort or discomfort in observing a lesion with a low likelihood of malignancy). In general, serial follow-up is acceptable for low-risk nodules in patients who find diagnostic uncertainty acceptable. For high-risk lesions, definitive diagnosis is required. In many institutions the need for open thoracotomy has been largely replaced by video-assisted thoracoscopic surgery (VATS) techniques. The accuracy of bronchoscopic or transthoracic needle techniques used to diagnose SPN varies widely based on the size of the lesion, its position in the chest, local practice patterns, and the practitioner's skill.[37]

Transthoracic needle aspiration (TTNA) is carried out under imaging guidance, commonly CT, but occasionally fluoroscopy or ultrasound. Overall the diagnostic yield is between 80% and 90%; however, the false-negative rate has been reported to be as high as 29%. The indications for TTNA are controversial but include tissue sampling in a patient with a presumed benign lesion,

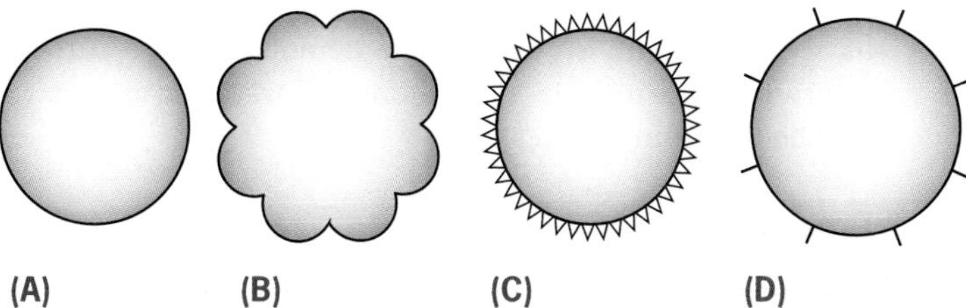

FIGURE 47–3 Margin of pulmonary nodules. Schematic representation of different patterns of the margin of pulmonary nodules. **(A)** Smooth. **(B)** Scalloped. **(C)** Corona radiata. **(D)** Spiculated. Redrawn with permission from Stark P. Computed and positron emission tomographic scanning of pulmonary nodules. In: *UpToDate*, Basow DS, ed. UpToDate, Waltham, MA 2010. Copyright © 2010 UpToDate, Inc. For more information visit www.uptodate.com.

the establishment of a diagnosis in patients who are high risk for VATS or surgery, and when there is a concern that the pulmonary nodule is a metastatic nonpulmonary tumor. Bronchoscopic sampling is of high yield when the tumor is central, when there is a clear airway leading up to the tumor, and when the tumor is large. Otherwise, VATS or surgical resection remains the standard of care for patients with SPN and a medium to high probability of malignancy.

Certain imaging modalities may be used to better evaluate the likelihood of malignancy. These are increasingly used as a frontline diagnostic method. They may be especially useful for lesions that are not amenable to nonsurgical sampling, when surgery is risky, or when the biospy result is negative. Contrast-enhanced CT scanning is based on the fact that malignant tissue is more metabolically active than nonmalignant tissue and therefore associated with greater blood flow. With the proper timing and rate of contrast bolus infusion, an enhancement of less than 15 Hounsfield units (HU) indicates a benign lesion in about 96% of cases; however, an enhancement of greater than 15 HU has only 56% to 78% specificity for malignancy.[39,40] In the latter situation, further diagnostic workup is usually indicated.

PET scanning with fluorodeoxyglucose (FDG) can be useful for the risk stratification of SPNs. Highly metabolically active tissues, such as tumors, should have the greatest affinity for glucose and hence should appear hot on PET scanning relative to normal tissue or benign nodules. PET scanning is usually used concomitantly with CT scan for anatomic correlation. The current mainstay of PET-CT scanning is for staging of known malignancies and for follow-up after treatment. Additionally, it can accurately characterize lesions larger than 15 mm as benign or malignant. However, the resolution of PET scanning deteriorates significantly for lesions smaller than 1 cm. PET scanning may be accurately used down to a lesion size of 7 mm. The specificity of PET scanning is on the order of 70% to 90%, because other lesions with infection or inflammation can be highly PET avid. There have not been any studies to date demonstrating a survival advantage in patients in whom PET was used as part of their screening process.[41]

Diagnosis

The diagnosis of bronchogenic cancer may be based on symptoms, the results of asymptomatic screening, or an incidental radiographic abnormality. Induced sputum is useful to reach a diagnosis in patients with a central lung mass on the chest radiograph. Sputum can be pooled over 24 hours, which increases the diagnostic yield of this study. Although the popularity of induced sputum as a diagnostic tool has declined in recent years, it is recommended in hospitals with adequate experience if it does not lead to prolonged delays in the diagnostic workup.

Bronchoscopy can be helpful in the workup of central and mediastinal lesions. Different biopsy techniques are available, depending on the location of the abnormality. **Transbronchial needle aspiration (TBNA)** is useful for biopsy of lesions close to the tracheobronchial tree, with diagnostic yields of 80% to 90% reported in skilled hands. Endobronchial biopsies can be performed for intrabronchial lesions, a technique also associated with excellent yields.[42] This also can be done with endoscopic ultrasound guidance.

An advance in the field of bronchoscopy is autofluorescence bronchoscopy for the detection of metaplasia and dysplasia in the tracheobronchial tree of individuals at risk. The laser-induced fluorescence emission (LIFE) system was developed to supplement standard bronchoscopy (white light) in the diagnosis of early malignant lesions in the central airways. Although one report suggests that LIFE can increase the absolute sensitivity of detection by as much as 46.9% over standard white light bronchoscopy, it has not been validated sufficiently for clinical use. LIFE therefore remains an investigational technique.[41,43]

RESPIRATORY RECAP

Diagnosis of Lung Cancer

- Sputum tests
- Bronchoscopy
- Mediastinoscopy
- Biopsy

Mediastinoscopy can be used for individuals with mediastinal lymphadenopathy (**Figure 47–4**). This technique is useful for diagnostic purposes if TBNA fails and for staging once the diagnosis of NSCLC has been established. The morbidity and mortality of mediastinoscopy are exceedingly low in most skilled hands. The risks and benefits of these invasive procedures must be considered based on the influence the result will have on patient management.[44,45]

Occasionally the diagnosis of metastatic bronchogenic cancer can be made on the basis of a biopsy of a remote lesion (e.g., cervical node, adrenal gland). In addition, pleural fluid may be sampled, and pleural biopsy

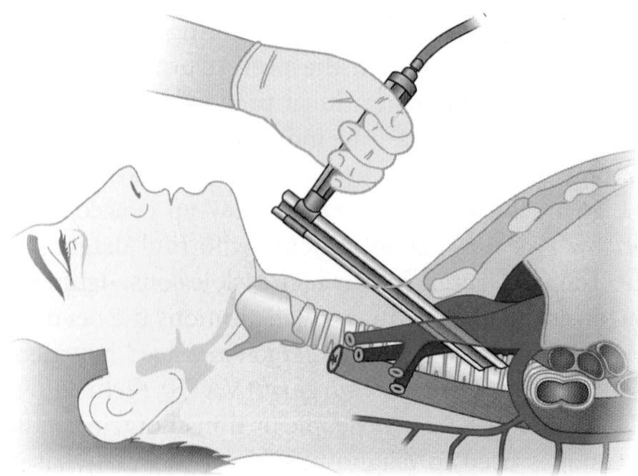

FIGURE 47–4 Mediastinoscope in place demonstrating the superior mediastinal plane. Adapted from Fishman AP. *Fishman's Pulmonary Diseases and Disorders*. 3rd ed. McGraw Hill; 1998.

can be performed for the diagnosis of malignant effusion. The advantage of pleural fluid sampling is that it can provide both diagnostic and staging information because the presence of a malignant effusion implies a lesion that disease is effectively metastatic with the stage being VI.

Workup and Staging

Once the diagnosis has been established, staging of disease is the next step. Knowledge of the staging system can help determine the necessary workup.[46,47] **Table 47–5** and **Table 47–6** reflect the current NSCLC staging classification advocated by the International Association for the Study of Lung Cancer (IASLC). **Table 47–7** illustrates survival according to the stage of lung cancer. As mentioned previously, the TNM staging system was revised and the revisions published in 2009. The major changes include downstaging T4 resulting from additional nodules in the same lobe to T3 and upstaging pleural dissemination and pericardial effusion from T4 to M1a.[48] Staging for SCLC can also be done by the TNM system advocated by the IASLC, which describes the extent and burden of disease more accurately than the Veterans' Affairs Lung Study Group

TABLE 47–5 TNM Descriptors

Descriptor	Criteria
T: Primary Tumor	
T0	No evidence of primary tumor
T1	Tumor ≤ 3 cm,* in greatest dimension, surrounded by lung or visceral pleura, not more proximal than the lobar bronchus
T1a	Tumor ≤ 2 cm*
T1b	Tumor > 2 but ≤ 3 cm*
T2	Tumor >3 but ≤ 7 cm* *or* tumor with any of the following:† invades visceral pleura; involves main bronchus ≥ 2 cm distal to the carina; atelectasis/obstructive pneumonia extending to hilum but not involving the entire lung
T2a	Tumor > 3 but ≤ 5 cm*
T2b	Tumor > 5 but ≤ 7 cm*
T3	Tumor > 7 cm *or* directly invading chest wall, diaphragm, phrenic nerve, mediastinal pleural or parietal pericardium *or* tumor in the main bronchus < 2 cm distal to the carina‡ *or* atelectasis/obstructive pneumonia of entire lung *or* separate tumor nodules in the same lobe
T4	Tumor of any size with invasion of heart, great vessels, trachea, recurrent laryngeal nerve, esophagus, vertebral body, or carina *or* separate tumor nodules in a different ipsilateral lobe
N: Regional Lymph Nodes	
N0	No regional node metastasis
N1	Metastasis in ipsilateral peribronchial and/or perihilar lymph nodes and intrapulmonary nodes, including involvement by direct extension
N2	Metastasis in ipsilateral mediastinal and/or subcarinal lymph nodes
N3	Metastasis in contralateral mediastinal, contralateral hilar, ipsilateral or contralateral scalene, or supraclavicular lymph nodes
M: Distant Metastasis	
M0	No distant metastasis
M1a	Separate tumor nodules in a contralateral lobe *or* tumor with pleural nodules or malignant pleural dissemination§
M1b	Distant metastasis
Special Situations	
TX, NX, MX	T, N, or M status not able to be assessed
Tis	Focus of in situ cancer
T1‡	Superficial spreading tumor of any size but confined to the wall of the trachea or main stem bronchus

*In the greatest dimension.

†T2 tumors with these features are classified as T2a if ≤ 5 cm.

‡The uncommon superficial tumor in central airways is classified as T1.

§Pleural effusions are excluded that are cytologically negative, nonbloody, transudative, and clinically judged not to be due to cancer.

Modified from Goldstraw P, Crowley J, Chansky K, et al. The IASLC Lung Cancer Staging Project: proposals for the revision of the TNM stage groups in the forthcoming (seventh) edition of the TNM classification of malignant tumours. *J Thorac Oncol.* 2007;2:706, Table 3. Reprinted with permission.

TABLE 47-6 TNM Elements Included in Stage Groups

Stage Groups	Descriptors T	N	M
IA	T1a, b	N0	M0
IB	T2a	N0	M0
IIA	T1a, b	N1	M0
	T2a	N1	M0
	T2b	N0	M0
IIB	T2b	N1	M0
	T3	N0	M0
IIIA	T1–3	N2	M0
	T3	N1	M0
	T4	N0,1	M0
IIIB	T4	N2	M0
	T1–4	N3	M0
IV	Tany	Nany	M1a, b

Adapted from Goldstraw P, Crowley J, Chansky K, et al. The IASLC Lung Cancer Staging Project: proposals for the revision of the TNM stage groups in the forthcoming (seventh) edition of the TNM classification of malignant tumours. *J Thorac Oncol.* 2007;2:706–714.

TABLE 47-7 Overall Survival by Clinical and Pathologic Stage

	Deaths/*N*	Median Survival Time (in months)	5-Year Survival (%)
Clinical Stage			
cIa	443/831	60	50
cIb	750/1284	43	43
cIIa	318/483	34	36
cIIb	1652/2248	18	25
cIIIa	2528/3175	14	19
cIIIb	676/758	10	7
cIV	2627/2757	6	2
Pathologic Stage			
pIa	1168/3666	119	73
pIb	1450/3100	81	58
pIIa	1485/2579	49	46
pIIb	1502/2252	31	36
pIIIa	2896/3792	22	24
pIIIb	263/297	13	9
pIV	224/266	17	13

Adapted from Goldstraw P, Crowley J, Chansky K, et al. The IASLC Lung Cancer Staging Project: proposals for the revision of the TNM stage groups in the forthcoming (seventh) edition of the TNM classification of malignant tumours. *J Thorac Oncol.* 2007;2:706–714.

(VALSG); however, it is of limited utility because there is considerable overlap in the prognosis for many of the stages. The TNM system is of most use for early-stage disease (stage I), when the disease is amenable to resection and adjuvant chemotherapy. Thus, the most commonly used staging system for SCLC remains the VALSG's limited versus extensive staging. Limited disease is defined as a case in which all disease lies within a single radiation port and is confined within one hemithorax (TNM stages I through IIIB). All other disease is classified as extensive disease.

The tests required after a diagnosis of lung cancer are controversial. A careful history and physical examination should be followed by tests of blood chemistry (serum calcium, alkaline phosphatase, aspartate aminotransferase, alanine aminotransferase, and lactate dehydrogenase levels, and a complete blood count) and CT scanning of the entire chest, extending caudally to the level of the adrenal glands. Additional tests that may be useful are CT or magnetic resonance imaging (MRI) scans of the head and a bone scan. However, the yield on these tests for metastasis is low if the patient has no symptoms; they are not generally indicated in such patients.

With SCLC, some advocate complete staging, including a head MRI, bone scan, and unilateral or bilateral bone marrow biopsies; others perform a sequential, symptom-based workup. With NSCLC, mediastinoscopy is recommended to assess the extent of mediastinal node involvement because PET and/or CT scanning can be misleading (false positives and false negatives) in the mediastinum. There has been a lot of interest in determining whether a preoperative PET and/or CT scan can obviate the need for mediastinoscopy. However, the data remain conflicting. The standard of care is to perform mediastinoscopy before any planned tumor resection for staging whenever possible. Further data on the use of PET-CT scanning may eventually change this.[49–52]

For patients who may be candidates for surgery, pulmonary function testing is useful to determine the patient's ability to undergo such a procedure. Ideally, a postoperative forced expiratory volume in 1 second (FEV_1) of 800 mL or 40% of predicted should be sought. However, this value is based largely on empiric data. In borderline cases a quantitative ventilation-perfusion scan can help estimate the amount of resection a patient can physiologically tolerate. Exercise testing also may help predict morbidity associated with thoracotomy; for example, patients with a maximum oxygen consumption under 10 mL/kg do poorly. On the other hand, if patients' predicted FEV_1 is less than 40% predicted, they can still safely undergo surgery if their exercise capacity is high. Improvements in surgical and anesthetic techniques and the reemergence of lung volume reduction surgery (LVRS) have helped lower the threshold for surgical resection of NSCLC.[53,54]

Treatment

Treatment options include surgery, **radiotherapy**, and **chemotherapy**. Newer options, although not the mainstays of treatment, include immunotherapy, brachytherapy, gene therapy, bronchoscopic treatments, and photodynamic therapy (PDT).[55] Because the individual chemotherapeutic agents and combinations of agents tend to change frequently, the underlying therapeutic principles in the treatment of lung cancer are emphasized here.

Small Cell Lung Cancer

Because of the aggressive nature of these tumors, most patients with SCLC who seek medical treatment have extensive disease at the time of diagnosis. Without treatment, patients with limited SCLC survive an average of 12 weeks; for extensive disease, survival is only 5 weeks. In addition to moderate improvements in survival, combination chemotherapy in some cases can lead to substantial improvements in the patient's quality of life.[56]

Chemotherapeutic agents have long been known to affect SCLC tumors in patients with both limited (90% of patients) and extensive disease (70% of patients). However, despite the sensitivity of these tumors to chemotherapeutic agents, relapse is the rule. There has been no substantial improvement in survival of this disease over the past 20 to 30 years. Commonly used agents include etoposide, platinum agents (e.g., cisplatinum, carboplatin), ifosfamide, vincristine, irinotecan, paclitaxel, and anthracyclines. Controversy exists regarding dose intensity, frequency, alternating therapies, sequential regimens, and bone marrow support, among other issues. In general, the platinum-based regimens are considered superior to non-platinum-based regimens, and cisplatin plus etoposide is the most frequently used combination based on its clinical activity and toxicity profile. In general, adding additional agents and using higher doses can lead to a higher response rate, but the regimens with the higher number of agents have a higher rate of toxicity.[57–60]

RESPIRATORY RECAP

Treatment of Lung Cancer

» Surgery
» Radiotherapy
» Chemotherapy

Patients with limited-stage SCLC treated with chemotherapy alone commonly develop local tumor progression. Studies have shown that the addition of thoracic radiotherapy reduces intrathoracic recurrence and provides a small but significant improvement in survival. Early administration of radiotherapy is superior to late radiation, especially in patients who are receiving etoposide and cisplatin chemotherapy. Delivering the radiotherapy in more intense but briefer doses (accelerated hyperfractionation) is superior to daily dosing. Furthermore, concurrent chemoradiotherapy is considered superior to sequential chemotherapy and radiotherapy in terms of survival. However, there may be some increased toxicity with the concurrent administration of chemoradiotherapy, and in patients who do not tolerate it, radiation can be delayed until chemotherapy is completed. Radiation therapy also can be used for treatment of metastatic disease. Radiotherapy has been shown to improve mortality in the treatment of patients with limited-stage SCLC. Another role for radiation in SCLC is in prophylactic cranial irradiation (PCI). Brain metastases are common in SCLC, even in patients who appear to have responded to systemic therapy; this may be because of poor penetration of chemotherapy through the blood–brain barrier.

Surgery traditionally has not been considered useful for SCLC because of the disease's systemic nature at the time of diagnosis. With improvements in chemotherapeutic regimens, however, there has been some improvement in control of systemic disease; consequently, local and regional recurrences have received increased attention. Surgical resection may improve survival after induction chemotherapy in patients with stage I to stage IIIB disease, and there may be a potential for benefit from surgery in early-stage disease, specifically, stage I or II. However, there are currently no prospective data to inform definitive recommendations. Surgical intervention can be considered for patients with early-stage SCLC but needs to be followed with adjuvant chemotherapy. If the surgical margins are positive or there is nodal disease, patients should also receive adjuvant radiotherapy.

Non-Small-Cell Lung Cancer

Several principles are important in the approach to treatment of patients with NSCLC. First, surgical resection is used much more commonly in NSCLC than in SCLC, particularly for early-stage disease. Second, the probability of achieving cure in early-stage NSCLC is quite good (5-year survival after surgery for stage I disease is 47%). Third, in multiple stages of the disease, there is an increasingly recognized role for multimodality therapy (i.e., **neoadjuvant therapy** and **adjuvant therapy** [chemotherapy and radiotherapy] followed by surgical resection).[61,62]

For early-stage NSCLC, surgical resection is the treatment of choice, with excellent long-term survival reported in several series (63% to 85% stage IA 5-year survival).[63] Most deaths that occur are caused by recurrent disease. Although largely based on empirical evidence, radiation therapy alone appears to provide inferior cure rates (approximately 30% for stage I and 20% for stage II). After resection there is now a clearly recognized role for adjuvant chemotherapy (i.e., after surgical resection in stage II disease, and possibly but less clearly so in stage IB disease).[64–69] Further, molecular profiling of tumors may be predictive of chemotherapeutic response, which would allow a priori prediction of which patients would benefit from additional or more aggressive therapy. It is unclear whether full lobectomy is always required for satisfactory resection of early-stage NSCLC. In older patients or those with small peripheral nodules or bronchoalveolar carcinoma histology, limited resection (wedge resection or segmentectomy) may offer equivalent survival. There is currently a trial under way examining this specific question, but enrollment has been sparse, likely because of bias toward one or the other approach by surgeons or patients.[70–74]

For patients who are not candidates for surgery due to comorbidities or who refuse surgery, several nonsurgical options exist. Definitive radiation, stereotactic radiation, heavy particle irradiation, and radiofrequency ablation are currently used. Definitive radiation is the most studied modality. Overall patient survival is 22% to 72% at 2 years. However, cancer-specific survival is better, at 54% to 93%, highlighting the poor health status of the patients receiving these therapies.[75,76] The lower survival of these patients might be partly related to understaging based on clinical assessment and radiologic imaging alone. The need for treatment advances remains and is highlighted by the fact that patients with breast, colon, and prostate cancer (the next three most common causes of cancer deaths) have better 5-year survival rates than patients with stage I NSCLC.

The treatment of locally advanced NSCLC with multimodality therapies has become increasingly popular. Stage III NSCLC has undergone the most changes in management over the course of the last decade. Curative intent remains the standard of care for this group of patients but is challenging to achieve, and treatment should be individualized. Surgery remains the standard of care for patients without N2 (mediastinal lymphadenopathy) disease. Formerly, patients with stage IIIA and nonbulky mediastinal lymphadenopathy were considered surgical candidates; however, it has become more recognized that cure is difficult to achieve even with surgery in this patient population, and multimodality therapy is now considered the standard of care. For stage III disease, neoadjuvant chemotherapy has been studied and is a controversial topic. Overall it offers no survival advantage when compared with postoperative (adjuvant) chemotherapy, although it may be used in cases of superior sulcus (Pancoast) tumors (in addition to preoperative radiation) or in cases of T4 disease with mediastinal invasion with curative intent to facilitate surgery.[77,78] Adjuvant chemotherapy offers a survival advantage after resection of stage III disease and is considered the standard of care.[79,80] Postoperative radiation therapy has been studied to reduce the risk of local recurrence. Although it was associated with a survival advantage in patients with N2 disease in a subset analysis, overall there does not seem to be a large survival advantage to postoperative radiotherapy because survival seems to be limited more frequently by distant metastases than by local recurrence.[81–84] Concurrent chemoradiation is considered the standard of care for nonresectable stage III NSCLC. Chemotherapy is usually with a platinum-based regimen. Data are emerging on the use of prophylactic cranial irradiation (similar to SCLC) to prevent the development of brain metastases, but these data have yet to be published.

For metastatic NSCLC, a number of trials have examined the role of palliative chemotherapy compared with best supportive care. Because these patients are essentially incurable, the goal of treatment is to prolong life without increasing suffering or side effects. Improvements in survival have been reported with the use of chemotherapy in this patient group. However, the optimum therapy for an individual patient must be carefully considered and discussed. There are data that indicate preservation of the quality of life and cost-effectiveness for those who undergo palliative chemotherapy in this setting. However, most of these clinical trials focused on younger patients with good performance status.

There has been a revolution in the world of cancer therapeutics with the advent of tyrosine kinase inhibitors. For advanced NSCLC, the endothelial growth factor receptor (EGFR) inhibitors erlotinib and gefitinib have been found to have dramatic responses in a subpopulation of patients. However, on average, when all patients with advanced NSCLC are treated with the EGFR inhibitors, the response rate is similar to second-line chemotherapeutic agents. There are clinical and molecular predictors of response. Clinical predictors include female sex, Asian ethnicity, nonsmoker status, and adenocarcinoma histology. Molecular predictors are specifically the presence of activating mutations in the tumor EGF receptor. The EGFR inhibitor gefitinib is now recommended as a frontline agent for patients with advanced NSCLC who have any clinical predictors or molecular predictors of response. For all other patients suitable for therapy, chemotherapeutic agents (namely, platinum-based agents) with the possible addition of other molecular agents such as cetuximab or bevacizumab are recommended. Bevacizumab increases the risk of bleeding and is contraindicated in patients with brain metastases and with hemoptysis. Cetuximab has been shown to have a small benefit in patients who express the EGFR by immunohistochemistry without carrying an activating mutation.[85]

Complications of Therapy

The complications of the individual chemotherapeutic drugs are beyond the scope of this chapter.[86] Roughly 1% of treatment-associated mortality is a result of chemotherapy itself. Several important general points can be made, as follows:

- In the week or two after chemotherapy, neutropenia can occur and greatly increases the risk of superimposed bacterial and opportunistic fungal pneumonias and sepsis. Growth factors can be used to prevent neutropenia in a susceptible or previously afflicted patient.

- Mucositis, which represents acute toxicity of the highly active lining cells of the gastrointestinal tract, leads to substantial discomfort and can increase infectious sequelae as a result of an increased risk of aspiration and altered gastrointestinal permeability.
- Various chemotherapeutic agents have acute or chronic pulmonary sequelae, which complicate the distinction between tumor spread or recurrence, infection, and drug toxicity; early invasive diagnostic attempts often are warranted in these cases. Fortunately the chemotherapeutic agents typically used for lung cancers do not, for the most part, have major pulmonary toxicities.
- Platinum-based chemotherapeutic drugs are commonly used in lung cancer and are frequently associated with neurologic toxicities, specifically peripheral neuropathy. This side effect can range from asymptomatic to nuisance to severe and disabling; therefore, it must be considered and discussed with patients undergoing chemotherapy.
- The tyrosine kinase inhibitors mentioned above are overall well tolerated. Rash and diarrhea are the most common side effects. Bevacizumab is associated with hemorrhage, poor surgical wound healing, and gastrointestinal perforation as less common but serious side effects.

Radiation damage to the lung parenchyma remains the limiting factor in chest radiotherapy. The complications of radiation therapy may be characterized as acute or chronic. The incidence of acute radiation pneumonitis is higher for patients receiving larger daily or cumulative doses and those receiving radiation to a larger amount of tissue. In addition, certain chemotherapeutic drugs used in lung cancer regimens, such as doxorubicin and vincristine, are radiosensitizers and can increase radiation-induced injury. Acute pneumonitis occurs within the first 6 months of therapy (mean is approximately 1 to 3 months) and is manifested by cough and dyspnea. It typically but not exclusively is confined to the radiation port, and the histopathology may be consistent with a lymphocytic alveolitis or diffuse alveolar damage. In addition, a nonspecific reaction, bronchiolitis obliterans with organizing pneumonia (BOOP), can occur in the lung in response to radiation injury. Corticosteroid therapy usually is given for acute pulmonary radiation toxicity, although human data are sparse.

Chronic complications of radiotherapy include injury to lung and mediastinal structures. Lung fibrosis can be seen 6 months after discontinuation of radiotherapy and manifests with progressive dyspnea and restrictive pulmonary function tests. Mediastinal radiotherapy has been associated with a number of complications, including mediastinal fibrosis, constrictive pericarditis, restrictive cardiomyopathy, accelerated coronary artery disease, and valvular fibrosis.[87]

With thoracotomy, mortality rates as low as 1% are now reported, a considerable improvement compared with 30 to 40 years ago. Smoking cessation at least 2 months before surgery has been associated with an improved outcome in elective coronary artery bypass patients. These data are generally extrapolated to thoracotomy patients as well.[88] Other preoperative measures, such as exercise, good nutrition, pulmonary rehabilitation, and deep breathing regimens, may help smooth the perioperative course. Meticulous attention must be paid to postsurgical pulmonary toilet to prevent and treat respiratory complications of atelectasis, lobar collapse, and pneumonia. Care after discharge from the hospital, through transitional care units and visiting nurses also are crucial in many cases. Late complications, such as post-thoracotomy pain syndromes, which occur in as many as 50% of patients, are somewhat underappreciated.

Prognosis

The prognosis for lung cancer is still quite poor; the 5-year survival rate is only 14%. The following are some useful prognostic variables:

- *Tumor stage, including size.* In addition to the tumor's stage, its size appears to linearly predict survival, with increasing mortality associated with larger size.
- *Weight loss.* As with many diseases and other cancers, weight loss is an important prognostic indicator. The poor outcome associated with patients with lung cancer who lose weight has prompted some to aggressively place percutaneous gastrostomy feeding tubes. Thus, even when oral intake is poor, caloric requirements can be met. Appetite stimulants such as megestrol acetate can help increase body weight. However, minimal outcome data support these approaches. Other systemic symptoms similarly predict a poor outcome.
- *Performance status.* The Karnofsky Performance Scale (**Table 47–8**) provides a quantitative measure of patient performance as a percentage of normal activities. As with many tumors, a lung cancer patient with good performance status has a much better outcome.
- *Histologic subtype.* In NSCLC, a few studies have suggested a superior outcome for squamous cell carcinoma compared with adenocarcinoma. However, several other studies have not shown important differences in survival or recurrence risk. Therefore, the histologic subtype probably is not a major prognostic factor in NSCLC. However, subtyping

RESPIRATORY RECAP

Prognosis for Lung Cancer

» The 5-year survival rate for lung cancer is only 14%.

TABLE 47-8 Karnofsky Performance Scale

Definition	Percentage	Criteria
Able to carry on normal activity and to work; no special care needed	100	Normal; no complaints; no evidence of disease
	90	Able to carry on normal activity; minor signs or symptoms of disease
	80	Normal activity with effort; some signs or symptoms of disease
Unable to work; able to live at home and care for most personal needs; varying amount of assistance needed	70	Cares for self; unable to carry on normal activity or do active work
	60	Requires occasional assistance but is able to care for most needs
	50	Requires considerable assistance and frequent medical care
Unable to care for self; requires equivalent of institutional or hospital care; rapid progression of disease possible	40	Disabled; requires special care and assistance
	30	Severely disabled; hospitalization indicated, although death may not be imminent
	20	Very sick; hospitalization necessary; active supportive treatment required
	10	Moribund; fatal processes progressing rapidly

of adenocarcinomas may be useful, because bronchoalveolar cell carcinoma may have an improved outcome compared with other adenocarcinomas.

- *Tumor differentiation*. Variable results have been published in different papers regarding the importance of this factor. Although some data suggest a worse outcome for patients with undifferentiated cancers, others report no important differences in survival on this basis.
- *Vascular or lymphatic invasion*. A resected tumor that demonstrates invasiveness may warrant more aggressive treatment than one that does not.
- *Molecular markers*. Molecular markers, such as K-ras mutations, have not yet had a major impact on prognostication or prediction of relapse, although early data from gene expression profiling is promising.[89] Tumor expression of the EGFR mutation predicts response to EGFR inhibitors as mentioned above.
- *Male gender*. Disease in men is associated with a worse outcome than disease in women.
- *African American race*. This factor is also associated with worse outcome for all stages of lung cancer. This appears to be at least partly related to less aggressive therapy in this population.[90]

Prevention

The most important cause of cancer death in North America is preventable. Prevention of lung cancer requires smoking cessation, avoidance of exposures, and early detection. Evidence clearly suggests a decline in the risk of lung cancer among former smokers compared with current smokers. Although statistics vary, the lung cancer risk falls by 5 years after smoking cessation and continues to decline thereafter. However, these individuals probably do not completely return to the baseline risk seen in those who have never smoked.

RESPIRATORY RECAP

Lung Cancer Prevention

» Smoking cessation
» Screening
» Interventions to prevent disease progression

Prevention generally is classified as primary, secondary, and tertiary in nature. *Primary prevention* refers to modification of potentially injurious behaviors. In the case of lung cancer, smoking cessation is the best defense. The onus is on the healthcare provider both to encourage and to facilitate the cessation of tobacco use. The modest success of tobacco control programs in North America should not distract health professionals from the huge problem of an estimated 1.1 billion smokers worldwide. For example, estimates suggest that 66% of all young men in China currently are smokers.[91] Primary prevention must target the problem on both a global and an individual level. Emphasis is placed on the need for repeated discussions with smokers and planned follow-up. Several attempts by patients and healthcare providers often are required to successfully overcome this addiction. Group or family therapy may be useful for some smokers.

Recent data support the usefulness of nicotine replacement therapies to facilitate smoking cessation. Bupropion (150 mg given orally twice a day) has been shown to facilitate withdrawal from nicotine. However, only 23.1% of participants in one study were tobacco free at 1 year, compared with 12.4% in the placebo group.[92,93] The combination of nicotine replacement and bupropion may have a higher probability of success. Varenicline (a nicotinic receptor partial agonist) is another first-line agent to help patients quit smoking. Compared with bupropion, it was found to be more efficacious.[93] Smoking cessation programs are cost-effective, particularly if they use personnel who are not physicians.[94,95]

Some limited data suggest the use of certain dietary supplements, especially antioxidants, to prevent lung and other cancers in high-risk groups. Randomized controlled trials of vitamin A and beta-carotene have yielded disappointing results, disproving any efficacy in primary prevention of disease.[96–100] There remains some evidence of a protective role for vitamins C and E. As it stands, however, the data are insufficient to recommend their use routinely in clinical practice.[101–103]

Secondary prevention refers to early detection or the screening of asymptomatic disease. Because lung cancer screening trials have thus far failed, secondary prevention is not generally recommended. Improvements in technology, with spiral CT scanning and possibly PET scanning, may make secondary prevention of lung cancer feasible. Although spiral CT scanning allows complete evaluation of the chest during a single breath hold, the possible cost for detection of false positives must not be overlooked. For example, a small peripheral granulomatous lesion that otherwise would have gone undetected may lead the patient to undergo open lung biopsy to exclude lung cancer. However, a number of reports have suggested that spiral CT scanning can detect early-stage lung cancers in at-risk populations with yields comparable to those of mammography in breast cancer. Currently, the precise role and ideal technique for lung cancer screening are unclear. A number of radiologic randomized control trials are under way that should help define the role of secondary prevention in lung cancer.[104]

Another example of secondary prevention is the use of molecular genetic analysis on bronchial biopsies or possibly sputum samples. By demonstrating genetic changes similar to those seen in lung cancer patients, individuals at high risk of developing lung cancer can be identified. These patients can then be followed closely or perhaps entered into clinical trials on chemoprevention. Technologic advances are being made in the early diagnosis and detection of lung cancer, but they must be evaluated for feasibility and cost-effectiveness before they can be widely recommended.

Tertiary prevention refers to interventions to prevent disease progression once a diagnosis has been made.

Future Directions

Worldwide smoking trends dictate that bronchogenic carcinoma will continue to be a major health problem in the foreseeable future. Current epidemiologic statistics likely will be eclipsed. Although advances in imaging, chemotherapy and radiotherapy, and genetics may produce some incremental benefit, prevention is the only secure answer. Primary prevention, through political and financial pressure on tobacco companies, would help limit the supply of tobacco and related products. Worldwide education programs through mass media could help limit the demand. Secondary prevention programs for early detection of lung cancer may benefit from advances in technology, such as spiral CT scanning. Gene therapy to manipulate proto-oncogenes and tumor suppressor genes may also come to fruition.[105,106]

CASE STUDIES

Case 1. Lung Cancer Screening

A 45-year-old man who smoked two packs a day for 20 years but who quit 2 years ago consults his physician. A friend of the patient recently has been diagnosed with lung cancer, and the patient is concerned that he might develop the same condition. He otherwise is healthy and has no diagnosed lung disease. The review of systems is negative for weight loss, chest pain, and hemoptysis. The patient is taking no medications, and his family history also is negative for cancer. The patient works in an office and has never been exposed to any dusts, fumes, or toxic chemicals. His physical examination is normal.

This individual, although asymptomatic, is clearly at risk of developing lung cancer, given his 40 pack year history of smoking. He has no additional risk factors from other exposures, from his family history, or from chronic obstructive pulmonary disease. He has no active symptoms or signs suggestive of lung cancer. However, this frequently is the case until the cancer becomes quite advanced. By the time a patient develops symptomatic lung cancer, the prognosis is quite poor because of the advanced disease. The emphasis thus has been placed on attempts at early diagnosis, before the onset of symptoms and signs.

Unfortunately, trials of screening for lung cancer in populations at risk have been largely unsuccessful. Sputum cytology and chest radiography have yielded some benefit in terms of increased detection of early-stage tumors but have had no substantial impact on patient outcome. Therefore, the general recommendation has been not to screen previous or current smokers. Similarly, there is no proven role for antioxidants or other secondary prevention strategies.

However, newer technologies may change this practice. Using spiral CT scanning has provided some encouraging preliminary data in this field. These scans can be performed quickly, with minimal radiation exposure, and at relatively low cost. However, false-positive results (e.g., identification of benign lesions that would not otherwise have been detected) could limit the utility of this technique. Further data are required before spiral CT scans can be generally recommended for lung cancer screening.

Case 2. Early-Stage Lung Cancer

A 63-year-old woman seeks medical attention after an abnormality is noted on a chest radiograph. She is a former smoker of 38 pack years who quit smoking 5 years ago. She otherwise is quite healthy and has no active medical problems. Her exposure history, social history, and family history are unremarkable, as is her physical examination. The chest radiograph shows a 2-cm peripheral lesion in the right upper lobe. No other abnormalities are seen on the film, specifically, no pleural effusion, no bony invasion, and no evidence of mediastinal adenopathy.

A transthoracic needle aspirate tests positive for squamous cell carcinoma. A CT scan of the chest to the level of the adrenal glands reveals no abnormalities apart from the 2-cm lesion. A complete blood count and serum calcium and liver enzyme values were all within normal limits. Mediastinoscopy revealed no evidence of adenopathy. Pulmonary function testing revealed an FEV_1 of 2.2 L (70% predicted). Because of the absence of symptoms, a bone scan and a CT scan of the head were not performed.

This patient has T1N0M0 disease, which represents stage IA non-small-cell lung cancer. The treatment of choice is surgical resection. The patient's pulmonary function tests are quite good and should easily allow resection of a single lobe. There is no proven role for postoperative chemotherapy or radiotherapy in this setting. The 5-year survival rate for this type of patient after resection is 70%. If this patient had a larger tumor (3 cm or more) and the presentation were otherwise identical, the clinical stage would be stage IB. Survival for this stage is lower, at about 58%. For this stage there is emerging data that postoperative chemotherapy may improve survival.

Case 3. Metastatic Lung Cancer

A 72-year-old man sees his physician because of new onset of headaches. The patient currently smokes and has smoked two packs of cigarettes a day for the past 40 years. His past medical history is remarkable for two myocardial infarctions. His medications include daily aspirin, atenolol, and captopril (all for his heart). His family history and social history are unremarkable. His physical examination is remarkable for marked gait instability and asymmetric deep tendon reflexes, which are consistent with a pathologic condition in the central nervous system.

His chest radiograph reveals a 5-cm mass in the right mid-lung zone with enlargement of the mediastinum, which is consistent with substantial adenopathy in the paratracheal region and the aorticopulmonary window. A right-sided pleural effusion also is present. A CT scan of the head reveals three intracranial lesions, a finding consistent with metastatic disease. A diagnostic thoracentesis yields a positive result for adenocarcinoma of the lung.

This patient has metastatic non-small-cell lung cancer. The staging would be T2N3M1. The T2 status is based on the 5-cm size of the tumor, whereas the N3 status is based on the radiographic evidence of contralateral mediastinal adenopathy. The metastatic lesion is evident from the pleural effusion and head CT scan. For diagnostic certitude, drainage of the pleural effusion should be performed; this will likely both confirm the diagnosis and stage the patient as stage IV.

The therapeutic goal in this situation should be palliation. The patient sought attention for his headaches, and cranial irradiation could be performed to control these symptoms. Because the patient has several intracranial metastases, surgical resection of these lesions is not recommended. Most would advocate offering chemoradiotherapy for palliative purposes. This decision is based on discussion with the patient and his family regarding his wishes. Although treatment would not offer a cure, there are data that suggest that survival is improved with chemoradiotherapy if a patient has a good performance status. However, the median survival still is likely to be less than 1 year.

KEY POINTS

- Lung cancer is common but preventable.
- A tissue-based diagnosis generally is required. This can be obtained by analysis of sputum or pleural fluid or of bronchoscopic, surgical, or needle biopsy specimens.
- Lung cancer generally is classified as small cell or non-small-cell cancer.
- Small cell lung cancer generally is treated with chemotherapy or radiotherapy or both but rarely with surgery.
- Surgical resection is the preferred treatment for early-stage non-small-cell lung cancer.
- Chemotherapy and radiotherapy in nonresectable non-small-cell lung cancer in patients with a good performance status is the standard of care.
- For patients with advanced disease and a poor performance status, supportive care and palliation remain the only options available.
- Prevention and early diagnosis are future areas of emphasis in lung cancer.

REFERENCES

1. Centers for Disease Control and Prevention. Lung cancer trends. Available at: http://www.cdc.gov/cancer/lung/statistics/trends.htm.
2. Ries LAG, Melbert D, Krapcho M, et al., eds. Section 15: lung and bronchus. In: *SEER Cancer Statistics Review, 1975–2004*. Bethesda, MD: National Cancer Institute; based on November 2006 SEER data submission, posted to the SEER website 2007. Available at: http://seer.cancer.gov/csr/1975_2004/results_merged/sect_15_lung_bronchus.pdf.
3. World Health Organization. Global cancer rates could increase by 50% to 15 million by 2020. Available at: http://www.who.int/mediacentre/news/releases/2003/pr27/en.
4. Osann K, Lowery J, Schell M. Small cell lung cancer in women: risk associated with smoking, prior respiratory disease, and occupation. *Lung Cancer*. 2000;28:1–10.
5. Molina JR, Yang P, Cassivi SD, Schild SE, Adjei AA. Non-small cell lung cancer: epidemiology, risk factors, treatment and survivorship. *Mayo Clin Proc*. 2008;83:584–594.
6. Andre F, Jacot W, Pujol JL, et al. Epidemiology, prognostic factors, staging, and treatment of non-small cell lung cancer. *Bull Cancer (Paris) Suppl*. 1999;3:17–41.

7. Christiani DC. Smoking and the molecular epidemiology of lung cancer. *Clin Chest Med.* 2000;21:87–93.
8. Mills NE, Fishman CL, Scholes J, et al. Detection of K-ras oncogenes mutations in bronchoalveolar lavage fluid for lung cancer diagnosis. *J Natl Cancer Inst.* 1995;87:1056–1060.
9. Komiya T, Hirashima T, Kawase I. Clinical significance of p53 in non-small cell lung cancer. *Oncol Rep.* 1999;6:19–28.
10. Pershagen G, Akerblom G, Axelson O, et al. Residential radon exposure and lung cancer in Sweden. *N Engl J Med.* 1994;330:159–164.
11. Churg A. Lung cancer cell type and asbestos exposure. *JAMA.* 1985;253:2984–2985.
12. Yngveson A, Williams C, Hjerpe A, et al. p53 mutations in lung cancer associated with residential radon exposure. *Cancer Epidemiol Biomarkers Prev.* 1999;8:433–438.
13. Saracci R. The interactions of tobacco smoking and other agents in cancer etiology. *Epidemiol Rev.* 1987;9:175–193.
14. Demiroglu H. Nonoccupational exposure to chrysotile asbestos and the risk of lung cancer. *N Engl J Med.* 1998;339:999–1000.
15. Du Y, Zhou BS, Wu JM. Lifestyle factors and human lung cancer: an overview of recent advances. *Int J Oncol.* 1998;13:471–479.
16. Jemal A, Travis WD, Tarone RE, et al. Lung cancer rates convergence in young men and women in the United States: analysis by birth cohort and histologic type. *Int J Cancer.* 2003;105:101–107.
17. Hubbard R, Venn A, Lewis S, et al. Lung cancer and cryptogenic fibrosing alveolitis: a population-based cohort study. *Am J Respir Crit Care Med.* 2000;161:5–8.
18. Yamasawa H, Ishii Y, Kitamura S. Concurrence of sarcoidosis and lung cancer: a report of four cases. *Respiration.* 2000;67:90–93.
19. Askling J, Grunewald J, Eklund A, et al. Increased risk for cancer following sarcoidosis. *Am J Respir Crit Care Med.* 1999;160:1668–1672.
20. Yanagawa H, Goto H, Maniwa K, et al. A case of resectable lung adenocarcinoma associated with sarcoidosis. *Med Oncol.* 1999;16:216–220.
21. Reich JM. Sarcoidosis and cancer revisited. *Eur Respir J.* 1999;14:482–483.
22. Rosenthal A, McLaughlin J, Gridley G, et al. Incidence of cancer among patients with systemic sclerosis. *Cancer.* 1995;76:910–914.
23. Bedimo R. Non-AIDS-defining malignancies among HIV-infected patients in the highly active antiretroviral therapy era. *Curr HIV/AIDS Rep.* 2008;5:140–149.
24. Engels EA, Biggar RJ, Hall HI, et al. Cancer risk in people infected with human immunodeficiency virus in the United States. *Int J Cancer.* 2008;123:187–194.
25. Patel A, Peters S. Clinical manifestations of lung cancer. *Mayo Clin Proc.* 1993;68:273–277.
26. Crapo JD, et al., eds. *Baum's Textbook of Pulmonary Disease.* 7th ed. Philadelphia: Lippincott Williams & Wilkins; 2004.
27. Arcasoy SM, Jett J. Superior pulmonary sulcus tumors and Pancoast's syndrome. *N Engl J Med.* 1997;337:1370–1376.
28. Yano S, Shimada K. Changes in superior vena cava pulsed Doppler flow patterns: possible indicator of improvement of superior vena cava syndrome due to lung cancer. *J Ultrasound Med.* 1997;16:707–710.
29. Kashitani N, Eda R, Masayoshi T, et al. Lobar extent of pulmonary lymphangitic carcinomatosis: Tl-201 chloride and Tc-99m MIBI scintigraphic findings. *Clin Nucl Med.* 1996;21:726–729.
30. Patel A, Davila D, Peters S. Paraneoplastic syndromes associated with lung cancer. *Mayo Clin Proc.* 1993;68:278–287.
31. Lennon V, Kryzer TJ, Griesmann G, et al. Calcium channel antibodies in the Lambert-Eaton syndrome and other paraneoplastic syndromes. *N Engl J Med.* 1995;332:1467–1474.
32. Sridhar K, Lobo C, Altman RD. Digital clubbing and lung cancer. *Chest.* 1998;114:1535–1537.
33. Strewler GJ. The physiology of parathyroid hormone-related protein. *N Engl J Med.* 2000;342:177–185.
34. Kagan A, Steckel R, Braun R. Asymptomatic peripheral lung nodule. *AJR Am J Roentgenol.* 1980;135:417–420.
35. Higgins GA, Shields TW, Keehn RJ. The solitary pulmonary nodule: 10-year follow-up of Veterans Administration Armed Forces Cooperative Study. *Arch Surg.* 1975;110:570–575.
36. Rubins JB, Rubins HB. Temporal trends in the prevalence of malignancy in solitary pulmonary lesions. *Chest.* 1996; 109:100–103.
37. Sagel S, Ferguson T, Forrest JV, et al. Percutaneous transthoracic aspiration needle biopsy. *Ann Thorac Surg.* 1978;26:399–405.
38. Swanson S, Jaklitsch M, Mentzer SJ, et al. Management of the solitary pulmonary nodule: role of thoracoscopy in diagnosis and therapy. *Chest.* 1999;116:523–524.
39. Swensen S, Silverstein M, Edell ES, et al. Solitary pulmonary nodules: clinical prediction model versus physicians. *Mayo Clin Proc.* 1999;74:319–329.
40. Swensen S, Viggiano R, Midthun DE, et al. Lung nodule enhancement at CT: multicenter study. *Radiology.* 2000;214:73–80.
41. Johnson DH. Cancer of the lung: non-small cell lung cancer and small cell lung cancer. In: Abeloff MD, et al., eds. *Abeloff's Clinical Oncology.* 4th ed. Philadelphia: Churchill Livingstone/Elsevier; 2008.
42. Prakash UB. Advances in bronchoscopic procedures. *Chest.* 1999;116:1403–1408.
43. Khanavkar B, Gnudi F, Muti A, et al. Basic principles of LIFE autofluorescence bronchoscopy: results of 194 examinations in comparison with standard procedures for early detection of bronchial carcinoma: overview. *Pneumologie.* 1998;52:71–76.
44. Preciado M, Duvall A, Koop SH. Mediastinoscopy: a review of 450 cases. *Laryngoscope.* 1973;83:1300–1310.
45. Trastek V, Pichler J, Pairolero PC. Mediastinoscopy. *Br Med Bull.* 1986;42:240–243.
46. Mountain C, Dresler C. Regional lymph node classification for lung cancer staging. *Chest.* 1997;111:1718–1723.
47. Mountain CF. Revisions in the International System for Staging Lung Cancer. *Chest.* 1997;111:1710–1717.
48. Zell JA, Ou SHI, Zioga A, Anton-Culver A. Validation of the proposed International Association for the Study of Lung Cancer non-small cell lung cancer staging system revisions for advanced bronchioloalveolar carcinoma using data from the California Cancer Registry. *J Thorac Oncol.* 2007;2:1078–1085.
49. Lau CL, Harpole D. Noninvasive clinical staging modalities for lung cancer. *Semin Surg Oncol.* 2000;18:116–123.
50. Kaplan D, Goldstraw P. New techniques in the diagnosis and staging of lung cancer. *Cancer Treat Res.* 1995;72:223–254.
51. Tasci E, Tezel C, Orki A, et al. The role of integrated positron emission tomography and computed tomography in the assessment of nodal spread in cases with non-small cell lung cancer. *Interact Cardiovasc Thorac Surg.* 2010;10:200–203.
52. Billé A, Pelosi E, Skanjeti A, et al. Preoperative intrathoracic lymph node staging in patients with non-small-cell lung cancer: accuracy of integrated positron emission tomography and computed tomography. *Eur J Cardiothorac Surg.* 2009;36:440–445.
53. Bae K, Slone R, Gierada DS, et al. Patients with emphysema: quantitative CT analysis before and after lung volume reduction surgery: work in progress. *Radiology.* 1997;203:705–714.
54. Lefrak S, Yusen R, Trulock EP, et al. Recent advances in surgery for emphysema. *Annu Rev Med.* 1997;48:387–398.
55. Sutedja G, Postmus P. Bronchoscopic treatment of lung tumors. *Lung Cancer.* 1994;11:1–17.
56. Johnson B, Patronas N, Hayes W, et al. Neurologic, computed cranial tomographic, and magnetic resonance imaging abnormalities in patients with small cell lung cancer: further follow-up of 6- to 13-year survivors. *J Clin Oncol.* 1990;8:48–56.
57. Pujol JL, Carestia L, Daures JP. Is there a case for cisplatin in the treatment of small-cell lung cancer? A meta-analysis of randomized trials of a cisplatin-containing regimen versus a regimen without this alkylating agent. *Br J Cancer.* 2000;83:8–15.

58. Murray N, Grafton C, Shah A, et al. Abbreviated treatment for elderly, infirm, or noncompliant patients with limited stage small cell lung cancer. *J Clin Oncol.* 1998;16:3323–3328.
59. Murray N, Livingston R, Shepherd FA, et al. Randomized study of CODE versus alternating CAV/EP for extensive stage small cell lung cancer: an Intergroup Study of the National Cancer Institute of Canada Clinical Trials Group and the Southwest Oncology Group. *J Clin Oncol.* 1999;17:2300–2308.
60. Jensen P, Sehestad M, Langer SW, et al. Twenty-five years of chemotherapy in small cell lung cancer sends us back to the laboratory. *Cancer Treat Rev.* 1999;25:377–386.
61. Rosell R, Gomez-Codina J, Camps C. Preresectional chemotherapy in stage IIIA non-small cell lung cancer: a 7-year assessment of a randomized controlled trial. *Lung Cancer.* 1999;26:7–14.
62. Rosell R. New approaches in the adjuvant and neoadjuvant therapy of non-small cell lung cancer, including docetaxel (Taxotere) combinations. *Semin Oncol.* 1999;26:32–37.
63. Reif M, Socinski M, Rivera MP. Evidence-based medicine in the treatment of non-small cell lung cancer. *Clin Chest Med.* 2000;21:107–120.
64. Arriagada R, Bergman B, Dunant A, et al. Cisplatin-based adjuvant chemotherapy in patients with completely resected non-small-cell lung cancer. *N Engl J Med.* 2004;350:351–360.
65. Waller D, Gowe N, Milroy MD, et al. The Big Lung Trial: determining the value of cisplatin-based chemotherapy for all patients with non-small cell lung cancer (NSCLC). Preliminary results in the surgical setting. *Proc Am Soc Clin Oncol.* 2003;22:639.
66. Scagliotti GV, Fossati R, Torri V, et al. Randomized study of adjuvant chemotherapy for completely resected stage I, II, or IIIA non-small-cell lung cancer. *J Natl Cancer Inst.* 2003;95:1453–1465.
67. Douillard JY, Rosell R, De Lena M, et al. Adjuvant vinorelbine plus cisplatin versus observation in patients with completely resected stage IB-IIIA non-small-cell lung cancer (Adjuvant Navelbine International Trialist Association [ANITA]): a randomised controlled trial. *Lancet Oncol.* 2006;7:719–727.
68. Winton T, Livingston R, Johnson D, et al. Vinorelbine plus cisplatin vs. observation in resected non-small-cell lung cancer. *N Engl J Med.* 2005;352:2589–2597.
69. Pignon JP, Tribodet H, Scagliotti GV, et al. Lung adjuvant cisplatin evaluation: a pooled analysis by the LACE collaborative group. *J Clin Oncol.* 2008;26:3552–3559.
70. El-Sherif A, Gooding WE, Santos R, et al. Outcomes of sublobar resection versus lobectomy for stage I non-small cell lung cancer: a 13-year analysis. *Ann Thorac Surg.* 2006;82:408–415.
71. Kodama K, Doi O, Higashiyama M, Yokouchi H. Intentional limited resection for selected patients with T1 N0 M0 non-small-cell lung cancer: a single institution study. *J Thorac Cardiovasc Surg.* 1997;114:347–353.
72. Lee W, Daly BD, DiPetrillo TA, Morelli DM. Limited resection for non-small cell lung cancer: observed local control with implantation of I-125 brachytherapy seeds. *Ann Thorac Surg.* 2003;75:237–243.
73. Nakata M, Sawada S, Saeki H, et al. Prospective study of thoracoscopic limited resection for ground-glass opacity selected by computed tomography. *Ann Thorac Surg.* 2003;75:1601–1606.
74. Yamato Y, Tsuchida M, Watanabe T, et al. Early results of a prospective study of limited resection for bronchioloalveolar adenocarcinoma of the lung. *Ann Thorac Surg.* 2001;71:971–974.
75. Rowell NP, Williams CJ. Radical radiotherapy for stage I/II non-small cell lung cancer in patients not sufficiently fit for or declining surgery (medically inoperable): a systematic review. *Thorax.* 2001;56:628–638.
76. Rowell NP, Williams CJ. Radical radiotherapy for stage I/II non-small cell lung cancer in patients not sufficiently fit for or declining surgery (medically inoperable). *Cochrane Database Syst Rev.* 2001;2:CD002935.
77. Bradbury PA, Shepherd FA. Chemotherapy and surgery for operable NSCLC. *Lancet.* 2007;369:1903–1904.
78. Attar S, Krasna M, Sonnett JR, et al. Superior sulcus (Pancoast) tumor: experience with 105 patients. *Ann Thorac Surg.* 1998;66:193–198.
79. National Comprehensive Cancer Network. NCCN clinical practice guidelines in oncology. Available at: www.nccn.org/professionals/physician_gls/f_guidelines.asp.
80. Pisters KM, Evans WK, Azzoli CG, et al. Cancer Care Ontario and American Society of Clinical Oncology adjuvant chemotherapy and adjuvant radiation therapy for stages I-IIIA resectable non small-cell lung cancer guideline. *J Clin Oncol.* 2007;25:5506–5518.
81. Lally BE, Zelterman D, Colasanto JM, et al. Postoperative radiotherapy for stage II or III non-small-cell lung cancer using the Surveillance, Epidemiology, and End Results database. *J Clin Oncol.* 2006;24:2998–3006.
82. Lally BE, Detterbeck FC, Geiger AM, et al. The risk of death from heart disease in patients with nonsmall cell lung cancer who receive postoperative radiotherapy: analysis of the Surveillance, Epidemiology, and End Results database. *Cancer.* 2007;110:911–917.
83. Douillard JY, Rosell R, De Lena M, et al. Adjuvant vinorelbine plus cisplatin versus observation in patients with completely resected stage IB-IIIA non-small-cell lung cancer (Adjuvant Navelbine International Trialist Association [ANITA]): a randomised controlled trial. *Lancet Oncol.* 2006;7:719–727.
84. Douillard JY, Rosell R, De Lena M, et al. Impact of postoperative radiation therapy on survival in patients with complete resection and stage I, II, or IIIA non-small-cell lung cancer treated with adjuvant chemotherapy: the Adjuvant Navelbine International Trialist Association (ANITA) randomized trial. *Int J Radiat Oncol Biol Phys.* 2008;72:695–701.
85. Azzoli CG, Baker S Jr, Temin S, et al. American Society of Clinical Oncology clinical practice guideline update on chemotherapy for stage IV non-small-cell lung cancer. *J Clin Oncol.* 2009;27:6251–6299.
86. Byhardt R, Scott C, Sause WT, et al. Response, toxicity, failure patterns, and survival in five Radiation Therapy Oncology Group (RTOG) trials of sequential and/or concurrent chemotherapy and radiotherapy for locally advanced non-small cell carcinoma of the lung. *Int J Radiat Oncol Biol Phys.* 1998;42:469–478.
87. Monson J, Stark P, Reilly JJ, et al. Clinical radiation pneumonitis and radiographic changes after thoracic radiation therapy for lung carcinoma. *Cancer.* 1998;82:842–850.
88. Warner MA, Offord K, Warner ME, et al. Role of preoperative cessation of smoking and other factors in postoperative pulmonary complications: a blinded prospective study of coronary artery bypass patients. *Mayo Clin Proc.* 1989;64:609–616.
89. Rom W, Hay JG, Lee TC, et al. Molecular and genetic aspects of lung cancer. *Am J Respir Crit Care Med.* 2000;161:1355–1367.
90. Bach P, Cramer LD, Warren JL, et al. Racial differences in the treatment of early stage lung cancer. *N Engl J Med.* 1999;341:1198–1205.
91. Zhang H, Cai B. The impact of tobacco on lung health in China. *Respirology.* 2003;8:17–21.
92. Hurt R, Sachs D, Glover ED, et al. A comparison of sustained-release bupropion and placebo for smoking cessation. *N Engl J Med.* 1997;337:1195–1202.
93. Gonzales D, Rennard SI, Nides M, et al. Varenicline, an a4b2 nicotinic acetylcholine receptor partial agonist, vs sustained-release bupropion and placebo for smoking cessation: a randomized controlled trial. *JAMA.* 2006;296:47–55.
94. Croghan I, Offord K, Evans RW, et al. Cost-effectiveness of treating nicotine dependence: the Mayo Clinic experience. *Mayo Clin Proc.* 1997;72:917–924.
95. Croghan I, Offord K, Patten CA, et al. Cost-effectiveness of the AHCPR guidelines for smoking. *JAMA.* 1998;279:836–837.
96. Omenn GS, Goodman GE, Thornquist MD, et al. Effects of a combination of beta carotene and vitamin A on lung cancer and cardiovascular disease. *N Engl J Med.* 1996;334:1150–1155.

97. The Alpha-Tocopherol Beta Carotene Cancer Prevention Study Group. The effect of vitamin E and beta carotene on the incidence of lung cancer and other cancers in male smokers. *N Engl J Med*. 1994;330:1029–1035.
98. Krinsky NI, Johnson EJ. Carotenoid actions and their relation to health and disease. *Mol Aspects Med*. 2005;26:456–516.
99. Ruano-Ravina A, Figueiras A, et al. Antioxidant vitamins and risk of lung cancer. *Curr Pharm Des*. 2006;2:599–613.
100. Lam WK. Lung cancer in Asian women: the environment and genes. *Respirology*. 2005;10:408–417.
101. Omenn G, Goodman G, Thornquist MD, et al. Risk factors for lung cancer and for intervention effects in CARET, the β-Carotene and Retinol Efficacy Trial. *J Natl Cancer Inst*. 1996;88:1550–1559.
102. Omenn G, Goodman G, Thornquist MD, et al. Effects of a combination of β-carotene and vitamin A on lung cancer and cardiovascular disease. *N Engl J Med*. 1996;334:1150–1155.
103. Omenn G, Goodman G, Thornquist M, et al. Chemoprevention of lung cancer: the β-Carotene and Retinol Efficacy Trial (CARET) in high-risk smokers and asbestos-exposed workers. *IARC Sci Publ*. 1996;136:67–85.
104. Field JK, Duffy SW. Lung cancer screening: the way forward. *Br J Cancer*. 2008;99:557–562.
105. Swisher S, Roth J, Nemunaitis J, et al. Adenovirus-mediated p53 gene transfer in advanced non-small cell lung cancer. *J Natl Cancer Inst*. 1999;91:763–771.
106. Dubinett S, Miller P, Sharma S, et al. Gene therapy for lung cancer. *Hematol Oncol Clin North Am*. 1998;12:569–594.

CHAPTER 48

Neonatal and Pediatric Respiratory Disorders

Sherry Barnhart

OUTLINE

Apnea of Prematurity
Respiratory Distress Syndrome
Bronchopulmonary Dysplasia and Chronic Lung Disease
Transient Tachypnea of the Newborn
Pneumonia in the Neonate
Meconium Aspiration Syndrome
Persistent Pulmonary Hypertension of the Newborn
Congenital Diaphragmatic Hernia
Air Leak Syndrome
Retinopathy of Prematurity
Bronchiolitis
Laryngotracheobronchitis
Epiglottitis

OBJECTIVES

1. List the factors that may predispose an infant or child to pulmonary disease.
2. Explain the underlying pathophysiology of pulmonary diseases affecting the newborn and child.
3. Identify the signs and symptoms of pulmonary diseases affecting the newborn and child.
4. Discuss diagnosis of pulmonary diseases affecting the newborn and child.
5. Recognize the radiographic appearance of various diseases of the newborn and child.
6. Integrate the history, physical examination, laboratory, and radiographic findings that are used in the diagnosis of diseases of the infant and child.
7. Discuss treatment options for pediatric pulmonary disease.
8. Explain the significance of monitoring oxygen at preductal and postductal sites.
9. Discuss the impact that hypoxia in a neonate has on the pulmonary vasculature.
10. Describe the development of retinopathy of prematurity.
11. Define apnea of prematurity and periodic breathing.
12. Differentiate between bronchopulmonary dysplasia and chronic lung disease.
13. Compare laryngotracheobronchitis and epiglottitis.

KEY TERMS

air leak syndrome
apnea of prematurity
bronchiolitis
chronic lung disease (CLD)
congenital diaphragmatic hernia (CDH)
epiglottitis
laryngotracheobronchitis (LTB)
meconium aspiration syndrome (MAS)
persistent pulmonary hypertension of the newborn (PPHN)
respiratory distress syndrome (RDS)
retinopathy of prematurity (ROP)
transient tachypnea of the newborn (TTN)

INTRODUCTION

Respiratory illness is the most common cause of infant and childhood morbidity in developed countries. There are many disorders that result in respiratory distress and place an infant or child at high risk of cardiopulmonary failure. Respiratory disease may begin early in life, even in utero, and remain a challenging problem that affects the infant's survival and quality of life. The causes are many. In utero abnormalities, such as congenital diaphragmatic hernia, can inhibit lung development. Maternal factors, such as medication or illicit drug use, often cause severe respiratory depression. Events at birth will affect the infant's respiratory status, as is found with transient tachypnea of the newborn and meconium aspiration syndrome. Premature birth with lungs that are unable to adequately support gas exchange may result in apnea and respiratory distress syndrome. Ironically, therapy for respiratory disorders can actually lead to more disease, which is what occurs with chronic lung disease, air leaks, and retinopathy of prematurity.

As for the child, acute respiratory tract infections may be mild or life threatening. Infections resulting in bronchiolitis, laryngotracheobronchitis, and epiglottitis are often cause for emergency department and hospital admissions. Although we have witnessed significant advances in the medical management of infants and children, the fact remains that all of the factors just described continue to have an impact on neonatal and pediatric respiratory care.

Apnea of Prematurity

The successful progression from fetal to neonatal life is dependent on complex physiologic changes that include moving from fetal respiratory activity to normal spontaneous breathing. When an infant is born premature, the immaturity of the central respiratory control center interrupts this normal transition and often leads to apnea. The standard definition of **apnea of prematurity** is the cessation of breathing for at least 20 seconds or for shorter periods if the apnea is followed by bradycardia, oxygen desaturation, cyanosis, or pallor.[1] Apnea of prematurity is different from the periodic breathing common to premature as well as some full-term infants. Periodic breathing is a respiratory pattern characterized by periodic pauses of breathing lasting between 5 and 10 seconds and then followed by regular breathing. It has no pathologic significance, does not result in bradycardia or cyanosis, and spontaneously resolves without the need for intervention.

Apnea of prematurity affects at least 85% of infants born at less than 34 weeks' gestation and 50% of infants of less than 1500 grams birth weight.[2] It is the most common cause of apnea in neonates, with peak incidence usually occurring between 2 and 7 days' postnatal age.

Pathophysiology and Etiology

Apnea of prematurity is largely due to immaturity of the medullary brain stem center that regulates breathing. This immaturity leads to impaired responses to hypoxia and hypercapnia, and an exaggerated inhibitory response to stimulation of airway receptors.

> **RESPIRATORY RECAP**
>
> **Apnea of Prematurity**
>
> » Cessation of breathing for at least 20 seconds
> » Caused by immaturity of the brain stem
> » Treated with respiratory stimulants, oxygen, CPAP, and mechanical ventilation
> » Home apnea monitor may be used

Apnea is traditionally classified as obstructive, central, or mixed, depending on the presence or absence of upper airway obstruction. No airflow, chest wall motion, or inspiratory efforts occur in central apnea. In obstructive apnea, inspiratory efforts and chest wall motion persist, but airflow is absent. Mixed apnea, the most common type associated with apnea of prematurity, has components of both central and obstructive apnea: inspiratory efforts with airway obstruction preceding or following central apnea.

Clinical Manifestations

In premature infants who are breathing spontaneously with no assistance, apnea usually occurs on the first or second day of life. If lung disease exists or the infant is receiving any form of mechanical ventilation, including continuous positive airway pressure (CPAP), apnea may be delayed or not present until the infant no longer needs ventilator assistance. The apneic episodes are typically accompanied by bradycardia, hypotension, cyanosis, pallor, and oxygen desaturation. Apnea of prematurity has usually resolved by 37 weeks' postconceptional age but may persist beyond term, especially in infants delivered at 24 to 28 weeks' gestation.[3] If apnea presents immediately after birth, first presents in a premature infant that is older than 2 weeks, or reoccurs after a 1- to 2-week period without apnea, it may signify an underlying pathophysiologic condition. Immediate investigation of possible causes is always warranted.

Diagnosis

A diagnosis of apnea of prematurity is made after other disorders have been considered and excluded. Several studies are routinely used to confirm the diagnosis. Laboratory studies performed when infection is suspected include a complete blood count, blood and spinal fluid cultures, and urinalysis. Electrolyte levels and glucose levels are tests useful in diagnosing a metabolic process. Chest radiographs and electrocardiograms (ECGs) are routine, whereas echocardiograms are obtained if symptoms are suggestive of cardiac disease. Imaging studies of the head and neck may be obtained if obstructive apnea is suspected. A swallow study or abdominal ultrasound is used to detect gastrointestinal problems.

Management

Clinical management includes cardiorespiratory monitoring and tactile stimulation. When apnea lasts for only a few seconds, stimulating the infant by patting the infant or flicking the feet is usually the only intervention needed. Pharmacologic treatment with methylxanthines, most often caffeine or theophylline, has been used since the 1970s to stimulate respirations, thereby reducing the frequency of apnea and need for mechanical ventilation. Caffeine is preferred over theophylline because it has a longer half-life that allows for once-daily dosing, a larger gap between therapeutic and toxic levels, and fewer side effects.[4]

Depending on the frequency and severity of the apneic episodes, oxygen therapy, CPAP, and intubation with assisted ventilation may be required. When apnea results in oxygen desaturation, oxygen is administered and manual ventilation applied if the apnea is prolonged. High-flow nasal cannula or CPAP is initiated when the apneic events continue or become more frequent in spite of methylxanthine therapy. If apnea with oxygen desaturation, bradycardia, or both continue, intubation

BOX 48–1

Protocol for Treating Apnea of Prematurity

1. Monitor with cardiorespiratory monitor and pulse oximeter.
2. Provide tactile stimulation and reposition head and neck.
3. Administer oxygen for bradycardia or oxygen desaturation.
4. Begin methylxanthine therapy (caffeine preferred).
5. Apply high-flow nasal cannula or nasal continuous positive airway pressure.
6. Intubate and begin mechanical ventilation.

BOX 48–2

Indications for Home Apnea Monitoring in Infants

Methylxanthine treatment at home
Bradycardia with methylxanthine use
GERD with apnea
Documented ALTE
Risk of central apnea
Twin or sibling with SIDS-related death*

*The American Academy of Pediatrics does not recommend home apnea monitoring to prevent SIDS.

GERD, gastroesophageal reflux disease; ALTE, apparent life-threatening event; SIDS, sudden infant death syndrome.

and mechanical ventilation may be indicated.[5] **Box 48–1** contains a suggested treatment protocol for apnea of prematurity. Although the time interval is not clearly established, methylxanthine therapy is discontinued when there have been no significant events for 7 to 14 days. The infant is discharged without methylxanthine treatment if no further events occur.

In some infants the apnea will reoccur, and medication is restarted. If the infant continues to need methylxanthines at discharge, an impedance monitor (apnea monitor) is provided for use at home. This monitor stores data and documents apneic, bradycardic, and tachycardic events. Parents and other caregivers receive training in cardiopulmonary resuscitation as well as observation and stimulation techniques. They also are instructed on monitor use, including how to apply monitor leads and correctly respond to alarms. The monitor can be safely discontinued after the infant has had no true and significant apneic and bradycardic events for 1 to 2 months after discharge home.[6] **Box 48–2** lists the indications for apnea monitoring at home.

Complications and Outcome

Apnea that leads to hypoxemia and bradycardia increases the risk of cerebral injury; however, treatment with caffeine decreases this risk.[7] Apnea due to prematurity is usually resolved by 44 weeks' conceptional age. Studies indicate that it does not cause an infant to be at a higher risk for sudden infant death syndrome (SIDS).[8]

Respiratory Distress Syndrome

Infants born before the 37th week of gestation are considered premature. The consequences of a premature birth are complex, with the earliest recognized complication being **respiratory distress syndrome (RDS)**. Previously referred to as hyaline membrane disease, RDS is the most common cause of respiratory distress in the premature infant and occurs most often in infants born at less than 28 weeks' gestation. RDS rarely occurs in term infants.[9]

Pathophysiology and Etiology

Box 48–3 lists factors that may predispose an infant to RDS. The risk of RDS may decrease if the mother has pregnancy-induced hypertension, prolonged rupture of membranes, or a history of narcotic addiction. It is believed that the stress of these situations helps the lungs to mature. Antenatal corticosteroid therapy to mothers with preterm labor accelerates maturation of the neonate's lung and significantly reduces the incidence of RDS and mortality.

RESPIRATORY RECAP

Respiratory Distress Syndrome

» Complication of prematurity
» Biochemical tests of amniotic fluid can be used to evaluate lung maturity
» Treatment includes oxygen, surfactant replacement, CPAP, mechanical ventilation, and supportive therapy

High surface tension and a lack of pulmonary surfactant in the lungs are responsible for the development of RDS in premature infants. Surfactant is a complex mixture of phospholipids and proteins that is produced by type II pneumocytes and stored in the lamellar bodies. Synthesis begins near 20 weeks of gestation and continues with accelerated production around 36 weeks. As surfactant spreads along the alveolar air–liquid interface, surface tension is decreased and lower pressures are

BOX 48–3

Risk Factors Associated with Respiratory Distress Syndrome

Male infant
Hypothermia
Premature birth
Maternal diabetes
Perinatal asphyxia
Multifetal pregnancy
Family history of respiratory distress syndrome
Caesarean delivery without labor

required to keep alveoli inflated. In the premature infant, immature type II alveolar cells produce less surfactant, causing alveoli to collapse.[10] The result is decreased compliance, reduced functional residual capacity (FRC), diffuse atelectasis, and increased airway resistance and dead space.[11] Well-perfused but poorly ventilated areas result in ventilation-perfusion ($\dot{V}/\dot{Q}$) mismatch with hypoxia and right-to-left shunting of blood. Because of the weak respiratory muscles and overly compliant chest that are characteristic of the premature neonate, work of breathing increases as lung compliance is reduced. Hypercarbia and respiratory acidosis quickly develop as the diaphragm and intercostal muscles fatigue. Prolonged hypoxemia leads to vasoconstriction of pulmonary arteries, decreased pulmonary blood flow, and direct damage to the respiratory epithelium, allowing plasma to leak into the alveoli, where hyaline membranes are formed, hence the term *hyaline membrane disease*.[12,13]

Clinical Manifestations

RDS is suspected in the premature infant who develops respiratory distress at or shortly after delivery. Tachypnea with respiratory rates of 60 or greater is often the initial symptom. Other hallmark clinical signs are nasal flaring, subcostal and intercostal retractions, and expiratory grunting. Grunting occurs as air is forced through the partially closed glottis in an attempt to increase the FRC. As the work of breathing continues, grunting becomes ineffective, and the alveoli collapse. Cyanosis and hypoxia are common, and breath sounds are diminished. Upon examination the infant may be inactive and have edema and decreased perfusion in peripheral extremities. Oxygen requirements and apnea often increase after birth, and within 48 hours the infant has rapidly progressed to respiratory failure with hypercarbia and respiratory acidosis. Extremely premature neonates with severe atelectasis and loss of compliance may have lungs so stiff that they are apneic before they leave the delivery room.

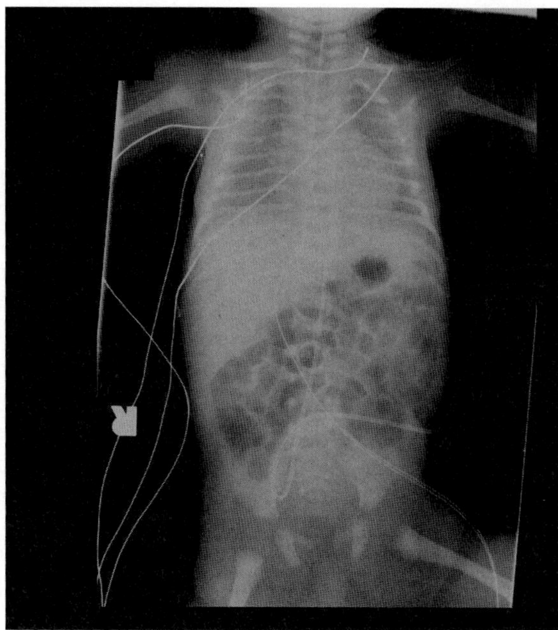

FIGURE 48–1 Chest radiograph of a preterm infant presenting with a bilateral diffuse fine granular (ground glass) appearance and reduced lung expansion, typical of respiratory distress syndrome.

Diagnosis

Clinical features and recognition of risk factors aid in the diagnosis, which is confirmed with physical findings, chest radiographs, and lab values consistent with RDS. A detailed history is also critical in the differential diagnosis. Details should include gestational age and maternal history. Age is important because RDS typically occurs in premature infants, unlike term infants affected by transient tachypnea or postterm infants with meconium aspiration syndrome. Information concerning labor and delivery is vital and should include fetal heart tracings, color and amount of amniotic fluid, method of delivery, and maternal temperature. Pneumonia due to β-hemolytic *Streptococcus* has been associated with rupture of membranes occurring more than 24 hours prior to delivery. Transient tachypnea of the newborn usually occurs in term infants following caesarean delivery without maternal labor.

Although the chest radiograph may not be typical in the first few hours after birth, RDS is characterized by a large thymus, markedly decreased lung expansion, atelectasis, and a diffuse symmetric reticulogranular (ground glass) appearance that extends to the periphery of the lungs. With severe disease, the chest radiograph may progress to complete "whiteout" that is difficult to distinguish from pneumonia (**Figure 48–1**).

Biochemical tests of lung maturity began in 1971 with the introduction of the lecithin-to-sphingomyelin (L/S) ratio. Lecithin and sphingomyelin are both phospholipids found in the amniotic fluid. Lecithin levels increase as the lung matures and begins producing surfactant, whereas the amount of sphingomyelin remains fairly constant. A calculated L/S ratio of 2 or more is considered an accurate indication that sufficient surfactant is being produced and the risk of RDS is low. The assessment of amniotic fluid for phosphatidylglycerol, first reported in 1976, was the next biochemical test developed to determine fetal lung maturity. The presence of phosphatidylglycerol is associated with a low risk for RDS.

Other biophysical tests to determine fetal lung maturity include the foam stability index, also known as the shake test, and the lamellar body count. The shake test consists of mixing a serial dilution of ethanol with amniotic fluid in a test tube. The tube is shaken, and a layer of foam forms at the surface. The tube with the highest concentration of ethanol in which the foam remains stable is reported as the foam stability index. An index of more than 0.47 is considered indicative of mature lungs. The lamellar body count is also used to anticipate RDS. Surfactant-containing lamellar bodies enter the amniotic fluid via the fetal mouth. Using a simple cell counter, this test determines lung maturity by the number of bodies in the amniotic fluid: the higher the count, the more mature the lung. A count of 30,000 to 50,000 per mL indicates lung maturity.[14]

Management

When there is a high risk of delivery occurring between 24 and 34 weeks' gestation, mothers are given tocolytics to delay delivery and then receive corticosteroids 24 to 48 hours before delivery. This has been shown to accelerate fetal lung maturation and surfactant production, thereby decreasing the incidence of RDS as well as intraventricular hemorrhage and neonatal mortality.[15]

After delivery, maintaining an airway and oxygenation is vital. Depending on the infant's clinical presentation, initial oxygen therapy is delivered using blow-by oxygen, a hood, or resuscitation bag and mask. In very low birth weight infants, attempts are made to maintain the fractional concentration of inspired oxygen (F_{IO_2}) to keep the oxygen saturation as measured by pulse oximetry (Sp_{O_2}) between 85% and 92% or the Pa_{O_2} at 50 to 80 mm Hg. For those infants who present with persistent pulmonary hypertension of the newborn (PPHN), oxygen is administered to keep the Sp_{O_2} greater than 95% or the Pa_{O_2} greater than 120 mm Hg. In some institutions, heated and humidified high-flow nasal cannula with flows greater than 2 L/min are used in place of CPAP. The high-flow therapy may prevent the need for intubation and mechanical ventilation, or it may be used to facilitate extubation.

Before the use of exogenous surfactant therapy, RDS was associated with significant morbidity and mortality. Following its introduction in the 1980s, surfactant replacement therapy for RDS has proven to be undoubtedly one of the greatest advances in neonatal care.[16] Today it is a standard of care for the infant with RDS; early administration is associated with a significant reduction in mortality, duration of mechanical ventilation, and incidence of air leaks.[17]

Two approaches have emerged in surfactant replacement therapy: prophylactic and rescue treatment.[18] In an attempt to replace surfactant before the development of severe RDS, prophylactic treatment consists of surfactant administration in the delivery room. It is given within 10 to 30 minutes following intubation and radiographic confirmation of RDS features. Studies have concluded that prophylactic surfactant replacement is associated with a lower incidence and severity of RDS and pulmonary air leaks.[19] One disadvantage to this approach is that some infants who might manage perfectly well on CPAP are unnecessarily treated with intubation and ventilation, increasing the risk of bronchopulmonary dysplasia.[20] This is avoided with rescue treatment, in which surfactant is administered only to those infants who have a diagnosis of RDS and are requiring mechanical ventilation. Rescue surfactant replacement is usually administered within the first 12 hours after birth. A criticism of rescue therapy is that the delay in surfactant replacement could result in progression of RDS.

Two types of surfactant preparations are used to treat RDS. The natural surfactants are derived from animal sources, including minced lung extracts from cows or pigs or surfactant extracted after lavage of cow lungs. The latest synthetic surfactants contain biologically active peptides or whole proteins that mimic the human surfactant protein.[21,22]

Prior to surfactant replacement, the infant must be intubated and the endotracheal tube placement confirmed with a chest radiograph. If needed, the infant is suctioned prior to instillation of surfactant. Suctioning is then avoided for at least 2 hours after surfactant administration unless airway compromise develops. A bolus or infusion of surfactant is administered through an adapter port on the proximal end of the endotracheal tube. Lung compliance can change rapidly following surfactant replacement and often necessitates adjusting ventilator and F_{IO_2} settings. Close monitoring of ventilator waveforms, transcutaneous CO_2 levels, blood gas values, and Sp_{O_2} is essential in determining safe and effective settings. To reduce the risk of pulmonary air leaks and hyperoxia, the F_{IO_2} is weaned and peak inspiratory pressures are reduced empirically by 1 to 2 cm H_2O within a few minutes following administration. Neonates often require two additional doses of surfactant.

With the clinical goal of maintaining FRC, CPAP applied to the stiff lungs of the infant with RDS results in improved lung compliance, alveolar inflation, and oxygenation, which in turn decrease intrapulmonary shunting and work of breathing. CPAP is indicated when the F_{IO_2} required is greater than 0.30 and the infant continues to have respiratory distress or whenever the required F_{IO_2} is greater than 0.40, regardless of the presence of respiratory distress. CPAP may be applied shortly after birth in an attempt to avoid the need for mechanical ventilation with prolonged intubation and thereby prevent ventilator-induced lung injury that may lead to chronic lung disease. Using binasal prongs or a nasal mask, administering pressures of 4 to 7 cm H_2O are usually adequate; however, pressures up to 8 cm H_2O may be necessary to improve alveolar recruitment in the infant with severely noncompliant lungs. It is believed that pressures greater than 8 cm H_2O provide no significant benefit and may in fact increase the risk of gastric insufflation. Extremely premature infants weighing less than 1000 g with a gestational age less than 28 weeks are typically intubated and begun on ventilator support immediately after delivery so they can receive preventive surfactant.[23,24]

CPAP may also be applied following mechanical ventilation. Extubation to CPAP stabilizes the airways and may decrease the risk of respiratory failure and need for reintubation. When the F_{IO_2} is weaned to less than 0.40, CPAP pressures can be decreased by increments of 1 cm H_2O until 4 cm H_2O is reached. At that point CPAP is discontinued and the infant provided oxygen therapy with an oxygen hood or low-flow nasal cannula.[25]

For some infants, CPAP alone cannot adequately support ventilation, especially in very low birth weight infants (<1000 g) or the extremely premature neonate with a gestational age of less than 26 weeks. Intubation and mechanical ventilation are indicated if the infant has an F_{IO_2} requirement greater than 0.40, more frequent or prolonged episodes of apnea, or hypercarbia and acidosis in spite of increased levels of CPAP. Initial ventilation settings typically include peak inspiratory pressures of 15 to 25 cm H_2O to maintain a tidal volume of 4 to 6 mL/kg, a rate of 30 to 60 breaths per minute, a positive end-expiratory pressure (PEEP) of 4 to 5 cm H_2O, and an inspiratory time between 0.3 and 0.5 second. The F_{IO_2} is adjusted to keep the appropriate S_{PO_2} levels (see oxygen therapy values).

If respiratory failure persists, high-frequency ventilation is implemented using high-frequency oscillatory ventilation (HFOV), high-frequency jet ventilation (HFJ), or high-frequency flow-interrupter (HFI). Studies report that infants treated with HFOV have a lower mortality rate and significantly reduced development of air leak syndrome, display fewer signs of bronchopulmonary dysplasia, and require fewer days of mechanical ventilation and lower oxygen concentrations. There is no clear evidence that choosing HFOV as the initial primary mode of ventilation or as rescue ventilation following conventional ventilation is more beneficial, except that there may be a small reduction in chronic lung disease when using HFOV. However, there is support of the use of HFOV over conventional ventilation in conjunction with nitric oxide therapy to treat PPHN.[26,27] Inhaled nitric oxide may be used to treat PPHN, but it is not administered to treat RDS alone.

To prevent hypothermia, which increases oxygen consumption, the infant is placed in a neutral thermal environment using either an incubator or a radiant warmer. Although it is vital to maintain minimal stimulation, it is necessary to constantly monitor the heart rate, respiratory rate, and S_{PO_2} and to obtain lab tests. Perfusion and blood pressure are monitored, and blood or volume expanders may be required. An echocardiogram is performed to diagnose a patent ductus arteriosus (PDA) and to determine the presence of pulmonary hypertension and congenital heart defects. Because it is difficult to distinguish between RDS and pneumonia at birth, infants receive empiric antibiotic therapy. Blood cultures are obtained, and antibiotics are discontinued after 2 to 4 days if cultures remain negative.

Complications and Outcome

Beginning in the 1980s, there has been a significant improvement in the prognosis for RDS, with survival to as low as 23 weeks' gestational age. This is believed to be a result of the administration of antenatal steroids to mothers with preterm labor, surfactant replacement, and gentler ventilation techniques. With adequate treatment, RDS usually resolves within 4 to 5 days in infants with a gestational age of more than 30 weeks. However, the more premature the infant, the greater the probability of requiring ventilator support for several weeks.

Acute complications of RDS, especially in infants who receive mechanical ventilation, include pneumothorax and pulmonary interstitial emphysema (PIE), intraventricular hemorrhage, necrotizing enterocolitis, PDA, and sepsis. With the increased survival of extremely premature infants, we can expect a higher incidence of long-term complications. Persistent RDS involving prolonged intubation and mechanical ventilation has a high incidence of chronic lung disease, retinopathy of prematurity, and neurologic impairment with learning disabilities. RDS also increases the incidence of wheezing, asthma, respiratory infection, and pulmonary function test abnormalities.[19,28]

Bronchopulmonary Dysplasia and Chronic Lung Disease

Bronchopulmonary dysplasia (BPD) and **chronic lung disease (CLD)** are both diseases of the premature infant characterized by respiratory failure, the need for supplemental oxygen and positive pressure ventilation, and a progressive deterioration of lung function that results in chronic lung injury. The wide variance in disease progression and severity of lung injury has led to distinct definitions and diagnostic criteria for each disease.

As the care of preterm infants has improved, there has been a dramatic decrease in mortality rates of extremely low birth weight infants. However, the incidence of BPD and CLD has not decreased. Instead, with more births and the increase in survival of more infants with gestational ages of less than 28 weeks and birth weights of less than 1 kg, the prevalence of long-term complications of prematurity has actually increased.[29,30]

Bronchopulmonary Dysplasia

When BPD was first described in 1967, mechanical ventilation of premature neonates was just beginning and infants with birth weights less than 1 kg rarely survived.[31] At that time BPD was considered a syndrome of severe lung injury in preterm infants with RDS who received high levels of supplemental oxygen and prolonged mechanical ventilation using high airway pressures. It was occasionally considered in term or near-term infants with pneumonia or aspiration syndromes who had also required oxygen and mechanical ventilation.[32] This classic BPD occurred in relatively larger preterm infants and was based on progressive radiographic changes. Exposure of the premature lung to mechanical ventilation and oxygen was considered the major factor in its development. Chest radiographs typically revealed areas of increased density, fibrosis, and marked hyperinflation and emphysema.

As practices and outcomes have changed, this severe form of BPD caused by injury to the immature lung has become less common. Instead, a new type of BPD has emerged in very low birth weight infants who quite often have received antenatal steroid therapy and surfactant replacement.[33] These infants may or may not have RDS, and their initial respiratory course is often mild. When required, oxygen is administered at low concentrations and ventilation is supported using low pressures. The BPD is typically triggered by infections and a PDA. Such infants require oxygen and mechanical ventilation, usually in the second or third week of life. As lung function progressively deteriorates, the need for mechanical ventilation and supplemental oxygen is prolonged. This form of BPD is characterized by less pulmonary hypertension and by radiographs revealing hazy lungs, cystic emphysema, less fibrosis, minimal hyperinflation, and more uniform inflation.

Chronic Lung Disease

CLD is believed to represent a disruption or arrest of lung development rather than the effects of severe lung injury and its repair. Although sometimes used interchangeably with BPD, CLD can be defined as the milder new form of BPD and is simply based on a continued oxygen requirement at 36 weeks' gestational age. It refers to the very low birth weight preterm infant with chronic lung disease who initially responded favorably to surfactant replacement and may or may not have a history of RDS. BPD is best described as CLD in the premature infant who requires prolonged mechanical ventilation and high oxygen concentrations to treat RDS and continues to be oxygen dependent at 28 postnatal days.[32]

Pathophysiology and Etiology

CLD is no longer believed to be predominantly a ventilator- and oxygen-induced injury but instead is multifactorial and includes inflammation, inadequate nutrition and fetal growth, infection, high oxygen levels that increase free radical exposure, mechanical ventilation with barotrauma and volutrauma, and genetic factors.[34] **Box 48–4** lists causes of CLD.

Lung inflammation is a major contributor to CLD and may actually begin prior to birth. It often continues after delivery if the infant requires mechanical ventilatory support or supplemental oxygen.

> **RESPIRATORY RECAP**
>
> **Chronic Lung Disease**
> - Occurs in premature infants with progressive deterioration of lung function
> - A milder form of bronchopulmonary dysplasia based on continued oxygen therapy at 36 weeks' gestation
> - Causes are multifactorial and include ventilator- and oxygen-induced injury
> - Treatment includes oxygen, mechanical ventilation, corticosteroids, and bronchodilators

Although it is possible for the immature lung to be damaged even if low levels of supplemental oxygen and ventilator pressures are used, injury is more likely due to a process that interferes with lung development. Limited fetal growth has been attributed to failure of the placenta to provide adequate oxygenation and nutrition, which can in turn interfere with alveolar and pulmonary artery development.[35] Any process that limits fetal growth has the ability to adversely affect lung growth after birth, making the lung more vulnerable to injury.

With supplemental oxygen, the lungs are exposed to toxic free radicals, ions that disrupt chemical bonds. Excessive free radical exposure further damages cell membranes and the already-injured pulmonary tissues. Because of inadequate concentrations of antioxidant enzymes, preterm infants are poorly equipped to handle

> **BOX 48–4**
>
> **Causes of Chronic Lung Disease**
>
> Prematurity
> Pneumonia and/or sepsis
> Aspiration syndromes
> Pulmonary hypoplasia
> Congenital heart disease
> Congenital diaphragmatic hernia
> Persistent pulmonary hypertension of the newborn

free radicals and are more susceptible to oxygen exposure injury.

The surfactant-deficient fetal lung is easily injured, with injury very likely occurring during resuscitation. Ventilating with lower tidal volumes minimizes the injury but may not prevent hypercarbia. As positive pressure ventilation inflates and stretches the lung, the walls and alveolar septa are damaged, triggering an inflammatory response.[33]

Prenatal infection is believed to be a risk factor for the development of CLD. The lungs of infants born before 30 weeks' gestation may be exposed to inflammation as a result of chorioamnionitis. *Ureaplasma urealyticum* and *Mycoplasma* are the most frequent contaminant organisms in amniotic fluid, and it is believed that the ascending intrauterine infection can inflame the infant lungs within hours.[36]

Clinical Manifestations and Diagnosis

Physical examination of the infant with CLD reveals tachypnea, tachycardia, wheezing, crackles, noisy breathing, and retractions. The infant is usually fussy and may be difficult to feed due to the increased work of breathing. The ECG and echocardiogram may reveal right ventricular hypertrophy and pulmonary hypertension. Chest radiographs vary widely, depending on the degree of lung injury. Typically there is a gradual progression from minimal findings to a picture of hyaline membranes with decreased lung volumes, areas of atelectasis and hyperexpansion, fine or coarse interstitial opacities, and a bubbly appearance with irregular dense areas (**Figure 48–2**). There is a medical history of prematurity, prolonged mechanical ventilation, and supplemental oxygen therapy. The diagnosis of CLD is based on clinical manifestations and radiographic changes.

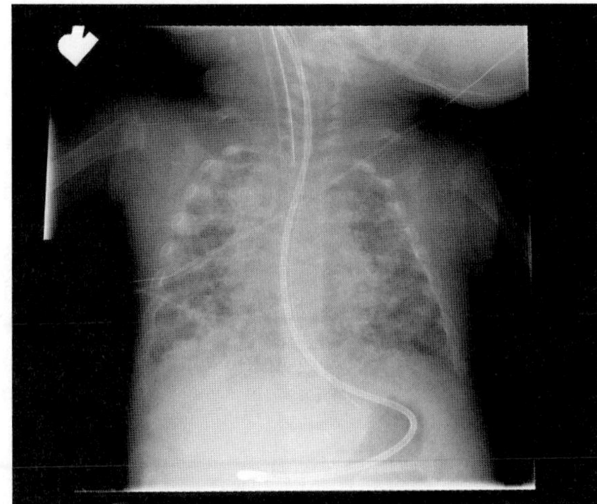

FIGURE 48–2 Chest radiograph of an infant with chronic lung disease showing areas of hyperaeration and reticular opacities with small cystic radiolucencies, giving a coarse, bubbly appearance.

Management

Management goals are to maintain adequate oxygenation, reduce inflammation, improve lung function, relieve symptoms, facilitate growth, and prevent further lung injury.

Supplemental oxygen is provided by nasal cannula or through mechanical ventilation and is weaned to maintain an oxygen saturation of 92% to 94%. Oxygen use is essential in preventing right ventricular hypertrophy (RVH), which often accompanies CLD. Because RVH resolves gradually, oxygen is maintained at a saturation greater than 94% and is often continued at home following discharge.[37] Infants with moderate to severe CLD are often difficult to wean from mechanical ventilation.

Inflammation is believed to be an important component in the pathogenesis of CLD. This led to treatment with systemic corticosteroids, primarily dexamethasone, which yielded several short-term benefits. However recent data indicate that the adverse effects of systemic corticosteroids outweigh the short-term benefits. These adverse effects include cerebral palsy, poor weight gain and brain growth, gastrointestinal bleeding and perforation, and hypertrophic obstructive cardiomyopathy. In view of these data, the American Academy of Pediatrics strongly discourages the routine use of systemic corticosteroids.[38] Inhaled corticosteroids, however, have been used and proven to reduce inflammation without the adverse effects of systemic administration.

It is believed that premature infants have enough bronchial smooth muscle to constrict, so it would appear logical to provide β-agonist therapy; however, this remains controversial. Use has not been proven to reduce F_{IO_2} requirements, number of days with mechanical ventilation, or mortality, and may actually cause $\dot{V}/\dot{Q}$ mismatch in some infants.[39] Administration may only be effective against acute bronchospasm, and routine use for prevention of CLD is not advised.

Multiple efforts should be made to prevent further illness. Doses of palivizumab given monthly between November and March have been shown to reduce hospital admissions for respiratory syncytial virus (RSV) and also to reduce hospital stays.[40] In the early fall, the influenza vaccine is given to those infants who are 6 months of age and older; siblings, parents, and caregivers are highly encouraged to also be vaccinated. Environmental control is essential in minimizing the risk of illness. Parents are advised to avoid day-care settings, large crowds, and people with respiratory infections; schedule elective medical procedures outside the viral season; eliminate exposure to tobacco smoke, dander-producing pets, and kerosene- or wood-burning stoves; wash hands frequently; and use liquid hand sanitizer prior to touching the infant.

CLD is a disease that must be outgrown, with clinical recovery and lung repair dependent on growth. Airways become larger and alveolarization continues up to 5 years of age. For this reason, optimal nutrition is essential. Unfortunately, the infant with CLD often experiences gastroesophageal reflux and oral aversion that leads to feeding intolerance. Hypoxemia, infections, and fluid or caloric restriction can also lead to growth failure, necessitating complex therapy in the home for several months or years. In addition to feeding supplies, respiratory equipment required by this technology-dependent child may include a home oxygen system, mechanical ventilator and humidifier, pulse oximeter, end-tidal CO_2 monitor, apnea monitor, and airway clearance devices. Parents and caregivers often require extensive education on how to care for their child and ongoing psychosocial support to help deal with the transition to home.

Complications and Outcome

The majority of infants with CLD will survive; however, they are at considerable risk for numerous pulmonary, cardiac, and neurologic impairments. Nearly 50% of these infants continue to wheeze or have asthma, and lung function tests are consistently abnormal in school-aged children with a history of CLD.[41] Most infants can be weaned off oxygen by age 2 years, but hospitalization rates remain high, with up to 50% of infants with CLD requiring readmission in the first year of life. Recurrent episodes of hypoxemia place these infants at risk of persistent RVH or pulmonary hypertension that may progress to heart failure if left untreated. Infants with CLD are at greater risk of cerebral palsy and have greater impairment of fine and gross motor skills, language, and academic delay. Growth failure is common and is likely due to frequent respiratory exacerbations, an elevated resting metabolic rate, feeding problems, fluid restriction, chronic oxygen desaturation during sleep, and aggressive weaning from oxygen.[41]

Adolescents and adults with a history of CLD are often smaller, but their growth is usually still within normal range. Lung function continues to be compromised and includes diminished airflow, obstructive lung disease, and reactive airways. Cough and wheeze are more common, and there is an increased risk of hospitalization for respiratory illness.[42,43]

Transient Tachypnea of the Newborn

In 1966, Mary Ellen Avery and her associates were the first to use the term **transient tachypnea of the newborn (TTN)** to describe those infants who shortly after birth present with rapid respirations that usually resolve within 24 to 48 hours.[44] Also known as transient RDS, type II RDS, wet lungs, and retained fetal lung liquid syndrome, TTN is a self-limiting disorder that most often affects term or near-term infants. TTN is considered the most common cause of neonatal respiratory distress, affecting approximately 11 in every 1000 births.[45]

Pathophysiology and Etiology

At term gestation, the fetal lung is filled with approximately 20 mL/kg fluid. This fluid is equivalent to the FRC of the newborn lung and is what distends the airways and alveoli. Rapid removal of this fluid is vital for a smooth transition from placental to pulmonary gas exchange.[46]

Production of lung fluid begins to decrease 2 to 3 days prior to labor. During labor, fluid is reduced through lymphatic drainage and pulmonary epithelial cell adsorption. Fluid is also removed with the thoracic squeeze that occurs during labor contractions. Fetal lung fluid is usually completely cleared within 24 hours after birth. When absorption of the fluid is delayed and fluid accumulates in fetal lung tissue, the resulting bronchiolar collapse causes air trapping and decreased lung compliance, resulting in TTN.[47]

TTN is particularly common in infants of mothers with a history of failure to progress in labor resulting in cesarean delivery. Other risk factors include male sex, maternal diabetes, maternal sedation, perinatal asphyxia, and macrosomia.[48] Maternal asthma also appears to increase the risk of TTN.[49]

Clinical Manifestations

Immediately after or within 2 hours of birth, the infant with TTN presents with respiratory rates of 60 to 100 breaths/min. Along with tachypnea, the clinical presentation can include grunting, intercostal retractions, cyanosis, and nasal flaring, with symptoms lasting for a few hours to days. Air trapping and hyperinflation may result in a barrel-shaped chest with the liver and spleen more palpable. Breath sounds are usually clear, and blood gas analysis may reveal a respiratory acidosis with mild to moderate hypoxemia.

> **RESPIRATORY RECAP**
>
> **Transient Tachypnea of the Newborn**
>
> » A self-limiting disorder of term and near-term infants
>
> » Respiratory rates of 60 to 100 common
>
> » Treatment: oxygen therapy

Diagnosis

The diagnosis is based on history, clinical and radiologic findings, and laboratory data. Because of the tachypnea, blood gas CO_2 levels are usually normal; however, if they begin to rise, the infant should be monitored closely for respiratory fatigue and failure. Should the infant's respiratory status worsen, blood gas analysis and chest radiographs are repeated to rule out complications or another diagnosis.

Chest radiography is the standard for diagnosis of TTN. It often reveals fluid in the interlobar fissures and perihilar streaking with alveolar edema presenting as fluffy, parenchymal infiltrates. There are no areas of consolidation, and the lungs may be hyperinflated, with

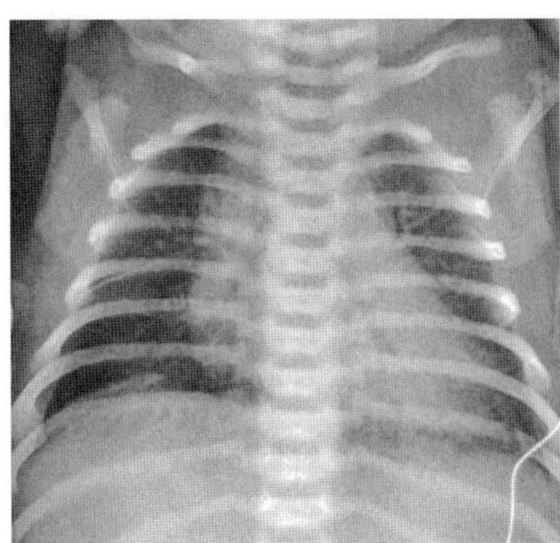

FIGURE 48–3 Transient tachypnea of the newborn is shown in this radiograph by flattened diaphragms, mild cardiomegaly, bulging intercostal spaces, and streaky perihilar markings.

widening of intercostal spaces and flattened diaphragms. Within 72 hours the findings are usually unremarkable except for perihilar markings, which may remain for up to 7 days (**Figure 48–3**).[50]

Other diagnoses to consider include RDS, meconium aspiration syndrome, pneumonia, PPHN, pneumothorax, pneumomediastinum, birth asphyxia, and congenital heart disease. Because it is often a diagnosis of exclusion, some infants may not be given a definitive diagnosis of TTN until the tachypnea has resolved.

Management

Because TTN is self-limited, treatment is directed at maintaining oxygenation and ventilation. Oxygen by hood at F_{IO_2} levels less than 0.50 is usually sufficient; however, CPAP may be indicated if the oxygen requirement increases. Although rare, a worsening clinical picture may require intubation and mechanical ventilation and be cause for concern that TTN is not the diagnosis. Ventilator settings at a rate of 20 with a tidal volume of 3 to 5 mL/kg and PEEP of 3 to 5 cm H_2O are usually adequate. Continuous monitoring of the oxygen saturation, respiratory rate, and heart rate is essential. Because it is initially difficult to rule out pneumonia, empiric antibiotics are given for the first 24 to 48 hours until blood cultures are negative. Until the respiratory rate improves enough to allow oral feeds, the infant is supported by intravenous fluids or gavage feedings. Supportive care also includes maintaining a neutral thermal environment with minimal stimulation. Although not common practice, corticosteroids may be given to the mother 48 hours before an elective cesarean section when the gestational age is greater than 36 weeks.

Complications and Outcome

Tachypnea due to TTN usually resolves within 72 hours of birth. Although air leaks may occur, few potential complications exist, and the prognosis is good.[51] There are reports that TTN has been associated with the later development of childhood asthma, especially among male infants.[52]

Pneumonia in the Neonate

The neonate is highly susceptible to infection, and when compared with the term infant has at least a 10-fold increase in the incidence of pneumonia. The World Health Organization estimates that 25% of neonatal deaths globally are caused by severe infections, with about one-third due to pneumonia.[53] Pneumonia in neonates is classified according to age at onset. Early-onset pneumonia presents at or within hours of birth through day 6 of life, while late-onset pneumonia occurs after 7 days of age.

Pathophysiology and Etiology

Pneumonia can occur at any gestational age and does not have an increased risk associated with sex, race, or ethnic group; however, premature infants are affected more often than term newborns. Immature mucociliary clearance, small conducting airways, and compromised host defense mechanisms render the fetus and neonate especially susceptible to infection. The pathologic findings in neonatal pneumonia are caused by invading microorganisms or foreign material that obstructs airways and increases airway resistance, mucus secretion, and inflammatory cells. In addition there is cell necrosis, damaged alveolar capillary epithelium, and disrupted alveolar capillary membrane permeability. The result is loss of surfactant activity, air trapping, atelectasis, consolidation, decreased lung compliance, and intrapulmonary shunting.

Neonatal pneumonia is divided into three categories: congenital, intrapartum, and postnatal. Congenital pneumonia is transplacentally acquired and is established before birth. The infant presents at birth or shortly after with clinical signs of pneumonia. In congenital pneumonia, infection from the mother is transmitted to the fetus in utero. This occurs when infection crosses the placenta or with intrauterine aspiration of amniotic fluid. Intrapartum pneumonia is acquired when the infant passes through the birth canal and aspirates infected maternal fluids, contaminated meconium, or blood. Symptoms usually occur a few hours after birth. Postnatal pneumonia originates after delivery. Infection is often acquired through invasive therapies, such as intravenous catheter insertion and intubation, or by aspiration of enteral feeds. Infection may also be transmitted through bacteria on the hands of hospital staff or parents.

Bacterial organisms are the most likely cause of neonatal pneumonia, with group B β-hemolytic *Streptococcus* (GBS) the cause of about 25% of cases of neonatal pneumonia, especially in the premature infant. GBS can also cause meningitis and sepsis. Also common among very low birth weight infants is infection with

Escherichia coli. Other bacterial pathogens responsible for pneumonia include *Listeria monocytogenes*, *Streptococcus pneumoniae*, *Haemophilus influenzae*, *Klebsiella*, and *Staphylococcus aureus*. Common viral causes include herpes simplex virus, enterovirus, and adenovirus. Congenital infection with cytomegalovirus and *Toxoplasma gondii* often presents within 24 hours of birth, whereas *Chlamydia* infection tends to develop several weeks later.

Clinical Manifestations

Fetal distress and tachycardia may present prior to delivery. Infected infants may present with respiratory distress immediately after birth, or symptoms may develop several hours later, usually within 8 to 10 hours. The initial signs of distress are similar to other respiratory disorders and include persistent tachycardia (respiratory rates greater than 60 breaths/min), grunting, use of accessory muscles, nasal flaring, and marked retractions. Airway secretions may be increased, and the skin and nails may be discolored or stained with meconium or blood. Other physical findings include abdominal distention, jaundice, cyanosis, and poor perfusion with low blood pressure. Early signs of infection can also include hypoglycemia or hyperglycemia, fever or hypothermia, poor feeding, irritability, lethargy, and seizures.

RESPIRATORY RECAP

Pneumonia

- Can occur at any gestational age
- Congenital, intrapartum, and postnatal forms
- Treatment is aimed at eradicating the infection and providing supportive care

Diagnosis

Box 48–5 lists radiographic findings associated with neonatal pneumonia. A chest radiograph with bilateral patchy alveolar densities is a common finding. Diffuse infiltrates resembling the ground glass pattern of RDS may be present, making it difficult to determine in the premature infant whether the findings are RDS or pneumonia. It may also be difficult to differentiate between pneumonia and meconium aspiration syndrome in term infants (**Figure 48–4**).[54]

Maternal history, chest radiographs, and clinical presentation can assist in the differential diagnosis of neonatal pneumonia (**Box 48–6**). Definitive diagnosis, however, is made with cultures identifying the infecting organism. Cultures of blood, urine, endotracheal and gastric aspirates, and cerebrospinal fluid should be performed when pneumonia is suspected. Results of cultures will facilitate the diagnosis of pneumonia and provide information necessary to determine what antibiotic should be used.

Management

Treatment of neonatal pneumonia is aimed at eradicating the infection and providing respiratory support to maintain adequate oxygenation and ventilation. Antibiotic or antiviral therapy is essential. Delays in treatment for infections, especially those caused by GBS, have potentially devastating consequences. Therefore, antibiotics are given to neonates with a clinical presentation or risk factors for pneumonia even though diagnosis is not

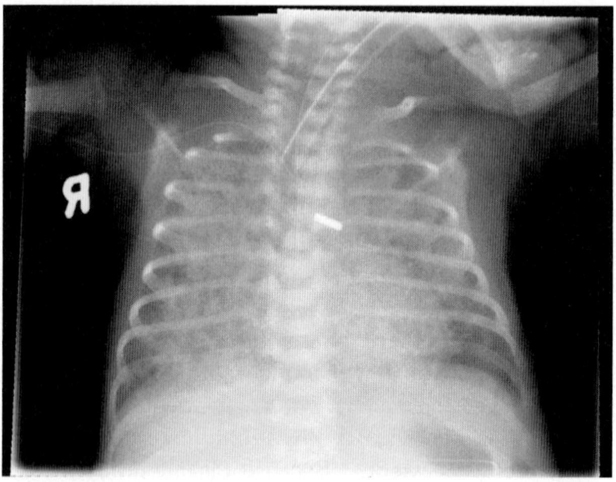

FIGURE 48–4 *Klebsiella* pneumonia in a neonate shows coarse and patchy opacity of the lung field and what appears to be some free air at the bases.

BOX 48–5

Radiographic Findings Associated with Neonatal Pneumonia

Cardiomegaly
Pneumatoceles
Pleural effusion
Air bronchograms
Pneumomediastinum
Thickened minor fissure
Bilateral patchy densities
Pulmonary interstitial emphysema
Diffuse granular pattern (ground glass)

BOX 48–6

Differential Diagnosis in Neonatal Pneumonia

Air leak syndrome
Respiratory distress syndrome
Meconium aspiration syndrome
Transient tachypnea of the newborn

BOX 48–7

Maternal Risk Factors for Group B *Streptococcus* Pneumonia

- Amniocentesis
- Premature labor
- Intrapartum fever
- Pelvic examinations
- Birth canal colonization
- Intrauterine catheter placement
- Premature rupture of membranes (longer than 18 hours before delivery)

confirmed. Ampicillin and gentamicin are recommended for initial empiric antibiotic therapy. Other agents may be used once the causative organism is identified.[55] Oxygen therapy is provided using an oxygen hood, nasal cannula, or CPAP. If oxygen requirements increase or respiratory failure is imminent, then endotracheal intubation and mechanical ventilation are indicated. Oxygenation and ventilation may be so compromised that the infant may require extracorporeal membrane oxygenation (ECMO). Screening for GBS and intrapartum antibiotic therapy are recommended in mothers with risk factors for early-onset GBS pneumonia. **Box 48–7** lists maternal risk factors for GBS infection.

Complications and Outcome

The clinical course of neonatal pneumonia depends strongly on the causative organism. Circulatory collapse, respiratory failure, and death within 24 hours of birth are most often associated with GBS and *Listeria monocytogenes*. Complications include pleural effusion, air leaks, septic shock, PPHN, hypoperfusion, BPD, and long-term ventilator dependency.

Meconium Aspiration Syndrome

Meconium is a viscous, dark green-black substance that constitutes the first intestinal discharge from a newborn infant. Passage usually occurs within 48 hours after birth but can also occur in utero, especially in term or post-term infants. Mixed with amniotic fluid, it is a sterile mixture of water, mucus, ingested lanugo hair, bile, and digestive enzymes, all toxic to the infant's lungs. Meconium passage in utero is associated with hypoxia, fetal distress, abnormal fetal heart tracings, fetal acidosis, and low Apgar scores.[56]

Meconium aspiration syndrome (MAS) occurs when the infant aspirates stained amniotic fluid prior to, during, or immediately after birth. Approximately 5% of infants born through meconium-stained fluid will develop MAS, with 30% to 50% of the affected infants requiring intubation and mechanical ventilation. The incidence of MAS may be decreasing and is thought to be due to changes in obstetric practice that have resulted in a reduction in postterm deliveries.[57,58]

BOX 48–8

Perinatal Risk Factors Associated with Meconium Aspiration Syndrome

- Preeclampsia
- Fetal distress
- Fetal hypoxia
- Oligohydramnios
- Chorioamnionitis
- Maternal diabetes
- Postterm delivery
- Maternal tobacco use
- Placental insufficiency
- Maternal hypertension
- Gestational age greater than 40 weeks
- Abnormal fetal heart tracings
- Meconium-stained amniotic fluid
- Maternal drug abuse, especially cocaine
- Meconium remaining in the airway prior to the first breath
- Positive pressure ventilation before clearing the airway of meconium

Pathophysiology and Etiology

Although meconium is sterile, within hours of aspiration it induces an inflammatory response that causes alveolar and parenchymal edema and a chemical pneumonitis. Protein leakage into alveoli inactivates surfactant and results in atelectasis and decreased lung compliance. The effect on surfactant is dose dependent: the more meconium present, the worse the effect. Aspiration of meconium may cause complete airway obstruction with regional atelectasis and $\dot{V}/\dot{Q}$ mismatch. Occurring more often is partial airway obstruction, in which the airways expand with air during inspiration but then collapse around meconium during expiration, trapping the air. This is commonly referred to as a ball-valve effect. The trapped air causes hyperinflation and may result in a pneumothorax, pneumomediastinum, or pneumopericardium. Pulmonary air leaks often develop during resuscitation of the infant with MAS. The lungs respond to the hypoxemia with thickening of the pulmonary vessels and pulmonary vasoconstriction, both of which may contribute to the PPHN that is often associated with MAS.[59] **Box 48–8** lists perinatal risk factors associated with MAS. Postterm delivery seems to be the greatest risk factor.

Clinical Manifestations

The infant with MAS is usually born at term or postterm and has a history of delivery through meconium-stained amniotic fluid. The fingernails, skin, and umbilical cord may have yellow-green staining. The postmature infant will have long fingernails and peeling skin with a wrinkled appearance. Meconium staining may be visible in the oropharynx, larynx, and trachea. Meconium pigment can be absorbed by the lung and excreted in urine, making the urine green. Some infants will have only mild symptoms, which may represent a smaller amount of aspirated meconium. Other infants will present with marked distress, including high oxygen requirements and respiratory failure requiring intubation and mechanical ventilation. The more pronounced symptoms may be due to a thicker or larger amount aspirated into the lungs. Symptoms include severe respiratory distress with tachypnea, grunting, nasal flaring, retractions, and cyanosis. With marked hyperinflation the infant may present with a barrel chest. Onset of respiratory distress may occur immediately after birth or several hours later. Breath sounds may be diminished, with rales and sometimes rhonchi. Results of arterial blood gas analysis will indicate hypoxemia and metabolic acidosis. Depending on the degree of distress, analysis may reveal hypercapnia and a mixed respiratory and metabolic acidosis. Mild symptoms will result in normal $Paco_2$ levels or hypocarbia if tachypnea is present.

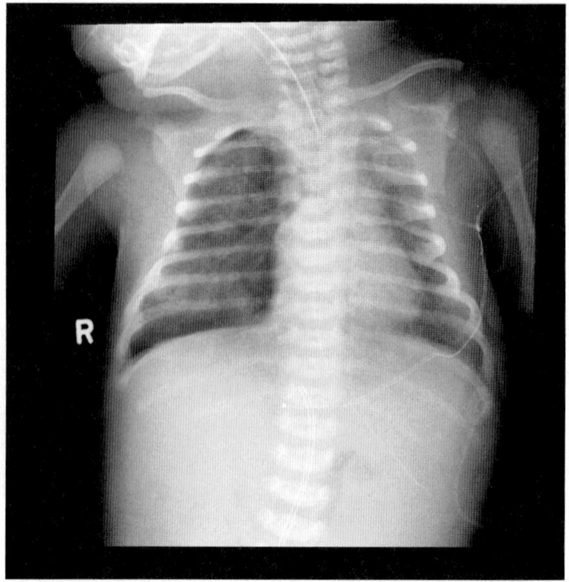

FIGURE 48–5 Chest radiograph of meconium aspiration syndrome with lung hyperexpansion, patches of atelectasis, and infiltrates that are more severe on the right.

Diagnosis

Chest radiographs vary depending on the degree of disease, with the severity of findings not predictive of the severity of illness. A contradictory combination of areas of hyperexpansion with areas of collapse is typical of MAS. Patchy and linear fluffy infiltrates are common, with diffuse, white areas indicative of atelectasis. Radiographs typically progress from atelectasis to widespread patchy opacification, hyperinflation, and atelectasis (**Figure 48–5** and **Figure 48–6**).

A diagnosis of MAS is suspected when an infant presents with respiratory distress after delivery through meconium-stained amniotic fluid. Diagnosis is confirmed by a chest radiograph with hyperinflation, variable areas of atelectasis, and flattened diaphragms.

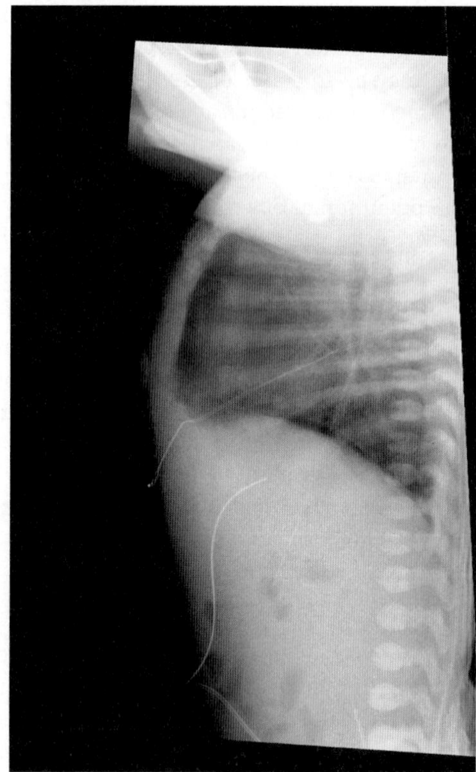

FIGURE 48–6 Lateral chest radiograph of an infant with meconium aspiration syndrome and lung hyperinflation.

Management

Since the 1970s, standard practice to prevent MAS in infants delivered through meconium-stained amniotic fluid has been to provide oropharyngeal and nasopharyngeal suctioning before the infant's shoulders are delivered. Unfortunately, intrapartum suctioning may cause vagal stimulation, postnatal fetal depression, and bradycardia. The efficacy of this procedure was debated after evidence suggested that meconium is aspirated in utero and not at the time of delivery.[60,61] Routine suctioning before delivery of the shoulders is no longer advised, and delivery is not delayed. Instead, the infant is evaluated immediately following delivery. If meconium is present and the infant has bradycardia with depressed respirations and muscle tone, then the trachea should be intubated and meconium suctioned from beneath the glottis. If the infant has a heart rate greater than 100 beats per minute, a strong respiratory rate, and good muscle tone, then selective intubation and tracheal suctioning is contraindicated.[62]

Oxygen administration is critical to the infant with MAS and should be provided at the first sign of respiratory distress. Once the diagnosis of MAS is established, the infant is maintained at a preductal Spo_2 greater than 95%. In some infants oxygen is the only therapy required. Nasal CPAP is considered if oxygen requirements exceed an Fio_2 of 0.4 to 0.5, while CO_2 levels remain stable. The infant in marked respiratory distress will require intubation and mechanical ventilation, often needing high Fio_2 and high pressures to maintain adequate gas exchange. With chronic hypoxia, pulmonary vasoconstriction and increased pulmonary resistance often lead to the development of PPHN. PPHN is confirmed with echocardiography and treated with oxygen, nitric oxide, and continued mechanical ventilation.

Inhaled nitric oxide is approved for use as a pulmonary vasodilator. High-frequency ventilation is used if conventional ventilation fails to meet the infant's respiratory requirements or if air leaks occur. When all other therapies have been exhausted, then ECMO is considered. The infant with MAS is easily agitated, which causes right-to-left shunting, hypoxia, and acidosis. Supportive care includes maintaining an optimal thermal environment with minimal stimulation.

RESPIRATORY RECAP

Meconium Aspiration Syndrome

- » Occurs when the infant aspirates stained amniotic fluid
- » Usually occurs in infants born at term or post-term
- » Treatment includes suctioning, oxygen therapy, mechanical ventilation, inhaled nitric oxide, extracorporeal membrane oxygenation, and surfactant replacement

Using the rationale that aspiration of meconium in the lungs causes surfactant to be altered or inactivated, surfactant replacement therapy has been used in infants with respiratory failure due to MAS. Studies suggest that surfactant administration may reduce the severity of the disease and the progression of respiratory failure to ECMO, but may also carry substantial risk.[63] Bolus therapy is analogous to surfactant replacement in infants with RDS. Surfactant is administered through an endotracheal tube using a 6-hour dosing interval, with infants receiving up to four doses. Airway lavage consists of instilling a small volume of dilute surfactant into the infant's airway and then suctioning the airway. This removes meconium debris but leaves behind surfactant.[64] Further studies are needed to determine the optimal surfactant concentration, dose, interval, frequency, and ventilator support as well as the efficacy compared with or in conjunction with other therapies, including inhaled nitric oxide and high-frequency ventilation.[63]

Complications and Outcomes

The clinical course of MAS is quite variable, with mild cases resolving within 2 to 4 days. However, infants with severe aspiration requiring mechanical ventilation, nitric oxide therapy, or ECMO have a more guarded recovery. Air leak syndromes further complicate the clinical course and often result in less favorable outcomes. Infants may have an increased incidence of infections during the first year of life. Unfortunately, those who have required more intensive therapy are at risk of developing BPD.[65] Infants who have developed severe parenchymal disease and PPHN have a mortality rate as high as 20%. Mortality risk factors include first-born infants, shock, air leaks, PPHN, renal failure, and resuscitation outside the hospital.[66]

Infants who had prenatal or postnatal hypoxia and acidosis are at increased risk of long-term neurologic deficits that include seizures, cerebral palsy, central nervous system damage, and mental retardation.[67] In spite of advances in treatment and early diagnosis, term infants with MAS continue to represent a high-risk population with significant morbidity.[67,68]

Persistent Pulmonary Hypertension of the Newborn

For postnatal survival, a dramatic cardiopulmonary transition must occur. Within minutes after birth, the lungs must fill with air and the pulmonary vasculature resistance (PVR) must fall. When this decrease in vascular tone does not occur, pulmonary blood flow is shunted to the systemic circulation. The resulting arterial hypoxemia, cyanosis, and severe respiratory distress are referred to as **persistent pulmonary hypertension of the newborn (PPHN)**. This syndrome has also been described as pulmonary vasospasm, neonatal pulmonary hypertension, persistent transitional circulation, and persistent fetal circulation. Recent estimates are that severe PPHN occurs in 2 per 1000 live births, with mortality at 20%. Although it may present without underlying pulmonary disease, it most often complicates the clinical course of infants with neonatal cardiorespiratory disorders, with approximately half of those having MAS.[69]

Pathophysiology

Prior to birth, pulmonary hypertension is a natural state, with the placenta serving as the gas exchange organ. Pulmonary vessels are constricted and pulmonary vascular resistance is high. This causes blood to be shunted through the foramen ovale and ductus arteriosus with only a small percentage of right ventricle blood flowing to the pulmonary circulation. When the umbilical cord is cut, the function of gas exchange is transferred from the placenta to the lungs and from fetal to neonatal circulation. Loss of the placenta elevates systemic vascular resistance and increases left atrium and ventricle pressures, leading to functional closure of the foramen ovale.

As the lungs expand with the first breath, mechanically compressed pulmonary vessels are physically pulled open, carbon dioxide tension drops, and oxygen tension increases, constricting the ductus arteriosus and ultimately dilating pulmonary vessels and reducing PVR. The greatest decline in resistance occurs within 24 hours of birth and continues for the next 2 weeks. The elevated systemic vascular resistance now directs blood to the low-resistance pulmonary circulation, leading to an 8- to 10-fold increase in pulmonary blood flow. Transition from fetal circulation has occurred.[70]

RESPIRATORY RECAP

Persistent Pulmonary Hypertension of the Newborn

- » Occurs when fetal circulation persists after birth
- » Echocardiography used to make the diagnosis
- » Treatment includes oxygen, mechanical ventilation, inhaled nitric oxide, extracorporeal membrane oxygenation, and supportive therapy

In PPHN the PVR remains elevated after birth and is equal to or greater than systemic vascular resistance. Fetal circulation persists, with blood continuing to flow through the foramen ovale and PDA. A right-to-left shunt develops, causing pulmonary perfusion to be inadequate. Arterial oxygen tension drops and the infant experiences significant and possibly refractory hypoxemia, cyanosis, and respiratory distress. When the heart must work harder to pump blood through this highly resistant vascular bed, the risk of right heart dilatation and failure is high.[71]

Etiology

Although the specific abnormality is unknown, there are three underlying etiologies most often associated with PPHN. The most common etiology is hypoxia associated with parenchymal lung disease (e.g., RDS, MAS, pneumonia). The second cause, often referred to as idiopathic PPHN, is associated with infants who have no evidence of lung disease and is most likely due to a structurally abnormal pulmonary vascular bed occurring secondary to chronic fetal stress. Intrauterine closure of the ductus arteriosus is also a form of idiopathic PPHN. Repeated closure may occur during the third trimester if the mother ingests nonsteroidal anti-inflammatory drugs (NSAIDs), such as ibuprofen and naproxen, or high doses of the prostaglandin inhibitor aspirin. After determining that selective serotonin reuptake inhibitor (SSRI) antidepressants also have this effect, the Food and Drug Administration (FDA) ordered that a warning be placed on SSRI labels stating that ingestion after the 20th week of pregnancy could increase the chance of PPHN. The third abnormality is underdeveloped pulmonary vasculature, as seen in pulmonary hypoplasia, congenital diaphragmatic hernia, and oligohydramnios syndrome.[72,73] **Box 48–9** lists both prenatal and antenatal conditions that may predispose an infant to PPHN.

BOX 48–9

Conditions That Predispose an Infant to Persistent Pulmonary Hypertension of the Newborn

Prenatal Conditions

Fetal hypoxia
Maternal asthma
Maternal obesity
Maternal diabetes
Poor prenatal care
Cesarean delivery
Maternal use of SSRI
Maternal use of NSAID
Abnormal fetal heart rate
Term or near-term gestation
Maternal tobacco smoke exposure
Maternal use of prostaglandin inhibitors

Antenatal Conditions

Sepsis
Pneumonia
Hypothermia
Polycythemia
Pneumothorax
Hypoglycemia
Birth asphyxia
Myocardial failure
Low Apgar score
Pulmonary hypoplasia
Large for gestational age
Respiratory distress at birth
Meconium aspiration syndrome
Transient tachypnea of the newborn

SSRI, selective serotonin reuptake inhibitor; NSAID, nonsteroidal anti-inflammatory drug.

Clinical Manifestations

Although PPHN may affect premature infants, it is most noted in term or postterm infants within 12 hours of birth. Early signs include cyanosis, tachypnea, and respiratory distress. The infant may have a gradual onset of distress with grunting, nasal flaring, tachycardia, and retractions that progressively worsen within 12 to 24 hours following birth. However, depending on the etiology, the infant may present at birth in severe distress with low Apgar scores, poor perfusion, and shock. Work of breathing may not be severe unless there is coincidental parenchymal lung disease. Typically, cyanosis and hypoxemia respond poorly to supplemental oxygen. The infant often experiences oxygen desaturation with any form of stimulation, such as feeds, diaper changes, noise, and suctioning. The worst cases require intubation and mechanical ventilation shortly after birth.[74]

Diagnosis

Diagnosis of PPHN is usually based on the clinical features. It should be suspected in the term infant who is in respiratory distress with cyanosis and who has a history that includes risk factors of PPHN. There should be an even higher index of suspicion when an infant presents with hypoxemia that is refractory to oxygen therapy and lung recruitment strategies, especially if there is a history of fetal hypoxia, birth asphyxia, or delivery through meconium-stained amniotic fluid.

The chest radiograph of an infant with idiopathic PPHN is typically clear with decreased vascular markings and a slightly enlarged heart. When PPHN is a result of an underlying lung disease, the radiograph will demonstrate abnormalities typical of that disorder. Scattered pulmonary parenchymal densities may be mild compared with the level of hypoxia.

Because the clinical presentation of PPHN mimics that of congenital heart defects, two-dimensional echocardiography is essential for diagnosing PPHN and excluding cyanotic heart disease. Findings characteristic of PPHN include right-to-left shunting across the foramen ovale or ductus arteriosus or both, right-to-left atrial septum deviation, right atrial enlargement, and tricuspid regurgitation. Diagnosis is confirmed by demonstrating right-to-left shunting at the ductal or atrial level and absence of a structural heart defect. The echocardiogram is also useful in assessing myocardial function, the severity of PPHN, and response to treatment. In the past, cardiac catheterization was used to monitor pulmonary artery pressures to diagnose PPHN; however, that is no longer needed and is not recommended.

Diagnosis may also be established by comparing preductal and postductal oxygen saturation values. By placing a pulse oximeter probe on a preductal extremity (right hand) and a second probe on a postductal extremity (right or left foot), the oxygen saturation values can be obtained simultaneously. The left hand should not be used as a site because it may be preductal or postductal. A preductal saturation value that is higher than the postductal saturation occurs when deoxygenated blood flows from the pulmonary circulation into the descending aorta by way of a PDA. Because the majority of right-to-left shunting in PPHN occurs through the ductus arteriosus, postductal oxygen saturations are lower than preductal values. Preductal oxygen saturation values higher than postductal values indicate a right-to-left shunt. If there is little to no difference when the values are compared, then ductal shunting is not present. When using Pa_{O_2} values for comparison, blood is drawn from an upper extremity artery (preductal) and compared with that from the umbilical artery catheter. A difference greater than 15 mm Hg indicates ductal shunting. Oxygen values obtained through transcutaneous monitoring may also be compared by placing a probe on the infant's right upper chest (preductal) and a lower extremity (postductal). The hyperoxia test may be considered to diagnose PPHN if two-dimensional echocardiography is not available, but it cannot be definitive because some congenital heart defects will produce results similar to PPHN.

Management

Treatment of PPHN is aimed at maintaining adequate oxygenation, lowering PVR, reversing right-to-left shunting, improving systemic blood pressure, correcting acidosis and hypercarbia, and minimizing complications. Continuous monitoring of blood pressure, oxygenation, and perfusion is essential.

To minimize hypoxia-induced pulmonary vascular constriction, treatment should always begin with administration of 100% oxygen and adjustments made to maintain adequate oxygenation.[75] Improvement in alveolar oxygenation reduces pulmonary vasoconstriction and improves pulmonary blood flow, factors that are especially important in infants with underlying parenchymal lung disease. Preductal and postductal oxygen saturation should be continuously monitored. It is important to know whether the ductus arteriosus has remained open because shunting blood through it allows the right ventricle to decompress. This reduces the work of the ventricle, ultimately preventing right heart failure. An indication that the ductus is constricted or closed is preductal desaturation in an otherwise stable infant. Confirmation by echocardiography would necessitate a trial of prostaglandin therapy to maintain a PDA. When hypoxia persists despite maximal administration of oxygen, then intubation with mechanical ventilation is indicated.

The goal of mechanical ventilation is to improve oxygenation using optimal lung volumes that minimize the risk of volutrauma lung injury. Lung recruitment strategies are dependent on the basis of underlying parenchymal lung disease. Treatment of idiopathic PPHN usually does not require pressures or volumes as high as those needed for ventilation of the infant with pneumonia or MAS. Infants with significant airspace disease or lung hypoplasia often require lung recruitment strategies attainable only through HFOV. Newborns with PPHN generally require sedation to achieve adequate mechanical ventilation. Although muscle paralysis can be used, adverse circulatory effects often occur, leading to overdistension of some areas of the lung and alveolar collapse in others.[76,77]

HFOV is used as rescue therapy for infants who are not improving or are showing signs of deterioration with conventional ventilation as well as infants who have developed air leaks. Response to HFOV depends on the underlying disease pathophysiology. HFOV has been shown in numerous studies to greatly improve the outcome in treatment of PPHN and to improve the response to inhaled nitric oxide in infants with severe lung disease.[78] The infant without significant lung disease may have a better response to inhaled nitric oxide when used with conventional mechanical ventilation than with HFOV.

Inhaled nitric oxide has proven to be a potent vasodilator with specific relaxation of pulmonary vasculature. In general the starting dose for treatment of PPHN is 20 ppm, which is then slowly lowered according to response and stability.[79] It is increasingly recognized that adequate lung inflation is needed to optimize delivery of nitric oxide within the lungs. Some infants with PPHN either do not respond to therapy or have only transient improvements in oxygenation. This tends to occur most often in infants with abnormalities of vascular development, especially those with congenital diaphragmatic hernia. Although inhaled nitric oxide has been shown to reduce the need for ECMO support, there is no proof that it reduces length of hospital stay, the risk of neurodevelopmental impairment, or mortality.[80,81] Approximately 30% of infants fail to respond to inhaled nitric oxide, and others experience rebound pulmonary hypertension when nitric oxide is discontinued.

Advances in the understanding of vasoactive mediators have led to the recent use of other pulmonary vasodilators. Sildenafil is a phosphodiesterase inhibitor that selectively reduces PVR. In 2005, the FDA approved the use of sildenafil in adults with pulmonary hypertension, which led to studies testing its effect in the treatment of PPHN. Studies have continued to demonstrate improved oxygenation and lower mortality with intravenous as well as oral sildenafil.[82,83]

ECMO support remains an effective rescue method and is considered in infants with PPHN who fail to maintain adequate oxygenation or systemic arterial pressure or who fail to wean from support with HFOV. By itself ECMO is purely supportive, allowing time for the lungs and pulmonary vasculature to recover. The usual criteria for ECMO use is a pH less than 7.15, oxygenation index (OI) greater than 40, and failure to respond to all available treatment. However, there are some cases in which it may be considered earlier.[84]

It is essential to maintain a neutral thermal environment to reduce oxygen consumption. Myocardial function is often poor, requiring volume replacement and inotropic agents to maintain systemic vascular resistance and improve cardiac output. Infants with PPHN are particularly vulnerable to medical procedures that involve handling and respond with a decrease in oxygenation. A minimum stimulation protocol dictates that infants be handled only when medically necessary. **Box 48–10** lists intervention strategies to facilitate minimal stimulation. Studies have proven that when a neonatal intensive care unit is altered for minimal light, noise, infant handling, and staff activity, there is a decrease in infant mean diastolic pressure and mean arterial pressure.[69,85]

BOX 48–10

Intervention Strategies for Minimal Stimulation

Place a sign at the bed announcing minimal stimulation.
Minimize frequency of baths.
Minimize positioning of the infant.
Suction only when absolutely necessary.
Decrease visual/auditory stimulation:

- Keep lights turned down low.
- Discourage loud talking at the bedside.
- Open incubator portholes quietly.
- Place phones away from beds.
- Place covers on incubators.
- Set equipment alarms at safest low level.
- Reduce fluid condensation in ventilator tubing.
- Carry out medical rounds away from bedside.
- Cluster activities.

Complications and Outcome

PPHN may last anywhere from 36 hours to several weeks after birth. There is no question that it contributes significantly to morbidity and mortality, regardless of the infant's gestational age. The use of inhaled nitric oxide and ECMO has led to a reduction in mortality rates, which were as much as 50% prior to the use of ECMO. Although ECMO support has improved overall survival to approximately 80%, the survival rate varies. Survival is highest in individuals with reversible parenchymal lung disease. Survival rates are as low as 50% in infants with congenital diaphragmatic hernia and as high as 90% in infants with MAS.[77,84]

In spite of advances in treatment and the remarkable decrease in mortality, survivors of PPHN remain at substantial risk for long-term disability. Complications are often a result of treatment; however, birth asphyxia and perinatal hypoxia are largely responsible for the neurodevelopmental impairments. Survivors of PPHN have an increased incidence of sensorineural hearing loss, motor disability, behavioral problems that include hyperactivity and conduct disorders, and reactive airway disease.

Congenital Diaphragmatic Hernia

Congenital diaphragmatic hernia (CDH) is an anomaly that occurs in about 1 in 2500 live births. It is a developmental abnormality in which the infant's diaphragm allows abdominal organs to protrude into the thoracic cavity during a period when bronchi and pulmonary arteries are undergoing branching. CDH is not just a hole in the diaphragm but a malformation with a complex pathophysiology that results in pulmonary hypoplasia and PPHN.

Pathophysiology and Etiology

Diaphragm development is still not completely understood but is believed to require the fusion of embryonic structures during the 8th to 10th weeks of gestation. Improper fusion prevents the diaphragm from completely closing and allows abdominal organs, most often the stomach and small intestine, to migrate into the chest cavity. Herniation of abdominal contents during gestation impedes normal development of the lung on the herniated side, resulting in hypoplasia. Although not as severe, hypoplasia can also occur on the unaffected side, possibly due to the mediastinal shift to that side. Pulmonary hypoplasia is characterized by a permanent reduction in the number of airways, fewer alveoli, and a small pulmonary artery and pulmonary vascular bed. Pulmonary hypoplasia causes inadequate gas exchange and contributes to the hypercarbia that is present. The reduced number of arterial branches in the pulmonary vascular bed, abnormal muscular hypertrophy, and thickening of the arterial walls increase vasoconstriction and PVR.[86] The size of the defect varies, ranging from very small to complete agenesis of the diaphragm.

> **RESPIRATORY RECAP**
>
> **Congenital Diaphragmatic Hernia**
>
> » Abnormality in which the infant's diaphragm allows the abdominal organs to protrude into the thorax
>
> » Treatment includes delivery room stabilization, mechanical ventilation, inhaled nitric oxide, extracorporeal membrane oxygenation, surgery, and supportive therapy

There are three basic types of hernias. The most common is the posterolateral Bochdalek hernia, representing approximately 90% of all hernias. These hernias are usually on the left side. It is thought that the left side is affected most because the liver may block herniation through the right side. With a left-sided hernia, there is herniation of the small and large intestine, stomach, and possibly liver into the thoracic cavity. The anterior Morgagni hernia represents only 5% to 10% of all cases, with 90% occurring on the right side. These infants are often asymptomatic. Usually only the liver and a portion of the bowel herniate on the right side. Bilateral hernia is rare and nearly always fatal. Hiatal hernia and diaphragmatic eventration are rare types of CDH.[87]

Clinical Manifestations

Within the first minutes or hours after birth, infants with CDH will typically develop severe respiratory distress and cyanosis that is unresponsive to supplemental oxygen. It is common for the infant to fail to respond to resuscitation immediately following delivery. The majority of infants who present with severe distress have left-sided hernias. Breath sounds are decreased or absent on the affected side, and chest movement is asymmetric secondary to the hypoplasia. Bowel sounds may be audible in the thorax on the affected side, and heart sounds are shifted to the unaffected side. As a result of abdominal organs in the chest cavity, the infant usually presents at birth with a scaphoid abdomen and possibly a barrel-shaped chest. The most severely affected infants will develop PPHN, and the hypoplastic lung places them at high risk of developing a pneumothorax on the unaffected side.

Diagnosis

Most cases of CDH are diagnosed prenatally on routine ultrasound scans or scans obtained following the discovery of polyhydramnios in the mother. Previously undiagnosed cases still occur, presenting at or very soon after birth depending on the severity of the hernia. By 15 weeks of gestation, prenatal diagnosis is possible using ultrasonography. CDH is confirmed when abdominal contents are visualized in the chest and there is a mediastinal shift away from the affected side. Defects on the right side are more difficult to diagnose and can be missed if the stomach is not in the thorax at the time of the scan. Gallbladder visualized in the chest is indicative of a right-sided hernia. However, the extent of pulmonary hypoplasia cannot be predicted with an ultrasound. A prenatal diagnosis is no indication for cesarean section delivery. Fetal hydrops may be noted as well as polyhydramnios, which tends to have a poorer prognosis. Low levels of maternal serum alpha fetoprotein have been associated with CDH and other defects. This is not considered a definitive test for CDH but calls for more investigation. Following delivery, diagnosis is confirmed by a chest radiograph that reveals air-filled loops of intestine in the thoracic cavity on the affected side with the mediastinum shifted to the unaffected side. The affected lung may be hypoinflated or hypoplastic (**Figure 48–7**, **Figure 48–8**, **Figure 48–9**, and **Figure 48–10**).

Management

Stabilization following delivery is critical. The infant is intubated immediately to avoid bag-mask ventilation and prevent stomach and bowel distention. Mechanical ventilation is implemented with an F_{IO_2} of 1.0, PEEP of 3 to 5 mm Hg, relatively high respiratory rates greater than 40 breaths per minute, and low peak inspiratory pressures not to exceed 25 mm Hg. An orogastric or nasogastric tube using low continuous suction is inserted

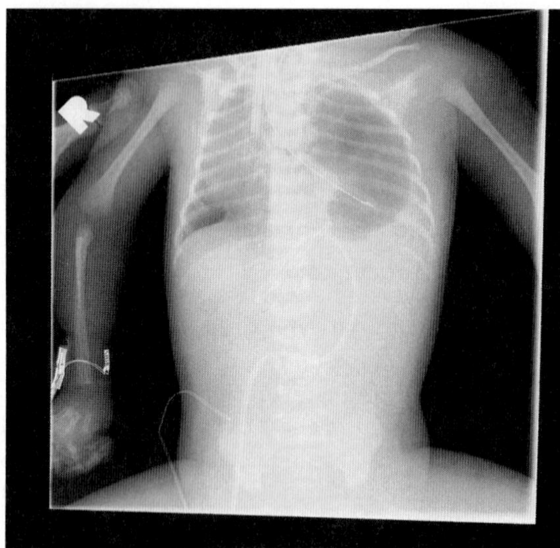

FIGURE 48–7 Chest radiograph of an infant with a left congenital diaphragmatic hernia showing herniation of bowel into the left hemithorax.

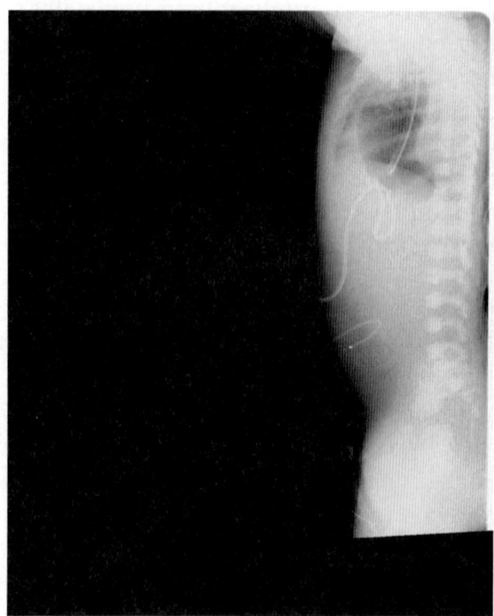

FIGURE 48–8 Lateral view of a left congenital diaphragmatic hernia.

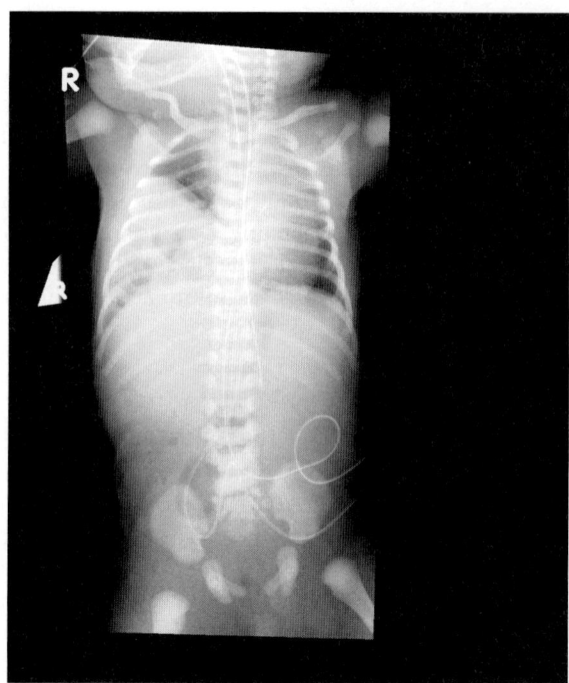

FIGURE 48–9 Chest radiograph of an infant with a right congenital diaphragmatic hernia. Gas-filled loops of bowel are in the right hemithorax, and there is a mediastinal shift to the left compressing the left lung.

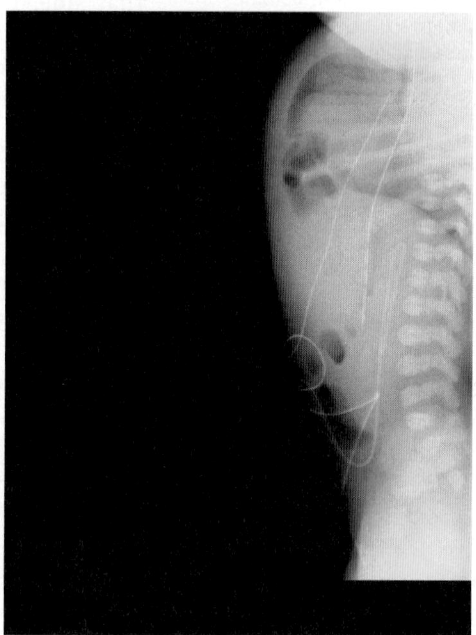

FIGURE 48–10 Lateral view of a right congenital diaphragmatic hernia showing bowel loops in the anterior mediastinum.

to decompress the stomach and avoid further lung compression.[88] Because air leak in either lung is highly possible, the infant is observed closely for signs of a pneumothorax, and a chest tube is immediately inserted if necessary. Care includes continuous monitoring of blood pressure and preductal and postductal oxygen saturation. It is important to monitor preductal oxygen because it reflects cerebral oxygenation. Successful delivery room resuscitation focuses on the avoidance of high airway pressures and an acceptable preductal saturation that is greater than 85%.

Although there is no single specific best strategy for mechanical ventilation of infants with CDH, mortality risk is reduced when ventilation is approached with the goals of lung protection, improved oxygenation, and decreased PVR. Gentle ventilation with strategies that avoid high peak pressures is recommended in an attempt to lower the risk of air leaks.[89,90] Although controversy still exists concerning the appropriate target for the $Paco_2$ level, more centers are using permissive hypercarbia to allow for ventilation at lower pressures and shorter inspiratory times.[91]

If a protocol tolerating hypercarbia is followed, the $Paco_2$ is maintained at 45 to 55 mm Hg and the pH at greater than 7.35, with bicarbonate administered if the pH drops below 7.35. HFOV is recommended when conventional ventilation is unable to prevent hypoxemia or hypercarbia. For many years treatment of CDH with HFOV was considered a rescue mode to be used only when hyperventilation with conventional ventilation had failed. Today institutions recommend HFOV as an early intervention strategy to avoid barotrauma when peak inspiratory pressures exceed 25 mm Hg with conventional ventilation.[92]

Nitric oxide has proven to be a powerful vasodilator and effective in reducing PVR and dilating the pulmonary vascular bed. Infants with CDH who present with PPHN, significant hypoxia, acidosis, and right ventricular failure may benefit from inhaled nitric oxide. Trials using inhaled nitric oxide in infants with PPHN have included infants with CDH; unfortunately, the latter was the group that responded least well, with no impact on survival or the use of ECMO.[93] Nitric oxide may be useful in providing short-term improvement in oxygenation to stabilize an infant during transport or as a bridge to ECMO.[88]

In spite of the use of nitric oxide, some infants with CDH will progress to refractory pulmonary hypertension. Using the same selection criteria as PPHN, ECMO should be considered when pH is less than 7.15, OI is greater than 40, preductal oxygen saturation is less than 85%, and all other support has been exhausted. The purpose of ECMO in the treatment of CDH is to serve as a lung-protective strategy during the preoperative period.[84,94]

Deferred surgery after stabilization with gentle ventilation and reversal of pulmonary hypertension remains the cornerstone of management. In the past, surgery was believed to be critical to reducing the hernia and allowing expansion of the unaffected lung. Understanding that CDH is not just a surgical disease and that the problems of pulmonary hypoplasia and PPHN are largely responsible for outcome has led to a delayed surgical approach. Removing abdominal contents from the chest cavity is no longer emergent; instead, time is allowed for respiratory and hemodynamic stabilization. Survival rates have been reported to be as high as 81% when the management of CDH includes delayed surgical repair, early postnatal HFOV, and selective referral for ECMO. Survival rates are favorable and respiratory morbidity just as low when treating isolated CDH with early HFOV and delayed surgery but excluding ECMO.[95,96]

It is critical that infants with CDH receive continuous monitoring. This includes preductal and postductal oxygen saturation monitoring with pulse oximetry and transcutaneous CO_2 monitoring to avoid hyperventilation. Arterial and central venous lines are placed for monitoring and fluid infusion. Umbilical arterial lines are placed for pressure monitoring and arterial blood gas analysis. Umbilical venous lines are needed for fluid resuscitation and fluid maintenance, although the umbilical venous line may be difficult to insert if there is liver herniation. In an effort to minimize the effects of PPHN, minimal-stimulation protocols should be in place and routine sedation and analgesia used.

BOX 48–11

Complications Associated with Congenital Diaphragmatic Hernia

- Scoliosis
- Hypotonia
- Hearing loss
- Oral aversion
- Failure to thrive
- Cortical atrophy
- Ventriculomegaly
- Chest asymmetry
- Chronic lung disease
- Patch-related infections
- Reactive airway disease
- Gastroesophageal reflux
- Small airway obstruction
- Limited pulmonary reserve
- Intraventricular hemorrhage
- Pectus, most often excavatum
- Learning and attention problems
- Recurrent pulmonary hypertension
- Lifelong limited exercise tolerance

Complications and Outcome

Infants with CDH are at considerable risk for long-term complications. The majority of these are due to pulmonary hypoplasia, respiratory failure, and PPHN and have very little to do with surgical repair of the defect. **Box 48–11** lists complications associated with CDH.[97,98]

Morbidity and mortality are largely dependent on three factors: the size of the defect and herniation, the degree of lung hypoplasia, and the severity of PPHN. Predictors of postnatal outcome prior to delivery are difficult, but extent of the herniation may be a reliable predictor. Simply stated, the more abdominal contents involved in the herniation, the poorer the prognosis. Occurrence of a left-sided CDH has a good prognosis if there is no herniation of the liver. Unfortunately, when liver herniation is present, survival rate is less than 50%. Nearly all infants with a right-sided defect will present with a portion of the liver in the chest cavity. Prognosis is worse if more than 50% of the liver is in the chest.[99,100]

Air Leak Syndrome

Pulmonary **air leak syndrome** comprises a group of clinically recognizable disorders that are characterized by the escape of air into tissue in which air is not normally present. These disorders include pulmonary interstitial emphysema, pneumothorax, pneumomediastinum, and pneumopericardium. Less common forms are subcutaneous emphysema and pneumoperitoneum. The incidence is greatest in premature infants who have existing lung disease. Term infants are also affected, especially those who had long periods of rupture of membranes prior to delivery or long durations of labor.[101] Although occurrence can be spontaneous, it is most often a complication of positive pressure mechanical ventilation. The decline in the incidence of air leak syndrome in newborns is believed to be due to surfactant replacement therapy and changes in ventilator management strategies. The use of shorter inspiratory times, lower peak inspiratory pressures, permissive hypercapnia, and the early introduction of CPAP are also believed to contribute to this decline.[91]

> **RESPIRATORY RECAP**
>
> **Air Leak Syndrome**
>
> » Includes pulmonary interstitial emphysema, pneumothorax, pneumomediastinum, and pneumopericardium
>
> » Transillumination used to make immediate diagnosis of pneumothorax

The common cause of the disorders comprising air leak syndrome is overdistention due to air trapping or uneven distribution of gas. As the volume in the lung exceeds its physiologic limit, tissue in the alveoli or terminal airspaces rupture and air leaks are created. The resulting disorders depend on where the free air is located. Clinical presentation is specific, and intervention varies for each condition. In every case definitive diagnosis is made with a chest radiograph.

Pneumothorax

Pneumothorax is the most common air leak and occurs most often in neonates. It refers to the presence of air in the pleural cavity between the visceral and parietal pleura. Air from ruptured alveoli moves toward the hilum, where blebs form and then dissect into the pleural space to develop a pneumothorax. With sufficient accumulation of air, a tension pneumothorax develops and the loss of intrapleural negative pressure causes lung collapse. Gas exchange is impaired as air accumulates and pressure increases, shifting mediastinal structures and compressing the uninvolved lung. Compression of the vena cava results in a decrease in venous return and consequently a decreased cardiac output that can emergently progress to hypotension, shock, and death. Risk factors for a pneumothorax include RDS, mechanical ventilation, MAS, pulmonary hypoplasia, and other air leak conditions. Although the majority of infants who develop a pneumothorax are receiving mechanical ventilation, healthy term infants can spontaneously develop a pneumothorax immediately after birth.

A pneumothorax should always be suspected if there is sudden deterioration in an infant's respiratory status, especially if the infant is receiving mechanical ventilation. Distress is often accompanied by nasal flaring, cyanosis, grunting, severe retractions, hypercarbia, and hypoxia. However, an infant may be asymptomatic or have only mild tachypnea, retractions, and grunting. Heart sounds are shifted and breath sounds are diminished on the affected side, although it may be difficult to appreciate breath sounds because they are so widely transmitted in the neonate's small thorax.[102]

In an emergent situation, transillumination of the chest is used for an immediate diagnosis. With lights lowered around the immediate area of the infant's bed, a fiberoptic light probe is held firmly against the infant's skin, about halfway down the chest and in line with the axilla. The side of the chest with the air leak transmits a bright light, whereas the lung is solid tissue and does not illuminate. Confirmation of a diagnosis of pneumothorax is provided with chest radiography, both anteroposterior (AP) and lateral views. Transillumination does not take the place of a chest radiograph. The affected lung will typically have increased lucency and decreased lung markings, with the free air appearing dark on the radiograph. As the leak increases, the affected lung is hyperinflated, with a flattened diaphragm and widened intercostal spaces (**Figure 48–11** and **Figure 48–12**).

A small pneumothorax usually resolves spontaneously without need for intervention. In an effort to resolve it more quickly, oxygen at an F_{IO_2} of 1.0 may be administered through a hood to a term infant with mild symptoms. This treatment should be carefully considered and closely monitored in the preterm infant who

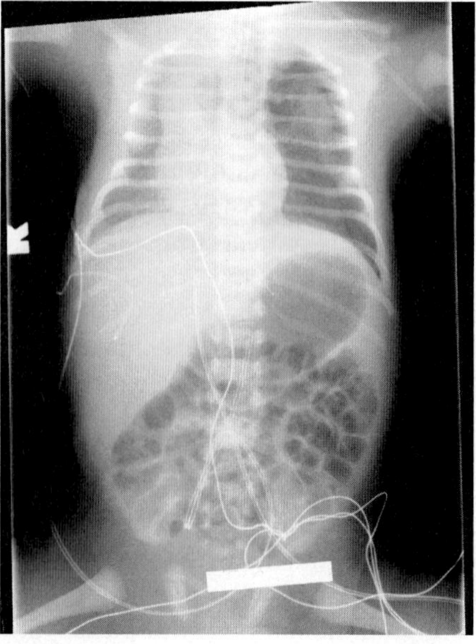

FIGURE 48–11 Chest radiograph showing large left pneumothorax.

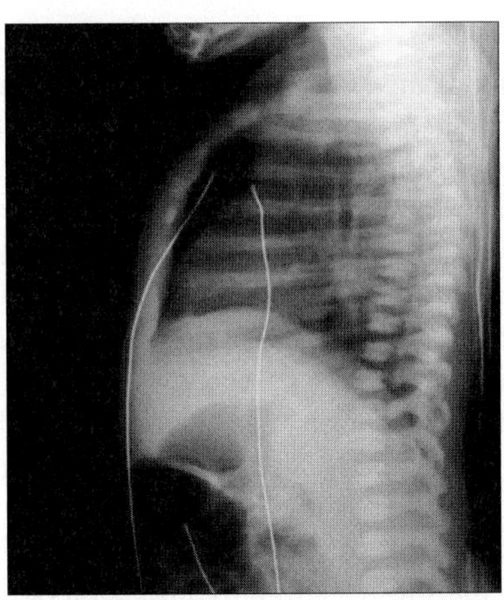

FIGURE 48–12 Lateral chest radiograph of a pneumothorax.

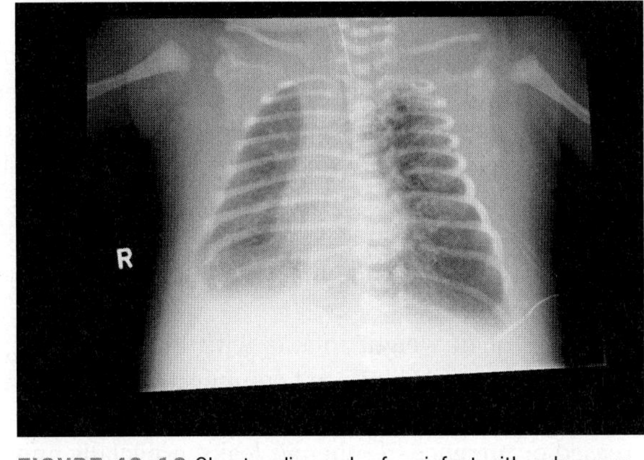

FIGURE 48–13 Chest radiograph of an infant with pulmonary interstitial emphysema on the left and granular appearance of the right lung consistent with respiratory distress syndrome.

is at risk of retinopathy of prematurity. Needle aspiration or thoracentesis is indicated if the pneumothorax is large, symptomatic, or under tension. If the infant has a tension pneumothorax and is receiving mechanical ventilation, chest tube placement will be needed.[103] With positive pressure ventilation and a large air leak, most of the air delivered by the ventilator may exit the lung through the bronchopleural fistula and not participate in gas exchange. When that occurs, HFV is often the only means to provide adequate ventilation and oxygenation.

Pulmonary Interstitial Emphysema

Pulmonary interstitial emphysema (PIE) begins with an air leak from the alveoli or terminal bronchioles that spreads into the pulmonary interstitium and perivascular tissues of the lungs. The air may form subpleural blebs that can rupture into the pleural space, resulting in a pneumothorax. Air does not rupture through the pleura. This development occurs usually, although not exclusively, in association with mechanical ventilation. If the resulting PIE affects only one lung, there is a mediastinal shift that compresses the normal adjacent lung. The extent of PIE is variable. It may involve one or both lungs and may have a diffuse or localized pattern within each lung. The more widespread the air leak, the more acute the respiratory distress. As trapped air compresses the pulmonary circulation, areas of healthy lung become atelectatic and pulmonary blood flow is reduced. The degree of air trapping and required ventilator pressures can decrease venous return and right ventricular outflow, increase PVR, and markedly reduce oxygenation. PIE that lasts longer than 1 week is referred to as persistent pulmonary interstitial emphysema.[104]

PIE often presents as hypotension and a slow, progressive deterioration of arterial blood gas values with increasing oxygen and ventilatory support requirements. In some cases the infant presents first with a pneumothorax, and PIE is not appreciated until after the collapsed lung is reexpanded. PIE is more common in infants of lower gestational age, typically occurring during the first week of life in preterm infants requiring mechanical ventilation or who have received late surfactant replacement therapy. Other conditions associated with PIE include MAS, aspiration of amniotic fluid or blood, low Apgar scores, resuscitation at birth, main stem intubation, and infection.

Diagnosis is based on chest radiography that typically demonstrates tubular or small bubblelike radiolucencies. They may be focal or diffuse, unilateral or bilateral, and may be described as "salt and pepper." When PIE is confined to one lung, there is hyperinflation with a mediastinal shift that compresses the contralateral lung. When this occurs, the compressed lung will look small and opaque. The heart looks smaller as intrathoracic pressure increases. If PIE involves both lungs, the mediastinum and cardiac silhouette will appear narrowed. The radiograph may look similar to that seen with BPD or may be confused with aspiration pneumonia, pulmonary edema, and air bronchograms similar to those seen with RDS (**Figure 48–13**).[105]

Treatment is mainly supportive, with HFOV or minimal pressure ventilation being the most successful interventions.[106] Lateral decubitus positioning is an easy and effective treatment for PIE if one lung is significantly more affected than the other. The infant is placed in the lateral decubitus position, lying on the side with the more severe PIE. This will help compress the lung, thereby decreasing leakage and possibly improving ventilation to the other lung.[107] Selective intubation and ventilation has been somewhat successful in treating infants with severe PIE who have failed conservative treatment. Intubation of the main bronchus and ventilation of the lung on the unaffected side decompresses the hyperinflated lung tissue in the affected lung, protecting it from high ventilator pressures and allowing time for the emphysema to regress. Once the air leak has stopped, which usually takes 24 to 48 hours, the endotracheal tube is pulled back and ventilation is provided again to both lungs. PIE may resolve over 1 or 2 days or it may persist on radiography for weeks, progressing into other air leak conditions.[108] A 3-day course of dexamethasone has been reported to provide significant clinical improvement in the treatment of PIE, possibly due to reduced airway obstruction, edema, and inflammation.[109] A lobectomy in which the hyperinflated lobe is removed is rare but may be indicated in the infant who fails all other medical interventions.

Very low birth weight infants with PIE have a high risk of mortality and significant complications, including CLD and intraventricular hemorrhage. There is also an increased occurrence of other air leaks, especially pneumothoraces and pneumomediastinum.

Pneumomediastinum

A pneumomediastinum occurs when ruptured alveolar air breaks through the visceral pleura into the connective tissue spaces of the mediastinum, neck, and scalp. Unlike a pneumothorax, the visceral pleura and parietal pleura remain in contact and the lungs remain inflated. The causes of pneumomediastinum are essentially the same as those for a pneumothorax. Known predisposing factors are lung diseases including pneumonia and MAS, mechanical ventilation, and other conditions of air leak syndrome; however, many infants develop a pneumomediastinum for no apparent reason.

Most cases of pneumomediastinum are completely asymptomatic. A preterm infant may experience mild to moderate respiratory distress with tachypnea and cyanosis and may also present with an increased AP diameter of the chest. Often preceded by PIE, pneumomediastinum should be suspected when heart sounds are distant or muffled during a routine newborn exam.

A chest radiograph with mediastinal air extending down and outlining the heart is diagnostic for pneumomediastinum. The thymus is often seen to be elevated, giving the appearance of a sail or angel wings. This is referred to as the thymic sail sign or spinnaker sign. In some cases pneumomediastinum is more obvious on the lateral view than on the AP view. A lateral decubitus film will rule out a pneumothorax if the AP film is unclear. Pneumomediastinum and pneumothorax can coexist, and some infants will be affected by both at the same time.[110]

A pneumomediastinum usually resolves spontaneously, and treatment is rarely required; however, the infant must be observed for other air leaks, especially a pneumothorax. HFOV may be indicated if the condition is severe or accompanied by other air leak conditions. Mortality and morbidity are generally attributed to underlying disease states.

Pneumopericardium

Pneumopericardium is a rare but potentially life-threatening form of air leak syndrome in which air is in the pericardial sac. It is the least common form of air leak syndrome and is almost exclusively preceded by other forms of air leak, most often PIE or a pneumothorax. It rarely occurs in an infant who is not requiring assisted ventilation. Although not well understood, it is believed that pneumopericardium is caused by air tracking along vascular sheaths, ending with dissection into the pericardium.

Clinical presentation of pneumopericardium varies from asymptomatic to life-threatening cardiac tamponade. An abrupt onset of tachycardia followed by severe cyanosis, hypotension, and bradycardia with distant heart sounds is the typical presentation of hemodynamic compromise due to cardiac tamponade. The first sign of pneumopericardium is often hypotension or a decreased pulse pressure.

Diagnosis is suspected when the infant experiences sudden clinical deterioration with acute circulatory collapse. It is confirmed with a chest radiograph or the return of air on pericardiocentesis. Pneumopericardium has the most classic radiograph of all the air leaks: the characteristic halo sign. Thin streaks of air may outline the left ventricle and right atrium or completely surround the heart with a radiolucent halo if there is a large amount of free air. Pneumomediastinum and pneumopericardium are not mutually exclusive and can occur together. Radiographs suggestive of both diagnoses should not be disregarded.

Treatment for pneumopericardium depends on the presence of cardiac tamponade and aortic blood pressure monitoring. Cardiac tamponade with a stable blood pressure requires minimal intervention. Symptomatic infants with a fall in aortic blood pressure should be treated emergently with pericardiocentesis and surgical insertion of a pericardial drain. The prognosis is dire and outcome fatal unless emergency treatment with pericardiocentesis is available.[111]

Retinopathy of Prematurity

Retinopathy of prematurity (ROP) is a complex disease that affects growth of the blood vessels needed to support the retina. Full-term infants have fully developed retinas and are not susceptible to ROP. It primarily affects premature infants with birth weights less than 1500 g. The severity is related to gestational age: the more premature the infant, the more severe the disease. Today ROP is the second most common cause of childhood visual impairment and blindness in premature infants. Of the approximately 28,000 infants who are born in the United States weighing less than 1250 g, about 14,000 to 16,000 have some degree of ROP, with 400 to 600 of these infants legally blind.[112] The incidence is greater in Caucasian infants than African American infants, and boys are more vulnerable than girls.

ROP was first described in 1942 and referred to as retrolental fibroplasia (RLF). Not coincidently, this was shortly after Julius Hess developed the "infant oxygen unit," an incubator that had a small porthole used for continuous oxygen administration.[113] In the decade that followed, thousands of children became blind. This was a direct result of abnormal blood vessel growth causing scarring and detachment of the retina. In 1951, Kate Campbell determined that there was a link between using oxygen and the development of this disease. Her suggestion was to avoid using oxygen except for treatment of cyanosis.[114] One year later strict guidelines were created to maintain oxygen concentrations at less than 40%.[115] As oxygen administration was controlled, this epidemic of blindness came to an end. In fact, in 1965 the incidence of RLF in the United States was only 4%, compared with 50% in 1950.[116] However, in the 1970s and 1980s, an increase in the survival rate of very low birth weight infants brought with it an increase in ROP. Today, with advanced technology and surfactant replacement therapy, the survival rates for infants with extremely low gestational ages and birth weights have markedly improved, placing these infants at the highest risk for ROP.

> **RESPIRATORY RECAP**
>
> **Retinopathy of Prematurity**
>
> » Affects growth of blood vessels needed to support the retina
>
> » Prevention is the best treatment: restrict oxygen therapy, use steroid therapy, reduce exposure to light, provide adequate nutrition

Pathophysiology

The function of the retina is to form images. Vessels that will support the retina begin to grow from the optic disk into the retina at approximately 16 weeks' gestation. Complete formation of the capillary bed occurs by 40 to 44 weeks' gestation. Once complete the vessels are no longer susceptible to injury.[117] When an infant is born prematurely, the retinal blood vessels have not had adequate time to mature, and normal vascular growth is terminated. These fragile retinal vessels are extremely vulnerable to injury.

The development of ROP begins when exposure to oxygen causes the delicate retinal vessels to constrict. Perfusion to the retina is interrupted, and capillary cells are destroyed. As the infant matures, the vessels grow, but unfortunately growth is excessive and abnormal. The result is hemorrhage, scar tissue formation, and retinal detachment with functional or complete blindness.

The most significant risk factors for ROP are extreme premature birth, low birth weight, and supplemental oxygen therapy. Genetic factors may contribute to ROP, which may be why it occurs in some premature infants who have not received oxygen therapy.[118] A number of other risk factors have been identified and include acidosis, intraventricular hemorrhage, *Candida* sepsis, mechanical ventilation, and twin pregnancy.[119]

Clinical Manifestations and Diagnosis

The progression of ROP is sequential; therefore, timely screening and treatment is necessary to reduce the risk of blindness.[120] To minimize the risk of retinal detachment and traumatic eye exams, the American Academy of Pediatrics (AAP) developed a policy statement that suggests a schedule be developed for timing eye examinations. This schedule is based on gestational and postnatal age.[121] The AAP's recommendation is to screen any infant with a birth weight of less than 1500 grams or gestational age of 32 weeks or less, or infants with an unstable clinical course who are believed to be at high risk for ROP. Retinal screening examinations are performed by a pediatric ophthalmologist and are done 4 to 6 weeks after birth, with repeat exams every 1 to 2 weeks. There is no need for a second exam if the initial examination shows that the retina in each eye is fully vascularized.

Because changes in the blood vessels cannot be visualized with the naked eye, the ophthalmologist uses a binocular with special lens for evaluation. Topical anesthetic eye drops are instilled 30 minutes prior to the examination. The infant is swaddled during the exam. The exam may cause reflex bradycardia, hypertension, and apnea; therefore, the infant should be relatively stable before an exam is performed.

An international classification of ROP was established in 1984.[122] It is based on the location, stage, and extent of the disease. Location and extent of the disease are described using zones.

Management

ROP is easiest to treat when it is caught early. Prevention remains the best treatment option. Possible preventive measures are restriction of oxygen therapy, use of steroid therapy, reduced exposure of the retina to light, and nutritional factors.[123] Current treatment begins with close monitoring of oxygen saturation levels. Although the ideal pulse oximetry range is debatable, most nurseries have policies in place that recommend a normal oxygen saturation range between 85% to 95%. Administration of vitamin E may help prevent ROP, along with covering the infant's eyes. This is accomplished by keeping nursery lights low and by placing a mask over the infant's eyes or placing a blanket on top of the incubator.

Usually infants with stages 1, 2, and 3 spontaneously resolve and surgical treatment is not needed. Two forms of surgery are available to stop the progression of ROP. Cryosurgery requires an incision into the conjunctiva. It consists of applying an extremely cold probe to the infant's eye and freezing hypoxic areas of the retina. This prevents the spread of abnormal vessels but has a high risk of visual complications, including retinal scarring and detachment. Laser photocoagulation is the newest surgical treatment. This technique involves applying a laser directly to the retina. It condensates protein material in the eye and destroys any abnormal blood vessels.

This treatment has less risk of tissue damage and only requires a topical anesthetic. Complications include scarring, intraocular hemorrhage, corneal haze, burns of the iris, and possibly cataracts. Most infants completely recover following treatment.[120,124]

Complications and Outcomes

Fortunately, ROP is of variable severity, and most infants recover with no lasting visual problems. However, it is impossible to accurately predict the outcomes. Some infants will progress to retinal scar formation or retinal detachment resulting in blindness. Strabismus, glaucoma, astigmatism, nystagmus, and amblyopia may also occur. Early screening and treatment for ROP along with surgical repair have improved long-term outcomes. In spite of limiting oxygen exposure, ROP remains a common problem in infants who weigh less than 1251 grams.[125]

BOX 48–12

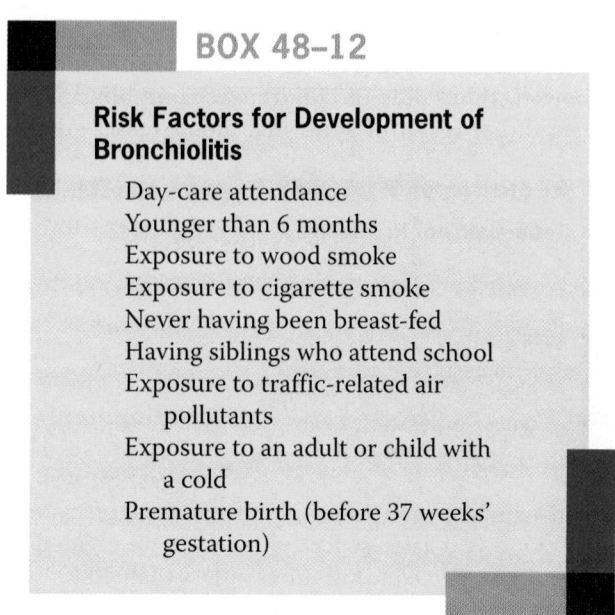

Risk Factors for Development of Bronchiolitis

- Day-care attendance
- Younger than 6 months
- Exposure to wood smoke
- Exposure to cigarette smoke
- Never having been breast-fed
- Having siblings who attend school
- Exposure to traffic-related air pollutants
- Exposure to an adult or child with a cold
- Premature birth (before 37 weeks' gestation)

Bronchiolitis

Bronchiolitis, defined as inflammation of the bronchioles, is an acute infectious disease that often occurs in epidemics. Although bronchiolitis may occur at any age, it usually affects children under the age of 24 months, with a peak incidence in infants 3 to 6 months old. It may be more prevalent in urban areas and occurs more frequently in males than females. Typically bronchiolitis is seasonal, appearing more frequently between November and April, and remains one of the most common reasons for an infant to be hospitalized during winter and early spring.[126]

Pathophysiology

Bronchiolitis begins with a viral infection in the upper respiratory tract and can spread to the terminal bronchiolar cells within 1 to 3 days. Pathologic changes begin 18 to 24 hours following the infection. The virus initiates an inflammatory response causing increased mucus production with bronchiolar and ciliated epithelial cell necrosis. The developing edema, airway debris, and sloughed epithelium cause partial or total obstruction to airflow. Airway narrowing during expiration produces a decrease in airflow along with air trapping that may lead to complete obstruction and atelectasis. Hypoxia is a result of $\dot{V}/\dot{Q}$ mismatch, and work of breathing is increased due to a decrease in lung compliance. The epithelial cells begin recovery after 3 to 4 days; however, it may take 2 or more weeks for cilia to regenerate.[127]

Etiology

Respiratory syncytial virus is the most common cause of bronchiolitis and may be responsible for 50% to 80% of all cases.[128] Less frequently identified viruses include adenovirus, influenza A and B, parainfluenza viruses, human metapneumovirus, rhinovirus, and measles virus. Some bacteria have been associated with bronchiolitis, including *Mycoplasma pneumoniae* and *Chlamydia pneumoniae.* RSV is so common that it is estimated that by the time infants are 12 months old, more than half of them have been exposed to the virus. Unfortunately, RSV is extremely contagious and is transmitted from person to person by inhaling airborne droplets of infected secretions or by direct contact with objects contaminated with respiratory secretions. These droplets can survive for several hours on contaminated objects, including bed rails and the hands of caregivers.

Box 48–12 lists risk factors that increase the likelihood that a child will develop bronchiolitis. Children at high risk of developing severe, life-threatening RSV infection include those with underlying cardiopulmonary disease, including congenital heart disease and BPD, infants younger than 6 weeks, and infants with congenital or acquired immunodeficiency. Multiple infections, such as RSV and metapneumovirus, also tend to result in more severe cases.[129]

Clinical Manifestations

RSV infection in older children and adults causes generally mild symptoms similar to the common cold. The bronchioles of an infant are much narrower than those of an adult, causing infants with RSV infection to present with more severe respiratory distress.

Bronchiolitis follows a variable course characterized by wheezing, tachypnea, and hypoxia. Clinical presentation typically begins with nasal congestion and rhinorrhea followed by mild coughing, and possibly a low-grade fever. The child may also have conjunctivitis or otitis media. Apnea may be the presenting feature of bronchiolitis, especially in younger infants with a history of premature birth. Over a period of 2 to 3 days, tachypnea develops with respiratory rates of up to 100 breaths/min in infants and 60 breaths/min in the older child. Audible wheezing with a prolonged expiratory phase is common, and fine inspiratory crackles are heard on auscultation. Dyspnea develops and symptoms progress to tachycardia, marked intercostal retractions, nasal flaring, grunting, and head bobbing with the use of accessory muscles. The infant may be irritable and appear anxious and toxic. Fever and tachypnea increase insensible fluid loss, while respiratory distress makes it difficult for an infant to take a bottle. This, along with a decreased appetite, can quickly lead to dehydration. The liver and spleen may be palpable from hyperinflation of the lungs and depression of the diaphragm. Persistent hypoxia and increased work of breathing lead to fatigue, more shallow respirations, and eventually respiratory failure.

> **RESPIRATORY RECAP**
>
> **Bronchiolitis**
>
> » Greatest incidence is in infants aged 3 to 6 months.
> » Respiratory syncytial virus is the most common cause.
> » Treatment includes nasotracheal suctioning, hydration, and oxygen.
> » Bronchodilator therapy is controversial.

Severe disease most often develops in toxic-appearing infants who are younger than 3 months and have an oxygen saturation of less than 95% on room air. Infants with respiratory rates greater than 70 breaths/min, apneic episodes, or chest radiographs with atelectasis are also at higher risk of developing acute respiratory distress.

Diagnosis

Bronchiolitis is diagnosed and the severity of the disease assessed on the basis of history and physical examination of the child. Although the clinical syndrome of bronchiolitis is well recognized, diagnosis can be supported by additional tests. Because hypoxia is common, oxygen saturation is monitored with pulse oximetry; no further testing is warranted when oxygen levels are normal. RSV rapid antigen testing is done using a nasal swab, and although it is diagnostic for RSV it is not generally necessary for disease management.

Laboratory tests and radiographs are not routinely recommended but may be useful in ruling out other disorders in children with complicating or worsening symptoms.[128,130] Although the white blood cell count is usually within normal limits, a complete blood count may be ordered if bacterial illness is suspected. If chest radiographs are indicated they should include AP and lateral views. Bronchiolitis typically presents as hyperinflation with flattened diaphragms, air bronchograms, peribronchial cuffing, and prominent hilar markings. Atelectasis and patchy infiltrates may be present as well as pneumonia (**Figure 48–14**).

When the child presents with atypical symptoms, additional tests are warranted and may reveal evidence of other diagnoses, including bronchitis, pneumonia, and congenital heart disease. Gastroesophageal reflux or dysphagia with aspiration of gastric contents may also present with a clinical picture similar to bronchiolitis. Foreign body aspiration should be considered when there is a history of sudden-onset wheezing without symptoms of upper respiratory tract infection. Asthma may present similarly but is much more likely to occur in a child who is older than 18 months. Vascular rings, tracheomalacia, and other anatomic airway abnormalities should be included in the differential diagnosis.

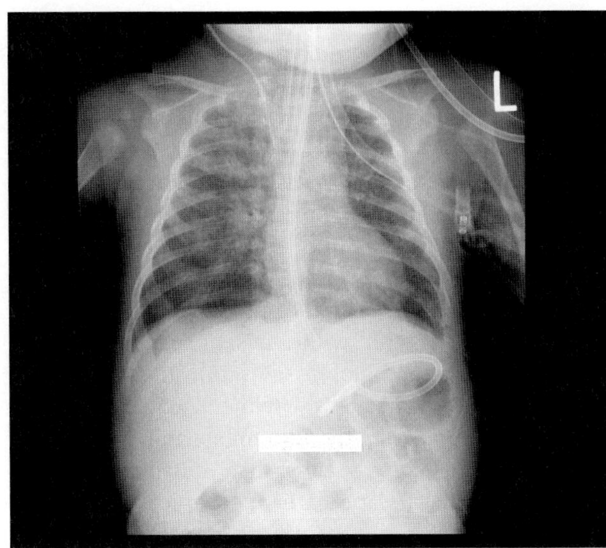

FIGURE 48–14 Chest radiograph with bilateral hyperinflation and widespread pulmonary infiltrates in an infant with bronchiolitis.

Management

In the majority of cases, bronchiolitis can be successfully treated in the outpatient setting. Indications for hospitalization include hypoxemia, tachypnea with respiratory rates greater than 60 breaths/min, retractions at rest, apnea, poor oral intake, and children with underlying cardiopulmonary disease or immunodeficiency. Many institutions use pathways or guidelines to standardize the management of bronchiolitis. There is mounting evidence that the use of pathways is associated with a decrease in unwarranted treatment, use of antibiotics, and hospital length of stays.[131,132] Because of the highly contagious nature of the virus, early efforts should be made to isolate infants confirmed to have RSV infection or who present with a clinical picture suggestive of bronchiolitis.

Nasopharyngeal suctioning is an effective component of the care of infants with bronchiolitis and should be used to clear nasal secretions. Saline drops may be instilled in the nose prior to suctioning. Parents and other caregivers must be proficient in bulb suctioning techniques to use at home and be educated on proper hand sanitation.

With oxygenation and hydration the primary goals, treatment is largely supportive and usually requires only fluids, oxygen, and suctioning of secretions. The risk of dehydration makes it essential that fluid intake and urine output be monitored. Frequent small feeds and IV fluid administration are used to maintain adequate hydration if the child's respiratory rate is greater than 80 breaths/min or the child has respiratory distress or oxygen desaturation during feedings.

Although not routinely recommended, supplemental oxygen is administered with a nasal cannula or oxygen hood if the oxyhemoglobin saturation of a previously healthy infant is persistently below 92%. Ventilation is assessed by monitoring the P_{CO_2} of arterial, capillary, or venous blood. A P_{CO_2} greater than 55 is an indication for high-flow nasal cannula or mechanical ventilation. Recurrent apnea requires intubation with mechanical ventilation. Oxygen may be discontinued when the S_{PO_2} is at or above 92%, the infant has adequate oral intake, and respiratory distress is at a minimum. Weaning oxygen in premature infants or infants with cardiopulmonary disease must be closely monitored.[133]

Bronchodilator use would seem to be the logical choice for treatment of wheezing; however, it continues to be controversial in the management of bronchiolitis. Recent guidelines from the AAP recommend that bronchodilators not be used routinely. A carefully monitored trial is an option, with use continued only if there is evidence of clinical improvement.[133] Chest physiotherapy is not recommended because no benefit has been documented and it may actually increase respiratory distress and irritability. Because bronchiolitis is viral in nature, antibiotics are ineffective and should not be administered unless there is evidence of concomitant bacterial infection (e.g., otitis media, pneumonia). Because clinical trials have reported that there is no benefit in using corticosteroids to treat bronchiolitis, routine use is not recommended.[134] There is recent evidence that nebulized hypertonic saline resulted in clinically significant reductions in hospital stay and is a safe and effective treatment for viral bronchiolitis.[135]

When first approved for use in the United States in 1986, the antiviral agent ribavirin was administered by continuous aerosol for 18 hours a day for 3 to 6 days.[136] Multiple studies since that time have criticized its application, concluding that there is marginal benefit from this expensive drug that requires a complicated aerosol delivery system and has the potential of teratogenic risks for pregnant caregivers. Present recommendations are that it not be used routinely and only be considered for treatment of documented RSV bronchiolitis in high-risk infants who may be immunocompromised or have underlying cardiopulmonary disease.[133] As of this date there is no RSV vaccine available for bronchiolitis. However, since its introduction in 1998, the humanized monoclonal antibody palivizumab (Synagis) has been shown to help protect high-risk infants from RSV infection and limit severity of the illness. The recommended dosage of palivizumab is 15 mg/kg body weight administered by a single intramuscular injection in five monthly doses during RSV season, usually beginning in November.[137] Recommendations made by the AAP currently limit its use to infants and children who are at high risk of developing severe disease from RSV. **Box 48–13** lists those who may benefit from palivizumab prophylaxis. Discharge is considered when the child is stable without supplemental oxygen, the respiratory rate is within normal range, and oral intake is adequate to maintain hydration.

BOX 48–13

Indications for Palivizumab Prophylaxis

- Infants born at 32 weeks' gestation or earlier
- Infants born between 32 and 35 weeks' gestation with at least two risk factors*
- Infants and children younger than 24 months with chronic lung disease
- Infants and children younger than 24 months with congenital heart disease

*Risk factors: day-care attendance, school-aged sibling, exposure to environmental air pollutants, congenital airway abnormalities, severe neuromuscular disease, acquired immunodeficiency.

Complications and Outcome

Complications of bronchiolitis are most severe in high-risk infants and children. Apnea often occurs in young infants or those with previous episodes of apnea. Severe respiratory distress may lead to respiratory failure and require intubation and mechanical ventilation. Although uncommon, a secondary bacterial pneumonia may occur. Although the association is controversial, there is some indication that infants hospitalized with bronchiolitis have increased risk for recurrent wheezing and development of early childhood asthma. Whether these children have an inherited asthma tendency that makes them more prone to bronchiolitis or whether bronchiolitis triggers asthma is uncertain.[138,139]

Most infants, regardless of the severity of illness, recover in 3 to 5 days. Wheezing, cough, and disruption in feeding and sleeping patterns often continue for 2 to 4 weeks. Although rare, death occurs most often in infants younger than 6 months and depends largely on comorbidities. The mortality rate is less than 1%, with this rate decreasing with increasing birth weight.

Laryngotracheobronchitis

Acute respiratory tract infections are common in the pediatric patient and are the number one reason for children under the age of 4 years to be hospitalized. Upper airway infections can be particularly severe because of the anatomy of the child's airway. Unlike an adult, whose glottis is the narrowest part of the airway, a child's narrowest airway segment is the subglottis. The subglottic area is cone-shaped, with the cricoid ring being the narrowest area. Because it is completely surrounded by the cricoid cartilage and loose connective tissue, a small amount of inflammation and edema of this subglottic tissue can result in significant airway obstruction.

Laryngotracheobronchitis (LTB), also referred to as croup, is the most common cause of infectious upper airway obstruction in children between the ages of 6 months and 3 years. It rarely occurs in children younger than 1 year or older than 6 years and is more prevalent in males than females. About 15% of affected children have a family history of LTB. It is epidemic by nature and occurs most often between early fall and late spring. The vast majority of children with LTB are not hospitalized but rather are treated at home with humidified air.[140]

Pathophysiology and Etiology

This disorder is termed laryngotracheobronchitis because it is characterized by diffuse inflammation that affects the airway from the larynx to the bronchus. It involves edema of the subglottic area and exudate in the airway, resulting in varying degrees of airway narrowing. It is usually due to a viral invasion, particularly parainfluenzae types 1 and 2. Although not as common, a number of other viruses have been reported, including influenza type A and B, adenovirus, rhinovirus, enterovirus, respiratory syncytial virus, herpes simplex type 1, measles, and varicella. A disruption in the laminar airflow through the constricted or partially obstructed airway during inspiration produces the characteristic harsh, brassy sound of stridor.

> **RESPIRATORY RECAP**
>
> **Laryngotracheobronchitis**
>
> » Most common cause of infectious upper airway obstruction in children between the ages of 6 months and 3 years
>
> » Treatment includes corticosteroids, racemic epinephrine, oxygen, heliox, and, in rare cases, intubation

Clinical Manifestations

The spectrum of disease severity is broad with LTB. The child typically presents with a several-day history of upper respiratory–type symptoms that include a low-grade fever, rhinorrhea, sore throat, and mild cough.[141] Over the next 2 to 3 days, the symptoms progress to hoarseness and the barking-seal cough that is characteristic of LTB. The cough often begins abruptly in the middle of the night and may occur in spasms. Stridor is heard mainly on inspiration, typically occurring when the child is irritated or crying. With more significant airway narrowing, it becomes audible even when the child is resting quietly and during both inspiration and expiration, which is referred to as biphasic stridor. Physical examination usually reveals an apprehensive-appearing child with mild fever, tachypnea, tachycardia, suprasternal and substernal retractions, head bobbing, and breath sounds that are mostly clear.

Diagnosis

The diagnosis of viral LTB is most often based on the characteristic clinical presentation. It does not require radiography in children with typical histories and mild symptoms that respond effectively to treatment. Lateral neck films typically reveal a normal epiglottis and supraglottic structures, an overdistended hypopharynx, and haziness within the subglottis with subglottic narrowing greater on inspiration. These films help confirm the diagnosis of LTB while ruling out other disorders, including epiglottitis, hemangioma, and congenital abnormalities such as a tracheal web or vascular ring (**Figure 48–15**). The AP view of the neck will demonstrate narrowing immediately below the vocal cords with the usual squared-shoulder appearance of the subglottic area replaced with airway narrowing referred to as a steeple sign or pencil-point sign. The absence of abnormalities, however, does not rule out the diagnosis of LTB, because radiographs may be normal in as many as 50% of children

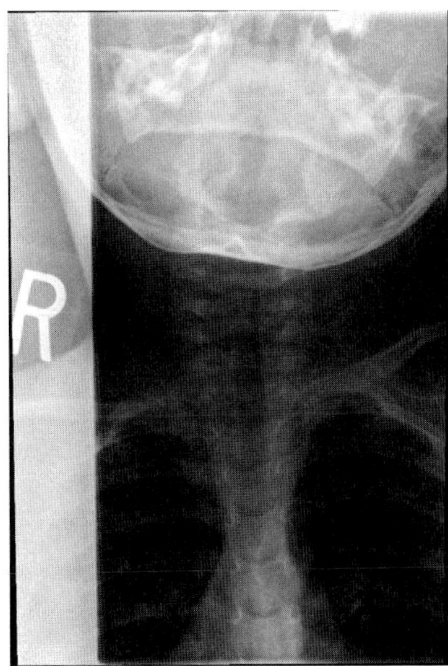

FIGURE 48–15 Chest radiograph of a child with laryngotracheobronchitis shows the pencil-point or steeple sign.

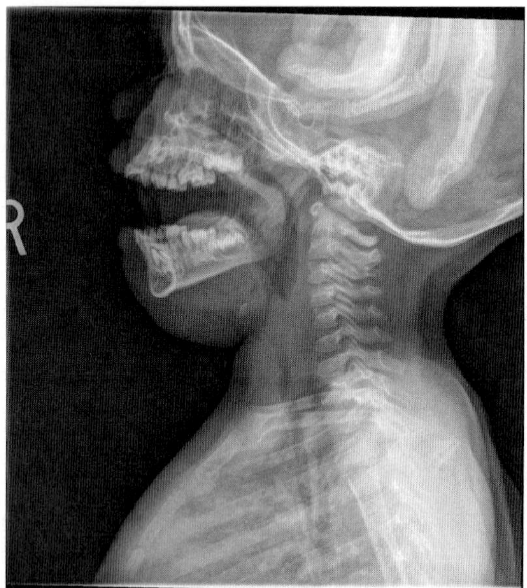

FIGURE 48–16 Lateral neck radiograph of a child with laryngotracheobronchitis shows a hypopharynx that is overdistended and subglottic haziness.

with LTB and diagnosis is made from history and clinical presentation alone (**Figure 48–16**).[141]

Management

For the majority of children, LTB is self-limiting and only supportive care is needed. Despite the lack of strong scientific evidence, there is anecdotal support for treating LTB at home with humidification using a humidifier or vaporizer at the bedside or sitting with the child in the bathroom with the door closed and a hot shower running. Although the benefit of such treatment may only be a placebo to make parents feel like they are helping their child, it is still used and even advised. However, it is not without risks, which may include scalding, unnecessary discomfort, and anxiety that worsens symptoms.[142]

Management of LTB has undergone dramatic changes, including the use of corticosteroids in both outpatient and inpatient settings. It is believed that the potent vasoconstrictive and anti-inflammatory properties of corticosteroids reduce mucosal edema and the inflammatory reaction. Use has been shown not only to reduce symptoms and the need for hospital admission but also to reduce the need for and duration of intubation.[143] Dexamethasone given orally at 0.6 mg/kg provides quick relief, with the effect lasting for at least 3 hours; many children responding to a single oral dose. Aerosolized budesonide is another option in delivering corticosteroid therapy in the treatment of LTB; however, it has not been proven to be more beneficial than dexamethasone and is currently more expensive to use.

Available in the United States since 1971, racemic epinephrine has a vasoconstrictive α-adrenergic effect on the vasculature mucosa that rapidly reduces upper airway edema. Upon presentation in the emergency department, children typically receive aerosolized racemic epinephrine by face mask with a hand-held nebulizer using a 2.25% solution diluted in normal saline. The amount of medication used is dependent on the child's response. Recommended dosage is 0.5 to 1.0 mg of a 2.25% solution diluted in normal saline to a total volume of 3.0 mL. The effect is short lived, though, usually lasting only 2 hours. For some children a single dose is all that is required to relieve symptoms, and they can be discharged home if they have been symptom free for 2 to 3 hours following the treatment.

For the child who has poor to no response to treatment in the emergency department, hospitalization is advised. Corticosteroid therapy is continued, and nebulized racemic epinephrine treatments may be given as often as every 30 minutes. Respiratory rate is the simplest predictor of hypoxemia in the child with LTB. To prevent the anxiety and crying that often triggers stridor and retractions, noninvasive monitoring with pulse oximetry is preferred over blood gas testing. Supplemental oxygen is provided only if the child's oxygen saturation is less than 92%. Because LTB is usually caused by a virus, antibiotics are not indicated unless the child has cultures suggestive of a bacterial infection.

Reports vary concerning the use of helium–oxygen (heliox) mixtures in the hospital management of LTB. Heliox has shown benefit as a useful alternative to intubation but also has been shown to have treatment efficacy equal to inhaled racemic epinephrine. With a density lower than oxygen, helium reduces turbulence in the airways, decreasing airway resistance and work of breathing. Premixed oxygen and helium are administered from a gas cylinder with oxygen-to-helium dilutions of 80:20 or 70:30. A close-fitting nonrebreathing mask or a mechanical ventilator should be used for gas delivery.[144]

On rare occasions a child will fail medical intervention and require endotracheal intubation. Because of the subglottic edema and narrowed airway, intubation should be with an endotracheal tube that is at least 1 mm smaller than the normal estimate. As airway edema and inflammation are resolved, an air leak will develop around the endotracheal tube, and extubation attempts are usually successful at that time. Close monitoring for the return of stridor and respiratory distress is necessary in the first 12 hours following extubation.

Complications and Outcome

Complications that develop from LTB are rare but can include dehydration as a result of tachypnea and increased respiratory distress or secondary infections of otitis media and pneumonia. LTB usually resolves within 72 hours of onset, although some cases last up to 7 days, with complete uncomplicated resolution. Some children have repeat episodes of LTB. Only 5% to 10% of LTB patients are hospitalized, with approximately only 2% of that group requiring intubation. Subglottic stenosis in the child with LTB is uncommon but is a possible complication if intubation is prolonged.[145]

Epiglottitis

The life-threatening bacterial infection known as **epiglottitis** is a true airway emergency. It was first described in 1878 and given the name epiglottitis, although today we appreciate that it is an infection that affects the supraglottic structures. These include the epiglottis, aryepiglottic folds, arytenoid soft tissue, and occasionally the uvula. It tends to occur in children aged 2 to 6 years, although cases have been reported in which the child is younger than 1 year, and may present at no particular season.

Pathophysiology and Etiology

> **RESPIRATORY RECAP**
>
> **Epiglottitis**
>
> » Epiglottitis is a life-threatening bacterial infection.
>
> » Common findings include drooling, dysphagia, dysphonia, and dyspnea.
>
> » Many cases respond to antibiotics and oxygen.
>
> » If epiglottitis is severe and intubation is indicated, it should be performed in the operating room.

Epiglottitis is purely a supraglottic lesion in which swelling pushes the epiglottis posteriorly and edema produces partial or complete airway obstruction. There is ballooning of the hypopharynx, thickened aryepiglottic folds, and circumferential narrowing of the subglottic portion of the trachea during inspiration. *Haemophilus influenzae* type b (Hib) is the most common causative organism; however, pneumococcus, group β-hemolytic *Streptococcus pneumoniae*, *Klebsiella*, and viruses such as herpes simplex 1 and parainfluenzae have also been implicated.[146]

Clinical Manifestations

Clinical findings include the classic four Ds of epiglottitis: drooling, dysphagia, dysphonia, and dyspnea. History is common for an abrupt onset of sore throat with refusal to eat, high fever (>38° C), irritability, and a muffled-sounding voice. The child is toxic appearing and drooling. In contrast to laryngotracheobronchitis, the respiratory pattern of the child with epiglottitis is one of very deliberate slow breaths with large tidal volumes. This is an effort to reduce turbulent airflow and airway resistance. Suprasternal and substernal retractions are evident, with nasal flaring and cyanosis if obstruction is severe. Typical presentation is in the tripod position: sitting upright supported by both hands and leaning forward with the neck extended in a "sniffing" position in an attempt to keep the airway open. Inspiratory stridor is heard but may diminish as airway obstruction worsens.

Diagnosis

Manipulation of the epiglottis with a tongue depressor, radiographs, and blood gas analysis are painful and anxiety-provoking procedures that greatly increase the risk of complete airway obstruction. For that reason they should be avoided if at all possible and diagnosis made by history and clinical presentation alone. However, if a diagnosis is in question, lateral neck films are valuable in confirming the diagnosis and ruling out other disorders, including LTB, foreign body aspiration, and retropharyngeal abscess. Patient age, clinical presentation, and radiographic findings can contribute to differentiation from LTB. **Table 48–1** lists those factors that assist in the differential diagnosis. The radiograph will typically reveal an enlarged epiglottis, described as the thumb sign, and a distended hypopharynx. It should be noted that if neck radiographs are performed, the child should never be left alone and must remain in an upright position during the study because the supine position may result in total airway obstruction.

Management

The overriding goal in treating the child with epiglottitis is to obtain and maintain a secure airway. Many patients will respond to intravenous antibiotics and supplemental

TABLE 48–1 Clinical Differentiation of Epiglottitis and Laryngotracheobronchitis

	Epiglottitis	Laryngotracheobronchitis
Age	2 to 6 years	6 months to 3 years
Gender	No prevalence	More prevalent in males
Onset	Sudden, within 4 to 8 hours	2- to 4-day history of cold symptoms
Seasons	All	Fall through spring
Fever	High	Low-grade
Respiratory rate	Bradypnea with deliberate, large tidal volumes	Late-onset tachypnea
Heart rate	Early-onset tachycardia	Late-onset tachycardia
Retractions	Severe	Mild to severe
Stridor	Inspiratory	Inspiratory and expiratory
Cough	Minimal	"Barking seal"
Voice	Muffled	Hoarse
Drooling	Yes	No
Dysphagia	Yes	No
Position	Supine worsens stridor	No effect on stridor
Appearance	Toxic, acutely ill	Irritable, restless
Radiograph	Lateral neck view: thumb sign	Anteroposterior view: steeple sign

oxygen and not require intubation but must be closely monitored in an intensive care setting.[147] If epiglottitis is severe and emergency intubation is indicated, it should be performed in an operating suite where an emergent tracheostomy can be performed if needed. After the patient is anesthetized, fiberoptic-assisted intubation is performed and airway specimens obtained for culture and sensitivity. As with LTB, intubation of the swollen airway will require an endotracheal tube that is one size smaller than that estimated for age and weight. Extubation should be attempted only after an air leak is noted and there is evidence of clinical improvement. A nasotracheal tube is preferred because it is more stable and better able to keep secured. If the child will need to be transported to another facility, the airway must be secured and the child should be sedated to prevent anxiety that can worsen airway compromise.[141]

Complications and Outcome

With a quick response to antibiotic therapy and corticosteroid administration, intubation is usually required for no more than 48 hours. Nearly half of all patients with epiglottitis will develop another infection, most often pneumonia and otitis media. Bacteremia can also lead to cellulitis and meningitis. Accidental extubation increases the risk of airway complications. Mortality rate can be as high as 10% when there is airway obstruction without intubation, in contrast to only 1% when intubation is performed. Introduction of the Hib vaccine in 1985 has led to a marked decrease in the number of cases of epiglottitis, with 41 cases reported per 100,000 children in 1987 compared with 1.3 cases per 100,000 children in 1997.[145,148]

KEY POINTS

- Apnea of prematurity is due to immaturity of the brain stem.
- Apnea of prematurity is treated with respiratory stimulants, oxygen, CPAP, and mechanical ventilation.
- Home apnea monitoring may be used with apnea of prematurity.
- Respiratory distress syndrome is a complication of prematurity.
- Biochemical tests of amniotic fluid can be used to evaluate lung maturity.
- Treatment of respiratory distress syndrome includes oxygen, surfactant replacement, CPAP, mechanical ventilation, and supportive therapy.
- Chronic lung disease occurs in premature infants with progressive deterioration of lung function.
- A milder form of bronchopulmonary dysplasia is based on continued oxygen therapy at 36 weeks' gestation.
- Causes of chronic lung disease in newborns are multifactorial and include ventilator- and oxygen-induced injury.
- Treatment of chronic lung disease in newborns includes oxygen, mechanical ventilation, corticosteroids, and bronchodilators.
- Transient tachypnea of the newborn is a self-limiting disorder of term and near-term infants.
- Pneumonia can occur at any gestational age and includes congenital, intrapartum, and postnatal forms.
- Treatment of neonatal pneumonia is aimed at eradicating the infection, along with supportive care.
- Meconium aspiration syndrome occurs when the infant aspirates stained amniotic fluid.
- Meconium aspiration syndrome usually occurs in infants born at term or post-term.
- Treatment of meconium aspiration syndrome includes suctioning, oxygen therapy, mechanical ventilation, inhaled nitric oxide, extracorporeal membrane oxygenation, and surfactant replacement.
- Persistent pulmonary hypertension of the newborn occurs when fetal circulation persists after birth.
- Echocardiography is used to make the diagnosis of persistent pulmonary hypertension of the newborn.
- Treatment of persistent pulmonary hypertension of the newborn includes oxygen, mechanical ventilation, inhaled nitric oxide, extracorporeal membrane oxygenation, and supportive therapy.
- Congenital diaphragmatic hernia is an abnormality in which the infant's diaphragm allows the abdominal organs to protrude into the thorax.
- Treatment of congenital diaphragmatic hernia includes delivery room stabilization, mechanical ventilation, inhaled nitric oxide, extracorporeal membrane oxygenation, surgery, and supportive therapy.
- Air leak syndrome in the newborn includes pulmonary interstitial emphysema, pneumothorax, pneumomediastinum, and pneumopericardium.
- Transillumination is used to make an immediate diagnosis of pneumothorax.
- Retinopathy of prematurity affects growth of blood vessels needed to support the retina.
- Prevention is the best treatment for retinopathy of prematurity and includes restriction of oxygen therapy, steroid therapy, reduced exposure to light, and adequate nutrition.
- The greatest incidence of bronchiolitis occurs in infants aged 3 to 6 months.
- Respiratory syncytial virus is the most common cause of bronchiolitis.
- Treatment of bronchiolitis includes nasotracheal suctioning, hydration, and oxygen.
- Bronchodilator therapy for the treatment of bronchiolitis is controversial.

- Laryngotracheobronchitis (LTB) is the most common cause of infectious upper airway obstruction in children between the ages of 6 months and 3 years.
- Treatment of LTB includes corticosteroids, racemic epinephrine, oxygen, heliox, and, in rare cases, intubation.
- Epiglottitis is a life-threatening bacterial infection.
- Common findings in epiglottitis include drooling, dysphagia, dysphonia, and dyspnea.
- Many cases of epiglottitis respond to antibiotics and oxygen.
- If epiglottitis is severe and intubation is indicated, it should be performed in the operating room.

REFERENCES

1. Finer NN, Higgins R, Kattwinkel J, et al. Summary proceedings from the apnea-of-prematurity group. *Pediatrics.* 2006;117:S47–S51.
2. Barrington K, Finer N. The natural history of the appearance of apnea of prematurity. *Pediatr Res.* 1991;29:372–375.
3. Eichenwald E, Aina A, Stark AR. Apnea frequently persists beyond term gestation in infants delivered at 24 to 28 weeks. *Pediatrics.* 1997;100:354–359.
4. Schmidt B. Methylxanthine therapy in premature infants: sound practice, disaster, or fruitless byway? *J Pediatr.* 1999;135:526–528.
5. American Academy of Pediatrics, Committee on Fetus and Newborn. Apnea, sudden infant death syndrome, and home monitoring. *Pediatrics.* 2003;111:914–917.
6. Sychowski SP, Dodd E, Thomas P, et al. Home apnea monitor use in preterm infants discharged from newborn intensive care units. *J Pediatr.* 2001;139:245–248.
7. Schmidt B, Roberts RS, Davis P, et al. Long-term effects of caffeine therapy for apnea of prematurity. *N Engl J Med.* 2007;357:1893–1902.
8. Hoffman HJ, Damus K, Hillman L, et al. Risk factors for SIDS. Results of the National Institute of Child Health and Human Development SIDS Cooperative Epidemiological Study. *Ann N Y Acad Sci.* 1988;533:13–30.
9. Hintz SR, Van Meurs KP, Perritt R, et al. Neurodevelopmental outcomes of premature infants with severe respiratory failure enrolled in a randomized controlled trial of inhaled nitric oxide. *J Pediatr.* 2007;151:e1–e3.
10. Ghodrat M. Lung surfactants. *Am J Health Syst Pharm.* 2006;63:1504–1521.
11. Rodriguez RJ. Management of respiratory distress syndrome: an update. *Respir Care.* 2003;48:279–287.
12. Pickerd N, Kotecha S. Pathophysiology of RDS. *J Paediatr Child Health.* 2009;19:153–157.
13. Cole FS. Defects in surfactant synthesis: clinical implications. *Pediatr Clin North Am.* 2006;53:911–927.
14. McGinnis KT, Brown JA, Morrison JC. Changing patterns of fetal lung maturity testing. *J Perinatol.* 2008;28:20–23.
15. NIH Consensus Development Panel. Effect of corticosteroids for fetal maturation on perinatal outcomes. *JAMA.* 1995;274:413–417.
16. Fujiwara T, Maeta H, Chida S, et al. Artificial surfactant therapy in hyaline-membrane disease. *Lancet.* 1980;1:55–59.
17. Ramanathan R. Surfactant therapy in preterm infants with respiratory distress syndrome and in near-term or term newborns with acute RDS. *J Perinatol.* 2006;26:S51–S56.
18. Kendig JW, Notter RH, Cox C, et al. A comparison of surfactant as immediate prophylaxis and as rescue therapy in newborns of less than 30 weeks' gestation. *N Engl J Med.* 1991;324:865–871.
19. American Academy of Pediatrics, Committee on Fetus and Newborn. Surfactant-replacement therapy for respiratory distress in the preterm and term neonate. *Pediatrics.* 2008;121:419–432.
20. Sweet DC, Halliday HL. The use of surfactants in 2009. *Arch Dis Child.* 2009;94:78–83.
21. Proquitte H, Dushe T, Hammer H, et al. Observational study to compare the clinical efficacy of the natural surfactants Alveofact and Curosurf in the treatment of respiratory distress syndrome in premature infants. *Respir Med.* 2007;101:169–176.
22. Moya F. Synthetic surfactants: where are we? Evidence from randomized, controlled clinical trials. *J Perinatol.* 2009;29: S23–S28.
23. Courtney SE, Barrington KJ. Continuous positive airway pressure and noninvasive ventilation. *Clin Perinatol.* 2007;34:73–92.
24. Morley CJ, Davis PG, Doyle LW, et al. Nasal CPAP or intubation at birth of very preterm infants. *N Engl J Med.* 2008;358:700–708.
25. DiBlasi RM. Nasal continuous positive airway pressure (CPAP) for the respiratory care of the newborn infant. *Respir Care.* 2009;54:1209–1235.
26. Lampland AL, Mammel MC. The role of high-frequency ventilation in neonates: evidence-based recommendations. *Clin Perinatol.* 2007;34:129–144.
27. Henderson-Smart DJ, Cools F, Bhuta T, et al. Elective high frequency oscillatory ventilation versus conventional ventilation for acute pulmonary dysfunction in preterm infants. *Cochrane Database Syst Rev.* 2007;3:CD000104.
28. Kovisto M, Marttila R, Saarela T, et al. Wheezing illness and rehospitalization in the first two years of life after neonatal respiratory distress syndrome. *J Pediatr.* 2005;147:486–492.
29. Thomas W, Speer CP. Prevention and treatment of bronchopulmonary dysplasia: current status and future prospects. *J Perinatol.* 2007;27:S26–S32.
30. Henderson-Smart DJ, Hutchinson JL, Donoghue DA, et al. Prenatal predictors of chronic lung disease in very preterm infants. *Arch Dis Child Fetal Neonatal Ed.* 2006;91:F40–F45.
31. Northway WH, Rosan RC, Porter DY. Pulmonary disease following respiratory therapy of hyaline membrane disease: bronchopulmonary dysplasia. *N Engl J Med.* 1967;276:357–368.
32. Truog WE. Chronic lung disease and randomized interventional trials: status in 2005. *Neoreviews.* 2005;6:e278.
33. Jobe AH. The new BPD. An arrest of lung development. *Pediatr Res.* 1999;46:641–643.
34. Peterson SW. Understanding the sequence of pulmonary injury in the extremely low birth weight, surfactant-deficient infant. *Neonatal Netw.* 2009;28:221–229.
35. Neerhof MG, Thaete LG. The fetal response to chronic placental insufficiency. *Semin Perinatol.* 2008;32:201–205.
36. Hernández-Ronquillo L, Téllez-Zenteno JF, Weder-Cisneros N. Risk factors for the development of bronchopulmonary dysplasia: a case-control study. *Arch Med Res.* 2004;35:549–553.
37. Kotecha S. Allen J. Oxygen therapy for infants with chronic lung disease. *Arch Dis Child Fetal Neonatal Ed.* 2001;87:F11–F14.
38. American Academy of Pediatrics, Committee on Fetus and Newborn. Postnatal corticosteroids to treat or prevent chronic lung disease in preterm infants. *Pediatrics.* 2002;109:330–338.
39. Deakins KM. Bronchopulmonary dysplasia. *Respir Care.* 2009;54:1252–1262.
40. Impact-RSV Study Group. Palivizumab, a humanized respiratory syncytial virus monoclonal antibody, reduces hospitalization from respiratory syncytial virus infection in high-risk infants. *Pediatrics.* 1998;102:531–537.
41. Broughton S, Thomas MR, Marston L, et al. Very prematurely born infants wheezing at followup: lung function and risk factors. *Arch Dis Child.* 2007;92:776–780.
42. Doyle L, Faber B, Callanan C, et al. Bronchopulmonary dysplasia in very low birth weight subjects and lung function in adolescence. *Pediatrics.* 2006;118:108–113.

43. Walter E, Ehlenbach W, Hotchkin D, et al. Low birth weight and respiratory disease in adulthood. *Am J Respir Crit Care Med.* 2009;180:176–180.
44. Avery ME, Gatewood DB, Brumley G. Transient tachypnea of the newborn: possible delayed resorption of fluid at birth. *Am J Dis Child.* 1966;111:380–385.
45. Guglani L, Lakshminrusimha S, Ryan R. Transient tachypnea of the newborn. *Pediatr Rev.* 2008;29:e59–e65.
46. Barker PM, Olver RE. Invited review: clearance of lung liquid during the perinatal period. *J Appl Physiol.* 2002; 93:1542–1548.
47. Jain L, Eaton DC. Physiology of fetal lung fluid clearance and the effect of labor. *Semin Perinatol.* 2006;30:34–43.
48. Riskin A, Abend-Weinger M, Riskin-Mashiah S, et al. Cesarean section, gestational age, and transient tachypnea of the newborn: timing is the key. *Am J Perinatol.* 2005;22:377–382.
49. Demissie K, Marcella SW, Breckenbridge MB, et al. Maternal asthma and transient tachypnea of the newborn. *Pediatrics.* 1998;102:84–90.
50. Jain L, Dudell GG. Respiratory transition in infants delivered by cesarean section. *Semin Perinatol.* 2006;30:296–304.
51. Al Tawil K, Abu-Ekteish FM, Tamimi O, et al. Symptomatic spontaneous pneumothorax in term newborn infants. *Pediatr Pulmonol.* 2004;37:443–446.
52. Birnkrant DJ, Picone C, Markowitz W, et al. Association of transient tachypnea of the newborn and childhood asthma. *Pediatr Pulmonol.* 2006;41:978–984.
53. The United Nations Children's Fund/World Health Organization. *Pneumonia: The Forgotten Killer of Children.* 2006. Available at: http://www.unicef.org/publications/files/Pneumonia_The_Forgotten_Killer_of_Children.pdf.
54. Haney PJ, Bohlman M, Sun CC. Radiographic findings in neonatal pneumonia. *Am J Roentgenol.* 1984;143:23–26.
55. Schrag S, Gorwitz R, Fultz-Butts K, et al. Prevention of perinatal group B streptococcal disease. *Morb Mortal Wkly Rep.* 2002;51:1–22.
56. Velaphi S, Vidyasagar D. Intrapartum and postdelivery management of infants born to mothers with meconium-stained amniotic fluid: evidence-based recommendations. *Clin Perinatol.* 2006;33:29–42.
57. Walsh MC, Fanaroff JM. Meconium stained fluid: approach to the mother and the baby. *Clin Perinatol.* 2007;34:653–665.
58. Yoder BA, Kirsch EA, Barth WH, et al. Changing obstetric practices associated with decreasing incidence of meconium aspiration syndrome. *Obstet Gynecol.* 2002;99:731–739.
59. Gelfand SL, Fanaroff JM, Walsh MC. Controversies in the treatment of meconium aspiration syndrome. *Clin Perinatol.* 2004;31:445–452.
60. Vain NE, Szyld EG, Prudent LM, et al. Oropharyngeal and nasopharyngeal suctioning of meconium-stained neonates before delivery of their shoulders: multicenter, randomized controlled trial. *Lancet.* 2004;364:597–602.
61. Wiswell TE, Gannon CM, Jacob J, et al. Delivery room management of the apparently vigorous meconium-stained neonate: results of the multicenter, international collaborative trial. *Pediatrics.* 2000;105:1–7.
62. ACOG Committee on Obstetric Practice. ACOG Committee Opinion No. 379. Management of delivery of a newborn with meconium-stained amniotic fluid. *Obstet Gynecol.* 2007;110:739.
63. El Shahed AI, Dargaville PA, Ohlsson A, et al. Surfactant for meconium aspiration syndrome in full term/near term infants. *Cochrane Database Syst Rev.* 2007;3:CD002954.
64. Kinsella JP. Meconium aspiration syndrome. Is surfactant lavage the answer? *Am J Respir Crit Care Med.* 2003;168:413–414.
65. Hamutcu R, Nield TA, Garg M, et al. Long-term pulmonary sequelae in children who were treated with extracorporeal membrane oxygenation for neonatal respiratory failure. *Pediatrics.* 2004;114:1292–1296.
66. Lin HC, Su BH, Lin TW, et al. Risk factors of mortality in meconium aspiration syndrome: review of 314 cases. *Acta Paediatr Taiwan.* 2004;45:30–34.
67. Beligere N, Rao R. Neurodevelopmental outcome of infants with meconium aspiration syndrome: report of a study and literature review. *J Perinatol.* 2008;28:s93–s101.
68. Singh BS, Clark RH, Powers RJ. Meconium aspiration syndrome remains a significant problem in the NICU: outcomes and treatment patterns in term neonates admitted for intensive care during a ten-year period. *J Perinatol.* 2009;29:497–503.
69. Walsh-Sukys MC, Tyson JE, Wright LL, et al. Persistent pulmonary hypertension of the newborn in the era before nitric oxide: practice variation and outcomes. *Pediatrics.* 2000;105:14–20.
70. Kinsella JP, Abman SH. Recent developments in the pathophysiology and treatment of persistent pulmonary hypertension of the newborn. *J Pediatr.* 1995;126:853–864.
71. Dakshinamurti S. Pathophysiologic mechanisms of persistent pulmonary hypertension of the newborn. *Paediatr Pulmonol Suppl.* 2005;39:492–503.
72. Hernandez-Diaz S, Van Marter LJ, Werler MM, et al. Risk factors for persistent pulmonary hypertension of the newborn. *Pediatrics.* 2007;120:e272–e282.
73. Ostrea EM, Villanueva-Uy ET, Natarajan G, et al. Persistent pulmonary hypertension of the newborn: pathogenesis, etiology, and management. *Paediatr Drugs.* 2006;8:179–188.
74. Jaillard S, Houfflin-Debarge V, Storme L. Higher risk of persistent pulmonary hypertension of the newborn after cesarean. *J Perinat Med.* 2003;31:538–539.
75. Sasidharan P. An approach to diagnosis and management of cyanosis and tachypnea in term infants. *Pediatr Clin North Am.* 2004;51:999–1021.
76. Berger S, Konduri GG. Pulmonary hypertension in children: the twenty-first century. *Pediatr Clin North Am.* 2006;53:961–987.
77. Konduri GG, Kim UO. Advances in the diagnosis and management of persistent pulmonary hypertension of the newborn. *Pediatr Clin North Am.* 2009;56:579–600.
78. Boden G, Bennett C. The management of persistent pulmonary hypertension of the newborn. *Curr Paediatr.* 2004;14:290–297.
79. Roberts JD, Fineman JR, Morin FC, et al. Inhaled nitric oxide and persistent pulmonary hypertension of the newborn. *N Engl J Med.* 1997;336:605–610.
80. American Academy of Pediatrics, Committee on Fetus and Newborn. Use of inhaled nitric oxide. *Pediatrics.* 2000;106:344–345.
81. Steinhorn RH. Nitric oxide and beyond: new insights and therapies for pulmonary hypertension. *J Perinatol.* 2008;28 (suppl 3):S67–S71.
82. Baquero H, Soliz A, Neira F, et al. Oral sildenafil in infants with persistent pulmonary hypertension of the newborn. *Pediatrics.* 2006;117:1077–1083.
83. Steinhorn RH, Kinsella JP, Pierce C, et al. Intravenous sildenafil in the treatment of neonates with persistent pulmonary hypertension. *J Pediatr.* 2009;155:841–847.
84. Betit P, Craig N. Extracorporeal membrane oxygenation for neonatal respiratory failure. *Respir Care.* 2009;54:1244–1251.
85. Slevin M, Farrington N, Duffy G, et al. Altering the NICU and measuring the infants' responses. *Acta Paediatrica.* 2007;89:577–581.
86. Clugston RD, Greer JJ. Diaphragm development and congenital diaphragmatic hernia. *Semin Pediatr Surg.* 2007;16:94–100.
87. Rottier R, Tibboel D. Fetal lung and diaphragm development in congenital diaphragmatic hernia. *Semin Perinatol.* 2005;29:86–93.
88. Bohn D. Congenital diaphragmatic hernia. *Am J Respir Crit Care Med.* 2002;166:911–915.
89. Chess PR. The effect of gentle ventilation on survival in congenital diaphragmatic hernia. *Pediatrics.* 2004;113:917.
90. Logan J, Cotten CM, Goldberg RN, et al. Mechanical ventilation strategies in the management of congenital diaphragmatic hernia. *Semin Pediatr Surg.* 2007;16:115–125.

91. Carlo WA. Permissive hypercapnia and permissive hypoxemia in neonates. *J Perinatol.* 2007;27:S64–S70.
92. Cacciari A, Ruggeri G, Mordenti M, et al. High-frequency oscillatory ventilation versus conventional mechanical ventilation in congenital diaphragmatic hernia. *Eur J Pediatr Surg.* 2001;11:3–7.
93. Finer NN, Barrington KJ. Nitric oxide for respiratory failure in infants born at or near term. *Cochrane Database Syst Rev.* 2001;4:CD000399.
94. Bryner BS, West BT, Hirschl RB, et al. Congenital diaphragmatic hernia requiring extracorporeal membrane oxygenation: does timing of repair matter? *J Pediatr Surg.* 2009;44:1165–1171.
95. Datin-Dorriere V, Walter-Nicolet E, Rousseau V, et al. Experience in the management of eighty-two newborns with congenital diaphragmatic hernia treated with high-frequency oscillatory ventilation and delayed surgery without the use of extracorporeal membrane oxygenation. *J Intensive Care Med.* 2008;23:128–135.
96. Bosenberg AT, Brown RA. Management of congenital diaphragmatic hernia. *Curr Opin Anaesthesiol.* 2008;21:323–331.
97. St. Peter SD, Valusek PA, Tsao K, et al. Abdominal complication related to type of repair of congenital diaphragmatic hernia. *J Surg Res.* 2007;140:234–236.
98. Cortes RA, Keller RL, Townsend T, et al. Survival of severe congenital diaphragmatic hernia has morbid consequences. *J Pediatr Surg.* 2005;40:36–45.
99. Gucciardo L, Deprest J, Done E, et al. Prediction of outcome in isolated congenital diaphragmatic hernia and its consequences for fetal therapy. *Best Pract Res Clin Obstet Gynaecol.* 2008;22:123–138.
100. Chiu PP, Sauer C, Mihailovic A. The price of success in the management of congenital diaphragmatic hernia: is improved survival accompanied by an increase in long-term morbidity? *J Pediatr Surg.* 2006;41:888–892.
101. Mirosh MD, Hayes B, Payton N. 187 risk factors associated with respiratory distress in term neonates with and without air leak. *Pediatr Res.* 2004;56:496.
102. Watkinson M, Tiron I. Events before the diagnosis of a pneumothorax. *Arch Dis Child Fetal Neonatal Ed.* 2001;85:F201–F203.
103. Litmanovitz I, Carlo W. Expectant management of pneumothorax in ventilated neonates. *Pediatrics.* 2008;122:e975–e979.
104. Phatak RS, Pairaudeau CF, Smith CJ, et al. Heliox with inhaled nitric oxide: a novel strategy for severe localized interstitial pulmonary emphysema in preterm neonatal ventilation. *Respir Care.* 2008;53:1731–1738.
105. Jabra AA, Fishman EK, Shehata BM, Perlman EJ. Localized persistent pulmonary interstitial emphysema: CT findings with radiographic-pathologic correlation. *Am J Roentgenol.* 1997;169:1381.
106. Clark RH, Gerstman DR, Null DM, et al. Pulmonary interstitial emphysema treated by high frequency oscillatory ventilation. *Crit Care Med.* 1986;14:926–930.
107. Schwartz AN, Graham CB. Neonatal tension pulmonary interstitial emphysema in bronchopulmonary dysplasia: treatment with lateral decubitus positioning. *Radiology.* 1986;16:351–354.
108. Chalek LF, Kaiser JR, Arrington RW. Resolution of pulmonary interstitial emphysema following selective left main stem intubation in a premature newborn: an old procedure revisited. *Paediatr Anesth.* 2007;17:183–186.
109. Fitzgerald D, Willis D, Usher R. Dexamethasone for pulmonary interstitial emphysema in preterm infants. *Biol Neonate.* 1998;73:34–39.
110. Bejvan SM, Godwin JD. Pneumomediastinum: old signs and new signs. *Am J Roentgenol.* 1996;166:1041–1048.
111. Carey BE. Neonatal air leaks: pneumothorax, pneumomediastinum, pulmonary interstitial emphysema, pneumopericardium. *Neonatal Netw.* 1999;18:81–84.
112. National Eye Institute. Retinopathy of prematurity. Available at: http://www.nei.nig.gov/health/rop/index.asp. Accessed January 23, 2010.
113. Terry TL. Extreme prematurity and fibroplastic overgrowth of persistent vascular sheath behind each crystalline lens. Preliminary report. *Am J Ophthalmol.* 1942;25:203–204.
114. Campbell K. Intensive oxygen therapy as a possible cause for retrolental fibroplasia: a clinical approach. *Med J Austr.* 1951;2:48–50.
115. Patz A, Hoeck L, DeLaCruz E. Studies on the effect of high oxygen administration in retrolental fibroplasia: nursery observations. *Am J Ophthalmol.* 1952;35:1248–1253.
116. Wheatley CM, Dickinson JL, Mackey DA, et al. Retinopathy of prematurity: recent advances in our understanding. *Arch Dis Child Fetal Neonatal Ed.* 2002;87:F78–F82.
117. Forrester JV, Dick AD, McMenamin PG, et al. Embryology and early development of the eye and adnexa. In: Forrester JV, Dick AD, McMenamin PG, et al., eds. *The Eye: Basic Sciences in Practice.* Philadelphia: Elsevier; 2002:99–113.
118. Holmstrom G, van Wijngaarden P, Coster DJ, et al. Genetic susceptibility to retinopathy of prematurity: the evidence from clinical and experimental animal studies. *Br J Ophthalmol.* 2007;91:1704–1708.
119. Karna P, Muttineni J, Angell L, et al. Retinopathy of prematurity and risk factors: a prospective cohort study. *BMC Pediatr.* 2007;26:371–378.
120. Harrell SN, Brandon DH. Retinopathy of prematurity: the disease process, classifications, screening, treatment, and outcomes. *Neonatal Netw.* 2007;26:371–378.
121. Section on Ophthalmology, American Academy of Pediatrics; American Academy of Ophthalmology; American Association for Pediatric Ophthalmology and Strabismus. Screening examination of premature infants for retinopathy of prematurity. *Pediatrics.* 2006;572–576.
122. International Committee for the Classification of Retinopathy of Prematurity. The international classification of retinopathy of prematurity revisited. *Arch Ophthalmol.* 2005;123:991–999.
123. DiBiasie A. Evidence-based review of retinopathy of prematurity prevention in VLBW and ELBW infants. *Neonatal Netw.* 2006;25:393–403.
124. Quiram PA, Capone A Jr. Current understanding and management of retinopathy of prematurity. *Curr Opin Ophthalmol.* 2007;18:228–234.
125. Good WV, Hardy RJ, Dobson V, et al. The incidence and course of retinopathy of prematurity: findings from the early treatment for retinopathy of prematurity study. *Pediatrics.* 2005;116:15–23.
126. Shay DK, Holman RC, Newman RD, et al. Bronchiolitis-associated hospitalizations among US children 1980–1996. *JAMA.* 1999;282:1440–1446.
127. Hall CB. Respiratory syncytial virus and parainfluenza virus. *N Engl J Med.* 2001;344:1917–1928.
128. Zorc JJ, Hall CB. Bronchiolitis: recent evidence on diagnosis and management. *Pediatrics.* 2010;125:342–349.
129. Karr CJ, Demers PA, Koehoorn MW, et al. Influence of ambient air pollutant sources on clinical encounters for infant bronchiolitis. *Am J Respir Crit Care Med.* 2009;180:995–1001.
130. Schuh S, Lalani A, Allen U, et al. Evaluation of the utility of radiography in acute bronchiolitis. *J Pediatr.* 2007;150:429–433.
131. Cheney J, Barber S, Altamirano L, et al. A clinical pathway for bronchiolitis is effective in reducing readmission rates. *J Pediatr.* 2005;147:622–626.
132. Wilson SD, Dahl BB, Wells RD. An evidence-based clinical pathway for bronchiolitis safely reduces antibiotic overuse. *Am J Med Qual.* 2002;17:195–199.
133. American Academy of Pediatrics, Subcommittee on Diagnosis and Management of Bronchiolitis. Clinical practice guide-

lines: diagnosis and management of bronchiolitis. *Pediatrics.* 2006;118:1774–1793.
134. Cade A, Brownlee KG, Conway SP, et al. Randomised placebo controlled trial of nebulised corticosteroids in acute respiratory syncytial viral bronchiolitis. *Arch Dis Child.* 2000;82:126–130.
135. Kuzik BA, Al Quadhi SA, Kent S, et al. Nebulized hypertonic saline in the treatment of viral bronchiolitis. *J Pediatr.* 2007;151:266–270.
136. Taber LH, Knight V, Gilbert BE, et al. Ribavirin aerosol treatment of bronchiolitis associated with respiratory syncytial virus infection in infants. *Pediatrics.* 1983;72:613–618.
137. Synagis (palivizumab) [package insert]. Full prescribing information. Gaithersburg, MD: MedImmune LLC; 2008.
138. Stein RT. Early-life viral bronchiolitis in the causal pathway of childhood asthma: is the evidence there yet? *Am J Respir Crit Care Med.* 2008;178:1097–1098.
139. Jartti T, Makela MJ, Vanto T, et al. The link between bronchiolitis and asthma. *Infect Dis Clin North Am.* 2005;19:667–689.
140. Kercsmar CM. Current trends in neonatal and pediatric respiratory care: conference summary. *Respir Care.* 2003;48:459–464.
141. Rotta AT, Wiryawan B. Respiratory emergencies in children. *Respir Care.* 2003;48:248–260.
142. Lavine E. Scolnik D. Lack of efficacy of humidification in the treatment of croup: why do physicians persist in using an unproven modality? *CJEM.* 2001;3:209–212.
143. Fitzgerald DA. The assessment and management of croup. *Paediatr Respir Rev.* 2006;7:73–81.
144. Myers TR. Use of heliox in children. *Respir Care.* 2006; 51:619–361.
145. Custer JR. Croup and related disorders. *Pediatr Rev.* 1993;14:19–29.
146. Sobol SE, Zapata S. Epiglottitis and croup. *Otolaryngol Clin North Am.* 2008;41:551– 566.
147. Glynn F, Fenton JE. Diagnosis and management of supraglottitis (epiglottitis). *Curr Infect Dis Rep.* 2008;10:200–204.
148. Centers for Disease Control and Prevention. Progress toward eliminating *Haemophilus influenzae* type b disease among infants and children—United States, 1977–1997. *MMWR.* 1998;47:993–998.

SECTION IV

Applied Sciences for Respiratory Care

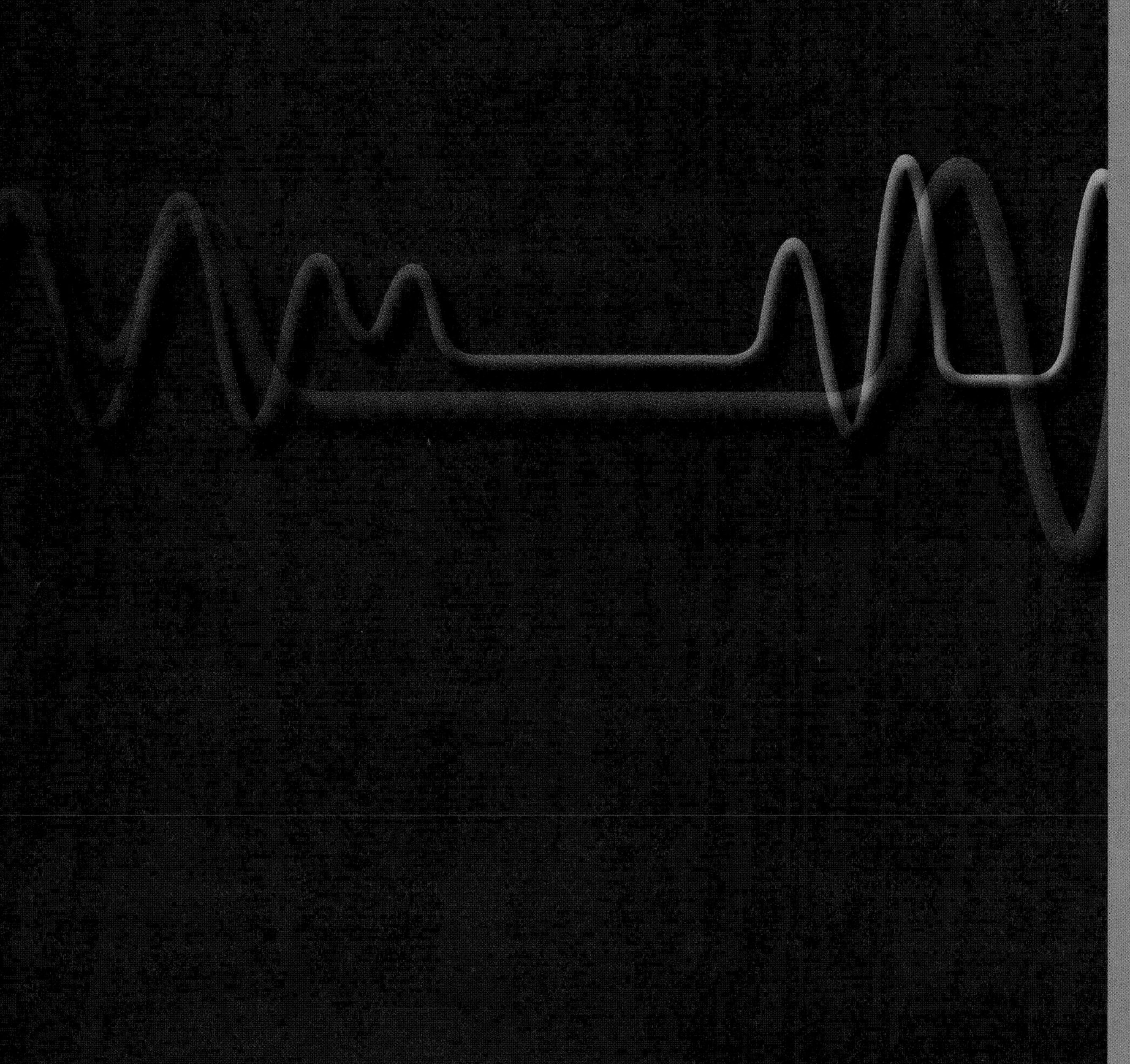

CHAPTER 49

Respiratory Care Research

Alexander B. Adams

OUTLINE

Design Factors
Statistical Issues
Study Types

OBJECTIVES

1. Describe and explain the purposes of study design factors.
2. Emphasize key points about statistics used in research.
3. Describe the types of medical study reports.

KEY TERMS

Bland-Altman plot
blinding
case control studies
case report
case series
cohort studies
continuous variable
correlation coefficients
crossover study
cross-sectional studies
descriptive statistics
incidence
inferential statistics
informed consent
institutional review board (IRB)
interventional study
Kaplan-Meier plot
matching
noncontinuous variables
observational study
prevalence
prospective studies
randomization
randomized controlled trial (RCT)
regression analysis
retrospective studies
standard deviation (SD)
surveys
type I error
type II error

INTRODUCTION

Advancements in the profession of respiratory care have been driven by supportive research. The practice of respiratory care is firmly based on principles described in other chapters of this text and on reports from research studies published in the medical literature. Uniquely, respiratory care has developed in parallel with advancements in pulmonary medicine, critical care, and technical devices. Research in respiratory care is reported in journals such as *Respiratory Care, Critical Care Medicine, Chest, American Journal of Respiratory and Critical Care Medicine,* and *Intensive Care Medicine.* To critically assess the investigations reported in these journals, a framework for evaluating their relevancy includes knowledge of design factors, basic statistics issues, and study types.

Design Factors

A number of factors must be considered when designing studies to answer research questions. To evaluate studies critically, a reader must be able to understand the purposes of study design factors. The methods section of a study report should address the general design issues, such as the number of study subjects, the study design factors, data collection methods, and a data analysis plan. As the study design is detailed in the methods section, a study's strengths and limitations should become apparent. The conclusions should be based on the study's success at answering the primary research questions within the constraints of the study design. The following are brief discussions of important design factors and other general study issues.

Controls

Study participants who do not receive the new treatment but receive instead the usual treatment, a placebo, or a sham treatment are the controls. A new treatment will be judged effective if it performs better in the treatment group than in the control group. Controls are studied in the same manner as the treatment group to guard against the investigators tricking themselves (or the public) into believing a new therapy is effective when nontherapy might be similar or safer or less costly.

Within the Acute Respiratory Distress Syndrome Network (ARDSnet) series of controlled studies of patients with acute respiratory distress syndrome (ARDS), treatment with ketoconozole,[1] methylprednisolone,[2] or lisophylline[3] did not reduce mortality in ARDS patients compared with controls. Even in carefully controlled studies, the syndrome or cases under study must be specifically defined, or findings from the report may not be conclusive. ARDS and sepsis have broad definitions that represent several routes to their current diagnostic definitions. For example, subgroups of ARDS patients might be responsive to methylprednisone in spite of the lack of benefit found in the large controlled ARDSnet trial.[2] In addition, one controlled study alone may provide evidence for an effect (or no effect), but one study alone will rarely prove the overall effectiveness or ineffectiveness of a therapy.

Matching

Controls must be similar, in most respects, to the treatment group. **Matching** may be necessary to prevent other factors (than the new treatment) from confounding or confusing the study results. For example, controls must not be allowed to enter a study sicker than the treatment group members, or the results may favor the treatment group for that reason. A common method of matching illness severity in critical care studies is to enroll patients with similar illness severity into the treatment and control groups. The APACHE (Acute Physiology and Chronic Health Evaluation) scoring system is used to quantify illness severity by assigning "severity" points to 12 routine physiologic measurements.[4] If treatment and control groups are well matched in APACHE scores, then differences between groups in results (positive, negative, or no difference) should be due to the treatment.

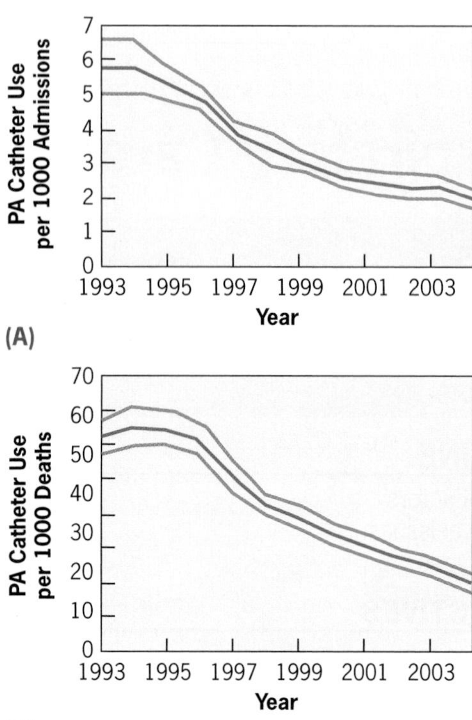

FIGURE 49–1 Pulmonary artery (PA) catheter use rate declined in all medical patients (**A**) and in medical patients who died (**B**) as studies revealed the increased risks and resources involved with PA catheter use. Blue lines indicate PA catheters placed per 1000 patients, and orange lines indicate 95% confidence intervals around the annual rate. From Wiener RS, Welch HG. Trends in the use of the pulmonary artery catheter in the United States, 1993–2004. *JAMA*. 2007;298:423–429. Reprinted with permission.

In a study reported in the *Journal of the American Medical Association* (*JAMA*) from 1996, elaborate matching of 5735 critically ill patients in nine disease categories found that pulmonary artery (PA) catheterization or Swan-Ganz catheter use was associated with increased mortality and increased use of resources.[5] Follow-up studies have supported this finding, and the use of PA catheterization has decreased since the original *JAMA* report (**Figure 49–1**).[6,7]

Randomization

To achieve a balance (similar patients, similar status) between treatment and control group members and to avoid investigator bias, a **randomization** process is used after enrollment to assign the patient to either the treatment or control limb of a study. This process can be completed by a simple coin flip or, preferably, by randomization software that is readily available via the Internet.[8]

Randomization is seemingly simple but potentially complex because a bias can be suspected when groups are not well matched if a truly random process for assigning treatment is not guaranteed. For example, with an assured randomization process in the ALVEOLI study of ARDS, patients were assigned to treatment groups using either a high or low positive end-expiratory pressure (PEEP). An unlucky randomization occurred because the high-PEEP group was 4 years older on average than the low-PEEP group, and age (as a factor) increases mortality in ARDS.[9] However, because the effect of age on ARDS mortality has been previously estimated, the results were statistically adjusted to account for this bad-luck randomization problem. Nevertheless, no statistical difference in mortality was found between the two PEEP strategies,[9] a finding that remains controversial.

RESPIRATORY RECAP

Design Factors for Avoiding Potential Investigator Biases

- » Controls
- » Matching
- » Randomization
- » Blinding
- » Crossover

Blinding or Masking

Whenever possible, investigators and participants should be unaware of the treatment being delivered (i.e., be blinded). If investigators or participants know who is receiving treatment, they might be able to affect the study outcome, even subconsciously, in a preferred direction. This tendency to alter a study is well known, and **blinding** can prevent this possible influence on the results. When both investigators and participants are blinded, the study is said to be *double blinded*. When the participants alone are unaware of their treatment status, the study is *single blinded*. For example, in medication studies, a new drug and the placebo are dispensed in coded bottles containing tablets that are identical in appearance and taste. Both the investigators and participants are unaware of, or blinded to, the real drug bottle and tablets. The bottles will be decoded by an independent investigator after the results are collected. Drug studies are frequently double blinded, whereas treatment studies usually cannot easily blind the investigators; however, the participants can often be blinded. A sham or fake treatment, like a placebo, can be administered to blind the study participants. Patients and investigators are usually unblinded or unmasked after the study is completed.

In a study of a new use for a medication, activated protein C (APC), a potent anti-inflammatory agent used in patients with sepsis, was tested in acute lung injury (ALI) patients. In this double-blinded, randomized, controlled study of 75 ALI patients who did not have sepsis, APC was unable to reduce mortality rates or increase ventilator-free days.[10] In a different study that blinded the participants only, volunteers judged the comfort of three ventilator modes. The use of a synchronized intermittent mandatory ventilation (SIMV) mode was associated with ventilator asynchrony and was rated uncomfortable by the volunteers blinded to the ventilator mode being tested.[11] The clinical relevance of this study is debatable because comfort has not been directly associated with other primary outcome variables such as mortality or ventilator-free days.

Crossover

As a method of matching controls to study patients and designing a more efficient study by reducing the number of subjects by 50%, the same patient can be assigned to both the treatment and control groups if the patient can cross over between therapies during the study. In a **crossover study**, the age, gender, disease state, and entire patient history are, of course, identical for both study limbs. The sequencing of the treatment-to-control or control-to-treatment crossover can be randomized or alternated, or, if possible, the participant can cross over back to the original therapy (double crossover) to avoid a sequencing effect.

As an example, in a controlled, randomized, blinded crossover study,[12] patients were ventilated with high-frequency oscillation (HFO) for 60 minutes without and then combined with tracheal gas insufflation (TGI) in random order. The sessions were repeated in inverse order within 24 hours. With the TGI-HFO combination, oxygenation improved and 28-day mortality was decreased. A study of the possible mechanisms for this effect seems warranted. In another crossover study that delivered sine-wave and triangular-wave high-frequency chest wall oscillation waveforms to 15 cystic fibrosis patients, airway clearance of mucus did not differ between the waveforms.[13] However, there was a reduction in air trapping and an increase in cough transportability with the use of the triangular waveform. A follow-up study of the secondary findings might be justified.

Observational Versus Interventional

An **observational study** does not change current practice but simply observes activities or results. Observational studies can be useful to report problems or to provide indices for quality assurance monitoring (e.g., timeliness of therapy or compliance with orders). Chart reviews are observational. Privacy rights must be considered even when reviewing charts or observing activities. External observations or reviews cannot be reported (without consent) if the person's identity might be determined by the report. In an observational study in which investigators were hidden, higher hand washing rates were observed for respiratory therapists than physicians or nurses.[14]

RESPIRATORY RECAP

Classification of Studies

- » Observational or interventional
- » Retrospective or prospective

An **interventional study** involves a change in care that is ordered by a physician with approval by the patient or relative via informed consent. Studies of major questions such as setting a safe tidal volume or a best PEEP require carefully planned interventions that are administered under tightly controlled conditions.

Prospective and Retrospective

Prospective studies are to be conducted in the future, whereas **retrospective studies** look back at records to analyze what has already happened. Retrospective data are susceptible to cherry picking (choosing the best data available and ignoring contrary data). Retrospective studies can also become fishing expeditions—looking for a discovery. There are no real controls in retrospective studies, but an attempt to match a control group to a cases group can be performed. There are lessons to be learned from retrospective analyses, but prospective studies are preferred because a carefully designed study can avoid most sources of investigator bias. Interventional studies are prospective. The ARDSnet studies of important clinical questions related to the treatment of ALI and ARDS patients have been prospective.[1–3,9,15,16] A number of retrospective analyses and discussions have been reported in association with the ARDSnet data sets because the ARDSnet studies were well controlled, with high compliance to the study protocol.[17–19]

Inclusion and Exclusion Criteria

Before candidates can be entered into or excluded from a study, clearly defined enrollment criteria must be decided upon—the inclusion criteria and exclusion criteria. In addition, conditions should be stated that would withdraw a patient from a study. Enrollment will typically require that patients are restricted to an age range (e.g., older than 16 years), an illness severity level (e.g., ventilated), a diagnosis (e.g., ALI, sepsis, chronic obstructive pulmonary disease [COPD]), or a combination of these. As a standard for studies of ALI, the criteria for enrollment or inclusion of an ALI patient require that the patient have a Pa_{O_2}/F_{IO_2} ratio below 300 mm Hg.[1,2,15] Patients in heart failure have been excluded if they display left atrial enlargement or their pulmonary capillary wedge pressure exceeds 18 mm Hg.[15]

> **RESPIRATORY RECAP**
>
> **Requirements for Conducting a Study**
> - » Inclusion and exclusion criteria
> - » Approval from an IRB
> - » Measurements
> - » Contingencies for dealing with missing values

Institutional Review Boards and Informed Consent

Human studies that are interventional must be approved by an **institutional review board (IRB)** before they can be conducted. The IRB is a committee of qualified, interested individuals who are often researchers. The IRB approves studies to ensure that participants are well informed of the possible risks of a new treatment, to assess whether the investigators are capable of conducting the study, and to judge whether the study has a reasonable probability of answering the study question. The IRB approves the **informed consent** form that must be signed by the patient, relative, or guardian to approve the participant's entry into the treatment or control group. As previously stated, retrospective or chart review studies may also require IRB approval if there is a risk of revealing a patient's identity by the reporting of results. Generally, most studies require IRB approval.

Measurements

The measured variables of prime interest in a study will, preferably, be common parameters (e.g., mortality, ventilator-free days, Pa_{O_2}, infection rates) with known degrees of accuracy and variability. The measurements must be part of an analysis plan that will be used to answer the study question. This plan also estimates a minimum number of participants (the sample size determination) required to obtain statistically significant results.

Incidence and Prevalence

Incidence is the number of new cases of a disease contracted or diagnosed in a given time period, usually a year. **Prevalence** is the number of individuals in a given population who have the disease or condition at a given time. The importance of these terms becomes relevant in studies of acute and chronic diseases. For example, approximately 40,000 deaths are caused by influenza each year in the United States.[20] Although millions may be contracting flu each year (the cases), the incidence of death due to the flu—the case fatality ratio—is the important metric for evaluating the severity of the influenza season each year. For chronic disease management, the prevalence rate measures the continuing burden of that disease on the healthcare system. For example, there are an estimated 13 million COPD patients in the United States, a prevalence associated with cigarette smoking that explains why COPD is the fourth leading cause of death.[21] Incidence and prevalence studies fall within the field of epidemiology, the branch of medicine involved with the transmission and control of diseases.

> **RESPIRATORY RECAP**
>
> **Incidence Versus Prevalence**
> - » *Incidence* is the number of new cases and usually refers to acute diseases.
> - » *Prevalence* is the number of people who currently have the disease and is a measure of chronic disease.

Missing Values and Dropouts

Even the best-designed studies conducted by meticulous investigators have problems with missing values or dropouts or both, because complete acquisition of clean data in any study is unusual. Fortunately, if there is no particular pattern to the missing values, they can be disregarded; if a pattern exists, statistical adjustments can be made to account for this problem. Studies over time (longitudinal studies) will frequently have missing data due to patients lost to follow-up.

A dropout rate can be a positive finding; for example, liberation from ventilator support is a success, as displayed in **Figure 49–2**.[22] The plot in this figure clearly shows that the use of a therapist-driven weaning protocol reduces ventilator hours when compared with the usual nonprotocolized weaning method. This type of graph, a **Kaplan-Meier plot**, is most often used to analyze survival rates in mortality studies. The Kaplan-Meier curves in **Figure 49–3** display mortality caused by lung cancer according to high or low depressive coping. The overall low survival rates in lung cancer have been strongly associated with cigarette smoking, and the coping behavior connection with survival may result from differing physical conditions rather than a beneficial psychological makeup such as high depressive coping.

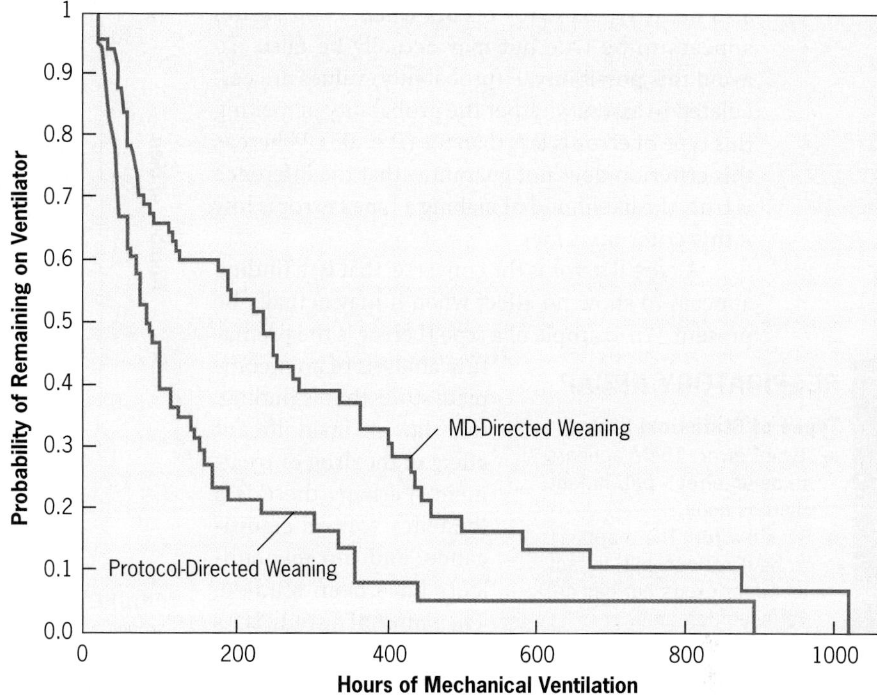

FIGURE 49–2 Kaplan-Meier analysis of the duration of mechanical ventilation after adjustment for the severity of illness at baseline (as measured by the APACHE II score), age, sex, race, location of the intensive care unit, and duration of intubation before enrollment. Mechanical ventilation was discontinued more rapidly in the therapist-driven protocol group than in the control group. From Ely EW, Baker AM, Dunagan DP, et al. Effect on the duration of mechanical ventilation of identifying patients capable of breathing spontaneously. *N Engl J Med.* 1996;335:1864–1869. © 1996 Massachusetts Medical Society. All rights reserved.

Statistical Issues

Statistics can be complex, and knowledge of statistics is essential to thoroughly evaluate the merit of research reports. Although there is no substitute for learning statistics in an organized program of study, the following are pointers that can aid in interpreting the statistical methods used in a study.

- Consider the purpose of the statistical analysis. **Descriptive statistics**, such as means with standard deviations of obtained variables, are often presented to provide an overview of the measurements from the study. Figures such as histograms, line graphs, scatter plots, and tables will display the data more clearly than descriptions within the narrative of the text. Statistics used to answer the study questions (i.e., to accept or reject the hypotheses) are known as **inferential statistics**, which require significance testing. A statistically significant result *infers* that the results can be applied to other settings (i.e., beyond the study itself).
- There are two important types of statistical errors (type I and type II errors) that can be committed when drawing conclusions from significance testing. The primary goal of statistics is to provide data to argue that a study has identified a truth that can be applied to other settings, but statistics can

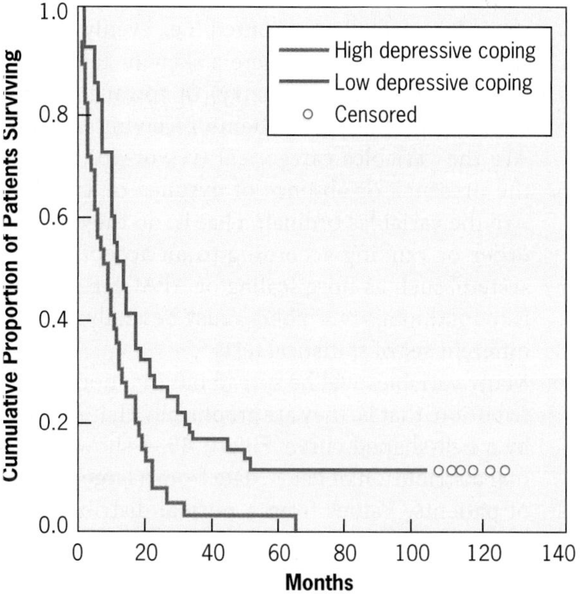

FIGURE 49–3 Kaplan-Meier survival curves showing probability of mortality over a 10-year follow-up period in lung cancer patients with high and low levels of depressive coping. From Faller H, Bülzebruck H. Coping and survival in lung cancer: a 10-year follow-up. *Am J Psychiatry.* 2002;159:2105–2107. Reprinted with permission from the *American Journal of Psychiatry*. Copyright © 2002 American Psychiatric Association.

also lie. A **type I error** occurs when a conclusion appears to be true but may actually be false. To avoid this possibility, *P* (probability) values are calculated to assess whether the probability of making this type of error is less than 5% ($P < .05$). Whereas this criterion does not guarantee that the inference is true, the likelihood of making a type I error is low if this criterion is met.

A **type II error** is the converse; that is, a finding appears to show no effect when it may actually be present. An example of a type II error is the premature analysis of an incomplete study that is finding, thus far, an insignificant effect of the drug or treatment. Perhaps there is a tendency toward significance, and too few subjects have been studied. The *power* of a study is its ability to detect a statistically significant difference between groups using some standard assumptions. Studies are usually powered to have a greater than 80% probability of finding significant results. If a study is negative, the therapy may be ineffective *or* the study may be underpowered (type II error) and more subjects are required to confirm an effect—possibly more subjects than the study can afford to enroll.

RESPIRATORY RECAP

Types of Statistical Errors

» Type I error: There appears to be an effect, but, in fact, there is none.

» Type II error: There appears to be no effect, but, in fact, an effect exists but has not yet been detected.

- Consider the measurements reported in a study. Are they **continuous variables**, such as Pao_2, plateau pressure, cardiac output, or forced expiratory volume in 1 second (FEV_1)? Are the continuous variables normally distributed (i.e., evenly on both sides of the mean)? Is there a skew or tail toward lower values (e.g., oximetry) or toward positive values (e.g., Pao_2 for patients receiving oxygen)? Are the variables categorical (yes-or-no), such as the presence or absence of dyspnea or cyanosis? Are the variables ordinal? That is, do they have an order or ranking according to an accepted scale system, such as Borg scaling or APACHE scoring? **Noncontinuous variables** must be analyzed by a different set of statistical tests.
- Many variables will be spread out in a normal distribution, that is, they are graphically characterized by a bell-shaped curve. **Figure 49–4** shows a normal distribution of $Paco_2$ data from a large number of patients. Values from a normal distribution of $Paco_2$ values have an average, or *mean*, of 40 mm Hg, displayed by the peak in the center. The dispersion of values about the mean is quantified by the **standard deviation (SD)**, where ±1 SD encompasses 68% of the values, ±2 SD encompasses 95% of the values, and ±3 SD encompasses 99% of the values. The *median* is defined as the midvalue where half the values are above and half are below that median; age distributions are often described by medians. The *mode* is the most frequent value; categorical and ordinal data are often described by modes. The mean, median, and mode are the same value in a normal distribution but differ when the data are skewed (i.e., there is a tail in the positive or negative direction). Depending on a variable's distribution, either a mean, median, or mode may best characterize the data.

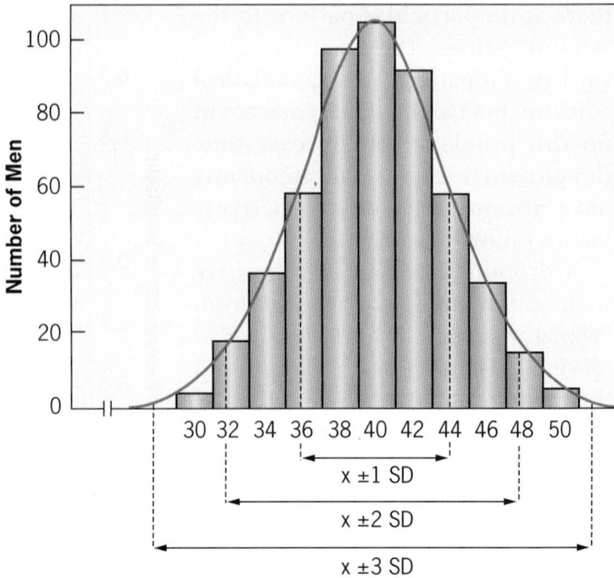

FIGURE 49–4 A normal frequency distribution of $Paco_2$ values around a mean of 40 mm Hg. The values are distributed about the mean in a bell shape. The standard deviation (SD) defines the width of the bell, with ±1 SD including 68% of the values, ±2 SD encompassing 95%, and ±3 SD encompassing 99% of the values.

- Associations are frequently the major findings from a study. **Correlation coefficients** indicate whether associations exist (+1 = positive or direct, −1= negative or indirect, 0 = no relationship). A **regression analysis** can definitively quantify the strength of the association or associations. For example, age and FEV_1 are negatively correlated, but **Figure 49–5** shows that FEV_1 declines about 20 to 25 mL for every year that we age. The measurement and interpretation of associations often require a statistician's assistance. Unfortunately, associations can be deceptive and may not tell us about causality. The classic example is the direct association between the number of churches in a city and the city's crime rate. Instead of concluding that churches cause crime, one must consider that the number of churches and crimes committed in a city are both associated with city size. Reports of associations should be further supported by reasonable causes for the associations or other supportive data, or both.
- Understand instrument evaluations. Respiratory therapists rely on measurements from monitors and instruments, and their accuracy is of

considerable interest. A new measurement instrument or method is frequently compared to the current gold standard instrument to assess its potential usefulness. A **Bland-Altman plot** is often used to display the values obtained by each method, easily illustrating the average differences (bias) and the variability (standard deviation of the differences) between the new and old instruments. In **Figure 49–6**, Bland-Altman plots display comparisons between CO_2 readings from arterial blood ($Paco_2$) and readings from a transcutaneous CO_2 monitor and an end-tidal CO_2 monitor.[23] The bias or average difference between the $Paco_2$ and transcutaneous values was +5.6 mm Hg, whereas the mean end-tidal CO_2 difference was −14.1 mm Hg. Variability of the differences was not great (3.4 and 7.4 mm Hg, respectively); therefore, the devices may be able to track $Paco_2$ changes while taking into account the bias. Bland-Altman plots also provide an easy way to evaluate where the devices differ (i.e., at higher or lower values).

- Be wary of multiple comparisons. As studies become more complex, several variables are frequently tested to detect any possible significant effects between the variables of interest. When a number of comparisons are made there is an increased risk of discovering chance relationships that may not be real. Statistical testing can be adjusted or changed to reduce this possibility. For example, if 20 factors are studied to assess weanability, one factor can be expected to be positive *due to chance* if the common criterion of $P < .05$ is used to define significance. Lowering the P value by a factor related to the number of comparisons will reduce the risk of this error.
- Understand statistical packages and methods. Simple calculations of means and standard deviations can be readily performed by available spreadsheets, as can the creation of figures. Meaningful inferential statistics must be calculated with the use of statistical packages such as SAS, SPSS, or R.[24] Increasingly, a statistician is becoming a critical member of the investigative team, and the statistician deserves coauthorship on most study reports.

The statistical findings with inferences often define the importance of a study. Ultimately, the importance of a study may not depend on the statistics but on the clinical relevance of the findings. Although an effect measured in a study may be statistically significant, it may

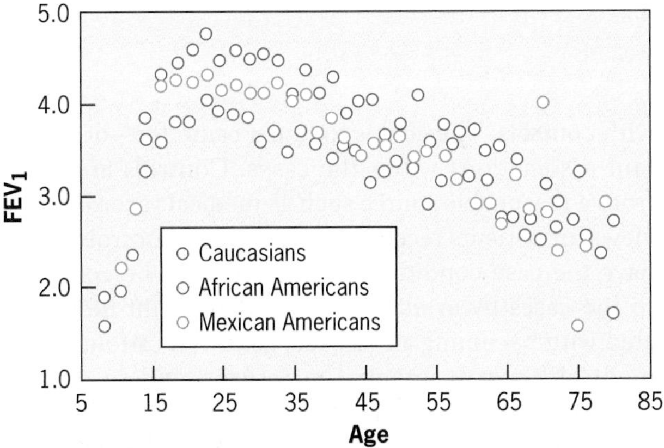

FIGURE 49–5 The association or regression of FEV_1 (y axis) with age (x axis) for men. Reprinted with permission of the American Thoracic Society. Copyright © American Thoracic Society. Modified from Hankinson JL, Odencrantz JR, Fedan KB. Spirometric reference values from a sample of the general U.S. population. *Am J Respir Crit Care Med.* 1999;159:179–187. Official Journal of the American Thoracic Society; Diane Gern, Publisher.

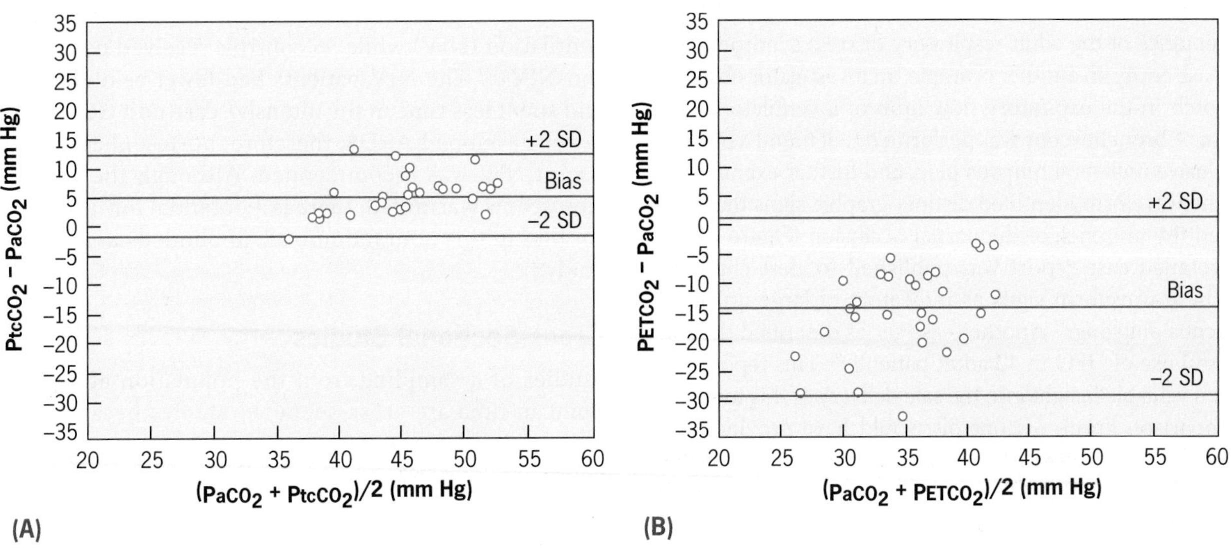

FIGURE 49–6 Bland-Altman plots of comparisons between $Paco_2$ and Pco_2 measured by a transcutaneous CO_2 monitor (**A**) and an end-tidal CO_2 monitor (**B**). The transcutaneous CO_2 monitor overestimates $Paco_2$, whereas the end-tidal CO_2 monitor underestimates $Paco_2$. From Stein N, et al. An evaluation of a transcutaneous and an end-tidal capnometer for noninvasive monitoring of spontaneously breathing patients. *Respir Care.* 2006;51:1162–1166. Reprinted with permission.

have minor clinical importance. In contrast, a small but statistically significant reduction in mortality can justify approval of a major new cardiovascular drug. Therefore, a reader must judge a study's relevance after considering the author's discussion and the overall relevance of the study for improving patient care.

Study Types

Case Reports and Case Series

A detailed description of an unusual, interesting case is known as a **case report**. Case reports can describe a condition that may be rare or an unusual treatment, or the report may make specific instructional points about a diagnostic procedure or therapy. Case reports do not provide data for testing of hypotheses. For example, an original case report in 1956 described a sleepy, overweight man who fell asleep after being dealt a full house in a poker game.[25] The report described his condition as Pickwickian syndrome based on a morbidly obese boy in a Charles Dickens novel, *The Pickwick Papers*. This case report was one of the original descriptions of obstructive sleep apnea syndrome—a current epidemic in the United States.

> **RESPIRATORY RECAP**
>
> **Case Reports and Case Series**
>
> » Case reports and case series are effective ways of reporting unusual observations or unique treatments, or emphasizing instructional points.

A **case series** will compile several cases to discuss a set of common signs or symptoms to describe a syndrome or to further characterize cases or a treatment. The expectation is that reports of cases or a case series will lead to studies that further clarify the disease, syndrome, or its treatment. Twelve severe lung injury cases were described by Thomas Petty in the journal *The Lancet* in 1970.[26] The common features of these patients led to an acceptance of the adult respiratory distress syndrome as a disease entity. In another example, an investigator observed a notch in the expiratory flow limb of a ventilator waveform. A bronchoscopy was performed that found a partially occlusive unilateral mucous plug, and further examination of the waveform identified distinct graphic signs that indicated the presence of the partial occlusion (**Figure 49–7**). A detailed case report was published to alert clinicians of these waveform signs as indicators of large unilateral mucous plugging.[27] Another case series described the successful use of HFO in 42 adult patients.[28] This report provided valuable insight into the safe delivery of this mode—a comparison group of controls would have provided evidence of effectiveness compared with usual care.

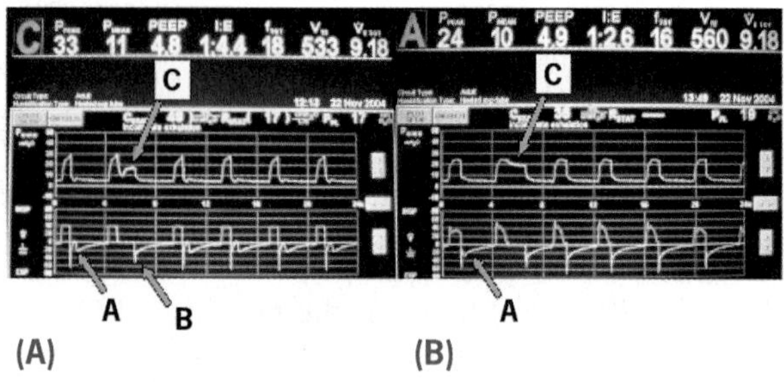

FIGURE 49–7 Airway pressure and flow tracings recorded (**A**) before and (**B**) after bronchoscopy. Arrow A in the prebronchoscopy panel indicates a flow stutter step that attenuates after clearance of plugs after bronchoscopy. Arrow B shows a normal exponential flow decay after a pause prior to bronchoscopy. The C arrows display an unusual rising plateau pressure before bronchoscopy when plugs are present that resolves to a normal plateau pressure display after plug clearance postbronchoscopy.

Case Control Studies

Case control studies, which are often retrospective, involve the accumulation of a number of disease cases that must meet a specific case definition to be compared with controls. The goal is to find a cause for—or important associations with—the cases. Controls are found from a reasonable source such as medical records, interviews, or patients receiving similar care. Controls do not have the case condition, but they should be compared to the cases by available factors that might be associated with becoming a case: age, gender, location, related medical history, potential exposures, and so on. The factors for the cases that the controls do not have are the associations with becoming a case (such as what was eaten or not eaten at a particular event). The associations will characterize the risk factors for becoming a case, but they may not reveal the actual cause or causes. Pathology, microbiology, or biochemical pathway studies are often required to determine causality. Case control studies can involve exhaustive medical record reviews.

In a case control study of esophagectomy patients, 36 consecutive patients (the cases) received noninvasive ventilation (NIV) while 36 controls received usual care (no NIV).[29] The NIV patients had fewer reintubations and spent less time in the intensive care unit (ICU), and fewer developed ARDS; therefore, postesophagectomy use of NIV was recommended. Although the conclusion seems warranted, there is a potential for investigator bias in this nonrandomized, unblinded case control study.

Cross-Sectional Studies

Studies of a sampling from the population at a given point in time are **cross-sectional studies** because they cut across the population. Cross-sectional data are generated by surveying or calculating parameters from existing data sets to determine a case rate (prevalence) or by measuring current values for a specific test or polling opinions. For example, the percentage of the United States population that smoked cigarettes in 2009 was 21% as determined by cross-sectional data from surveys,[30] compared with a 42% rate in 1961. The drop in smoking rates over time helps to explain the recent stabilization in COPD prevalence and lung cancer incidence rates.

Spirometry standards, or normal predicted values according to age, gender, and height, are based on a large cross-sectional study of persons with normal lungs in 1999.[31] This data set was generated by performing spirometry using a standardized technique on 16,000 normal individuals. From this study (HANES III), mean values and regression equations for FEV_1, FEV_6, and vital capacity were determined to become the basis for predicting normal spirometric values (according to one's age, height, and gender). Predicted values would be more confidently based on spirometry testing from the same people as they age throughout their lives—a cohort study.

Cohort Studies

Cohort studies attempt to answer important questions about the cause, treatment, progression, or prevention of a disease. These studies enroll large numbers of participants (the cohort) and follow them over years, even decades. The research team will test, treat, or monitor the cohort with the goal of detecting insights into disease progression and the effects of treatment as the participants age. Cohort studies require a continual effort to track participants. Follow-up is often difficult, and dropouts can be a serious problem. The Scandinavian countries are known for conducting meticulous cohort studies. The Framingham heart studies have followed individuals in Framingham, Massachusetts, (the cohort) over decades to identify factors associated with many diseases, particularly coronary heart disease.[32] The Framingham data have documented the important role of primary care such as cholesterol reduction and blood pressure control in the reduction of cardiovascular disease. In a study of COPD in the Framingham cohort, investigators reported that smoking increases the rate of lung function decline and that quitting smoking has a beneficial effect at any age, but that the benefit is more pronounced in earlier quitters.[33] Although these results seem logical, this type of solid evidence continues to emphasize and confirm the detrimental effects of smoking.

Animal Studies

The use of animals in medical research is controversial, but nearly all significant advancements in medicine have been made possible through discoveries from animal studies. There are strict regulations in the United States governing the use of animals in research to guarantee their humane treatment, including the avoidance of pain or discomfort. Investigators who conduct animal research are monitored by an Animal Care and Use Committee that is directed by *The Guide for the Care and Use of Laboratory Animals*.[34]

To study lung disease, several animal models have been developed to simulate the human diseased state. Models of ARDS (a frequently fatal syndrome) can be caused by oleic acid infusion, high airway pressures or ventilator-induced lung injury, saline lavage to wash out surfactant, or instillation of bacteria to cause a severe pneumonia. The procedures are often 4 to 12 hours in duration and are designed to study pressing critical care questions. Generally, the animals studied most frequently in research are small animals such as mice and rats, while swine or sheep often serve as models for the human cardiopulmonary system. Limiting factors to large animal studies are the short-term nature of the studies and minor anatomic differences from humans; generally, however, their cardiopulmonary physiology is similar to humans. In an animal study of recruitment maneuvers (RM), the effectiveness of three types of lung RMs were tested in three swine injury lung models.[35] Pressure control ventilation (PCV) was superior to sustained inflation at improving oxygenation, and sustained inflation had a greater detrimental effect on cardiac output compared with PCV in the pneumonia model of lung injury (**Figure 49–8**).

Equipment Evaluations

The innovation of industry continues to develop machines and instruments for use in the treatment, monitoring, and diagnosis of illnesses. Devices that are similar to a previously tested device (the predicate device) do not require additional testing and can be marketed as is. But as technology progresses, newly introduced instruments must be compared in some manner to a gold standard measurement, as discussed earlier in the section on statistics. If an equipment evaluation study of a new instrument provides comparable values to the gold standard device or if the instrument is more accurate, more efficient, less expensive, or safer, the instrument will be adopted. Although some comparisons can be made easily in the laboratory, convincing comparisons should be made in the clinical setting to fairly assess the safety and accuracy of the instrument.

> **RESPIRATORY RECAP**
>
> **Equipment Evaluations**
>
> » Equipment that is similar to previous devices can be marketed as is and does not require additional studies.
>
> » New devices are studied by comparing their measures to gold standard measurements from established devices.

Examples of situations in which equipment evaluations have been used follow. When Swan-Ganz catheters are not placed, the cardiac output ($\dot{Q}c$) measure is unavailable but $\dot{Q}c$ is still of interest. Arterial pressure can be deceptive as an indicator of $\dot{Q}c$ if systemic resistance is elevated or changing. Alternative methods of estimating $\dot{Q}c$ by analysis of the arterial pressure waveform[36] or by a partial rebreathing method in ventilated patients[37] have been developed. Evaluations

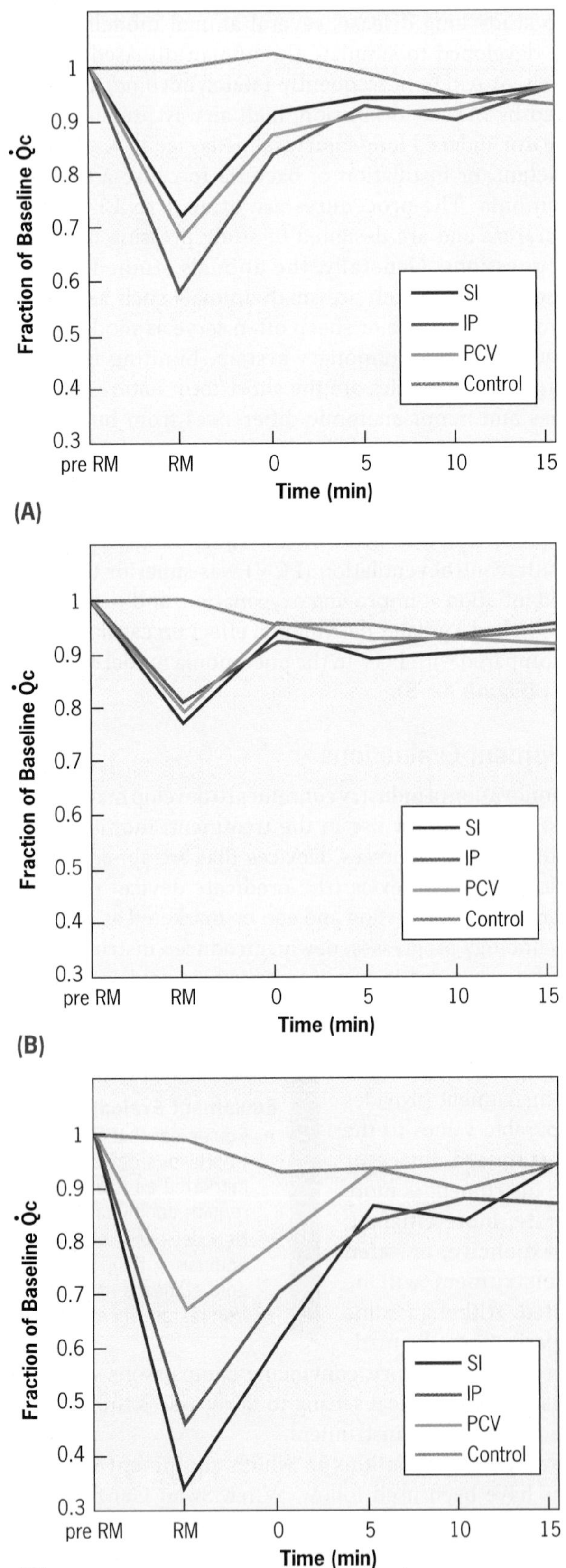

FIGURE 49–8 Oxygenation and cardiac output declines during recruitment maneuvers in (**A**) oleic acid injury (OAI), (**B**) ventilator-induced lung injury (VILI), and (**C**) pneumonia (PNM) injury models. SI, sustained inflation; IP, incremental positive end-expiratory pressure; PCV, pressure control ventilation; control, no recruitment maneuver. From Lim S, et al. Transient hemodynamic effects of recruitment maneuvers in three experimental models of acute lung injury. *Crit Care Med.* 2004;32:2378–2384. Reprinted with permission.

of their accuracy in comparison to the gold standard thermodilution technique have been favorable.[36,37]

An innovative technique for measuring functional residual capacity (FRC) in ventilated patients has become available. Patients with lung injury have a decreased FRC that may be recruitable with PEEP or a specific ventilation strategy, but FRC has been difficult to measure in a ventilated patient. A gas wash-in/washout technique for measuring FRC that is integrated into the ventilator has been favorably evaluated.[38,39] New techniques and machines are often tested, initially, under normal conditions, but their reliability must be determined under abnormal or challenging conditions to learn limitations to their use.

Surveys

Surveys use questionnaires or a set of questions sometimes called an *instrument* to obtain results. A survey goal may be to determine opinions, practice patterns, or purchasing intentions. Surveys or polling can be carefully conducted to be more accurate by using small samples that are highly representative of the target group. Surveys are not interventional. In a survey of clinicians involved with the ARDSnet studies, the investigators attempted to determine barriers to implementing a lung-protective ventilatory strategy.[40] Lung-protective strategies include reduced tidal volume (V_T) settings to reduce pressure exposure. The potentials for tachypnea, discomfort, hypoxemia, and acidosis were important concerns or barriers to implementing a lung-protective or lower-V_T ventilator strategy.[40]

Randomized Controlled Trials

The **randomized controlled trial (RCT)** is the most important type of study of medical interventions in clinical care. Proposed changes in care must undergo the scrutiny of RCTs to investigate a change in treatment or a new treatment in the clinical setting through comparison with the current (or usual) therapy. In the FDA approval process of new medications, phases of an investigational drug are formalized (in phases I through III) to examine a drug's safety, effectiveness, and applicability to human use. Most RCTs are lengthy (1 to 3 years) and expensive and are often investigations of new medications. An RCT is interventional, prospective, randomized, and blinded (if possible), and the treatment group will, it is hoped, randomly match with the control group.

> **RESPIRATORY RECAP**
> **Randomized Controlled Trials**
> » RCTs are the primary means of testing the safety and effectiveness of new medications or therapies.

RCTs conducted within the ARDSnet collaboration of hospitals have produced important discoveries in the treatment of ARDS. This consortium is a disciplined group of investigative teams that have recruited ARDS patients into RCTs to study tidal volume settings, PEEP, fluid resuscitation, and methylprednisone, ketoconazole, and lisophylline use. The first decisive RCT study of 887 ARDS patients found that high VT compared with low VT (12 vs. 6 mL/kg) was associated with increased mortality.[1] In another RCT, 550 patients tested the use of high versus low PEEP and found no difference in mortality between the PEEP settings.[3]

KEY POINTS

- A study design is a plan for conducting the study that avoids bias and attempts to answer the study question or questions.
- Statistics are necessary to describe and display results and to show that the study's conclusions apply elsewhere.
- Studies are reported in a range of formats that reflect the design features and the overall importance of the findings.

REFERENCES

1. The ARDS Network Authors for the ARDS Network. Ketoconazole for early treatment of acute lung injury and acute respiratory distress syndrome. A randomized controlled trial. *JAMA*. 2000;283:1995–2002.
2. Steinberg KP, Hudson LD, Goodman RB, et al. Efficacy and safety of corticosteroids for persistent acute respiratory distress syndrome. *N Engl J Med*. 2006;354(16):1671–1684.
3. The ARDS Clinical Trials Network. Randomized, placebo-controlled trial of lisofylline for early treatment of acute lung injury and acute respiratory distress syndrome. *Crit Care Med*. 2002;30(1):1–6.
4. Knaus WA, Wagner DP, Draper EA, et al. The APACHE III prognostic system. Risk prediction of hospital mortality for critically ill hospitalized adults. *Chest*. 1991;100:1619–1636.
5. Connors AF Jr, Speroff T, Dawson NV, et al. The effectiveness of right heart catheterization in the initial care of critically ill patients. *JAMA*. 1996;276:889–897.
6. Wiener RS, Welch HG. Trends in the use of the pulmonary artery catheter in the United States, 1993–2004. *JAMA*. 2007;298:423–429.
7. Pinsky MR, Vincent JL. Let us use the pulmonary artery catheter correctly and only when we need it. *Crit Care Med*. 2005;33:1119–1122.
8. Institute for Medical Informatics, Statistics and Documentation. Randomizer: web-based patient randomization service for multicenter clinical trials. Available at: http://www.randomizer.at.
9. Brower RG, Lanken PN, MacIntyre NR, et al. Higher versus lower positive end-expiratory pressures in patients with the acute respiratory distress syndrome. *N Engl J Med*. 2004;351:327–336.
10. Liu KD, Levitt J, Zhuo H, et al. Randomized clinical trial of activated protein C for the treatment of acute lung injury. *Am J Respir Crit Care Med*. 2008;178:618–623.
11. Russell WC, Greer JR. The comfort of breathing: a study with volunteers assessing the influence of various modes of assisted ventilation. *Crit Care Med*. 2000;28:3645–3648.
12. Mentzelopoulos SD, Roussos C, Koutsoukou A, et al. Acute effects of combined high-frequency oscillation and tracheal gas insufflation in severe acute respiratory distress syndrome. *Crit Care Med*. 2007;35:1500–1508.
13. Kempainen RR, Williams CB, Hazelwood A, et al. Comparison of high-frequency chest wall oscillation with differing waveforms for airway clearance in cystic fibrosis. *Chest*. 2007;132: 1227–1232.
14. Donowitz LG. Handwashing technique in a pediatric intensive care unit. *Am J Dis Child*. 1987;141:683–685.
15. The Acute Respiratory Distress Syndrome Network. Ventilation with lower tidal volumes as compared with traditional tidal volumes for acute lung injury and the acute respiratory distress syndrome. *N Engl J Med*. 2000;342:1301–1308.
16. The National Heart, Lung and Blood Institute Acute Respiratory Distress Syndrome (ARDS) Clinical Trials Network. Pulmonary artery versus central venous catheter to guide treatment of acute lung injury. *N Engl J Med*. 2006;354:2213–2224.
17. Hough CL, Kallet RH, Ranieri VM, et al. Intrinsic positive end-expiratory pressure in Acute Respiratory Distress Syndrome (ARDS) Network subjects. *Crit Care Med*. 2005;33:527–532.
18. Schoenfeld DA, Bernard GR. Statistical evaluation of ventilator free days as an efficacy measure in clinical trials of treatment for acute respiratory distress syndrome. *Crit Care Med*. 2002;30:1772–1777.
19. Brower RG, Matthay MA, Bernard GR. Questions about ARDS Network trial of low tidal volume. *Am J Respir Crit Care Med*. 2003;167:1717–1718.
20. Dushoff J, Plotkin JB, Viboud C, et al. Mortality due to influenza in the United States—an annualized regression approach using multiple-cause mortality data. *Am J Epidemiol*. 2006;163:181–187.
21. Halbert RJ, Isonaka S, George D, et al. Interpreting COPD prevalence estimates: what is the true burden of disease? *Chest*. 2003;123:1684–1692.
22. Girard TD, Bernard GR. Mechanical ventilation in ARDS. *Chest*. 2007;131:921–929.
23. Stein N, Matz H, Schneeweiss A, et al. An evaluation of a transcutaneous and an end-tidal capnometer for noninvasive monitoring of spontaneously breathing patients. *Respir Care*. 2006;51:1162–1166.
24. R Development Core Team. R: a language and environment for statistical computing. 2007. R Foundation for Statistical Computing. Available at: http://www.R-project.org.
25. Bickelmann AG, Burwell CS, Robin ED, et al. Extreme obesity associated with alveolar hypoventilation: a Pickwickian syndrome. *Am J Med*. 1956;21:811–818.
26. Petty TL, Ashbaugh DG. The adult respiratory distress syndrome. Clinical features, factors influencing prognosis and principles of management. *Chest*. 1971;60:233–239.
27. Zamanian M, Marini JJ. Pressure-flow signatures of central-airway mucus plugging. Case report. *Crit Care Med*. 2006; 34:223–226.
28. David M, Weiler N, Heinrichs W, et al. High-frequency oscillatory ventilation in adult acute respiratory distress syndrome. *Intensive Care Med*. 2003;29:1656–1665.
29. Michelet P, D'Journo XB, Seinaye F, et al. Non-invasive ventilation for treatment of postoperative respiratory failure after oesophagectomy. *Br J Surg*. 2009;96:54–60.
30. U.S. Department of Health and Human Services, Centers for Disease Control and Prevention, National Center for Health Statistics. *Health, United States, 2008*. Available at: http://www.cdc.gov/nchs/data/hus/hus08.pdf#063.
31. Hankinson JL, Odencrantz JR, Fedan KB. Spirometric reference values from a sample of the general U.S. population. *Am J Respir Crit Care Med*. 1999;159:179–187.
32. Preis SR, Hwang SJ, Coady S, et al. Trends in all-cause and cardiovascular disease mortality among women and men with and without diabetes mellitus in the Framingham Heart Study, 1950 to 2005. *Circulation*. 2009;119:1728–1735.
33. Kohansal R, Martinez-Camblor P, Agusti A, et al. The natural history of chronic airflow obstruction revisited: an analysis of the Framingham offspring cohort. *Am J Respir Crit Care Med*. 2009;180:3–10.
34. Institute of Laboratory Animal Resources. *Guide for the Care and Use of Laboratory Animals*. Washington, DC: National Academies Press; 1996.
35. Lim SC, Adams AB, Simonson DA, et al. Intercomparison of recruitment maneuver efficacy in three models of acute lung injury. *Crit Care Med*. 2004;32:2371–2384.

36. Mehta Y, Chand RK, Sawhney R, et al. Cardiac output monitoring: comparison of a new arterial pressure waveform analysis to the bolus thermodilution technique in patients undergoing off-pump coronary artery bypass surgery. *J Cardiothorac Vasc Anesth.* 2008;22:394–399.
37. Odenstedt H, Stenqvist O, Lundin S. Clinical evaluation of a partial CO_2 rebreathing technique for cardiac output monitoring in critically ill patients. *Acta Anaesthesiol Scand.* 2002;46:152–159.
38. Chiumello D, Cressoni M, Chierichetti M, et al. Nitrogen washout/washin, helium dilution and computed tomography in the assessment of end expiratory lung volume. *Crit Care.* 2008;12:R150.
39. Heinze H, Sedemund-Adib B, Heringlake M, Meier T, Eichler W. Changes in functional residual capacity during weaning from mechanical ventilation: a pilot study. *Anesth Analg.* 2009;108:911–915.
40. Rubenfeld GD, Cooper C, Carter G, et al. Barriers to providing lung-protective ventilation to patients with acute lung injury. *Crit Care Med.* 2004;32:1289–1293.

CHAPTER 50

Physical Principles

Peter Bliss
Alexander B. Adams

OUTLINE

Basic Physics
Gas Laws
Gas Mixtures and Partial Pressures
Humidity, Water Vapor, and Evaporation
Gases in Solution, Diffusion, and Osmosis
Conversion of Gas Volumes
Conservation of Energy
Flow of Gases and Other Fluids
Application of Physical Principles to Measurement and Physiology

OBJECTIVES

1. Identify the physical principles that are most important to respiratory physiology and respiratory care.
2. Explain the behaviors of fluids at various pressures, volumes, temperatures, and flows.
3. Describe units of measurement, molecules, and states of matter.
4. Discuss physical principles affecting force, stress, pressure, and work.
5. Describe compliance, elastance, and resistance and their relationships to work of breathing.
6. Describe surface tension and its relationship to lung function.
7. Discuss Boyle's, Charles's, and Gay-Lussac's laws and the ideal gas law and explain how changes in pressure, temperature, and volume affect the behavior of gases.
8. Describe applications of physical principles to monitoring, measurement, and assessment of the lung.

KEY TERMS

Bernoulli principle
Boyle's law
Charles's law
compliance
Dalton's law
density
elastance
Fick's law
flow
force
Gay-Lussac's law of combining volumes
Gay-Lussac's law of pressure and temperature
Graham's law
gravity
Hagen-Poiseuille equation
humidity deficit
hydrostatic pressure
ideal gas law
joule
laminar flow
mass
Ohm's law
pascal
percentage of body humidity (%BH)
pressure
resistance
Reynolds number
strain
stress
surface tension
Système International d'Unités (SI system)
temperature
time constant
turbulent flow
velocity
Venturi principle
viscosity
work

INTRODUCTION

Respiratory therapy lies at an intersection of the clinical and physical sciences. Respiratory therapists must understand the physical principles important to respiratory physiology and the practice of respiratory care, particularly the behavior of gases and liquids under varying conditions of pressure, temperature, and flow. Physical forces have primary effects on gas movement, ventilation of the lungs, and perfusion. Some of the equations and relationships presented in this chapter simplify the physics and physiology, but a simplified approach provides insight into the usefulness of these important concepts.

Basic Physics

Molecules and States of Matter

Atoms, molecules, and compounds are the building blocks of all matter. The periodic table displays all known atoms, the elemental units of matter. Molecules are composed of two or more atoms. A molecule may be a pure element, in which the atoms are the same, or a compound of different atoms. Molecular oxygen (O_2) is composed of two atoms of the same element (oxygen), whereas carbon dioxide (CO_2) is a compound—a molecule with different atoms, made up of one carbon atom and two oxygen atoms.

Molecular theory describes three states of matter: solid, liquid, and gas. The amount of kinetic energy present and interactions among molecules determine the physical state that molecules assume. For example, water can exist as a solid, liquid, or gas (**Figure 50–1**). A solid is a condensed structure in which strong intermolecular bonds determine a definite shape and volume. Solids do not move and are difficult to compress. A liquid, which is composed of molecules that move freely, has a definite volume without definite shape. Liquids are denser than gases. Like solids, liquids are difficult to compress. The intermolecular bonds of a gas, on the other hand, are weak. A gas is compressible and completely fills an enclosed space. Both gases and liquids are considered fluids, that is, substances that can flow.

RESPIRATORY RECAP

Three States of Matter

- » Solid
- » Liquid
- » Gas

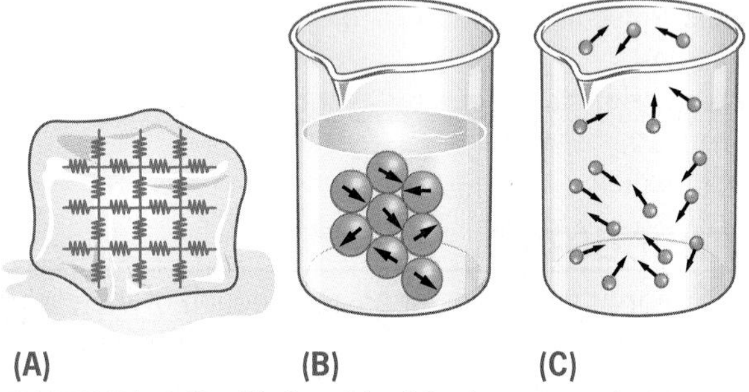

(A) (B) (C)

FIGURE 50–1 Simplified models of the three states of matter. (**A**) Solid. (**B**) Liquid. (**C**) Gas. Adapted from Nave CR, Nave BC. *Physics for the Health Sciences*. 3rd ed. WB Saunders; 1985.

All three states of matter have a characteristic elasticity, or reversible deformability. An ideal gas may be considered perfectly elastic: when the molecules collide with the wall of a vessel or with each other, no energy is lost. Gases in the real world are not quite ideal, but for our purposes they are close enough to ideal to be analyzed as if they were.

Units of Measurement

A common system of measurement is important to establish clear, consistent communication. Unfortunately, several units of measure are used in respiratory physiology. The **Système International d'Unités (SI system)** is an international system of measurement that is universally accepted but not always used. SI units are preferred, particularly in scientific and healthcare settings; however, for some measures both SI and clinical units are used. In the SI system the **pascal** (Pa; 1 newton/m^2) is the primary unit of pressure (**Table 50–1**); for ease of calculation, the kilopascal (kPa; 1000 Pa) is commonly used because the pascal is too small in the physiologic range. However, in the clinical setting, the more common units of measurement for pressure are cm H_2O for gases and mm Hg for liquids. **Table 50–2** shows these conversions.

Familiarity with the symbols used in respiratory physiology is essential to understand common terminology. The symbols of respiratory physiology have particular meanings and may be modified by characters placed above the symbol and by superscripts or subscripts below. A dot over a symbol indicates the rate of change (i.e., distance over time or velocity), whereas two dots indicate the change in the rate of change (i.e., change in velocity over time, acceleration). For example, V indicates volume, and $\dot{V}$ is flow or change in volume over time. A bar over a symbol indicates a mean quantity. **Table 50–3** lists commonly used symbols.

Mass, Force, Stress, Pressure, and Work

Mass is the amount of a substance determined by the number and type of molecules. The molecular mass of a substance is a number of moles (mol) of a substance, and 1 mole is Avogadro's number (6.023×10^{23}) of atoms or molecules of that substance.

TABLE 50–1 International System (SI) Base and Derived Units

SI Base Units			SI Derived Units			
Measurement	*Unit*	*Abbreviation*	*Measurement*	*Unit*	*Abbreviation*	*Derivation*
Length	Meter	m	Force	Newton	N	$kg \times m \times s^{-2}$
Mass	Kilogram	kg	Pressure	Pascal	Pa	$N \times m^{-2}$
Time	Second	s	Work	Joule	J	$N \times m$ ($L \times kPa$)
Temperature	Kelvin	K	Frequency	Hertz	Hz	s^{-1}

Force is a mechanical energy applied to a body. In mathematic terms, force is the product of mass times acceleration. *Weight* describes the force due to the acceleration of **gravity** acting on a mass (**Equation 50–1**). The acceleration of gravity is approximately 9.8 m/s^2. **Density** (ρ) is mass per unit volume, or m/V. The product of density times volume times the acceleration of gravity also is weight.

TABLE 50–2 Common Conversions in Units of Measurement

Measurement	Unit of Measure	Conversions*
Pressure	1 kilopascal (kPa)	7.5 mm Hg 10.2 cm H_2O 0.00987 atm 10^4 dyne × cm^{-2}
	1 millimeter of mercury (mm Hg)	1 torr 0.133 kPa 1.36 cm H_2O 1.33 × 10^3 dyne × cm^{-2}
	1 atmosphere	101.3 kPa 760 mm Hg 1033 cm H_2O 10 m seawater
Work	1 joule	0.239 calories 1 L × kPa
Power	1 watt	1 J × s^{-1}

*Atmospheres (atm) and millimeters of mercury (mm Hg) are not International System (SI) units, but they are in common use.

TABLE 50–3 Symbols and Modifiers Commonly Used in Respiratory Physiology

Symbol	Meaning	Modifier*	Meaning
V	Volume	I	Inspired
V_T	Tidal volume	E	Expired
$\dot{V}$	Flow	A	Alveolar
$\dot{V}_E$	Ventilation	a	Arterial
Q	Volume of liquid	v	Venous
$\dot{Q}$	Blood flow, perfusion	atm	Atmospheric
S	Saturation	rc	Rib cage
F	Fraction	cw	Chest wall
P	Pressure	pl	Pleural
T	Temperature	es	Esophageal
C	Compliance		
E	Elastance		
R	Resistance		
T	Time		
F	Frequency (respiratory rate)		

*A modifier usually is expressed as a subscript or suffix.

Stress is a force applied to an area. Force applied at an angle generates shear stress. **Pressure** (force per unit area) is the same concept applied to fluids, including gases (**Equation 50–2**). Examples include the pressure of the atmosphere (barometric pressure) and the pressure measured in an airway during a respiratory cycle. Force is the product of pressure and area.

Strain is the physical deformation or change in shape of a structure or substance—usually caused by stress. Elasticity is the amount of *reversible* deformability that can be generated by a stress yet allow the structure or substance to return to its original shape. A gas is highly elastic, which means that its volume can be compressed relatively easily. Other fluids, such as liquids, are less elastic and behave as if incompressible. **Viscosity** is the resistance to movement between adjacent fluid molecules. Solids lack elasticity compared with gases or liquids. A stress applied to solid materials can alter the strength or soundness of a substance without changing its apparent shape.

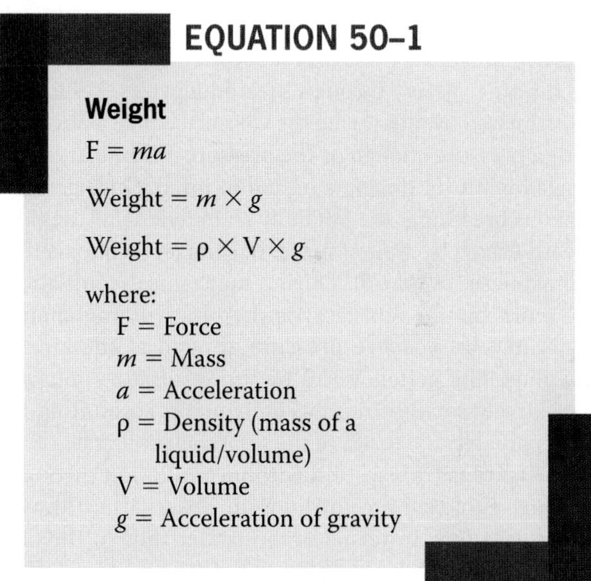

EQUATION 50–1
Weight
$F = ma$
$Weight = m \times g$
$Weight = \rho \times V \times g$
where:
F = Force
m = Mass
a = Acceleration
ρ = Density (mass of a liquid/volume)
V = Volume
g = Acceleration of gravity

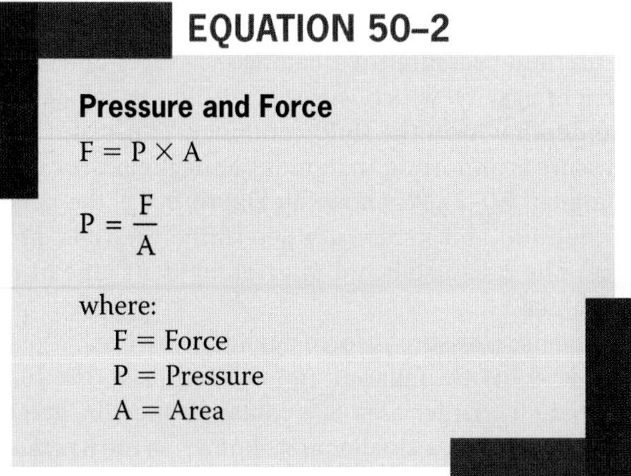

EQUATION 50–2
Pressure and Force
$F = P \times A$
$P = \frac{F}{A}$
where:
F = Force
P = Pressure
A = Area

A stress that stretches the lungs may not seem to permanently change the size or shape of the lung, but it may affect lung integrity. The lungs are elastic structures that respond in an elastic manner to stress and strain. The normal stress on the lungs is a changing transpulmonary pressure (the difference between alveolar pressure and the driving pressure generated outside the lungs—the negative pleural pressure). The strain on the lungs is the movement of the lungs during a breath, or tidal volume (VT), compared with its resting volume, or functional residual capacity (FRC). Excessive stresses and strains can damage the lungs, which can become a serious concern when positive pressure ventilators become the driving pressure for ventilation.

A force causing displacement of matter does **work**. For gases, a force can be measured as pressure, and the displacement is the volume change to the lungs. Using SI units, work is expressed in newton meters (N · m) or **joules** (J) or joules per liter. Table 50–2 presents conversion factors between units (note: atm > mm Hg > cm H_2O > kPa).

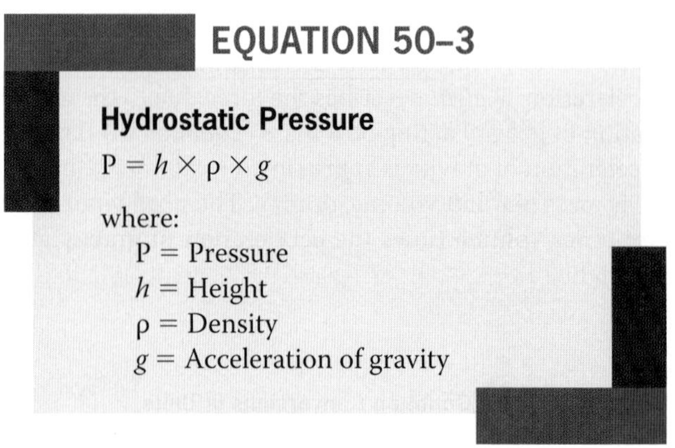

EQUATION 50–3

Hydrostatic Pressure

$$P = h \times \rho \times g$$

where:

P = Pressure
h = Height
ρ = Density
g = Acceleration of gravity

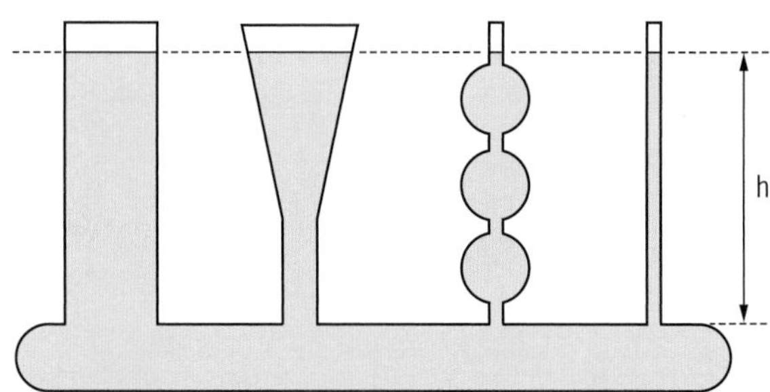

FIGURE 50–2 Pascal's law. Liquid pressure depends only on the height (h) of the vessel and not on the vessel's shape or the total volume of liquid. Adapted from Nave CR, Nave BC. *Physics for the Health Sciences*. 3rd ed. WB Saunders; 1985.

Work of Breathing

Work of breathing (WOB) is the work necessary to move air (or other gases) through breathing cycles. WOB can be estimated by measuring the volume change associated with a pressure change or the pressure-volume area of a single breath (or during a period of time). During spontaneous breathing, the WOB by an individual is the tidal breath driven by pleural pressure changes (referenced to atmospheric pressure). During mechanical ventilation, the work by the ventilator is the lung volume change generated by positive pressure applied at the airway opening. The actual WOB by the respiratory muscles is relatively small in normal individuals, accounting for approximately 2% to 4% of the total metabolic rate.

Pressure is transmitted without reduction throughout any enclosed static fluid, an observation known as *Pascal's law*. In terms of molecular theory, the collisions of molecules with one another and the wall of their containing vessel will generate pressure. If conditions are at equilibrium, pressure is constant throughout the fluid if the pressure caused by the weight of the fluid itself is neglected. The weight of a fluid generates static fluid pressure (**hydrostatic pressure**) due to the force of gravity, which varies according to the density and depth within the fluid container. This static fluid pressure is important in liquids but negligible for gases (**Equation 50–3**). As shown in **Figure 50–2**, the height of the fluid and its density determine the fluid pressure. The pressure is not affected by the shape of the container.

Because pressure is force applied to an area, if pressure is equal throughout an enclosed fluid, the force exerted on a larger area of a container must be greater than the force at a smaller area, known as the *hydraulic press principle*. Given two syringes of different diameters, the syringe with the larger diameter can generate greater force than the syringe with the smaller diameter. Because work is the product of force and distance, the distance the syringe with the smaller diameter (less force) moves is greater than the distance that the larger-diameter syringe moves. If equal force is applied simultaneously to syringes of different diameters, a greater pressure will be generated in the syringe of lesser cross-sectional area.

Atmospheric (barometric) pressure is an example of static fluid pressure. Atmospheric pressure is the pressure generated by the weight of atmospheric gas above the barometer at any particular altitude. As elevation increases, atmospheric pressure decreases. The decrease in atmospheric pressure at a higher altitude can be understood to be caused by a shorter column of atmospheric gas. At a fixed altitude, comparatively minor changes in barometric pressure such as those witnessed in low- and high-pressure systems can cause major differences in weather.

The volume change to spherelike structures such as lungs or alveoli caused by a pressure change is the **compliance**, or stiffness, of the sphere (**Equation 50–4**). A balloon that is difficult to blow up is an example of a low-compliance sphere. Commonly, the compliance of the respiratory system is a composite

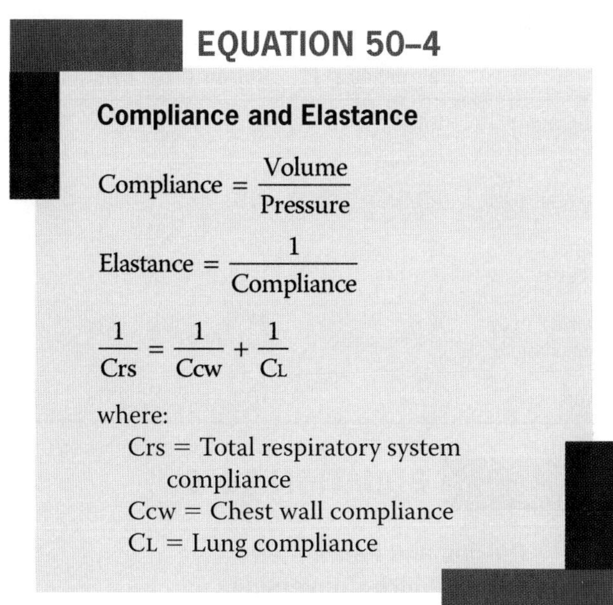

EQUATION 50–4

Compliance and Elastance

$$\text{Compliance} = \frac{\text{Volume}}{\text{Pressure}}$$

$$\text{Elastance} = \frac{1}{\text{Compliance}}$$

$$\frac{1}{C_{RS}} = \frac{1}{C_{CW}} + \frac{1}{C_L}$$

where:

Crs = Total respiratory system compliance
Ccw = Chest wall compliance
CL = Lung compliance

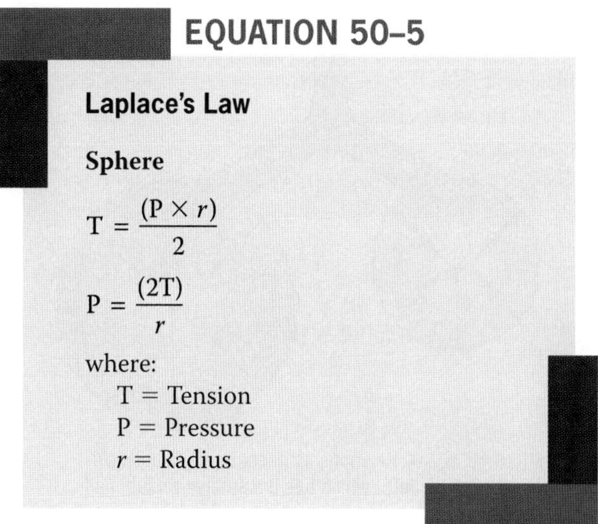

EQUATION 50–5

Laplace's Law

Sphere

$$T = \frac{(P \times r)}{2}$$

$$P = \frac{(2T)}{r}$$

where:

T = Tension
P = Pressure
r = Radius

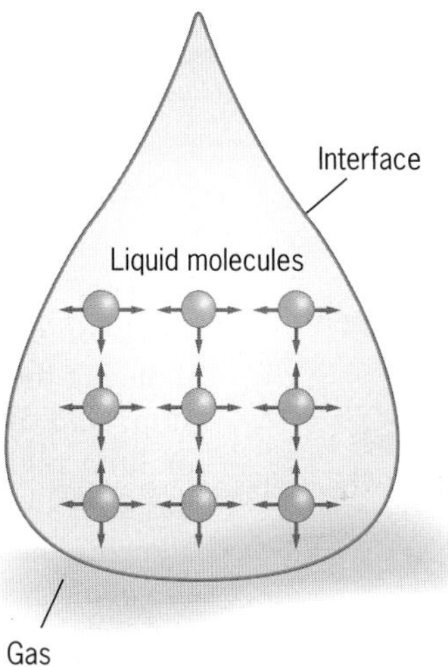

FIGURE 50–3 The force of surface tension in a drop of liquid. Cohesive force (arrows) attracts molecules inside the drop to one another. Cohesion can pull the outermost molecules inward only, creating a centrally directed force that tends to contract the liquid into a sphere. Adapted from Scanlan CL, et al. *Egan's Fundamentals of Respiratory Care.* 7th ed. Mosby; 1999.

of two compliances, lung compliance and chest wall compliance—springs pulling in opposite directions. The reciprocal of respiratory system compliance is the addition of the reciprocals of lung and chest wall compliance (refer to Equation 50–4). **Elastance** (pressure per unit volume) is the reciprocal of compliance; therefore, respiratory system elastance is the addition of the lung and chest wall elastances. Compliance of the respiratory system is routinely monitored in ventilated patients during a tidal breath to track the stiffness of the lungs. Because injured lungs can be functionally smaller, compliance can be referenced to *specific compliance* (total compliance divided by actual lung size) to account for the lung size reduction due to injury.

Wall Tension and Surface Tension

Although Pascal's law states that pressure is equal throughout a containing structure (ignoring hydrostatic pressure), the tension at the boundary of a structure—the wall tension—varies. Laplace's law describes the tension of the wall of a sphere or cylinder (**Equation 50–5**). Wall tension increases with radius.

However, a smaller structure (r) generates a greater inward pressure (P), resulting in a tendency to collapse due to surface tension. Surface tension is not the same as wall tension. **Surface tension** describes the property of a liquid that tends to reduce the surface of a liquid toward a minimum, pulling the surface molecules inward. This is what causes water to bead up on a surface rather than spread out. Surface tension is not the stretch between molecules of the wall structure itself (such as in a sheet of rubber) but rather the force acting at the boundary surface between two regions, such as the boundary between the liquid coating the lung tissue and the adjoining air (**Figure 50–3**). The force generated across the wall of a structure is a combination of wall and surface tension.

A surfactant is a fluid that reduces surface tension. Soap is a common example of a surfactant. In the lung, surfactant reduces the pressure required to expand an alveolus. Surfactant also reduces the pressure differences between alveoli of different diameters. Without surfactant, smaller alveoli would empty into larger ones because of the greater surface tension in the smaller alveoli (**Figure 50–4**). Surfactant is necessary for normal lung function

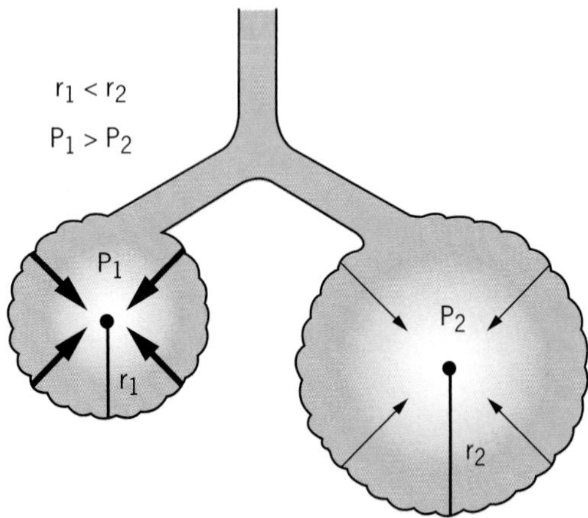

FIGURE 50–4 Relationship described by Laplace's law. Bubble A (left), which has the smaller radius, has the greater inward or deflating pressure and is more prone to collapse than is bubble B (right). Because the two bubbles are connected, bubble A would tend to deflate and empty into bubble B. Conversely, because of bubble A's greater surface tension, it would be harder to inflate than bubble B. Adapted from Scanlan CL, et al. *Egan's Fundamentals of Respiratory Care*. 7th ed. Mosby; 1999.

RESPIRATORY RECAP

Surface Tension and Surfactant

- » Surface tension tends to reduce the surface of a liquid to a minimum.
- » Surfactant reduces surface tension.

because it reduces the work of breathing (by reducing the surface tension) and allows alveoli or lung regions of various sizes to remain open, allowing the equalization of volumes and pressures between regions.

Temperature

Temperature describes the amount of heat, or thermal energy, present in a system. Three temperature scales are in common use. The Fahrenheit and Celsius scales are used in healthcare and are calibrated in reference to the freezing and boiling points of water—distinct points of reference (**Table 50–4**). The Fahrenheit scale divides the temperature range between freezing and boiling into 180 gradations, or degrees, whereas the Celsius scale uses 100 gradations. In scientific settings, the scales are referenced to 0° or absolute zero (without minus degrees) and are the Kelvin scale, which uses Celsius units, and the Rankin scale, which uses Fahrenheit units; the Rankin scale is rarely used, however.

RESPIRATORY RECAP

Temperature Scales

- » Fahrenheit (F)
- » Celsius (C)
- » Kelvin (absolute) (K)

The formula for converting Celsius to Fahrenheit takes into consideration the difference in zero points (32°) and the ratio of the two degree sizes because Celsius degrees are 1.8 times larger than Fahrenheit degrees (**Equation 50–6**).

TABLE 50–4 Temperature Scales

	Fahrenheit (° F)	Celsius (° C)	Kelvin (K)
Absolute zero	–460	–273	0
Oxygen boils	–297	–183	90
Water freezes	32	0	273
Normal body temperature	98.6	37	310
Water boils	212	100	373

EQUATION 50–6

Celsius and Fahrenheit Temperature Conversions

Conversion from Celsius to Fahrenheit

Fahrenheit = 32 + (Celsius degrees × $\frac{9}{5}$)

Conversion from Fahrenheit to Celsius

Celsius = (Fahrenheit degrees − 32) × $\frac{5}{9}$

TABLE 50–5 Changes in the State of Matter

Type of Change	Conversion	Example
Exothermic Change (Energy Given Up)		
Condensation (liquefaction)	Gas to liquid or solid	Water condensing on a cold glass
Freezing (crystallization)	Liquid to solid	Ice forming
Endothermic Change (Energy Added)		
Sublimation	Solid to gas	Dry ice
Melting (fusion)	Solid to liquid	Ice melting
Evaporation (vaporization)	Liquid to gas	Water boiling

Thermodynamics and Heat Exchange

Thermodynamics describes changes in the thermal state of a system by adding or removing energy, such as when changes in pressure, volume, or temperature alter the state of the substance. When a change of state requires the addition of energy, the process is called *endothermic*. An *exothermic* process gives off energy. **Table 50–5** lists common endothermic and exothermic processes as the states of matter change between gas, liquid, and solid states. Substances usually condense into liquids before becoming solids.

Gas Laws

Solids and liquids follow the same basic principles but do not exhibit the perfectly elastic intermolecular behavior of an ideal gas. Theoretical, or ideal, gases obey gas laws and behave precisely the same at all temperatures and pressures. Real gases act ideal but are not ideal under all conditions; however, under the relatively low pressure and temperature conditions encountered in respiratory physiology, their behavior can be predicted quite well by ideal gas laws.

The **ideal gas law** defines a relationship between pressure, volume, temperature, and the number of molecules of a gas (**Equation 50–7**). Pressure and volume are inversely related, whereas temperature is directly proportional to volume or pressure (**Figure 50–5**):

$$PV = nRT$$

The term n in the ideal gas law accounts for the number of gas molecules present. The universal gas constant, R, expresses the force (or work) required to move a quantity of ideal gas. This has a value of 8.1314 joules × degrees $\text{Kelvin}^{-1} \times \text{moles}^{-1}$. From the ideal gas law, several other important relationships can be derived. If one or more quantities change, the others must also change to compensate and keep the equation in balance. In particular, if the amount and makeup of a gas stays constant, then the quantity PV/T must remain constant, although these three quantities may each change within their fixed relationship.

Gay-Lussac's law of combining volumes states that volumes of gases combine chemically in volumetric proportions that are small whole numbers (**Equation 50–8**). This observation confirms that under equivalent conditions, equal volumes of ideal gases contain an equal number of molecules. Under standard conditions of 0° C and barometric pressure of 1 atmosphere (1 atm), 1 mol of an ideal gas has a volume of 22.4 L.

Boyle's law states that pressure is inversely proportional to volume (**Equation 50–9**); therefore, the product of pressure and volume may be expressed as a constant, k. Boyle's law predicts the relationship of a volume of gas to a pressure change. If the volume of a gas is halved, pressure will double, given a constant mass and temperature. A pressure change important in pulmonary function testing is the change in lung pressure while attempting to pant against a blocked airway. This application of Boyle's law allows a calculation of lung volume in body plethysmography studies.

Charles's law predicts the effect of temperature on a fixed amount of dry gas. At constant pressure, gas

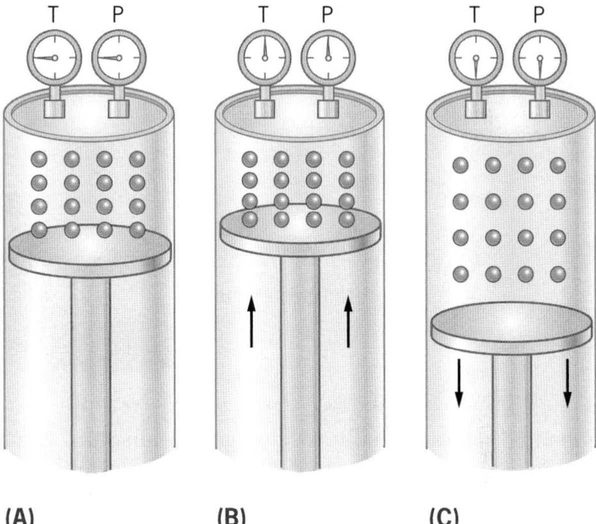

FIGURE 50–5 (**A**) A mass of gas in the resting state exerts a given pressure at a given temperature in a cylinder. (**B**) As the piston compresses the gas, the molecules are crowded closer together, and the increased energy of molecular collisions increases both the temperature and the pressure. (**C**) Conversely, as the gas expands, molecular interaction diminishes and the temperature and pressure fall. Adapted from Scanlan CL, et al. *Egan's Fundamentals of Respiratory Care*. 7th ed. Mosby; 1999.

EQUATION 50–7

Ideal (Combined) Gas Law

$$\frac{(P_1 \times V_1)}{T_1} = \frac{(P_2 \times V_2)}{T_2}$$

where:

P = Pressure
V = Volume
T = Absolute temperature

$$PV = nRT$$

where:

P = Pressure
V = Volume
n = Number of moles
R = Gas constant
T = Absolute temperature

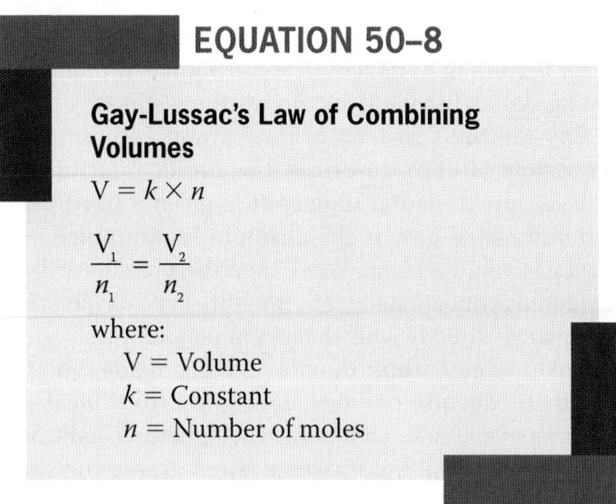

EQUATION 50–8

Gay-Lussac's Law of Combining Volumes

$$V = k \times n$$

$$\frac{V_1}{n_1} = \frac{V_2}{n_2}$$

where:

V = Volume
k = Constant
n = Number of moles

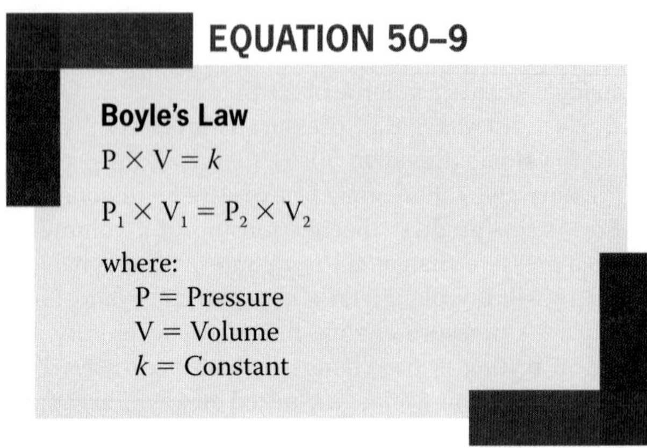

EQUATION 50–9

Boyle's Law

$$P \times V = k$$

$$P_1 \times V_1 = P_2 \times V_2$$

where:
P = Pressure
V = Volume
k = Constant

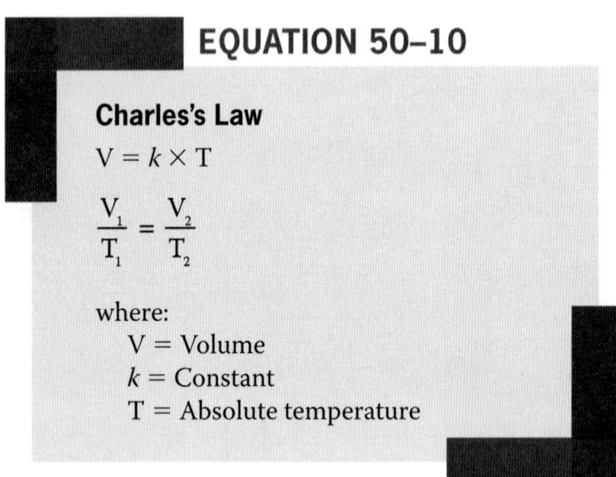

EQUATION 50–10

Charles's Law

$$V = k \times T$$

$$\frac{V_1}{T_1} = \frac{V_2}{T_2}$$

where:
V = Volume
k = Constant
T = Absolute temperature

expands proportionally to changes in absolute temperature (**Equation 50–10**). A constant multiplied by temperature predicts volume; for example, an ideal gas expands 37.5% when heated from 0° C to 100° C. For this reason, a volume of inhaled gas at room temperature expands when inhaled into a 37° C body. When exhaled, the volume will remain proportionally larger according to its temperature; pulmonary function testing systems account for this warming effect.

> **RESPIRATORY RECAP**
>
> **Gas Laws**
> » Gay-Lussac's law of combining volumes
> » Boyle's law
> » Charles's law
> » Gay-Lussac's law of pressure and temperature
> » Ideal (combined) gas law

Gay-Lussac's law of pressure and temperature (**Equation 50–11**) describes the direct relationship between pressure and temperature given a fixed mass and volume of gas. If the absolute temperature of a fixed gas volume is increased, then the pressure will be increased proportionally. The pressure in an oxygen tank will change directly with changes in temperature.

Gases (e.g., carbon dioxide, nitrous oxide, volatile anesthetic agents) can deviate slightly from ideal gas behavior even under commonly encountered conditions. For example, ideal gases assume purely elastic collisions between molecules. Nonideal gases require quantitative

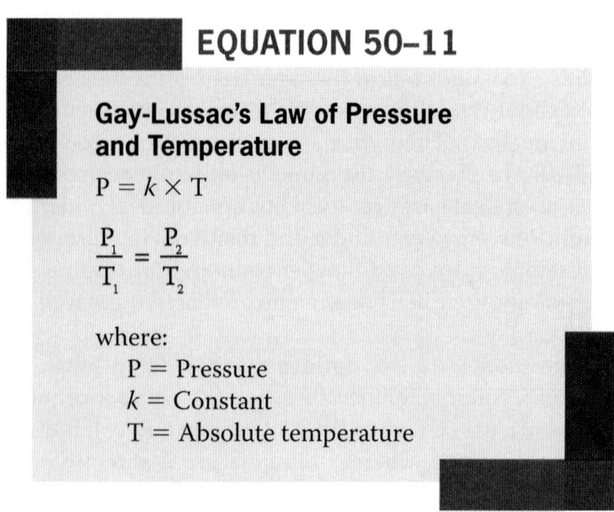

EQUATION 50–11

Gay-Lussac's Law of Pressure and Temperature

$$P = k \times T$$

$$\frac{P_1}{T_1} = \frac{P_2}{T_2}$$

where:
P = Pressure
k = Constant
T = Absolute temperature

modifications of the classic gas laws to describe their behavior. For example, under standard conditions, the volume of 1 mole of carbon dioxide is 22.2 L rather than 22.4 L. Factors that describe attraction or repulsion between molecules (e.g., Van der Waals forces) attempt to predict these differences from ideal behavior.

Gas Mixtures and Partial Pressures

Dalton's law of partial pressures describes the behavior of physical mixtures of gases and vapors. In these mixtures, each separate gas acts according to the ideal gas law as if it were alone. The partial pressure of each particular gas is equal to the fractional concentration times the total atmospheric pressure. Oxygen accounts for approximately 21% of atmospheric air, a percentage that can be expressed as a fractional oxygen content of inspired air (F_{IO_2}) of 0.21. At 1 atm (760 mm Hg), the partial pressure of oxygen is therefore 159.6 mm Hg (**Equation 50–12**). Nitrogen, which accounts for approximately 78% of air, has a partial pressure that can be similarly calculated to be 592.8 mm Hg at 1 atm.

Physical combinations of gases mix uniformly. Gases are continuously in motion, are at equilibrium, and are evenly distributed in any particular confined space. The same fractions of oxygen and nitrogen are present in Death Valley (86 m below sea level) as on Mount Everest (elevation 8850 m), although their partial pressures vary greatly according to the respective altitude.

Humidity, Water Vapor, and Evaporation

Most gases encountered in physiologic conditions are combinations of various dry gases, but they also contain water vapor (gas), which combines with the other gases according to Dalton's law of partial pressures. Water is particularly important as a vapor under conditions encountered in respiratory care.

EQUATION 50–12

Dalton's Law

Pressure of Oxygen at 1 Atmosphere

$P_{IO_2} = F_{IO_2} \times Patm$

$P_{IO_2} = 0.21 \times 760$ mm Hg $= 159.6$ mm Hg

Pressure of Nitrogen at 1 Atmosphere

$P_{IN_2} = F_{IN_2} \times Patm$

$P_{IN_2} = 0.78 \times 760 = 592.8$ mm Hg

P_{IO_2} = Partial pressure of inspired oxygen
F_{IO_2} = Fractional oxygen content of inspired gas
Patm = Atmospheric pressure
P_{IN_2} = Pressure of inspired nitrogen
F_{IN_2} = Fractional nitrogen content of inspired gas

Evaporation and Condensation

A water surface emits molecules of vapor continuously by evaporation. As vapor molecules hit the surface of a liquid, some are absorbed into the liquid by condensation. The net change due to evaporation or condensation depends on which is greater—the rate of condensation or the rate of evaporation. Above 100° C at atmospheric pressure, water is largely a vapor. Below 0° C, water is a solid. Between those temperatures, where we generally live, there is a saturation pressure (or partial pressure of water) at any given temperature at which water will condense (**Figure 50–6**). Temperature defines a limit to the maximum amount of water vapor that can be contained in air at that temperature.

Humidity can be quantified by partial pressure of water (P_{H_2O}), absolute humidity, or relative humidity. *Absolute humidity* (**Equation 50–13**) is the amount of water vapor in the air or the mass of water present in a volume of gas, usually measured in milligrams per liter. Humidity is most often expressed as *relative humidity*, or the total water content in a gas, such as air, compared with the capacity for water content at that temperature. A sample of gas having a relative humidity of 50% at 20° C has a vapor pressure of 8.75 mm Hg (0.5 × 17.5 mm Hg). At the usual body temperature of 37° C, 50% relative humidity has a water vapor pressure of 23.5 mm Hg, or one-half the maximum of 47 mm Hg.

If temperature is decreased and vapor pressure (and absolute humidity) remains the same, condensation occurs.

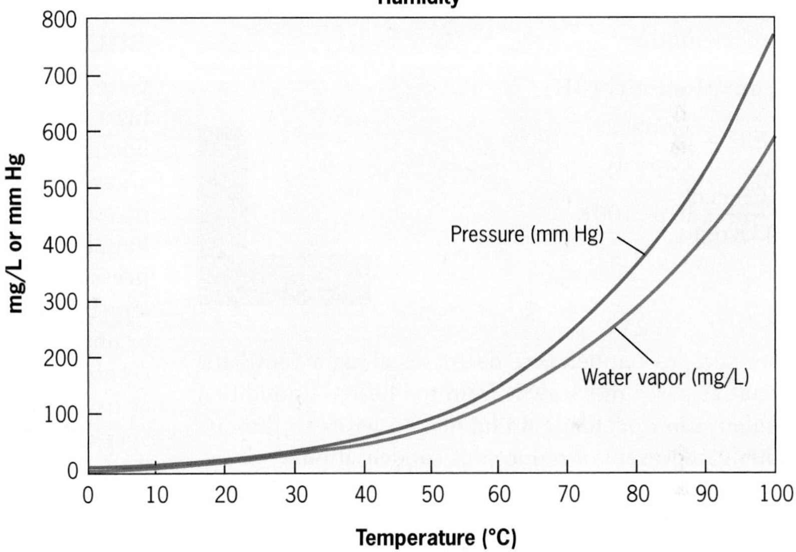

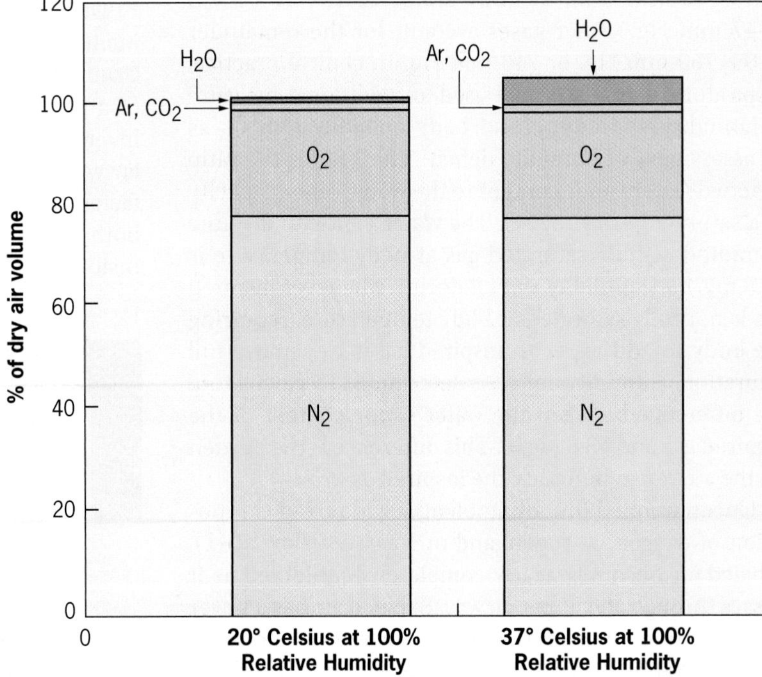

FIGURE 50–6 Absolute humidity and water vapor pressure as a function of temperature.

EQUATION 50–13

Calculating Humidity

Absolute Humidity

Absolute humidity = $(16.42 - 0.73T) + 0.04T^2$

where:

T = temperature (Celsius)

Relative Humidity

% Relative humidity =

$$\left(\frac{\text{Absolute humidity}}{\text{Humidity capacity}}\right) \times 100\%$$

Humidity Deficit

Humidity deficit = Content − Capacity at 37° C = Content − 43.8 mg/L

Body Humidity (BH)

$$\%BH = \frac{\text{Content}}{\text{Capacity}} \times 100\% = \frac{\text{Content}}{43.8 \text{ mg/L}} \times 100\%$$

Therefore, as temperature decreases along a ventilator circuit as gases move away from the heated humidifier, condensation occurs. Adding heated wires to the circuitry can prevent or reduce this condensation.

When conditions such as pressure and temperature are constant, a vapor can be analyzed in the same manner as any gaseous substance. At 1 atm, fully humidified or saturated air at body temperature has a P_{H_2O} of 47 mm Hg. Other gases account for the remainder of the 760 mm Hg, or 713 mm Hg. In clinical practice, respiratory therapists have used an additional measure of humidity—**percentage of body humidity (%BH)**—as an assessment of humidity deficit. The %BH is the ratio of actual water vapor content to the water vapor capacity in a saturated gas at 37° C. The water content (absolute humidity) of fully saturated gas at body temperature is 43.8 mg/L. A **humidity deficit** occurs whenever inspired gas is not fully saturated at body temperature, requiring the body to add water to inspired gases to achieve full saturation. Humidity deficit is determined by calculating the difference between the water vapor content of the inspired gas and 43.8 mg/L. This difference is the burden on the airway to humidify the inspired gas.

Unconditioned (dry or ambient) air is a fixed composition of oxygen, nitrogen, and other gases (**Box 50–1**). Inhaled air becomes nearly completely humidified as it passes through the upper airway. Exhaled air has a lower concentration of oxygen (by approximately 5%, or about 16%), a significant concentration of carbon dioxide of approximately 5% and exhaled air remains humidified.

BOX 50–1

Composition of Unconditioned Dry Air

Nitrogen: 78.08%
Oxygen: 20.95%
Carbon dioxide: 0.03%
Argon: 0.93%
Trace gases: 0.01%

Water vapor at 20° C and 50% relative humidity accounts for 1.1% of air volume.

Gases in Solution, Diffusion, and Osmosis

Gases dissolve in a liquid in a predictable manner according to Henry's law and the solubility coefficient of the liquid. *Henry's law* states that at a constant temperature, a gas dissolves in solution in proportion to its partial pressure. The solubility coefficient, or the capacity of a liquid to carry a gas (mass dissolved per unit of partial pressure) decreases as temperature increases. Constituents in the blood affect the solubility coefficient. For example, Henry's law does not predict whether a gas will combine chemically with a constituent of the fluid, such as oxygen combining with hemoglobin, and the blood is very capable of carrying CO_2. Although carbon dioxide has a lower partial pressure than oxygen in air and blood, CO_2 is approximately 19 times more soluble than oxygen due to its high solubility coefficient or large carrying capacity in blood.

Diffusion is the process of intermingling and movement of molecules as a result of their random motion. **Graham's law** predicts the rate of diffusion or movement of a gas (**Equation 50–14**). The velocity of diffusion is inversely proportional to the square root of the molecular weight of a substance; therefore, lighter gases diffuse faster than heavier gas molecules. In a liquid medium, both Graham's law and Henry's law affect the rate of diffusion of gases.

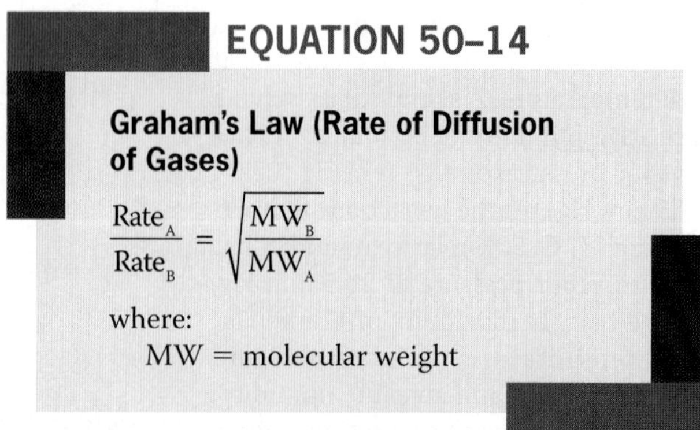

EQUATION 50–14

Graham's Law (Rate of Diffusion of Gases)

$$\frac{\text{Rate}_A}{\text{Rate}_B} = \sqrt{\frac{MW_B}{MW_A}}$$

where:

MW = molecular weight

Osmosis is the movement of a solvent by diffusion, primarily, through a semipermeable membrane that does not permit movement of larger solute molecules. A solvent diffuses across the membrane from an area of lesser to greater concentration. **Fick's law** (**Equation 50–15**) relates the factors that affect the transmembrane transfer of solute during osmosis. The total diffusion rate of a gas across a barrier (such as the alveolar membrane in the lung) is directly proportional to the cross-sectional area available for diffusion (lung size), to the difference in concentration gradients of the diffusing gases, and to the perpendicular distance of that cross-sectional area (thickness of the alveolocapillary membrane).

Conversion of Gas Volumes

Pressure, temperature, and humidity have important effects on gas volume. Several sets of conditions are commonly encountered in respiratory therapy because of the conditions under which certain gases are stored (dry) or measured (body temperature, humidified). These are (1) standard temperature and pressure, dry (STPD); (2) body temperature and pressure, saturated (BTPS); (3) atmospheric temperature and pressure, dry (ATPD); and (4) atmospheric temperature and pressure, saturated (ATPS) (**Table 50–6**). Gas is transformed from ATPD to BTPS on inspiration, causing volume changes due to warming and humidifying. Similarly, although gas may be collected and measured under BTPS conditions, measurement of gas exchange (such as oxygen consumption) usually is reported at STPD, or 1 atm and 0° C. **Equation 50–16** shows conversions between

EQUATION 50–15

Fick's Law

$$V_{gas} = \frac{A}{T} \times D_{gas}(P_1 - P_2)$$

where:

V_{gas} = Volume of gas diffusing across a membrane
A = Surface area for diffusion
T = Thickness of the membrane
$(P_1 - P_2)$ = Pressure gradient
D_{gas} = Diffusibility of the gas (solubility coefficient/density)

$$Do_2 = \frac{0.023}{\sqrt{32/22.4}} = 0.0192$$

$$Dco_2 = \frac{0.51}{\sqrt{44/22.4}} = 0.364$$

The diffusibility of carbon dioxide (Dco_2) is 19 times greater than that of oxygen (Do_2).

EQUATION 50–16

Gas Conversion Formulas

$$V_{BTPS} = V_{ATPS} \times \frac{Patm - PH_2O(T)}{Patm - PH_2O(37)} \times \frac{273 + 37}{273 + T}$$

$$V_{STPD} = V_{ATPD} \times \frac{Patm}{Patm(standard)} \times \frac{273}{273 + T}$$

$$V_{BTPS} = V_{STPD} \times \frac{Patm(standard)}{Patm - PH_2O(T)} \times \frac{310}{273}$$

$$V_{STPD} = V_{ATPS} \frac{273}{273 + T} \times \frac{Patm(standard)}{Patm - PH_2O(T)}$$

where:

V_{BTPS} = Volume at body temperature and pressure, saturated
V_{ATPS} = Volume at atmospheric temperature and pressure, saturated
Patm = Atmospheric pressure
PH_2O = Partial pressure of water
T = Temperature
V_{STPD} = Volume at standard temperature and pressure, dry
V_{ATPD} = Volume at atmospheric temperature and pressure, dry
Patm(standard) = Standard pressure

TABLE 50-6 Common Sets of Conditions Affecting Gas Volume

Condition	Description	Temperature (° C)	Atmospheres (atm)	Relative Humidity (%)
STPD	Standard temperature and pressure, dry	0	1 (760 mm Hg)	0
BTPS	Body temperature and pressure, saturated	37	1	100
ATPD	Atmospheric temperature and pressure, dry	Ambient (≈ 25)	Ambient	0
ATPS	Atmospheric temperature and pressure, saturated	Ambient (≈ 25)	Ambient	100

EQUATION 50–17

Gas Constant

$$(760 - 47) \div \left(\frac{273}{310} \times \frac{713}{760}\right) = 863$$

$$\text{mm Hg} - \text{mm Hg} \div \left(\frac{^\circ\text{K}}{^\circ\text{K}} \times \frac{\text{mm Hg}}{\text{mm Hg}}\right)$$

This constant is the standard partial pressure of dry gas (partial pressure of vapor pressure subtracted from standard atmospheric pressure) divided by the ratio of standard temperature and body temperature in degrees Kelvin (273 and 310 degrees, respectively) multiplied by the ratio of the partial pressure of humidified gas at body temperature to dry gas at 1 atmosphere (760 mm Hg). It is used to express moles of carbon dioxide (CO_2) production in terms of volumes measured at standard temperature and pressure, dry (STPD). Units of temperature cancel.

Expressing $PaCO_2$ in mm Hg and CO_2 production in mL/min, the gas constant is 0.863:

$$Paco_2 = \frac{\dot{V}co_2 \times 0.863}{\left(1 - \frac{V_D}{V_T}\right) \times \dot{V}_E}$$

where:

$Paco_2$ = Partial pressure of arterial carbon dioxide
$\dot{V}co_2$ = Carbon dioxide production
V_D = Dead space
V_T = Tidal volume
$\dot{V}_E$ = Minute ventilation

conditions of BTPS, STPD, and ATPD. Although tables and conversions are readily available, the basis of these equations must be understood, and some conversion factors should be committed to memory.

A frequently needed conversion is between STPD and BTPS. The *gas constant* (which is different from the universal gas constant) is used to convert between the standard temperature and pressure of 1 atm and 0° C and body temperature and pressure of 37° C and 1 atm (**Equation 50–17**). This conversion is important in the calculation of dead space from measurements of carbon dioxide production and minute ventilation. Production of CO_2 is measured in STPD, whereas minute ventilation is directly measured in BTPS.

Conservation of Energy

When analyzing a system, one can assume that the total energy of that system is constant. Energy may change forms, but the total amount of energy must remain the same. There are many types of energy, but for the purposes of respiratory care, important types include the following:

- Potential (e.g., a ball on a shelf)
- Kinetic (e.g., a moving ball)

Subtypes of energy are as follows:

- Thermal (e.g., kinetic energy of molecules in hot water)
- Chemical (e.g., potential energy of molecules in unburned fuel)
- Pressure (e.g., potential energy of molecules in a fluid, especially a compressible gas)

When a ball falls off a shelf, its potential energy (a product of its mass and height) is converted to kinetic energy (a function of its mass and velocity), but the same total energy must exist. If chemical energy in the form of fuel is released by burning (oxidization) and heats a pot of cold water, the temperature of the water will increase, or convert to thermal energy. The temperature of the water, or thermal energy, is actually a manifestation of the kinetic energy of the water molecules. The total energy of the system remains the same, with less chemical energy and greater thermal energy. Some of the thermal energy will undoubtedly be lost to increasing the temperature (kinetic energy) of the surrounding air.

Flow of Gases and Other Fluids

Flow is the movement of a specified volume of fluid (gas or liquid) in a particular period of time. Both liquids and gases can flow. The flow of gas through tubes is a key physical phenomenon in respiratory physiology, whether in reference to the flow of air into and from the lungs or the flow of gas through a ventilator circuit. Flow is central to other areas of physiology as well, such as blood flow through vessels.

The rate of flow can be determined mathematically by dividing volume change by time. That is, the rate of volume change determines the rate of flow. A volumetric spirometer is one measuring device that uses this technique. Alternatively, volume can be calculated by multiplying a constant flow rate by time.

Principle of Continuity

If any liquid flows through a rigid pipe, the mass of fluid entering a tube must equal the mass leaving the tube. This concept is the principle of continuity (**Equation 50–18** and **Figure 50–7**). Considering geometry alone, during flow conditions any thin segment of fluid moves a particular distance in a set time. This movement of fluid over a time period is flow **velocity**. The product of velocity and the area of the tube defines the volume of fluid moving over time. If the diameter (hence area) of a section of tube

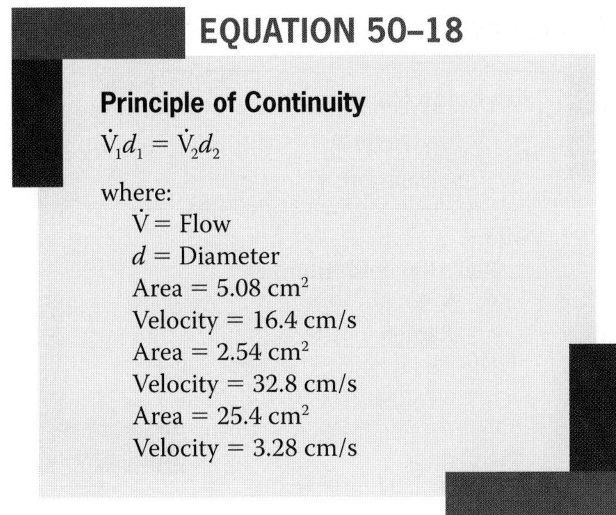

EQUATION 50–18

Principle of Continuity

$\dot{V}_1 d_1 = \dot{V}_2 d_2$

where:

$\dot{V}$ = Flow
d = Diameter
Area = 5.08 cm^2
Velocity = 16.4 cm/s
Area = 2.54 cm^2
Velocity = 32.8 cm/s
Area = 25.4 cm^2
Velocity = 3.28 cm/s

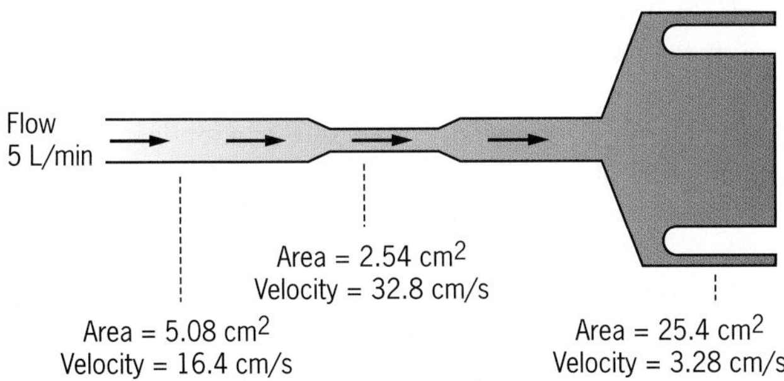

FIGURE 50–7 Principle of continuity. Note that fluid velocity is related inversely to the cross-sectional area. Adapted from Nave CR, Nave BC. *Physics for the Health Sciences*. 3rd ed. WB Saunders; 1985.

increases, the velocity decreases through that segment because the same mass entering must equal the mass exiting the tube. Diameter and velocity therefore are inversely related.

Bernoulli and Venturi Principles

The **Bernoulli principle** generally describes the pressure in a fluid as the velocity changes. The Bernoulli principle can explain the lift caused by airplane wings. More specific to respiratory care, if a fluid flowing into a tube reaches a section where the diameter is reduced or constricted, the velocity must increase according to the law of continuity. In the high-velocity section, pressure will be reduced. This occurs because energy must be conserved. In the large-diameter section, velocity is lower, so most of the energy is associated with the pressure. When the diameter is reduced and velocity increases, kinetic energy increases. Because the total energy must remain the same, the pressure energy must decrease as velocity increases. If the diameter of the tubing returns to its original size, the reverse energy shift occurs: kinetic energy will exchange again for pressure energy, and the pressure will return to its original value. This is ideally true, but not strictly true, because real fluids have viscosity and there is some loss of energy due to viscous friction between the tubing and the fluid and within the fluid itself. But especially for gas flows (with low viscosity), this analysis is approximately correct.

This phenomenon is particularly important in respiratory care. For instance, in a constricted airway, the reduced pressure will cause a narrow airway to collapse even further. Similarly, vessels tend to collapse with increased flow of blood in constricted or partially occluded vessels. The Bernoulli principle is used in some nonrespiratory fields of flow measurement because simple pressure measurements at two diameter points in a tube can estimate a reading of flow; however, these types of devices are not often seen in respiratory care applications.

The **Venturi principle** is an application of the Bernoulli principle and the law of continuity that explains the entrainment of fluids through an open port in a tube. A common misconception is that air entrainment oxygen delivery masks (so-called Venturi masks) operate according to the Bernoulli principle. This is not correct, because such masks operate by entraining a flow of gas through an orifice. The system is open, and, therefore, regions of different diameters will not attain the pressure changes expected from the Bernoulli principle effect. These devices use the converging funnel half of the Venturi tube, increasing the velocity of flow as the same amount of gas moves through a reduced diameter. The higher-velocity gas traveling through the narrowed tube interacts with stagnant ambient air. Molecules of gas exiting the jet collide with molecules in the surrounding air and drag them along, entraining air molecules into the forward flow of gas. The pressure drop across a narrowed section that allows entrainment can be restored if the postsection angle of divergence is less than 15 degrees.

Viscosity

All real fluids, both gases and liquids, have the property of viscosity, which is not accounted for by the Bernoulli principle. The Bernoulli principle assumes that fluids have zero viscosity. Viscosity can be described as the internal friction of a fluid and is independent of the density of a fluid. Molecules of a liquid flowing through a tube collide with the walls and reduce the overall velocity of the liquid. For gas movement, viscosity increases with temperature because the frequency of collisions between molecules is greater at higher temperatures. Viscosity in liquids, however, is increased at lower temperatures. For a viscous fluid such as molasses or oil, viscosity is highly dependent on temperature.

Viscosity most frequently refers to dynamic, or molecular, viscosity. A fluid in motion may be viewed as a set of thin parallel layers that move past each other. Dynamic viscosity is the stickiness between the layers. If a constant force pushes against an upper layer while the lower one is fixed, the upper layer moves with a flow velocity. The

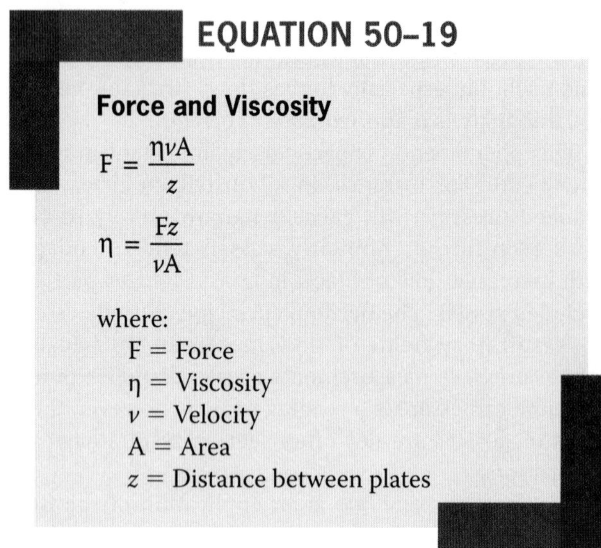

EQUATION 50–19

Force and Viscosity

$$F = \frac{\eta v A}{z}$$

$$\eta = \frac{Fz}{vA}$$

where:
F = Force
η = Viscosity
v = Velocity
A = Area
z = Distance between plates

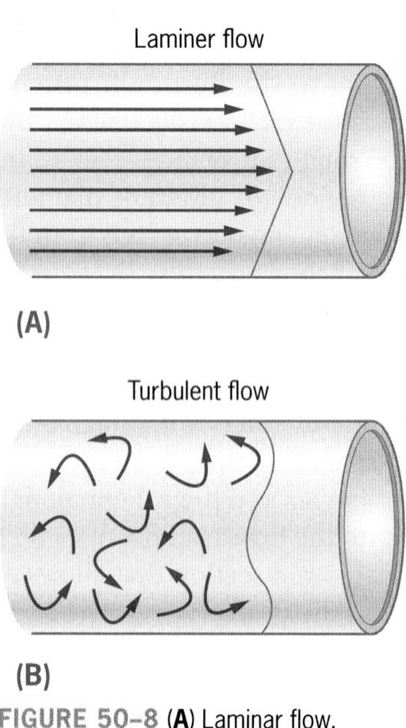

FIGURE 50–8 (**A**) Laminar flow. (**B**) Turbulent flow.

required force to achieve a velocity depends on the area of the layer, the viscosity, and the distance between layers (**Equation 50–19**). Measurement of viscosity using SI units is in pascal-seconds, a unit without a specific name. The poise (dyne · second · cm^{-2}) is a non-SI unit for viscosity that remains in frequent use. A poise is approximately one-tenth the unnamed SI unit. Typically, a gas is less viscous than a liquid. Air is approximately 50 times less viscous than water.

Laminar and Turbulent Flow

Flow of any fluid can be characterized as laminar or turbulent. **Laminar flow** is the orderly flow of a fluid through a straight tube as a series of concentric cylinders slide over one another (**Figure 50–8**). Laminar flow creates a parabolic distribution of velocities from the wall (slower velocity) to the center (faster velocity) of a tube. *Turbulence*, however, describes the circumstances in which this orderly flow is disrupted. **Turbulent flow** is a jumbled mixture of velocities across the section of tube. Friction also has a prominent effect on flow, which is decreased during laminar flow and, conversely, friction is increased during turbulent flow.

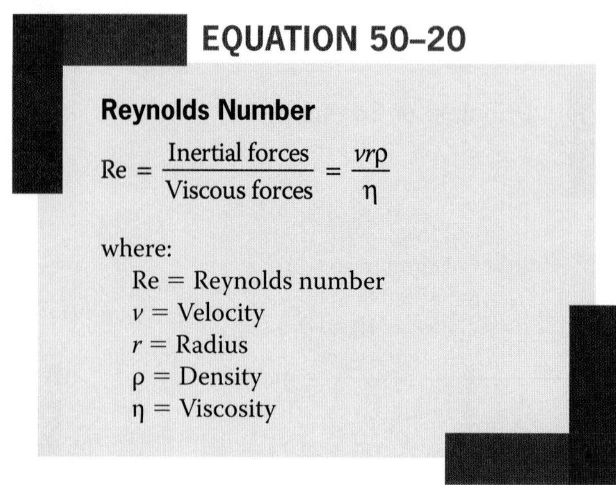

EQUATION 50–20

Reynolds Number

$$Re = \frac{\text{Inertial forces}}{\text{Viscous forces}} = \frac{vr\rho}{\eta}$$

where:
Re = Reynolds number
v = Velocity
r = Radius
ρ = Density
η = Viscosity

The **Reynolds number** (**Equation 50–20**) describes factors associated with the generation of laminar or turbulent flow. The Reynolds number is a dimensionless number because the units of measure cancel one another in its calculation. Flow tends to be more turbulent at high velocity, through large-diameter conduits, and with high-density and low-viscosity fluids. The equation shows that density and viscosity are independent factors affecting turbulence. Whereas viscosity is inversely related to the Reynolds number, the fluid density, velocity, and conduit radius are directly related. On a qualitative basis, Reynolds numbers describe a ratio of inertial forces to viscous forces. A fluid with significant inertia (the tendency to continue in the direction of movement) is more likely to be turbulent. A low Reynolds number (under 2000) in smooth tubes with a length substantially longer than the diameter indicates laminar flow, whereas a high number (more than 3000) indicates turbulent flow.

RESPIRATORY RECAP

Types of Flow

- » Laminar
- » Turbulent

Hagen-Poiseuille Equation

If a viscous fluid is flowing without turbulence through a tube (i.e., is laminar), the layer of fluid next to the wall of the tube (the boundary layer) has low velocity due to friction, whereas the layer at the center of the tube has the maximum velocity. The different flow rates create fronts with parabolic configurations. Because of viscosity, analysis beyond the principle of continuity and the Bernoulli principle must be applied. The force required to push flow through a tube is the product of the pressure difference and the area of the tube.

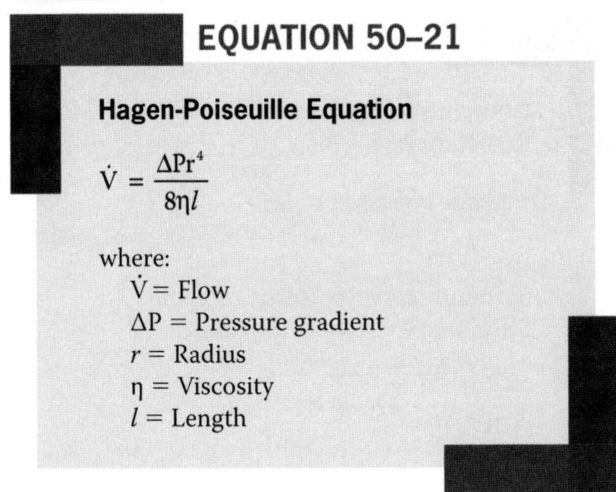

EQUATION 50–21

Hagen-Poiseuille Equation

$$\dot{V} = \frac{\Delta P r^4}{8\eta l}$$

where:
$\dot{V}$ = Flow
ΔP = Pressure gradient
r = Radius
η = Viscosity
l = Length

After several mathematic transformations, the **Hagen-Poiseuille equation** can be derived (**Equation 50–21**). A most relevant factor is that flow or pressure drop is related to the fourth power of the radius. Flow is inversely related to the viscosity of the fluid and the length of the tube through which the fluid passes and directly related to the pressure gradient. If these variables remain constant, the pressure gradient over the length of the tubular structure is directly proportional to flow. Most importantly, differential pressure pneumotachographs within ventilators use this principle to measure flow.

The relationship between pressure and a tube's radius is very important in respiratory care. A change in the inside diameter of a tracheal tube from 6 mm to 5 mm increases the pressure drop across the tube by a factor of 2.1 if constant flow is maintained. Endotracheal tube size can have a dramatic effect on work of breathing.

In contrast to laminar flow, turbulent flow varies directly with the square of flow rate and carries a term for friction, implying greater resistance at equivalent flows. Density rather than viscosity is a more prominent fluid characteristic. These differences explain the use and possible effectiveness of ventilating with helium–oxygen mixtures when the upper airways are narrowed. Although the viscosities of helium, oxygen, and air are not markedly different, helium is much less dense. **Equation 50–22** describes the effects of density when flow is turbulent. Flow velocity is greater in the upper airway and trachea than in the more numerous small airways, as explained by the principle of continuity. The total area of the smaller airways is greater; thus, velocity is less.

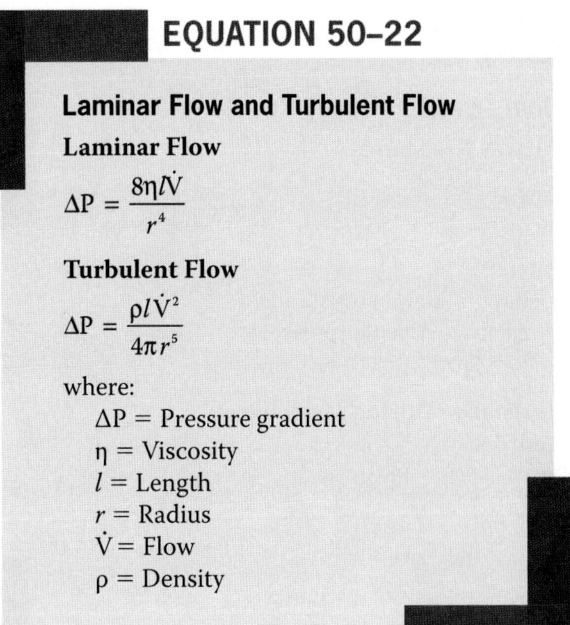

EQUATION 50–22

Laminar Flow and Turbulent Flow

Laminar Flow

$$\Delta P = \frac{8\eta l\dot{V}}{r^4}$$

Turbulent Flow

$$\Delta P = \frac{\rho l\dot{V}^2}{4\pi r^5}$$

where:
ΔP = Pressure gradient
η = Viscosity
l = Length
r = Radius
$\dot{V}$ = Flow
ρ = Density

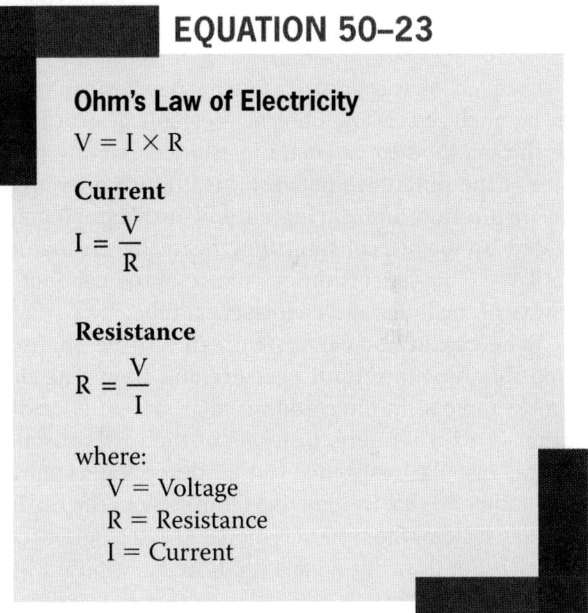

EQUATION 50–23

Ohm's Law of Electricity

$$V = I \times R$$

Current

$$I = \frac{V}{R}$$

Resistance

$$R = \frac{V}{I}$$

where:
V = Voltage
R = Resistance
I = Current

Flow, Resistance, and Pressure

An analysis of flow/pressure and resistance relationships assumes linear relationships without the loss of thermal energy or effects of turbulence. This analysis allows application of easily measured quantities, such as resistance, to other circular systems of single or connected circuits in which measurements may be more technically difficult. The more general expression of **Ohm's law** involving electrons flowing in electrical circuits describes the relationships among voltage, current, and resistance (**Equation 50–23**).

In physiologic terms, voltage correlates with pressure differences, current with flow rate, and electrical resistance with airflow resistance. Ohm's law gives a general expression for **resistance**, the ratio of pressure gradient to flow. This relationship may be used to calculate airway resistance. Using a body plethysmography box, the subject pants or breathes with a small tidal volume. The alveolar pressure change during each inspiratory effort is associated with a flow measurement. Airway resistance is then calculated from the measurement of instantaneous airflow and pressure changes (**Equation 50–24**).

EQUATION 50–24

Ohm's Law for Airway Resistance

Airway Resistance

$$\text{Raw} = \frac{\Delta \text{Palv}}{\dot{V}}$$

where:

Raw = Airway resistance
ΔPalv = Alveolar pressure
$\dot{V}$ = Flow

Resistance During Mechanical Ventilation

$$\text{Raw} = \frac{\text{PIP} - \text{Pplat}}{\dot{V}}$$

where:

Raw = Airway resistance
PIP = Peak inspiratory pressure
Pplat = Plateau pressure

EQUATION 50–25

Ohm's Law for Vascular Resistance

$$\text{Vascular resistance} = \frac{\Delta \text{P}}{\dot{Q}\text{c}}$$

Systemic Vascular Resistance and Pulmonary Vascular Resistance

$$\text{SVR} = \frac{\text{MAP} - \text{CVP}}{\dot{Q}\text{c}}$$

$$\text{PVR} = \frac{\text{MPAP} - \text{PAWP}}{\dot{Q}\text{c}}$$

where:

SVR = Systemic vascular resistance
MAP = Mean arterial pressure
CVP = Central venous pressure
$\dot{Q}$c = Cardiac output
PVR = Pulmonary vascular resistance
MPAP = Mean pulmonary artery pressure
PAWP = Pulmonary artery wedge pressure

Alternatively, airway pressures during passive inspiration can be analyzed. Many current mechanical ventilators use this method to calculate resistance. Airway resistance is the difference between inspiratory pressure at end-inspiration and during an end-inspiratory pause divided by the set constant flow from the mechanical ventilator. This reflects the resistance of the conducting airways of the lungs and endotracheal tube.

The cardiovascular system can also be analyzed using this relationship of pressure and flow. The flow of most interest in the cardiovascular system is cardiac output ($\dot{Q}$c). Therefore, in terms of the cardiovascular system, vascular resistance can be described as shown in **Equation 50–25**. By applying Ohm's law to the cardiovascular system, the system is modeled as a single circuit in which the flow out equals the flow in, opposed by a single resistance over a particular section of the circuit. For example, systemic vascular resistance is estimated by subtracting right atrial (central venous) pressure from mean arterial pressure and dividing that quantity by $\dot{Q}$c. Similarly, pulmonary vascular resistance is estimated by subtracting pulmonary artery occlusion (or wedge) pressure from mean pulmonary pressure and dividing that quantity by $\dot{Q}$c.

Application of Physical Principles to Measurement and Physiology

Principles of Measurement

Any measurement device will convert a physical entity into a number or signal. Even a water column manometer converts a pressure existing somewhere in a system of interest into a column of water height that can be measured. Electronic transducers are in common use for the purposes of measurement. Important considerations in the ability of measurement devices to record physical signals faithfully include: linearity, the proportional output of a system including hysteresis (i.e., a difference between responses to increasing and decreasing pressure), drift, or the long-term shift in the system output in response to a constant signal, and dynamic response, or distortion of the signal caused by the way the physical signal reaches the transducer.

An analog meter or gauge measures by a physical continuous scale, such as a spring (mechanical) or voltage range (electronic). Passing the signal into a suitable circuit allows simple manipulation of the signal (e.g., integration, differentiation). A digital meter, on the other hand, measures the signal of interest not continuously but at regular, discrete intervals. Digital analysis of a signal permits a more flexible and complicated analysis but must sample the signal at a sufficiently rapid frequency to reproduce it faithfully.

Noise is unwanted effects detected by the recording system. Noise may be intrinsic, such as oscillations or physical movements occurring in a catheter system attached to a pressure manometer, or extrinsic, such as electrical interference occurring between a transducer and an amplifier. A goal is to maximize the signal-to-noise ratio.

Calibration refers to the process by which the output of a measurement system is adjusted to a known input. Calibration may be passive, in which the output is compared with a static input signal (such as a particular set pressure) or dynamic, which compares the system output with a forcing function or probe in which a varying signal is used for calibration.

Common Methods of Measuring Flow in Respiratory Systems

Devices that measure flow are capable of faster responses to changes than are devices that directly measure volume. This limitation in frequency response, or ability to faithfully reflect changes in volume over short periods, has restricted the use of volumetric spirometers. Therefore, most volume measurement devices in wide use today measure flow and calculate volume by integration.

The following device types are found in mechanical ventilators, spirometers for measurements of pulmonary function, and other specialty devices.

- *Pneumotachometer:* A device that actually measures a pressure difference between two sides of a resistance element. As flow increases, the pressure drop across the element also increases due to viscous forces. If the flow is laminar (nonturbulent), the change in pressure versus flow is nearly linear (i.e., a doubling in flow results in a doubling of pressure). An element can be inserted to laminarize the flow, such as a screen, filter paper, or an array of smaller-diameter tubes—also known as a laminar flow element.
- *Fixed orifice meter:* A variant on the pneumotachometer uses a fixed orifice that is not linear because the flow is generally turbulent. This is a simple device that is resistant to fouling with secretions or humidity but requires more sophisticated software to calculate the actual flow. Generally, the total resistance at the highest flow rate will be higher than that measured by a linear pneumotachometer.
- *Thermal meter:* As flow increases, so does convective heat transfer (think of wind chill). Devices heat an element electrically and measure the power required to maintain a particular temperature. Hence, some method of measuring the temperature of the heated element is also required. One common thermal meter is a hot-wire anemometer.
- *Ultrasonic meter:* This type of meter operates similar to sonar or radar by measuring the speed of sound as affected by flow toward and away from an ultrasonic signal. The difference represents the gas velocity.
- *Rotating vane anemometer (Wright respirometer):* This uses a rotating vane set in a tube with oblique slots through which air enters. This device is not linear at low flows because gas can enter the tube before the vanes rotate.

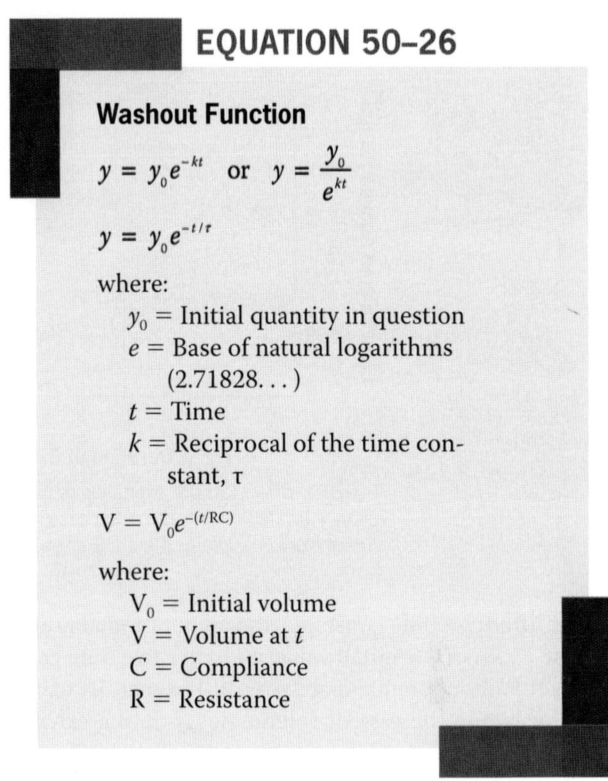

EQUATION 50–26

Washout Function

$$y = y_0 e^{-kt} \quad \text{or} \quad y = \frac{y_0}{e^{kt}}$$

$$y = y_0 e^{-t/\tau}$$

where:

y_0 = Initial quantity in question
e = Base of natural logarithms (2.71828. . .)
t = Time
k = Reciprocal of the time constant, τ

$$V = V_0 e^{-(t/RC)}$$

where:

V_0 = Initial volume
V = Volume at t
C = Compliance
R = Resistance

The most straightforward method of flow measurement is direct, timed collection of volume (e.g., of blood or gas); however, this method cannot be applied to a closed system. Any measurement applied must add minimal resistance and generate a signal that is linear over the range of expected flows. Devices used to measure the flow of some liquids include electromagnetic flow meters, which rely on a conductor moving through a magnetic field; ultrasonic flow meters, in which frequency changes of reflected sound waves are measured (the Doppler frequency shift principle); radioactivity counting devices; and direct volume measurement, in which a volume change is directly measured when outflow is occluded for a set period. All these methods have been used to determine blood flow, but the underlying principles do not apply (electromagnetic, ultrasound techniques) or are impractical (plethysmography) to measure airflow.

Expiratory Flow

Expiratory flow demonstrates a physical principle important to respiratory physiology because volume is exhaled in a manner that decays at a rate that can be analyzed. The passive exhalation tracing of volume is an example of a washout function. In this case the function is associated with lung impedance. Other pertinent examples of washout functions include the change in P_{AO_2} after an F_{IO_2} change or the change in P_{aCO_2} after a change in minute ventilation. In these cases the decrease in a quantity is proportional to the amount of quantity remaining (**Equation 50–26**). After one time period, called the **time constant**, the amount remaining is approximately 37% of its initial

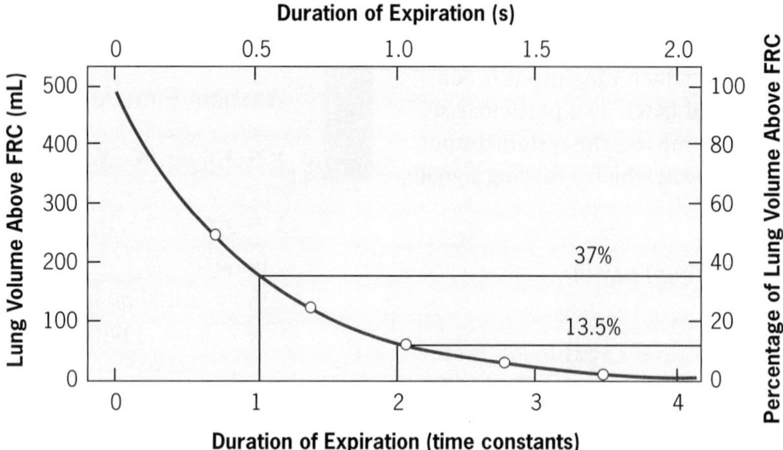

FIGURE 50–9 Passive expiration of one breath washout function. The points on the curve indicate the passage of successive half lives. Adapted from Nunn JF. *Nunn's Applied Respiratory Physiology*. 4th ed. Butterworth-Heinemann; 1993.

value. After two time constants, the amount remaining is $1/e^2$, or 13.5% of the initial value, and after five time constants the amount remaining is $1/e^5$, or less than 1% of the initial value. In the case of volume decay during exhalation, the time constant is a function of the product of compliance and resistance. Thus, the tidal volume remaining in the lungs at any point during exhalation is determined by the resistance and compliance of the respiratory system (refer to Equation 50–26 and **Figure 50–9**).

KEY POINTS

- Molecular theory describes physical entities and their response to physical forces by describing atoms and molecules and the interactions between them.
- Work of breathing may be estimated by measurement of volume change and the associated pressure change.
- Pascal's law describes the way in which pressure is transmitted without reduction throughout any enclosed static fluid; this law is the basis for manometric measurements.
- Laplace's law describes the tension of the wall of a sphere or cylinder (wall tension) and is useful for understanding pressures in an alveolus.
- Surface tension describes the property of liquid that tends to reduce the surface of a liquid toward a minimum, pulling the surface molecules inward.
- Surfactant is necessary for normal lung function because it reduces surface tension.
- The ideal gas law states that pressure and volume are inversely related, whereas temperature is directly proportional to volume or pressure.
- Common conditions for reporting of gas volumes are STPD, BTPS, ATPD, and ATPS.
- A humidity deficit occurs whenever inspired gas is not fully saturated at body temperature.
- Graham's law predicts the rate of diffusion of a gas as inversely proportional to the gram molecular weight of the gas.
- Fick's law describes the transfer of a solute by diffusion.
- The Bernoulli principle describes the pressure drop when fluid passes through a constriction in a rigid tube.
- The Venturi principle states that a pressure drop across an obstruction can be restored, provided the angle of divergence is less than 15 degrees.
- The Hagen-Poiseuille equation states that flow is related to the fourth power of the radius, the viscosity of the fluid, the length of the tube, and the pressure gradient.
- The Reynolds number is a dimensionless number used to describe laminar or turbulent flow.
- Ohm's law describes the relationship among pressure, flow, and resistance.
- Expiratory flow is an example of a washout function, in which the decrease in quantity is a function of the initial volume and a time constant associated with respiratory system impedance.

CHAPTER 51

Chemistry for Respiratory Care

Carl F. Haas
Allan G. Andrews

OUTLINE

Basic Chemistry
Inorganic Molecules
Organic Molecules
Fluid Balance
Metabolic Pathways

OBJECTIVES

1. Describe the structure of the atom.
2. Compare ionic, covalent, and hydrogen bonds.
3. Describe synthesis, decomposition, and exchange reactions.
4. List factors that affect the solubility of solutions.
5. Compare methods used to state concentrations of solutions.
6. List colligative properties of solutions.
7. Compare organic and inorganic compounds.
8. Describe the physical and chemical properties of water, oxygen, carbon dioxide, and electrolytes.
9. Describe the chemical properties of acids, bases, buffers, and salts.
10. Discuss the biologic importance of carbohydrates, lipids, proteins, nucleic acids, vitamins, hormones, cytokines, and enzymes.
11. Explain the biologic basis of fluid balance.
12. Describe the energy-producing metabolic pathways.

KEY TERMS

acid
adenosine triphosphate (ATP)
adsorption
allele
amino acid
anabolism
anions
atom
atomic mass unit (amu)
atomic number
atomic weight
base
boiling point
buffers
carbohydrate
catabolism
cations
cholesterol
chromosome
citric acid (Krebs) cycle
colligative properties
colloid
compound
concentrated
covalent bond
crenation
cytokine
deoxyribonucleic acid (DNA)
dilute
eicosanoid
electrolytes
electrons
electron transport system
element
enzyme
freezing point
genotype
glucose
glycolysis
heat of vaporization
hemolysis
Henderson-Hasselbalch equation
hormone
hydrogen bond
hydrophilic
hydrophobic
hypertonic
hypotonic
ionic bond
ions
isotonic
isotope
lipid
mass number
matter
milliequivalent
molar solution
mole
neutrons
nucleic acid
osmosis
osmotic pressure
oxidative phosphorylation
peptide
percent solution
periodic table
pH
phenotype
phospholipids
polar
precipitate
proteins
protons
ribonucleic acid (RNA)
saturated
saturated fatty acid
semipermeable membrane
solute
solution
solvent
specific heat
steroids
suspension
triglycerides
unsaturated fatty acid
valence electron
vapor pressure
vitamin

INTRODUCTION

Chemistry is the science of the composition, structure, properties, and reactions of matter. An understanding of basic chemistry is essential to the practice of respiratory care. This chapter covers basic chemistry, the chemistry of inorganic and organic molecules, fluid balance, and metabolic pathways.

Basic Chemistry

Matter

Anything that occupies space and has mass is **matter**. Matter is classified as an element or a compound. An **element** cannot be broken down into two or more substances; it is a pure substance containing only one type of atom. Although oxygen is a good example of an element, most living materials are not composed of pure elements but rather are a combination of elements. When two or more elements join to form a chemical combination, the result is a **compound**. Three important examples of compounds in the human body are water (H_2O), in which two hydrogen atoms combine with one oxygen atom; carbon dioxide (CO_2), in which one carbon atom combines with two oxygen atoms; and glucose ($C_6H_{12}O_6$), in which six carbon atoms combine with twelve hydrogen and six oxygen atoms.

> **RESPIRATORY RECAP**
>
> **Components of the Atom**
> » Protons
> » Neutrons
> » Electrons

The **atom** often is called the building block of the universe. It is the smallest portion of an element that retains all the properties of the element. Each atom is composed of a small, heavy, corelike nucleus with particles surrounding it at relatively great distances. The three fundamental particles that make up the atom are the proton, the neutron, and the electron. **Protons** have a positive electrical charge (+1) and are located in the nucleus. **Neutrons** have no net electrical charge and are also located in the nucleus. **Electrons** have a negative electrical charge (−1) and are located outside the nucleus (**Figure 51–1**). This gives the atomic nucleus a positive charge and the surrounding electron cloud a negative charge.

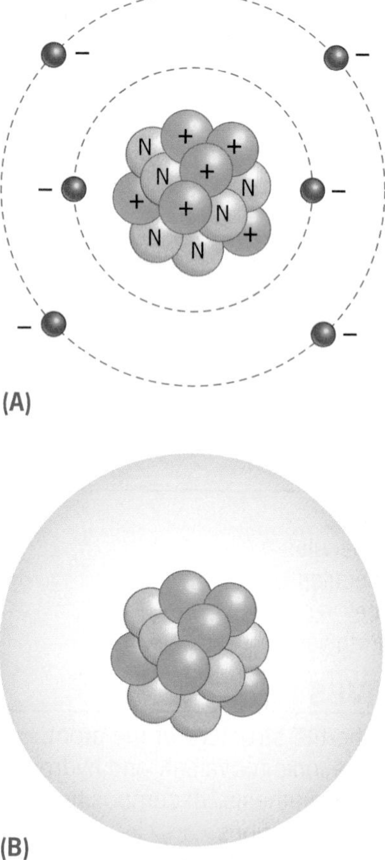

FIGURE 51–1 Model of the atom. (**A**) The nucleus contains protons (+1 change) and neutrons (0 charge). Electrons (−1 charge) occupy the outer regions, which are called electron shells. This figure represents the carbon atom, which has six protons and six neutrons in the nucleus and six electrons orbiting the nucleus. Two electrons are in the first electron shell, and the remaining four are in the outer shell. (**B**) The outer shells can be thought of collectively as an electron cloud.

The number of protons in the nucleus defines the element and is known as the **atomic number**. Because all atoms are electrically neutral, the number of protons is the same as the number of electrons. The sum of the protons and neutrons determines the atom's **mass number**. The naturally occurring sodium atom has an atomic number of 11 and a mass number of 23, indicating 11 protons and electrons and 12 neutrons. The relative weight of an atom is its **atomic weight**, a term often used interchangeably with *mass number*. The carbon atom, which has a mass number of 12 (carbon-12), has been assigned the weight of 12 **atomic mass units (amu)**, to which all other atoms are referenced.

Each element has a unique atomic number, suggesting a specific and unchanging number of protons in the nucleus, but not necessarily the same mass number. **Isotopes** are atoms with nuclei that have the same number of protons (atomic number) but a different number of neutrons (mass number). All elements have isotopes. Oxygen has three isotopes, each having eight protons and eight electrons but 8, 9, or 10 neutrons (99.8% of atmospheric oxygen is composed of oxygen-16, 0.04% is oxygen-17, and 0.16% is oxygen-18). Isotopes of the same element have the same basic chemical properties because they have the same number of electrons and protons, but they have different physical properties because they differ in the number of neutrons. Most isotopes are stable and do not break up, particularly the lighter elements. Isotopes of some of the heavier unstable elements give off radiation when they break up and are referred to as being *radioactive*.

Each element has a symbol that represents not only the element but also one atom of the element. The symbol "O" stands for one oxygen atom. As of 2006, 117 chemical elements had been confirmed. There are 94 naturally occurring elements; the others are synthetic elements produced artificially in particle accelerators. These elements can be arranged into a table containing seven rows, known as the **periodic table**. **Figure 51–2** shows the first four rows of the periodic table. Note in each box that the large letter represents the element symbol, the number above the symbol is the atomic number, and the number below the symbol is the mass number.

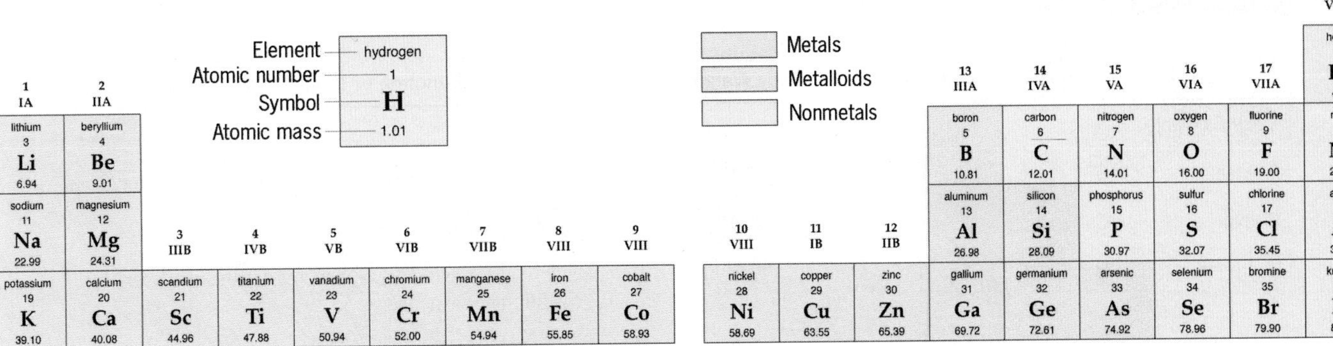

FIGURE 51–2 The first 36 elements of the periodic table of the elements.

For example, carbon has a symbol of C, an atomic number of 6, and a mass number of 12.01. Elements in a vertical column belong to the same *group*. They have similar chemical properties because they have the same number of electrons in their outer shell. For example, each element in column IA has one electron in its outer shell, whereas elements in column VIIA have seven electrons. Elements in a horizontal row belong to the same *period*. It is interesting that 23 of the first 36 elements on the periodic table are found in the body. **Table 51–1** lists elements that are important to the functioning of the human body.

Electrons are arranged in a definite order in the atom. They occupy various principal energy levels, or *shells*, which can be thought of as a volume occupied by an electron cloud. Each level can hold a maximum number of electrons, which is defined by the formula $2n^2$, where n is the number of energy levels or orbits from the nucleus. The first level can hold 2 electrons, the second, 8; the third, 18, and so on. Each element in a given period (row) in the periodic table has the same number of energy levels, or orbitals. For example, the elements in the first row have one orbital for their electrons, the elements in the second row each have two energy levels, and so on. Currently the maximum number of orbitals or shells is seven.

Each energy level has sublevels, called *subshells*. As the energy level increases, so does the number of subshells. The atoms of known elements have four types of subshells, labeled *s*, *p*, *d*, and *f*. In "excited atoms," electrons may occur in subshells labeled *g*, *h*, *i*, and so on, but further detail is beyond the scope of this discussion. The number of subshells is equal to the shell (energy level) number. The first energy level has one subshell, the *s* subshell, which contains 2 electrons (one pair). The second energy level has two subshells: an *s* subshell (2*s*) containing 2 electrons, and a *p* subshell (2*p*) that has 6 electrons (three pairs). The third energy level has an *s* subshell (3*s*) with 2 electrons, a *p* subshell (3*p*) with 6 electrons, and a *d* subshell (3*d*), which holds 10 electrons (five pairs). The fourth energy level has the *s*, *p*, *d* subshells and an *f* subshell, which can hold 14 electrons (seven pairs). Electrons fill shells in an orderly manner: first the orbital 1*s*; then 2*s*; then 2*p* and 3*s*; then 3*p* and 4*s*; then 3*d*, 4*p*, and 5*s*; then 4*d*, 5*p*, and 6*s*; then 4*f*, 5*d*, 6*p*, and 7*s*; followed by 5*f*, 6*d*, and 7*p*. Overlapping of shells begins with the transition from shell 3 to shell 4.

The number of electrons in the various energy levels and a notation referred to as the *electron configuration* can represent the subshells of an element. For example, the electron configuration for the element sodium (Na, atomic number 11) is $1s^2 2s^2 2p^6 3s^1$. This representation indicates that the 1*s* subshell has two electrons, the 2*s* subshell has two electrons, the 2*p* subshell has six electrons, and the 3*s* (outermost) subshell has one electron. **Table 51–2** shows the electron configuration for the first 20 elements.

Chemical Bonding

The outermost electron shell is most important to determine an element's chemical properties, because these orbitals are involved in the formation of chemical bonds and in chemical reactions. An electron dot structure, known as a *Lewis dot structure*, often is used to represent the structure of an atom. The nucleus and all the filled energy levels are represented by the element's symbol; the symbol is surrounded by dots equal to the number of electrons in the outer shell. These electrons are known as **valance electrons**. The Lewis dot structures for the first 20 elements are included in Table 51–2. The gases helium, neon, and argon, which are known as *noble gases*, have full outer shells (helium has only two electrons because it is filling only the 1*s* orbital, whereas the others have eight electrons). Eight electrons in the outer energy level correspond to filled *s* and *p* orbitals, which in turn leads to great stability. This tendency to fill the *s* and *p* levels is known as the *octet rule*. Elements with the same number of valance electrons are in the same column in the periodic table. They belong to the same group or family and have similar chemical properties.

> **RESPIRATORY RECAP**
>
> **Chemical Bonds**
>
> » Ionic bond
> » Covalent bond
> » Hydrogen bond

TABLE 51-1 Important Elements Found in the Body

Element	Symbol	Atomic Number	Percentage of Body Weight	Function or Importance
Major Elements				
Oxygen	O	8	65.0	Cellular respiration; a component of water and organic compounds
Carbon	C	6	18.5	Backbone of organic molecules
Hydrogen	H	1	9.5	Component of water and most organic molecules; necessary for energy transfer and respiration
Nitrogen	N	7	3.3	Component of all proteins and nucleic acids
Calcium	Ca	20	1.5	Component of bones and teeth; necessary for certain enzymes, nerve and muscle function, hormonal action, cellular motility, and blood clotting
Phosphorus	P	15	1.0	Main component of nucleic acids; required for bones and teeth; important in energy transfer and for phospholipids and some proteins
Potassium	K	19	0.4	Main positive intracellular ion; important in muscle and nerve function
Sulfur	S	16	0.3	Component of most proteins and some organic compounds
Sodium	Na	11	0.2	Important positive ion surrounding cells; important in muscle and nerve function and in fluid balance
Chlorine	Cl	17	0.2	Important negative ion surrounding cells
Magnesium	Mg	12	0.1	Component of many energy-transferring enzymes
Trace Elements				
Silicone	Si	14	<0.1	—
Aluminum	Al	13	<0.1	—
Iron	Fe	26	<0.1	Critical component of blood hemoglobin and many enzymes
Manganese	Mn	25	<0.1	Requirement for many enzymes
Fluorine	F	9	<0.1	Requirement for bones and teeth; inhibitor of certain enzymes
Vanadium	V	23	<0.1	—
Chromium	Cr	24	<0.1	Relationship to action of insulin
Copper	Cu	29	<0.1	Requirement for many enzymes, for the synthesis of hemoglobin, and for normal bone formation
Boron	B	5	<0.1	—
Cobalt	Co	27	<0.1	Assistance to vitamin B_{12} in blood clot production
Zinc	Zn	30	<0.1	Requirement for many enzymes; related to action of insulin; essential for normal growth and reproduction
Selenium	Sn	34	<0.1	Close relationship to action of vitamin E
Molybdenum	Mo	42	<0.1	Key component of many enzymes
Tin	Sn	50	<0.1	—
Iodine	I	53	<0.1	Component of thyroid hormone

Dashes (—) denote that the exact function is unclear or unknown.

TABLE 51-2 Electron Representations of the First 20 Elements

Element	Atomic Number	Electron Configuration	Lewis Dot Structure
H	1	$1s^1$	H·
He	2	$1s^2$	He:
Li	3	$1s^2 2s^1$	Li·
Be	4	$1s^2 2s^2$	Be:
B	5	$1s^2 2s^2 2p^1$	B̈·
C	6	$1s^2 2s^2 2p^2$	·C̈·
N	7	$1s^2 2s^2 2p^3$	:Ṅ·
O	8	$1s^2 2s^2 2p^4$	:Ö·
F	9	$1s^2 2s^2 2p^5$	:F̤̈·
Ne	10	$1s^2 2s^2 2p^6$	:N̤̈e:
Na	11	$1s^2 2s^2 2p^6 3s^1$	Na·
Mg	12	$1s^2 2s^2 2p^6 3s^2$	Mg:
Al	13	$1s^2 2s^2 2p^6 3s^2 3p^1$	Äl·
Si	14	$1s^2 2s^2 2p^6 3s^2 3p^2$	·S̈i·
P	15	$1s^2 2s^2 2p^6 3s^2 3p^3$	·P̈·
S	16	$1s^2 2s^2 2p^6 3s^2 3p^4$	:S̈·
Cl	17	$1s^2 2s^2 2p^6 3s^2 3p^5$	:C̤̈l·
Ar	18	$1s^2 2s^2 2p^6 3s^2 3p^6$	:Ä̤r:
K	19	$1s^2 2s^2 2p^6 3s^2 3p^6 4s^1$	K·
Ca	20	$1s^2 2s^2 2p^6 3s^2 3p^6 4s^2$	Ca:

H, hydrogen; He, helium; Li, lithium; Be, beryllium; B, boron; C, carbon; N, nitrogen; O, oxygen; F, fluorine; Ne, neon; Na, sodium; Mg, magnesium; Al, aluminum; Si, silicon; P, phosphorus; S, sulfur; Cl, chlorine; Ar, argon; K, potassium; Ca, calcium.

Such elements tend to form similar compounds and often substitute for each other.

Atoms bond in such a way that each atom participating in the chemical bond either acquires a completed outer shell and attains the configuration of the closest noble gas to satisfy the octet rule or obtains at least a spin pair of electrons in the outer shell. Stable configurations are achieved by the transfer of electrons (**ionic bond**) or by the sharing of electrons (**covalent bond**). Elements with only one, two, or three valence electrons tend to give them up, thereby becoming positive **ions**. Positively charged ions are known as **cations**. Sodium (Na) loses its one valance electron and takes on a +1 charge (11 protons and 10 electrons); aluminum (Al) loses its three valance electrons and takes on a +3 charge (13 protons and 10 electrons) (**Equation 51–1**). Elements with six or

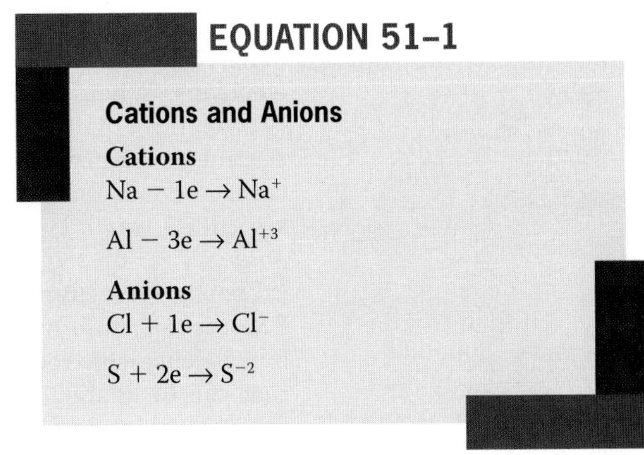

EQUATION 51–1

Cations and Anions

Cations

$Na - 1e \rightarrow Na^+$

$Al - 3e \rightarrow Al^{+3}$

Anions

$Cl + 1e \rightarrow Cl^-$

$S + 2e \rightarrow S^{-2}$

seven valance electrons tend to gain electrons to reach stability. Chlorine (Cl), which has seven valance electrons, gains one electron to fill its outer shell, thereby taking on a −1 charge and becoming a negative ion. Similarly, sulfur (S) takes on two electrons to fill its outer shell and becomes an ion with a −2 charge. Negatively charged ions are also known as **anions**.

Ions of opposite charge are attracted to each other. When a sodium atom (Na) combines with a chlorine atom (Cl) to form a sodium chloride molecule (NaCl), the sodium atom loses (or donates) an electron, and the chlorine atom gains (or accepts) the electron. In the process a positive sodium cation (Na^+) and a negative chloride (Cl^-) anion are formed. The two opposite-charged ions are held together by electrostatic attraction of their opposite charges to form a sodium chloride molecule:

$$Na^+ + Cl^- \rightarrow NaCl$$

Compounds having ionic bonds, called *ionic compounds*, share some characteristics, such as high melting and boiling points and the ability to conduct electricity in the gaseous or liquid state. Ions are very important in the chemistry of the body, especially as electrolytes and minerals.

Another type of bonding involves the sharing of one or more pairs of electrons to achieve a stable electron configuration. When each of the two bonding atoms shares one of its valance electrons, the bond is referred to as a *covalent bond*. When one of the atoms shares two of its valance electrons with another atom, the bond is called a *dative bond*. Once formed, both covalent and dative bonds produce a shared pair of electrons and therefore have identical structures. The molecular orbital theory is used to describe the sharing of electrons and the overlap of atomic orbitals. When the atomic orbital of one atom overlaps with the atomic orbital of another atom, two new molecular orbitals are formed that encompass both nuclei. Each molecular orbital can hold one spin pair of electrons, which is the property of the whole molecule, not just the atoms forming the bond. This molecular arrangement is more stable than a combination in which each nucleus retains its own electrons.

Ethane (C_2H_6) single bond (sharing 2 e^-)

H–C–C–H (each carbon also bonded to two H)

Ethylene (C_2H_4) double bond (sharing 4 e^-)

$H_2C{=}CH_2$

Acetylene (C_2H_2) triple bond (sharing 6 e^-)

H–C≡C–H

FIGURE 51-3 Formation of carbon–carbon single, double, and triple bonds.

Atoms often share more than one pair of electrons. When one, two, or three pairs of electrons are shared, the covalent bonds formed are called *single* (–), *double* (=), or *triple* (≡) bonds, respectively. The carbon atom has four valence electrons that can be shared to form covalent bonds (**Figure 51-3**). It uses all three types of covalent bonds when bonding with another carbon atom, often with the remaining valence electrons single bonded with hydrogen atoms.

The covalent bond is particularly important in physiology because the major elements of the body (carbon, oxygen, hydrogen, and nitrogen) almost always share electrons to form bonds. Carbon, nitrogen, and oxygen form covalent bonds using atomic orbitals of the second principal energy level (elements in the second row on the periodic table). Table 51–2 shows that oxygen (atomic number 8) has six valence electrons and that the two unpaired electrons in the 2*p* subshell are available to form covalent bonds. Oxygen exists naturally as a diatomic molecule (O_2), which uses a double covalent bond to form. When two oxygen atoms unite to form molecular oxygen, each oxygen atom shares its two unpaired 2*p* electrons.

In addition to covalent and ionic bonds, which form molecules, a third type of bond can exist within or between biologically important molecules. The **hydrogen bond** is a weak bond and requires much less energy to break than a covalent or ionic bond. It forms as the result of unequal charge distribution on a molecule rather than from sharing or transfer of electrons. This type of molecule is called a **polar** molecule. Water is a polar molecule; although it is electrically neutral, it has a partial positive charge on the hydrogen side and a partial negative charge on the oxygen side. Hydrogen bonds weakly attach the negative (oxygen) side of one water molecule with the positive (hydrogen) side of an adjacent water molecule. This ability of water to form hydrogen bonds makes water an ideal medium for the chemistry of life. Hydrogen bonds also help maintain the three-dimensional structure of proteins and nucleic acids.

Chemical Reactions

Chemical reactions involve the formation or breaking of chemical bonds between atoms and molecules. The three basic types of chemical reactions are synthesis reactions, decomposition reactions, and exchange reactions (**Equation 51-2**). *Synthesis reactions* combine two or more substances (reactants) to form a different, more complex substance (product). Energy is required for this reaction to occur and the new product to be formed.

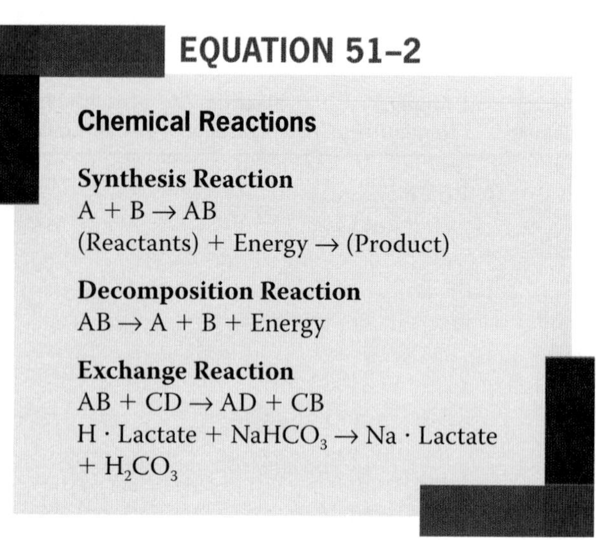

EQUATION 51-2

Chemical Reactions

Synthesis Reaction
$A + B \rightarrow AB$
(Reactants) + Energy → (Product)

Decomposition Reaction
$AB \rightarrow A + B$ + Energy

Exchange Reaction
$AB + CD \rightarrow AD + CB$
H · Lactate + $NaHCO_3$ → Na · Lactate + H_2CO_3

Decomposition reactions break down complex substances into two or more simpler substances. During this reaction chemical bonds are broken, and energy is released. The energy can be released in the form of heat energy, or it can be captured and stored for future use. An example of a decomposition reaction is the breakdown of a complex nutrient in a cell to release energy for other cellular functions. The products of such reactions are ultimately waste products. Synthesis and decomposition reactions are opposites: synthesis forms chemical bonds and builds up, whereas decomposition undoes bonds and breaks down. Often the two opposite processes are coupled in such a way that the energy released through decomposition is used to drive a synthesis reaction.

RESPIRATORY RECAP

Chemical Reactions
- » Synthesis reaction
- » Decomposition reaction
- » Exchange reaction

An *exchange reaction* allows two reactants to exchange components and to form two new products. Exchange reactions break down two compounds and synthesize two new compounds. An example of such a reaction in the blood is the reaction of lactic acid with sodium bicarbonate to form sodium lactate and carbonic acid.

Liquid Mixtures

Most chemical reactions in the body take place in a liquid environment. Water is the primary liquid in the body, making up about 45% to 80% of the human body. Every cellular process takes place in a watery environment, and water is essential to the processes of digestion, circulation, elimination, and regulation of body temperature.

Water allows substances and particles to get into a liquid form as one of three types: a solution, a suspension, or a colloid.

A **solution** is a homogeneous mixture of two or more substances, meaning that the substances mix evenly and occupy the entire volume of the solution in equal proportions. A liquid solution consists of two parts: the **solute**, which is the solid, liquid, or gaseous material being dissolved, and the **solvent**, which is the liquid material into which the solute is dissolved. Water is the most common solvent in the body. Common nonbody solvents are alcohol, which forms the basis of medicinal tinctures, and ether, which dissolves fats and oils.

Solutions have several common characteristics: they have a variable concentration; they are transparent; they are homogeneous; they do not settle; they may be separated by physical means; and they can pass through filter paper. When a salt crystal is dropped into a glass of water and stirred, the crystal dissolves and the solution remains clear. The same thing occurs when sugar is mixed with water. If more salt or sugar (solute) is mixed into the water (solvent), the solution becomes more concentrated but remains clear. If the solution is poured into a funnel with filter paper, the solute particles pass though, indicating that solute particles in a solution are very small. If the glass is left undisturbed for a time, the solute particles do not settle out, provided evaporation does not occur. Should the solvent evaporate, the solute particles would be left behind.

The degree to which solute particles can dissolve into a solvent is referred to as the *solubility of the solution*. A high solubility indicates that the solvent allows many solute particles to be dissolved. The following factors affect solubility.

- *The nature of the solute*: A physical characteristic of matter that determines how certain substances dissolve in a solvent.
- *The nature of the solvent*: In general, polar liquids (such as water, methyl alcohol, and ethyl alcohol) dissolve polar compounds (such as sodium chloride and potassium iodide), and nonpolar solvents (such as benzene, ether, and carbon tetrachloride) dissolve nonpolar compounds (such as oils and waxes).
- *Temperature*: Most solids become more soluble as temperature increases (i.e., the solubility of solids is directly related to temperature), although sodium chloride shows little change; gases become less soluble as temperature increases (the solubility of gases is inversely related to temperature).
- *Pressure*: The solubility of a gas is directly related to pressure, although pressure has little effect on solid or liquid solutes.
- *Surface area*: Although the actual solubility is not changed, the rate of dissolution is directly related to surface area, which explains the rationale for a powder solute.
- *Agitation*: Stirring a solution brings solute particles in contact with fresh solvent more quickly, which increases the rate of dissolution but not the actual solubility.

The relative concentration, or strength, of a solution is classified as dilute or concentrate. **Dilute** means that the solution contains a small amount of solute. As more solute is added, the solution becomes more **concentrated**. No specific point exists at which dilute becomes concentrated; these are relative terms, used only in a comparative sense, and do not provide a specific quantitative meaning. The term **saturated** means that the maximum amount of solute is dissolved for given conditions. If conditions such as temperature or pressure change, the maximum amount of solute that a given volume of solvent can dissolve also changes. An unsaturated solution contains fewer solute particles than it maximally could under normal conditions. A supersaturated solution contains more solute particles than it normally does under specific conditions. Such a solution is formed by the addition of solute as a mixture is heated, until the solution is saturated. On slow cooling, if the solution is not disturbed, excess solute remains in solution. Such a solution is very unstable, and any physical disturbance causes the excess solute to crystallize and form a solid, or **precipitate**, at the bottom of the container.

The terms related to saturation are relative and do not indicate the quantity of solute in solution. In hospitals, chemical laboratories, and industry it is important to be specific; therefore, more precise terms must be used. A **molar solution** is defined as a solution that contains 1 mole (mol) of solute per liter of solution. One **mole** of a substance is equal to its gram molecular weight, which has 6.02×10^{23} atoms (Avogadro's number). Carbon-12 has an atomic weight of 12 amu; therefore, the gram molecular weight of carbon-12 is 12 g. One mole of carbon-12 weighs 12 g. When 1 mole of an element combines with 1 mole of another element, the result is 1 mole of a new molecule or substance. For example, a mole of potassium chloride (KCl) contains 1 mole of potassium (K) atoms and 1 mole of chlorine (Cl) atoms, or 6.02×10^{23} KCl molecules. Therefore the weight of KCl (74.4 g) is the sum of the gram molecular weights of K (39 g) and Cl (35.4 g).

The concept of molarity is commonly used in chemistry to quantify solute in solutions. It reflects the number of moles of a solute per volume of solvent:

$$\text{Molarity (M)} = \frac{\text{Number of moles (mol)}}{\text{Liter (L)}}$$

Given the weight (grams) and the gram molecular weight of a solute, it is possible to determine the number of moles (**Equation 51–3**) and therefore the molarity of a solution (**Equation 51–4**).

In clinical situations, a **percent solution** is used more often. *Percent* implies "parts per hundred," so *percent*

EQUATION 51–3

Calculation of Moles

$$\text{Number of moles} = \frac{\text{Number of grams}}{\text{Gram molecular weight}}$$

Example: Calculate the number of moles in 8 grams of carbon (the gram molecular weight of carbon is 12 g).

$$\frac{8\text{ g carbon}}{12\text{ g carbon/mol}}$$

$$8\text{ g carbon}\ \frac{1\text{ mol}}{12\text{ g}} = 0.75\text{ mol carbon}$$

EQUATION 51–4

Calculation of Molarity

Example: Calculate the molarity of a 150-mL solution containing 10 g of NaCl.

Step 1: Determine the weight of 1 mol of NaCl. (The gram molecular weight of sodium is 23 g and that of chloride is 35 g.)

$$1\text{ mol NaCl} = 23\text{ g} + 35\text{ g} = 58\text{ g}$$

Step 2: Determine the number of moles of NaCl in 10 g.

$$10\text{ g}\left(\frac{1\text{ mol}}{58\text{ g}}\right) = 0.172\text{ mol}$$

Step 3: Convert 150 mL to liters

$$150\text{ mL}\left(\frac{1\text{ L}}{1000\text{ mL}}\right) = 0.15\text{ L}$$

Step 4: Determine the molarity.

$$M = \frac{0.172\text{ mol } H_2O}{0.15\text{ L}} = 1.15\text{ M}$$

EQUATION 51–5

Weight/Weight Percent Solutions

$$\text{w/w\%} = \frac{\text{Grams of solute}}{\text{Grams of solute} + \text{Grams of solvent}} \times 100$$

Example: Calculate the percent solution containing 2.5 g of sugar in 47.5 g of water. Because both the solute and solvent are expressed as weights, the weight/weight percent method is used.

$$\text{w/w\%} = \frac{2.5\text{ g sugar}}{2.5\text{ g sugar} + 47.5\text{ g } H_2O} \times 100 = 5\%\text{ (w/w)}$$

EQUATION 51–6

Weight/Volume Percent Solutions

$$\text{w/v\%} = (\text{Grams of solute/mL of solution}) \times 100$$

Example: What percent solution is the bronchodilator albuteral if its concentration is 2.5 mg/0.5 mL?

$$\text{w/v\%} = (2.5\text{ mg/0.5 mL}) \times 100$$
$$= 500\text{ mg/mL}$$

Then convert to grams:

$$= (500\text{ mg/mL})\ (1\text{ g/1000 mg})$$
$$= 5\%\text{ (w/v)}$$

solution specifies the number of parts of solute present per 100 parts of solution. The three commonly used percent measurements are weight/weight percent, weight/volume percent, and volume/volume percent.

The weight/weight percent method (w/w%) describes the relative weight of the solute (in grams) compared with the total weight of the solution (**Equation 51–5**). The weight/volume percent method (w/v%) describes the weight of the solute with the relative volume of solution (in mL) and is commonly used in clinical situations and in pharmacology (**Equation 51–6**). The volume/volume percent method (v/v%) describes the volume of solute compared with the total volume of solution and is commonly used with liquid solutes (such as in expressions of the alcohol content of beer or wine) (**Equation 51–7**).

RESPIRATORY RECAP

Concentration of a Solution

- Molar
- Percent
  - Weight/weight
  - Weight/volume
  - Volume/volume
- Ratio
- Normal

EQUATION 51–7

Volume/Volume Percent Solutions

v/v% =
(mL of solute/mL of solution) × 100

Example: A 0.5-L bottle of wine contains 60 mL of ethanol. What is the percentage (v/v%) of ethanol in this aqueous solution?

v/v% = (60 mL/500 mL) × 100

= 12% (v/v)

EQUATION 51–8

Ratio Concentrations

Example: How much solute (active drug) of isoproterenol is contained in 0.5 mL of a 1:200 solution?

Step 1: Determine the concentration of a 1:200 solution.

1:200 = 1 g/200 mL = 1000 mg/200 mL
= 5 mg/mL

Step 2: Calculate the amount of solute.

0.5 mL isoproterenol (5 mg/1 mL) =
2.5 mg solute

EQUATION 51–9

Dilution of Stock Solutions

$V_1C_1 = V_2C_2$

where V_1 and V_2 are the initial and final volumes, and C_1 and C_2 are the initial and final concentrations, respectively.

Example: Prepare 5 mL of a 10% solution, given a 20% stock solution. Given C_1 (20%), C_2 (10%), and V_2 (5 mL), solve for V_1 (x mL of stock solution).

x mL stock solution × 20% = 5 mL × 10%

$20x$ = 50 mL

x = 2.5 mL

To prepare the solution, take 2.5 mL of the 20% stock solution and add 2.5 mL of water to dilute it to a final 5-mL 10% solution.

Simple ratios are sometimes used to describe the concentration of certain drugs. A ratio of 1:100 indicates that 1 g of solute is dissolved in 100 mL of solvent (**Equation 51–8**). In clinical medicine it often is necessary to prepare a weaker solution from a stronger (stock) solution. This usually is done by the addition of water or 0.9% NaCl to the stock solution (**Equation 51–9**).

Gram equivalent weight is the mass of a substance that will supply or react with one mole of hydrogen ions (H^+) in an acid-base reaction. The gram equivalent weight of a compound can be calculated by dividing the gram molecular weight by the number of positive or negative electrical charges that result from the dissolution of the compound. The normality of a solution is the number of gram equivalent weights in a liter of solution. A 1 normal (N) solution contains 1-gram equivalent weight in 1 L of solution.

The properties of a pure solvent are different from those of a solution. The term **colligative properties** refers to the properties of solutions that depend on the number of solute particles dissolved and not on chemical properties. Such properties include vapor pressure, boiling point, freezing point, and osmotic pressure. When a solute is added to a solvent, the solute dilutes the solvent and displaces some of the solvent particles at the surface of the solution. This displacement allows fewer solvent particles to escape in the form of gas particles, thereby reducing the **vapor pressure** of the solution. As a result of the lower vapor pressure, a higher temperature is required to raise the vapor pressure to atmospheric pressure. The solute particles in effect raise the **boiling point** of the solution compared with a pure solvent. For every mole of solute particles added per kilogram of water (1 kg of water has a volume of 1 L), the boiling point is raised 0.52° C. Solute particles also reduce the likelihood that water will enter the solid state and freeze, effectively reducing the **freezing point** of the solution. This is why salt is added to water when pasta is boiled (to raise the boiling point) and why salt is added to ice on sidewalks or antifreeze is added to radiators (to reduce the freezing point).

RESPIRATORY RECAP

Colligative Properties of Solutions

- » Depress vapor pressure
- » Depress freezing point
- » Elevate boiling point
- » Elevate osmotic pressure

Another colligative property of solutions involves osmosis. **Osmosis** is the process by which water molecules are transferred through a semipermeable membrane. A **semipermeable membrane** allows water but not other molecules to pass through it. Osmosis is very important in the maintenance of water balance between intracellular and extracellular fluid. It involves the movement of water from an area of high concentration of water to an area of low concentration in an attempt to make the concentrations equal. As an example,

Figure 51–4 shows the effect of the placement of equal volumes of 20% NaCl and 40% NaCl in a U-tube container, with the two sides separated by a semipermeable membrane. Because the concentration of NaCl is higher on the right, the concentration of water must be lower on that side. Water therefore moves from an area of high water concentration (the left side) to an area of low concentration (the right side). This net movement of water results in both sides of the membrane having equal concentrations of solution, but because the membrane did not allow solute particles to pass through, the volume of fluid on the right is now much greater than on the left. The increased volume raises the height of the column of fluid, which exerts a pressure. External pressure (hydrostatic) can be applied to the right side of the column to push the higher column down and make the sides equal again. The externally applied pressure that would just stop the flow of solvent through the membrane is called the **osmotic pressure**. The osmotic pressure of pure water is always zero, whereas the osmotic pressure of a solution is directly related to the number of solute particles in solution. The greater the concentration of the solution, the greater the osmotic pressure the solution exerts.

Cells in the body can be harmed if the concentrations of solutes in the body fluids are not carefully maintained.

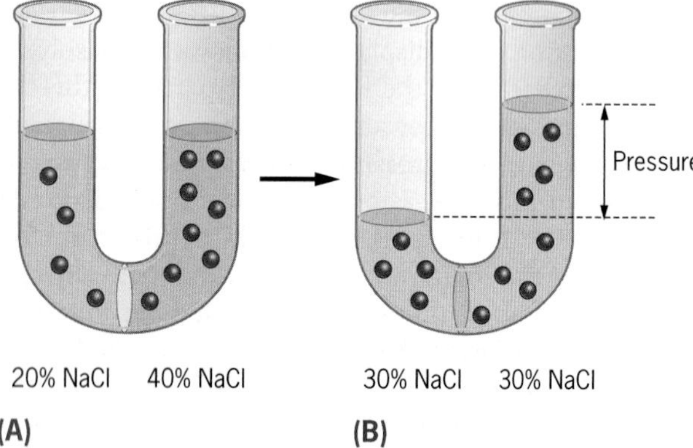

FIGURE 51–4 Osmotic pressure. (**A**) A U-shaped tube divided by a semipermeable membrane has a 20% sodium chloride (NaCl) solution on the left side of the membrane and an equal volume of 40% NaCl solution on the right side. As time passes, water moves from the area of the high-solvent (water) and the low-solute (NaCl) concentration (left side) to the area of low-solvent and high-solute concentration (right side). (**B**) Because the membrane allows movement only of the solvent and not of the solute, the volume on the right side increases. The difference in the height of the water column creates back pressure, which helps stop the flow of water.

If the concentration of water outside a red blood cell is less than that inside the cell (i.e., the osmotic pressure is higher outside the cell), water leaves the cell, causing it to shrivel, a process called **crenation**. In the reverse situation, when the water concentration is higher outside the cell (i.e., the osmotic pressure is lower outside the cell), water passes into the cell and may burst it, a process called **hemolysis**.

When intravenous fluids are administered, the composition of the fluid must be carefully considered. Solutions with an osmotic pressure equal to that found inside the cell are **isotonic**. A 0.9% sodium chloride solution and a 5.5% glucose solution are considered isotonic. Solutions with an osmotic pressure less than that inside the cell are considered **hypotonic**. Distilled water, tap water, and 0.45% sodium chloride are all hypotonic solutions. Solutions with an osmotic pressure greater than that inside the cell are **hypertonic**. Examples of hypertonic solutions include 5% sodium chloride and 10% glucose solutions.

A second type of liquid mixture is a **suspension**. Whereas particles in solutions consist of ions and molecules, particles in suspensions consist of large clumps of molecules. Properties of suspensions include the following: they consist of an insoluble substance dispersed in a liquid; they are heterogeneous (not the same throughout); they are not clear; they settle out over time; and they do not pass through filter paper or membranes. Certain medications are dispensed as solutions, such as milk of magnesia. Water often is the suspending medium, although oils can also be used, as is the case with certain antibiotics. An aerosol is an example of a liquid suspended in a gas.

A third type of liquid mixture, a **colloid**, consists of tiny particles suspended in a liquid. Although similar to suspensions, colloids have entirely different properties. Colloids do not settle; they can pass through filter paper but not through membranes; they adsorb (hold) particles on their surface; they have electrical charges, owing to the adsorption of charged particles (ions); and they exhibit the Tyndall effect and brownian movement, which are discussed later. **Table 51–3** compares the properties of colloids, solutions, and suspensions.

The particles in a colloid are larger than those in a solution (<1 nm) but smaller than those in a suspension (>100 nm); colloid particles therefore are small enough to pass though filter paper but too large to pass through a membrane. Colloids have a vast surface area because they consist of so many tiny particles. The property of adsorption is due to this tremendous surface area. **Adsorption** is defined as the ability to hold substances

TABLE 51–3 Comparison of the Properties of Solutions, Suspensions, and Colloids

	Size	Passes Through Filter Paper	Passes Through Membranes	Settles	Adsorbs	Charged
Solution	<1 nm	Yes	Yes	No	No	No
Suspension	>100 nm	No	No	Yes	No	No
Colloid	1–100 nm	Yes	No	No	Yes	Yes

to a surface. Most colloids have selective adsorption, or the ability to adsorb only certain substances. Colloidal charcoal adsorbs large amounts of gas. Coconut charcoal selectively adsorbs poisonous gas but not ordinary gas, which is why it is used in gas masks. Colloids can selectively adsorb ions and take on an electrical charge. If a colloidal mixture consists of like charges, the particles repel each other and have minimal likelihood of coming together to form larger particles that would settle. On the other hand, if colloids of opposite charges come in contact, they attract each other and settle out. When the poison bichloride of mercury ($HgCl_2$) is swallowed, it forms a positive colloid in the stomach. Drinking egg white, a negative colloid, is the antidote. These two opposite-charged colloids neutralize each other and coagulate in the stomach. The coagulate must be pumped out of the stomach before the egg white is digested, which would expose the body to the poison again.

When a beam of light is passed through a colloid, the beam reflects off the colloidal particles and scatters. Such a beam passes directly through a solution without scattering because the particles are so small. This phenomenon, referred to as the *Tyndall effect*, is used as a way to distinguish between colloids and solutions. Colloids also exhibit a haphazard, irregular motion, known as *brownian movement*, that never ceases. This movement is thought to be due to constant bombardment of the colloid particles by the molecules of the suspending medium, which are in continuous, random motion.

Colloidal dispersions can be **hydrophilic** (water attracting) or **hydrophobic** (water repelling). Systems in which a strong attraction exists between the colloidal particles and water (hydrophilic systems) are called *gels*. Gels, such as gelatin, are semisolid or semirigid and do not flow easily. When little attraction exists between the colloid and water (hydrophobic systems), the system is referred to as a *sol*. Such a dispersion in air is called an *aerosol*; when it is in water, it is called a *hydrosol*. When a gel is heated, it turns into a sol, which returns to a gel on cooling. Protoplasm has the ability to change from gel to sol and vice versa.

Several clinical applications use the concept by which solutions and colloids are passed through membranes. Dialysis involves the separation of solute particles from colloid particles with a semipermeable membrane. Peritoneal dialysis involves bathing of the gut with a solution, after which water-soluble waste particles are allowed to pass through the semipermeable intestinal wall. Hemodialysis involves passing blood by a semipermeable membrane, where soluble waste products are removed and the blood cells and plasma proteins retained. Antitoxins are prepared by placement of an impure material inside a membrane suspended in running water. The soluble impurities are washed out, leaving the pure antitoxin. Low-sodium milk is produced by a similar method.

Inorganic Molecules

The compounds that make up living organisms can be divided into two broad categories: organic compounds and inorganic compounds. Organic compounds generally are composed of molecules containing carbon–carbon (C—C) or carbon–hydrogen (C—H) covalent bonds. Inorganic compounds do not have any C—C or C—H bonds, although several inorganic compounds do contain carbon. Organic compounds usually are larger and more complex than inorganic compounds. The human body contains both types of compounds. As shown in Table 51–1, the body is made up of 26 important elements. Eleven are considered major elements, and the remaining 15 are referred to as *trace elements*. More than 96% of body weight is made up of oxygen, carbon, hydrogen, and nitrogen; oxygen alone is responsible for 65% of the body's weight. The most abundant molecule in the body is water (H_2O).

Water

The importance of water in the human body is evidenced by the fact that the body can stay alive for several weeks without food but only a few days without water. Water is essential for existence. As mentioned earlier, water accounts for 45% to 80% of the total weight of the human body and is essential for proper digestion, circulation, elimination, and regulation of body temperature. Every activity in each cell in the body takes place in a watery environment.

Pure water is colorless, odorless, and tasteless. Many physical constants are based on water as a reference. The freezing point (0° C or 32° F) and the boiling point (100° C or 212° F) of water at 1 atmosphere of pressure are the standard reference points for the measurement of temperature. The calorie is defined as the amount of heat required to change the temperature of 1 g of water 1° C. The metric standard of weight, the gram, is equal to the weight of 1 mL of water at 4° C (its maximum density). The concept of specific gravity is based on water and is defined as the weight of a substance compared with the weight of an equal volume of water.

The atomic structure of water results from the combination of two covalent bonds between a single oxygen atom and two hydrogen atoms. The water molecule is not arranged in a straight line (such as HOH) but rather in a nonlinear manner, with the angle between the hydrogen atoms being approximately 105 degrees (**Figure 51–5**). The shared electrons between the hydrogen and oxygen are attracted to the oxygen more than the hydrogen, which results in a slight negative charge at the oxygen end of the molecule and a slight positive charge at the hydrogen end. This polar nature of water is what makes it such an effective solvent. As a polar solvent, water has a tendency to ionize substances in solution. This allows large compounds to be broken into smaller, more reactive particles (ions), getting them ready for chemical reactions to occur.

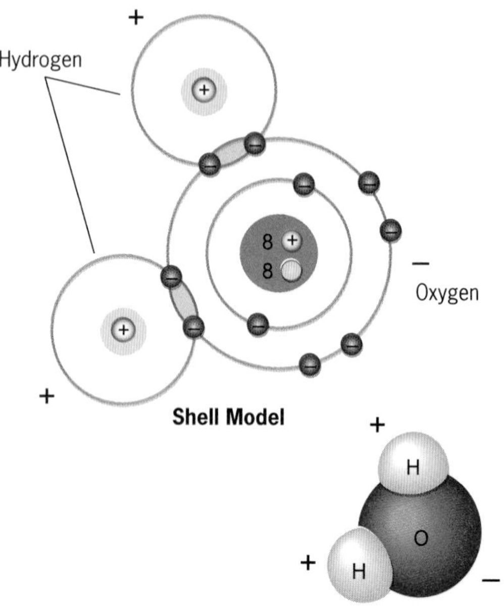

FIGURE 51–5 Structure of the water molecule.

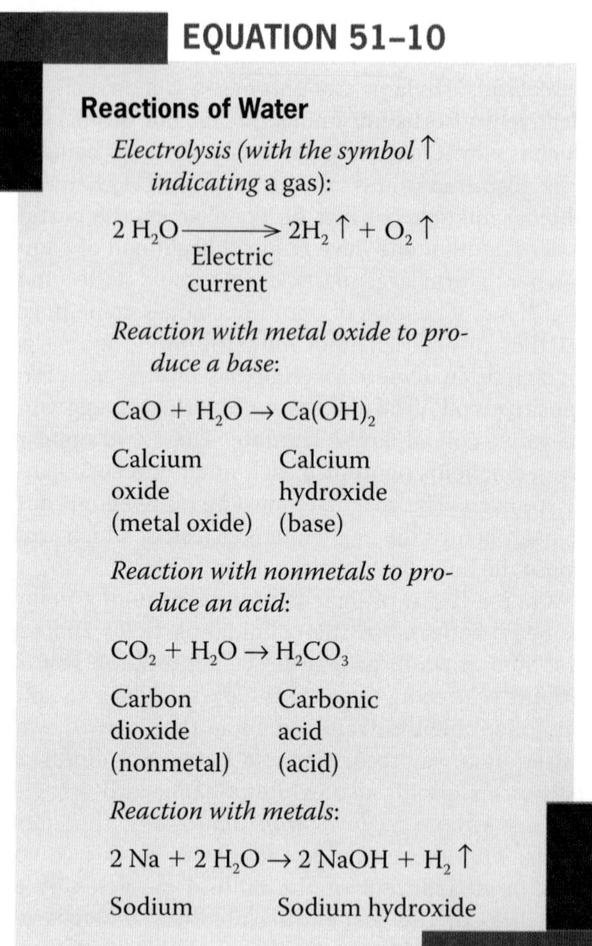

EQUATION 51–10

Reactions of Water

Electrolysis (with the symbol ↑ indicating a gas):

$$2\,H_2O \xrightarrow[\text{current}]{\text{Electric}} 2H_2\uparrow + O_2\uparrow$$

Reaction with metal oxide to produce a base:

$$CaO + H_2O \rightarrow Ca(OH)_2$$

Calcium oxide (metal oxide)	Calcium hydroxide (base)

Reaction with nonmetals to produce an acid:

$$CO_2 + H_2O \rightarrow H_2CO_3$$

Carbon dioxide (nonmetal)	Carbonic acid (acid)

Reaction with metals:

$$2\,Na + 2\,H_2O \rightarrow 2\,NaOH + H_2\uparrow$$

Sodium	Sodium hydroxide

Water also has several chemical properties worth noting (**Equation 51–10**). When an electric current is passed through water, it undergoes electrolysis and forms hydrogen gas (H_2) and oxygen gas (O_2). Water is extremely stable; when it boils and turns into a gas (steam), it does not decompose, even at extreme temperatures (≈0.3% decomposition at 1600° C). When water reacts with a metal oxide (metals are found on the left side of the periodic table), it forms a compound known as a *base*. When water reacts with a nonmetal (nonmetals are found on the right side of the periodic table), it forms a compound known as an *acid*. When water reacts with active metals, such as sodium or potassium, a vigorous reaction occurs and hydrogen gas is formed.

Water plays a crucial role in the transport of many essential materials in the body. For example, by dissolving oxygen and food substances in the blood, water enables these materials to enter and leave the blood capillaries in the lungs and digestive organs and eventually to enter cells in every area of the body. Water then transports waste products from the place where they are produced to the excretory organs, where they are eventually eliminated.

Water's ability to absorb and give up heat slowly gives it a major role in another unique and important bodily function—maintaining a relatively constant temperature. Chemists refer to water's ability to lose and gain large amounts of heat with little change in temperature as its high **specific heat**. Because the body has a large water content, it can resist sudden changes in temperature. For example, it can transport the heat produced by muscle contraction during exercise to the surface of the body to be evaporated, with little change in core temperature.

Another important physical property of water is its high **heat of vaporization**; this refers to the fact that a significant amount of heat must be absorbed to change water from a liquid to a gas (specifically, 540 calories per gram). The energy is used to break the hydrogen bonds holding adjacent water molecules together in the liquid state. When water is placed on the skin, the heat required to make it evaporate comes from the skin. In this manner the skin loses heat and is cooled. In a similar manner, the skin is cooled by the evaporation of perspiration.

Oxygen and Carbon Dioxide

Oxygen and carbon dioxide are inorganic substances that play an important role in cellular respiration (**Figure 51–6**). Oxygen is required to complete the decomposition reactions required for the release of energy from nutrients burned by the cells. Carbon dioxide is a waste product of these same decomposition reactions and is important to acid–base homeostasis of the body.

Electrolytes

Electrolytes constitute another large group of inorganic compounds. They include acids, bases, and salts. **Electrolytes** are substances that break down, or dissociate,

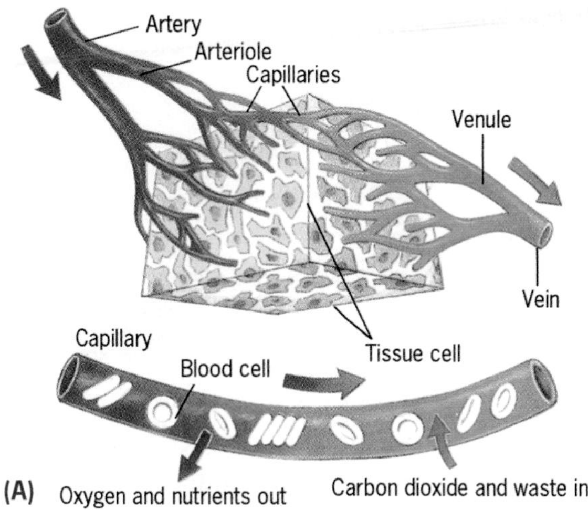

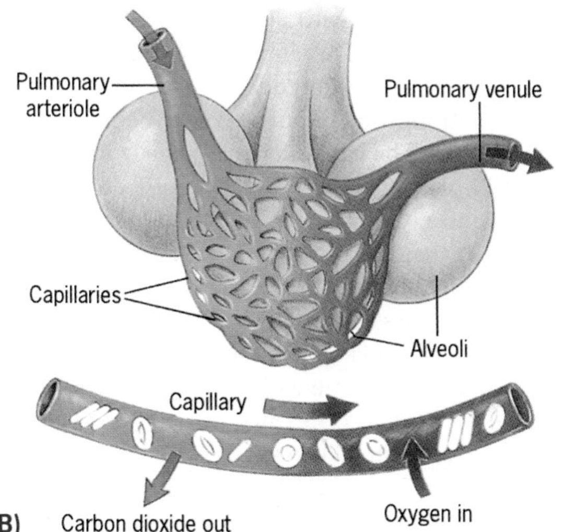

FIGURE 51–6 Transport of carbon dioxide (CO_2) and oxygen (O_2) at the (**A**) tissue and (**B**) lung levels. Note that the process of CO_2 uptake and O_2 release at the tissue level is reversed at the lung level (O_2 uptake and CO_2 release).

in solution to form ions. As stated earlier, positively charged ions are called *cations* and negatively charged ions are called *anions*. In solution, electrolytes are capable of carrying an electrical current.

The unit of measurement for electrolytes is the number of milliequivalents per liter of solution (mEq/L). **Milliequivalents** measure the number of ionic charges or electrovalent bonds in a solution and therefore are an accurate measure of the chemical combining power, or reactivity, of the electrolyte solution. The number of milliequivalents can be determined from the weight of the ion in 100 mL of the solution (mg%) (**Equation 51–11**).

EQUATION 51–11

Calculation of mEq/L

$$\text{mEq/L} = \frac{\text{mg/100 mL} \times 10 \times \text{Valence}}{\text{Atomic weight}}$$

Example: Convert 16 mg% of potassium to mEq/L, given potassium's atomic weight = 39 and valence = 1.

$$\text{mEq/L} = \frac{16 \times 10 \times 1}{39} = \frac{160}{39} = 4.1$$

Acids, Bases, and Buffers

An **acid** is a compound that donates, or yields, a hydrogen ion (H^+) in an aqueous solution. Acid solutions have a sour taste. Citric acid gives a sour taste to lemons and grapefruits, acetic acid gives a sour taste to vinegar, and lactic acid makes milk taste sour. Because a hydrogen ion is the result of the hydrogen atom losing its only electron, it becomes a single proton, since it has no neutron in its nucleus. Actually, an aqueous hydrogen ion, H^+ (aq), is not a bare proton but rather a proton chemically bonded to water as H_3O^+ (aq). According to the Brönsted-Lowry theory, an acid is the species that donates a proton in a transfer reaction. An acid, then, can also be thought of as a substance that donates protons.

Some common acids are hydrochloric acid (HCl), sulfuric acid (H_2SO_4), nitric acid (HNO_3), carbonic acid (H_2CO_3), phosphoric acid (H_3PO_4), and acetic acid (CH_3CO_2H). Acids yield ions when placed in water (**Equation 51–12**). Strong acids (such as HCl, HNO_3, and H_2SO_4)

EQUATION 51–12

Acid Reactions

Reactions in Water

Acids with a single ionizable hydrogen ionize into one cation and one anion:

$HCl \rightarrow H^+ + Cl^-$

$HNO_3 \rightarrow H^+ + NO_2^-$

Acids with multiple ionizable hydrogen atoms donate their protons in stages:

Stage 1: $H_2SO_4 \rightarrow H^+ + HSO_4^-$

Stage 2: $HSO_4^- \rightarrow H^+ + SO_4^{-2}$

that can be combined and represented as:

$H_2SO_4 \rightarrow 2\,H^+ + SO_4^{-2}$

Reactions with Metal Oxides and Hydroxides to Form Water and a Salt

$H_2SO_4 + 2\,NaOH \rightarrow 2\,H_2O + Na_2SO_4$

almost completely ionize in solution to form H^+ ions, whereas weak acids (such as H_2CO_3) dissociate very little and therefore produce few excess H^+ ions. Acids react with metal oxides and hydroxides to form water and a salt.

The water molecule dissociates continually in a reversible reaction to form hydrogen ions and hydroxide ions (OH^-):

$$H_2O \leftrightarrow H^+ + OH^-$$

The single unpaired valence electron makes hydrogen unstable, and by losing or donating the electron, it becomes more stable. This is why the dissociation of water occurs. Rather than share its electron with oxygen, hydrogen would just as soon give up its electron to OH to maintain stability. In pure water the balance between the two ions is equal, but when an acid, such as HCl, dissociates into H^+ and Cl^-, it shifts the H^+/OH^- balance in favor of H^+ ions, increasing the acidity level.

RESPIRATORY RECAP

Acids and Bases

- *Acid*: donates hydrogen ions
- *Base*: accepts hydrogen ions
- *Buffer*: minimizes change in the hydrogen ion concentration
- *Salt*: produced by a reaction between an acid and a base

A **base** is a solution that yields a hydroxide ion (OH^-) in an aqueous solution. The base, or alkaline compound, shifts the H^+/OH^- balance in favor of OH^-, as shown in the ionization reaction of sodium hydroxide (**Equation 51–13**). A base can also be thought of as the substance that accepts the proton in a transfer reaction. With this definition the bicarbonate ion (HCO_3^-) also is a base because it can accept a proton. Basic solutions feel slippery and soapy and have a bitter, biting taste. A strong base has a high hydroxide concentration and is corrosive to tissues because of its ability to react with proteins and fats.

The concentration, or strength, of an acid or base is expressed as pH. The **pH** indicates the hydrogen ion concentration $[H^+]$ in a solution and is mathematically defined as the negative logarithm of the hydrogen ion concentration:

$$pH = -\log[H^+]$$

EQUATION 51–13

Chemical Reactions Involving Bases

The ionization reaction of sodium hydroxide to yield OH^-:

$$NaOH \rightarrow Na^+ + OH^-$$

Reactions that accept a proton:

$$\underset{\text{Base}}{HCO_3^-} + \underset{\text{Proton}}{H^+} \rightarrow H_2CO_3$$

EQUATION 51–14

The pH of a Solution

$$pH = -\log [H^+]$$

A solution with a $[H^+]$ of 10^{-7} mol/L has a pH of 7:

$$pH = -\log[H^+] = -\log 10^{-7} = -(^-7) = 7$$

Because a logarithm is an exponent, the logarithm (log) of 100, or 10^2, is 2, and log 10^{-4} is -4 (10^{-4} is 0.0001). Therefore, a solution with a $[H^+]$ of 10^{-7} mol/L has a pH of 7 (**Equation 51–14**). The sum of $[H^+]$ and $[OH^-]$ is always 10^{-14}; therefore, when the concentration of one increases, the concentration of the other must be reduced by an equal amount. The values for pH range from 0 to 14. For example, a pH of 0 indicates a $[H^+]$ mol/L of 10^0 mol/L (or 1 mol/L) and a $[OH^-]$ of 10^{-14} mol/L. A pH of 14 indicates a $[H^+]$ of 10^{-14} mol/L and a $[OH^-]$ of 10^0 mol/L. A pH of 7 indicates a neutral solution, because the concentrations of the two ions are the same, 10^{-7}. A pH above 7 indicates a base, whereas a pH below 7 indicates an acid. Because of its logarithmic relationship, a difference of 1 pH unit represents a tenfold difference in strength. This means that an acid solution with a pH of 5.5 is 10 times as strong as one with a pH of 6.5 and that a base with a pH of 9.0 is 10 times as strong as one with a pH of 8.0.

Buffers maintain a relative constant pH when a strong acid or a strong base is added. Blood is an effective buffer. For the bicarbonate buffer system, the degree to which the pH changes depends on the ratio of base bicarbonate to carbonic acid. A ratio of 20:1 produces a pH of 7.4. This is mathematically expressed by the **Henderson-Hasselbalch equation**, which includes the ionization constant for carbonic acid:

$$pH = 6.1 + \log \frac{[HCO_3^-]}{[P_{CO_2} \times 0.03]}$$

The ratio of HCO_3^- to H_2CO_3 for a pH of 7.4 is 20:1. If the ratio goes up by means of an elevation in bicarbonate or a reduction in the partial pressure of carbon dioxide (P_{CO_2}), the pH increases, or become more basic or alkaline. Either a reduction in the bicarbonate or an increase in P_{CO_2} causes the pH to decrease and become more acidic.

Salts

When an acid and a base react, the result is a salt. When the result is a salt and water, the reaction is known as a *neutralization reaction* (**Equation 51–15**). Although acids (H^+) and bases (OH^-) all have an ion in common,

TABLE 51–4 Common Inorganic Salts in the Body

Salt	Chemical Formula	Electrolyte Combination	Medicinal Use
Sodium chloride	$NaCl$	$Na^{+} + Cl^{-}$	Replacement therapy, irrigation, diluent
Calcium chloride	$CaCl_2$	$Ca^{+2} + 2\ Cl^{-}$	Reduction in blood clotting time
Sodium bicarbonate	$NaHCO_3$	$Na^{+} + HCO_3^{-}$	Antacid, buffering agent
Potassium chloride	KCl	$K^{+} + Cl^{-}$	Potassium replacement therapy
Sodium sulfate	Na_2SO_4	$2\ Na^{+} + SO_4^{-2}$	Cathartic agent
Calcium carbonate	$CaCO_3$	$Ca^{+2} + CO_3^{-2}$	Antacid
Calcium phosphate	$Ca_3(PO_4)_2$	$3\ Ca^{+2} + 2\ PO_4^{-3}$	Replacement therapy
Magnesium sulfate	$MgSO_4$	$Mg^{+2} + SO_4^{-2}$	Cathartic agent, anticonvulsant, laxative
Potassium iodide	KI	$K^{+} + I^{-}$	Expectorant, antitussive

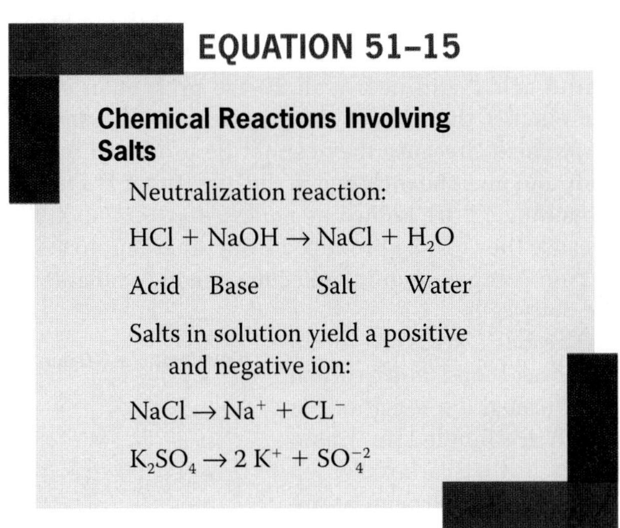

EQUATION 51–15

Chemical Reactions Involving Salts

Neutralization reaction:

$HCl + NaOH \rightarrow NaCl + H_2O$

Acid Base Salt Water

Salts in solution yield a positive and negative ion:

$NaCl \rightarrow Na^{+} + CL^{-}$

$K_2SO_4 \rightarrow 2\ K^{+} + SO_4^{-2}$

salts do not. Salts in solution yield a positive and negative ion. Many of the major and trace minerals listed in Table 51–1 are derived from inorganic salt sources, which are common in many body fluids and specialized tissue such as bone. Often, these elements can exert a full physiologic effect only when present as an ion in solution. **Table 51–4** lists some common inorganic salts.

Organic Molecules

Organic chemistry is the chemistry of carbon compounds. Carbon compounds have a separate category because although there are tens of thousands known inorganic compounds, there are millions of known organic compounds. Some important organic compounds in the body are carbohydrates, lipids, proteins, nucleic acids, vitamins, hormones, and enzymes. Other common materials that contain organic compounds include drugs, wool, silk, cotton, linen, nylon, rayon, Dacron, perfumes, dyes, flavors, soaps, detergents, plastics, gasoline, and oils.

TABLE 51–5 Comparison of Common Characteristics of Most Organic and Inorganic Compounds

Organic Compounds	Inorganic Compounds
Complex structure	Simpler structure
Flammability	Nonflammability
Low melting point	High melting point
Low boiling point	High boiling point
Solubility in nonpolar liquids	Insolubility in nonpolar liquids
Insolubility in water	Solubility in water
Covalent bonds	Ionic bonds
Reactions usually formed between molecules	Reactions usually formed between ions
Generally many atoms	Usually relatively few atoms

Organic compounds are different from inorganic compounds in many ways. **Table 51–5** lists some of the most important differences. One of the unique characteristics of carbon is its ability to bond other carbon atoms to itself to form very large, complex atoms. The carbon atoms may form continuous or branched chains, creating substances known as *aliphatic compounds*. Carbon atoms also can form in the shape of a ring. If the ring is formed of all carbon atoms, the compound is called a *cyclic* or *aromatic compound*; if another element, such as nitrogen, is substituted for one of the carbon atoms in the ring, the compound is called a *heterocyclic compound*.

RESPIRATORY RECAP

Biologically Important Organic Molecules

- » Carbohydrates
- » Lipids
- » Proteins
- » Nucleic acids
- » Vitamins
- » Hormones
- » Enzymes

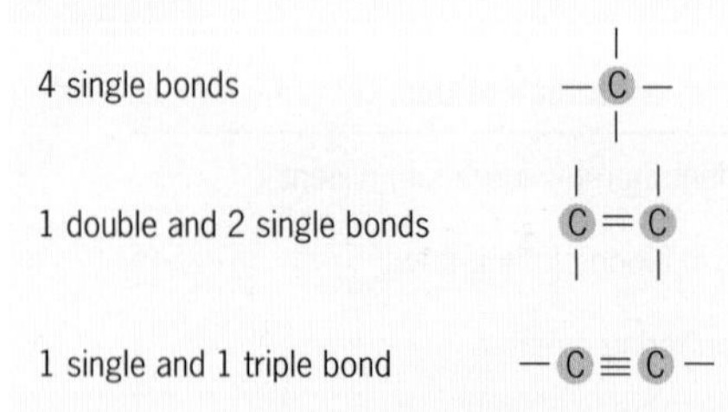

FIGURE 51–7 Covalent bonds formed by carbon. Each dash represents a pair of shared electrons.

Because the carbon atom has four valence electrons and needs four more to reach a full shell of eight electrons, carbon can form up to four covalent bonds. This requirement can be satisfied by its bonding to four separate atoms by use of four single bonds; to three atoms by use of two single bonds and one double bond; or to two atoms by use of one triple bond and one single bond (**Figure 51–7**). The three atoms most commonly bound with carbon are hydrogen, which needs one electron to fill its outer shell and can form only one bond; oxygen, which forms two bonds; and nitrogen, which forms three bonds. With this brief overview, let us move on to the four major groups of organic substances most important in the human body: carbohydrates, proteins, lipids, and nucleic acids.

Carbohydrates

All **carbohydrate** molecules contain the elements carbon, hydrogen, and oxygen; the word *carbohydrate* literally means "carbon and water." The carbon atoms are linked to form chains of varying lengths. Sugars and starches are carbohydrates and the primary sources of chemical energy required by each cell in the body. Carbohydrates are divided into four groups based on the length of the carbon chain: monosaccharides (simple sugars), disaccharides (double sugars), oligosaccharides (few sugars), and polysaccharides (complex sugars).

The basic unit of the carbohydrate molecule is the monosaccharide. **Glucose** (dextrose), the most important monosaccharide, is a six-carbon sugar with the formula $C_6H_{12}O_6$. Because it is a six-carbon molecule, it is referred to as a *hexose* (*hexa* means "six"). Glucose is present in a straight chain in the dry state but forms a cyclic compound when in solution. Glucose is the primary source of energy for the cells. Fructose and galactose are other important hexoses. Some monosaccharides consist of five-carbon atoms and are referred to as *pentoses*. Two important pentoses are ribose and deoxyribose, which are integral to the formation of the nucleic acids ribonucleic acid (RNA) and deoxyribonucleic acid (DNA).

Disaccharides are composed of two simple sugars bonded together through a synthesis reaction that involves the removal of water. Examples of disaccharides include sucrose (table sugar from cane or beet sugar), maltose (grain sugar), and lactose (milk sugar). Each consists of two linked monosaccharides. The combining of glucose and fructose forms sucrose. After they are eaten, these important dietary disaccharides are broken down into monosaccharides so that the cells can use them.

Oligosaccharides are made up of 3 to 20 monosaccharides linked together. They are often bound to proteins on the outer surface of cell membranes as a "self" antigen. Having "self" antigens on our own cells allows the immune system to recognize antigens that are "non-self."

Polysaccharides are made up of many chemically linked monosaccharides. Glycogen is the body's most important polysaccharide. It sometimes is referred to as *animal starch*. Because it has a molecular weight of several million atomic mass units, it is considered a macromolecule. When excess glucose is present in the blood, it is converted to glycogen by the liver and stored in liver and muscle cells for later use.

Proteins

Proteins are very large molecules composed of carbon, hydrogen, oxygen, and nitrogen. The molecular weight of a protein usually ranges to several million atomic mass units. The basic protein unit or building block is the **amino acid**. Proteins are composed of 20 such amino acids, and nearly all 20 are present in every protein. Of the 20, only 8 are considered *essential amino acids* because they cannot be produced by the body and must be included in the diet (**Box 51–1**). The remaining 12 are known as *nonessential amino acids* because they can be produced from other amino acids or from simple organic molecules readily available to the body cells.

The basic structure of an amino acid consists of a carbon atom (called the α-carbon) to which are bonded an amino group (NH_2), a carboxyl group (COOH), a hydrogen atom, and a side chain (**Figure 51–8**). The side chain is a group of elements denoted by the letter R. It is the side chain that constitutes the unique and identifying characteristic of an amino acid.

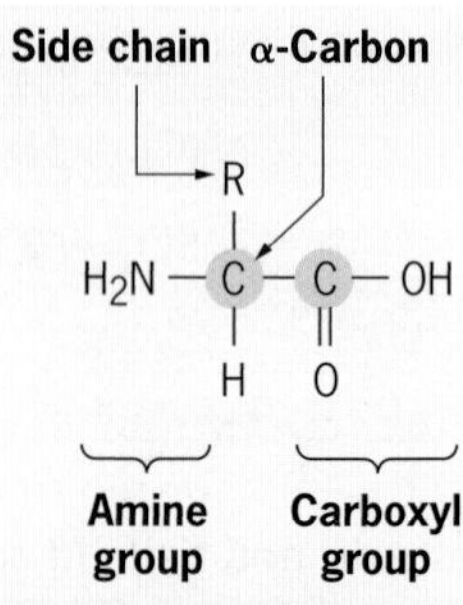

FIGURE 51–8 Basic structure of an amino acid.

BOX 51–1

Essential Amino Acids

Histadine
Isoleucine
Leucine
Methionine
Phenylalanine
Theonine
Tryptophan
Valine

To link amino acids, the OH from the carboxyl group of one amino acid and the H from the amine group of another amino acid split off to form water plus a new compound called a **peptide**. A long chain of peptides is called a *polypeptide*, and the compound is finally considered a protein when the chain reaches about 50 amino acids or more in length.

The shape of a protein molecule determines its function, and there are two main classes of proteins: fibrous and globular. Fibrous proteins are long linear chains of amino acids that are usually water insoluble. Examples of fibrous proteins are collagen (in skin) and keratin (in hair). Globular proteins are usually soluble in water and are highly folded, spherical in shape. Examples of globular proteins include hormones, hemoglobin, antibodies, and enzymes. Proteins can also bind with other organic compounds to form mixed molecules, such as a glycoprotein (sugar with a protein) or a lipoprotein (a lipid and a protein).

Lipids

A **lipid** is an organic biomolecule that is soluble in nonpolar organic solvents, such as ether, alcohol, or benzene. Lipids are not soluble in water. Lipids are composed primarily of carbon, hydrogen, and oxygen, although nitrogen and phosphorus are also used. The proportion of oxygen is much lower in lipids than it is in carbohydrates. The different lipid categories include triglycerides (fats), phospholipids, steroids, and eicosanoids.

Lipids have critically important biologic functions. They provide energy (they yield more energy per unit of weight than carbohydrates or proteins); structure (phospholipids and cholesterol are required components of cell membranes); essential nutrients in the form of vitamins (fat-soluble vitamins include vitamins A, D, E, and K); protection (fat surrounds and protects organs); insulation (skin fat minimizes heat loss; fatty tissue, or myelin, covers nerve cells and electrically insulates them); and regulation (steroid hormones such as estrogen, testosterone, and eicosanoids regulate many physiologic processes).

Triglycerides are the most abundant lipids and function as the body's most concentrated source of energy. Fats and oils are both triglycerides; fats are solid at room temperature (e.g., butter, lard), and oils are liquid (e.g., corn oil, olive oil). The basic building blocks of the triglyceride are a glycerol molecule and three fatty acids. The glycerol unit is the same for all triglycerides; the specific type of fatty acid determines the identity and chemical nature of the fat.

Naturally occurring fats have long fatty acid chains, consisting of an even number of carbons that range from 12 to 24 carbons long. A **saturated fatty acid** is one in which all available bonds of the hydrocarbon chain are filled with hydrogen atoms. The chain has all single carbon–carbon bonds. **Unsaturated fatty acids** have one or more double carbon–carbon bonds in their hydrocarbon chain because not all of the chain carbon atoms are saturated with hydrogen atoms. The degree of saturation determines the physical and chemical properties of fatty acids. Fats become more oily and liquid as the number of unsaturated double bonds increases. Double bonds cause the chain to bend or kink, thereby keeping the molecules from fitting closely together. For example, animal fats such as lard are saturated, whereas vegetable oils are not.

Phospholipids are similar to triglycerides in structure but do not store energy. Instead of three fatty acids attached to a glycerol, one of the fatty acid chains is replaced by a chemical structure containing phosphorus and nitrogen. The shape of the phospholipid molecule resembles a head with two tails: the head is the phosphorus and nitrogen group, and the tails are the two fatty acids. The head is hydrophilic (attracts water), whereas the tails are hydrophobic (repel water). This unique property allows the phospholipid molecule to bridge or join two different chemical environments—for example, a water environment on one side and a lipid environment on the other. Phospholipids are a primary component of cell membranes, of pulmonary surfactant (a surface tension–reducing agent in the lungs), and of myelin.

Steroids are an important lipid group. They are widely distributed throughout the body and are involved in many important structural and functional roles. **Cholesterol** is a steroid lipid that combines with phospholipids in the cell membrane to help stabilize the membrane's bilayer structure. The body also uses cholesterol as a starting point for making steroid hormones such as estrogen, testosterone, and cortisol and for bile salts used in digestion.

Eicosanoids are signaling molecules made by oxidation of three different 20-carbon essential fatty acids (EFA): eicosapentaenoic acid (EPA), arachidonic acid (AA), and dihomo-gamma-linolenic acid (DGLA). Eicosanoids are not stored within cells, but are synthesized as required. Some of the most complex pathways in the human body depend on eicosanoids. The four families of eicosanoids are prostaglandins (PG), prostacyclins (PGI2), thromboxanes (TX), and leukotrienes (LT).

Prostaglandins are lipids composed of a 20-carbon unsaturated fatty acid that has a 5-carbon ring. They are often referred to as *tissue hormones.* Sixteen types of prostaglandins have been classified into nine broad categories, labeled PGA through PGI. Prostaglandins are produced by cell membranes in almost every body tissue. They are formed and released in response to specific stimuli. Once released, they have a very local effect and are then inactivated. Prostaglandins help regulate blood pressure and the secretion of digestive juices, enhance the immune system and inflammatory response, play an important role in blood clotting, and help regulate the effects of several hormones. The use of prostaglandin and prostaglandin inhibitor drugs is gaining attention

TABLE 51–6 Physiologic Actions of Prostaglandins

Constriction or dilation in vascular and bronchial smooth muscle cells	Sensitize spinal neurons to pain
Aggregation or disaggregation of platelets	Decrease intraocular pressure
Regulate inflammatory mediation	Regulate calcium movement
Control hormone regulation	Control cell growth
Regulates gastric acid secretion	Stimulates release of insulin from pancreas

for the treatment of conditions ranging from relief of menstrual cramps to treatment of asthma, high blood pressure, and ulcers. Because prostaglandins have a short half-life, their effect is felt primarily locally or within the cell of origin. **Table 51–6** summarizes some of the physiologic actions of prostaglandins.

Prostacyclin also has a short half-life. Prostacyclin is an inhibitor of platelet aggregation and a potent vasodilator. *Thromboxanes* have an effect opposite to that of prostacyclin. They facilitate platelet aggregation and have a contractive effect on a variety of smooth muscle. *Leukotrienes* play an important role in asthma and allergic reactions and sustain inflammatory reactions. As multifunctional mediators, leukotrienes probably play a role in other diseases. The role of leukotrienes in cardiovascular and neuropsychiatric illnesses is actively being investigated.

Nucleic Acids

The two principal forms of **nucleic acid** are **deoxyribonucleic acid (DNA)** and **ribonucleic acid (RNA)**. The basic building blocks of nucleic acids are nucleotides. Just as proteins are made from chains of amino acids, nucleic acids are made from chains of nucleotides. Each nucleotide consists of a phosphate group, a five-carbon sugar, and a nitrogenous base. The sugar component in DNA is deoxyribose, whereas ribose is used in RNA. The five nitrogenous bases are uracil (U), thymine (T), cytosine (C), guanine (G), and adenosine (A). Both DNA and RNA use the bases cytosine, guanine, and adenosine; DNA also uses thymine, and RNA also uses uracil.

DNA molecules are the largest molecules in the body. They are composed of two long polynucleotide chains that run parallel to each other (**Figure 51–9**). The sugar–phosphate part of the molecule faces toward the outside, and its bases point inward, toward the bases of the other chain. Each base in one chain is joined to a base in the other chain by hydrogen bonds, forming a base pair. DNA base pairs always consist of A with T and G with C. The double chains coil around each other to form a double helix. The DNA molecule looks like a twisted ladder, with the rails of the ladder being the sugar–phosphate backbone of the nucleotide chain and the rungs of the ladder the base pairs connected by hydrogen bonds.

Although a DNA molecule contains only two types of base pairs (A—T and G—C), millions of them are present in each DNA molecule. The millions of base pairs occur in the same sequence in all of the DNA molecules in the body, but in a different sequence in the DNA of another person's body. In other words, the base pair sequence in DNA is unique to each individual.

The genetic code consists of three-letter words called *codons* formed from a sequence of three nucleotides in the DNA. The codons make up a *gene*, and each unique form of a gene is called an **allele**. Mutations are random changes in genes and can create new alleles. Alleles are present in pairs, one on each of a **chromosome** pair. Human somatic cells (body cells) are diploid, having two sets of 23 chromosomes (46 total), one from the mother and one from the father. Gametes, or reproductive cells, are haploid and have one set of chromosomes. One of the 23 pairs of chromosomes determines sex, and diseases transmitted on this pair of chromosomes are called *sex-linked*. Examples include hemophilia and Duchenne muscular dystrophy. The other 22 pairs of chromosomes are called *autosomal*.

Homozygous refers to having identical alleles for a single trait, whereas *heterozygous* refers to having two different alleles for a single trait. If one allele overrides the instructions from another, it is called the *dominant allele*, and the allele that is overridden is called the *recessive allele*. For a recessive trait to be expressed, its allele must be present on both chains of DNA. Individuals with one dominant allele and one recessive allele are called *carriers*. The visible traits of an organism are called its **phenotype**, and the genes responsible for those traits are called its **genotype**. Genetic disorders are diseases that are caused by a single allele of a gene and are inherited in families. An example is cystic fibrosis, which is caused by a single recessive gene called CFTR. Disruptions in the normal chromosomal content of a cell results in diseases such as Down syndrome, which is caused by an extra copy of chromosome 21 (trisomy 21).

A single-nucleotide polymorphism (SNP) is a DNA sequence variation occurring when a single nucleotide in the genome differs from paired chromosomes in an individual. Genetic polymorphism is the recurrence of two or more discontinuous genetic variants of a specific trait. The occurrence of SNP and genetic polymorphism is increasingly recognized as important in diseases such as asthma, chronic obstructive pulmonary disease, and acute lung injury.

The function of genes is to provide the information needed to make proteins. The codon in a nucleic acid sequence specifies a single amino acid. In this way, the genotype is translated into the phenotype of the individual. DNA carries the genetic information necessary for synthesis of proteins specific for a given species, but RNA acts as the machinery for this process. RNA is used

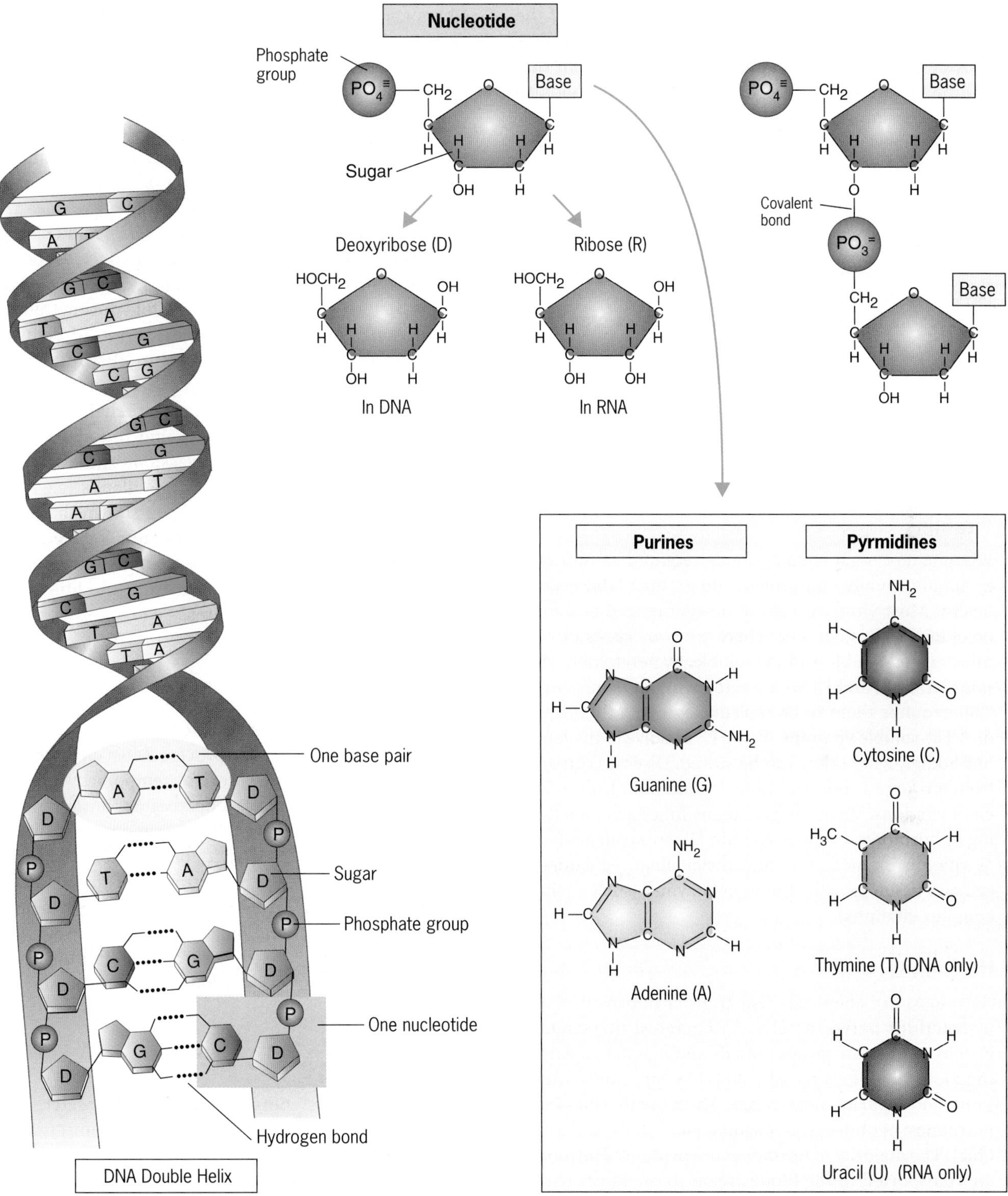

FIGURE 51–9 Structure of the DNA molecule.

to translate the genetic information stored in DNA into protein structures. RNA consists of a single strand of a polynucleotide and occurs in three basic forms: messenger RNA (mRNA), transfer RNA (tRNA), and ribosomal RNA (rRNA).

Tiny cellular particles called *ribosomes* are the sites of protein synthesis. They consist of numerous proteins and three to four rRNA molecules. In addition to providing a surface for protein synthesis, ribosomes contain enzymes that catalyze the process. An mRNA molecule diffuses about the cell and attaches itself to a ribosome, where it acts as a pattern for protein synthesis. A sequence of three base pairs in an mRNA molecule acts as the code for a particular amino acid. This sequence is called a *codon*, and each codon represents one of the 20 different amino acids. The attached mRNA codons provide the sequence of amino acids for a protein that will be synthesized. A tRNA molecule then bonds to a particular amino acid and carries it to a ribosome. It attaches itself to an mRNA codon through base pairing. Once the sequence of amino acids is complete, a termination codon signals the end of the polypeptide, and the finished product, a protein, is released from the ribosome.

In addition to their role in DNA and RNA, nucleotides have other important biologic functions. Most notable is their role in the production of high-energy triphosphate, or **adenosine triphosphate (ATP)**, which is the main molecule used to store energy. Another important nucleotide group is the cyclic nucleotides, such as cyclic 3′5′-adenosine monophosphate (cAMP), which, among other functions, is involved in relaxation of the smooth muscles of the airways (bronchodilation).

Vitamins

Vitamins are organic compounds required as nutrients in minute amounts for growth and for maintaining good health. Most vitamins cannot be synthesized and must be obtained through diet. There are two classes of vitamins: water soluble and fat soluble. Water-soluble vitamins (A, D, E, and K) are excreted without being stored. This requires them to be replenished regularly through diet. Fat-soluble vitamins (B and C) dissolve in the fats of our bodies, where they can be stored. Diseases can arise from too large a concentration of vitamins or from a deficit of vitamins. Vitamins have many functions, functioning as hormones (such as vitamin D), antioxidants (such as vitamin E), mediators of cell signaling, regulators of cell and tissue growth, and as coenzymes (such as the B complex vitamins).

Hormones

Hormones are chemicals that transfer information and instructions between cells. As chemical messengers, hormones regulate growth and development, control the functions of various tissues, support reproductive functions, and regulate metabolism. There are two classes of hormones: peptides (water soluble) and steroids (fat soluble). The majority of hormones are peptides. Hormones are transported in the bloodstream to the target tissue, which contains a specialized protein called a *receptor*. Typically, the water-soluble peptide uses a receptor on the surface of the target tissue. The fat-soluble steroid hormones pass through the cell membrane to receptors in the cytoplasm. When the compatible receptor and hormone bind, both molecules undergo structural changes that activate mechanisms within the cell. These mechanisms produce the desired effect dictated by the hormone. Hormonal effects are complex. Some hormones change the permeability of the cell membrane. Others can alter enzyme activity, and some hormones stimulate the release of other hormones.

Cytokines

Cytokines are substances that carry signals between cells and thus have an effect on other cells. They encompass a large and diverse family of polypeptide regulators that are produced widely throughout the body. Cytokines are classified as lymphokines, interleukins (IL), and chemokines. Hormones circulate in nanomolar concentrations, whereas some cytokines circulate in picomolar concentrations that can increase up to 1000-fold during trauma or infection. The widespread distribution of cellular sources for cytokines is another feature that differentiates cytokines from hormones. Virtually all nucleated cells (especially endothelial cells, epithelial cells, and macrophages) produce IL-1, IL-6, and tumor necrosis factor-α (TNF-α). In contrast, classic hormones, such as insulin, are secreted from discrete glands (e.g., the pancreas). In recent years, it has been shown that lung injury, such as may occur with ventilator-induced lung injury, can result in increased release of cytokines from the lungs. The cytokines released from the lungs can induce downstream organ failures.

Enzymes

Enzymes are proteins secreted by cells that act to speed up (catalyze) chemical changes in other substances while they remain unchanged in the process. Most enzymes are globular proteins. Enzymes work by temporarily binding to one or more reactants, thus decreasing the amount of activation energy needed for reactions and increasing the rate of the reaction. The activity of enzymes is affected by temperature, pH, the concentration of the reactant, and inhibitors such as drugs and poisons. Enzymes have a wide variety of functions, including signal transduction and cell regulation, muscle contraction, acting as ion pumps involved in active transport, and creating metabolic pathways.

Fluid Balance

The human body is composed primarily of water. The weight of a newborn infant is 75% to 80% water; that of a woman, 45% to 50%; and that of a man, 55% to 60%. These percentages vary depending on gender, age, and weight. People with a higher fat content have lower water content per kilogram of body weight. Women have relatively less total water content than men primarily because of their higher percentage of fat.

Water in the body is functionally distributed between two major areas: the intracellular compartment and the extracellular compartment. Intracellular fluid is a solvent in the cells that facilitates intracellular chemical reactions. Extracellular fluid serves the dual roles of providing a relatively constant environment for cells and

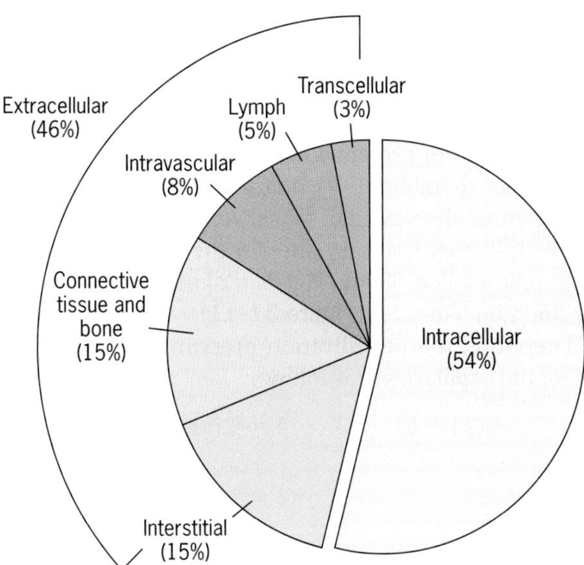

FIGURE 51–10 Fluid compartments of the body.

TABLE 51–7 Electrolyte Concentrations of Body Fluids

Electrolyte	Intravascular Concentration (mEq/L)	Interstitial Concentration (mEq/L)	Intracellular Concentration (mEq/L)
Cations			
Sodium (Na^+)	142	145	10
Potassium (K^+)	4	4	158
Magnesium (Mg^{+2})	3	2	35
Calcium (Ca^{+2})	5	3	2
Total	154	154	205
Anions			
Chloride (Cl^-)	103	115	2
Bicarbonate (HCO_3^-)	27	30	8
Phosphate (PSO_4^{-2})	2	2	140
Sulfate (SO_4^{-2})	1	1	—
Protein ($Prot^-$)	16	1	55
Organic acids	5	5	—
Total	154	154	205

transporting substances to and from the cell. Approximately 54% of the body's water is intracellular and 46% is extracellular (**Figure 51–10**). The extracellular fluid compartment is composed of five areas: the interstitial compartment, which accounts for the fluid outside or between the cells (15% of total body water); the intravascular (plasma) compartment, which accounts for the fluid in the heart and blood vessels (8%); dense connective tissue, cartilage, and bone (15%); lymph (5%); and the transcellular compartment, which includes the fluid in the salivary glands, thyroid gland, gonads, mucous membranes of the respiratory and gastrointestinal tracts, kidneys, liver, pancreas, cerebrospinal fluid, joint fluid, and the fluid in the spaces of the eyes (3%). The interstitial and intravascular compartments are the extracellular areas most involved with fluid balance.

The normal daily water intake is 2400 to 2500 mL, which is offset by an equal amount of fluid output. Fluid is taken in primarily through daily food (≈700 mL) and drink (≈1500 mL), but some also comes from body metabolism (≈200 mL a day). In the oxidation of food, about 14 mL of water is produced for every 100 kcal of energy released. The type of energy substrate oxidized determines the volume of water produced: 100 g of carbohydrate produces 55 g of water; 100 g of fat produces 107 g of water; and 100 g of protein produces 41 g of water.

Fluid loss occurs as a sensible loss through the kidneys as urine (≈1400 mL/day) and through the gastrointestinal tract as feces (≈200 mL/day) or as an insensible loss through the skin as perspiration (≈450 mL/day) or from the lungs as expired water vapor (≈350 mL/day). The volume of insensible loss is higher with vigorous muscular exercise; with an increased respiratory rate; in a hot, dry environment; with a fever; or with severe skin burns.

The various compartments are separated by semipermeable membranes that allow certain fluids and solutes to move freely between them. The movement of water between compartments is maintained by a dynamic equilibrium among five interdependent factors: intake and output, osmotic and hydrostatic pressure, hormones, electrolyte concentration, and the cardiovascular system.

An important concept in fluid balance is that the amount of fluid taken in must equal the amount of fluid leaving the body. If this does not occur, the fluid level in the various compartments must change. The body's primary mechanism to maintain total body fluid volume is adjustment in the amount of fluid leaving the body through the volume of urine excreted. Although it is difficult for the body to control the amount a person eats or drinks, it can influence the desire to do so through thirst and hunger.

The composition of the solutions in the different compartments has a major effect on fluid balance. The principal difference in the composition of the intracellular, intravascular, and interstitial fluids is the difference in the protein and salt concentrations. As shown in **Table 51–7**, the electrolyte concentration of the extracellular compartments is very similar, with the major cation being sodium and the major anions being chlorine and bicarbonate. The intravascular compartment has a much higher protein concentration than the interstitial compartment, thereby generating an osmotic pressure that helps keep fluid in the vascular space and out of the interstitial space. Extracellular and intracellular fluids are more unlike chemically than they are similar. The primary intracellular cation is potassium, and the major anion is phosphate; the protein content is highest in the cells.

One important mechanism used to control extracellular fluid (ECF) volume is the electrolyte concentration, particularly sodium. The phrase "Where sodium goes, water soon follows" can aid in remembering this concept. The arterial blood pressure declines when the ECF and blood volume are reduced from lack of fluid intake. This stimulates pressure receptors (baroreceptors) in the hypothalamus and thorax to stimulate the adrenal cortex to increase secretion of the hormone aldosterone. Aldosterone increases resorption of sodium in the kidney tubule, which leads to an increase in kidney tubule resorption of water and a reduction in urine volume. The reduced urine volume increases the ECF volume and steers it back toward a normal balance.

Stimulation of the hypothalamus also triggers the pituitary gland to secrete antidiuretic hormone (ADH). ADH functions to reduce the amount of water excreted by promoting resorption of water into the circulation at the renal tubules. The pituitary gland can also trigger secretion of ADH after receiving a signal from the baroreceptors in the aortic bodies that the blood pressure is low.

Two factors working together determine urine volume: the kidney glomerular filtration rate and the rate of water resorption by the renal tubules. Except under abnormal conditions, the filtration rate is fairly constant and is not a major factor in urine excretion. The rate of tubular resorption, on the other hand, fluctuates considerably. During the course of a single day, the kidneys filter 190 L of water, yet reabsorb 189 L. As already discussed, the amounts of the hormones secreted by the pituitary gland (ADH) and the adrenal cortex (aldosterone) regulate water resorption.

Another important mechanism that regulates the water and electrolyte levels in the extracellular fluid is the pressure gradient. According to the physical laws governing filtration and osmosis, hydrostatic pressure tends to push fluid out of its compartment, whereas osmotic pressure tends to pull water into its compartment. English physiologist Ernest Starling proposed a mechanism that controls movement across capillary membranes (**Equation 51–16**).

Because the intravascular compartment contains a larger number of proteins than the interstitial compartment (refer to Table 51–7), a larger osmotic pressure is generated in the vascular space. At the arterial end of tissue capillaries, normal values for the various pressures are as follows: Pch, 35 mm Hg; Pco, 24 mm Hg; Pih, 2 mm Hg; and Pio, 0 mm Hg (**Figure 51–11**).

Therefore, the net filtration pressure at the arterial end of the capillaries is as follows:

$$(35 - 2) - (24 - 0) = 33 - 24 = 9 \text{ mm Hg}$$

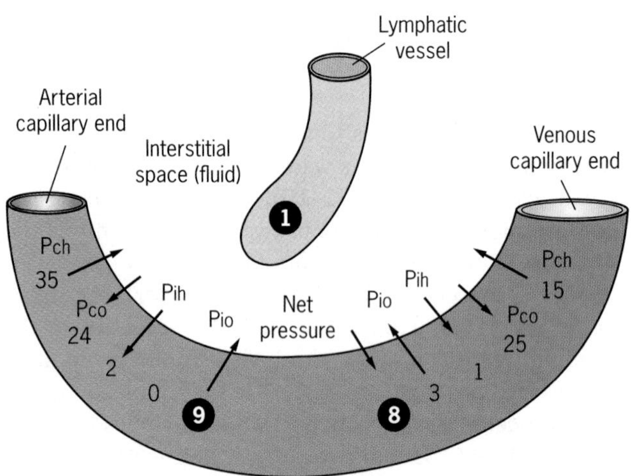

FIGURE 51–11 Starling's law governs the movement of fluids between the capillary and interstitial compartments based on hydrostatic (capillary [Pch] and interstitial [Pih]) and osmotic (capillary [Pco] and interstitial [Pio]) pressure differences.

EQUATION 51–16

Starling's Law

Starling's law is expressed as

$$Q_f = K_1\,(Pch - Pih) - K_2\,(Pco - Pio)$$

where:

Q_f = Effective filtration pressure between blood and interstitial fluid, which determines the bulk or net outward flow of fluid from the capillaries
Pch = Capillary hydrostatic pressure
Pih = Interstitial hydrostatic pressure
Pco = Capillary osmotic pressure
Pio = Interstitial osmotic pressure
K_1 = Capillary permeability coefficient for fluids and electrolytes
K_2 = Capillary permeability coefficient for proteins

This suggests that a net positive pressure of 9 mm Hg tends to push fluids from the vascular space at the arterial end of the capillaries.

At the venous end of the tissue capillaries, normal pressures are as follows: Pch, 15 mm Hg; Pco, 25 mm Hg; Pih, 1 mm Hg; and Pio, 3 mm Hg. The net filtration pressure of the venous end of the capillaries is as follows:

$$(15 - 1) - (25 - 3) = 14 - 22 = -8 \text{ mm Hg}$$

This suggests that a net negative pressure of 8 mm Hg tends to pull fluids in toward the vascular space at the venous end of the capillaries. As blood flows through the capillary tissue bed, the tendency is for fluid to be pushed out into the interstitial space at the arterial end (net outward pressure of 9 mm Hg) and pulled back into the capillaries from the interstitial space at the venous end (–8 mm Hg). Interstitial fluid that is not pulled back into the capillaries is drained via the lymphatic system.

Of the three main body compartmental fluids, interstitial fluid varies the most. Plasma volume usually fluctuates only slightly and briefly. If an abnormally large amount of fluid shifts to the interstitial (and eventually to the intercellular) tissue space, the condition is known as *edema*. Edema can be caused by any of the factors governing the movement of fluids between the vascular and interstitial compartments, including (1) retention of electrolytes (especially sodium) in the extracellular fluid as a result of increased aldosterone secretion or after serious renal disease; (2) an increase in capillary hydrostatic pressure, as is seen in congestive heart failure caused by left ventricular failure; and (3) a decrease in plasma proteins because of a low overall protein concentration, such as that caused by poor nutrition (reflected in a low serum albumin level) or because of increased capillary permeability, such as that caused by infection, burns, or shock. Increased capillary permeability allows protein molecules to leak out of the vascular space into the interstitial space, where they exert an osmotic pressure and pull fluid toward that area.

Metabolic Pathways

Food is broken down into nutrients that are used by the body to promote growth, maintenance, and repair. The six classes of nutrients are carbohydrate, fat, protein, vitamins, minerals, and water.

The word *metabolism* is derived from the Greek word *meta*, meaning "change." Metabolism involves the processes by which these nutrients are used after they are ingested, digested, absorbed, and circulated to the cells of the body. It uses them in two ways: as an energy source to drive vital functions (carbohydrates, fat, and protein are the energy nutrients) or as the ingredients to make complex chemical compounds. Before nutrients can be used, catabolism must occur. **Catabolism** involves reactions in which large molecules are broken down to smaller ones that can be used by the cells, where they undergo many chemical changes. The process by which the nutrients are used to build more complex biomolecules is **anabolism**.

Catabolism is a decomposition process involving the oxidation of nutrient molecules. It releases energy (exergonic metabolism) in two forms: as heat or as chemical energy. Heat energy helps maintain the homeostasis of body temperature, but it cannot be used as a form of energy by the cells. Chemical energy, on the other hand, can be used by the cells, but it must first be transferred to high-energy bonds of ATP molecules. These bonds break more easily than other types of chemical bonds and therefore give up their energy more readily. ATP is one of the crucial compounds of the biologic world because it supplies energy directly to the energy-using reactions of all cells in all kinds of living organisms, from one-celled plants to trillion-celled human beings. The end products of catabolism include such molecules as lactic acid, ethanol, CO_2, urea, ammonia, and water.

RESPIRATORY RECAP

Metabolic Pathways

- Glycolysis
- Citric acid (Krebs) cycle
- Electron transport

Anabolism is a synthesis process that assembles precursor molecules, such as amino acids, sugars, fatty acids, and nitrogenous bases, into cell macromolecules such as proteins, polysaccharides, lipids, and nucleic acids. This process requires energy (endergonic metabolism), which is supplied by the ATP generated during catabolism.

These two metabolic processes occur simultaneously in the cell in that some of the energy released and the products produced during catabolism are immediately used in the process of anabolism. The cell manages the conflicting demands of concomitant catabolism and anabolism in two ways. First, the cell maintains a tight and separate regulation of both processes through the use of literally hundreds of enzymatic reactions organized into discrete pathways. Second, the metabolic pathways are localized in different cellular compartments. For example, the enzymes responsible for fatty acid biosynthesis are found in the cytosol, whereas the fatty acid oxidation process takes place in the mitochondria.

The pathways of catabolism converge to a few end products, and the process consists of three stages (**Figure 51–12**). Stage 1 involves the breakdown of protein, polysaccharide, and lipid macromolecules into their respective building blocks. Proteins give up their 20 component amino acids; polysaccharides break down to carbohydrate units that are ultimately converted to glucose; and lipids produce glycerol and fatty acids. The cells prefer glucose as their primary energy fuel and therefore catabolize most of the carbohydrates absorbed and anabolize a relatively small portion of it. Fats and proteins are catabolized only when the amount of glucose entering cells is inadequate for their energy needs.

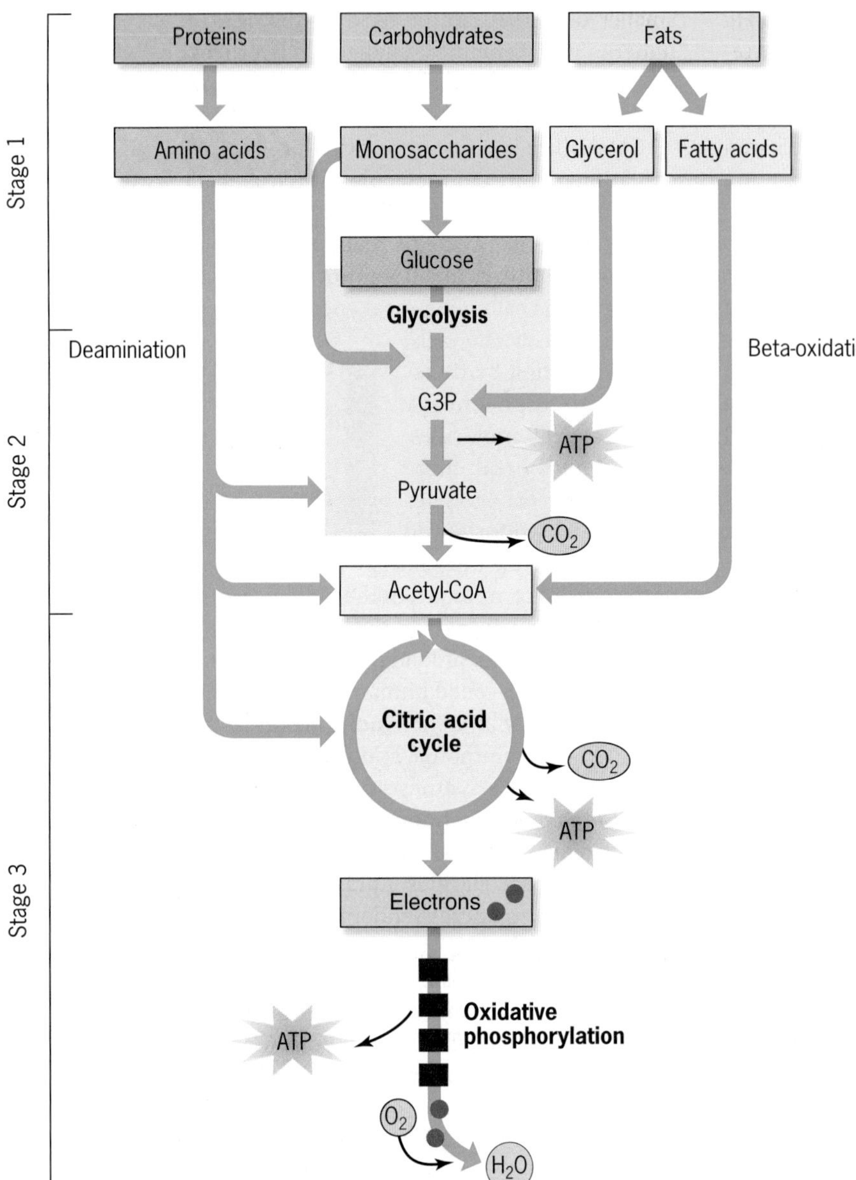

FIGURE 51–12 Three stages of catabolism. CoA, coenzyme A.

Stage 2 converts the products from stage 1 into an even more limited set of simpler metabolic by-products. Fatty acids break down into two-carbon units of acetyl coenzyme A (acetyl-CoA). Glucose and the glycerol from lipids generate the three-carbon α-keto acid pyruvic acid (pyruvate), which breaks down into acetyl-CoA in the presence of oxygen (aerobic metabolism) or to lactic acid when oxygen is absent (anaerobic metabolism). Amino acids give rise to pyruvate, acetyl-CoA, or intermediates fed directly into the citric acid cycle of stage 3. Stage 3 involves the combustion of the acetyl groups of acetyl-CoA by the citric acid cycle and oxidative phosphorylation to yield CO_2, water, and ATP molecules.

As stated previously, carbohydrates are the primary source of energy. Glucose metabolism begins with the breakdown of a six-carbon glucose chain ($C_6H_{12}O_6$) to two three-carbon pyruvate (pyruvic acid) molecules by means of a process called **glycolysis**. Glycolysis takes place in the cytosol of the cell. It is an anaerobic process in that it does not use oxygen and as such is the only process that provides cells with energy when the oxygen supply is inadequate or even absent. Glycolysis releases about 5% of the energy stored in the glucose molecule, releasing some energy as heat and the rest as energy transferred to ATP molecules and to reduced nicotinamide adenine dinucleotide (NAD) molecules (NADH). For every glucose molecule undergoing glycolysis, a net of two ATP molecules is formed. Although only a small amount of energy is released during glycolysis, it is an essential process because it prepares glucose for the second step in catabolism, namely the citric acid cycle.

The **citric acid (Krebs) cycle** converts two pyruvic acid molecules into six CO_2 molecules and six water molecules. The citric acid cycle takes place in the presence of oxygen in the mitochondria of the cell. Before pyruvic acid molecules enter the mitochondria, they combine with coenzyme A to split off CO_2 and a pair of high-energy electrons to form acetyl-CoA. Coenzyme A then detaches from acetyl-CoA, leaving a two-carbon acetyl group to enter the citric acid cycle. The citric acid cycle consists of a series of eight reactions, the first of which is the formation of citric acid from the combination of the two-carbon acetyl group with the four-carbon oxaloacetic acid (which was formed as a product in the eighth step of the cycle). Citric acid is also known as *tricarboxylic acid (TCA)*, and the citric acid cycle therefore is also known as the *TCA cycle*; it is also called the *Krebs cycle* because Sir Hans Krebs deciphered the cyclic nature of pyruvate oxidation, earning the 1935 Nobel Prize for his work on this metabolic pathway. In addition to eight acids, the citric acid cycle produces CO_2, a small amount of ATP, a small amount of reduced flavin adenine dinucleotide (FAD), and a large amount of reduced NAD (NADH).

The energy produced during glycolysis and the TCA cycle is not enough to sustain life. The high-energy electrons removed during the first two processes in the form of reduced FAD and NAD enter a chain of carrier molecules that is embedded in the inner membrane of the mitochondria. This process, known as the **electron transport system**, is responsible for the production of 90% of the ATP formed during carbohydrate catabolism.

The most important fact about electron transport is that as electrons move down the carrier chain, they release small bursts of energy to pump protons between the inner and outer membranes of the mitochondria. The diffusion of the protons into the matrix in the inner compartment drives a process called **oxidative phosphorylation**, which refers to the joining of a phosphate group to adenosine diphosphate (ADP) to form ATP. At the end of the electron transport chain, oxygen serves as the final electron receptor to form water:

$$NADH + H^+ + ½O_2 \rightarrow NAD^+ + H_2O$$

The NAD^+—NADH system can be viewed as a shuttle that carries electrons released from catabolic substrates to the mitochondria, where they are transferred to oxygen, the ultimate electron acceptor in catabolism. In the process, the free energy is trapped in ATP molecules. The net result of oxidation of glucose is as follows:

$$\text{Glucose} + 38\ ADP + 38\ HPO_4^{-2} + O_2 \rightarrow 6\ CO_2 + 38\ ATP + 44\ H_2O$$

Certain drugs can disrupt the coupling of electron transport and ATP synthesis. Cyanide poisoning is an example of such an uncoupler. Rather than producing ATP, the energy released in electron transport is dissipated as heat, oxygen is not consumed, and death eventually occurs.

KEY POINTS

- Atoms consist of protons, neutrons, and electrons.
- Atoms join to produce ionic, covalent, and hydrogen bonds.
- Chemical reactions involve the forming or breaking of chemical bonds.
- The degree to which solute particles dissolve into a solvent is called *solubility*.
- The concentration of a solution can be stated as moles, percent, ratio, or mEq/L.
- Colligative properties are the properties of a solution that depend on the number of dissolved solute particles.
- Living organisms are composed of organic and inorganic compounds.
- Electrolytes include acids, bases, and salts.
- Acids are hydrogen ion or proton donors, bases are hydrogen ion or proton acceptors, buffers minimize the change in hydrogen ion concentration, and salts are the result of reactions between acids and bases.
- Carbohydrates can be monosaccharides, disaccharides, oligosaccharides, or polysaccharides.
- Proteins are composed of amino acids.
- Triglycerides, phospholipids, steroids, and eicosanoids are lipids.
- DNA and RNA are nucleic acids.
- DNA carries the genetic information (genes) for protein synthesis.
- Fluid and electrolyte balance is normally maintained within a narrow range.
- Glycolysis, the citric acid (Krebs) cycle, and electron transport are responsible for energy production in the cell.

SUGGESTED READING

Berg JM, Tymoczko JL, Stryer L. *Biochemistry*. 6th ed. New York: WH Freeman; 2007.

Jones A. *Chemistry: An Introduction for Medical and Health Sciences*. West Sussex, England: John Wiley & Sons; 2005.

Lieberman M, Marks AD. *Mark's Basic Medical Biochemistry: A Clinical Approach*. 3rd ed. Baltimore: Lippincott Williams & Wilkins; 2009.

Malley WJ. *Clinical Blood Gases: Assessment and Intervention*. 2nd ed. Philadelphia: WB Saunders; 2005.

Murry RM, Granner DK, Rodwell VW. *Harper's Illustrated Biochemistry*. 27th ed. New York: Lange Medical Books/McGraw-Hill; 2006.

Nelson DL, Cox MM. *Lehniger Principles of Biochemistry*. 4th ed. New York: WH Freeman; 2005.

Raymond KW. *General, Organic, and Biological Chemistry: An Integrated Approach*. 2nd ed. Hoboken, NJ: John Wiley & Sons; 2008.

Sackheim GI, Lehman DD. *Chemistry for the Health Sciences*. 8th ed. Upper Saddle River, NJ: Prentice-Hall; 1998.

Scanlon VC, Sanders T. *Essentials of Anatomy and Physiology*. 4th ed. Philadelphia: FA Davis; 2003.

CHAPTER 52

Respiratory Microbiology

Ruben D. Restrepo
Marcos I. Restrepo

OUTLINE

Bacteria
Viruses
Fungi
Parasites
Common Respiratory Infections
Sampling Methods
Microbiology Techniques
Antimicrobial Resistance

OBJECTIVES

1. Identify the major microorganisms causing respiratory infections.
2. Compare bacteria, viruses, fungi, and parasites.
3. List the most common pathogens infecting the upper airway and lower respiratory tract.
4. Compare the techniques of sputum induction, bronchoscopy, and bronchoalveolar lavage.
5. Describe microbiology techniques to identify pathogens.
6. Discuss the mechanisms of antibiotic resistance.

KEY TERMS

acid-fast bacilli (AFB)
aerobe
anaerobe
antibiotic resistance
antigen detection
bacilli
bacteria
biofilm
bronchoalveolar lavage (BAL)
bronchoscopy
cocci
culture
fungi
Gram-negative bacteria
Gram-positive bacteria
Mantoux test
microbiology
multiresistant
mutation
normal flora
parasites
purified protein derivative (PPD)
spirochetes
sputum induction
transtracheal aspiration (TTA)
virologic studies
viruses

INTRODUCTION

The respiratory therapist encounters patients with upper and lower airway infections every day. The pathogens responsible for these common illnesses are diverse, representing essentially the entire spectrum of **microbiology**, from bacteria to viruses, fungi, and occasionally parasites.

Bacteria

Bacteria are a large group of unicellular microorganisms first observed by Antonie van Leeuwenhoek in 1676.[1] Their name derives from the Greek word *baktērion*, which means "small staff."

Bacterial Microbiology

Bacteria typically measure between 0.5 and 5 μm in diameter. However, *Mycoplasma*, a very important bacterium in respiratory infections, only measures 0.3 μm. The human body contains approximately 10 times more bacterial cells than human cells. Most of these bacteria reside on the skin and in the gastrointestinal tract. Bacteria are classified as prokaryotes. Unlike the larger eukaryotes and other animal cells that contain a fully differentiated nucleus, prokaryotic bacterial deoxyribonucleic acid (DNA) forms only in a single, circular chromosome (a nucleoid) that is not bound by a membrane. Like animals and plants, bacteria use ribosomes to translate ribonucleic acid (RNA) into protein products. Bacteria (excluding the mycobacteria) are surrounded by both a cell membrane and a rigid cell wall. Eukaryotes lack a cell wall. **Figure 52–1** shows a schematic diagram of a typical bacterium.

Bacteria are free-living organisms that vary in their survival requirements. Oxygen is a variable of particular clinical importance. An **aerobe** requires oxygen for survival, an **anaerobe** requires the absence of oxygen, and a *facultative anaerobe* has limited oxygen tolerance. Bacteria are ubiquitous but are found preferentially in certain sites. For example, anaerobes such as *Clostridium* are found in soil, where oxygen concentrations are lower, explaining why soil-contaminated wounds are more prone to tetanus infection and gas gangrene (*C tetani* and *C perfringens*, respectively; both are anaerobes). Because *Pseudomonas aeruginosa* commonly colonizes the leaves of plants, live flowers are frequently banned from ventilator and burn units.

> **RESPIRATORY RECAP**
>
> **Bacterial Shape Classification**
>
> » Cocci: round
> » Bacilli: rod
> » Spirochetes: spirals

Bacteria display a wide variety of morphologies, as seen in **Figure 52–2**. Most bacterial species are either spherical (**cocci**) or rod-shaped (**bacilli**). Some are comma shaped (vibrio), spiral shaped (spirilla), or coiled (**spirochetes**). These different shapes can influence the ability of bacteria to acquire nutrients, swim through liquids, attach to surfaces, and escape predators. Some bacteria also associate in characteristic patterns: *Streptococcus* forms pairs or chains, *Staphylococcus* forms clusters like grapes, and *Neisseria* forms pairs.

Bacterial cell walls are made of peptidoglycan. This wall is essential to the survival of many bacteria. Penicillin kills bacteria by inhibiting synthesis of peptidoglycan. According to the reaction of the cell wall to the Gram stain, bacteria can be classified as Gram positive and Gram negative. **Gram-positive bacteria** retain the crystal violet dye when washed in a decolorizing solution, whereas **Gram-negative bacteria** do not retain the crystal violet dye in the Gram staining protocol.

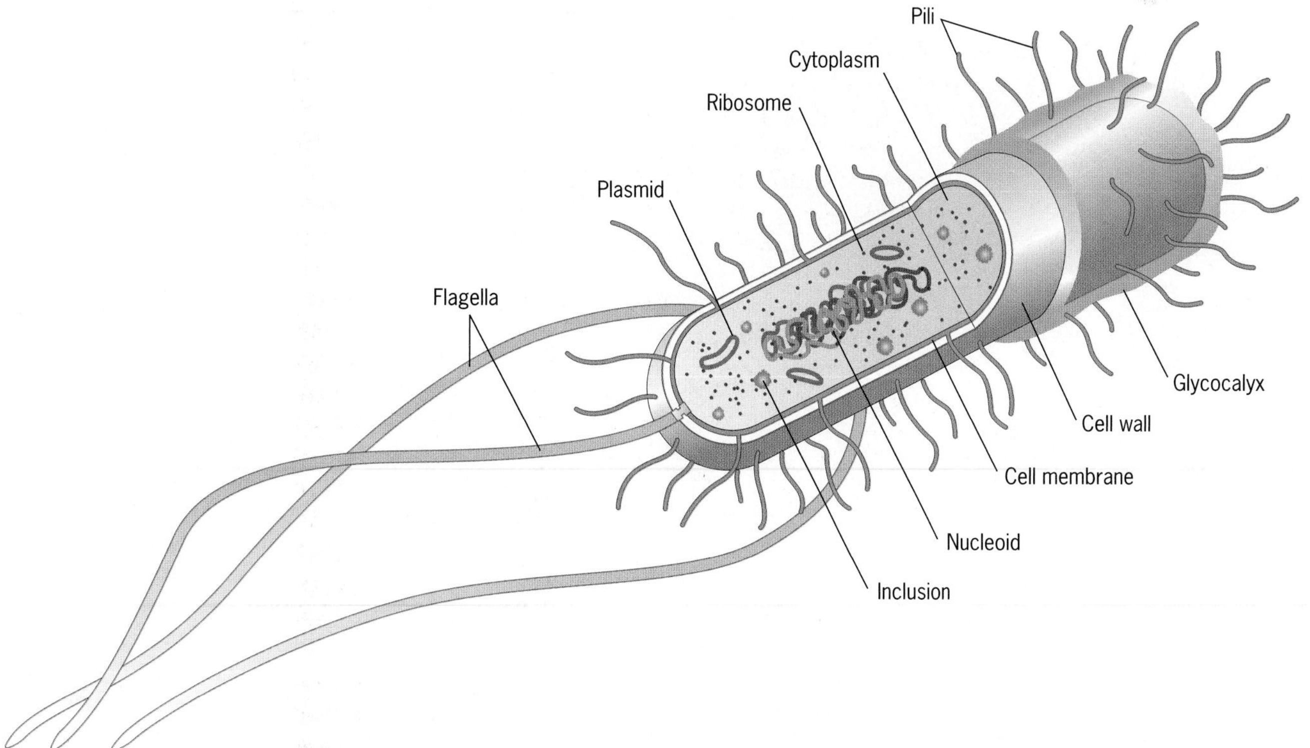

FIGURE 52–1 A typical bacterium.

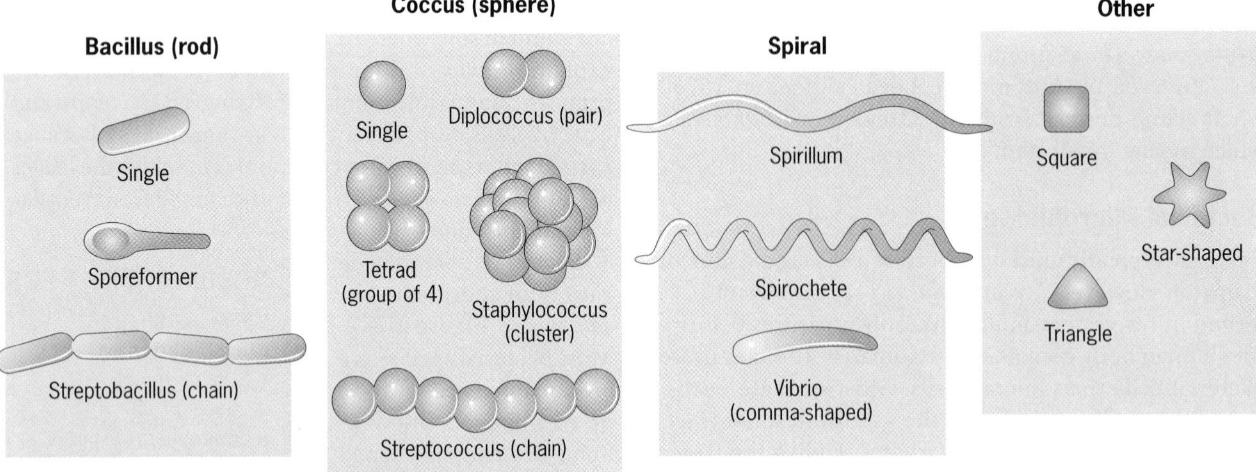

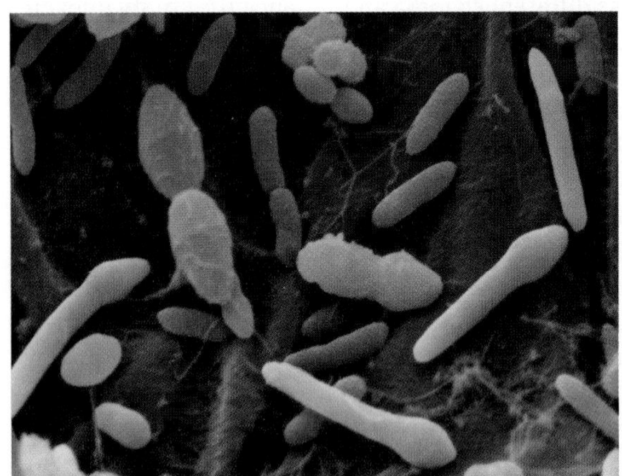

FIGURE 52–2 Basic bacterial shapes.

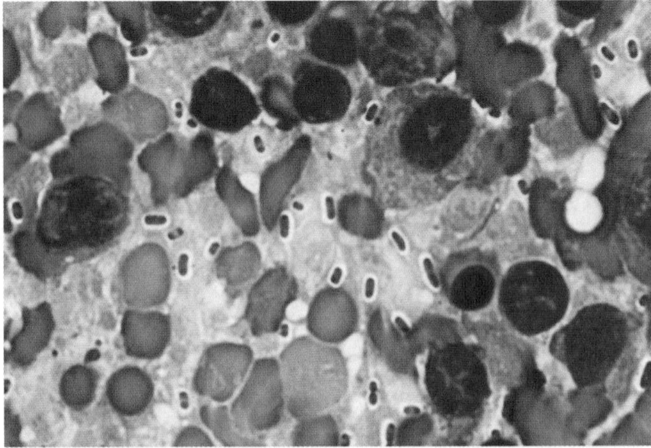

FIGURE 52–3 Electron micrograph of Gram-negative bacilli (*Klebsiella pneumoniae*).

A safranin counterstain that is added after the crystal violet is washed out is responsible for coloring all Gram-negative bacteria pink or red (**Figure 52–3**).

Gram-positive bacteria have a thick cell wall, whereas Gram-negative bacteria have a thin cell wall with a few layers of peptidoglycan surrounded by a lipid membrane. This difference is one of the most important criteria used to classify bacteria and to determine antibiotic susceptibility. **Figure 52–4** schematically illustrates typical cell walls of Gram-positive and Gram-negative bacteria.

> **RESPIRATORY RECAP**
>
> **Bacterial Reaction to Gram Staining**
>
> » *Gram-positive bacteria*: peptidoglycan in cell wall; stains violet
> » *Gram-negative bacteria*: no violet stain; pink appearance due to safranin counterstain

Although bacteria may be free floating (exhibiting planktonic behavior), they are capable of forming complex and stable aggregate communities, also known as bacterial mats or **biofilms**. These biofilms attach to any surface, liquid or solid. Once formed, biofilms may be virtually impossible to remove from the surface to which they attach and may be 100 times more resistant to antibiotics than bacterial cells exhibiting planktonic behavior.

Bacteria grow to a fixed size and then reproduce by binary fission, a form of asexual reproduction whereby each bacterium makes two identical cloned bacterial cells. Because this process is asexual, the ability of bacteria to vary their genetic traits is limited. Given an environment that provides unlimited nutrients, binary fission produces rapid bacterial growth. Because the number of bacteria doubles with each division, the pattern of growth is exponential (logarithmic). Each bacterium has a characteristic doubling time under ideal conditions. Although it can be as fast as 9.8 minutes (for *Pseudomonas natriensis*),[2] it typically ranges from 20 minutes (for *Escherichia coli*) to 24 hours (for *Mycobacterium tuberculosis*). Under ideal conditions, a single *E coli* bacterium can yield over 50 million bacteria in 8 hours. Within 24 hours the bacterial growth would fill a patient's room.

Because nutrients are limited in natural environments, however, bacteria cannot continue to reproduce at these fast rates. Adaptation to this low-nutrient environment is described by three different growth stages:

7. *Lag phase*: Period of slow growth when cells are adapting to the new environment.

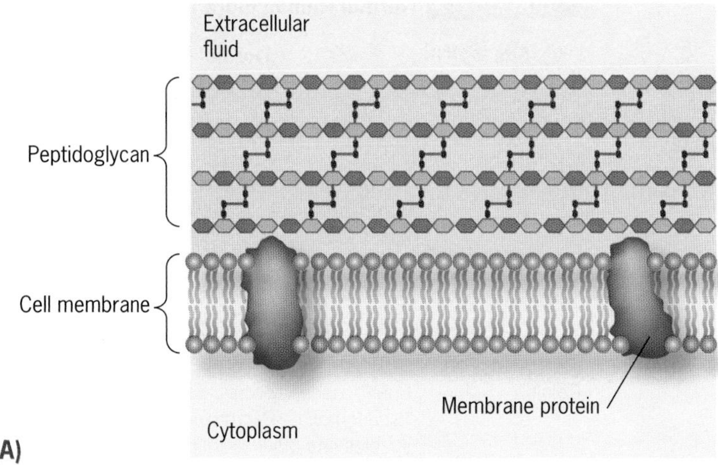

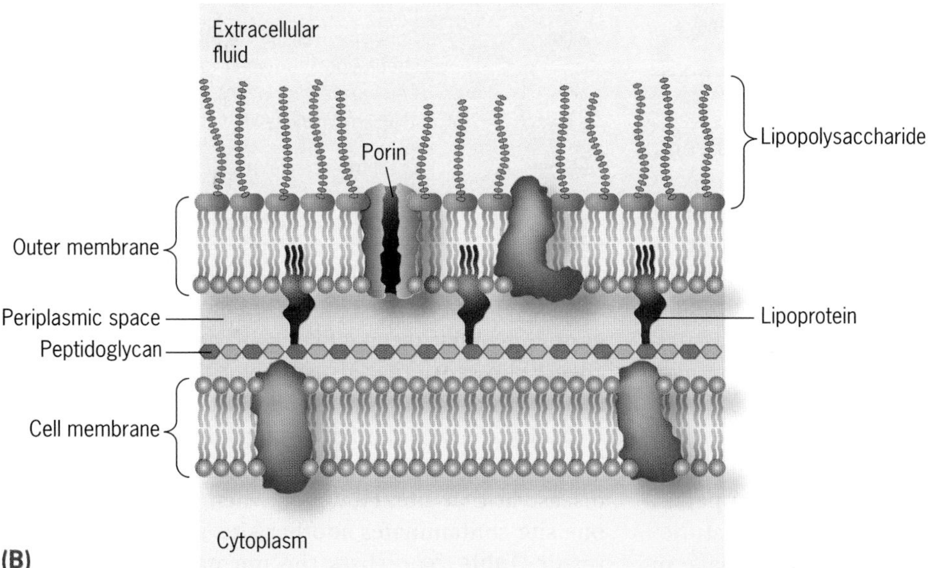

FIGURE 52–4 Gram-positive and Gram-negative bacteria. (**A**) A Gram-positive bacterium has a thick layer of peptidoglycan. (**B**) A Gram-negative bacterium has a thin peptidoglycan layer and an outer membrane.

8. *Log (logarithmic) phase*: Rapid exponential growth. Nutrients are metabolized at maximum speed until depleted.
9. *Stationary phase*: Nutrients are locally depleted, and waste products accumulate, growth rate slows, and the population reaches a steady state. The cells consume nonessential cellular proteins.

If conditions continue to deteriorate, bacterial counts begin to decline to low levels. This phase occurs in abscesses or as a consequence of immune system activity.

Gene transfer between bacterial cells is important in understanding antibiotic resistance. It occurs in three ways: mutation, conjugation, and transduction. **Mutation**, or transformation, is a genetic alteration that can result from the uptake of foreign DNA. This genetic material is added to or replaces part of a bacterium's DNA. Although some mutations are repaired and most produce nonfunctional genes, an occasional fortuitous mutation occurs, producing an improved gene. This altered gene then is passed on as the bacterium divides. If the new gene imparts a survival advantage, bacteria carrying it may come to predominate over normal, wild-type bacteria. In bacterial *conjugation*, the DNA is transferred through direct cell contact, a process also known as horizontal gene transfer. *Transduction* involves the integration of a virus that infects bacteria (a bacteriophage) introducing foreign DNA into the chromosome. When viruses are released, they carry this DNA to newly infected bacteria.

Bacteria cause disease through three major mechanisms: toxin formation, direct damage, and inflammatory response. In addition to the endotoxin contained in the cell walls of Gram-negative bacteria, many bacteria secrete exotoxins, potent substances recognized as the primary virulence factor. These toxins are capable of damaging the plasma membrane of eukaryotic cells, inhibiting their protein synthesis or altering cellular proteins without killing the intoxicated cell. **Table 52–1** lists some important examples of toxins. Toxic illness does not require invasion of the bacteria into tissue or even the presence of viable bacteria. Particularly in foodborne illnesses, preformed toxins may be ingested even when all bacteria have been killed during brief cooking. Cooking or sterilization must produce high enough temperatures for sufficient duration to break down toxins as well as kill bacteria.

> **RESPIRATORY RECAP**
>
> **Bacterial Growth**
> » Lag phase
> » Log phase
> » Stationary phase

Although some bacterial illnesses are due solely to toxins, most bacteria cause direct tissue damage by tissue invasion. Once in tissue, bacteria deplete nutrients and produce toxins that damage host tissues. More important, many bacteria produce substances that cause damage to adjacent tissues, facilitating bacterial spread. Examples include the collagenase and hyaluronidase

TABLE 52-1 Common Disease-Causing Toxins

Toxin	Producer	Effect
Toxic shock	*Staphylococcus aureus*	Causes fever, rash, shock, tissue necrosis
Diphtheria	*Corynebacterium diphtheriae*	Inhibits protein synthesis, causing cell death
Erythrogenic	*Streptococcus pyogenes*	Causes scarlet fever rash
Tetanus	*Clostridium tetani*	Inhibits release of the neurotransmitter glycine, causing muscle spasm and rigidity
Botulism	*Clostridium botulinum*	Blocks release of the neurotransmitter acetylcholine, causing paralysis and flaccidity
Enterotoxin	*Escherichia coli*	Stimulates adenylate cyclase, increasing fluid secretion into the gut and causing diarrhea

produced by *Streptococcus pyogenes*, which digest components of the intercellular matrix. *Staphylococcus aureus* produces coagulase, which forms a fibrin clot around the site of infection, protecting *S aureus* from immune attack. New strains of methicillin-resistant *S aureus* (MRSA) acquired in the community produce the Panton-Valentine leukocidin toxin, which is associated with tissue necrosis, abscess formation, and a high mortality.[3–5]

Immune responses to bacterial invasion are responsible for clinical manifestations that include fever, hypotension, muscle aches, malaise, loss of appetite, confusion, and temporary liver and heart dysfunction. Immune cells also cause local tissue damage in their attempt to directly kill bacteria. This damage can manifest in pyogenic or granulomatous patterns. With the pyogenic pattern the predominant immune cells are neutrophils. Intense activity kills bacteria and host cells, producing a collection of neutrophils and dead tissue called *pus*. A cavity called an *abscess* may form where tissue has been destroyed. Because immune cells tend to travel along tissue surfaces, bacteria may survive within the center of an abscess unless it is drained. Some bacteria, of which *Mycobacterium tuberculosis* is the archetype, stimulate the formation of granulomas, which are collections of macrophages arranged in a palisade, or wall, around a focus of infection. The macrophages are surrounded by T lymphocytes, a formation that tends to wall off the infection, preventing its spread. Organisms then are phagocytized (ingested) by the macrophages. The interior of a granuloma may become filled with dead cells, forming a cheesy substance that gives these granulomas the name *caseating necrotizing granulomas.*

RESPIRATORY RECAP

Mechanisms of Bacterial Disease

- Toxin formation by bacteria
- Direct local tissue damage from bacteria
- Damage as a result of the immune response (pyogenic or granulomatous)

TABLE 52-2 Normal Human Flora by Body Site

Site	Normal Flora
Pharynx and upper gastrointestinal tract	*Moraxella catarrhalis*; *Staphylococcus epidermidis* and *S aureus*; α-hemolytic streptococci; viridans group streptococci; *Streptococcus pneumoniae*; *Peptostreptococcus*, *Lactobacillus*, and *Fusobacterium* species; *Actinomyces israelii*; *Haemophilus influenzae* and *parainfluenzae*; *Corynebacterium* species; *Neisseria meningitidis*, *Bacteroides* species, and other anaerobes; and *Candida* (yeast) species
Colon	*Enterococcus* species; *Escherichia coli*; *Pseudomonas*, *Bacteroides*, and *Clostridium* species and other Gram-negative bacilli and anaerobes; also *Candida* (yeast) species; organisms known as coliforms or enteric bacteria because of their location in the colon
Skin	*Staphylococcus epidermidis* and *S aureus*; streptococci; *Corynebacterium* species; *Clostridium perfringens*; *Propionibacterium aenes*; *Candida* (yeast) species
Lower respiratory tract	Essentially sterile; possibility of colonization when illness or structural lung disease compromises immune function

Many areas of the body normally contain bacteria, known as the **normal flora**, that do not usually cause disease at that site. However, when normal flora from one site contaminates another site, serious illness may result. **Table 52–2** lists the normal flora of several important sites.

Common Bacteria Associated with Respiratory Disease

Streptococcus pneumoniae

Streptococcus pneumoniae, or pneumococcus, is a Gram-positive, α-hemolytic (turns blood agar green) facultative anaerobe. It is also known as *Diplococcus pneumoniae* because of its characteristic appearance in Gram-stained sputum (**Figure 52–5**). *S pneumoniae*'s polysaccharide capsule is variably resistant to phagocytosis, which determines its virulence, prevalence, and extent of drug resistance. This bacterium is normally found in the nasopharynx of 20% to 40% of healthy children and 5% to 10% of healthy adults. However, its count may be higher in environments where people are in close proximity to each other for long periods of time, such as day-care centers and hospitals. Although *S pneumoniae* causes respiratory infections such as pneumonia, acute sinusitis, and otitis media, it is also responsible for causing endocarditis, pericarditis, osteomyelitis, and bacteremia.

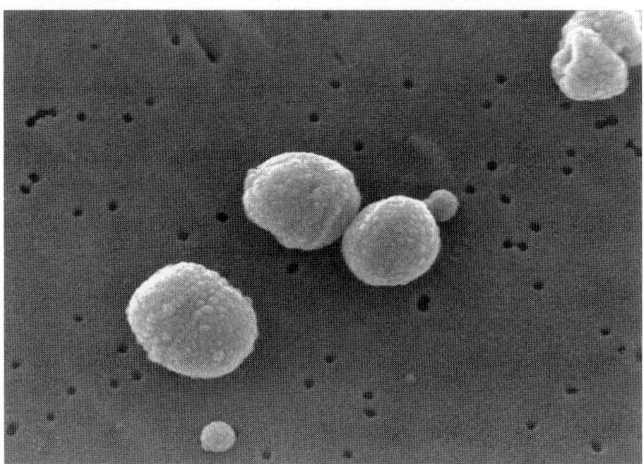

FIGURE 52–5 Electron micrograph of *Streptococcus pneumoniae* showing its characteristic appearance in pairs.

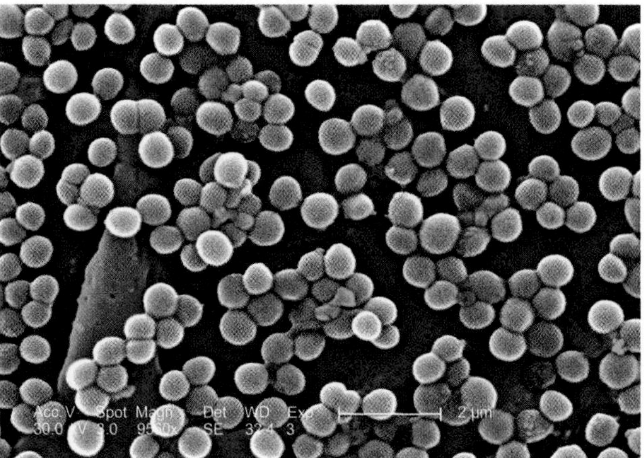

FIGURE 52–6 Electron micrograph depicting numerous grapelike clusters of *Staphylococcus aureus*.

S pneumoniae is the most common cause of bacterial meningitis in children and adults. It spreads to the bloodstream from the site of original infection.

A heptavalent pneumococcal conjugate vaccine (PCV-7) is recommended for all children aged 2 to 23 months and for at-risk children aged 24 to 59 months. Immunization with the PCV is suggested for those at highest risk of infection, including those 65 years or older.

Staphylococcus aureus

Staphylococcus aureus is a spherical Gram-positive coccus, a facultative anaerobe bacterium that appears as grapelike clusters under the microscope (**Figure 52–6**). It forms round, golden (*aureus* in Latin) colonies when grown on blood agar. *S aureus* is primarily coagulase positive; therefore, it causes clot formation. Some strains of *S aureus* carry the Panton-Valentine leukocidin (PVL) toxin, which is responsible for increased virulence and resistance to antibiotics. This toxin is associated with severe necrotizing pneumonia in children. Nearly 25% to 30% of otherwise healthy people carry *S aureus* on the skin or in the nose. *S aureus* can cause a range of

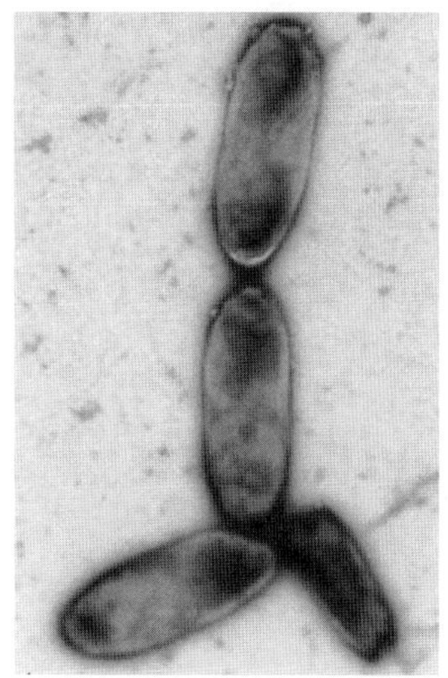

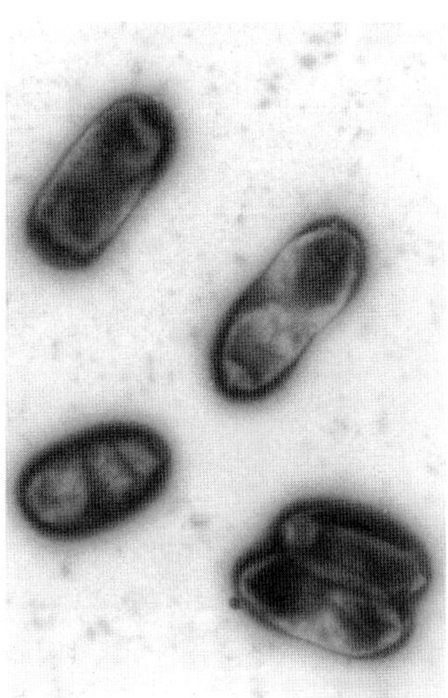

FIGURE 52–7 Electron micrographs of *Haemophilus influenzae*.

illnesses, from minor skin infections to life-threatening diseases such as pneumonia, meningitis, osteomyelitis, endocarditis, toxic shock syndrome (TSS), and septicemia. It is one of the four most common causes of nosocomial infections and is responsible for most postsurgical wound infections.

Nosocomial and healthcare-associated *S aureus* bacteremia are more likely to be caused by methicillin-resistant *Staphylococcus aureus* (MRSA). MRSA is a strain of *S aureus* resistant to a large group of antibiotics called the β-lactams, which include the penicillins and the cephalosporins. Patients with open wounds, invasive devices, and weakened immune systems are at greater risk for infection by MRSA than the general public. Patients with community-associated MRSA (CA-MRSA) pneumonia may require hospitalization or admission to the intensive care unit (ICU). MRSA is easily transferred from patient to patient if hospital isolation protocols are not rigorously followed. Either linezolid or vancomycin can be used for the treatment of MRSA pneumonia.[6]

Haemophilus influenzae

Haemophilus influenzae is a nonmotile, Gram-negative coccobacillus with two defined strains: encapsulated and nonencapsulated (**Figure 52–7**). There are six types of *H. influenzae:* a, b, c, d, e, and f. The encapsulated type b (Hib) is seen in conditions such as epiglottitis. Similar to *S aureus*, the capsule makes *H influenzae* resistant to phagocytosis. Most strains of *H influenzae* are opportunistic bacteria. Since 1990, the routine use of the Hib conjugate vaccine has dramatically reduced the rate of severe meningitis and pneumonia in young children. Non–b type *H influenzae* cause otitis media, sinusitis, conjunctivitis, and pneumonia. Ampicillin has been the drug of choice for strains that do not produce β-lactamase, whereas a third-generation cephalosporin is used for strains that do.

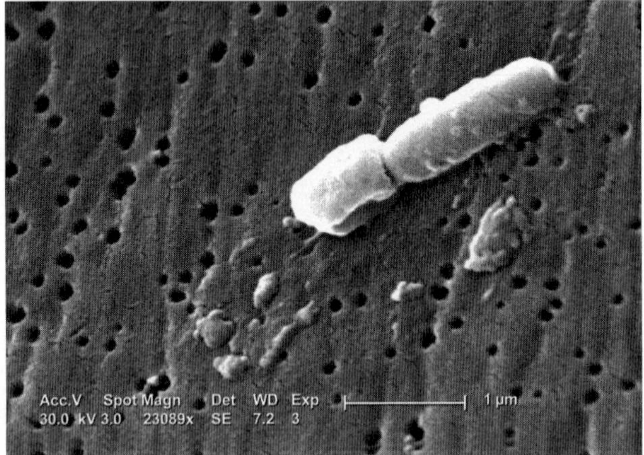

FIGURE 52–8 Electron micrograph of *Klebsiella pneumoniae.*

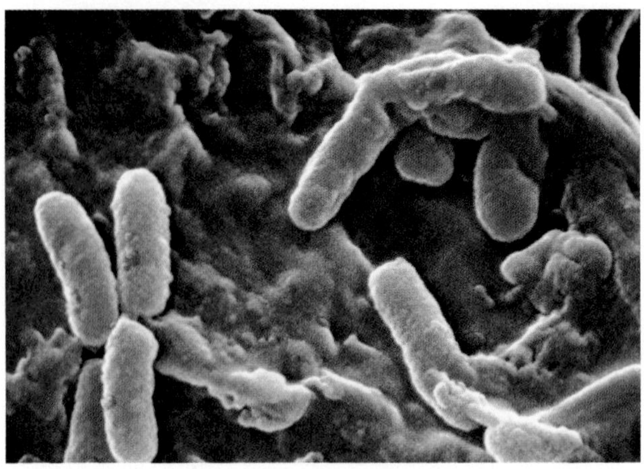

FIGURE 52–9 Electron micrograph of *Pseudomonas aeruginosa.*

Klebsiella pneumoniae

Klebsiella pneumoniae is a Gram-negative, nonmotile, encapsulated, facultative anaerobic bacillus (**Figure 52–8**). It causes some of the most common Gram-negative infections seen worldwide. *K pneumoniae* is commonly associated with hospital-acquired urinary tract and wound infections, particularly in immunocompromised and malnourished individuals. It causes bacterial pneumonia, typically as a result of aspiration in alcoholics, and is a common opportunistic pathogen for patients with chronic obstructive pulmonary disease (COPD) and diabetes. Pneumonia caused by *K pneumoniae* is associated with necrotic, inflammatory, and hemorrhagic changes in the lung parenchyma that produce the characteristic "red-currant jelly" sputum.

K pneumoniae contains a β-lactamase that confers a resistance to ampicillin. Although *Klebsiella* bacteria remain largely susceptible to aminoglycosides and cephalosporins, the emergence of infections due to multidrug-resistant Gram-negative pathogens in the ICU has resulted in a more frequent use of colistin.

Pseudomonas aeruginosa

Pseudomonas aeruginosa is a Gram-negative aerobic bacillus (**Figure 52–9**). It is considered an opportunistic human pathogen that typically causes infection of the respiratory tract, urinary tract, burns, and wounds, as well as causing other blood infections. It is the most common cause of infections in burned patients and the most common pathogen found in invasive medical devices such as catheters. *P aeruginosa* can cause community-acquired pneumonia, healthcare-associated pneumonia, and ventilator-associated pneumonias. Patients with cystic fibrosis are frequently predisposed to respiratory infections caused by *P aeruginosa.*

Laboratory sensitivity studies rather than empiric antibiotic therapy should guide treatment of *P aeruginosa* infections. Some of the antibiotics considered active against *P aeruginosa* are aminoglycosides (gentamicin, amikacin, and tobramycin) or quinolones (ciprofloxacin and levofloxacin but *not* moxifloxacin) in combination with cephalosporins (ceftazidime and cefepime but *not* cefuroxime, ceftriaxone, or cefotaxime); ureidopenicillins (piperacillin or ticarcillin; *P aeruginosa* is intrinsically resistant to all other penicillins); carbapenems (meropenem, imipenem, and doripenem but *not* ertapenem); polymyxins (polymyxin B and colistin); and monobactams (aztreonam).

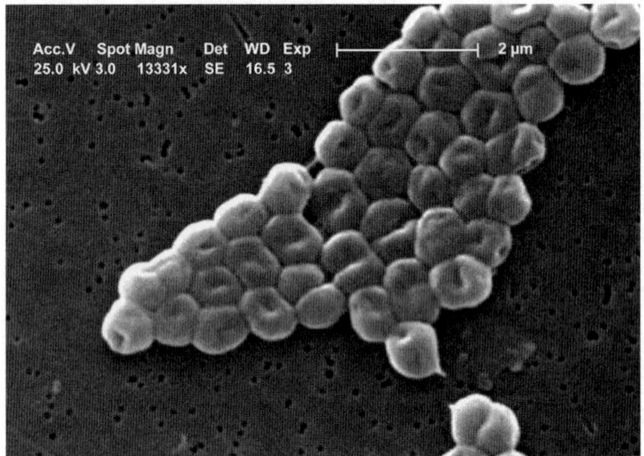

FIGURE 52–10 Electron micrograph of a highly magnified cluster of Gram-negative, nonmotile *Acinetobacter baumannii* bacteria.

Acinetobacter baumannii

Acinetobacter baumannii is a Gram-negative aerobic bacillus similar in appearance to *H influenzae* on the Gram stain (**Figure 52–10**). *A baumannii* is associated with opportunistic infections and enters the body through catheters, endotracheal tubes, and open wounds. It has emerged as a very important pathogen among wounded soldiers. *A baumannii* commonly colonizes irrigation solutions and intravenous fluids. Healthcare workers can become carriers of *Acinetobacter* and be responsible for hospital-acquired infections. Prolonged hospitalization

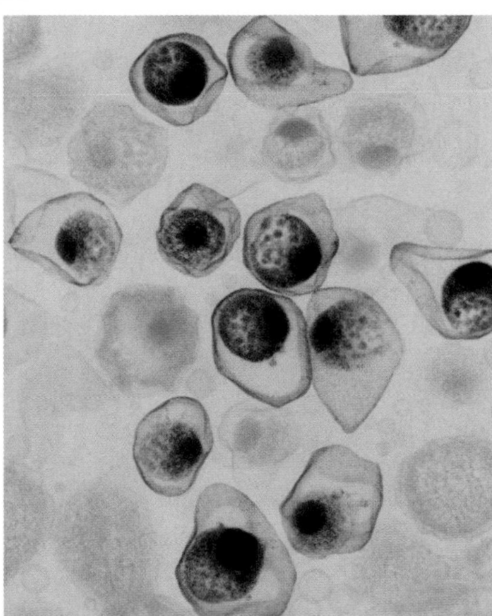

FIGURE 52–11 Electron micrograph of chlamydial particles (pear-shaped cells) of *Chlamydophila pneumoniae.*

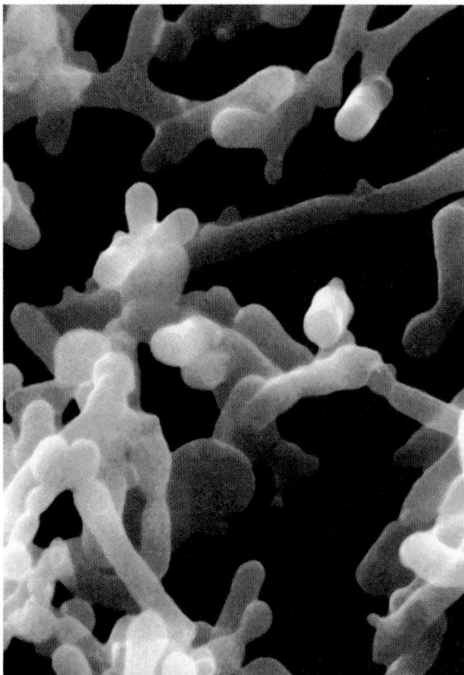

FIGURE 52–12 Electron micrograph showing *Mycoplasma pneumoniae.*

or antibiotic therapy is known to predispose to *Acinetobacter* colonization. *Acinetobacter* pneumonias usually occur as a consequence of colonized respiratory support equipment or fluids. Bacteremia may be associated with mortality rates as high as 75%. *A baumannii* is a multiresistant bacillus sensitive to relatively few antibiotics. Multidrug-resistant strains are frequently treated with imipenem and polymyxins.[7–9]

Chlamydophila pneumoniae

Chlamydophila (formerly *Chlamydia*) *pneumoniae, Mycoplasma pneumoniae,* and *Legionella pneumophila* are known as atypical bacteria because they do not appear in standard culture and staining techniques. *C pneumoniae* is an obligate intracellular Gram-negative bacterium that belongs to the genus *Chlamydia* (**Figure 52–11**). *C pneumoniae* is an airborne organism. Chlamydiae commonly cause pharyngitis, bronchitis, and atypical pneumonia. There is increasing evidence to support an association between atypical bacterial infection—particularly with *C pneumoniae* and *M pneumoniae*—and stable asthma and asthma exacerbations.[10] The clinical presentation of *C pneumoniae* infection is indistinguishable from other causes of pneumonia and includes dry cough, fever, and dyspnea. Several medications have been used to treat patients with *C pneumoniae* infection, including tetracyclines, macrolides, and fluoroquinolones.

Mycoplasma pneumoniae

Mycoplasma bacteria are the smallest free-living organisms, with diameters as small as 0.3 μm, similar to large viruses (**Figure 52–12**). These bacteria lack a cell wall.[11] Without a cell wall, they are unaffected by many common antibiotics such as penicillin or other β-lactam antibiotics that target cell wall synthesis. Several species are pathogenic in humans, including *Mycoplasma pneumoniae,* which is the most common cause of atypical pneumonia and among the most common causes of pneumonia in children and young adults. *M pneumoniae* is spread through respiratory droplet transmission, causing pharyngitis, bronchitis, and pneumonia. The atypical pneumonia caused by *M pneumoniae* is characterized by its relatively slow progression of symptoms, lack of sputum production, and a positive blood test for cold hemagglutinins in 50% to 70% of patients after 10 days of infection. The most sensitive and rapid test to diagnose *M pneumoniae* infection in children is a combination of oropharyngeal polymerase chain reaction (PCR) and IgM enzyme immunoassay.[12,13] Second-generation macrolide antibiotics, doxycycline, and fluoroquinolones are effective antimicrobials against infections caused by *Mycoplasma* species.

Legionella pneumophila

Legionella pneumophila is a flagellated, noncapsulated, aerobic Gram-negative bacillus that produces β-lactamase (**Figure 52–13**). *L pneumophila* is the etiologic agent of legionellosis or Legionnaire disease. *Legionella* is transmitted via inhalation of mist droplets containing the bacteria. *Legionella* earned its name after an outbreak of illness among people at a convention of the American Legion in Philadelphia in 1976. Legionnaire disease is a form of pneumonia that often goes undiagnosed and is difficult to distinguish from other

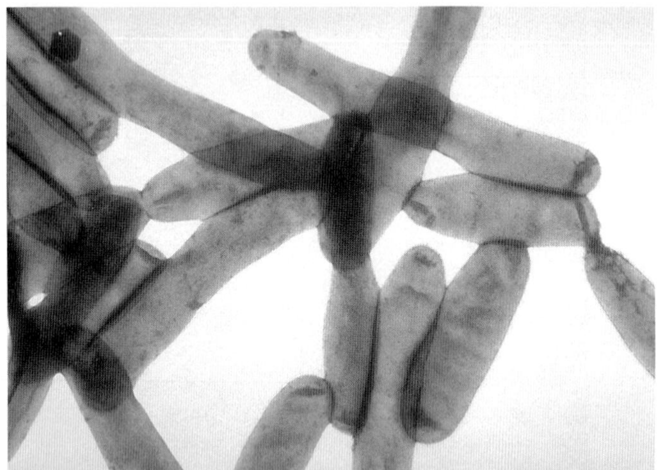

FIGURE 52–13 Electron micrograph of *Legionella pneumophila.*

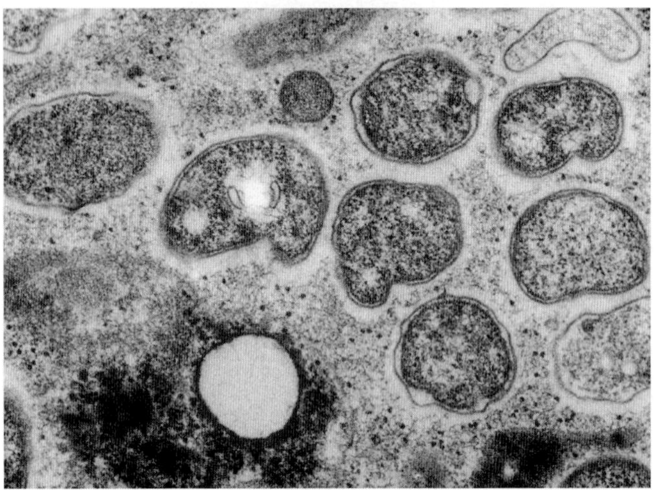

FIGURE 52–14 Electron micrograph of *Rickettsiae prowazeki* inside host cells.

types of pneumonia. It is typically not harmful except in elderly individuals or those with an immunocompromised system. On the other hand, hospital-acquired *Legionella* pneumonia carries a mortality rate as high as 28%. Current therapy for Legionnaire disease includes quinolones and newer macrolides such as azithromycin, clarithromycin, and roxithromycin.[14]

Rickettsiae

Like chlamydiae, rickettsiae are small bacteria that are obligate intracellular organisms. Rickettsiae are maintained within a mammalian reservoir (humans in the case of *Rickettsia prowazekii*). However, rickettsiae are transmitted to humans indirectly, through the bite of specific arthropods (lice, mites, fleas, or ticks) that have previously encountered an infected mammal (**Figure 52–14**). The agent causing Q fever, originally named *Rickettsia burnetii* but recently renamed *Coxiella burnetii,* is an exception to this pattern; *C burnetii* is spread by aerosol emitted directly from cats, dogs, sheep, cattle, and goats. Aerosolization from the surface of the placenta is particularly

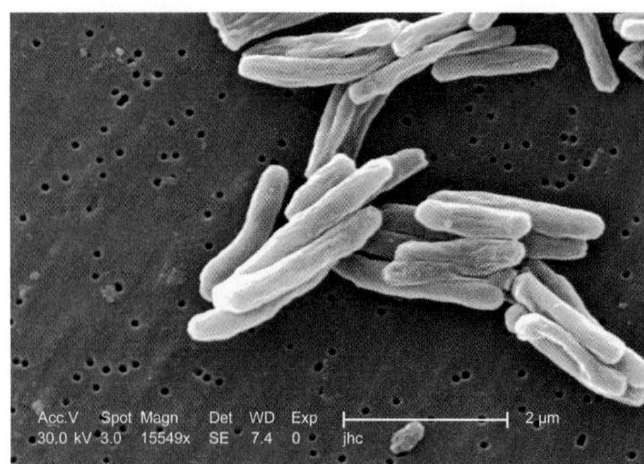

FIGURE 52–15 Electron micrograph depicting numerous clusters of *Mycobacterium tuberculosis.*

effective, so attendance at an animal birth is a risk factor for infection.

Rickettsial diseases manifest as fever, severe headache, and influenza symptoms. Rickettsial diseases with important pulmonary manifestations include Q fever (*C burnetii*), epidemic typhus (*R prowazekii*), endemic typhus (*Rickettsia typhi*), and scrub typhus (*Rickettsia tsutsugamushi*). Cell culture is possible but not commonly used. Diagnosis is based on serology, that is, the detection of a specific antibody response to the organism. Serology may not show positive results for up to 2 weeks after infection. The majority of *Rickettsia* bacteria are susceptible to antibiotics of the tetracycline group.

Mycobacteria

Mycobacteria are rod-shaped bacteria distinguished by an unusual staining pattern in response to the Ziehl-Nielsen stain. Because mycobacteria's cell walls retain red carbolfuchsin stain despite rinsing with hydrochloric acid, they are called **acid-fast bacilli (AFB)**. The cell wall is neither truly Gram negative nor positive, and it is resistant to a number of antibiotics, such as penicillin, that work by destroying bacterial cell walls.[11]

Mycobacterium tuberculosis (MTB) causes most cases of tuberculosis (**Figure 52–15**). Nontuberculous mycobacteria (NTM) are a large group of mycobacteria that includes *Mycobacterium avium-intracellulare* (MAI) and *Mycobacterium intracellulare*—together called *Mycobacterium avium* complex (MAC)—*Mycobacterium gordonae, Mycobacterium kansasii, Mycobacterium fortuitum, Mycobacterium chelonae, and Mycobacterium abscessus*; the last three are also known as rapid growers. Mycobacteria causing primarily nonpulmonary disease include *Mycobacterium marinum, Mycobacterium leprae, Mycobacterium bovis* (used to produce bacille Calmette-Guérin [BCG] vaccine for tuberculosis), and *Mycobacterium scrofulaceum.*[15] Mycobacteria are slow-growing obligate aerobes that cause a slowly progressive, wasting disease over months to years.

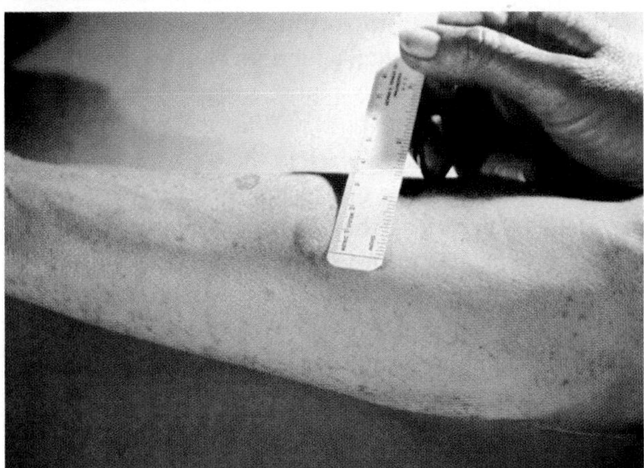

FIGURE 52–16 A 48-hour purified protein derivative (Mantoux or tuberculin) test being measured.

Tuberculosis (TB) is spread through the air when people who have the disease cough, sneeze, or spit. One-third of the world's population has been infected with *M tuberculosis*; however, most of these infections remain asymptomatic or latent. New infections occur at a rate of one per second.[16] The typical symptoms of tuberculosis include fever, night sweats, chronic cough with blood-tinged sputum, and weight loss. Chest radiography, the tuberculin skin test, blood tests, and microscopic examination and microbiological culture of bodily fluids are the most commonly used diagnostic tools. Immunofluorescence has largely replaced actual acid-fast staining for AFB. This technique uses antibodies that bind specifically to mycobacteria and are joined to a molecule that fluoresces under ultraviolet light. The presence of fluorescence is evaluated microscopically. Like staining, this technique is limited by the very small numbers of organisms present in most cases of active disease. Therefore these techniques, although rapid, are insensitive. Additionally, neither test distinguishes MTB from other species of mycobacteria. Mycobacterial culture remains essential to reliably detect the presence of mycobacteria, identify the species, and determine the pattern of susceptibility to antibiotics. The major drawback to mycobacterial culture is the slow growth rate of mycobacteria; even with newer, rapid-growth techniques, results may take longer than 1 week.

Placement of **purified protein derivative (PPD)** subcutaneously, called the **Mantoux test** or tuberculin skin test, detects the presence of an immune response to mycobacteria by eliciting a delayed-type hypersensitivity response. This response manifests as induration of the injection site within 72 hours (**Figure 52–16**).[17] A positive test is defined as an induration of 5 to 15 mm in diameter, depending on the population group (**Table 52–3**), representing exposure to mycobacteria at some time in the past, but not necessarily infection. Once converted to a positive PPD status, most patients remain positive indefinitely.

TABLE 52–3 Criteria for Purified Protein Derivative (PPD) Test Positivity

Threshold for Positive Test (Diameter of Induration at 48 to 72 Hours)	Group
5 mm	Recent TB exposure, chest radiograph suggestive of TB, immunocompromised because of disease (e.g., HIV infection) or drugs (e.g., corticosteroids)
10 mm	High-prevalence groups: born in a country with high prevalence of TB; poor access to healthcare; persons who live or spend time in certain facilities (e.g., nursing homes, prisons, shelters); persons who inject drugs High-risk groups: children younger than 4 years; close contact with infectious TB; chest radiograph suggestive of old TB; PPD conversion to positive in the past 2 years; certain medical conditions (diabetes, silicosis, prolonged therapy with corticosteroids, immunosuppressive therapy, leukemia, Hodgkin disease, head and neck cancers, severe kidney disease, malnutrition)
15 mm	General population

TB, tuberculosis; HIV, human immunodeficiency virus.

Some patients fail to demonstrate an immune response even after exposure and are termed *anergic*. The BCG vaccine rarely produces an induration greater than 15 mm into adulthood, so Mantoux tests can be useful in this population and should be read as if no prior BCG vaccination had been applied. However, the Mantoux test should not be applied to patients who have received BCG vaccine recently or to patients known to be PPD positive, because a vigorous immune response may produce tissue damage at the test site.[18] A positive Mantoux test may be produced by exposure to any *Mycobacterium* species.

In the past few years, drug-resistant strains of MTB leading to multidrug-resistant TB (MDR-TB) and extensively drug-resistant TB (XDR-TB) have emerged, carrying a high mortality, especially in developing countries. Drug-resistant tuberculosis is transmitted in the same way as regular TB. Multidrug-resistant TB is typically resistant to at least two first-line drugs (isoniazid [INH] and rifampin [RFP]) used to treat all persons with TB. Extensively drug-resistant TB is a relatively rare disease defined as TB resistant to INH and RFP plus resistant to any fluoroquinolone and at least one of three injectable second-line drugs (i.e., amikacin, kanamycin, or capreomycin).[19] Healthcare providers can help prevent

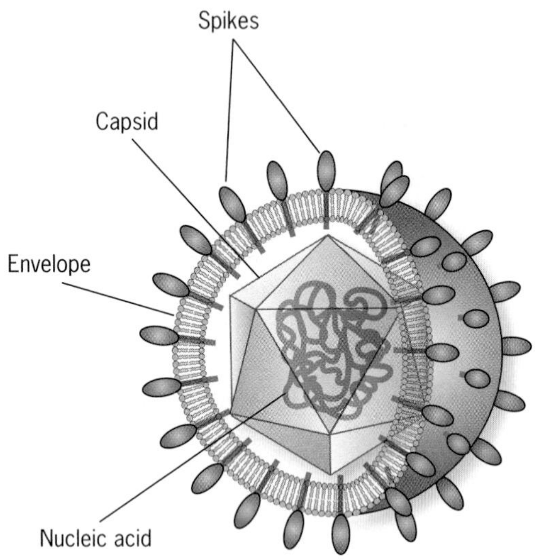

FIGURE 52–17 Diagrammatic view of a virus depicting its parts. Adapted from Kaiser GE. Viruses. In: *Microbiology Lecture Guide*. Community College of Baltimore County, Catonsville Campus; 2006.

MDR-TB by quickly diagnosing cases, following recommended treatment guidelines, monitoring patients' response to treatment, and making sure therapy is completed. Healthcare providers should avoid exposure to patients who have TB in closed or crowded places and should consult infection control or occupational health experts to determine environmental procedures for preventing exposure to TB. A DNA-based test known as nucleic acid amplification (NAA) that can quickly diagnose drug-resistant forms of tuberculosis eliminates the several weeks it typically takes to detect TB and MDR-TB, cutting the time down to 4 to 7 hours.[20] This test looks at the genetic sequence of the organism to identify mutations in the genome of MDR-TB.[21] The Centers for Disease Control and Prevention (CDC) has published updated guidelines for the use of NAA in the diagnosis of tuberculosis.

Viruses

With the exception of prions, **viruses** are the smallest and simplest class of pathogens. They are about 100 times smaller than bacteria, ranging in size from 0.02 to 0.3 μm. Viruses consist of genetic material, either RNA or DNA, surrounded by a protein coat called a *capsid*. Some viruses also are surrounded by a lipoprotein membrane called an *envelope* (**Figure 52–17**).

Viruses are infectious agents that are unable to grow or reproduce outside a host cell. After gaining entry into a host, viruses attach themselves selectively to certain host cells; for example, rhinovirus infects the upper airway mucosa, whereas human immunodeficiency virus (HIV) has a predilection for CD4+ lymphocytes. This specificity is imparted by different proteins embedded in the outer surface of the capsid or, in enveloped viruses, by glycoproteins embedded in the envelope. These proteins or glycoproteins bind to specific cell surface receptors, and the virus then is taken up into the host cell and sheds its capsid or envelope to expose its genetic material, a process known as *uncoating*. Whereas replication of most DNA viruses takes place in the cell's nucleus, RNA viruses replicate in the cytoplasm. A reverse transcribing virus is any virus that forms DNA from an RNA template. The Baltimore classification places viruses into one of seven groups depending on a combination of their nucleic acid (DNA or RNA), strandedness (single stranded or double stranded), genome type, and method of replication.

Viruses themselves are metabolically inactive, but once inside a cell they use the host cell metabolism to replicate. The mechanism of viral replication varies, depending on the type of virus, but its goal is always to produce messenger RNA (mRNA), from which viral proteins are translated by the host cell. Most positive-polarity RNA viruses simply use their genome directly as mRNA, whereas negative-polarity RNA viruses carry their own RNA-dependent RNA polymerase to transcribe their genome into positive-polarity mRNA. Some RNA viruses—the retroviruses, of which the best known is HIV—first transcribe their RNA into DNA (**Figure 52–18**).

Because eukaryotic cells lack the reverse transcriptase necessary for DNA production from RNA, the retroviruses must carry a copy of their own reverse transcriptase. The resulting viral DNA then is transcribed by the host cell's RNA polymerase to produce mRNA. The genome of DNA viruses is transcribed directly into mRNA by the host cell RNA polymerase. Regardless of the mechanism used, the host cell eventually fills with newly synthesized virions—sometimes clustered together as a recognizable inclusion body—and then ruptures, releasing the virus into the environment.

It is believed that viruses produce clinical disease by causing host cell rupture and death; by causing host cell dysfunction, including fusion with other cells to produce multinucleate giant cells; by malignant transformation; and by stimulating the body's cellular host defenses against infection. Although local disease is mediated by cell dysfunction and death, the final mechanism (stimulation of cellular host defenses) is responsible for many systemic symptoms associated with viral infection, including fever, malaise, loss of appetite, and increased mucus production. Because viruses use the host cell to reproduce and then reside within them, they are difficult to eliminate without killing the host cell. Despite their limitations, vaccinations and antiviral drugs continue to be the most effective therapies against viral infections.[22]

Because a large number of virus species exist, they are usually considered in groups; **Table 52–4** lists some of the more important viral respiratory pathogens. Respiratory syncytial virus (RSV), rhinovirus, influenza virus, and the severe acute respiratory sydrome–associated coronavirus (SARS-CoV) cause respiratory infections

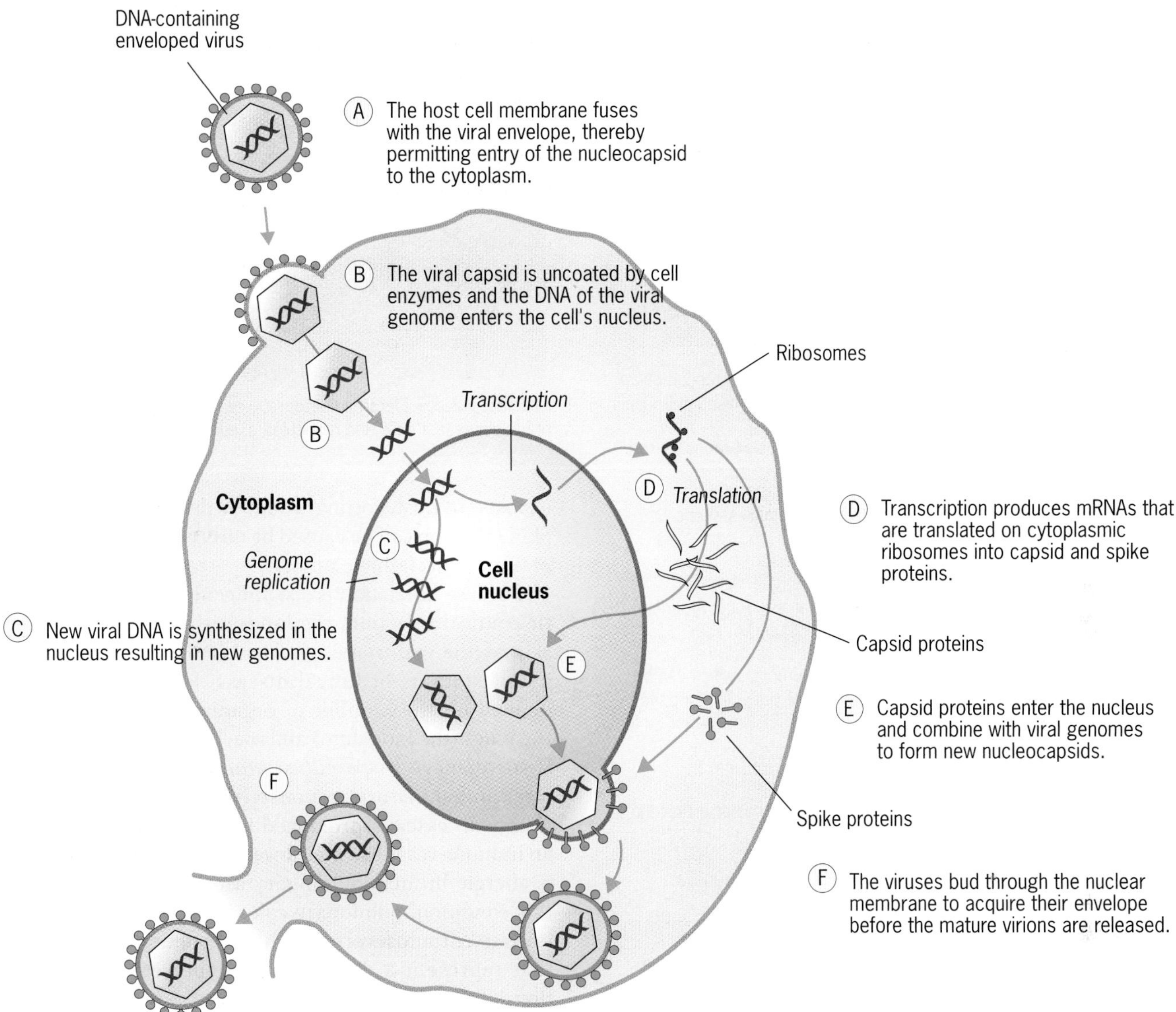

DNA-containing enveloped virus
A The host cell membrane fuses with the viral envelope, thereby permitting entry of the nucleocapsid to the cytoplasm.
B The viral capsid is uncoated by cell enzymes and the DNA of the viral genome enters the cell's nucleus.
Ribosomes
Transcription
B
Cytoplasm
D Translation
D Transcription produces mRNAs that are translated on cytoplasmic ribosomes into capsid and spike proteins.
C
Genome replication
Cell nucleus
C New viral DNA is synthesized in the nucleus resulting in new genomes.
Capsid proteins
E
E Capsid proteins enter the nucleus and combine with viral genomes to form new nucleocapsids.
F
Spike proteins
F The viruses bud through the nuclear membrane to acquire their envelope before the mature virions are released.

FIGURE 52–18 Process of viral replication from viral attachment to the cell to release of viral particles to infect the other cells.

that affect the practice of respiratory care around the world due to their widespread epidemiologic and clinical impact. RSV is the most common cause of bronchiolitis and pneumonia in children younger than 1 year.[23] A very contagious disease, RSV infection is spread as a result of direct or indirect contact with nasal or oral secretions from infected persons. There seems to be an association between asthma diagnosed at early school age and severe viral infections caused by RSV and group C human rhinoviruses.[24–26]

Influenza virus is responsible for seasonal flu epidemics that result in the deaths of hundreds of thousands annually. In severe cases, influenza causes life-threatening pneumonia, particularly in young children and the elderly. The highly recommended trivalent influenza vaccine contains material from two influenza A virus subtypes and one influenza B virus subtype.[27] The CDC has identified several subtypes of influenza A and B virus resistant to neuraminidase inhibitors (oseltamivir and zanamivir).[28,29]

Severe acute respiratory syndrome (SARS) is a respiratory disease caused by the SARS-CoV that reached almost a pandemic state between late 2002 and early 2003, when the infection spread over 37 countries around the world with a mortality rate of nearly 10%.[30] Other than isolation and supportive measures, no therapy has been found to be effective against SARS-CoV infection. Although it is considered a rare viral infection today, its legacy has been much stricter infection control policies to protect the public, healthcare workers, and patients around the world.

Fungi

Fungi differ from the other organisms in that they are eukaryotic and thus share many features with human cells. This homology makes difficult the development of antifungal therapy that is nontoxic to humans. Fungal structure differs in the following two important ways

TABLE 52-4 Viruses Important in Human Respiratory Disease

Virus	Resulting Disease
Rhinoviruses, adenoviruses, coronaviruses	Common cold
Herpes simplex virus (HSV)	Herpetic skin lesions; infection of the lungs and brain, causing pneumonia and encephalitis (e.g., in immunocompromised individuals)
Varicella-zoster virus (VZV)	Chickenpox and shingles, both of which may involve the lung and central nervous system
Cytomegalovirus (CMV)	Systemic infection, including pneumonia, usually in immunocompromised individuals
Epstein-Barr virus (EBV)	Infectious mononucleosis ("mono")—rare in lungs
Retroviruses (including HIV)	Diverse respiratory manifestations resulting from HIV
Flaviviruses (including yellow fever and dengue viruses)	Yellow fever and dengue, diseases common in Central and South America—rare involvement of lungs
Orthomyxoviruses	Influenza (flu); pneumonia, which can be fatal, particularly for the young and the elderly
Paramyxoviruses	Measles, mumps, parainfluenza
Respiratory syncytial virus (RSV)	Bronchiolitis in infants; milder disease in children and adults
Togaviruses	Diverse illnesses, including rubella
Hantavirus	Hantavirus pulmonary syndrome (HPS) from rodents
SARS-CoV	Severe acute respiratory syndrome (SARS)

HIV, human immunodeficiency virus; SARS-CoV, severe acute respiratory syndrome–associated coronavirus.

from human cells: (1) the fungal cell membrane contains ergosterol and zymosterol instead of cholesterol, and (2) fungi have a rigid cell wall composed of chitin (unlike the peptidoglycan cell wall of bacteria). Fungi occur in two forms. The majority of species grow as multicellular filaments called *hyphae,* forming a mycelium; some fungal species also grow as single cells or yeasts (**Figure 52–19**). Although individual yeasts are approximately 4 µm each, mycelia can be quite large, covering up to 1500 acres, and are claimed to be the world's largest organisms.[31] Some fungi are dimorphic, existing as molds in soil but forming yeasts at human body temperatures. All fungi reproduce by spore formation, which may occur either sexually or asexually, depending on the species.

With the exception of *Candida,* which is part of the normal human flora, fungi are found naturally in soil, bird feces, and other decaying material. Therefore, they often produce disease after an individual has been

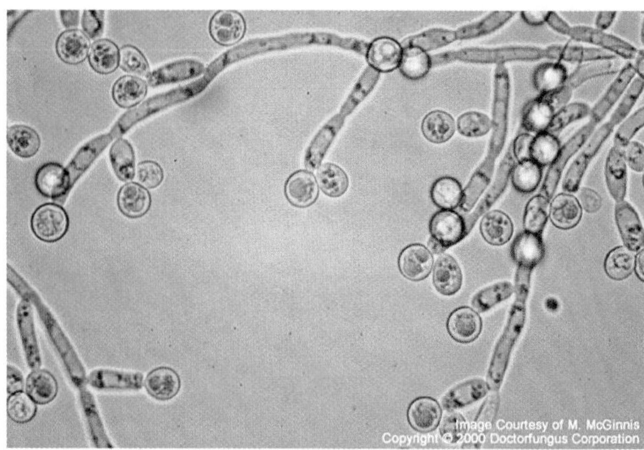

FIGURE 52–19 Electron micrograph of *Candida* showing clusters of budding yeast cells and branching pseudohyphae.

exposed to dust, rotting wood, or dried bird droppings. Skin infection can be caused by direct contact, as in cases of tinea pedis (athlete's foot).

Because inhalation is a significant route for transmitting fungal infection, the lungs are second only to the skin as the major site of fungal infection. The clinical manifestations of fungal disease, known as mycosis, depend on the number of organisms introduced into the lungs (the inoculum) and mechanisms such as direct tissue damage (*Aspergillus, Mucor,* and *Rhizopus* species), inflammatory response (*Candida albicans*), and allergy. In cases of prolonged infection or colonization, an immune response may develop. An excellent example is allergic bronchopulmonary aspergillosis (ABPA). In this condition, pulmonary colonization with aspergillus leads to chronic fevers, cough, and pulmonary infiltrates that represent a delayed-type hypersensitivity reaction (allergy) and not a direct effect of the aspergillus. Because the aspergillus cannot be eradicated, treatment requires immune suppression such as steroids and itraconazole. **Table 52–5** lists important fungal respiratory pathogens in normal hosts, whereas **Table 52–6** lists mycoses known as *opportunistic* because they generally occur in response to lowered host immune activity.

Fungi may be cultured by special techniques but grow more slowly than bacteria. Diagnosis can be made either by cytology or microscopic observation after treatment with potassium hydroxide (KOH), which dissolves most tissue but leaves the chitinous fungal wall intact. Serology is often useful, but its utility is limited in endemic areas, where the majority of healthy individuals may be seropositive. Latex agglutination is frequently used as a rapid detection test for cryptococci in cerebrospinal fluid.

Pneumocystis jiroveci

Pneumocystis jiroveci was previously known as and is still often referred to as *Pneumocystis carinii.* Little was known about *Pneumocystis jiroveci* before the era of the acquired immunodeficiency syndrome (AIDS), and it

TABLE 52–5 Important Fungal Respiratory Pathogens in Normal Hosts

Organism	Disease	Comments
Coccidioides immitis, Coccidioides posadii	Coccidioidomycosis	Commonly found in the arid regions of the southwest United States (Arizona, central California, and Texas). It causes "valley fever," bilateral pneumonia, and may later form thin-walled pulmonary cavities.
Histoplasma capsulatum	Histoplasmosis	Commonly found along the Mississippi and Ohio River valleys. A high, inhaled *Histoplasma* inoculum may cause acute fever and pneumonia. Some patients develop disseminated infection, often causing skin lesions. In rare cases, fibrosis of the mediastinum may result. Most residents of endemic areas have had asymptomatic infection, causing elevated antibody titers, and often one or more calcified granulomas are visible on chest radiographs.
Blastomyces dermatitidis	Blastomycosis	Commonly found in the central United States. The disease varies from mild fever and pulmonary infiltrates to severe illness, nodular pulmonary infiltrates, and dissemination.
Paracoccidioides brasiliensis	Paracoccidioidomycosis	Occurring in Central America, this clinical disease is similar to mild coccidioidomycosis.

TABLE 52–6 Opportunistic Fungal Respiratory Pathogens

Organism	Disease	Comments
Candida albicans	Candidiasis (thrush, esophagitis, intertrigo)	Organism is commonly found in infants and the elderly and also in HIV-infected and critically ill patients. Thrush also may be precipitated by inhaled steroid deposition in the mouth. True candidal pneumonia is rare.
Aspergillus species	Aspergillosis	Disease causes otitis externa in normal hosts; may infect skin, sinuses, or lung of immunocompromised individuals and can disseminate, with extremely high mortality. Preexisting lung cavities from tuberculosis or emphysema are particularly prone to infection, with formation of a "fungus ball" inside.
Cryptococcus neoformans	Cryptococcosis	Organism is found in kitten feces and causes pneumonia and meningitis.
Mucor and *Rhizopus* species	Mucormycosis	Organism can infect the sinuses, lungs, or gut, forming a black eschar. Treatment is difficult, often requiring surgical debridement.

HIV, human immunodeficiency virus.

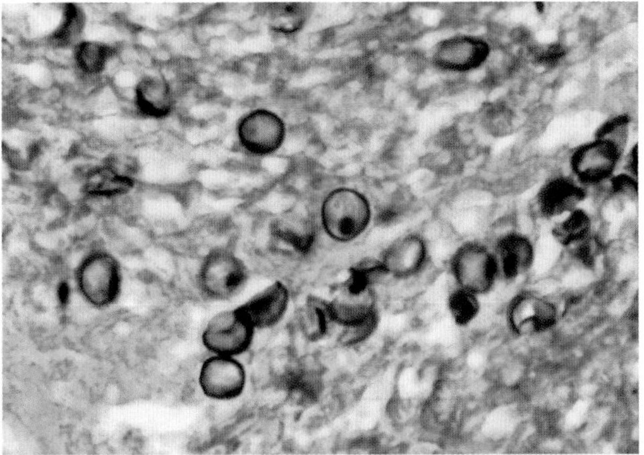

FIGURE 52–20 Methenamine silver stain showing cysts of *Pneumocystis jiroveci* in AIDS.

has only recently been classified as a fungus, based on genetic studies. *P jiroveci* is dimorphic, existing as trophozoites and cysts (**Figure 52–20**).

Pneumocystis carinii pneumonia (PCP) was a common opportunistic infection during the first decade of AIDS and remains an important complication, although its incidence has dropped since the institution of trimethoprim-sulfamethoxazole (TMP-SMX) or aerosolized pentamidine prophylactic therapy. PCP caused by *P jiroveci* is common among people with weakened immune systems, such as patients on medium- to high-dose long-term corticosteroids, those receiving transplants, premature or severely malnourished children, the elderly, and especially AIDS patients, in whom it is most commonly observed today.[32] The risk of PCP increases when CD4 levels are less than 200 cells/μl. Symptoms of PCP include fever, nonproductive cough, dyspnea on exertion, night sweats, and weight loss. The disease causes marked thickening of the alveolar septa and alveoli, leading to significant hypoxia. A hallmark of PCP is that the patient's degree of hypoxia often is greater than expected based on the chest radiographic findings. A Pa_{O_2} of less than 70 mm Hg is an indication for systemic corticosteroids, which have significantly reduced mortality.[33] Pathologic identification of the organism in induced sputum or bronchial washings obtained by bronchoscopy via coloration by toluidine blue or immunofluorescence assay will show characteristic cysts. *Pneumocystis* infection can also be diagnosed by immunofluorescent or histochemical staining of the specimen. Molecular analysis of PCR products, comparing DNA samples, is one of the most recent diagnostic tools.

The most commonly used medication is trimethoprim-sulfamethoxazole. Alternative medications include pentamidine, trimetrexate, dapsone, atovaquone, primaquine, and clindamycin. Treatment is usually for a period of about 21 days.

Parasites

A **parasite** is defined as a plant or animal that lives with or on another, deriving benefit from the association but having a detrimental effect on the host. Those that live inside the host are called *endoparasites*, and those that live on the host's surface are called *ectoparasites*. Essentially any pathogen can be considered a parasite by this definition, but in practical usage the term *parasite* is usually limited to protozoa and helminths (worms). Parasites are an important cause of disease in developing countries but are rare pulmonary pathogens in developed countries and thus will be discussed in this chapter only briefly. Examples of pulmonary parasites include *Entamoeba histolytica* (amebiasis), *Paragonimus westermani* (paragonimiass), and *Echinococcus multilocularis/ Echinococcus granulosus* (echinococcosis: hydatid cysts). *Plasmodium falciparum* (malaria) may cause pulmonary manifestations in 3% to 10% of individuals.

The single-celled protozoa usually cause pulmonary disease through abscess formation or stimulation of a vigorous inflammatory response in the lungs. The multicellular helminths frequently produce focal lesions in the lungs—cysts or larvae—and usually are easily visible on chest radiographs. Manifestations are most frequently malaise, fever, cough, and dyspnea. Chest pain may be present, and eosinophilia is a frequent occurrence.

Common Respiratory Infections

Upper Respiratory Tract Infections

Otitis and Sinusitis

The nasopharynx is surrounded by several airspaces in the skull that drain into it via channels. These airspaces include the middle ear, which drains into the posterior nasopharynx via the eustachian tube, along with the frontal, sphenoid, and maxillary sinuses, which drain into the nasopharynx through ostia located above the superior turbinate and under the middle turbinate. In addition, two collections of small air cells are present in the skull: the ethmoid air cells above the nose and the mastoid cells behind the ears. Because the drainage passages to the middle ear and sinuses are vulnerable to obstruction by mucosal swelling, thick secretions, or mechanical obstruction by tubes or nasal polyps, these spaces can become essentially closed spaces, prone to infection. Anatomic differences in the child's eustachian tube predispose it to obstruction, explaining the higher incidence of otitis media in children.

The organisms that cause upper respiratory tract infections (URTIs) may be acquired by inhalation of infected aerosol drops, as with *S pneumoniae* and viruses. However, infection frequently represents an overgrowth of local flora after normal drainage of the airspace is compromised, explaining why sinusitis frequently follows a viral URTI that has caused mucosal edema. The most common organisms causing otitis and sinusitis therefore reflect the normal flora of the nasopharynx to a great extent. In decreasing order of frequency, they are *S pneumoniae, S aureus, H influenzae,* and *Moraxella catarrhalis.*

RESPIRATORY RECAP

Upper Respiratory Pathogens: Viruses

- *Streptococcus pneumoniae*
- *Haemophilus influenzae*
- *Moraxella catarrhalis*

Pharyngitis, Parapharyngeal Abscess, Epiglottitis, and Tracheitis or Tracheobronchitis (Croup)

The trachea and posterior pharynx are also frequent sites of infection. Infections in these regions are primarily acquired via aerosol spread. Examples include group A β-hemolytic streptococci (*S pyogenes*) and *C diphtheriae.* Infection of the pharynx rarely causes respiratory complications, although the thick gray peel of necrotic mucosa generated in cases of diphtheria can cause airway obstruction. Infection of the trachea can be more severe, especially in infants, in whom even minor mucosal swelling can significantly narrow the airway. Croup, the viral tracheobronchitis that causes stridor and brassy cough in infants, can produce respiratory failure in severe cases. Infection and swelling of the epiglottis (acute epiglottitis) can rapidly produce severe airway compromise in young children and represents a true emergency because acute airway obstruction may occur. If the infection spreads to the soft tissues around the pharynx and trachea (parapharyngeal abscess), local swelling can compress the airway. Alternatively, the deep tissue planes of the neck may facilitate the rapid spread of infection down into the mediastinum (Ludwig's angina).

Lower Respiratory Tract Infections

The lungs may become infected by two major routes: aspiration of secretions, and inhalation of infected aerosols. Infection also may be carried to the lung by the bloodstream (hematogenous spread). Up to 98% of the cardiac output flows through the pulmonary capillary bed, which is the first filter encountered by organisms or objects returning to the heart from the body via the venous system of the body. Nevertheless, hematogenous infection is much less common than aspiration or inhalation.

Lower respiratory infections are thought to originate from the person's own flora, which gain access to the lung by aspiration of secretions, usually from the pharynx and upper digestive tract. Organisms from the upper digestive tract find their way to the pharynx via gastroesophageal reflux, which occurs nearly universally in healthy individuals. Once organisms are present in the pharynx, they are readily aspirated into the lower respiratory tract. Up to 45% of healthy individuals aspirate small amounts of secretions (microaspiration).[4] Weakened hospitalized patients, spending long periods of time flat and often with nasogastric tubes traversing the pharynx, experience an even greater incidence of aspiration. Intubated, mechanically ventilated patients are believed to universally aspirate.

RESPIRATORY RECAP

Mechanisms of Infection

- » Overgrowth of normal flora
- » Aspiration of oral and gastric flora
- » Aerosol inhalation
- » Hematogenous spread
- » Direct contact (rare except during instrumentation)

The aspirated organisms generally represent the normal flora, but illness and extensive exposure to antibiotics may modify the flora substantially, as is particularly evident in the increasing role of Gram-negative organisms in healthcare-associated pneumonia.

Risk factors that increase pharyngeal colonization with potentially pathogenic Gram-negative bacteria are as follows: depressed level of consciousness (e.g., alcoholism, coma, hypotension), compromised immune function (e.g., acidosis, alcoholism, azotemia, diabetes mellitus, leukocytosis, leukopenia), anatomic alteration of the respiratory system (e.g., nasogastric or endotracheal tubes, preexisting pulmonary disease), exposure to antibiotics, and extreme age (either very young or very old).

Aerosol spread is another common route of lower respiratory infection. Coughing and sneezing project large quantities of aerosol a surprising distance, but even quiet breathing produces aerosol capable of spreading infection. In the case of fungi, large numbers of organisms may be present in the general environment. Aerosol transmission can occur in the hospital, although isolation of patients with pneumonia is not a common practice. An important exception is tuberculosis, which requires immediate respiratory (aerosol) isolation as soon as a reasonable suspicion of the disease is present.

Direct contact rarely causes pneumonia but is believed to be a common mode by which bacteria are spread between patients and caregivers. These bacteria often include antibiotic-resistant and unusual organisms, such as MRSA and vancomycin-resistant enterococcus (VRE). Once spread to a new individual, these bacteria frequently reside in the nasopharynx, skin, and digestive tract, where they displace normal flora. From these locations, they infect the lower respiratory tract, providing a reason why hand washing is an effective and essential technique used to limit the spread of infectious agents in the healthcare setting. Direct contact does become an important mechanism of infection when instrumentation is introduced into the lower respiratory tract.

BOX 52–1

Etiologic Agents of Community-Acquired, Hospital-Acquired (HAP), Healthcare-Associated (HCAP), Ventilator-Associated (VAP), and Nosocomial Pneumonias

Community-Acquired Pneumonia

- *Streptococcus pneumoniae*
- *Mycoplasma pneumoniae*
- Viruses
- *Chlamydophila pneumoniae*
- *Haemophilus influenzae*
- *Legionella* species
- *Staphylococcus aureus*
- *Mycobacterium tuberculosis*
- Fungi (*Histoplasma, Coccidioides, Blastomyces* species)
- Gram-negative bacilli, nonpseudomonal (*Klebsiella*, enteric species)
- *Pseudomonas* species
- Gram-negative bacilli, nonpseudomonal

Nosocomial (HAP/HCAP/VAP) Pneumonia

- Not multidrug resistant
  - *S pneumoniae*
  - *H influenzae*
  - Gram-negative rods
- Multidrug resistant
  - *S aureus* (MRSA)
  - *P aeruginosa*
  - Extended-spectrum β-lactamases (ESBLs)
  - *Acinetobacter* species

The cause of lower respiratory tract infections (LRTIs) varies with age and setting. Community-acquired pneumonia (CAP) originates outside a healthcare setting and must be distinguished from nosocomial pneumonia and ventilator-associated pneumonia (VAP). Nosocomial pneumonia (defined as pneumonia diagnosed more than 48 hours after hospital admission) is hospital acquired, whereas VAP is a subset of nosocomial pneumonia occurring in patients who are mechanically ventilated for more than 48 hours. **Box 52–1** lists the microorganisms commonly responsible for all types of pneumonia.[34,35] A term recently added to the literature is *healthcare-associated pneumonia* (HCAP), which is caused by the pathogens often seen in nosocomial pneumonia. Risk factors for HCAP are residence in nursing homes or long-term care facilities; recent hospitalization for more than 2 days in the previous 3 months; infusion therapy; hemodialysis; and having contact with family members with MDR pathogens.

Anaerobes are as important in nosocomial pneumonia and VAP as they are in community-acquired pneumonia. Identifying the causative organisms in nosocomial pneumonia—and especially VAP—may be difficult because of the high rate of lower respiratory tract colonization. Pathogen identification is important in order to define susceptibility and determine and quickly initiate the most appropriate antimicrobial therapy.

Sampling Methods

Respiratory therapists are often responsible for obtaining respiratory specimens for different diagnostic studies. Adequate sampling using methods such as bronchoscopy, tracheal aspiration, and nonbronchoscopic bronchoalveolar lavage is critical to the diagnosis and management of respiratory infections.

Sputum Induction

When a patient is unable to produce sputum for analysis, the sample can be obtained as an endotracheal aspirate or after inhalation of nebulized 3% saline. The hypertonic saline increases the tonicity of the fluid layer lining the airways, both drawing fluid into these secretions and stimulating an irritant cough response. In the patient who is able to produce sputum spontaneously, induction does not improve sensitivity. Care must be taken during **sputum induction** in a patient with suspected contagious illness, especially tuberculosis, to prevent transmission of the disease to the respiratory therapist and other healthcare providers. Because some patients may experience severe bronchospasm after a sputum induction, a bronchodilator must be at hand to relieve induced bronchospasm.[36]

Acceptable Sputum Specimens

The collection of sputum specimens from which microbiologic diagnoses can be made is quite difficult, accounting for the low percentage of pneumonias identified by sputum alone (less than half). Three criteria must be met to obtain a useful sputum specimen. First, the specimen must be collected in a sterile container and handled with sterile technique. Second, the specimen must be transported to the laboratory promptly. Some respiratory pathogens are very sensitive to bacterial overgrowth, which may occur if the sputum remains unprocessed for long periods of time. Finally, the sample must be screened to verify that it is in fact sputum from the lower respiratory tract and not saliva, which is accomplished by counting the number of squamous epithelial cells per microscopic low-power field (lpf). Because these cells originate from the oropharynx, a large number of them (>25/lpf) indicates a specimen that is unacceptably contaminated with oral secretions. Sputum with less than 25 squamous epithelial cells and more than 10 polymorphonuclear leukocytes per low-power field is considered a good specimen.

RESPIRATORY RECAP

Acceptable Sputum Specimens

- Less than 25 squamous cells per low power field
- More than 10 polymorphonuclear leukocytes per low power field

Bronchoscopy

Fiberoptic **bronchoscopy** is a powerful technique that enables the collection of many sample types from the lower airways. The working channel is generally contaminated with upper airway secretions, so simple suctioned specimens yield unreliable cultures. This problem has been addressed with the protected specimen brush (PSB), also called the protected brush catheter (PBC). A sterile brush is passed through the working channel into the bronchus. The brush is advanced from the catheter and worked back and forth to collect secretions and cells before it is withdrawn into the protective sheath and retrieved for culture. The reported sensitivity of PSB varies from 47% to 54%, with specificity of 87% to 100%.[37–40]

Another common technique used to diagnose pneumonia is **bronchoalveolar lavage (BAL)**. The bronchoscope is positioned as far distally as possible in the airway leading to the site of interest. Aliquots of 20 to 50 mL of sterile saline, usually on the order of 100 mL, are introduced via the working channel. This saline migrates distally, mixing with secretions, and each aliquot then is suctioned back and collected in a sterile trap. Bronchoalveolar lavage is a sensitive technique and is used to detect organisms that are not reliably isolated from sputum, including nontuberculous mycobacteria, cytomegalovirus, and *Pneumocystis* species, for which sensitivities may be more than 90%, with near-100% specificity. When used to diagnose acute nosocomial pneumonia, BAL has been reported to produce a sensitivity between 55% and 91% and a specificity of between 63% and 100%.[41–48]

Regardless of the technique used for specimen collection, quantitative culture is superior to standard, qualitative culture techniques because of its increased ability to distinguish contaminants from true infection.

Biopsy of the lung parenchyma is useful for diagnosis of pneumonia, especially fungal and granulomatous infections, and is accomplished bronchoscopically by tearing of small pieces of tissue (approximately 1 mm) from the lung parenchyma with small grasping biopsy forceps that are placed through the working channel. For bacterial pneumonia, transbronchial biopsy (TBB) has a reported sensitivity of 57% and specificity of 100%.[49] Because the technique appears to offer little advantage over PSB and BAL and carries a much higher risk of hemorrhage and pneumothorax, TBB is not often used to diagnose acute pneumonia.

Transtracheal Aspiration

Transtracheal aspiration (TTA) is a sputum-collection technique designed to bypass the upper airway, with its potential contaminants. The method begins with a careful skin preparation of the anterior neck, followed by the insertion of a sterile needle directly into the trachea through the cricothyroid membrane. Proper position is ensured by aspiration of air from the needle, and tracheal secretions are aspirated. The obvious disadvantage of this procedure is its invasive nature, which explains why it is no longer used in clinical practice.

Nonbronchoscopic Bronchoalveolar Lavage

Bronchoalveolar lavage can be performed with a blind, nonbronchoscopic technique in mechanically ventilated patients. With this technique a catheter is advanced through the endotracheal tube until resistance is felt in the distal airways of the (usually) right lower lobe, usually at a distance of 50 to 60 cm. Aliquots of sterile saline are instilled and suctioned. In studies in the same patients, the reported sensitivities of nonbronchoscopic BAL (NB-BAL) and traditional bronchoscopic BAL (B-BAL) were 73% and 93%, respectively; specificities were 96% and 100%, respectively.[50] Although B-BAL is superior to NB-BAL, the nonbronchoscopic technique is useful because of its ease of performance and substantially lower cost. It is also a method that can be available at all times without the need of a bronchoscopist. Respiratory therapists can be effectively trained to perform this procedure.

Pleural Fluid Analysis

The presence of significant pleural fluid usually demands sampling and analysis of the fluid to determine its nature, unless a cause is readily apparent. Pleural fluid analysis may address two principal issues. First, the measurement of fluid characteristics, such as cell type, pH, protein, amylase, lactate dehydrogenase, and others, may provide clues to the effusion's cause. For example, demonstration of increased adenosine deaminase in the fluid, a predominance of lymphocytes in the white blood cell differential, and a paucity of mesothelial cells (which make up the pleural surface and are usually found in abundance) all suggest tuberculosis as a potential cause.

A second issue is frequently addressed when a pleural effusion is adjacent to an area of pneumonia. These parapneumonic effusions are at risk for becoming secondarily infected from the pneumonia. When pus is present, this is known as *empyema*. If organisms are cultured from the normally sterile pleural space, this technique usually identifies the cause of the pneumonia. Parapneumonic effusions also tend to be highly proteinaceous, prone to developing loculations and forming peels around the adjacent lung, permanently limiting its expansion. For this reason, parapneumonic effusions are most frequently drained completely at the time of sampling.

Microbiology Techniques

Once a good respiratory specimen is obtained, different diagnostic techniques allow identification of the pathogen. These techniques include cultures and virologic antigen identification.

Sputum Culture

After Gram stains are used on the specimen, the sputum or tracheal aspirate is cultured. A microbiological **culture** is one of the primary methods to diagnose bacterial infection. It is a method in which microorganisms are allowed to reproduce in a predetermined culture media under controlled laboratory conditions. To distinguish contamination from colonization and from active infection, the number of colony-forming units (CFUs) per milliliter is counted from the culture; this is called a *quantitative culture*. Colony-forming units measure viable bacterial cells and therefore the microbiologic load that correlates with the magnitude of the infection. After pathogens are isolated, the in vitro testing of bacterial cultures with antibiotics is performed to determine the bacteria's susceptibility to specific antibiotic therapy. Specimens containing more than 10 epithelial cells per low-power field are considered inappropriate for culture and are rejected. Typically, only one sputum specimen per patient is cultured per day. A preliminary report is given in 24 hours, but the final report takes between 48 and 72 hours.

Respiratory Tract Culture

Evaluation of sputum cultures does not examine for *Legionella pneumoniae*, *Chlamydophila pneumoniae*, or *Mycoplasma pneumoniae*, since these pathogens require specialized testing. Adequate samples for culture, excluding sputum, can be obtained from bronchoalveolar lavage, bronchial wash, lung aspirates, sinus aspirates, and quantitative bronchoalveolar lavage. Specimens from nasal passages may be cultured to determine the presence of MRSA or *Neisseria meningitidis* carrier status. A preliminary report is typically available in 24 hours and the final report in 72 hours.

Virologic Studies

Culture

Respiratory specimens for **virologic studies** such as culture include nasopharyngeal washes or aspirates, sputum, bronchial wash, BAL, and lung tissue. Viruses are grown in cell culture, where they produce recognizable cytopathic changes, a process that can take up to 2 weeks. A rapid shell vial culture technique is used to obtain a diagnosis of cytomegalovirus (CMV) infection within 48 hours and is frequently performed on respiratory secretions and bronchoscopy specimens. Certain viruses, especially CMV and Epstein-Barr virus, produce characteristic microscopically visible inclusion bodies in infected cells. Virus culture tests for the presence of RSV, influenza A and B, adenovirus, and parainfluenza 1, 2, and 3.

Viral Antigen Detection

Detection of the influenza A and B antigen is possible through optical immunoassay of nasal specimens. However, the test should not be part of therapeutic decision making because of the insufficient negative predictive value of the test. A result is available in 30 to 60 minutes. RSV **antigen detection** also requires the use of an optical immunoassay and direct fluorescent antibody. Specimens of choice are nasopharyngeal aspirates and washes.

Antimicrobial Resistance

Antibiotic resistance is the ability of bacteria and fungi to withstand the effects of antibiotics that would normally kill them or limit their growth. The widespread and increased use of antimicrobials in humans, animals, and agriculture has resulted in many microorganisms developing resistance to these powerful drugs. Antibiotic resistance is a growing concern worldwide and has become a major problem, especially in environments that are constantly exposed to antibiotics, such as hospitals, where resistant bacterial strains can become a dominant part of the endogenous flora.

Microorganisms adapt to their environment and change to ensure their survival. Antibiotic resistance is a complex process of adaptation that evolves as the result of mutation, gene transfer, and selective process. With each replication, genetic mutations may help an individual microorganism survive exposure to an antibiotic. Once such a resistant gene is generated, microorganisms can transfer or acquire this new genetic material via plasmid exchange. In the presence of an antibiotic, bacteria are killed unless they carry resistance genes. These survivors then become the dominant type throughout the microbial population. When a microorganism possesses several resistance genes, it is called **multiresistant**, or a *superbug*.

The most important mechanism of resistance to penicillins and cephalosporins is the production of β-lactamases, which digest the β-lactam ring structure of these antibiotics. The most important mechanisms of resistance to aminoglycosides and chloramphenicol are the production of various inactivating enzymes.

The activity of antibiotics may be improved by modification of their targets, which usually involves a change in the chromosomal genes of the microorganism. The second-most-important mechanism of resistance to penicillins and cephalosporins is modification of the penicillin-binding proteins in the bacterial cell membrane to which the drugs attach. Resistance to aminoglycosides, macrolides, sulfonamides, fluoroquinolones, and rifampin is imparted by mutations in the bacterial ribosomes or enzymes that make up the targets of these antibiotics.

Resistance to aminoglycosides, tetracyclines, and isoniazid results from decreased permeability of the cell wall and membrane to the antibiotic, reducing the antibiotic levels inside the bacterium. Antibiotics also may be actively transported from the bacteria by an enzymatic pump, which is usually plasmid encoded. Resistance to tetracyclines and sulfonamides is also accomplished by active transport of the antibiotic from the bacteria.

Gram-negative ventilator-associated pneumonia in critically ill patients is associated with substantial morbidity, longer ICU stays, prolonged mechanical ventilation, and higher mortality. Aerosolized aminoglycosides may play a valuable role as adjunct therapy in selected patients with multidrug-resistant Gram-negative organisms.[51–53]

KEY POINTS

- Respiratory infections are caused most frequently by typical and atypical bacteria and by viruses. Some species of rickettsiae, mycobacteria, and fungi also are commonly encountered.
- Bacteria are classified by three major characteristics: oxygen requirement, Gram staining, and shape.
- Normal flora bacteria are generally present in certain areas of the body but are major causes of respiratory infection when they overgrow in the upper airway or are introduced to the normally near-sterile lower airways.
- The modes of infection and the most common respiratory pathogens vary significantly, depending on an individual's age and setting.
- Among normal adults the major pathogens of upper airway infection are *Streptococcus pneumoniae, Haemophilus influenzae*, and *Moraxella catarrhalis*. The most common community-acquired lower respiratory pathogens are *S pneumoniae*, viruses, and *H influenzae*. *Mycoplasma pneumoniae, Chlamydophila pneumoniae*, and assorted Gram-negative bacteria are also common.
- Aspiration represents the major route of pulmonary infection, especially among hospitalized patients. However, a wide variety of respiratory care equipment has been implicated in the spread of infection.
- Viruses are responsible for a variety of seasonal respiratory infections, are highly contagious, and require strict adherence to infection control policies.
- Induced sputum is frequently useful for diagnostic purposes, but some infections are much more reliably diagnosed with bronchoscopy or nonbronchoscopic bronchoalveolar lavage.
- Selection of an adequate sampling method and obtaining an acceptable sputum specimens are

critical elements for the diagnosis and management of respiratory infections.

- A large number of antibiotics are available to treat respiratory infections, each with toxicities that must be considered. Use of nebulized antibiotics can reduce toxicity.
- Antibiotic resistance is now a common phenomenon and has necessitated use of multiple antibiotics for some infections, such as tuberculosis and *Pseudomonas* pneumonia.

REFERENCES

1. Porter JR. Anthony van Leeuwenhoek: tercentenary of his discovery of bacteria. *Bacteriol Rev*. 1976;40:260–269.
2. Eagon R. *Pseudomonas natrienses*, a marine bacterium with generation time of less than 10 minutes. *J Bacteriol*. 1962;83:736–737.
3. Jahamy H, Ganga R, Al Raiy B, et al. *Staphylococcus aureus* skin/soft-tissue infections: the impact of SCCmec type and Panton-Valentine leukocidin. *Scand J Infect Dis*. 2008;40:601–606.
4. Garnier F, Tristan A, François B, et al. Pneumonia and new methicillin-resistant *Staphylococcus aureus* clone. *Emerg Infect Dis*. 2006;12:498–500.
5. Brulé N, Jaffré S, Chollet S, et al. Necrotizing pneumonia due to *Staphylococcus aureus* producing Panton-Valentine toxin. *Rev Mal Respir*. 2008;25:875–879.
6. Ganesan A. Methicillin-resistant *Staphylococcus aureus* bacteremia and pneumonia. *Dis Month*. 2008;54:787–792.
7. Gerischer U, ed. *Acinetobacter Molecular Biology*. Norfolk, England: Caister Academic Press; 2009.
8. Joshi SG, Litake GM, Satpute MG, et al. Clinical and demographic features of infection caused by *Acinetobacter* species. *Indian J Med Sci*. 2006;60:351–360.
9. Robenshtok E, Paul M, Leibovici L, et al. The significance of *Acinetobacter baumannii* bacteraemia compared with *Klebsiella pneumoniae* bacteraemia: risk factors and outcomes. *J Hosp Infect*. 2006;64:282–287.
10. Cosentini R, Tarsia P, Canetta C, et al. Severe asthma exacerbation: role of acute *Chlamydophila pneumoniae* and *Mycoplasma pneumoniae* infection. *Respir Res*. 2008;30:9–48.
11. Ryan KJ, Ray CG, eds. *Sherris Medical Microbiology*. 4th ed. McGraw Hill; 2004:409–412.
12. Ferwerda A, Moll HA, de Groot R. Respiratory tract infections by *Mycoplasma pneumoniae* in children: a review of diagnostic and therapeutic measures. *Eur J Pediatr*. 2001;500:483–491.
13. Nilsson AC, Björkman P, Persson K. Polymerase chain reaction is superior to serology for the diagnosis of acute *Mycoplasma pneumoniae* infection and reveals a high rate of persistent infection. *BMC Microbiol*. 2008;8:93.
14. Yu VL, Stout JE. Community-acquired Legionnaires' disease: implications for underdiagnosis and laboratory testing. *Clin Infect Dis*. 2008;46:1365–1367.
15. Parish T, Brown A, eds. *Mycobacterium: Genomics and Molecular Biology*. Norfolk, England: Caister Academic Press; 2009.
16. World Health Organization. Tuberculosis. Fact sheet no. 104. March 2010. Available at: http://www.who.int/mediacentre/factsheets/fs104/en/index.html.
17. ATS: diagnostic standards and classification of tuberculosis in adults and children. *Am J Respir Crit Care Med*. 2000;501:1376–1395.
18. Hoft DF, Tennant JM. Persistence and boosting of bacille Calmette-Guerin-induced delayed-type hypersensitivity. *Ann Intern Med*. 1999;131:32.
19. Dye C. Doomsday postponed? Preventing and reversing epidemics of drug-resistant tuberculosis. *Nat Rev Microbiol*. 2009;7:81–87.
20. el-Sayed Zaki M, Abou-el Hassan S. Clinical evaluation of Gen-Probe's amplified *Mycobacterium tuberculosis* direct test for rapid diagnosis of *Mycobacterium tuberculosis* in Egyptian children at risk for infection. *Arch Pathol Lab Med*. 2008;132:244–247.
21. Sekiguchi J, Miyoshi-Akiyama T, Augustynowicz-Kopeć E, et al. Detection of multidrug resistance in *Mycobacterium tuberculosis*. *J Clin Microbiol*. 2007;45:179–192.
22. Dimmock NJ, Easton AJ, Leppard K. *Introduction to Modern Virology*. 6th ed. Malden, MA: Blackwell Publishing; 2007.
23. Centers for Disease Control and Prevention. Respiratory syncytial virus infection. Available at: www.cdc.gov/rsv/index.html. Accessed February 17, 2009.
24. Stensballe LG, Simonsen JB, Thomsen SF, et al. The causal direction in the association between respiratory syncytial virus hospitalization and asthma. *J Allergy Clin Immunol*. 2009;123:131–137.
25. Miller EK, Edwards KM, Weinberg GA, et al. A novel group of rhinoviruses is associated with asthma hospitalizations. *J Allergy Clin Immunol*. 2009;123:98–104.
26. Jackson DJ, Gangnon RE, Evans MD, et al. Wheezing rhinovirus illnesses in early life predict asthma development in high-risk children. *Am J Respir Crit Care Med*. 2008;178:667–672.
27. Horwood F, Macfarlane J. Pneumococcal and influenza vaccination: current situation and future prospects. *Thorax*. 2002;57(suppl 2):1124–1130.
28. Centers for Disease Control and Prevention. FluView: 2008–2009 influenza season week 53 ending January 3, 2009. Available at: http://www.cdc.gov/flu/weekly. Accessed February 17, 2009.
29. Stephenson I, Democratis J, Lackenby A, et al. Neuraminidase inhibitor resistance after oseltamivir treatment of acute influenza A and B in children. *Clin Infect Dis*. 2009;48:389–396.
30. Smith RD. Responding to global infectious disease outbreaks: lessons from SARS on the role of risk perception, communication and management. *J Soc Sci Med*. 2006;63:3113–3123.
31. Carrier R, ed. *Guinness Book of World Records*. New York: Bantam Books; 1999:236.
32. Aliouat-Denis CM, Chabé M, Demanche C, et al. *Pneumocystis* species, co-evolution and pathogenic power. *Infect Genet Evol*. 2008;8:708–726.
33. Fishman JA. Treatment of infection due to *Pneumocystis carinii*. *Antimicrob Agents Chemother*. 1998;42:1309–1314.
34. Community-acquired pneumonia in adults: guidelines for management. *Clin Infect Dis*. 2007;44:S27–S72.
35. Guidelines for the management of adults with hospital-acquired, ventilator-associated, and healthcare-associated pneumonia. *Am J Respir Crit Care Med*. 2005;171:388–450.
36. Paggiaro PL, Chanez P, Holz O, et al. Sputum induction. *Eur Respir J*. 2002;37(suppl):3s–8s.
37. Ramirez P, Valencia M, Torres A. Bronchoalveolar lavage to diagnose respiratory infections. *Semin Respir Crit Care Med*. 2007;28:525–533.
38. Marquette CH, Copin MC, Ballet F. Diagnostic tests for pneumonia in ventilated patients: prospective evaluation of diagnostic accuracy using histology as a diagnostic gold standard. *Am J Respir Crit Care Med*. 1995;151:1878–1888.
39. Papazian L, Autillo Touati A, Thomas P. Diagnosis of ventilator-associated pneumonia: an evaluation of direct examination and presence of intracellular organisms. *Anesthesiology*. 1997;87:268–276.
40. Meduri GU, Reddy RC, Stanley T, El-Zeky F. Pneumonia in acute respiratory distress syndrome: a prospective evaluation of bilateral bronchoscopic sampling. *Am J Respir Crit Care Med*. 1998;158:870–875.
41. Fagon JY. Diagnosis and treatment of ventilator-associated pneumonia: fiberoptic bronchoscopy with bronchoalveolar lavage is essential. *Semin Respir Crit Care Med*. 2006;27:34–44.
42. Torres A, El-Ebiary M. Bronchoscopic BAL in the diagnosis of ventilator-associated pneumonia. *Chest*. 2000;117:198S–202S.

43. Ioanas M, Ferrer R, Angrill J, et al. Microbial investigation in ventilator-associated pneumonia. *Eur Respir J.* 2001;17: 791–801.
44. Kirtland SH, Corley DE, Winterbauer RH. The diagnosis of ventilator-associated pneumonia: a comparison of histologic, microbiologic and clinical criteria. *Chest.* 1997;112:445–457.
45. Clec'h C, Jauréguy F, Hamza L, et al. Agreement between quantitative cultures of postintubation tracheal aspiration and plugged telescoping catheter, protected specimen brush, or BAL for the diagnosis of nosocomial pneumonia. *Chest.* 2006;130:956–961.
46. Baughman RP. Nonbronchoscopic evaluation of ventilator-associated pneumonia. *Semin Respir Infect.* 2003;18:95–102.
47. Leo A, Galindo-Galindo J, Folch E, et al. Comparison of bronchoscopic bronchoalveolar lavage vs blind lavage with a modified nasogastric tube in the etiologic diagnosis of ventilator-associated pneumonia. *Med Intensiva.* 2008;32:115–120.
48. Goldberg AE, Malhotra AK, Riaz OJ, et al. Predictive value of broncho-alveolar lavage fluid Gram's stain in the diagnosis of ventilator-associated pneumonia: a prospective study. *J Trauma.* 2008;65:871–876.
49. Rao VK, Ritter J, Kollef MH. Utility of transbronchial biopsy in patients with acute respiratory failure: a postmortem study. *Chest.* 1998;114:549–555.
50. Pugin J, Auckenthaler R, Mili N, et al. Diagnosis of ventilator-associated pneumonia by bacteriologic analysis of bronchoscopic and nonbronchoscopic "blind" bronchoalveolar lavage fluid. *Am Rev Respir Dis.* 1991;143:1121–1129.
51. Mohr AM, Sifri ZC, Horng HS, et al. Use of aerosolized aminoglycosides in the treatment of Gram-negative ventilator-associated pneumonia. *Surg Infect (Larchmont).* 2007;8:349–357.
52. Dhand R. The role of aerosolized antimicrobials in the treatment of ventilator-associated pneumonia. *Respir Care.* 2007;52:866–884.
53. Michalopoulos A, Fotakis D, Virtzili S, et al. Aerosolized colistin as adjunctive treatment of ventilator-associated pneumonia due to multidrug-resistant Gram-negative bacteria: a prospective study. *Respir Med.* 2008;102:407–412.

CHAPTER 53

Cardiopulmonary Anatomy and Physiology

Joseph Buhain
Avi Nahum

OUTLINE

The Heart
Circulatory System
Gross Anatomy of the Respiratory System
Anatomy of the Thorax
Microanatomy of the Respiratory System
Functional Characteristics of the Respiratory System

OBJECTIVES

1. Describe the gross and functional anatomy of the heart and circulatory system.
2. Describe the gross and functional anatomy of the respiratory system.
3. Describe the anatomy of the upper airway.
4. Describe the anatomy of the tracheobronchial tree.
5. Discuss the relationship between the bony elements of the thorax.
6. Compare the roles of the diaphragm, accessory inspiratory muscles, and abdominal muscles.
7. Discuss the pulmonary and bronchial circulations.
8. Describe how breathing is controlled by the pons and medulla.
9. Describe innervation of the lungs.
10. Describe the visceral pleura, parietal pleura, and pleural space.
11. Describe the anatomy of the mediastinum.
12. Describe the mucociliary apparatus.
13. Describe the smooth muscle function of the airways and the pulmonary circulation.
14. Compare macrophages and dendritic cells found within the respiratory system.
15. Compare alveolar type I and type II cells.
16. Describe the interstitial space within the lungs.
17. Describe the role of airway resistance and respiratory system compliance on the pressures generated during the respiratory cycle.
18. Compare the distribution of ventilation and blood flow within the lungs.
19. Discuss the importance of the ventilation-perfusion ratio.
20. Describe oxygen uptake from the lungs.

KEY TERMS

abdominal muscles
accessory muscles
alveoli
atrioventricular (AV) node
atrium
bronchi
channels of Lambert
compliance
conchae
coronary artery
coronary sinus
dead space volume
dendritic cells
diaphragm
diffusion capacity
epiglottis
glottis
hilum
laryngopharynx
larynx
lobes
macrophages
mast cells
mediastinum
mucociliary apparatus
nasopharynx
oropharynx
parietal pleura
pericardium
phrenic nerve
pleural space
pores of Kohn
pulmonary arteries
resistance
segments
sinoatrial (SA) node
thorax
trachea
type I cells
type II cells
ventilation-perfusion ratio
ventricle
visceral pleura
work of breathing

INTRODUCTION

Knowledge of the functional anatomy of the heart and lungs is essential for understanding the extent and course of cardiopulmonary disorders. The anatomical and physiological details of the cardiopulmonary system provide the basis for monitoring changing pathology and response to treatment. This chapter will discuss the basic anatomy and physiological principles related to the cardiopulmonary system.

The Heart

The major function of the heart is to generate pressure that will propel blood through the lungs and the systemic circulation. In addition, minor movements of the heart may help distribute gas within the lungs through cardiogenic oscillations. The heart is located within the pericardial sac, which contains a small amount of fluid that allows the heart to move freely. The muscular structure of the heart consists of three parts: the epicardium, myocardium, and endocardium. The epicardium, a thin membrane, lines the outside of the heart. The innermost lining of the heart is the endocardium, composed of endothelial cells. Finally, the myocardium consists of cardiac muscle, serving the primary pumping function of the heart. Most cardiac cells are contractile, but some make up the electrical conduction system of the heart.

Although the heart is considered a single pump, it functions as two pumps involving flow through four chambers: the right **atrium** and **ventricle** and the left atrium and ventricle (**Figure 53–1**). An interventricular septum separates the two ventricles. The right atrium of the heart receives blood from the inferior and superior vena cavae and the **coronary sinus**. The right ventricle generates pressures of approximately 25 mm Hg over the central venous pressure to drive deoxygenated blood into the **pulmonary arteries** toward the lungs. The tricuspid valve prevents blood from flowing back into the right atrium. The pulmonic valve closure then maintains a pressure of about 25/10 mm Hg in the pulmonary artery to allow blood runoff through the lungs. After traveling through the pulmonary capillaries, oxygenated blood drains via the pulmonary veins into the left atrium and through the mitral valve into the left ventricle. The contraction of the left ventricle generates pressures of approximately 120 mm Hg over the pulmonary capillary wedge pressure; this pressure head drives blood into the aorta, which dispenses the blood into the systemic circulation at a pressure of about 120/80 mm Hg. Strategic placement of the valves within the heart allows the movement of blood only in one direction, thus filling and emptying the chambers of the heart in a choreographed manner during systole and diastole. Valves can leak (regurgitate) or can narrow from disease; in either case, pressures will increase in the preceding chambers and vessels.

The electrical conduction system of the heart consists of specialized cells (**Figure 53–2**). The major pacemaker of the heart, the **sinoatrial (SA) node**, is located in the upper right atrium. A conduction system throughout the atria coordinates propagation of electrical signals that cause a weak contraction of the two atrial chambers. Impulses travel to the ventricles after being received by the **atrioventricular (AV) node**. The impulse is then carried via the bundle of His down the right and left bundle branches along Purkinje fibers that innervate both ventricular muscles. When the ventricles contract via this pathway, they contract simultaneously with greatest efficiency. Impulses traveling retrograde via irregular pathways are, typically, inefficient (e.g., premature ventricular contractions).

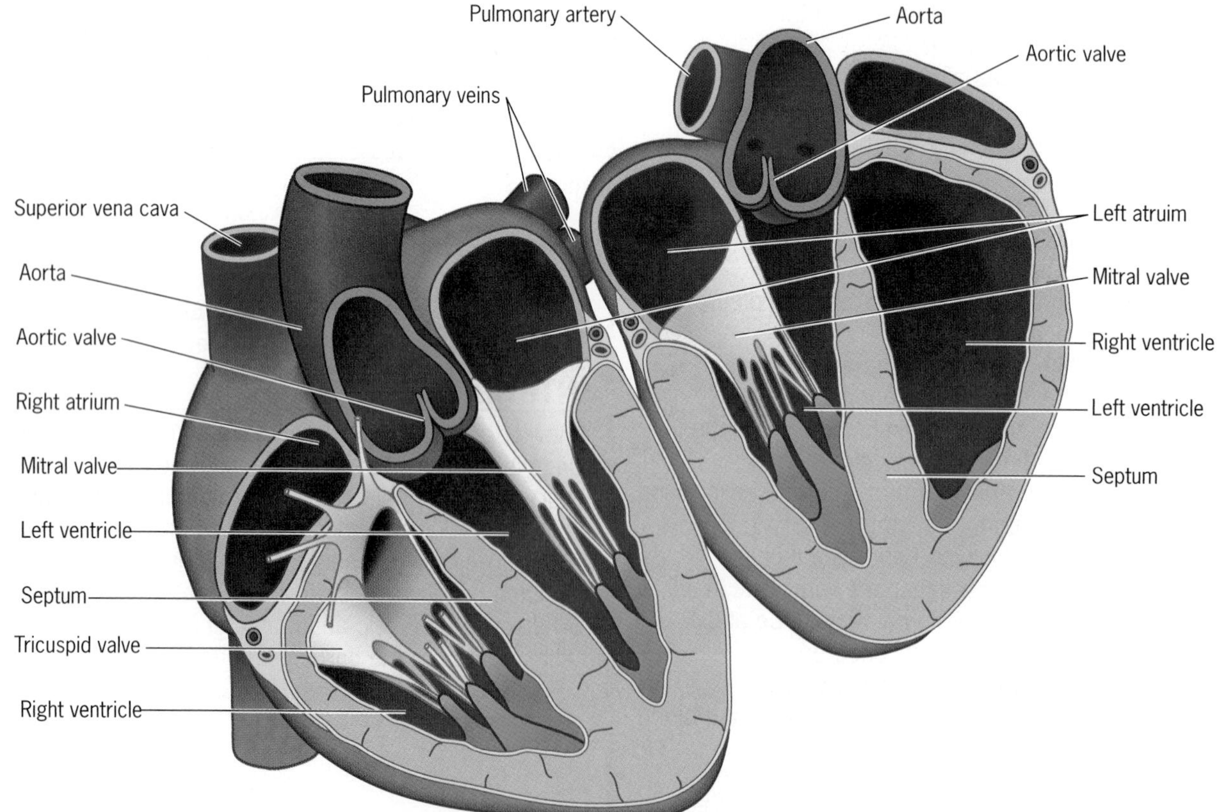

FIGURE 53–1 The heart and great vessels presented in a medial plane that slices the structures in half.

The blood supply to the heart, the coronary circulation, arises from the ascending aorta (**Figure 53–3**). The right **coronary artery** passes anteriorly over the heart until it reaches the inferior surface, where it connects with the terminal branch of the left coronary artery. Major branches of the right coronary artery include the artery to the SA node, the intraventricular artery supplying the septum, and the rest of the electrical conduction system of the heart. The left main coronary artery divides into the left anterior descending and circumflex arteries. The former

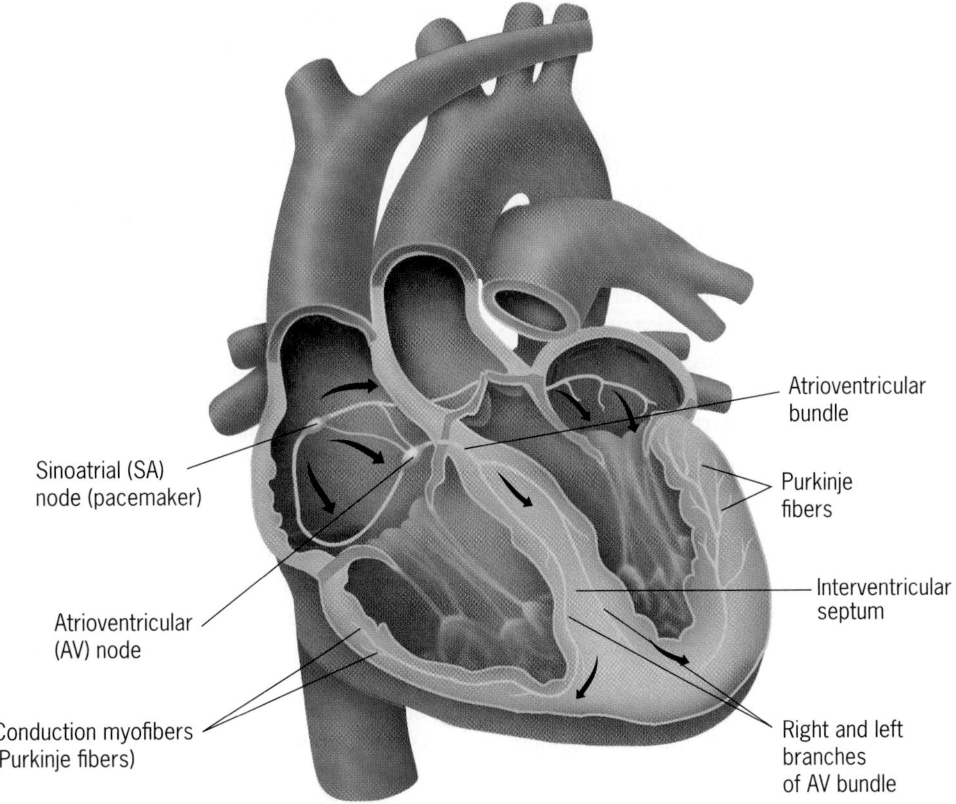

FIGURE 53–2 The electrical conduction system of the heart.

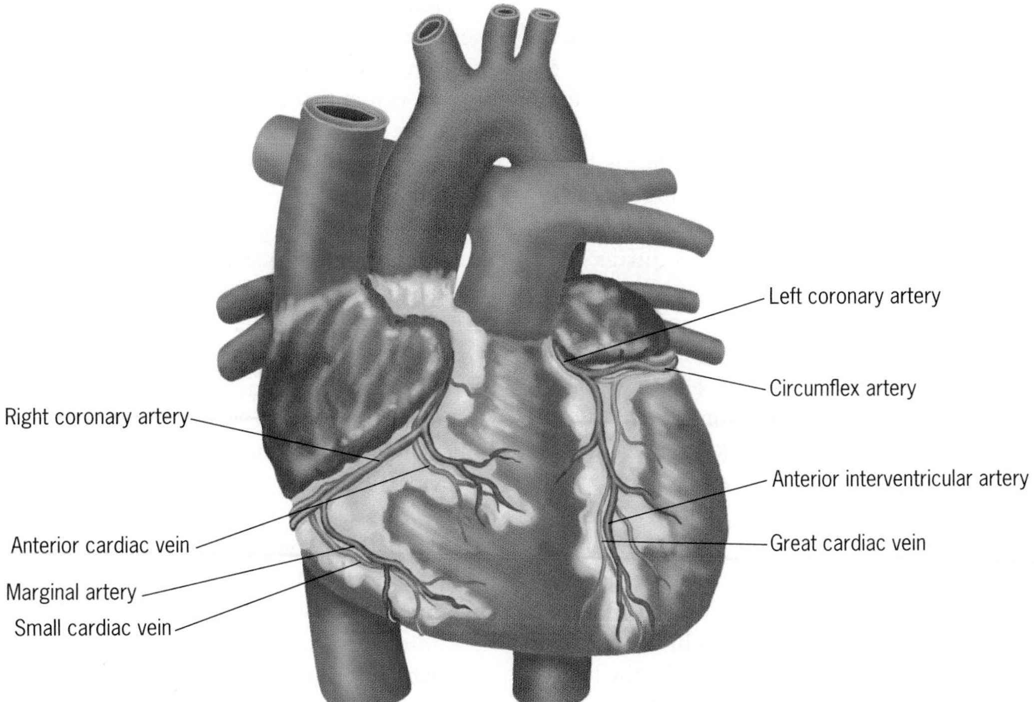

FIGURE 53–3 Coronary circulation.

supplies blood to the walls of both ventricles and the interventricular septum. A branch of the left descending artery forms the diagonal artery that supplies blood to the left ventricular wall. The circumflex artery, a continuation of the left coronary artery, follows the surface of the heart to the inferior portion of the heart. Venous drainage of the heart accompanies the major branches of the coronary arteries and finally drains into the coronary sinus, where blood is returned to the right atrium.

Innervation of the heart is via the autonomic nervous system. The sympathetic supply is from the upper thoracic segments of the spinal cord, through the sympathetic trunk. These fibers join the cardiac plexus beneath the arch of the aorta and innervate the SA and AV nodes, the myocardium, and the coronary arteries. The parasympathetic innervation is from the vagus nerves. Stimulation of the sympathetic nervous system increases heart rate, cardiac contractility, and stroke volume. Stimulation of the parasympathetic nervous system does the opposite—that is, decreases heart rate, contractility, and stroke volume.

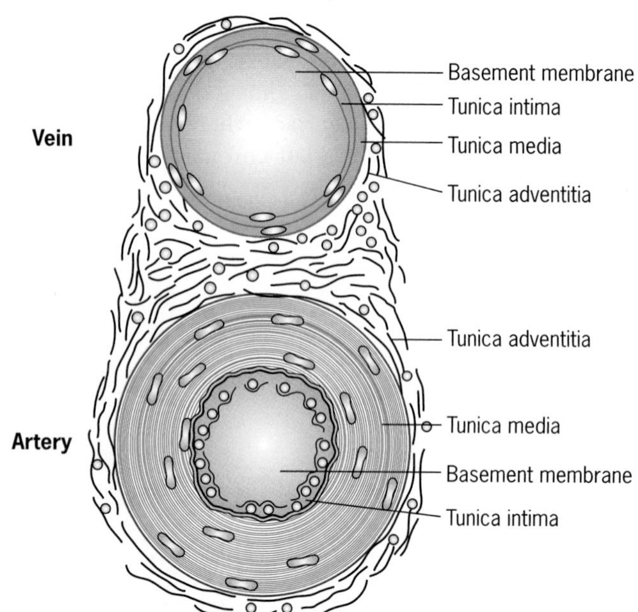

FIGURE 53–4 Structure of a vessel.

Circulatory System

The circulatory system has the task of providing nutrients, particularly oxygen, to all of the cells in the body. The arterial system is a branching series of vessels that carries blood from the heart to the capillary beds and subsequently to the cells of the lungs and body. The venous drainage system collects the blood from those capillary beds and returns the entire volume of blood to the heart. Unless there is a cut or rupture in either system, blood remains within vessels and, therefore, circulates. The basic physiologic concept of circulation was initially described and detailed by William Harvey in 1628.

There are several important reasons for interest in the circulatory or cardiovascular system. Primarily, an uninterrupted flow of oxygen must continue to the tissues of the body throughout life, but the circulatory system is susceptible to injuries and diseases that can be rapidly fatal. Also, in care settings, access to arteries and veins allows caregivers to monitor cardiovascular pressures, obtain blood specimens for analysis, and administer medications rapidly into veins.

> **RESPIRATORY RECAP**
>
> **Gross Anatomy of the Circulatory System**
>
> » The heart muscle
> » Valves, chambers, and pressures
> » Arteries, veins, and capillaries
> » Conduction system
> » Coronary circulation
> » Innervation

The circulating volume of blood in the body is about 5 liters in an adult, which is only about 10% to 15% of the 40 liters of fluid in the body. The rest lies within the cells or in the interstitial space between the cells. The average cardiac output is 5 L/min; therefore, a blood volume equal to the entire blood quantity is ejected by the heart every minute. However, blood flow is not circulated evenly throughout the body; in fact, there is an elaborate control system for routing blood to organs and tissues that require more oxygen or nutrients according to varying needs. Normally, blood flow proportionally favors the brain and kidneys. During exercise, cardiac output can increase markedly (as much as six times normal) to over 30 L/min as the additional output (with its oxygen) is sent to the working muscles.

The vessels have characteristics that relate to their role within the circuitry; that is, they have an anatomic structure to withstand pressures, avoid leaks, and control distribution of flow and contain valves to send blood in the right direction. The vessels have layers: a basement membrane is innermost, followed by the tunica intima, tunica media, and tunica adventitia (**Figure 53–4**). Arteries are thicker and flexible to withstand the higher pressures required to drive blood to and through major organs. Veins are thinner because their role is more passive as conduits for returning blood to the heart. However, the driving pressures within the arteries are not adequate to deliver blood to the capillary beds *and* to push the blood back to the heart. Thus, many veins (primarily in the legs) have one-way valves aimed toward the heart to allow muscular contraction to help nurse blood back to the heart. Stagnant blood tends to clot and form thrombi—a risk that is greatest in the legs. The tunica media of the arteries is larger and is composed of elastic fibers and longitudinal muscles. The control of these muscles is autonomic; that is, sympathetic and parasympathetic nerves control the tone of the longitudinal muscles that line the arteries. Medications with specific autonomic effects (i.e., sympathomimetic) can be administered to control blood pressure.

A circulatory model for blood movement within the body is used to help understand the mechanisms of

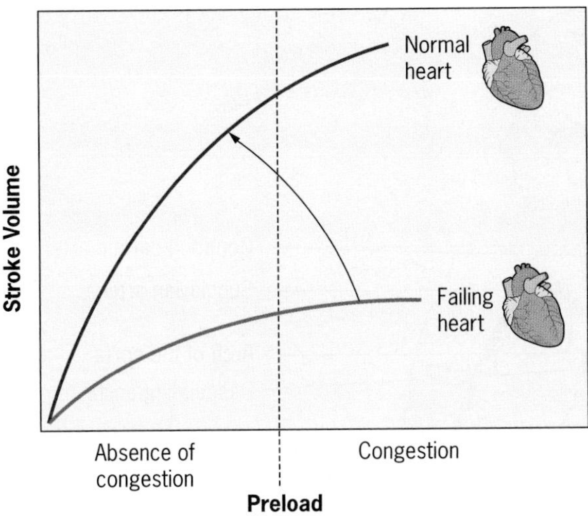

FIGURE 53–5 Frank-Starling curve.

cardiac performance, blood pressure control (or blood delivery to the capillary beds), and venous drainage. Basically, the heart is the pump that ejects blood with a certain force—its contractility. The strength of the heart's contractility can be increased by medications that have primarily that effect. The arterial system receives blood from the heart as it runs off to the capillaries. The arteries as they branch create a back pressure that affects afterload—the pressure encountered by the left ventricle to eject blood during systole. Afterload is increased by medications or stiffened arteries and may be decreased by medications or disease such as sepsis. The heart is a pump that must be primed with enough liquid (blood) to pump properly. The blood volume at end-diastole available for ejection by the heart is called the *preload*. Preload can be controlled by fluid administration, fluid restriction, or fluid withdrawal, as in the use of diuretics. Cardiac performance can be described (and affected) in terms of contractility, afterload, and preload. The relationship of blood volume to cardiac performance is graphically displayed by the Frank-Starling curve (**Figure 53–5**).

Arteries of the body (**Figure 53–6**) tend to be deeper, but blood pressure can be felt or palpated on the skin surface if circulation is adequate. Normal arterial pressure is relatively uniform at about 120/80 mm Hg throughout the arterial system. The major arteries—the aorta, subclavian, and abdominal aorta—are deep. Palpation is usually possible at several sites, such as the radial, brachial, dorsalis pedis, carotid, and femoral arteries. Blood pressure is measured, most often, with a sphygmomanometer from the brachial artery. Catheters can be inserted into the radial, brachial, or femoral arteries to monitor arterial pressure and allow sampling of arterial blood for blood gas analysis. The radial artery is the usual site for intermittent arterial blood sampling.

The arterial system is vulnerable to disease as a result of consuming substances (such as high-cholesterol foods or cigarette smoke) that are associated with the formation of plaques on the inner walls of major arteries. Occlusions or strictures of the coronary arteries are extremely dangerous; therefore, they are promptly treated with stents, vessel-widening balloons, and transplanted vessels to route blood around the lesions. The carotid arteries are bypassed when they are narrowed or occluded. Arterial grafts can be implanted to replace other large damaged vessels.

The veins of the body (**Figure 53–7**) tend to be near the surface of the skin and are more numerous than arteries. Venous blood samples can be obtained for most diagnostic testing purposes. A light tourniquet on the upper arm will cause veins to stand out, including the easily accessible antecubital vein. An intravenous catheter can usually be placed in the forearm to ensure continual access for medication delivery. When venous access is required in patients with unreliable circulation, a central venous catheter is placed via the internal jugular, subclavian, or femoral veins. Thrombi that form in the venous system present the risk of breaking free and becoming emboli, which tend to lodge in the lungs. Medications are available to prevent thrombi formation and to actively dissolve the clots. Large thrombi can be trapped by an implanted vascular umbrella or physically extracted if necessary.

Gross Anatomy of the Respiratory System

The respiratory system can be divided into the upper and lower respiratory tracts. The upper respiratory system (tract) includes the nasal cavity, paranasal sinus, pharynx, tongue, epiglottis, soft and hard palates, oral cavities, laryngopharynx, and portions of the trachea. The lower respiratory tract extends from the trachea to the alveoli.

The air conditioning goals of the upper airway begin as air enters the upper respiratory tract (**Figure 53–8**). The air enters through two external openings in the nose called nostrils. The nostrils open to two nasal cavities made of bone and cartilage. Mucus-coated epithelial membranes line the cavities. Their main function is to filter, warm, and humidify the inspired air. The nasal **conchae**, also known as turbinates, are bony ridges that laterally project into the nasal cavity. Within the cavities, sensory neurons allow smell (via the olfactory nerve) and initiate reflexes that cause sneezes or a sense of breathlessness.

As air travels through the nasal passages, it continues downward toward the pharynx, which combines with the inner ear canals. The pharynx has three regions: the nasopharynx, oropharynx, and laryngopharynx. The **nasopharynx** is a passageway lined with ciliated epithelial and goblet cells and is reserved for air movement only; the remainder of the pharynx serves to carry air and food. The **oropharynx** is distal to the mouth and is lined with stratified squamous epithelium that is continuous with the oral cavity. Tonsils are two masses in the back

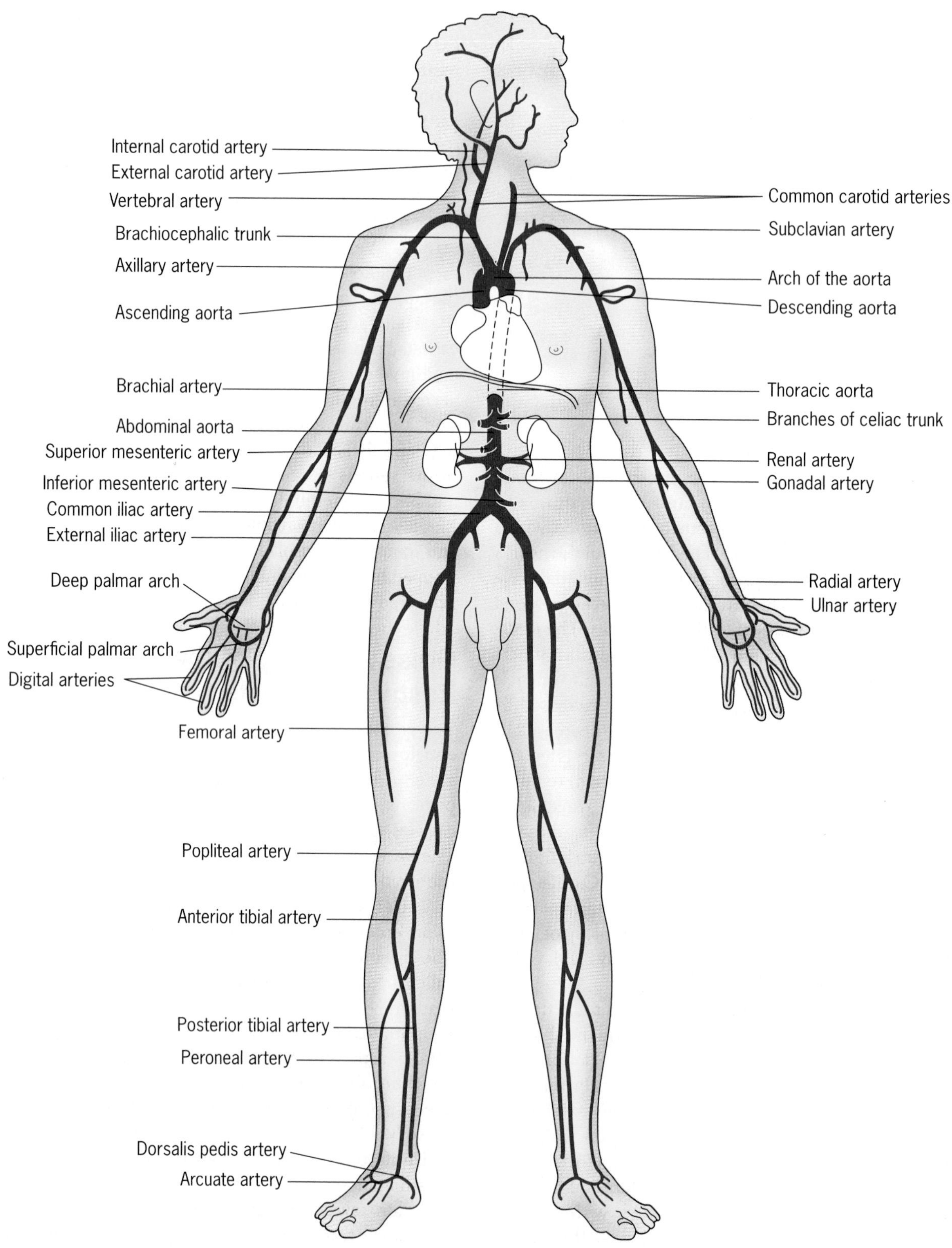

FIGURE 53–6 Arteries.

of the throat. Adenoids are a single pharyngeal tonsil located high in the throat behind the nose and the roof of the mouth (soft palate) and are not visible through the mouth. The uvula is the visible projection of the middle of the soft palate—easily seen in an open mouth. Enlargement of these structures may impede breathing, especially during sleep. The **laryngopharynx** is the most inferior portion of the pharynx. In the pharynx, actually a muscular tube, the air and food passages coincide below the oral cavity. Air is directed to the larynx by the negative thoracic pressure generated primarily by the diaphragm, and food is directed posterior into the

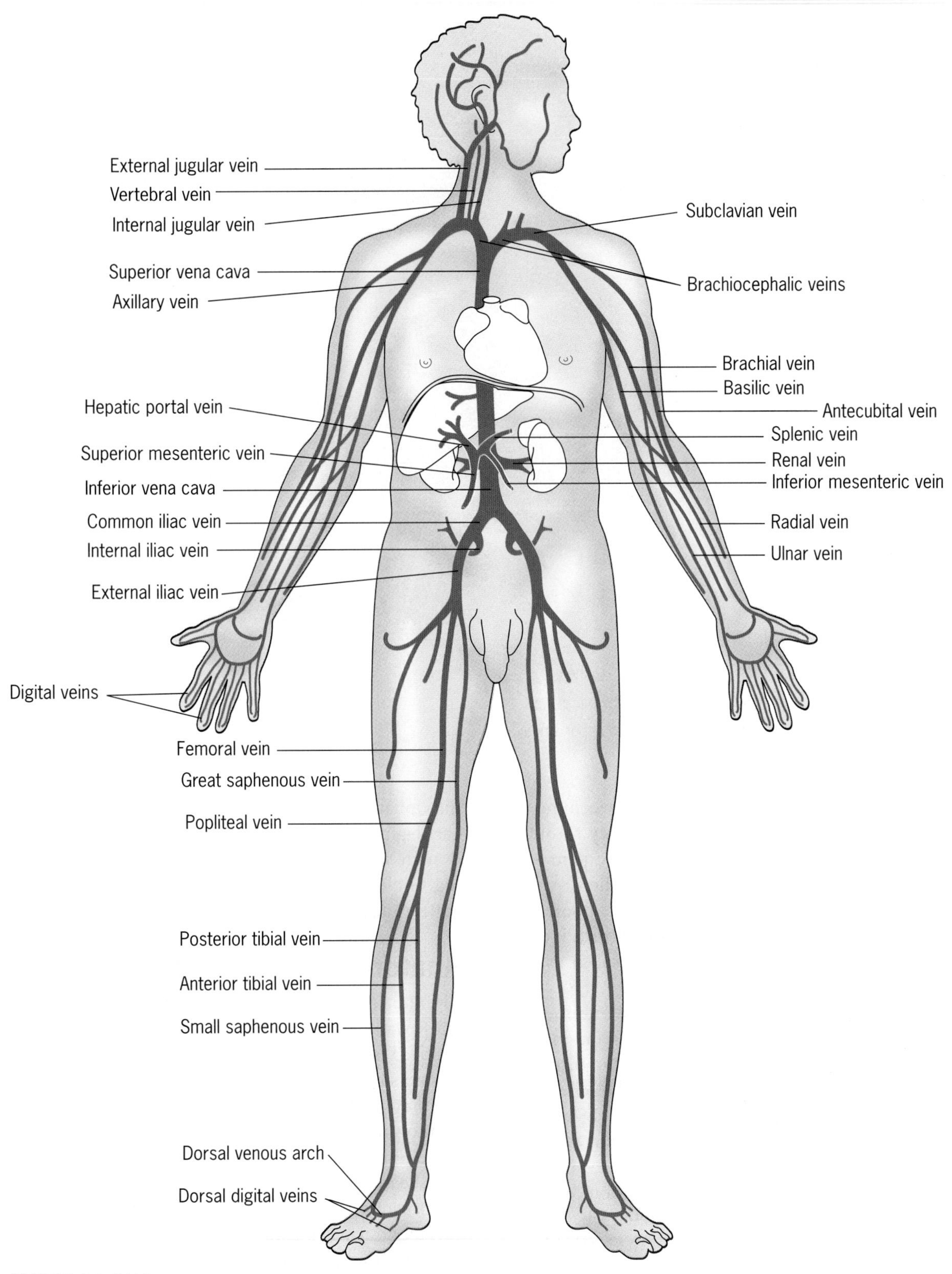

FIGURE 53–7 Veins.

esophagus by a complex coordination of muscles during swallowing. The **epiglottis**, a valvelike structure, can close the entry to the larynx, preventing aspiration of food particles.

The **larynx** is a cartilaginous structure that serves as the passageway for air between the pharynx and trachea. The hyoid bone is seated above the larynx. The epiglottis is the uppermost cartilage of the larynx. The largest cartilage of the larynx is the thyroid cartilage, which protrudes more prominently in men (the Adam's apple). The only complete-ring cartilage around the airway is the cricoid cartilage, which is located below the thyroid

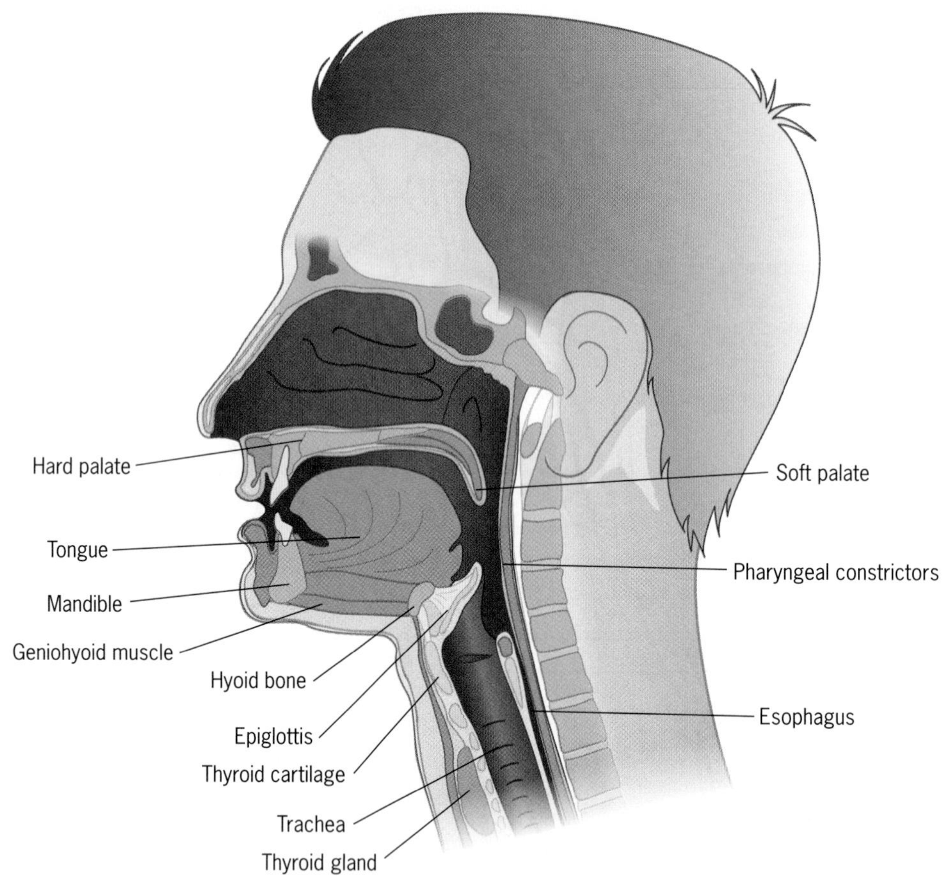

FIGURE 53-8 Anatomy of the upper airway.

cartilage. The cricothyroid membrane (between the two cartilages) can be opened in an emergency to obtain access to the lower airways. Small cartilage pairs—the corniculates and arytenoids—complete the posterior larynx. The vocal cords are mucosal folds supported by elastic ligaments; the opening between the cords is called the **glottis**. When air moves through the vocal cords, they can be vibrated to create sounds.

The **trachea**, commonly called the windpipe, is a large hollow tube that bifurcates at the carina into the two primary **bronchi**. The trachea marks the beginning of the conducting system, often called the tracheobronchial tree. The trachea measures 10 to 13 cm in length. It is protected and supported by 16 to 20 C-shaped pieces of cartilage, which keep the trachea open even during the negative thoracic pressures of inspiration. An adult trachea is about 2.0 to 2.5 cm in diameter. The mucosa that lines the trachea and a majority of the tracheobronchial tree is pseudostratified ciliated columnar epithelium. Smoking has been known to destroy the cilia that line the airways. The trachea bifurcates asymmetrically, with the right main stem bronchus branching out at a smaller angle (20 to 30 degrees from vertical) than the left (45 to 55 degrees). Therefore, foreign bodies are aspirated mainly into the right bronchus, and endotracheal suction catheters will commonly advance into and aspirate from the right lung. The main bronchi branch into lobar and then segmental bronchi, all of which have cartilaginous support for their walls. Bronchi continue to branch sequentially 23 times, or generations, terminating in clusters of **alveoli**, air sacs that have a grapelike appearance.

Anatomy of the Thorax

The **thorax** contains an infrastructure composed of the chest wall and the vertebrae within which major organs reside. The chest wall (i.e., skin, ribs, intercostal muscles) protects the lungs from injury. Thoracic muscles such as the **diaphragm** perform the work of breathing. A serous membrane called the **parietal pleura** adheres firmly to the chest wall, whereas the **visceral pleura** covers the surface of each lung. Fluid within the pleural cavity prevents friction and allows smooth sliding between the two surfaces during respiration.

The thorax has three regions: the mediastinum, a right pleural cavity, and a left pleural cavity. The **mediastinum** contains major blood vessels, the esophagus, and the heart, whereas the pleural cavities contain the lungs.

Bony Thorax

The bony elements provide support and protection for the heart and lungs. The elements that make up the thorax include the sternum, ribs, thoracic vertebrae, clavicles, and scapulae. The vertebrae allow movement, rotation, and elevation of the thoracic ribs. The sternum, which anchors the ribs to the front of the chest wall, is subdivided into three parts: the manubrium, the body, and the xiphoid process. The manubrium connects to the first two ribs, and the body of the sternum connects directly to the third through seventh ribs. The xiphoid process forms the tip of the sternum. These bony elements protect the contents of the thorax, help to expand and relax the chest via contraction of respiratory muscles during inspiration and expiration, and stabilize the chest wall during changes in intrapleural pressure.

> **RESPIRATORY RECAP**
>
> **Bony Elements of the Thorax**
> - Sternum
> - Ribs
> - Thoracic vertebrae
> - Clavicles
> - Scapulae

The twelve pairs of ribs correspond to their vertebrae of origin. The first through seventh ribs play an important function in ventilation. These ribs lift like bucket handles (outward and upward), while the sternum rises like a pump handle. In contrast, the lower ribs rotate toward the back. Obstructive lung disorders such as chronic bronchitis or emphysema limit the expansion. Normally, the anterior-to-posterior (AP) diameter is much less than the chest width, but with obstructive disease, air trapping expands the lungs and increases the AP diameter of the chest, forming the so-called barrel chest.

Respiratory Muscles

Various muscles contracting in synchrony help to maintain the elasticity and ease of lung movement. Contraction of a coordinated set of muscles of respiration helps to move air into the lungs, leading to inspiration. Although exhalation is typically passive, thoracic muscles can fix the chest, and **abdominal muscles** can contract to force air out of the lungs, most dramatically in coughing or sneezing. The diaphragm and external intercostals are the primary muscles of inspiration. The diaphragm typically is shaped like a dome. During inspiration, the diaphragm contracts and becomes flat, causing lung expansion. During exhalation, the elastic recoil of the lungs and relaxation of the diaphragm allow the lungs to return to their end-expiratory volume and position.

The diaphragm is a large muscle that provides the primary force for the **work of breathing**. The diaphragm attaches to the large vertebrae, the ribs, and the xiphoid process. Fibers of the diaphragm connect to a broad connective sheet called the *central tendon*. During tidal breathing, the diaphragm moves approximately 1.5 cm. At high levels of stress and movement with increasing work of breathing, the diaphragm can move up to 6 to 10 cm with each tidal breath. The diaphragm produces an important mechanical effect that draws air into the airways and lungs. When diaphragmatic contraction draws the central tendon down, flattening the diaphragm, intrathoracic pressure is decreased, creating a pressure differential with atmospheric pressure.

> **RESPIRATORY RECAP**
>
> **Muscles of Ventilation**
> - Diaphragm
> - Accessory muscles of inhalation
> - Accessory muscles of exhalation

The diaphragm receives its major nerve supply from the **phrenic nerve** that exits the cervical region at C3–C5. A hiccup, a reflex, is a spasm of the diaphragm caused by an irritation of the phrenic nerve. Cervical fractures between C1 and C5 are likely to affect the phrenic nerve and disrupt or impair the ability to breath.

During exercise, **accessory muscles** can be recruited on inspiration and expiration to increase the respiratory effort. Accessory muscles are coordinated with diaphragm movement during inspiration. The external intercostals, located between each rib pair, assist with inspiration by lifting the ribs; the internal intercostals aid with expiration by fixing the chest wall (**Figure 53–9**). Other accessory muscles of inspiration that expand the chest wall are the scalenes, sternocleidomastoids, pectoralis majors, and trapezius. A way to evaluate whether subjects are in respiratory distress is to observe a retraction at the notch above the clavicles during inspiration. The accessory muscles of expiration (which is normally passive) help exhalation if resistance to expiration is significant or demands on ventilation greatly increase, as with exercise. These muscles include the rectus abdominis, external abdominis oblique, internal

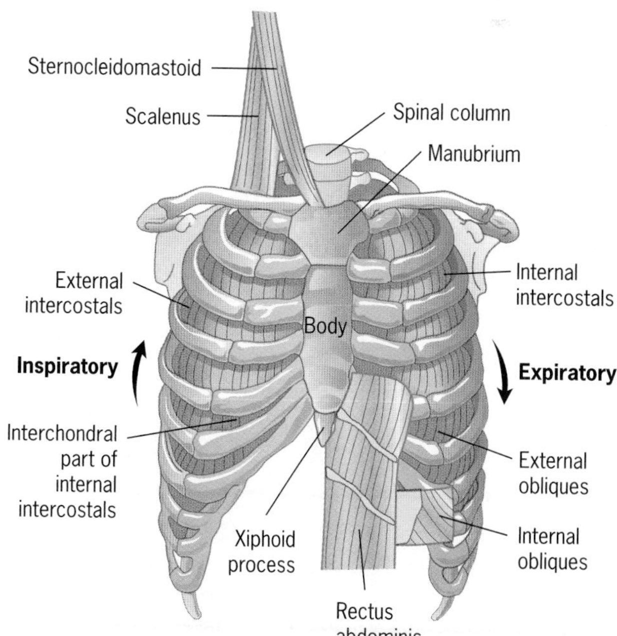

FIGURE 53–9 Bony components and muscles of the chest wall involved in ventilation. The red portions represent the costal cartilage and associated ribs. Arrow pointing upward represents the muscles that are active during respiration. Arrow pointing downward denotes muscles that contribute to forced expiratory maneuvers.

abdominis oblique, transversus abdominal, and internal intercostal muscles. Consequently, active exhalation can be observed if contraction of the abdomen is apparent. In patients with severe obstructive disease with increased work of breathing, both inspiratory and expiratory accessory muscles are often active.

Lungs

The lungs are cone shaped, with a broad and concave base surrounded by the thoracic ribs and diaphragm. There are five **lobes** and 18 lung **segments** between the right and left lungs (**Figure 53–10**). The average pair of adult lungs weighs about 800 g and contains about 90% gas and 10% tissue. The tops of the lungs are called the *apices* and extend from above the clavicle to the first vertebra. During quiet breathing, at end-expiration, the anterior portion of the lung borders the sixth rib. The medial portion of each lung is adjacent to the mediastinum and contains an opening called the **hilum**—a region where the bronchi and the pulmonary vessels enter the lungs. Each lung is divided into lobes, which are separated by fissures; each lobe is divided into segments according to the branching of the tracheobronchial tree (**Table 53–1**).

The right lung is larger (and therefore heavier) than the left lung, which shares a larger portion of its hemithorax with the heart than the right lung. The right lung is divided into upper, middle, and lower lobes that are separated

RESPIRATORY RECAP

Anatomy of the Lungs

» Airways and alveoli
» Lobes and segments

TABLE 53–1 Lobes and Segments of the Lungs

Lung	Lobe	Segments
Right	Upper	Apical
		Anterior
		Posterior
	Middle	Lateral
		Medial
	Lower	Superior
		Anterior basal
		Posterior basal
		Lateral basal
		Medial basal
Left	Upper	Apical posterior
		Anterior
		Superior lingular
		Inferior lingular
	Lower	Superior
		Anterior medial basal
		Lateral basal
		Posterior basal

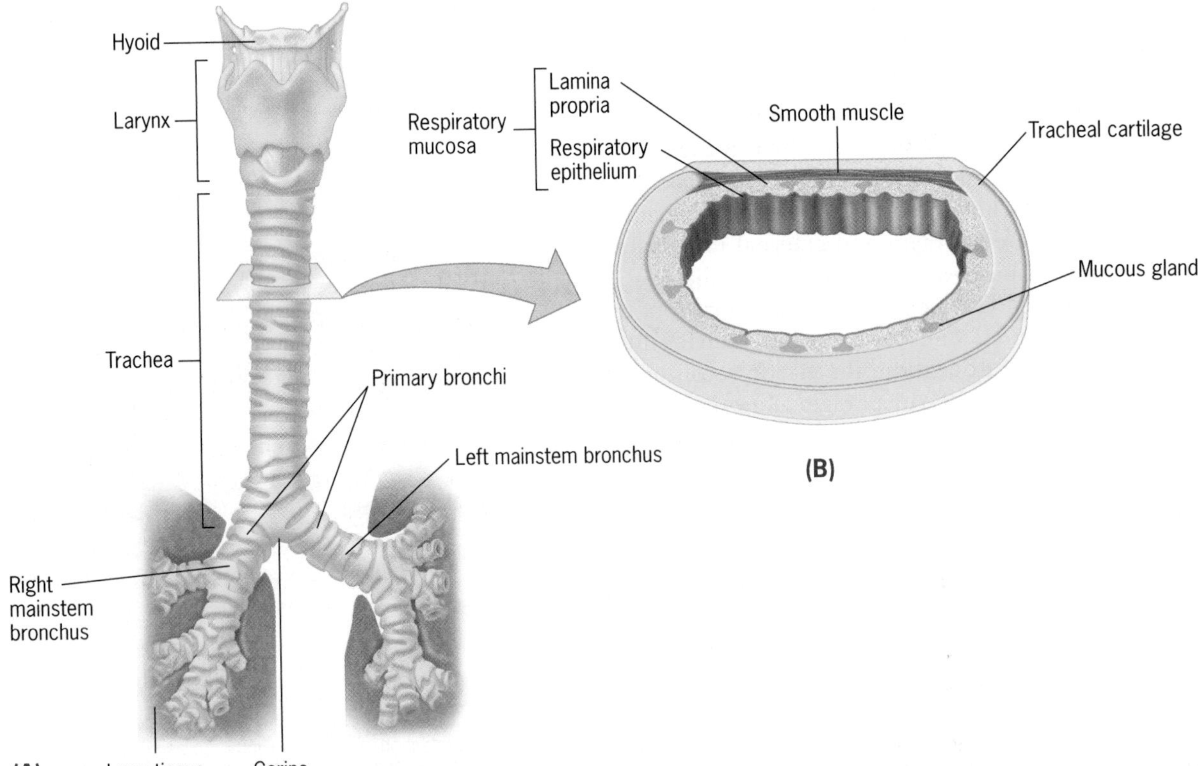

FIGURE 53–10 **(A)** Frontal view of the trachea and major bronchi, with designations of the major lung lobes to which they conduct air. **(B)** A schematic cross-sectional view of the trachea.

by horizontal and oblique fissures. The horizontal fissure extends horizontally, separating the middle and upper lobes. The oblique fissure separates the middle and lower lobes. The left lung is divided into two lobes (upper and lower) separated by an oblique fissure. Knowledge of lobe and segment anatomy is required of bronchoscopists and those assisting in the procedures.

The lungs consist of two major anatomic divisions: the airways and the parenchyma (the functional part of an organ). Within the lung parenchyma, adults have approximately 300 million alveoli. Each alveolus is between 200 and 300 microns in diameter. Small pulmonary capillaries that provide perfusion to the alveoli cover about 85% to 90% of the alveolar surface area. The alveolar sacs originate from a single terminal bronchiole referred to as a *primary lobule*. There are about 130,000 primary lobules in the lung, each containing 2000 alveoli. Capillary blood and alveolar gas are separated by vascular endothelium, interstitial space, and alveolar epithelium. Gas exchange occurs via diffusion across the alveolocapillary membrane encompassing the alveolar sacs (**Figure 53–11**).

The alveolar epithelium is composed of two principal cell types: type I and type II cells. **Type I cells** are the structural squamous pneumocytes that cover 90% to 95% of the alveolar surface. They are the major sites of alveolar gas exchange. Their thickness ranges from 0.1 to 0.5 microns. **Type II cells** cover the remaining 5% to 10% of the alveolar surface. Small and cuboidal in shape, they are the primary source of surfactant production. Surfactant helps to inflate the alveoli and prevent collapse by reducing the surface tension of the air–fluid interface within the alveoli.

Adjacent alveoli communicate through connections called the **pores of Kohn** and **channels of Lambert**. Alveolar macrophages, or type III cells, play a defensive role by removing bacteria from the acini or lung units. The interstitium (the space between cells) contains a gel-like substance made up of acid molecules that are contained in two major compartments: tight space and loose space. Collagen (a connective tissue protein) surrounds the interstitium and is believed to limit the alveolar distention beyond hazardous limits. Tight space is the area in the alveoli between the alveolar epithelium and the pulmonary capillary endothelium. Loose space surrounds the bronchioles, respiratory bronchi, alveolar ducts, and alveolar sacs.

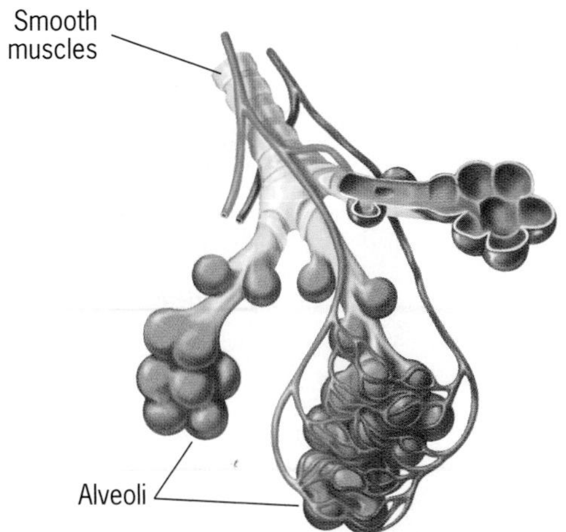

FIGURE 53–11 The terminal bronchioles, alveolar ducts, alveolar sacs, and alveoli that make up the acinus. These intrapulmonary structures are directly associated with gas exchange.

The lungs and their covering, the pleura, also are well endowed with lymphatic circulation and lymph nodes. The open-ended lymphatic vessels are found superficially around the lungs just beneath the visceral pleura. The primary function of the lymphatic vessels is to remove excess fluid and protein molecules that leak from the capillaries. Lymphatic drainage also allows lungs to defend against bacteria or foreign products and helps achieve homeostasis in the lungs. The lymphatic vessels exit the lungs at the hilum, and lymph (i.e., a clear or milky fluid called chyle) drains away from the lung toward the mediastinal lymph nodes. The mediastinal nodes are the storage sites for lymph fluid, which eventually returns to the circulatory system via the thoracic duct.

Blood Supply to the Lungs

The lungs are well perfused, receiving nearly all of the cardiac output. The pulmonary arteries originate from the right ventricle and deliver deoxygenated blood to the lungs and the visceral pleura. These are the only arteries in the human body that carry deoxygenated blood. (Remember that arteries carry blood away from the heart, whereas veins carry blood toward the heart.) Unlike the systemic arteries, the pulmonary arteries operate at low pressures. Consequently, pulmonary arteries are less muscular, with a lower resistance to blood flow and a higher compliance, than systemic arteries.

Control of Breathing

Respiratory centers in the midbrain control ventilation in response to emotional, physical, and chemical changes or stimuli. Muscles of respiration are controlled via the motor nerves that arise from the spinal cord at C3–C5. The partitioning of a tidal breath between inspiration and expiration is controlled primarily by the medulla oblongata and the pons. The medulla, the primary control center, is composed of ventral and dorsal respiratory groups where inspiratory and expiratory neurons are intermingled; there are no discrete inspiratory or expiratory centers. The pons is above the medulla in the brain stem and contains the pneumotaxic and apneustic centers. The pneumotaxic center coordinates the fine tuning of respiratory cycle timing. The apneustic center prevents apneusis—prolonged inspiratory efforts interrupted by expiratory gasps.

Changes in $Paco_2$ and pH, metabolic changes, stress, or hypoxia influence the breathing centers. Chemoreceptors within the medulla oblongata respond to changes in pH primarily. Cerebral spinal fluid (CSF) bathes the midbrain; the pH of CSF is readily affected by CO_2 levels because CO_2 diffuses quickly into the CSF. Other chemoreceptors that are more sensitive to Po_2 are located in the carotid bodies. Their sensory impulses respond via the glossopharyngeal nerve (cranial nerve IX) and vagus nerve (cranial nerve X). Baroreceptors located in the carotid arteries and aortic arch sense the stretching of vessels or blood pressure, which can elicit a *baroreflex,* that is, a feedback effect on vascular resistance to increase or decrease blood pressure.

Innervation of the Lungs

The nerve supply of the lung involves all the organ's components—the airways, parenchyma, and vasculature. The vagus nerves and the upper four to five thoracic sympathetic ganglia contribute fibers to nerves that supply the bronchi and veins. Adrenergic, primarily β_2-adrenergic, receptors are present on airway smooth muscles. Epinephrine released by the adrenal medulla and β_2-specific drugs may stimulate these receptors and cause bronchodilation. Parasympathetic innervation via the vagus nerve and parasympatholytic medications can also markedly affect bronchial muscle tone. The pulmonary vessels have both parasympathetic and sympathetic innervation, but vasomotor tone is influenced more by changes in the composition of alveolar gases (hypoxia and hypercapnia) than by stimulation of these nerves.

The lung contains a number of receptors associated with respiratory reflexes. These reflexes influence the way subjects control their ventilation. An extensive network of free nerve fiber endings called *C-fibers* are located in the conducting airways, blood vessels, and interstitial tissue between the pulmonary capillaries and alveolar wall. C-fibers located near the alveolar capillaries are called *J-type receptors* or *juxtapulmonary–capillary receptors.* An example of J-receptor response is rapid shallow breathing in response to pulmonary congestion, pulmonary edema, lung deflation, or chemical inhalation injury.

RESPIRATORY RECAP

Innervation of the Lungs

» Parasympathetic (cholinergic)
» Sympathetic (adrenergic)

Other reflexes that influence breathing response are as follows.

- *Herring Breuer (inflation) reflex.* A response generated from the visceral pleura and the walls of the bronchi and bronchioles when overinflation occurs.
- *Irritant reflex.* Inhalation of noxious gases or accumulated mucus secretions causes a vagal response. Such responses include an increased respiratory rate, coughing, sneezing, and bronchoconstriction.
- *Peripheral proprioceptor reflex.* When muscles, tendons, joints, and pain receptors are stimulated, that triggers a neural impulse to the medulla, which affects respiration.
- *Hypothalamic control.* Emotional triggers can activate sympathetic centers in the hypothalamus, which can alter respiration.
- *Cortical controls.* Breathing patterns can, of course, be controlled voluntarily.

A minor reflex is yawning. Most people yawn when they are tired or bored, but the stimulus for yawning is unknown.

Pleurae

Each lung is covered with a lining, the visceral pleura, whereas the chest wall is lined by the parietal pleura. The visceral pleura covers the surface of the lungs, extending into the fissures between the lobes. On the medial surface of the lung, the visceral pleura is reflected onto the mediastinum to become part of the parietal pleura. Thus, the pleurae isolate the right and left lungs from the heart, which sits within its own container, the **pericardium**. Ciliated mesothelial cells line both pleurae.

Between the two pleurae is the **pleural space** (**Figure 53–12**), a cavity containing a small amount of thin fluid (<20 mL) that has a low protein concentration. Regulation of the fluid volume within the pleural space involves balancing of leakage from systemic and pulmonary capillaries and drainage by lymphatic vessels located in the pleurae. The lymphatic vessels involved in reabsorption of fluid have a relatively high capacity of approximately 700 mL per day. The fluid in the pleural space is vital in allowing frictionless sliding between the visceral and parietal pleurae and maintaining a tight

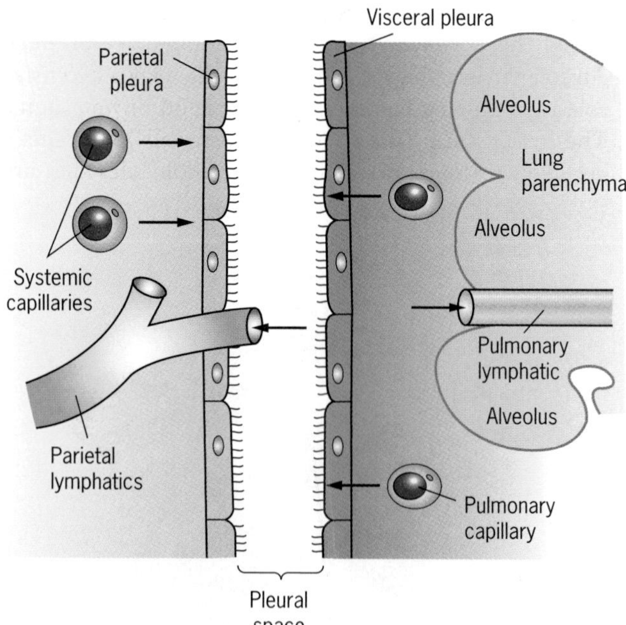

FIGURE 53–12 Diagram of the structures making up the pleurae and the pleural space. The pleurae are lined with mesothelial cells containing microvilli that face the pleural space. The arrows denote the direction for filtration and reabsorption of pleural fluid. This fluid emanates from capillaries and is predominantly reabsorbed by the lymphatics.

junction between the lungs and chest wall. An analogy is a drop of water between two glass slides. The water allows the slides to be moved slightly, but separation of the slides is difficult. In addition, the opposing mechanical forces between the lungs and chest wall—the lungs tending to collapse and the chest wall tending to expand—helps ensure a negative pressure (below atmospheric pressure) within the pleural space. Intrapleural pressure was first measured through placement of a catheter within the pleural space. Intrapleural pressure is currently estimated through measurement of the pressure in the lower esophagus using an esophageal balloon.

Innervation of the visceral pleura is by the vagus nerve, whereas intercostal and phrenic nerves supply the parietal pleura. Importantly, irritation of the visceral pleura does not result in pain sensation because it has no nerves of general sensation, whereas the parietal pleura is extremely sensitive to irritation. Severe pain that may be referred to the root of the neck and over the shoulder occurs in pleurisy as sensed in the parietal pleura.

> **RESPIRATORY RECAP**
>
> **Pleurae**
>
> » Visceral pleura
> » Parietal pleura
> » Pleural space

The mediastinum is the area between the two pleural sacs and is divided into superior and inferior as well as anterior, middle, and posterior regions. All structures within the thorax except the lungs and pleurae are located in the mediastinum. The superior mediastinum contains the thymus, great vessels associated with the heart, esophagus, trachea, and thoracic duct, and numerous nerves, including the vagus and esophageal plexus. Within the other regions are located the heart (within the pericardium), main bronchi, great vessels, phrenic nerves, and portions of the thymus and esophagus.

Microanatomy of the Respiratory System

The main function of the lung is to provide adequate gas exchange. The following sections describe the microanatomy of the respiratory system as it relates to maintaining a balanced ventilation-perfusion relationship while providing normal mucus transport to remove debris and particles from the airways.

Mucociliary Clearance

As air moves in and out of the lungs, gas exchange in the alveoli maintains adequate homeostasis in the body. While a normal tidal volume is approximately 500 mL, ventilation of between 12,000 and 24,000 liters of air per day can expose the lungs to damaging agents, including pollutants, viruses and bacteria, and organic agents such as antigens. Responses to foreign body inhalation can lead to respiratory compromise. The body reacts to these exposures by coughing, sneezing, bronchoconstriction, and increasing mucus production to expel or avoid damaging effects from these inhaled agents.

The primary defense mechanism within the conducting airways is the bed of pseudostratified ciliated columnar epithelium that lines the airways and serves as an escalator of mucus from the lungs (**Figure 53–13**). Goblet cells secrete mucus, which catches the inhaled debris. The trachea contains both ciliated and nonciliated epithelial cells as the proportion of ciliated cells increases down the bronchi. Immediately bathing the epithelial cells is a watery fluid (sol) where the cilia beat, on top of which sits a mucous (gel) layer. In the bronchioles are also cuboidal cells and secretory Clara cells. Under the ciliated cell bed is a layer of fibroblasts, nerves, lymphatics, and smooth muscle cells extending from the nose to the bronchioles. The ratio of ciliated cells to goblet

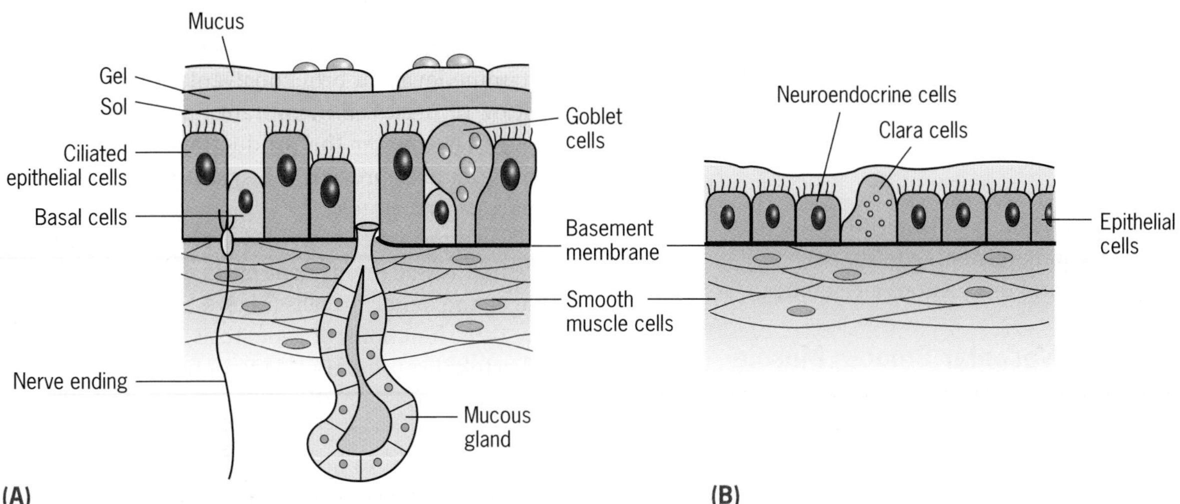

FIGURE 53–13 Cells that contribute to the mucociliary clearance apparatus in (**A**) large and (**B**) small airways. Basal cells are thought to be stem or progenitor cells that give rise to epithelial and goblet cells when the epithelium is damaged.

cells is about 4:1. Each ciliated cell contains about 200 to 250 cilia, with each cilium in the trachea having a length of about 6 μm and a diameter of about 2 μm. Ciliary beat frequency is between 1000 and 1500 per minute, with faster rates in larger airways. Boluses of mucus that move in a rhythmical fashion upward will lead to expulsion from the airway to be, most often, swallowed.

It is important for the **mucociliary apparatus** to maintain a fluid homeostasis. Dehydration prevents the ability of patients to adequately produce secretions. The volume of expelled tracheobronchial secretions in a normal subject has been estimated to be between 10 and 100 mL/day. Smoking and other lung conditions impede the function of the mucociliary apparatus yet stimulate the production of secretions. The viscosity of mucosal secretions is mainly attributed to mucoglycoproteins.

RESPIRATORY RECAP

Mucociliary Apparatus

» Contains a mucous layer
» Contains cilia that move the mucous layer

Many factors and conditions adversely affect mucociliary transport and clearance. One significant disease process known to impair ciliary transport is bronchiectasis. Cystic fibrosis (CF) is the most prevalent lung disorder associated with bronchiectasis; severe CF can be life threatening. Although CF is caused by chloride channel transport malfunction, increasing production of mucus, altered mucus properties, and impaired ciliary function as well as digestive problems are characteristic of CF. Another lung condition that often has an impaired mucociliary apparatus is status asthmaticus—asthma that does not respond to treatment. Mucous plugging of airways due to severe bronchoconstriction during status asthmaticus can be lethal.

The paranasal sinuses (air cavities in the maxillae, frontal sphenoid, and ethmoid bones) are lined with ciliated epithelium. When infections occur, mucus often drains from these sinuses into the nasal cavities. This postnasal drip can cause local irritation at the level of the larynx and is one of the common causes of a chronic cough.

General and specific medications that also can impair mucociliary clearance are as follows:

- Narcotics
- Ethyl alcohol
- Atropine
- Acetylsalicylic acid (aspirin)
- Beta-adrenergic antagonists
- Inhaled and intravenous anesthetics

Airway and Vascular Smooth Muscle

Both the airways and pulmonary vasculature are lined with smooth muscle cells. Smooth muscle control is involuntary. When smooth muscles contract, the cells become shorter and wider. When stimulated, airways, pulmonary vasculature, mast cells, and epithelial cells can alter smooth muscle tone.

Smooth muscle within the pulmonary vasculature, especially the pulmonary artery bed, is scarcer than that found in systemic arteries. Moreover, vascular tone in the pulmonary vessels is low, as are pressure and resistance compared with the systemic circulation. Smooth muscles direct blood flow within the lung parenchyma by changing the caliber of pulmonary vessels. Thus, factors that influence smooth muscle tone affect regional lung perfusion.

Chemicals that affect vascular tone are produced locally or metabolized by endothelial cells, nerves, and mast cells, or by other organs. Nerve endings within the pulmonary vasculature can release acetylcholine and norepinephrine. Finally, mast cells produce histamine and leukotrienes. Pulmonary vascular tone is potently affected by changes in surrounding gas concentrations and acid–base status. Thus, hypercapnia, a decrease in pH, and particularly hypoxia cause vascular vasoconstriction. Hypoxia acts directly on smooth muscle cells. The significance of changes in alveolar gases affecting pulmonary vasomotor tone is the need to match alveolar ventilation and perfusion and therefore maximize gas exchange.

Mast Cells, Dendritic Cells, and Macrophages

Mast cells range from 10 to 20 μm in diameter and may be oval or more irregularly shaped. They frequently are located in the respiratory mucosal surfaces and alveolar septa. A major feature of mast cells is the presence of abundant granules. Mediators released from mast cell granules are one of three classes: (1) granule-associated mediators, such as histamine and serotonin; (2) membrane-derived lipid mediators, such as leukotrienes; and (3) cytokines. In individuals with asthma, mast cell numbers in bronchial and alveolar tissue are elevated, as are protease and histamine levels in bronchoalveolar lavage fluid. Stabilization of mast cell membranes and administration of drugs that counter the production or activity of these mediators help prevent the symptoms manifested during an asthma attack.

RESPIRATORY RECAP

Mast Cells, Dendritic Cells, and Macrophages

» Mast cells: cells that release mediators
» Dendrites: antigen-presenting cells
» Macrophages: phagocytic cells

Two types of cell derived from bone marrow stem cells that reside in different parts of the lung are macrophages and dendritic cells (**Figure 53–14**). **Macrophages** have three functions: phagocytosis, antigen presentation, and cytokine production. Macrophages engulf and digest bacteria, viruses, or other foreign material (phagocytosis). Antigen presentation is the transfer and display of antigen "shapes" to other immune system cells that can launch an antibody response. Macrophages also produce cytokines, the most significant being interleukine-1 (IL-1) and tumor necrosis factor (TNF).

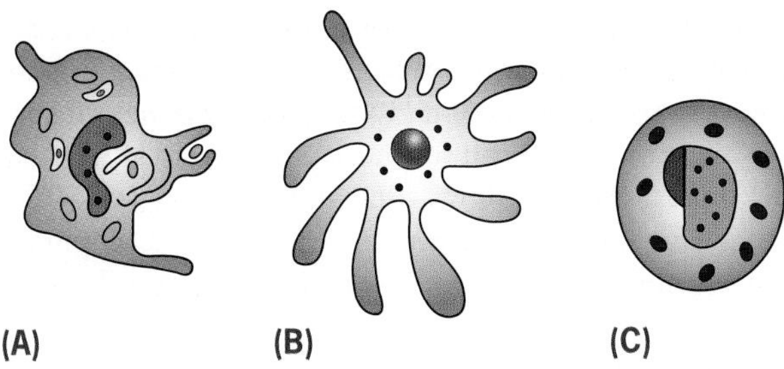

FIGURE 53–14 A schematic representation of an (**A**) alveolar macrophage, (**B**) dendritic cell, and (**C**) mast cell.

Dendritic cells are mobile cells with irregular shapes and long processes. Normally they are found in small numbers within the airway epithelium and lung parenchyma. Their major function in the lung is as antigen-presenting cells. When exposed to antigens, dendritic cells phagocytose antigens and process them, migrate to lung-draining lymph nodes, and present the antigens to T lymphocytes, thus activating T lymphocytes. If an individual is chronically exposed to inhaled irritants, the number of dendritic cells within the lung increases dramatically. Inhaled or systemically administered steroids reduce the number of dendritic cells within the lung.

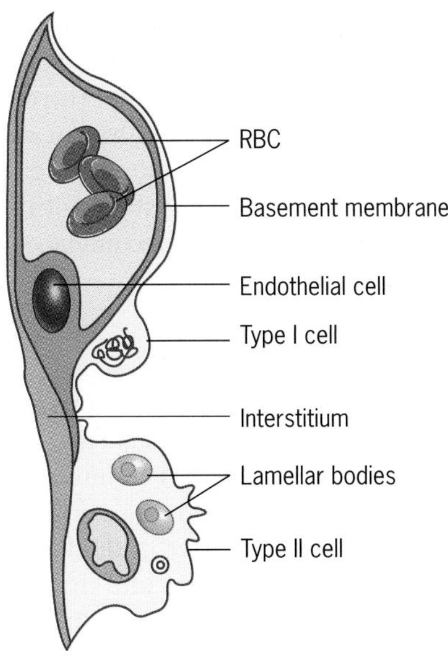

FIGURE 53–15 A schematic representation of the alveolocapillary complex showing the structural relationships between type I and type II cells and endothelial cells that make up the pulmonary capillaries. RBC, red blood cells (within the pulmonary capillary).

Alveolar Cells

As previously discussed, the most distal functional units of the lungs arising from bronchioles are the air sacs known as alveoli. There are millions of alveoli in each lung. The alveolocapillary division outlines two alveolar epithelial cells (type I and type II), a basement membrane, an interstitial space, and endothelial cells that make up the pulmonary capillaries that contain red blood cells (**Figure 53–15**).

Alveolar type I pneumocytes are the smallest, most abundant cells covering the alveoli. Type I pneumocytes are extremely flat and cover about 95% of the alveolar surface. Type I cells have a mean thickness of approximately 0.1–0.5 μm. Gases move easily across these cells' walls. Type I cells are sensitive to injury, including high levels of O_2, bacteria, bleomycin, cyclophosphamide, and particulates.

> **RESPIRATORY RECAP**
>
> **Alveolar Cells**
>
> » Type I: cover greatest surface area
>
> » Type II: produce surfactant

Alveolar type II cells, or granular pneumocytes, are cube shaped and cover only 5% of the alveolar surface. They are located predominantly in corners of alveolar sacs and form tight junctions with type I cells, which helps impede the movement of excess fluid into the alveolar spaces. Type II cells exhibit a number of functions, including the production of surfactant, differentiation into type I cells when the latter have been damaged, and transport of sodium and water toward the endothelial cells and blood to help minimize fluid accumulation in the alveolar space.

Type II cells are larger and more irregularly shaped than type I cells. The surfactants produced by type II cells contain lipoproteins that coat the inner surface of the alveoli and lower the surface tension at end-expiration, preventing alveolar collapse. Pulmonary surfactant is composed of 90% phospholipids and 10% protein. The primary surface tension–lowering chemical in the pulmonary surfactant is phospholipid dipalmitoyl phosphatidylcholine (DPPC). DPPC contains hydrophobic (water-insoluble) and hydrophilic (water-soluble) substances. The average surface tension of the alveolus varies from 5 to 15 dynes/cm (small) to about 50 dynes/cm (large or fully distended alveolus). As the radius gets smaller, surface tension decreases. As the radius grows larger, surface tension increases. As the alveolar area decreases, the surfactant molecules are crowded together and begin to repel one another.

Absence of pulmonary surfactant can cause collapse of the alveoli, resulting in atelectasis. Pulmonary complications are often seen when there is a reduction in surfactant. Several conditions are associated with a deficiency in surfactant or type II cell instability:

- Infant respiratory distress in premature births
- Congenital surfactant deficiency
- Pulmonary alveolar proteinosis

The following safety factors within the alveolocapillary complex help prevent fluid accumulation within the alveoli:

- Tight junctions that exist between alveolar cells
- Transport of water from the alveolar spaces into the pulmonary vessels as hydrostatic pressure within the pulmonary vasculature is low

- Surfactant and its associated proteins, which help repel water
- An active defense system within the alveolar sacs that helps prevent injury to alveolar membranes, thus maintaining their structural integrity
- An extensive lymphatic system within the lung that helps drain fluid that accumulates within the interstitial space.

Interstitial Space

Broadly speaking, the pulmonary interstitium is the "space" between the alveolar epithelial and the endothelial cells lining the vasculature. The interstitium serves as mechanical support, containing various cell types associated with the maintenance of fluid balance in the lung. The interstitium is a continuum that pervades the entire lung, from the visceral pleura to the hilum, where it is connected to the mediastinum. Cells within the interstitium include fibroblasts, myofibroblasts, smooth muscle cells, pericytes, lymphatic endothelial cells, and inflammatory/immune cells such as lymphocytes, mast cells, and macrophages. Structural components that form the matrix within the interstitium include collagens, elastic fibers, proteoglycans, and fibronectin.

In pulmonary interstitial lung diseases there is a marked increase in the number of cells that reside in the interstitium, with an increase in its thickness. These components consist of elastin and collagen fibers, fibronectin, proteoglycans, and constituents of the epithelial and endothelial basement membranes. The scaffolding that forms the alveolar walls and septa consists primarily of collagen and elastin fibers. Collagen represents 15% to 20% of lung dry weight. Elastin fibers form a three-dimensional network that contributes to the elastic recoil characteristics of the lung. Although normally the adult lung features very little elastin turnover, the presence of elastases or a deficiency of α_1-antitrypsin can lead to considerable lung damage.

Functional Characteristics of the Respiratory System

The preceding sections have emphasized the structural characteristics of the lung, with some comments directed at function. This section uses the structural components of the lung at the gross anatomic and microanatomic levels to help understand the ways they contribute to (1) the system's mechanical characteristics, (2) the distribution of ventilation, and (3) gas exchange within the respiratory system.

Airflow into and from the Lungs

The major purpose of the lungs and the chest wall is to generate pressure gradients to allow air to flow into and from the lung. Before a breath is taken, no airflow exists; therefore, the pressure within the lung, or the alveolar pressure, is equal to atmospheric pressure. The atmospheric pressure can be considered a reference pressure and is designated as 0 cm H_2O. Within the pleural space the pressure is below atmospheric (e.g., –3 cm H_2O) due to the opposing forces of the lung and the chest wall. When the respiratory muscles contract, especially the diaphragm during normal breathing, the pleural pressure becomes more negative, the pressure within the alveoli becomes negative, and a pressure gradient is created between the atmosphere and the alveolar compartment. Driven by this pressure gradient, air will flow into the lungs. For air to leave the lungs, the pressure within the lung must become greater than atmospheric. With a relaxed diaphragm the passive elastic recoil of the lung generates a positive pressure within the lung that is greater than atmospheric pressure; consequently, air flows from the lung.

Pressures within the pleural space were measured originally by introduction of a catheter attached to a pressure transducer within the pleural space, but this technique led to the development of pneumothoraces (collapse of the lung). Currently, a catheter with a balloon on its end is introduced into the lower third of the esophagus, and the pressure measured thereby is used to approximate pleural pressure. A pressure transducer attached to a mouthpiece measures pressure at the mouth, reflecting alveolar pressure at end inspiration and/or end expiration.

Through evaluation of pleural pressure, alveolar pressure, volume changes, and airflow rate, mechanical characteristics of the respiratory system may be determined. A primary consideration is to measure the elastic recoil of the lung, chest wall, and the entire respiratory system. The elastic recoil is analogous to the transmural pressure, or the pressure within a structure minus that outside the structure. For example, the alveolar pressure minus the pleural pressure determines the transmural pressure across the lung (called the *transpulmonary pressure*). The transmural pressure across the chest wall is determined by subtraction of atmospheric pressure (which is assumed to be 0 cm H_2O) from the pleural pressure. Thus, the transmural pressure across the chest wall is equal to the pleural pressure. Finally, the transmural pressure across the entire respiratory system is equal to the alveolar pressure minus atmospheric pressure, or simply the alveolar pressure.

> **RESPIRATORY RECAP**
>
> **Mechanics of Breathing**
>
> » Resistance to flow through airways
>
> » Compliance of the lungs and chest wall

Physiologically, the greater the elastic recoil of the lung, the more work is needed by the respiratory muscles to stretch the lungs and the more rapidly and forcefully they tend to deflate. This increase in elastic recoil occurs in pulmonary fibrosis, decreased surfactant production, or congestive heart disease when more fluid than normal is contained within the pulmonary vasculature. The opposite occurs when the lung parenchyma have been destroyed, as in emphysema, where lack of elastin and collagen result in a reduction of lung elastic recoil.

Compliance and Resistance

Two mechanical parameters, compliance and resistance, can be calculated when the pressure, volume, and flow characteristics of the respiratory system are known. **Compliance** is determined by measuring the change in lung volume divided by the corresponding change in pressure. Because compliance is influenced by lung volume, another parameter can be calculated, the specific compliance, which is compliance as referenced to total lung volume.

Figure 53–16 shows the static pressure–volume curves for the lungs, chest wall, and respiratory system. The slope of the pressure–volume curve is compliance. Note that the pressure–volume curve is sigmoidal, or S-shaped. The compliance is low at both low and high lung volumes.

Aside from an evaluation of lung compliance, compliance may be determined for the chest wall and the entire respiratory system. In fact, the relationship between chest wall (Ccw), lung (CL), and total respiratory system (Crs) compliance may be calculated with the following formula:

$$\frac{1}{\text{Crs}} = \frac{1}{\text{C}_\text{L}} + \frac{1}{\text{Ccw}}$$

The **resistance** to airflow is associated primarily with the size and patency of the airways as well as the relative turbulence of airflow. Airway resistance (R) is inversely proportional to the fourth power of the radius. Thus, physiologic factors that decrease airway radius will markedly increase resistance. Such factors include allergens that cause constriction of airway smooth muscles, edema in the airway, excess mucus production, or tumors within or impinging on airways. In emphysema, airway resistance increases because the elastic fibers holding open the airways are weaker or destroyed. Thus, during normal breathing and especially during a forced expiratory maneuver, these airways can dynamically collapse.

Another factor that may increase airway resistance is turbulent flow. As airflow rate increases, turbulence increases, as does airway resistance. Thus, in contrast to the airway diameter effect on resistance, turbulence causes resistance to be higher in the nose, upper airways, and larger conducting tubes (trachea and bronchi) than in the smaller airways. Resistance elements in a common tube, such as the nose and larger airways, are in series and are additive. Consequently, as flow rate increases during exercise, turbulence and resistance increase to the point where breathing switches from the nose to the mouth. Flow in smaller airways is more laminar. Thus, in the smaller airways, turbulence does not play as prominent a role in increasing resistance. Furthermore, because smaller airways are arranged in parallel, the total resistance is equal to the sum of the inverse of the individual resistances.

Airway resistance is determined by dividing airway opening pressure minus alveolar pressure by the flow rate. In most measurements, airway resistance due to the nose is discounted. Also, resistance differs between inspiration and expiration; in fact, resting expiratory

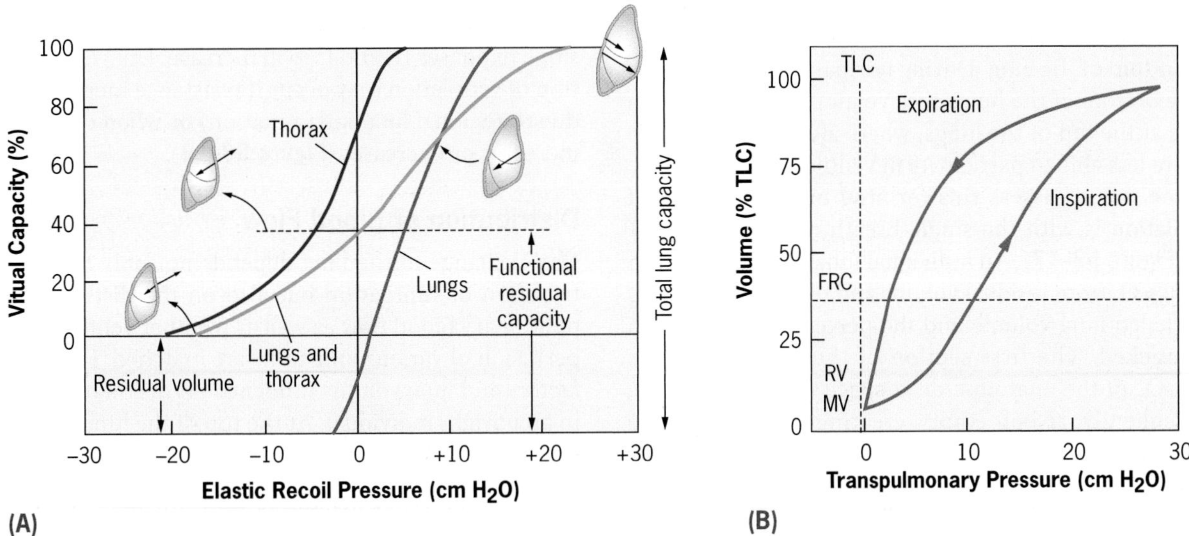

FIGURE 53–16 **(A)** Pressure–volume curves for the lungs, chest wall, and respiratory system. Note that the respiratory system curve is the sum of those for the lungs and the chest wall and that the respiratory system compliance is greatest at functional residual capacity (FRC). **(B)** Pressure–volume curve of the respiratory system. The difference between the inspiratory and expiratory curves represents hysteresis. TLC, total lung capacity; RV, residual volume; MV, minimum volume. **(A)** Modified from Beachey W. *Respiratory Care Anatomy and Physiology*. Mosby; 1998. **(B)** Modified from Berne RM, Levy MN. *Physiology*. 3rd ed. Mosby; 1993.

resistance exceeds inspiratory resistance, accounting for an efficient normal inspiration-to-expiration (I:E) ratio of 1:2.

The work of breathing is a small portion of total body O_2 consumption (1% to 3%). During quiet breathing in a healthy individual, most of the work is used to overcome the elastic recoil properties of the respiratory system associated with inspiration. Only 25% of the work of breathing is needed to counter the effects of airway resistance. Increasing ventilation during exercise increases both the elastic and the resistive components. In individuals with lung disease, work of breathing is markedly increased, assuming a greater proportion of total O_2 consumption that may contribute to the hypoxia and eventually hypercapnia caused by the lung disease.

Distribution of Ventilation

An inspired tidal volume is distributed to the conducting airways and alveoli. The volume of the conducting airways does not participate in gas exchange and is called **dead space volume**. Only the alveolar volume can participate in gas exchange. During disease some alveoli may be ventilated but not perfused. These alveoli contribute to dead space and are referred to as *alveolar dead space*. A pulmonary embolus is an example of a dead space producing disease. Alveolar dead space requires increases in minute ventilation to maintain constant alveolar ventilation.

For optimal gas exchange, ventilation must be distributed to match perfusion throughout the lungs. The distribution of ventilation may be uneven because of gravitational forces acting on the lung in the upright position. Thus, a pleural pressure gradient exists from the apex (top) to the base of the lung, with the pleural pressure being more negative at the apex than at the base. Therefore, transpulmonary pressure is greater at the top of the lung, where alveoli will be more open than those at the bottom of the lung. During normal breathing, alveoli at the bottom of the lungs receive more ventilation than those at the top of the lungs, where alveoli remain open but are less able to participate in ventilation.

One way to assess this (or any) maldistribution of ventilation is with the single-breath nitrogen washout test (**Figure 53–17**). An individual inhales a single breath of 100% O_2 from residual volume and then slowly exhales as exhaled lung volume and the percentage of nitrogen are tracked. The first section of the washout comes from O_2 in the anatomic dead space (phases I and II). Subsequently, alveoli empty, creating the stable phase III. Superimposed on this tracing are regular oscillations caused by rhythmic contraction of the heart that may help distribute gas within the alveoli. Finally, nitrogen from the alveoli at the very top of the lung empties, whereas the alveoli at the bottom of the lungs remain closed, known as phase IV, or the closing volume. As ventilation becomes more unequal due to respiratory diseases, such as chronic obstructive pulmonary disease (COPD), the

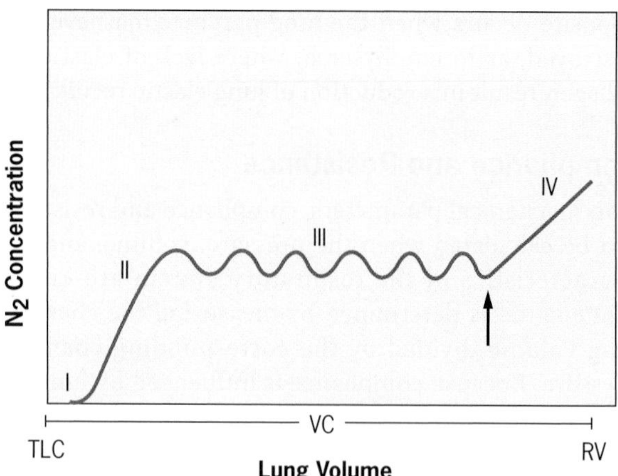

FIGURE 53–17 The components of the single-breath nitrogen washout test. Numbers I through IV represent different phases of the test. The arrow indicates the onset of the closing volume. TLC, total lung capacity; VC, vital capacity; RV, residual volume; N_2, nitrogen.

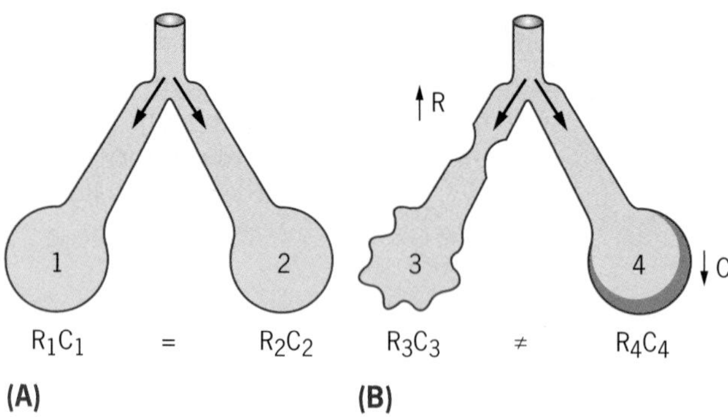

FIGURE 53–18 A diagrammatic representation of two lung units exhibiting (**A**) equal and (**B**) unequal resistance (R) and compliance (C) values. In lung A, airflow would be distributed equally to units 1 and 2. In lung B, distribution of airflow may be unequal due to increased resistance (3) or decreased compliance (4).

slope of phases III and IV will increase. Uneven distribution of ventilation may occur if resistance increases (e.g., due to regional lung inflammation) or when compliance increases or decreases (**Figure 53–18**).

Distribution of Blood Flow

Gas exchange in the lung depends not only on the distribution of ventilation but also on the distribution of pulmonary blood flow as well as whether ventilation and perfusion of various lung units are matched. Hydrostatic factors and lung volume influence perfusion of the lungs in an upright individual. At the top of the lungs, alveolar pressure is greater than pulmonary vascular pressure, resulting in no blood flow (dead space), called *West zone 1*. At the bottom of the lungs, pulmonary vascular pressure is greater than alveolar pressure, called *West zone 3*. In West zone 2, between zones 1 and 3, blood flow is determined by the difference between pulmonary vascular pressure and alveolar pressure. Thus, blood flow at the top of the lung is less than that at the bottom.

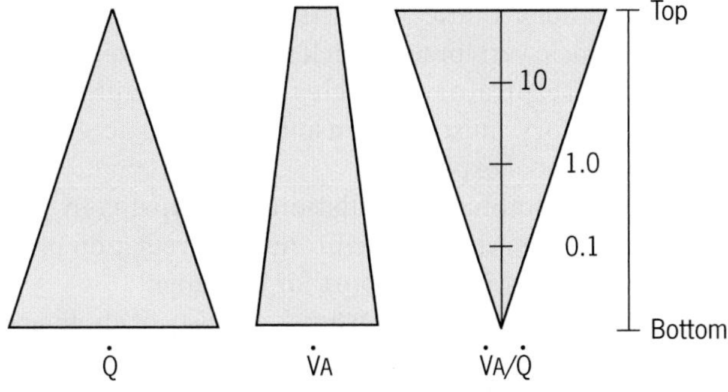

FIGURE 53–19 Ventilation-perfusion matching. A schematic representation of the relative distribution of perfusion (Q̇), alveolar ventilation (V̇A), and the ratio of V̇A/Q̇ throughout the lung of an upright individual breathing at functional residual capacity. Top denotes alveoli and capillaries in the hilar regions of the lung, and bottom denotes these structures at the base of the lung.

The lowest resistance to blood flow in the lung is at functional residual capacity (FRC)—resistance increases at either total lung capacity or residual volume. Thus, perfusion of the lung is markedly affected by ventilation, particularly positive pressure ventilation. In diseased areas of the lung that receive less ventilation, perfusion will become decreased as hypoxia causes constriction of vascular smooth muscles. The major purpose of this mechanism is to match ventilation to perfusion and optimize overall gas exchange.

Ventilation-Perfusion Ratio

The **ventilation-perfusion ratio** (V̇/Q̇) ideally should be nearly equal to ensure the most effective gas exchange (**Figure 53–19**). Overall V̇/Q̇ is normally 0.8, as alveolar ventilation is 4 L/min and cardiac output is 5 L/min. A healthy individual will have a vertical distribution of V̇/Q̇ ratios within the lung. Most lung units have a V̇/Q̇ close to 1. With shunt (perfusion without ventilation), the V̇/Q̇ is zero. At the opposite extreme (dead space), the V̇/Q̇ is infinity. In individuals with pathologic processes of the lung, the distribution of V̇/Q̇ exhibits more and more heterogeneity, leading to poor gas exchange. Arterial gas values in these individuals display hypoxemia and possibly hypercapnia. Anatomic abnormalities, fluid in the alveolar spaces, or atelectasis (collapse of lung units) can give rise to shunts. In these situations, blood bypasses the lung and no gas exchange occurs, adding greatly to arterial hypoxemia.

Normally, the alveolocapillary membrane is thin, devoid of excess fluid either in the interstitium or in the alveolar sacs, and patent. Factors that thicken the alveolocapillary complex (edema, fibrosis, or increased number of type II cells) increase the distance that O_2 needs to transverse, decreasing the gas exchange barrier for O_2 to cross. Transport of O_2 also is influenced by the O_2 gradient. The mixed venous partial pressure for oxygen ($P\bar{v}O_2$) is 40 mm Hg in a healthy young person at sea level, whereas alveolar PaO_2 is approximately 95 mm Hg. Thus, the PO_2 gradient across the lung is 55 mm Hg. As this gradient decreases, for instance, at high altitude (alveolar PO_2 being only 59 mm Hg in La Paz, Bolivia) or in the case of lung disease, less O_2 is likely to diffuse into the lung. In contrast to O_2, the high diffusibility of the lung for CO_2 (20 times the rate of O_2) necessitates only a partial pressure gradient of 5 mm Hg. Thus, in individuals with lung disease, hypoxemia generally occurs before hypercapnia.

RESPIRATORY RECAP

Ventilation-Perfusion Ratio
- » Ideal: 1.0
- » Normal: 0.8
- » Shunt: 0
- » Dead space: infinity

Oxygen Uptake and Diffusion Capacity

Another factor that influences gas exchange is the time that a red blood cell (RBC) needs to transit the pulmonary capillary. In a resting individual, the transit time for an RBC to travel through the pulmonary capillary is 0.75 second (**Figure 53–20**). As cardiac output increases during exercise, transit time may decrease to 0.25 second. In a healthy person this time is adequate for O_2 diffusion, but in a person with lung disease or living at a high altitude this decrease in time profoundly decreases O_2 diffusion across the lung and can lead to hypoxemia. Thus, exercise in an individual with lung disease and without additional inhaled O_2 can lead to marked dyspnea.

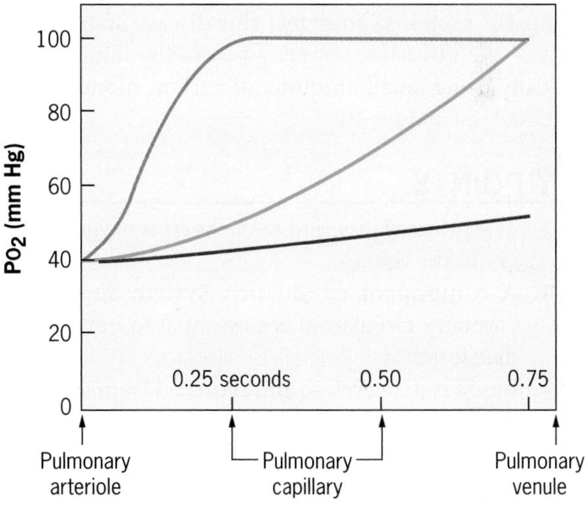

FIGURE 53–20 Changes in the partial pressure of oxygen (PO_2) of blood as it enters the pulmonary capillary from a pulmonary arteriole and reaches a pulmonary venule. The orange line represents increasing levels of PO_2 as blood transverses the capillary in an individual with a normal diffusion capacity. The green and red lines denote the effects of progressively poorer diffusion capabilities of individuals with lung disease on PO_2 levels in blood moving across the pulmonary capillary. At rest in a healthy individual living at sea level, the red blood cell transverses the pulmonary capillary by 0.75 second and picks up all the oxygen possible. This scenario is also true for the person with mild lung disease. But for the person with severe lung disease during exercise (arrow at 0.25 second), the effects of impaired diffusion capacities are magnified due to the decreased transit time.

The number and characteristics of RBCs influence gas exchange across the lung. The greater the number of RBCs, the more sites for gas exchange are available. Without RBCs, which contain hemoglobin (a molecule that can carry four O_2 molecules), the amount of O_2 in the blood would depend on the solubility of O_2 in plasma. The amount of dissolved O_2 in plasma at sea level is 0.003 mL/100 mL of blood per mm Hg of O_2. Thus, arterial blood contains 0.3 mL of O_2 for every 100 mL of blood. The amount of O_2 potentially bound to hemoglobin is about 20 mL for 100 mL of blood. The amount of O_2 bound to hemoglobin depends on the amount of hemoglobin present, the reactivity of O_2 with hemoglobin, and the percent saturation, which is related to the arterial Po_2 and the biochemical characteristics of the hemoglobin. For example, the biochemical characteristics of hemoglobin may be altered by genetic abnormalities (sickle cell anemia), exposure to carbon monoxide or drugs, hypoxemia (which elevates 2,3-diphosoglycerate levels in RBCs), and developmental changes (fetal to adult hemoglobin). In a normal person, 5 L of blood pass through the lung per minute, and the O_2 uptake is approximately 250 mL of O_2 per minute.

Some individuals with normal lung mechanics exhibit hypoxemia for another reason. Their lung tests may not indicate the presence of obstructive or restrictive disease. In this case there may be thickening of the alveolocapillary membrane that impairs gas exchange as a result of a number of possible causes presented earlier in the "Mast Cells, Dendritic Cells, and Macrophages" and "Interstitial Space" sections. To detect this disease state, evaluation of the **diffusion capacity** across the lung is done clinically using small amounts of carbon monoxide, as discussed in Chapter 10.

KEY POINTS

- The primary function of the heart is oxygen delivery to the tissues.
- A component conduction system and patent coronary circulation are essential to normal cardiac function.
- Blood is delivered to and returned from the heart within a network of arteries and veins.
- The primary function of the lungs is gas exchange.
- The upper airway consists of the nose, nasopharynx, oropharynx, laryngopharynx, and larynx.
- The lungs consist of the airways and alveoli.
- The bony thorax consists of the sternum, ribs, thoracic vertebrae, clavicles, and scapulae.
- The respiratory muscles are the diaphragm, accessory muscles of inspiration, and accessory muscles of expiration.
- The pulmonary circulation participates in gas exchange, whereas the bronchial circulation provides nutritional support for the lungs.
- The innervation of the lungs consists of cholinergic and adrenergic components.
- The visceral pleurae surround the lungs, and the parietal pleurae line the chest wall; the pleural space is between the visceral and parietal pleurae.
- The mediastinum is the area between the two pleural sacs and contains the heart, great vessels, esophagus, and thymus.
- The mucociliary apparatus clears inhaled agents from the lower respiratory tract.
- Important cells in the lower respiratory tract include mast cells, macrophages, and dendritic cells.
- The alveolus is composed of type I and type II cells.
- The interstitial space is located between the alveolar epithelia and the vascular endothelia.
- The mechanics of airflow into and from the lungs is influenced by resistance and compliance.
- The $\dot{V}/\dot{Q}$ ratio is normally 0.8 but can range in disease states from zero (shunt) to infinity (dead space).

SUGGESTED READING

Des Jardins T. *Cardiopulmonary Anatomy and Physiology: Essentials for Respiratory Care*. 5th ed. Clifton Park, NY: Delmar; 2008.

Huether S, McCrane K. *Understanding Pathophysiology*. 4th ed. St. Louis, MO: Mosby; 2004.

Loengenbaker S. *Understanding Human Anatomy and Physiology*. 6th ed. New York: McGraw Hill; 2008.

Murray JF. *The Normal Lung*. 2nd ed. Philadelphia: WB Saunders; 1986.

Netter FH. *Atlas of Human Anatomy*. 2nd ed. East Hanover, NJ: Novartis; 1997.

Scanlon V, Sander T. *Essentials of Anatomy and Physiology*. 5th ed. Philadelphia: FA Davis; 2007.

Schneeberger EE. Alveolar type I cells. In: Crystal RG, West JB, Barnes PJ, et al., eds. *The Lung: Scientific Foundations*. 2nd ed. New York: Raven Press; 1991:229–234.

Shier D, Butler JL, Lewis R. *Hole's Essentials of Human Anatomy and Physiology*. 9th ed. New York: McGraw Hill; 2006.

Standring S. *Gray's Anatomy: The Anatomical Basis of Clinical Practice*. 40th ed. New York: Elsevier Churchill Livingstone; 2008.

CHAPTER 54

Respiratory Pharmacology

Kelly Sioris
Kristin Engebretsen

OUTLINE

OBJECTIVES

1. Discuss the different routes of administration for medications.
2. Explain the principles of pharmacokinetics and pharmacodynamics.
3. Explain the mechanisms of action for drugs used to treat respiratory diseases.
4. Describe the drugs used for airway and ventilator management goals.
5. Describe types of drugs used in hemodynamic management.
6. Describe the mechanism of action of diuretics.

KEY TERMS

anticholinergic
antihistamine
anti-immunoglobulin E
benzodiazepine
corticosteroid
diuretic
inhalation
intramuscular (IM)
intraosseous (IO)
intravenous (IV)
leukotriene modifiers
long-acting β_2-agonist (LABA)
mast cell stabilizer
methylxanthine
neuromuscular blocking agent
opiate
parenteral
pharmacodynamics
pharmacokinetics
short-acting β_2-agonist (SABA)
subcutaneous (SQ)
vasopressor

INTRODUCTION

The list of medications that affect the respiratory system or treat respiratory diseases continues to expand significantly both in terms of new mechanisms of action and variety of dosage forms. It is important that healthcare professionals understand the epidemiology, pathophysiology, and pharmacologic treatments not only of asthma and chronic obstructive pulmonary disease (COPD) but also of other respiratory diseases. This chapter provides an overall review of the most important aspects of drug therapy facing respiratory therapists.

Routes of Delivery

Drugs may be delivered to a patient by five main routes: oral, inhalational, parenteral, transcutaneous, and intraosseous. Oral medications are not commonly used to treat respiratory diseases but are often prescribed for patients who cannot tolerate or do not respond to inhaled medications. In general, respiratory medications administered via **inhalation** have less adverse side effects than medications administered orally.

Most respiratory drugs are delivered through the inhalation route. The smaller the particle size of the drug, the more easily it is delivered to the lungs.[1,2] Inhalation is the only way to deliver some drugs, such as cromolyn sodium and tiotropium, and is the preferred method of acute drug delivery for β-agonists and chronic use of corticosteroids and β-agonists. Delivery of drugs via inhalation bypasses the need for gastrointestinal absorption, limits first-pass effects (a phenomenon in which the amount of drug delivered to the systemic circulation is significantly reduced secondary to the drug undergoing hepatic metabolism), and results in less adverse effects. Higher concentrations of drug can be delivered directly to the lung, while using smaller amounts and avoiding the general systemic circulation. Common devices used to deliver drugs by inhalation include pressurized metered dose inhalers (pMDIs), dry powder inhalers (DPIs), and nebulizers.

Intravenous (IV), **intramuscular (IM)**, and **subcutaneous (SQ)** drugs are used to treat respiratory diseases. These routes of delivery constitute **parenteral** delivery and are commonly used in severely ill patients who cannot tolerate oral or inhaled drugs. Parenteral routes tend to have a quicker onset of action but also lead to more systemic side effects than the inhaled route. IM and SQ medications are placed into muscle or tissue beds and still require absorption into the bloodstream. Absorption of drugs from the IM or SQ route varies depending on the drug. In general, the SQ route tends to be faster in onset than the IM route, but SQ is more limited in the volume that can be administered.[1]

RESPIRATORY RECAP

Routes of Drug Delivery

» Inhalational
» Oral
» Parenteral

Intraosseous (IO) delivery involves administration of medications directly into the bone marrow. This route is only used if IV access cannot be established or other parenteral routes of drug administration are not available. There are currently no resuscitation drugs for which IO administration is contraindicated.[3] The main concern regarding IO administration of medications is extravasation leading to necrosis and rare cases of osteomylitis.[3,4]

Principles of Pharmacotherapy

Pharmacokinetics

Understanding pharmacokinetics is required to be able to select and dose a respiratory medication appropriately. **Pharmacokinetics** is best described as the complex process that governs drug disposition—in other words, the effect the human body has on a given drug. The most important of these concepts are drug absorption, distribution, metabolism, and elimination. To further understand this process, we must first define these terms and other important pathophysiologic variables involved in the process.

Absorption is the process in which a drug transverses biological membranes and enters into the systemic circulation or target tissues. Bioavailability denotes the fraction of drug that reaches the systemic circulation. It takes into consideration the amount of drug that is absorbed and bypasses any first-pass elimination. Distribution occurs after absorption and delineates the transfer of drug within the body. Distribution of a drug throughout the body is not uniform and should generally be considered as existing in multiple compartments with varying concentrations instead of a single compartment with a steady-state concentration. Compartments may consist of blood, tissue, fat, organs, and so on. When a drug distributes to the tissues, blood, organs, and other parts of the body and exhibits different concentrations within these areas, the drug is considered to be multicompartmental.

Volume of distribution is a concept that may be difficult for students to comprehend. It is not an actual measured volume but a constant that relates the amount of drug in the body to the concentration of drug in the serum or plasma. It is the *theoretical* volume needed to contain the total amount of drug in the body and produce a particular concentration measured in the serum or plasma. In general, drugs with large volumes of distribution compartmentalize into tissues beyond serum or plasma.

RESPIRATORY RECAP

Pharmacokinetics

» Absorption
» Bioavailability
» Volume of distribution
» Clearance
» Half-life

Clearance is the body's way of eliminating a particular drug. This may encompass excreting the drug changed or unchanged in the urine or via metabolism through other organs in the body or by a combination of these processes. Clearance is directly affected by the degree of blood flow to those organs. It is considered the most important pharmacokinetic parameter, because it allows one to correlate the amount of drug in the body to a calculated steady-state serum concentration.[1]

Half-life ($T_{1/2}$) describes the amount of time it takes for the plasma drug concentration to decrease by 50%.

Dosing regimens in respiratory medications are frequently based on a drug's half-life. In first-order kinetics, drug concentration is cut in half after each half-life (that is, ½, ¼, ⅛, 1/16, and so on). Most respiratory medication dosing intervals are based on the order of one half-life. In general, a drug is considered eliminated from the body after approximately five half-lives.

When discussing how medications are eliminated from the body, different orders of kinetics are frequently cited. Zero-order kinetics defines a process in which the rate of drug elimination is constant. A constant amount of drug is eliminated from the body over time, and increasing the amount of drug in the body will not increase the amount of drug eliminated. Zero-order kinetics is independent of drug concentration. Theophylline is an example of a drug that may exhibit zero-order kinetics at higher doses. As the drug concentration increases, the body still eliminates it at a constant rate, thus increasing serum levels of the drug and causing toxicity. Alcohol may be used as another example to better understand zero-order kinetics. A person will metabolize alcohol at a constant rate, so when a person continues to consume alcohol, he or she becomes intoxicated because the body is not able to metabolize all of the alcohol. First-order kinetics depends on drug concentration. The greater the amount of drug in the body, the greater the rate of drug elimination. Most drugs follow first-order kinetics.

Saturation kinetics describes the process in which the enzyme pathways become saturated and can no longer increase elimination at the same rate as concentration increases. Thus, the drug changes from first-order kinetics to zero-order kinetics. Theophylline, as stated previously, is a good example of a drug that exhibits saturation kinetics. The drug is initially metabolized through first-order kinetics, but if the dose is increased and all of its elimination enzymes are saturated while metabolizing the drug, the drug turns to zero-order metabolism and serum theophylline levels will increase.

Pharmacodynamics

Whereas pharmacokinetics defines what the body does to a drug, **pharmacodynamics** describes what a drug does to the body. Potency describes how much drug is needed to cause an effect. Some drugs are more potent than others, meaning that less drug is needed to cause the same effect. This explains why drugs have different doses. A drug that causes an effect with a dose of 3 mg is more potent than a drug that requires a dose of 100 mg to cause the same effect.[5,6]

Most drugs produce their clinical effects by binding to receptors. Medications produce effects by either stimulating a receptor (agonists) or by blocking the receptor (antagonists). However, some drugs may weakly stimulate a receptor while preventing it from being more strongly stimulated by other agonists.[5,6] These agents are called partial agonists. **Table 54–1** lists receptors important in respiratory care pharmacology. β_2-Receptors are located in the lungs, pancreas, liver, and arteriolar smooth muscle. When stimulated, these receptors cause bronchodilation and vasodilation. β_1-Receptors are located in the heart and increase heart muscle contraction; β_1-blockers decrease cardiac contraction and are used in the treatment of hypertension. α-Receptors cause arteriolar smooth muscle contraction. Epinephrine has α, β_1, and β_2 effects. Isoproterenol has β_1 and β_2 effects. Inhaled bronchodilators such as albuterol have short-acting selective β_2 effects. The muscarinic receptors M_1, M_2, and M_3, which are located in bronchial tissue, cause bronchoconstriction when stimulated and bronchodilation when inhibited. The M_3 receptor also causes mucus secretion through its action on mucous glands.

RESPIRATORY RECAP

Receptors

- » β-Receptors
  - » β_1: heart
  - » β_2: lungs and blood vessels
- » α-Receptors: blood vessels
- » Muscarinic receptors: bronchial tissue

Pharmacologic Therapies

Anaphylaxis

Epinephrine is considered the first-line treatment for anaphylaxis. However, administration of fluids, antihistamines, β-agonists, and corticosteroids may be required in severe reactions. Epinephrine has both α- and β-adrenergic activity. α-adrenergic effects of epinephrine promote vasoconstriction both in the periphery and in the lung, decreasing capillary leakage. Epinephrine's β-adrenergic effects relax bronchial smooth muscle, increase heart rate and cardiac contractility, and inhibit further release of inflammatory mediators. Epinephrine 1:1000 should be administered at a dose of 0.01 mg/kg IM (maximum dose 0.5 mg in adults) into the anterolateral thigh muscle as soon as possible. Intramuscular dosing is preferred over subcutaneous dosing because IM dosing has been shown to have faster absorption and produce higher plasma epinephrine levels. Doses may be repeated every 15 to 20 minutes if no clinical signs of improvement are seen. Preloaded epinephrine syringes are available for patients in the outpatient setting and come in both junior and adult doses.

RESPIRATORY RECAP

Treatment of Anaphylaxis

- » Epinephrine
- » Antihistamines
- » Corticosteroids

Antihistamines are considered second-line agents to epinephrine and should never be given without epinephrine for anaphylaxis. Antihistamines are helpful in reducing allergic symptoms such as itching and angioedema. Studies have shown combination treatment with both an H_1 and H_2 antagonist to be more effective than with an H_1 antagonist alone.[7]

TABLE 54–1 Receptors Affecting Respiratory Function

Receptor	Type	Respiratory Effects	Heart and Vascular Effects	Other Effects
α_1	Adrenergic	Bronchoconstriction	Vasoconstriction	Bladder contraction, glycogenolysis, potassium release by the cells, platelet aggregation
α_2	Adrenergic		Vasoconstriction	
β_1	Adrenergic		Increased heart rate (chronotropy) and pumping force (inotropy)	
β_2	Adrenergic	Bronchodilation, increased edema clearance	Vasodilation	Sphincter relaxation, glycogenolysis, tremor
H_1	Histamine	Bronchoconstriction; increases secretions and airway edema by direct stimulation and by increasing vascular permeability		
H_2	Histamine	Possible bronchodilation (minimal)		Primary effects on gastric acid secretion
H_3	Histamine	Bronchoconstriction		
M_1	Cholinergic			
M_2	Cholinergic			
M_3	Cholinergic	Enhanced mucus production, bronchoconstriction		

Corticosteroids have a delayed onset of action of 4 to 6 hours, which is too long to make them effective as first-line agents for anaphylaxis. However, corticosteroids have made their way into the treatment algorithms for anaphylaxis as preventive agents for possible biphasic reactions, which may occur anywhere from 1 to 72 hours after the initial reaction. The effect of corticosteroids on altering the course of the biphasic reaction has not been determined.[8]

β-Agonists

β-agonists have been used for thousands of years, but more recently, selective β_2-agonist drugs have been developed for use in respiratory diseases due to the discovery of β_2-receptors in the lungs.[9] They are the most prescribed bronchodilator and are the most effective medication for bronchodilation.[9] β-agonists are available in the inhaled dosage form and have long-acting and short-acting formulations. Short-acting formulations are limited to use for rescue treatment. The short-acting β_2-agonists include albuterol, pirbuterol, and levalbuterol. Other short-acting β-agonists, such as metaproterenol and terbutaline, are nonselective in their pharmacologic action and are not used as often because of their associated side effects.

Short-acting β_2-agonists (SABAs) are most commonly used to treat asthma and COPD. They are also used before exercise to prevent exacerbations. The mechanism of action of the SABAs is bronchodilation through relaxation of the bronchial smooth muscle.[9] There has been controversy regarding the use of SABAs and their possible enhancement of disease progression. However, this risk has not been shown to be clinically significant, and the benefits of their use still far outweigh their risks.[9] All of the short-acting β_2-agonists have similar side effects.

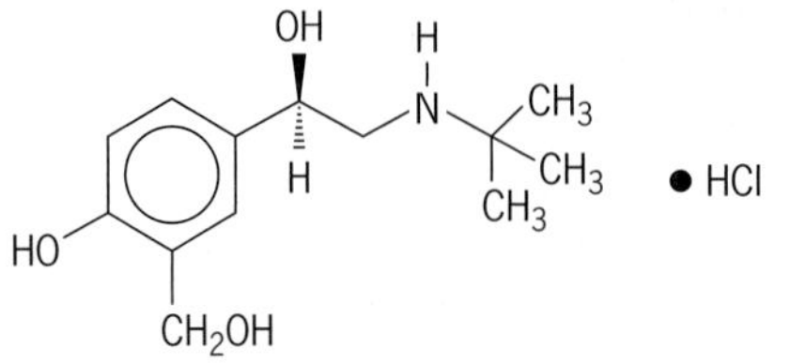

FIGURE 54–1 Albuterol structure.

Albuterol is currently the most commonly used SABA. Albuterol is a racemic mixture of the S- and R-enantiomers (**Figure 54–1**), whereas levalbuterol is only the R-enantiomer (**Figure 54–2**). The R-enantiomer is responsible for bronchodilation, but the effects of the S-enantiomer are still unknown.[10] It has been suggested that levalbuterol has more selectivity for the R-enantiomer and fewer side effects associated with its use, but the difference in side effect profiles of the two medications has not been shown to be clinically important in clinical trials. Levalbuterol is more expensive than albuterol. Albuterol's onset of action is approximately

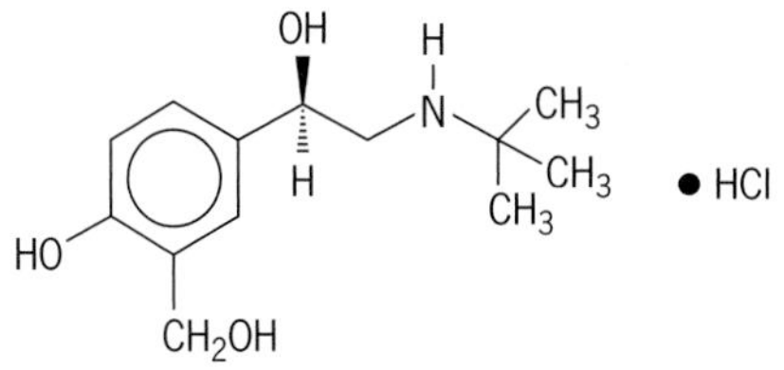

FIGURE 54–2 Levalbuterol structure.

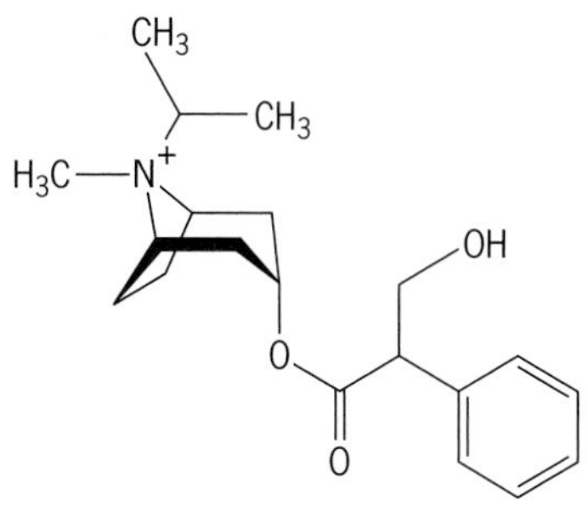

15 minutes, and it lasts for about 5 to 8 hours. The most common side effects from these drugs are palpitations, tachycardia, hypertension, and tremor.[9–12] Intravenous doses of SABAs are available for patients who do not respond to inhaled SABAs, but this route is rarely used. Albuterol dosing for the IV formulation is 0.2 to 0.4 mL (0.1–0.2 mg) infused slowly over at least 1 to 2 minutes.[9]

Long-acting β_2-agonists (LABAs) have multiple indications, including moderate to severe asthma and COPD, maintenance bronchodilation, and control of nocturnal symptoms.[9] LABAs include salmeterol and formoterol. They are more commonly used as maintenance therapy, since their duration of action is about 12 hours. Formoterol has an onset of action similar to that of the SABAs.[11] LABAs are not used as first-line therapy for asthma, but are prescribed adjunctively with steroids when steroid maintenance and SABA rescue therapy have not been effective. In steroid-naïve patients with mild to moderate persistent asthma, initiation of treatment with a LABA–steroid combination does not reduce the rate of exacerbations and does not reduce the use of SABAs as compared with those started on steroid therapy alone.[13] The combination improves lung function in regard to an increase in forced expiratory volume in 1 second (FEV_1) and increases the number of symptom-free days.[14]

Recent concerns regarding LABAs' ability to increase the risk of asthma-related mortality has limited the role of salmeterol to adjunctive treatment, but the evidence is not conclusive.[15] Formoterol is given with the corticosteroid budesonide as a DPI, and salmeterol is given with the corticosteroid fluticasone as a DPI or pMDI. The formoterol/budesonide maintenance dosing may be adjusted, whereas the salmeterol/fluticasone dosing is fixed. The two combination products are similar in their effects of preventing asthma symptoms and increasing lung function at fixed doses and in their use of rescue medications, but the formoterol–budesonide combination has been shown to reduce hospitalization rates compared with the salmeterol/fluticasone combination.[16–18] Other studies have found that salmeterol/fluticasone use results in more symptom-free days, a reduction in exacerbation rates, and a higher quality of life.[19,20]

Anticholinergics

Only two **anticholinergic** inhaled drugs are commonly used in the treatment of respiratory diseases: ipratropium and tiotropium. Ipratropium is a short-acting

FIGURE 54–3 Ipratropium structure.

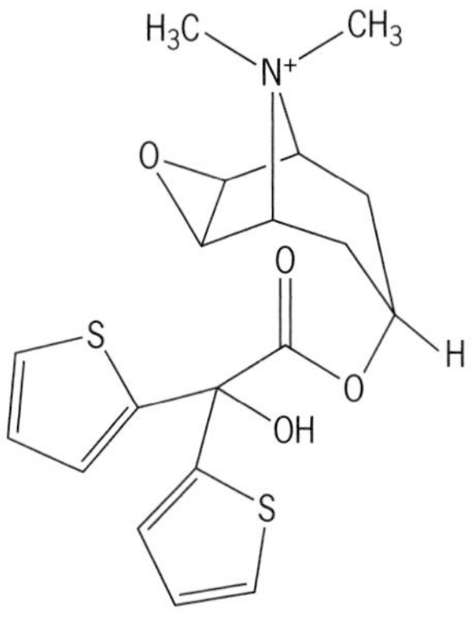

FIGURE 54–4 Tiotropium structure.

anticholinergic, whereas tiotropium is a long-acting anticholinergic.[21] Both are used for maintenance therapy in COPD, chronic bronchitis, and emphysema. These anticholinergic drugs exhibit their mechanism of action at the muscarinic receptors M_1, M_2, and M_3, which are located in bronchial tissue.[22] The receptors can stimulate bronchoconstriction, but when inhibited, they cause relaxation of the bronchial smooth muscle. The M_3 receptor also mediates mucus secretion through its location on mucous glands.[22]

Ipratropium (**Figure 54–3**) is a nonselective anticholinergic that blocks all of the muscarinic receptors equally.[23] Tiotropium (**Figure 54–4**) dissociates slowly at the M_1 and M_3 receptors, allowing for once-daily dosing. Because it dissociates quickly at the M_2 receptor, it may be of benefit in decreasing acetylcholine release.[24] Acetylcholine is the main component of the cholinergic system in the central nervous system (CNS), which causes excitability and bronchoconstriction. Ipratropium has a shorter duration of action and is dosed four times daily. It does not cross the blood–brain barrier, leading to fewer side effects associated with its use. Ipratropium is formulated as an MDI, and each dose

RESPIRATORY RECAP

Medications for Respiratory Disease

- β-Agonists
- Anticholinergics
- Corticosteroids
- Methylxanthines
- Leukotriene modifiers
- Mast cell stabilizers
- Magnesium
- Antimicrobials
- Secretion modifiers

delivers 42 μg of ipratropium to the lungs. The recommended initial dose for COPD is 2 inhalations four times daily. The maximum daily dose is 12 inhalations daily. Ipratropium is not typically recommended for use in asthma exacerbations, but is often used in emergency departments when symptoms do not fully resolve with a SABA and systemic steroid.[23] Combination therapy containing both albuterol and ipratropium may be found in an MDI formulation named Combivent and in the nebulizer solution DuoNeb.

Tiotropium has been shown to be more effective than salmeterol and ipratropium for decreasing exacerbations and hospitalizations in patients with moderate to severe COPD. However, it has not been shown to have a stronger effect on FEV_1.[22,24,25]

Corticosteroids

Corticosteroids are used for numerous respiratory diseases and are now considered a first-line treatment for asthma.[26] Although corticosteroids come in oral, IV, and inhaled dosage forms, the inhaled and IV routes of delivery are preferred for respiratory diseases. It has been shown that inhaled steroids reduce hospital admission rates of asthmatic patients.[27] They do no not cure the underlying disease, but are used for controlling inflammation.

Corticosteroids have a potent anti-inflammatory action by inhibiting cytokines and proinflammatory cells in the airway. They have also been shown to decrease mucus secretion. The most common side effects with inhaled corticosteroids are bruising, adrenal suppression, and decreased bone mineral density.[26] The most common side effects with parenteral steroids include osteoporosis, arterial hypertension, diabetes, obesity, cataracts, glaucoma, bruising, and muscle weakness.[28] Because of the severity of these side effects, it is recommended that oral and parenteral steroids not be used for long-term maintenance of asthma.

Inhaled corticosteroids have a wide margin of safety, but should be used with caution in children. Long-term use of inhaled corticosteroids may lead to growth suppression in children, especially with larger doses.[29] Other common side effects that may be seen include sore throat, hoarseness, and potential oral thrush (*Candida* infection). Patients should be advised to rinse their mouth after use and also to keep their inhaler mouthpiece clean to avoid thrush.

Corticosteroids are commonly used for maintenance treatment, but IV steroids in high doses are reserved for use in emergency departments for acute exacerbations.[30] Inhaled steroids are the most effective drugs for preventing asthma exacerbations.[26] Inhaled steroids are typically used for maintenance treatment in adults, but studies also have shown them to be effective in the acute setting with children.[31] Fewer adverse effects are associated with inhaled steroids than with steroids via oral or IV routes. Inhaled corticosteroids typically show benefits in adults at doses equivalent to 400 μg of budesonide daily. Dosing for pediatric patients is equivalent to about 100 to 200 μg of budesonide daily.[32] A study found that oral steroids are not effective in small children with upper respiratory infections.[33] Another study found that high-dose inhaled steroids had minimal benefit over placebo, but that the children treated with steroids had a smaller gain in height and weight than children treated with placebo.[34] Failure to control asthma exacerbations in patients on low-dose corticosteroids should prompt treatment with an alternative class of medication. However, in some cases of severe asthma, higher doses of corticosteroids may be of benefit.[27] Currently prescribed inhaled steroids include fluticasone, budesonide, beclomethasone, and mometasone.

Methylxanthines

Methylxanthines were commonly prescribed for treatment of asthma and other respiratory diseases; however, because of their inherent toxicity and the recent availability of safer and more effective options such as the inhaled bronchodilators and glucocorticoids, these drugs are not currently commonly prescribed.[26] The class of drugs known as methylxanthines consists of aminophylline, theophylline, and dyphylline. These agents are only available in the oral and IV routes. Although these drugs do have therapeutic benefits, their narrow therapeutic range, risks of toxicity, and side effects limit their therapeutic use. Methylxanthines produce direct relaxation of airway smooth muscle. Methylxanthines also have significant cardiac effects, leading to an increased potential for side effects that include tachycardia, palpitations, and arrhythmias. Toxicity from methylxanthines includes hypokalemia, tachycardia, dysrhythmias, and seizures.[35] Theophylline exhibits its anti-inflammatory effects by inhibiting cytokines and expression of inflammatory genes.

In pediatric patients, aminophylline has been shown to increase lung function as an additive therapy to β_2-agonists and glucocorticoids in acute exacerbations, but does not decrease symptoms, hospital length of stay, or the number of nebulized treatments.[36]

Leukotriene Modifiers

Leukotrienes are mediators of inflammation and stimulate bronchoconstriction, mucus production, mucosal edema and inflammation, eosinophil airway infiltration, and dendritic cell maturation that prepares for allergic response. Leukotriene inhibitors are not only involved in allergy and exercise asthma but also may be of benefit in treating asthma symptoms and improving lung function.

Leukotriene modifiers are the most recent class of asthma medications available in the oral tablet or chewable (montelukast) form. The antileukotrienes include montelukast, zafirlukast, and zileuton. They are dosed once or twice daily and have a wide margin of safety.[37] They are commonly prescribed for children with asthma, but also may be used in adults with asthma or allergic rhinitis.[37–39] Leukotriene modifiers are considered a second line to corticosteroids for the treatment of asthma. They are considered beneficial as add-on therapy in patients with moderate to severe asthma whose symptoms are not controlled with low- or high-dose corticosteroid treatment.[40,41] Leukotriene modifiers have been shown to cause bronchodilation, reduce coughing symptoms, improve lung function, and reduce airway inflammation and exacerbations. The most potent antileukotriene is zafirlukast. Both montelukast and zafirlukast are antagonists at the type 1 leukotriene receptor. Zileuton is a 5-lipoxygenase inhibitor. Zileuton may result in hepatoxicity, so liver enzyme levels should be monitored when this drug is used.

Mast Cell Stabilizers

Sodium cromoglycate (cromolyn) is a **mast cell stabilizer**. Although this drug has been available for many years, it is not commonly used in the treatment of asthma.[42] It is only for maintenance treatment and should not be used for acute asthma exacerbations. Corticosteroids have been shown to be much more effective in asthma than the mast cell stabilizers. If adverse side effects from inhaled corticosteroids are of concern, mast cell stabilizer treatment may be considered.[43] Mast cell stabilizers have been shown to improve asthma symptoms, bronchial responsiveness, and peak expiratory flow and to reduce infiltration of eosinophils into the bronchial mucosa.[44] Although the exact mechanism of action is unknown, cromolyn appears to stabilize mast cells and suppress inflammatory cells, including eosinophils.[45]

Anti-Immunoglobulin E

Omalizumab (Xolair) is currently the only drug in the **anti-immunoglobulin E** category available in the United States. It has been on the market since 2003. It is commonly used for the treatment of allergy-related asthma in patients with an elevated serum immunoglobulin E (IgE) level.[46,47] IgE has been found to play an important part in airway inflammation, obstruction, and hyperresponsiveness.[48] Omalizumab works by binding to IgE and preventing it from binding to its receptor. It has also been shown to inhibit production of proinflammatory cytokines, growth factor, and nitric oxide.[47] It is not recommended as a first-line therapy, but is indicated for patients with severe asthma who have not responded to combination steroid and β-agonist therapy. Omalizumab differs from other asthma medications in that it is delivered subcutaneously. The monthly dose is 0.016 mg/kg, with a maximum dose at each injection site of 150 mg. If the calculated dose exceeds 300 mg, it is recommended to divide the monthly dose by half, rounding to the nearest 75 mg and administering half of the dose at 2-week intervals.[47] Omalizumab is not recommended for patients weighing more than 150 kg due to its weight-based dosing and the maximum daily dose, but a study involving children above 150 kg showed that they had improvement of their asthma symptoms receiving the maximum daily dose.[49] It is not necessary to taper or gradually increase doses. It may take up to 4 weeks to see initial effects from omalizumab, and maximum benefit may not be seen for up to 16 weeks.

A black-box warning exists for omalizumab because of concern regarding anaphylaxis. Patients most likely to benefit from omalizumab include patients who have had emergency asthma treatment in the past year, use high-dose inhaled corticosteroids, and have an FEV_1 of 65% or less. Omalizumab is only indicated in patients who have an elevated serum IgE of 30 IU/mL or greater, and dosing should be based on the serum level. Serum IgE is not used as a monitoring parameter because serum IgE levels may still be elevated during treatment and remain elevated 1 year after treatment has been discontinued. Body weight should be monitored and dosing adjusted upon significant weight changes.

Magnesium

Intravenous magnesium was first recommended in 1923 for acute asthma exacerbations.[50] Although there is some controversy about whether magnesium actually changes outcome in these patients, it is fairly routine to see magnesium (2–4 g IV) used in the emergency department for severe asthma attacks. Magnesium is known to be a relaxant of smooth muscle. When given intravenously, peripheral vasodilation, systolic hypotension, flushing, nausea, and phlebitis at the infusion site can occur. Because of these adverse effects, studies have examined the use of inhalational administration of magnesium but have shown mixed results.[50] Inhaled isotonic magnesium sulfate is available as an adjuvant to albuterol in patients with severe asthma exacerbations but is rarely used. Inhaled magnesium with albuterol has shown no benefit over albuterol alone in patients with mild to moderate asthma exacerbations.[50]

Antimicrobial Therapy

The only antibiotics that may be administered in aerosolized form are amikacin, tobramycin, and colistin.[51] These agents are typically reserved for use in patients with cystic fibrosis or multidrug-resistant gram-negative pneumonia.[51] Tobramycin is the most commonly used antibiotic via inhalation. One ampule (300 mg) is administered by nebulizer twice daily.[52] Colistimethate is also administered by inhalation in serious multidrug-resistant gram-negative bacterial infections. It must be reconstituted from the injectable form for inhalation. After reconstitution, it is only good for 24 hours.[53]

Ribavirin is an antiviral agent for inhalation.[54,55] It is only recommended to be administered through a small-particle aerosol generator (SPAG). The recommendation is to administer continuous aerosolization for 12 to 18 hours per day for 3 to 7 days. Use of ribavirin has been shown to reduce total ventilator and hospital days but has not been proven to be cost-effective because of ribavirin's high price. Its effects on mortality, respiratory deterioration, and long-term pulmonary function are not clear, and more studies are needed.[56]

Amphotericin B is an antifungal medication that has been in use for many years. It is considered the gold-standard treatment for multiple fungal infections, but is specifically used for invasive aspergillosis (IA) infections. It comes in inhaled and parenteral dosage forms. The parenteral form is often used for treatment of fungal infections, whereas the inhaled dosage form is used more often for prophylaxis of IA in immunocompromised patients. The recommended dose for inhalation can range from 5 to 20 mg per inhalation session two to three times daily. There are few data on the efficacy of the inhaled dosage form of amphotericin B, but its use is still increasing.[57] Severe adverse effects may occur with injectable amphotericin B use, but those side effects have not been reported as frequently in patients taking the inhalation form. The most common adverse effects seen with the injectable form include abdominal pain, nausea, vomiting, diarrhea, chills, impaired renal function, and electrolyte imbalance. Amphotericin B has a narrow margin of safety and these adverse effects may be severe, which is why the inhaled dose form is preferred over the injectable form.

Pentamidine is an aerosolized antibiotic that has been a second-line treatment for the prophylaxis of *Pneumocystis carinii* pneumonia (PCP) in patients infected with the human immunodeficiency virus. Like amphotericin B, it also is available in a parenteral formulation, but the aerosolized formulation is used for prophylaxis. Although this medication is typically well tolerated by patients, cough and bronchospasm may occur during nebulization. If symptoms occur, they are treated with bronchodilators.

Although most antibiotics are not administered via inhalation, they are commonly prescribed for patients admitted to the hospital. Some patients are on antibiotics that cover multiple organisms (broad spectrum), whereas others are on antibiotics that cover only a few organisms (narrow spectrum). The most important antibiotics for a respiratory therapist to know about are those used to treat community-acquired pneumonia (CAP) or hospital-acquired pneumonia in the intensive care unit (ICU). Different organisms cause different types of pneumonia, so it is important to have the patient on the correct antibiotic.

Several categories of antibiotics exhibit similar mechanisms of action. **Table 54–2** shows the common classes of antibiotics and the most commonly prescribed agents. The most common antibiotics used for CAP are β-lactam antibiotics (specifically cefotaxime, ceftriaxone, or ampicillin/sulbactam) with azithromycin.

Secretion Modifiers

Abnormal volume or thickness (or both) of respiratory secretions is a hallmark of some pulmonary diseases, particularly cystic fibrosis and other forms of bronchiectasis. In fact, secretion clearance remains one of the truly challenging problems in pulmonary medicine. The anticholinergics reduce secretion volume but may thicken the secretions; antihistamines have a similar effect. These two classes of drugs have been effective in the treatment of cystic fibrosis, but unfortunately their use for other diseases, such as chronic bronchitis and pneumonia, has not produced definite benefit.

The antihistamines are commonly used to reduce the volume of secretions, especially upper airway secretions, associated with upper respiratory infections and allergies. Although they are effective in this role, they are rarely used for lower respiratory tract secretions. The most common indication for antihistamines in pulmonary medicine is the treatment of chronic cough caused by postnasal drip. The antihistamine diphenhydramine (Benadryl) has both H_1- and H_2-blocking activity. Its principal disadvantage is significant sedation. A new group of nonsedating antihistamines that includes cetirizine (Zyrtec), fexofenadine (Allegra), and loratadine (Claritin) is becoming quite popular. These drugs have selective activity for the H_1 receptor.

Use of anticholinergics as bronchodilators was discussed earlier in this chapter. Other anticholinergics occasionally are used to reduce secretions. They are most commonly used to facilitate procedures, although long-term use is a treatment for weakened patients who have difficulty with secretion control. Like ipratropium, atropine has bronchodilating properties but is more commonly used for its ability to reduce the volume of secretions by blocking the muscarinic M_3 receptors. This affects primarily the aqueous (watery) portion of the secretions. Consequently, secretions may thicken as their volume is reduced. Because atropine penetrates the central nervous system, it is associated with more of the typical anticholinergic side effects than ipratropium. Glycopyrrolate is similar to atropine in its effects and clinical use. The CNS side effects associated with glycopyrrolate are less severe than those of atropine. Scopolamine also has anticholinergic properties; it is used as a transdermal patch in patients with excessive oral secretions (sialorrhea).

N-acetyl-L-cysteine, commonly known as acetylcysteine, is the classic mucolytic agent. It is most commonly thought of as the antidote for an acetaminophen overdose. Acetylcysteine has been shown to reduce the viscosity of airway secretions by breaking the bonds between the sulfide compounds in the secretions. Inhaled acetylcysteine may cause bronchospasm.

TABLE 54–2 Common Antibiotics, Mechanisms, Spectra of Activity, and Toxicities

Class	Examples	Spectrum of Activity	Toxicity
Antibacterials			
Penicillins	Penicillin, amoxicillin, amoxicillin-clavulanate, piperacillin, ticarcillin, sulbactam, tazobactam	G+, G−, and anaerobic activities increasing with successive generations	Hypersensitivity, GI intolerance, hepatitis with prolonged use
Cephalosporins	First generation: cefazolin, cephalexin Second generation: cefuroxime, cefaclor, cefotetan Third generation: ceftriaxone, cefotaxime Fourth generation: ceftazidime, cefepime	Same as penicillins; third and fourth generation used against *Pseudomonas aeruginosa*	Rare cytopenias
Carbapenems	Imipenem, meropenem, ertapenem, doripenem	Broad G+, G−, anaerobic coverage	Seizure, GI intolerance, occasional cytopenias
Monobactams	Aztreonam	G−, anaerobic coverage	Similar to penicillins, except nephrotoxicity
Aminoglycosides	Gentamicin, tobramycin (TOBI), amikacin	G− rods	Nephrotoxicity, ototoxicity, rare paralysis; levels require monitoring
Tetracyclines	Tetracycline, doxycycline, minocycline	G+, atypicals	Tooth and bone defects, phototoxicity, GI intolerance, benign intracranial hypertension, mild hepatitis
Sulfonamides	Trimethoprim/sulfamethoxazole (TMP/SMX)	G+, G−, *Pneumocystis jiroveci, Nocardia*	Hypersensitivity, possible trigger of hemolysis in G6PD deficiency
Fluoroquinolones	Ciprofloxacin, levofloxacin, moxifloxacin, norfloxacin, clinafloxacin, gemifloxacin	G−, G+, atypical, TB/NTM	Not administered in children, except those with cystic fibrosis
Macrolides	Erythromycin, clarithromycin, azithromycin, roxithromycin, dirithromycin	G+, some G−; good atypical coverage, including *Legionella* species; TB/NTM	GI intolerance
Others	Vancomycin	G+, including MRSA; *Enterococcus faecalis* species; anaerobes	Hypotension and rash with infusion, ototoxicity, nephrotoxicity
	Metronidazole	Anaerobes, parasites	Ethanol intolerance, seizures, peripheral neuropathy
	Chloramphenicol	G+, many G−, anaerobes, rickettsiae	Aplastic anemia
	Clindamycin	G+ and anaerobes	*Clostridium difficile* colitis or diarrhea
	Linezolid	G+, including MRSA	Diarrhea, headache, nausea, thrombocytopenia
	Daptomycin	G+ only	Gastrointestinal adverse effects, headache, rash
	Tigecycline	G+, G−, anaerobes, MRSA and multidrug-resistant *Acinetobacter baumannii*	Diarrhea, nausea, vomiting
Antifungals			
Imidazoles	Miconazole, ketoconazole, clotrimazole, econazole	*Aspergillus, Blastomyces,* and *Histoplasma* species, onychomycosis	Hepatotoxicity
Triazoles	Fluconazole, itraconazole, ravuconazole, posaconazole, voriconazole	Yeasts, molds, and dimorphic fungi	Hypertension, hypokalemia, edema, headache and alterations in mental status are seldom observed; hepatotoxicity is rare
Polyenes	Amphotericin, natamycin, candicin, nystatin	Preferred for severe infections; nystatin for *Candida* infection only	Fever, rigors, hypotension with infusion, nephrotoxicity, hypersensitivity, hepatotoxicity, cytopenias
Allylamines	Terbinafine, amorolfine, naftifine, butenafine	Dermatomycoses (*Tinea pedis*)	Headache, rash, GI upset
Echinocandins	Anidulafungin, caspofungin, micafungin	*Candida* species, *Aspergillus, Blastomyces, Histoplasma*	
Antivirals			
	Acyclovir, famciclovir, valacyclovir	HSV, VZV, CMV	Headache, nausea
	Amantadine, rimantadine	Influenza A	Reversible neurotoxicity
	Ganciclovir, valacyclovir, famciclovir	CMV	Cytopenias, impaired male fertility
	Foscarnet	HSV, VZV, CMV, EBV	Nephrotoxicity in most patients, electrolyte abnormalities, seizures, anemia
	Ribavirin	RSV	Clogging of ventilator valves, bronchospasm, rash, hemolytic anemia
	Oseltamivir	Treatment and prevention of influenza A and B virus	Nausea, vomiting, diarrhea, abdominal pain, and headache
	Zanamivir (inhalation)	Treatment and prophylaxis of influenza A and B virus	Bronchospasm, psychiatric problems
	Peramivir	Hospitalized patients with known or suspected H1N1 influenza	Diarrhea, nausea, vomiting, leukopenia
Antituberculous			
	Rifampin, rifabutin	G+, G−, MTB, NTM	Flulike syndrome, hepatotoxicity
	Isoniazid (INH)	MTB	Hepatotoxicity, neurotoxicity, hypersensitivity
	Ethambutol (EMB)	MTB, NTM	Optic neuritis, peripheral neuropathy
	Pyrazinamide (PZA)	MTB	Hepatotoxicity, hyperuricemia
	Streptomycin	MTB, G−, NTM	Hypersensitivity, ototoxicity, neurotoxicity

G+, gram-positive bacteria; G−, gram-negative bacteria; GI, gastrointestinal; TB, tuberculosis; NTM, nontuberculous mycobacteria; G6PD, glucose-6-phosphate dehydrogenase; MRSA, methicillin-resistant *Staphylococcus aureus*; HSV, herpes simplex virus; VZV, varicella-zoster virus; CMV, cytomegalovirus; EBV, Epstein-Barr virus; RSV, respiratory syncytial virus; MTB, *Mycobacterium tuberculosis*.

Dornase alfa is commonly used in cystic fibrosis. This drug has theoretic value for other patients with purulent secretions (it is not effective against mucoid secretions because they lack significant amounts of DNA), but its efficacy has not been proven in diseases other than cystic fibrosis. Hypertonic saline (3% to 7%) is also used in patients with cystic fibrosis for airway clearance.

Drug Compatibility

Respiratory therapists may be asked to administer various aerosolized medications and are often faced with the challenge of the compatibility of these drugs when mixed together. A guide for aerosolized medications can be used to determine whether various drugs, when mixed together in a nebulizer, are compatible (**Figure 54–5**).

Drugs for Airway and Ventilator Management

Neuromuscular Blocking Agents

Neuromuscular blocking agents are used in intubation, during mechanical ventilation, and to help prevent increased intracranial pressure. They are typically divided into two categories: depolarizing and nondepolarizing agents. Depolarizing agents inhibit nicotinic cholinergic receptors, resulting in depolarization and muscle fasciculation, which lasts approximately 40 seconds until the muscles become flaccid and paralyzed. Succinylcholine is the only depolarizing agent currently used. Succinylcholine is contraindicated in patients with major burns or crush injuries (after 48 hours), severe abdominal sepsis, denervation syndromes, spinal cord injuries, malignant hyperthermia, or hyperkalemia.

The nondepolarizing agents are competitive antagonists at the nicotinic muscarinic receptor sites. Examples include vecuronium, rocuronium, pancuronium, and cisatracurium These drugs produce paralysis of all striated skeletal muscles, including the diaphragm and all accessory respiratory musculature. It is important to realize that neuromuscular blocking agents have minimal effect on smooth muscle, including bronchial smooth muscle, and that therefore the underlying disease exacerbation still needs to be treated. The most common adverse effect from these drugs is weakness, and patients may have prolonged weakness after the drug is discontinued, especially patients receiving vecuronium.[58] Finally, even though the patient's skeletal muscles are paralyzed, the patient will remain fully conscious. Therefore it is critical that an induction agent be used for anxiolytic and amnestic sedation prior to administration of the neuromuscular blocking agents.

Induction Agents

Etomidate is an ultra-short-acting nonbarbiturate hypnotic and is currently considered the preferred induction agent in rapid sequence intubation (RSI). It has a rapid onset of action, short duration of action, does not release histamine, and has unique advantages in patients prone to hemodynamic instability. Among all the induction agents, etomidate may have the best cardiovascular profile in patients with coronary artery disease, cardiomyopathy, cerebral vascular disease, or hypovolemia because it has the least effect on blood pressure and heart rate and decreases myocardial oxygen consumption without affecting coronary perfusion pressure.[59] The main adverse effects of etomidate include nausea and vomiting. However, even a single induction dose of etomidate will inhibit adrenal production of cortisol for up to 24 hours and inhibit the adrenocortical stress response.[60–62]

> **RESPIRATORY RECAP**
>
> **Drugs Used for Airway Management**
>
> » Neuromuscular blocking agents
> » Induction agents
> » Propofol
> » Dexmedetomidine
> » Opiates

Benzodiazepines have been used as induction agents and during mechanical ventilation for their amnestic and anxiolytic effects and are considered quite safe and effective. Midazolam is considered the benzodiazepine of choice as an inductive agent because it has the shortest onset of action. However, its time to onset of action is still 2 to 5 minutes, which may be too long if administered concomitantly with succincholine. This delay in onset does not allow for the patient to be adequately anesthetized prior to paralysis if midazolam is given immediately prior to succincholine.[62] For this reason, midazolam is considered second to etomidate as an induction agent.[60] There are many other benzodiazepines that may be used while a patient is mechanically ventilated. Long-acting benzodiazepines may be preferred because they require less dosing, but short-acting benzodiazepines may be preferred if the patient's neurologic status must be assessed periodically. The two most common benzodiazepines used for sedation in mechanically ventilated patients are midazolam and lorazepam. The concern regarding lorazepam is propylene glycol toxicity. Propylene glycol is the diluent for lorazepam. When large doses or prolonged infusions are used, accumulation of propylene glycol may cause metabolic acidosis or renal injury.

Delirium continues to be a concern regarding patients sedated in the ICU, especially in patients who require prolonged mechanical ventilation. Delirium has been associated with an increase in hospital stay, mortality, and hospital costs.[63] Up to 80% of patients experience delirium during their stay in the ICU. Studies have shown that benzodiazepines have been associated with more delirium and longer hospital stays compared with dexmedetomidine. Dexmedetomidine has been associated with less delirium, less time on a ventilator, and less tachycardia and hypertension.[63,64]

	Albuterol	Arformoterol[a]	Epinephrine[b]	Formoterol	Levalbuterol[c]	Metaproterenol[d]	Budesonide	Cromolyn[e]	Ipratropium	Acetylcysteine[f]	Colistimethate[g]	Tobramycin[h]	Sodium Chloride Solutions	Dornase Alfa
Albuterol		NI	NI	NI	NI	NI	C	C	C	NI	C	C	NI	X
Arformoterol	NI		NI	NI	NI	NI	C	NI	C	C	NI	NI	NI	X
Epinephrine	NI	NI		NI	NI	NI	NI	C	NI	NI	NI	NI	NI	X
Formoterol	NI	NI	NI		NI	NI	C	NI	NI	NI	NI	NI	NI	X
Levalbuterol	NI	NI	NI	NI		NI	C	C	C	NI	NI	NI	NI	X
Metaproterenol	NI	NI	NI	NI	NI		NI	C	C	NI	NI	NI	NI	X
Budesonide	C	C	NI	C	C	NI		C	C	C	NI	X	NI	X
Cromolyn	C	NI	C	NI	C	C	C		C	C	NI	X	NI	X
Ipratropium	C	C	NI	NI	C	C	C	C		C	NI	C	NI	X
Acetylcysteine	NI	C	NI	NI	NI	NI	C	C	C		C	NI	NI	X
Colistimethate	C	NI	NI	NI	NI	NI	NI	NI	NI	C		CD	NI	X
Tobramycin	C	NI	NI	NI	NI	NI	X	X	C	NI	CD		NI	X
Sodium Chloride Solutions	NI	NI	NI	NI	NI	NI	NI	NI	NI	NI	NI	NI		X
Dornase Alfa	X	X	X	X	X	X	X	X	X	X	X	X	X	

FIGURE 54–5 Compatibility guide for commonly used inhalation solutions and suspensions. Dark green shading with corresponding letter C indicates that there is evidence in the form of clinical studies confirming the stability and compatibility of the particular admixture. Light green shading with corresponding letter C indicates that there is evidence from manufacturers' reports confirming the stability and compatibility of a particular admixture; in many instances, these studies were unavailable for review and were confirmed either by reference in the package insert or direct communication with the manufacturer. Red shading with corresponding letter X indicates that there is evidence confirming or suggesting that a particular admixture is not compatible. Yellow shading with corresponding letters NI indicates that there is insufficient evidence to evaluate compatibility and should be avoided unless future evidence becomes available. Blue shading with corresponding letters CD indicates that there are conflicting data regarding compatibility of the combination. Consider the following information when determining the feasibility of preparing drug combinations for inhalation: (1) all admixtures should be prepared from formulations that do not contain preservatives; (2) the United States Pharmacopeia requirements state that the particle size of the delivered drug must be carefully controlled and the average diameter must be <5 μm; (3) physical and chemical compatibilities do not describe possible effects on aerodynamic behavior; (4) decreases in temperature can occur in certain nebulizers, and the effect of such decreases on compatibility has not been studied; (5) mixing solutions or suspensions increases total volume, and the relationship between the volume fill, total mass output, and inhaled mass of nebulized drug must be considered; and (6) if admixtures are to be stored, sterility issues must be addressed. References should be consulted to verify drug concentrations are compatible.

[a] No safety and efficacy studies available for admixtures of arformoterol with other drugs. Physical and chemical compatibility studies with acetylcysteine, ipratropium, budesonide, and tiotropium have indicated compatibility of concentrations studied.

[b] Epinephrine is readily destroyed by oxidizing agents or alkali (e.g., sodium bicarbonate, halogens, permanganates, chromates, nitrates, nitrites) and by salts of easily reducible metals (e.g., iron, copper, zinc).

[c] No safety and efficacy studies available for admixtures of levalbuterol with other drugs. Physical and chemical compatibility studies with budesonide, cromolyn, and ipratropium have indicated compatibility of concentrations studied.

[d] No safety and efficacy studies available for admixtures of metaproterenol with other drugs available from manufacturer.

[e] Compatibility of cromolyn with albuterol, fenoterol, metaproterenol, and terbutaline confirmed by manufacturer.

[f] Acetylcysteine has been reported to be compatible with netilmicin or betamethasone. The manufacturer reports that acetylcysteine is incompatible with amphotericin B, tetracyclines, erythromycin, or ampicillin. Also incompatible with any oxiding agent, iodized oil, trypsin, chymotrypsin, and hydrogen peroxide.

[g] Colistimethate sodium (available as an injectable formulation in the United States; dosage expressed in terms of colistin) is not approved for inhalation via a nebulizer. A case of acute respiratory failure and subsequent death of a cystic fibrosis patient who received premixed colistimethate sodium via nebulization has been reported. The prescribing information for a formulation available outside of the United States states that precipitation may occur in admixtures with other nebulized antibiotics.

[h] Tobramycin solution for oral inhalation should not be diluted or mixed with other drugs in the nebulizer. Based on protocols used in clinical studies evaluating tobramycin solution for oral inhalation in cystic fibrosis patients, it has been recommended that patients receive doses of inhaled bronchodilators first, then dornase alfa, then chest physiotherapy, and then tobramycin.

[i] Admixtures of albuterol, cromolyn, and ipratropium appear to be stable with ipratropium as the limiting component.

[j] Albuterol and ipratropium are available as a combination solution for nebulization.

[k] Albuterol containing benzalkonium chloride (1 mL) mixed with 1 mL colistin resulted in immediate cloudiness, which was believed to be due to interaction of benzalkonium chloride with colistin (effect on aerodynamics unknown). Colistin mixed with preservative-free unit-dose albuterol inhalation solution was chemically stable for one hour. No additional information available from manufacturer.

[l] Manufacturer of budesonide stated that cloudiness occurred in mixtures of budesonide with cromolyn, but information is not included in the prescribing information or corroborated by studies.[3]

[m] Prescribing information for ipratropium states that it should not be mixed with cromolyn because precipitation can occur. It has been reported that cromolyn mixed with ipratropium instantly produced cloudiness, which was attributed to the effect of an unknown excipient in the cromolyn formulation. The manufacturer attributed the cloudiness to benzalkonium chloride in the formulation. However, ipratropium mixed in a nebulizer with cromolyn sodium solution for oral inhalation also has been reported to be stable for one hour.

[n] Acetylcysteine sodium solution (10%) for oral inhalation and colistin 37.5 mg/mL have been reported to be compatible, with immediate use recommended.

Originally published in Burchett DK, Darko W, Zahra J, et al. Mixing and compatibility guide for commonly used aerosolized medications. *Am J Health-Syst Pharm.* 2010;67:227–230. (R1018)

Ketamine is a phencyclidine derivative and produces a unique anesthetic state different from those of etomidate or the benzodiazepines. It produces a rapid onset of sedation, with potent analgesic and amnestic effects. Ketamine is able to produce a dissociative state in which patients may be under complete sedation but look awake, exhibiting involuntary limb movements and having their eyes open. Ketamine has bronchodilatory effects, making it an excellent choice for patients exhibiting or at high risk for bronchoconstriction. Adverse effects of ketamine include increased mucus production, tachycardia, hypertension, and emergence phenomenon. The emergence phenomenon is characterized by terrifying dreams, fear, anxiety and the inability to calm or reassure the patient as he or she is awakening from the medication. This phenomenon tends to occur more in adults than in children and may be mitigated or lessened by calmly talking to patients and having them focus on a pleasant thought as the medication is administered and as they wake up. Ketamine is mostly used in the pediatric population. Midazolam and atropine had been used in combination with ketamine in the past, but more recently ketamine has been used alone, with midazolam administered only if an emergence phenomenon occurs.[65,66]

Propofol

Propofol is now the most commonly used parenteral anesthetic in the United States.[60] Propofol has an ultrashort onset of action and a short duration of action. Propofol has become popular because it can be used in the emergency department for short procedures without the need for intubation. Propofol can be used as an RSI agent and can maintain sedation in intubated patients in the ICU. The main disadvantages of propofol include its lipid formulation, which can cause hyperlipidemia and is susceptible to bacterial contamination. Propofol contains both egg and soy products; therefore, it should be avoided in patients with these food allergies. Major adverse effects of propofol include hypotension, bradycardia, and respiratory depression; these effects are dose related. Small boluses can be given approximately every 5 minutes for short procedures. An infusion is better if longer-term anesthetic maintenance is desired. Infusion rates should be titrated to patient response. Prolonged maintenance at high doses is not recommended because of concern about propofol infusion syndrome, which may result in metabolic acidosis, hypotension, cardiovascular dysrhythmias and collapse, rhabdomyolysis, hyperlipidemia, and hypertriglyceridemia.[67]

Dexmedetomidine

Dexmedetomidine is a sedative, anesthetic, and analgesic medication that is known for the cooperative state of sedation it produces, in which patients are still able to communicate and interact with healthcare providers.[68] Dexmedetomidine is used in the ICU in patients who are in need of sedation without respiratory depression. Dexmedetomidine is a short-acting α_2-agonist that decreases norepinephrine release into the presynapse of neurons, therefore decreasing the intensity of CNS excitation. Dexmedetomidine should be avoided in patients who are dependent on an adrenergic response to maintain vascular tone. The mechanism of action of dexmedetomidine is very similar to that of clonidine. Therefore, the most common side effects of dexmedetomidine are hypotension and bradycardia. These effects are dose dependent and not as prominent with smaller doses.[69] A study found that dexmedetomidine reduced ventilation time and delirium compared with midazolam.[65] Although expensive, this drug may be considered cost-effective because it decreases the overall amount of time spent in the ICU.

Opiates

Opiates are potent medications prescribed for analgesia. They have mild anxiolytic effects but do not have amnestic effects. Therefore, if an opioid is used in RSI, it is usually used in combination with a benzodiazepine. Opiates are divided into two classifications—natural or synthetic derivates of morphine—and exhibit their effect by stimulating the mu, delta, and kappa receptors in the brain and spinal cord. Fentanyl is the most commonly used opioid in management of the airway and mechanical ventilation because of its short onset of action and tendency to produce less histamine release and less hypotension than other opiates. Although the opiate class of medication may be extremely beneficial in pain management, opiates may also induce respiratory depression, resulting in hypoventilation, apnea, and potentially death. Naloxone is the antidote for opiate overdose and should be administered immediately if respiratory depression from an opiate is suspected.[70,71]

Diuretics

Diuretics stimulate urine flow and commonly are used in the ICU to promote loss of excess body water and salt. There are five classes of diuretics: thiazides, loop, potassium-sparing, osmotics, and carbonic anhydrase inhibitors. Diuretics are indicated for multiple disease states, the most common being hypertension, heart failure, renal failure, and pulmonary edema. Each class of diuretics exhibits its own mechanism of action on different parts of the kidney (**Figure 54–6**).

> **RESPIRATORY RECAP**
>
> **Classes of Diuretics**
> » Thiazides
> » Loop
> » Potassium-sparing
> » Osmotic diuretics
> » Carbonic anhydrase inhibitors

The most common class of diuretics used in an ICU is the loop diuretics, which include furosemide, torsemide, and bumetanide. They act by inhibiting sodium, potassium, and calcium reabsorption in the loop of Henle in the kidney, thereby causing their excretion. Bumetanide is the most potent loop diuretic and furosemide the least potent.

The second most commonly prescribed class of diuretics is the thiazide diuretics, which include chlorothiazide, hydrochlorothiazide, chlorthalidone, and metolazone. These medications inhibit the sodium chloride transport in the distal convoluted tubule, thus enhancing excretion of sodium. The thiazide diuretics also enhance reabsorption of calcium. All of the thiazide diuretics are available in oral dosage forms, but chlorothiazide is the only one available in the parenteral dosage form.

Another class of diuretics is the potassium-sparing diuretics, which include triamterene, spironolactone, amiloride, and eplerenone. They can be classified into two groups as aldosterone antagonists (spironolactone, eplerenone) and sodium channel blockers (triamterene and amiloride). The aldosterone antagonists competitively inhibit the binding of aldosterone to mineralocorticoid receptors. The sodium channel blockers inhibit sodium reabsorption in the collecting tubules of the kidney. Potassium levels should consistently be monitored for hyperkalemia while patients are on these medications.

Mannitol is the most commonly prescribed osmotic diuretic. It blocks water transport in the proximal tubule, hence blocking the descending limb of the loop of Henle. Doses higher than 200 g per day are not recommended because they can cause acute renal failure.

The last class of diuretics is the carbonic anhydrase inhibitors. These medications include acetazolamide and dorzolamide, but dorzolamide is only available as an ophthalmic solution. Carbonic anhydrase is an enzyme that breaks down carbon dioxide and water into bicarbonate and hydrogen. By blocking this enzyme, the amount of bicarbonate is decreased and there is an increase in excretion of water.

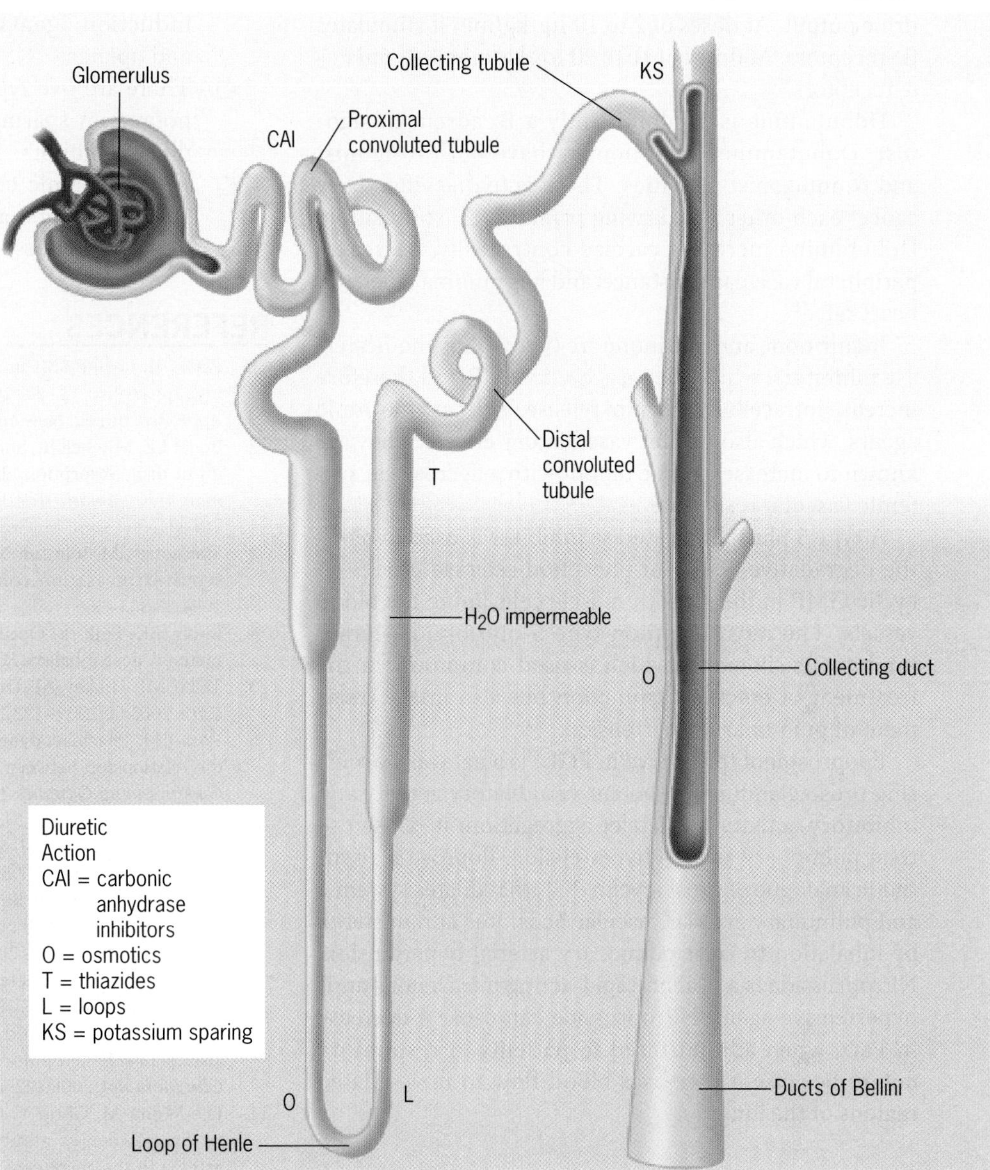

FIGURE 54–6 Overview of renal function and diuretic activity.

Hemodynamic Control

Vasopressors are a group of medications that exhibit vasoconstriction on the blood vessels, causing an increase in mean arterial pressure. The most commonly used vasopressors are epinephrine, norepinephrine, and vasopressin. These medications all work at the adrenergic receptors (refer to Table 54–1).

> **RESPIRATORY RECAP**
>
> **Hemodynamic Control**
>
> » Vasopressors
> » Dopamine
> » Dobutamine
> » Phosphodiesterase inhibitors
> » Prostacyclin
> » Nitroprusside

Dopamine is another medication that is commonly used for hemodynamic control. Its action is dose dependent. At doses of 0.5 to 2 μg/kg/min, the drug stimulates dopamine receptors, which cause vasodilation in renal vessels, increasing blood flow to the kidney and increasing urine output. At doses of 2 to 10 μg/kg/min it stimulates β_1-receptors. At doses of 10 to 20 μg/kg/min it stimulates α-receptors.[72]

Dobutamine is predominantly a B_1 adrenegic agonist. Dobutamine's enantiomers have both α-agonist and α-antagonist activities. These activities effectively cancel each other out, leaving primarily B_1 stimulation. Dobutamine increases cardiac contractility, decreases peripheral vascular resistance, and has minimal effect on heart rate.[72]

Inamrinone and milrinone are type 3 phosphodiesterase inhibitors, which increase cyclic AMP and therefore increase intracellular calcium release. They are inotropic agents, which also exhibit vasodilatory effects. They are known to increase cardiac output with a decrease in systemic vascular resistance.

A type 5 phosphodiesterase inhibitor is used to block the degradative action of phosphodiesterase type 5 on cyclic GMP in the smooth muscle cells lining the blood vessels. The most common type 5 phosphodiesterase inhibitor is sildenafil, which is used commonly in the treatment of erectile dysfunction but also in the treatment of pulmonary hypertension.

Epoprostenol (prostacyclin PGI_2) is a naturally occurring prostaglandin with potent vasodilatory activity and inhibitory activity of platelet aggregation; it is used to treat pulmonary arterial hypertension. Iloprost is a synthetic analogue of prostacyclin PGI_2 that dilates systemic and pulmonary arterial vascular beds. It is administered by inhalation to treat pulmonary arterial hypertension. Nitroprusside is a potent, rapid-acting intravenous antihypertensive agent. Nitroprusside can cause a decrease in Pao_2 when administered to patients in respiratory failure because it increases blood flow to unventilated regions of the lungs.

KEY POINTS

- Routes for administering medications include inhalation, oral, and parenteral.
- The inhalational route treats the lungs directly, incurring fewer systemic effects.
- Pharmacokinetics describes how the body handles a drug as influenced by absorption, bioavailability, distribution, volume of distribution, clearance, and half-life.
- Pharmacodynamics describes the effect of a medication on the body as determined by potency and receptor sites.
- Categories of therapeutic agents to treat the lungs include β-agonists, anticholinergics, corticosteroids, methylxanthines, leukotriene inhibitors, mast cell stabilizers, anti-IgE, magnesium, nonsteroidal anti-inflammatory agents, antimicrobials, and secretion modifiers.
- Drugs used in airway and ventilator management include neuromuscular blocking agents, induction agents, propofol, dexmedetomidine, and opiates.
- There are five types of diuretics: loop, thiazides, potassium-sparing, mannitol, and carbonic anhydrase inhibitors.
- Hemodynamic control drugs include vasopressors, dopamine and dobutamine, phosphodiesterase inhibitors, prostacyclin, and nitroprusside.

REFERENCES

1. Peters JI, Levine SM. Introduction to pulmonary function testing. In: DiPiro JT, ed. *Pharmacotherapy: A Pathophysiologic Approach*. 6th ed. New York: McGraw-Hill; 2005.
2. Benet LZ, Mitchell JR, Sheiner LB. Pharmacokinetics: the dynamics of drug absorption, distribution, and elimination. In: *Goodman and Gilman's The Pharmacological Basis of Therapeutics*. 9th ed. New York: McGraw-Hill; 1996.
3. Simmons CM, Johnson NE, Perkin RM, Van Stralen D. Intraosseous extravasation complication reports. *Ann Emerg Med*. 1994;23:363–366.
4. Rubin BK, Fink JB. Optimizing aerosol delivery by pressurized metered-dose inhalers. *Respir Care*. 2005;50:1191–1200.
5. Telko MJ, Hickey AJ. Dry powder inhaler formulation. *Respir Care*. 2005;50:1209–1227.
6. Ross EM. Pharmacodynamics: mechanisms of drug action and the relationship between drug and concentration and effect. In: *Goodman and Gilman's The Pharmacological Basis of Therapeutics*. 9th ed. New York: McGraw-Hill; 1996.
7. Liberman DB, Teach SJ. Management of anaphylaxis in children. *Pediatr Emerg Care*. 2008;24:861–867.
8. Tole JW, Lieberman P. Biphasic anaphylaxis: review of incidence, clinical predictors, and observation recommendations. *Immunol Allergy Clin North Am*. 2007;27:309–326.
9. Op't Holt TB. Inhaled beta agonists. *Respir Care*. 2007;52:820–832.
10. Tripp K, McVicar WK, Nair P, et al. A cumulative dose study of levalbuterol and racemic albuterol administered by hydrofluoroalkane-134a metered-dose inhaler in asthmatic subjects. *J Allergy Clin Immunol*. 2008;122:544–549.
11. Lee-Wong M, Chou V, Ogawa Y. Formoterol fumarate inhalation powder vs albuterol nebulizer for the treatment of asthma in the acute care setting. *Ann Allergy Asthma Immunol*. 2008;100:146–152.
12. Blake K, Madabushi R, Derendorf H, Lima J. Population pharmacodynamic model of bronchodilator response to inhaled albuterol in children and adults with asthma. *Chest*. 2008;134:981–989.
13. Camargo CA Jr, Spooner CH, Rowe BH. Continuous versus intermittent beta-agonists for acute asthma. *Cochrane Database Syst Rev*. 2003;4:CD001115.
14. Ni Chroinin M, Greenstone IR, Ducharne FM. Addition of inhaled long-acting beta2-agonists to inhaled steroids as first line therapy for persistent asthma in steroid-naïve adults. *Cochrane Database Syst Rev*. 2008;3:CD005307.
15. Nelson SH, Weiss ST, Bleecker ER, et al. The Salmeterol Multicenter Asthma Research Trial: a comparison of usual pharmacotherapy for asthma or usual pharmacotherapy plus salmeterol. *Chest*. 2006;129:15–26.
16. Fitzgerald JM, Boulet LP, Follows RM. The CONCEPT trial: a 1-year, multicenter, randomized, double-blind, double-dummy comparison of a stable dosing regimen of salmeterol/fluticasone propionate with an adjustable maintenance dosing regimen of formoterol/budesonide in adults with persistent asthma. *Clin Ther*. 2005;27:393–406.
17. Blais L, Beauchesne MF, Forget A. Acute care among asthma patients using budesonide/formoterol or fluticasone propionate/salmeterol. *Respir Med*. 2009;103:237–243.

18. Bousquet J, Boulet LP, Peters MJ, et al. Budesonide/formoterol for maintenance and relief in uncontrolled asthma vs. high-dose salmeterol/fluticasone. *Respir Med.* 2007;101:2437–2446.
19. Boonsawat W, Goryachkina L, Jacques L, Frith L. Combined salmeterol/fluticasone propionate versus fluticasone propionate alone in mild asthma: a placebo-controlled comparison. *Clin Drug Invest.* 2008;28:101–111.
20. Price DB, Williams AE, Yoxall S. Salmeterol/fluticasone stable-dose treatment compared with formoterol/budesonide adjustable maintenance dosing: impact on health-related quality of life. *Respir Res.* 2007;8:46.
21. Drescher GS, Carnathan BJ, Imus S, Colice GL. Incorporating tiotropium into a respiratory therapist-directed bronchodilator protocol for managing in-patients with COPD exacerbations decreases bronchodilator costs. *Respir Care.* 2008;53:1678–1684.
22. Barr RG, Bourbeau J, Camargo CA, Ram FS. Tiotropium: for stable chronic obstructive pulmonary disease: a meta-analysis. *Thorax.* 2006;61:854–862.
23. Wellington K. Ipratropium bromide HFA. *Treat Respir Med.* 2005;4:215–220.
24. Keam SJ, Keating GM. Tiotropium bromide: a review of its use as maintenance therapy in patients with COPD. *Treat Respir Med.* 2004;3:247–268.
25. Barr RG, Bourbeau J, Camargo CA, Ram FSF. Tiotropium for stable chronic obstructive pulmonary disease. *Cochrane Database Syst Rev.* 2005;2:CD002876.
26. Bateman ED, Hurd SS, Barnes PJ, et al. Global strategy for asthma management and prevention: GINA executive summary. *Eur Resp J.* 2008;31:143–178.
27. Edmonds ML, Camargo CA Jr, Pollack CV Jr, Rowe BH. Early use of inhaled corticosteroids in the emergency department treatment of acute asthma. *Cochrane Database Syst Rev.* 2003;3:CD002308.
28. O'Byrne PM. Acute asthma intervention: insights from the STAY study. *J Allergy Clin Immunol.* 2007;119:1332–1336.
29. Guevara JP, Ducharme FM, Keren R, et al. Inhaled corticosteroids versus sodium cromoglycate in children and adults with asthma. *Cochrane Database Syst Rev.* 2006;2:CD003558.
30. Starobin D, Bolotinsky L, Or J, et al. Efficacy of nebulized fluticasone propionate in adult patients admitted to the emergency department due to bronchial asthma attack. *Israel Med Assoc J.* 2008;10:568–571.
31. Sorkness CA, Lemanske RF, Mauger DT, et al. Long-term comparison of 3 controller regimens for mild-moderate persistent childhood asthma: the pediatric asthma controller trial. *J Allergy Clin Immunol.* 2007;119:64–72.
32. Pauwels RA, Pedersen S, Busse WW, et al. Early intervention with budesonide in mild persistent asthma: a randomized, double-blind trial. *Lancet.* 200;361:1071–1076.
33. Panickar J, Lakhanpaul M, Lambert PC, et al. Oral prednisolone for preschool children with acute virus-induced wheezing. *N Engl J Med.* 2009;360:331–338.
34. Ducharme FM, Lemire C, Noya FJ, et al. Preemptive use of high-dose fluticasone for virus-induced wheezing in young children. *N Engl J Med.* 2009;360:339–353.
35. Hoffman RJ. Methylxanthines and selective beta-2 adrenergic agonists. In: Flomenbaum N, et al., eds. *Goldfrank's Toxicologic Emergencies.* 8th ed. New York: McGraw-Hill; 2006.
36. Bassler MA, Lasserson WK, Ducharme FM. Intravenous aminophylline for acute severe asthma in children over two years receiving inhaled bronchodilators. *Cochrane Database Syst Rev.* 2005;2:CD001276.
37. Walia M, Lodha R, Kabra SK. Montelukast in pediatric asthma management. *Indian J Pediatr.* 2006;73:275–282.
38. Virchow JA, Bachert C. Efficacy and safety of montelukast in adults with asthma and allergic rhinitis. *Respir Med.* 2006;100:1952–1959.
39. Nayak A, Langdon RB. Montelukast in the treatment of allergic rhinitis: an evidence-based review. *Drugs.* 2007;67:887–901.
40. Ducharme FM, Schwartz Z, Kakuma R. Addition of anti-leukotriene agents to inhaled corticosteroids for chronic asthma. *Cochrane Database Syst Rev.* 2004;2:CD003133.
41. Ducharme FM, Di Salvio F. Anti-leukotriene agents compared to inhaled corticosteroids in the management of recurrent and/or chronic asthma in adults and children. *Cochrane Database Syst Rev.* 2004;2:CD002314.
42. Sridhar AV, McKean M. Nedocromil sodium for chronic asthma in children. *Cochrane Database Syst Rev.* 2006;3:CD004108.
43. Zielen S, Rose MA, Bez C, et al. Effectiveness of budesonide nebulising suspension compared to disodium cromoglycate in early childhood asthma. *Curr Med Res Opin.* 2006;22:367–373.
44. Yoshihara S, Kanno N, Yamada Y, et al. Effects of early intervention with inhaled sodium cromoglycate in childhood asthma. *Lung.* 2006;184:63–72.
45. Miyatake A, Fujita M, Nagasaka Y, et al. The new role of disodium cromoglycate in the treatment of adults with bronchial asthma. *Allergol Int.* 2007;56:231–239.
46. D'Amato G. Role of anti-IgE monoclonal antibody (omalizumab) in the treatment of bronchial asthma and allergic respiratory diseases. *Eur J Pharmacol.* 2006;533:302–307.
47. Hendeles L, Sorkness CA. Anti-immunoglobulin E therapy with omalizumab for asthma. *Ann Pharmacother.* 2007;41:1397–1410.
48. Hansen I, Klimek L, Mosges R, Hormann K. Mediators of inflammation in the early and the late phase of allergic rhinitis. *Curr Opin Allergy Clin Immunol.* 2004;4:159–163.
49. Kwong KY, Jones CA. Improvement of asthma control with omalizumab in 2 obese pediatric asthma patients. *Ann Allergy Asthma Immunol.* 2006;97:288–293.
50. Hughes R, Goldkorn A, Masoli M, et al. Use of isotonic nebulised magnesium sulphate as an adjuvant to salbutamol in treatment of severe asthma in adults: randomized placebo-controlled trial. *Lancet.* 2003;361:2114–2117.
51. O'Riordan TG. Inhaled antimicrobial therapy: from cystic fibrosis to the flu. *Respir Care.* 2000;45:836–845.
52. Chuchalin A, Csiszér E, Gyurkovics K, et al. A formulation of aerosolized tobramycin (Bramitob) in the treatment of patients with cystic fibrosis and pseudomonas aeruginosa: a double-blind, placebo-controlled, multicenter study. *Pediatric Drugs.* 2007;9(suppl 1):21–31.
53. Michalopoulos A, Fotakis D, Virtzili S, et al. Aerosolized colistin as adjunctive treatment of ventilator-associated pneumonia due to multidrug-resistant gram-negative bacteria: a prospective study. *Respir Med.* 2008;102:407–412.
54. Murata Y. Respiratory syncytial virus infection in adults. *Curr Opin Pulmonary Med.* 2008;14:235–240.
55. Checchia P. Identification and management of severe respiratory syncytial virus. *Am J Health Sys Pharm.* 2008;65(23 suppl 8):S7–S12.
56. Ventre K, Randolph A. Ribavirin for respiratory syncytial virus infection of the lower respiratory tract in infants and young children. *Cochrane Database Syst Rev.* 2007;1:CD000181.
57. Mohammad RA, Klein KC. Inhaled amphotericin B for prophylaxis against invasive aspergillus infections. *Ann Pharmacother.* 2006;40:2148–2154.
58. Murray MJ, Cowen J, DeBlock H, et al. Clinical practice guidelines for sustained neuromuscular blockade in the adult critically ill patient. *Crit Care Med.* 2002;30:142–156.
59. Holder A, Paladino L. Sedation. *Emedicine.* June 4, 2006.
60. Avers AS, Crowder CM, Balser JR. General anesthetics. In: *Goodman and Gilman's The Pharmacological Basis of Therapeutics.* 11th ed. New York: McGraw-Hill; 2006.
61. Wagner RL, White PF. Etomidate inhibits adrenocortical function in surgical patients. *Anesthesiology.* 1984;61:647–651.
62. Wagner RL, White PF, Kan PB, et al. Inhibition of adrenal steroidogenesis by the anesthetic etomidate. *N Engl J Med.* 1984;310:1415–1421.

63. Skrobik Y. Delirium prevention and treatment. *Crit Care Clin.* 2009;25:585–591.
64. Riker RR, Fraser GL. Altering intensive care sedation paradigms to improve patient outcomes. *Crit Care Clin.* 2009;25:527–538.
65. Wathen JE, Roback MG, Mackenzie T, et al. Does midazolam alter the clinical effects of intravenous ketamine sedation in children? A double-blind, randomized controlled emergency department trial. *Ann Emerg Med.* 2000;36:579–588.
66. Filandrinos D, Harris CR. Ketamine. In: Harris CR, ed. *Emergency Management of Selected Drugs of Abuse.* Dallas, TX: American College of Emergency Physicians; 2000.
67. Rajda C, Dereczyk D, Kunkel P. Propofol infusion syndrome. *J Trauma Nurs.* 2008;15:118–122.
68. Gerlach AT, Dasta JF. Dexmedetomidine: an updated review. *Ann Pharmacother.* 2007;41:245–254.
69. Carollos DS, Nossaman BD, Ramadhyani U. Dexmedetomidine: a review of clinical applications. *Curr Opin Anaesthesiol.* 2008;21:457–461.
70. Pattinson KT. Opioids and the control of respiration. *Br J Anaesthesia.* 2008;100(6):747–758.
71. Benyamin R, Trescot AM, Datta S, et al. Dexmedetomidine vs midazolam for sedation of critically ill. *Pain Physician.* 2008;11:S105–S120.
72. Kee VR. Hemodynamic pharmacology of intravenous vasopressors. *Crit Care Nurse.* 2003;23:79–82.

SECTION V

The Respiratory Care Profession

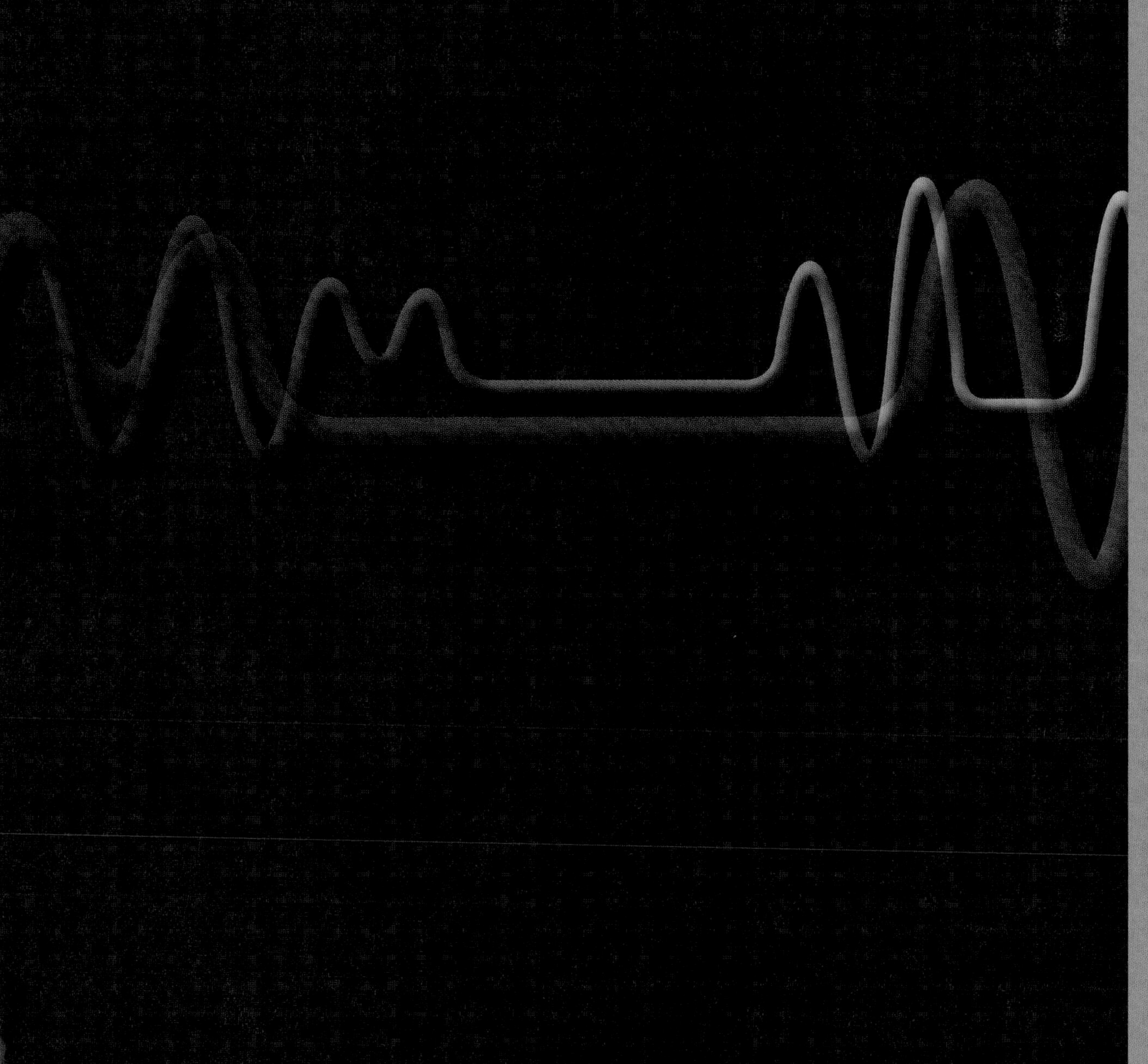

CHAPTER 55

History of the Respiratory Care Profession

Jeffrey J. Ward

OUTLINE

OBJECTIVES

1. Identify early philosophers, scientists, inventors, and physicians whose discoveries were important to the evolution of Western medicine.
2. Note key events and pioneers in the areas of medical gases, aerosol medications, airway care, resuscitation, and mechanical ventilation.
3. Trace the evolution of the professional, credentialing, and educational organizations involved in the infrastructure of the respiratory care profession.
4. Identify current major trends that are likely to shape the future of respiratory care.

INTRODUCTION

A historical review provides beginning respiratory care practitioners with a perspective on the evolution of both clinical practice and the related professional organizations. We are all travelers in history. An understanding of the past may allow an explanation for the present. It also can provide insight into what lies ahead. This chapter notes major events and trends that became important milestones. Behind these milestones are personal contributions. It would be impossible to note them all. However, respiratory care is a relatively young field. A few of the pioneers are still with us! Although the focus of this chapter is on respiratory care practice as it developed in North America, international connections will be placed in context. Events that occurred following World War II are highlighted. More comprehensive coverage is available both in books and on the Internet.[1–6]

Historical Events and Key Advances in Medical-Related Sciences

Respiratory care has its roots in a diverse history that includes the unraveling of key scientific concepts in chemistry, physics, biology, and pharmacology. A long list of pioneers allowed concurrent development of impressive technology, a medical infrastructure, and insights into the ethics, art, and science of clinical practice. **Table 55–1** summarizes major historical contributors to the background and clinical science related to respiratory care.

Ancient Times

The earliest records of practical medicine are from ancient Egypt and Mesopotamia, dating before 3000 BC. Their medicine was highly advanced for the time and included simple surgery, setting of bones, and an extensive pharmacy. Medical texts specified a rational, stepwise approach to diagnosis and treatments. These beliefs were synergistic with mysticism and religion. Egyptians developed a theory of channels that carried air, water, and blood to the body.

By 2000 BC the ancient Chinese had developed a part-philosophic and part-physiologic concept of breathing. They believed that what was breathed from the air was transmitted to the soul. They developed rituals for taking a pulse. They also practiced moxibustion, burning substances on the skin. Medicines included herbal teas, such as ephedra (ma huang, from the plant *Ephedra sinica*) for asthma and hay fever. The ancient Indian pharmacopeia had even more extensive antiasthma drugs, including ginger. The Bible's Old Testament records the story of the prophet Elisha's resuscitating a Shunammite child by relieving a tracheal obstruction (II Kings 4:34).[2–6] In early history, the East and Middle East were well ahead of the West in medical sciences and practice. About 430 BC the Sinhalese royalty (modern-day Sri Lanka) appeared to be the first governance to provide dedicated institutions for their sick.

A key part of Western medicine's scientific heritage began with the Greeks, who felt such knowledge had both altruistic and practical value. Pythagoras (580–489 BC) defined life's four elements as being earth, fire, water, and air. Hippocrates of Cos II (460–370 BC; **Figure 55–1**) is considered the father of medicine. He established medicine as a separate discipline, aligned with philosophy and science and incorporating professional attributes that continue today. He felt that diseases were not punishments from the gods but rather were disorders of essential humors. This promoted a lucid approach of careful examination and identification of physical signs. For example, Hippocrates is given credit for the first description of digital clubbing (Hippocratic fingers), an important diagnostic sign in chronic suppurative lung disease, lung cancer, and cyanotic heart diseases. Aristotle (384–322 BC) is likely to have recorded the first respiratory physiology experiment when he observed that animals died when kept in air-tight chambers. He believed the heart to be the source of the body's heat and nervous center. Erasistratus (304–250 BC), a Greek anatomist who worked in the school of anatomy in Alexandria, Egypt, felt respiration involved the lungs passing air into the left ventricle and then to the body using air-filled arteries.

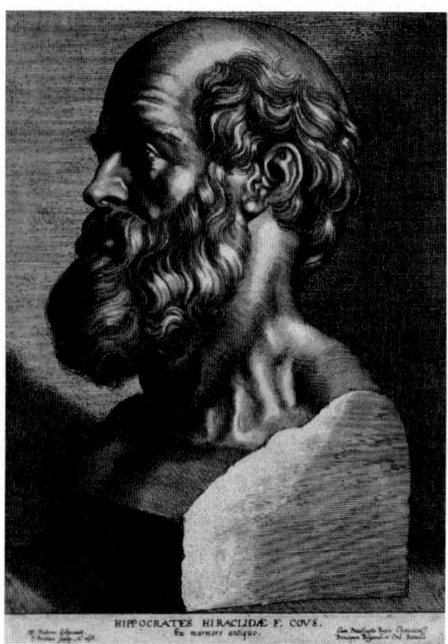

FIGURE 55–1 Hippocrates of Cos II, the father of Western medicine (460–ca. 370 BC).

Galen of Pergamum (130–199 AD) was a prominent Roman physician and probably the most accomplished medical researcher of the Roman period. His theories dominated Western medicine for over a millennium. He believed blood carried "pneuma" from inspired air via a pulmonary and then via an arterial circulation. By dissection of animals and observation of gladiators' injuries, he demonstrated that nervous control originated in the brain and spinal cord. The Romans established the importance of physicians on the battlefield. The Romans also established the value of public health measures to prevent and control epidemics.[2–6]

The Middle Ages

Little scientific or medical investigation was done in Europe after Galen. During the early Middle Ages (400–500 AD), the collapse of the Roman Empire and invasion by Germanic tribes threatened both written records and civilized infrastructure. The survival of some medical texts from Rome, Greece, and Persia is credited to monastic communities in Ireland, France, and Italy that preserved and transcribed original documents.[7] The works of ancient Greek and Moslem scientists and philosophers were reintroduced into the Western world. These works provided new intellectual material for European scholars.

TABLE 55-1 Major Contributors to Medical Sciences and Respiratory Clinical Medicine

Contributor	Country; Birth and Death Dates	Contribution
Ancient Period		
Hippocrates	Greece; 460–370 BC	Early guidelines for medical profession; importance of observation and diagnostic logic
King Pandukabhaya	Sri Lanka; 437–367 BC	Founded first institutions specifically dedicated to the care of the sick (other than religious temples)
Aristotle	Greece; 384–322 BC	Animal experiments; observed suffocation
Early Renaissance		
Leonardo da Vinci	Italy; 1578–1657	Human dissection; inflation of lungs caused by subatmospheric intrapleural pressures
Andreas Vesalius	Belgium; 1514–1564	Experiments with respiration in animals; early resuscitation
William Harvey	England; 1578–1657	Elucidated arterial and venous systemic and pulmonary circulations
Antonie van Leeuwenhoek	Netherlands; 1632–1723	Development of microscope lenses and discovery of single-cell organisms
Isaac Newton	England; 1643–1727	Mathematics and physics, especially motion and gravitation
18th Century		
Daniel Bernoulli	Holland and Switzerland; 1700–1782	Aerodynamics and hydrodynamics
Joseph Black	Scotland; 1728–1799	Discovery of carbon dioxide
Carl Scheele	Sweden; 1742–1786	Manufacture and discovery of oxygen
Joseph Priestley	England; 1733–1804	Discovery of oxygen
Antoine Lavoisier	France; 1743–1794	Discovery of role of oxygen and carbon dioxide in metabolism
Thomas Beddoes	England; 1760–1808	Clinical use of supplemental oxygen
Jacques Alexandre César Charles	France; 1746–1823	Gas law
Rene Laennec	France; 1781–1826	Invention of the stethoscope
Joseph Louis Gay-Lussac	France; 1778–1850	Gas law
Edward Jenner	England; 1749–1832	Microbiology; smallpox vaccination
19th Century		
John Dalton	England; 1766–1844	Gas pressure and atomic theory
William Henry	England; 1775–1836	Absorption of gases in fluids
Thomas Graham	Scotland; 1805–1869	Diffusion of gases through membranes
Louis Pasteur	France; 1822–1895	Bacteriology; germ theory
Robert Koch	Germany; 1843 1910	Bacteriology; discovery of cause of tuberculosis
Eduard Pfluger	Germany; 1829–1910	Oxygen consumption; respiratory quotient
Christian Bohr	Denmark; 1855–1911	Oxyhemoglobin dissociation curve
Adolf Fick	Germany; 1828–1901	Cardiac output measurement; contact lenses
Florence Nightingale	England; 1820–1910	Nursing care, hygiene, and sterile technique; medical statistics
Clara Barton	United States; 1821–1912	Battlefield evacuation; distribution of medical resources; American Red Cross
William Roentgen	Germany; 1845–1923	Discovered the x-ray
20th Century		
Karl Albert Hasselbalch	Denmark; 1874–1962	Blood oxygen physiology and acid–base chemistry
John Scott Haldane	England; 1980–1936	Hemoglobin oxygen physiology; regulation of breathing; gas therapy devices
Lawrence J. Henderson	United States; 1878–1942	Blood oxygen physiology and acid–base chemistry
Willem Einthoven	Holland; 1860–1927	Cardiac electrophysiology; invented the electrocardiogram
Ernest Henry Starling	England; 1866–1927	Cardiac muscle physiology; Frank-Starling law
Otto Frank	Germany; 1865–1944	Isotonic contractile behavior of cardiac muscle
Gerhard Domagk	Germany; 1895–1964	Antimicrobials; sulfanilamide
Alexander Fleming	Scotland; 1881–1955	Discovered penicillin
Selman Waksman	Russia, United States; 1888–1973	Antituberculosis use of streptomycin
Edward Kendall and Philip Hench	United States; 1886–1972 and 1896–1965	Isolated the corticosteroid cortisone
Carl Gottfried von Linde	Germany; 1842–1934	Manufacture of oxygen by fractional distillation
Alvan Barach	United States; 1895–1977	Oxygen and helium–oxygen therapy; constant positive pressure breathing (CPPB)
Linus Pauling	United States; 1901–1994	Chemistry and molecular biology; oxygen analysis using paramagnetic qualities
Chevalier Jackson	United States; 1865–1958	Endoscopy; tracheal intubation and tracheotomy
Leland C. Clark Jr.	United States; 1918–2005	Membrane oxygen electrochemical analysis
Philip Drinker	United States; 1894–1972	Coinventor of the iron lung
John H. Emerson	United States; 1907–1997	Inventor of iron lung and early volume-controlled mechanical ventilator
Forrest M. Bird	United States; 1921–	Inventor of Bird Mark-7 and Baby Bird ventilators
Virginia Apgar	United States; 1909–1974	Developed the Apgar score for newborn infants
Willam Ganz	United States; 1919–	Codeveloper of balloon-tip pulmonary artery catheter
John Severinghaus	United States; 1922–	Membrane pH and carbon dioxide electrochemical analysis
Harold James C. (Jeremy) Swan	United States; 1922–2005	Codeveloper of balloon-tip pulmonary artery catheter
Peter Safar	Austria and United States; 1924–2003	Modern CPR procedures; intensive care units and critical care education
Mary Ellen Avery	United States; 1927–	Furthered understanding of perinatal lung pathophysiology
Thomas Petty	United States; 1932–	Coauthored landmark work on ARDS, PEEP, and long-term oxygen therapy
Takuo Aoyagi	Japan; 1936–	Reported findings leading to development of pulse oximeter

CPR, cardiopulmonary resuscitation; ARDS, adult respiratory distress syndrome; PEEP, positive end-expiratory pressure.

The first hospital incorporated into an organized component for clinical education of physicians was the Academy of Gudishapur (Persia) in late 400 AD. However, in Europe, medical care was mostly limited to some monasteries. The monasteries incorporated almshouse for the poor, infirmaries, leprosaria, and hospices open to both clergy and lay populations. The term *hospital* is derived from the Latin *hospes*, which is also the root for the English words *hospitality*, *hostel*, and *hotel*.

A series of more than nine major Crusades occurred from 1092 through the 13th centuries. Although undertaken with Christian religious purpose, there was significant brutality and intolerance of both Moslem and other minorities. Over the course of 200 years, some 2 million Europeans died in the Middle East Crusades. However, there was some benefit. Much knowledge in areas such as science, medicine, and architecture was transferred from the Islamic to the Western world during the Crusade era. There also was a resurgence of commerce in the 1300s. By the 14th century, the Crusades had decreased the centralized power of the papacy. This kindled the foundation of modern nation-states in Europe.

RESPIRATORY RECAP

Key Events That Influenced Respiratory Care Today

» Ancient Times
» The Middle Ages
» Renaissance periods
» The 18th century
» The 19th century

Populations became more concentrated in cities, and problems with public health became significant. A series of pandemic plagues occurred, which began in Asia and reached Europe during the mid and late 14th century, where it was known as the Black Death (bubonic plague). It is estimated that one-fourth of the European population (20 million) died. Initially the disease was blamed on comets, or on scapegoats such as lepers or Jews. The actual cause of the plague was the bacteria *Yersinia pestis*, which inhabited the intestines of fleas. The impact of the plague was most significant in killing off old-school physicians. This allowed those with new ideas regarding medicine to establish practice.

The Renaissance: The 14th to 17th Centuries

The period beginning in the late 14th century and spanning to the 17th century reflected a general revival of learning based on classical sources and widespread educational reform, which included the arts and sciences. Men such as Leonardo da Vinci (1452–1519) took up human dissection to better understand human physiology. He was the first to report that subatmospheric pressures were required to inflate mammalian lungs. In 1543, Andreas Vesalius (1514–1564) published his masterful anatomy text, *De Humani Corporis Fabrica* ("On the artistry of the human body"), which dispelled many of Galen's premises (**Figure 55–2**). The record shows that Vesalius performed a thoracotomy on a live pig. He then documented pneumothorax, subsequent ventricular fibrillation, and recovery after ventilation via a primitive tracheostomy tube.

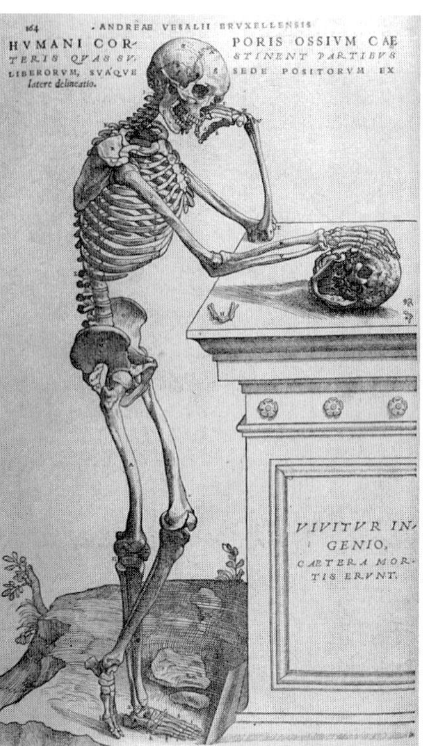

FIGURE 55–2 Illustration from Vesalius's *De Humani Corporis Fabrica*, 1543.

Educational reform was not without setbacks due to the Western Roman Catholic Church, which suppressed scientific theories or practices (such as autopsy and dissection) that it saw as heresy. Spanish anatomist Michael Servetus (1509–1553) was burned at the stake after his revolutionary anatomy text stated that blood in the pulmonary circulation, once it mixed with air from the lungs, returned to the left heart. It was another 75 years (1628) before English physician William Harvey (1578–1657) correctly described details of the arterial and venous circulations.[2–6]

Advances in understanding the primary and physical sciences continued throughout Europe during the 17th century. In Italy, Evangelista Torricelli (1608–1647; **Figure 55–3**) and associates made the first barometer by 1650. In France, Blaise Pascal (1623–1662) documented the relationship between barometric pressure and altitude. Irish theologian, alchemist, and gentleman scientist Robert Boyle (1627–1691; **Figure 55–4**) is regarded as one of the founders of modern chemistry. He received credit for espousing the inverse relationship between gas volumes and pressure, a hypothesis that was originally formulated by Henry Power in 1661. A multitalented assistant of Boyle, Robert Hooke (1635–1703), played important roles in the scientific revolution. He built vacuum pumps for Boyle's experiments, as well as telescopes and microscopes. Hooke is known principally for his law of elasticity but is also acknowledged

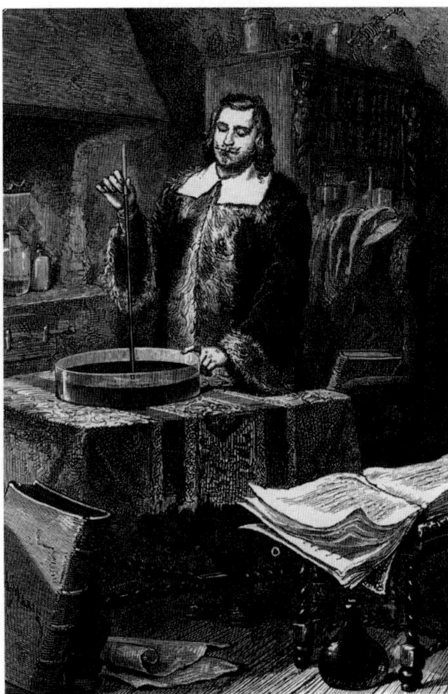

FIGURE 55-3 Evangelista Torricelli with his mercury barometer (circa 1640).

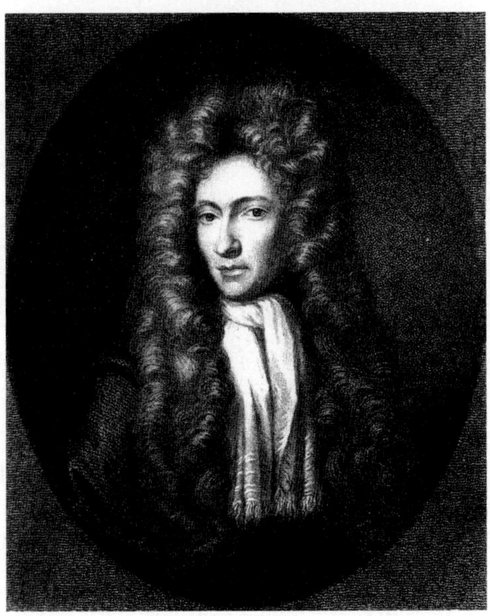

FIGURE 55-4 Robert Boyle, Irish chemist, physicist, and inventor, best known for the formulation of Boyle's law.

as a father of microscopy. It is believed that Hooke coined the word *cell* to describe the basic unit of biological life.

In the Netherlands, cloth merchant Antonie van Leeuwenhoek (1632–1723) was intrigued after reading Robert Hooke's book on microscopes in the mid-1600s. Van Leeuwenhoek's skill in glass making and lens grinding allowed him to improve on the early microscope. His revolutionary findings about single-celled organisms were published in 1673. This period in history would not be complete without mentioning the major contribution of Sir Isaac Newton (1643–1727). His work in mathematics, physics, the mechanics of motion, and gravitation, as well as light and optics, suggests that he was one of the most influential scientists in human history.

The 18th Century

During the 1700s, advances continued in the understanding of physical and chemical sciences. Daniel Bernoulli (1700–1782), a Dutch-Swiss mathematician, studied mechanics especially fluid and gas hydrodynamics. Bernoulli's principle was critical in the area of aerodynamics. In addition, his statistical-epidemiologic work was notable in his 1766 analysis of smallpox morbidity and mortality data to demonstrate the efficacy of vaccination. This was prior to Edward Jenner's 1796 findings.

The identification of respiratory gases that occurred during this period provided valuable insight into scientific competition, publication, and communication. Priority for discovery of a respiratory gas implies both preparation and identification. But it also involves communication of the work (oral or written) to other scientists and publication in either a book or journal. This sequence remains true today. Scotsman Joseph Black (1728–1799) is credited with the discovery of carbon dioxide (which he called "fixed air") by heating limestone in 1754. However, this discovery was earlier reported by Flemish chemist Baptiste van Helmont (1580–1644). He was the first to understand that there are distinct gases within atmospheric air and reported that carbon dioxide ("gas sylvestre") was given off by burning charcoal, which he felt was the same gas as produced during fermentation.

For some time, English theologian-scientist and politician Joseph Priestley (1733–1804) was credited with the discovery of oxygen ("dephlogisticated air"). These findings were communicated in September of 1774. However, he later confessed that he had no clear comprehension of oxygen. Priestley published his findings in November 1775. He felt this work would defend German scientist George Stahl's phlogiston theory and disprove the new chemical revolution of atomic theory. The former believed that combustible substances consumed phlogiston, which had negative mass when burned. Rejection of atomic theory eventually left Priestley isolated within the scientific community.

Swedish apothecary Carl Scheele (1742–1786) appears to have generated oxygen ("fire air") by heating magnesium oxide with sulfuric acid in June of 1771, three years ahead of Priestley. He communicated these findings by letter to Antoine Lavoisier in October 1774 and later in his book *Air and Fire* in August 1777. Of interest is that Scheele also discovered the element molybdenum and a method to mass-produce phosphorus. He likely died prematurely due to exposure to mercury from heating mercuric oxides.

In France, a third scientist, Antoine Lavoisier (1743–1794; **Figure 55-5**) capitalized on the work of

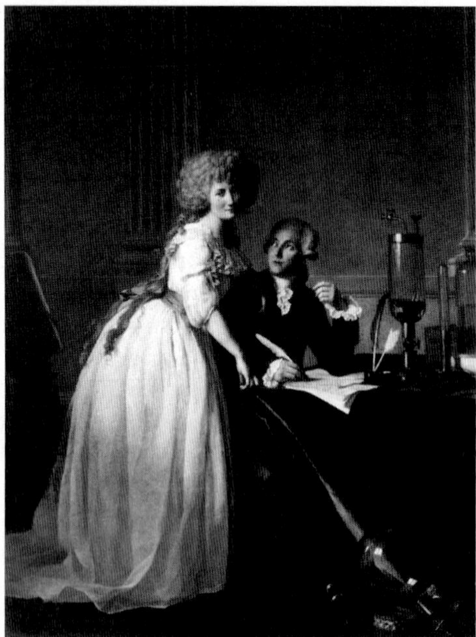

FIGURE 55-5 Marie and Antoine Lavoisier.

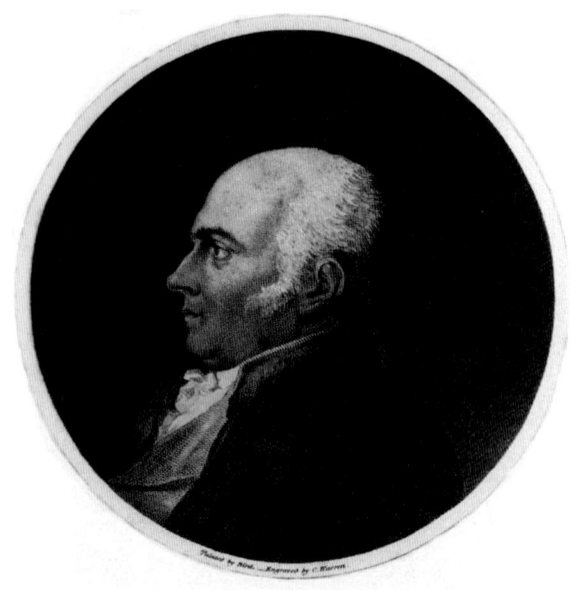

FIGURE 55-6 Thomas Beddoes (1760–1808), father of respiratory therapy.

Scheele and Priestley. He too has strong claims to the discovery of the gas that he termed "oxygen" (Greek *oxys* = sharp [acid] + *genes* = begetter), a description of which he published in May 1775. Lavoisier dispelled the phlogiston theory. His research included some of the first quantitative chemical analysis, which supported the law of conservation of mass, which he was the first to state. His later work confirmed that oxygen was consumed by the body, that carbon dioxide and water vapor were primary components of exhalation, and that nitrogen was essentially unchanged in the breathing process. Unfortunately, knowledge that his laboratory was supported by the French royalty resulted in his death by guillotine in the prime of his career.

In summary, Scheele probably has priority for actual chemical manufacture of oxygen. As for written communication of the discovery, Priestley and Scheele seem to have equal priority. The criterion of earliest publication by the individual scientist of his own work would give Priestley an edge. However, the criteria of earliest publication by other than the original investigator and a true understanding of the discovery's physiologic significance would give Lavoisier the credit.[8] Similar issues relate to Charles's law of gases. The law was first published in 1808 by Joseph Louis Gay-Lussac (1778–1850), but he referenced to an earlier unpublished work by fellow Frenchman Jacques Alexandre César Charles (1746–1823) around 1787.

Thomas Beddoes (1760–1808; **Figure 55-6**) deserves special mention for his scholarly contribution and for being the first clinician to implement therapeutic use of medical gases, as well as nitrous oxide. In 1784, his multilingual skills were employed as he translated Scheele's *Chemical Essays* from German to English. He then reviewed Priestley's work and visited Lavoisier.

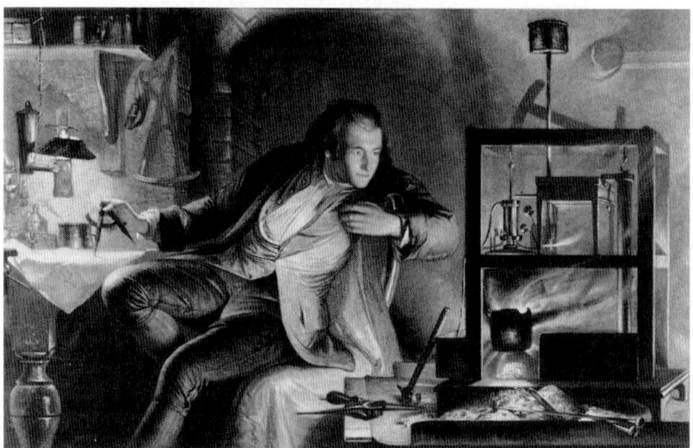

FIGURE 55-7 The Pneumatic Institute's early apparatus to generate medical gases, invented by James Watt.

He may be considered the father of respiratory therapy because he applied and investigated the "medical powers of factitious airs and gases." He solicited funds from a wide intellectual circle of friends. He gained technical support to generate gases from the inventor James Watt. In 1798 a Pneumatic Institute was established at Clifton, overlooking Bristol, England.[9] The facility was a spa-like environment incorporating a dispensary (clinic), hospital, and laboratory (**Figure 55-7**). The latter was supervised by Sir Humphrey Davy (1778–1829), who used oxygen and nitrous oxide to treat a number of conditions, including dyspnea, asthma, scrofulous infections, and congestive heart failure. However, the pneumatic component was overshadowed by demand for general care due to a typhus epidemic in 1800. The institute was largely abandoned by 1801.

The East developed understanding of immunology centuries before Italian Fracastoro Girolamo (1478–1553) proposed that epidemic diseases were caused by

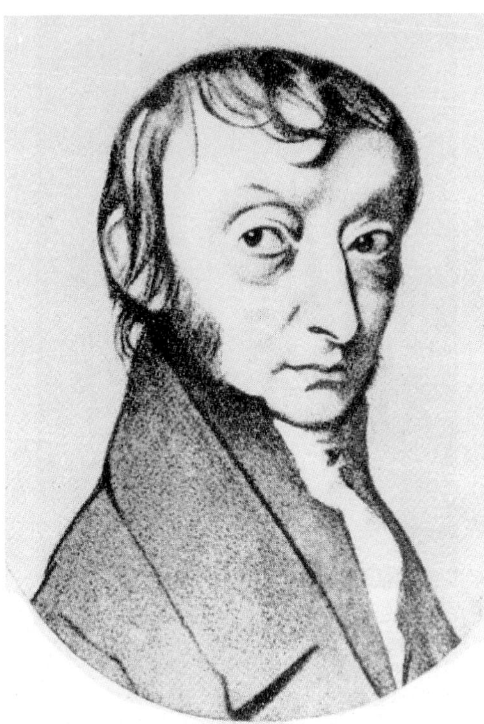

FIGURE 55–8 Amedeo Avogadro, who in 1811 published *Essay on Determining the Relative Masses of the Elementary Molecules of Bodies and the Proportions by Which They Enter These Combinations.*

tiny particles or spores that could transmit infection. Fellow Italian Agostino Bassi (1773–1856) is often credited with having stated the germ theory of disease for the first time, based on his observations. Englishman Edward Jenner (1749–1832) published his findings on smallpox vaccination in 1789.

The 19th Century

Italian savant Lorenzo Romano Amedeo Carlo Avogadro di Quaregna e di Cerreto (1776–1856; **Figure 55–8**) was educated in law, but then dedicated himself to mathematics and physics. In 1811 he proposed what is now known as Avogadro's hypothesis. He stated that at the same temperature and pressure, equal volumes of gases contain the same number of molecules or atoms. This was a radical statement at the time and was not widely accepted for 50 years. Avogadro developed this hypothesis after Joseph Louis Gay-Lussac had published his law in 1808 on volumes and combining gases. Of interest is that Avogadro had not resolved the question of whether molecules were made up of atoms.[2–6] John Dalton (1766–1844), an English chemist and meteorologist, is best known for his pioneering work in the development of modern atomic theory. In 1803 Dalton published his work on his principles of gas partial pressures, which constitute Dalton's law. Fellow English chemist William Henry (1775–1836) quantified the absorption of gases by water at different temperatures and under different pressures. This later became known as Henry's law.

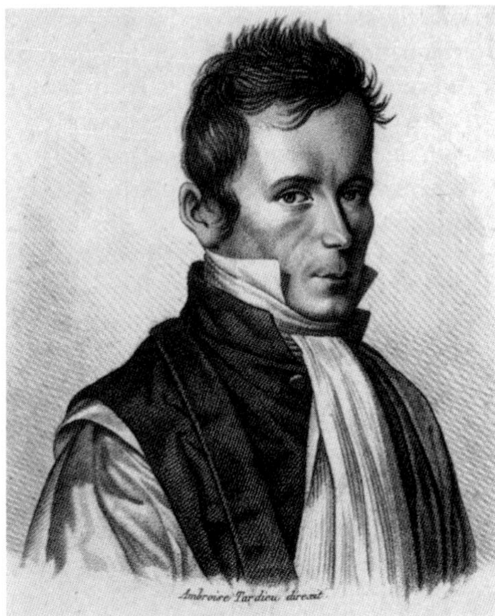

FIGURE 55–9 Rene Laennec, who developed the science of auscultation and is credited with inventing the stethoscope (Greek *stethos*, meaning "chest," and *skopos*, meaning "to look at").

Closely related to concepts about the physics of gases was the understanding of factors that govern diffusion through membranes. This was first quantitated by Scotsman Thomas Graham (1805–1869) in 1831. Heinrich Gustav Magnus (1802–1870) was a German-born chemist and physicist who studied under Gay-Lussac in Paris. Between the 1830s and 1860s he is credited with extending the understanding of vapor pressures of water, electrolysis, the conduction of heat in gases, and the thermal effects produced by condensation. He is credited with the first quantitative analysis of arterial and venous O_2 and CO_2 content.

Advances in science likely promoted initial acceptance of the metric system in 1875 in an international treaty known as the Convention du Mètre. The idea of a metric system has been attributed to John Wilkins, first secretary of the Royal Society of London in 1668. French abbot and scientist Gabriel Mouton proposed a decimal system of linear measurement based on the circumference of the earth in 1670. He then suggested a system of subunits, dividing successively by factors of 10 into the centuria, decuria, virga, virgula, decima, centesima, and millesima.

Paris became a center of modern medicine in the first half of the 19th century. Based on recent understanding of physics and chemistry, its institutions used a scientific approach based on experiment and observation. French physicians who provided clinical-related advances included Jean-Nicolas Corvisart, who assessed heart disease by tapping on the chest, and Rene T. H. Laennec (1781–1826; **Figure 55–9**), inventor of the stethoscope (a 2-cm by 25-cm hollow wooden tube) in 1819. There is conjecture as to whether his skill as a flutist, his interest in preventing the embarrassment of direct ear-to-chest contact with the opposite sex, or his desire to distance himself from patients' body odor and lice prompted this invention. French chemist Charles Fredrick Gerhardt was the first to prepare acetylsalicylic acid in 1853, which was patented under the name Aspirin in 1899.

The sciences of microbiology/bacteriology and immunology also advanced rapidly toward the middle of the 19th century. French chemist and microbiologist Louis Pasteur (1822–1895) continued work on germ theory and bacteriology. He conducted experiments in the mid-1800s that clearly validated the concepts of spoilage of beer, wine, and milk. By 1862 he and Claude Bernard showed that treating fluids with heat could kill bacteria. This process became known as pasteurization. Pasteur's immunology work, initially done on chicken cholera, led to a patent for his vaccination against anthrax in 1870. German Heinrich Hermann Robert Koch also studied cholera and anthrax. His most important contribution was the discovery of *Mycobacterium tuberculosis* in 1882, for which he was awarded a Nobel Prize in 1905. Both he and Pasteur are regarded as the fathers of germ theory and bacteriology.

In England, surgeon John Hutchinson (1811–1861) developed a spirometer to measure the effect of disease on lung volumes. He coined the term *vital capacity*. In 1846 he published results of vital capacities of over 2000 subjects (at autopsy and live patients). He found decreased volumes in those with tuberculosis or heart failure and in coal miners.[10]

By the mid-1800s education in medicine was promoted by French and German universities. Religion no longer dominated the curriculum, and education became increasing more accessible for all students. The German approach became an international model because a university could support both basic sciences as well as clinical medicine. German scientists are credited with development of the laryngoscope, ophthalmoscope, and cystoscope. William Roentgen discovered x-rays in 1895. German physiologist Eduard Pfluger (1829–1910) noted that oxygen consumption in tissues was proportional to their needs and devised the term *respiratory quotient*. By 1885 his laboratory also revealed that hypoxemia and hypercarbia both stimulated ventilation. Miescher-Rusch showed that carbon dioxide was the more potent stimulator.[11]

Danish physician-physiologist Christian Bohr (1855–1911; **Figure 55–10**) constructed the oxyhemoglobin-hemoglobin dissociation curve in 1886 and in 1891 characterized dead space. German physiologist and biophysicist Adolf Eugene Fick (1828–1901; **Figure 55–11**) made contributions in gas diffusion and described the direct method for measuring cardiac output in 1870. He also is credited with inventing contact lenses. About 1860, Bunsen and Kirchhoff invented the spectroscope. Later, Georg Gabriel Stokes realized that hemoglobin's absorption of oxygen changed its color. The first effort to monitor human blood oxygenation was reported by Karl von Vierordt (1818–1854), a German physiologist in 1874. He noted that red light diminished when tissues became ischemic.

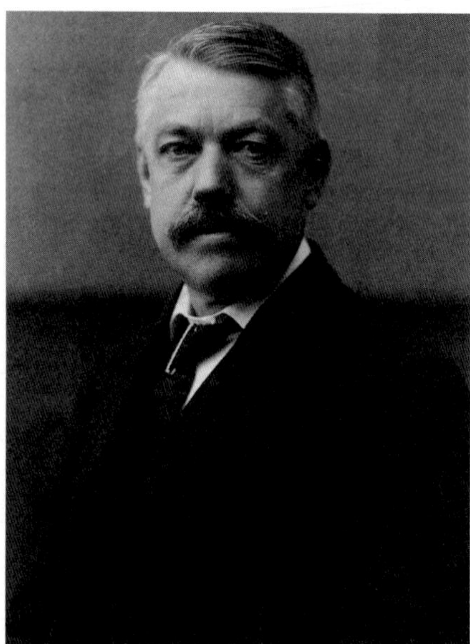

FIGURE 55–10 Danish physician Christian Bohr was educated at the University of Leipzig, Germany, and is credited with describing physiologic relationships involving oxygen–hemoglobin dissociation and dead space ventilation.

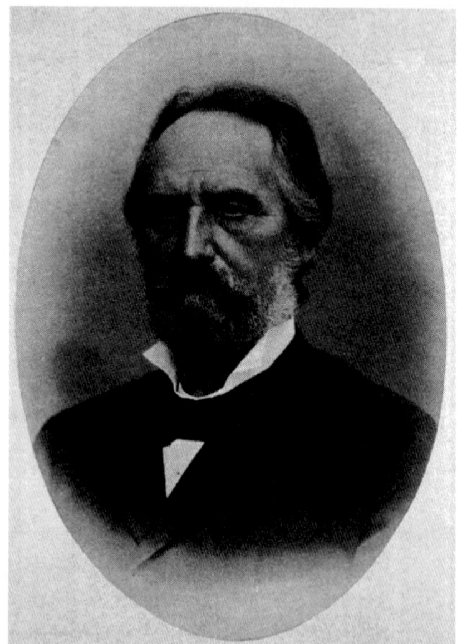

FIGURE 55–11 Adolf Fick, a German physiologist, is credited with the invention of contact lenses as well as an explanation of the diffusion of gases across a membrane and a method for determining cardiac output.

Warfare during the 19th century provided some positive benefit to medicine in spite of its human and economic devastation. Napoleon realized the importance of medical care. His army physicians began the practice

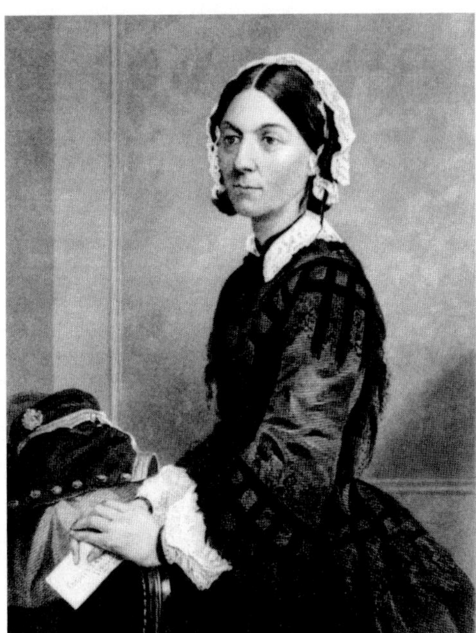

FIGURE 55–12 Florence Nightingale was a pioneering nurse who reduced the mortality of British soldiers in the Crimean War. She also was an early medical statistician.

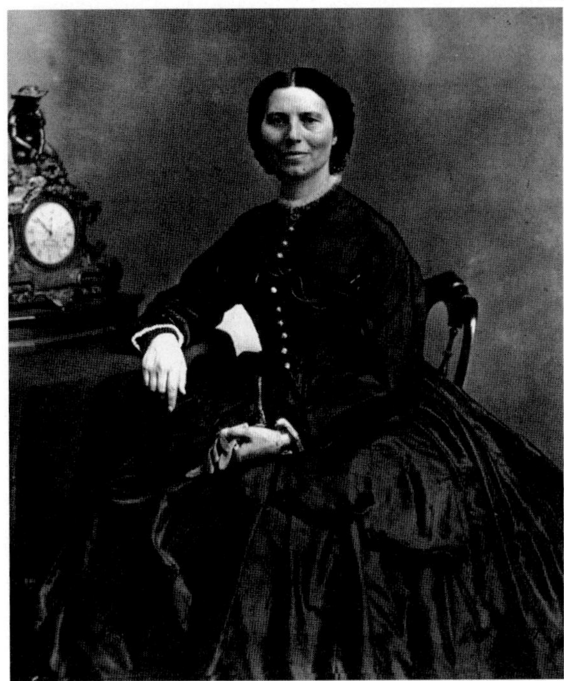

FIGURE 55–13 Clara Barton served as a nurse in the American Civil War and was instrumental in establishing the American Red Cross.

of triage. Advances in surgery, including limb amputation, elevated the competency of battlefield surgeons, who returned to civilian practice after the Napoleonic wars (1803–1815). Newspaper correspondents during the Crimean War (1853–1856) reported the scandalous treatment of soldiers in British field hospitals. Deaths due to typhus, typhoid, cholera, and dysentery were ten times as frequent as those from battlefield wounds. This prompted the advancement of nursing care of the wounded by Florence Nightingale (1820–1910; **Figure 55–12**). Her introduction of clean and sterile techniques and emphasis on the importance of diet and activity reduced death rates from 42% to 2%. She also had skills in mathematics and statistics, using pie charts to document causes of mortality and the effects of sanitation practices.[12]

The American Civil War (1861–1865) provided a similar grisly lesson for American physicians, with a total death count of about 620,000. Union soldier deaths exceeded 360,000, with approximately 70% from nonbattlefield causes. Many soldiers were left on the battlefield or died from communicable diseases. Union physician Jonathan Letterman developed a more modern system of first aid stations. He used a triage system with mobile field hospitals connected by ambulance corps.

Women's roles in medicine advanced slowly in the United States. Elizabeth Blackwell became the first woman to earn a medical degree in 1849, but she was banned from practice in most hospitals. She trained nurses for the Union. However, the requirements of the Civil War did allow Dr. Mary Edwards Walker (1832–1919) to become the first woman U.S. Army surgeon. She received the Medal of Honor for her service. Clara Barton (1821–1912; **Figure 55–13**) served as a nurse on Union Civil War ambulances behind enemy lines. She was also an organizer to improve distribution of medical supplies. She became involved in the International Red Cross movement. By 1873, she helped establish the American Red Cross, which had a scope broader than war crises.

Anesthesia was available at the time of the Civil War in the form of chloroform, and analgesia in the form of opium or morphine. In 1842, American medical student William Clark used diethyl ether during a tooth extraction for its anesthetic properties. It also was used during a surgical operation by a country physician in Georgia, Dr. Crawford Long, in that same year. The first public demonstration of ether for surgery was conducted in 1846 by William Thomas Green Morton in Boston. This provided the documentation that established anesthesia internationally. In that same year Morton used the anesthetic gas nitrous oxide for a dental extraction. However, Thomas Beddoes's chemist associate Humphrey Davy had used nitrous oxide for recreational purposes in 1799.[13]

Evolution of Respiratory Care in the 20th and 21st Centuries

The 20th century ushered in a wave of advancements. Medical practice was affected by international contributions in the fields of human physiology, pathophysiology, and technology. In the area of cardiopulmonary physiology,

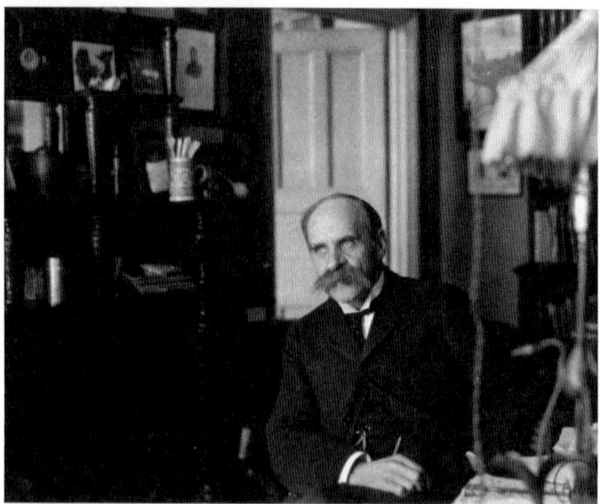

FIGURE 55–14 John Scott Haldane was a Scottish physiologist and biochemist whose work included research on respiration at extremes of pressure, exposure to toxic gases, and hemoglobin's interaction with oxygen and carbon dioxide, as well as the development of gas masks and oxygen delivery systems.

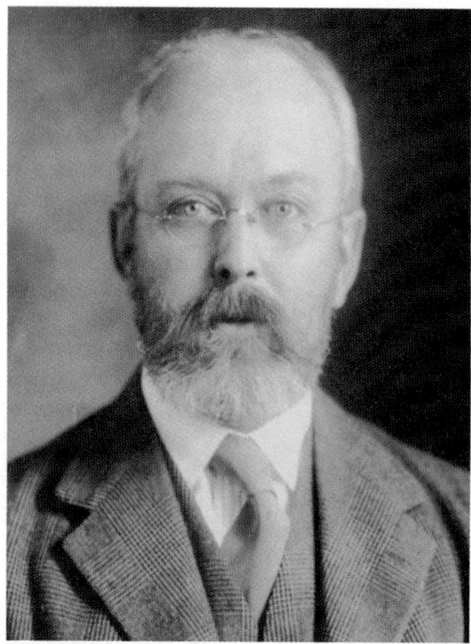

FIGURE 55–15 Lawrence J. Henderson investigated acid–base regulation, finding that acid–base balance is regulated by buffer systems of the blood (hemoglobin), in complex coordination with respiration, and the kidneys.

Christian Bohr, Karl Albert Hasselbalch (1874–1962), Joseph Barcroft (1882–1947), and August Krogh (1874–1949) made major contributions. Legendary research was conducted by John Gillies Priestley (1880–1941), Yandell Henderson (1873–1944), and John Scott Haldane (1980–1936; **Figure 55–14**). In 1898, Haldane created his gas analysis apparatus to measure oxygen content in blood. He also worked on regulation of breathing. Haldane discovered the effect of oxygen on hemoglobin dissociation of CO_2 (the Haldane effect). His interests included study of respiration under both hypobaric and hyperbaric conditions. The latter resulted in U.S. expedition to Colorado in 1911 where he conducted high-altitude research on Pikes Peak. His interest in mining disasters in the United Kingdom promoted study of carbon monoxide, hydrogen sulfide, and dust (silica) exposure. His work prompted his development of a gas mask for use in World War I.[14]

In the United States, physiologist-biochemist Lawrence J. Henderson (1878–1942; **Figure 55–15**), while working at Harvard, calculated the oxygen dissociation constants for oxygenated and reduced hemoglobin. He also calculated the law of mass action for the CO_2/bicarbonate buffer system. Karl Albert Hasselbalch was the first to determine the pH of blood. In 1916, he converted Henderson's 1908 equation to logarithmic form, which is now known as the Henderson-Hasselbalch equation. In 1920, August Krogh was awarded the Nobel Prize in Physiology or Medicine for the discovery of the mechanism of capillary blood flow regulation in skeletal muscle. Wallace O. Fenn (1893–1917) contributed primary research in understanding the mechanics of breathing and became the founder of the *Journal of Applied Physiology*. He and Herman Rahn devised a diagram for displaying alveolar gas information.[15]

Cardiac physiology also experienced a rapid evolution. Dutch physician Willem Einthoven (1860–1927; **Figure 55–16**) invented the electrocardiogram in 1903 as well as methods for understanding rhythm disturbances. For that work, he received the Nobel Prize for Medicine in 1924. German physiologist Otto Frank (1865–1944) studied the isotonic contractile behavior of heart muscle. His collaboration with Englishman Ernest Henry Starling (1866–1927) resulted in the Frank-Starling law of the heart, which was first presented in 1915.

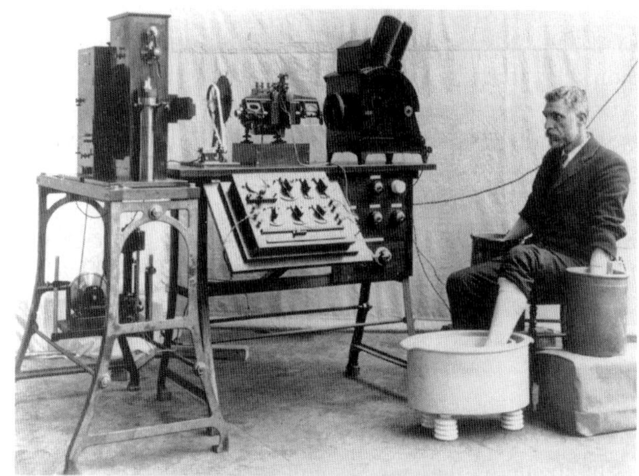

FIGURE 55–16 Willem Einthoven invented the electrocardiogram and methods to evaluate cardiac electrophysiologic disturbances.

World War I provided yet another horrific lesson for both surgeons and internists. Tanks, machine guns, and gas warfare replaced antiquated cavalry and cannons. Nonbattlefield problems included typhus, trench foot, and shell shock (what is now termed post-traumatic stress disorder [PTSD]). Some advances included use of tetanus antitoxin to prevent or treat gangrenous infections. Gunshot wounds were treated with Dakin's solution (sodium hypochlorite). The Spanish influenza pandemic followed the end of hostilities in 1918. Influenza A virus, which probably originated at the Fort Riley, Kansas, U.S. Army training camp, later evolved to a more virulent strain in France. The Spanish flu resulted in the death of approximately 680,000 Americans and 22 to 40 million people worldwide. This was 2% to 5% of the world population at that time. The virus elicited a storm of macrophage-derived chemokines and cytokines, which resulted in the lungs becoming infiltrated by inflammatory cells, causing severe pulmonary hemorrhage.[16]

By 1921 the cause of diabetes had been elucidated. Insulin was isolated by a research team in Toronto, Canada, led by Dr. Fredrick Banting. The antibiotic era began as German chemist Gerhard Domagk (1895–1964) discovered the antimicrobial properties of an industrial dye that was converted to sulfanilamide in the body. He received the Nobel Prize for Medicine in 1939 for his work. He was forced by the Nazi regime to refuse the prize and was arrested by the Gestapo.

While serving in World War I, Scottish physician-pharmacist Alexander Fleming (1881–1955) saw the devastation of septicemia and the limited value of antiseptics. The lack of cleanliness in his lab's sinks led to the accidental discovery of penicillin. He shared the Nobel Prize for Medicine with Howard Florey and Ernst Chain in 1945 for the discovery of penicillin. Biochemist and microbiologist Selman Waksman (1888–1973) immigrated to the United States from Russia in 1910 to work at Rutgers University, where he isolated the antituberculosis agent streptomycin in 1944. Mayo Clinic chemists Edward Kendall and Philip Hench isolated the steroid hormone cortisone, for which they later received the Nobel Prize for Medicine in 1950.[17] This allowed the treatment of Addison disease and rheumatologic disorders.

Historical Events That Signaled the Evolution of Respiratory Care

Clinical Oxygen Therapy

Earlier in this chapter, the work of Thomas Beddoes during the late 1700s was noted. He applied the chemical discovery of Scheele, Priestley, and Lavoisier to patients. The first oxygen devices began appearing as modified anesthetic masks made of oiled canvas, velveteen leather, mouth pipes, and cheek pieces (**Figure 55–17**). Fresh oxygen was manufactured on location using electrolysis in local apothecaries. By 1868, copper cylinders were developed to store and transport oxygen.[18]

Only gradually did the medical community embrace oxygen therapy, after significant strides were made in understanding the physiology of oxygen transport by Bohr, Krogh, Haldane, and Barcroft (**Figure 55–18**).[17,18] The first reports of potentially toxic effects of sustained breathing of oxygen at high concentrations also began

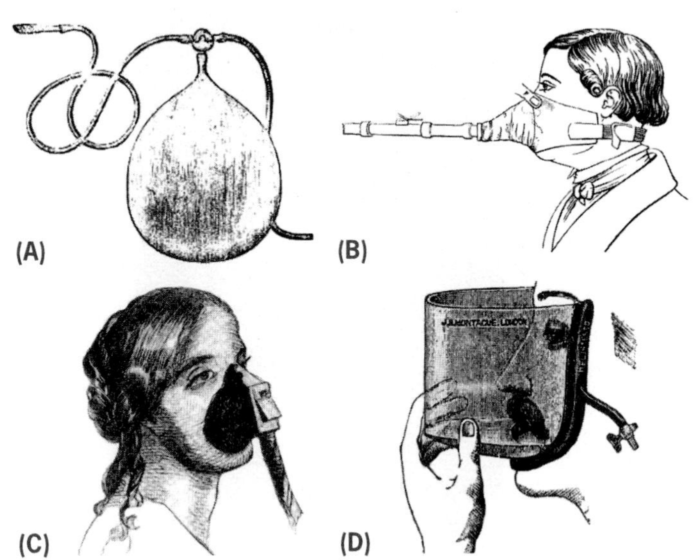

FIGURE 55–17 (**A**) Oxygen (mouthpiece) inhaler after design of Beddoes and Watt (circa 1796). (**B**) Oxygen face-piece mask of canvas and oiled silk (circa 1847). (**C**) Leaden mask covered with leather and velveteen (circa 1847). (**D**) Open face-tent originally used for nitorous oxide (circa 1899).

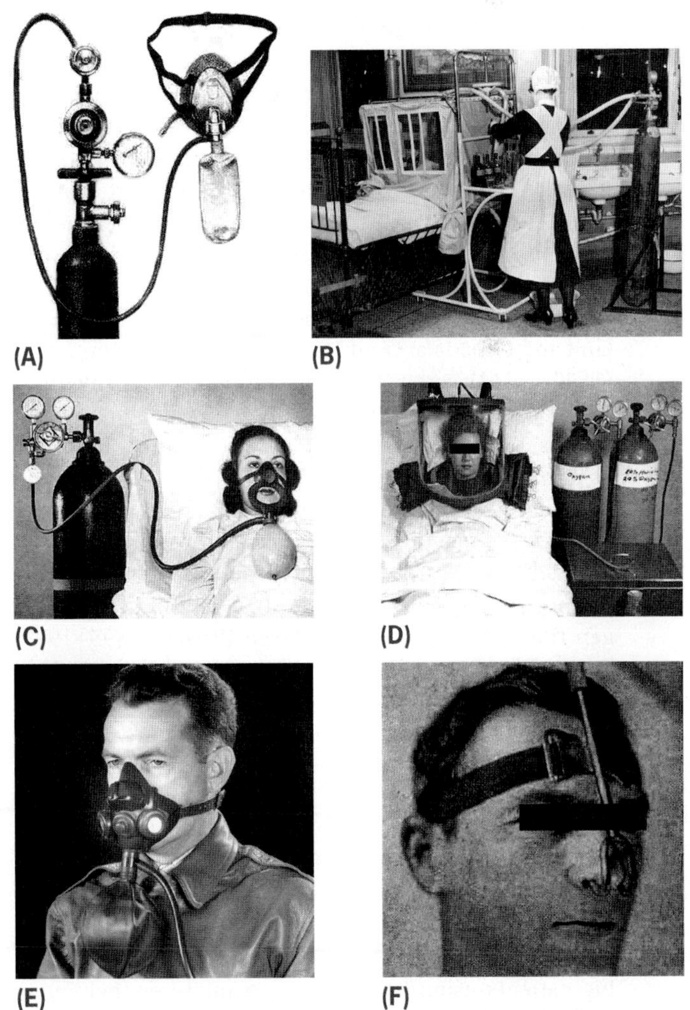

FIGURE 55–18 (**A**) Haldane's reservoir oxygen mask (circa 1919). (**B**) Apparatus for supplying patients with oxygen (circa 1950). (**C**) Barach's "mix-o-mask." (**D**) Barach's heliox constant positive airway pressure device. (**E**) World War II aviator with BLB mask. (**F**) Metallic nasal cannula.

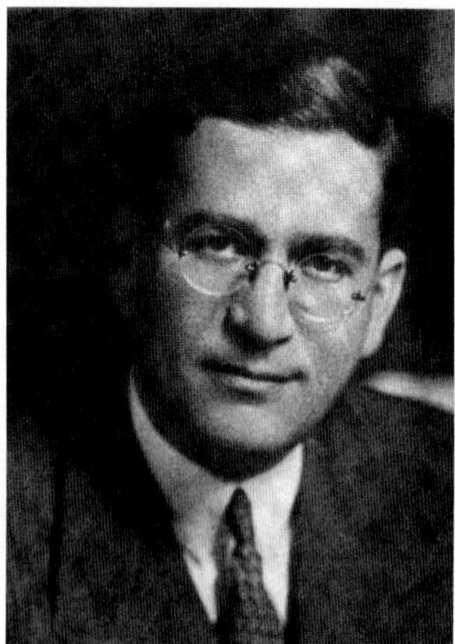

FIGURE 55–19 Dr. Alvan Barach (1895–1977).

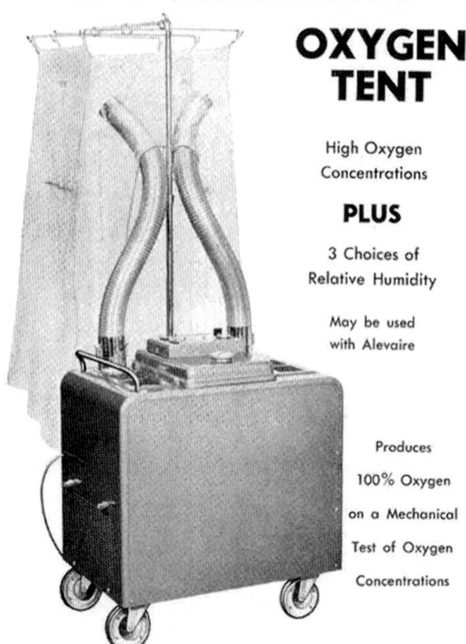

RV-3 REFRIGOMATIC
OXYGEN TENT
High Oxygen Concentrations
PLUS
3 Choices of Relative Humidity
May be used with Alevaire
Produces 100% Oxygen on a Mechanical Test of Oxygen Concentrations
Write for details today
THE JOHN BUNN CORPORATION
163 Ashland Avenue • Buffalo 22, N. Y.

FIGURE 55–20 Electrically powered refrigerated oxygen tent (circa 1956).

to appear in the literature. Sir Arbutot Lane introduced the nasal catheter using simple rubber tubing in 1907. He first used these nasal catheters for sick children and adult victims of World War I gas poisoning. Haldane developed an oxygen mask with a 2-liter reservoir bag to extend the performance of the catheter to treat soldiers with pulmonary edema due to chlorine gas poisoning (refer to Figure 55–18A). Haldane and Barcroft exposed themselves to subambient (15%) oxygen in experimental chambers to simulate hypoxia, in addition to their work at altitude.

Oxygen enclosures for clinical use appeared in England and Canada around 1910. Carl Gottfried von Linde (1842–1934) was a German engineer who invented technologies for refrigeration, which facilitated cooling for gas separation by fractional distillation. There had been much demand for CO_2 in European breweries. He was successful in generating oxygen in 1895, and the process was quickly commercialized. A U.S. patent was granted in 1903, and the Linde Air Products Company was formed by 1907. By 1926, U.S. physician and oxygen therapy proponent Dr. Alvan Barach (1895–1977; **Figure 55–19**) saw to the development of closed-system oxygen tents, which removed CO_2 with calcium chloride and used chunk ice for cooling (refer to Figure 55–18B).

American inventors Thomas Midgley and Charles Kettering developed Freon® for refrigeration in 1928; oxygen tents soon took advantage of that technology (**Figure 55–20**). Barach and Haldane both developed types of meter masks with diluting valves to allow specific entrainment of room air (refer to Figure 55–18C).[19] Barach also conducted trials with spontaneously breathing patients using helium–oxygen mixtures (heliox) as well as heliox with constant positive airway pressure (CPAP) hoods in 1934 (refer to Figure 55–18D).[20,21]

World War II provided incentive for engineers to develop planes that could fly at greater altitudes to avoid antiaircraft artillery. This prompted further study of oxygen physiology at low barometric conditions. A group of physicians (William Boothby, W. Randolph Lovelace, and Arthur Bulbulian) with the Mayo Clinic's Aero Medical Unit developed a partially valved reservoir mask capable of providing 80% to 100% oxygen in 1938. Later they termed this the BLB mask. It was made commercially available by Ohio Chemical (refer to Figure 55–18E). The Mayo Aero Medical Unit was also instrumental in creating the G-suit, which allowed external compression of a pilot's legs and abdomen to prevent hypotension-induced blackouts during conditions of high gravitational forces on the circulation. Metal cannulas became available as an alternative to the nasal catheter (refer to Figure 55–18F).

In the late 1940s, the ability to administer oxygen to premature infants in warming enclosures (**Figure 55–21**) resulted in an epidemic of retrolental fibroplasia (RLF), later named retinopathy of prematurity (ROP). Theodore Terry was the first to hypothesize that indiscriminate use of supplemental oxygen was a potential cause.[22]

Both increasing complications and increased demand for clinical use of supplemental oxygen escalated work in the pathophysiology and new technology of oxygen therapy. At this time, there were no simple methods to measure oxygen levels in inspired gas or blood. Efforts to provide this technology began with Heinrich Danneel and Walther Nernst, who determined the electrochemical reduction of oxygen in 1897. Polarographic characteristics were accidently discovered by Jaroslav Heyrovsky

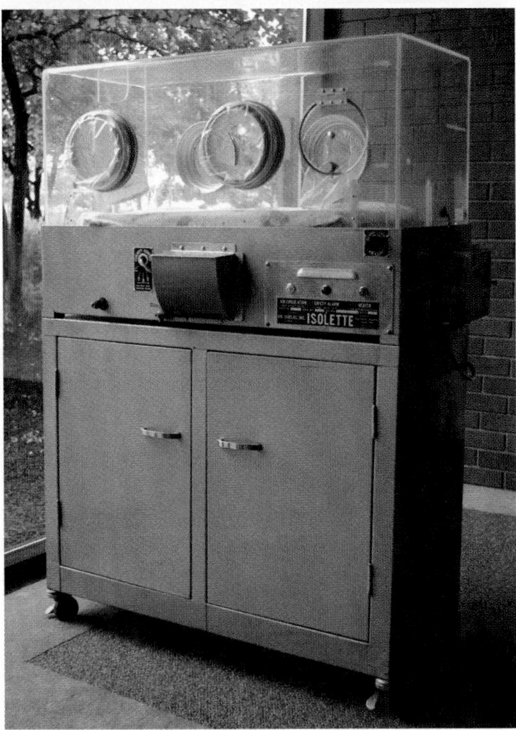

FIGURE 55–21 Infant warmer-incubators (Isolette brand) were fitted with adaptors to provide supplemental oxygen.

in 1922 using platinum cathodes. In 1935, German physiologist Kurt Kramer (1906–1985) used photocells to measure oxygen saturations using an in vivo cuvette in dogs. American Glen Millikan (1906–1947) capitalized on Karl Matthes's (1905–1962) work by using two hemoglobin absorption wavelengths for his external ear oximeter. Linus Pauling (1901–1994) exploited the characteristic that increased oxygen enhanced a magnetic field. The Arnold Beckman Company developed the D-2 oxygen analyzer in 1945 in collaboration with Pauling.

By this time demand for gas supplies and knowledgeable personnel to support physicians and nurses in a 24-hour-per-day service heralded the beginning of organized inhalation therapy departments. In 1954, Leland C. Clark Jr. (1918–2005) was credited with developing the first membrane oxygen electrode that was not poisoned by blood proteins.[23] By the mid-1960s, commercially available arterial blood gas (ABG) electrodes developed by Clark and John Severinghaus (1922–) allowed analysis of Pa_{O_2}, Pa_{CO_2}, and pH. Their operation often became incorporated within the clinical services of respiratory therapy departments. Arterial blood collection and interpretation skills were one more skill set added to the growing list of job functions. Millikan's ear oximeter was made clinically available by 1974, and by the early 1980s ABG-type electrodes had been miniaturized so they could be applied transcutaneously. In 1974, Japanese bioengineer Takuo Aoyagi published an abstract of his serendipitous discovery of pulse oximetry. His discovery occurred while working on an ear probe densitometer for recording dye dilution curves for cardiac output.[24] The pulse oximeter has become a standard device for monitoring patient oxygenation in emergency departments, operating rooms, intensive care units, and hospital floors.

The goal of improving titration of oxygen levels to patients, especially those with chronic obstructive pulmonary disease (COPD), led E. J. Moran Campbell to develop the Venturi mask in 1960. It was similar in function to Barach's meter mask and provided high-flow controlled F_{IO_2} to meet the inspiratory demands of tachypneic patients while minimizing the risk of induced carbon dioxide retention.[25] Reliable air–oxygen blenders became commercially available by the mid-1970s and were quickly put into use in nurseries and intensive care units. They were also incorporated into mechanical ventilators. The oxygen concentrator and portable liquid systems also became available by the mid-1970s. Conserving devices such as reservoir masks or cannulas, demand pulse units, and transtracheal catheters were developed in response to a growing demand for out-of-hospital oxygen therapy. The benefit of that approach was made clear in 1980 as the Nocturnal Oxygen Therapy Trial (NOTT) group published its findings. These investigators showed a positive mortality benefit when oxygen was continuously used for hypoxic patients with COPD.[26]

By the 1990s oxygen therapy had evolved to require significant skills in assessing patients' medical requirements, recommending care, and evaluating its effects. Therapist-driven protocols (TDPs) were now required to better define the science and patient applications. It was not surprising that oxygen therapy became the subject of one of the first in a series of clinical practice guidelines (CPGs) developed by the American Association for Respiratory Care.[27,28]

Medicated Aerosols

For the purposes of reviewing the history of clinical aerosols, the concept should also include use of mists, fogs, vapors, or fumes. The practice of inhaling sulfuric vapors from the slopes of Mt. Vesuvius was mentioned by Galen (130–201 AD). The practice of inhaling burning medicinal substances from smoking pipes goes back thousands of years. The leaves and roots of *Datura ferrox* were used to treat asthma. Jimsonweed (*Datura stramonium*) was also used for its added psychotropic effect. Commercially produced antiasthma cigarettes (e.g., Asmador) were available until 1992, when they were withdrawn because of the potential for abuse. Heated vapors (**Figure 55–22**) and sprays from either thermal spa waters or antiseptics for tuberculosis were popular throughout the 19th century.

In 1912, adrenaline to treat asthma was made available and delivered with perfume-type squeeze-ball atomizers. By 1940, more sophisticated pneumatic nebulizers evolved from work by Lucien Dautrebande and others, which improved these devices with baffling designs. High-velocity jet-type nebulizers were applied via self-inflating bags, intermittent positive pressure breathing (IPPB) devices, and volume-controlled mechanical ventilators, for both humidification and medication delivery. The most commonly used β-agonist in 1940 was isoproterenol (Isuprel), which became appreciated for its robust bronchodilation. It also was known for its tendency to produce tachycardia. Ultrasonic nebulizers were made available in 1949, first used as room humidifiers. Later physicians added medications and directed them by masks.[29]

Pharmacologic research provided medications that targeted specific airway receptors. The first introduced was Bronkosol, which was available by 1951. A proliferation of more specific β-agonists, anticholinergics, and corticosteroid medications subsequently occurred. Chlorofluorocarbon (CFC)–powered metered dose inhalers (MDIs) were developed in 1956 and became the most commonly used devices because of their low cost, simplicity, and ability for self-administration. Dry powder inhaler (DPI) use began in the United States with delivery of cromolyn sodium via the Spinhaler in 1973. Concerns about the environmental effects of CFCs on the earth's ozone layer resulted in international cooperation to discontinue the use of CFC propellants, including those in MDIs, by 2009. In response, other propellants have been introduced. Use of MDIs and DPIs has increased, especially for nonacute care application.

For many years, antimicrobial agents have been administered by pneumatic nebulizers. Evidence for their efficacy occurred in the treatment of cystic fibrosis patients with *Pneumocystis carinii* infections. That patient group has also been treated with rhDNase aerosols to diminish the viscosity of pulmonary secretions.[29] Aerosol therapy has continued to advance in terms of new devices using technologies such as porous mesh and medications such as insulin.[30]

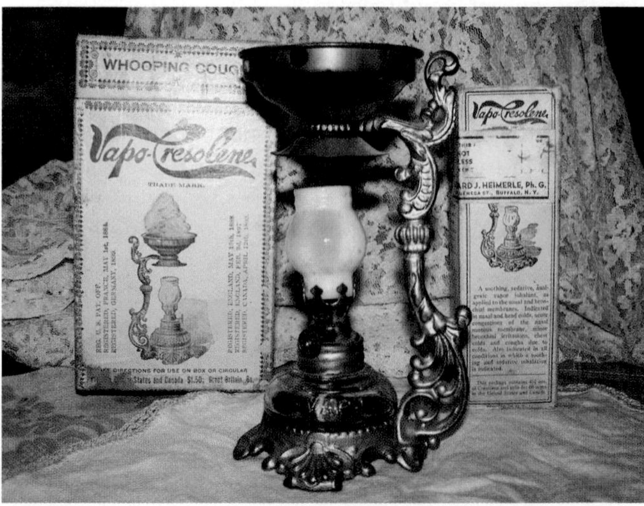

FIGURE 55–22 Vaporizers were commonly used for home therapy. An alcohol- or kerosene-lamp burner heated liquid medication in a chamber to be vaporized into a room or inhaled directly.

Airway Management and Resuscitation

Tracheotomy is an ancient medical procedure. Its use was first recorded in Hindi and Egyptian literature from about 3600 to 2000 BC. Homerus of Byzantium wrote that Alexander the Great performed the procedure with a sword to treat an ailing soldier in about 1000 BC. Hippocrates campaigned against the tracheotomy because of serious and frequent complications from vascular damage, as well as unsterile instruments. In 1542 Andreas Vesalius performed a tracheotomy on a pig on which he had previously performed a thoracotomy, using a reed for the tracheostomy tube. Once ventilation was applied, he observed its recovery from (presumed) ventricular fibrillation following a pneumothorax. The procedure was first named tracheotomy in 1718. Until the early 1900s, it was largely regarded as a last-ditch effort or considered only in emergency situations.

The first tracheal intubation for anesthesia was reportedly done by German surgeon Fredrich Trendelenburg in 1869. He introduced the tube through a temporary tracheostomy. In 1878, the Scottish surgeon William MacEwan reported the first elective oral intubation. During World War I, Drs. Ivan Magill and Robert Macintosh advanced the procedure for direct tracheal intubation. American laryngologist Chevalier Jackson (1865–1958; **Figure 55–23**) is credited with inventing the first anesthetic laryngoscope in 1913. This then was modified by Magill, Miller, and Macintosh. Jackson largely invented the science of endoscopy of the upper airway and esophagus by refining procedures to reduce complications and

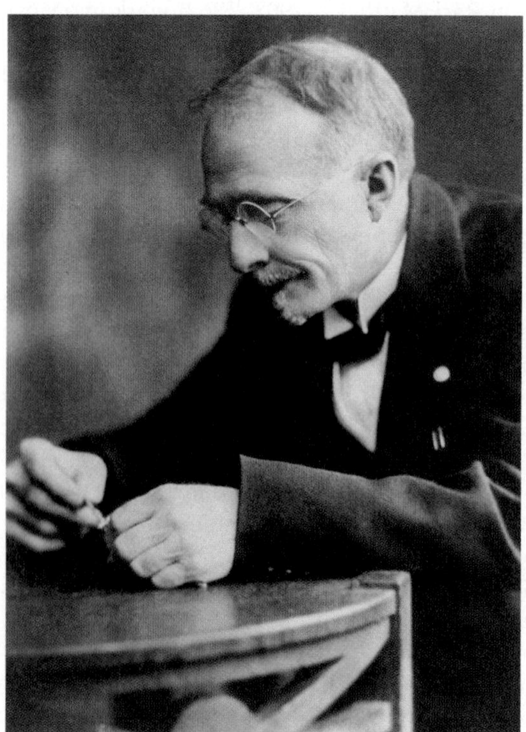

FIGURE 55–23 Dr. Chevalier Jackson was a pioneer in laryngoscopy, bronchoscopy, and endoscopy. He refined the procedures for tracheotomy and endotracheal intubation.

improve physician training. A model of metallic tracheostomy tube still bears his name. Subsequent advances included blind nasal intubation, described by Magill in 1930, and catheters for secretion removal, described by F. J. Murphy in 1941.[31] The polio pandemic renewed interest in tracheostomy. With the dwindling availability of the costly iron lungs, tracheostomy allowed positive pressure ventilation. This was often applied by simple hand-powered bag systems.

The modern techniques of resuscitation were developed from the late 1940s to the 1960s. Impetus came from experiences with mobile army surgical hospital (MASH) units during the Korean War. By 1955, successful open and closed-chest heart defibrillation had been documented by Claude Beck and Paul Zoll. In 1958, Peter Safar (1924–2003; **Figure 55–24**) and colleagues published their work on mouth-to-mouth resuscitation compared with the older Silvester arm-lift technique.[32] In 1960, Kouwenhoven documented the success of closed-chest cardiac massage.[33] Airway management procedures, manual or mechanical ventilation, and closed-chest circulation methods were integrated and advocated by Peter Safar's landmark publication in 1961, and the first national cardiopulmonary resuscitation (CPR) guidelines were published.[34,35]

Modern CPR became an international standard of practice necessary for hospital personnel, not just emergency squads. Initially, resuscitation tools were only used by rescue teams (outside the hospital). Special procedures such as intubation or mechanical ventilation were not performed outside the operating or recovery room. Safar collaborated with Åsmund Laerdal to have a Norwegian card and toy manufacturer produce the Resusi® Anne manikin to allow simulator training for medical personnel and the lay public. Advances in the science of and effective instrumentation for cardiac defibrillation with direct current closely followed.[36] Safar and others recognized the need for specialized resuscitation equipment and skills in critical care to be made rapidly available to any hospitalized patient. He developed both the first intensive care unit and intensivist physician training program in the United States. He also was active in early medical disaster planning.[37]

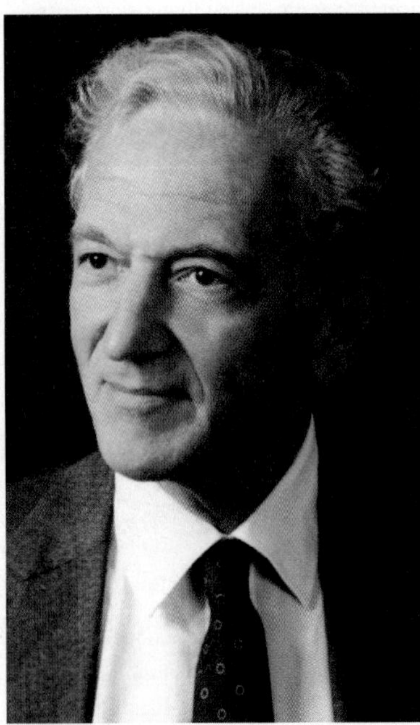

FIGURE 55–24 Dr. Peter Safar is recognized as the father of CPR for his research, promotion, and teaching of both cardiopulmonary resuscitation and intensive care practice.

Direct oral endotracheal intubation became an essential skill and the advanced airway of choice following bag-mask ventilation. More frequent and larger numbers of intubated patients resulted in significant complications from high-pressure cuffs. Improved design and plastic compounds quickly reduced the occurrence of this complication.

Dr. Archie Brain developed the laryngeal mask airway in the mid-1980s. He also developed the Mallampati system for identifying potentially difficult intubation candidates. These concepts were incorporated into the American Society of Anesthesiology's first publication of a difficult airway algorithm in 1993.[38,39] In 1985, a variant of the standard surgical tracheotomy was presented that could be performed in an intensive care setting.[40]

Mechanical Ventilation

A complete historical review of mechanical ventilation is beyond the scope of this introductory chapter.[41–43] Mechanical ventilating devices that were more than fireplace bellows began appearing in the mid-1800s. Most early devices, such as Woillez's 1876 Spirophone (**Figure 55–25**), followed a physiologic approach, using a body-enclosing chamber and bellows to create subatmospheric pressure. The head was allowed to protrude. A sealing membrane around the neck allowed pressure to be applied only to the chest. The problems of providing and maintaining an artificial airway were avoided. Because problems of patient access prevented using such devices for any surgical application, German surgeon Ernst Sauerbruch developed a negative pressure operating chamber in 1904.

The difficulty of transporting negative pressure devices prompted early development of positive pressure resuscitators for use by rescue squads. The operating room and the ambulance became the early incubators for positive pressure ventilator development. The Fell-O'Dwyer apparatus (circa 1888; **Figure 55–26**) combined a metallic laryngeal tube and a foot-operated bellows. In 1907, German inventor Heinrich Dräger patented

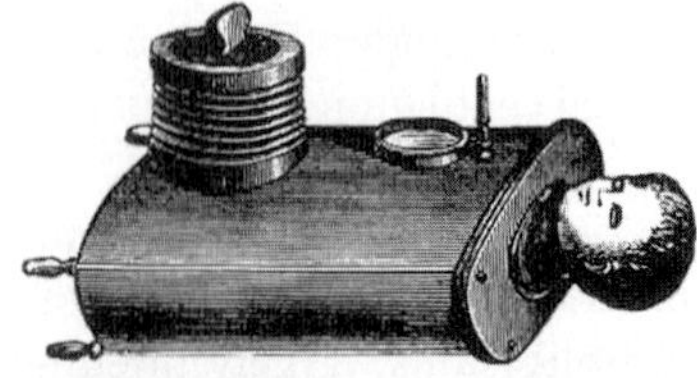

FIGURE 55–25 Woillez's Spirophone negative pressure ventilator (circa 1876). This article was published in Morch ET. History of mechanical ventilation. In Kirby RR, Banner MJ, Downs JB, eds. *Clinical Applications of Ventilatory Support.* Copyright Elsevier (Churchill Livingstone) 1990.

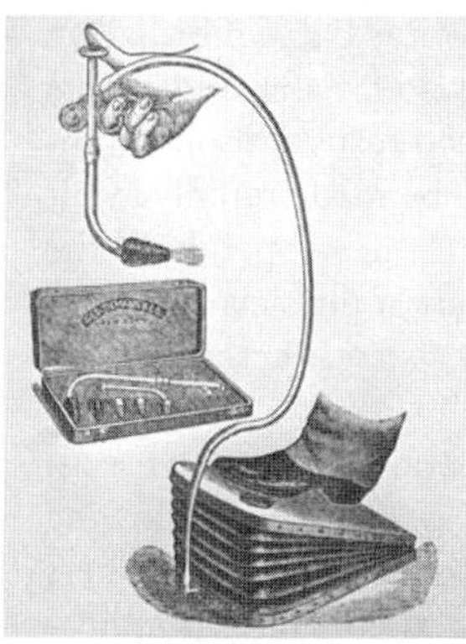

FIGURE 55–26 Fell-O'Dwyer bellows and endotracheal intubating device (circa 1888). This article was published in Morch ET. History of mechanical ventilation. In: Kirby RR, Banner MJ, Downs JB, eds. *Clinical Applications of Ventilatory Support.* Copyright Elsevier (Churchill Livingstone) 1990.

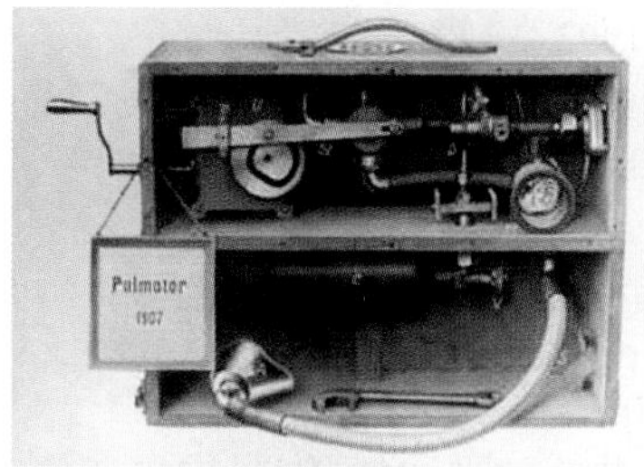

FIGURE 55–27 Drager Pulmotor (circa 1907).

his Pulmotor (**Figure 55–27**). Henry Janeway constructed an anesthesia machine capable of automatic ventilation by 1910.[41–43]

The poliomyelitis pandemic signaled both the heyday of the iron lung and its demise. A variable pattern of polio events occurred in America and Europe (**Figure 55–28**). An early epidemic in New York in 1916 prompted Philip Drinker, Charles McKhann, and Louis Shaw to develop the first iron lung at Harvard in Boston by 1928 (refer to Figure 55–28B). It became the most widely used iron lung, costing $1500 (the price of a modest home in those days). In 1932, John H. Emerson constructed his version, which had an optional transparent dome to provide positive pressure ventilation while the device was opened for patient care (refer to Figure 55–28A).

Significant numbers of polio patients developed respiratory muscle paralysis with or without bulbar involvement. Many urban hospitals were faced with caring for long-term patients. Facilities such as Rancho Los Amigos Rehabilitation Center were established (**Figure 55–29**). The Scandinavian countries were hit hard by polio in the early 1950s. The main hospital serving Copenhagen, Denmark, which previously had only three negative pressure devices, was faced with ventilating up to 70 patients daily during the summer of 1952. Physicians such as Drs. Bjorn Ibsen and H. C. Lassen were pioneers in abandoning the iron lung in place of anesthesia methods of positive pressure ventilation with artificial airways (cuffed tracheostomy). Lassen's simple device incorporated a humidifier, a canister of soda lime for CO_2 absorption, and valves for administration of 50% oxygen from a high-pressure gas cylinder (**Figure 55–30**). A rubber bag allowed manual ventilation by personnel such as medical students.

The experience with long-term ventilators for polio patients underscored the importance of preventing pulmonary complications, largely pneumonia. Secretion clearance in the form of suctioning, frequent turning, and postural drainage was used to prevent pneumonia.

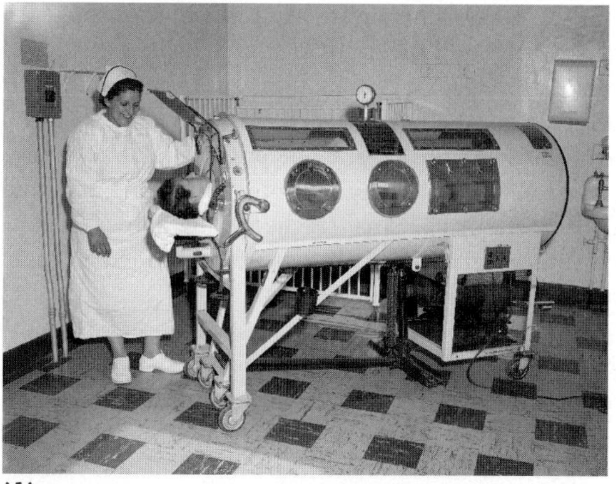

(A)

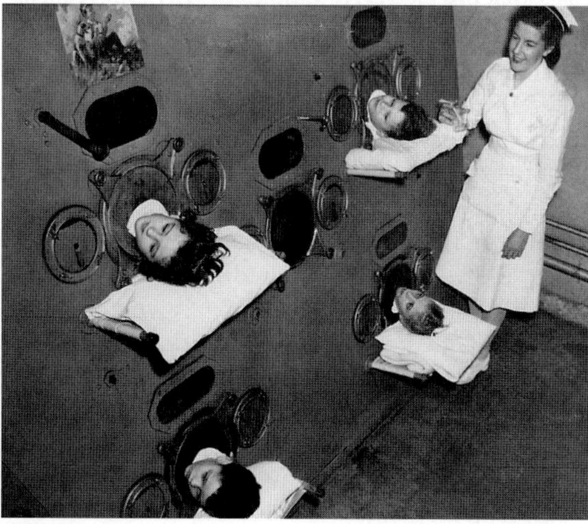

(B)

FIGURE 55–28 (**A**) Emerson iron lung. (**B**) A nurse at Children's Hospital in Boston, Massachusetts, in 1938 shown tending to young polio patients lying in a 4-place iron lung room, which was developed by Philip Drinker. Their bodies were contained inside the room, falling then rising pressure allowed their lungs to inhale and exhale respectively.

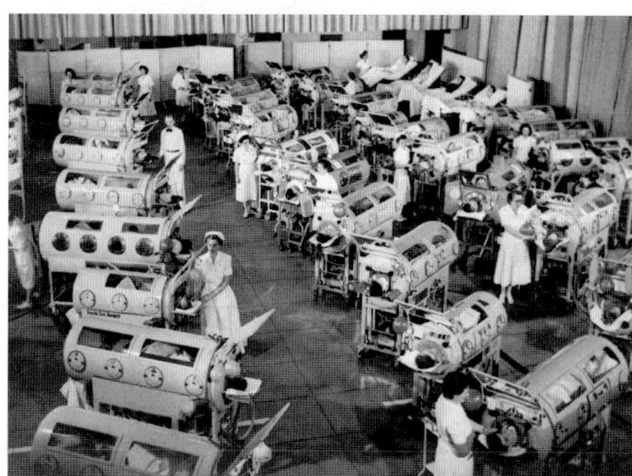

FIGURE 55–29 Polio ward at Rancho Los Amigos Rehabilitation Center, California (circa 1952). Various-sized Drinker iron lungs can be seen. The angled plates above patient's heads contained a mirror to allow patients to observe their surroundings.

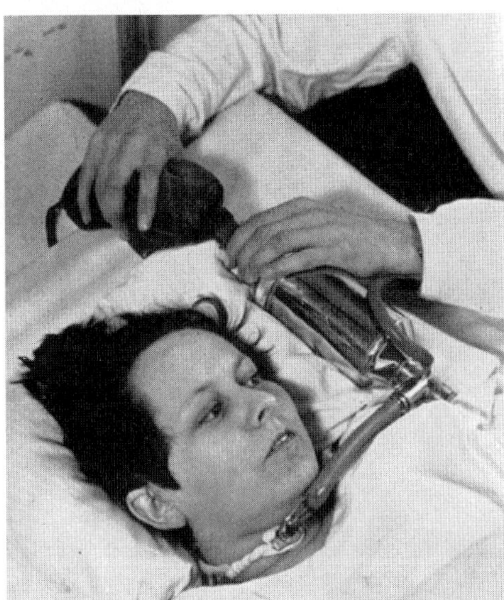

FIGURE 55–30 H.C. Lassen's manual positive pressure ventilation was used for polio patients in Copenhagen, Denmark, when negative pressure became unavailable.

Skin care and frequent turning helped prevent pressure ulcers. In Europe and America, automated ventilators were developed rapidly. Besides interest in their use in long-term care, there was increasing interest in their use in the operating room. Positive pressure ventilation was also used for prophylactic postoperative care following thoracic and cardiac surgery.[44]

During the German occupation of Denmark in 1942, Dr. Ernst Trier Mørch developed a piston device using scavenged sewer pipe for the cylinder. After World War II, he immigrated to the United States, where his refined designs were manufactured in Chicago by Mueller, Inc., by 1953. The Mørch III (**Figure 55–31**) maintained his original rotary piston design, fitting under the bed in a polio ward. It also was adapted for use in the ICU. In Denmark, Dr. C. Bang developed a ventilator that used a solenoid valve that cycled to interrupt minute volume gas flow to provide a tidal volume.[41,45,46] Around this same time, the Swedish Engstrom ventilator was developed for application in either the operating room or respiratory unit. In Germany, the Dräger Company developed the Poliomat in 1951 and the Spiromat by 1958. British anesthesiologists adept at mechanical tinkering came up with a range of devices in the early 1950s, including the Beaver, Blease, Radcliffe, and Clevedon ventilators. The polio experience also allowed physiologic research to help guide selection of ventilatory parameters.[47] The Radford nomogram provided a scientific basis for estimating initial selection of tidal volume and rate. Radford predicted tidal volumes in the 7 to 8 mL/kg range for polio patients that typically had normal lung mechanics.[48]

In contrast to the Europeans, who used a mechanical approach with pistons or concertina bags, Americans initially favored positive pressure using pressure valves often spawned from World War II military applications

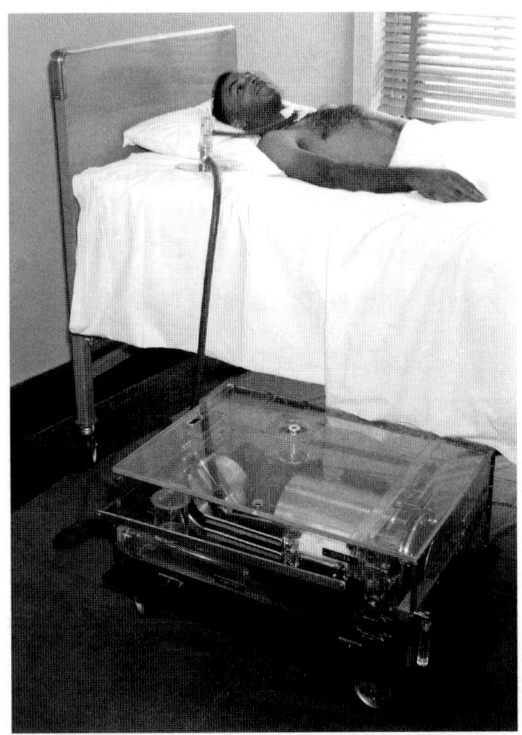

FIGURE 55–31 Mørch III piston ventilator (circa 1953).

(**Figure 55–32**). V. Ray Bennett's (refer to Figure 55–32A) Ben X-2 flow-sensing valve had been used to deliver oxygen in unpressurized aircraft. He incorporated the valve into the TV-2P assister and BA-2 anesthesia machine in 1948. Dr. Forrest Bird (refer to Figure 55–32B) introduced the clinical magnetic respirator in 1951. With the addition of automatic cycling mechanisms, the Bird Mark 7 and the Mark 4 anesthesia version were available in 1955 and 1959, respectively. The Bennett PR-1 and PR-2 were in large-scale production after 1961. The Bird and Bennett positive pressure ventilators were often the first post–iron lung ventilators in newly formed inhalation therapy departments in the United States.

The importance of volume-controlled ventilation became a dominant theme about the same time that intensive care units were undergoing their rapid growth phase in the 1960s. J. H. Emerson (**Figure 55–33**) took the lead in 1964 with the manufacture of his rotary piston volume- and time-controlled 3-PV ventilator. A fleet of American ICU workhorses soon followed, including the Puritan Bennett MA-1 (1967), Ohio 560 (1968), Ohio/Monaghan 225 (1972), and Bourns Bear I (1975). By the mid- to late 1960s arterial blood gas electrodes had become available in most hospitals. This technology provided the ability to monitor both ventilation and oxygenation. Anesthesiologists developed a new awareness of the effects of intraoperative atelectasis, which was initially treated by increasing tidal volume to 10 to 15 mL/kg. Unfortunately, that approach was indiscriminately transferred to the ICU for all patients, including those with diseased or injured lungs.[49,50] The Vietnam

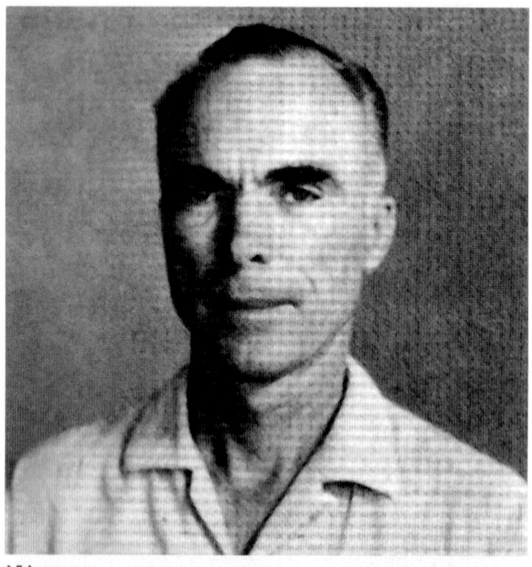

(A)

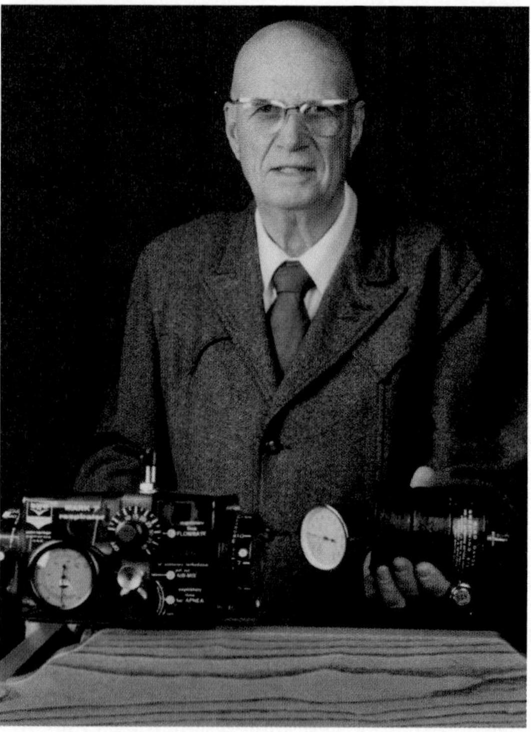

(B)

FIGURE 55–32 **(A)** V. Ray Bennett, developer of the flow-sensitive valve used on early Puritan-Bennett assistors and anesthesia machines. **(B)** Dr. Forrest Bird, shown holding his original magnetic device (right) and a Bird Mark 7 (left).

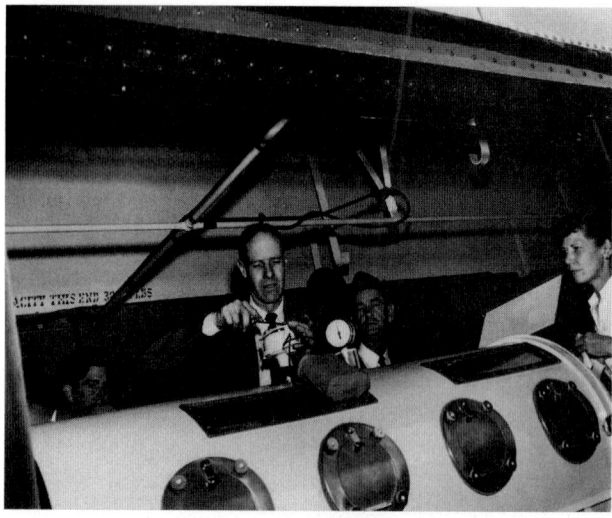

FIGURE 55–33 J. H. (Jack) Emerson was a notable inventor of mechanical ventilators. He is shown working on his version of the iron lung (circa 1932), which was less costly and lighter weight than the Drinker. He also invented an early positive pressure piston-driven (3-PV) ventilator in 1964 that became one of the early "workhorses." He later modified that device for IMV in the 1970s.

War provided further insight into critical care medicine. Drs. David Ashbaugh, Thomas Petty (**Figure 55–34**), and Boyd Bigelow published their landmark paper on acute respiratory distress syndrome (ARDS) in 1967, and the use of positive end-expiratory pressure (PEEP) soon followed.[51,52]

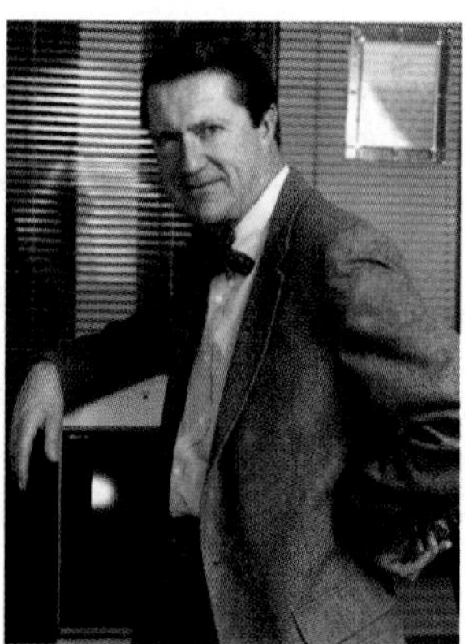

FIGURE 55–34 Dr. Thomas Petty, pulmonologist who coauthored the initial publications on acute respiratory distress syndrome, positive end-expiratory pressure, and the benefits of long-term oxygen therapy.

In perinatal and pediatric medicine, Dr. Virginia Apgar (1909–1974; **Figure 55–35**) developed her scoring system for newborns in 1955. In the 1970s, research on fetal lambs elucidated the cause of respiratory distress syndrome in infants. Soon CPAP systems were promoted by Gregory.[53] Exogenous surfactant therapy followed. Ventilators specifically designed for infants began to appear. In 1964, Bourns Inc. developed a linear piston-driven infant volume ventilator, the LS104-150. However, intermittent mandatory ventilation with PEEP/CPAP, developed by Kirby, evolved to be the standard of practice. Kirby collaborated with Bird in the development of the Baby Bird in 1971. Similar ventilators, such as the Bourns PB-200, Bear Cub, and Sechrist IV-100B, became familiar sights in neonatal ICUs, along with respiratory therapists with specialized skills.[54]

Adult and perinatal/pediatric mechanical ventilators have evolved steadily (**Table 55–2**). Technology advancements, first in printed circuits and later in microprocessors, have allowed manufacturers to usher in new operational characteristics (modes), improved valve response, and enhanced monitoring and alarm capabilities. The 1960s classification system devised by Mushin

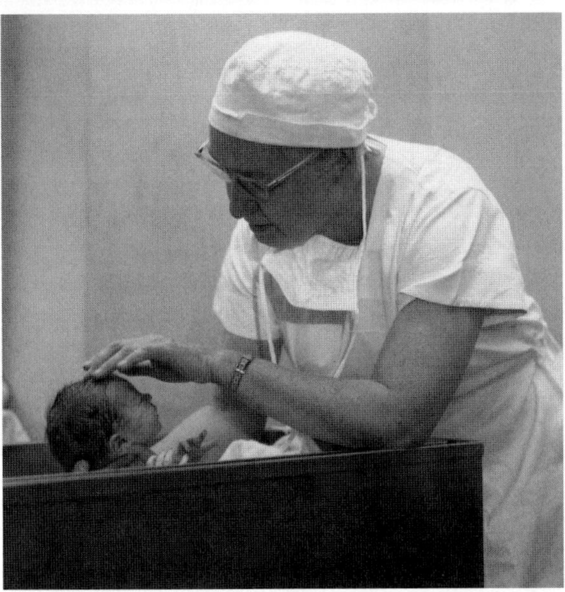

FIGURE 55–35 Dr. Virginia Apgar developed a newborn infant scoring system based on physical assessment to aid in guiding care in the delivery room.

was updated by respiratory therapist Rob Chatburn.[55] In contrast to the many modes of ventilation, there have been few changes that have translated into decreased morbidity and mortality.

In the mid-1980s, the use of noninvasive ventilation (NIV) for patients with either acute exacerbations of COPD or neurologic respiratory failure was proposed. Over time, NIV modes have become the standards of practice. In addition, improved diagnosis of sleep-disordered breathing resulted in a phenomenal increase in the use of nasal CPAP for obstructive sleep apnea (OSA) and of NIV for patients with a central component. Advances in mask design, CPAP generators, and ventilators to meet those needs have rapidly occurred in the past few years.[56,57] Alternative ventilator modes, such as airway pressure release ventilation (APRV), first appeared in 1987.[58] Ventilator manufacturers have aggressively marketed newer modes. Dual-control models permit switching from pressure or volume control. Weaning modes include auto mode, proportional assist ventilation (PAV), adaptive support ventilation (ASV), and auto tube compensation (ATC).[59]

> **RESPIRATORY RECAP**
>
> **Historical Developments in Respiratory Care**
>
> » Clinical oxygen therapy
> » Medicated aerosol therapy
> » Airways and intubation
> » Mechanical ventilation

Animal studies and a multicenter human study by the Acute Respiratory Distress Syndrome Network (ARDSnet) resulted in a major rethinking of tidal volume size during mechanical ventilation.[60,61] Reducing the traditional tidal volume from 10 to 12 mL/kg to 6 mL/kg can provide a lung-protective strategy and reduce mortality. Use of high-frequency modes such as high-frequency oscillatory ventilation (HFO) has seen greater acceptance for use with premature infants.[62] Its use for adults with ARDS has not demonstrated significant outcome differences. Adjuncts such as prone positioning and the use of inhaled nitric oxide have shown some benefit to improve oxygenation in ARDS patients. Research continues to better identify which patients might benefit most.[63]

Milestones in the Organizations Within the Respiratory Care Profession: Beginning Years

In 1943, Chicago-based otolaryngologist Albert H. Andrews (**Figure 55–36**) wrote a monograph entitled *Manual of Oxygen Therapy Techniques* in which he proposed that formal hospital departments of inhalation therapy should be established. Inhalation therapy departments would function under the medical direction of a knowledgeable staff physician. Pulmonologist Edwin R. Levine and anesthesiologist Max Sadov (refer to Figure 55–36) joined Andrews to teach every 2 weeks for a 9-month period. They realized the importance of both scientific background and a well-organized inhalation therapy hospital department. Early oxygen technicians were employed through central supply or the orderly staff. Their job was to ensure that oxygen cylinders with functioning regulators and flow meters were available on demand for the bedside care of postsurgical patients who needed masks or oxygen tents.

A core group formed, consisting of Chicago-based oxygen technicians from Michael Reese and Alexian Brothers Hospitals and nurse anesthesia students from area schools. The founders organized the Inhalational Therapy Association (ITA) on July 13, 1946, at the University of Chicago Hospital. It became apparent that much work was needed to gain financial support and to devise a systematic approach for developing an infrastructure for a national organization, an educational system, and a method for awarding a credential. On April 5, 1947, articles of incorporation for chartering this nonprofit organization were filed with the Illinois secretary of state. The mission statement, which suggested fostering a cooperative relationship with physicians and the need to advance the art and science of inhalation therapy through education, is summarized here:

- To promote higher standards in methods and the professional advancement of members of the association
- To create mutual understanding and cooperation among the technicians, physicians, and all others working in the interest of individual or public health
- To advance the knowledge of inhalation therapy through institutes, lectures, and other means under the sponsorship of physicians
- To grant certificates of qualification to individuals who have completed educational requirements

TABLE 55–2 Adult and Infant Ventilator Development

Year Introduced	Brand/Model	Year Introduced	Brand/Model
1907	Drager Pulmotor	1982	Bear Medical Bear 2
1948	Bennett TV-2P	1983	Biomed IC-5 Microprocessor
1951	Engstrom 150	1984	Puritan Bennett 7200
1953	Drager Poliomat	1984	Sechrist Adult 2200B
1953	Thompson portable	1985	Bear Medical Bear 5
1954	Morch III	1985	Ohmeda CPU
1955	Bird MK-7	1986	Hamilton Veolar
1956	Emerson Assistor	1986	Bird 6400 ST
1958	Drager Spiromat	1986	Infrasonics Infant Star
1961	Bennett PR-1	1988	Bear Medical Bear 3
1963	Air Shields 1000	1988	Hamilton Amadeus
1964	Emerson Post-op 3-PV	1988	Bird 8400 ST
1964	Bourns LS104-150	1988	Respironics S/T D-30
1967	Puritan-Bennett MA-1	1989	Bunnell Life Pulse
1968	Ohio 560	1989	PPG Irisa/Drager Evita
1968	Engstrom ER 300	1989	Infrasonics Adult Star
1970	Veriflow CV 2000	1991	Siemens Servo 300
1970	Hamilton Standard PAD-1	1993	Bear Medical Bear 1000
1971	Siemens 900	1993	Drager Evita
1972	Monaghan 225 fluidic	1996	Respironics Vision
1972	Baby Bird	1997	Drager Evita 2 Dura
1972	Bird IMV	1998	Hamilton Galileo
1973	Chemtron Gill 1	1998	Buritan Bennett 840
1974	Emerson 3-MV	2001	Siemens Servo
1974	Searle VVA	2001	Respironics Esprit
1974	Ohio 550 fluidic	2001	Viasys/Cardinal Health Vela
1975	Bourns Bear I	2001	Drager Savina
1976	Forreger 210	2001	Newport e500
1978	Puritan Bennett MA-2 & MA-2+2	2001	Pulmonetics LTV 1000
1980	Engstrom Erica	2002	Viasys/Cardinal Health Avea
1980	Respironics BiPAP	2003	Drager Evita XL
1982	Siemens 900C	2005	GE Datex-Ohmeda Engstrom Carestation

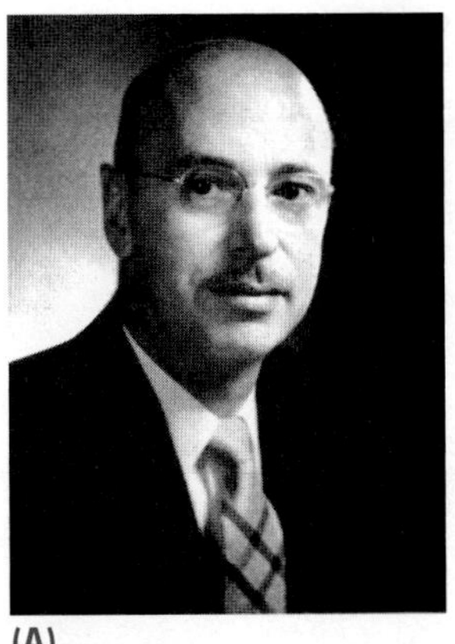
(A)

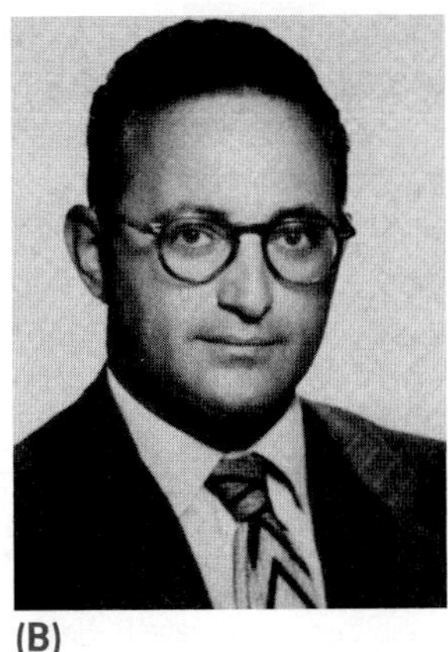
(B)

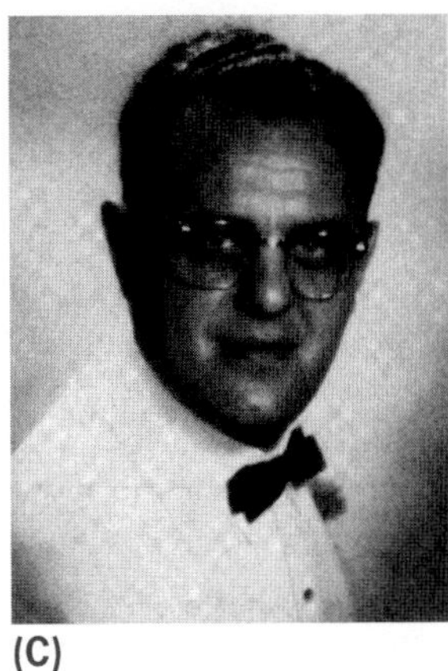
(C)

FIGURE 55–36 **(A)** Dr. Albert Andrews Jr., **(B)** Dr. Edwin Levine, and **(C)** Dr. Max Sandov were physicians in the Chicago metropolitan area who promoted education for those who provided oxygen therapy.

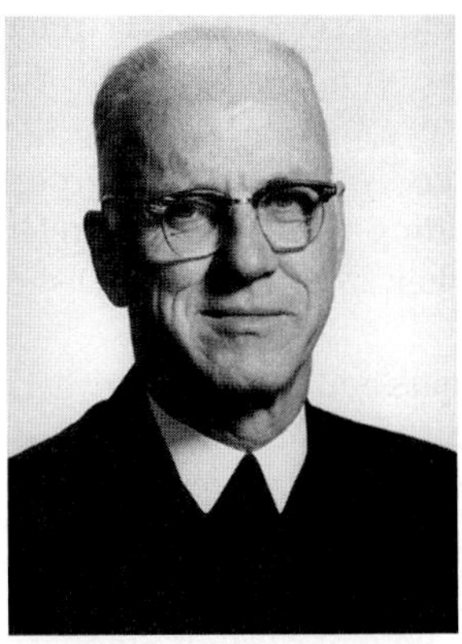
FIGURE 55–37 Brother Roland Maher was the second president of the Inhalational Therapy Association (ITA). He worked at Alexian Brothers Hospital in Chicago. He served as president from 1949 to 1951 and from 1953 to 1954.

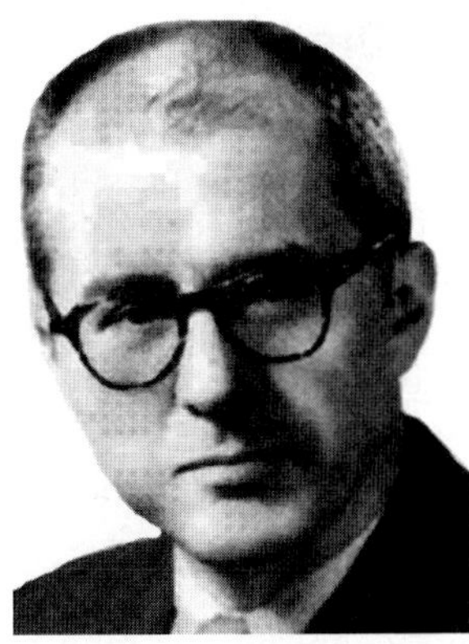
FIGURE 53–38 Albert Carrière, first executive director of the AIT (from 1955 to 1966).

There were 59 charter members, including pharmacists, nurse anesthetists, nurses, inhalation therapy department managers, an attorney, a member of the oxygen medical industry, and nine physicians. George A. Kneeland served as chairman. Brother Roland Maher, a nurse anesthetist, served as assistant chairman (**Figure 55–37**). Drs. Andrews, Levine, and Sadov served as medical advisors for the next 9 years.[1]

In 1948, the fledgling group changed its name to the Inhalation Therapy Association. To act on its mission statement, a quarterly newsletter entitled the *ITA Bulletin* was published from 1950 to mid-1954 and sent to 1500 U.S. hospitals free of charge. Also in 1950, the ITA began sponsoring a series of lectures and workshops. The first glimpse of credentialing was the awarding of 31 certificates to those who had attended 16 of the workshops. In the following year, a more formal 5-day workshop was cosponsored with the American College of Chest Physicians (ACCP).

In 1954 membership grew to over 200 members, representing 14 states. The national scope was reflected in a name change to the American Association of Inhalation Therapists (AAIT). Because of the increasing need for administrative management, in 1955 the association's president, Sister Mary Borromea, OSF, CRNA, hired a public relations firm to manage the association's business affairs. Albert Carrière (**Figure 55–38**), a principal in the firm, was named the first executive director of the AAIT and served until 1967. The profession established a code of ethics in 1958. To broaden the base of governance, in 1966 the AAIT established its House of Delegates. In 1972 the association changed its name to the American Association for Respiratory Therapy (AART) to better reflect changing medical practice, which had come to include pulmonary and cardiovascular diagnostics. In 1982, the professional association changed its name to the American Association for Respiratory Care (AARC).

The initial mission of the AAIT was not only to establish an infrastructure to serve as a professional association but also to provide national standards for education and a formal credentialing system. However, these were daunting tasks for one organization and also set up a potential for conflicts of interest. This set the stage for two other independent organizations to assist the AAIT as part of an educational system and credentialing board. Education took a step forward when Drs. Alvan Barach, Edwin Emma, and Vincent Collins published formalized minimum standards for training programs in 1950. They received support from the Committee on Public Health Relations of the New York Academy of Medicine. In the document, they specified a curriculum and conditions of training. They noted that in most medical schools, inhalation therapy was rarely part of the curriculum.[64,65]

The first hospital-based training programs were in place by 1960. However, it was apparent that a system of school accreditation would be required. The Board of Schools (BOS) was formed under the American Medical Association (AMA) Council on Medical Education and Hospitals (CMEH) in 1963. The board was composed of two members from each of the sponsoring physician organizations (the ACCP and the American Society of Anesthesiologists [ASA]) and three representatives from the AAIT. In early 1964, the first survey teams began evaluating training programs. Over the years the accreditation group has evolved; currently, that function is the mission of the Commission for Accreditation of Respiratory Care (CoARC).

By November of 1960, the credentialing portion of the tripartite system was formalized. A core group of three ITA members along with three physicians formed

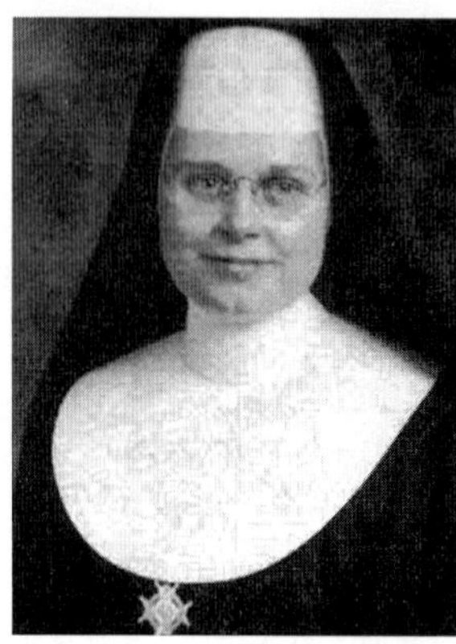

FIGURE 55–39 Sister Mary Yvonne Jenn, BS, RN, first registrar of the American Registry of Inhalation Therapists (ARIT) and registered therapist number 1.

the American Registry of Inhalation Therapists (ARIT). The initial plan was for a written exam and a set of two oral exams. The group's exam standards were purposely quite rigorous because of the modest educational requirements compared with other allied health professions. The rigor was also attributed to the significant responsibility a respiratory therapist has for a patient's life. The first executive group consisted of Dr. Albert Andrews, president; Dr. Duncan Holiday, vice president; Sr. Mary Yvonne Jenn (**Figure 55–39**), registrar; and Jim Whitacre, secretary. Twelve candidates passed the first pilot exam in 1960. Because the ARIT was not legally incorporated until January 1961, the first group of 28 registered respiratory therapists (RRTs) was awarded their credentials after a second session of examinations in April of that year. Like the AIT, the ARIT has had a series of name changes. In 1975 it became the National Board for Respiratory Therapy (NBRT). In 1983 it took its current title as the National Board for Respiratory Care (NBRC).

Professional Publications

Since the early days of the quarterly *ITA Bulletin* (1950–1954), the professional association has supported publications for its members to stay informed of association news. Its news magazine, *AARC Times*, began in 1978. Its peer-reviewed scientific journal is *Respiratory Care*, which was initially called *Inhalation Therapy* and published its first issue in February 1956 (**Figure 55–40**). It featured original research, special articles, journal symposia proceedings, case reports, and teaching cases. The first editor was James Whitacre, MS, RRT (refer to Figure 55–40A), who served until 1967. In 1971 the journal was renamed *Respiratory Care.* Over time the editor's key role has been served by an important group of respiratory therapists, including Phil Kittredge (refer to Figure 55–40B), Pat Brougher, and physician David Pierson, MD.

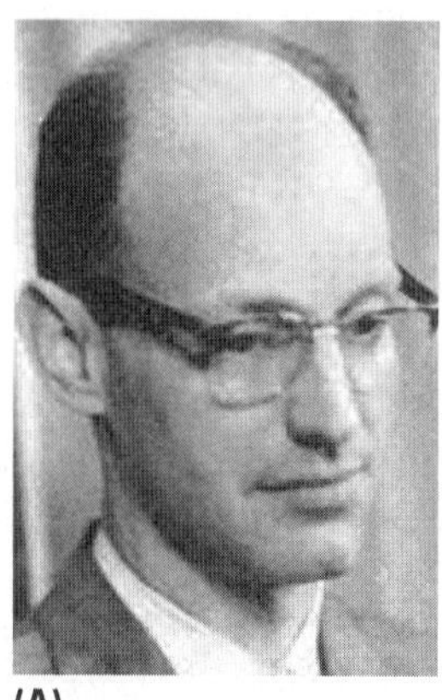

(A)

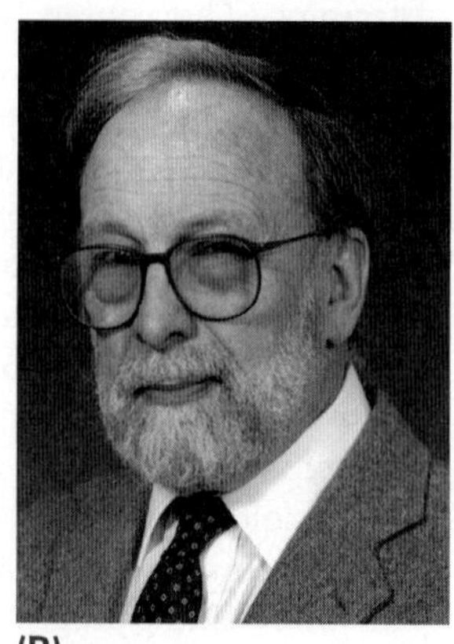

(B)

FIGURE 55–40 **(A)** James F. Whitacre, MS, RRT, first secretary of the American Registry of Inhalation Therapists (ARIT) and first editor of *Inhalation Therapy: Journal of the American Association of Inhalation Therapists.* **(B)** Phil Kittredge, BA, RRT, second editor of *Respiratory Care* (1968–1986). He coedited with Ms. Pat Brougher, BA, RRT, from 1987 to 1989.

TABLE 55–3 Past Editors of the AARC's Scientific Journal *Respiratory Care*

Years	Editor(s)
1956–1967	James F. Whitacre, MS, RRT
1968–1986	Philip Kittredge, BA, RRT
1987–1989	Philip Kittredge, BA, RRT, and Pat Brougher, BA, RRT
1990–1997	Pat Brougher, BA, RRT
1998–2007	David J. Pierson, MD
2008–	Dean R. Hess, PhD, RRT

Table 55–3 records the journal's editors and their years of service. The journal is a major international publication that is focused on respiratory care. Its special proceedings and consensus conferences publish the work of world-class experts in specific content areas. These have tremendous value to the entire field of cardiopulmonary medicine. In 2000, the journal was included in Index Medicus. This validates the increasing level of scholarship and scientific research within the respiratory care profession. The journal also has facilitated research from a broad base of practitioners through its sponsorship of Open Forum abstract-poster presentations at the annual AARC International Congress meeting.

History of the Credentialing Organization and State Licensure

Credentialing is a generic term that refers to recognition of individuals who have attained a specified level of competency in an occupation. The two major forms of credentialing are by voluntary national certification/registry and by state licensure. The NBRC is the nationally recognized, voluntary credentialing body in respiratory care. Through its examination systems, therapists demonstrate competency. Each state legislature, or state medical board, typically determines laws that define the right to practice, provide title recognition, or require registration/listing of practitioners. At present, all U.S. states have licensure/registration provisions except Alaska. Puerto Rico also has licensure. In addition to documentation of successful completion and graduation from an accredited respiratory care program, state licensure (in most states) is based on completion of the certified respiratory therapist (CRT) credentialing exam administered by the National Board for Respiratory

Care. The registered respiratory therapist (RRT) credential requires completion of a second written exam, as well as a clinical simulation exam.

The history of the profession's two-tiered CRT and RRT system is the source of some controversy and continued discussion. In the 1960s, the leadership of the AARC (then the AAIT) and NBRC (then the ARIT) originally envisioned one registry credential, to be provided via the latter organization. However, in 1968, AAIT president John R. Julius appointed Louise H. Julius to head a committee to undertake the process of both educating and granting a credential for certified inhalation therapy technicians (CITT). It appears there was pressure within the AAIT membership to have some recognition for those who were not able to complete the more rigorous registry exams. It was thought that this could help maintain employment by having a credential (for the future) if pending state licensure acts were enacted. By the fall of 1969, the AAIT had established a Technician Certification Board (TCB) and established a training process and programs. It administered its first pilot exam to 100 practitioners. This concept was not originally supported by the ARIT.

After significant deliberations, in 1972 the AARC (then the ARRT) transferred the TCB's credentialing role to the ARIT. By 1975 the latter began administering its version of the CITT exam. During this time, the U.S. Department of Health, Education, and Welfare conducted a survey of the profession of respiratory therapy.[66] Not surprisingly, the study found significant overlap in the tasks performed by those with technician and therapist credentials. By 1978 a national job analysis by the NBRC (then NBRT) found a similar employment pattern. With support from the AART, the NBRC agreed to develop an initial written examination that would reflect the tasks and competency level required of all candidates for entry to practice. Successful completion would allow certification. After a 6-month interval, completion of a second set of exams (written and clinical simulation) would allow the registry credential for the advanced practitioner graduates of therapist-level programs. This hierarchical certified-to-registered system was put into place in 1983.

Over the next 20 years, as most states implemented licensure systems, completion of the entry-level (CRT) examination became the criterion. However, over that same time, as job responsibilities became more complex, there has been a gradual decline in the employment demand for CRTs. Currently there are no longer technician-only training programs. Therefore, a decision made in 1968 has resulted in a two-tiered system becoming embedded into the licensure process, even though it was not originally intended by the profession's original leaders in credentialing.[1]

In addition to the CRT and RRT credentials, the NBRC currently provides specialty board exams in pulmonary function diagnostics, perinatal/pediatrics, and sleep diagnostics. **Table 55–4** identifies current examinations and credentials.

TABLE 55–4 National Board for Respiratory Care Examinations

Examinations	Credentials
Primary Examinations	
Entry level	Certified respiratory therapist (CRT)
Advanced practitioner	Registered respiratory therapist (RRT)
Specialty Examinations	
Entry-level pulmonary function	Certified pulmonary function technologist (CPFT)
Advanced pulmonary function	Registered pulmonary function technologist (RPFT)
Neonatal/pediatric respiratory care	Certified neonatal/pediatric specialist (CRT-NPS) or registered neonatal/pediatric specialist (RRT-NPS)
Sleep disorders	Certified respiratory therapist–sleep disorders specialist (CRT-SDS) or registered respiratory therapist–sleep disorders specialist (RRT-SDS)

History of Respiratory Care Education and Program Accreditation

The Board of Schools (BOS) was charged with reviewing applications for new training programs and conducting site visits to grant approval status. The original members of the BOS were four therapists and three physicians. In 1967, the new guidelines of the AMA's Council on Medical Education mandated a minimum program length of 18 months of training. At that time, schools were primarily based in hospitals. The Board of Schools was disbanded in 1969 because of some resistance to orienting programs with academic institutions, problems with funding site visits, and continued concerns about the quality of the school accreditation process. Its replacement, the Joint Review Committee for Respiratory Therapy Education (JRCRTE) was incorporated in 1970. It was approved by the AMA's Council on Medical Education for its role in national program accreditation of respiratory care programs. The first chairman was H. Fred Helmholz Jr., MD (**Figure 55–41**), a representative of the ACCP. He was an experienced cardiopulmonary physiologist, having worked in the Mayo Aero Medical Unit during World War II.

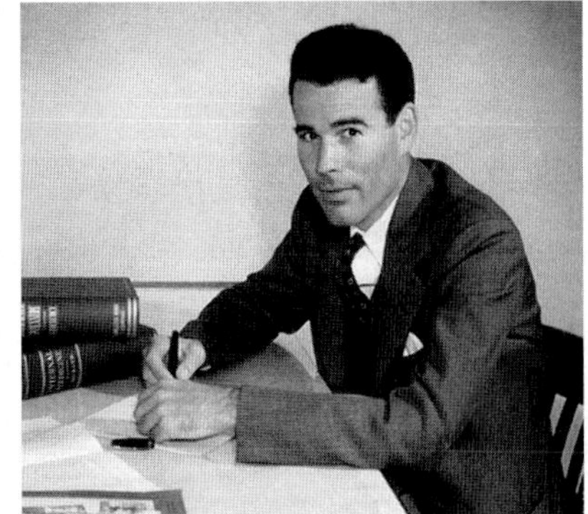
FIGURE 55–41 Dr. H. F. Helmholz Jr. (circa 1942), first chairman of the Joint Review Committee for Respiratory Therapy Education, 1970 to 1976.

During this time, all programs were required to be sponsored by a formally accredited academic institution.

When the AMA CME withdrew as an overseer of allied health education, the JRCRTE became one of the 25 other review committees under the "umbrella accreditor," the Committee on Allied Health Education and Accreditation (CAHEA). Upon Dr. Helmholz's retirement in 1976, the office was moved from Rochester, Minnesota, to the Dallas, Texas, area. Over the years, the process of accreditation has continued to evolve. In 1986, the JRCRTE became the first allied health programmatic accrediting committee to support a focus on outcomes of education. This shift focused on board exam performance rather than the training process. The Essentials and Guidelines have gone through multiple updates to reflect the escalating demands of education and clinical practice experiences.

Following recommendations by a Pew Commission Report, the CAHEA accreditation system was restructured into the Commission on Accreditation of Allied Health Education Programs (CAAHEP) in 1994. In 1994, the AARC experienced difficulties with JRCRTE in the matter of accreditation and withdrew its sponsorship. It temporarily set up a separate Respiratory Care Accreditation Board (RCAB). The concerns were resolved by 1996, and as a result the JRCRTE was renamed the Commission on Accreditation for Respiratory Care (CoARC). In an effort to provide broader and more responsive accreditation service to programs, CoARC withdrew from CAAHEP in 2009 and established itself as an independent accrediting agency under the Council for Higher Education Accreditation (CHEA). Besides members at large and the lay public, other sponsor and representative organizations of CoARC include the AARC, ASA, ATS, ACCP, Association of Schools of Allied Health Professions (ASAHP), National Network of Health Career Programs in Two-Year Colleges (NN2).

Respiratory care educators have maintained a pragmatic approach in terms of teaching strategies, blending classroom, laboratory, and clinical practicums. However, the scope of practice, responsibilities, and technology continued to escalate. Recognizing the need to plan for future change, during 1992 and 1993 the AARC sponsored two educational consensus conferences and supported research on the future scope of the practice and education of therapists.[67,68] The first conference documented those practice demands and the difficulty in providing entry-level education in less than an associate degree's 2-year time frame. The second conference's recommendations resulted in the AARC, JRCRTE, and NBRC all agreeing to set the associate degree as the minimum academic entry level in 2002. This resulted in the decline and eventual closure of training programs at the CRT-only level.

RESPIRATORY RECAP

Achievements of the Beginning Years of the Respiratory Care Profession

- » Circulation of the foundational documents
- » Creation of the professional organization
- » Establishment of the professional journal
- » Development of the credentialing organization
- » Establishment of a system for accreditation of respiratory educational programs

Throughout this period, the demand for therapists exceeded the supply, and the pressure to meet workforce needs may have maintained the lower-division academic degree as compared with other health professions. Respiratory care has evolved from conducting limited, task-based technical functions in 1947 to performing an array of services requiring more complex cognitive abilities and patient management skills in the 21st century. In 2008, the AARC sponsored the first of a three-part series to again look at how the education and credentialing systems can prepare to meet the evolving roles of the respiratory therapist.[69] Data presented at this conference documented that respiratory therapists have become more involved in public health, end-of-life and palliative care, smoking cessation, home care, and sleep diagnostics. Because of increasing pressures to reduce medical costs, responsibility for outpatient case management will likely become a major new role for therapists for patients with asthma, COPD, cystic fibrosis, lung cancer, and pulmonary interstitial fibrosis as well as cardiovascular diseases. Therapists are, and will continue to be, more involved in providing patient education and in coordinating care in cost-effective approaches and multiple settings.

To meet these future needs, educational programs will likely respond by expanding both didactic curricula and clinical practicums beyond the traditional settings. These new responsibilities require professional competencies. The roles of both outpatient case manager and respiratory consultant to interdisciplinary hospital teams demand higher levels of communication, assessment abilities, and integrative critical thinking skills to operate within protocols and best-practice consensus guidelines. Besides applying a scientific approach, therapist recommendations need to be individualized based on economic and humanistic (ethical and moral) dimensions.[67–69] Department managers will also need therapists who are multicompetent—bedside caregivers who have added abilities to assist in management tasks, patient and staff development and education, and research. These trends may be reflected in the increasing number of baccalaureate degree programs, which have grown from 7 in 1970 to approximately 60 in 2009. There also is more interest in developing postgraduate residency programs, following models of physician and pharmacy education.[70–72]

Respiratory Care Science: Contemporary and Future

This chapter has chronicled the history of respiratory care prior to the establishment of the profession, as well as the past 60 years since it officially began in 1947. The original AIT mission statement of caring for patients and supporting the art and science of respiratory care has not changed. However, the technology, scope of practice, and level of responsibility of today's respiratory care practitioners hardly resemble that of the original respiratory therapists who were oxygen orderlies. It is difficult to imagine practicing respiratory care without medical gas supplies, sterile techniques, full-ranging pharmaceuticals, microprocessor-based mechanical ventilators, and Internet communication.

In the United States, medical education took a huge step forward with the Carnegie Foundation–commissioned Flexner report.[73] After studying every school in the United States, Abraham Flexner found several different approaches (apprenticeship, proprietary, and university) and vastly different curricula (e.g., scientific, homeopathic, botanical, physiomedical, spiritual). His study revealed some good schools but also many deplorable schools with incompetent faculty, dismal laboratories, and haphazard clinical experiences, all of which contributed to ill-prepared graduates.

A lack of a scientific approach, without much research-based science, was notable in the early days of inhalation therapy education and practice in spite of school standards and early textbooks on inhalation/respiratory therapy by Drs. Alvan Barach, Peter Safar, and Donald Egan.[74–79] This was clearly identified in 1974 by the first Conference on the Scientific Basis of Respiratory Therapy, supported jointly by the then-National Heart and Lung Institute (NHLI) and the American Thoracic Society (ATS), held at Temple University Conference Center at Sugarloaf in Philadelphia.[77] Prominent scientists nationwide reviewed available evidence (or lack of evidence) for oxygen therapy, aerosol therapy, physical therapy, and IPPB therapy. IPPB therapy, a major clinical task of the 1960s and early 1970s, was scrutinized, and the evidence suggested a vast enterprise of abuse in spite of good science that showed no value of IPPB for conditions such as emphysema.[78] The lesson was clear: the scientific method needed to be applied, not tradition. Physicians and therapists needed to assess patients and perform only justified care with identifiable, measureable outcomes and individualized needs.

This premise was clearly promoted in 1988 in the journal *Respiratory Care*.[79] By 1992 the term *evidence-based medicine (EBM)* began to appear in the literature.[80] The clinical practice of respiratory care paralleled this theme by using committees of therapist and physician experts to systematically review therapeutic and diagnostic care. In 1996, the AARC began publication of clinical practice guidelines (CPGs) in *Respiratory Care*. They have subsequently been categorized as evidence-based or expert panel guidelines. CPGs for over 50 types of care are available via *Respiratory Care*'s website.[81] Similar approaches have been used by major groups to provide guidelines for the care of patients with COPD and asthma, as well as the American Heart Association's standards for CPR.[82–84] In addition to use of EBM, there has been an evolution of therapist-driven protocols (TDPs). TDPs allow respiratory therapy, nursing, and physician staff to use algorithm-like decision plans to choose therapy based on assessment and individual needs.[85]

The healthcare system in the United States and internationally is positioned for dramatic changes. To continue its successful evolution, the AARC is facilitating a process similar to the Carnegie Foundation's support of Flexner's study. The results of the three-part 2015 and Beyond conferences should be valuable to guide future directions. In 2007, the profession of respiratory care celebrated its 60th year. Since 1947 the number of respiratory therapists practicing in the United States has grown from a handful to 145,117.[86] There also is a considerable representation internationally. From a group of 28 in 1963, as of 2008 there were 115,883 registered and 93,000 certified therapists credentialed by the NBRC. Informal hospital conferences have evolved into over 400 accredited respiratory therapy educational programs at colleges and universities. A final quote from medical historian Henry Sigerist should set the theme for those who practice respiratory care into the future: "Medical history teaches us where we came from, where we stand in medicine at the present time, and what direction we are marching. It's the compass that guides us into the future. If our plan is not to be hap-hazard but to follow a well-laid plan, we need the guidance of history, and it is not by accident that all great medical leaders were fully aware of historical studies."[87]

KEY POINTS

- Key scientists helped establish the foundation for respiratory care modalities and treatments.
- A variety of discoveries in math, science, and engineering contributed to the development of respiratory care as an allied health profession.
- Several key individuals, organizations, and events led to the establishment of respiratory care as an allied health profession.
- Throughout history and up to the current time, many organizations have promoted, supported, sponsored, and funded the respiratory care profession.
- Certain organizations have very specific and limited missions, whereas others are more diverse in purpose and mission.
- The goals of each supporting organization ultimately improve the scope, practice, education, credentials, quality, and professional growth of respiratory care, which ultimately benefits society through health and wellness.
- The American Association of Respiratory Care (AARC) and related professional organizations enhance the entire respiratory care profession, with far-reaching effects beyond each organization's membership.

- Membership in the AARC should be considered an integral part of a respiratory care professional's identity.
- Knowing the history of the profession serves as a guide and compass, pointing individuals and organizations into the future.

REFERENCES

1. Smith GA, ed. *Respiratory Care: Evolution of a Profession*. Lenexa, KS: Applied Measurement Professionals; 1989.
2. Loudon I, ed. *Western Medicine: An Illustrated History*. New York: Oxford University Press; 1997.
3. Magner LN. *A History of Medicine*. 2nd ed. New York: Informa Healthcare; 2005.
4. Bynum WF. *The History of Medicine: A Very Short Introduction*. New York: Oxford University Press; 2008.
5. National Institutes of Health. History of medicine. Available at: http://www.nlm.nih.gov/hmd. Accessed January 14, 2009.
6. Perkins JF. Historical development of respiratory physiology. In: Fenn WO, Rahn H, eds. *Handbook of Physiology: Respiration*. Washington, DC: American Physiological Society; 1964:1–58.
7. Cahill T. *How the Irish Saved Civilization*. New York: Doubleday; 1996.
8. Cassebaum H, Schufle JA. Scheele's priority for the discovery of oxygen. *J Chem Ed*. 1975;52(7):442–444.
9. Gottlieb LS. Thomas Beddoes, MD, and the pneumatic institution at Clifton, 1798–1801. *Ann Intern Med*. 1965;63:530–533.
10. Petty TL. John Hutchinson's mysterious machine revisited. *Chest*. 2002;121(5 suppl):219S–223S.
11. Colice GL. Historical perspective on the development of mechanical ventilation. In: Tobin MJ, ed. *Principles and Practice of Mechanical Ventilation*. New York: McGraw-Hill; 1994.
12. Miracle VA. The life and impact of Florence Nightingale. *Dimensions Crit Care Nursing*. 2008;27(1):21–23.
13. Bergman NA. *The Genesis of Surgical Anesthesia*. Park Ridge, IL: Wood Library–Museum of Anesthesiology; 1998.
14. Haldane JS. *Respiration*. New Haven, CT: Yale University Press; 1922.
15. Helmholz HF. Professional champions (1900–1940). In: Smith GA, ed. *Respiratory Care: Evolution of a Profession*. Lexena, KS: Applied Measurement Professionals; 1989.
16. Kobasa D, Takada A, Shinya K, et al. Enhanced virulence of influenza A viruses with the haemagglutinin of the 1918 pandemic virus. *Nature*. 2004;431(7009):703–707.
17. Perkins JF. Historical development of respiratory physiology. In: Fen WO, Rahn H, eds. *Handbook of Physiology*. Vol. 3. Washington, DC: American Physiological Society; 1964.
18. Leigh JM. The evolution of the oxygen therapy apparatus. *Anaesthesia*. 1974;29:462.
19. Barach AL. Symposium: inhalation therapy historical background. *Anesthesiology*. 1962;23:407.
20. Barach AL. Use of helium as a new therapeutic gas. *Proc Soc Exp Biol Med*. 1934;32:462.
21. Barach AL. The therapeutic use of helium. *JAMA*. 1936;107:1273.
22. Terry TL. Extreme prematurity and fibroblastic overgrowth of persistent vascular sheath behind each crystalline lens. *Am J Opthalmol*. 1942;25:203–204.
23. Severinghaus JW, Astrum PB. History of blood gas analysis: IV. Leland Clark's oxygen electrode. *J Clin Monit*. 1986;2:125.
24. Severinghaus JW, Honda Y. History of blood gas analysis: VII. Pulse oximetry. *J Clin Monit*. 1987;3:135
25. Campbell EJM. A method of controlled oxygen administration which reduces the risk of CO_2 retention. *Lancet*. 1960;1:12.
26. Nocturnal Oxygen Therapy Trial Group. Continuous and nocturnal oxygen therapy in hypoxic chronic obstructive lung disease: a clinical trial. *Ann Intern Med*. 1980;93:931.
27. AARC clinical practice guideline: oxygen therapy in the acute care hospital. *Respir Care*. 1991;36:1410.
28. AARC clinical practice guideline: oxygen therapy in the home or extended care facility. *Respir Care*. 1992;37:918.
29. Dessanges JF. A history of nebulization. *J Aerosol Med*. 2001; 14(1):65–71.
30. Dehand R. Nebulizers that use a vibrating mesh or plate with multiple apertures to generate aerosols. 2002;47(12):1406–1416.
31. Stoller JK. History of intubation, tracheostomy and airway appliances. *Respir Care*. 1999;44:595–603.
32. Safar P, Escarraga LA, Elam JO. A comparison of the mouth-to-mouth and mouth-to-airway methods of artificial respiration with the chest pressure arm-lift methods. *N Engl J Med*. 1958;258:671–677.
33. Kouwenhoven WB, Jude JR, Knickerbocker GG. Closed-chest cardiac massage. *JAMA*. 1960;173:1064–1067.
34. Safar P, Brown T, Holtey W, Wider R. Ventilation and circulation with closed-chest massage in man. *JAMA*. 1961;176:574–576.
35. Ad Hoc Committee on Cardiopulmonary Resuscitation of the Division of Medical Sciences, National Academy of Sciences–National Research Council. Cardiopulmonary resuscitation. *JAMA*. 1966;198:138–145.
36. Lown B, Neuman J, Amarasingham R, Berkovits BV. Comparison of alternating current with direct current electroshock across the closed chest. *Am J Cardiol*. 1962;10:223.
37. Hilberman M. Evolution of intensive care units. *Crit Care Med*. 1975;3(4):159.
38. Brain AIJ. The laryngeal mask: a new concept in airway management. *Br J Anaesthesia*. 1983;55(8):801–806.
39. Mallampati SR, Gatt SP, Gugino LD, et al. A clinical sign to predict difficult tracheal intubation: a prospective study. *Can Anaesth Soc J*. 1985;32(4):429–434.
40. ASA Task Force on Management of the Difficult Airway. Practice guidelines for management of the difficult airway. *Anesthesiology*. 1993;78:597–602.
41. Ciaglia P, Firsching R, Syniec C. Elective percutaneous dilatational tracheostomy. A new simple bedside procedure; preliminary report. *Chest*. 1985;87(6):715–719.
42. Mørch ET. History of mechanical ventilation. In: Kirby RR, Banner MJ, Downs JB, eds. *Clinical Applications of Ventilatory Support*. New York: Churchill Livingstone; 1990.
43. Mushin WW, Rendel-Baker L, Thompson PW, Mapleson WW. *Automatic Ventilation of the Lungs*. 3rd ed. London: Blackwell Scientific; 1980.
44. Colice G. Historical background. In: Tobin MJ, ed. *Principles and Practice of Mechanical Ventilation*. New York: McGraw-Hill; 2002.
45. Lassen HCA. A preliminary report on the 1952 epidemic of poliomyelitis in Copenhagen—with special reference to the treatment of acute respiratory insufficiency. *Lancet*. 1953;1(6749):37–41.
46. Rosenberg H, Axelrod JK. Ernst Trier Mørch: inventor, medical pioneer, heroic freedom fighter. *Anesth Analg*. 2000;90:218.
47. Avery EE, Mørch ET, Benson DW. Critically crushed chests, a new method of treatment with continuous mechanical hyperventilation to produce alkalotic apnea and internal pneumatic stabilization. *J Thoracic Surg*. 1956;32:291–309.
48. Radford EP. Ventilation standards for use in artificial respiration. *J Appl Physiol*. 1955;7:451.
49. Hedley-Whyte J, Pontoppidan H, Morris MJ. The response of patients with respiratory failure and cardiopulmonary disease to different levels of constant volume ventilation. *J Clin Invest*. 1966;45:1543–1554.

American Association for Respiratory Care

The AARC is the national association that represents the respiratory care profession to communities of interest. A profession is described by its advancing science, technology, and practice; continuing education; active participation of its members; credentials; leadership; research; and innovation. The AARC was organized in 1946 as the Inhalation Therapy Association (ITA). As the profession progressed, the name changed and the organization evolved into the professional entity it is today.

The art and science of respiratory care are supported by the publications of the AARC, which include **Respiratory Care**, ***AARC Times***, *Education Annual*, and others published by specialty sections. The editorial board for the scientific journal, *Respiratory Care*, comprises researchers who are also respiratory therapists or physicians. The AARC has various standing and special committees to support the profession.

Funding for operations of the AARC is derived from member dues, advertising, and revenues from educational programs and conventions throughout the year. The AARC has a membership of over 48,000, with approximately 40,000 active members as of January 2009. The AARC also offers student, associate, life, and honorary memberships. The AARC has consistently provided some of the highest member benefits found in the health professions while maintaining nearly the lowest dues of all national healthcare organizations. The AARC has 10 specialty sections that support major subsets of therapists, including management, education, perinatal/pediatrics, adult critical care, home care, subacute care, transport, diagnostics, sleep, and continuing care and rehabilitation. Many AARC members belong to different specialty sections based both on their work activities and on their professional interests.

RESPIRATORY RECAP

Description of a Profession

- » Advancing science and technology
- » Evolving practice, scope, credentialing, and accreditation
- » Advanced degrees and continuing education
- » Active participation by members
- » Leadership, research, and innovation

TABLE 56-1 Common Acronyms in Respiratory Care Related to Professional Organizations

Acronym	Organization or Credential
AARC	American Association for Respiratory Care
AAE	Association of Asthma Educators
AASM	American Academy of Sleep Medicine
AE-C	Certified asthma educator
BOMA	Board of Medical Advisors
BRPT	Board of Registered Polysomnographic Technologists
BOD	(AARC) Board of directors
CoARC	Commission on Accreditation for Respiratory Care
HOD	(AARC) House of Delegates
NBRC	National Board for Respiratory Care
NAECB	National Asthma Educator Certification Board
NAMDRC	National Association for Medical Direction of Respiratory Care
ACCP	American College of Chest Physicians
AAP	American Academy of Pediatrics
ACAAI	American College of Allergy, Asthma, and Immunology
ATS	American Thoracic Society
ALA	American Lung Association
RCP	Respiratory care professional
ASA	American Society of Anesthesiologists
RPSGT	Registered polysomnographic technologist
SCCM	Society of Critical Care Medicine

The AARC in 2009

The AARC comprises several governance and advisory bodies, including the Board of Directors, House of Delegates, Board of Medical Advisors, and executive office, located in Irving, Texas.[1]

Board of Directors

The executive government of the AARC is composed of the **Board of Directors (BOD)** of at least 17 active members consisting of five officers, at least six directors-at-large, and section chairs serving as a director from each specialty section of at least 1000 active members of the association. The officers consist of the president, immediate past president, vice president for internal affairs, vice president for external affairs, secretary-treasurer, and, in alternate years, president-elect.[1] So long as the number of section chairs serving as directors is at least six, the number of at-large directors is equal to the number of section chairs serving as directors. If the number of section chairs serving as directors is less than six, the number of at-large directors is increased to ensure a minimum of 17 members of the Board of Directors. The significance of the section chairpersons is magnified by their inclusion as BOD directors (provided that section has more than 1000 members), which allows growth of the AARC through the potential inclusion of new associations and specialties that relate to the profession. Therefore, the specialty section chairpersons can serve a dual role as both a section chair and BOD director.

In general, the AARC term of office is 3 years. Up to one-third of the at-large directors are elected each year, and the term of office for all directors begins following the annual business meeting. The immediate past speaker of the House of Delegates (HOD), chair of the President's Council, and current chairperson of the Board of Medical Advisors serve 1-year terms as nonvoting members of the BOD.[1]

> **RESPIRATORY RECAP**
>
> **Responsibilities of the Board of Directors**
>
> » The Board of Directors is the governing body of the AARC, with fiduciary responsibility for the professional organization and its members.

The current executive director of the AARC serves as an advisor to the BOD, reporting to the current AARC president. In addition, the incoming AARC president appoints a parliamentarian to the BOD to help with parliamentary procedures for BOD activities before, during, and between board meetings. The BOD meets three times per year, usually during March, directly after the AARC Summer Forum and directly preceding the AARC International Congress in the fall. The BOD and HOD meet simultaneously during the summer and fall meetings, facilitating communications, costs, and actions required by bylaws that govern some activities of the budget, nominations, and joint members of various BOD and HOD committees.

There are currently seven standing committees: bylaws, elections, executive, finance, judicial, program, and strategic planning. This structure significantly streamlines the committee structure and has helped unravel some of the previously overlapping lines of authority. In addition, the combination of the treasurer and secretary positions reflects the reality that the AARC executive office provides much of the support for these functions, with a controller for financial activities and an administrative assistant who records and distributes the minutes of all BOD meetings.

> **RESPIRATORY RECAP**
>
> **AARC Standing Committees**
>
> » Bylaws
> » Elections
> » Executive
> » Finance
> » Judicial
> » Program
> » Strategic planning

House of Delegates

The **House of Delegates (HOD)** is a representative body for the chartered affiliate's societies to contribute to the growth, existence, governance, and future of the respiratory care profession. The general membership can bring wishes and concerns to the national organization through local representatives in the HOD. The HOD further serves as a communication bridge, reporting activities, data, information, and needs to the AARC chartered affiliates and members. Its structure, organization, and function are similar to the United States Congress. The HOD is an advisor to the BOD. The HOD helps govern the AARC through approval of bylaws, budgets, nominations, and audits and through consideration of resolutions and motions forwarded to the BOD for consideration.[1] Any AARC member can bring issues to his or her state delegation, which in turn broaches the issue in a resolution or motion for consideration by the entire HOD.

The current HOD meets preceding the annual business meeting of the association and at such other times as called by its speaker or by the majority vote of the House of Delegates.[1] The HOD is composed of one to three members from each chartered affiliate. Currently, 50 delegations represent 48 states. A two-state delegation comprises Vermont and New Hampshire. One state-and-district combination is composed of Maryland and the District of Columbia. The territory of Puerto Rico has its own delegation. The HOD elects officers, including the speaker-elect, speaker, immediate past speaker, treasurer, and secretary. The speaker appoints the parliamentarian for a 1-year term. As with the BOD, HOD officers also serve 1-year terms, with the exception of the 3-year term as speaker-elect, speaker, and past speaker.

> **RESPIRATORY RECAP**
>
> **House of Delegates**
>
> » Each chartered affiliate of the HOD elects active members of the AARC (from their respective affiliates) to represent the membership of the professional association.

Board of Medical Advisors

The **Board of Medical Advisors (BOMA)** consists of professional medical societies that provide significant input to the art and science of the profession of respiratory care. The current societies include the American Society of Anesthesiologists (ASA), the American College of Chest Physicians (ACCP), the American Thoracic Society (ATS), the American Academy of Pediatrics (AAP), the American College of Allergy, Asthma, and Immunology (ACAAI), the National Association for Medical Directors of Respiratory Care (NAMDRC), and the Society of Critical Care Medicine (SCCM). BOMA consists of no less than 12 individual members nominated from each society, who serve staggered terms.[1] BOMA provides medical guidance in the art and science of respiratory

> **RESPIRATORY RECAP**
>
> **Medical Societies Composing the Board of Medical Advisors**
>
> » American Society of Anesthesiologists (ASA)
> » American College of Chest Physicians (ACCP)
> » American Thoracic Society (ATS)
> » Society for Critical Care Medicine (SCCM)
> » American Academy of Pediatrics (AAP)
> » American College of Allergy, Asthma, and Immunology (ACAAI)
> » National Association for Medical Directors of Respiratory Care (NAMDRC)

care through service to the AARC. The BOMA chairperson is designated in a rotation so that each society has a representative serve as chair.

Specialty Sections

AARC **specialty sections** consist of members with special interests in specific areas of respiratory practice. Like AARC membership, specialty section membership is voluntary. Members of a section pay special dues over and above their annual AARC dues. The current membership in the specialty sections ranges from approximately 450 to 1900 members. Each section has a chairperson, chair-elect, and various committee chairpersons and committee members. Each section publishes an electronic newsletter approximately six times per year, with a circulation to the section's members. Many AARC professionals are members of multiple specialty sections.

The specialty sections usually meet during the Summer Forum and the International Respiratory Care Congress. The sections may introduce recommendations directly to the BOD through their liaison, and the board takes action on such reports during meetings. The AARC vice president for internal affairs serves as the liaison between the specialty sections and the BOD. In response to the fast pace of healthcare policy and practice changes, specialty sections are popular and play a broadened role in governing the AARC.

> **RESPIRATORY RECAP**
>
> **AARC Specialty Sections**
> - Management
> - Education
> - Adult acute care
> - Perinatal/pediatrics
> - Long-term care
> - Home care
> - Diagnostics
> - Continuing care and rehabilitation
> - Transport
> - Sleep

President's Council

The **President's Council** was formed in 1971. The council is composed of past presidents of the AARC who have been elected to membership by the council. The President's Council serves as an advisory body to the Board of Directors and performs other duties assigned by the Board of Directors.[1] This council has significant experience and wisdom gained through its members' experiences as elected officials of the AARC. The chair of the President's Council is elected by the members to serve a 1-year term and presides at meetings of the council. The chair also serves as a nonvoting member of the AARC Board of Directors.

> **RESPIRATORY RECAP**
>
> **President's Council**
> - The President's Council comprises past presidents of the AARC who advise the current Board of Directors and other duties as assigned by the BOD.

Executive Office

The executive office is composed of those individuals employed on behalf of the AARC. The BOD, HOD, and BOMA are composed of professional volunteers who meet membership requirements and work on behalf of the profession. Members of the executive office are hired to focus on the daily activities of the AARC. The executive offices are located in Irving, Texas.

The AARC executive office has an executive director who reports to the president of the AARC. In addition, associate executive directors and staff members support the membership, *Respiratory Care* journal, and educational functions of the AARC. The AARC has an in-depth website (http://www.aarc.org). Users can access membership and respiratory care information, special articles, and announcements at the website. Members can visit a special members-only section of the website for specific information and services.

The AARC in 2015 and Beyond

The profession is involved in a strategic planning process to direct its activities for the future by identifying the clinical and nonclinical skills, attributes, and characteristics of the respiratory therapist for 2015 and beyond. The planning process is projecting the future role of the profession based on the expected needs of the public, patients, profession, and the evolving healthcare system. The AARC and its many allied organizations are keenly interested in the findings of these consensus conferences so that organizational and functional changes can be made as needed. Changes in the profession reflect the changes in healthcare, science, technology, education, and communications. Consequently, the AARC continuously examines its structure, organization, and operations. The AARC continually assesses its relationships to its members, current practices, and communities of interest. The AARC also addresses larger societal changes to advocate and enhance the professionalism of respiratory therapists.

American Respiratory Care Foundation

The **American Respiratory Care Foundation (ARCF)** is a not-for-profit organization. It was formed to support research, education, and charitable activities. ARCF activities include the funding of clinical and economic research, granting educational recognition awards, supporting educational activities, granting literary awards, and supporting scholarly publications. The ARCF is committed to health promotion, disease prevention, and improving the quality of the environment. The ARCF also educates the public about respiratory health and assists in the training and continuing education of healthcare providers.

National Board for Respiratory Care

The **National Board for Respiratory Care (NBRC)** is a voluntary health-certifying board founded in 1960 for the evaluation of the professional competence of respiratory therapists.[2] The organization first was named the American Registry of Inhalation Therapists (ARIT) to reflect the designation of the profession at that time. The primary purpose of the NBRC and its board of trustees is to provide high-quality voluntary credentialing examinations for respiratory therapists.

The NBRC has established standards for the **credentialing** of practitioners who work under medical direction and cooperates with accrediting agencies to support respiratory therapy education. The NBRC supports the ethical and educational standards of respiratory care. The NBRC also publishes an electronic newsletter called *NBRC Horizons* as well as a directory of credentialed individuals.

RESPIRATORY RECAP

National Board for Respiratory Care

» The NBRC is the national credentialing organization for respiratory therapists.

To date, the NBRC has issued more than 318,000 professional credentials to more than 193,000 individuals and currently tests nearly 18,000 candidates per year.[2] The NBRC has established itself as a credible credentialing organization. Its respiratory therapy examinations are used as the standard for **licensure** or **certification** in the current 48 states that regulate the profession. The national offices of the NBRC have been located in the greater Kansas City area since 1974, when the ARIT and the technician certification board of the AARC merged to form a single, independent credentialing organization. The offices are currently located in Olathe, Kansas.

The NBRC is accredited by the National Commission for Certifying Agencies (NCCA) and is a member of the National Organization for Competency Assurance (NOCA). The NBRC is sponsored by the AARC, ACCP, ASA, and ATS. Each sponsoring organization appoints members who serve on the 31-member NBRC board of trustees. The three physician groups and the National Society for Pulmonary Technology appoint 5 members each, and the AARC appoints 10 members; a public member also is added.

The NBRC uses periodic assessments of the practice of respiratory care through direct profiles of current practice provided by active practitioners. The board's credentialing examinations are consistent with the federal government's Uniform Guidelines on Employee Selection Procedures. The credentialing examinations are also consistent with the American Psychological Association's standards for job-relatedness, validity, and criterion-referenced passing points. The clinical simulation examination was one of the first credentialing examinations of its kind in the United States. All credentialing examinations are developed, prepared, and administered through Applied Measurement Professionals, Inc. (AMP), a wholly owned subsidiary of the NBRC. All NBRC examinations are administered by computer.

TABLE 56–2 National Board for Respiratory Care (NBRC) Respiratory Care Credentials

Credential	Acronym
Registered respiratory therapist	RRT
Certified respiratory therapist	CRT
Registered pulmonary function technologist	RPFT
Certified pulmonary function technologist	CPFT
Perinatal/pediatric respiratory care specialist	RRT-NPS or CRT-NPS
Sleep disorders specialist	RRT-SDS or CRT-SDS

Examinations

All NBRC examinations have a common education requirement that includes graduation from a program recognized by the Commission on Accreditation for Respiratory Care. **Table 56–2** provides an overview of the different professional **credentials** awarded by the NBRC.

NBRC examinations are graded with a minimum pass level (MPL) preestablished by the examination committee using a modified Angoff procedure. This accepted psychometric procedure uses the judgments of content experts to determine the number of correct answers required to achieve a passing score for the examination.[3] Canadian registered respiratory therapists (RRTs) may be admitted as candidates for the certification examination (certified respiratory therapists) and seek reciprocity for their credential in the United States by successful completion of the clinical simulation section of the registry examination. All NBRC credentialing examinations have specific admittance criteria for applicants, which may be reviewed through applications available from the NBRC website at http://www.nbrc.org. Examinations are administered in over 43 countries around the world through AMP.

The NBRC also offers examinations for respiratory care practitioners in Spanish. The Latin American Board for Proficiency Certification in Respiratory Therapy partners with the NBRC to offer credentialing exams. Registrants can attempt the Professional Certification in Respiratory Therapy exam, which is recognized by members of the Latin American Board. Other countries are in the initial stages of creating their own versions of respiratory therapy proficiency examinations with the assistance of the NBRC.

Certified Respiratory Therapist

The certified respiratory therapist (CRT) examination is the entry-level credential for practice in respiratory care. Candidates for the CRT exam must be 18 years of age and graduates of an accredited associate's degree program in respiratory therapy. The graduate respiratory therapist must attempt and successfully complete the CRT exam before attempting any portion of the registry exam. Competence exhibited through successful completion of the CRT exam is the primary credential used for licensure by state licensure boards that regulate respiratory care practice.

Registered Respiratory Therapist

The Registry Examination System was developed to objectively measure essential knowledge, skills, and abilities required of advanced respiratory therapists. The RRT examination contains two parts, the written registry exam (WRRT) and the clinical simulation examination (CSE), which may be taken on the same day or at separate times. The WRRT uses a multiple-choice question format. The clinical simulation exam presents layered clinical problems that can be solved successfully in many ways. On the written registry examination, the graduate therapist demonstrates a sufficient factual database of information. The clinical simulation examination focuses on the graduate's ability to critically think and to assess patient data in clinical practice components. Candidates for the RRT exam must possess the CRT credential and have satisfied other degree or semester-hour requirements.

Certified Pulmonary Function Technologist

The certified pulmonary function technologist (CPFT) examination is an entry-level certification exam for pulmonary function technologists. It is designed to validate a core competency in pulmonary function testing, data analysis, equipment, and instrumentation. Candidates must be 18 years old, have an associate's degree from an approved program, or be a CRT or RRT. Another way to attain eligibility is to complete 62 semester hours of college credit, including college credit–level courses in biology, chemistry, and mathematics. A minimum of 6 months of clinical experience in the field of pulmonary function technology under the direction of a medical director of a pulmonary function laboratory is also required prior to applying for the examination.[3]

Registered Pulmonary Function Technologist

The registered pulmonary function technologist (RPFT) examination is for advanced practice credentialing in pulmonary function technology. The areas of core competency are the same as for the CPFT exam, but at a higher level of practice. Candidates must meet the common eligibility requirements and must possess the CPFT credential.

Perinatal/Pediatric Respiratory Care Specialist

The perinatal/pediatric specialty certification examination recognizes advanced practice in perinatal, neonatal, and pediatric respiratory care. The successful candidate must demonstrate advanced practice knowledge desirable by employers seeking to hire individuals to perform primary duties. The exam validates competency in core areas of clinical data, equipment, and therapeutic procedures. Candidates must meet the common eligibility requirements and hold the RRT or the CRT credential, plus 1 year of clinical experience in perinatal/pediatric respiratory care after attaining NBRC certification.

Sleep Disorders Specialist

The specialty certification for sleep disorders recognizes respiratory therapists performing sleep disorders testing and therapeutic interventions. The successful candidate must demonstrate advanced practice knowledge desirable by employers seeking to hire individuals to perform sleep-testing duties. Admission eligibility includes being a CRT or RRT who has graduated from an accredited respiratory therapy program including a sleep add-on track, or who has achieved either the CRT credential plus 6 months of full-time clinical experience or the RRT credential plus 3 months of full-time clinical experience. Required clinical experience for this specialty credential must be in a sleep diagnostics and treatment setting under medical supervision. The examination covers five major content areas: pretesting, sleep disorders testing, study analysis, administrative functions, and treatment plan. Candidates are given 4 hours to complete this examination, and should expect to find polygraphic tracings based on old and new recording guidelines in the examination.

Commission on Accreditation for Respiratory Care

The **Commission on Accreditation for Respiratory Care (CoARC)** is located in Bedford, Texas. The initial composition of CoARC included board members from each organization, with sponsorship from the AARC, ACCP, ASA, ATS, the Association of Schools of Allied Health Professions, and the National Network of Health Career Programs in Two-Year Colleges. CoARC was preceded by the Committee on Accreditation for Respiratory Care, which made recommendations to the Commission on Accreditation of Allied Health Education Programs (CAAHEP). The CoARC board of directors made a decision to proceed with the option of leaving the CAAHEP and becoming a freestanding **accreditation** agency of respiratory therapy education programs. The Commission

RESPIRATORY RECAP

Commission on Accreditation for Respiratory Care

» CoARC is the national accreditation body for respiratory care education programs.

on Accreditation for Respiratory Care came into being on November 12, 2009.

Under CAAHEP and the current CoARC, the accrediting body meets similar standards of excellence required for all allied health education programs. CoARC evaluates the accreditation findings of respiratory care programs and makes all accreditation decisions.

Accreditation is voluntary, but failure to submit to the accreditation process may be construed as a program's failure to meet the standards and expectations set forth for all allied health education programs. Furthermore, the NBRC requires graduation from an accredited educational program for eligibility for its credentialing examinations. More information about CoARC may be found at http://www.coarc.com.

Accreditation Process

Respiratory care educational programs prepare for the critical CoARC on-site survey visit by following the commission's manual of policies and procedures detailing the expectations for accreditation of a program.[4] The standards by which CoARC measures programs include sponsorship, outcome orientation, resources, student disclosure, instructional planning, and program evaluation. Each critical area has objective standards of expectation established through careful scrutiny of successful high-quality programs. The manuals, policies, procedures, and written information provided by the prospective program for the accreditation decision process are confidential. The confidentiality requirement protects the hard work of each program's educators in their preparation for accreditation. CoARC uses periodic written reviews, reports, and evaluations with an on-site visit by a team of accreditation experts to determine the worthiness of an applicant program for accreditation.

The on-site review process ensures that policies and procedures submitted before an on-site visit reflect the reality of the educational experience at any prospective school. In addition, the accreditation and review process provides a measurable benchmark by which all such programs can be compared. The on-site evaluation team is composed of two individuals, such as one physician and one respiratory therapist, both of whom have completed a site-visitor training program. Either member may serve as the team captain during the site visit. The assignment process for CoARC site-visit teams ensures that any on-site visit team members do not have any potential or real conflicts of interests. Avoidance of potential or actual conflicts of interest ensures objectivity.

CoARC publishes on-site team behavioral expectations so that the program directors are aware of the expectations of on-site accreditation visitors. The policies and procedures create a formal matrix that guides the on-site team in its objective consideration of the quality of a prospective program. The accreditation process allows outsiders, prospective students, and government educational oversight groups an objective measure of a program's accomplishments and the quality of respiratory care education.

The on-site survey team provides its written findings to the referee for the program's accreditation process, and a final written report is provided to the program. The assigned program referee provides a report following the site visit with proposed accreditation recommendations. The analytic report of CoARC findings indicates any potential or actual violations of the accreditation standards. The prospective program also provides written evaluation feedback about the on-site survey team, which provides CoARC with information about the objectivity, knowledge, and demeanor of its on-site team members. Up until November 2009, CoARC submitted written recommendations to CAAHEP regarding initial accreditation and reaccreditation of educational programs every 5 to 10 years. Since then the Commission on Accreditation for Respiratory Care has become a freestanding accreditor of respiratory therapy educational programs.

National Association for Medical Direction of Respiratory Care

The **National Association for Medical Direction of Respiratory Care (NAMDRC)** has existed for over 30 years. The mission of NAMDRC is to educate its members and address regulatory, legislative, and payment issues that relate to the delivery of healthcare to patients with respiratory disorders.[5] NAMDRC's national offices are located in Vienna, Virginia. Currently, NAMDRC's members comprise the medical directors at more than 2000 hospitals. Medical direction of respiratory care departments has been described in many states and through the Joint Commission as most appropriate for those physicians with special training and background in respiratory disease and management. Therefore, NAMDRC members provide respiratory care medical direction consistent with the guidelines of most oversight agencies.

Most frequently, medical direction for respiratory care has stemmed from pulmonary medicine physicians, as well as anesthesiologists and a small percentage of individuals in other medical specialties, including sleep specialists. NAMDRC seeks to provide support across a full range of cardiopulmonary services, including respiratory care, critical care, ventilator management, cardiopulmonary rehabilitation, pulmonary physiology assessment, respiratory home healthcare services, hyperbaric oxygen therapy, and sleep disorders. More extensive information about NAMDRC may be obtained through its publications or its website at http://www.namdrc.org.

Publications

NAMDRC prints several publications, including *Washington Watchline*, *The Presidential Update*, *The Clinical and Management Quarterly Newsletter*, *Understanding Oxygen Therapy*, and *The Medical Director's Handbook*. The *Washington Watchline* is a monthly publication that keeps NAMDRC membership current on legislative and reimbursement issues associated with pulmonary care.

NAMDRC also publishes and distributes position and policy statements in *The Medical Director's Handbook.* Examples of pertinent position statements for respiratory care include "The Delivery of Hospital Respiratory Care and Duties" and "Responsibilities of the Medical Director of Respiratory Care Services and Pulmonary Function Laboratories." In many cases, related organizations use these position statements when certain issues require a respected physician perspective. For example, the AARC may use the position statement entitled "The Delivery of Hospital Respiratory Care" as a basis for the promotion of the respiratory therapist as the best provider of high-quality respiratory care. The related professional organization may have members in multiple roles, such as NAMDRC or BOMA members or representatives of a sponsoring organization.

American College of Chest Physicians

The ACCP provides resources for the worldwide improvement of cardiopulmonary health and critical care. Its primary mission is to promote prevention and treatment of diseases of the chest through membership, leadership, education, research, communication, and government relations. Communication occurs through publication of *Chest: The Cardiopulmonary and Critical Care Journal,* clinical practice guidelines, and consensus statements. Philanthropy is achieved via the Chest Foundation.

The ACCP, established in 1935, is located in Northbrook, Illinois. Up-to-date information about its conferences, new initiatives, and current publications is available at http://www.chestnet.org.

Membership

Membership includes more than 16,000 physicians and other professionals in this unique multidisciplinary society dedicated to the advancement of research, teaching, and clinical practice of cardiopulmonary medicine, surgery, and critical care. The designation Fellow College of Chest Physicians (FCCP) indicates recognition as a specialist in the field.

Allied health professionals who provide direct patient care, department supervision at a hospital, practice administration, or engage in clinical, academic, or research activities are eligible for ACCP membership as allied members. The ACCP also grants the FCCP designation to nonphysicians, specialists, and scientists with distinguished accomplishments in cardiopulmonary research, teaching, and clinical practice.

> **RESPIRATORY RECAP**
>
> **Physician Organizations That Provide Resources for Respiratory Therapists and Offer Membership as Affiliate Members**
>
> » American College of Chest Physicians
> » American Thoracic Society
> » American Society for Anesthesiologists
> » American Academy for Sleep Medicine

Educational Offerings

The ACCP offers and sponsors a large array of educational materials through meetings, video, audiotapes, compact discs, hands-on workshops, and online self-study. The ACCP is accredited for physician continuing medical education, holding large seminars or meetings and cosponsoring educational meetings with professional organizations such as the AARC. The Health and Science Policy Committee of the ACCP is a leading resource for the assessment of the science and development of clinical policy in cardiopulmonary medicine and critical care. Its mission is to oversee and monitor significant developments in the scientific and clinical arenas of cardiopulmonary health and critical care, to transfer research findings to clinical practice, and to provide scientific conferences. A major goal of the scientific conferences is to discuss research initiatives for future research activities.

Relationship with Respiratory Care

The ACCP is a sponsor of the AARC, NBRC, and CoARC, providing board members to these organizations. The ACCP also provides leadership for the AARC by naming ACCP members to BOMA.

American Thoracic Society

The American Thoracic Society (ATS) was founded in 1905 by a small group of physicians desiring to improve the care of tuberculosis patients. The ATS was originally formed as the American Sanatorium Association. Later, it was renamed the American Trudeau Society in 1938, which became the ATS in 1960. Today, it is an international professional and scientific society focusing on respiratory and critical care medicine. Currently the society has about 15,000 members. The primary mission of the ATS is the prevention and treatment of respiratory disease. Through education, research, and patient care, the ATS works to decrease morbidity and mortality associated with respiratory disease.

The ATS has a long history of cooperation and advocacy through the American Lung Association (ALA), for which the ATS serves as the medical section. The ALA's mission is to promote lung health and prevent lung disease. In the past decade, the ATS has become more active in critical care medicine and in the prevention, control, and treatment of diseases such as pneumonia, tuberculosis, and human immunodeficiency virus (HIV) infection. Recently, the ALA and ATS have severed their organizational ties. More information about the ATS may be obtained at http://www.thoracic.org.

Primary Missions

Research

The ATS promotes research through discovery of new knowledge related to respiratory and critical care medicine in health and disease. The ATS accomplishes this through assistance to the ALA in peer review process and interaction with agencies and organizations that fund new research. In addition, the ATS helps in the creation of new research funds through philanthropic organizations.

Education

Educational initiatives at the ATS promote the dissemination of new scientific information. ATS education encourages high standards for training, education, research, and clinical practice and facilitates rapid transfer of new scientific information to practice. The ATS also synthesizes new information for the public through the ALA.

The ATS publishes the *American Journal of Respiratory and Critical Care Medicine*, the *American Journal of Respiratory Cell and Molecular Biology*, and *Proceedings of the American Thoracic Society*. Each is highly respected and used worldwide by pulmonary and critical care practitioners.

Patient Care

Patient care initiatives include promotion of the highest standards for quality in healthcare, establishment of partnerships between pulmonary and critical care medicine, and evaluation of the relationship between cost and quality in the delivery of healthcare.

Advocacy

The ATS encourages growth in programs and methods that provide high-quality care. In addition, the ATS advises and promotes cooperation by and between governmental and nongovernmental agencies for matters of common interest. For example, the ATS sponsors the AARC, which includes activities in BOMA, NBRC, and CoARC.

American Society of Anesthesiologists

The ASA is an educational, research, and scientific association of physicians organized in 1905 to raise and maintain the standards of anesthesiology and improve patient care. Contact with respiratory care usually involves postsurgical care, most prominently in the area of critical care. The anesthesiologist maintains analgesia and life functions during the surgical procedures in the operating suite. After surgery, the anesthesiologist maintains contact with the patient's care team to ensure a comfortable and stable recovery after surgery.

Members of ASA must be doctors of medicine who are licensed practitioners and have successfully completed a training program approved by the Accreditation Council for Graduate Medical Education (ACGME). Members may also be doctors of osteopathy who have successfully completed training approved by the American Osteopathic Association (AOA). Currently more than 43,000 practitioners are ASA members. The ASA is currently located in Park Ridge, Illinois, a suburb of Chicago. More information is available at http://www.asahq.org.

Relationship with Respiratory Care

The ASA is currently a sponsoring member of the AARC, NBRC, and CoARC. Through clinical expertise, provision of members to BOMA for AARC and other support mechanisms, the ASA contributes to the practice and science of respiratory care. The ASA supports AARC activities and professional issues, developing position statements and clinical practice guidelines to denote the need for respiratory therapy personnel in all areas of clinical practice. The anesthesiologist is the perioperative physician who provides medical care to the patient throughout his or her surgical experience.

True to this definition, the anesthesiologist may order preoperative testing, including arterial blood gases and pulmonary function studies, to determine the current health status of the patient. In addition, the anesthesiologist may order respiratory care procedures to help promote a higher level of lung function in preparation for surgery. Since 1970 the number of deaths attributed to anesthesia have dropped from 1 in 10,000 to 1 in 250,000.[6]

Mission

The ASA supports the world's largest educational program for anesthesiology practice and science. The annual meeting of ASA provides up-to-date research, science, and continuing education to its members. The ASA sponsors the self-education and evaluation (SEE) program and publishes its own monthly peer-reviewed journal, *Anesthesiology*.

Governmental Affairs

The ASA's Office of Governmental Affairs (OGA), located in Washington, DC, monitors legislative activities and regulations at the state and federal levels to ensure the continuance of high-quality care in all areas of healthcare. Examples include Medicare and Medicaid. The ASA works closely with others groups, such as the AMA and AARC, on clinical practice issues of regulation that may influence anesthesiology and respiratory care.

Governance

The ASA's governance structure is similar to that of the AARC. The ASA has a House of Delegates distributed by geographic region that meets at the ASA annual meeting. Officers, past presidents, the editor in chief of *Anesthesiology*, and chairs of sections for education and residency all contribute to the practice, governance, and direction of anesthesiology.

Society of Critical Care Medicine

The SCCM, formed in 1970, is the youngest organization related to the practice of respiratory care. The SCCM was formed to further a multidisciplinary and multiprofessional approach to the care of the critically ill patient. Currently the society boasts more than 14,000 members in over 80 countries. The SCCM's membership is evidence of its multiprofessional approach. Members include intensivists, nurses, respiratory therapists, pharmacists, pharmacologists, scientists, researchers, bioengineers, critical care industry executives, and other interested allied health professionals.

The use of a multidisciplinary approach to research and patient care promotes a continuum of care. This continuum begins at the moment of injury or illness and proceeds through full recovery. Critical care may be practiced at the site of an accident or in the perioperative setting. However, most activity involving the respiratory therapist occurs in the emergency and intensive care areas. More information may be found at http://www.sccm.org.

Journals and Relationship with Respiratory Care

The SCCM publishes *Critical Care Medicine*, a monthly journal dedicated to the science and treatment of critically ill patients. As a multidisciplinary organization, SCCM is engaged in respiratory care in ways similar to previously described medical groups and professional organizations. The SCCM is directly involved in the AARC through BOMA and as a BOD member during its rotation as BOMA chair. SCCM sponsors AARC, NBRC, and CoARC, providing a valuable multiprofessional perspective to advances in care and regulatory issues affecting respiratory care.

The Joint Commission

The Joint Commission (TJC) is the nation's predominant standards-setting and accrediting body in healthcare. This organization changed its name in 2007 from the Joint Commission on Accreditation of Health Care Organizations to The Joint Commission. The central office is located in Oakbrook Terrace, Illinois, with a satellite office in Washington, DC. The Joint Commission is an independent, not-for-profit organization.

Since 1951, TJC has maintained state-of-the-art standards that focus on improving the quality and safety of care provided by healthcare organizations. TJC evaluates and accredits more than 15,000 healthcare organizations and programs in the United States. Joint Commission certification is recognized nationwide as a symbol of quality that reflects an organization's commitment to meeting certain performance standards. To earn and maintain certification, an organization must undergo an on-site survey by a Joint Commission survey team at least every 3 years.

TJC also awards disease-specific care certification to health plans, disease management service companies, hospitals, and other care delivery settings that provide disease management and chronic care services. TJC also has a healthcare staffing services certification program. It is developing a certification program for transplant centers and healthcare services.

Mission

The mission of TJC is to continuously improve the safety and quality of care provided to the public through the provision of healthcare accreditation and related services that support performance improvement in healthcare organizations.[7] Programs that are accredited by TJC include not only hospitals but also home care, laboratory services, assisted living, long-term care, and office-based surgery. Requirements and survey guides are provided for all these program-specific certifications on the Commission's website at http://www.jointcommission.org.

Relationship to Respiratory Care

Respiratory therapists are directly involved with Joint Commission surveyors when their facility or program is under review. Technical directors of respiratory care services are responsible for the core performance measures of patient care related to respiratory care in the hospital or home care setting. The AARC also appoints members to TJC to provide input and influence professional and technical advisory committees (PTACs). The Joint Commission PTACs are designed to assist in important matters pertaining to its accreditation programs. Periodically, TJC seeks input from respiratory therapists to comment on proposed standards. A recent proposal on medication management in acute care settings is an example of how respiratory therapists add value to this organization.

National Asthma Educator Certification Board

The **National Asthma Educator Certification Board (NAECB)** was established in 2000 as a result of over 50 stakeholder groups coming together to discuss the need for an asthma certification exam. The mission of the NAECB is to promote optimal asthma management and quality of life among individuals with asthma, their families, and communities by advancing excellence in asthma education through the certified asthma educator (AE-C) process.[8] The 17-member board represents the multiple disciplines involved in asthma education, including allergy/immunology, behavioral science, emergency medicine, nursing, patient advocacy, environmental health, health education, medicine, pediatrics, pharmacy, public health, pulmonary medicine, and respiratory therapy. The NAECB plans to incorporate the latest Expert Panel Report of the National Asthma Education Prevention Program guidelines for control and treatment of asthma in 2009.

Certified Asthma Educator

An AE-C is an expert in teaching, educating, and counseling individuals with asthma and their families in the knowledge and skills necessary to minimize the impact of asthma on their quality of life.[8] The

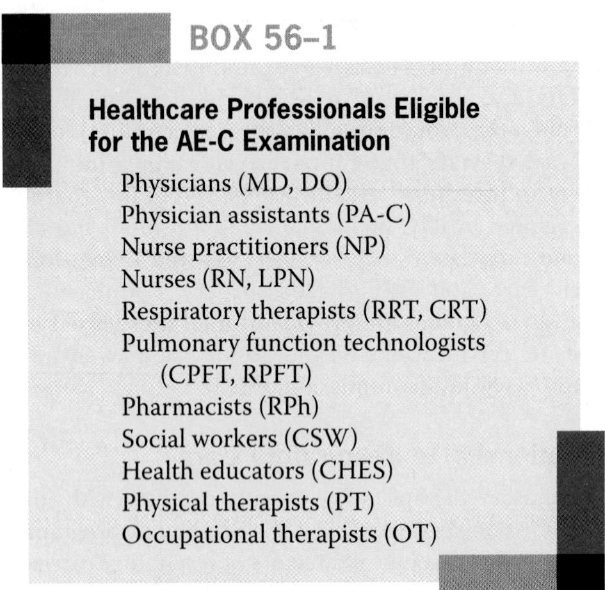

BOX 56–1

Healthcare Professionals Eligible for the AE-C Examination

Physicians (MD, DO)
Physician assistants (PA-C)
Nurse practitioners (NP)
Nurses (RN, LPN)
Respiratory therapists (RRT, CRT)
Pulmonary function technologists (CPFT, RPFT)
Pharmacists (RPh)
Social workers (CSW)
Health educators (CHES)
Physical therapists (PT)
Occupational therapists (OT)

AE-C possesses comprehensive, current knowledge of asthma pathophysiology and management, including developmental theories, cultural dimensions, the impact of chronic illness, and principles of teaching and learning. Respiratory therapists make ideal asthma educators because they are very knowledgeable on the optimal use of medications and delivery devices. Respiratory therapists are particularly good at explaining technical concepts to individuals in language each can understand.

Other roles and duties of the AE-C include assessments of individuals and families to identify strengths and resources as well as negative psychological factors, the social and economic impact of asthma, educational needs, and barriers to optimal health care and self-management.[8] The educator works with an individual with asthma, his or her family, and other healthcare professionals to develop, implement, monitor, and revise an asthma action plan customized to the individual's needs, environment, disease severity, and lifestyle to optimize the individual's self-management skills.

AE-C Examination

The NAECB administers the AE-C exam in a manner similar to the process used by the NBRC. The exam is administered by Applied Measurement Professionals. Registrants can apply for the exam if they meet eligibility requirements, which include being a licensed or credentialed healthcare professional. **Box 56–1** lists the healthcare professions eligible for the AE-C. Individuals who are not licensed but who have provided professional asthma education and counseling with a minimum of 1000 hours experience in these activities also can register to take the exam.

The examination is based on seven major content areas. Content areas are outlined in detail in the candidate handbook, including the exam matrix. As of October 31, 2008, there were 2492 individuals certified, with a national pass rate of 68.5%. Recertification by examination is required every 7 years and costs $245. Information regarding the AE-C exam and the NAECB can be found at http://www.naecb.org.

Association of Asthma Educators

The **Association of Asthma Educators (AAE)** is an interdisciplinary professional organization with the goal of raising the competency of individuals who educate patients and families affected by asthma.[9] Formed in 1998, the majority of AAE members are asthma educators who do not have prescribing privileges. One of the AAE's primary goals is to be the leading resource for asthma educators to help improve health outcomes for individuals and families affected by asthma. An annual conference is held each year. The AAE also offers a review course program by CD to prepare participants to take the AE-C exam. Other programs available are listed on the organization's website at http://www.asthmaeducators.org. Membership is open to all licensed healthcare professionals. Associate and student memberships are also available.

American Academy of Sleep Medicine

Established in 1975 as the Association of Sleep Disorders Centers, the **American Academy of Sleep Medicine (AASM)** is the only professional society that is dedicated exclusively to the medical subspecialty of sleep medicine. The AASM sets standards and promotes excellence in healthcare, education, and research. The AASM serves its members and advances the field of sleep healthcare by setting the clinical standards for sleep medicine; advocating for the recognition, diagnosis, and treatment of sleep disorders; educating professionals to provide optimal sleep healthcare; and fostering the development and application of scientific knowledge.[10]

Publications

The journal *Sleep* is a publication of the Associated Professional Sleep Societies, LLC, which is a joint venture of the AASM and the Sleep Research Society. *Sleep* was the first journal published that was dedicated exclusively to sleep. As the official publication of the AASM, the *Journal of Clinical Sleep Medicine* publishes applied sleep science of clinical trials, clinical reviews, case series and reports, and commentaries and debates. It also publishes reports, news, and updates from the AASM.[10]

Membership

The AASM membership consists of more than 7000 physicians, researchers, and other healthcare professionals. These members specialize in studying, diagnosing, and treating disorders of sleep and daytime alertness such as insomnia, narcolepsy, and obstructive sleep apnea. Respiratory therapists are eligible to join for affiliate membership if they have special training in sleep disorders. Special training includes sleep technologists or sleep center managers who are active in the clinical or research aspects of sleep medicine.

Board of Registered Polysomnographic Technologists

The **Board of Registered Polysomnographic Technologists (BRPT)** is an independent, nonprofit certification board that seeks to cultivate the highest professional and ethical standards for polysomnographic technologists. Established in 1978 to benefit the developing field of polysomnographic technology and set credentialing standards for technologists, the BRPT developed the registry examination for polysomnographic technology (RPSGT). The BRPT also maintains and administers the RPSGT exam. There are more than 13,000 registered polysomnographic technologists.

RPSGT Examination

The RPSGT credential indicates that the technologist has a level of experience and competence aligned with an international standard. There are three pathways to become eligible for the exam: (1) completing an 18-month polysomnographic (PSG) experience through on-the-job training, (2) having 6-month PSG experience (credentialed health professionals), or (3) as a graduate of a CAAHEP-accredited polysomnographic technology program. After July 1, 2012, to be eligible for the RPSGT exam, applicants must complete a comprehensive training program accredited by the CAAHEP, Accreditation of Educational Programs in Polysomnographic Technology, or CoARC.[11]

KEY POINTS

- Many organizations sponsor and support the profession of respiratory care.
- Certain organizations have very specific and limited missions, whereas others are more diverse in purpose and mission.
- The goals of each supporting organization ultimately improve the scope, practice, education, credentials, quality, and professional growth of respiratory care.
- The AARC provides various forms of education and educational opportunities through meetings, publications, grants, awards, fellowships, activities, and services for its members to facilitate continued growth of the profession.
- Although some supporting organizations are restricted to physician membership, many are not, providing numerous opportunities for participation by respiratory therapists.
- The AARC and related professional organizations enhance the entire respiratory care profession, with far-reaching effects beyond each organization's membership.
- Membership in the AARC should be considered an integral part of a respiratory care professional's identity.

REFERENCES

1. American Association for Respiratory Care. *AARC Bylaws*. Irving, TX: AARC; 2007.
2. National Board for Respiratory Care. About the National Board for Respiratory Care. Available at: http://www.nbrc.org/Home/AboutNBRC/tabid/73/Default.aspx. Accessed August 2, 2010.
3. National Board for Respiratory Care. *Candidate Handbook and Application*. Olathe, KS: National Board for Respiratory Care; 2010.
4. Commission on Accreditation of Respiratory Care. *CoARC Accreditation Policies and Procedures Manual*. Available at: http://www.coarc.com/31.html. Accessed August 2, 2010.
5. National Association for Medical Direction of Respiratory Care. Welcome to NAMDRC. Available at: http://www.namdrc.org. Accessed August 2, 2010.
6. American Society for Anesthesiology. Anesthesia information for patients. Available at: http://www.asahq.org/patientEducation.htm. Accessed August 2, 2010.
7. The Joint Commission. Home page. Available at: http://www.jointcommission.org. Accessed August 2, 2010.
8. National Asthma Education Certification Board. Home page. Available at: http://www.naecb.org. Accessed August 2, 2010.
9. Association of Asthma Educators. Home page. Available at: http://www.asthmaeducators.org/index.htm. Accessed August 2, 2010.
10. American Academy of Sleep Medicine. Home page. Available at: http://www.aasmnet.org. Accessed August 2, 2010.
11. Board of Registered Polysomnographic Technologists. Eligibility requirements. Available at: http://www.brpt.org/Exam_info/eligibility.htm. Accessed August 2, 2010.

CHAPTER 57

Healthcare Trends and Evolving Roles of Respiratory Therapists

Shelley C. Mishoe
Kathleen M. Hernlen

OUTLINE

Healthcare Trends
Traditional Roles of Respiratory Therapists
Nontraditional Roles for Respiratory Therapists

OBJECTIVES

1. Describe the six major forces affecting healthcare trends in the United States.
2. Discuss the historical and traditional role of the respiratory care therapist.
3. Describe how current trends in the U.S. healthcare delivery system influence the future of healthcare and respiratory care.
4. Discuss why nontraditional roles for respiratory therapists are emerging.
5. Describe the roles of respiratory therapists across the continuum of healthcare, wellness and disease prevention programs, case management, industry, and research.
6. Discuss the role of respiratory therapists as physician extenders.
7. Explain how the respiratory therapy profession must evolve within changing healthcare delivery systems.

KEY TERMS

case manager
diagnosis-related group (DRG)
diagnostics
fee-for-service system
home healthcare
managed care
Medicaid
Medicare
physician extender
prospective payment system (PPS)
provider
pulmonary rehabilitation
subacute care
wellness programs

INTRODUCTION

This chapter introduces students and respiratory therapists to current and future trends in healthcare, including forces changing the healthcare delivery system in the United States. It discusses traditional and new roles for respiratory therapists and presents possibilities and tactics for respiratory therapists to work across the range of patient care. The chapter also discusses careers in industry, education, management, research, and other areas. Respiratory therapists will continue to play major roles in healthcare and an important role in the changes being made to healthcare delivery. With education, experience, credentials, and documented value, respiratory therapists can continue to assume leadership roles in healthcare systems.

Healthcare Trends

Between World War II and the late 1970s, the U.S. healthcare system remained stable. Doctors and nurses delivered healthcare through small, local, and nonprofit organizations. In time, other specialists, including respiratory therapists, emerged. These new professions thrived. An unlimited insurance system was based on fees for service. The level of healthcare was unequaled, but healthcare costs continued to rise at an increasing rate. Care was delivered without documentation of quality improvements, access, or effectiveness. The 1990s witnessed unique changes in healthcare in the United States and was one of the most dynamic decades ever faced by the nation's health professionals. The rate of healthcare reform continues to gather speed in an effort to improve healthcare in this country. The U.S. healthcare system will continue to change as it responds to the challenge of delivering high-quality care and making good use of its resources. To do this, respiratory therapists must always consider how they best add value to the delivery of health services.[1]

Healthcare reform has centered around four main issues: decreasing costs, improving quality, evaluating usefulness with measurable outcomes, and improving resource allocation, including access to healthcare. The ultimate goal is to improve use of healthcare resources. More people should receive better healthcare for the least possible cost. There are many opinions as to how to achieve this goal. Policymakers, federal and state governments, insurers, **providers**, scholars, administrators, educators, special interest groups, and the public have voiced their opinions in many ways. All agree that many forces have shaped healthcare. Economic factors have often received the greatest attention.

> **RESPIRATORY RECAP**
>
> **Major Healthcare Reform Issues**
>
> » Decreasing cost of healthcare
> » Improving quality of healthcare
> » Evaluating effectiveness using outcomes measures
> » Improving access and resource allocation

Factors in both the private and public sectors have changed the emphasis from hospitals to other healthcare settings. Private-sector factors have included **managed care**. Another factor was the emergence of healthcare as a major social issue. Public-sector policy changes to the **Medicaid** and **Medicare** systems had great impacts on the delivery of healthcare. In the traditional system, the acute care hospital provided most healthcare. This was replaced by a system with a widened range of care. This new system values **subacute care** facilities and home health agencies. It also values disease prevention and wellness programs. In the future, patients may spend more time in nontraditional settings than in the hospital.

Changes to the healthcare system are occurring quickly. Healthcare professions must adapt and be flexible. This section briefly describes the six major forces affecting healthcare and healthcare reform in the United States.

Economic

With the creation of Medicare and Medicaid in the 1960s, healthcare flourished. The reimbursement policies allowed consumers to choose their own providers in a fee-for-service agreement. Under the **fee-for-service system**, an individual or an insurance carrier made payment to healthcare providers when services were given. These payments occurred after the service was provided and were thus called *retrospective payments*. The use and costs of healthcare suddenly increased significantly in the United States. There were few limits under the fee-for-service system. This payment system greatly affected inflation. Healthcare costs consumed greater amounts of the gross domestic product. Medicare is now the nation's largest payer for health services, covering approximately 40 million beneficiaries.[2]

Innovation and technology also grew under the fee-for-service system. Healthcare providers, including physicians and nurses, became more specialized. The respiratory care profession began in the 1940s and grew during this time. Eventually, healthcare in the United States became the envy of other nations.[3] However, quality healthcare came at a price. At the end of the century, American healthcare had become the most expensive in the world. Powerful public and private efforts emerged to drastically alter the delivery and financing of healthcare.

The healthcare system has come under demands from the public and from private payers, who are no longer willing to financially support this system. It continues to have high inflationary costs, which fueled the managed care industry and created lengthy debates on national healthcare reform. Employers have decreased the amount of money they are willing to spend for employee health benefits. Consequently, insurers are finding ways to offer the same services at lower costs.

Managed care developed to put constant pressure on healthcare providers to restrain costs and control use. Managed care requires doctors, nurses, and ancillary service providers to reorganize their work and modify duties. Managed care uses systems to reduce duplicate services and facilities, which leads to lower costs. The goals of managed care are to maximize the value of health benefits and coordinate healthcare management.[4]

Prospective payment systems (PPSs) evolved and replaced fee-for-service agreements. Managed care companies such as health maintenance organizations (HMOs) and preferred provider organizations (PPOs) evolved. These provide enrollees with medical and hospital care in exchange for an agreed-upon fee. The goal is to make sure that patients will receive adequate care in the appropriate healthcare setting. Utilization reviews determine and assess requirements for continued stay for each healthcare setting. When a patient no longer meets the acuity level required, the patient is transferred to a less costly setting. With managed care, the hospital receives a set fee per diagnosis on each patient covered (a prospective payment). If healthcare providers can provide care for less cost than this set fee, they make a profit. If the cost of care exceeds the set fee, the healthcare provider takes a loss.

Prospective payment systems have become increasingly popular as a replacement for the more traditional fee-for-service system. With a PPS, healthcare professionals provide whatever care they feel is appropriate. The fee in a PPS often is based on the diagnosis, using the federal government's Medicare **diagnosis-related groups (DRGs)**. The payment can also be based on a fee per day of hospitalization (the per diem method). Payment also can be based on a fixed amount of reimbursement per person, per year, in a geographic area. This type of fixed payment is called *capitated payment.* In these systems, the healthcare provider has an incentive to carefully analyze the way in which services are delivered.

Managed care is becoming increasingly popular among Medicare and Medicaid patients. Twenty percent of eligible Medicare patients in 2007 used managed care. More than 29 million Medicaid recipients participated in managed care programs in 2006.[5] At the same time, home health and subacute care have seen decreases in payments for respiratory services. These factors have brought additional change to the healthcare delivery system.

For-profit corporations became a powerful new influence on the way hospitals and practices operate. Today, the U.S. healthcare system is in a constant state of change. With these changes come both rewards and liabilities for society. The system is becoming more efficient in its use of resources. However, it has disenfranchised over 47 million people who do not have health insurance, public or private.[6]

Demographic

The factor that will have the most impact in the future of the delivery of healthcare is the changing demographic makeup of the United States. Significant changes continue to occur in the age, ethnicity, economic status, and geographic distribution of the population. These changes have a direct influence on healthcare systems by altering the population groups who seek healthcare services and the diseases for which they seek care. Population growth and changing demographics contribute to the increased use of healthcare as well as to increasing costs.

A growing number of people are using healthcare services. The U.S. population is expected to continue to grow until the year 2038, when it is expected to peak.[7] The population is also getting older and living longer. The percentage of the population 75 years or older is expected to increase from 6% in 2006 to 12% in 2050.[7] The over-85 population is the fastest-growing segment of our society. Society refers to this change as the "graying of America." Expectations are that the number of people needing respiratory care will increase with the aging demographics. Caring for the very old will place additional burdens on healthcare systems and will require further innovation in the use of healthcare resources.

> **AGE-SPECIFIC ANGLE**
>
> The over-85 population is the fastest-growing segment of the American society.

Ethnicity is also changing and influencing healthcare needs. Birth rates and immigration rates determine the ethnicity of the U.S. population. Hispanics, African Americans, and other ethnic groups will represent greater percentages of the U.S. population. There is an increasing need for healthcare services directed at specific ethnic groups. Efforts will be needed to improve access and quality of care without increasing the cost of care.

Imbalances in healthcare also exist between urban and rural communities. Many rural areas experience a shortage of physicians and other providers. Physicians are not distributed equally across the country.[7] Healthcare reform is focused on ways to improve the access and quality of health care The focus will turn to rural, inner city, and ethnic groups and the aging population.

Epidemiologic

Another reason for the development and expansion of outpatient and subacute care is the number and types of patients. Many of these patients have chronic problems and lifestyle-related illnesses. Cigarette smoking is an important health risk that contributes to increased incidences of cancer, heart disease, and chronic obstructive pulmonary disease (COPD). Current trends show that tobacco use will cause more than 8 million deaths annually by 2030. An estimated 20.8% of all adults (45.3 million people) smoke cigarettes in the United States.[8] COPD is the fourth leading cause of death in the United States and is projected to be the third leading cause of death for both males and females by the year 2020.[9] An estimated 12 million people have undiagnosed COPD and still continue to smoke. This group represents a need for respiratory care in the future.[1] Influenza and pneumonia are the eighth leading cause of death in the United States.[10]

Asthma affects 22 million people in the United States. As many as 4000 to 5000 people die from asthma each year.[11] Another disease that is often undiagnosed is obstructive sleep apnea. There may be as many as 18 million people with obstructive sleep apnea,[12] which greatly affects the overall health of these individuals. The prevalence of diseases such as asthma, chronic bronchitis, pneumonia, and congestive heart failure, especially among the elderly, will remain a challenge for respiratory care therapists in the 21st century.

Sociological

Sociological factors affect the way individuals and society think, feel, and act about all aspects of life, including health and healthcare delivery. Access to high-quality healthcare is a priority for most Americans. However, access is determined by the individual's economic status. This usually involves the individual's education and value to society. Minority Americans are at higher risk of living in poverty, being uninsured, and having poorer health status indicators.[11]

U.S. healthcare has achieved great success, in part, because of advances in biomedical science. The advances have allowed practitioners to confront the challenges of specific diseases. However, there is a growing recognition that other challenges to healthcare are equally important. There is a demand for a more integrated approach to care that takes into account the multiple factors that interact to promote health or cause illness. Society now realizes that healthcare requires individual responsibility for one's health. Society also recognizes its responsibility for the health of the population at large.

The focus of healthcare can no longer be on specific illnesses of individual patients. New concepts in health focus on the patient's experience, which includes many variables, such as psychological, sociological, spiritual, and biological variables. These deepened perspectives on health and illness will shape care in the future. As people live longer with chronic diseases, this concept promotes a more humane approach to healthcare. It encourages practitioners to help people, even those with incurable illnesses or those who are dying, to live as wholly functional as possible.[13] We no longer refer to our patients in terms of their disease or their status as patients. We realize that healthcare involves real people.

More emphasis is being placed on patient satisfaction, wellness, and quality of life, which have become important determinants of healthcare outcomes. In turn, healthcare outcomes have become determinants of effective healthcare. The respiratory therapist should incorporate outcomes in his or her care. It is important that students and respiratory therapists think of their work in terms of whole people. Respiratory therapists also must think of their work in terms of the broader society. Respiratory therapists should not think strictly in terms of diseases, treatments, and individual patients.

Technological

It is hard to imagine, but many believe that the advances in medical technology over the next decade will make our current healthcare practices seem primitive. Technological influences include drugs, devices, and medical and surgical procedures. Advances in information technology will merge with biomedical technology to produce care management technology. Telemedicine will be used even more in the future. These technologies will allow patients to be more directly connected to healthcare knowledge.[1] Technological advances, such as vaccinations, organ transplants, and mechanical ventilation, have greatly contributed to health. The evolution of the respiratory care profession has been tied to technology. Changing technologies will create new health professionals. The respiratory therapist of the future will need to be even more sophisticated concerning technology.

The year 2000 announced the mapping of the human genome, which had profound and dramatic implications for healthcare. Knowledge of the genome holds implications for new screening and treatment strategies for chronic cardiopulmonary diseases such as cystic fibrosis, asthma, and emphysema, as well as for infectious diseases such as tuberculosis and human immunodeficiency virus (HIV) infection. **Box 57–1** lists many advances that have had a technological influence on healthcare.

BOX 57–1

Technological Advances in Healthcare

- Diagnostics
- Therapeutics
- Drug delivery technologies
- Gene therapies
- Organ transplants
- Laser surgeries
- Biosensors and implants
- Computer technology
- Automated systems for information systems, artificial intelligence, and robotics

In respiratory care, advances in technology have influenced how we manage patients. Examples include those with acute respiratory distress syndrome (ARDS) or asthma. Advances in technology have contributed to improved ventilators. Ventilator graphics in turn have led to improved management of patients. This has taken the guesswork out of many of our strategies for oxygenation and ventilation, which is critical with the most difficult patients. Improvements in drug delivery devices have altered our uses and recommendations for aerosol therapies. These changes have come at such a fast pace it can be difficult to keep up. Technological advances have enormous educational implications. They require advanced and continued training so healthcare professionals can safely and effectively use the latest devices and methods.

Technology also indirectly influences educational needs by its impact on society's view of health and healthcare. For example, patients increasingly use the Internet as a source of medical information. The public no longer thinks of physicians or other healthcare providers as the experts. Consumers have increased access to global information. These changes have probably contributed to the growth of complementary medicine, including Eastern and homeopathic approaches to healthcare.

Technological advances also have influenced the ways in which healthcare professionals interact with their patients and clients. They often now provide patient education via computer, including the Internet. Technological advances will continue to flourish in the next century and will continue to have an impact on the way healthcare is provided.

Educational

As society continues to redefine its understanding of health and healthcare, several questions arise. How can healthcare practitioners change their approach to patient care to match these new and evolving healthcare trends? How can education programs develop practitioners who approach patient care in ways that address the complex processes in health and illness? How can educational programs address values and beliefs in patient care? How can the regulatory systems for healthcare practices be reinvented? How can new systems remove barriers? How can systems ensure the highest level of professional practice? How can accreditation of educational programs be improved to ensure public safety? How can licensing of healthcare professionals ensure safety but remove artificial constraints? The healthcare professions and public and private sectors continue to grapple with these and many other questions.

Current literature consistently points to the need for reforms in education. These reforms will prepare professionals with the skills and traits required for future healthcare systems.[14–17] These changes include managed care, seamless care, and patient-focused care as well as numerous new models and settings for delivering healthcare. Prospective payment has also changed healthcare education by changing how healthcare providers plan, manage, and think about healthcare.[18] As a result, the roles, skills, and traits expected from healthcare professionals have also changed.

It is no longer sufficient for healthcare professionals to have specialized clinical skills. They must now be educated at a higher level and must have professional competence exceeding technological or clinical skills. They must also have advanced technical skills.[1] These changes in healthcare delivery have been experienced by all healthcare professionals. Employers, educators, and patients of respiratory therapists argue that practitioners need more than medical knowledge and technical skills. They need professional competencies and characteristics to work in the changing healthcare system. Technical knowledge alone does not equal professional competence.[19]

The National Consensus Conference on Respiratory Care Education identified and ranked the 41 most important areas in the scope of practice for the respiratory therapist.[20] The American Association for Respiratory Care (AARC) established a task force to look ahead to 2015 and beyond.[1] The goal was to analyze the future roles of respiratory therapists. The task force looked specifically at new responsibilities and focused on the value added to patients. Evolving changes in healthcare include rising costs and an aging population. There is more attention on chronic disease management. Technology is rapidly changing. Consumers are becoming increasingly involved in healthcare. The 2015 task force agreed that evidence-based medicine will be more important and that biomedical inventions will mandate more "sophistication" of respiratory therapists.[1] Future sessions will focus on changes needed in the education of future respiratory therapists.

> **RESPIRATORY RECAP**
>
> **Changes Increasing the Need for Respiratory Therapy**
>
> » An aging American population
> » Increased life expectancy
> » Increased incidence of chronic pulmonary diseases
> » Steady rate of cigarette smokers
> » Other lifestyle-related risk factors
> » Technological advances
> » Increased focus on health promotion, wellness, and disease management
> » Better-informed public
> » Greater access to medical information
> » Focus on patient education
> » Patient-centered care

According to a report by the National Commission on Allied Health, curricula should emphasize rural and urban health, aging, maternal and child health, and minority health in new ways. These changes should result in measurable improvements in the quality of care.[21] Community-based healthcare, patient and family education, and care at alternate sites also need to be added to the curricula.[15]

Box 57–2 lists 21 competencies that the Pew Commission recommends for the preparation of allied health professionals for the 21st century.[22] Curricula should be modified to prepare respiratory therapists for the current and future healthcare markets. This will allow the respiratory care profession to continue to thrive.[15]

Healthcare Reform

The previous sections described the various factors influencing healthcare reform in this country and described some of the changes. Prior sections detailed the numerous problems with the U.S. healthcare system and how healthcare delivery has undergone rapid and perpetual change. However, this chapter would be incomplete if it failed to mention some of the problems with healthcare reform. While the nation has been preoccupied with transforming the health delivery system to managed care, others trends have occurred at the same time.[7] These healthcare trends include the declining ability of healthcare providers to deliver uncompensated care, the declining proportion of people with private insurance, and the continued

BOX 57-2

Allied Health Competencies for the 21st Century

1. Embrace a personal ethic of social responsibility and service.
2. Exhibit ethical behavior in all professional activities.
3. Provide evidence-based, clinically competent care.
4. Incorporate the multiple determinants of health in clinical care.
5. Apply knowledge of the new sciences.
6. Demonstrate critical thinking, reflection, and problem-solving skills.
7. Understand the role of primary care.
8. Rigorously practice preventive healthcare.
9. Integrate population-based care and services into practice.
10. Improve access to healthcare for those with unmet health needs.
11. Practice relationship-centered care with individuals and families.
12. Provide culturally sensitive care to a diverse society.
13. Partner with communities in healthcare decisions.
14. Use communication and information technology effectively and appropriately.
15. Work in interdisciplinary teams.
16. Ensure care that balances individual, professional, system, and societal needs.
17. Practice leadership.
18. Take responsibility for quality of care and health outcomes at all levels.
19. Contribute to continuous improvement of the healthcare system.
20. Advocate for public policy that promotes and protects the health of the public.
21. Continue to learn and help others learn.

From Kacmarek RM, Barnes TA, Walton JR. Creating a vision for respiratory care in 2015 and beyond. *Respir Care*. 2009;54(3): 375–388. Reprinted with permission.

RESPIRATORY RECAP

Additional Healthcare Reform Issues

» More people are without access to healthcare systems.
» Providers have a declining ability to provide uncompensated healthcare.
» Patients frequently change providers based on insurance criteria.
» Professionals, patients, and policymakers are experiencing growing dissatisfaction.
» There is a lack of coordination within and across the healthcare delivery system.
» Managed care does not reduce the costs of healthcare as intended.
» The healthcare system is struggling to reduce costs and improve quality.

growth in the total number of uninsured people.[6,7] There have also been increases in the rate of inflation in healthcare costs, and budget reductions in Medicare and Medicaid.[7] The failure of healthcare reform to effectively address the multifaceted problems of our healthcare system continues to make healthcare a national concern. Respiratory therapists are increasingly involved in contributing to the improvements in healthcare. We face growing challenges not only as healthcare providers but also as healthcare consumers.

Traditional Roles of Respiratory Therapists

History

Respiratory therapy has a long and interesting history that led to its evolution as a health profession. Respiratory therapists can trace their roots to the modern use of oxygen at the turn of the 20th century. During the first two decades of the century, oxygen devices such as oxygen tents, nasal catheters, and oxygen masks were developed. Increasingly, they were used in clinical settings. Modern uses of oxygen created a need for knowledgeable people who could administer oxygen. Thus, the field of respiratory therapy was born. Today, the government recognizes respiratory therapy as a health profession according to the definition found in the Public Health Service Act, title VII, section 701.[23]

In the 1940s, a group of physicians and "oxygen technicians" in Chicago began meeting to discuss oxygen therapy. These discussions led to the creation of the Inhalational Therapy Association in 1946.[24] Over the next few years, the number of members grew; in 1954, the group was renamed the American Association of Inhalation Therapists (AAIT).

The 1970s saw even more advancements in respiratory therapy. Air–oxygen blenders, pulse oximetry, oxygen concentrators, portable liquid oxygen systems, and intermittent mandatory ventilation (IMV) were developed. These and other inventions were incorporated into clinical practice. In 1978, the National Board for Respiratory Care (NBRC) developed an entry-level concept that set the standards for entry into the field. In 1979, the NBRC administered the first clinical simulation exam for advanced practitioners. This exam replaced the previously used oral exam.[25]

Technology continued to improve in the 1980s and 1990s, which led to advancements in the profession. These included the development and use of pressure control ventilation and continuous flow ventilation. Advances in extracorporeal membrane oxygenation (ECMO) and home care ventilators also occurred. The respiratory care profession saw tremendous growth, especially among specialty fields. The certified pulmonary function exam was first administered in 1984. This was followed in 1987 by the advanced pulmonary function exam, and in 1991 by the first perinatal/pediatric exam. In 2008, the NBRC offered the first sleep disorders specialty exam for certified and registered respiratory therapists with experience in sleep diagnostics and treatment.[26]

The profession emphasized the importance of providing respiratory care by trained, qualified persons. Educational programs and respiratory care departments evolved and expanded. Eventually, respiratory therapists assumed roles as managers and educators. As new trends in healthcare emerged, respiratory therapists quickly responded. They worked to best meet patients' needs and establish the new profession. This adaptability has been an asset as healthcare continues to rapidly change. The profession began to require respiratory therapists with advanced education and experience in clinical decision making and critical thinking.[19,20,22] Respiratory therapy departments capitalized on the therapists' skills in clinical decision making, leading to the implementation of protocol-based care.[4]

RESPIRATORY RECAP

Evolution of Respiratory Therapy

- » Respiratory therapy can trace its roots to oxygen therapy, which began in the early 20th century.
- » A professional organization was established in 1946 as the Inhalational Therapy Association, which was renamed the American Association of Inhalation Therapists in 1956.
- » The first certification exam for inhalation therapy was administered in 1969.
- » Entry-level standards for the profession were established in 1978.
- » Protocol-based care began in the early 1980s.
- » Respiratory therapy was recognized as a profession by the government in the 1990s.
- » Respiratory therapy has continued to evolve into the 21st century.

TABLE 57–1 Traditional Respiratory Care Services Provided by Respiratory Therapy Departments

Services	Percentage Providing Service in 1992
Oxygen therapy	100
Mechanical ventilation	96
Chest physiotherapy	96
Bland aerosol therapy	81
IPPB therapy	93
Intermittent mask CPAP	63
Incentive spirometry	96
Aerosol bronchodilator therapy	100
MDI bronchodilator therapy	82
MDI steroid therapy	66
Pulse oximetry	98
Blood gas analysis	83
Pulmonary function testing	96
Pulmonary rehabilitation	43
Home care and/or durable medical equipment	32

IPPB, intermittent positive pressure breathing; CPAP, continuous positive airway pressure; MDI, metered dose inhaler.

From Mishoe SC, MacIntyre NR. Expanding professional roles for respiratory care practitioners. *Respir Care*. 1997;42:71. Reprinted with permission.

Traditional Services Provided by Respiratory Therapists

The primary or traditional setting for the delivery of respiratory therapy has been in the hospital. Typically, a centralized respiratory therapy department provides a variety of respiratory services (**Table 57–1**). Services provided are usually divided into two major areas: general patient care and critical care. The categories of services provided by respiratory therapists include oxygen therapy, other respiratory therapies, physiologic monitoring, ventilation, and specialized skills. Oxygen therapy involves routine oxygen administration, transport, and hyperbaric oxygen administration. Other respiratory therapies include jet nebulization, metered dose inhalers, intermittent positive pressure breathing, and chest physiotherapy. Physiologic monitoring encompasses more techniques and procedures, including arterial blood gas sampling and interpretation, pulmonary function testing, and pulse oximetry and capnography. Ventilator management includes adult, pediatric, infant, and noninvasive ventilation. Specialized skills such as transports, CPR, and airway care also are part of respiratory therapy's scope of practice. Respiratory therapists deliver many of these services in both general care and critical care. Other services, such as ventilator management, are only in critical care.

> **RESPIRATORY RECAP**
>
> **Traditional Respiratory Therapy Services**
>
> » Centralized respiratory therapy departments
> » General care and critical care (primarily provided in hospitals)
> » Oxygen therapy
> » Medication delivery and airway clearance
> » Physiologic monitoring
> » Ventilator management
> » Specialized skills

Formal programs educated students to work in hospitals, providing acute care in the treatment of cardiopulmonary disease. During the past decade, the traditional role and career expectations have dramatically changed. This change has coincided with the changes in healthcare delivery. Today, educational programs and continuing education must prepare respiratory therapists to work in nontraditional roles. They must be prepared to work in numerous sites, in addition to acute care in hospitals.

Why Nontraditional Roles Are Emerging for Respiratory Therapists

The past few years have seen many changes in the delivery of healthcare. The traditional delivery system, the acute care hospital, has been replaced with a system that has broadened the continuum of care. Subacute care facilities, home health agencies, and prevention/wellness programs have evolved and become important.

The changes in reimbursement strategies and the aging population challenged hospitals, which had to develop means to decrease their costs. Recent changes include decreasing the levels of management and decentralizing respiratory care departments. Labor substitution and alternative or contract employees have been used. Patient-focused care has become more popular. The use of protocols emerged, which allowed respiratory therapists to expand their skills. They are now able to provide assessments and treatment plans for patients.

On the other hand, nurses and others began to assume selected respiratory therapist duties in some settings. This led to concerns about the basic, technical skills of these personnel. Studies have shown that respiratory therapists exhibit better technique in the delivery of respiratory procedures than other providers.[4,27,28] Hospitals that employ respiratory therapists and use protocol-directed care have less overuse of respiratory therapy treatments.[29] Routine assessments and patient education make a difference in the delivery of healthcare. Who provides these services will also make a difference in the recovery of the patient.

The cost of caring for patients is greater in the acute care setting because of the number of fixed costs, such as staff and equipment. This has led to the development of postacute care delivery sites. These sites include home health, subacute care, and outpatient programs. The cost of caring for patients is lower in these facilities: studies have found that it costs 40% to 60% less to care for patients in subacute care facilities than in acute facilities.[30] Today, more procedures are provided on an outpatient basis. The length of stay in acute care facilities also has shortened.

Respiratory therapists have had to change as the healthcare system changed, and they have benefited from new ways of thinking. Respiratory therapists have strong, specialized backgrounds in the diagnosis, treatment, and prevention of cardiopulmonary diseases, which make up a large portion of the high cost of chronic diseases. Respiratory therapists have strong assessment skills and the ability to create treatment plans. These plans can lower the cost of caring for chronic pulmonary patients. Respiratory therapists have the necessary skills needed to thrive under managed care.

Respiratory therapists are the experts on respiratory equipment, products, and medications. Because of their knowledge of cardiopulmonary diseases, respiratory therapists make excellent patient educators. They can make use of their assessment, communication, and critical thinking skills in disease management. Programs such as pulmonary rehabilitation and asthma management allow respiratory therapists to educate their patients. This education can help improve patient involvement in their care plans for better outcomes.

> **RESPIRATORY RECAP**
>
> **Why Respiratory Therapists Are Qualified for New Roles**
>
> » Strong clinical backgrounds
> » Experts in cardiopulmonary disease
> » Technology specialists with computer skills
> » Patient assessment skills
> » The ability to create effective treatment plans
> » Patient education abilities
> » Patient-centered care is a strong point
> » Excellent candidates for new technologies and emerging practices
> » Education and credentialing are adapting to expanded scope of practice
> » Scope of practice is adapting to meet patient needs

Respiratory therapists have been using their strong clinical backgrounds and assessment skills to create new careers in nontraditional settings. Although 80% of all respiratory therapists are employed in hospitals, many of the job opportunities for respiratory therapists will be in nontraditional settings.[1] To work in these new areas, respiratory therapists must add to their existing competencies. They must prove they can save their employers money. They must adapt to new practice settings. They must focus on dealing with the chronic aspects of disease management. They must be willing to take on new tasks and be open to risks.[4] Respiratory therapists will need to advance their skills in communication and patient education.

They will need to know more about managed care and reimbursement.

Respiratory therapists are valued for their expertise and management of respiratory diseases. Working in nontraditional roles requires different skills. What is important in an acute care setting may not be as important in a subacute care setting. The skills required usually change with the environment. This constant change requires flexibility, problem solving, and continued learning. Respiratory therapists must be able to provide effective care and must be able to document their worth in this competitive healthcare system.

Nontraditional Roles for Respiratory Therapists

The growth of nontraditional arenas for healthcare offers new, challenging opportunities. Respiratory therapists have taken advantage of this larger range of care to create new roles for themselves, expanding into areas such as cardiopulmonary diagnostic testing and polysomnography. Nontraditional roles include home health, diagnostics, subacute care, wellness/disease management, and case management. There are also roles for respiratory therapists in industry, including research, sales, technical development, and medical writing. Roles in education and management continue to be available. Since the beginning of the field, respiratory therapists have benefited from strong relationships with physicians. They have created new roles by becoming physician extenders. The role of the respiratory therapist as physician extender continues to evolve. However, current reimbursement limits may restrict this role to acute care settings.

The future has promise for exciting new opportunities. Respiratory therapists must continue to evolve. They must build on the base started by innovative founders. **Box 57–3** lists nontraditional roles of respiratory therapists. The following sections explain these nontraditional roles.

BOX 57–3

Evolving Scope of Practice for Respiratory Therapy

- Mechanical ventilation management and life support systems
- Invasive and noninvasive cardiodiagnostics and cardiopulmonary monitoring, cardiac monitoring, arterial lines, indwelling catheters
- Traditional basic therapies (e.g., oxygen therapy, aerosol therapy, humidity therapy, incentive spirometry)
- Management
- Pulmonary function testing
- Treatment assessment/outcome assessment
- Home care
- CPR/resuscitation
- Respiratory care of neonatal and pediatric patients
- Arterial blood gases
- Rehabilitation/cardiopulmonary rehabilitation
- Patient and family education
- Protocols
- Health promotion and disease prevention
- Smoking cessation/nicotine intervention
- Hyperbaric oxygenation
- ECLS and other life support techniques
- Management
- Discharge planning
- Sleep studies
- Research
- Medication administration
- Stress and exercise testing
- Alternate-site care delivery
- Bronchoscopy
- Infection control
- Electrolyte analysis
- Geriatrics
- Quality and performance assessment
- Case management
- EEG/neurodiagnostics
- Computerization/information management
- Transport/trauma in-flight specialist
- Metabolics
- ACLS, PALS, NRP
- Mechanical cardiac support
- Ethics
- Teaching and team management with other health professions
- Patient-focused care
- Technology assessment
- Charting and record keeping

CPR, cardiopulmonary resuscitation; ECLS, extracorporeal life support; EEG, electroencephalography; ACLS, advanced cardiac life support; NRP, neonatal resuscitation program; PALS, pediatric advanced life support.

From Mishoe SC, MacIntyre NR. Expanding professional roles for respiratory care practitioners. *Respir Care.* 1997;42:71. Reprinted with permission.

Diagnostics

Respiratory therapists have intense education and training in **diagnostics**. This training includes blood gas analysis; nutritional, cardiac, pulmonary, exercise, and sleep assessments; chest radiology; bronchoscopy; pulmonary function testing; and hemodynamics and gas exchange monitoring. The following sections highlight some of the nontraditional roles for respiratory therapists in diagnostics.

Cardiopulmonary Diagnostics

Cardiopulmonary diagnostics is an area with potential for the expansion of the role of the respiratory therapist.[20] The technology used for diagnostics has increased in hospitals and alternative sites. Pulmonary function testing, blood gas analysis, and cardiac testing are already performed by respiratory therapists in acute care. However, the growing trend is to perform these tests in outpatient settings. This can be done by private, contract services. Many subacute care facilities do not have laboratories on site. They contract with outside labs for these services.

Respiratory therapists are ideal for working with the latest cardiopulmonary diagnostics. New monitoring devices are moving from the research laboratory to the bedside. Examples of these are optoelectronic plethysmography, electrical impedance tomography, and acoustic thoracic monitoring.[1] Many therapists have started their own labs, which offer services such as pulmonary function and sleep study testing. They have contracted with managed care companies to provide services for clients enrolled in their programs. Other respiratory therapists have provided diagnostic testing in industrial settings. Federal law requires employers to provide safe workplaces for employees. Many tests are required for industries by the Occupational Safety and Health Administration (OSHA). These tests include fit testing for respirators, asbestosis testing, and audiometric testing for noise levels.

RESPIRATORY RECAP

Opportunities and Rewards of Cardiopulmonary Diagnostics

- » Expansion of the scope of practice for respiratory therapists
- » Satisfaction of helping with the diagnosis of disease and treatment planning
- » Opportunities to use clinical, computer, creative, and business skills
- » Expanded markets with potential to establish new business ventures
- » Opportunities for consult and contract work

Skills and Rewards of Cardiopulmonary Diagnostics

Respiratory therapists working in diagnostic testing require outstanding technical abilities. They should enjoy working with and maintaining equipment. They also need strong computer skills, especially with hardware, software, and telecommunication processes. They should be familiar with the various groups that sanction laboratories. They should have knowledge of government rules involved with labs. Respiratory therapists who service industries will need to be familiar with OSHA standards and testing requirements. They may need to complete further continuing education courses to meet OSHA compliance levels.

Many respiratory therapists involved in diagnostics enjoy the satisfaction of providing needed services. They enjoy the aspect of diagnosis of a disease. As prospects for new ventures expand, some respiratory therapists have fulfilled their dreams of owning their own businesses. Diagnostics has expanded new markets for these respiratory therapists. It has allowed them to use their creative skills and business savvy.

Polysomnography

During the last three decades, polysomnography has observed great growth. The public and medical professionals have become more aware of the importance of sleep and of the costs of sleep deprivation. Centers that perform special testing in sleep-related diseases have become more important in recent years. Sleep studies include two main tests: polysomnography and the multiple sleep latency test (MSLT). Testing helps the diagnosis of sleep disorders such as narcolepsy, sleep apnea, and restless leg syndrome.

Sleep testing requires the use of various types of equipment to monitor body movement. Typical sleep studies involve placing electroencephalographic electrodes on the scalp to monitor brain activity for sleep staging, and electrodes to monitor eye movement. Electromyographic electrodes are used to monitor limb movement, and belts or strain gauzes to monitor abdominal and chest wall movement. Nasal or oral air flow transistors are also used. In addition, pulse oximeters monitor oxygen saturation levels, and electrocardiographic electrodes monitor cardiac rate/rhythms. Many hospitals have developed their own sleep labs. However, the equipment is expensive and requires specialized personnel. Therefore, some hospitals contract with independent sleep laboratories. The majority of sleep tests are performed in the outpatient setting. Many labs now perform sleep studies in the patient's home.

Skills and Rewards of Polysomnography

Respiratory therapists interested in polysomnography should be skilled in performing and evaluating diagnostic procedures, specifically sleep studies. They also should have the ability to operate a variety of equipment. They should be able to work night shifts and enjoy quiet environments. Many patients feel uncomfortable with someone watching them sleep. The testing procedure itself is threatening to patients because it involves the use of electrodes and monitors to the body. The polysomnographer needs strong people skills to calm patients so that they feel at ease, allowing the polysomnographer to obtain a valid test.

Many respiratory therapists have the basic background needed to begin working in sleep laboratories.

> **RESPIRATORY RECAP**
>
> **Opportunities and Rewards of Polysomnography**
>
> » Many respiratory therapists have the basic backgrounds needed to begin working in sleep laboratories.
>
> » The Board of Registered Polysomnographic Technologists offers a credentialing exam to assess the competence of individuals performing polysomnography.
>
> » Further education allows one to score sleep studies.
>
> » Opportunities exist to work independently in sleep centers and patients' homes.
>
> » The ability to assist with the diagnosis and development of effective care plans yields the self-satisfaction of dramatically improving patients' quality of life.

Additional training in the equipment and procedures related to sleep testing is required. Respiratory therapists have a variety of educational programs available to receive education in polysomnography. These range from 2-year programs to 1- to 2-week courses on sleep-related subjects. Advancing in the field requires more education. This allows one to score sleep studies. Scoring a study requires interpretation of data, which can be done any time after the test is completed. Many sleep labs employ polysomnographers who provide scoring services only. This allows some polysomnographers to work during the day.

The Board of Registered Polysomnographic Technologists offers an exam designed to assess the ability of those performing polysomnography. Individuals earn the credential of Registered Polysomnographic Technologist (RPSGT) when they pass this exam. Exam candidates must either complete 18 months of experience in polysomnography or 12 months of experience if they are credentialed in a health-related field.

Probably the biggest reward of polysomnographers is the ability to correctly diagnose sleep disorders. They also participate in the development and implementation of effective care plans. Effective treatment of sleep disorders has a great impact on patients' quality of life. Polysomnographers find this aspect of the job satisfying. Please refer to Chapter 12 for a complete chapter on this topic.

Home Healthcare

Home healthcare is a formal, regulated program of care that is delivered by a variety of healthcare professionals in the patient's home. At the turn of the 20th century, doctors and nurses provided the majority of healthcare in the home. Soon technology advanced and it seemed that it was no longer possible to provide healthcare in the home. Hospitals became the choice site of healthcare. During the past century, most patients recovered from illnesses in acute care hospitals. Patients did not return to their homes until they were able to care for themselves. There has been a recent change in this thinking. Managed care companies realized that it is cheaper to care for patients in the subacute care or home setting. The future of medicine may see a return to more patients treated in their homes. Reimbursements and costs will factor into this trend.[1]

> **RESPIRATORY RECAP**
>
> **Types of Home Healthcare Services**
>
> » Home health agencies
>
> » Hospice
>
> » Home medical equipment
>
> » Home infusion therapy
>
> » Homemaker/private-duty nursing

Today, healthcare professionals can provide home health services. Patients may have acute illnesses or exacerbations of chronic illnesses. Some may have long-term disabilities. Home health services fall into five different categories: home health agencies, hospice, home medical equipment, home infusion therapy, and homemaker services or private-duty nursing.

Skills and Rewards of Home Healthcare

A typical day in home care may take the respiratory therapist from the most expensive subdivision to a government housing project. Respiratory therapists must be adaptable and ready to work in any environment, with a variety of people. They should work with patients in a nonjudgmental manner. This helps build the relationship between the patient and the therapist. Many patients have difficulty adjusting to the permanence of the oxygen equipment. Others have issues about needing lifelong medications. Respiratory therapists may not truly appreciate the reality of chronic cardiopulmonary disease until they work in home healthcare.

One of the biggest rewards may be the ability to offer suggestions for dealing with potential problems, such as helping patients plan outings so that they will have an adequate supply of oxygen. Often patients decide not to wear their oxygen or take their medications because they feel better. They may be in denial that they still have problems. Respiratory therapists must use their persuasive powers to educate such patients. They need to partner with patients about the many costs of their choices. Some costs are financial, but others are from decreased health and wellness.

> **RESPIRATORY RECAP**
>
> **Opportunities and Rewards of Home Healthcare**
>
> » Ability to work in various environments
>
> » Educate patients and family members dealing with chronic cardiopulmonary diseases
>
> » Gain ongoing knowledge of reimbursement policies
>
> » Opportunities could increase if respiratory therapy were included in the reimbursement for skilled visits

Therapists in the home healthcare setting also need a strong knowledge of reimbursement policies. They need to be experts in case management. Physicians may order drugs or treatments for patients thinking they are using the most cost-effective means, but there may be less costly alternatives. For example, a metered dose inhaler (MDI) may be the most cost-effective method of delivering bronchodilator therapy in the hospital, but it may not be the most cost-effective in the home. In some states, Medicare may not pay for the MDI, but will pay for the unit dose of albuterol via mobilization. The role of the respiratory therapist is critical in reducing the cost of care for the healthcare provider as well as the patient.

Despite the reimbursement concerns, home health therapists find their jobs rewarding. Many enjoy the flexibility of being able to set their own schedule. They also report that the job is less stressful than acute care work. They do not have to deal with frequent emergencies. Home health respiratory therapists enjoy personal interaction with their patients. They are able to build stronger relationships with patients and their families. Being able to follow a patient for a significant amount of time is another reward. The chance to teach patients about their disease, equipment, and improving their quality of life is one of the most rewarding aspects of home healthcare.

Subacute Care

As hospitals look for ways to decrease the number of patient days per stay, postacute care has become more popular. Subacute care attributes its growth to the Medicare prospective payment system. Managed care sets limits to the money provided to hospitals for patient care. It also uses strict review criteria for patients to meet requirements for acute care. Subacute care has become a viable alternative. Subacute care often involves a partnership between the acute care hospital and home healthcare with the goal of returning the patient to the home. The rise of managed care has shown a trend for more use of subacute care. More patients are being discharged from acute care hospitals more quickly than before the employment of managed care. If this trend continues, the number of long-term acute care facilities and rehabilitation hospitals will increase. This will provide more opportunities for respiratory therapists.

> **RESPIRATORY RECAP**
>
> **Differentiating Between SNFs and LTACs**
>
> » Long-term acute care facilities (LTACs) are licensed hospitals.
>
> » LTACs are exempt from the Medicare prospective payment system as long as they keep their average patient length of stay greater than 25 days.
>
> » Skilled nursing facilities (SNFs) are identified beds certified by the CMS to participate in the Medicare program for its long-term care benefits.
>
> » SNFs may be freestanding or hospital based.

There has been some confusion in the healthcare delivery system regarding the criteria for subacute care. Subacute care patients are stable and do not require acute care services. At the same time they are too sick to return home or to a nursing home. They usually need rehabilitation or monitoring.[31] Medicare reimbursement policies add to the confusion. Most reimbursement for subacute care is paid by Medicare, Medicaid, and managed care. Sixty-eight percent of patients using subacute care have Medicare.[7]

The type and amount of respiratory therapy services provided at subacute care facilities vary depending on the type of facility and the acuity of the patients. The Joint Commission has identified respiratory care as a necessary component for accreditation as a subacute care facility.[4,31] If ventilator management is offered in the subacute facility, respiratory therapists are available 24-7. If ventilator management is not a part of care, respiratory therapists may be available daily. Whereas respiratory therapists working in hospitals have become more specialized, respiratory therapists working in subacute care have become more generalized. Ironically, administrators of subacute care facilities value respiratory therapists for their specialization.

Services may be complex and often are similar to duties performed by therapists in hospitals. These services include assessment, treatment, care planning, and airway care. They also include monitoring, diagnostics, and other traditional therapies. Respiratory therapists provide most of the airway care, such as trach care and suctioning. The patients in subacute care are generally medically stable. They do not require broad diagnostic workups. There is thus less emphasis on diagnostic procedures and a greater reliance on assessment and monitoring. There is less interaction with physicians in subacute care. Respiratory therapists usually use protocols for oxygenation, ventilator management, and other therapies.

The interdisciplinary team is essential for effective subacute care delivery. Team members include nurses, physical therapists, occupational therapists, speech pathologists, and others depending on the patient's needs. Critical members of the team are the patient and the patient's family, who play a vital role in the planning and implementing of care plans. Working closely with other disciplines helps to ensure that patients have information to help achieve their treatment goals.

Types of Subacute Care

Different types of subacute care facilities exist, including long-term acute care (LTAC) facilities, skilled nursing facilities (SNFs), specialty hospitals, and rehabilitation hospitals. There are also respiratory units within acute care hospitals. The Centers for Medicare and Medicaid Services (CMS), previously known as the Health Care Financing Administration (HCFA), defines the types of postacute care setting by the following criteria: nursing hours per day, rehabilitation requirements, length of stays, and cost within a particular institution.

LTAC facilities are licensed hospitals that are exempt from the Medicare prospective payment system if they meet certain criteria. They must keep their average patient length of stay greater than 25 days. Long-term hospitals receive payment from Medicare on a reasonable-cost basis. LTAC hospitals usually specialize in patients who have pulmonary problems or medially complex problems. The patients no longer require extensive diagnostic workups, but do need additional therapy and nursing support. If the LTAC has ventilator patients, respiratory therapy is offered 24 hours per day. Patients usually stay an average of between 10 and 60 days.

Skilled nursing facilities are identified beds certified by the CMS. They participate in the Medicare program for servicing its long-term care benefits. One way to distinguish SNFs from LTACs is to look at the number and amount of services provided. SNFs generally provide fewer services than LTACs and offer an average of 2 to 3 nursing hours per day. Occupational therapy, physical therapy, and respiratory therapy are offered on an as-needed basis. The length of stay for patients in an SNF averages 60-plus days. Skilled nursing facilities may be freestanding or hospital based. As a rule, the cost of caring for a patient is higher in a hospital-based SNF.

Many hospitals have created their own SNFs to deal with patients who require long-term ventilation or who have medically complex problems. These units were among the first subacute care programs in the country.[4] These SNFs have been proven to be cost-effective in many cases. Patients in subacute care settings do not require as much skilled nursing care as patients in acute care facilities. By moving these patients to subacute care facilities, savings can be incurred. One study suggests that Medicare could save at least $142 million per year if clinically stable ventilator-dependent patients were treated in SNFs rather than acute care facilities.[4]

The AARC authorized a study to determine the cost-effectiveness of respiratory therapists who provide services to Medicare patients with respiratory diagnoses in skilled nursing facilities. The study reviewed outcomes and costs and looked at two groups of patients. One group received respiratory services provided by respiratory therapists. The other group received respiratory services provided by non-respiratory therapists. The study revealed that patients treated by respiratory therapists had better outcomes. They also had lower costs than those not treated by respiratory therapists.[32] Patients who were treated by respiratory therapists had a shorter length of stay, leading to cost savings in the millions to Medicare.[32] Patients treated by non-respiratory therapists required later services in a hospital emergency room or outpatient setting. Medicare spent 23% more to treat these patients.[32]

RESPIRATORY RECAP

Benefits of Respiratory Therapists in Skilled Nursing Facilities

- Patients had a 3.6-day shorter length of stay.
- Mortality of patients was reduced by 42%.
- Medicare cost savings were $97.9 million.

Skills and Rewards of Subacute Care

Many of the same skills used in subacute care settings are used by respiratory therapists in traditional hospital settings. There are some important differences. Respiratory therapists who work in subacute settings have less physician interaction, so they must be self-directed. They must be able to use protocols and reimbursement criteria. They should be willing and able to make decisions, and able to implement treatment plans for their patients. They must be aware of costs and reimbursement requirements so that the care they provide is covered. Respiratory therapists must possess strong clinical, disease management, critical thinking, and problem-solving skills plus experience working with protocols and care plans before working in subacute care.

Subacute care respiratory therapists find there is more of an educational component involved in their job. They must have excellent communication and teaching skills. Subacute care places an emphasis on interdisciplinary care planning and teamwork. In addition to working independently, the respiratory therapist must also function as a team member. A good knowledge of the skills and services provided by other allied health professionals is essential, and a cooperative nature and strong communications skills are needed. A good background in the development and implementation of care plans, outcomes assessment, and discharge planning is needed.

The rewards of working in subacute care differ from the intrinsic motivators involved in acute care. Many patients in subacute settings are long-term or chronic patients. Being able to wean a patient from mechanical ventilation who has been ventilated for weeks, or months, is just one of the rewards. Other respiratory therapists enjoy being able to become more involved and spend more time with patients. They find satisfaction from improving their patients' quality of life. They may enjoy the less hurried one-on-one contact with their patients. Many respiratory therapists who work in subacute care enjoy getting to know not only the patients, but their family members as well. They feel this helps them see the patient as a whole person. Other respiratory therapists enjoy the opportunity to be self-directed by the use of protocols. Respiratory therapists are able to assess their patients and implement the care they

RESPIRATORY RECAP

Opportunities and Rewards of Subacute Care

- Working with interdisciplinary teams
- Opportunities to develop and use protocols and care plans to provide and evaluate care
- Rewards from focusing on the whole person for holistic care
- Addressing the emotional and physical impact of chronic disease
- Improving quality of life of patients with chronic disease

feel is needed. The opportunity to work closely with other disciplines also appeals to respiratory therapists who work in subacute care.

Disease Prevention and Wellness Management Programs

Society is changing its concept of health and healthcare. Wellness and disease prevention are becoming more important. The following section overviews the increasingly important role of respiratory therapists in disease prevention and wellness programs.

Pulmonary Rehabilitation

A greater emphasis on education and the prevention of diseases has come about as a means of controlling costs. Many hospitals have developed pulmonary rehabilitation centers and wellness programs for chronic diseases. Pulmonary rehabilitation has become more important in recent years. **Pulmonary rehabilitation** has several goals: it works to alleviate and control symptoms of respiratory diseases, helps to restore functional capabilities as much as possible, and improves the patient's quality of life. An interdisciplinary team of specialists works with the patient to achieve these goals.[33]

The goals of pulmonary rehabilitation are to help patients increase their activity through exercise training and education. Pulmonary rehabilitation programs are usually divided into three phases. Phase I is the pretesting portion of the program. The patient performs tests such as pulmonary function studies, a stress test, and the 6- to 12-minute walking test. Patients usually complete questionnaires that assess their nutritional, psychological, lifestyle, and vocational needs.

The second phase of the program includes education and exercise. Educational topics include lung anatomy, breathing and pulmonary hygiene techniques, and nutritional guidelines. Medications, equipment, and the importance of exercise conditioning are also covered. Exercise is introduced during phase II. Respiratory therapists monitor patients for oxygen saturation levels, breathing techniques, pulse, rhythm rates, and blood pressure while patients perform exercise. The exercise may be very simple, such as walking or riding a stationary bike. As the patient progresses through the program, the workload is gradually increased. The final phase of the program includes follow-up care and long-term maintenance.

> **AGE-SPECIFIC ANGLE**
>
> Respiratory therapists working in pulmonary rehabilitation should have a strong background in geriatrics.

Skills and Rewards of Pulmonary Rehabilitation

A good understanding of cardiopulmonary physiology and pathophysiology is important to work in pulmonary rehabilitation. Respiratory therapists must be able to perform and understand pulmonary function tests. They need strong interpersonal and communication skills. They should be able to motivate people. Respiratory therapists working with pulmonary rehabilitation should have a strong background in geriatrics.

Respiratory therapists who work in pulmonary rehabilitation and wellness programs enjoy building positive relationships with their patients and their families. They often have the opportunity to get to know their patients as individuals much better than traditional therapists do. They become the primary source of health education for patients and their families. A strong bond may become established. Making a difference in the quality of life of patients rewards therapists working in pulmonary rehabilitation.

> **RESPIRATORY RECAP**
>
> **Opportunities and Rewards of Pulmonary Rehabilitation**
>
> » Controlling costs for patients suffering from chronic lung disease
> » Assessment, education, exercise training, and long-term maintenance
> » Using a multidisciplinary approach for evaluation, education, and care
> » Focusing on the psychosocial and quality of life aspects of chronic pulmonary diseases

Wellness Programs

Managed care has placed an emphasis on providing education and programs for individuals who are healthy in order to maintain their good health. This approach is an attempt to decrease the long-term costs of providing healthcare services. Healthy people require less healthcare.

To accomplish the goal of keeping people healthy, hospitals and managed care companies have set up **wellness programs**. Wellness programs include classes that educate consumers so that they can maintain, and possibly even improve, their quality of life. Wellness programs cover topics such as the benefits of diet, good sleep habits, and relaxation techniques. Other programs include routine exercise, diagnostic screenings, and the psychosocial aspects of health. The emphasis is placed on preventing disease and on establishing and maintaining healthy habits for life. Because paying for healthcare has become a stressor, wellness programs can and should focus on access and reimbursement issues related to acute and chronic care.

Hospitals are not the only companies offering wellness programs. Managed care companies offer wellness programs as a means to keep hospital readmissions low. By reducing admissions to hospitals, managed care companies benefit financially. At the same time they improve the health of their clients. Many managed care companies now employ respiratory therapists as disease mangers, or **case managers**. Respiratory therapists can provide expert education to clients with asthma, COPD, and other pulmonary diseases. This approach addresses the chronic aspect of the disease, and it provides patients with individual treatment plans and an expert to help guide them in their care.

Disease specialists develop treatment plans with physicians for enrollees. They monitor the enrollee's progress, either by telephone or during home visits. They evaluate the enrollee's progress and offer moral support and expert education.

Respiratory therapists have welcomed these opportunities and challenges. They can either work for managed care companies or start their own businesses. Many respiratory therapists have marketed educational programs to managed care companies or directly to physicians. Many physicians do not have the time or up-to-date information to provide for their patients' education. Respiratory therapists have been able to step into the role created by this need.

Skills and Rewards of Working in Disease Management and Wellness Programs

Respiratory therapists who work in pulmonary rehabilitation or wellness programs require well-developed educational skills. They need to have strong backgrounds in the lifestyle changes that promote good health as well as a good understanding of the pathophysiology and treatment of pulmonary diseases.

These therapists strive to motivate individuals to make positive lifestyle changes to improve their health. An added benefit is that in the process of this work the respiratory therapists themselves may become healthier. They are able to provide hope and encouragement to people who have seen their lives change due to chronic illnesses. Many rehabilitation therapists enjoy their job because the patients are committed to learning and want to benefit from the program. They are not there because of acute care needs. They want to learn how to stay healthy by preventing or managing disease. Helping individuals achieve and maintain the highest possible quality of physical, emotional, and social life is a primary reward of working with wellness programs.

RESPIRATORY RECAP

Opportunities and Rewards of Working in Wellness Programs

» Respiratory therapists working in these programs have the opportunity to work with healthy people and focus on prevention of disease.
» An added benefit may be that respiratory therapists working with disease prevention and wellness may themselves adopt a healthier lifestyle.
» Managed care has created greater demand for respiratory therapists to work in pulmonary rehabilitation and wellness programs.
» Entrepreneurial opportunities and rewards exist.
» Managed care companies that employ respiratory therapists in wellness and disease prevention programs have been able to reap financial rewards.
» Helping individuals achieve the highest possible quality of physical, emotional, and social life is a primary reward.

Case Management

Case management has become an essential component of all healthcare professions. There are two elements of case management related to respiratory care. The first is inclusion of case management into the daily activities of respiratory therapists. The second is respiratory therapists acting in the capacity of case managers for patients.

Many hospitals, insurance companies, HMOs, and PPOs use respiratory therapists as case mangers. This provides a way to be cost-effective in supplying respiratory care. Respiratory therapists have experience in patient assessment, patient education, care planning, and the implementation, monitoring, and evaluation of the course of therapy.[31] This makes them highly qualified for this role. The number of respiratory therapists functioning in the role of case manager has increased.

Many respiratory therapy case managers deal with patients who have chronic pulmonary diseases, which are often difficult to supervise under managed care. Respiratory therapists are experts in dealing with patients with chronic pulmonary problems because they know the equipment and services needed to treat these diseases.

Respiratory therapists have added case management to their duties as a routine part of their daily work.[3] Case management will continue to be a vital role in the respiratory therapist's job. Case management can save resources. More hospitals have incorporated disease management programs into the services provided by respiratory therapy departments.

Another way respiratory therapists have used case management is through protocol-based care. Hospitals have seen the benefit of using protocols. Protocols lead to a reduction of length of stay and bring about costs savings when treating patients with pulmonary diseases.[3] Hospital-based case mangers have varied job duties. They must work closely with insurance companies to ensure the patient still meets the requirements for acute care. Case managers perform clinical reviews of the patient on a daily basis. Case managers must coordinate discharge planning and function almost as social workers in working with patients and their families. They also may be involved in the prevention aspect of the disease, because one of their goals is to decrease readmissions to the hospital.

HMOs that employ respiratory therapists as case mangers use them for education and clinical services.[3] Nursing homes and home health organizations are four times more likely to use respiratory therapists as case mangers than hospitals.[4] These case managers also review hospital daily censuses to identify case management patients. They work with the hospital-based case manager to coordinate discharge planning. Managed care case managers are responsible for confirming patient eligibility. They also authorize referrals for home healthcare and equipment.

Physicians have also seen the benefits of having respiratory therapists as case managers in their offices. Physicians who participate in managed care plans often have their outcomes monitored by the managed care companies. If their outcomes are not appropriate, they could be in jeopardy of losing managed care contracts. This has led some physicians and physician groups to hire respiratory therapists as case managers. The respiratory therapists can help them decide which pulmonary tests might be beneficial for each patient. Physicians have also used respiratory therapy case managers to help with the education of their patients. Patient education might focus on topics such as disease processes and medication delivery.

Skills and Rewards of Respiratory Therapy Case Managers

Respiratory therapist entry into case management requires a bachelors degree and RRT credential. Respiratory therapists who want to be case managers should have strong clinical backgrounds. They should have knowledge of the diagnosis and treatment of pulmonary diseases. They need outstanding patient assessment skills. They should also have effective social, organizational, and communication skills. They must be able to balance the needs of the patient and family with the needs of the managed care company. They often meet with family members to update them on the plans for the patient. They become the liaison between the family members and the physician and the managed care company.

> **RESPIRATORY RECAP**
>
> **Opportunities and Rewards of Case Management**
>
> » Assisting providers to be cost-effective
> » Coordinating total care of patients, not solely cardiopulmonary care
> » Developing long-term relationships with patients and their families
> » Acting as a liaison between the patient and the healthcare industry
> » Directly contributing to controlling healthcare costs
> » Promoting fiscal responsibility
> » Promoting appropriate allocation of finite healthcare resources
> » Assisting consumers with the complex healthcare delivery system

In addition, respiratory therapists working as case managers should have a good knowledge of reimbursement and health plan benefits. They should be familiar with patient care settings, support services, and current legislation. They serve as the intermediary between the insurance company and the physician. Effective communication is essential! Respiratory therapist case managers must be able to work independently and prioritize.

Respiratory therapists working as case managers must be able to deal with many different healthcare disciplines. They must look at the patient as a whole. They cannot focus on just the respiratory illness. Case management entails social work, discharge planning, and disease management. The respiratory therapy case manger must be able to wear different hats and juggle many aspects of the job.

Rewards of case management include working with patients to help improve their quality of life through effective education and utilization of services. Patients often develop strong relationships with their case managers. This relationship can help patients to make changes in their lives. Case managers serve as motivators. Another reward is coordinating the total care of the patient instead of only the cardiopulmonary component of care.[4] Most important, case managers find rewards in helping individuals and the larger society. They help to effectively and responsibly use expensive and finite healthcare resources.

Physician Extender

The role of respiratory therapists is evolving from that of a task performer to that of functioning as a mutual decision maker and **physician extender**. Another avenue recently opened to respiratory therapists is as physician extenders in nontraditional settings, such as physician offices. Managed care emphasizes treating the patient before acute situations occur. The best place to do this is the physician's office. Major goals are to decrease emergency department visits and hospital admissions. Some respiratory therapists have the necessary clinical background and expertise needed to fill the role of physician extender.[23] Physician practices can be reimbursed for primary care and education provided by respiratory therapists during office visits.

Respiratory therapists working in physician offices perform many of the same acute care duties as hospital-based respiratory therapists. They also have the opportunity to advance their clinical skills. In particular, there is more opportunity for primary care. Physician extenders spend a large portion of their time providing patients with education. Patient education includes discussing their diseases, treatment techniques, and medications. They have more time to spend with the patients than the physicians do. Respiratory therapists often follow up with patients about their care. They become an important liaison between the patient and the physician. They may also be involved with the arrangement of home care services. They participate in negotiations with HMOs and insurance companies for providing care. They also provide certification of care.

Skills and Rewards of Respiratory Therapists Working as Physician Extenders

Respiratory therapists who wish to function as physician extenders should have excellent clinical competencies. They must have primary care skills. They also should have several years of experience in the acute care setting. They should possess strong educational skills. They need the ability to teach at all levels of education because a good portion of their time will involve educating patients and their families. Although physician extenders work under the authority of a physician, they enjoy a large degree of autonomy.

Respiratory therapists working as physician extenders can assume a variety of duties. Many of these duties overlap with other healthcare professionals. Licensure laws are nonrestrictive in most states. This means that scopes of practice for providing healthcare services are not restricted to any single healthcare profession. A respiratory therapist working as a physician extender may perform duties that include medical technology, radiological services, and nursing and physician assistant tasks. These duties are performed under the direction and authority of physicians. State laws regulating physicians, nurses, and other healthcare personnel will factor into what roles respiratory therapists can assume.

RESPIRATORY RECAP

Opportunities and Rewards of Respiratory Therapists as Physician Extenders

» Opportunity to advance skills by providing clinical services not provided as traditional therapists
» Large portion of time spent providing patients with education about their disease, treatment techniques, and medications
» Ability to make a greater or positive impact on the lives of patients

Respiratory therapists as physician extenders should feel comfortable working independently. They need good organizational skills to function in a busy medical practice. Above all, they need high levels of professionalism because they function as an extension of physicians.

Respiratory therapists who work as physician extenders enjoy the opportunity to expand their skills. They also see a chance to expand their profession as well. They report the ability to make a positive impact on the lives of patients as one of the best rewards of the job. One of the benefits of being a physician extender is the chance to spend more time with patients. Many respiratory therapists enjoy the added autonomy of working as a physician extender.

Industry

Many respiratory therapists are employed by different types of industry. Companies are now using respiratory therapists more than ever before. Jobs in industry include technological design, consulting, product development, and marketing and sales. Management, education, research, and medical writing are also industry-related jobs. Companies realize that respiratory therapists should be involved in the planning, design, and marketing of respiratory therapy equipment. These fields realize the importance and potential that respiratory therapists can have for their industries. They offer opportunities for the future growth of respiratory therapy.

Pharmaceutical and biotechnical corporations hire respiratory therapists to aid in product design and development, market development, marketing, education, research, technical writing, and sales. Respiratory therapists with strong backgrounds in healthcare, anatomy, physiology, and cardiopulmonary disease management can benefit these companies. Companies involve respiratory therapists in the market analysis of new or existing products. Marketing positions often involve sales. Travel is required with marketing and sales positions. The territories can cover several hundred miles, across several states. International travel may also be required.

Respiratory therapists in industry assess the market by communication with physicians, researchers, and respiratory therapists. They educate physicians and research scientists about the company's current products. They provide current research outcomes and studies. They interact with the medical community to determine the research necessary for a product and assist in the recruitment of research participants. Consultants often coordinate educational programs. They can present lectures at educational programs. In return, clinicians share their opinions on the need for future products.

When an industry finds a healthcare need, respiratory therapists work with engineers to design the product. They must design a product that meets the user's needs. It must also meet regulatory issues such as Food and Drug Administration (FDA) guidelines. Once the FDA approves a product, respiratory therapists often help with the marketing. Respiratory therapists provide the clinical expertise to the sales force. Respiratory therapists are important members of the sales force. They can provide technical education about the product and assist in the marketing of the product. Respiratory therapists also may be involved in contract negotiations with distributors and purchasing groups.

Skills and Rewards of Industry-Related Positions

Respiratory therapists who work in industry need strong backgrounds in the basic sciences. Their education should have an emphasis on anatomy, physiology, physics, and math. Industry consultants must know the geographic area they cover in terms of the experts in their field. They must have extensive knowledge of research methodologies and know the research performed on their products. They must also identify proposed research needs. Respiratory therapy industry consultants enjoy autonomy in their work. They must be self-directed and motivated. They should have strong organizational and prioritization skills. They also must have well-developed time management skills. They must be aware of the different environments posed by industry. The hours are usually long and irregular. Traveling often is required. Although there is often little patient contact, they need strong clinical backgrounds. They also need the ability to translate the knowledge they have gained from their clinical backgrounds into visions of the future.

RESPIRATORY RECAP

Opportunities and Rewards of Working in Industry

- » Looking at patient care from a different angle to improve healthcare for many
- » Assisting with the identification, development, marketing, and sales of new products that improve respiratory care and health
- » Directly contributing to the growth of the profession and others' professional development
- » Opportunity to travel and network with others
- » Rewards of using creative talents in innovative ways

Respiratory therapists involved in the design and development of technology find it rewarding to examine patient care from a different angle. These respiratory therapists enjoy the ability to make a difference in the lives of patients and fellow respiratory therapists. They also enjoy the prospect of making sure the products used are the best for the patient. They directly add to advances within the profession.

Research and Medical Writing

Most of the research reported today by respiratory therapists resulted from questions that came from their day-to-day practice. Respiratory therapists should be interested in research because it validates the care they provide. Research supports and promotes the growth of the profession.

Respiratory therapists interested in conducting research should start small. They can begin with their daily activities. What questions do respiratory therapists have concerning the outcomes or the cost-effectiveness of therapies? They should choose research in an area in which they have some clinical expertise. The prospects for performing research are greater in colleges, universities, and large teaching hospitals. Research can and has been performed at all levels of care. Managed care has influenced the demand for outcomes research and evidence-based medicine. Managed care often funds studies to promote cost-containment strategies.

Before undertaking a research project, the novice should find a mentor. The mentor should be someone who has experience in conducting and presenting research. Research mentors should be experienced with research techniques and publication. Even seasoned researchers benefit from contact with others who can provide constructive feedback, questions, insights, suggestions, and ideas. Experienced researchers often suggest that new researchers begin with an abstract presentation. These take less time and effort. Abstracts may be case reports, device evaluations, or original studies. Another research option is to write critical reviews or clinical papers for submission to peer-reviewed journals.

Most research conducted at this level does not need funding. If funding is needed, several sources are available. Often, industries will provide funding for limited or preliminary projects. In some cases, industry will fund projects with larger scope and budgets. Researchers should negotiate a contract before the project starts. The contract ensures that the corporation cannot withdraw funding if disappointed with the preliminary results. Other organizations, such as the American Association for Respiratory Care, the American Respiratory Care Foundation, and the American Lung Association, offer competitive grants and monetary awards to promote research.

There is a vast need for research proving the effectiveness of respiratory care. Research is needed to show the value of respiratory therapists in all aspects of the healthcare industry. Outcomes research to provide objective evidence of the value of respiratory therapists and the care they give is the best way to ensure continued growth of the profession.

Skills and Rewards of Research and Medical Writing

Many respiratory therapists feel they need advanced degrees to enter the research field. This is not always the case. However, a background in statistics is helpful. Research in all aspects of respiratory therapy is needed. The main requirement is a background in the area of your research. Research is time consuming. It can take months to years to conduct a study. You must review the literature, design a study, collect data, analyze findings, and publish. Respiratory therapists interested in research must be willing to make a time commitment. Research often means working on your own time.

RESPIRATORY RECAP

Opportunities and Rewards of Research and Medical Writing

- » The ability to demonstrate the value of respiratory therapists
- » The opportunity to show the effectiveness of respiratory therapists
- » Contributions to the growth and development of the profession
- » Personal and professional sense of achievement
- » Working in a variety of venues
- » New opportunities for patient education
- » Creating clinical pathways and protocols
- » Documenting outcomes measured by research

Respiratory therapists interested in conducting research must be self-motivated. They must be able to sustain and persevere throughout all phases of a study. Most respiratory therapists performing research are doing so either in conjunction with their full-time jobs or as independent efforts. Respiratory therapist researchers should also be able to withstand criticism and rejection. Research undergoes extensive peer review. The peer review process involves many degrees of criticism before publishing. Ideally, the criticism is constructive and detailed. It is not uncommon for an article to be rejected or to require several rewrites before it is published.

Researchers must be skilled writers because their work must be published in peer-reviewed journals in order to benefit anyone. Another avenue open to respiratory therapists is the field of medical writing. Medical writers are not the actual researchers of an original study. Respiratory therapists have broad backgrounds in cardiopulmonary anatomy and pathophysiology. This makes them ideal candidates for medical writing. Medical writers may write in a variety of venues, including journal articles, research articles, and textbooks. Medical writers not only write their own material but also assist authors in their writing or serve as editors. They also create and edit tables, graphs, and present statistical information.

Medical writers are needed to write and edit information presented at professional conferences, such as pamphlets, brochures, slides, and handouts. Medical writers also serve in the process of obtaining FDA approval of drugs. Before the FDA approves a drug, extensive documentation must be presented. Medical writers are charged with the task of completing the application, which requires extensive writing skills. Managed care has created new opportunities for medical writers to educate patients, create clinical pathways, and document outcomes. These outcomes are measured by research.

Respiratory therapists interested in medical writing need a good background in the English language and its rules. A master's degree is preferred. Medical writers must be able to work alone. Computer skills are necessary. Respiratory therapists who are interested in medical writing should contact the American Medical Writers Association (AMWA), which offers certification programs and education.

KEY POINTS

- Numerous forces are affecting healthcare and healthcare reform in the United States.
- Healthcare costs continue to escalate.
- Documentation of improvements in the quality, access, or effectiveness of healthcare is inadequate.
- This past decade has witnessed unprecedented change in healthcare in the United States.
- Managed care evolved to put constant pressure on healthcare providers to restrain healthcare costs and control utilization.
- Managed care includes HMOs and PPOs.
- Healthcare reform has centered around four main issues: decreasing costs, improving quality, using measurable outcomes for effectiveness, and improving resource allocation.
- Improving resource allocation involves reductions in healthcare costs and utilization.
- The ultimate goal of healthcare reform is to improve the way healthcare resources are used.
- The goal is for more people to receive better healthcare at the least possible cost.
- Healthcare trends include a declining ability of healthcare providers to deliver uncompensated care, a declining proportion of people with private insurance, continued growth in the total number of uninsured people, continued increase in the rate of inflation in healthcare costs, and budget reductions in Medicare and Medicaid.
- The profession must provide the appropriate education to prepare respiratory therapists for the current healthcare markets.
- Current healthcare markets include nontraditional roles and new opportunities for respiratory therapists.
- New opportunities include diagnostics, home healthcare, subacute care, disease management and health promotion, case management, industry, research, and medical writing.
- The role of the respiratory therapist as physician extender is expanding in acute care, physician practices, and nontraditional healthcare settings.
- Respiratory therapists will continue to play a major role in healthcare and in the changes occurring in healthcare delivery.

REFERENCES

1. Kacmarek RM, Barnes TA, Walton JR. Creating a vision for respiratory care in 2015 and beyond. *Respir Care.* 2009;54:375–388.
2. Centers for Medicare and Medicaid Services. 2006 Medicare state enrollment. Available at: http://www.cms.hhs.gov/MedicareEnRpts/Downloads/06All.pdf. Accessed March 24, 2009.
3. Ward JJ, Hemholtz HF. Roots of the respiratory care profession. In: Burton GG, Hodgins JE, Ward JJ, eds. *Respiratory Care: A Guide to Clinical Practice.* 4th ed. Philadelphia: Lippincott Williams & Wilkins; 1997.
4. American Association for Respiratory Care. *Lewin Group Report: Respiratory Care Practitioners in an Evolving Health Care Environment.* Dallas, TX: AARC; 1999.
5. Centers for Medicare and Medicaid Services. 2006 Medicare managed care enrollment report: summary statistics as of June 30, 2006. Available at: http://www.cms.hhs.gov/MedicaidDataSourcesGenInfo/Downloads/mmcer06.pdf. Accessed March 24, 2009.
6. Johnson TD. Census Bureau: number of U.S. uninsured rises to 47 million Americans are uninsured: almost 5 percent increase since 2005. *Nations Health.* 2007;37(8).
7. National Center for Health Statistics. *Health, United States, 2007 with Chart Book on Trends in the Health of Americans.* Hyattsville, MD: U.S. Department of Health and Human Services; 2007. Available at: http://www.cdc.gov/nchs/data/hus/hus07.pdf. Accessed March 25, 2009.
8. Department of Health and Human Services. Smoking and tobacco use: fast facts. Available at: http://www.cdc.gov/tobacco/data_statistics/fact_sheets/fast_facts/index.htm#toll. Accessed March 26, 2009.
9. U.S. Department of Health and Human Services, National Institutes of Health. COPD. Available at: http://www.copd-international.com/library/statistics.htm. Accessed March 26, 2009.
10. Kung HC, Hoyert DL, Xu J, Murphy SL. Deaths: final data for 2005. *Natl Vital Stat.* 2008;56(10).
11. U.S. Census Bureau. *Population Projections of the United States by Age, Sex, Race and Hispanic Origin: 1995–2050.* U.S. Bureau of the Census, Current Population Reports P25-1130. Washington, DC: U.S. Government Printing Office; 1999. Available at: http://www.census.gov/prod/1/pop/p25-1130. Accessed March 28, 2009.
12. Peters RW. Obstructive sleep apnea and cardiovascular disease. *Chest.* 2005;127:1–3.

13. Flowers J. The futures of respiratory care are powered by cost pressures, new technologies and consumer demands. RT Magazine.com. http://www.rtmagazine.com/issues/articles/2006-07_05.asp. Accessed March 30, 2009.
14. Merendino D, Wissing DR. New roles for respiratory therapists: expanding the scope of practice. *Respir Care Clin North Am.* 2005;11:543–555.
15. Shelledy DC, Wiezalis CP. Education and credentialing in respiratory care: where are we and where should we be headed? *Respir Care Clin North Am.* 2005;11:517–530.
16. Douce FH. Bachelor of science degree education programs: organization, structure, and curriculum. *Respir Care Clin North Am.* 2005;11:401–415.
17. Ari A, Goodfellow LT, Rau JL. Characteristics of a successful respiratory therapy education program. *Respir Care Clin North Am.* 2005;11:371–381.
18. PricewaterhouseCoopers' Health Research Institute. *HealthCast 2020: Creating a Sustainable Future.* 2005. Available at: http://www.pwc.com/us/en/healthcast/past-reports.jhtml. Accessed March 29, 2009.
19. Mishoe SC. Critical thinking in respiratory care practice: a qualitative research study. *Respir Care.* 2004;48:500–516.
20. Cullen DL, Sullivan JM, Bartel RE, et al. *Year 2001: Delineating the Educational Direction for the Future Respiratory Care Practitioner. Proceedings of a National Consensus Conference on Respiratory Care Education.* Dallas, TX: American Association for Respiratory Care; 1992.
21. U.S. Department of Health and Human Services. *Report of the National Commission on Allied Health.* Rockville, MD: U.S. Government Printing Office; 1995.
22. O'Neil EH, Pew Health Professions Commission. *Recreating Health Professional Practice for a New Century.* San Francisco: Pew Health Professions Commission; December 1998.
23. Mishoe SC, MacIntyre NR. Expanding professional roles for respiratory care practitioners. *Respir Care.* 1997;42:71–85.
24. Weilacher R. History of the respiratory therapy profession. In: Hess D, MacIntyre N, Mishoe SC, et al., eds. *Respiratory Care: Principles and Practice.* St. Louis, MO: Harcourt Health Science; 2001.
25. Gaebler G. History of the respiratory therapy professional organizations. In: Hess D, MacIntyre N, Mishoe SC, et al., eds. *Respiratory Care: Principles and Practice.* St. Louis, MO: Harcourt Health Science; 2001.
26. National Board for Respiratory Care. Sleep Disorders Specialty Exam. 2008. Available at: https://www.nbrc.org/Examinations/SDS/tabid/92/Default.aspx. Accessed June 5, 2009.
27. Song WS, Mullon J, Regan NA, Roth BJ. Instruction of hospitalized patients by respiratory therapists on metered-dose inhaler use leads to decrease in patient errors. *Respir Care.* 2005;50:1040–1045.
28. Chopra N, Oprescu N, Fask A, Oppenheimer J. Does introduction of new "easy to use" inhalational devices improve medical personnel's knowledge of their proper use? *Ann Allergy Asthma Immunol.* 2002;88:395–400.
29. Kollef MH, Shapiro SD, Clinkscale D, et al. The effects of respiratory therapist-initiated treatment protocols on patient outcomes and resource utilization. *Chest.* 2000;117:467–475.
30. Cheek M, Tumlinson A, Blum J. *Keeping Pace: Trends, Options and Opportunities in Long Term Care.* Washington, DC: American Health Care Association; 2005.
31. National Association of Subacute/Post Acute Care. *NASPAC Frequently Asked Questions.* Washington, DC: National Association of Subacute/Post Acute Care; 2006.
32. Muse and Associates. Executive summary. In: *A Comparison of Medicare Nursing Home Residents Who Receive Services from a Respiratory Therapist with Those Who Did Not.* Washington, DC: Muse and Associates; 1999:1–3.
33. Heuer AJ, Scanlan CL. Respiratory care in alternative settings. In: Wilkins RL, Stoller JK, Kacmarek RM, eds. *Egan's Fundamentals of Respiratory Care.* St. Louis, MO: Mosby; 2009:1255–1285.

CHAPTER 58

Critical Thinking in Respiratory Care

Shelley C. Mishoe

OUTLINE

OBJECTIVES

1. Develop a personal definition of critical thinking.
2. List, define, and give examples of the essential skills for critical thinking in respiratory care practice.
3. Describe abilities and characteristics of critical thinkers.
4. Describe problem-based learning (PBL).
5. Compare traditional teaching methods and PBL for the teaching of critical thinking.
6. Explain why self-directed and lifelong learning is essential for respiratory therapists.
7. Discuss ways to facilitate critical thinking in respiratory care practice.

KEY TERMS

analytical paradigm
anticipating
communicating
critical thinking
decision making
negotiating
prioritizing
problem-based learning (PBL)
reflecting
troubleshooting

INTRODUCTION

Respiratory therapists often hear that they must be critical thinkers and have critical thinking skills. Respiratory therapists read articles and reports that highlight the importance of critical thinking. Licensing and accrediting agencies emphasize critical thinking and problem solving. Patients ask practical questions that challenge conventional practices. How does critical thinking relate to job performance? What is the importance? What is the personal significance? Processing information and making decisions are at the core of clinical practice. Respiratory therapists need to develop essential critical thinking skills and traits to be effective in practice. By the end of this chapter, you should be able to derive your own personal definition of critical thinking. Your definition should be unique to a clinical setting and applicable to the many situations you encounter in respiratory care practice.

What Is Critical Thinking, and Why Is It Important for Respiratory Therapists?

The respiratory care profession emphasizes the need to prepare practitioners who can gather information and make appropriate clinical decisions using critical thinking. This emphasis can be seen in the National Board for Respiratory Care (NBRC) credentialing examinations for the advanced respiratory care practitioner, the registered respiratory therapist (RRT). It is evident in the outcome-oriented essentials for respiratory therapy educational programs accredited by the Commission for Accreditation of Respiratory Care (CoARC). The NBRC clinical simulation examinations are examples of commercially available critical thinking assessment tools that are domain specific.[1]

Additional emphasis on the need to prepare respiratory care practitioners with developed critical thinking skills has been described in a Delphi study by the American Association for Respiratory Care (AARC),[2] the AARC Board of Directors' 2001 report on the respiratory care practitioner,[3] the proceedings of the AARC's education consensus conferences,[4] and the AARC's Task Force 2015 and Beyond.[5] The goal of the latest task force was to analyze the future roles of respiratory therapists. The task force looked specifically at new responsibilities as well as evolving changes in healthcare, including rising costs and an aging population. Recent trends include a focus on chronic disease management, rapid changes in technology, and increased involvement by consumers. The 2015 task force agreed that evidence-based medicine will gain in importance and that biomedical inventions will mandate more "sophistication" of respiratory therapists. Clearly, it is important to prepare and develop respiratory care practitioners with critical thinking skills for the present and the future.

To be effective on the healthcare team, respiratory therapists need more than knowledge. Because of the dynamic and expanding nature of medical knowledge, the average professional cannot rely on information gained in school. Healthcare professionals must have the ability to think independently and to adapt to changes in practice. They must continuously learn new approaches to patient care. Mastering the thinking skills for processing both old and new knowledge is the most important requirement for today's respiratory therapist. Respiratory therapists must be critical thinkers who are self-directed, lifelong learners. Respiratory therapists who are critical thinkers will have a vital role in healthcare that extends from the present into the future.

Critical thinking merges principles of logical reasoning, problem solving, and reflection.[6] Complex thinking involves various intellectual activities that encompass creative and critical aspects. The creative aspect of thinking allows the origin of ideas and alternatives. The critical aspect enables the testing and evaluation of the products of creative thinking. Judgment, decision making, scientific reasoning, and lifelong learning are highly related. These terms are often used synonymously to mean critical thinking. The term *critical thinking* has become widely and loosely used, with interpretations that are based on personal agendas, purposes, beliefs, biases, and perspectives. One leading critical thinking expert argues that one should not put too much emphasis on any particular definition because each has limitations.[7] **Table 58–1** shows common definitions of critical thinking.

TABLE 58–1 Common Definitions of Critical Thinking

Definition	Source (Ref. No.)
"political awareness and personal development"	Brookfield, 2004 (19)
"cognitive problem solving"	Dressel & Mayhew, 1954 (38)
"effective thinking" to encompass the relationships among thinking skills, the dispositions to think and discipline content	Eljamal et al., 1998 (39)
"logical reasoning"	Hallet, 1984 (40)
"rational and purposeful attempt to use thought to move toward a future goal"	Halpern, 2003 (41)
"discipline-specific knowledge, skills and attitudes to solve real problems"	McPeck, 1990 (42)
"logical reasoning, problem solving and reflection"	Mishoe, 2003 (9)
"an understanding of and an ability to formulate, analyze, and assess the elements of thought"	Paul & Elder, 2008 (37)

The Essential Skills for Critical Thinking in Practice

The process of critical thinking involves numerous thoughts and activities, each of which usually has many steps. The size and complexity of the events that trigger critical thinking determine the direction and extent of activities. Research regarding critical thinking has been conducted mainly with college students. Therefore, it is not surprising that critical thinking is most often associated with intellectual abilities. However, focusing on cognitive abilities does not fully grasp the ways in which practitioners think and behave. Also, the extent to which critical thinking in an academic setting transfers to professional practice is unclear. Although the intellectual aspects are essential, there is also a practical aspect to critical thinking.

What we know about critical thinking in healthcare comes primarily from studies in medicine and nursing.

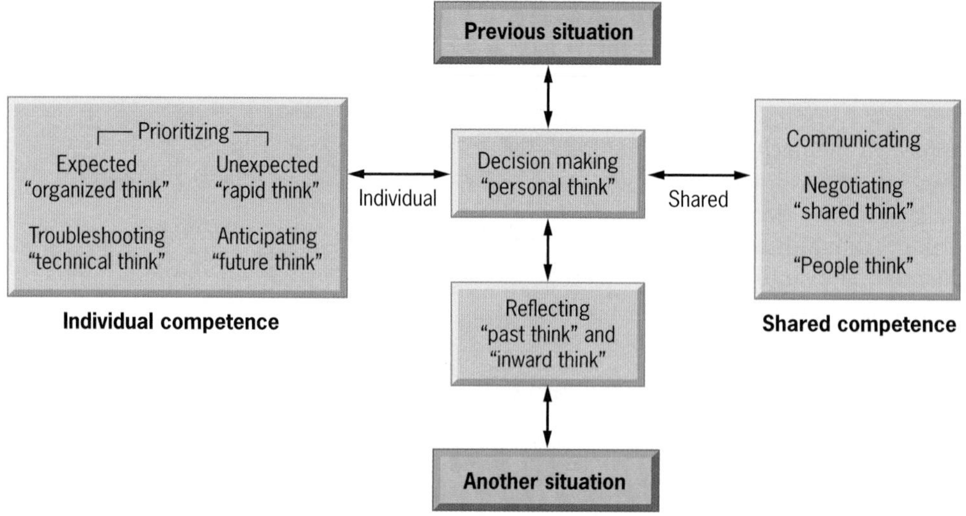

FIGURE 58–1 Interrelationship of the skills for critical thinking in practice. From Mishoe SC, Martin S. Critical thinking in the laboratory. *Learning Laboratorian Series*. 1994;6(4):1–63. Reprinted with permission from the American Association of Bioanalysts.

However, one study in respiratory care describes the actual critical thinking skills and traits that are important to respiratory care practice. The skills needed for critical thinking in respiratory care practice include prioritizing, anticipating, troubleshooting, communicating, negotiating, decision making, and reflecting.[8–10] This section describes these skills, and **Figure 58–1** shows the interrelationship among these skills, the individual, and other healthcare professionals.

Prioritizing

Prioritizing is the ability to arrange work according to importance. Prioritizing may be defined as "organized think" and "rapid think."[8–10] The work that is already scheduled or expected requires "organized think"; the unexpected or emergency work requires "rapid think." Respiratory therapists perform many routine tasks, but they must also respond to emergencies. Both types of work cause conflicting demands. These demands require respiratory therapists to quickly make judgments on the importance of tasks and situations. After an initial judgment has been made, adjustments must be performed. The effective therapist must accommodate the highest priority.

> **RESPIRATORY RECAP**
>
> **Critical Thinking Skills**
> » Prioritizing
> » Anticipating
> » Troubleshooting
> » Communicating
> » Negotiating
> » Decision making
> » Reflecting

In a busy intensive care unit, a respiratory therapist may be drawing an arterial blood gas sample on a patient receiving mechanical ventilation. At the same time, a nearby patient may suddenly go into respiratory arrest, requiring intubation. The respiratory therapist must quickly seek help from another team member, who should either intubate the arrested patient or complete the arterial blood gas measurement. This adjustment allows the respiratory therapist to provide optimal patient care. Additional work may be required for the resuscitation and stabilization of the patient. At the same time, the respiratory therapist's pager may indicate that a patient is having a severe asthma attack in the emergency department (ED). A few minutes later, another patient's computed tomographic scan is complete, and the respiratory therapist is notified that the patient can be transported back to the intensive care unit. During this time, multiple trauma patients from a car accident also may arrive in the ED. This respiratory therapist must quickly prioritize responsibilities and tasks so that all these patients receive optimal care. The respiratory therapist must also communicate quickly and effectively with others, including nurses, physicians, and other respiratory therapists. These other people must either assist or be aware of any delays in patient care. Patient lives may depend on the ability of the respiratory therapist to prioritize work.

Anticipating

Anticipating involves the ability to think ahead and envision possible problems. Anticipating is "future think."[8–10] This activity pertains to the continuous and total approach to resolving a situation. It includes the ability to see the big picture. Anticipating differs from prioritizing in that the emphasis in prioritization is to respond quickly to a problem, whereas anticipation seeks to avoid a problem. However, both skills are interrelated. The ability to anticipate influences the therapist's ability to prioritize. Respiratory therapists are better able to prioritize and respond appropriately when they are also able to anticipate what might happen. What might happen is often a result of actions or decisions. On the other hand, the ability to prioritize allows the therapists to use their time more effectively. Consequently, respiratory therapists can have greater opportunity to avoid problems through anticipation.

Anticipating occurs when respiratory therapists make some modification in patient care; are expecting a new patient or facing a new situation; plan ahead for the equipment needs and actions they will take; prepare what they intend to discuss with physicians; and when they notice subtle changes in their patients that might indicate a problem. Anticipating involves the respiratory therapist's ability to continuously and holistically assess the patients, the data, the technology, and the situation to prevent problems and come up with early solutions.

Anticipating requires global or gestalt thinking, which aims at having a grasp of the whole situation. Then, the therapist can effectively come up with solutions to prevent problems. Students can develop the skill of anticipating by working through "what if" types of questions, especially during clinical rotations.

Troubleshooting

Respiratory care is a highly technical healthcare profession. At the same time, respiratory care requires significant interaction with patients and other healthcare providers. Respiratory therapists are intimately involved in patient care diagnostics, therapeutics, and education. Therefore, respiratory care can be described as "high tech" and also "high touch." The technical aspects of respiratory care require the critical thinking skill of troubleshooting.

Troubleshooting involves the ability to locate, correct, and process technical problems. Troubleshooting is "technical think."[8–10] Respiratory therapists should be able to introduce new equipment and methodologies. They need to be able to modify and adapt new technology for particular needs and situations. Respiratory therapists must identify and correct equipment malfunctions or breakdowns. Logical thinking and problem solving are integral components of troubleshooting. Respiratory therapists are assisted in this process by many resources, including their training, manufacturers' manuals, online technical assistance, and others who are familiar with the equipment.

Troubleshooting may range from simple (Is the machine turned on?) to complex (Why does an error message continue after proper corrective steps have been taken?). Respiratory therapists are expected to properly maintain and use the equipment they require for therapy and diagnostics. Proper maintenance and quality controls (part of anticipating) help to avoid an equipment malfunction. Developing troubleshooting skills is an important part of respiratory therapy students' training. However, students should not rely solely on their instructors. Students must gain independent skills. They must learn how to figure out and use resources to troubleshoot technology. For example, students should be encouraged to use instruction manuals and computer help menus. They need to figure out technological problems whenever possible. Rather than rely on the instructor to solve equipment problems during labs or clinical rotations, independent troubleshooting should be practiced.

Communicating

The reflective dimension includes the communicative aspect of critical thinking that guides beliefs, decisions, and actions within a social context. Critical thinking in practice is dependent on communications with others as a primary means for giving and receiving information needed for patient care. **Communicating** is "people think."[8–10]

Cognitive skills are important. However, information gathering is not merely selecting data from a list of possibilities as presented on a clinical simulation exam. Respiratory therapists must be able to communicate effectively to gather the appropriate information to interpret, analyze, evaluate, infer, judge, or explain. If a respiratory therapist cannot communicate effectively, he or she will be unable to think critically during a situation in clinical practice. Critical thinking in practice is not likely unless the person is able to access and share information with others.

Effective communication is dependent on working relationships. Therefore, critical thinking in practice not only involves the skill of communicating, but is also affected by personal traits.[8] The personal traits that facilitate critical thinking are discussed in more detail later in this chapter.

Respiratory therapists need to be able to share information with members of the healthcare team. If respiratory therapists cannot properly communicate patient information, care may be limited or even jeopardized. Respiratory therapists may obtain abnormal or conflicting laboratory results. This may indicate the need to speak with a physician or nurse to inquire about the patient's clinical status. If respiratory therapists cannot communicate competently, they will be unable to think critically in actual practice.

The goal in communicating is to obtain more information or to give others information. If insufficient information is due to a lack of communication, the respiratory therapist may not be able to interpret, analyze, evaluate, infer, judge, or explain. For example, a respiratory therapist may be able to critically analyze laboratory data or troubleshoot technical errors. If that individual cannot communicate, however, he or she cannot perform critical thinking in actual practice because prompt access to needed information will be missing. This situation is similar to a person who tries to work a puzzle without all the pieces.

> **RESPIRATORY RECAP**
>
> **The Importance of Communication**
>
> » Respiratory therapists must be able to communicate effectively to gather the appropriate information to interpret, analyze, evaluate, infer, judge, or explain. If a respiratory therapist cannot communicate effectively, he or she will be unable to think critically during a specific situation in clinical practice.

Communicating in practice is practitioner specific and situation specific.[8,9] Communication style, duration, and frequency vary greatly depending on the key players involved. Key players include other therapists, physicians, nurses, patients, and family members. Communication is essential to educate patients and their families, reassure or explain care to patients, function as part of the broader healthcare team, and mentor respiratory therapy students and other new clinicians. Communication is such an important aspect of practice that an entire chapter is devoted to this topic (see Chapter 60).

Negotiating

Critical thinking in practice also requires respiratory therapists to be able to negotiate regarding patient care. This involves negotiating medical orders and responsibilities. **Negotiating** is "initiating discussion in an attempt to influence others." *Negotiating* is an umbrella term that can encompass teamwork, using your influence, making recommendations, accepting verbal orders, and contacting physicians to discuss a patient. Practitioners must negotiate to do what they believe is best in a given situation. Negotiating is also involved in patient care when interacting with patients and their families.

Negotiating does not necessarily mean conflict, confrontation, or difficulty. Negotiating takes into account the diversity of roles and opinions that exist in the real world. It also includes the ways professionals must interact to maximize efforts for better patient care outcomes. Negotiating is "shared think."[8–10]

Negotiating patient care responsibilities and medical orders is essential to collectively solve problems. If respiratory therapists are unable to negotiate, then there will be limited access to the therapists' professional expertise and cognitive critical thinking skills. Respiratory therapists must be skilled negotiators to participate in decision making and influence medical orders. This is most important in the management of respiratory care.

There is an intimate relationship between the skills of communicating and negotiating. Although negotiating requires communication skills, all communicating is not negotiating. Negotiating differs from communicating in that the intent is to impart information and ask questions to influence others' decisions and actions. Cognitive performance on a clinical simulation exam requires respiratory therapists to make the "right" clinical decision after assessing appropriate data. However, in practice respiratory therapists must negotiate power through the medical order. This permits the opportunity to do what they believe is right or best for the patient under specific circumstances. To negotiate effectively, respiratory therapists need good communication skills and the ability to make judgments.[8–10] They must also be able to explain how they came to their conclusions and explain their suggestions.

> **RESPIRATORY RECAP**
>
> **Importance of Negotiation**
>
> » Negotiating does not mean conflict. Negotiating is an umbrella term that can include teamwork, using your influence, making recommendations, and discussing verbal orders.
>
> » Respiratory therapists must be skilled negotiators to participate in decision making and influence patient care medical orders for respiratory care. If the respiratory therapist is unable to negotiate, there will be limited access to that therapist's expertise.

Successful negotiators often phrase their suggestions as questions. They make indirect implications and inferences about possible alternative actions.[9] The ability to effectively communicate enhance therapists' opportunities to negotiate patient care decisions. Through negotiations, respiratory therapists can expand their opportunities for improving patient care based on their unique expertise.

The criteria for negotiating in respiratory care practice include the extent to which a particular solution is evident; the need to clarify medical orders or obtain assistance; the particular physician or physician service; the seriousness of the patient's problem; whether there is a cardiopulmonary problem; the therapist's feelings at the time; and the therapist's confidence in his or her abilities.[9] Physicians have the final authority for medical orders and decisions.

Respiratory therapists should understand their responsibility to make appropriate recommendations. However, they should also realize their limitations. Physician support, teamwork, critical thinking, and professionalism are essential for effective respiratory care practice.[10,11] Practitioners should not shy away from negotiating. They must learn how to negotiate. Students and novices can develop their communication and negotiation skills through direct observation and interaction with effective models.

Decision Making

Decision making is the ability to reach a conclusion. Decision making is "personal think."[8–10] Respiratory therapists often have the opportunity to participate in clinical decision making. Respiratory therapists can make decisions about their own work flow, work patterns, and work space by practicing three of the previously described aspects of critical thinking.

The terms *reasoning, problem solving, decision making,* and *critical thinking* are closely related. The skills and tasks involved overlap.[11–16] Some authors claim that "making a decision is the end point of using critical thinking and scientific reasoning in problem resolution."[15] This view is acceptable if critical thinking is conceived as solely cognitive activity. However, clinical practice also involves emotive, practical, and social aspects of critical thinking. Consequently, critical thinking can be described in terms of skills, abilities, and traits. These skills and traits are in addition to, and as a result of, cognitive skills.

The development of cognitive skills can enhance clinical reasoning for effective decision making. Reasoning involves the review of evidence against, as well as in favor of, a position. Inaccurate decision making can result when conflicting evidence is discounted. Inaccurate decision making also occurs when disconfirming evidence is ignored. When biases determine explanations, they can also limit decision making. Studies of decision making demonstrate that physicians who are inaccurate with medical diagnoses tend to discount evidence that contradicts a favored hypothesis.[14,15]

Physicians who make accurate medical assessments pay attention to information that contradicts as well as supports a diagnosis. Furthermore, practitioners should be able to recognize and avoid fallacies (errors or mistakes in thinking). For example, the degree to which one values an outcome can be confused with the probability that it will occur.[15] Avoiding formal and informal fallacies can enhance clinical reasoning and decision making in clinical practice.

When respiratory therapists seek input from other healthcare professionals, the process can result in conflicting evidence, recognition of biases, and multiple alternatives. Expert respiratory therapists should be able to appreciate multiple perspectives. They must be willing to reconsider when presented with conflicting alternatives. These traits contribute to improved clinical reasoning and decision making because the therapist can avoid fallacies and improve reasoning abilities.

Research suggests that cognitive skills can be enhanced. Improving cognitive skills can result in improved decision making. Clinical decision making can be improved by increasing content and procedural knowledge, as well as clear thinking skills. Clinicians can benefit from improved judgmental processes using scientific reasoning and clear thinking skills. People have difficulty integrating diverse sources of information. Furthermore, the fact that experts may make the same mistakes as novices when confronting unfamiliar problems suggests the need for cognitive skills and metacognitive strategies.

Developing critical thinking in respiratory therapy students has been proposed as a method for improving clinical decision making. At least two studies demonstrate that there is a relationship between general critical thinking and decision making in respiratory care; these studies compared data from the Watson Glaser Critical Thinking Appraisal (WGCTA, Psychological Corporation, San Antonio, Tex.) and the Clinical Simulation Self Assessment Examinations (CSSAE, developed by the National Board for Respiratory Care) to measure decision making.[16,17] Respiratory therapy students with developed critical thinking made better clinical decisions on clinical simulations.

In practice, respiratory therapists must be able to provide reasons when sharing decision making. This is particularly important when negotiating medical orders. Improved cognitive skills can facilitate critical thinking. However, cognitive skills alone are insufficient for critical thinking. To be effective in practice, respiratory therapists also must have practical skills. They must be able to communicate and negotiate effectively. Furthermore, respiratory therapists must reflect on their decisions, beliefs, and actions to further develop critical thinking skills and traits.

Reflecting

Reflecting is the ability to think about thinking. It is a form of metacognition. Reflecting invites the exploration of assumptions, opinions, biases, and decisions. Reflecting may be considered introspective or "inward think."[8–10] If retrospective thinking is considered as part of reflecting, it becomes "past think."[8–10] Respiratory therapists may reflect on their work, patients, decisions, and profession. Reflection helps respiratory therapists to learn from previous mistakes and problems. Reflection helps therapists to gain satisfaction from their work and to handle the regret caused by errors in judgment. It helps therapists to understand their contribution to healthcare and their profession.

Reflection changes as respiratory therapists grow in their careers and assume different roles and responsibilities.[9] As respiratory therapists become more experienced, they make fewer errors. They begin to reflect more on the wider context of their profession and healthcare. One of the most profound outcomes of reflection is that practitioners recognize the existence of multiple perspectives. They begin to understand that there are gray areas of decision making. They can recognize the many levels of interpretations. In other words, there is usually more than one correct translation of reality. Therefore, reflection is important for respiratory therapists to develop the disposition of a critical thinker, which is important for the implementation of critical thinking in practice.

Abilities and Characteristics of Critical Thinkers

Researchers have explored the relationships between thinking skills, the disposition to think, and the discipline content. Not only do critical thinkers have certain abilities, but also they show distinct characteristics. No matter which definition of critical thinking is used, certain common attributes emerge. These attributes help distinguish the critical from the uncritical thinker. The critical thinker has acquired the ability to examine, command, and perfect the elements of thought.[8] The critical thinker has an understanding of and an ability to formulate, analyze, and assess the elements of thought as shown in **Box 58–1**. The uncritical thinker, however, is usually perceived as unclear, imprecise, vague, shallow, illogical, unreflective, superficial, inconsistent, inaccurate, or trivial.[7,18–20]

> **RESPIRATORY RECAP**
>
> **Characteristics of Critical Thinkers**
>
> » Inquisitive
> » Alert
> » Well informed
> » Open-minded
> » Honest
> » Flexible
> » Reasoned

Critical thinkers also show common qualities. These are called affective traits, characteristics, or dispositions.[1,18] The critical thinker is characterized as someone who has a general approach to living that includes inquisitiveness and being well informed. Critical thinkers are alert to opportunities to use critical thinking. They trust in the process of reasoning inquiry. They have

BOX 58–1

Affective and Cognitive Strategies That Promote Critical Thinking for Effective Problem Solving

Refining generalizations and avoiding oversimplifications
Comparing analogous situations
Evaluating credibility of sources and information
Generating solutions
Comparing and contrasting ideals with actual practice
Noting similarities and differences
Examining or evaluating assumptions
Distinguishing relevant from irrelevant facts
Making plausible inferences, predictions, and interpretations
Recognizing contradictions
Exploring consequences and implications
Giving reasons and evaluating evidence and alleged facts
Considering multiple perspectives
Suspending judgment
Drawing conclusions
Making a decision and/or taking an action
Reflecting on a decision or action

self-confidence in their ability to reason. Critical thinkers are open-minded and flexible. They understand others' opinions. They are fair-minded and honest. Critical thinkers are prudent in suspending judgment and are willing to reconsider. These traits or dispositions can be taught, learned, and continuously developed.

In the healthcare professions, a study of expert respiratory therapists revealed the following traits related to critical thinking in practice: willingness to reconsider; appreciation of multiple perspectives; willingness to challenge someone else regardless of the power structures; understanding of how other therapists' behavior affects them and their profession; responsibility for their own learning and understanding; and openness to continuing change in their personal and professional lives.[8,9] These traits were evident in a sample of expert respiratory therapists who were nominated by their peers and supervisors as displaying critical thinking. This sample of expert respiratory therapists displayed the characteristics of critical thinkers as described in the literature.

No matter the profession, a broad listing of characteristics seems to indicate that there are differing degrees of critical thinking. Most adults possess some of the attributes, qualities, and abilities of critical thinkers.[18–21] Respiratory therapists are challenged to foster development of their own critical thinking skills and the dispositions to be critical thinkers in their personal and professional lives.

Teaching Critical Thinking

Learning critical thinking should be fundamental to the educational experience of every respiratory therapist.[6,22–24] The teaching of critical thinking may occur in a variety of educational settings. In recent years, critical thinking has been officially recognized. Critical thinking may be included as part of a formal curriculum program. New graduates may have had some training in using critical thinking skills. Some students may have heard the term *critical thinking* but may have had no opportunities to apply and practice these skills. Critical thinking skills can be enhanced if they are incorporated as part of an educational program. The setting may be a technical school or college, undergraduate or graduate program, or in-service or continuing education. Faculty shares the responsibility for developing students' thinking skills and cultivating the dispositions to use them.

Professions undergo rapid and perpetual change. Textbooks can be outdated before they are published. Traditional curricula have emphasized factual knowledge and rote skills, not thinking and reasoning skills. Practitioners emerge from educational programs and may not be prepared to handle the day-to-day problems of their profession. Handling situations effectively and safely is more important than the ability to state some facts. Respiratory therapists need critical thinking skills and traits. They need to apply these across the many settings where respiratory care

RESPIRATORY RECAP

Characteristics of Traditional Teaching Methods

- » The instructor retains control over students' learning by using learning objectives and lectures to convey scientific knowledge derived from research, task analysis, and expert opinion.
- » Traditional education places students in passive roles, with the emphasis being on teaching rather than learning.

is practiced today. The context in which the respiratory therapist works greatly influences the opportunities for critical thinking.[25] Gradually, the goals of respiratory care education have been shifting from teaching "what to think" to teaching "how to think."

Traditional Teaching Methods

In the past, educational programs were designed to convey scientific and medical knowledge from research. Accomplishment of specific learning objectives was the focus. This traditional method of teaching is often called the **analytical paradigm**.

In the analytical paradigm, the instructor retains control over the learning process. This includes setting objectives, delivering content, and determining evaluation. Learners remain in passive roles. They are assumed to be receptive to new information. Educational experiences are highly structured. The dominant instructional strategy is the lecture method. Coursework is organized according to competencies. Course content is based on research, expert opinion, and task analysis.

The Role of Faculty in Traditional Curricula

Traditional education places more emphasis on faculty teaching than on student learning. Faculty assumes the major responsibility for determining the content, sequence, pace, emphasis, and evaluation of students' learning. Some faculty may rely too heavily on textbook sources and lecture notes, even though the information may be dated or unnecessarily biased. Controversial aspects of practice are not usually discussed. Sometimes the teacher might mention that the topic is "controversial" or "under investigation." Some instructors may discourage questions from students or even refuse to answer questions. They may find questions distracting to the lecture.

The traditional approach perpetuates the assumption that there is one correct answer and implies that the teacher is the expert. Naturally, the expert has all of the answers. Of course, in actual practice there are usually multiple approaches to patient care. There are numerous possibilities to address regarding what is best for each patient. It is rare in healthcare today that any one person has all the answers. Faculty use of lectures does little to give students a role model. It does not give experience with the skills and traits needed for professional practice.

In healthcare today, the team approach is emphasized and required. The team approach gives patients the benefits of the collective expertise of specialists in medicine and the other healthcare disciplines.

The Role of Students in Traditional Curricula

Students have become accustomed to passive roles. They sit passively while the teacher lectures to convey medical knowledge. In traditional education, the role of students is to listen to lectures. Students take notes and use the learning materials required by the teacher. Students memorize facts to regurgitate on tests. Although students may have been rewarded with passing grades, they may actually understand little about the subject. Generally, students taught by the lecture method cannot apply their knowledge to solve problems or make decisions. Little of the classroom teaching is actually learned by the student. Later, students cannot apply what they learned to the clinical setting.

Students trained by the analytical model surrender their own responsibility for learning to the "expert teacher." Consequently, students are unable to grasp their discipline as a whole.[26] They also do not fully understand their role in practice.

Traditional teaching does not expect students to research topics of interest. It does not ask them to independently review areas of weakness. Furthermore, students do not bring up topics for discussion. They do not bring up related clinical cases or something relevant that they previously learned. The traditional method does not allow much deviation from the lesson plan.

Evaluation of Students in Traditional Curricula

Students have been rewarded for demonstrating their ability to recall factual knowledge on course examinations. Little attention has been placed on the development and assessment of students' reasoning and problem-solving skills. Communication and other professional skills and attitudes may not be addressed at all. There may not be adequate evaluation of the students' professional development.

Traditional evaluation methods perpetuated the notion that there is always a "right answer." Such a view suggests that making good grades on course exams is sufficient. However, it is a tremendous leap to assume that because someone knows information, they will perform well on the job. Yet surprisingly, that assumption is often found with traditional curricula.

Traditional teaching may also incorporate laboratory and clinical experiences to coincide with lecture-based courses. In these types of courses, students have more active roles. However, even then the learning environment is structured. The emphasis is often placed on acquisition of respiratory therapy content and psychomotor skills. Sufficient attention must be given to developing and evaluating students' reasoning, decision-making, and communication skills. Students must also practice troubleshooting, anticipating, and prioritizing.

In practice, healthcare professionals must be able to seek information and answers to patient problems. They need to use a variety of resources. Respiratory therapists must have the skills to effectively solve clinical problems. They must interact with others and adapt to change.

Respiratory therapists need the experience and skills to seek information and alternatives to solve work-related problems in the real world. Listening to lectures does not contribute to students' abilities to critically read, write, speak, or think. Therefore, traditional approaches do not adequately prepare healthcare professionals to acquire skills that can transfer to clinical practice. Consequently, newer approaches are being incorporated to foster critical thinking skills and traits for respiratory care practice today and in the future.

Problem-Based Learning

Problem-based learning (PBL) is a teaching/learning model that is designed to facilitate critical thinking. Over the past few decades, schools of medicine[26–32] and some respiratory therapy programs[33–35] have adopted PBL as a method specifically designed to facilitate students' clinical decision making.[21–25] The problem-based curriculum is built on research into the problem-solving skills of physicians and the principles of educational psychology.[27] PBL has been advocated as a useful way to educate allied health practitioners for the future and has been used in clinical psychology, nursing, occupational therapy, physical therapy, respiratory therapy, and physician assistant programs.[6,26–34] PBL also has been applied to other disciplines, including business education, biology, chemistry, physics, general education, architecture, and calculus.[30]

RESPIRATORY RECAP

Problem-Based Learning

» Uses student-centered, self-directed, small-group discussions whereby students are facilitated by faculty to solve clinical problems similar to the ones they will encounter in respiratory care practice

PBL is student-centered rather than teacher-centered. It allows individualization of instruction. PBL assumes that students are self-directed learners. It permits them to have some influence over the direction, speed, and depth of their learning. The setting for PBL is usually a small group (6 to 10 students) with a faculty tutor. A skilled facilitator may be able to handle a larger group discussion. However, as the number of people in a group increases, the ability for equal participation can be jeopardized. Equal participation of students promotes self-directed learning. It also enhances students' abilities to develop their reasoning and communication skills. Therefore, maintaining small groups is recommended.

Implementation

During PBL courses, students are given a clinical problem. The problem gradually unfolds over multiple group sessions. Group sessions are often face to face, but online methods are increasingly being incorporated. Technology today permits high degrees of group interaction that can cross time and place. Each session may last from 2 to 4 hours, depending on the clinical problem, learning issues, size of the group, and students' abilities.

Someone from the group is the "reader," who reads aloud the clinical problem given by the facilitator. The group may decide to read one line, one paragraph, or one page at a time. Someone else from the group is the "scribe." The scribe records the discussions of the group on a blackboard, overhead projector, or computer with projection in such a way that everyone can see the group's notes. The scribe makes five columns to record information from the group discussions on what the group knows, needs to know, hypothesizes, need to learns, and recommends (**Table 58–2**). The medical model for PBL uses three or four columns. However, I suggest adding a column to include respiratory therapy recommendations, as shown in Table 58–2. The recommendations column will help prepare students for the NBRC clinical simulation examinations. Graduates are expected to make and evaluate respiratory care recommendations throughout each simulation. Furthermore, the professional role of respiratory therapists requires clinicians to make recommendations and give feedback for management of patients with cardiopulmonary disease.[10]

RESPIRATORY RECAP

Discussing Clinical Problems in Problem-Based Learning

» What we know
» What we need to know
» What we hypothesize
» What we recommend
» Learning issues

Students evaluate what they know about the problem, what they need to know, and what they hypothesize. Based on the group discussions, students determine

TABLE 58–2 Format for Recording a Group's Problem-Based Learning Discussion

Biological		Clinical		Psychosocial
What do we know?	*What do we need to know?*	*What do we hypothesize?*	*What do we recommend?*	*What topics will we research? (Learning issues)*

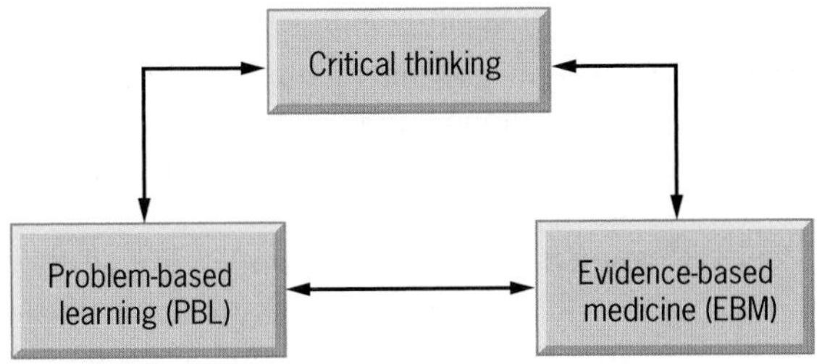

FIGURE 58–2 Supporting relationships of critical thinking, problem-based learning, and evidence-based medicine.

their recommendations for respiratory care. The group also collectively determines its learning issues. Students decide their learning issues when the group realizes it needs to review or investigate a topic further to understand the clinical problem in the case. The learning issues are essentially the subject areas and questions that require further research. Research is done whenever the group is lacking information or the knowledge base to make further clinical decisions. Students are informed that resources for their research include textbooks, journal articles, indexes, dictionaries, medical experts on and off campus, the Internet, and the faculty.

Students should receive instruction on how to locate, evaluate, and use various forms of evidence when researching their learning issues. An understanding of the basics of research is essential to being an informed consumer of medical literature. Students should be encouraged to apply evidence-based approaches to respiratory care. Students and respiratory therapists should use the highest levels of evidence to make their decisions. In addition, critical thinking skills and traits develop further whenever we closely examine and reflect on the basis for our thoughts and actions. Evidence-based practice is a large component of critical thinking. **Figure 58–2** shows the relationships among critical thinking, evidence-based medicine, and problem-based learning. The topic is so important that an entire chapter is devoted to evidence-based medicine (refer to Chapter 62).

At the end of each group discussion, members of the group negotiate who will research each learning issue. Each group member assumes responsibility to research the assigned learning issue and report back to the group at the next session. Students choose learning issues to research. Then they gather data to resolve the problem (either individually or in smaller groups). When the group reconvenes, each member presents learning issues and provides handouts. Each student contributes information for the group to present solutions. Students must indicate the sources of their information so that the group can evaluate the accuracy, validity, and relevance of the information for solving the clinical problem. Group interaction and discussion are vital to the success of this approach. Therefore, facilitator and peer evaluations of each student's performance in the group are recommended.

Goals

PBL enables students to direct their own learning by using a variety of resources to manage and solve work-related problems. The clinical problems are similar to the realistic problems they will encounter in professional practice. Students are encouraged to discuss and evaluate the biological, clinical, and psychosocial issues related to the clinical problems.

Biological issues include application of knowledge from the basic sciences that explains physiology and pathophysiology. Clinical issues include various aspects of the prevention, diagnosis, treatment, and long-term management of disease. Psychosocial issues include patient understanding, education, compliance, and self-management, as well as societal factors such as cost and access, which influence healthcare.

Emphasis is placed on the students' development of skills such as analysis, synthesis, and hypothesis generation. These skills are needed for the successful completion, assessment, and evaluation of the learning sequence. PBL also gives students experience discussing and evaluating the issues in the diagnosis and management of cardiopulmonary disease.

The PBL approach requires students to draw on their abilities to work collaboratively, to manage time and resources, and to develop the skills and characteristics of critical thinkers. Most important, students have the opportunity to interact with faculty mentors who role-model critical thinking. Role modeling is perhaps one of the best strategies for the development of critical thinkers.[5,16]

> **RESPIRATORY RECAP**
>
> **Goals of Problem-Based Learning**
>
> » Acquire a body of knowledge that is better retained, retrieved, and used in the clinical setting
> » Develop the ability to use knowledge effectively in the evaluation and care of patients' health problems
> » Develop skills and attitudes of a critical thinker and lifelong learner
> » Gain experience discussing and evaluating the biological, clinical, and psychosocial issues in cardiopulmonary disease and respiratory care practice

Role of the Facilitator

PBL facilitators are guides and coaches, not lecturers or resources. PBL places emphasis on learning rather than teaching. Although each facilitator has a personal style, the role is to promote student-centered learning and critical thinking. Facilitators do this by posing non-directive questions at appropriate times to encourage analytical thought and aid group process. The facilitator also helps to handle conflict within a group. The facilitator promotes professional debate on controversial issues. The facilitator also provides feedback on individual and group performance. The facilitator provides direction to enhance group learning.

Challenges for Students

Students' major challenge with PBL is to learn to rely on their own abilities to understand, discover, and apply knowledge and skills that can transfer to the real world. A major obstacle from the student's perspective is the degree to which he or she has been taught to rely on the "expert." Students are naturally curious and eager to solve problems. However, traditional learning methods have often stifled these natural tendencies. PBL shifts the role of student from "passive student" to "active learner." PBL works best when faculty shift from teachers to mentors, and students shift to a primary role as learners. Students may initially be reluctant to assume so much responsibility for their learning.[36] They may not know how to do the research to prepare for class discussions. However, every student has a responsibility to come prepared to participate fully.

Some students are naturally reserved or quiet. They may be hesitant to join group discussions. This is counterproductive in PBL. It is the different experiences, knowledge, perceptions, and ways of thinking applied in active discussions that make PBL a powerful learning method.[35] Speaking up in a group is the only way you can test your ideas. Testing ideas is a hallmark of critical thinking. If you do not express your own thinking and understanding, you miss the opportunity to test the accuracy and validity of your ideas. Group participation provides the opportunity to learn how to communicate, negotiate, and reflect on your ideas, beliefs, and actions. Quietness in a group discussion can also be misinterpreted as ignorance. Each student must participate. Faculty tutors and group members can assess how well you understand the group discussions. They also can assess how much you have learned.

RESPIRATORY RECAP

Challenges for Students

» Problem-based learning shifts the role of respiratory therapy students from "passive" listeners to "active" learners.

» Group participation provides the opportunity to learn how to communicate, negotiate, and reflect on your ideas, beliefs and actions. Speaking up in a group discussion is the major way that you can test the validity and accuracy of your ideas, which is the hallmark of critical thinking.

Evaluation of Students

The evaluation methods for PBL should include an assessment of students' abilities to summarize issues clearly; offer information from diverse sources; use information from previous cases, including clinical experiences; and reconsider hypotheses and decisions. PBL assessment techniques can include oral and written examinations, course assignments or projects, research papers related to the problems or clinical cases, development of concept maps, clinical simulations (computerized or written text), group discussion, group interaction, and peer evaluation. Discussion questions relevant to the cases are particularly useful. These can assess students' grasp of the content, as well as their problem-solving abilities. PBL evaluations should also provide feedback on learners' skills, learning issues, peer teaching, and critical thinking.

Peer evaluation is an important aspect of PBL. It should be incorporated into the course, lab, or clinical grade. Peers should have the opportunity to evaluate their classmates' presentation of learning issues, incorporation of resources, preparedness for group discussion, and participation in group discussion. Peer evaluation should address both the quantity and quality of each group member's participation. Forms can be used to obtain peer scores and comments. These should be incorporated into each student's evaluation for grading purposes. Grading of specific assignments can be determined by an overall score or pass/fail. Course grades can also be assigned by a numeric or letter grade or some form of pass/fail.

RESPIRATORY RECAP

Peer Evaluation

» Peers should have the opportunity to evaluate their classmates' presentation of learning issues, incorporation of resources, preparedness for group discussion, and the quantity and quality of group participation.

Curriculum Changes to Facilitate Critical Thinking

Most respiratory care curricula are already overburdened with professional courses. Present curricula cannot accommodate new courses. Neither can educators rely on general technical school or college curricula to meet the learning needs of critical thinkers. Courses that are already a part of the curriculum, such as introductory management, education, and ethics courses, can easily accommodate the teaching of critical thinking. By changing methods to include strategies for learning critical thinking, the curriculum itself does not need to change. The teaching of critical thinking can also be taught by incorporating PBL in courses that are traditionally "hard science" courses.

Teaching critical thinking requires innovative teaching approaches. It requires dynamic learning experiences and creative evaluation strategies. A variety of methods should be incorporated. These may include PBL, discussion, debate, case study, puzzles, games, logic analyses, troubleshooting, observations, journal writing, case presentations, writing papers, group projects, research studies, clinical apprenticeships, and clinical simulations.[6,17]

Evaluation of Critical Thinking

There is no overall consensus on the definition of critical thinking and the process of critical thinking.[36] It is dependent on the individual and the circumstances. Therefore, the measurement of critical thinking is a controversial topic. Many authors point out that having a disposition toward critical thinking is a key issue. However, measuring for this is extremely difficult in any testing format, particularly multiple choice. Furthermore, the tendency to think critically is affected by circumstances. These factors cannot be accounted for by most standardized tests. The organizational climate can either promote or limit opportunities for critical thinking in the workplace. Critical thinking in respiratory care practice is facilitated when there is a supportive medical director, strong department leadership, a progressive climate, and specific role delineations in practice.[9,25]

There are dozens of critical thinking assessment tests. Some tests focus on general critical thinking skills or cognitive ability. Other tests focus on critical reading or writing. A few instruments assess the dispositional traits of a critical thinker. No test is comprehensive in measuring all the abilities or affective characteristics of a critical thinker. Each test has its own unique strengths and weaknesses.

Most aspects of professional education, including evaluation mechanisms, require professionals to make individual decisions. The ways that professionals earn formal degrees and credentials involve individual competencies of the practitioner. However, shared cognition and decision making are characteristic features of critical thinking in the real world. In practice, it is common to see patients managed collectively by a variety of professionals. Shared competence involves decision making, communicating, and negotiating. Therefore, evaluation mechanisms should assess respiratory therapy students' abilities in these areas.

In respiratory care education it is important to use a variety of evaluation methods to assess respiratory therapy students' cognitive, psychomotor, and affective abilities. It is equally important to assess respiratory therapists' critical thinking skills and traits, including logical reasoning, problem solving, reflection, and the dispositions of a critical thinker.

KEY POINTS

- Fostering critical thinking is an important issue for respiratory therapists.
- Awareness and education can enhance the capacity to improve critical thinking.
- Developing a personal definition of critical thinking may be helpful to improve your own critical thinking.
- Respiratory therapists who aspire for career advancement need to expand their capacity for critical thinking.
- Individual traits and work context influence opportunities for critical thinking in respiratory care practice.
- The essential skills for critical thinking in practice include prioritizing, anticipating, troubleshooting, communicating, negotiating, decision making, and reflecting.
- Critical thinkers exhibit certain characteristics. Attributes for respiratory therapists include problem solving, common sense, initiative, judgment, critical evaluation, objective decision making, motivation, inquisitiveness, and lifelong learning.
- Teaching of critical thinking can be accomplished through a variety of methods, including a problem-based learning (PBL) approach.
- In the PBL curriculum, students are active learners who confront questions, problems, and situations using critical thinking skills and dispositions.
- The teaching of critical thinking may be performed in any setting or any course: formal degree programs; science, technical, or medical courses; management or education courses; practical experiences; continuing education; or in-service settings.
- Technology and online learning methodologies can be effectively used for small-group learning to enhance critical thinking.
- Dozens of commercially available tests are available to measure various aspects of critical thinking.
- The emphasis placed on critical thinking in respiratory care practice will continue to increase.
- The essential skills, dispositions, educational strategies, and assessment of critical thinking will continue to be topics for discussion into the future.

REFERENCES

1. Facione PA. Critical thinking: a statement of expert consensus for purposes of educational assessment and instruction. ERIC Document Reproduction Service No. ED 315 423, 1990.
2. O'Daniel CO, Cullen DL, Douce FH, et al. The future educational needs of respiratory care practitioners: a Delphi study. *Respir Care.* 1992;37:65–78.
3. Dunne P. Shaping a vision of the future respiratory care practitioner. *AARC Times.* 1992;16(4):8–30.
4. Cullen DL, Sullivan JM, Bartel RE, et al., eds. *Year 2001: Delineating the Educational Direction for the Future Respiratory Care Practitioner. Proceedings of a National Consensus Conference on Respiratory Care Education.* Dallas, TX: American Association for Respiratory Care; 1992.
5. Kacmarek RM, Durbin CG, Barnes TA, et al. Creating a vision for respiratory care in 2015 and beyond. *Respir Care.* 2009;54(3):375–389.
6. Mishoe SC. Critical thinking, educational preparation and development of respiratory care practitioners. *Distinguished Papers Monograph.* 1993;1(2):29–43.
7. Paul RW. *Critical Thinking: Basic Theory and Instructional Structures Handbook.* Rohnert Park, CA: Foundation for Critical Thinking; 2000.
8. Mishoe SC, Courtenay B. Critical thinking in respiratory care practice. In: *Proceedings of the 35th Annual Adult Education Research Conference.* Knoxville: University of Tennessee; 1994:276–281.
9. Mishoe SC. Critical thinking in respiratory care practice: a qualitative research study. *Respir Care.* 2003;48:500–551.
10. Mishoe SC. Critical thinking in respiratory care practice. *Respir Care.* 1996;41:958.

11. Mishoe SC, MacIntyre NR. Expanding professional roles for respiratory care practitioners. *Respir Care.* 1997;42:71–91.
12. Gambrill E. *Critical Thinking in Clinical Practice: Improving the Quality of Judgments and Decisions.* 2nd ed. Hoboken, NJ: John Wiley & Sons; 2005.
13. Bandman EL, Bandman B. *Critical Thinking in Nursing.* 2nd ed. Norwalk, CT: Appleton & Lange; 1995.
14. Elstein AS, Shulman LS, Sprafka SA. Medical problem-solving: a ten year retrospective. *Evaluation Health Professions.* 1990;13:5–36.
15. Elstein AS. Cognitive processes in clinical inference and decision making. In: Turk DC, Salovey P, eds. *Reasoning, Inference and Judgment in Clinical Psychology.* New York: Free Press; 1988.
16. Mishoe SC, Dennison FH, Thomas-Goodfellow L. A comparison of respiratory therapy students' critical thinking abilities with performance on the clinical simulation examinations. *Respir Care.* 1997;42:1078.
17. Hill TV. The relationship between critical thinking and decision-making in respiratory care students. *Respir Care.* 2002;47:571–577.
18. Facione PA, Facione NC. *The Critical Thinking Disposition Inventory (CCTDI) and CCTDI Test Manual.* Millbrae, CA: California Academic Press; 1992.
19. Brookfield SD. *The Power of Critical Theory: Liberating Adult Learning and Teaching.* San Francisco: Jossey-Bass; 2004.
20. Mishoe SC, Martin S. Critical thinking in the laboratory. *Learning Laboratorian Series.* 1994;6(4):1–63.
21. Goodfellow LT. Respiratory therapists and critical-thinking behaviors: a self-assessment. *J Allied Health.* 2001;30:20–25.
22. Facione N, Facione PA. Critical thinking and clinical judgment. In: *Critical Thinking and Clinical Reasoning in the Health Sciences: A Teaching Anthology.* Milbrae, CA: Insight Assessment/California Academic Press; 2008.
23. Mishoe SC, Hernlen K. Teaching and evaluating critical thinking in respiratory care. *Respir Care Clin North Am.* 2005;11:477–488.
24. Mishoe SC. Educating respiratory care professionals: an emphasis on critical thinking. *Respir Care.* 2002;47(5):568.
25. Mishoe SC. The effects of institutional context on critical thinking in the workplace. In: *Proceedings of the 36th Annual Adult Education Research Conference.* Edmonton, Alberta: University of Alberta; 1995:221–228.
26. Nosich GM. *Learning to Think Things Through: A Guide to Critical Thinking in the Curriculum.* 3rd ed. Englewood Cliffs, NJ: Prentice Hall; 2009.
27. Barrows HS. *How to Design a Problem-Based Curriculum for the Preclinical Years.* New York: Springer Verlag; 1985.
28. Savery J. Overview of problem-based learning. *Interdisciplinary J Problem-based Learning.* 2006;1(1).
29. Bruhn JG. Problem-based learning: an approach toward reforming allied health education. *J Allied Health.* 1992;21:161–173.
30. Wilkerson L, Gijselaers W, eds. *Bringing Problem-Based Learning to Higher Education: Theory and Practice.* New Directions for Teaching and Learning 68. San Francisco: Jossey-Bass; 1996.
31. Teshima DY. Outcome measurement of problem-based learning. *Clin Lab Sci.* 2001;14:68–69.
32. Curtis JA, Indyk D, Taylor B. Successful use of problem-based learning in a third-year pediatric clerkship. *Ambulatory Pediatr.* 2001;1:132–135.
33. O'pt Holt TB. A first year experience with problem-based learning in a baccalaureate cardiorespiratory care program. *Respir Care Educ Annu.* 2000;9:47–58.
34. Beachey WD. A comparison of problem-based learning and traditional curricula in baccalaureate respiratory therapy education. *Respir Care.* 2007;52:1497–1506.
35. Mishoe SC. Problem-based learning: any influence in respiratory care? *Respir Care.* 2007;52:1457–1459.
36. Barrows HS. *What Your Tutor May Never Tell You: A Guide for Medical Students in Problem-Based Learning.* Springfield, IL: Southern Illinois University School of Medicine; 1997.
37. Paul R, Elder L. *Critical Thinking Concepts and Tools.* Dillon Beach, CA: Foundation for Critical Thinking; 2008.
38. Dressel P, Mayhew LB. *General Education: Explorations in Evaluation. Final Report of the Cooperative Study of Evaluation in General Education.* Washington, DC: American Council on Education; 1954.
39. Eljamal MB, Sharp S, Stark JS, et al. Listening for disciplinary differences in the faculty goals for effective thinking. *J Gen Education.* 1998;47:117–148.
40. Hallet GL. *Logic for the Labyrinth: A Guide to Critical Thinking.* Washington, DC: University Press of America; 1984.
41. Halpern DF. *Thought and Knowledge: An Introduction to Critical Thinking.* 4th ed. Hillside, NJ: Lawrence Erlbaum Associates; 2003.
42. McPeck JE. T*eaching Critical Thinking: Dialogue and Didactic.* New York: Routledge; 1990.

CHAPTER 59

Ethics of Healthcare Delivery

Douglas E. Masini

OUTLINE

Definition of Ethics
Foundations of Ethical Thinking
Ethical Versus Legal Behavior
Ethical Theories
Ethical Principles
Role of Professional Organizations in Ethics
Ethics Committees
Case Studies

OBJECTIVES

1. Define ethics.
2. Describe methods by which an ethical orientation is formed.
3. Distinguish between ethical and legal behavior.
4. Describe an ethical dilemma.
5. State the role of ethics in the delivery of effective respiratory care.
6. Define common ethical theories.
7. Describe the way the analysis method is used to solve ethical dilemmas.
8. Identify and explain eight contemporary ethical principles.
9. List components of the Patient Care Partnership.
10. List ways in which managed care has affected basic ethical principles.
11. Discuss the way technology has increased the incidence of confidentiality violations.
12. Describe key components of the American Association for Respiratory Care's statement of ethics and professional conduct.
13. Discuss the role of ethics committees and the respiratory therapist.
14. Describe common ethical dilemmas associated with the delivery of respiratory care.

KEY TERMS

AARC Code of Ethics
advance directive
analysis method
attitudinal orientation
autonomy
beneficence
bias
capacity
Comfort Measures Only (CMO)
confidentiality
deontological theory
Do Not Intubate (DNI)
Do Not Resuscitate (DNR)
durable medical power of attorney
ethics
ethics committees
fidelity
informed consent
justice
living will
moral philosophy
nonmaleficence
optimum care committees
Patient Care Partnership
personal belief system
personal value system
prejudice
proxy
surrogate
teleological theory
veracity

INTRODUCTION

Increasingly, respiratory therapy literature has called for respiratory therapists to take on new roles and have new levels of autonomy and independence in decision making, especially in the context of respiratory care protocols. The new student and the seasoned therapist must recognize that such a paradigm shift requires not only experience and technical training but also enhanced communication skills to promote their knowledge of professional ethics and ethical considerations in the delivery of respiratory care. In other words, we have to walk the walk and talk the talk when we discuss the ethical practice of respiratory therapy with other caregivers.

Definition of Ethics

Every working day, the respiratory therapist is faced with ethical dilemmas and new questions that have to be answered. For example, how can respiratory therapists continue to provide quality patient care while departmental staffing is undergoing a reduction in force? How can therapists maintain patient confidentiality in the information age? Is there a place for the respiratory therapist on the community ethics or optimal care committee? What role do respiratory therapists play in assisting families with the difficult decision to use life support equipment or agree to Do Not Resuscitate orders for their loved ones? Should advanced and expensive monitoring, intravascular lines, and heroic mechanical ventilation be used in every critical care situation?

These ethical questions confront both students and clinicians every day. Ethical discussions and decisions are never easy. With ethical questions in particular, answers are rarely black or white and often lie within gray zones. Ethical decisions depend on the specific value systems and decisions of the individuals involved.

Although discussions about medical ethics have increased in recent years, the topic is not a new one. Medical ethics have been discussed since the days of ancient Greece. The Hippocratic Oath, established in the fourth century BC, outlined ethical guidelines and behaviors for physicians, who vowed "to keep their patients from harm and injustice."[1] The oath contained other provisions that addressed confidentiality for patients and the role of the physician. These and other ethical issues in patient care have transcended time, but society continues to reestablish, refine, and redefine its code of ethics for healthcare. This chapter teaches the respiratory therapist how to model and communicate the ethical practice of respiratory care.

RESPIRATORY RECAP

Ethics

- » Ethical principles have long been a part of medical practice, dating back to the time of Hippocrates.
- » Ethics is a decision-making process, and in that process societies and individuals make decisions regarding what is right and wrong.

The World Medical Association defines **ethics** as "the study of morality—careful and systematic reflection on and analysis of moral decisions and behavior, whether past, present or future."[2] The study of ethics is not specifically the determination of right or wrong answers, but rather the study of the ways in which individuals come to the judgment that their decisions are right or wrong; ethics is the study of the decision-making pathway one takes in determining what one believes is right or wrong.

Two important variables worthy of discussion when we talk about personal or clinical decision making are bias and prejudice. **Bias** is defined as "[a] preference or an inclination, especially one that inhibits impartial judgment," or "an unfair act or policy stemming from prejudice."[3] Allport defined **prejudice** as "[a] judgment formed before due examination and consideration of the facts—a premature or hasty judgment."[4] Both bias and prejudice inform clinical decision making, and both the student and seasoned clinician must confront their own biases and prejudices prior to making decisions. Conflict-of-interest statements, signed by the speaker or presenter, have become standardized as documentation that the speaker or presenter has reflected on his or her professional relationships and influences and considered any possible bias or prejudice prior to presentation of information to a larger audience. For example, one must identify specific conflict-of-interest relationships such as remuneration, travel expenses, or honoraria that one has received from vendors, manufacturers, or pharmaceutical companies. These relationships have the potential to skew a presentation, which in turn could bias or prejudice the opinions or decisions made by individual respiratory therapists.

No individual is born knowing what is right or wrong. Ethics are based in part on values individuals develop as they mature. Many times these values are influenced by gender, geographic location, social and economic standards, religious convictions, family members, ethnicity, prejudice and bias, political beliefs, education, life experience, and culture.

Foundations of Ethical Thinking

Personal Belief System

As individuals experience life and are educated in the morals and mores of our society, they develop a set of personal beliefs, or **personal belief system**. These beliefs are not necessarily right or wrong and are certainly not objective, yet they are deeply ingrained in an individual's thoughts and decision-making processes.

Attitudinal Orientation

Attitudinal orientation is the outward expression of an individual's personal belief system. It is what a person says and how that person behaves and is based on what the individual believes. Attitudes have a large effect on behavior; this is most evident when an individual is confronted with an ethical dilemma.

Personal Value System

A **personal value system** is formed when the decision is made to continue to believe and express a conviction even when a person or event challenges it. For example, having a particular belief about the death penalty is easy, as is expression of this belief when no opposition exists. However, maintaining a belief and defending it to others becomes more difficult in the face of opposition, especially if a person's bias or prejudice is without evidence or merit. When an individual is willing to maintain

RESPIRATORY RECAP

Personal Value Systems

- » Personal beliefs include the mores and morals of our society.
- » Attitudinal orientation is the outward expression of a personal belief system.
- » A personal value system is formed when beliefs become convictions.
- » An individual's moral philosophy can be viewed as a behavioral code.

a belief in the face of opposition, that belief becomes a conviction. When the individual integrates convictions into a personal value system and maintains them in the face of opposition, they become personal principles. This progression is an important step in the formation of an individual's ethical orientation because personal principles influence that individual's ethical orientation and decision making.

Moral Philosophy

An individual's **moral philosophy** can be viewed as a behavioral code. Morals define what individuals will or will not do in a given situation, and moral philosophy is based on the individual's previously adopted personal principles. Ethics can be viewed as a work in progress, and ethical principles often reflect the current society. As a society evolves and changes, so will its ethical beliefs; two timely examples are abortion and the death penalty. Changes in the way society views these issue are reflected in newer laws governing these practices.

Ethical Versus Legal Behavior

Ethical Orientation

A discussion of ethical behavior is difficult without at least an allusion to legal behavior. Legal behavior in this sense simply means abiding by the law. Sometimes the line between the ethical and the legal is fine, sometimes that line disappears and the behaviors merge, and at other times the gap between the two widens. A given behavior can be described as both ethical and legal, and it often has the same foundation. Ethical and legal behaviors differ primarily in the individual freedom allowed for decision making. For example, an individual may be free to adhere to a given ethical code but required to abide by the legal code under the threat of punishment by law.

Legal Standards

Ideally, behavior would always be both ethical and legal. In reality, however, that standard is not always met. Several reasons exist for the discrepancy between the legal and the ethical, the primary reason being that neither ethical behavior nor legal requirements are static standards. Ethical and legal standards of behavior change as society grows and changes.

In recent history abortion is a classic example that demonstrates the way major societal issues influence both ethical and legal standards. Before 1973, when the Supreme Court's *Roe v. Wade* decision was handed down, abortion was clearly illegal. Needless to say, the Supreme Court did not decide in a vacuum on that day to legalize abortion. Instead, the argument had grown over the previous decades that not all abortions should be illegal. It may not have been stated as such, but this view marked a gradual change in society's ethical orientation. Although not every American citizen agreed that abortion should be legalized, at the time of the Supreme Court decision society's ethical orientation had shifted so significantly that the Court's interpretation was inevitable. Some legal scholars might argue that the Court simply interpreted the Constitution and that the ruling had nothing to do with society's ethical orientation. However, constitutional interpretation is usually related to society's ethical orientation. Take, for example, the Supreme Court's decisions on the death penalty and slavery. The legal decisions handed down by courts, whether deemed positive or negative, reflect society's orientation at specific times in history.

A major ethical and legal shift in the area of death and dying is pending. The right to die appears to have gained a growing acceptance from an ethical standpoint. Customary in these kinds of shifts is for legal standards to lag behind ethical development. For example, Jack Kevorkian, a Michigan pathologist, was found legally responsible for the death of one of his patients. Close examination of the opinions surrounding his work reveals a subtle shift from the view that his work is ethically wrong to one of recognizing a right to die. This shift in ethical viewpoints in the United States toward euthanasia is primarily evident in the nonscientific literature.[5] However, in 1997 Oregon introduced the Death with Dignity Act to legalize physician-assisted suicide, and 22 other states have proposed similar legislation. Respiratory therapists practicing today and in the future will no doubt confront the ramifications of this type of legislation in their daily practice.[6,7]

RESPIRATORY RECAP

Ethical Versus Legal Behavior

- » Legal behavior simply means abiding by the law, whereas ethical behavior involves personal beliefs, attitudinal orientation, and moral philosophy.
- » Legal and ethical behaviors are not static.
- » Ideally, behavior would always be both ethical and legal.
- » A major pending shift in ethical and legal behavior is presently happening in areas concerning death and dying.

The preceding discussion on legal standards and ethical orientation may appear unrelated to ethics for the respiratory therapist. However, it is important in helping respiratory therapists to understand the dynamics of ethical dilemmas. Ethical dilemmas are not static issues that remain constant; they change as society changes. Thus, the most important point for the therapist to learn is how to deal with ethical dilemmas in situational settings.

The respiratory therapist may encounter many ethical dilemmas, ranging from dramatic life support and end-of-life issues to the basic staffing and level of care issues prevalent in today's managed care environment. In fact, most dilemmas the average therapist faces are the less dramatic ones. However, that these dilemmas are less dramatic does not make them less important.

Ethical Theories

Two main theories are used to describe the decision-making process an individual undertakes in deriving an ethical conclusion to a dilemma. Teleological and deontological theories guide ethical decision making. In addition to these two major ethical theories, the analysis method is used, which combines teleological and deontological theory, recognizing that most ethical decisions require systematic analysis.

Teleological Theory

Teleological theory is based on consequences: the right or wrong of an action is judged on the outcomes or consequences of predicted outcomes. The most common type of consequential theory is utilitarianism, in which an individual chooses the act that brings about the best outcome. To determine the best outcome the individual must follow a system of steps, during which the problem first is described, all solutions then are listed, and the solutions finally are compared with the good each can provide. The correct answer is the most useful solution and becomes the best outcome. For example, enough money is available for either a heart transplant for one patient or vaccines for hundreds of infants. Using the teleological theory, the consequences of helping hundreds would be better than helping one patient. Therefore, the best outcome would be to use the money to buy the vaccines. Patient triage is another example of utilitarianism. In today's fast-paced respiratory care department, triage skills are critical when, simply put, the right person must give the right therapy to the right patient at the right time.

> **RESPIRATORY RECAP**
>
> **Teleological Theory**
>
> » Teleological theory is consequential theory—that is, based on consequences.
>
> » The most common type of consequential theory is known as utilitarianism.
>
> » Utilitarianism looks for the best outcome.

Deontological Theory

Deontological theory is based on duty and states that an act is right or wrong based on its intrinsic character rather than on its consequences. Although deontological theory is concerned with doing the best thing, it also tries to do the right thing. The philosophical works of Immanuel Kant, as well as many religions, are examples of this type of theory.

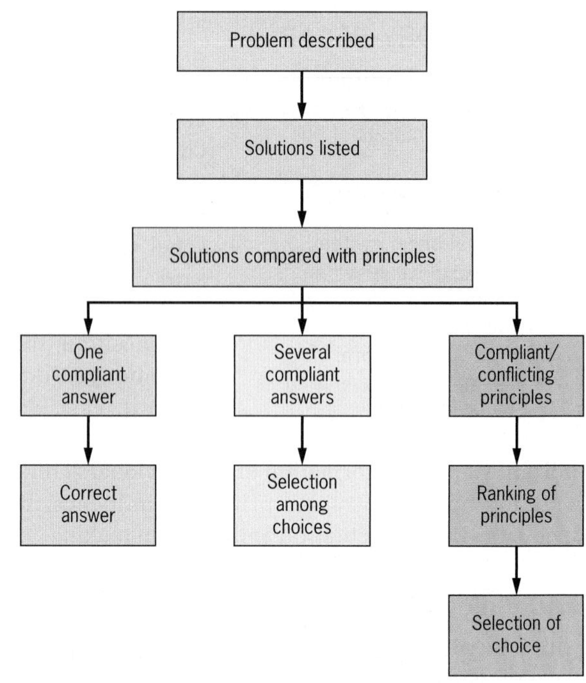

FIGURE 59–1 Deontological theory of reasoning.

The steps involved in deontological theory are much more complicated than those in teleological theory and are outlined in **Figure 59–1**.

> **RESPIRATORY RECAP**
>
> **Deontological Theory**
>
> » Deontological theory is an ethical theory based on duty.
>
> » An act is either right or wrong based on its intrinsic character (one's duty) rather than on its consequences.
>
> » The philosophical works of Immanuel Kant, as well as many religions, are examples of this type of theory.

Analysis Method

One other theory used in ethics is the **analysis method**, which combines key components from teleological and deontological theories. It recognizes that in the final analysis, most ethical decisions are made by a systematic analytic process devised by the individual.[8]

Fletcher and coworkers established a case method of moral problem solving using clinical pragmatism in the spirit of John Dewey's pragmatic philosophy. In their method they suggested the following steps: assessment, moral diagnosis, goal setting, and evaluation. The case method of moral problem solving asks many incisive questions; it evaluates a patient's medical condition, relevant contextual factors, the patient's capacity for decision making, patient preferences, needs of the patient as a person, preferences of the patient's family or surrogate decision maker, interests other than and potentially competing with those of the patient, and issues of power or conflict in the interactions of the key actors in the case that need to be addressed. This method asks whether all the parties have had the opportunity to be heard and whether all institutional factors contributing to the problems posed by the case have been addressed.[9]

Analysis methodology became increasingly popular in the 21st century. Most ethical dilemmas were solved with the analysis method, which combines the best of the ethical theories, as judged by an individual's ethical orientation, with critical thinking and problem-solving skills. The actual process varies but includes the following steps:

> **RESPIRATORY RECAP**
>
> **Analysis Method**
>
> » The analysis method combines key components from teleological and deontological theories.
>
> » Health professionals resolve most ethical dilemmas using the analysis method.

1. Identification of the problem
2. Clarification of the problem
3. Formulation of possible solutions
4. Testing of possible solutions against consequences, feasibility, and sense of right and wrong, with each individual free to place a different emphasis on each test
5. Selection and application of a solution

Ethical Principles

Using ethical theories, society has developed several principles or standards of behavior to help determine right or wrong actions. These principles change over time as societies change. Eight ethical principles considered important in contemporary medicine are beneficence, capacity, nonmaleficence, veracity, autonomy, confidentiality, justice, and role fidelity.

Beneficence

Beneficence means charity or mercy. This principle imposes on the clinician the responsibility to seek good for the patient under all circumstances. The healthcare professional should do only what will benefit the patient.

Healthcare workers enter their professions with the genuine desire to help patients and receive intrinsic rewards by helping and caring for those who need their expertise. Beneficence has long played a role in the delivery of healthcare. Hippocrates wrote, "I will apply dietetic measures for the benefit of the sick according to my ability and judgment."[1] This desire to provide care to benefit patients has been a continuing principle. Healthcare and professional organizations recognize the need for continued education to foster growth and competence in healthcare.

However, determining what is good is a difficulty encountered with beneficence. If beneficence means seeking good for the patient, who will decide what is good? Will the patient make the determination or the healthcare worker? Just as individuals have different values, so will patients have different opinions as to what will benefit them the most.

Beneficence is becoming increasingly more difficult to determine in today's advanced technologic world. For example, the technology now exists to prolong lives that would have been lost just two decades ago. At the same time the question remains of whether this technology should be used to save every life. An individual with terminal cancer could be kept alive for months on life support. Should technology be used in this case? Would it benefit the patient? Is it good for the patient? Is it good for the family?

> **RESPIRATORY RECAP**
>
> **Beneficence**
>
> » Beneficence imposes the responsibility to seek good for the patient under all circumstances.
>
> » Determining what is good can be difficult.
>
> » Beneficence is becoming increasingly more difficult to determine in today's advanced technologic world.

Patients Who Refuse Intubation and Ventilation

Advance directives, which are addressed in greater detail later in this chapter, communicate patients' wishes to their physicians and caregivers. They may be modified to assert a patient's wishes, that is, what he or she wants done and does not want done. Of particular importance to respiratory therapists is whether patients do not wish to have an artificial airway placed.

Mehta and Hill examined the use of noninvasive positive pressure ventilation (NIV) in patients who did not wish to be intubated. In some NIV patients who have declined or are reluctant to undergo intubation, NIV is used to lessen dyspnea, preserve patient autonomy, and permit verbal communication with loved ones. However, this indication is controversial and may in theory prolong the dying process and lead to inappropriate utilization of scarce resources. The authors believed that the use of NIV for patients who are not to receive invasive ventilation is justifiable if the patient understands that NIV is being used as a form of life support, and there is the potential for reversal of the acute process.[10]

Nava found that in European respiratory intermediate and high-dependency care units, the most common end-of-life practices were withholding treatment, the use of noninvasive mechanical ventilation as the ceiling of therapy, and provision of a Do Not Resuscitate or Do Not Intubate order. The author concluded that patients, when competent, and their families, together with nurses, were most often involved in reaching these key decisions.[11]

Levy stated that when determining the overall value of NIV at the end of life, physicians should ask patients whether they mean that they do not wish to be intubated because they do not want the discomfort of an endotracheal intubation or a mechanical ventilator, or whether they mean that they do not want any intervention and are prepared to die. When patients say they do not want to be intubated, they may simply mean that they do not wish to be subjected to the discomfort of an endotracheal tube or mechanical ventilator, but they might be willing to receive NIV.[12]

Kacmarek wrote that the most critical issues with regard to NIV for patients with Do Not Intubate and Comfort Measures Only orders were patient and family education and informed consent. The respiratory therapist must ask whether the risks and potential benefits of NIV have been clearly discussed and whether the patient agrees to accept the risks. Data from terminal cancer patients suggest that factors that are important to patients are retaining control over their end-of-life care decisions and having adequate time to prepare for their death. If control over care decisions is ensured, NIV may be able to reverse acute respiratory failure that was not necessarily a life-terminating event, and improve patient comfort and sustain life until the patient can put his or her affairs in order.[13]

Capacity

Capacity is the determination by one or more principal caregivers, based on the best evidence available, that the patient is capable of making a sound decision to accept or to withhold care. Fletcher noted that "the capable patient has a duty implied within the context of shared decision making . . . to articulate as clearly as possible what motivates a decision to refuse (or accept) treatment. Such a decision may be motivated by coherent personal reasons, religious beliefs, social or political ideology, or emotions." Fletcher went on to say that "treatment refusals by capable patients are valid when the elements of informed consent has been satisfied. The patient must demonstrate the following: (1) understanding of his/her medical condition, (2) understanding of the consequences of his/her decision, and (3) voluntariness."[9]

Roth and colleagues described competency testing, an indicator of capacity, as including "evidencing a choice—a very low-level test, most respectful of autonomy, looking only for consent or denial; reasonable outcome of choice; choice based upon rational reasons; ability to understand; and actual understanding, the highest test. In cases where there is doubt as to the patient being capable, psychiatric or neurologic consultants would be a valued asset in the case."[14] The establishment of capacity may be clouded by the influence on the patient in question of severity of injury, blood loss or shock, medications, cardiopulmonary or neurologic decompensation, or by pressures from family members, caregivers, or others who are directly or indirectly involved. The recognition of such influences and the ability to evaluate their impact on capacity are important roles for the caregiving team.

> **RESPIRATORY RECAP**
> **Capacity**
> » The determination that the patient is capable of making a sound decision to accept or withhold care
> » Essential components that must be met: an understanding of his/her medical condition, an understanding of the consequences of his/her decision, and voluntariness

Nonmaleficence

Nonmaleficence is the principle that requires therapists to avoid or refrain from harm. It is often viewed as the opposite of beneficence. This principle is outlined in the Hippocratic Oath with the words "I will keep them from harm and injustice."[1] Violations of this principle are the basis for most lawsuits.

> **RESPIRATORY RECAP**
> **Nonmaleficence**
> » Nonmaleficence is the principle that requires clinicians to avoid or refrain from harm.
> » The principle of double effects occurs when the benefit (or beneficence) of a treatment is accompanied by undesirable side effects that could cause harm.

As with beneficence, nonmaleficence can be seen as a double-edged sword. Often the benefits (or beneficence) of a treatment are accompanied by undesirable side effects that could cause harm, known as the *principle of double effects*. A common example of this dilemma is the use of narcotics to relieve pain. Although use of narcotics may relieve a patient's pain (beneficence), the patient also may suffer respiratory depression (nonmaleficence).

Clinicians use these guidelines to deal with the principle of double effects:[15]

- The action taken must be good, or at least morally neutral.
- The good must not follow as a consequence of the secondary harmful effects.
- The harm must never be intended, but rather be tolerated as casually connected with the good intended.
- The good must outweigh the harm.

Veracity

Veracity means truth. This principle implies that clinicians should tell patients the truth at all times and is based on the belief that healthcare is best served in a relationship of trust in which clinicians and patients are both bound by truth.

Veracity has not always been the norm in medical practice. A few decades ago, doctors made decisions about what their patients should or should not be told about their conditions. In a 1961 study, 90% of the 219 physicians surveyed stated that they would not disclose a diagnosis of cancer to a patient, believing that the patient would not be able to handle the news or would give up. A similar study was done 20 years later; of 264 phy-sicians surveyed, 97% stated that they would disclose a diagnosis of cancer.[16] Research has also demonstrated that patient attitudes concerning veracity have changed in recent years. Patients are more knowledgeable about medical treatments and more active in the decision-making process involving their healthcare, and they expect that healthcare providers will be truthful with them.

Truth in medicine serves several purposes. By telling patients the truth about their medical condition, an important bond is created between the public and the medical community. Without trust, many patients would not seek medical attention or would make uninformed decisions about their condition. The absence of veracity can result in legal action. Before undergoing procedures or participating in research studies, health professionals must give patients adequate information about the procedure or research. Patients must then have an opportunity to ask questions and understand the risks involved, or to decline the procedure.

Although the medical community realizes the importance of veracity, it also recognizes that in certain instances a physician not telling the patient the truth is equally important. Benevolent deception is the view that a physician can withhold information from a patient for that patient's own good. For instance, telling the patient the truth could result in psychological or physiologic harm in certain situations; at other times, patients may not wish to know everything about their medical conditions. Some patients do not want to know all the possible side effects or risks involved in a procedure and may rely on the principle that ignorance is bliss.

RESPIRATORY RECAP

Veracity

- » This principle states that clinicians should tell patients the truth at all times.
- » Benevolent deception is the view that a clinician can lie to a patient for that patient's own good.
- » Veracity has not always been the norm in medical practice.

The value of veracity often is culture specific. Asian cultures, for example, may not regard the truth as we know it to be as important as it is in the American culture. Family members with this type of cultural background may ask that information such as a terminal condition be kept from the patient. This situation requires patience, tact, and respect for cultural differences, and the healthcare professional must work closely with the family to establish the best course for the patient.

Autonomy

Autonomy is the right and the ability to govern one's self. In medical terms, it allows patients to make decisions about the medical treatment they will receive and decide which treatments they do not wish to receive. In the past, physicians took a more paternalistic role in the delivery of care, making the treatment choices for their patients, and were rarely questioned. Patients viewed doctors as the experts who would take care of them.

With recent advancements in medical science and telecommunications, patients have become more aware of treatment options and more vocal about making decisions regarding their health. The Patient Care Partnership and informed consent are the results of this changing view of autonomy.

The Patient Care Partnership

The American Hospital Association established the **Patient Care Partnership** in 2003 to outline the rights and responsibilities that patients have regarding their medical care (**Box 59–1**). The Partnership was previously called the Patient's Bill of Rights. Provisions of the Patient Care Partnership state that patients have the right to know about all aspects of their care, including their diagnosis, who is treating them, potential outcomes, and financial issues, and that the patient may refuse treatment to the extent permitted by law. Patients should also be informed of the medical consequences of their actions if they accept or refuse treatment.[17]

Informed Consent

Informed consent includes disclosure, understanding, voluntarism, competence, and permission. Before undergoing or refusing treatments, a patient must be provided with all relevant information. The Patient Care Partnership has a provision dealing specifically with informed consent, in which a patient has the right to receive information necessary to give consent. The patient also has the right to know about significant medical alternatives and the names of the individuals responsible for the treatment or procedure.[17]

Refusal of Treatment

The patient has the right to refuse treatment or to go against medical authority in any situation. The caregiver should attempt to evaluate the patient's capacity at the time of refusal, document the same, and attempt to assess the patient's understanding of the nature of his or her condition and the consequences of various options. The patient should have the mental capacity, or competency, to process the information required to make these decisions, which must be within the law.

Increasingly, caregivers are considering their right to refuse to participate in medical procedures or treatments that go against their ethical or religious values. Controversial topics that are frequently discussed in the medical and popular literature include the gathering and use of stem cells, the morality of late-term abortion, and assisted suicide. While several states have looked at legislation regarding assisted suicide, only Oregon has a statute in place, the Death with Dignity Act, which allows a patient at the point of medical futility to take a prescribed lethal dose of medication. Caregivers in Oregon may be concerned about their legal status if they are involved in caring for a patient who chooses to end his or her own life. In Oregon, the Death with Dignity statute says, in part, that "Except as provided in Oregon Revised Statutes (ORS) 127.890.1 . . . No person shall be subject to civil or criminal liability or professional disciplinary

BOX 59–1

The Patient Care Partnership

What to Expect During Your Hospital Stay

High-Quality Hospital Care

Hospital care, when needed, is provided with skill, compassion, and respect. You have the right to know the identity of doctors, nurses, and others involved in your care, and you have the right to know when they are students, residents, or other trainees.

A Clean and Safe Environment

The hospital works hard to keep a patient safe. Special policies and procedures are aimed at preventing mistakes and keeping you free from abuse and neglect. If anything unexpected and significant happens during your hospital stay, you will be told what happened, and any resulting changes in your care will be discussed with you.

Involvement in Your Care

You and your doctor often make decisions about your care before you go to the hospital. Other times, especially in emergencies, those decisions are made during your hospital stay. When decision-making takes place, it should include the following.

Discussing your medical condition and information about medically appropriate treatment choices

To make informed decisions with your doctor, you need to understand:

- The benefits and risks of each treatment
- Whether your treatment is experimental or part of a research study
- What you can reasonably expect from your treatment and any long-term effects it might have on your quality of life
- What you and your family will need to do after you leave the hospital
- The financial consequences of using uncovered services or out of network providers

Please tell your caregivers if you need more information about treatment choices.

Discussing your treatment plan

When you enter the hospital you sign a general consent to treatment. In some cases, such as surgery or experimental treatment, you may be asked to confirm in writing that you understand what is planned and agree to it. This process protects your right to consent to or refuse a treatment. Your doctor will explain the medical consequences of refusing recommended treatment. It also protects your right to decide if you want to participate in research study.

Getting information from you

Your caregivers need complete and correct information about your health and coverage so that they can make good decisions about your care. That includes:

- Past illnesses, surgeries or hospital stays
- Past allergic reactions
- Any medicines or dietary supplements (such as vitamins and herbs) that you are taking
- Any network or admission requirements under your health plan

Understanding your health care goals and values

You may have health care goals and values or spiritual beliefs that are important to your well-being. They will be taken into account as much as possible throughout your hospital stay. Make sure your doctor, your family, and your care team know your wishes.

Understanding who should make decisions when you cannot

If you have signed a health care power of attorney stating who should speak for you if you become unable to make health care decisions for yourself, or a "living will" or "advance directive" that states your wishes about end-of-life-care, give copies to your doctor, your family, and your care team. If you or your family need help making difficult decisions, counselors, chaplains and others are available to help.

(continues)

Box 59–1 *(continued)*

Protection of Your Privacy
We respect the confidentiality of your relationship with your doctor and other caregivers, and the sensitive information about your health and health care that are part of that relationship. State and federal laws and hospital operating policies protect the privacy of your medical information. You will receive a Notice of Privacy Practices that describes the ways that we use, disclose, and safeguard patient information and that explains how you can obtain a copy of information from our records about your care.

Preparing You and Your Family for When You Leave the Hospital
Your doctor works with hospital staff and professionals in your community. You and your family also play an important role in your care. The success of your treatment often depends on your efforts to follow medication, diet, and therapy plans. Your family may need to help care for you at home.

You can expect us to help you identify sources of follow-up care and to let you know if your hospital has a financial interest in any referrals. As long as you agree that we can share information about your care with them, you will coordinate our activities with your caregivers outside the hospital. You can also expect to receive information and, where possible, training about the self-care you will need when you go home.

Help with Your Bill and Filing Insurance Claims
Our staff will file claims for you with health care insurers or other programs such as Medicare and Medicaid. They also will help your doctor with needed documentation. Hospital bills and insurance coverage are often confusing. If you have questions about your bill, contact our business office. If you need help understanding your insurance coverage or health plan, start with your insurance company or health benefits manager. If you do not have health coverage, we will try to help you and your family find financial help or make other arrangements. We need your help with collecting needed information and other requirements to obtain coverage or assistance.

Courtesy of the American Hospital Association. *The Patient Care Partnership*. Chicago: American Hospital Association; 2003.

action for participating in good faith compliance with ORS 127.800 to 127.897. This includes being present when a qualified patient takes the prescribed medication to end his or her life in a humane and dignified manner."[18] Many caregivers may not feel comfortable about caring for patients who have made decisions about assisted suicide, chemical contraception, or abortion, and some clinicians will have misgivings about participating in practices that violate their own ethical, moral, or spiritual beliefs.

With the exception of three states (Alabama, New Hampshire, and Vermont), state statutes known as protection of rights of conscience laws exist to protect individuals engaged in medical and allied health practice.[19] Respiratory therapists and other clinicians are not bound to participate in acts they believe are outside their moral or religious beliefs. An example of such a statute in Florida states, "The provisions of this section shall not be interpreted so as to prevent a physician or other person from refusing to furnish any contraceptive or family planning service, supplies, or information for medical or religious reasons; and the physician or other person shall not be held liable for such refusal."[20] Individuals concerned about rights of conscience laws in their state should consult their state respiratory care board and the practice act, and read the statutes concerning rights of conscience in their state.

Advance Directives

An **advance directive** is one or more documents that communicate a person's foresight and planning and document his or her thoughts, ideas, and wishes concerning what the individual wants done in the event he or she is unable to verbally or otherwise direct his or her medical treatment, resuscitation, nutritional support, or other specifics related to his or her health and welfare. Such documents are generally designed by knowledgeable case managers, social workers, legal entities, or healthcare agencies.

People should discuss the content of their advance directives with their spouse, children, family members, and a legal advisor if desired. Likewise, people should speak with their primary healthcare provider about the content of their advance directive. Advance directives communicate people's wishes to those they would like to speak for them, interpret their documents, consult, or be physically present when they are in an extreme or incapacitated state. A well-designed advance directive gives clear instructions that detail many health-related issues. Some forms, such as those published by several state attorneys general, incorporate a living will; pain management directives; acceptance or rejection of nutritional support and hydration; designation of a healthcare proxy; and **Do Not Intubate (DNI), Do Not Resuscitate (DNR)**, or **Comfort Measures Only (CMO)** forms into the published state-sponsored advance directive document (**Appendix 59–1**).

A frequently discussed advance directive is a DNR order. Advance directives do not routinely include a DNR order, and a patient can have a DNR order without other advance directives. Generally, a patient speaks with his or her family and physician to have a DNR inserted into the medical record. The order would clearly state that if the patient's heart stops beating or he or she stops breathing, he or she would not receive cardiopulmonary resuscitation, no effort to institute an airway, no assisted breathing, and no chest compressions, formerly called external cardiac massage. Advance directives may specify Do Not Intubate or No Tracheostomy, or other types of limited resuscitation. However, it is important to clarify exactly what the patient wants done, and not confuse the staff regarding the patient's true code status. Unusual practices or variations in resuscitation status, such as the Show Code or Slow Code, are widely discussed in the literature and strongly discouraged.[21,22]

Advance directive documents do not come in a one-size-fits-all format, and even the best advance directive document needs to be customized for the individual patient and reviewed carefully, because the value of resuscitation or medical intervention may change as a person grows older or acquires a new diagnosis. The **living will** is a document that details the types of medical treatments and life-prolonging measures that one does or does not want performed if one were to be incapacitated. Designating a **surrogate** decision maker, or **durable medical power of attorney**, requires a legal document allowing someone to serve as your decision maker, or **proxy**, in the event you are incapable of making a decision. Any and all facets of the advance directive can be modified or terminated if there is a change in the health of the patient. Likewise, advance directives enabling a durable medical power of attorney do not restrict or involve matters of ownership of property or finance.

RESPIRATORY RECAP

Autonomy

- Autonomy is the ability and right to govern oneself.
- The Patient Care Partnership outlines the rights and responsibilities of patients regarding their medical care.
- For a patient to refuse treatment, that individual must understand the nature of the condition and the consequences of various options.
- Advance directives, living wills, and medical power of attorney specify which treatments patients desire.

Regardless of the sophistication of the family and the level of advance directive preparation, decision making at the end of life is difficult for all parties, including medical clinicians. A physician wrote an account of the difficult experience of acknowledging his mother's desire to discontinue intravenous antibiotics and of supporting her wish to expedite her death by stopping all hydration and nutrition.[23] Ganzini and associates studied nurses who worked with hospice patients who had decided to expedite their death by stopping food and fluids. These nurses reported that they felt the quality of the process of dying for most patients was good, and the authors suggested that caregivers evaluate the standards of care and policies when caring for these special types of patients.[24]

Advance directives grew from efforts by the courts and government to resolve ethical dilemmas. In 1990 the U.S. Supreme Court, in an attempt to determine whether a patient has a right to refuse medical treatment, handed down a landmark decision in *Cruzan v. Director, Missouri Dept. of Health* that recognized a competent patient's right to refuse medical treatment.[25] Although the decision clarified the rights of competent patients, it raised many questions about informed consent, which is based on the ethical principle of autonomy. An opposing ethical principle no longer considered valid is the principle of paternalism, which stems from the word *parent* and assumes that an individual with more knowledge, in this case the healthcare professional, is more capable than the patient of making decisions for the patient.

As a result of the Court's decision and the autonomy/paternalism conflict related to informed consent, Congress passed the Patient Self-Determination Act, effective December 1991.[26] The act requires healthcare facilities receiving Medicaid or Medicare reimbursement to inform patients of their right to refuse treatment and of the availability of advance directives. Because these facilities depend financially on Medicaid and Medicare reimbursement, all states immediately passed statutes recognizing advance directives.

Pain Management

Patients' perception of their pain is a critical facet of providing comfort at the end of life. Kay Miller discussed the improved comfort of her husband, an anesthesiologist, after working with a palliative care team's respiratory therapist, who recommended nebulized morphine sulfate by aerosol inhalation.[27] Moneymaker suggested that patients may include a set of orders in their advance directive that specify comfort measures only when the patient notes the following: a cure or prolongation of life is no longer a reachable goal, and comfort is the patient's priority; when the expected quality of the rest of the patient's life is at a level that is not acceptable to the patient; and when the durable power of attorney for healthcare indicates that comfort is a priority in this situation.[28]

When a patient is in pain, the alleviation of pain becomes an important goal regardless of the patient's stage of life. The Joint Commission has encouraged patients to discuss pain management goals as well as other health issues through a national campaign entitled Speak Up. The Speak Up initiative provides a framework that urges patients to take a more active and involved role in their care. The mnemonic Speak Up represents the following:[29]

- **S**peak up if you have questions or concerns, and if you don't understand, ask again. It's your body and you have a right to know.
- **P**ay attention to the care you are receiving. Make sure you're getting the right treatments by the right healthcare professionals. Don't assume anything.
- **E**ducate yourself about your diagnosis, the medical tests you are undergoing, and your treatment plan.
- **A**sk a trusted family member or friend to be your advocate.
- **K**now what medications you take and why you take them. Medication errors are the most common healthcare errors.
- **U**se a hospital, clinic, surgery center, or other type of healthcare organization that has undergone a rigorous on-site evaluation against established state-of-the-art quality and safety standards, such as that provided by the Joint Commission.
- **P**articipate in all decisions about your treatment. You are the center of the healthcare team.

Specific issues related to pain management are addressed in a brochure entitled *What You Should Know About Pain Management*, which encourages patients to ask their caregivers specific questions about pain medication, including the doses and times at which medication should be taken, the side effects, how long the medication will take to work, and what to do if the medication does not work.[30]

Confidentiality

Confidentiality ensures that the information entrusted to healthcare professionals in the line of duty is not revealed to others except when necessary to carry out their duties. This principle has a long past and is included in the Hippocratic Oath, which states, "What I may see or hear in the course of treatment . . . I will keep to myself holding such things shameful to be spoken aloud."[1] The principle of confidentiality remains one of the most cherished medical ethical principles, and the Patient Care Partnership guarantees confidentiality by stating, "We respect the confidentiality of your relationship with your doctor and other caregivers, and the sensitive information about your health and health care that are part of that relationship."[17]

Need for Confidentiality

Maintaining confidentiality is important because it contributes to necessary trust in the practice of medicine. Patients often reveal personal or embarrassing information in the course of receiving medical treatment. If this information is not guarded, patients will lose this trust and may not provide healthcare professionals with the information they need to be properly diagnosed and treated. Many laws have been passed to protect patient confidentiality, including the Privacy Act of 1974, the Conditions of Participation for Hospitals in Medicare and Medicaid Programs, the Conditions of Participation for Long Term Care Facilities, and the Uniform Health Care Information Act.

RESPIRATORY RECAP

Confidentiality

- » Confidentiality ensures that the information entrusted to healthcare professionals in the line of duty is not revealed to others except when necessary to carry out such duties.
- » Maintaining confidentiality is important because it contributes to the trust patients need in the medical community.
- » Confidentiality has become more difficult to maintain due to technologic advances.

Violations of Confidentiality

Confidentiality is the most violated of the ethical principles. As the medical system has expanded in recent years, so has the number of individuals with access to medical records. Estimations are that more than 75 individuals see a medical chart during a patient's hospital stay.[15] Confidentiality has become more difficult to maintain due to technologic advances; although fax machines, cellular phones, and computers have made healthcare jobs easier, they also have helped decrease patient confidentiality.[31] For example, celebrity medical records have been viewed by unauthorized personnel, videos and pictures of accident victims have been taken using cell phone cameras, patient records have been faxed accidentally to restaurants, and conversations concerning patients have been overheard in elevators and nursing stations.

Computers offer even faster and more dangerous access to medical records. Databases can be accumulated containing information gathered legitimately by businesses. For example, drug companies may enter prescription purchases into a billing database; if an insurance company obtained these records, they could screen potential clients for high-risk conditions and deny them coverage.

Breaking Confidentiality

Although respect for confidentiality is an important tenet, at times healthcare professionals must break confidentiality. In such situations the clinician must balance the need to protect others from foreseeable harm with the need to protect confidentiality. For example, if a patient threatens to harm someone, the healthcare worker has a responsibility to warn the individual potentially in danger.

An example is the case of *Tarasoff v. Regents of the University of California*.[32,33] In this case, a psychologist had reason to believe that one of his patients would kill a woman whose name was Tatiana Tarasoff. The psychologist had the campus police arrest his patient, but the police later released the man when he assured them he would not contact Tarasoff. Neither the campus police nor the psychologist warned Tarasoff of the potential danger to her, and the man in question later killed Tarasoff. The woman's family brought a lawsuit against the University of California, resulting in an important decision in which the courts ruled that healthcare providers have a duty to warn individuals of foreseeable danger.

Breaking confidentiality is often necessary when the public's welfare may be jeopardized. Many states have laws requiring certain diseases, such as tuberculosis or sexually transmitted diseases, to be reported to public health agencies so that others who might have been exposed to the disease can be informed and can receive the necessary treatment. Most states have laws requiring healthcare workers who suspect child or elder abuse to file confidential reports. In such cases a concern exists for the public's welfare, so confidentiality may be violated. Most state licensure boards and hospital codes of ethics provide guidance for clinicians who observe what they believe is an ethical violation or potentially dangerous situation; this is covered in most human resources departmental orientations.

RESPIRATORY RECAP

Breaking Confidentiality

- » When confidentiality is broken, one must balance the need to protect others from foreseeable harm with the need to protect confidentiality.
- » Confidentiality may be broken when a concern exists for the public's welfare.

Justice

Justice is the principle that deals with fairness and equity in the distribution of scarce resources, such as time, services, equipment, and money. Although this concept may seem simple, in reality it is one of the most difficult principles to implement, creating numerous questions. For example, which criteria should be used to decide who receives life-saving organ transplants? Should a person's lifestyle (e.g., being overweight, smoking, drinking) be considered? Researchers have suggested that a patient's lifestyle choices, particularly smoking, should be considered prior to the prescription of home oxygen therapy. The danger to the patient and others, such as housemates and neighbors, from an oxygen-accelerated house fire should be considered and inform a physician's decision to prescribe or withhold domiciliary oxygen for active smokers.[34–37]

Theories of Justice

How should limited healthcare resources be distributed? Several theories deal with this question, with the egalitarian theory stating that all individuals should have equal access to goods and services. However, this theory does not always translate neatly into reality. For instance, healthcare availability in rural areas of the country is not the same as availability in metropolitan areas.

Other theories approach the question from different angles. The utilitarian theory of justice states that the distribution of resources should be such that it achieves the greatest good for the greatest number of individuals. The libertarian theory emphasizes personal rights to society and economic liberty. Another theory is the maximin principle of justice.[38] Using this theory, the individual maximizes the minimum, even if doing so does not maximize the total amount of good done. In other words, the individual needing the resources is helped the most, even if others are not helped. Another way to look at this theory is that the maximum amount of healthcare would go to a minimum number of patients (i.e., the most needy or critical).

With healthcare resources stretched these days, decisions about who gets the resources are never easy decisions. This question has created robust discussions in Congress, public rallies, and at the supper table in homes nationwide. The distribution of healthcare can be seen in changes in payment structures for Medicare and insurance companies, which have influenced the country's healthcare system. The distribution of justice affects all levels of healthcare and remains one of the more problematic ethical principles facing healthcare professionals today.

RESPIRATORY RECAP

Justice

- » Justice is the principle that deals with fairness and equity in the distribution of scarce resources, such as time, services, equipment, and money.
- » The egalitarian theory of justice states that all individuals should have equal access to goods and services.
- » The utilitarian theory of justice states that the distribution of resources should be such that it achieves the greatest good for the greatest number of individuals.
- » The maximin principle states that the individual most needing the resources should be helped, even if others are not helped.

Managed Care and Justice

The implementation of managed care has changed the distribution of medical resources. Managed care uses a variety of techniques that influence the clinical behavior of healthcare providers and patients. These techniques, including utilization restraints and preapproval criteria, often integrate the payment and delivery of healthcare and are used with the overall goal of cost efficiency.

To keep costs down, managed care reduces resources such as time spent with patients, medications, tests, and treatments and offers incentives to physicians who are cost-effective. Many physicians receive bonuses if they stay within the guidelines of the managed care provider. Those who are not cost-efficient may be penalized with reduced income or receive peer pressure from superiors to become more cost-efficient.

> **RESPIRATORY RECAP**
>
> **Managed Care and Justice**
>
> » Managed care uses techniques that influence the clinical behavior of healthcare providers and patients.
> » To meet efficiency goals, managed care companies often offer incentives to physicians who control costs.
> » As managed care grows, so will the ethical dilemmas associated with justice.

The distribution of healthcare resources often is debated, but managed care has fueled this controversy as efforts to contain the rising costs of healthcare compete with its fair distribution. Companies and policies, instead of healthcare professionals, often dictate the decisions as to how resources are distributed. As managed care continues to expand, healthcare professionals will continue to face more ethical dilemmas, particularly those dealing with justice.

Role Fidelity

Fidelity to Patients

Fidelity implies an obligation or faithfulness to duty. Each member of the healthcare team has a role with specific tasks and responsibilities, or a scope of practice, that is usually set by tradition or the state legislature that regulates healthcare practice. Each clinician has a duty to practice within this role (role fidelity). Keeping within the scope of practice is considered in the best interests of the patient. The American Association for Respiratory Care (AARC) has made this preference clear in its statement on ethics, as shown in **Box 59–2**: "Respiratory therapists shall perform only those procedures or functions in which they are individually competent and that are within the scope of accepted and responsible practice."[39] The nature of this role is one in which a relationship is established between the healthcare provider and the patient and in which the patient expects truth and loyalty from the provider. Patients place trust in their providers to perform their duties to the best of their abilities and refrain from duties not in their expertise.

BOX 59–2

AARC Position Statement of Ethics and Professional Conduct

In the conduct of professional activities the Respiratory Therapist shall be bound by the following ethical and professional principles. Respiratory Therapists shall:

- Demonstrate behavior that reflects integrity, supports objectivity, and fosters trust in the profession and its professionals
- Actively maintain and continually improve their professional competence and represent it accurately
- Perform only those procedures or functions in which they are individually competent and that are within the scope of accepted and responsible practice
- Respect and protect the legal and personal rights of patients they treat, including the right to privacy, informed consent and refusal of treatment
- Divulge no protected information regarding any patient or family unless disclosure is required for the responsible performance of duty authorized by the patient and/or family, or required by law
- Provide care without discrimination on any basis, with respect for the rights and dignity of all individuals
- Promote disease prevention and wellness
- Refuse to participate in illegal or unethical acts
- Refuse to conceal, and will report, the illegal, unethical, fraudulent, or incompetent acts of others
- Follow sound scientific procedures and ethical principles in research
- Comply with state or federal laws which govern and relate to their practice
- Avoid any form of conduct that is fraudulent or creates a conflict of interest, and shall follow the principles of ethical business behavior
- Promote health care delivery through improvement of the access, efficacy, and cost of patient care
- Encourage and promote appropriate stewardship of resources

From American Association for Respiratory Care. *AARC Statement of Ethics and Professional Conduct.* Effective December 1994; revised December 2007 and July 2009. Available at: http://www.aarc.org/resources/position_statements/ethics.html. Reprinted with permission.

Fidelity to Colleagues

Role fidelity also exists among colleagues, with an obligation of loyalty to coworkers and the profession. At times this loyalty may interfere with loyalty to the patient, and loyalty to colleagues does have exceptions. For example, most state license boards and professional organizations have ethical codes that require members to report incompetent or dishonest practices or impaired colleagues. In such cases, loyalty to the patient would outweigh loyalty to colleagues. The AARC states in its position statement that the respiratory therapist "shall refuse to conceal illegal, unethical or incompetent acts of others."[39]

Conflicts with Fidelity

Role fidelity creates a number of problems. In many cases, roles that once were clearly established by tradition are now changing. Managed care and a desire for cost efficiency have created overlapping jobs. Various professionals now perform tasks that were once assigned to one particular profession, creating conflicts with role fidelity.

Other practices, such as joint ventures and referrals, have added to the fidelity question. Joint ventures involve physicians who have investments in healthcare services to which they may refer their patients (e.g., a physician who owns a radiology center and refers all of his patients to that facility for radiographs). Referrals also create problems with role fidelity. For instance, a therapist refers or recommends a home health company or equipment company to a patient and then collects a finder's fee from that company. To deal with this problem, the AARC issued a statement regarding the ethical performance of therapists and prohibiting this type of conduct. In some states, self-referral and finder's fees are illegal, resulting in legal violations in addition to ethical misconduct.

RESPIRATORY RECAP

Role Fidelity

- » Fidelity implies an obligation or faithfulness to duty.
- » Each clinician has a duty to practice within the role that is set by tradition or by the state legislature that regulates healthcare practice.
- » Problems with role fidelity occur more often today because of changes in traditional roles, conflicts of interest, and referrals.

Role of Professional Organizations in Ethics

Need for Professional Ethics

Professional medical organizations recognize the need for guidelines in helping their members maintain high ethical standards. The respiratory care profession, although still new compared with other professions, has established a code of ethics for its members. New professions must establish themselves as entities that embrace guidelines and standards and are willing to set direction and provide some degree of self-governance for their members. Along the same lines, new professionals must establish themselves as responsible clinicians who adhere to guidelines and standards. Important characteristics of a professional include the abilities to operate with integrity and demonstrate self-governance and direction.

RESPIRATORY RECAP

Professional Organizations' Role in Ethics

- » Professional medical organizations recognize the need for guidelines in helping their members maintain high ethical standards.
- » The AARC Code of Ethics tends to the legal and professional growth needs of the profession.

AARC Code of Ethics

The **AARC Code of Ethics**[39] has evolved through several revisions over the life of the respiratory therapy profession. In its present form (refer to Box 59–2), it closely resembles the ethical theories and principles discussed in this chapter and embraces the major legal concerns that all professionals face today in the performance of their professional duties. The following discussion analyzes each of the code's discrete components.

Item 1: Demonstrate behavior that reflects integrity, supports objectivity, and fosters trust in the profession and its professionals

Item 1 of the statement addresses the need for integrity, objectivity, trust, and role fidelity for respiratory care professionals. These traits can be incorporated into the principle of veracity, or truth. By fostering integrity, healthcare clinicians demonstrate that in performing their duties, they adhere to unimpaired standards of care that are free of flaws. Fidelity is upheld as long as clinicians work within their professional competence.

A common trait is that all professionals adhere to a community standard of care. *Community* in this case may refer to both the profession as well as a physical community, such as a state or region of the country. Adherence to a community standard of care can be extremely important when clinicians are required to defend themselves in legal actions. Objectivity in the delivery of care ensures that the clinician does not discriminate on any basis—ethnicity, gender, or type of disease. The objective clinician simply delivers the best care possible to whoever needs it. Public trust in the professional is essential both to establish and maintain professional status and to maximize adherence to the service and directions of the professional.

Item 2: Seek educational opportunities to improve and maintain their professional competence and document their participation accurately

Item 3: Perform only those procedures or functions in which they are individually competent and that are within the scope of accepted and responsible practice

Items 2 and 3 reflect the need for research and continuing education, along with the requirement for professionals to self-govern themselves by acknowledging their own limitations. These items also address fidelity in reflecting the need for continuing education because the therapist's scope of practice will grow. Therapists must continue to enhance their education by learning about new procedures, treatments, and equipment. With continual learning, beneficence and nonmaleficence are served; therapists will be better able to treat their patients and provide them with the best care while avoiding unnecessary therapy or harm.

Item 4: Respect and protect the legal and personal rights of patients they treat, including the right to privacy, informed consent and refusal of treatment

Item 4 of the AARC statement emphasizes the need for informed consent, which relates to autonomy, the patient's right to decide care. This item respects the patient's right to make decisions regarding care, including the right to refuse treatments.

Item 5: Divulge no protected information regarding any patient or family unless disclosure is required for the responsible performance of duty authorized by the patient and/or family, or required by law

Item 5 refers to one of the oldest and best-established ethical principles, confidentiality, a mainstay of healthcare delivery. The respiratory therapist has a duty to uphold the confidentiality of information shared in the course of treatment unless sharing the information is required to perform the job or disclosure is required by law.

Item 6: Provide care without discrimination on any basis, with respect for the rights and dignity of all individuals

Item 6 refers to the principles of justice and autonomy. The distribution of healthcare resources should be provided without discrimination. At the same time, respiratory therapists must respect the autonomy and dignity of the patient.

Item 7: Promote disease prevention and wellness

Item 7 supports the principles of role fidelity, justice, beneficence, and nonmaleficence. Role fidelity is addressed by the need for respiratory therapists to educate the public about disease prevention and wellness. Because therapists are the allied health experts, their involvement in the cardiopulmonary aspect of health is vital. By educating individuals about disease prevention and wellness, the public may become healthier, thus lowering the demand for respiratory resources. Justice can be served by provision of these services to those who need them. Through education, clinicians can provide good to their patients and prevent harm, thus serving beneficence and nonmaleficence.

Item 8: Refuse to participate in illegal or unethical acts

Item 9: Refuse to conceal, and will report, the illegal, unethical, fraudulent, or incompetent acts of others

Item 12: Avoid any form of conduct that is fraudulent or creates a conflict of interest, and shall follow the principles of ethical business behavior

Items 8, 9, and 12 discuss the importance of fidelity and veracity. With fidelity, patients expect loyalty from their therapists, a trait evident in competent, ethical respiratory therapists. Therapists also have a duty to the profession to identify members of the profession who are not maintaining competency and ethical behavior, thus enforcing nonmaleficence.

Item 10: Follow sound scientific procedures and ethical principles in research

Item 11: Comply with state or federal laws which govern and relate to their practice

Items 10 and 11 again deal with fidelity. State and federal laws dictate the scope of practice, and respiratory therapists should be familiar with these laws, particularly state laws. Item 10 also addresses the need for ethical research, which has led to many breakthrough discoveries and enhanced beneficence. Ethical standards must be maintained so that patients can benefit from research, not be harmed by it.

In addition, sound research includes veracity. Research subjects must be informed of the risks of any research and have the opportunity to ask questions and receive truthful answers. Individuals have the right to refuse to participate in research studies without any adverse effects or discontinuance of their healthcare.

Item 13: Promote health care delivery through improvement of the access, efficacy, and cost of patient care

Item 14: Encourage and promote appropriate stewardship of resources

Items 13 and 14 deal with justice. The current distribution of resources in the United States is imperfect and unequal. To deal with this problem, the AARC has stated that every respiratory therapist has a duty to try to improve the principle of justice.[39] Respiratory therapists should be aware of the distribution of healthcare resources and constantly seek measures to improve their delivery and access. They should be conscious of the cost of the care provided and seek cost-efficient, effective ways to deliver care.

Ethics Committees

In 1991, the Joint Commission on Accreditation of Healthcare Organizations (JCAHO), now the Joint Commission (TJC), adopted guidelines requiring each accredited organization to establish a mechanism to consider ethical issues in patient care and education for healthcare clinicians. Most facilities responded by establishing **ethics committees** (sometimes called **optimum care committees**), the composition, duties, and activities of which vary widely from institution to institution. A typical committee is composed of approximately 12 members, including medical staff, administration, and various service departments. A member of the clergy also may serve on the ethics committee, along with a medical ethicist (often an ethics professor or researcher) and representatives of the community. Townsend noted that "[t]oleration of and receptivity to divergent viewpoints, important for cultural diversity and understanding, can also serve to win the trust of various constituencies."[40] Thus, committee members should exhibit these characteristics. The knowledge and insight of the respiratory therapist regarding advanced resuscitation, life support, and weaning procedures, particularly terminal weaning,[41] would be critical and useful resources to any ethics or optimal care committee.

Committees may develop policies and procedures, sponsor educational activities, and serve as clearinghouses for the distribution of information on ethical issues. The committee may consider specific ethical dilemmas, but when ethics committees become involved in patient care, their only goal is to issue a recommendation. Further research on the outcomes and effectiveness of ethics committees is recommended, because ethics committee are now being strongly recommended or required by accreditation agencies such as the Joint Committee.

RESPIRATORY RECAP

Ethics Committees

» Ethics committees were formed to consider ethical issues in patient care and education for the healthcare professional.
» Ethics committees may develop policies and procedures, sponsor educational activities, and serve as clearinghouses for the distribution of information on ethical issues.

Adherence to ethical standards improves patient outcomes, decreases the likelihood that a facility will encounter accountability problems, and assures patients that they can trust their healthcare system. Given the current state of healthcare accountability, it is more important than ever that healthcare providers, including respiratory therapists, take every precaution possible to ensure that the services they provide meet the highest ethical standards.

CASE STUDIES

Case 1. A Fifty for Your Trouble

Bernie is a student in clinical training, based in a large metropolitan hospital. He has been on the floor for 3 weeks and twice previously cared for an older gentleman with chronic obstructive lung disease, named Mr. Meehan. Today, after he delivered a medicated aerosol treatment to Mr. Meehan, he was washing his hands and his clinical instructor had just stepped out of the room to answer a page. Mr. Meehan's wife approached and put a $50 bill in Bernie's pocket, stating, "I know you students have a tough time financially, and my husband just wanted to say 'Thank you' for the excellent care you have been giving him. Let's just keep this our little secret." What would you have done and why would you (or would you not) do it?

Bernie's future as a therapist would be compromised by accepting money for performing duties that will be documented and billed by the hospital. A caregiver should gently but firmly tell Mrs. Meehan that accepting gifts or money is strictly forbidden because accepting this gift creates a conflict of interest. The AARC has suggested that respiratory therapists avoid any conflict of interest, and a student accepting a gift of money from a patient would also be a breach of the principles of ethical business behavior.[39] The student is duty bound to reveal anything outside the ordinary that occurs while under the instructor's supervision, because a student's role fidelity requires that he or she not conceal information from the instructor.

Case 2. A Double-Edged Sword

Beth is a respiratory therapist working in a regional burn center. One of her patients has second-degree burns on his lower extremities and is in considerable pain. He is crying and thrashing about in his bed, begging Beth, "Please give me something for the pain!" Beth is concerned that the patient will pull out his intravenous tube and hurt himself if he doesn't stop thrashing. The intern on call orders more morphine, but Beth is concerned that the additional morphine could depress the patient's respiratory drive. Should the additional morphine be given?

Using the guiding principles presented in this chapter, delivery of the narcotic would be beneficial for the patient because it would relieve his pain and keep the patient from dislodging his intravenous catheter. The narcotic is administered for a good purpose, the relief of pain, and the undesirable side effect of respiratory depression is not intended. In this particular case, pain relief outweighs the possibility of respiratory depression. The morphine was given and the patient should be carefully monitored for any potential undesirable side effects.

Case 3. To Intubate or Not to Intubate

Mrs. Schuster is 68 years old and has a history of chronic obstructive pulmonary disease, congestive heart failure, and renal disease. She has been admitted to the hospital numerous times in the past 3 years, and the respiratory therapy staff members know her well. On previous admissions, she stated to several respiratory therapy staff members that she never wanted to be intubated or placed on mechanical ventilation.

Mrs. Schuster's current admission is for pneumonia. The respiratory therapist assigned to give Mrs. Schuster her nebulizer treatments receives a stat page; on arrival in the patient's room, the therapist finds Mrs. Schuster's daughter and physician in a discussion outside. Mrs. Schuster is unresponsive and in impending respiratory failure. The physician explains that the antibiotics have not had time to treat Mrs. Schuster's pneumonia and that without mechanical ventilation, she will suffer respiratory failure and die.

The physician says that they must decide whether to intubate Mrs. Schuster. The daughter insists, "I want everything done for my mother! Put her on the breathing machine!" The physician agrees with the daughter and asks the respiratory therapist to intubate and ventilate the woman per the respiratory care protocol. The therapist informs the physician of Mrs. Schuster's previous requests regarding intubation and mechanical ventilation, but the physician angrily states, "Mrs. Schuster doesn't have an advance directive. It is the daughter's decision to make. We can treat the pneumonia and then probably extubate her." Should Mrs. Schuster be intubated and placed on mechanical ventilation? Which ethical principles are involved? What decision-making processes are the respiratory therapist and physician each using to make their judgments?

This case involves several ethical principles, including autonomy, beneficence, and nonmaleficence. The respiratory therapist, knowing that Mrs. Schuster previously requested not to be intubated or placed on mechanical ventilation, may think that Mrs. Schuster's autonomy is being compromised with intubation. Although the patient did not formally put her wishes in writing, she made her wishes well known to the respiratory staff members. Whether the patient fully understood the nature of her condition and the consequences of this decision are not known. These two criteria are required for a patient to make an autonomous decision to refuse therapy. If she understood that her medical condition could at some point in time require intubation with mechanical ventilation and that refusing this therapy could result in her death, then she made a conscious decision invoking her autonomy. She had the right to make this decision for herself.

The physician's decision to intubate could be based on the principle of beneficence, which involves the performance of procedures and treatments to benefit the patient. The assumption may be made that Mrs. Schuster did not inform the physician of her past decision to refuse intubation and mechanical ventilation. The physician believes the pneumonia can be treated and that Mrs. Schuster will be extubated. By performing these procedures, the physician thinks that in the long run, the patient will benefit and that beneficence must be upheld in this matter. From this viewpoint, not treating Mrs. Schuster would result in harm.

The physician is guided by a consequential, or teleological, theory and is basing the decision to intubate on the possible consequences or outcomes of the actions. If the patient is not placed on mechanical ventilation, the physician believes she will die. If she is placed on mechanical ventilation and treated for her pneumonia, the physician believes that recovery and subsequent extubation are likely. According to the physician's beliefs, the consequences or likely outcomes of this situation should direct the decision making. Based on this reasoning, the physician has sufficient reason to intubate.

The respiratory therapist is guided by the principle of duty, or deontology, in the decision to inform the doctor of Mrs. Schuster's wishes. The therapist believes in a duty to the patient to abide by previously stated wishes and that the patient's autonomous decision should be upheld, despite her daughter's wishes. Because the therapist appears to have known Mrs. Schuster and has discussed intubation with her in the past, the respiratory therapist may be aware of possible psychological or financial impacts on Mrs. Schuster if her autonomy is not upheld. By refusing to uphold the patient's autonomous decision regarding life support, the therapist may believe that the principle of nonmaleficence is being violated and that intubating the patient against her wishes would harm her.

This situation is not uncommon in today's medical practice. The absence of advance directives and poor communication among family members and attending physicians often leads to ethical dilemmas in which all parties involved in the patient's care must balance the beneficence of an action with its nonmaleficence.

Case 4. Nosy Therapists

Connor and Christine are respiratory therapists working in a hospital. They have discovered that they can uncover personal information about their coworkers by using the hospital computer. They already have learned that two of their coworkers are living together and that one of these individuals has a history of psychological problems. In addition, they have discovered that the husband of another coworker, Denise, recently tested positive for human immunodeficiency virus (HIV) and are concerned that Denise, who frequently draws patients' blood for arterial blood gas measurements, may be HIV positive and could be a risk to patients. They wonder whether they should inform their boss.

In this case, two employees have learned to use the computer for some dangerous snooping. In the process they have not only most likely violated hospital policy regarding computer access but also violated patient confidentiality. They have learned that one of their coworkers has been exposed to HIV, are concerned about patient risk, and are making some assumptions regarding that coworker, including the assumption that their boss does not know about her husband's positive HIV test. This may not be the case. They also are assuming that Denise has tested HIV positive, which may not be true. Furthermore, none of these matters involves them because they are not supervisors, and neither has a right or need to know the information in question. From a deontological viewpoint, Connor and Christine could argue they should inform their boss of their discovery. They believe that patients are at risk for harm and that they have a duty to protect their patients. Informing their supervisor could protect Denise's patients from potential harm.

A teleological view of this scenario involves listing all of the consequences. Connor and Christine believe that if they do not tell their boss, Denise could be placing her patients at risk. They could tell their boss but would most likely have to admit how they gained this information, which would place them both at risk for punishment. Connor and Christine would have to decide which consequence would have the best outcome.

Case 5. You Can Tell Mom

A patient has been admitted to the hospital with an acute myocardial infarction. The respiratory therapist on duty receives a phone call from his mother, who works with the patient's wife. The respiratory therapist's mother asks the therapist to ensure that the physicians are telling the patient's wife the full story, which she also wants to know.

In this case the respiratory therapist would violate patient confidentiality if he provided his mother with this information. He has a duty to respect the confidentiality of the patient by not revealing anything about the case to his mother. Although his mother's intentions may be good, they do not justify a breach of confidentiality. The therapist should inform his mother why he is not able to give her this information.

Case 6. Who Gets the Therapy?

Tom is a respiratory therapy supervisor at a large metropolitan hospital. When he arrives to start his shift, the departing supervisor notifies him that two members on his shift have called in sick for the night and that replacements for both are unavailable. The hospital is extremely busy that night, with each staff member already taking a full load of patients, and performance of all of the respiratory therapy procedures needed is impossible. Tom must decide how to distribute the available resources.

Policy states that patients who are either in the intensive care unit (ICU) or on mechanical ventilation receive priority over those receiving general floor therapy. Tom knows that several ventilator patients are stable and have not been weaned in several weeks. However, several asthmatic patients cannot afford to be without therapy. He also knows that the nurses in the ICU are educated in respiratory therapy procedures and in a better position to help with treatments than the nurses in the general nursing units.

He could decide that all patients will receive one less treatment during this shift. For instance, a patient who was scheduled to receive three jet nebulizer treatments would receive only two treatments. He also could decide that several patients will not receive any therapy so that the others who need their treatments the most will receive therapy as ordered. Furthermore, he could assign all the procedures and allow his staff members to decide who receives the therapy. What should Tom do?

In making his decision, Tom may choose to look at issues from several viewpoints. If he decides to reduce the therapy received by all patients, he would be taking an egalitarian position. This theory states that all individuals should have equal access to goods and services. In this case, he could argue that all patients would be treated fairly in that they all would receive reduced services.

Tom may choose to assume a maximin position of justice. This theory states that justice would be served if the therapists maximized the minimum. In other words, Tom and the staff would provide therapy to those who need it most. Tom would not deliver therapy to some patients but instead would concentrate his resources on those with the greatest need.

In this case, an institutional respiratory care policy exists that addresses the way in which care should be delivered during a shortage of staff members: respiratory care should be prioritized to treat patients in the ICU first. However, Tom does not think this policy fairly distributes the resources. If Tom were to approach the problem with a utilitarian theory, he would look at the consequences of all the possible alternatives and decide on the choice that maximizes the total amount of good done, regardless of who benefits. Because Tom believes the patients with asthma have the greatest need for respiratory care, he could use the utilitarian theory to support his decision to perform the treatments on the asthmatic patients instead of the stable ventilated ICU patients. According to Tom's values, the asthmatic patients would receive the greatest good from the treatments and thus should receive therapy.

By making a decision in opposition to hospital policy, Tom is placing his values above those of the hospital. By violating policy as a supervisor, he is setting a poor example for his staff members. Failure to follow policies can result in detrimental actions not only to the individual disregarding the policy but also to the hospital. The hospital could face legal action if policies are not followed and patients suffer ill consequences. Tom will have to deal with any consequences that occur as a result of his actions. If he believes the policy is incorrect, he should address this issue with his superiors.

Case 7. A Couple of Beers

After a busy evening shift, respiratory therapist Ryan is glad when Tim arrives to relieve him. While giving his report, Ryan smells alcohol on Tim's breath and notices that Tim's speech is slurred. Ryan knows that Tim had mentioned he was going to watch the football game at a bar with some friends before coming in to work the night shift. Ryan suspects that Tim might have had some alcohol and might not be in shape to work. He decides to question him about his suspicion. Tim admits, "I had a couple of beers. It's no big deal." Ryan asks him whether he is competent to do his job, and Tim replies, "Be a friend. Don't make so much out of this. Don't worry; I can do my job." Ryan is not convinced but is unsure what to do. He doesn't want to jeopardize his friendship with Tim, but he is concerned that Tim could harm a patient. What should Ryan do?

Ryan is torn between fidelity to his patients and fidelity to his coworker. He can allow his colleague to maintain his autonomy and do nothing. However, Ryan is not convinced his colleague has the capacity to make that decision because he believes Tim is impaired by alcohol.

Ryan believes that his patients could be at risk if Tim were allowed to care for them. Following this line of thinking, he believes that fidelity to his patients and nonmaleficence take precedence. The respiratory therapy code of ethics also states he has a duty to the profession to report incompetence among fellow members. Thus,

Ryan would do best to report the incident to his supervisor immediately so that managerial decisions about staffing for the shift can be made.

Case 8. Two Lives Inseparable

Anne is the daughter of the respiratory therapy department director, a seasoned registered respiratory therapist who has been involved in healthcare for many years. Anne is a beautiful young lady who was stricken with systemic lupus erythematosus (SLE) at the age of 17. Within 3 years of diagnosis, Anne quickly developed lupus cerebritis, pericardial and pleural effusions, and renal failure and a commitment to hemodialysis. Anne survived multiple critical care admissions, mechanical ventilation, exploratory craniotomy, *C. difficile* colitis, and long-term anticonvulsant therapy. Anne's serum complement and immune system were delicate, with no detectable immunoglobulin (Ig) A, and declining levels of IgM and IgG. In spite of the many volunteers from a long list of family, friends, and the extended donor community, her immune system problems complicated the search for a compatible donor. Anne remained on continuous cycling peritoneal dialysis (CCPD) and continuous ambulatory peritoneal dialysis (CAPD) for 4.5 years.

Anne and her family discussed and documented what she wanted done at the time of her death, including funeral and burial arrangements, disposition of her estate, and in particular the care of her beloved cats. At 17 years of age, Anne, a deeply spiritual young lady, made peace with her God and decided that if she continued on dialysis therapy and ceased to breathe on her own, or her heart stopped, she declined to be intubated or resuscitated. Her father and family agonized over the dilemma of honoring Anne's wishes for a Do Not Resuscitate advance directive. Having worked for many years in critical care, her father knew that patient outcomes in end-stage renal disease differed, especially in young patients, and that Anne's compliance with regimen made her an excellent transplant candidate once a donor was located. How could her father, mother, and brother stand by and not aggressively resuscitate and care for this precious daughter and sister?

Anne's desire to work with empirical and experimental therapy for the sequelae of lupus led her to participate in research protocols requiring chemotherapy, and in spite of the resulting nausea and side effects, she was a highly compliant patient. Late one evening, Anne received a call from the regional organ transplant coordinator, noting that she had a near-perfect match with a 3-year-old donor, and it was time to go to the hospital and receive her transplant. The transplantation was a success, and after many challenges, Anne initiated contact with the donor family through the regional donor organization. Since her surgery, the two families have enjoyed a warm friendship and regular visits. Anne is married, teaches school, and has had no issues with renal function since 1998.

All of the modern miracles of medicine came together to bring this story to a happy ending. This is an exemplary case to show that any and all facets of the advance directive can be modified or terminated if there is a change in the health of the patient. After Anne's recovery, her father relinquished durable medical power of attorney. The joy of Anne's receiving the transplant is tempered by the reality of the situation, and the death of the 3-year-old has weighed heavily on everyone involved. Anne's father keeps a photo of the child donor on his desk, never forgetting the courage of her parents in making the decision to donate their child's organs or their child's role in uniting these families, two lives made inseparable by the gift of organ donation.

KEY POINTS

- Ethics is the study of the ways individuals and societies make judgments regarding right and wrong.
- Many factors affect decisions about right and wrong, including prejudice and bias, culture, religion, morals, and societal mores.
- Eight important ethical principles help guide healthcare: beneficence, capacity, nonmaleficence, veracity, autonomy, confidentiality, justice, and role fidelity.
- Beneficence is the principle that imposes on the healthcare professional the responsibility to seek good for the patient.
- Capacity is the measureable capability of a patient to make an informed decision that accepts, changes, or withholds therapy, treatment, or medical care.
- Nonmaleficence is the principle that the healthcare professional must refrain from harming the patient.
- Veracity requires the healthcare professional to tell the patient the truth.
- Confidentiality ensures that information revealed to the healthcare professional is not revealed to others except when necessary to perform duties or when silence may result in harm to an individual or the public.
- Justice deals with the fair and equitable distribution of healthcare resources.
- Role fidelity refers to one's faithfulness to duty.
- The Patient Care Partnership defines what a patient can expect prior to and during a hospital admission.
- Professional organizations such as the AARC recognize the need to establish guidelines for professional ethical behavior.
- The AARC Code of Ethics describes ethical behaviors for respiratory therapists that guide professional practice.
- Hospitals have established ethics committees or optimal care committees to deal with ethical issues in patient care and educate healthcare professionals.

- Each respiratory therapist has a duty and responsibility to provide quality healthcare guided by legal and ethical principles.

ACKNOWLEDGMENTS

A special thank you is extended to Kathleen M. Hernlen and Charles Carroll, who developed the framework for this chapter in the first edition of the textbook; to Shirley Masini and Anne Masini Cox for their story and editorial assistance; to Anne Hanne for her proofreading; and to the Office of Constituent Services of the Arizona Attorney General's Office and the Department of Health of the State of Tennessee for permission to use their advance directive forms.

REFERENCES

1. Hippocrates. The oath. In: Jones WHS, trans. *Hippocrates*. Vol. 1. Cambridge, MA: Harvard University Press; 1923:299–301.
2. World Medical Association. *Medical Ethics Manual*. 2009:8–9. Available at: http://www.wma.net/en/30publications/30ethicsmanual/pdf/ethics_manual_en.pdf. Accessed October 8, 2009.
3. *The American Heritage Dictionary of the English Language*. 4th ed. Boston: Houghton Mifflin; 2006.
4. Allport GW. *The Nature of Prejudice*. Reading, MA: Perseus Publishing; 1979.
5. Evans RW. The physician-assisted-killing fallacy. *Life Adv*. 1999;13(6).
6. Sullivan AD, Hedberg K, Fleming K. Legalized physician-assisted suicide in Oregon—the second year. *N Engl J Med*. 2000;342:598–604.
7. Oregon.gov. Death with Dignity Act: records and report data on the act. Available at: http://www.oregon.gov/DHS/ph/pas. Accessed October 8, 2009.
8. Carrol C. Ethical theories and methods. In: Carrol C. *Legal Issues and Ethical Dilemmas in Respiratory Care*. Philadelphia: FA Davis; 1996:68–74.
9. Fletcher JC, Lombardo PA, Marshall MF, Miller FG. *Introduction to Clinical Ethics*. 2nd ed. Hagerstown, MD: University Publishing Group; 1997:30–31, 71–81.
10. Mehta S, Hill NS. Noninvasive ventilation. *Am J Respir Crit Care Med*. 2001;163:540–577.
11. Nava S, Sturani C, Hartl S, et al. End-of-life decision-making in respiratory intermediate care units: a European survey. *Eur Respir J*. 2007;30:156–164.
12. Levy M, Tanios MA, Nelson D, et al. Outcomes of patients with do-not-intubate orders treated with noninvasive ventilation. *Crit Care Med*. 2004;32:2002–2007.
13. Kacmarek RM. Should noninvasive ventilation be used with the Do-Not-Intubate patient? *Respir Care*. 2009;54:223–229.
14. Roth LH, Meisel A, Lidz CW. Tests of competency to consent to treatment. *Am J Psychiatry*. 1977;134:279–284.
15. Edge RS, Groves JR. *Basic Principles of Healthcare Ethics: A Guide for Clinical Practice*. Albany, NY: Delmar; 1994:38.
16. Hebert PC, Hoffmaster B, Glass KC, et al. Bioethics for clinicians: truth telling. *Can Med Assoc J*. 1997;156:225–228.
17. American Hospital Association. *Patient Care Partnership*. Available at: http://www.aha.org/aha/issues/Communicating-With-Patients/pt-care-partnership.html. Accessed October 8, 2009.
18. Oregon Revised Statutes (Death With Dignity Act), 127.885 s.4.01. Immunities; basis for prohibiting health care provider from participation; notification; permissible sanctions. Available at: http://www.consciencelaws.org/conscience-laws-usa/Conscience-Laws-USA-05.html#Oregon. Accessed October 8, 2009.
19. Protection of Conscience Laws, United States. American state protection of conscience laws. Available at: http://www.consciencelaws.org/conscience-laws-usa/Conscience-Laws-USA-01.html. Accessed October 8, 2009.
20. The 2009 Florida Statutes. Title XXIX, §381.0051. Public health general provisions: family planning. Available at: http://www.leg.state.fl.us/Statutes/index.cfm?App_mode=Display_Statute&Search_String=&URL=Ch0381/SEC0051.HTM&Title=-%3E2009-%3ECh0381-%3ESection%200051#0381.0051. Accessed October 8, 2009.
21. Gazelle G. The slow code: should anyone rush to its defense? *N Engl J Med*. 1998;338:467–469.
22. Hardin JD. The slow code: an ethics case conference. *P & S Med Rev*. 1998;5(2). Available at: http://cpmcnet.columbia.edu/news/review/archives/medrev_v5n2_0002.html. Accessed September 30, 2009.
23. Eddy D. A conversation with my mother. *JAMA*. 1994;272:179–181.
24. Ganzini L, Goy ER, Miller LL, et al. Nurses' experiences with hospice patients who refuse food and fluids to hasten death. *N Engl J Med*. 2003;349:359–365.
25. *Cruzan v. Director, Missouri Dept. of Health*, 497 U.S. 261 (1990).
26. Logue BJ. *Last Rights: Death Control and the Elderly in America*. New York: Macmillan; 1993.
27. Miller KL. Pain management from the other side of the mountain. *Am Soc Anesthesiol Newsletter*. August 1997;61(8). Available at: http://www.asahq.org/Newsletters/1997/08_97/PainMgmt_0897.html. Accessed September 30, 2009.
28. Moneymaker KM. Comfort measures only. *J Palliative Med*. 2005;8(3):688.
29. Powers K. The Joint Commission urges patients to Speak Up about pain. Available at: http://www.jointcommission.org/NewsRoom/NewsReleases/nr_pain_management.htm. Accessed October 8, 2009.
30. The Joint Commission. *What You Should Know About Pain Management*. Available at: http://www.jointcommission.org/PatientSafety/SpeakUp/Speak_up_pain_managment.htm.
31. Dodek DY, Dodek A. From Hippocrates to facsimile: protecting patient confidentiality is more difficult and more important than ever. *Can Med Assoc J*. 1997;156:847–852.
32. *Tarasoff v. Regents of the University of California*, 529 P.2d 553; 118 Cal Rpt 129 (1974).
33. *Tarasoff v. Regents of the University of California*. Reargued. 17 Cal.3d 425; 551 P.2d 334; 131 Cal Rpt 333 (1976).
34. Lacasse Y, LaForge J, Maltais F. Got a match? Home oxygen therapy in current smokers. *Thorax*. 2006;61:374–375.
35. U.S. Veteran's Administration National Ethics Teleconference. *Home Oxygen for Patients Who Smoke: Prescription vs. Proscription*. Teleconference minutes of October 23, 2001. Available at: http://www.ethics.va.gov/ETHICS/docs/net/NET_Topic_20011023_Home_Oxygen_For_Smokers.doc. Accessed September 30, 2009.
36. McDonald CF, Crockett AJ, Young I. Adult domiciliary oxygen therapy. Position statement of the Thoracic Society of Australia and New Zealand. *Med J Austr*. 2005;182:621–626.
37. Lambert AEC. Adult domiciliary oxygen therapy: a patient's perspective. *Med J Austr*. 2005;183:472–473.
38. Rawls J. *A Theory of Justice*. Cambridge, MA: Harvard University Press; 1999.
39. American Association for Respiratory Care. AARC position statement of ethics and professional conduct. Available at: http://www.aarc.org/resources/position_statements/ethics.html. Accessed September 30, 2009.
40. Townsend T. Health care ethics committees. In: Roberts LW, Dyer AR, eds. *Ethics in Mental Health Care*. Arlington, VA: American Psychiatric Publishing; 2004:295–311.
41. Keene S, Samples DA, Masini DE, Byington R. Ethical concerns that arise from terminal weaning procedures of a ventilator dependent patient: a respiratory therapist's perspective. *Internet J Law Healthcare Ethics*. 2007;4(2). Available at: http://www.ispub.com/ostia/index.php?xmlFilePath=journals/ijlhe/vol4n2/weaning.xml. Accessed September 30, 2009.

GENERAL INSTRUCTIONS: Use this Durable Health Care Power of Attorney form if you want to select a person to make future health care decisions for you so that if you become too ill or cannot make those decisions for yourself the person you choose and trust can make medical decisions for you. Talk to your family, friends, and others you trust about your choices. Also, it is a good idea to talk with professionals such as your doctor, clergyperson and a lawyer before you sign this form.

Be sure you understand the importance of this document. If you decide this is the form you want to use, complete the form. **Do not sign this form until** your witness or a Notary Public is present to witness the signing. There are further instructions for you about signing this form on page three.

1. Information about me: (I am called the "Principal")

My Name: ____________________ My Age: ____________________
My Address: ____________________ My Date of Birth: ____________________
____________________ My Telephone: ____________________

2. Selection of my health care representative and alternate: (Also called an "agent" or "surrogate")

I choose the following person to act as my representative to make health care decisions for me:

Name: ____________________ Home Telephone: ____________________
Street Address: ____________________ Work Telephone: ____________________
City, State, Zip: ____________________ Cell Telephone: ____________________

I choose the following person to act as an alternate representative to make health care decisions for me if my first representative is unavailable, unwilling, or unable to make decisions for me:

Name: ____________________ Home Telephone: ____________________
Street Address: ____________________ Work Telephone: ____________________
City, State, Zip: ____________________ Cell Telephone: ____________________

3. What I AUTHORIZE if I am unable to make medical care decisions for myself:

I authorize my health care representative to make health care decisions for me when I cannot make or communicate my own health care decisions due to mental or physical illness, injury, disability, or incapacity. I want my representative to make all such decisions for me except those decisions that I have expressly stated in Part 4 below that I do not authorize him/her to make. If I am able to communicate in any manner, my representative should discuss my health care options with me. My representative should explain to me any choices he or she made if I am able to understand. This appointment is effective unless and until it is revoked by me or by an order of a court.

The types of health care decisions I authorize to be made on my behalf include but are not limited to the following:

- To consent or to refuse medical care, including diagnostic, surgical, or therapeutic procedures;
- To authorize the physicians, nurses, therapists, and other health care providers of his/her choice to provide care for me, and to obligate my resources or my estate to pay reasonable compensation for these services;
- To approve or deny my admittance to health care institutions, nursing homes, assisted living facilities, or other facilities or programs. By signing this form I understand that I allow my representative to make decisions about my mental health care except that generally speaking he or she cannot have me admitted to a structured treatment setting with 24-hour-a-day supervision and an intensive treatment program – called a "level one" behavioral health facility – using just this form;

Developed by the Office of Arizona Attorney General
TERRY GODDARD
www.azag.gov
1
Updated December 3, 2007
(All documents completed before December 3, 2007 are still valid)
DURABLE HEALTH CARE POWER OF ATTORNEY

- To have access to and control over my medical records and to have the authority to discuss those records with health care providers.

4. DECISIONS I EXPRESSLY DO NOT AUTHORIZE my Representative to make for me:

I do not want my representative to make the following health care decisions for me (describe or write in "not applicable"):

____
____
____
____
____

5. My specific desires about autopsy:

NOTE: Under Arizona law, an autopsy is not required unless the county medical examiner, the county attorney, or a superior court judge orders it to be performed. See the General Information document for more information about this topic. Initial or put a check mark by one of the following choices.

_____ Upon my death I DO NOT consent to (want) an autopsy.
_____ Upon my death I DO consent to (want) an autopsy.
_____ My representative may give or refuse consent for an autopsy.

6. My specific desires about organ donation: ("anatomical gift")

NOTE: Under Arizona law, you may donate all or part of your body. If you do not make a choice, your representative or family can make the decision when you die. You may indicate which organs or tissues you want to donate and where you want them donated. Initial or put a check mark by A or B below. If you select B, continue with your choices.

_____ **A.** I DO NOT WANT to make an organ or tissue donation, and I do not want this donation authorized on my behalf by my representative or my family.
_____ **B.** I DO WANT to make an organ or tissue donation when I die. Here are my directions:

1. **What organs/tissues I choose to donate:** (Select a or b below)
_____ **a.** Any needed parts or organs.
_____ **b.** These parts or organs:
1.) ____________________
2.) ____________________
3.) ____________________

2. **What purposes I donate organs/tissues for:** (Select a, b, or c below)
_____ **a.** Any legally authorized purpose (transplantation, therapy, medical and dental evaluation and research, and/or advancement of medical and dental science).
_____ **b.** Transplant or therapeutic purposes only.
_____ **c.** Other: ____________________

3. **What organization or person I want my parts or organs to go to:**
_____ **a.** I have already signed a written agreement or donor card regarding organ and tissue donation with the following individual or institution: (Name) ____________________
____
_____ **b.** I would like my tissues or organs to go to the following individual or institution: (Name) ____________________
_____ **c.** I authorize my representative to make this decision.

Developed by the Office of Arizona Attorney General
TERRY GODDARD
www.azag.gov
2
Updated December 3, 2007
(All documents completed before December 3, 2007 are still valid)
DURABLE HEALTH CARE POWER OF ATTORNEY

7. Funeral and Burial Disposition: (Optional)

My agent has authority to carry out all matters relating to my funeral and burial disposition wishes in accordance with this power of attorney, which is effective upon my death. My wishes are reflected below:

Initial or put a check mark by those choices you wish to select.
_____ Upon my death, I direct my body to be buried. (As opposed to cremated)
_____ Upon my death, I direct my body to be buried in ____________________
____________________. (Optional directive)
_____ Upon my death, I direct my body to be cremated.
_____ Upon my death, I direct my body to be cremated with my ashes to be ____________________
____________________. (Optional directive)
_____ My agent will make all funeral and burial disposition decisions. (Optional directive)

8. About a Living Will:

NOTE: If you have a Living Will and a Durable Health Care Power of Attorney, **you must attach** the Living Will to this form. A Living Will form is available on the Attorney General (AG) web site. Initial or put a check mark by box A or B.

_____ **A.** I have SIGNED AND ATTACHED a completed Living Will in addition to this Durable Health Care Power of Attorney to state decisions I have made about end of life health care if I am unable to communicate or make my own decisions at that time.
_____ **B.** I have NOT SIGNED a Living Will.

9. About a Prehospital Medical Care Directive or Do Not Resuscitate Directive:

NOTE: A form for the Prehospital Medical Care Directive or Do Not Resuscitate Directive is available on the AG Web site. Initial or put a check mark by box A or B.

_____ **A.** I and my doctor or health care provider HAVE SIGNED a Prehospital Medical Care Directive or Do Not Resuscitate Directive on paper with ORANGE background in the event that 911 or Emergency Medical Technicians or hospital emergency personnel are called and my heart or breathing has stopped.
_____ **B.** I have NOT SIGNED a Prehospital Medical Care Directive or Do Not Resuscitate Directive.

HIPAA WAIVER OF CONFIDENTIALITY FOR MY AGENT/REPRESENTATIVE

_____ **(Initial)** I intend for my agent to be treated as I would be with respect to my rights regarding the use and disclosure of my individually identifiable health information or other medical records. This release authority applies to any information governed by the Health Insurance Portability and Accountability Act of 1996 (aka HIPAA), 42 USC 1320d and 45 CFR 160-164.

SIGNATURE OR VERIFICATION

A. I am signing this Durable Health Care Power of Attorney as follows:

My Signature: ____________________ Date: ____________________

B. I am physically unable to sign this document, so a witness is verifying my desires as follows:

Witness Verification: I believe that this Durable Health Care Power of Attorney accurately expresses the wishes communicated to me by the principal of this document. He/she intends to adopt this Durable Health Care Power of Attorney at this time. He/she is physically unable to sign or mark this document at this time, and I verify that he/she directly indicated to me that the Durable Health Care Power of Attorney expresses his/her wishes and that he/she intends to adopt the Durable Health Care Power of Attorney at this time.

Developed by the Office of Arizona Attorney General
TERRY GODDARD
www.azag.gov
3
Updated December 3, 2007
(All documents completed before December 3, 2007 are still valid)
DURABLE HEALTH CARE POWER OF ATTORNEY

Witness Name (printed): ____________________
Signature: ____________________ Date: ____________________

SIGNATURE OF WITNESS OR NOTARY PUBLIC:

NOTE: At least one adult witness OR a Notary Public must witness the signing of this document and then sign it. The witness or Notary Public CANNOT be anyone who is: (a) under the age of 18; (b) related to you by blood, adoption, or marriage; (c) entitled to any part of your estate; (d) appointed as your representative; or (e) involved in providing your health care at the time this form is signed.

A. Witness: I certify that I witnessed the signing of this document by the Principal. The person who signed this Durable Health Care Power of Attorney appeared to be of sound mind and under no pressure to make specific choices or sign the document. I understand the requirements of being a witness and I confirm the following:

- I am not currently designated to make medical decisions for this person.
- I am not directly involved in administering health care to this person.
- I am not entitled to any portion of this person's estate upon his or her death under a will or by operation of law.
- I am not related to this person by blood, marriage or adoption.

Witness Name (printed): ____________________
Signature: ____________________ Date: ____________________
Address: ____________________

Notary Public (NOTE: If a witness signs your form, you DO NOT need a notary to sign):

STATE OF ARIZONA) ss
COUNTY OF ____________________)

The undersigned, being a Notary Public certified in Arizona, declares that the person making this Durable Health Care Power of Attorney has dated and signed or marked it in my presence and appears to me to be of sound mind and free from duress. I further declare I am not related to the person signing above by blood, marriage or adoption, or a person designated to make medical decisions on his/her behalf. I am not directly involved in providing health care to the person signing. I am not entitled to any part of his/her estate under a will now existing or by operation of law. In the event the person acknowledging this Durable Health Care Power of Attorney is physically unable to sign or mark this document, I verify that he/she directly indicated to me that this Durable Health Care Power of Attorney expresses his/her wishes and that he/she intends to adopt the Durable Health Care Power of Attorney at this time.

WITNESS MY HAND AND SEAL this ___ day of ____________, 20___.
Notary Public ____________________ My Commission Expires: ____________________

OPTIONAL:
STATEMENT THAT YOU HAVE DISCUSSED
YOUR HEALTH CARE CHOICES FOR THE FUTURE
WITH YOUR PHYSICIAN

NOTE: Before deciding what health care you want for yourself, you may wish to ask your physician questions regarding treatment alternatives. This statement from your physician is not required by Arizona law. If you do speak with your physician, it is a good idea to have him or her complete this section. Ask your doctor to keep a copy of this form with your medical records.

Developed by the Office of Arizona Attorney General
TERRY GODDARD
www.azag.gov
4
Updated December 3, 2007
(All documents completed before December 3, 2007 are still valid)
DURABLE HEALTH CARE POWER OF ATTORNEY

On this date I reviewed this document with the Principal and discussed any questions regarding the probable medical consequences of the treatment choices provided above. I agree to comply with the provisions of this directive, and I will comply with the health care decisions made by the representative unless a decision violates my conscience. In such case I will promptly disclose my unwillingness to comply and will transfer or try to transfer patient care to another provider who is willing to act in accordance with the representative's direction.

Doctor Name (printed): ____________________
Signature: ____________________ Date: ____________________

FIGURE 59A–1 State of Arizona: Durable Health Care Power of Attorney. Instructions and form. Developed by the Office of Arizona Attorney General, Terry Goddard. www.azag.gov.

(continues)

Instructions: Competent adults and emancipated minors may give advance instructions using this form or any form of their own choosing. To be legally binding, the Advance Care Plan must be signed and either witnessed or notarized.

I, ______________________________, hereby give these advance instructions on how I want to be treated by my doctors and other health care providers when I can no longer make those treatment decisions myself.

Agent: I want the following person to make health care decisions for me:

Name: ____________________ Phone #: ____________ Relation: ____________
Address: ____

Alternate Agent: If the person named above is unable or unwilling to make health care decisions for me, I appoint as alternate:

Name: ____________________ Phone #: ____________ Relation: ____________
Address: ____

Quality of Life:

I want my doctors to help me maintain an acceptable quality of life including adequate pain management. A quality of life that is unacceptable to me means when I have any of the following conditions **(you can check as many of these items as you want):**

- ☐ **Permanent Unconscious Condition:** I become totally unaware of people or surroundings with little chance of ever waking up from the coma.
- ☐ **Permanent Confusion:** I become unable to remember, understand or make decisions. I do not recognize loved ones or cannot have a clear conversation with them.
- ☐ **Dependent in all Activities of Daily Living:** I am no longer able to talk clearly or move by myself. I depend on others for feeding, bathing, dressing and walking. Rehabilitation or any other restorative treatment will not help.
- ☐ **End-Stage Illnesses:** I have an illness that has reached its final stages in spite of full treatment. Examples: Widespread cancer that does not respond anymore to treatment; chronic and/or damaged heart and lungs, where oxygen needed most of the time and activities are limited due to the feeling of suffocation.

Treatment:

If my quality of life becomes unacceptable to me and my condition is irreversible (that is, it will not improve), I direct that medically appropriate treatment be provided as follows. **Checking "yes" means I WANT the treatment. Checking "no" means I DO NOT want the treatment.**

☐ ☐ Yes No	**CPR (Cardiopulmonary Resuscitation):** To make the heart beat again and restore breathing after it has stopped. Usually this involves electric shock, chest compressions, and breathing assistance.
☐ ☐ Yes No	**Life Support / Other Artificial Support:** Continuous use of breathing machine, IV fluids, medications, and other equipment that helps the lungs, heart, kidneys and other organs to continue to work.
☐ ☐ Yes No	**Treatment of New Conditions:** Use of surgery, blood transfusions, or antibiotics that will deal with a new condition but will not help the main illness.
☐ ☐ Yes No	**Tube feeding/IV fluids:** Use of tubes to deliver food and water to patient's stomach or use of IV fluids into a vein which would include artificially delivered nutrition and hydration.

PLEASE SIGN ON PAGE 2 Page 1 of 2

Other instructions, such as burial arrangements, hospice care, etc.: ______________________________

(Attach additional pages if necessary)

Organ donation (optional): Upon my death, I wish to make the following anatomical gift (please mark one):
☐ Any organ/tissue ☐ My entire body ☐ Only the following organs/tissues: ____________

SIGNATURE

Your signature should either be witnessed by two competent adults or notarized. If witnessed, neither witness should be the person you appointed as your agent, and at least one of the witnesses should be someone who is not related to you or entitled to any part of your estate.

Signature: ______________________ (Patient) DATE: ____________

Witnesses:

1. I am a competent adult who is not named as the agent. I witnessed the patient's signature on this form. ______________________ Signature of witness number 1

2. I am a competent adult who is not named as the agent. I am not related to the patient by blood, marriage, or adoption and I would not be entitled to any portion of the patient's estate upon his or her death under any existing will or codicil or by operation of law. I witnessed the patient's signature on this form. ______________________ Signature of witness number 2

This document may be notarized instead of witnessed:

STATE OF TENNESSEE
COUNTY OF ____________

I am a Notary Public in and for the State and County named above. The person who signed this instrument is personally known to me (or proved to me on the basis of satisfactory evidence) to be the person who signed as the "patient". The patient personally appeared before me and signed above or acknowledged the signature above as his or her own. I declare under penalty of perjury that the patient appears to be of sound mind and under no duress, fraud, or undue influence.

My commission expires: ____________ ______________________ Signature of Notary Public

WHAT TO DO WITH THIS ADVANCE DIRECTIVE

- Provide a copy to your physician(s)
- Keep a copy in your personal files where it is accessible to others
- Tell your closest relatives and friends what is in the document
- Provide a copy to the person(s) you named as your health care agent

Approved by Tennessee Department of Health, Board for Licensing Health Care Facilities, February 3, 2005
Acknowledgement to Project GRACE for inspiring the development of this form.

Page 2 of 2

FIGURE 59A–2 Advance Care Plan. Approved by the Tennessee Department of Health, Board for Licensing Health Care Facilities, February 3, 2005. Acknowledgment to Project GRACE for inspiring the development of this form.

I, ______________________________, give my agent named below permission to make health care decisions for me if I cannot make decisions for myself, including any health care decision that I could have made for myself if able. If my agent is unavailable or is unable or unwilling to serve, the alternate named below will take the agent's place.

Agent:	Alternate:
Name	Name
Address	Address
City State Zip Code	City State Zip Code
( ) Area Code Home Phone Number	( ) Area Code Home Phone Number
( ) Area Code Work Phone Number	( ) Area Code Work Phone Number
( ) Area Code Mobile Phone Number	( ) Area Code Mobile Phone Number
Patient's name (please print or type) Date	Signature of patient (must be at least 18 or emancipated minor)

To be legally valid, **either** block A **or** block B must be properly completed and signed.

Block A Witnesses (2 witnesses required)

1. I am a competent adult who is not named above. I witnessed the patient's signature on this form. ______________________ Signature of witness number 1

2. I am a competent adult who is not named above. I am not related to the patient by blood, marriage, or adoption and I would not be entitled to any portion of the patient's estate upon his or her death under any existing will or codicil or by operation of law. I witnessed the patient's signature on this form. ______________________ Signature of witness number 2

Block B Notarization

STATE OF TENNESSEE
COUNTY OF ____________

I am a Notary Public in and for the State and County named above. The person who signed this instrument is personally known to me (or proved to me on the basis of satisfactory evidence) to be the person whose name is shown above as the "patient." The patient personally appeared before me and signed above or acknowledged the signature above as his or her own. I declare under penalty of perjury that the patient appears to be of sound mind and under no duress, fraud, or undue influence.

My commission expires: ____________ ______________________ Signature of Notary Public

Approved by Tennessee Department of Health, Board for Licensing Health Care Facilities, February 3, 2005

FIGURE 59A–3 Appointment of Health Care Agent (Tennessee). Approved by the Tennessee Department of Health, Board for Licensing Health Care Facilities, February 3, 2005.

I, ______________________ (**Designated Physician**) made the decision to appoint ______________________ (**Name of Surrogate**) as surrogate for ______________________ (**Name of Patient**).

Surrogate Contact Information: Home: ____________
Work: ____________
Cell Phone: ____________

Reasons for Appointment (check all that apply):

___ Knows patient's wishes	___ Demonstrates care and concern
___ Knows patient's best interest	___ Visits patient regularly during illness
___ Had regular contact with patient	___ Engages in face-to-face contact with caregiver
___ Available and willing to serve	___ Participates in decision making process

______________________ **Physician Signature** **Date/Time**

If designated physician is to act as surrogate, one of the following signatures must be obtained:

______________________ **Ethics Committee Representative Date** or ______________________ **Concurring Second Physician Date**

Any individuals in disagreement? Yes ___ No ___
If yes, please explain ______________________________

ACCEPTANCE OF SURROGATE SELECTION

I accept the appointment as surrogate for ______________________ (**Patient**)
and understand I have the authority to make all medical decisions.

______________________ **Signature of Surrogate** **Date/Time**

Approved by Tennessee Department of Health, Board for Licensing Health Care Facilities, May 3, 2005

FIGURE 59A–4 Appointment of Surrogate (Tennessee). Approved by the Tennessee Department of Health, Board for Licensing Health Care Facilities, February 3, 2005.

Appendix 59–1 *(continued)*

COPY OF FORM SHALL ACCOMPANY PATIENT WHEN TRANSFERRED OR DISCHARGED

Physician Orders for Scope of Treatment (POST)	Patient's Last Name
This is a Physician Order Sheet based on the medical conditions and wishes of the person identified at right ("patient"). Any section not completed indicates full treatment for that section. When need occurs, first follow these orders, then contact physician.	First Name/Middle Initial
	Date of Birth

Section A — *Check One Box Only*

CARDIOPULMONARY RESUSCITATION (CPR): Patient has no pulse and/or is not breathing.

☐ **Resuscitate (CPR)** ☐ **Do Not Attempt Resuscitate (DNR/no CPR)**

When not in cardiopulmonary arrest, follow orders in **B, C,** and **D.**

Section B — *Check One Box Only*

MEDICAL INTERVENTIONS. Patient has pulse and/or is breathing.

☐ **Comfort Measures** Treat with dignity and respect. Keep clean, warm, and dry. Use medication by any route, positioning, wound care and other measures to relieve pain and suffering. Use oxygen, suction and manual treatment of airway obstruction as needed for comfort. **Do not transfer to hospital for life-sustaining treatment. Transfer only if comfort needs cannot be met in current location.**

☐ **Limited Additional Interventions** Includes care described above. Use medical treatment, IV fluids and cardiac monitoring as indicated. Do not use intubation, advanced airway interventions, or mechanical ventilation. **Transfer to hospital if indicated. Avoid intensive care.**

☐ **Full Treatment.** Includes care above. Use intubation, advanced airway interventions mechanical ventilation, and cardioversion as indicated. **Transfer to hospital if indicated. Include intensive care.**

Other Instructions: ____________

Section C — *Check One Box Only*

ANTIBIOTICS – Treatment for new medical conditions:

☐ **No Antibiotics**

☐ **Antibiotics**

Other Instructions: ____________

Section D — *Check One Box Only in Each Column*

MEDICALLY ADMINISTERED FLUIDS AND NUTRITION. Oral fluids and nutrition must be offered if medically feasible.

☐ **No IV fluids** (provide other measures to assure comfort)	☐ **No feeding tube**
☐ **IV fluids for a defined trial period**	☐ **Feeding tube for a defined trial period**
☐ **IV fluids long-term if indicated**	☐ **Feeding tube long-term**

Other Instructions: ____________

Section E — *Must be Completed*

Discussed with:	**The Basis for These Orders Is:** (Must be completed)
☐ Patient/Resident	☐ Patient's preferences
☐ Health care agent	☐ Patient's best interest (patient lacks capacity or preferences unknown)
☐ Court-appointed guardian	☐ Medical indications
☐ Health care surrogate	☐ (Other) ____________
☐ Parent of minor	
☐ Other: ________ (Specify)	

Physician Name (Print)	**Physician Phone Number**	**Office Use Only**
Physician Signature (Mandatory)	**Date**	

COPY OF FORM SHALL ACCOMPANY PATIENT WHEN TRANSFERRED OR DISCHARGED

HIPAA PERMITS DISCLOSURE OF POST TO OTHER HEALTH CARE PROFESSIONALS AS NECESSARY

Signature of Patient, Parent of Minor, or Guardian/Health Care Representative

Significant thought has been given to life-sustaining treatment. Preferences have been expressed to a physician and/or health care professional(s). This document reflects those treatment preferences.

(If signed by surrogate, preferences expressed must reflect patient's wishes as best understood by surrogate.)

Signature	Name (print)	Relationship (write "self" if patient)

Contact Information

Surrogate	Relationship	Phone Number	
Health Care Professional Preparing Form	Preparer Title	Phone Number	Date Prepared

Directions for Health Care Professionals

Completing POST

Must be completed by a health care professional based on patient preferences, patient best interest, and medical indications.

POST must be signed by a physician to be valid. Verbal orders are acceptable with follow-up signature by physician in accordance with facility/community policy.

Photocopies/faxes of signed POST forms are legal and valid.

Using POST

Any incomplete section of POST implies full treatment for that section.

No defibrillator (including AEDs) should be used on a person who has chosen "Do Not Attempt Resuscitation".

Oral fluids and nutrition must always be offered if medically feasible.

When comfort cannot be achieved in the current setting, the person, including someone with "Comfort Measures Only", should be transferred to a setting able to provide comfort (e.g., treatment of a hip fracture).

IV medication to enhance comfort may be appropriate for a person who has chosen "Comfort Measures Only".

Treatment of dehydration is a measure which prolongs life. A person who desires IV fluids should indicate "Limited Interventions" or "Full Treatment".

A person with capacity, or the surrogate of a person without capacity, can request alternative treatment.

Reviewing POST

This POST should be reviewed if:

(1) The patient is transferred from one care setting or care level to another, or
(2) There is a substantial change in the patient's health status, or
(3) The patient's treatment preferences change.

Draw line through sections A through E and write "VOID" in large letters if POST is replaced or becomes invalid.

Approved by Tennessee Department of Health, Board for Licensing Health Care Facilities, February 3, 2005

COPY OF FORM SHALL ACCOMPANY PATIENT WHEN TRANSFERRED OR DISCHARGED.

DO NOT ALTER THIS FORM !

FIGURE 59A–5 Physician Order Scope of Treatment (POST). Approved by the Tennessee Department of Health, Board for Licensing Health Care Facilities, February 3, 2005.

CHAPTER 60

Communication Skills

William F. Galvin

OUTLINE

OBJECTIVES

1. Identify common miscommunication problems.
2. Identify and explain the basic concepts of communication, including commonly used expressions, levels of communication, principles and assumptions, and a working definition.
3. List and explain the factors that affect communication, including environmental factors, emotional and sensory factors, verbal expressions, nonverbal cues, intrapersonal factors, and physical appearance and status.
4. Identify barriers to communication.
5. State the true purpose and four major subgoals of communication.
6. Explain the importance of conveying believability.
7. Identify and explain skills of the sender.
8. Identify and explain skills of the receiver.
9. List and discuss the characteristics and qualities of a nurturing relationship.
10. Identify and explain questioning strategies and techniques.
11. Illustrate the effective use of questioning strategies and techniques in the practice of respiratory care.

KEY TERMS

channel
clarification
closed-ended questions
communication
compound questions
confidentiality
confrontation
decoding
dialogue
emotional filters
empathy
empowerment
encoding
facilitation
feedback
grapevine
jargon
kinesics
leading questions
medium
message
mind-set
mutuality
nonverbal communication
nonverbal cues
open-ended questions
paralinguistics
personal space
proxemics
transactional
verbal expression
"white lab jacket" phenomenon

INTRODUCTION

The intention of this chapter is to enhance and strengthen the interpersonal communications among respiratory therapists and physicians, nurses, allied health professionals, patients, and family members. Practical and everyday examples of miscommunication are provided, along with a wide array of definitions and perspectives, and an extensive list of factors affecting communication is discussed. The major goals and the purpose of communication are highlighted, along with the importance of the conveyance of believability. This chapter addresses the skills of the sender and receiver and provides an overview of questioning strategies and techniques, concluding with examples of the ways these communication strategies and techniques apply to respiratory care practice.

Miscommunication: The Case for Effective Communication Skills

Communication is a complex and dynamic process at the heart of all human interaction. It is universally applicable and has been identified as one of the most formidable and ubiquitous problems individuals face in any encounter. The importance of its effectiveness cannot be overstated, underestimated, or trivialized; communication is clearly one of the most vital of the basic life skills. If communication is not mastered and used effectively, it can result in misunderstanding, disagreement, conflict, and, in the case of healthcare, significant medical errors.

The urgent and critical nature of healthcare renders it markedly more vulnerable to the devastating consequences and repercussions of poor communication. Respiratory therapists use communication skills in healthcare assessment, disease management, patient education, and multidisciplinary collaboration. Communication has been identified an as essential component of future respiratory care curricula.[1] Little doubt remains as to its central role in the practice of respiratory care.

One way to make the case for effective communication skills is to provide examples of communication blunders. Some rather amusing yet pointed examples illustrate the serious nature and magnitude of the problem. It has been suggested that any interaction should entail adherence to the 5 Cs of communication, namely, that communication should be complete, clear, concise, courteous, and cohesive.[2] Although all five elements are important, the first two are especially problematic and are highlighted in the five examples given in this section, which comprise a selection of general and healthcare-related scenarios.

RESPIRATORY RECAP

Five Cs of Communication

» Complete
» Clear
» Concise
» Courteous
» Cohesive

Miscommunication 1: One Thousand Times the Prescribed Dosage of Heparin

On November 18, 2007, the 2-week-old newborn twins of actor Dennis Quaid and his wife, Kimberly, were among three patients accidentally administered 1000 times the common and prescribed dosage of the blood thinner heparin.[3] The twins were receiving intravenous medications, and the heparin was used to flush the catheters to prevent clotting. The twins mistakenly received vials containing 10,000 units per milliliter instead of the appropriate and prescribed dosage of 10 units per milliliter.

Although none of the overdose victims suffered any ill effects, the incident brought back to the forefront the alarming and disturbing findings of a previous landmark report, *To Err Is Human*,[4] regarding the severe and significant problem of medical mistakes within the healthcare community. In short, the report indicated that approximately 44,000 patients experience a medical mistake or misadventure every year in the United States, which would make medical mistakes the eighth leading cause of death in the United States. The specific root causes for these problems are complicated and complex, yet communication has been cited as a significant factor associated with the problem. In the case of the Quaid twins, improvement in drug labeling as well as more effective communication and interaction among healthcare professionals (physicians, nurses, and pharmacists) might have prevented the problem.

Miscommunication 2: Watch the Borders!

A story is circulating through the federal government regarding the famous and feared former director of the Federal Bureau of Investigation, J. Edgar Hoover. Its authenticity and origin are mysterious and sketchy, but its message is quite powerful. According to the story, Hoover asked his secretary to type an important memo to all his high-level, worldwide regional directors. The content of the memo is insignificant, but after the memo was typed and returned to Hoover, he wrote on the bottom of the memo the words *Watch the borders!* The memo then was copied and circulated to all the recipients. The directors read and interpreted the memo to mean that they were to increase security and surveillance at their respective regional borders. However, it was later determined that what Hoover meant with the words *Watch the borders!* was that his secretary should reduce the size of the margins of the memo's page.

Whether real or contrived, this story does bring home a message. The communication pitfalls were misinterpretation and a lack of rapport between Hoover and his secretary. Hoover was not addressing geographic borders but rather the physical borders of the memo. He was concerned that the margins of the text were either too narrow or too broad, but his ruthlessness, short temper, and feared personality prevented his secretary from seeking clarification to prevent the ensuing calamity. The consequence could have been a costly outlay of additional funds to satisfy personnel expenses for what was thought to be a need for more security and surveillance at the borders of these regions.

Miscommunication 3: Orson Welles's *War of the Worlds*

Perhaps one of the most famous radio broadcasts was the 1938 version of the *War of the Worlds*. The talented actor Orson Welles narrated a spell-binding and convincing broadcast over national radio on Halloween Eve, telling a story of the United States being invaded by Martians. Although the broadcast began with a disclosure that the story was purely fictitious and merely presented as a form of entertainment, listeners were captivated and convinced of its truth because Welles told the story with considerable conviction and a tremendous sense of reality. The audience was terrified, and the results were nearly catastrophic. As the story goes, a number of listeners from a small New Jersey community were so convinced of its authenticity that they fetched their guns and passed through the streets looking to confront what they believed were invaders from Mars. What was the problem?

This story represents a classic example of an incomplete message and how incomplete facts can have potentially serious consequences. Simply stated, much of the audience did not hear those opening remarks about the story being fiction. The power of the speaker and the circumstances surrounding the broadcast (Halloween Eve) were so convincing that the listening audience actually believed it to be true. So convincing was the broadcast that some listeners were prepared to go to battle. The message is a simple one: be certain that you hear or observe the entire message and monitor your emotions before jumping to conclusions.

Miscommunication 4: Put This Blood Gas on Ice!

A new respiratory therapy student was attending to his first-ever cardiac arrest. He was all eyes and ears and eager to help. During the resuscitation, the senior therapist drew an arterial blood gas sample and asked that it be sent to the lab immediately. The sample was handed back to the new student, and with it, directions to immediately put it on ice and take it to the stat laboratory. The student went down the corridor to the ice machine, secured a cup of ice, took the cap off the syringe, and instilled the blood into the cup before he ran it down to the laboratory. What is the problem?

Besides the young student being placed in a totally inappropriate situation, gross assumptions were made that commonly used medical **jargon** was understood by this inexperienced, aspiring practitioner. Although any seasoned therapist would have understood the instructions, the new student's placement in this situation was grossly unfair and unacceptable. The student obviously was unfamiliar with medical language, and although willing and eager to help and make a good impression, he was asked to perform a task without proper education, supervision, and training. The case may appear extreme and even amusing, but it nonetheless makes the point about assumptions regarding the understanding of commonly used medical expressions.

Miscommunication 5: Know Bronchodilators!

A respiratory therapy student just starting out in the program visited the office of her program director to complain about the fairness of her first respiratory pharmacology examination. The director initially was reluctant to listen because previous experience had taught him that many students make unfair accusations about the difficulty and validity of exams. However, being somewhat familiar with the student's mild manner and studious work ethic, he decided to engage her in further discussion. The student stated that during the course of the exam review session the faculty member indicated the students should "know bronchodilators." The student stated that she had studied for hours and hours thereafter. She arrived early for the morning of the exam, feeling confident and well prepared, and progressed through the exam, at one point noting five or six questions on albuterol, salmeterol, and other bronchodilating agents. Believing these to be normal pharmacology questions, the director nodded affirmatively. However, with this nodding the student became distraught and even enraged. She began to raise her voice in displeasure and said, "But that's not fair; we were told that bronchodilators would not be on the exam." The director appeared perplexed and said, "Clearly you have to agree that questions on bronchodilators are obviously appropriate for an exam in respiratory pharmacology." The student then responded, "But he said *no bronchodilators*!" The director then realized that the student was interpreting the statement to mean *no* instead of *know*.

> **RESPIRATORY RECAP**
>
> **Importance of Communication**
>
> » Communication is complex and dynamic and is considered one of the biggest problems and challenges facing society.

Although the story is alarming, it also reflects a significant finding within schools—an increase in the cultural diversity of the student body and the potential for misunderstanding or misinterpretation of language. The message is that the obvious cannot be assumed, and virtually all communications occurring with students from different cultures requires care, diligence, and attention to detail. Continual efforts must be made to enhance students' understanding of language and cultural norms.

Some of the previously discussed miscommunication stories are amusing, but they nonetheless reflect serious flaws and problems in the transmittal and receipt of messages. Medicine leaves little margin for error. The medical literature is replete with examples in which a misplaced decimal point hurriedly transcribed by a healthcare practitioner has resulted in the death of a patient. Other patients have had the wrong limbs amputated; angry managers have been frustrated by staff members who seemingly disregard their directives; and patients can appear noncompliant with treatment regimens designed and developed by healthcare professionals to meet their specific needs. At the heart of these issues is a complex process that entails considerable complication. An appreciation of the concepts involved in communication can help the healthcare professional alleviate the complexity.

Basic Concepts of Communication

Commonly Used Expressions

Communication can be expressed in a variety of ways. As a form of small talk, or chit-chat, in a social context, it follows a pattern of social amenities in which prescribed rules, ceremonies, or customs are observed. When a therapist says *hello* to a colleague or patient, it is a simple greeting that abides by a socially acceptable custom. Often this small talk encompasses mundane topics and simply wastes time, tests reactions, avoids involvement, or serves as a bridge to more significant conversation.[5] The exchange of information informally and spontaneously between friends and colleagues is sometimes called the **grapevine** and is often viewed as merely gossip, rumors, half-truths, and even distorted or inaccurate information; nonetheless, it is a normal growth of organizational life and a fulfillment of the desire to be "in the know."[6]

Communication also can be expressed in the form of a **dialogue**, which involves purposeful, reciprocal, and close or intimate expression between participants.[5] Dialogue is particularly significant and valuable in healthcare settings, in which meaningful communication must occur between therapist and patient or therapist and healthcare professional. This is in contrast to a *monologue*, in which one party speaks and dominates the conversation. A monologue can obviously be highly ineffective and limit interaction. On the other hand, it may be appropriate in a crisis situation, such as in an emergency department, where one party must take control and direct emergent medical treatment.

Levels of Communication

Communication exists on five different levels, which are summarized in **Table 60–1** and discussed briefly in this section.[7–9]

Level 5 communication (cliché conversation) is considered the lowest level of human interaction and is characterized by meaningless statements and clichés. No genuine human sharing takes place at this superficial level. For example, you pass a casual friend and say, "Hi. How are you?" At this point you expect the response "I'm fine. How are you?" Nothing meaningful occurs, but each party abides by expected social niceties. However, if the acquaintance responds by saying, "I feel terrible. I have a bad cold, the kids are sick, and my wife is angry with me," that individual is trying to enter into a higher level of communication. Such a detailed response is generally frowned on because the expectation is a simple "I'm fine." As the initiator of the message, you can either express concern and encourage further dialogue or simply say "Oh! That's too bad" while looking down at your watch and hurriedly walking away. In choosing the latter, you are essentially communicating, "I don't want to hear your problems. I was just trying to be friendly." Your intention was to engage in a level 5 communication.

Level 4 communication (fact reporting) is still a relatively shallow form of interaction in which neutral topics are discussed and small talk ensues. It entails such issues as the news, the weather, or sports scores. Neither party shares anything personal, and the interaction remains safe and noncontroversial. An example of level 4 communication is a situation in which you are waiting outside the conference room for a lecture to begin, you see a familiar medical student, and you say "Hi! How are you?" The student may respond, "Fine, thanks" (a level 5 communication), after which a silence ensues as you both continue to wait for the conference door to open. If you choose to enter level 4 communication, you say, "What a beautiful day outside." Although still shallow and without risk, this conversation is more engaging and entails a higher level of communication. The medical student has the option of engaging you in level 4 conversation or providing a short response that essentially says, "I don't want to talk to you," in which he chooses to stay at level 5.

If a person enters into a level 3 interaction (personal ideas or judgments), that individual begins to share personal ideas, opinions, or judgments. The information is usually guarded and closely monitored; in fact, if the listener indicates disapproval, boredom, or confusion, the sender may become anxious or hesitate to continue. In level 3 communication, the participants take more risk and engage in self-disclosure to begin to build a relationship, which also requires some degree of trust and time to develop. A level 3 exchange requires both parties to participate. If you begin expressing your views while the other person either remains silent or evades the issue, you may be at level 3 while the other person is still at level 4. At this point you may want to end the conversation or move back up to level 4. Level 3 communications, for example, can occur between you and a fellow therapist when you are both willing to share personal views on controversial health-related issues, such as termination of life support.

If the relationship continues, you can enter into a level 2 communication (feelings and emotions), in which more self-disclosure ensues and both parties begin to share the more personal and emotional aspects of their lives. The second level of

TABLE 60–1 Five Levels of Communication

Level	Type	Characteristics
5	Cliché conversation	No genuine sharing; shallow, simple, superficial; standard answers expected
4	Reporting facts	Some sharing; neutral topics; nothing personal; safe, nonconfrontational topics
3	Personal ideas or judgments	Beginning of self-disclosure; some risk; guarded and closely monitored; usually reserved for coworkers and social friends
2	Feelings and emotions	Used within atmosphere of trust and mutual respect; reserved for very close friends and family
1	Peak communication	Highest level; intimate; reserved for select few such as marriage partner, immediate family, and extremely close and intimate friends

Data from Purtilo R. *Health Professional and Patient Interaction*. 4th ed. Philadelphia: WB Saunders; 1990.

BOX 60–1

Principles of Communication

Each communication situation is unique.
The key to successful communication is feedback.
Face-to-face communication is most effective.
Distractions can garble your message.
The more people involved, the more complex communication becomes.
Every message contains both information and emotion.
Words are symbols used to express thoughts, and are always open to interpretation.
Selective perception can distort the message.
People communicate according to their expectations of a situation.
If they don't trust you, they won't understand you.

Data from Dellinger S, Deane B. *Communicating Effectively: A Complete Guide for Better Managing.* Radnor, PA: Chilton Book; 1980.

communication is characterized by individuals who have spent a considerable amount of time together; shared their innermost thoughts, fears, joys, and emotions; developed a solid foundation of trust; and enjoy true friendship.

The last and highest level of communication is level 1 (peak communication), which is limited to a select few and generally restricted to married partners, family members, and intimate friends. This level of communication is characterized by significant sharing, empathy, and the mastery of a deep relationship.

Although the five levels of communication do not apply universally to all healthcare encounters, they have been addressed in the literature and have value in therapeutic relationships.[8] In any therapeutic relationship, the respiratory therapist must go beyond levels 4 and 5 to establish a rapport, encourage the patient to "open up," and gain trust and cooperation. Attaining these levels can be especially tricky during the interview and physical assessment process because the therapist must maintain a professional demeanor but not be too distant or impersonal, which would impede the flow of valuable health-related information. Equally important is the therapist's need to avoid displaying any inappropriate emotion (level 2). When faced with a hostile or emotionally charged encounter, the therapist should stick to the facts and not succumb to useless name-calling or derisive discourse. Finally, development and maintenance of a good rapport among other members of the healthcare team can be invaluable in the creation of a congenial, productive, and satisfying work climate. The important point is to develop and maintain relationships built on honesty, trust, and respect.

Principles and Assumptions

Box 60–1 provides a comprehensive list of the underlying principles of communication.[9] These principles, along with the assumptions that follow, are used to develop a working definition to be used throughout this chapter.

Multidimensional Communication

Communication has a content dimension and a relationship dimension, meaning that any encounter entails the words, language, and information (content dimension), as well as the perceived relationship of one communicant to another (relationship dimension), which involves attitudes, feelings, and emotions.[10] For example, a therapist says to a patient, "Please take this treatment." Those words represent the content dimension and are fairly straightforward, whereas the relationship dimension refers to how the two "get along" or how they perceive their association. Is the relationship one of support, care, concern, compassion, and mutual respect? Or is it strained, distant, hierarchical, directive, contemptuous, or disrespectful?

Other authors have alluded to this issue by identifying communication as having a cognitive dimension (thoughts) and an affective dimension (emotions).[9,11,12] **Figure 60–1** is a graphic view of this phenomenon in which the cognitive dimension (thoughts) is represented by the head and the affective dimension (feelings or emotions) by the heart. Both the relationship dimension and the affective

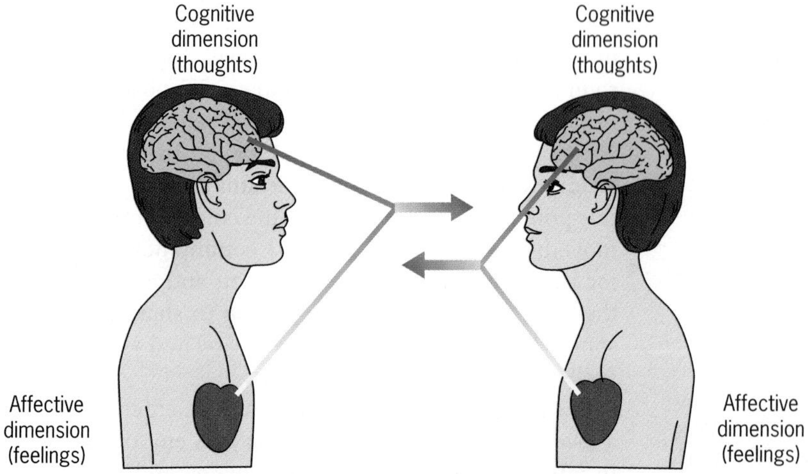

FIGURE 60–1 Cognitive and affective dimensions of communication. Adapted from Balzer-Riley JW. *Communication in Nursing.* 4th ed. Mosby; 2000.

dimension are critical for successful communication. An amicable relationship built on honesty and trust goes a long way toward a patient adhering to suggested treatment regimens, a subordinate following directives, or peers cooperating and collaborating as a team.

Transactional Communication

To say the communication is **transactional** simply means that each party is both a sender and a receiver. A reciprocal relationship, a give and take, exists in which each alternates between these two roles. When senders speak, they also receive messages from the listener; likewise, the listener does more than simply receive a message but also sends a message. This constant sending and receiving takes the form of feedback and can be done verbally or nonverbally. **Figure 60–2** illustrates a transactional relationship.

The Process of Communication

Virtually every source on the topic of communication explains communication as a process that involves separate and distinct components that are essential for successful communication.[10–16] One author expresses this process as consisting of seven components, which are graphically represented in **Figure 60–3** and expressed in the following statement: "The *sender* transmits the *message,* which is *encoded* and sent through the *channel* for *decoding* by the *receiver* who then sends *feedback*."[16]

The sender, or source, is the person or group initiating the interaction. The sender can be a single individual serving as a manager and attempting to direct a department; a patient educator communicating valuable advice or guidance to a patient or family member; a clinician or diagnostician attempting to collaborate with a physician, nurse, or fellow healthcare practitioner; or an institution or organization communicating its mission or philosophy. The **message** consists of the information, facts, data, ideas, thoughts, feelings, or attitude conveyed. It is the content to be communicated. The message is encoded in the form of words, symbols, actions, pictures, numbers, or gestures and transmitted through a **channel**, or **medium**, which can be verbal or nonverbal and involves the senses. Messages can be transmitted through sound (speaking and listening), sight (seeing), touch (feeling), smell, and taste. **Decoding** is similar to **encoding** and entails interpretation of the words, symbols, actions, pictures, numbers, or gestures back into the thought, feeling, or attitude.

The receiver is the recipient of the sender's message or the person or group for which the communication was intended. The receiver can be a student learning an important concept or principle; an employee receiving direction from a superior regarding workload; or a patient or family member receiving information, education, or training regarding treatment. **Feedback** is the final component in the process and occurs when the receiver and sender verify their perception of the message. The receiver encodes a return message either verbally or nonverbally through gestures.

With regard to the channel, the therapist must be aware of the extensive and increasing use of electronic media. Memos, letters, directives, bulletin boards, and

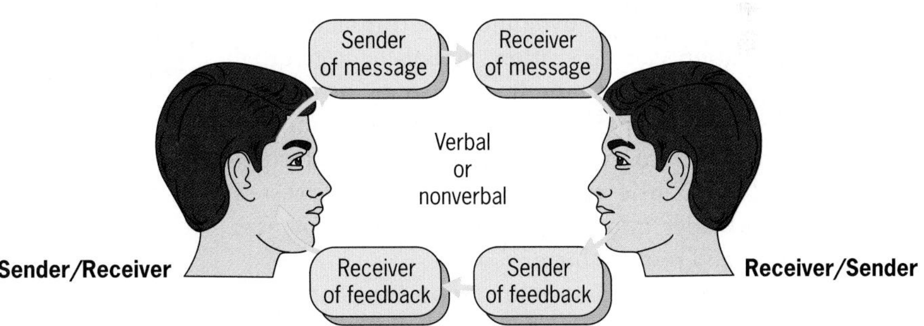

FIGURE 60–2 Transactional dimension of communication. Adapted from Schuster P. *Communication: The Key to the Therapeutic Relationship.* FA Davis; 2000:5.

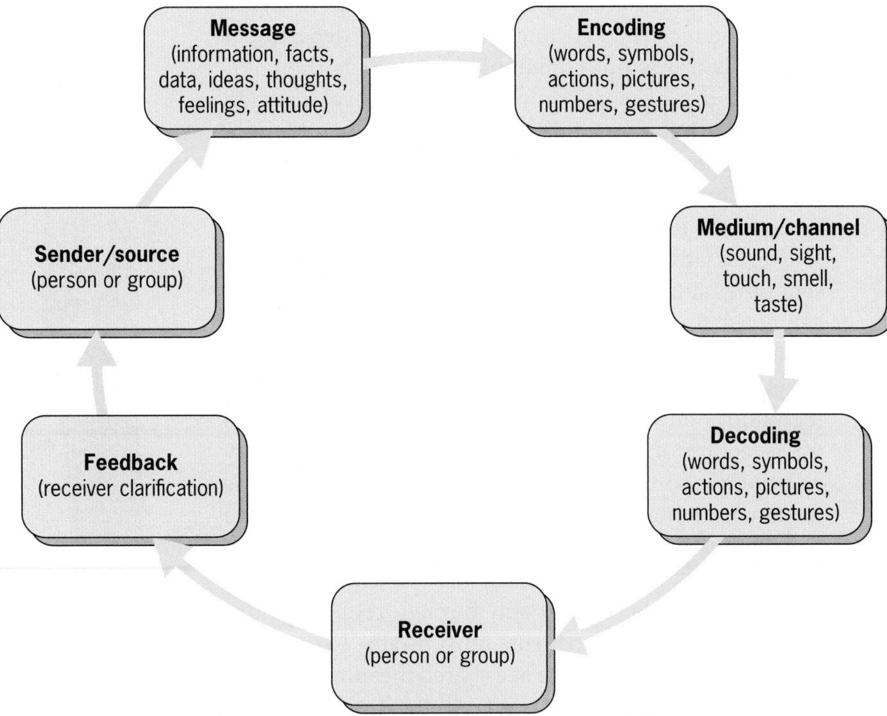

FIGURE 60–3 The communication process.

other written formats are being replaced by voice mail, email, texting, and other electronic vehicles that offer real and significant advantages in speed and cost. When using such media, the wise therapist follows the KISS acronym (keep it short and simple). However, the most important point is to pick and choose the medium most appropriate for the circumstances and situation at hand. *Short* and *simple* do not apply to every type of interaction. Therapists must recognize the importance of face-to-face communication, in which verbal and **nonverbal communication** can help clarify meaning and nurture relationships.

Communication Defined

Communication has been defined as the sending and the receipt of a message[11] and in terms of encoding and decoding, in which information in the form of words, symbols, actions, pictures, numbers, and gestures are transformed into ideas and feelings.[5] Communication is clearly an interactive process[13] that uses a set of common rules.[10] It is continuous, dynamic, and transactional.[10] Communication can be written, verbal, or nonverbal and can even be therapeutic in that it may involve an exchange that culminates in a person being helped to overcome stress, anxiety, fear, or other emotional experiences. Therapeutic communication also expresses support, provides information and feedback, corrects distortions, and restores hope.[12]

Although all these issues are important considerations in any understanding of the complexity of communication, any working definition must incorporate a common understanding between sender and receiver. With this view in mind, this chapter refers to effective communication as having a "shared meaning" between sender and receiver.[10] Posting a memo on the department bulletin board is not communication, nor is the common practice of emailing information to every person on an institution's mailing list. The obvious problem in both such cases is that the sender receives no assurance that the intended recipient actually read the memo or received the email.

The classroom and the patient-teaching setting represent other situations in which communication problems can occur. Teachers often use written examinations and clinical competency assessments to ensure this shared meaning, and patient education uses simple questioning techniques and return demonstration. Teachers often use a lecture or presentation to communicate a theory or principle to their students (or patients) and provide demonstration and observation in clinical situations to communicate the proper performance of a procedure. In reality, subject matter understanding and clinical competency mastery are ensured only through return demonstration. Students and patients must be able to convince the teacher of the existence of a shared meaning between the information that was taught and the knowledge that was learned. In summary, communication is not effective unless and until both the sender and the receiver share the same meaning.

Factors Affecting Communication

Why do managers complain about their subordinates not following through with directives, teachers become frustrated with their students' inability to recall information recently covered in class, or practitioners disturbed by their patients' inability to perform a repeatedly taught procedure? Why was a message sent not received? The answer is complex and tied to a multitude of factors.[11,14,15,17] The major categories of factors affecting communication are listed in **Box 60–2** and illustrated in **Figure 60–4**.

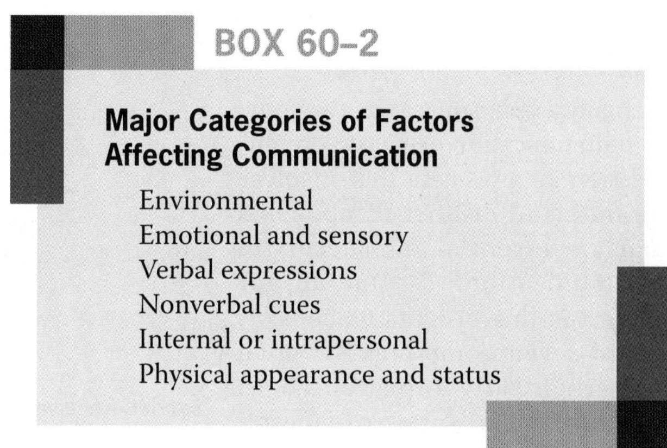

BOX 60–2

Major Categories of Factors Affecting Communication

- Environmental
- Emotional and sensory
- Verbal expressions
- Nonverbal cues
- Internal or intrapersonal
- Physical appearance and status

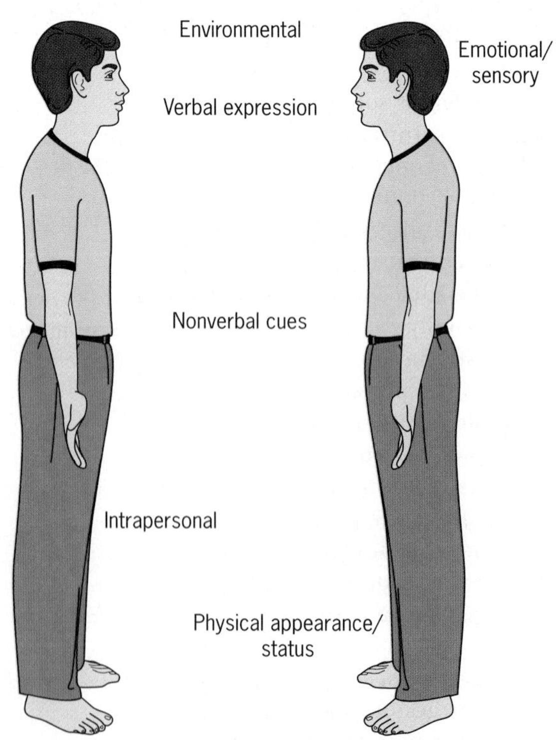

FIGURE 60–4 Factors influencing interpersonal communication. Adapted from Balzer-Riley JW. *Communication in Nursing*. 4th ed. Mosby; 2000.

Environmental Factors

Environmental factors can include physical surroundings (such as lighting, noise, temperature, and climate), a sense of formality, a lack of warmth, little privacy, unfamiliarity with the surroundings, feelings of urgency and stress, loss of personal freedom, excessive constraints, uncomfortable distance or spacing between people, overcrowding, and uncomfortable or obstructed seating arrangements.

> **RESPIRATORY RECAP**
>
> **Environmental Factors Affecting Communication**
>
> » Lighting
> » Noise
> » Temperature
> » Climate
> » Formality
> » Warmth
> » Privacy
> » Familiarity
> » Feelings of constraint
> » Physical distance between people
> » Mood
> » Architecture
> » Furniture arrangement

When patients are treated in a hospital, clinic, or extended care facility, they are not in familiar surroundings. Intensive care units are busy, noisy, and crowded places, and the medical personnel working in them are absorbed in the urgency of their jobs and may unconsciously be abrupt and impatient. Couple these facts with the formality of stark white lab jackets and a person could clearly feel a degree of "coolness" in the environment. The sense of urgency is exacerbated by the continuous sound of monitors and alarms and the near-steady beams of bright fluorescent lights. Moving to a less critical area of the hospital is not likely to cause this feeling to abate because hospital wards and clinics often feature lack of privacy, lack of freedom, and a significant degree of constraint.

Privacy issues stem from cloth curtains that serve as the only barrier between the patient and other people. History and physical assessments are performed and personal and intimate questions asked with merely a single drawn curtain separating the patient from others in the room. The meager size of the room does not allow for many personal possessions, and intravenous lines and electrocardiographic leads limit patients' mobility and anchor them to the bed.

In addition, space and distance can impede communication and threaten the comfort and openness of the conversation. Space and distance are particularly important because the therapist must avoid violations of personal space and the consequence of serious communication impairment. **Personal space** is considered to be within 1.5 to 4 feet of an individual; the boundaries themselves and reactions to breaches of them vary according to the individual's culture and background. The four major space or distance zones are identified in **Table 60–2** and illustrated in **Figure 60–5**.[8] A therapist who invades a patient's personal space should expect to see crossed legs, folded arms, little eye contact, and obvious movement from the sender. The offending therapist must discern the invasion of space and take appropriate measures to correct the situation, including moving slowly away, talking calmly, and exhibiting genuine concern, care, and compassion.

TABLE 60–2 Major Space/Distance Zones

Zone	Number of Feet	Characteristic Findings
Public space	12–25	Lecture halls or presentation areas; no physical contact; little eye contact
Social space	4–12	Typical business and work settings; more formal business and social occasions
Personal space	1.5–4	Generally an arm's length; personal conversation with close friends; one-on-one patient education activities
Intimate space	Within 1.5	Limited to more intimate relationships in which healthcare measures or procedures are performed to comfort the patient

Data from Purtilo R. *Health Professional and Patient Interaction.* 4th ed. Philadelphia: WB Saunders; 1990.

These environmental factors are not limited to just patients. Students attempting to listen to lectures in overcrowded classrooms or engage in meaningful interaction during medical rounds are equally subject to communication problems. Distractions from their peers, uncomfortable seating, and obstructed views of the blackboard and audiovisual materials all can impair reception of important information and impede effective communication.

Managers and supervisors attempting to interview new employees or conduct performance appraisals also are subject to environmental obstacles. The ringing of a telephone or the constant interruption of drop-in visitors seeking guidance and advice can wreak havoc on an interview session between a manager and a potential employee. The physical location and layout of administrative areas should be such that these obstacles and interruptions are minimized or prevented. Additionally, uncomfortable seating and the arrangement of furniture can serve as barriers between managers and subordinates and interfere with open and meaningful dialogue.

That environmental issues are significant in setting the stage for effective interaction should be apparent. Respiratory therapists and managers must be astute in identifying such factors and adept in correcting or optimizing them to enhance the relationships among subordinates, peers, and patients.

Emotional and Sensory Factors

A second major category affecting communication is emotional and sensory factors, which can consist of fear, stress, anxiety, and pain, as well as limited or

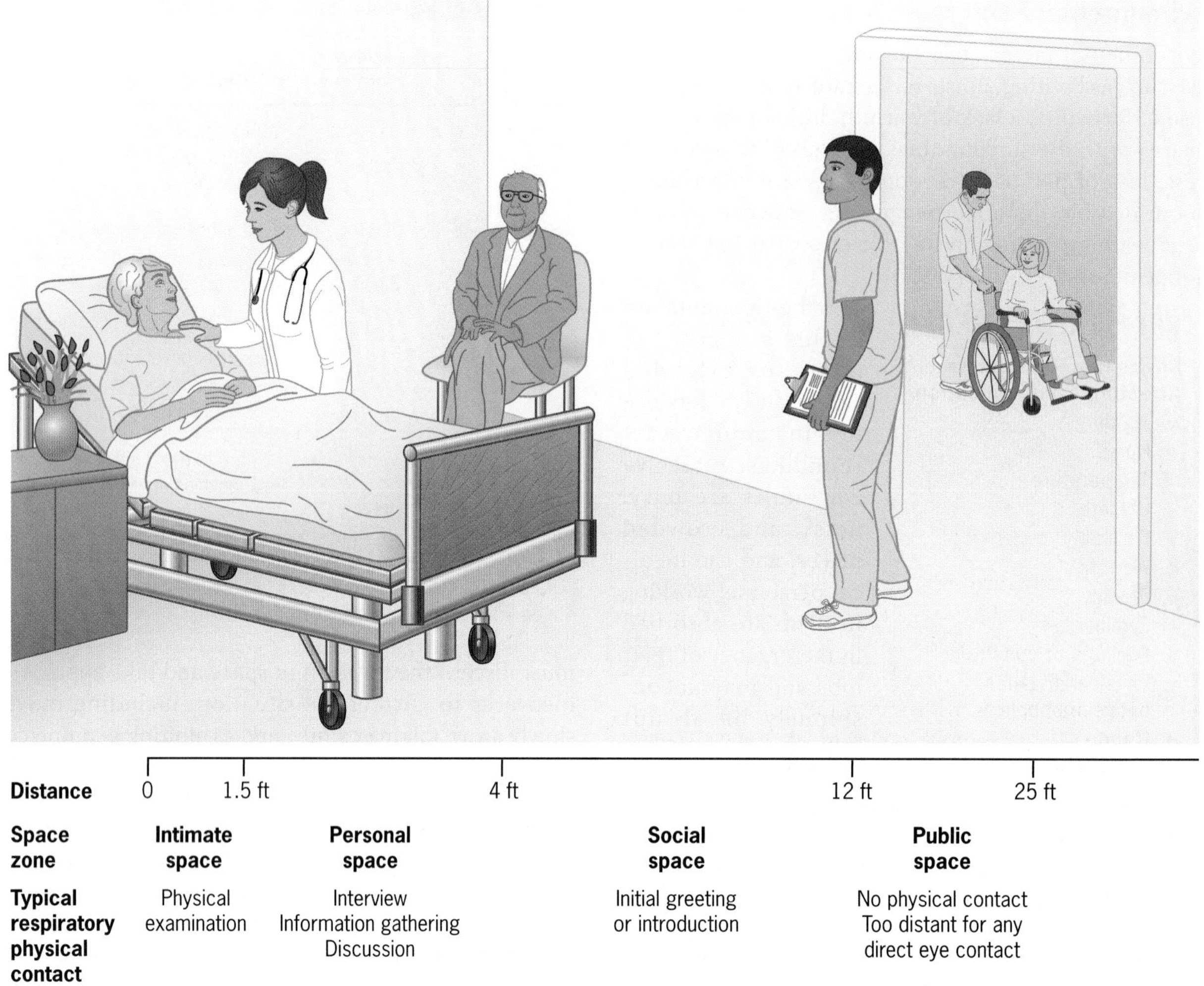

FIGURE 60–5 Public, social, personal, and intimate spaces of the patient requiring healthcare. Adapted from Wilkins RL, et al. *Clinical Assessment in Respiratory Care*. 4th ed. Mosby; 2000.

compromised mental acuity, sight, hearing, or speech. The healthcare environment involves considerable stress and anxiety, and patients, students, practitioners, and other healthcare providers can exhibit these emotions because of loss of control, frustration, low self-esteem, or feelings of inadequacy. Patients often demonstrate fear for their own well-being or that of their family members. A patient suspecting lung cancer may be so distraught about the thought of imminent death and the inability to care for loved ones that the ability to communicate can be significantly impaired.

The stress and tension of heavy treatment loads also can significantly affect the therapist's ability to effectively interact with the patient. Wanting to do a good job and knowing that many others require treatment raises tensions, anxiety, and frustration in the mind of the conscientious therapist. Students are not immune to such feelings and are under considerable pressure to satisfy classroom assignments and demonstrate clinical competency. In addition, pain can distract a person from conversation. Significant degrees of physical pain and the numbing effects of medications may make communication less than optimal. Therapists attempting to instruct postoperative patients in the correct use of their incentive spirometer must be mindful and sensitive to incisional pain, which can interfere with the reception of instructions. Other patients may be seriously impaired or limited in hearing, speaking, or thinking. Respiratory therapists must be vigilant in recognizing these obstacles and be prepared to adapt their behavior to ensure effective communication.

RESPIRATORY RECAP

Sensory and Emotional Factors Affecting Communication

- » Fear
- » Stress
- » Anxiety
- » Pain
- » Compromised mental acuity, sight, hearing, or speech

Sensory communication issues, whether in patient care or the classroom, can be overcome when the sender uses multiple senses in sending messages. Multiple-sense learning may entail pictures (visual) and explanations with words (auditory). **Box 60–3** represents the relative percentage of remembering and learning from the use of various senses.

BOX 60–3

Learning and Remembering

We Learn . . .	We Remember . . .
1% through taste	10% of what we read
1.5% through touch	20% of what we hear
3.5% through smell	30% of what we see
11% through hearing	50% of what we see *and* hear
83% through sight	80% of what we say
	90% of what we say *and* do

Verbal Expressions

A third major category affecting effective communication is **verbal expression**, which involves language, jargon, choice of words or questions, voice tone and quality, and feedback. Language is the basis of communication, and words are the tools or symbols for the exchange. For instance, highly technical medical jargon is rarely appropriate for patient–therapist interaction. Although the use of medical jargon has the potential to increase patient confidence and credibility,[8] the loss of information and missed opportunity to build a rapport far outweigh such potential. In addition to medical terms such as *stat, prn,* and *NPO,* administrative terminology also must be explained. The student or young graduate may be unfamiliar with jargon, such as *FTE, HMO,* or *DRG* because such issues are not always taught in school.

> **RESPIRATORY RECAP**
>
> **Verbal Expression That Affect Communication**
> - Language
> - Jargon
> - Choice of words or questions
> - Voice tone and quality
> - Feedback

Additionally, verbal expression entails the rate and volume of the spoken word. A depressed patient generally speaks slowly at a low pitch and tolerates longer periods of silence. Aggressive individuals generally speak loudly and rapidly, enunciate precisely, often interrupt, and may ridicule, tease, joke, and even insult.[5] Care must be exercised to avoid this latter style of communicating. Verbal expression also involves feedback, an important tool to ensure understanding and build rapport. For example, vague responses or squinting gestures with the eyes may indicate uncertainty, which the therapist must note and follow up with additional communication.

Nonverbal Cues

Nonverbal cues are defined as a form of communication without words and include messages created through body motion (**kinesics**), the use and interpretation of space (**proxemics**), the use of sounds (**paralinguistics**), and touch.[10] Nonverbal communication is powerful but learned. Individuals are not born knowing these cues but develop them through modeling or imitating the actions or gestures of parents and peers. Recognizing and interpreting such messages can be tricky, but nonverbal communication is considered an extremely reliable index of the real meaning of what is being said or communicated, because a person generally is unable to exert as much conscious control over this aspect of behavior.[2] Body positions or posture can send particular messages. An instructor at the front of the classroom with hands on the hips may be sending a nonverbal message—"Knock it off and pay attention!"—just as a hand under the chin represents thinking or mulling over.

> **RESPIRATORY RECAP**
>
> **Nonverbal Cues That Affect Communication**
>
> **Body Motion (Kinesics)**
> - Gestures
> - Position/posture
> - Facial expression
> - Eye movement
> - Smiles
>
> **Use and Interpretation of Space (Proxemics)**
> - Distance zones (personal space)
>
> **Sounds (Paralinguistics)**
> - Giggling, laughing, belittling
> - *Ahs* and *ums*
> - Knuckle cracking
> - Silence
>
> **Touch**
> - Handshake
> - Squeeze, sharp pinch
> - Gentle touch

Facial expressions are perhaps the most prominent nonverbal cue. **Figure 60–6** graphically depicts a variety of facial expressions and the corresponding emotion each represents.[10] Masking or hiding one's true thoughts or feelings is difficult because facial expressions are thought to be a stronger representation of inner thoughts than are words. A smile is a universal sign of friendship

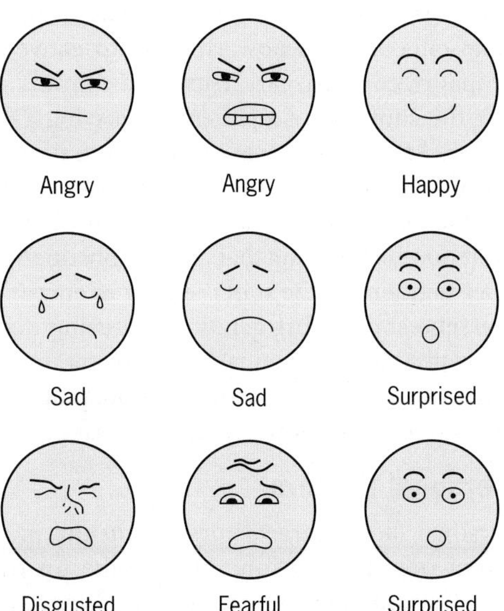

FIGURE 60–6 Common facial expressions and corresponding emotional meanings. Modified from Harrison RP. *Beyond Words: An Introduction to Nonverbal Communication.* Prentice-Hall; 1974:120.

and goes a long way to open the door to communication. Eye contact is another nonverbal cue, whether it consists of a wink, gaze, or movement of the eyebrow.

A patient who raises his or her head and eyebrows to the side when the therapist enters the room to administer a metered dose inhaler (MDI) treatment may be indicating discontent with the treatment. Words for such emotions might sound like this: "Oh no, not another one!" An appropriate reaction by the therapist might be to engage the patient in a dialogue to accurately interpret the meaning of such gestures. The therapist must never create hostility or conflict but rather must identify the reason for the sentiment, which may be as simple as the patient desiring to spend that particular moment with a visiting friend. Suggesting a return in 10 to 15 minutes may help win that patient's cooperation. Another finding regarding the eyes is that dilation conveys excitement or pleasure, whereas constriction generally reflects unpleasantness. In the United States, good eye contact is extremely important and considered to reflect a positive self-concept.[5] In contrast to this finding, some Eastern cultures consider eye contact disrespectful.

Sound is another nonverbal cue—giggling, laughing, cracking knuckles, *ah*s and *um*s, or even silence. Although knuckle cracking may simply be irritating, silence or giggling when a person enters a room can create discomfort. Walking into a room and having a few colleagues instantaneously stop talking may make a person feel that colleagues are hiding something or talking behind his or her back.

Touching—a gentle squeeze, a firm handshake, or a sharp pinch—is another form of nonverbal expression. Slapping a person on the back is demeaning and insulting, except, of course, in sports in which such practice is common and considered a means to motivate or acknowledge a job well done. In medicine, touching must be done judiciously; when done appropriately, it can be an effective and powerful way to convey closeness, empathy, concern, care, trust, and comfort. Lightly touching the shoulder of a patient and saying, "I'm here to help you, Mrs. Jones" goes a long way in demonstrating care and compassion and enhancing the relationship. Nonverbal communication should never be taken lightly because it may be *the* thing that gets the obstinate patient to take a treatment or the staff member to stay and work that overtime shift. Being genuine and using nonverbal cues appropriately helps enhance the respiratory therapist's effectiveness; it is not only important what the therapist says but also how the therapist says it.

Intrapersonal Factors

Intrapersonal factors are factors *within* the individual that affect communication. They make up the person's constitution and thus indirectly influence medical choices and decisions, but are not necessarily heard or seen. Although intrapersonal factors are present in both the sender and the receiver, this discussion focuses primarily on these factors as they pertain to the patient. The specific intrapersonal factors of interest are developmental stage, language mastery, previous experiences, attitudes, values, cultural heritage, religious beliefs, convictions, preoccupations, feelings, interest, and relative state of health.

Generally speaking, a person's developmental stage entails cognitive abilities and psychosocial development, for example, the ability to think and comprehend, reading level, attention span, maturity, and independence. The developmental stage of the very young requires them to receive assistance from family members. The elderly also may need assistance because mental acuity diminishes over time. However, it should be noted that 20% of American adults are illiterate, and another 34% are functionally illiterate.[18] Couple this fact with the average reading level of the adult population in the United States, the eighth-grade level,[18] and it becomes questionable whether patients understand what is being communicated at all.

RESPIRATORY RECAP

Intrapersonal Factors Affecting Communication

- » Developmental stage
- » Language mastery
- » Previous experiences
- » Attitudes/values
- » Cultural heritage
- » Religious beliefs and convictions
- » Preoccupations
- » Feelings
- » Interests
- » Relative state of health

Language mastery is another concern because many patients do not use English as their primary language, a cultural diversity issue that is becoming significant, with 2009 census data indicating that more than 35% of the U.S. population is minority.[19] In addition, the belief systems of these diverse groups can be considerably different. Western cultures are largely biomedical in healthcare beliefs, whereas Eastern cultures may adhere to magic, religion, or natural healing.[18] Eastern cultures are generally male dominated in hierarchy, have a strong family structure, and demonstrate considerable respect for their elderly. Communication between the therapist and such culturally diverse groups regarding terminating the ventilator of an elderly parent or a decision to use institutional care versus home care for an ailing family member is significantly affected by these values and beliefs. Interacting with patients from different cultures can be challenging because eye contact, words such as *no* and *yes*, and touch can all have different meanings. **Table 60–3** provides some guidelines to help therapists in cultural interactions.[18]

The Joint Commission recognizes that communication is a critical element of patient safety and quality care.[20] It makes provisions within its standards to address the need for effective communication by stating that hospitals must provide information in a manner tailored to the patient's age, language, and ability to understand. The Joint Commission goes on to include the need for interpretive and translation services as necessary for patients

TABLE 60–3 Guidelines to Facilitate Communication with Individuals from Other Cultures

Cultural Group	Guidelines
Asian Americans	Nonverbal communication important No eye contact; no touch May be hesitant to verbalize feelings or ask questions
Chinese Americans	Shame and embarrassment are common reactions when unable to do a task Especially avoid touching the head
Japanese Americans	Avoid the use of the word *no* by asking open-ended questions Will avoid conflict
Vietnamese Americans	*Yes* indicates respect but may not indicate agreement May avoid giving negative answer because it is not respectful or is confrontational An upward palm is considered an insult
Native American Indians	Avoid eye contact and pointing May answer *yes* to please questioner Sensitive to nurse taking notes
African Americans	May use own language variations, with some words meaning opposite (e.g., *bad* may mean *good*) Use a great deal of nonverbal communication with verbal communication Eye contact usually acceptable
Hispanic Americans	Touch is a dominant means of expression; women use more than men Smiling and hand-shaking are part of established trust Self-disclosure is difficult

Modified from Boyd MD, Gleit CJ, Graham BA, Whitman NI. *Health Teaching in Nursing Practice: A Professional Model.* 3rd ed. 1998. Electronically reproduced by permission of Pearson Education, Inc., Upper Saddle River, New Jersey.

with limited English proficiency. It suggests that organizations assess the language and communications needs of the population they serve and determine the type and assortment of language services to provide. A means of addressing language barriers include interpreters for oral communication; translators for converting written materials into language other than English; communication boards developed in languages needed by an organization's patient population; and signage to aid the patient population in navigating the physical environment.

Additionally, a person's attitude regarding a previous unpleasant experience, such as a 5-hour wait in the hospital emergency department, could leave that person with a bad feeling and impair future communication. Other patients may simply be too physically ill to focus on any communication. Preoccupation with family matters or with the gravity of an illness can wreak havoc on any communication encounter.

Consider the following example. You (the therapist) enter the room of a 42-year-old man to teach him the proper use of his MDI. Minutes before, his attending physician gave him the bad news that his wife has cancer. What are the chances you can engage him in any meaningful patient education? The answer is obvious: the patient no doubt will be preoccupied with the dreadful news. Respiratory therapists must be mindful of both the magnitude and the impact that these interpersonal factors can have on communication.

Physical Appearance and Status

Physical appearance and status involve age, gender, race, body size and shape, body movements, posture, dress, hair, body adornments, body smell, role, position, organizational status and influence, and professionalism.

Communication should always be age-appropriate. In general, the elderly require slower, more deliberate communication, with written materials enlarged and presented in bold print. Children are usually strong auditory communicators but respond more favorably to less formal, more casual interactions; they are more comfortable with technology and thrive on media that involve pictures, games, and simulations. With regard to gender, many patients are shy and uncomfortable in dealing with members of the opposite sex. A considerable amount of sensitivity should be exercised whenever communication and interaction occurs across genders. Although blatantly inaccurate, many patients, especially the elderly, perceive that men are physicians and women are nurses.

With regard to body size and shape, many individuals perceive that large physical size conveys dominance, power, authority, and control. Posture and body movement also factor into communication because acting stern, distant, and holding the body rigid can send a message of being unapproachable. Posture and body movement also can convey openness and receptiveness, such as freely walking around the room, extending an arm, or sitting back in a chair with the hands behind the head.

Dress is an especially important point because people generally judge others based on attire. If a therapist were to enter a patient's room in soiled scrubs, old, oil-stained sneakers, and 2 or 3 days of facial hair growth, that therapist would not likely make a positive impression. On the other hand, if the therapist were attired in a shirt and tie and a heavily starched white lab jacket with the name embroidered over the front pocket, that therapist may well receive immediate attention and credibility. Fair or not, patients and other healthcare professionals do respond more favorably to a positive professional appearance. Therapists are advised to remain well groomed with minimal body adornments. Long

RESPIRATORY RECAP

Physical Appearance and Status Factors Affecting Communication

- » Age, gender, and race
- » Body size and shape
- » Body movements and posture
- » Dress
- » Hair
- » Body adornments
- » Body smell
- » Role/position
- » Organizational status and influence
- » Professionalism

nails, heavily scented perfume, and large, ornate jewelry are not considered in good taste or likely to set a professional tone.

Regarding role, position, and organizational status and influence, physicians and upper-level healthcare administrators are considered to live at a higher socioeconomic level than the general population. This higher level or status can be problematic and intimidating to patients and subordinates, who may curtail or refrain from any purposeful communication. Both of these groups must be especially sensitive and make concerted efforts to remove this barrier. A related issue is the **"white lab jacket" phenomenon**, which essentially means that a white lab jacket generally creates an aura of instant credibility, acceptance, recognition, and stature that affords the wearer the opportunity to ask intimate questions and perform physical assessments. Departmental managers and supervisors also benefit from their elevated positions in the hierarchy of the institution, a situation fraught with advantages and disadvantages. For instance, some department members operate under a "we versus them" mentality in which they view the goals of the institution as inharmonious with their own. Such a climate creates strained relationships and communication difficulties. Physical appearance and status have a significant bearing on communication.

Barriers to Effective Communication

Box 60–4 is a general list of approaches and techniques that interfere with helpful communication between therapists and patients, family members, subordinates, and peers.[5] The choice of words should always be carefully considered. Abstract words, slang, and medical jargon create confusion and misunderstanding. Separation of emotional feelings from communication also is important. Anger, anxiety, and frustration are apparent in an individual's nonverbal communication and impair the interaction. Inappropriate facts, unrelated information, glib statements, and clichés such as "You'll be OK" are irrelevant and may be annoying to the recipient. Being too opinionated, giving advice, and expressing unnecessary approval or undue disapproval can curtail the exchange, as can probing, requiring explanations, and belittling the person's feelings. Being defensive, interrupting the person, and interpreting behavior are also destructive tendencies. Efforts should always be directed toward relationship enhancement and satisfaction of the purpose of the communication.

BOX 60–4

Barriers to Communication

- Using the wrong words
- Conveying your feelings of anxiety, anger, strangeness, denial, isolation, lack of control, or lack of physical health
- Failing to realize that the person's reluctance to make a message clear can prevent therapeutic communication
- Making inappropriate use of facts, introducing unrelated information, offering premature explanation or counseling, wrong timing, saying something important when the person is upset or not feeling well and thus unable to hear what is really said
- Making glib statements, offering false reassurance
- Using clichés, stereotyping responses, trite expressions, and empty verbalisms
- Being too strongly opinionated
- Expressing unnecessary approval
- Expressing undue disapproval
- Giving advice, stating personal experiences, opinion, or value judgments, giving pep talks, telling another what should be done
- Probing, persistent, pointed, or "yes/no" questioning
- Requiring explanations, demanding proof, challenging or asking "why"
- Belittling the person's feelings
- Making only literal responses
- Interpreting the person's behavior or confronting him or her
- Interrupting or abruptly changing the subject
- Defending or protecting someone or something

Data from Murray RB, Zentner JP. *Nursing Concepts for Health Promotion.* 3rd ed. Englewood Cliffs, NJ: Prentice-Hall; 1985.

Basic Goals and Purpose of Communication

Four Major Goals

In the definition of communication, the phrase *shared meaning* is highlighted and stressed. Although the transmission of a message from one person to another that is mutually understood is a vital function of the communication process, the process does not stop there. The real purpose of mutual understanding is to influence the other to change.[11] The sender attempts to persuade the receiver

> **RESPIRATORY RECAP**
>
> **Sender's Expectations from Receiver**
> » Understanding
> » Action
> » Information
> » Comfort

to respond to the sender's request. Requests from senders may be for understanding, action, information, or comfort.[11] Requests can be either direct or indirect. For example, you enter the room of a patient with documented asthma that physiologically requires an aerosolized bronchodilator. You observe that he is tachypneic and gasping for air, and he asks you, "When did I receive my last treatment?" His direct request is for *information* about when he had his last treatment. His indirect request is for *understanding* and *action*; he wants another treatment. You give him the treatment, and he is *comforted*.[11]

Conveying Believability

As noted previously, the real goal in communication is to influence the other person to affect change,[11] which is perhaps most obvious when a respiratory therapist communicates with a physician to have an order changed or when a respiratory manager must convince his or her staff of the benefits of a new protocol or when the therapist must convince an asthmatic patient of the value of monitoring peak flows. Being able to speak convincingly and persuasively is a valuable skill because where there is no belief, there can be no action.[21] The question then becomes: How can a person convey believability in communication? The answer lies in the consistency or inconsistency of the message, and more specifically with the harmony between the three Vs—the verbal, vocal, and visual elements of the message.

According to Albert Mehrabian's landmark publications on nonverbal communication, the verbal component represents a mere 7% of the communication, the vocal 38%, and the visual a hefty 55%.[22,23] In other words, appearance and body language (visual) account for 55% of the way in which a message is interpreted; tone of voice (vocal) accounts for 38% of the message; and the actual spoken words (verbal) have the least importance, representing a meager 7%.[10] The implication is that 93% of the way communication is interpreted deals with the nonverbal element, or the delivery of the message, whereas 7% deals with the content. Furthermore, Mehrabian's research indicates that when the message is inconsistent, the receiver is more inclined to believe the visual and vocal rather than the verbal.[22]

> **RESPIRATORY RECAP**
>
> **Three Vs of Communication**
> » *Verbal* represents 7% of communication.
> » *Vocal* represents 38% of communication.
> » *Visual* represents 55% of communication.

For example, if a therapist asks the physician to change an order from q2h to qid and in his nonverbal communication reflects uncertainty and quivering in his posture and gestures, hesitation, and an abundance of qualifiers (*ah*s and *um*s) in his voice, the physician may interpret these cues to mean that the therapist may not know what to do or at least that he is uncertain of his recommendation; thus, the physician may refuse to modify treatment. Although therapists undoubtedly must know the science of respiratory care, it is equally important that they can communicate with conviction, confidence, and believability. Remember the old saying: Actions speak louder than words.

> **BOX 60–5**
>
> **Methods for Effective Therapeutic Communication**
>
> Use thoughtful silence to encourage the person to talk.
> Be accepting.
> Help the person strengthen self-identification in relation to others.
> Suggest collaboration and a cooperative relationship.
> Use open-ended, generalized leading questions.
> Ask related questions.
> Place events in time sequence.
> State observations that you perceive about the person.
> Encourage description of behavior or observation.
> Restate or repeat the main idea expressed.
> Reflect by paraphrasing feelings, questions, ideas, and key words.
> Verbalize the implied.
> Attempt to translate feelings into words.
> Clarify.
> Reintroduce reality.
> Offer information.
> Seek consensual validation.
> Encourage evaluation of the situation by the person.
> Encourage formulation of a plan of action.
> Summarize.
>
> Data from Murray RB, Zentner JP. *Nursing Concepts for Health Promotion*. 3rd ed. Englewood Cliffs, NJ: Prentice-Hall; 1985.

Effective Communication

Given the concepts and definitions provided thus far, it is obvious that communication is not a science. It is not governed by a strict set of scientific laws or theories. It is an art that entails skills that can be learned, developed, and, with appropriate practice, mastered. Mastery of effective communication skills is a primary goal of this chapter. **Box 60–5** provides some general methods for effective therapeutic communication,[5] but specific communication skills related to both the sender and the receiver are identified and discussed in the following sections.

Skills of the Sender

To be an effective sender, the therapist should be aware of six simple measures that can enhance this aspect of the communication. The acronym SENDER can help recall the six measures: (1) set the stage, (2) enunciate clearly, (3) notify the receiver of the importance, (4) demand feedback, (5) eliminate the unnecessary, and (6) receiver-orient the message.[9]

Setting the stage simply means that before commencing, the sender should decide what information is desired and decide on a time and an appropriate setting for the interaction. For example, if the occasion is a patient education session, the intention is to assess learning needs, provide instruction, and evaluate understanding and performance. The choice of time and setting should entail a time free of interruptions and distractions in a quiet, comfortable room furnished with appropriate resources (e.g., blackboard, audiovisual aids, written materials). Such an environment may be the patient's room or a designated conference area. The same would hold true for a new employee interview, a staff performance appraisal, or a student clinical competency assessment.

RESPIRATORY RECAP

Skills of the Sender

- » Set the stage.
- » Enunciate clearly.
- » Notify the receiver of the importance of the message.
- » Demand feedback.
- » Eliminate the unnecessary.
- » Receiver-orient the message.

The second measure is to enunciate clearly. Frequently the therapist is under considerable pressure and has limited time at the patient's bedside. Avoiding fast talk and garbled, inaudible, or inarticulate speech is particularly important. This issue is especially problematic for the elderly, who may need added time to absorb and process information. Equally important is that the therapist does not speak too softly; he or she should try to energize the delivery.

A third measure is to notify the receiver of the importance of the communication. For example, before a patient education session, the wise therapist would inform the patient of his or her imminent hospital discharge and stress that the patient must self-administer the MDI thereafter. This statement is a strong motivating factor for the patient to learn the procedure, and the therapist is more likely to gain that patient's attention and cooperation. Additionally, the therapist may indicate the estimated length of the exchange and keep the patient informed about the time throughout the process. Finally, a summary of the key points of the exchange may help highlight important considerations.

Soliciting feedback also facilitates communication. Again using the patient education session example, the therapist may open the dialogue with a general statement inviting the patient to stop the instruction at any point with a question or concern. Periodic queries about whether the patient understands can help. Requiring a return demonstration from patients is an extremely effective way to obtain assurance of mastery and secure feedback.

The fifth measure is to eliminate the unnecessary. Research has found that most people use 30% more words than necessary.[6] The therapist should be as clear and concise as possible, and when in doubt, should say something and wait for feedback. Further information can always be provided as needed. The previously discussed acronym KISS is appropriate—keep it short and simple.

Finally, the speaker should orient the message for the receiver. The sender's focus should not be *me* but *we*. This focus helps instill an attitude of collaboration rather than one of superiority and authority. Whenever possible, information should be *shared* rather than *told.*

Skills of the Receiver

At one time or another every person has walked away from a conversation only to say, "I have no idea what was just said." The volume and tone of the sender were more than adequate, so the message was heard. The problem was not hearing, but listening. Hearing is a physical act that acknowledges sound, whereas listening is an intellectual and emotional act that includes understanding and requires active involvement. With this information in mind, the following section addresses the five skills of the active listener: (1) listen to the content, (2) listen to the intent, (3) assess the sender's nonverbal communication, (4) monitor nonverbal communication and **emotional filters**, and (5) listen without judgment and with empathy.[24]

RESPIRATORY RECAP

Skills of the Receiver

- » Listen to the content.
- » Listen to the intent.
- » Assess the sender's nonverbal communication.
- » Monitor personal nonverbal communication and emotional filters.
- » Listen without judgment and with empathy.

Listening to the content means giving full attention to the speaker. A listener should eliminate internal and external distractions and, if needed, be prepared to take notes and physically move closer to the sender. A listener should not prepare responses while the sender is communicating but should stop talking and simply listen.

Listening to the intent is a challenging skill. It means attempting to hear the whole message, not just what is implied. The intent includes the content, the nonverbal cues, the sender's background and biases, and any other factors that affect the issue at hand. For example, a patient says, "I'm not taking my treatment today because my brother told me not to. I started to shake last night when he was here, and he said that it could be due to the medication." The therapist in this case must not prematurely turn off the conversation. A busy and harried therapist may hear only the first part of the communication and prematurely pass judgment that the patient is trying to stop treatment. Listening to the intent means listening to *why* the patient says something rather than just *what* is being said. The listener may need to paraphrase or seek clarification of the sender's intention but should not use emotions to interpret the intent.

The third skill is the ability to assess the sender's nonverbal communication, which involves body language and tone of voice and represents more than 90% of the message. Nonverbal elements also represent the *how* rather than the *what*, and are considered a true reflection of the sender's innermost thoughts. When incongruity exists between what is seen and heard (the nonverbal) versus what is reflected in the verbal, the nonverbal is almost always the correct interpretation. Astute therapists note such inconsistency and seek clarification. For example, a respiratory manager asks for a volunteer to work an overtime shift, and a staff member responds, "Sure, I'll do it." The nonverbal interpretation is the more critical component of the message because the staff member may be genuine or may raise the eyes and head (a visual indicator of sarcasm) and emphasize the word *sure* (a vocal inflection signifying, "no way!").

Skillful listeners monitor their own nonverbal cues and control their emotional filters, meaning simply that just as the sender sends nonverbal messages, so does the receiver. The receiver's messages may be supportive and encouraging, such as, "Yeah, I follow you; go on" or just the opposite, such as, "Yeah, right (*sarcasm*); no way that could be true." Nonverbal signs of disapproval or rejection should not be used to discourage communication; the listener must maintain neutrality so as to hear the whole message. With emotional filters, both the sender and the receiver have a particular **mind-set** developed over years, consisting of personal biases, experiences, and expectations. Each person has these deep-seated feelings and beliefs and should control them. A mind-set may sound like this: "Nursing is a feminine job, and homosexuals are effeminate males; therefore, a male nurse is a homosexual." Although this statement is obviously ridiculous, it does reflect the fact that a person's mind-set stems from the particular culture in which that individual was raised. The listener should check emotional filters and not allow them to interfere with listening to the whole message.

Empathetic listening simply means the return of feedback that reflects care about the receiver and the importance of that individual's message. Being nonjudgmental means being open-minded and not entering a situation with one's mind already decided. In essence, the listener reflects on the whole message and at the same time says, "I am here for you."

Bridges to the Relationship

The respiratory therapist must understand the importance of exhibiting qualities and characteristics compatible with effective therapeutic relationships. Six qualities or characteristics are considered essential to nurture the relationship: care, empowerment, trust, empathy, mutuality, and confidentiality.[25]

Caring is an intentional human action characterized by commitment and a sufficient level of knowledge and skill to allow the therapist to support the needs of the patient.[26] It entails offering a presence, attending, affiliating, and empowering.[27] **Empowerment** involves the provision of the proper tools, resources, and environment to build, develop, and increase the ability and effectiveness of others to set and reach goals for individual and social ends.[28]

Trust is present when individuals feel that they can rely on others. Building trust requires that communication be descriptive rather than evaluative, problem-oriented rather than control-oriented, spontaneous rather than strategic, empathetic rather than neutral, equal rather than superior, and provisional rather than certain.[10]

Empathy describes individuals mutually imagining themselves in the shoes of others and then verbally conveying that understanding.[11] **Mutuality** simply means that the therapist and patient agree on the health problems and the means to resolve them.[25] Finally, **confidentiality** involves an assurance on the part of both parties that the other will not divulge private information. The sole purpose of confidentiality is to protect the patient from unauthorized disclosures. All six qualities are essential ingredients for any successful therapist–patient interaction, and their value in the nurturing of a relationship is best represented by the following saying: Patients don't care how much you know, until they know how much you care.

> **RESPIRATORY RECAP**
>
> **Qualities or Characteristics of a Nurturing Relationship**
>
> » Care
> » Empowerment
> » Trust
> » Empathy
> » Mutuality
> » Confidentiality

Questioning Techniques

Questioning techniques in respiratory care can be used between the therapist and his or her superiors, subordinates, professional colleagues, peers, or patients during physical assessments, patient interviews, employee appraisals, student clinical assessments, or progressive discipline sessions, to name a few instances. Regardless of the purpose or motive, questioning techniques are a powerful way to obtain information, clarify uncertainties, facilitate learning, and resolve conflicts. Some of the more important questioning strategies and techniques used by the respiratory therapist are closed-ended questions, open-ended questions, clarification,

> **RESPIRATORY RECAP**
>
> **Questioning Strategies and Techniques**
> » Closed-ended questions
> » Open-ended questions
> » Clarification
> » Leading questions
> » Compound questions
> » Facilitation
> » Confrontation
> » Silence
> » Support and reassurance

leading questions, compound questions, facilitation, confrontation, silence, and support or reassurance.[5,10,12,29]

Closed-ended questions help obtain specific information, yield a limited number of possible answers, and generally can be answered with a simple *yes* or *no*. Although they are valuable in certain focused questioning sessions, they have limited value during the initial patient interview or assessment. Examples include "Have you ever had TB?" or "How many puffs of your inhaler do you use every day?"

Open-ended questions are considered the most valuable form of questioning during the initial patient assessment. They yield the broadest amount of information and allow for more freedom of response. They generally involve short probes followed by periods of silence in which the interviewee is permitted more in-depth and personal responses. Such questions almost always begin with the words *what*, *why*, or *how*. Examples include "What brings you to the hospital?" or "How do you use your inhaler?" or "Tell me about your shortness of breath."

Clarification attempts to correct ambiguity and clear up the meaning of confusing responses. Patients may be asked to elaborate on an ambiguous or uncertain issue. Examples of clarifying questions include "What do you mean by the statement that you have a cold?" or "What exactly do you mean by shortness of breath?"

Leading questions are those phrased so that a predetermined or expected response is inevitable. Such questions reflect the bias of the interviewer and should not be asked because they can produce useless, unreliable, or inaccurate responses. Examples include "You've never smoked, have you?" or "You're feeling better today, aren't you?"

Compound questions ask more than one question at a time and do not allow adequate time for each answer. They are confusing and generally result in a response to the last part of the question only. Examples include "Tell me about yourself. How old are you? Are you married? What do you do for a living?" or "Have you ever had TB, HIV, asbestos exposure, used drugs, or smoked cigarettes?" The interviewee is likely to hear "What do you do for a living?" and "Have you ever smoked?" In short, the interviewee is likely to answer the very last part of the question, which garners the interviewer little information about the other issues.

Facilitation is actually a technique whereby words, postures, or actions encourage more detail. Facilitation is a skill that must be performed with sincerity and genuineness, with examples including "Please go on . . ." or "uh huh." Nonverbal actions that display sincerity, genuine interest, and attentiveness can include sitting forward or touching the patient.

Confrontation can be very tricky because the therapist, for example, would not want to close off communication and yet needs to be honest and bring a patient's behavior or emotional state to that individual's conscious awareness. Examples include "You said your breathing was fine, yet I noticed your respiratory rate was quite high and your breathing is labored" or "You said you are not angry, yet I observed you raising your voice and clenching your fist."

Silence allows time for reflection and is an effective way for the patient to organize thoughts and feelings. Although silence takes many forms,[5] the interviewer must learn to deal with the difficulty of prolonged periods of utter stillness. Significant delays in speech are naturally difficult between two people. Because healthcare is an area foreign and mysterious to the patient, that person may simply need time to process and think through the information.

Finally, support and reassurance are valuable techniques in questioning. When the therapist expresses sensitivity and sincere understanding regarding the patient's reactions, that is demonstrating support. The most important aspect of this technique is to be genuine and sincere. Even with sincerity and genuineness, the therapist is still likely to receive a curt rebuttal stating, "You have no idea what I am going through." As difficult as this response may be, a continued display of warmth, hope, dignity, empathy, and reassurance is recommended. The hope should not be false hope but should be directed at having the patient come to some degree of acceptance and peace of mind. Feelings of sympathy are feelings of sorrow *for* someone, whereas empathy describes feelings of sorrow *with* a person, meaning that the empathizer too has had similar experiences.

Examples in Respiratory Care

Patient Interview

You are a respiratory therapist (RT) working in a pulmonary rehabilitation department and have been asked to provide support and assistance to Mr. Ryan, a 59-year-old man referred to you by his physician for pulmonary rehabilitation. He was recently diagnosed with chronic obstructive pulmonary disease (COPD). Your initial interview with him follows.[29]

RT: Hello, Mr. Ryan. My name is Beth Fallon. I am a respiratory therapist and am working with your lung doctor, Dr. Connor. Before performing a physical exam, I'd like to ask you a few questions.

Patient: *[nods and acknowledges the introductory remarks]*

Question Session 1

RT: I have your records and know some of your medical history. However, could you tell me in your own words why you are here?

Patient: Sometimes I have a lot of trouble breathing.

Question Session 2

RT: Trouble breathing?

Patient: Yes. When I walk up the steps to the bathroom, I can't seem to catch my breath. It scares me.

Question Session 3

RT: You seem worried about this.

Patient: Well, yes. My dad died from lung disease, and he was only 61. *[starts to cry]*

Question Session 4

RT: *[hands box of tissues to patient}*

Question Session 5

Patient: Thanks. My dad was a great guy, and I think of him all the time.

RT: I'm sorry to hear of your loss. I lost my dad 4 years ago. Although relationships between people can sometimes be different, I *think* I can understand how you must feel. This must have been a very difficult moment for you.

Question Session 6

Patient: Ever since my dad died, I've taken care of my mom and frankly I'm worried about her as well. I don't want her to worry about my illness.

RT: How do you feel about your illness?

Question Session 7

Patient: I'm scared to death. I don't know much about my disease and whether I will be able to take care of both of us.

RT: I'm glad you were able to tell me this. It's natural for you to feel this way. I'm here to help you. I will teach you how best to cope with your COPD.

Question Session 8

Patient: Thanks. I'm glad I came.

RT: Can you tell me a little more about your COPD? Does your shortness of breath occur when you go up flights of steps or just a few steps?

Question Session 9

Patient: Flights of steps.

RT: Can you tell me approximately how many steps?

Question Session 10

Patient: Approximately 12.

RT: I noted in your records that you produce about a cup of sputum every day. Can you tell me whether it is thick and discolored? Explain it in your own words.

Discussion

The questioning techniques used in the previous scenario are as follows.

Question Session Number	Question Technique, Strategy, and Discussion
1	*Open-ended questioning*: This is a very appropriate use of the open-ended questioning technique, allowing the patient to express his own feelings in his own words.
2	*Facilitation*: By repeating the patient's statement, the therapist helps the patient better express his condition.
3	*Confrontation*: The therapist picks up on an emotional feeling and confronts the patient in a nonthreatening manner.
4	*Silence*: The therapist allows the patient to regain composure and sympathetically addresses his emotional need.
5	*Support*: The therapist genuinely expresses both sympathy and empathy. The relationship appears to strengthen through this interaction.
6	*Open-ended question*: The therapist continues to focus on the emotional needs of the family and to bring out the patient's feelings about his condition.
7	*Support and reassurance*: The therapist strengthens the bond by approving the openness of the relationship and provides hope, indicating that specific intervention is available to address the condition.
8	*Closed-ended question*: The therapist tries to obtain some specific information regarding how far the patient can move before the onset of his shortness of breath.
9	*Clarifying question*: The therapist asks the patient to clarify his ambiguous response.
10	*Elaboration*: The therapist picked up on statements in the patient's record and asked him to provide more detail.

New Hire

The director of the respiratory care department for a 400-bed tertiary care facility has an 8 AM interview with a new graduate from the local college program for a full-time staff position on the 3 to 11 PM shift. The candidate, Christine Meehan, arrives promptly, and the director greets her in the human resources conference room. The employment interview with her follows.

Question Session 1

Director: Hello and welcome to University Hospital. Should I call you Ms. Meehan or would you prefer something else?

Candidate: Christine would be just fine. *[appears nervous]*

Question Session 2

Director: Well, welcome Christine. My name is Timothy Sean and you can call me Tim. *[pleasant smile]* I am the director of respiratory care services, and I will be doing the initial interview with you this morning.

Candidate: [nods and smiles but still appears nervous]

Question Session 3

Director: I see that you are a graduate of the respiratory care program at Gwynedd Mercy College. We've had a number of their graduates and have been very pleased with their performance. It's a very good program.

Candidate: Yes, I graduated just this past month. I'm glad you have been pleased.

Question Session 4

Director: Christine, tell me a little about yourself.

Candidate: Well, as you know I graduated from Gwynedd Mercy this past May. I am single, live at home with my parents, did well in school, and am a hard worker.

Question Session 5

Director: Why would you like to work at University Hospital?

Candidate: University is only 4 miles from my home, and I've heard very good things about the hospital.

Question Session 6

Director: What have you heard?

Candidate: Well, I grew up in the area, and my family came here whenever we needed to be hospitalized. But more importantly, I know it is a large teaching hospital and that you have an active open-heart surgery program and a wide array of cardiorespiratory services.

Question Session 7

Director: Open-heart program? *[followed by pause]*

Candidate: I have an interest in working in critical care medicine. I enjoy this kind of environment and believe it will help me with my registry. I want to go as far as I can in the profession.

Question Session 8

Director: You are a member of the AARC, aren't you? *[voice inflection at end]*

Candidate: Well, yes. *[a slight hesitancy in voice]* I ah, I ah, *[stammering a bit]* think it's very important for one to be involved in their profession. I joined as a student and have every intention of maintaining membership. *[genuine and sincere tone of voice]*

Question Session 9

Director: I'm glad to hear you feel that way. *[more mild and affirming tone of voice]* You said you want to work in critical care medicine. Have you worked with the Servo Is, the Draegers, and 840s?

Candidate: Yes, I worked with the 840 all through my clinical rotations.

Question Session 10

Director: I'm sorry. I confused you. What about the Servo? *[waits for response]*

Candidate: Yes, I did work with the Servo while rotating through my clinicals. We also were exposed to the Servo in the laboratory.

Director: How about the Draeger?

Candidate: Yes, I have experience with the Draeger.

Question Session 11

Director: Is there anything else you would like to share with me?

Candidate: I would really like to work at University. It is close to my home, and I could be available for call-outs. I feel I could fit in well with the staff. I believe my program prepared me for this kind of opportunity. And I want to provide quality patient care. I really care about my patients and will make a commitment to the institution.

Discussion

The questioning techniques used in the previous scenario are as follows.

Question Session Number	Question Technique, Strategy, and Discussion
1	*Closed-ended questioning/clarification*: The director poses a focused question that allows only a limited response, setting the stage for the candidate to determine the degree of formality.
2	*Support/clarification*: The director recognizes the candidate's nervousness and tries to build rapport while clarifying the purpose of the meeting.
3	*Reassurance*: The director continues to use the first 2 to 3 minutes to build rapport and provide reassurance, attempting to decrease the candidate's anxiety so that she will be more comfortable and "open up" to express her true self. *[appears to be successful]*
4	*Open-ended question*: The director allows the candidate considerable freedom to provide information she feels is important.

(*continues*)

Question Session Number	Question Technique, Strategy, and Discussion
5	*Open-ended questioning*: Once again the director tries to get the candidate to express herself to identify her motivation for wanting to work at University Hospital.
6	*Clarification*: The director probes to see what specifically she means by the statement, her depth of understanding.
7	*Facilitation/silence*: The director seeks elaboration on what this candidate sees as an "open-heart program." His comment is followed by a pause and silence, which the candidate immediately fills with elaboration.
8	*Leading question*: Although the director tries to identify this candidate's degree of commitment to the profession, this question is not effective. Her qualifying statement substantiates her claim in a convincing way. However, had she stopped after the word *yes*, the director would have doubts. More important, he makes the candidate feel defensive and runs the risk of not getting to really know her.
9	*Compound question*: This question is not well structured because the candidate answered only the last part, a common response to such questions. An open-ended question, such as "Which ventilators have you worked with?" would be better.
10	*Clarification/closed-ended question*: Recognizing his error and the confusion created, the director repeats his questions one at a time. He receives the feedback he was originally seeking.
11	*Open-ended question*: The director demonstrates an excellent use of open-ended questioning, effectively allowing his candidate to open up and share her innermost feelings.

KEY POINTS

- Miscommunication can include misinterpretation of the message, incomplete messages, inappropriate use of medical terminology or expressions, and cultural influences in language.
- Communication involves accepted social customs and amenities, as well as more formal dialogue.
- Communication has a content dimension (language and information) and a relationship dimension (perceived relationship between communicants).
- Communication has a cognitive dimension (thoughts) and an affective dimension (feelings and emotions).
- Communication involves a reciprocal transaction in which each communicant alternates between the roles of sender and receiver.
- Communication is simply defined as a shared meaning.
- Environmental factors, emotional and sensory factors, verbal expressions, nonverbal cues, internal or interpersonal factors, and physical appearance and status all affect communication.
- The degree of believability of the message is a result of congruence among the verbal, vocal, and visual components of the message.
- The vocal and visual components made up 93% of the communication.
- Effectiveness in any communication requires sending skills and receiving skills.
- Care, empowerment, trust, empathy, mutuality, and confidence are important ingredients to nurture any relationship.
- Effective questioning strategies and techniques include the appropriate use of open-ended questions, closed-ended questions, clarification, facilitation, confrontation, silence, support, and reassurance.

REFERENCES

1. Barnes TA, Gale DD, Kacmarek RM, Kaegler WV. Competencies needed by graduate respiratory therapists in 2015 and beyond. *Respir Care.* 2010;55(5):604.
2. Wilkes M, Crosswait CB. *Professional Development: The Dynamics of Success.* Orlando, FL: Harcourt Brace Jovanovich; 1991.
3. Ornstein C. Quaids recall twins' drug overdose. *Los Angeles Times.* January 15, 2008.
4. Kohn L, Corrigan JM, Donaldson MS, eds. *To Err Is Human: Building a Safer Health System.* Committee on Quality of Health Care in America, Institute of Medicine. Washington, DC: National Academies Press; 2000.
5. Murray RB, Zentner JP. *Nursing Concepts for Health Promotion.* 3rd ed. Englewood Cliffs, NJ: Prentice-Hall; 1985.
6. Haimann T. *Supervisory Management for Health Care Organizations.* 3rd ed. St. Louis, MO: The Catholic Health Association of the United States; 1984.
7. Powell JSJ. *Why Am I Afraid to Tell You Who I Am*? Chicago: Argus Communications; 1969.
8. Purtilo R. *Health Professional and Patient Interaction*. 4th ed. Philadelphia: WB Saunders; 1990.
9. Dellinger S, Deane B. *Communicating Effectively: A Complete Guide for Better Managing.* Radnor, PA: Chilton Books; 1980.
10. Northouse LL, Northouse PG. *Health Communication: Strategies for Health Professionals.* 3rd ed. Stamford, CT: Appleton & Lange; 1998.
11. Balzer-Riley JW. *Communication in Nursing.* 4th ed. St. Louis, MO: Mosby; 2000.
12. Van Servellen G. *Communication Skills for the Health Care Professional: Concepts and Techniques.* Gaithersburg, MD: Aspen; 1997.
13. Schuster PM. *Communication: The Key to the Therapeutic Relationship.* Philadelphia: FA Davis; 2000.
14. Scanlon CL, Wilkins RL, Stoller JK. *Egan's Fundamentals of Respiratory Care.* St. Louis, MO: Mosby; 1999.
15. Burton GG, Hodgkin JE, Ward JJ. *Respiratory Care: A Guide to Clinical Practice.* Philadelphia: Lippincott Williams & Wilkins; 1997.
16. Fink JB, Fink AK. *The Respiratory Therapist as Manager.* Chicago: Year Book; 1986.

17. Wilkins RL, Krider SJ, Sheldon RL. *Clinical Assessment in Respiratory Care*. 4th ed. St. Louis, MO: Mosby; 2000.
18. Boyd M, Graham B, Gleit C, et al. *Health Teaching in Nursing Practice: A Professional Model*. 3rd ed. Stamford, CT: Appleton & Lange; 1998.
19. Yen H. US minority population could be majority by mid-century Census shows. *Huffington Post*. Available at: http://www.huffingtonpost.com/2010/06/10/us-minority-population-co_n_607369.html. Accessed October 5, 2010.
20. The Joint Commission. *Advancing Effective Communication, Cultural Competence, and Patient- and Family-Centered Care: A Roadmap for Hospitals*. Oakbrook Terrace, IL: The Joint Commission; 2010.
21. Decker B. *The Art of Communicating: Achieving Interpersonal Impact in Business*. Los Altos, CA: Crisp Publications; 1988.
22. Mehrabian A, Williams M. Nonverbal communication of perceived and intended persuasiveness. *J Pers Social Psych*. 1969; 13:37.
23. Mehrabian A. *Silent Messages*. Belmont, CA: Wadsworth; 1971.
24. Dugger J. *Listen Up: Hear What's Really Being Said*. West Des Moines, IA: American Media Publishing; 1995.
25. Arnold E, Boggs K. *Interpersonal Relationships: Professional Communication Skills for Nurses*. 2nd ed. Philadelphia: WB Saunders; 1995.
26. Clarke J. A view of the phenomenon of caring in nursing practice. *J Adv Nurs*. 1992;17:1283–1290.
27. Clayton G. Connecting: a catalyst for caring. In: Chin P, ed. *Anthology of Caring*. New York: NLN Press; 1991.
28. Hawks J. Empowerment in nursing education: concept analysis and application to philosophy, learning and instruction. *J Adv Nurs*. 1992;17:609–618.
29. Ballweg R, Stolberg S, Sullivan EM. *Physician Assistant: A Guide to Clinical Practice*. Philadelphia: WB Saunders; 1994.

SUGGESTED READING

Axtell RE. *Gestures: The Do's and Taboos of Body Language Around the World*. New York: John Wiley & Sons; 1998.

Bone D. *The Business of Listening: A Practical Guide to Effective Listening*. Los Altos, CA: Crisp Publications; 1988.

Mehrabian A. *Nonverbal Communication*. Chicago: Aldine-Atherton; 1972.

Mindell P. *A Woman's Guide to the Language of Success: Communicating with Confidence and Power*. Englewood Cliffs, NJ: Prentice Hall; 1995.

Tamparo CD, Lindh WQ. *Therapeutic Communications for Allied Health Professions*. Albany, NY: Delmar; 1992.

CHAPTER 61

Healthcare Reimbursement

Karen Stewart
William F. Galvin

OUTLINE

OBJECTIVES

1. Explain the four major functions of the healthcare delivery system.
2. Explain the role of the major stakeholders in healthcare delivery.
3. Discuss the forces influencing healthcare change and costs.
4. Describe the general healthcare payment systems.
5. Explain the history and evolution of managed care.
6. Explain the types of managed care organizations.
7. Describe the more popular reimbursement methodologies.
8. Discuss the future of healthcare financing.
9. Discuss the implications of reimbursement for the respiratory therapist.

KEY TERMS

all-patient refined diagnosis-related groups (APR-DRGs)
bundled charges
capitation
case mix
Centers for Medicare and Medicaid Services (CMS)
copayment
diagnosis-related group (DRG)
exclusive provider organization (EPO)
fee-for-service system
health maintenance organization (HMO)
indemnity insurance plan
insurance
managed care organization (MCO)
Medicaid
Medicare
minimum data set (MDS)
pay for performance (P4P)
point-of-service plan (POS)
preferred provider organization (PPO)
prospective payment system (PPS)
resource-based relative value scale (RBRVS)
resource intensity
retrospective payment system (RPS)
risk of mortality
severity of illness
skilled nursing facility (SNF)
third-party payer

INTRODUCTION

The economic climate of today's healthcare system in the United States is precarious, extremely volatile, and unpredictable. Forces are at play within the private and public sector that are attempting to shape it and minimize the deleterious effects of spiraling healthcare costs. While the healthcare system is constantly evolving and undergoing change, the way in which it reimburses has a profound impact on its delivery and practice. Reimbursement and economic considerations are central issues for healthcare executives. In fact, some would say that the present healthcare system in the United States is driven almost exclusively by the dollar. Although such a statement may sound cold, greedy, impersonal, and even callous, the wise respiratory therapist must recognize the paramount importance placed on reimbursement methodologies and sources. Converting care and services into financial returns to the provider has become critical to survival, and economic pressures are not likely to change in the foreseeable future.

The problem is that respiratory therapy schools and departments have not done an especially good job in helping students and practitioners understand the critical importance of the reimbursement process and the underlying economic principles guiding the system. This chapter identifies and discusses the basic functions of healthcare, provides an overview of the forces driving the system, identifies and explains the role of the major stakeholders, provides a basic and simplified view of the history and various forms of reimbursement, and explains the role and function of the respiratory therapist within this system. The theme of the chapter is that the respiratory therapist can no longer limit his or her involvement to simply the provision of quality care. Today's healthcare environment demands that respiratory therapists be a valued-added member of the healthcare team and be savvy with regard to healthcare economics.

Basic Healthcare Delivery Functions

The four major functions of the healthcare system in the United States are financing, insurance, delivery, and payment.[1] Although this chapter focuses on insurance and payment, all four are discussed to set the stage for a better understanding of how the system works. **Table 61–1** depicts the four major functions, their roles, and the group or organization that is associated with each.

The first major function in healthcare delivery is *financing*, which involves the purchase of insurance and serves as the means to pay for the healthcare services consumed by the patient or client. Employers generally finance healthcare as a fringe benefit. The federal, state, and local government also can provide it.

Strictly speaking, the **insurance** function entails protection of the patient, client, or consumer against catastrophic risk. *Insurance* also refers to the administration of the customer's benefits package and is provided by an insurance company or managed care organization (MCO) that serves as an intermediary between the purchaser and the recipient or consumer. Interestingly, providers (especially hospitals) contract directly with employers to provide healthcare services.

TABLE 61–1 Four Major Functions of Healthcare

Function	Role	Affected Group or Organization
Financing	Purchase of health insurance	Private sources: employers, individuals Public sources: federal, state, and local governments
Insurance	Protection against risk	Commercial insurance companies: Aetna US Healthcare, Met Life, Prudential, others Blue Cross/Blue Shield Quasi-fraternal organizations: AARP, managed care groups
Delivery	Provision of services	Physicians and other healthcare practitioners, hospitals, alternative care sites
Payment	Determination of reimbursement methodology and disbursement of funds	Commercial insurance companies Blue Cross/Blue Shield Third-party claims processors

Healthcare *delivery*, the third major function, involves the provision of services by the physician or other healthcare provider to the patient or consumer. *Delivery* also can refer to the hospital, skilled nursing home, clinic, or home care company. The respiratory therapist is closely involved in this function.

Perhaps the most complex function of the system is *payment*, a major focus of this chapter that is addressed in detail in subsequent sections. The respiratory therapist must understand that payment deals specifically with reimbursement and disbursement of funds. It is an infinitely complicated process that undergoes continuous change and ceaseless revision. Payers are constantly searching for ways to optimize their profits and work the system.

> **RESPIRATORY RECAP**
>
> **Basic Healthcare Delivery Functions**
> » Financing
> » Insurance
> » Delivery
> » Payment

The sources of these funds for disbursement are employers; the federal, state, and local governments; fraternal organizations; MCOs; and self-pay. These disbursements take the form of premiums or entitlement payments. The insurance company is the intermediary providing payment to the provider orchestrated by way of a consumer claim. The provider or patient submits the claim to the intermediary, which settles or processes it. Payment can be made for the entire amount or for a designated portion identified by the plan and addressed during contract negotiations. With managed care the patient may simply pay a small copayment, deductible, or out-of-pocket amount. More detail regarding payment is addressed in the "Reimbursement Methodologies" section.

The respiratory therapist should recognize that the U.S. healthcare system is not a well-oiled, finely tuned machine with components interconnected in such a way that duplication, inconsistency, and inadequacy are prevented. Regrettably, the system is fragmented, duplicative, and disjointed, with a lack of integration among the system's four major functions. Additionally, coordination, collaboration, and integration among the major stakeholders (purchasers, insurers, payers, patients, and providers) is poor. The result is a system that is loosely connected, without central oversight, brimming with confusion, and undergoing near-constant change.

Stakeholders in Healthcare Reimbursement

Providing and delivering healthcare services involves many stakeholders. Historically, three major players existed: the patient (primary party), the provider (secondary party), and the insurer (commonly referred to as the **third-party payer**). Over the years the system has become increasingly more complicated and complex.

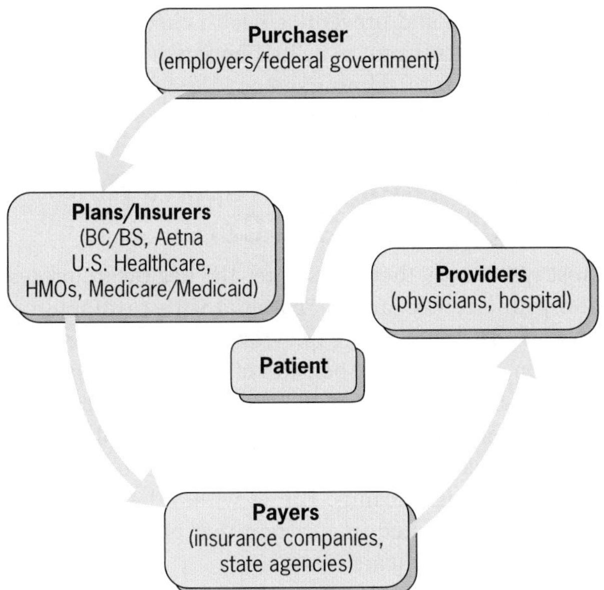

FIGURE 61–1 Stakeholders in healthcare reimbursement.

Roles and functions of participants have expanded so that the following five significant stakeholders are involved in today's healthcare system: purchasers, plans, providers, payers, and patients (**Figure 61–1**).

At times the role and function of each overlaps, often clouding the lines of distinction. Purchasers are generally employers or the federal, state, or local governments and presently subsidize much of the cost of healthcare. Employers are purchasers in the form of employee-benefit packages, whereas the government funds healthcare in the form of entitlement and shared assistance programs. Employers began providing this benefit early in the 20th century to provide an added benefit to their employees' compensation packages. Medical coverage was viewed as a way to safeguard both the employee and the company from catastrophic healthcare losses. In addition, it was viewed as a way to add a benefit without having to incur a more direct expense in the form of salary increases. The federal government entered healthcare reimbursement by instituting Medicare and Medicaid in 1965 to assist the elderly and the poor. In recent years, purchasers have become increasingly concerned with financial risk. Their expenses have soared, and thus employers are interested in getting out of the business of providing benefits and the federal government desires to exercise better control of costs.

RESPIRATORY RECAP

Stakeholders in Healthcare Reimbursement

» Purchasers
» Plans
» Providers
» Payers
» Patients

The organizations or groups that provide healthcare plans to purchasers make up the second group of stakeholders, generally insurance companies or insurers. The insurer can be from the public or private sector and thus can be the federal government, a commercial insurance company, or an MCO. Examples of healthcare insurers include Blue Cross/Blue Shield, Aetna US Healthcare, and Kaiser Permanente. The healthcare insurer is an intermediary that negotiates and administers the healthcare coverage. This role was established to take the responsibility of oversight from the employer. Healthcare economics grew so complex that employers simply wanted to rid themselves of the responsibility of day-to-day administration and management of such issues. The healthcare plan serves in this capacity; the plan is the policy, and the entity is the organization that administers the plan.

The third major stakeholder in healthcare delivery is the provider, which can be the hospital and all its associated healthcare practitioners—respiratory therapists, nurses, medical technologists, physical therapists, and others. Long-term care facilities, such as psychiatric facilities and nursing homes, and skilled nursing facilities are other providers, along with the medical community—primary care physicians, pulmonologists, cardiologists, surgeons, and others. Others in this category include agencies that provide home nursing care and homemaker services and companies that provide medical equipment and services to patients in their homes. Essentially, any healthcare professional, agency, company, or service involved in the diagnosis, care, management, or treatment of the patient is considered a provider.

The provider community recently has been placed in the precarious position of being considered most responsible for increases in costs. Waste, fraud, abuse, unproductive activities, and unnecessary and inappropriate treatment and services often are cited as major factors contributing to escalating healthcare costs. Considerable pressure has been placed on providers to decrease costs, including downsizing, decentralizing, restructuring, and reengineering.

The fourth stakeholder is the payer, the group or organization that processes the claim and disburses the funds. The payer can be an insurance company or a health maintenance organization (HMO), and thus the payer and the plan (or insurer) can be one and the same, the distinction being simply with regard to function. The health plan or insurer performs the insurance function, whereas the payer provides payment or disbursement. The payer holds considerable power and influence because it can accept or reject the claim; it also is known as the *third-party administrator* (*TPA*).

Patients are perhaps the easiest group to explain and understand. They are the consumers, the recipients of the care and services provided by the healthcare system. In healthcare delivery, and specifically healthcare economics, patients have been a rather passive group, simply interested in receiving quality and affordable healthcare. Their passivity stemmed from their historically employer-provided healthcare coverage in the form of a benefit or package that could cost the employer an additional 25% to 35% of the employee's salary—a figure that continues to increase annually. However, consumer passivity is beginning to change as a result of increased consumer financial obligation. Employers are simply unable to sustain the added expense and burden of escalating healthcare premiums and still compete in a global economy; the escalating healthcare premiums are ravaging operating budgets and cutting into company profits. Consequently, employers have begun to shift some of these expenses to employees in the form of copayments, deductibles, out-of-pocket expenses, and curtailed healthcare coverage. Consumers are increasingly responsible for their healthcare costs today.

Currently all five stakeholders are attempting to limit their risk of exposure to financial harm. **Figure 61–2** depicts a theoretic view of the amount of risk incurred by the major stakeholders during various time periods. The most recent events in healthcare have exposed the provider network to considerably more risk. Employers (purchasers) simply wish to unload any risk by contracting and negotiating with the insurers (the plans/payers). Insurers are attempting to distance themselves from risk by placing more and more pressure on providers to increase productivity, cut staff members, improve patient satisfaction, eliminate inefficiency, and decrease use. Providers seem to have taken the brunt of the responsibility, with the consumer (patient) assuming the role of the silent stakeholder. Speculation is that hospitals and physicians (providers) will continue to carry the pressure and burden for change to improve the system.

Today, the consumer (patient) can be pulled into the conflict and required to participate more significantly because of the demand for patients to incur additional significant financial burdens or hardships in the form of copayments, increased deductibles, or reduced services. Additionally, patients may be held more accountable for their health practices and required to participate more actively and responsibly in their own care. In some scenarios, rationing has been discussed, with a reward-and-punishment system enacted to stimulate or motivate healthy lifestyle behaviors and practices. For example, significantly reduced premiums, copayments, or deductibles can be provided to consumers who choose not to smoke or who engage in healthy lifestyle behaviors that include regular exercise, annual vaccinations or immunization, and preventive health checkups. Participating in regular exercise by joining a gym or health club can translate into reimbursement for a portion of the health club membership fee.

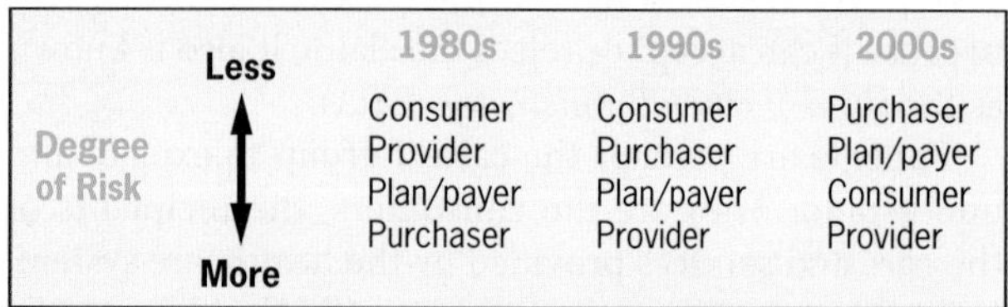

FIGURE 61–2 Theoretic view of risk incurred by major stakeholders in healthcare. Data from U.S. Department of Health and Human Services, Centers for Medicare and Medicaid, Office of Information Services.

The Respiratory Therapist's Role: Balancing Cost and Care

Most respiratory therapists enter the healthcare profession primarily to care for patients with cardiopulmonary needs. In short, respiratory therapists' primary function is to serve as bedside clinicians and, as such, the nonphysician experts in cardiorespiratory care and management. Although little has changed with regard to this primary purpose, the system in which it occurs has changed significantly. Forces within the system and society have resulted in a system that places increasing emphasis on healthcare costs.

Respiratory therapists now compete with other healthcare providers for the broad array of procedures and modalities that once were considered their exclusive domain. The system is beginning to question the need and efficacy of care. Additionally, pressure is increasing to address the burgeoning increase in healthcare needs and costs that is outstripping what companies and consumers want to pay. **Figure 61–3** provides a graphic display of the exponential growth of healthcare expenditures. Healthcare is simply becoming too costly, and cost containment is a particularly important concern to the respiratory therapist, who must learn the business of healthcare, develop a better understanding of the financial considerations associated with the decisions that relate to patient care, and learn to strike a balance between care and costs.

Forces Influencing Healthcare Costs

Commencing in March 2008 and currently in progress is the American Association for Respiratory Care's (AARC) consensus conference, Creating a Vision for Respiratory Care in 2015 and Beyond.[2] Although the intent of the conference was broad in scope, the issue of drivers of healthcare change was addressed. Five interrelated drivers were hypothesized as shaping the healthcare landscape over the next decade and a half: cost of care, demographics, shift in disease burden, technology, and healthcare consumers. The issue of cost of care is particularly troublesome because the United States spends more than 16% of its gross domestic product on healthcare and clearly has the most expensive healthcare system in the world. Healthcare is

RESPIRATORY RECAP

Drivers of Healthcare Change

- » Cost of care
- » Demographics
- » Shift in disease burden
- » Technology
- » Healthcare consumers

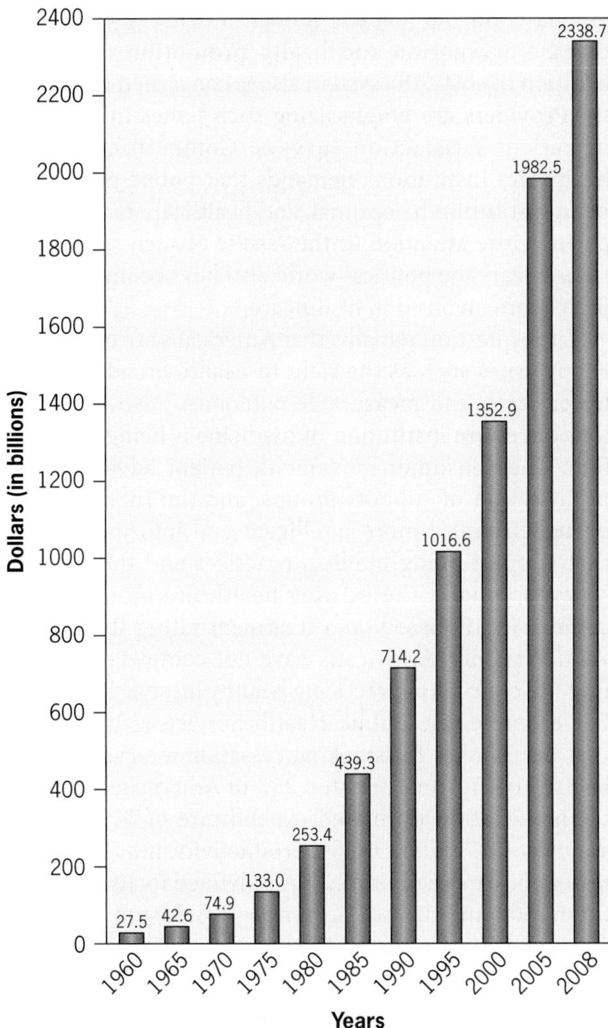

FIGURE 61-3 Healthcare expenditures for selected years. Data from Centers for Medicare and Medicaid. National health expenditure data. Available at: http://www.cms.gov/NationalHealthExpendData/02_NationalHealthAccountsHistorical.asp.

the largest portion of the public budget and amounts to approximately $2 trillion per year. Of particular concern is speculation that the funds that pay for Medicare will be exhausted in approximately 10 years. Additionally, the corporate world, which funds the bulk of private health insurance, has been reducing coverage and shifting the cost burden to the employee in the form of copayments and deductibles.

In a previous conference entitled Emerging Health Care Delivery Models and Respiratory Care,[3] the AARC provided the respiratory care community with critical information about the future of healthcare delivery and the ways it might affect respiratory care practice. A recurring theme once again was the emphasis placed on escalating healthcare costs, particularly that healthcare costs were surpassing general inflation at a threefold to fourfold pace during the 1970s and 1980s. But what were the reasons for escalating costs? Four broad factors had been identified: general inflation, population growth and its demographics, medical price inflation, and service intensity.[3]

Healthcare consultants and industry leaders have identified service intensity as the major area of focus to effect change and curtail costs. Service intensity is influenced by technology, exemption from market forces, fragmentation, excess capacity, supplier control of demand, lack of efficacy and quality of care information, administrative costs, unnecessary care and defensive medicine, productivity costs, growth in the number of uninsured individuals, and growth in specialization.[3]

> **RESPIRATORY RECAP**
>
> **Factors Influencing Growth in Healthcare Costs**
>
> » General inflation
> » Population growth and its demographics
> » Medical price inflation
> » Service intensity

Growth in technology has added significantly to the problem because new technology is expensive, is demanded by the public or providers or both, and drives up cost. Advances in diagnostics, monitoring, and mechanical ventilation have driven the cost of such equipment to unprecedented levels. Mechanical ventilators and their accoutrements—namely monitoring and graphics packages—can cost more than $30,000. Furthermore, today's healthcare consumer expects to benefit from advances in medicine and the latest in technology, and the system has encouraged providers to use such advances to improve patient care, achieve higher degrees of patient satisfaction, and increase revenues. In this sense, technology has been at least partially responsible for the proliferation of specialization and in some cases the performance of unnecessary or questionable procedures or services.

Under a third-party insurer payment system the patient is insulated from costs, and little incentive exists for the primary party (patient) or secondary party (provider) to contain costs. In many cases, insurance is provided by either the employer or the federal, state, or local governments, and the patient does not pay at all or pays only a minimum amount in the form of a copayment or deductible. The patient has little understanding or appreciation of the value of the healthcare benefit. In addition, unless the insurance plan uses restraining measures, the physician (provider) is free to order diagnostic studies and therapeutic interventions with little regard to cost. The system was created on an incentive system whereby the physician was economically

> **RESPIRATORY RECAP**
>
> **Factors Influencing Service Intensity**
>
> » Technology
> » Exemption from market forces
> » Fragmentation
> » Excess capacity
> » Supplier control of demand
> » Lack of efficacy and quality of care information
> » Administrative costs
> » Unnecessary care and defensive medicine
> » Productivity costs
> » Growth in number of uninsured
> » Growth in specialization

rewarded for ordering more services and generating more income for that physician and the hospital. Historically, the patient and provider have essentially been without the incentive to be cost-conscious, resulting in the mentality that the insurance company will cover everything. Patients and providers only recently have begun to appreciate the costs of healthcare services, and some of the new reimbursement methodologies are beginning to address these issues.

Traditionally, delivery and payment mechanisms have not been integrated or well coordinated; the system is fragmented. When patients are moved from one practice site to another (e.g., physician offices to acute care, then to subacute or home care sites), services are duplicated considerably. Blood gas measurements often are repeated, as are electrocardiograms and pulmonary function studies, resulting in excessive and unnecessary services. Practice variations are considerable, and only recently have the disparities in the effectiveness of care begun to be addressed. Benchmarking, practice guidelines, protocols, and best practices have given rise to evidence-based medicine, whereby conclusive, scientific evidence drives the clinical decision-making process.

Conflict continues to exist between appropriate and necessary care and the overordering of unnecessary, nonessential care, often driven by defensive medicine. Physicians are concerned about the risk of litigation and malpractice suits and consequently may order services of questionable value to protect their interests, resulting in waste and, equally disconcerting, fraud and abuse. Fraud entails a knowing disregard for the truth and generally occurs in the form of fraudulent billing claims or fraudulent delivery but can also include a practitioner's knowingly providing unnecessary or excessive services and receiving remuneration in exchange for a referral of services. Regrettably, the home care market has been especially suspect regarding such concerns, especially regarding durable medical equipment. A provider referring a patient to any company with which that provider is associated or in which the provider holds a financial interest is simply inappropriate and illegal. Such practice is considered a kickback and is subject to prosecution.

The increase in the elderly population also has added significantly to medical costs inflation because the elderly consume considerably more healthcare services than other age group. In fact, in 2004, Medicare expenditures for the elderly averaged $14,797 per beneficiary, versus $4511 per capita for all Americans.[4] In addition, considerable cost is associated with the uninsured and the underinsured, with the number of uninsured growing steadily and reaching 47 million in 2007. This figure correlates to approximately 15.7% of the population being uninsured at any one time,[5] a significant figure that places tremendous burden on the system.

Other factors affecting costs and driving changes in healthcare include quality and access, politics, the demystification of medicine, and the disproportionate emphasis on the medical model of delivery versus the disease prevention and health promotion model. In addition to costs, the system also is concerned with quality. Providers are emphasizing such issues in the form of patient-satisfaction surveys. Competition among healthcare institutions demands that public perception of an institution be optimal, and healthcare facilities are paying close attention to the results of such surveys. In recent years the political world also has become exceedingly more involved in healthcare.

Little question remains that Americans are concerned about issues such as the right to health, broader access, lower costs, and measurable outcomes. Also evident is that the entire institution of medicine is being demystified. The consumer movement, patient advocacy, the proliferation of support groups, and the Internet have brought about a more intelligent and informed public that is questioning medical practices and the costs of services. Finally, the existing healthcare model in this country is still based on a treatment rather than a prevention model. Americans have not completely bought into the concept of practicing healthy lifestyle behaviors. For example, the Public Health Service estimates the cost per smoker for smoking cessation interventions to be $165.61. Yet an estimated 25% of Americans continue to smoke, at an estimated expenditure of $193 billion annually ($97 billion in lost productivity and $96 billion in healthcare expenditures).[6] A redefined focus on health promotion and disease prevention would add considerably to healthcare cost reductions.

Financing Healthcare: A Brief History and Overview

Payment for healthcare services in the form of reimbursement is crucial to the survival of any healthcare institution, facility, or provider. There are limited instances of self-pay, out-of-pocket, or direct pay in which the patient deals directly with the provider. The more common practice entails a third party, possibly an insurance company, the government, or an MCO. Reimbursement models and methodologies are constantly evolving, and hybridization is becoming the norm. Nonetheless, an attempt to simplify and eliminate some of the complexity is provided in the sections to follow. Certain liberties are exercised in this discussion, and healthcare finance is addressed in terms of three general payment systems: the **retrospective payment system (RPS)**, the prospective payment system, and capitation.[7]

Retrospective Payment

Traditional Health Insurance

The origins of American health insurance are rooted in the historical inability of individuals and their families to sustain the expense and resulting debt incurred by extensive medical care. Medical care, in the form of extended hospital stays or repeated office visits to the family physician, was unaffordable to most individuals. Community hospitals and family doctors recognized that some means to finance healthcare was required to prevent the inevitable consequences of unpaid medical bills, personal destitution, catastrophic bankruptcy, and ultimate economic disaster for the patient, physician, and hospital. Out of this concern grew the concept of health insurance, whereby individuals pooled their limited and yet manageable amount of funds and distributed the risk of illness among a larger group. Thus grew the concepts of shared risk and shared losses.

The true beginning of modern private health insurance was in 1929 when a group of teachers made a contract with Baylor Hospital in Dallas, Texas, to provide coverage against certain hospital expenses. This event was considered the birth of the first Blue Cross plan.[8] Blue Cross and Blue Shield plans, considered service plans, historically reimbursed providers for the total costs of covered benefits. This system is in contrast to an **indemnity insurance plan**, commercial in nature, that provided a benefit only if and when a medical event occurred. Indemnity plans provided payment of a fixed sum for a covered benefit.

RESPIRATORY RECAP

Three General Payment Systems

- Retrospective payment system (RPS)
- Prospective payment system (PPS)
- Capitation

Around this period, employers were equally concerned with the health and well-being of their workers. World War II was under way, and businesses and industries, such as the railroad, steel, aluminum, and shipbuilding, needed assurance that the workforce could maintain productivity and sustain the war effort. Coupled with this desire to sustain a consistent, dependable, and healthy workforce was the desire to optimize company profits and provide additional employee incentives and rewards, the latter being especially true after the war as employers wanted to provide their employees with additional, small fringe benefits and yet avoid the costly burden of salary increases. Providing healthcare coverage was the perfect solution, and this benefit enhancement became a reality endorsed and sanctioned by hospitals, physicians, and employers.

Government Involvement

In 1965, the federal government entered the healthcare reimbursement scene with the U.S. Congress legislating and amending the Social Security Act of 1935 and establishing the Medicare (Title XVIII) and Medicaid (Title XIX) entitlement programs. **Medicare** provides health insurance for the elderly, whereas **Medicaid** helps states pay for the healthcare of the poor and certain other groups, such as the elderly, infants and children, and the blind and other disabled people. In 1973, additional legislation extended Medicare coverage to other groups, including persons with disabilities and end-stage renal disease requiring dialysis or kidney transplant.

The Medicare program consisted of Parts A and B. Medicare Part A is considered hospital coverage, and Part B is considered supplemental outpatient coverage. Part A pays the institutional provider for inpatient hospital care, care in a **skilled nursing facility (SNF)**, home health services, and hospice services provided to enrolled recipients. Part A covers all inpatient hospital care, including semiprivate room, meals, regular nursing services, operating and recovery room costs, intensive care, drugs, laboratory tests, x-rays, and all other medically necessary services and supplies. However, it does not cover physician fees, because it was designed solely as hospital insurance. **Box 61–1** addresses the specifics of Part A as they pertain to eligibility, the benefit period, coverage, copayments, SNFs, and hospice services.

Medicare Part B is a voluntary, supplemental insurance program that covers services not provided under Part A. Part B pays for covered physician services, such as diagnostic tests, medical and surgical services, approved ambulatory services, drugs that cannot be self-administered, home health, durable medical equipment, and outpatient services. **Box 61–2** addresses the specifics of Part B as they pertain to cost sharing, deductibles, and coverage of home medical and home respiratory equipment. **Box 61–3** details the specific Part B coverage requirements for home respiratory equipment that a patient must meet for Medicare reimbursement.

In 2005 Medicare initiated **pay for performance (P4P)** with the intent of encouraging increased quality in healthcare for the recipients of Medicare. This initiative crossed all venues of care, from inpatient hospital care to physician offices. Initially, this was done with demonstration projects that encouraged participation from healthcare providers by giving increased payment for top performance. Eventually, acceptance of evidence-based care led to improvements in care such as preventing community-acquired pneumonia via strict attention to the type of antibiotics used and the timely delivery of antibiotics. As pay for performance evolves, there will be payment penalties for patient care that does not follow evidence or for a health provider who does not perform to a set level.[9]

As stated previously, Medicaid provides medical assistance for certain individuals and families with low incomes and resources. It is a jointly funded cooperative venture between the federal and state governments to assist states in the provision of adequate medical care to eligible needy persons. Within broad national guidelines set by the federal government, each state establishes its own eligibility standards; determines the type, amounts, duration, and scope of services; sets the rate of payment

BOX 61–1

Medicare Part A: Financing, Eligibility, Coverage, and Benefits

Financing

Mandatory employer and employee payroll taxes are collected under Social Security—1.45% from each—paid by all working individuals, including the self-employed. The employer must match the 1.45%, for a total of 2.9%.

Eligibility

The benefits usually are provided automatically to persons 65 years of age or older, most people who are disabled for at least 24 months, and those who have end-stage renal disease.

Coverage

Hospital inpatient services, care in a skilled nursing facility (SNF), home health visits, and hospice care are covered.

Premiums*

No premium is required if the individual or spouse has worked for at least 10 years in Social Security/Medicare-covered employment. Other eligible individuals can purchase coverage at a monthly premium of $254 to $461 (depending on coverage status). Medicare Part B premiums range from $96.40 to $110.50 based on income.

Deductibles/Copayments*

A cost-sharing deductible of $1100 is assessed per benefit period. No copayments are required for the first 60 days of hospitalization, with a copayment of $275 per day for days 61 through 90 and $550 per day for days 91 through 150. No copayments are assessed for skilled nursing for the first 20 days, with $137.50 per day for days 21 through 100. No copayments are required for home health visits, whereas small copayments are assessed for drugs through hospice care.

Benefits

The benefit period is defined as the period beginning when the beneficiary first enters the hospital and ending when the beneficiary has been out of the hospital or other facility for 60 concurrent days. Benefit periods cannot exceed 90 days of inpatient hospital care, but the number of benefit periods is unlimited. If the 90 days of inpatient hospital care are exhausted, the beneficiary can draw from a nonrenewable "lifetime reserve" of up to 60 additional days. Skilled nursing care pays up to 100 days only if it follows within 30 days of a hospitalization of 3 or more days and is certified as medically necessary. Home care through a home health agency is covered when a beneficiary is homebound and requires intermittent or part-time skilled nursing or rehabilitation care. No limits exist for time or visits for home health care. Hospice services to the terminally ill with life expectancy of 6 months or less also are covered.

*Premium, deductible, and copayment information current as of April 2010. Values are subject to change.

Data from U.S. Department of Health and Human Services. Medicare premium and coinsurance rates for 2010. Medicare.gov. Updated April 12, 2010. Available at: http://www.medicare.gov/navigation/medicare-basics/medicare-benefits/part-a.aspx.

for services; and administers its own program. Thus, Medicaid varies considerably from state to state.

Medicare and Medicaid have been heralded as perhaps one of the most massive and sweeping social welfare initiatives undertaken by the federal government, targeting whole segments of the population and successfully improving the health and quality of life for millions of seniors, people with disabilities, and the poor and indigent of society. **Table 61–2** reflects Medicare data for selected years, and **Table 61–3** represents Medicaid data for selected years.

Prospective Payment

The **prospective payment system (PPS)** arose because of increasing pressure from employers and the federal government to curtail spiraling healthcare costs. It was initiated in 1983 and involves reimbursement that establishes fixed and preestablished payment for the actual primary reason for admission. The rates are determined annually by the plan administrator, who may be the federal government (under the direction of the **Centers for Medicare and Medicaid Services [CMS]**,

BOX 61–2

Medicare Part B: Financing, Eligibility, Coverage, and Benefits

Financing

The voluntary program is financed by general tax revenues and requires individual premium contributions. General federal tax revenues support approximately 75% of the costs, with the remaining 25% financed through individuals choosing to enroll and pay the premiums.

Eligibility

All resident citizens over 65 years of age, even those who are not entitled to Part A services, and disabled beneficiaries entitled to Part A are eligible.

Coverage

Part B coverage is optional. Coverage of home medical equipment requires that the item be used in the home, medically useful, able to stand up to repeated use, and reasonable and necessary for the treatment of illness or injury or the improvement of function. (Equipment that satisfies this criteria is considered durable medical equipment [DME].) To be reimbursed, the supplier must have a physician's order for the items and in some cases a certificate of medical necessity (CMN).

Premiums*

Beneficiaries must pay a monthly premium of $50 per month, which in most cases is automatically deducted from the Social Security payment.

Deductibles*

An annual $155 deductible and a coinsurance payment of 20% of most allowable charges are assessed.

Benefits

Covered physician services include (excluding routine physical exams) emergency department services, outpatient surgery, diagnostic tests and laboratory services; outpatient physical, occupational, and speech therapy; outpatient mental health services; ambulance; renal dialysis; blood transfusion and blood components; medical equipment and supplies; rural health clinic services; and some limited preventive services (for example, Pap smears, mammography, and influenza shots).

*Premium and deductible information current as of April 2010. Values are subject to change.

Data from Centers for Medicare and Medicaid Services. *Medicare and You 2010*. Available at: http://www.medicare.gov/Publications/Pubs/pdf/10050.pdf.

TABLE 61–2 Medicare Data for Selected Years

Year	Beneficiaries (Millions)	Expenditures (Billions)
1970	20.5	$7.7
1980	28.5	$37.5
1990	34.3	$111.5
1999	39.5	$212.0
2008	45.2	$462.0

Data from U.S. Department of Health and Human Services, Health Care Financing Administration, Office of Information Services. 2008 data from Boards of Trustees, Federal Hospital Insurance and Federal Supplementary Medical Insurance Trust Funds. *2009 Annual Report.* Available at: http://www.cms.gov/ReportsTrustFunds/downloads/tr2009.pdf.

TABLE 61–3 Medicaid Data for Selected Years

Year	Beneficiaries (Millions)	Expenditures (Billions)
1970	17.6	$5.3
1980	21.6	$26.1
1990	25.3	$75.3
1999	41.4	$190.7
2008	42.7	$227.6

Data from U.S. Department of Health and Human Services, Health Care Financing Administration, Office of Information Services. 2008 data from Boards of Trustees, Federal Hospital Insurance and Federal Supplementary Medical Insurance Trust Funds. *2009 Annual Report.* Available at: http://www.cms.gov/ReportsTrustFunds/downloads/tr2009.pdf.

BOX 61–3

Medicare Part B: Coverage of Home Respiratory Equipment

Medicare has set very specific eligibility and qualifying requirements for all durable medical equipment used in the home. That a physician prescribes a certain item is no guarantee that Medicare will pay for it. The majority of private insurers and many managed care organizations also follow the Medicare guidelines in determining eligibility and reimbursement.

Oxygen

Medicare pays a flat monthly amount for oxygen, the same whether provided from cylinders, a concentrator, or a liquid source and regardless of the liter flow. This rental fee is all-inclusive, covering the oxygen, equipment, most disposable supplies, and all services, such as delivery, maintenance, and repair.

In addition, Medicare has no required standards of service specific to providers of oxygen therapy. The supplier is not required to be accredited, perform any type of initial instruction or ongoing follow-up, or employ respiratory therapists. Suppliers who do provide these services are reimbursed at the same level as those who do not.

To qualify for home oxygen under Medicare Part B the patient must have a diagnosis of pulmonary or cardiac disease, which in the opinion of the attending physician will likely improve with the administration of oxygen. In addition, Medicare has established very specific levels of hypoxemia that the patient must demonstrate through arterial blood gases (ABGs) or pulse oximetry under specified conditions ($Pao_2 \leq 55$ mm Hg or $Sao_2 \leq 88\%$ breathing room air at rest, on exercise, or during sleep). The company providing the oxygen cannot do the testing, which must be performed by an objective third party, such as an independent laboratory, a hospital, or a physician.

Continuous Positive Airway Pressure

This intervention, more commonly known as CPAP, is covered if the patient has obstructive sleep apnea that has been documented during studies done in a sleep laboratory and demonstrates at least 30 episodes of apnea, each lasting a minimum of 10 seconds, during 6 to 7 hours of recorded sleep. Bilevel devices also qualify for reimbursement for treatment of obstructive sleep apnea, but only if the patient meets all of the previous criteria and CPAP has been tried without success.

Noninvasive Ventilation and Respiratory Assistive Devices

Since 1999 these devices have been covered for chronic obstructive pulmonary disease (COPD), restrictive thoracic disorders, central sleep apnea, and obstructive sleep apnea when specific qualifying awake ABGs, nocturnal oximetry, and certain other criteria are met.

Ventilators

Ventilators, either positive- or negative-pressure types, are covered if the patient has a diagnosis of neuromuscular disease, thoracic restrictive disease, or chronic respiratory failure due to COPD.

Suction Machine

A device for nasal, oral, or tracheal suctioning is covered only if the patient has difficulty raising and clearing secretions secondary to cancer or surgery of the throat, dysfunction of the swallowing muscles, unconsciousness or obtundent state, or tracheostomy.

previously know as the Health Care Financing Administration [HCFA]) or commercial insurance carriers such as Blue Cross or Aetna US Healthcare. The year 1983 began a multiyear phase-in of the PPS for hospital reimbursement through Medicare.

Physician reimbursement under the PPS is based on a methodology known as the **resource-based relative value scale (RBRVS)**. A relative value scale is a reimbursement methodology developed by a Harvard research team that assigned values to physician services based on the resource costs of providing those services.[10] The RBRVS was implemented on January 1, 1992, by HCFA as a fee schedule for physicians who participate in Medicare Part B. It is based on a national fee schedule and replaces the previous payment method outlining "usual, customary, and reasonable charges." The RBRVS assigns a relative value to each current procedural terminology (CPT) code. The relative value units are based on the time, skill, and **resource intensity** it takes to provide a service, and the actual reimbursement is derived from a complex formula. Relative values were designed with the objective of narrowing the gap between the incomes of specialists and generalists.[1]

Capitation

Capitation is a prepaid, fixed amount negotiated in advance by the payer or plan and the provider. It involves payment for each eligible person for a particular time period regardless of the care or services provided and also is known as the *per-member, per-month* (*PMPM*) system, which represents or reflects the amount paid by each participating member each month enrolled in the plan. Managed care programs for primary care providers commonly use capitation, but specialists (e.g., pulmonologists) are still more likely to be paid under a negotiated fee schedule.

The Era of Managed Care

Managed care is actually a generic term for a payment system alternative to traditional insurance plans, such as fee-for-service or indemnity plans. The concept of managed care is considered similar to managed costs, but a distinction should be made between the techniques of care and costs management versus the organization that performs those functions. Managing care or costs may involve a variety of techniques, such as health promotion, disease prevention, wellness, disease management, patient education, and utilization control, to name a few. These are strategies or techniques and should not be confused with managed care organizations, which can implement these strategies but mainly are responsible for delivering and financing health services. In other words, managed care organizations are more than just the claims payers; they actively manage the delivery of the care.

A **managed care organization (MCO)** is an integrated network of doctors, hospitals, and other healthcare providers that delivers health services to an insured population. In the past 15 years, managed care became the predominant form of healthcare in most parts of the United States. More than 70 million Americans have enrolled in health maintenance organizations (HMOs), and almost 90 million have been part of preferred provider organizations (PPOs).[11] Overall enrollment numbers in HMOs peaked in 2001 and are declining substantially in almost every area, but managed care generally remains a dominant type of healthcare coverage (**Table 61–4**).

RESPIRATORY RECAP

Types of Managed Care

- Health maintenance organization (HMO)
- Preferred provider organization (PPO)
- Exclusive provider organization (EPO)
- Point-of-service plan (POS)

The four different types of MCOs are HMOs, PPOs, exclusive provider organizations (EPOs), and point-of-service plans (POSs). These are discussed individually in the following sections.

TABLE 61–4 Breakdown of Enrollment by Plan Type, 2008

Plan Type	Percentage
Managed Care	
Health maintenance organization (HMO)	20
Preferred provider organization (PPO)	58
Point-of-service plan (POS)	12
Non-Managed Care	
High-deductible health plan	8
Conventional/indemnity	2

Data from The Kaiser Family Foundation and Health Research and Educational Trust. *Employer Health Benefits 2009 Annual Survey.* Available at: http://ehbs.kff.org.

Health Maintenance Organizations

Contrary to popular opinion, managed care models have been around for almost a century. The first cited example of an MCO was the Western Clinic in Tacoma, Washington, a prepaid group practice begun in 1910 to provide a broad range of medical services to lumber mill owners and their employees. These eligible individuals were provided services for a premium payment of a mere 50 cents per member per month, dating PMPM's history back 90 years. A number of additional examples can be cited, such as the rural workers' cooperative in Elk City, Oklahoma; the Kaiser Foundation Health Plan of Southern California; the Group Health Association of Washington, DC; the Health Insurance Plan of Greater New York; and the Group Health Cooperative of Puget Sound.

Managed care plans developed relatively slowly. However, in 1973 they received a major boost with the passage of the federal HMO Act, which reflected concern with the fee-for-service system that rewarded healthcare providers for increased volume of services. Little in the way of checks and balances were in place under this system, and the incentives encouraged overuse. The HMO movement is considered the brainchild of Dr. Paul Ellwood, who spearheaded the effort and is often referred to as the "father of the modern HMO movement." Because of Ellwood's expertise, President Nixon asked him to devise ways to curtail the spiraling healthcare costs in Medicare.

The **health maintenance organization (HMO)** model of health care is uniquely different from the traditional model. Rather than pay for care when the individual is ill, it provides service to maintain health—thus the term *health maintenance*—placing considerable emphasis on preventive

RESPIRATORY RECAP

General Characteristics of an HMO

- Emphasis on preventive services
- Provision of a complete range of services for a fixed fee
- Requirement that all care be provided by participating providers
- Adherence of services to established standards of quality

services encouraging wellness and healthy lifestyle practices. It also provides a wide array of services for a fixed fee per month, use of which is coordinated and managed by the HMO. This type of managed care is an attempt to address the fragmentation of basic healthcare delivery functions alluded to previously. Under the HMO model, the subscriber must secure all services from providers participating in the plan or must pay a higher amount for using a nonparticipating provider. Finally, services are provided according to established standards of quality.[1]

HMOs have four general models: the staff model, group model, network model, and independent practice association (IPA) model. Their distinction from one another is based on the way the organization relates to its participating physicians.

RESPIRATORY RECAP

General Types of HMOs

- Staff model
- Group model
- Network model
- Independent practice association (IPA) model

The staff model entails the provision of physician services through a salaried staff of physicians employed by the HMO. The physicians in this model work exclusively for the HMO and provide care to its enrollees only. The HMO exercises considerable control over physician practice, and thus the physician's performance and practice are subject to restrictions and bonuses for curtailed costs. In the staff model the HMO assumes the financial risk, as opposed to the physician. The staff model is considered the least popular of the four.

In the group model the HMO contracts with a multispecialty group practice. The physicians are not employees of the HMO but rather employees of the group. This model can provide more choice to the consumer when compared with the staff model, and if the practice enjoys a high degree of notoriety and respect, the HMO gains popularity and credibility with its enrollees.

The network model entails the HMO contracting with more than one physician group and generally is more likely to occur when a large population of enrollees requires medical services. This model is more attractive to the enrollee because the number of physicians involved in the network can be quite significant, providing increased choice.

The IPA model is unique in that the association serves as an intermediary, or buffer, between the HMO and physicians, handling the logistics of arranging physician services. The responsibility for administrative issues is shifted to the IPA and not the HMO. The IPA is paid a capitated amount, reimburses the physicians based on a methodology determined by both parties, and assumes some of the risk. The IPA's degree of control over physician practices varies widely, but enrollee choice is enhanced.

Preferred Provider Organizations

Preferred provider organizations (PPOs) date back to the late 1970s. PPOs differ from traditional HMOs in that services are provided at a discounted fee-for-service basis, usually 25% to 35% below competitors or below the usual, customary, and reasonable fees. In other words, PPOs use a discounted fee-for-service system, and HMOs use capitation. Additionally, enrollees are required to use a particular group of physicians and hospitals that the PPO has preselected. Enrollees are free to choose physicians or hospitals outside the system, but nonpreferred providers constitute additional charges. Thus, PPOs encourage enrollees to use their preferred providers, who have agreed to abide by the PPO's guidelines.

Point-of-Service Plans

Point-of-service plans (POSs) entered the market in the late 1980s and are a hybrid of HMOs and PPOs. They represent features of both organizations, attempting to provide the tight use controls of the HMO and the ability to choose a nonparticipating provider at the point (time) at which service is received, thus the phrase *point of service*. The POS addresses the unpopular feature of limited or restricted choice that continues to plague the industry. Simply stated, a significant number of Americans insist on choosing their physician and hospital, and the POS models satisfy this need.

Exclusive Provider Organizations

Exclusive provider organizations (EPOs) are the most affordable of the managed care models. However, they are clearly the most restrictive. Enrollees must use the physician and hospital stipulated in the plan, completely eliminating the element of choice. The advantage is the purchaser's considerable cost savings.

The distinction among the various plans is beginning to blur, becoming less obvious. Considerable hybridization has occurred as the plans attempt to optimize their models to satisfy purchaser and consumer demands.

Reimbursement Methodologies

Reimbursement and its methodologies involve payment for healthcare delivery. Intermediaries or third-party payers generally perform this function and are responsible for determining the method and amount of reimbursement, as well as the actual disbursement of funds. Examples of intermediaries are the federal government, MCOs, and insurance companies.

The methodologies for reimbursement are numerous. **Box 61–4** lists a number of models for reimbursing hospitals. However, the four most popular hospital reimbursement methodologies by HMOs are fee schedule (or fee for service), per diem, diagnosis-related groups (DRGs), and capitation.[12] The more popular physician methodologies are fee-for-service systems and capitation.

Fee for Service

The **fee-for-service system** is simply a reimbursement methodology in which the provider establishes the fee for each distinct service. Billing is based on an itemized

BOX 61–4

Models for Reimbursing Hospitals

- Charges
- Discounts
- Per diems
- Sliding scales for discounts and per diems
- Differential by day in hospital
- Diagnosis-related groups (DRGs)
- Differential by service type
- Case rates
  - Institutional only
  - Package pricing or bundled rates
- Capitation
- Percentage of premium revenue
- Contact capitation (uncommon)
- Bed leasing (very uncommon)
- Periodic interim payments or cash advances
- Performance-based incentives
  - Quality and service incentives
  - Penalties and withholds
- Ambulatory patient groups (APGs) and ambulatory payment classifications (APCs) for outpatient care

From Kongsvedt P. *Essentials of Managed Care.* 5th ed. Jones & Bartlett Learning; 2007:145.

account of each service provided. For example, the pulmonologist could submit a claim for a physical examination, chest radiograph, and pulmonary function test in which each service would constitute a separate charge.

Initially, the insurer paid fee-for-service reimbursement after care was delivered (retrospectively), without any restrictions or limitations. However, insurers eventually adopted a "usual, customary, and reasonable" charge methodology, which limited the fee to a standard determined through regional or statewide surveys. If the provider-determined charge exceeded the usual, customary, and reasonable amount, either the patient or the contracted provider was responsible for the difference. Some managed care plans, notably PPOs, adopted a discounted fee-for-service methodology. The main drawback to this method is that providers are rewarded for providing additional services, with less incentive to be cost-conscious. In fact, providers could increase their income by overordering unnecessary and costly services.

RESPIRATORY RECAP

Popular Types of Physician Reimbursement

» Fee for service
» Capitation

Cost Plus or Charge Minus

In another methodology, rates are preestablished on a cost-plus or charge-minus basis. The cost-plus method was used by the federal government in its Medicare and Medicaid programs to establish inpatient rates for hospitals, nursing homes, and home healthcare. The institution was required to submit a cost report to the third-party payer detailing the total costs that facility incurred. Complicated formulas were used to determine the per diem rate. This methodology was tied directly to costs of providing services, number of services provided, and length of stay. Historical data were essentially used to determine the amount to be paid in future years. As with the fee-for-service methodology, cost plus also presented an incentive for providers to order costly and unnecessary services. This indiscriminate practice eventually led to the initiation of the PPS.

Prospective Reimbursement

The PPS was introduced by the federal government in 1983 under Part A of its Medicare program to curtail costs. Reimbursement was fixed at a preestablished amount in advance of the services rendered, still established annually by the CMS. Prospective payment was applied to SNFs in 1998, and provisions were made to implement this system for hospital outpatient services and home health agencies through the Balanced Budget Act of 1997.

Diagnosis-Related Groups

The **diagnosis-related group (DRG)** system is based on a classification of patients into approximately 500 different groupings, all entailing a predetermined amount of reimbursement. DRGs establish a rate based on bundled services for a particular diagnosis established at the time of admission. The provider receives this amount regardless of the medical care provided.

This system provides an incentive for providers to decrease overuse, misallocation, and inefficiency. Each DRG assumes that all patients with the same diagnosis require the same care and receive the same services. Differences in DRG reimbursement are provided for the following extenuating circumstances: variations in regional employee wages, location of institution, existence of residency programs, and provision of care to the indigent. Institutions located in an urban environment may require higher employee salaries, involve teaching requirements for medical training, and have a disproportionately high number of low-income patients. Such variables allow for adjustment to the fixed rates. Additionally, extensive lengths of stay and costs for extraordinary circumstances, classified as outliers, allow for higher rates.

TABLE 61–5 Common Respiratory-Related Diagnosis-Related Groups (DRGs)

DRG Code	Description
88	Chronic obstructive pulmonary disease
79	Pulmonary infections and inflammations, age > 17 with comorbid condition
98	Bronchitis and asthma, age 0 to 17
475	Respiratory system diagnosis with ventilator support
87	Pulmonary edema and respiratory failure
82	Respiratory neoplasms
482	Tracheostomy for face, mouth, and neck diagnosis
83	Major chest trauma with comorbid condition
78	Pulmonary embolism
462	Rehabilitation
90	Simple pneumonia and pleurisy, age > 17 without comorbid condition
143	Chest pain
495	Lung transplantation

Data from Centers for Medicare and Medicaid Services. List of Diagnosis Related Groups (DRGS), Fiscal Year 2005. Available at: http://www.cms.gov/MedicareFeeforSvcPartsAB/Downloads/DRGDesc05.pdf.

The DRG system, based on total inpatient stay, is in direct contrast to the per diem methodology, which is based on a daily charge. The DRG methodology is an attempt to place risk and reward solely on the hospital (provider). If the hospital provides the service for less than the predetermined DRG reimbursement rate, that facility profits. If the hospital's costs exceed the predetermined allotment, the facility incurs a loss. One concern of the DRG system is underprovision of care and services because limits on the amount of services can result in increased profits. **Table 61–5** lists examples of common respiratory-related DRGs.

All-Patient Refined Diagnosis-Related Groups

Originally, DRGs were created to support the intensity of care and the resources consumed to care for a patient with a particular diagnosis. Over time, there has been a need to refine the system to more accurately describe the patient's condition. In particular, a patient classification system was needed for the following:

- Comparison of hospitals across a wide range of resource and outcome measures
- Evaluation of differences in inpatient mortality rates
- Implementation and support of critical pathways
- Identification of continuous quality improvement projects
- Serving as the basis of internal management and planning systems
- Serving as the management of capitated payment arrangements

To meet these changing needs, the system needed to incorporate more information regarding the **severity of illness** and the **risk of mortality** while maintaining a measurement for resource intensity.

All-patient refined diagnosis-related groups (APR-DRGs) were created and now include four subclasses to each original DRG to address the severity of illness and the risk of mortality. This requires more specific documentation in the medical record for each patient, including details about the illness and possible complications of the patient. The four subclasses represent minor, moderate, major, or extreme severity of illness and risk of mortality.[13]

Resource-Based Relative Value Scale

The RBRVS, mentioned previously, is an initiative to reimburse physicians according to services provided. It replaces the fee-for-service methodology and was intended to narrow the disparity in reimbursement figures between specialists and general practitioners. In reality, it merely pays for the intensity of services rendered. Pulmonologists have done fairly well under this system, whereas cardiologists have experienced a 20% to 40% reduction in gross income. The scale is based on the time, skill, and intensity of the services provided. The RBRVS, developed by the federal government under the Medicare fee schedule (MFS), is composed of more than 7000 covered services. To compute the physician's payment, the relative value unit is adjusted for geographic area and then multiplied by a conversion factor, a monetary amount set annually by the federal government.

Bundled Charges

Bundled charges describe a type of packaged pricing, a form of reimbursement in which a number of related services are grouped together and provided in one fee. An example of a bundled charge would be the provision of pulmonary rehabilitation. Rather than charge separately for each component, all the services falling under this service, such as education and training in pursed-lip breathing, chest physiotherapy, and pulmonary hygiene, are packaged or bundled together and a single price charged.

Managed Care Approaches

Managed care approaches consist of the HMO, PPO, POS, and EPO. The HMO plan provides or arranges for a comprehensive array of services through a defined network of providers for a monthly fee. Members are required to stay within the network of physicians, outpatient providers, and hospitals. Coverage restrictions

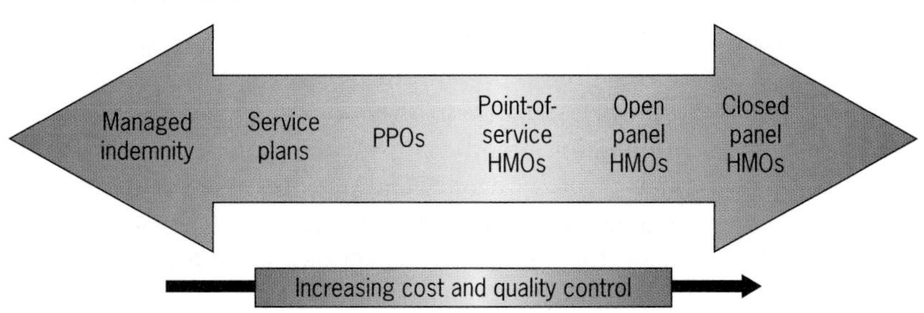

FIGURE 61–4 Continuum of cost control in U.S. healthcare. From Kongsvedt P. *Essentials of Managed Care.* 5th ed. Jones & Bartlett Learning; 2007:22

apply to services provided outside the network, except in certain emergencies or when specific approval is provided in advance of care. The HMO receives a monthly premium in advance for each member, who then has unlimited use of most of the health plan's services as long as such services are considered medically necessary. Each member usually pays a limited fee for each physician visit, prescription, or other service stipulated in the plan, referred to as a **copayment**, or *copay*.

Figure 61–4 depicts the relative level of patient choice and provider control (particularly of costs) for a variety of plans.[12] As one moves from one end of the continuum to another, one adds greater degrees of control and accountability and greater or lesser degrees of cost and quality. The more restrictive plans are on the right-hand side of the continuum. They offer fewer choices and greater restrictions, but yield lower costs. The managed care approaches are variations of a common theme, all focusing on cost containment.

Case Mix

Case mix is a relatively new form of reimbursement that refers to the overall intensity of conditions requiring medical and nursing intervention. It involves extensive assessment of the patient's condition, followed by a determination of specific services or procedures considered necessary or essential to effectively manage the patient. The case mix approach is used extensively in SNFs and is driven by the **minimum data set (MDS)**, which consists of a core of screening elements that are assessed for each patient admitted to the facility. These elements focus on patient care; function, health, and mental status; and treatment.

The Future of Healthcare Funding

The ability to forecast the future would certainly provide considerable advantage to executives in the healthcare financial industry. Change appears to be the only constant in a financial market that has evolved exponentially over the past century. Interestingly enough, the futurists do not anticipate any significant change in the sources of healthcare funding for the immediate future, meaning that the purchasers will remain relatively constant. However, the Centers for Disease Control and Prevention has reported that the number of Americans with private health insurance is at an all-time low, with only 65% of nonelderly persons carrying such insurance. This is a decrease from 67% in 2008. Additionally, there are 40 to 46 million Americans with no coverage at all.[14]

Little question remains that employers want to absolve themselves of this role or at least limit their financial exposure. However, employer-based insurance most likely will continue to serve as a major source of health insurance in the foreseeable future, with the public sector (in the form of the federal government's Medicare and Medicaid programs) clearly taking on a new (albeit still undefined) role.

Perhaps less predictable is the type of healthcare funding that will exist in the future. Employers have been successful in enticing their employees to move from the traditional indemnity plans and adopt the less expensive and more cost-effective features of the managed care programs. This movement resulted from a considerable concern for significant increases in healthcare premiums. Employees are concerned with out-of-pocket expenses and thus are attracted by the lower premiums, lower deductibles, and absence of copayments. Cost sharing (sharing of the escalating costs between employer and employee) is a strong incentive for employees to join managed care programs, such as HMOs, PPOs, or POSs, and shift from indemnity plans, which expose them to greater risk for out-of-pocket expenses.

Reimbursement and the Respiratory Therapist

So what does the changing face of healthcare reimbursement mean for respiratory therapists? In short, significant reasoning supports the theory that managed care will continue to evolve and dominate the market. Under such a design, respiratory therapists must address three key points to effectively contribute to such a system: documenting the care they provide, ensuring its appropriateness and quality, and demonstrating value.

Documenting Care: Charting

The old adage "If it's not charted, it wasn't done" rings especially true in a system that is attempting to reduce or curtail healthcare spending. Respiratory therapists must recognize that payers are looking for opportunities to deny reimbursement. Therefore, therapists must document every procedure and service so that the medical coder can capture the appropriate charge and reimbursement rate.

Three Rights

Ensuring appropriateness of care can be represented by adherence to the three rights of healthcare delivery: provision of the right care, in the right setting, by the right provider.

Providing the right care is analogous to a balance between overuse and underuse of services. Therapists must recognize that they are rewarded for appropriate care, not for either too little or too much. Under former reimbursement methodologies, overuse of services was rewarded, in that respiratory therapy departments were revenue generators. An increase in services meant increased revenue for the institution. In today's system, which is heavily based on capitation, DRGs, and per diems, institutions are paid on a fixed-income structure, effectively eliminating the incentives or rewards to provide additional services. In fact, providing too many services results in a loss of revenue for an institution.

Conversely, although underuse may at first glance appear to result in significant profit for an institution, too little healthcare can result in persistence of the problem and costly readmission and reentry into the system. A lack of adequate therapeutic interventions to the acutely ill asthmatic patient can result in a second trip to the emergency room 8 to 10 hours after a premature discharge, resulting in a more ill patient who perhaps requires more intensive and costly therapeutic interventions. The answer lies in appropriate care.

In addition to providing the right care, respiratory therapists must understand the importance of providing care in the right setting. Critical care areas represent the most expensive settings in which to provide healthcare services. The estimated daily charge for 1 day of admission to an intensive care unit (ICU) is approximately three to five times greater than the charge for a non-ICU ward. The number, intensity, and critical nature of services in an ICU are extremely costly and labor intensive. Respiratory therapists must recognize this fact and make every effort to assist in decision making regarding the transfer of patients to less costly and less intensive settings. Theoretically, the costs of care in a routine medical/surgical environment may represent per diem charges of approximately $1200. The costs of an SNF or extended care facility may result in per diems of $500. Providing care in the home could reduce costs even further, to approximately $250 per day. In addition, patients prefer the comforts and familiarity of the home to the formal and impersonal nature of healthcare institution. Clearly, compelling evidence suggests that the home, when feasible, is the most desirable and cost-effective environment for the provision of healthcare services. Every effort should be made to move the patient to the most appropriate care site.

Equally important is that the healthcare provider possesses the appropriate skill, training, and education to appropriately care for the patient, satisfying professional credentialing standards and matching education and skill appropriately. A highly paid provider who routinely performs relatively low-level skills is neither economical nor cost-effective. In other words, a neurosurgeon should not be routinely performing phlebotomies. Nor should the nursing aide be performing chest tube insertions. These situations simply do not make good economic sense. Providers should perform services and skills appropriate to their levels of training and education. Minimizing blood gas measurements, effectively using pharmacologic agents, and appropriately using ventilator management (all in the form of protocols) can earn the respiratory therapist respect and value as a member of the healthcare team. An experienced and knowledgeable therapist well versed in the art and science of respiratory care is indispensable in the critical care environment.

Demonstrating Value

Much has been written about the future role of the respiratory therapist, with potential roles including clinician, diagnostician, patient advocate, technical expert, consultant, counselor, and educator. Convincing and growing evidence suggests that respiratory therapists are best suited for these various roles. However, the bottom line is that therapists must demonstrate value.

Demonstrating value, central to the success of any professional, can occur clinically at the bedside, diagnostically in the pulmonary function laboratory, in consultation with the physician, nurse, or other healthcare provider, and in counseling and education as a patient advocate and educator. Although physicians, nurses, other healthcare professionals, and especially patients have heralded respiratory therapists as significant contributors to quality care, therapists must continue to provide evidence through randomized controlled trials that respiratory care achieves positive outcomes. The challenge is to expand the scientific literature and document the value of the respiratory therapist in reducing costs and improving quality of care.

KEY POINTS

- The four major functions of the healthcare delivery system in the United States are financing, insurance, delivery, and payment.
- Managed care is an attempt to integrate and coordinate the various functions of healthcare and create a system that functions effectively and efficiently.
- The five major players in the healthcare system are the patients, purchasers, plans, payers, and providers.
- Cost is the primary force driving healthcare in the United States, and is joined by demographics, shift in disease burden, technology, and the behavior of the healthcare consumer.
- Escalating costs in healthcare are the result of general inflation, growth in the elderly population, a medical price index that is higher than general inflation, and unique features regarding service intensity.
- The retrospective payment system uses a per diem methodology for inpatient hospital

reimbursement and a fee-for-service system and "usual, customary, and reasonable" fee schedule for physician services.

- Employer-based insurance is the dominant model among most consumers, who traditionally have not been very involved or motivated to curtail costs.
- The federal government is a major player in healthcare reimbursement through Medicare and shares responsibility with the states through Medicaid.
- Diagnosis-related groups (DRGs) are an attempt to curtail escalating costs with a fixed reimbursement rate based on a predetermined formula for inpatient hospital admissions.
- The all-patient refined DRG (APR-DRG) was added to the reimbursement mix to address the severity of illness and the risk of mortality.
- The resource-based relative value scale (RBRVS) has replaced the "usual, customary and reasonable" fee payment methodology and is used to pay physicians under Medicare Part B.
- The capitated system entails a per-member, per-month payment methodology.
- The four major types of managed care are the health maintenance organization, preferred provider organization, point-of-service plans, and exclusive provider organizations.
- Managed care emphasizes prevention, provides a complete range of services for a fixed fee, requires participants to use designated providers, and adheres to established standards of quality.
- The more popular methodologies used in healthcare reimbursement are fee for service, cost plus or charge minus, prospective payment, DRGs, resource-based relative value scales, bundled charges, multiple managed care approaches, and case mix.

REFERENCES

1. Shi L, Singh DA. *Delivering Health Care in America: A Systems Approach.* 3rd ed. Sudbury, MA: Jones & Bartlett Learning; 2004.
2. Kacmarek R, Durbin CG, Barnes TA, et al. Creating a vision for respiratory care in 2015 and beyond. *Respir Care.* 2009;54:375–389.
3. Fox Stoller T. What is driving change in health care delivery today? *Respir Care.* 1997;42:20–27.
4. Centers for Medicare and Medicaid Services. National health expenditure fact sheet. Available at: http://www.cms.gov/NationalHealthExpendData/25_NHE_Fact_Sheet.asp.
5. Johnson TD. Census Bureau: number of US uninsured rises to 47 million Americans are uninsured: almost 5 percent increase since 2005. *Nations Health.* 2007;37(8). Available at: http://www.medscape.com/viewarticle/567737.
6. Centers for Disease Control and Prevention. Smoking and tobacco use: fast facts. Available at: http://www.cdc.gov/tobacco/data_statistics/fact_sheets/fast_facts/index.htm.
7. Abdelhak M, Grostick S, Hanken MA, et al. *Health Information: Management of a Strategic Resource.* 3rd ed. St. Louis, MO: Saunders/Elsevier; 2007.
8. Williams SJ, Torrens PR. *Introduction to Health Services.* 5th ed. Albany, NY: Delmar; 1999.
9. Centers for Medicare and Medicaid Services. Medicare "pay for performance (P4P)" initiatives. January 31, 2005. Available at: http://www.cms.gov/apps/media/press/release.asp?Counter=1343.
10. Kimball AM, Miller EK. *Making Sense of Managed Care.* Vol. 1. San Francisco: Jossey-Bass; 1997.
11. London A. Models of managed health care delivery in the United States. *Respir Care.* 1997;42:30–38.
12. Kongstvedt P. *Essentials of Managed Health Care.* 5th ed. Sudbury, MA: Jones & Bartlett Learning; 2007.
13. Averill RF, Goldfield N, Hughes JS, et al. *All Patient Refined Diagnosis Related Groups (APR-DRGs): Methodology Overview.* Version 20.0. Wallingford, CT, and Murray, UT: 3M Health Information Systems; 2003. Document GRP–041.
14. Associated Press. CDC: percentage of Americans with private health insurance hits 50-year low. Fox News.com. Available at: http://www.foxnews.com/story/0,2933,529821,00.html.

CHAPTER 62

Evidence-Based Respiratory Care

Dean R. Hess

OUTLINE

What Is Evidence-Based Respiratory Care?
Hierarchy of Evidence
Evidence for a Diagnostic Test
Evidence for a Therapy
Meta-Analysis
Finding the Evidence
Narrative Reviews and Systematic Reviews
Clinical Practice Guidelines

OBJECTIVES

1. Define evidence-based medicine.
2. List the hierarchy of evidence.
3. Use the tools of evidence-based medicine to evaluate the evidence for a diagnostic test and for a therapy.
4. Describe the details of a forest plot resulting from a meta-analysis.
5. Use techniques to identify the best evidence.
6. Compare narrative and systematic reviews.
7. Use the recommendations of clinical practice guidelines.

KEY TERMS

clinical practice guideline (CPG)
evidence-based medicine
forest plot
likelihood ratio (LR)
meta-analysis
***N*-of-1 randomized controlled trial**
receiver operating characteristic curve
sensitivity
specificity
systematic review

INTRODUCTION

One of the more important movements affecting healthcare practice in the 21st century is the emergence of **evidence-based medicine**. Respiratory care practice demands evidence for the accuracy of diagnostic tests, as well as the efficacy and safety of treatments. The principles of evidence-based medicine provide the tools to incorporate the best evidence into everyday respiratory care practice. Research evidence has a short doubling time—perhaps 10 years or less. Thus, it can be a challenge for clinicians to stay abreast of the newest research findings. The evolving research evidence replaces currently accepted diagnostic tests and treatments with new ones that are more powerful, more accurate, more efficacious, and safer. The availability of evidence is not sufficient, however. It is increasingly recognized that the translation of evidence into practice is often slow.[1] This chapter reviews the principles of evidence-based medicine as it applies to respiratory care practice.

What Is Evidence-Based Respiratory Care?

Evidence-based respiratory care is the integration of individual clinical expertise with the best available research evidence from systematic research and a patient's values and expectations.[2] The best evidence is not static, but rather changes when better evidence becomes available. Evidence-based medicine does not devalue clinical skills and clinical judgment. To the contrary, evidence-based medicine demands a high level of clinical skill and judgment. The practice of evidence-based medicine requires us to apply the evidence to the right patient, at the right time, in the right place, at the right dose, and using the right resources. We need to recognize the correct patient diagnosis before applying the evidence to the care of the patient. For example, the best evidence for management of asthma may not apply to a patient with chronic obstructive pulmonary disease (COPD).

Research evidence comes from real clinical research among intact patients. Animal studies do not trump patient studies. That is not to say that animal studies are not important to test proof of concept or to explore physiologic mechanisms. However, care must always be taken when extrapolating animal studies to patient care. The findings of properly conducted studies in a relevant patient population should never be discarded in favor of the findings from an animal study. No number of animal studies can outweigh the findings of even a single well-done human study.

Patient values and expectations are an important part of evidence-based medicine. For example, there is a compelling body of high-level research evidence supporting the use of noninvasive ventilation (NIV) in patients with an exacerbation of COPD.[3] However, the patient with COPD exacerbation may choose not to accept NIV. Another example relates to the choice of an aerosol delivery device. The evidence shows that similar outcomes result from the use of a nebulizer and a metered dose inhaler (MDI) with valved holding chamber.[4] A patient may reject the use of the MDI in favor of the nebulizer. Although this may contradict the bias of the clinician, the patient's choice should be respected; moreover, the nebulizer may result in better compliance if it better meets the expectations of the patient.

Evidence-based respiratory care is not cookbook medicine or cost-cutting care. The best evidence needs extrapolation to the patient's unique pathophysiology and values. With the implementation of evidence-based medicine, costs may increase, decrease, or remain unchanged.

Hierarchy of Evidence

A hierarchy of evidence can be used to assess the strength upon which clinical decisions are made (**Box 62–1**).[5] Respiratory therapists should seek the highest available evidence from this hierarchy. Evidence always exists, but sometimes it may be weak. The best available evidence may be the unsystematic observation of a single clinician or a generalization from physiologic studies.

BOX 62–1

Hierarchy of Evidence

- *N*-of-1 randomized trial
- Meta-analysis of randomized trial
- Single randomized controlled trial
- Systematic reviews of observational study
- Single observational study
- Physiologic studies
- Unsystematic clinical observations

RESPIRATORY RECAP

Evidence-Based Medicine

» Evidence-based medicine is the integration of individual clinical expertise with the best available research evidence from systematic research and a patient's values and expectations.

» A hierarchy of evidence can be used to assess the strength upon which clinical decisions are made.

Note that randomization is an important attribute of higher levels of evidence. The highest level of evidence is an **N-of-1 randomized controlled trial** (RCT). In the *N*-of-1 RCT, an individual patient undertakes pairs of treatment periods in which the patient receives a target treatment in one period of each pair and a placebo or alternative in the other. The order of the target treatment and the control is randomized, and quantitative ratings are made for each treatment. The *N*-of-1 RCT continues until both the patient and clinician conclude that there is, or is not, benefit from the intervention. For example, imagine that a decision is made to try flutter therapy for a patient with cystic fibrosis. The clinician and patient agree that a clinically useful outcome measure is sputum production. A 12-week trial is designed. For 1 week, the only sputum clearance technique used is huff coughing. For a second week, flutter therapy in addition to huff coughing is used. For a third week, sham therapy is used. The order of treatments is randomized (the patient flips a coin), and the sequence is repeated four times. Each day, the sputum produced during the therapy session is weighed. A diary is also kept in which events such as chest infections are logged. At the end of 12 weeks, the results are analyzed (this may include statistical analysis), reviewed together by the clinician and patient, and a collaborative decision is made regarding the benefit of the therapy. In this manner, an objective decision is made regarding the benefits of this therapy for this individual patient.

There are some therapies for which there has not been a randomized trial, and one might argue that a randomized trial is either unethical or unnecessary. For example, it is unlikely that a randomized trial will ever be conducted to study the survival benefit of mechanical ventilation in patients with apnea, transfusion for massive blood loss, or antibiotics for bacterial pneumonia. In such cases, the benefit of therapy is overwhelmingly obvious and a randomized controlled trial is unnecessary. In respiratory care, some therapies are unproven. In other words, the evidence to support their use is weak. Because a therapy is unproven does not mean that it is wrong, but it also does not mean that it is right.

Evidence for a Diagnostic Test

In respiratory care, diagnostic tests are commonly used to make clinical decisions. Using the tools of evidence-based medicine, metrics are calculated such as sensitivity, specificity, receiver operating characteristic curves, and likelihood ratios (**Figure 62–1**).

Sensitivity and Specificity

Sensitivity is the proportion of patients who have a disorder and are correctly identified by the test. **Specificity** is the proportion of patients who are free of a disorder and are correctly identified by the test.

Likelihood Ratio

Likelihood ratio (LR) is used for assessing the value of performing a diagnostic test.

- An LR of 1 indicates that the posttest probability is exactly the same as the pretest probability. Thus, diagnostic tests with an LR of 1 are not helpful.
- An LR greater than 1 increases the probability that the target condition is present, and an LR less than 1 decreases the probability that the target condition is present.
- An LR greater than 10 or less than 0.1 generates large and conclusive changes in the probability of a given diagnosis.
- An LR in the range of 5 to 10 or 0.1 to 0.2 generates moderate and usually useful shifts in pretest to posttest probability.
- An LR in the range of 2 to 5 or 0.5 to 0.2 generates small, but sometimes important, changes in pretest probability.
- An LR in the range of 1 to 2 or 0.5 to 1.0 alters the probability of a given condition to a small and rarely important degree.

The rapid shallow breathing index (RSBI) can be used to illustrate the use of these statistical metrics.[6,7] Meade et al. suggest an LR of 1.58 and 0.22 for positive and negative predictions, respectively.[6] An LR of this magnitude generates a small change in pretest probability. A nomogram can be used to derive posttest probabilities from the pretest probability and the likelihood ratio. Imagine an intubated 30-year-old patient following multiple trauma. In your clinical experience, 80% of similar patients extubate successfully following resolution of the chest trauma (the pretest probability of successful extubation is 80%). Suppose that the patient's RSBI is 85 (test is positive for extubation). As shown in **Figure 62–2**, the likelihood ratio produces a posttest probability of successful extubation that differs little from the pretest probability. However, if the RSBI is 120 (test is negative for extubation), the posttest probability of successful extubation does change the pretest probability.

Imagine an 85-year-old patient with resolving COPD exacerbation. In your experience, only 20% of similar

		Reference Standard	
		Positive	Negative
Test Result	Positive	a	b
	Negative	c	d

True Positive = a
True Negative = d
False Positive = b
False Negative = c
Sensitivity = a/(a + c)
Specificity = d/(b + d)
Likelihood Ratio for Positive Test (LR+) = sensitivity/(1– specificity)
Likelihood Ratio for Negative Test (LR–) = (1 – sensitivity)/specificity
Positive Predictive Value (PPV) = a/(a + b)
Negative Predictive Value (NPV) = d/(c + d)
Diagnostic Accuracy = (a + d)/(a + b + c + d)

(A)

		Extubation	
		Successful	Unsuccessful
Rate/Tidal Volume Ratio	<100	32	12
	>100	1	19

True Positive = 32
True Negative = 19
False Positive = 12
False Negative = 1
Sensitivity = 32/(32 + 1) = 97%
Specificity = 19/(12 + 19) = 61%
Likelihood Ratio for Positive Test (LR+) = 0.97/(1 – 0.61) = 2.49
Likelihood Ratio for Negative Test (LR–) = (1 – 0.97)/0.61 = 0.05
Positive Predictive Value (PPV) = 32/(32 + 12) = 0.73
Negative Predictive Value (NPV) = 19/(1 + 19) = 0.95
Diagnostic Accuracy = 51/64 = 0.80

(B)

FIGURE 62–1 (**A**) Statistical tests commonly used to assess a diagnostic test. (**B**) Comparison of the results of a diagnostic test (ratio of rate to tidal volume) with the results of a reference standard (successful spontaneous breathing trial), assuming that a ratio less than 105 indicates successful extubation. Data from Yang KL, Tobin MJ. A prospective study of indexes predicting the outcome of trials of weaning from mechanical ventilation. *N Engl J Med.* 1991;324:1445.

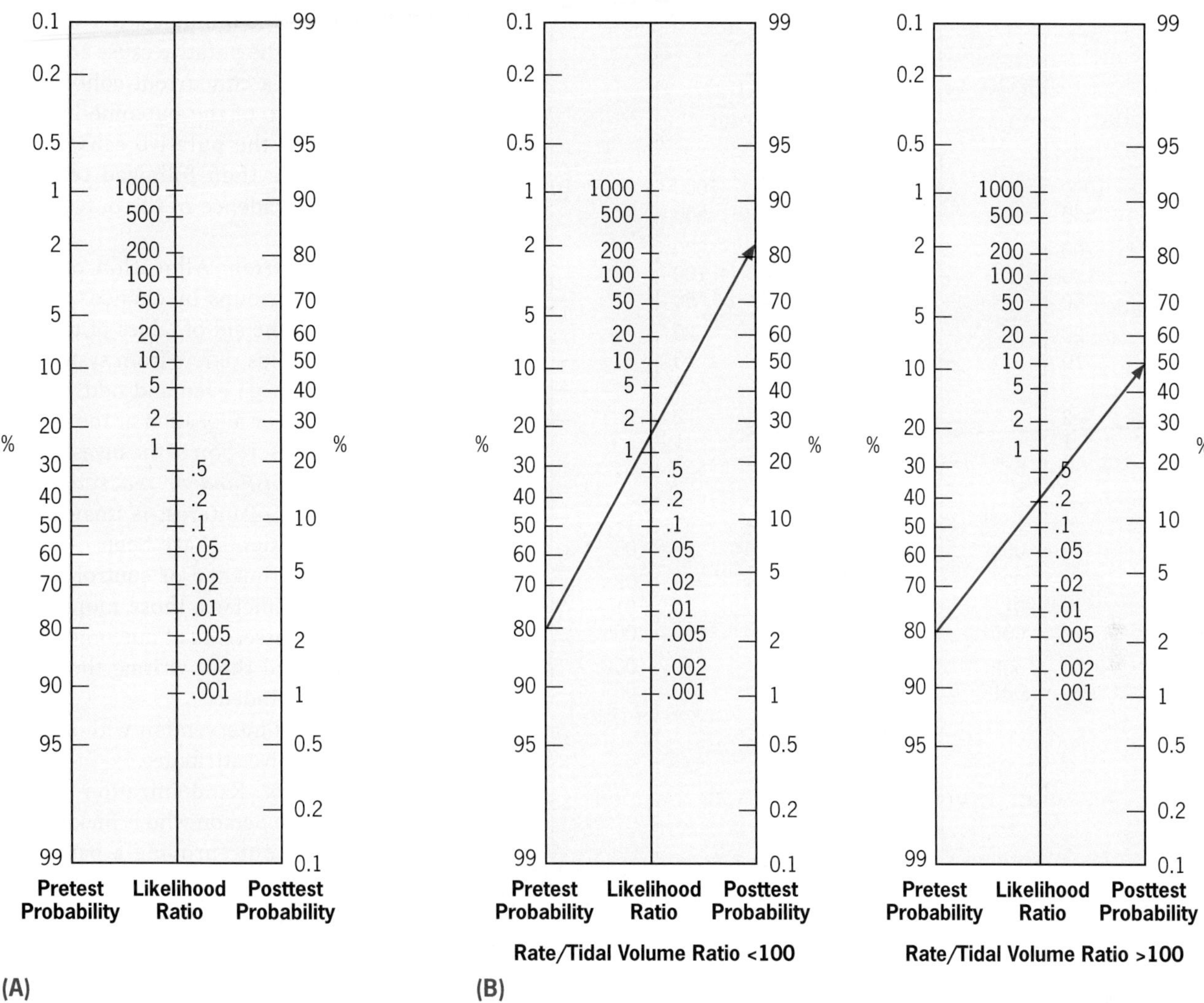

FIGURE 62–2 (**A**) A nomogram to determine posttest probability from pretest probability and likelihood ratio. (**B**) Patient recovering from acute respiratory distress syndrome (ARDS) with 80% pretest probability of ventilator liberation. The solid line represents the likelihood ratio. (**C**) Patient recovering from chronic obstructive pulmonary disease (COPD) with 20% pretest probability of ventilator liberation. The solid line represents the likelihood ratio. Data from Meade M, et al. Predicting success in weaning from mechanical ventilation. *Chest.* 2001;120:400S–424S. (*continues*)

patients extubate successfully following resolution of the COPD exacerbation (the pretest probability of successful extubation is 20%). Suppose that this patient's RSBI is 85. As shown in Figure 62–2, using the likelihood ratio produces a posttest probability of successful extubation that increases the pretest probability, but not by a lot. However, if the RSBI is 120, the posttest probability of successful extubation is extremely low.

> **RESPIRATORY RECAP**
>
> **Evidence for a Diagnostic Test**
>
> » Sensitivity and specificity
> » Likelihood ratio
> » Receiver operating characteristic curve

Receiver Operating Characteristic Curve

The **receiver operating characteristic curve** is a figure showing the power of a diagnostic test. It plots the true-positive rate (sensitivity) on the vertical axis and the false-positive rate (specificity) on the horizontal axis for different cut points, thus dividing a positive from a negative test. For a perfect test, the area under the curve is 1.0. For a test that performs no better than chance, the area under the curve is 0.5. In **Figure 62–3**, note that the modest area under the curve (0.70) demonstrates that the RSBI has no more than modest accuracy in predicting extubation readiness.[6]

Evidence for a Therapy

Increasingly, studies are being published related to respiratory therapy. It is important to assess the validity of such studies. High-level studies are prospective, randomized, blinded, placebo controlled, concealed allocation, and of parallel design and assess patient-important outcomes.

- *Prospective study*: Prospective investigation of the factors that might cause a disorder in which a cohort of individuals who do not have evidence

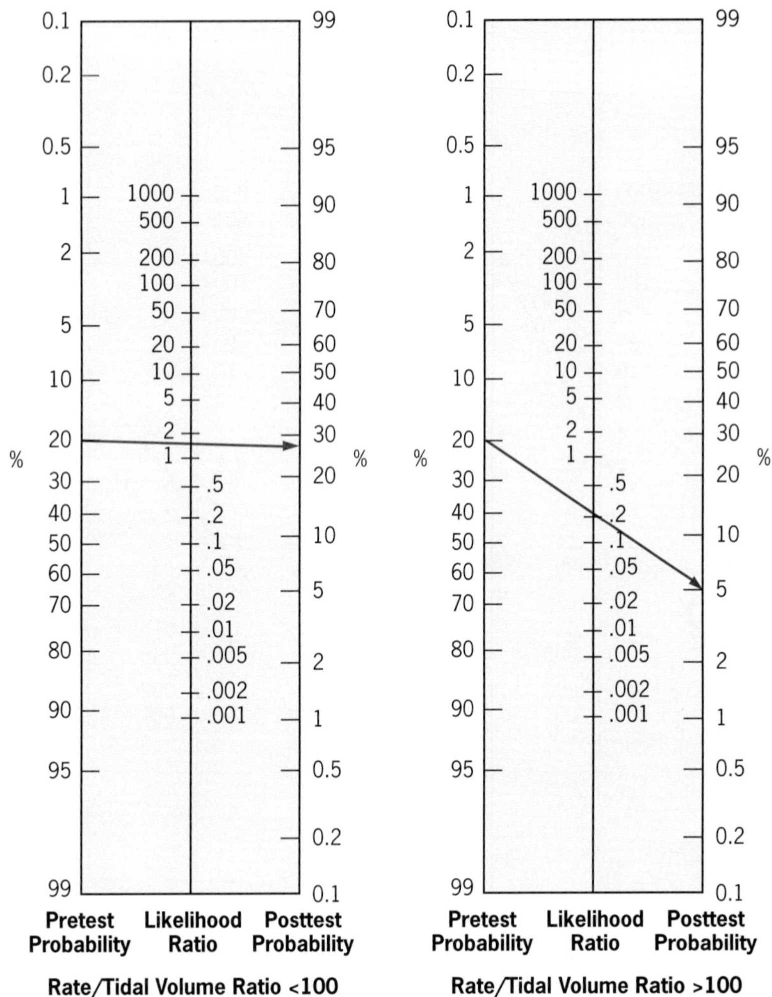

FIGURE 62–2 (*Continued*).

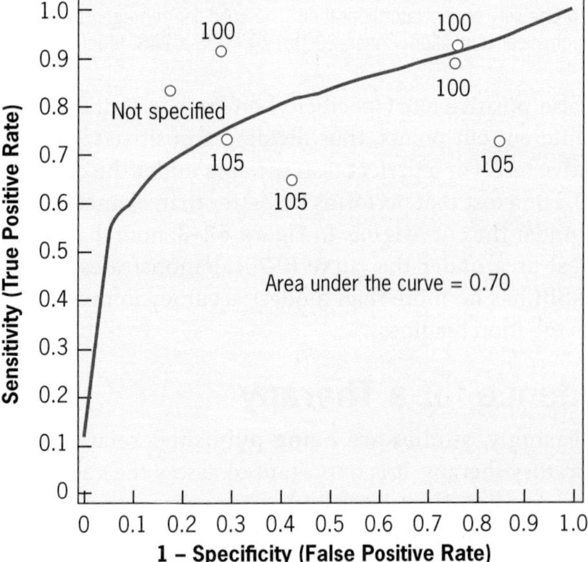

FIGURE 62–3 Summary receiver operating characteristic curve for the rapid shallow breathing index (RSBI) predicting successful extubation. The numbers in the figure represent the RSBI cut points from the various studies. From Meade M, et al. Predicting success in weaning from mechanical ventilation. *Chest.* 2001;120:400S–424S. Copyright 2001. American College of Chest Physicians. Reproduced with permission of American College of Chest Physicians in the format Textbook via Copyright Clearance Center.

of an outcome of interest but who are exposed to the putative cause are compared with a concurrent cohort who are also free of the outcome but not exposed to the putative cause. Both cohorts are then followed to compare the incidence of the outcome of interest.

- *Randomization*: Allocation of individuals to groups by chance, usually done with the aid of tables of random numbers. This differs from systematic allocation (e.g., even and odd days of the month) or allocation at the convenience or discretion of the investigator.
- *Blind (or blinded or masked)*: The participant of interest is unaware of whether patients have been assigned to the experimental or control group. Patients, clinicians, those monitoring outcomes, assessors of outcomes, data analysts, and those writing the paper can all be blinded.
- *Placebo*: An intervention without biologically active attributes.
- *Concealment*: Randomization is concealed if the person who is making the decision about enrolling a patient is unaware of whether the next patient enrolled will be entered in the treatment or control group.
- *Parallel design*: With a parallel study design, subjects are randomly assigned to the treatment or control group, an intervention is applied, and the outcome is identified for each subject. This is different from a crossover study, in which subjects receive both the treatment and control intervention.

Depending on the type of study, some of these criteria cannot be applied. For example, blinding is not possible with studies of aerosol delivery devices. Placebo-controlled studies of noninvasive ventilation are difficult to implement.

When assessing a therapy, it is important to evaluate a patient-important outcome. Clinicians are often interested in physiologic outcomes such as an improvement in arterial blood gas results. Patients, on the other hand, are more interested in outcomes such as survival. There are a number of examples in which an improvement in physiologic outcomes does not correlate with patient-important outcomes. For patients with acute respiratory distress syndrome (ARDS), inhaled nitric oxide improves Pa_{O_2}, but not mortality.[8] High tidal volumes in patients with ARDS improve the Pa_{O_2}, but mortality is lower for small tidal volumes.[9]

Using the tools of evidence-based medicine, metrics such as event rate, relative risk, relative risk reduction, absolute risk reduction, number needed to treat, and odds ratio can be calculated.

- *Event rate*: The proportion of patients in a group in whom an event is observed. *Control event rate* and *experimental event rate* refer to this metric in control and experimental groups of patients, respectively.
- *Relative risk*: The ratio of the risk of an event among an experimental group to the risk among the control group. A relative risk less than 1 means benefit, a relative risk greater than 1 means harm, and a relative risk equal to 1 means the intervention has no effect.
- *Relative risk reduction*: An estimate of the proportion of baseline risk that is removed by the therapy.
- *Absolute risk reduction*: The difference in the absolute risk (percentage or proportion of patients with an outcome) in the exposed (experimental event rate) versus the unexposed (control event rate) group.
- *Number needed to treat*: The number of patients who need to be treated to prevent one bad outcome.
- *Odds ratio*: The ratio of the odds of an event in an exposed group to the odds of the same event in a group that is not exposed.
- *Survival curve*: Survival analysis involves the modeling of time to event data. In this context, death or failure is considered an event in the survival analysis literature. Survival analysis asks questions such as "What is the fraction of a population that will survive past a certain time?" In medicine, a typical application might involve grouping patients into categories and then determining whether one group dies more quickly than the other.
- *Confidence interval*: The range of values within which it is probable that the true value lies for the whole population of patients from which the study patients were selected. The confidence interval is affected by sample size and effect size (i.e., the difference in outcomes between the intervention and control groups divided by some measure of variability, typically the standard deviation). A larger sample size narrows the range of the confidence interval, increasing the precision of the study results. A larger sample size also decreases the risk of a type II (beta) error, in which the study fails to detect an important difference. High-level studies conduct a power analysis as part of the study design so that an appropriate sample size can be determined a priori.

The Acute Respiratory Distress Syndrome Network (ARDSnet) study can be used as an example (**Figure 62–4**).[9] In this study, 861 patients with ARDS or acute lung injury (ALI) were randomly assigned to be mechanically ventilated with a tidal volume of 12 mL/kg or 6 mL/kg. The primary outcome was mortality. Mortality for the control group (12 mL/kg tidal volume) was 39.8%, and mortality for the experimental group (6 mL/kg tidal volume) was 31%. The relative risk of mortality was lower for the 6-mL/kg group (0.787), with a relative risk reduction of 0.213 compared with the 12-mL/kg group. The absolute risk reduction for mortality was 8.8%, resulting in a number needed to treat of 11 patients. In other words, for every 11 mechanically ventilated patients with ALI or ARDS who receive a tidal volume of 6 mL/kg (rather than 12 mL/kg), one additional life will be saved. The survival curves from this study are shown in **Figure 62–5**.

		Outcome	
		Present	Absent
Treatment	Present	a	b
	Absent	c	d

Controlled Event Rate (CER) = c/(c + d)
Experimental Event Rate (EER) = a/(a + b)
Relative Risk (RR) = EER/CER = [a/(a + b)] / [c/(c + d)]
Relative Risk Reduction (RRR) = 1 – RR
Absolute Risk Reduction (ARR) = c/(c + d) – a/(a + b)
Number Needed to Treat (NNT) = 1/ARR
Odds Ratio (OR) = (a × d) / (c × b)

(A)

		Outcome	
		Death at 28 days	Alive at 28 days
Treatment	6 mL/kg tidal volume	134	298
	12 mL/kg tidal volume	171	259

Controlled Group Mortality (12 mL/kg) = 171/(171 + 259) = 0.398
Experimental Group Mortality (6 mL/kg) = 134/(134 + 298) = 0.31
Relative Risk (RR) = 0.31/0.398 = 0.787
Relative Risk Reduction = 1 – 0.787 = 0.213 (21.3%)
Absolute Risk Reduction = 0.398 – 0.31 = 0.088 (8.8%)
Number Needed to Treat = 1/0.088 = 11
Odds Ratio = (134 × 259) / (171 × 298) = 0.68

(B)

FIGURE 62–4 **(A)** Statistical tests commonly used to assess a therapy. **(B)** The results of the ARDSnet study. Data from The Acute Respiratory Distress Syndrome Network. Ventilation with lower tidal volumes as compared with traditional tidal volumes for acute lung injury and the acute respiratory distress syndrome. *N Engl J Med.* 2000;342:1301–1308.

RESPIRATORY RECAP

Evidence for a Therapy

» Event rate
» Relative risk
» Relative risk reduction
» Absolute risk reduction
» Number needed to treat
» Odds ratio
» Survival curve

Meta-Analysis

Clinical trials related to respiratory care are often expensive, and it may be difficult to recruit an adequate sample size to avoid a beta error. A **meta-analysis** uses statistical methods to combine the results of several studies

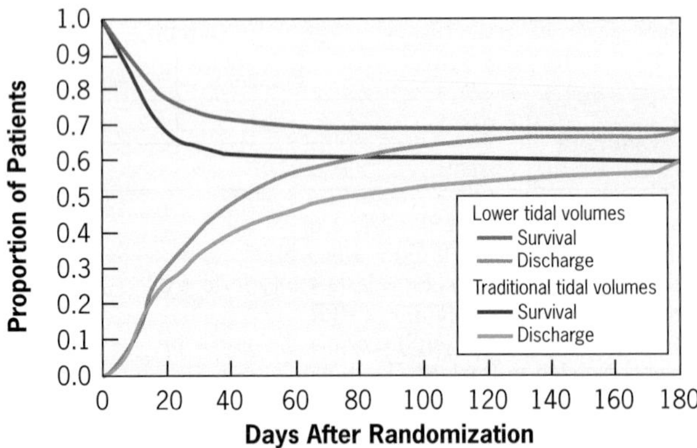

FIGURE 62–5 Probability of survival and of being discharged home and breathing without assistance during the first 180 days after randomization in patients with acute lung injury and the acute respiratory distress syndrome. Reproduced from The Acute Respiratory Distress Syndrome Network. *N Engl J Med.* 342;(2000):1301–1308.

into a single pooled metric. Meta-analysis is a statistical approach that combines the results of several independent studies. As with any study design, the question asked will influence the design and the method of meta-analysis. Because it is usually based on a literature review, the meta-analysis is observational rather than experimental in nature. The person conducting the meta-analysis has limited control over the availability of the data reported in individual studies. The studies included in the meta-analysis should be comparable, but the degree of comparability is subjective and determined by the person conducting the meta-analysis. Included studies should be identified from a comprehensive review of the literature, and unpublished data should ideally be included to reduce the risk of publication bias. Ideally, the meta-analysis will be conducted from the discrete data from the included studies, but more commonly it is conducted using summary data published in the individual studies.

The results of a meta-analysis are often displayed as a **forest plot**. The name refers to the forest of lines produced. Forest plots are commonly presented with two columns (**Figure 62–6**). The left-hand column lists the

First Author	Early Tracheostomy n/N	Late Tracheostomy n/N	Odds Ratio (random) (95% CI)	Odds Ratio	95% CI
Blot	30/61	31/62		0.97	0.48–1.96
Dunham	20/34	20/40		1.43	0.57–3.59
Rumbak	3/60	15/60		0.16	0.04–0.58
Saffle	21/21	22/23		2.87	0.11–74.28
Total	74/176	88/185		0.76	0.28–2.05

Heterogeneity: tau = 0.59, chi-square = 8.43, degrees of freedom = 3, P = .04, I^2 = 64%

Test for overall effect: P = .58

0.01 0.1 1 10 100

Favors Experimental | Favors Control

(A)

First Author	Early Tracheostomy n/N	Late Tracheostomy n/N	Odds Ratio (random) (95% CI)	Odds Ratio	95% CI
Blot	12/61	15/62		0.77	0.33–1.81
Dunham	0/0	0/0		Not calculable	Not calculable
Rumbak	19/60	37/60		0.29	0.14–0.61
Saffle	4/21	6/23		0.67	0.16–2.79
Total	35/142	58/145		0.49	0.25–0.97

Heterogeneity: tau = 0.13, chi-square = 3.11, degrees of freedom = 2, P = .21, I^2 = 36%

Test for overall effect: P = .04

0.01 0.1 1 10 100

Favors Experimental | Favors Control

(B)

FIGURE 62–6 An example of a forest plot as used to display meta-analysis results. This meta-analysis is of high-quality studies of early versus late tracheostomy. (**A**) Pneumonia rate. (**B**) Mortality. From Durbin CG Jr, Perkins MP, Moores LK. Should tracheostomy be performed as early as 72 hours? *Respir Care.* 2010:55(1):81. Reprinted with permission.

names of the studies, commonly in chronological order from the top downward. The right-hand column is a plot of the measure of effect for each of these studies, often represented by a square, incorporating confidence intervals represented by horizontal lines. The graph often is plotted on a logarithmic scale when using ratio-based effect measures, so that the confidence intervals are symmetrical about the means from each study. The size of each square is proportional to the study's weight in the meta-analysis. The overall measure of effect is commonly plotted as a diamond, the lateral points of which indicate confidence intervals for this estimate. A vertical line representing no effect is also plotted. If the confidence intervals for individual studies overlap with this line, it demonstrates that their effect sizes do not differ from no effect.

RESPIRATORY RECAP

Meta-Analysis

» Uses statistical methods to combine the results of several studies
» Results are often displayed as a forest plot

Finding the Evidence

Finding the evidence begins with a question.[10,11] There are two types of questions: background questions and foreground questions.[5] Background questions are those that might be answered by referring to a textbook or performing a basic Internet search. Examples include the following:

- How many lobes are in the right lower lobe?
- What are normal blood gas values for a newborn?
- How does a noninvasive ventilator work?

Foreground questions are asked by more seasoned clinicians and require the ability to find the evidence, assess its validity, and determine whether it applies to the unique patients seen by the clinician. Examples of foreground questions are as follows:

- What is the current role of inhaled steroid therapy in patients with COPD?
- How should positive end-expiratory pressure be set when ventilating a patient with ARDS?
- Should NIV be used in patients with hypoxemic respiratory failure?

Internet Search

The Internet is a confederation of networks around the world that allows computers connected to the Internet to communicate with other computers across the Internet. Browsers such as Internet Explorer and Safari access documents called Web pages that are linked to each other via hyperlinks.

A common method to find information is a basic Web search. Many search engines are available free of charge, and the choice of one over the other is based on personal preference. A commonly used search engine is Google (www.google.com). Because Google returns only Web pages that contain all the words in the query, refining or narrowing the search is done by adding more words to the search terms. The result is a smaller subset of the pages found by Google for the original broad query. It is important to choose key words carefully.

- Try the obvious words first. For information on noninvasive positive pressure ventilation, enter "noninvasive ventilation" rather than "mechanical ventilation."
- Use words that are likely to appear on a website with the information you want. "BiPAP" gets more specific results than "equipment for noninvasive ventilation."
- Choose key words that are as specific as possible. "Noninvasive positive pressure ventilation" gets more relevant results than "positive pressure ventilation."

Conducting a Web search is a quick way to find lots of information. In fact, the amount of information obtained can be overwhelming and involve a considerable amount of time filtering through Web pages and hypertext links. It is not unusual to follow a link to a page that is no longer available (dead link). Much of the information that is found may be irrelevant. Moreover, the validity of information may be suspect. Information posted on the Web may be outdated or incorrect; it is almost never subjected to peer review.

RESPIRATORY RECAP

Finding the Evidence

» Internet search
» Google Scholar
» PubMed
» Web of Science
» Ovid
» Journal websites

Google Scholar

Google Scholar (http://scholar.google.com) is a freely accessible Web search engine that indexes the full text of scholarly literature across an array of publishing formats and disciplines. Scholarly searches appear using the references from full-text journal articles, technical reports, preprints, theses, books, and other documents that are deemed to be scholarly.

PubMed

PubMed (www.pubmed.gov) provides access to citations to medical journals dating to the mid-1960s and includes links to many sites that provide full-text articles and other related resources. To search PubMed, enter search terms in the site's query box (**Figure 62–7**). The search rules are straightforward:

- Enter one or more search terms.
- Enter author names in the format "Hess DR" (initials are optional).
- Enter journal titles in full or using abbreviations.

A search strategy helps identify the information needed. First, identify the key concepts and search those terms. Then consider alternative terms and search those. It may

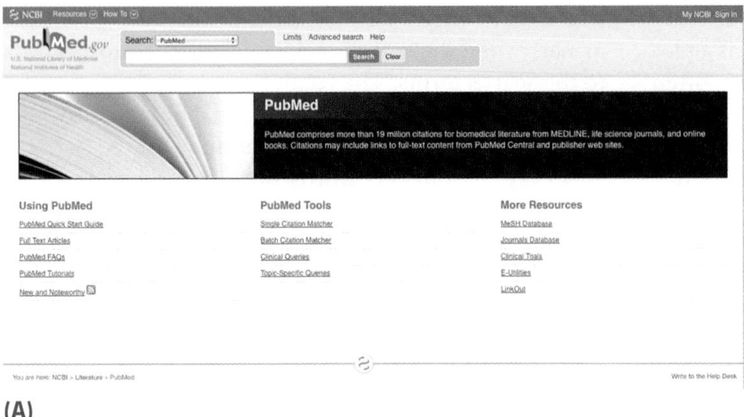

(A)

(B)

(C)

FIGURE 62–7 (**A**) The PubMed home page. (**B**) The results of a PubMed search. (**C**) When a citation is clicked, note the "Related citations" links on the side of the window.

then be useful to refine the search to dates, study groups, and other limits as appropriate. The Boolean operators "AND," "OR," and "NOT" can be used to refine the search. There is no right or wrong way to do a search. Search strategies differ according to personal choice, and efficient searching requires practice and a systematic approach.

Note that PubMed provides some suggestions for additional searches to the right of the screen. This can be helpful to refine your search. Using the Limits feature of PubMed, one can limit the search to citations in English. Using the Advanced feature, one can search for papers in a specific journal. Clicking on the citation opens a window with the abstract. The icon next to the citation also identifies whether the article is available as a full text. A direct link between PubMed and the journal allows easy access to the full-text article if it is available. PubMed also provides links to related papers.

Cumulative Index to Nursing and Allied Health Literature

The Cumulative Index to Nursing and Allied Health Literature (CINAHL) is a comprehensive resource for nursing and allied health literature. Although there is considerable overlap between PubMed and CINAHL, there are a number of nursing and allied health journals listed in CINAHL that are not found in PubMed.

Web of Science

Web of Science is an online academic service with access to seven databases, the most important of which is the Science Citation Index. Its multidisciplinary content covers over 10,000 of the highest-impact journals worldwide. It covers the sciences, social sciences, arts, and humanities.

Ovid

Ovid provides medical information services to individuals in medical schools, hospitals, and academic institutions. Ovid offers content in more than 3000 ebooks, more than 1200 peer-reviewed journals, and more than 100 bibliographic and full-text databases.

Journal Websites

Most medical journals are available online. You can access the journal's content via the journal website, although a subscription is usually required for the most recent content. The website for *Respiratory Care* (www.rcjournal.com) is typical. Many journal websites provide the opportunity to receive email notifications of the journal's table of contents, which allows you to survey the most recent content for papers of interest.

Narrative Reviews and Systematic Reviews

Review papers are commonly published in medical journals and summarize in detail the literature related to a subject matter.[12] Narrative reviews are limited by incomplete searches of the literature, intentional or unintentional bias by the authors, and failure to account for the quality of individual publications. Additionally, narrative reviews typically fail to effectively deal with studies that have conflicting results. Narrative reviews by experts are notoriously biased because experts tend to rely on their own expertise and experience rather than on the available evidence.

A **systematic review** is different from a narrative review in purpose and process. A systematic review details the methods by which papers were identified in the literature. This includes the search terms and the search engines utilized. A systematic review uses predetermined criteria for selection of papers to be included in the review. Explicit methods for appraising the literature are used to evaluate the quality and validity of individual studies. Many systematic reviews include a quantitative review of the literature in the form of a meta-analysis. The Cochrane Collaboration (www.cochrane.org) is a good source of high-level systematic reviews and meta-analyses.

Clinical Practice Guidelines

Clinical practice guidelines (CPGs) are systematically developed statements to help clinicians deliver appropriate care in specific clinical circumstances.[13] Well-designed CPGs help to fill the gap between evidence and practice. Although the CPGs are not treatment protocols per se, they do provide a context within which specific policies and protocols can be developed. Evidence-based CPGs have two components: the evidence component and the detailed instructional component. The detailed instructional component is expressed in the form of recommendations. Furthermore, the strength of a recommendation is given a grade based on the strength of the supporting evidence.

The Grading of Recommendations Assessment, Development, and Evaluation (GRADE) system classifies the quality of evidence using four levels: high, moderate, low, and very low.[14,15] The highest-quality evidence is generally considered to arise from randomized controlled trials. However, the GRADE system allows even an RCT to be downgraded in strength if there are important study limitations (e.g., inconsistency of results, indirectness of evidence, reporting bias, imprecision). Observational studies are usually graded as low quality, but can be upgraded if the magnitude of the treatment effect is very large, if there is evidence of a dose–response relationship, or if all biases would increase the magnitude of a treatment effect. The GRADE system uses two grades of recommendations, strong and weak. A strong recommendation is given when desirable effects clearly outweigh undesirable effects. When the tradeoffs are less certain, either because of low-quality evidence or because evidence suggests that the desirable and undesirable effects are similar, a weak recommendation is given. Many professional societies have adopted GRADE for writing clinical practice guidelines.

> **RESPIRATORY RECAP**
>
> **Reviews and Clinical Practice Guidelines**
>
> » Narrative reviews are often incomplete and biased.
>
> » A systematic review uses explicit methods to search and appraise the literature.
>
> » Clinical practice guidelines provide recommendations for care.

A number of CPGs have been published by the American Association for Respiratory Care and can be found at www.rcjournal.com. The National Guideline Clearinghouse (www.guideline.gov) is a comprehensive database of evidence-based CPGs and related documents produced by the U.S. Department of Health and Human Services Agency for Healthcare Research and Quality. Several sources can be searched for evidence-based systematic reviews and clinical practice guidelines. PubMed can be searched using the limits of "meta-analysis" or "practice guideline."

KEY POINTS

- Evidence-based respiratory care is the integration of individual clinical expertise with the best available research evidence from systematic research and a patient's values and expectations.
- A hierarchy of evidence can be used to assess the strength upon which clinical decisions are made.
- To evaluate a diagnostic test, metrics such as sensitivity, specificity, receiver operating characteristic curves, and likelihood ratios are calculated.
- High-level studies are prospective, randomized, blinded, placebo controlled, concealed allocation, and of parallel design, and assess patient-important outcomes.
- When assessing a therapy, it is important to evaluate a patient-important outcome.
- To evaluate a therapy, metrics such as event rate, relative risk, relative risk reduction, absolute risk reduction, number needed to treat, and odds ratio can be calculated.
- A meta-analysis uses statistical methods to combine the results of several studies into a single pooled metric.
- A number of electronic search strategies can be used to find the best evidence.
- A systematic review details the methods by which papers were identified in the literature, uses predetermined criteria for selection of papers to be

included in the review, and uses explicit methods for appraising the literature based on the quality and validity of individual studies.

- Clinical practice guidelines are systematically developed statements to help clinicians deliver appropriate care in specific clinical circumstances.

REFERENCES

1. Pierson DJ. Translating evidence into practice. *Respir Care.* 2009;54:1386–1401.
2. Hess DR. What is evidence-based medicine and why should I care? *Respir Care.* 2004;49:730–741.
3. Nava S, Hill N. Non-invasive ventilation in acute respiratory failure. *Lancet.* 2009;374:250–259.
4. Dolovich MB, Ahrens RC, Hess DR, et al. Device selection and outcomes of aerosol therapy: evidence-based guidelines—American College of Chest Physicians/American College of Asthma, Allergy, and Immunology. *Chest.* 2005;127:335–371.
5. Guyatt G, Drummond R, Meade M, Cook D. *Users' Guides to the Medical Literature: Essentials of Evidence-Based Clinical Practice.* 2nd ed. New York: McGraw-Hill; 2008.
6. Meade M, Guyatt G, Cook D, et al. Predicting success in weaning from mechanical ventilation. *Chest.* 2001;120:400S–424S.
7. Yang KL, Tobin MJ. A prospective study of indexes predicting the outcome of trials of weaning from mechanical ventilation. *N Engl J Med.* 1991;324:1445–1450.
8. Adhikari NK, Burns KE, Friedrich JO, et al. Effect of nitric oxide on oxygenation and mortality in acute lung injury: systematic review and meta-analysis. *BMJ.* 2007;334:779.
9. The Acute Respiratory Distress Syndrome Network. Ventilation with lower tidal volumes as compared with traditional tidal volumes for acute lung injury and the acute respiratory distress syndrome. *N Engl J Med.* 2000;342:1301–1308.
10. Hess DR. Information retrieval in respiratory care: tips to locate what you need to know. *Respir Care.* 2004;49:389–400.
11. Chatburn RL. How to find the best evidence. *Respir Care.* 2009;54:1360–1365.
12. Callcut RA, Branson RD. How to read a review paper. *Respir Care.* 2009;54:1379–1385.
13. Hess DR. Evidence-based clinical practice guidelines: where's the evidence and what do I do with it? *Respir Care.* 2003;48:838–839.
14. Guyatt GH, Oxman AD, Vist GE, et al. GRADE: an emerging consensus on rating quality of evidence and strength of recommendations. *BMJ.* 2008;336:924–926.
15. Restrepo RD. AARC clinical practice guidelines: from "reference-based" to "evidence-based." *Respir Care.* 2010;55:787–788.

Glossary

A

a wave On the central venous pressure tracing, the a wave is due to the increased atrial pressure during right atrial contraction. It correlates with the P wave on an electrocardiogram.

AARC Code of Ethics Professional policy document of the American Association for Respiratory Care that describes ethical behaviors for respiratory therapists that should guide professional practice.

AARC Times The premier news and feature magazine of the respiratory care profession, which includes management tips, educational articles, human interest features, how-to articles, profiles of leaders in the profession, reports on current government trends, and job opportunities nationwide.

abdominal muscles Muscles in addition to those directly involved in respiration that nevertheless aid in expiration, including the rectus abdominis, external and internal oblique muscles, and the transversus abdominis muscles, which depress the lower ribs, increase intra-abdominal pressure, and flex the thoracic spine.

absorption The incorporation of a substance in one state into another of a different state, such as liquids being absorbed by a solid or gases being absorbed by a liquid.

accessory muscles Muscles outside the principal respiratory muscles that nevertheless affect inspiration, including the pectoralis minor and major (innervated by C5 through C8 and T1), the serratus anterior (innervated by C5 through C7), and the erector spinae, which all help raise ribs, push the sternum forward and upward, and straighten the concavity of the thoracic spine.

accreditation Voluntary process intended to help establish and maintain the standards and expectations for all allied health education programs; although accreditation is voluntary, the National Board for Respiratory Care requires graduation from an accredited educational program for eligibility for its credentialing examinations for individual professionals.

acid Compound that donates or yields a hydrogen ion (H^+) in an aqueous solution; a substance that donates a proton in a proton-transfer reaction.

acid maltase deficiency Type II glycogen storage disease that arises because of a deficiency of the lysosomal enzyme responsible for the hydrolysis of glycogen.

acid-fast bacilli (AFB) Bacteria in which the cell wall, because of the presence of waxes such as mycolic acid, retains red carbolfuchsin stain despite rinsing with hydrochloric acid, making these bacteria acid fast; acid-fast bacteria are considered neither gram positive nor gram negative.

activated partial thromboplastin time (aPTT) Direct way of evaluating overall coagulation status; used to assess the intrinsic clotting pathway, especially the early stages involving factors XII, XI, IX and VIII; often used to monitor patients on heparin therapy.

active cycle of breathing Breathing maneuver that combines breathing control, thoracic expansion control, and forced expiration technique.

active errors Errors that occur at the point of contact between a human and some aspect of a larger system (e.g., a human–machine interface). They are generally readily apparent (e.g., pushing an incorrect button, ignoring a warning light) and almost always involve someone at the front line.

active humidifier Humidification device in which energy (heat) is used to add water to the inspired gas.

acute lung injury (ALI) Respiratory disorder characterized by the abrupt onset of respiratory distress; associated with severe hypoxemia and diffuse pulmonary opacities on chest radiograph that are not caused by congestive heart failure or volume overload; $PaO_2/FIO_2 < 300$ mm Hg.

acute respiratory distress syndrome (ARDS) Respiratory disorder characterized by the abrupt onset of respiratory distress; associated with severe hypoxemia and diffuse pulmonary opacities on chest radiograph that are not caused by congestive heart failure or volume overload; $PaO_2/FIO_2 < 200$ mm Hg.

adaptive pressure control A volume feedback mechanism for pressure-controlled or pressure-supported breaths; the desired tidal volume is set and the ventilator adjusts the inspiratory pressure to deliver the set minimal target tidal volume.

adaptive support ventilation A mode of ventilation in which the ventilator automatically selects tidal volume and frequency for mandatory breaths and the tidal volume for spontaneous breaths on the basis of the respiratory system mechanics and target minute ventilation.

adenocarcinoma Any one of a large group of malignant epithelial cell tumors.

adenosine triphosphate (ATP) High-energy triphosphate that is the main molecule used to store energy; supplies energy directly to the energy-using reactions of all cells in all kinds of living organisms.

adjuvant Substance, especially a drug, added to a prescription to assist in the action of the main ingredient; also, an additional treatment or therapy.

adsorption Ability to hold substances to a surface.

advance directive Document to be used on a patient's behalf, in the absence of competency, specifying what treatments the patient does or does not want in such a case and sometimes, in some states, specifying a surrogate to make decisions in the event that the patient cannot (see *medical power of attorney*).

advanced cardiovascular life support (ACLS) Postarrest treatment after a cardiac arrest; includes (1) maintaining the airway with equipment and advanced techniques, (2) monitoring electrocardiogram and recognizing dysrhythmias, (3) using conventional defibrillators, (4) administering supplemental oxygen and drugs via parenteral or endotracheal routes.

aerobe Free-living organism that requires oxygen for survival.

aerobic Pertaining to the presence of air or oxygen.

aerosol A suspension of solid or liquid particles in a gas.

affective domain The area of learning involved in appreciation, interests, and attitudes. This domain describes the way people react emotionally and their ability to feel another person's pain or joy.

afterload Resistance in the circulation against which the ventricle must eject blood during contraction; the load that opposes myocardial shortening.

air bronchogram Radiographic abnormality in the image of the bronchi occurring when the alveolar airspaces become filled with fluid, causing increased contrast between the air-filled bronchi and adjacent fluid-filled lung parenchyma, rendering the bronchi lucent and projecting them as branching tubular air-filled structures.

air leak syndrome The movement of gas from the lungs into spaces where it is not normally present; includes pneumothorax, pneumomediastinum, pneumopericardium, pneumoperitoneum, pulmonary interstitial emphysema, and subcutaneous emphysema.

air-to-oxygen blender A mechanical device designed to proportion air and oxygen to a specific concentration.

air-to-oxygen mix ratio The proportion of oxygen and air required to produce a specific oxygen concentration.

air trapping Condition in the lung in which air is not exhaled because of decreased lung elasticity and increased expiratory airway resistance; accompanied by hyperinflation.

air-entrainment mask An oxygen delivery device in which air is entrained proportional to oxygen flow for a fixed oxygen concentration delivered to the patient.

airborne precautions Actions used to prevent the transmission of infectious agents over a long distance when they are suspended in the air.

airway cuff An inflatable balloon that surrounds the endotracheal tube (or tracheostomy tube) near its distal end to seal the airway for mechanical ventilation and to minimize aspiration.

airway hyperresponsiveness Marker associated with asthma that is responsive to both specific and nonspecific factors (such as environment, exercise, allergens, and viral infections), whereby the airways constrict too easily and frequently.

airway inflammation Condition that exacerbates asthmatic reactions by the release of mediators, including mast cells, eosinophils, macrophages, epithelial cells, and T lymphocytes, resulting in recurrent exacerbations that manifest as wheezing, progressive shortness of breath, chest tightness, and coughing; may be classified as acute, subacute, or chronic.

airway pressure release ventilation A mode of ventilation that is time cycled and pressure-controlled, with an active exhalation valve that allows the patient to breathe spontaneously throughout the ventilator-imposed pressures; it is often used with a long inspiratory:expiratory timing pattern.

airway resistance (Raw) Pressure difference developed per unit flow as gas flows into or out of the lungs; normally, < 2.4 cm H_2O/L/s at 0.5 L/s. Measurements of Raw can complement other tests evaluating airway responsiveness to bronchial provocation or bronchodilation.

airway stent An endobronchial device designed to maintain patency of the airway in the presence of central airways obstruction due to benign or malignant causes.

alarm event Any condition or occurrence on a ventilator that requires the clinician's awareness or action.

algorithm Specific protocol that provides explicit rules for solving a healthcare problem.

all-patient refined diagnosis-related groups (APR-DRGs) An enhancement of the original diagnostic related groups (DRGs), designed to apply to a population broader than that of Medicare beneficiaries and that include four subclasses to each original DRG to address the severity of illness and the risk of mortality.

allele Either of a pair of alternative forms of a gene.

Allen test Test performed before radial arterial puncture or cannulation to ascertain whether there is adequate ulnar artery perfusion to the hand.

allergen Common triggering mechanism for asthmatic reactions; can be indoor factors (e.g., mold, animal dander, cleaning chemicals, cockroach antigen, dust mites) or outdoor factors (e.g., noxious fumes, grass, tree pollens).

α_1-antitrypsin (AAT) deficiency α_1-Antitrypsin is a plasma protein produced in the liver that inhibits trypsin and other proteolytic enzymes; deficiency is associated with the development of emphysema.

alpha-stat hypothesis A hypothesis that states that the degree of ionization (alpha) of the imidazole groups of intracellular proteins remains constant despite change in temperature.

alveoli Small sacs through which gas exchange takes place between alveolar gas and capillary blood; composed of type I and type II cells.

American Academy of Sleep Medicine (AASM) A professional society dedicated exclusively to the medical subspecialty of sleep medicine that sets standards; it promotes excellence in healthcare, education, and research.

American Association for Respiratory Care (AARC) Primary professional organization for respiratory care. The AARC and related organizations contribute to the scientific basis, governance, stature, and future growth of respiratory care; assist chartered affiliates in their efforts to pursue meaningful, nonrestrictive licensure; and promote the sequential functions of higher education: research, archiving, and dissemination of knowledge.

American Registry of Inhalation Therapists (ARIT) Organization established to oversee the processing and registration of inhalation therapists, and maintenance of the registry; the organization that preceded the American Association for Respiratory Care.

American Respiratory Care Foundation (ARCF) Trusteeship administering awards, education recognition, fellowships, and grants as well as providing financial support of the consensus and special proceedings conferences of the American Association for Respiratory Care (AARC).

American Standard Safety System This system uses a combination of the following factors specific for each gas or gas combination: diameter of the outlet, number of threads per inch, whether the outlet has right-handed or left-handed threads, whether the threads are external or internal, and the shape of the mating nipple on the corresponding regulator.

amino acid Basic protein unit or building block of proteins. The basic structure of an amino acid consists of a carbon atom (called the *alpha carbon*) to which are bonded an amino group (NH_2), a carboxyl group (COOH), a hydrogen atom, and a side chain that constitutes the unique and identifying characteristic of the amino acid.

amplifier Any device that changes (usually increases) the amplitude of a signal. An amplifier multiplies an input signal with a constant, which is usually in the range of 2 to 1000. The amplification factor is referred to as gain and can be expressed as V_{out}/V_{in}.

amyotrophic lateral sclerosis (ALS) Progressive neurodegenerative disorder of both upper and lower motor neurons leading to a loss of skeletal muscle strength, including the respiratory muscles.

anabolism Synthesis process that assembles precursor molecules, such as amino acids, sugars, fatty acids, and nitrogenous bases into cell macromolecules such as proteins, polysaccharides, lipids, and nucleic acids.

anaerobe Free-living organism that requires an absence of oxygen; thought to be a minor cause of community-acquired pneumonia but becomes increasingly important in nosocomial pneumonia and ventilator-associated pneumonia.

anaerobic bacterial pneumonia Pneumonia, usually multimicrobial, caused by anaerobic pathogens such as *Peptostreptococcus* species, *Bacteroides melaninogenicus, Fusobacterium necrophorum, Bacteroides asaccharolyticus, Porphyromonas endodontalis,* and *Porphyromonas gingivalis.*

analysis method Ethics theory that combines key components from teleological and deontological theories, asserting that in the final analysis, most ethical decisions are made by a systematic analytic process devised by the individual.

analytical paradigm Traditional teaching method designed to convey scientific and medical knowledge, derived from research, through the accomplishment of specific, set learning objectives. The instructor retains control over the learning process, from setting objectives to determining evaluation. Learners remain in largely passive roles for a highly structured educational experience that emphasizes the lecture method and competency- or performance-centered course work based on research, expert opinion, and task analysis.

angina Choking, crushing, painful feeling most often associated with cardiac pain caused by hypoxia of the myocardium.

animal studies Use of animals for medical research to establish and study models or simulations of human disease.

anion Negatively charged ion that is attracted to the positive electrode (anode) in electrolysis; negatively charged atom, molecule, or radical.

anion gap Difference between the concentrations of serum cations and anions such that the anion gap = $([Na^+] + [K^+]) - ([HCO_3^-] + Cl^-])$. If the anion gap exceeds 12 mmol/L, excessive unmeasured anions are likely present. Because its concentration is normally low, $[K^+]$ is often omitted from this calculation.

anteroposterior (AP) projection A chest radiographic view in which the x-ray beam passes through the chest from the front to the back.

anthropometry Study of human body measurements and components, including measurement of height, weight, body mass index, midarm muscle circumference, skinfold thicknesses, and skeletal breadths.

antibiotic Chemical substance capable of inhibiting the growth of, or killing, certain microorganisms but generally nontoxic enough to be used chemotherapeutically in the treatment of infectious diseases.

antibiotic resistance The ability of bacteria and fungi to withstand the effects of antibiotics that would normally kill them or limit their growth.

anticholinergic agent Any agent that blocks the parasympathetic nerves; often used as bronchodilators, delivered by inhalation (e.g., ipratropium bromide for chronic obstructive pulmonary disease).

anticholinergic Class of bronchodilators that decrease both bronchial and upper airway secretions. Pertains to a blockade of acetylcholine receptors that results in the inhibition of the transmission of parasympathetic nerve impulses; the drug functions by competing with the neurotransmitter acetylcholine for its receptor sites at synaptic junctions.

anticipating Key skill used in critical thinking; involves the ability to think ahead and envision possible problems; sometimes referred to as "future think."

anticoagulation Use of an agent that prevents or delays coagulation of the blood.

antiemetic Substance or procedure that prevents or alleviates nausea or vomiting.

antigen detection See *antigen detection and polymerase chain reaction (PCR).*

antigen detection and polymerase chain reaction (PCR) Technique that is applied to sputum samples to help in the rapid identification of pathogens that may be difficult to culture or pathogens scarcely growing due to prior antibiotic treatment; can be applied to sputum, serum, urine, and body fluids; most valuable in the diagnosis of difficult-to-culture organisms such as *Mycoplasma pneumoniae, Legionella pneumophila, Chlamydophila pneumoniae,* and viral pneumonias. See also *polymerase chain reaction (PCR).*

antihistamine Drug or substance capable of reducing the physiologic and pharmacologic effects of histamine, including a wide variety of drugs that block histamine receptors.

anti-immunoglobulin E Class of antibody that is a pharmacologic therapy used to treat respiratory disease.

Apgar score A system used to assess heart rate, respiratory effort, muscle tone, reflex irritability, and color in newborns.

apical lordotic A chest radiographic view that provides a good view of the lung apex, lingula, and right middle lobe.

apnea Absence of spontaneous respiration.

apnea of prematurity Category or type of cessation of airflow in a premature infant's breathing; resolution may be determined more by the maturation of the respiratory control center than by an underlying disease process; prevalence is higher at lower gestational ages and may be the result of an immature respiratory control system; manifested by frequent periodic breathing, a decreased ventilatory response to CO_2, and a depression of respiration produced by hypoxemia.

arousal index Value derived from the data gathered during a polysomnogram: the number of arousals divided by the total sleep time, expressed in arousals per hour, which normally should be less than 15.

arousals Sudden changes from sleep to wakefulness or from a deeper stage of non–rapid eye movement (NREM) sleep to a lighter stage, characterized by an abrupt shift in electroencephalographic frequency.

arterial blood gas Blood component whose primary measurements (Po_2, Pco_2, and pH) provide important information about oxygenation, ventilation, and acid–base status.

arterial blood pressure One of the four vital signs; monitoring techniques range from intermittent manual determinations using sphygmomanometry to automated noninvasive devices or an indwelling arterial catheter providing continuous measurement and waveform graphics.

artificial nose Passive humidifier, also known as a *heat and moisture exchanger (HME),* that captures exhaled heat and moisture and transfers part of that heat and humidity to the next inspired breath; can include condensers, hygroscopic condensers, and hygrophobic condensers.

assessment In the patient education context, the systematic and thorough collection of data relevant to the teaching process; the process of documenting, usually in measurable terms, knowledge, skills, attitudes, and beliefs.

assisted ventilation A ventilator's function, occurring whenever airway pressure (i.e., ventilator pressure) rises above baseline during inspiration; thus the breath is said to be assisted, independent of other breath characteristics (i.e., whether the breath is classified as spontaneous or mandatory). Not to be confused with the meaning of the word *assist* in specific names of modes of ventilation (e.g., assist/control mode) sometimes used by ventilator manufacturers for modes without regard to consistency or theoretical relevance.

Association of Asthma Educators (AAE) A professional society that promotes asthma education as an integral component of a comprehensive asthma program to raise the competence of healthcare professionals who educate individuals and families affected by asthma, and to raise the standard of care and quality of asthma education delivered to those with asthma.

asthma Chronic inflammatory disorder of the airways in which many cells and cellular elements play a role, in particular, mast cells, eosinophils, T lymphocytes, macrophages, neutrophils, and epithelial cells; causes recurrent episodes of wheezing, breathlessness, chest tightness, and coughing, particular at night or in the early morning.

asthma education program Plan implemented by clinicians to ensure patient and caregiver compliance, thereby minimizing exacerbations and healthcare costs by providing maximum understanding of current asthma treatment and management.

asthma trigger Any mechanism that can cause asthmatic reactions, including allergens, pollution, food and drug additives, and viral agents.

atelectasis Incomplete expansion of the lung or the collapse of previously expanded lung tissue, a common noninfectious pulmonary complications after surgery; may be due to many factors, including small, monotonous tidal volumes and inadequate lung distending forces, airway obstruction with gas absorption, and reduction in surfactant levels.

atom The smallest portion of an element that retains all the properties of the element.

atomic mass unit Unit for expressing masses of atoms or molecules.

atomic number Number of protons contained inside the nucleus of an atom, determining the actual element.

atomic weight Relative weight of an atom; often used interchangeably with the term *mass number*.

atrioventricular (AV) node Located in the septal wall of the right atrium, the AV node receives impulses from the SA node and transmits them to the AV bundle for eventual symmetric distribution throughout the ventricle.

atrium Chamber of the heart; the left atrium receives blood from the pulmonary veins and delivers it to the left ventricle.

attitudinal orientation The outward expression of an individual's personal belief system. What a person says and how that person behaves, based on what the individual believes.

atypical organisms Strains of unusual type; for example, *Legionella* species, *Mycoplasma pneumoniae, Chlamydia psittaci, Chlamydophila pneumoniae,* and *Coxiella burnetii.*

atypical pneumonia Pneumonia caused by any strain of unusual type (see *atypical organisms*) and characterized by a flulike disease with prodromal symptoms, dry cough, myalgia, malaise, rhinorrhea, and moderate fever; usual pathogens in atypical pneumonia include *Mycoplasma pneumoniae, Chlamydia psittaci, Coxiella burnetii, Chlamydophila pneumoniae,* and respiratory viruses.

auscultation Most commonly used physical assessment technique, involving listening to sounds produced by the body with the aid of a stethoscope placed on bare skin.

authentication (1) Process used to verify that a medical record entry is complete, accurate, and final, including identification of the date and the author. (2) The identification of an individual with the highest degree of confidence; usually provided through trusted third parties and systems that can vouch for the individual's identity even though the individual may not be physically present.

auto-PEEP End-expiratory alveolar pressure that is greater than the pressure at the proximal airway, which results from high airways resistance and a short expiratory time.

auto-positive airway pressure (APAP) A feature on some devices for continuous positive airway pressure (CPAP) that actively monitor one or more airway variables during sleep and respond to upper airway changes by automatically adjusting the pressure.

autogenic drainage Technique that aims to achieve the highest possible airflow in the different generations of bronchi to move secretions.

automated external defibrillator (AED) A portable device capable of diagnosing life-threatening cardiac arrhythmias and using electrical therapy to reestablish an effective rhythm.

automatic resuscitator A device designed to replace the need for manual ventilation.

autonomy Right and ability to govern one's self, particularly in regard to medical treatment and personal and financial care.

B

baby boomers The generation born between 1946 and 1964.

bacilli Rod-shaped bacteria.

backup ventilator In situations in which patients need ventilator support most or all of the hours of the day at home, a primary ventilator is usually provided at the bedside, and a secondary ventilator, the backup ventilator, may be provided, often mounted on the patient's wheelchair. The backup ventilator performs two functions: it facilitates patient mobility and can be used in the event the primary ventilator fails.

bacteria Large group of unicellular, prokaryote microorganisms.

bactericidal A method of killing bacteria.

bag technique Procedure used to minimize the likelihood of cross-contamination as a clinician travels from house to house. Bag technique requires the clinician to remove all needed care supplies from the bag with clean hands and to clean all used items prior to returning them to the bag.

barrel chest Chest configuration in which the individual's anteroposterior chest is equal to the lateral diameter.

basal metabolic rate (BMR) Amount of energy required to maintain the most basic bodily functions, expressed as kilocalories per day and having a fixed relationship with gender, weight, height, and age.

base Solution that yields a hydroxide ion (OH^-) in an aqueous solution; species accepting the proton in a proton-transfer reaction.

basic life support (BLS) Primary patient assessment and treatment procedure to be taken to stabilize the emergency patient, including preliminary actions such as assessing unresponsiveness and conducting the primary ABCD survey.

Beck's triad Three classic symptoms or signs of cardiac tamponade: hypotension, distended neck veins, and distant heart sounds.

Becker muscular dystrophy An X-linked recessive inherited disorder characterized by slowly progressive muscle weakness that primarily affects males.

Beer-Lambert law Law defining the relationship between the concentration of a substance and the amount of light (I) transmitted through it: $I_{out} = I_{in}\ e^{-A}$ and $A = L \times C \times \varepsilon$, where L is the optical path length, C is the concentration of the substance, and ε is the absorption of the particular wavelength used.

behavior modification The use of basic learning techniques, such as conditioning, biofeedback, reinforcement, or aversion therapy, to alter human behavior.

behavioral contracting Teaching technique creating a higher level of learner accountability and responsibility and calling on one's own integrity and autonomy.

benchmarking Process of peer comparison that includes all efforts to determine not the average utilization of a particular diagnosis but the most medically appropriate utilization per diagnosis. This process is foundational to the standardization of healthcare delivery and the maximization of its benefits.

beneficence Charity or mercy toward a patient. This principle imposes on the practitioner the responsibility to seek good for the patient under all circumstances.

benign Noncancerous.

benzodiazepine A class of drugs that possess sedative, hypnotic, anxiolytic, anticonvulsant, muscle relaxant, and amnesic actions, which may useful in critically ill mechanically ventilated patients.

Bernoulli principle First law of fluid dynamics, used in 1738 by David Bernoulli to describe the relationship of fluid flow through a tube and thus to explain the pressure drop when fluid passes through a constriction in a rigid tube by showing how potential energy, kinetic energy, and pressure energy interact.

bias A preference or an inclination that inhibits impartial judgment. Bias may result in an unfair act or policy stemming from prejudice.

bicarbonate buffer system System influenced by the independent and direct effect of P_{CO_2} on $[HCO_3^-]$; made up of two components—hydration of CO_2 into carbonic acid (H_2CO_3) and the dissociation of carbonic acid into HCO_3^- and hydrogen ion.

bilirubinemia The presence of excess bilirubin in the blood.

biofilm Complex aggregation of microorganisms that adhere to each other or to a surface, or both.

Biot respirations Pattern of breathing symptomatic of elevated intracranial pressure and meningitis; characterized by a short burst of uniform, deep respirations followed by a period of apnea lasting 10 to 30 seconds.

bite block Device that is placed between the teeth to prevent the patient from biting an orotracheal airway or the tongue or lips, causing bleeding and trauma to the mouth; also used during bronchoscopy.

bland aerosol therapy Humidification therapy using inspired gas consisting of water, saline solution, or other substances without important pharmacologic action; used primarily to humidify, liquefy, or otherwise change the character of thick secretions.

Bland-Altman plot A method of displaying the level of agreement between two measurement methods.

blinding Research technique for ensuring that the investigators or the participants or both are as unaware as possible of the treatment being studied to avoid any tendency to prefer a specific outcome (bias).

blood urea nitrogen (BUN) Most common nonprotein nitrogenous compound in the blood; measurement used to assess renal function in the adult. Normal values for BUN are between 7 and 21 mg/dL.

blunt trauma Any traumatic injury that occurs due to a force that does not penetrate the body of the patient. Common mechanisms of blunt trauma include motor vehicle crashes, falls, and being struck by an automobile.

blunted costophrenic angle A finding on chest x-ray consistent with pleural effusion.

Board of Directors (BOD) One of several governance and advisory entities of the American Association for Respiratory Care, composed of an executive committee consisting of the president, president-elect, immediate past president, vice president, treasurer, secretary, immediate past speaker of the House of Delegates, and chairperson of the Board of Medical Advisors.

Board of Medical Advisors One of several governance and advisory entities of the American Association for Respiratory Care (AARC); consists of four AARC sponsoring professional medical societies that provide significant input concerning the art and science of the profession of respiratory care.

Board of Registered Polysomnographic Technologists (BRPT) An independent, nonprofit certification board that oversees a program of competency-based testing for sleep technicians and technologists.

body plethysmography Diagnostic tool that is used to achieve measurements of airway resistance (Raw), airway conductance (Gaw), and static lung volumes, based on Boyle's law. In practice, the patient is placed inside a fixed-volume, air-sealed body box in which the effects of excursion of the chest wall can be measured by small pressure changes in the box and airway.

Bohr effect The relationship between hydrogen ion concentration and hemoglobin affinity for oxygen. An increase in hydrogen ion concentration decreases the affinity of hemoglobin for oxygen.

boiling point Temperature required to raise the vapor pressure of a solution to atmospheric pressure; a colligative property of a solution.

Borg Scale of Perceived Exertion Numeric scale for assessing dyspnea, from 0 (representing no dyspnea) to 10 (maximal dyspnea).

botulism Rare disorder caused by toxin produced by *Clostridium botulinum*, often ingested via improperly cooked food, wound contamination by the organisms, or absorption of the toxin from the gastrointestinal tract, particularly in infants; GI symptoms predominate initially, followed by neurologic impairment.

Bourdon gauge flow meter Flow control device with a fixed outlet orifice that allows an adjustable inlet pressure.

Boyle's law Observation credited to Robert Boyle, early in the 18th century, that predicts the relation of a volume of a fixed mass of gas to a pressure change; in short, with temperature constant, volume is inversely related to pressure.

brachytherapy Radiotherapy treatment that involves applying an ionizing radiation source near the body area being treated; in respiratory treatment, this usually entails the endobronchial placement of encapsulated radionuclide in close proximity to an endobronchial malignancy.

bradypnea Slow respiratory rate.

brain natriuretic peptide (BNP) Also known as B-type natriuretic peptide; a polypeptide secreted by the ventricles of the heart in response to excessive stretching of heart muscle cells.

breathing retraining A component of pulmonary rehabilitation, consisting of pursedlip breathing and diaphragmatic breathing.

bronchi Larger air passages of the lungs.

bronchial artery embolization (BAE) Method used to occlude or restrict blood flow within the bronchial artery; the therapy of choice when bleeding is from the bronchiectatic airways.

bronchial breath sounds Auscultation sounds normally heard over the trachea, at the manubrium anteriorly and between the scapulae posteriorly; heard over the periphery of the lungs, this suggests consolidation of lung tissue.

bronchial challenge testing Use of either methacholine or histamine to measure responsiveness to general stimuli, usually administered in a pulmonary function lab and followed (usually within 15 minutes) with a short-acting β-agonist that results in a 12% to 15% increase in a patient's forced expiratory volume in 1 second (FEV_1).

bronchiolitis Inflammation of the bronchioles caused by infection.

bronchiolitis obliterans with organizing pneumonia (BOOP) Acute interstitial lung disease that appears to be a response of the lung to a variety of injuries affecting the smaller airways and alveoli as a unit, including infections, exposures to toxic gases, radiation therapy, drug toxicity, eosinophilic pneumonia, Wegener granulomatosis, and hypersensitivity pneumonitis.

bronchoalveolar lavage (BAL) Procedure for collecting an alveolar specimen by use of a bronchoscope or other hollow tube through which saline is instilled into distal bronchi and then withdrawn; also used to describe the specimen thus obtained.

bronchogenic carcinoma A malignant lung tumor that originates in the bronchi.

bronchophony Auscultation sound typical in consolidation of lung tissue, meaning that the normally aerated tissue has been filled with fluid, mucus, pus, or cellular debris; in bronchophony, the patient's repetition of "99" becomes easily audible, as opposed to its normal muffling.

bronchopulmonary dysplasia Chronic iatrogenic lung disease caused by oxygen toxicity and barotrauma resulting from positive pressure ventilation; incidence is greater in premature infants, perhaps related to the increased requirement for oxygen therapy and mechanical ventilation in this patient population.

bronchoscopic brushing A technique in which a brush is introduced into the airway via a bronchoscope to collect cells or microorganisms for diagnostic purposes.

bronchoscopic washing Technique designed to sample the airway, rather than the alveolar space, particularly in cytologic sampling when a patient has an exophytic lesion obstructing a lobar or segmental orifice.

bronchoscopy Examination using a bronchoscope that enables inspection of the interior of the tracheobronchial tree, and related diagnostic and therapeutic maneuvers, including taking specimens for culture, biopsy, and removal of foreign bodies.

bubble humidifier System in which dry gas is directed toward the bottom of a water-filled reservoir, where the stream of gas is broken into bubbles that gain humidity as they rise through the water.

bubonic plague This term is often used synonymously for the plague caused by the bacteria Yersinia pestis, commonly transmitted from the bite of an infected flea.

buffer Substances that maintain a relatively constant pH level when strong acids or strong bases are added.

bullae Airspace enlargements greater than 1 cm; can progressively enlarge and compress adjacent lung tissue, impairing respiratory function.

bullectomy Removal of giant bullae (airspace enlargements that occupy one-third of a hemithorax), a reversible cause of pulmonary decompensation, particularly in patients with emphysema.

bundled charges A single comprehensive group of related charges. Payments for bundled charges have become the norm in recent years, and unbundled services are investigated closely by the Health Care Financing Administration (HCFA) and other payers for evidence of fraud.

C

C-reactive protein (CRP) A protein found in the blood, the levels of which rise in response to inflammation.

CABD survey Primary patient assessment and treatment steps to be taken in emergency or resuscitation situations, including **c**irculation, **a**irway, **b**reathing, and **d**efibrillation, focusing on basic CPR and defibrillation.

calcium channel blocker Drug that inhibits the flow of calcium ions across smooth muscle cell membranes, thus relaxing smooth muscles and reducing muscle spasm risk.

capacity The measureable capability of a patient to make an informed decision that accepts, changes, or withholds therapy, treatment, or medical care.

capitation Prepaid and fixed amount that is negotiated in advance by the payer or plan and the provider; involves payment for each person for a particular period of time regardless of the care or services provided.

capnogram Assessment of gas at the proximal airway that plots CO_2 on the vertical axis and time or volume on the horizontal axis.

capnography Noninvasive technique that measures carbon dioxide levels in inspired and expired gas and displays a capnogram.

capnometry Numeric display of CO_2 measurements taken from the proximal airway.

carbogen Oxygen–carbon dioxide mixture, usually consisting of 90% O_2 and 10% CO_2 or 95% O_2 and 5% CO_2.

carbohydrate Organic compound containing the elements carbon, hydrogen, and oxygen.

carbon dioxide (CO_2) A gas that is an end product of metabolism and cannot support life.

carbon dioxide production The amount of CO_2 produced by the tissues and excreted by the lungs each minute; normally about 200 mL/min in adults.

carbonic acid (H_2CO_3) Product of the hydration of carbon dioxide (CO_2) that ionizes to H^+ and bicarbonate; carbonic acid then forms bicarbonate.

carboxyhemoglobin (COHb) Compound produced by exposing hemoglobin to carbon monoxide, usually inhaled into the lungs and subsequently bound to hemoglobin in the blood, blocking the sites for oxygen transport.

cardiac arrhythmia A condition in which the heart beat may be too fast or too slow, and may be regular or irregular.

cardiac catheterization Invasive means to quantify valvular stenosis and regurgitation and assess coronary artery blood flow.

cardiac enzymes Group of enzymes that are released from myocardial tissue and appear in the serum during myocardial injury (usually ischemia).

cardiac failure A complex clinical syndrome that can result from any structural or functional cardiac disorder that impairs the ventricle from filling with or ejecting blood.

cardiac output ($\dot{Q}c$) Volume of blood expelled by the heart's ventricles, equal to the amount of blood ejected at each beat multiplied by the heart rate (in beats per minute).

cardiac tamponade Life-threatening complication of penetrating wounds to the heart, most often characterized by Beck's triad (distention of neck veins, muffled heart sounds, and hypotension) and often by elevated central venous pressure; compression of the heart by fluid or blood within the pericardial space. This increase in pressure generated by an increase in fluid volume may prevent blood return to the heart.

cardiomyocytes Muscle cells that make up the heart.

cardiomyopathy Any disease that affects the heart's structure and function.

cardiopulmonary exercise testing (CPET) A relatively noninvasive test that measures respiratory gas exchange (oxygen uptake and carbon dioxide output, minute ventilation, and anaerobic threshold), electrocardiography, blood pressure, and pulse oximetry during maximal exercise tolerance.

cardiopulmonary resuscitation (CPR) A formalized approach to maintain blood flow of individuals who have had a sudden cessation of heartbeat or respiration to delay or prevent death due to lack of oxygen for cellular function.

care management Umbrella term referring to the coordination of patient interventions, comprising many loosely related terms: component management, demand management, case management, and disease management.

case control studies Studies that involve, initially, the accumulation of a number of cases that are then matched as much as possible with those that do not have that condition so that both the cases and noncases (controls) can be studied for differences that may account for why the cases contracted the disease.

case management Collaborative process that assesses, plans, implements, coordinates, monitors, and evaluates the options and services required to meet an individual's health needs, using communication and available resources to promote quality, cost, and effective outcomes.

case manager Works with people to help improve their quality of life through effective education, coordination and utilization of healthcare services, which can reduce costs and improve outcomes.

case mix Relatively new form of reimbursement that refers to the overall intensity of conditions requiring medical and nursing intervention. It involves extensive assessment of the patient's condition followed by a determination of specific services or procedures considered necessary or essential to manage the patient effectively.

case report Detailed, observational report of an unusual, interesting case. Case reports are observational and can be reported easily.

The disease described in the case may be rare, the treatment may be unusual, or there may be specific instructional points.

case series Several case reports presented over time.

catabolism Process of releasing chemical energy from food molecules in a decomposition process involving the oxidation of nutrient molecules, releasing energy (exergonic metabolism) in two forms, as either heat or as chemical energy.

cation Positively charged ion; one of the most common serum electrolytes.

cell-mediated immunity Primary component of the immune system involving lymphocytes; adversely affected by protein-calorie malnutrition.

Centers for Medicare and Medicaid Services (CMS) Previously known as the Health Care Financing Administration (HCFA); branch of the U.S. Department of Health and Human Services that administers the Medicare and Medicaid programs.

central apnea Loss of diaphragmatic and other respiratory muscle function, resulting in the cessation of respiratory effort; stemming from central nervous system.

central venous pressure (CVP) Pressure measured in the superior vena cava or right atrium and used to estimate intravascular volume status.

cepacia syndrome Rapid clinical decline characterized by fever and frank sepsis at some point after initial infection by *Burkholderia cepacia*. The precise pathogen and host factor(s) that trigger this dramatic decompensation are unknown.

certification Verification from a professional organization that a person is able to competently complete a job or task, usually by the passing of an examination.

channel A course or pathway through which information is transmitted.

channels of Lambert Anatomic connections between alveoli and adjacent terminal bronchioles that allow collateral ventilation (along with the pores of Kohn).

Charles's law Principle that predicts the effect of temperature on a fixed amount of dry gas, such that, at constant pressure, gas expands proportionally to changes in temperature, thus describing, at least at a qualitative level, the effect of kinetic energy on volume; in short, with pressure constant, volume and temperature vary directly.

chemical agent Any chemical power, active principle, or substance that can produce an effect in the body by interacting with various body substances.

chemotherapy Treatment of cancer, infections, and other diseases with chemical agents.

chest compressions The rhythmic application of pressure on the lower half of the sternum to facilitate blood flow by compressing the heart during CPR.

chest physiotherapy (CPT) Technique used to help remove mucus and fluid from the lungs. Conventional CPT consists of postural drainage, percussion, and vibration.

chest radiograph An image produced by x-ray beams passing through the thorax.

Cheyne-Stokes breathing Breathing consisting of a repeating pattern in which the rate and depth of breathing increases to a peak, followed by a decrease in the rate and depth of breathing, followed by a period of apnea.

cholesterol Steroid lipid that combines with phospholipids in the cell membrane to help stabilize its bilayer structure; also used by the body as a starting point in making steroid hormones such as estrogen, testosterone, and cortisol.

chromosome A strand of DNA in the cell nucleus that carries the genes.

chronic bronchitis Type of chronic obstructive pulmonary disease (COPD) defined by the presence of cough and sputum production for 3 or more months in 2 successive years in patients who do not have other causes of cough.

chronic lung disease Any lung disease that progressively damages lung tissue and airways over a period of years, ultimately resulting in a depletion of ventilatory reserves.

chronic obstructive pulmonary disease (COPD) Progressive, irreversible condition characterized by dyspnea and difficulty exhaling, and sometimes including chronic cough.

citric acid (Krebs) cycle Aerobic process in stage 3 catabolism that converts two pyruvic acid molecules into six carbon dioxide molecules and six water molecules, taking place within the mitochondria of the cell.

clarification A therapeutic active listening strategy designed to aid in understanding the message of the client by asking for more information or for elaboration on the client's point.

Clark electrode Po_2 electrode, consisting of a platinum cathode and a silver anode immersed in a dilute, buffered potassium chloride solution; measures Po_2 using the principle of polarography.

cleaning Removal of visible soil from surfaces of equipment.

client education The use of the educational process for individuals who are partners in the health education effort.

Clinical Laboratory Improvement Amendment (CLIA) Federal law regulating general aspects of laboratory quality control.

clinical practice guideline (CPG) Statement to assist clinicians with appropriate healthcare for specific clinical circumstances developed by professional associations and related clinical groups.

clinical respiratory services A term used by some accrediting agencies to describe the services provided by a respiratory care practitioner or respiratory therapist, usually within the patient's home.

closed-ended questions Questions that can be answered with yes, no, or other one-word answers.

closed-loop control Means of mechanical system control in which information about output is used to modify input, which in turn improves the output; also called feedback control or servo control.

clubbing Enlargement of the distal phalanges, particularly the fingers.

CO oximetry Means for measuring carboxyhemoglobin levels in inhalation injury. CO oximetry is also the standard technique used to measure hemoglobin oxygen saturation and methemoglobin.

cocci Spherical bacteria.

Cochrane Library Database of controlled trials, systematic reviews of the effects of care, and critical assessments of effectiveness.

cognitive domain The area of learning involved in knowledge, comprehension, and critical thinking.

cohort study Study that attempts to definitively answer an important question about the cause, treatment, or prevention of disease by enrolling a large number of participants and following them over time so that the study participants are measured, tested, or treated and followed up for years.

collagen vascular disease Any of a group of diseases that can present with interstitial lung disease, including progressive systemic sclerosis, systemic lupus erythematosus, polymyositis and dermatomyositis, Sjögren syndrome, and mixed connective tissue disease; clinical presentation and histopathologic features are comparable to that of idiopathic pulmonary fibrosis with additional features of lymphoid hyperplasia, cellular interstitial pneumonitis, lymphoid interstitial pneumonitis, diffuse alveolar damage, and bronchiolitis obliterans with organizing pneumonitis.

colligative property Property of a solution that depends on the number of solute particles dissolved and not on chemical properties.

colloid Liquid mixture that consists of tiny particles suspended in a liquid.

Comfort Measures Only (CMO) Measures taken when a cure or prolongation of life is no longer a reachable goal and the quality of the patient's life is at a level not acceptable to the patient, so that comfort becomes the priority.

Commission on Accreditation for Respiratory Care (CoARC) Constituency group that makes the final accreditation decisions for respiratory therapy educational programs.

communicating The ability to interact with others orally and in writing to give, receive, and confirm information and feelings.

communication An interpersonal activity involving the transmission of messages by a source to a receiver for the purpose of influencing the receiver's behavior; a complex composite of verbal and nonverbal behaviors integrated for the purpose of sharing information.

community-acquired pneumonia (CAP) Pneumonia acquired outside the hospital.

complex sleep apnea syndrome Sleep apnea that displays both obstructive and central characteristics.

compliance Lung characteristic that, with resistance, serves as a determinant in the mechanics of airflow in and out of the lungs; the ratio of volume change and pressure change.

component management Method of controlling healthcare costs that focuses on limiting the use of resources or services such as therapeutic procedures, diagnostic tests, medications, or hospital lengths of stay.

compound A substance formed by the reaction of two or more chemical elements

compound questions Questions that ask several points, ideas, or issues simultaneously and might require different answers.

Compressed Gas Association (CGA) Industry technical trade organization that has developed numerous safety standards involving cylinders, fittings, and connections.

compressed gas system Oxygen stored in a high-pressure cylinder, usually at 2000 to 3000 pounds per square inch; gas is regulated to the patient through a pressure-reducing valve with a flow metering device

compressible volume The volume of gas compressed in the ventilator circuit and thus not delivered to the patient.

computed tomographic angiography (CTA) A technique used to examine the pulmonary arteries to detect pulmonary embolism.

computed tomography (CT) Radiographic technique that produces a film representing detailed cross sections of tissue using an array of detectors in a variety of angles and a collimated beam of x-rays that rotates in a continuous 360-degree motion around the patient to create cross-sectional images.

concentrated Solution that contains a large amount of solute relative to the amount that could dissolve.

conchae Three curled bony plates or turbinates that project downward from the walls of the nasal cavity and greatly enlarge the surface area of the nose, move mucus toward the nasopharynx, and warm and humidify incoming air.

confidentiality The legally protected right afforded to (and duty required of) specifically designated healthcare professionals not to disclose information discerned or communicated during consultation with a patient, except in cases of suspected abuse, commission of a crime, or threat of harm to self or others.

confrontation Coming face to face with someone; in a counseling context, entails telling a person about inconsistencies that he or she may not yet have spotted.

congenital diaphragmatic hernia Condition associated with a left posterolateral diaphragmatic defect and the failure of closure of the pleuroperitoneal canal early in gestation (5th to 10th week of fetal life), resulting in compression of the developing lung by abdominal organs.

conscious sedation Use of sedative medications by properly trained healthcare providers to enhance relaxation while maintaining adequate spontaneous respiratory efforts by the patient during an invasive procedure.

consolidation A condition in which alveoli become filled with fluid, infection and inflammatory exudate, as with pneumonia.

consumer education The use of the educational process by an individual or group of individuals who are independent decision makers.

contact precautions Used to prevent transmission of infectious agents that are spread by direct or indirect contact with a patient or the patient's environment.

continuous mandatory ventilation (CMV) System for delivering a set tidal volume (or pressure) and a minimum respiratory rate in which the patient can trigger additional breaths above the minimal rate, but the set volume or pressure is constant at the preset level.

continuous positive airway pressure (CPAP) A ventilation method by which a constant pressure greater than atmospheric pressure is applied to the airway through the respiratory cycle.

continuous variable A variable for which any value within a range is possible; that is, there are no clear cut breaks between values.

continuous-flow oxygen (CFO) The traditional method of oxygen delivery in which oxygen is metered to the patient continuously via a delivery system. The amount of oxygen a patient receives is determined by the flow rate and patient inspiratory time.

contractility Feature of muscle tissue, especially cardiac muscle, that allows it to contract by shortening the sarcomeres.

control circuit Drive mechanism in a ventilator that transmits or transforms energy in a predetermined manner to assist or replace the patient's muscles in performing the work of breathing.

control variable Factors that determine what controls breath delivery from a ventilator, such as pressure, volume, flow, and sometimes inspiratory and expiratory times.

controller medication Any of a number of pharmacologic interventions whose goal is to maintain normal (or near normal) lung function, including inhaled corticosteroids, nonsteroidal antiinflammatory agents, long-acting β-agonists, methylxanthines, and leukotriene modifiers.

controls Study participants who do not receive the new treatment being studied but receive instead the usual treatment, a placebo, or sham treatment.

copayment Limited fee paid by enrollees of managed care organizations for each physician visit, prescription, or other service stipulated in the plan.

cor pulmonale Hypertrophy and dilatation of the right ventricle.

coronary angiography Direct imaging of the coronary arteries using cardiac catheterization and subsequent injection of contrast dye; can identify atherosclerotic lesions as well as coronary anomalies, areas of spasm, and acute thrombi.

coronary artery Vessels that provide blood supply to the heart muscle.

coronary artery bypass surgery Surgical procedure that can improve myocardial function by reducing ischemia after restoration of normal blood flow. An area of obstruction in a coronary artery is bypassed.

coronary sinus Veins that drain deoxygenated blood from the myocardium into the right atrium.

correlation coefficient Statistical parameter used to measure the strength of the relationship between two variables.

corticosteroid Major class of antiinflammatory drug that generally produces two types of effect: the *glucocorticoid effect*, which reduces inflammation, increases blood glucose, and generally induces a catabolic state; and the *mineralocorticoid effect*, which is active primarily at the kidney, promoting sodium conservation.

cough etiquette The procedure whereby one covers the nose and mouth when coughing/sneezing, uses tissues to contain respiratory secretions and disposes of them in the nearest receptacle after use, and performs hand hygiene after having contact with respiratory secretions or contaminated objects

covalent bond Stable atomic configuration accomplished when each of the two bonding atoms shares one of its valance electrons.

crackles Fine, high-pitched, discontinuous sounds heard during auscultation of the lungs.

creatinine Substance formed from creatine metabolism and measured in blood and urine as an indicator of kidney function; creatinine levels are a function of skeletal muscle breakdown, and most creatinine is filtered in the glomeruli with little reabsorption.

credentialing Formal identification of professionals who meet predetermined standards of professional skill or competence; can include both licensure and certification.

credentials An attestation of qualification, competence, or authority issued to an individual by a third party with relevant or assumed competence. Examples of credentials include diplomas, academic degrees, certifications, security clearances, and powers of attorney.

crenation Process in which water leaves a cell, causing it to shrivel, as a result of greater osmotic pressure outside that cell.

cricothyrotomy Incision into the larynx between the cricoid and thyroid cartilages, usually done emergently when no other airway access is available.

critical care ventilator Full-featured ventilators designed for use with critically ill patients in respiratory failure.

critical illness polyneuromyopathy Disease affecting several areas of the peripheral nervous system at once; diagnosis is confirmed by electromyographic studies, showing primary axonal polyneuropathy rather than demyelination as suggested by the reduction in the amplitude of the compound action potential without significant prolongation of the conduction latency period; may be caused by hyperglycemia causing nerve ischemia by endovascular shunting or nerve toxins generated from multiple organ failure.

critical pathway (CP) Description of the probable sequence of events during a patient's course of healthcare; outlines all the tests, procedures, treatments, and teaching services that patients may use during a length of stay.

critical thinking Merges the principles of logical reasoning, problem solving, and reflection, although there is no single agreed-upon definition.

crossover study Research studies in which each patient is randomized to either a treatment or control group and, after measurements are made, each patient is then restudied in the other group (control or treatment).

cryptography Type of technical control process for information security that involves writing the information in a code.

cuirass Type of body ventilator that consists of a lightweight rigid dome that fits over the anterior chest wall and connects to a negative pressure generator; also called a chest shell or turtle shell.

culture In context of microbiology, a method of multiplying microorganisms by letting them reproduce in predetermined culture media under controlled laboratory conditions.

culture of safety A term referring to a commitment to safety that permeates all levels of an organization, from frontline personnel to executive management.

cyanosis Bluish hue to the skin that suggests hemoglobin is poorly saturated with oxygen.

cycle In respiration, an inspiration followed by an expiration; period of time between the beginning of one breath and the beginning of the next.

cycle time Ventilatory period; the reciprocal of ventilatory frequency (that is, 60 seconds per minute divided by the number of breaths per minute).

cystic fibrosis Disorder that is inherited in an autosomal recessive pattern and affects the exocrine glands, resulting in abnormally thick secretions of mucus.

cystic fibrosis transmembrane conductance regulator (CFTR) The gene responsible for cystic fibrosis.

cystic fibrosis–related diabetes (CFRD) Type of diabetes associated with cystic fibrosis and characterized by insidious onset, failure to gain or maintain weight despite nutritional intervention, poor growth, or an unexplained chronic decline in pulmonary function.

cytokines Small proteins that are secreted by cells and carry signals between cells.

D

Dalton's law Principle of partial pressures that describes the behavior of physical mixtures of gases and vapors such that each separate gas acts as predicted by the combined gas law, as if it were present alone; in such a mixture, the partial pressure of each particular gas is proportional to the fractional concentration of that gas and equal to the product of fraction concentration and total atmospheric pressure.

dead space The part of the tidal volume that does not participate in gas exchange; ventilation without perfusion.

decannulation The removal of a tracheostomy tube.

decision making The ability to reach a conclusion and make up one's mind using evidence and various techniques, including problem solving.

decoding The activity of making clear or converting information from one format into another.

deep sulcus sign Distinctive radiographic appearance of a pneumothorax in patients in the supine position, with free air in the pleural space rising to the highest portion of the thorax, usually the anterior costophrenic sulcus, and projecting over the upper abdomen and diaphragm.

deep vein thrombosis (DVT) Blood clotting in the legs and pelvis, which usually occurs as a result of venostasis; common in surgical patients and with other causes of immobility, damage to the endothelial wall of the blood vessels, and hypercoagulability states.

defibrillation Use of an electrical current passed through the heart in an attempt to eliminate the chaotic asynchronous activity of ventricular fibrillation by depolarizing cardiac cells and repolarizing them in a uniform manner with resumption of coordinated cardiac contraction; indicated for ventricular fibrillation, pulseless ventricular tachycardia, and asystole (with the possibility that the rhythm is actually fine ventricular fibrillation).

delta waves Electroencephalographic activity with a frequency less than 4 Hz. Conventionally, in sleep stage scoring, the minimum criteria for scoring delta waves are 75-μV (peak-to-peak) amplitude, and 0.5-second duration (2 Hz).

demand delivery device A system of oxygen delivery that responds to the patient's inspiratory effort and cycles off on the expiratory signal. Some demand systems (hybrid) provide a higher flow of oxygen initially yet return to a set base flow during the inspiratory cycle.

demand management Any organized effort or program designed to guide healthcare consumers into the most appropriate level of healthcare service by involving them in their own care.

density Mass per unit volume.

deontological theory Ethical theory based on duty, asserting that an act is either right or wrong based on its intrinsic character rather than consequences.

deoxyribonucleic acid (DNA) Nucleic acid in which the sugar component is deoxyribose; largest molecule in the body, composed of two long polynucleotide chains running parallel to each other; carries the genetic information necessary for synthesis of proteins specific for a given species.

Department of Transportation (DOT) Government agency that regulates cylinder manufacture and the testing and the transporting of hazardous materials, including compressed gases and cryogenic liquids.

descriptive statistics Data or raw information obtained from conducting a study whose results are often presented more clearly and efficiently in tables, graphs, or figures.

diabetic ketoacidosis Buildup of ketones in the blood due to the breakdown of stored fats for energy; a potentially life-threatening complication in patients with diabetes mellitus.

diagnosis-related groups (DRGs) Form of hospital reimbursement based on a patient classification system consisting of approximately 500 different groups, all entailing a predetermined amount of reimbursement. DRGs establish a rate based on bundled services for a particular diagnosis established at the time of admission. The provider receives this amount regardless of the medical care provided.

diagnostic bronchoscopy A procedure involving the direct observation of the airways using a bronchoscope to elucidate the cause of a pulmonary abnormality.

diagnostics A function that incorporates aspects of assessment and testing that include (1) blood gas analysis; (2) nutritional, cardiac, pulmonary, exercise, and sleep assessments; (3) chest radiology; (4) bronchoscopy; (5) pulmonary function testing; and (6) hemodynamics and gas exchange monitoring.

dialogue A conversation between two or more persons; an exchange of ideas or opinions with a view to reaching an amicable agreement or settlement.

Diameter Index Safety System (DISS) One of three indexed safety systems for medical gas distribution station outlets. In this system, a female nut and nipple is manually tightened onto the outlet until contact is made with the plunger, moving it forward until it seats on the stem, thus allowing gas to flow from the piping system.

diaphragm Membranous muscle separating the abdomen and thorax and serving as a major inspiratory muscle.

diaphragmatic pacing Use of a radio frequency transmitter and an antenna that discharges signals to a surgically implanted receiver to transmit electrical impulses to a surgically implanted electrode placed over the phrenic nerve to ensure stimulation of all phrenic nerve roots.

diastole Part of the cardiac cycle that consists of a period of relaxation during which venous blood returns to the heart.

diastolic Pertaining to the diastole; the nadir of a blood pressure measurement.

diastolic dysfunction Impaired ventricular filling, recognized increasingly as a cause of congestive heart failure symptoms.

diet-induced thermogenesis An increase in metabolic rate of 10% to 15% that occurs after eating as a result of the energy cost of digesting and storing nutrients.

diffusing capacity Number of milliliters of gas that transfer from the lungs across the alveolocapillary membrane into the bloodstream each minute, for each 1 mm Hg difference in the pressure across the membrane.

diffusion defect A deficiency in the ability of gases to cross the alveolocapillary membrane.

dilute Relative concentration or strength of a solution indicating that it contains a small amount of solute.

disaster management plan A predetermined plan for responding to disaster.

disease management Approach to patient care that emphasizes coordinated, comprehensive care along the continuum of disease and across healthcare delivery systems.

disinfection A process that eliminates pathogenic microorganisms except bacterial spores.

distal intestinal obstruction syndrome Blockage of the intestines by thickened stool that occurs in individuals with cystic fibrosis.

diuretic Drug used to stimulate urine production.

Do Not Intubate (DNI) Clearly written orders in the advanced directive that stipulate that no intratracheal, endotracheal, or tracheostomy tube be used during a resuscitation.

Do Not Resuscitate (DNR) An advanced directive order that states that if the patient's heart stops beating or he or she stops breathing, he or she should not receive cardiopulmonary resuscitation, no effort to institute an airway, no assisted breathing, and no chest compressions.

documentation Recording or charting individual patient education, including date and time of intervention, subject matter or content addressed, method of instruction, and response of learner or results of the learning.

Doppler echocardiography Echocardiography that uses ultrasound to detect the velocity of blood.

DRG See *diagnosis-related group.*

droplet precautions Used to prevent transmission of pathogens spread through close respiratory or mucous membrane contact with respiratory secretions.

dry powder inhaler (DPI) Device that creates aerosols by drawing air through a dose of powdered medication. DPIs produce aerosols in which most of the drug particles are in the respirable range.

Duchenne muscular dystrophy Hereditary familial muscle disease transmitted via an X-linked recessive gene, although about one-third of cases may be caused by spontaneous mutation; early presenting symptoms are gait disturbances and delayed motor development, as well as limb-girdle muscle weakness and pseudohypertrophy of the calf muscles.

durable medical equipment (DME) companies Companies that provide products to aid in the care of the patient at home, including, but not limited to, mobility aides (wheelchairs, walkers, electric or semielectric hospital beds); respiratory equipment (apnea monitors, bilevel and continuous positive airway pressure devices, home oxygen therapy, mechanical ventilators); enteral products (pumps and enteral formula); and wound and skin care products (lymphedema pumps, special seating and mattresses).

durable medical power of attorney Document that names an individual or agent who can make decisions specifically related to healthcare for another individual.

dynamic airway compression Condition occurring as a result of decreased lung elasticity and leading to increased expiratory airway resistance, which ultimately results in air trapping and hyperinflation.

dynamic hyperinflation An increase in lung volume secondary to air trapping.

dyspnea Shortness of breath or breathlessness; distressing feeling of inability to breathe or great effort required to breathe.

E

echocardiography Diagnostic and assessment tool using ultrasound to examine the heart structures and function by transmission of high-frequency ultrasound waves through the chest and calibrating the velocity of sound waves in the medium under examination.

EEG rhythms See *electroencephalographic rhythms.*

egophony Auscultation sound typical in consolidation of lung tissue, meaning that the normally aerated tissue has been filled with fluid, mucus, pus, or cellular debris; in egophony, *e* sounds like *a*.

eicosanoids Naturally occurring substances derived from 20-carbon polyunsaturated fatty acids; they include the prostaglandins, thromboxanes, leukotrienes, and epoxyeicosatrienoic acids and function as hormones.

ejection fraction Percentage of blood pumped from the ventricle during a single cardiac contraction; normal left ventricular ejection fraction is greater than 50%.

elastance Ratio of pressure change to volume change (i.e., the reciprocal of compliance).

elastic recoil The tendency of a structure to return to its resting position after it is stretched.

electrical impedance tomography (EIT) A medical imaging technique in which an image of a part of the body is inferred from surface electrical measurements. Conducting electrodes are attached to the skin, and small alternating currents are applied to the electrodes. The resulting electrical potentials are measured, and the process may be repeated for numerous different configurations of applied current.

electrically powered portable ventilator A portable ventilator that requires a battery or external power source for operation; a pneumatic gas source may not be required.

electrocardiography (ECG) A test for the evaluation of the electrical activity of the heart.

electroencephalogram (EEG) Recording through the scalp of electrical potentials (activity) from the brain and the changes in these potentials.

electroencephalographic rhythms Combined waveforms that are generally classified according to their frequency, amplitude, and shape, as well as the sites on the scalp at which they are recorded. The most familiar classification uses EEG waveform frequency divided into rhythms such as beta, alpha, theta, delta, and mu.

electrolytes Any substance containing free ions that make the substance electrically conductive.

electromyogram (EMG) Recording of electrical activity from the muscular system.

electron Particle with a negative charge (–1) located outside the nucleus of an atom.

electron transport system Movement of high-energy electrons (removed during glycolysis and the tricarboxylic acid cycle in the form of reduced FAD and NAD) down a chain of carrier molecules imbedded in the inner membrane of the mitochondria, resulting in the production of some 90% of the adenosine triphosphate (ATP) formed during carbohydrate catabolism.

electronic health record (EHR) An individual patient's medical record in digital format. Electronic health record systems coordinate the storage and retrieval of individual records with the aid of computers. See also *electronic medical record (EMR)*.

electronic medical record (EMR) A medical record in digital format. In health informatics, an EMR is considered by some to be one of several types of electronic health records (EHRs), but in general usage *EMR* and *EHR* are synonymous.

electronic signature Unique code or password that verifies the individual creating the entry and creates an individual signature on the record, then stores it on magnetic, optical, or some other computer storage media. A legally recognized electronic means that indicates that a person adopts the contents of an electronic message.

electrooculogram (EOG) Recording of voltage changes resulting from shifts in position of the eyeball—possible because each globe is a positive (anterior) and negative (posterior) dipole. Sleep recordings use surface electrodes placed near the eyes to record the movement of the eyeballs. Rapid eye movements in sleep indicate a certain stage of sleep (usually REM sleep).

element A pure chemical substance consisting of one type of atom, distinguished by its atomic number.

emergency plan A plan developed by the home care therapist, the patient, and the patient's family that includes an analysis of the most likely emergencies the patient and family may experience, based on the patient's medical needs, the home environment, and the geographical area in which the patient lives in.

emotional filter Nonverbal, internal interpretation of another's actions or communication as seen in light of a judgment, emotional reaction, or opinion of the listener.

empathy Characteristic essential to nurturing a relationship: envisioning oneself in the place of another and then verbally conveying that you understand what it must feel like to be in that person's situation.

emphysema Type of chronic obstructive pulmonary disease occurring in patients who experience damage to the lung parenchyma; results in histopathologic evidence of alveolar wall destruction without fibrosis and physiologic evidence of decreased lung elastic recoil, resulting in bullae that eventually enlarge and compress adjacent lung tissue, impairing respiratory function.

empowerment Characteristic essential to nurturing a relationship: providing the proper tools, resources, and environment to build, develop, and increase the ability and effectiveness of others to set and reach goals for individual and social ends.

EMS portable ventilator A ventilator used in patient transport, typically in emergency care via ambulance.

encoding Sender's act of assigning form to a message in either words, symbols, actions, pictures, numbers, or gestures.

end-tidal P_{CO_2} P_{CO_2} at end-exhalation (P_{ETCO_2}).

endobronchial biopsy Method for sampling endoscopically visible exophytic central tumors or mucosal ulceration, irregularity, or infiltration.

endotracheal intubation Establishment of an artificial airway by placing a tube through the mouth or nose, through the glottis, and into the trachea.

endotracheal tube Large-bore tube inserted through the mouth or nose and into the trachea.

enteral Oral route (PO) of drug administration, passing into the gastrointestinal system.

enteral nutrition Provision of nutrients through the gastrointestinal tract when the patient is unable to chew or swallow.

enteral tube feeding (ETF) Nutrition administration via direct access to the gastrointestinal tract, bypassing the mouth and throat in a patient who cannot eat but who has adequate gastric motility and emptying.

enzymes Proteins that are produced by cells and act as catalysts in specific biochemical reactions.

eosinophilic granuloma Rare, predominantly pulmonary disorder that occurs almost exclusively in smokers or ex-smokers between 10 and 40 years old; likely an inflammatory response by Langerhans cells to a component of tobacco smoke.

epidemic An event that occurs when new cases of a certain disease, in a given human population and during a given period, substantially exceed what is expected.

epidural hematoma A traumatic brain injury resulting in the accumulation of blood between the skull and the outer covering of the brain (dura mater).

epiglottis Cartilaginous structure overhanging the entrance to the larynx to prevent food or foreign material from entering the larynx and trachea while swallowing.

epiglottitis Rapidly progressing inflammation of the epiglottis and surrounding tissue that can result in severe airway obstruction

equipment management services The provision of durable medical equipment, usually to the patient's home, in order to aid in the patient's home care. These services include helping the patient and family select the proper equipment for the patient's needs, ensuring the adequacy of the home environment for the intended equipment, delivering and setting up the equipment, training the patient and family on how to safely and properly use the equipment, and the appropriate maintenance of the equipment.

equipment surveillance A quality assurance program in which cultures of equipment are processed to ensure that high-level disinfection or sterilization is effective.

eschar Scab or dry crust that develops after trauma, such as a thermal or chemical burn, infection, or excoriating skin disease.

escharotomy Surgical incision into necrotic tissue resulting from a severe burn to prevent edema from generating sufficient interstitial pressure to impair capillary filling, causing ischemia.

ethics The study of morality; a careful and systematic reflection on and analysis of moral decisions and behavior, whether past, present, or future.

ethics committees Committees consisting of physicians, administrators, service department members, clergy, a medical ethicist, and community members brought together to consider divergent viewpoints related to the ethical issues in patient care. When involved in patient care, their goal is to issue a recommendation.

evaluation In the patient education context, entails monitoring the ongoing process of teaching effectiveness, the teaching process, and the learner's response.

evidence-based medicine (EBM) An approach to incorporate the best current evidence based on scientific methods, which is then integrated in the decision-making process with the needs of an individual patient to achieve the best outcome of medical treatment.

exacerbation Sudden worsening of respiratory symptoms accompanied by deteriorating lung function; most often, patients will present with increased dyspnea, cough, and changes in the quality or quantity of sputum.

exclusion criteria Stipulations made before a study begins to determine how a subject or patient is to be excluded from or withdrawn from a study.

exclusive provider organization (EPO) Managed care model in which choice is completely eliminated and enrollees must employ the physician and hospital stipulated in the plan; the most affordable but most restrictive of the managed care models.

exercise assessment An assessment that performs two functions: (1) it quantitates the level of disability and provides information for setting initial exercise loads and program expectations, and (2) provides insight into the various cardiorespiratory factors that are involved in functional disabilities.

exercise capacity The ability to perform behaviors such as activities of daily living.

exercise training One of the key components of pulmonary rehabilition.

exercise-induced asthma Form of asthma characterized by transient airway obstruction, typically occurring 5 to 15 minutes after strenuous exertion; prevalent in 90% of individuals with asthma.

exertional dyspnea Shortness of breath that occurs during exercise.

exhaled nitric oxide Marker of airway inflammation, particularly useful in both acute and chronic asthma in both children and adults.

expiratory flow time Interval from the start of expiratory flow to the end of expiratory flow.

expiratory pause time Interval from the end of expiratory flow to the start of inspiratory flow; used to measure auto-PEEP.

expiratory phase Respiration period during which all mechanics from the start of expiratory flow to the end of expiratory flow occur, including those associated with expiratory hold or pause, until the start of inspiratory flow.

expiratory positive airway pressure (EPAP) Pressure applied to the airway during the expiratory phase with ventilators designed for noninvasive ventilation; synonymous with positive end-expiratory pressure (PEEP).

expiratorytime Timeintervalfromthestartofexpiratoryflowtothestart of inspiratory flow; components include expiratory flow time and expiratory pause time.

extracellular fluid (ECF) Body fluid comprising interstitial fluid and blood plasma.

extracorporeal life support (ECLS) Management technique for improving oxygenation and reducing ventilating pressures in selected full-term neonates through cannulation of the right heart; blood is drained from this cannula into a circuit containing a membrane oxygenator and a pump so that oxygen circulates through one side of the membrane and blood is pumped through the other side of the membrane, leading to oxygen diffusion into the blood and carbon dioxide elimination from the blood for its reinfusion into the infant.

extrinsic asthma Asthma associated with external allergens.

extubation Process of removal of an endotracheal tube.

exudative A classification of pleural fluid based on laboratory findings suggesting an inflammatory or malignant etiology of the effusion.

F

face shield Apparatus used to provide emergency exhaled-gas ventilation; not as effective as masks, with or without nonrebreathing valves.

facilitation Technique in which words, postures, or actions encourage more detail if delivered with sincerity and genuineness.

fascioscapulohumeral muscular dystrophy Autosomal dominant, slow-progressing dystrophy that affects primarily the face and the proximal portion of the upper extremities, caused by a defective gene.

fee-for-service system A system of payment whereby an individual or an insurance carrier makes payment to healthcare providers when services are given.

feedback The response given by a receiver to a sender about a message.

fetal hemoglobin Hemoglobin F; has higher affinity to O_2 than adult hemoglobin (hemoglobin A), which can be attributed to the replacement of β-chains in hemoglobin A by γ-chains.

fiberoptic plethysmography Rib cage or abdominal displacements stretch an elastic belt, which changes light transmission through the fibers result.

Fick equation Equation that relates $\dot{V}o_2$ to cardiac output and arterial and mixed venous oxygen content, where $\dot{V}o_2$ is the product of the cardiac output and the arteriovenous oxygen content difference.

Fick's law Description of transfer by diffusion, demonstrating that the diffusion rate across a barrier is directly proportional to the cross-sectional area available for diffusion and the difference in concentration gradient per unit distance perpendicular to that cross section.

fidelity Principle dealing with one's faithfulness to duty.

flail chest Multiple rib fractures on one side or from two or more rib fractures in two or more places, from sternal fracture, or from costochondral separation. The term *flail* refers to the paradoxic motion of the chest resulting from loss of chest wall stability.

flexible fiberoptic bronchoscope A bronchoscope constructed with a fiberoptic light conduit to allow for visualization of the airways through the bronchoscope.

flow Movement of a specified volume of fluid (gas or liquid) in a specific period of time.

flow restrictor Specific-sized orifice that allows a specific flow of gas to pass through a flow control device, provided the inlet pressure is a constant 50 psig.

flow triggering Alternative to pressure triggering, in which the ventilator responds to a change in flow rather than a pressure drop at the airway.

flow-inflating bag Manual resuscitator that requires a continuous flow from an external gas source; pressure is determined by the flow and the pressure release valve.

fluid resuscitation Intravascular fluid administration to treat shock.

Food and Drug Administration (FDA) Agency of the Department of Health and Human Services (HHS) that enforces regulations and standards concerning drugs.

force Mechanical energy applied to a body.

forced expiratory technique Breathing maneuver that consists of one or two forced expirations or huffs, combined with a period of controlled breathing.

forced vital capacity Test of pulmonary function that measures the maximal volume of gas that can be expelled forcibly after full inspiration.

foreign body obstruction Presence of any object lodged in any part of the airway, interfering with the individual's ability to breathe and causing sudden choking.

forest plot A graphical display designed to illustrate the relative strength of treatment effects in multiple quantitative scientific studies addressing the same question.

forward heart failure Heart failure causing poor organ perfusion.

fractional distillation of liquefied air Process by which the two major components of air (oxygen and nitrogen) are produced in bulk commercial quantities.

frailty The state of being weak in health or body (especially from old age).

freezing point Temperature at which a liquid will enter the solid state and freeze (0° C or 32° F at 1 atmosphere of pressure for water).

fungal respiratory infections Respiratory infection caused by fungi and including the following: histoplasmosis, blastomycosis, coccidioidomycosis, cryptococcosis, aspergillosis, and *Candida* respiratory infection.

fungi Large group of eukaryotic organisms that includes microorganisms such as yeasts and molds, as well as the more familiar mushrooms.

G

Gay-Lussac's law of combining volumes States that volumes of gases combine chemically in volumetric proportions that are small whole numbers.

Gay-Lussac's law of pressure and temperature Describes the direct relationship between pressure and temperature given a fixed mass and volume of gas.

genotype The genetic makeup of an organism.

geometric standard deviation (GSD) Measure of the magnitude of variation in particle size distribution; for example, a monodisperse aerosol in which all particles are basically the same size has a GSD less than 1.2, whereas a heterodisperse aerosol, with a wider range of particle sizes, has a GSD higher than 1.2.

glossopharyngeal breathing A technique involving the use of oropharyngeal muscles to inject air into the trachea and thus augment ventilation to provide short periods of spontaneous ventilation, improve effective cough, and increase the volume of the voice; also known as frog breathing.

glottis The opening in the larynx where the vocal cords reside that separates the upper and lower airways.

glucose Six-carbon sugar with the formula of $C_6H_{12}O_6$, found in fruits and other foods; primary source of energy for cells.

glycolysis Anaerobic process necessary for glucose metabolism that begins with the breakdown of a 6-carbon glucose chain ($C_6H_{12}O_6$) to two 3-carbon pyruvate (pyruvic acid) molecules in the cytosol of the cell; prepares glucose for the second step in catabolism, the citric acid cycle.

glycosuria The presence of sugar in the urine.

go-bag A carefully prepared bag that includes the equipment and supplies a patient may need when away from home (such as a resuscitation bag, a metered dose inhaler adapter, a list of important phone numbers, a copy of the prescribed ventilator settings, and a flashlight). It is helpful if the bag is kept always stocked and ready so that crucial items are not forgotten should a last-minute excursion occur.

goiter Enlargement of the thyroid gland.

Graham's law Principle predicting the rate of diffusion of a gas as inversely proportional to the square root of its density.

Gram stain Test that stains microorganisms with crystal violet dye, followed by an iodine solution, decolorizing, and then counterstaining with safranin. The retention of either the violet color of the stain or the pink color of the counterstain serves as a primary means of identifying and classifying bacteria by revealing details of the cell wall structure; gram-positive stains blue and gram-negative stains pink.

gram-negative bacteria Bacteria that have a cell wall composed of a thin layer of peptidoglycan covered by an outer membrane of lipoprotein and lipopolysaccharide and which lose the stain or are decolorized by alcohol in Gram staining; examples include *Haemophilus influenzae, Moraxella catarrhalis, Pseudomonas aeruginosa, Klebsiella* species, *Escherichia coli, Enterobacter* species, *Serratia* species, *Acinetobacter* species, and *Proteus mirabilis*.

gram-positive bacteria Bacteria whose cell walls are composed of a thick layer of peptidoglycan with attached teichoic acids and which retain the stain or resist decolorization by alcohol in Gram staining; examples include *Streptococcus pneumoniae, Staphylococcus aureus,* and *Enterococcus* species.

grapevine The informal transmission of information, gossip, or rumor from person to person.

gravitational sedimentation Deposition of aerosol particles due to gravity.

gravity The force of attraction between all masses in the universe.

ground circuit detector An inexpensive device that, when plugged into an electrical outlet, identifies whether the electrical outlet is properly grounded.

ground glass appearance A hazy increased attenuation of the lungs, with preservation of bronchial and vascular margins.

grunting A sound heard in newborns with respiratory distress. It occurs when the glottis is closed in an attempt to maintain lung volume.

Guillain-Barré syndrome (GBS) Acute idiopathic polyneuritis usually presenting as an ascending symmetric paralysis associated with absent tendon reflexes.

gum elastic bougie Endotracheal tube introducer used to assist intubation, generally used when a difficult intubation is encountered.

H

Hagen-Poiseuille equation Relates flow to the fourth power of the radius, directly and inversely related to the viscosity of the fluid and the length of the tube through which the fluid passes, while directly related to the pressure gradient; if these variables are kept constant, the pressure gradient over the length of the tubular structure in question is directly proportional to flow.

Haldane effect Influence of O_2 on the CO_2 dissociation curve; ensures that the CO_2 content of deoxygenated blood is greater than oxygenated blood at any Pco_2.

Hampton hump A wedge-shaped peripheral infiltrate that may be seen after a pulmonary embolus that occludes distal vessels in the pulmonary arterial tree

hand hygiene Hand washing with soap and water for 15 to 20 seconds or using alcohol-based gels, foams, or rubs that do not require water.

handoff A transfer of responsibility for a patient from one caregiver to another. The goal of a handoff is to provide timely, accurate information about a patient's care plan, treatment, current condition, and any recent or anticipated changes.

hard stops Fields in electronic charting of medical information in which clinicians are required to enter data or complete the field in order to progress or commit the record to the electronic medical record.

health belief model Theory focusing on prevention of disease and asserting that taking action depends on one's perception of four issues: one's level of susceptibility to the condition, the degree of severity of the consequences that might result from contracting the condition, the potential benefits of the health action in preventing or reducing susceptibility, and the barriers or costs related to starting or continuing the proposed behavior.

Health Insurance Portability and Accountability Act (HIPAA) A group of federal laws that establish rights, protections, and other standards of care for working people with preexisting medical conditions.

health maintenance organization (HMO) Type of group healthcare practice that provides basic and supplemental health maintenance and treatment services to voluntary enrollees who prepay a fixed periodic fee that is set without regard to the amount or kind of services received.

health promotion Individual's voluntary adoption of a wellness model and choice to gain an awareness or knowledge of healthy lifestyle practices, incorporate such practices into the daily routine, and ultimately reach a higher level of well-being and wellness.

healthcare utilization The use of heath-related resources such as drugs, devices, and hospitalization.

healthcare-associated infection (HAI) Infection associated with the delivery of healthcare in any setting.

heart rate The number of heart beats in a minute.

heat of vaporization The amount of heat required to convert a liquid into a gas at constant temperature and pressure.

heliox Gas mixture of helium and oxygen; used clinically because of its low density.

helium (He) An inert gas with a lower density than either air or O_2.

helium dilution One of the most commonly used methods for measuring functional residual capacity (FRC).

helmet An interface for noninvasive ventilation (NIV) or continuous positive airway pressure (CPAP) that fits over the entire head of the patient.

hematocrit Proportion of whole blood that is red blood cells (the hemoglobin-carrying cells).

hemoglobin Iron-containing globular protein consisting of two pairs of polypeptides; primary function is the transport of oxygen from the lungs to the tissues.

hemolysis Process in which water passes through a cell, possibly bursting it, as occurs when the water concentration is higher outside the cell.

hemothorax Blood trapped in the pleural space, causing a space-occupying lesion; source of blood is typically from fractured ribs lacerating the intercostal blood vessels or lacerating the lung.

Henderson-Hasselbalch equation Assertion that the pH of a buffer is determined by the ratio of the concentration of base to the concentration of weak acid.

heparin Drug used to prevent further clot formation.

hepatojugular reflux Inappropriate elevation of a usually normal jugular venous pressure (JVP) when the abdomen is compressed for 1 minute over the liver.

hepatosplenomegaly Enlarged liver and spleen.

hertz (Hz) Unit of measure for wave frequency; equal to 1 cycle per second.

high-flow nasal cannula A delivery device in which humidified oxygen in excess of 6 L/min is delivered to the nares via well-fitted nasal prongs.

high-flow/fixed-performance devices Oxygen delivery devices that provide a premixed oxygen concentration at flows that meet or exceed a patient's inspiratory demand.

high-frequency chest wall compression An airway clearance technique that uses a vest to compress the chest externally with short, rapid expiratory flow pulses, and relies on chest wall elastic recoil to return the lungs to functional residual capacity.

high-frequency chest wall oscillation An airway clearance technique that uses a chest cuirass to generate biphasic changes in transrespiratory pressure difference.

high-frequency flow interrupter ventilation (HFFIV) One of four general types of high-frequency ventilation; delivers inspiratory flow to the patient in short bursts via a rotating ball valve or microprocessor-controlled solenoid valve, producing breath rates of 2 to 22 Hz (1 Hz = 60 breaths/min); inspiration and exhalation are both active.

high-frequency jet ventilation (HFJV) One of four general types of high-frequency ventilation; delivers short pulses of gas directly into the trachea through a narrow-bore cannula or jet injector.

high-frequency oscillatory ventilation (HFOV) One of four general types of high-frequency ventilation; essentially an airway vibrator, usually using piston pumps or a vibrating diaphragm that operates at frequencies ranging from 3 to 15 Hz; both inspiratory and expiratory phases are active.

high-frequency positive-pressure ventilation (HFPPV) Conventional positive pressure ventilation at high breath rates (>150 per min) and small tidal volumes with short inspiratory time to facilitate the increased respiratory rate; exhalation is passive.

high-frequency ventilation (HFV) Widely accepted mode of mechanical ventilation in neonatal and pediatric critical care; positive pressure ventilation at rates greater than 150 breaths/min and tidal volumes approximating anatomic dead space, with an ability to deliver an adequate minute volume with a lower airway pressure—often when conventional mechanical ventilation has failed.

high-reliability organizations Organizations or systems that operate in hazardous conditions but have fewer than their fair share of adverse events. The features of high-reliability organizations include a preoccupation with failure; a commitment to resilience; sensitivity to operations; and a culture of safety, in which individuals feel comfortable drawing attention to potential hazards or actual failures without fear of censure from management.

hilum Depression in the lung where the vessels and nerves enter.

HITECH Act Health Information Technology for Economic and Clinical Health Act—legislation created to stimulate the adoption of electronic health records (EHRs). The act stipulates that, beginning in 2011, healthcare providers will be offered financial incentives for demonstrating meaningful use of EHR. Incentives will be offered until 2015, after which time penalties may be levied for failing to demonstrate such use. The act also establishes grants for training centers for the personnel required to support a health information technology infrastructure.

home healthcare Provision of services and equipment to the patient in the home for the purpose of restoring and maintaining his or her maximal level of comfort, function, and health; home health services fall into five different categories: home health agencies, hospice, home medical equipment, home infusion therapy, and homemaker services/private duty nursing.

home medical equipment (HME) companies See *durable medical equipment (DME) companies.*

home respiratory care Those prescribed respiratory care services provided in a patient's personal residence; these may include patient assessment and monitoring, as well as diagnostic and therapeutic modalities and providing education regarding respiratory equipment, disease management, and health-promoting behaviors for the patient and the family caregiver(s).

honeycomb appearance The presence of cystic airspaces with thick fibrous walls lined by bronchiolar epithelium.

hormone A chemical substance produced in the body that controls and regulates the activity of certain cells or organs.

hospital-acquired pneumonia Pneumonia that develops after hospital admission, excluding any infection that is incubating at the time of admission.

Hounsfield units (HU) A system used in computed tomography, in which air is given a value of −1000 and water is given a value of 0, causing most soft tissues to have values ranging from −100 to 100 and bone to range from 600 to over 2000.

House of Delegates (HOD) One of several governance and advisory entities of the American Association for Respiratory Care (AARC).

huff coughing Forced expiratory technique (FET) that is performed by sharply exhaling from high- to mid-lung volumes through an open glottis; used for patients unable to generate an effective cough.

human immunodeficiency virus (HIV) A retrovirus that causes acquired immune deficiency syndrome (AIDS) by infecting helper T cells of the immune system.

humidity deficit Occurs whenever inspired gas is not fully saturated at body temperature, requiring the body to add water to inspired gases to achieve full saturation

humidity therapy A respiratory therapy that delivers water vapor or aerosol.

hybrid stent An airway stent composed of a nitinol frame and a silicone or polyurethane sheath.

hydrogen bond Connection holding adjacent water molecules together in a liquid state and requiring a significant amount of heat to be absorbed to change this water from a liquid to a gas.

hydrophilic Water-loving; describes molecules that tend to be attracted to, and mix well with, water molecules.

hydrophobic Water-hating; describes molecules that tend to be repelled by, and to repel, water molecules.

hydrostatic pressure Static water pressure, generated by the water's weight and varying on the basis of the density of the fluid and its height, reflecting the force of gravity; with other fluids, this pressure is called manometric pressure.

hydrostatic testing Process that measures the expansion characteristic of the cylinder when exposed to internal pressures two-thirds greater than normal; performed by totally suspending the cylinder in a tank of water and pumping water into the cylinder.

hyperbaric oxygen therapy Treatment modality in which a patient breathes 100% oxygen intermittently while the pressure of the treatment chamber is increased to a point higher than sea-level pressure.

hypercalcemia Increased calcium serum levels characterized by anorexia, vomiting, polyuria, mental confusion, obtundation, and death.

hypercapnia Excess carbon dioxide in the blood; can be caused by hypoventilation, increased dead space, and increased CO_2 production.

hypercarbia Elevation of $Paco_2$ above 40 mm Hg.

hyperchloremia Excessive chloride in the blood.

hyperinflation Condition in the lung in which air is not easily exhaled, resulting from decreased lung elasticity and subsequent increased expiratory airway resistance and air trapping as a result of dynamic airway compression.

hyperkalemia Serum potassium levels above normal; can produce hyporeflexia and muscle weakness; paralysis can occur in severe cases, but death because of cardiac arrhythmias usually takes place before this occurs.

hypermagnesemia High serum magnesium levels.

hypernatremia High serum sodium levels.

hyperosmolar An osmolar concentration of the body fluids that is abnormally increased.

hyperphosphatemia High serum phosphorus levels.

hyperpnea Rapid, deep, labored breathing.

hyperresonant The quality of a sound, often produced in percussion technique, that is loud, low pitched, and long; often heard over an emphysematous lung.

hypersomnolence A condition characterized by excessive sleepiness.

hypertonic Property existing in a solution with an osmotic pressure greater than that within the cell.

hyperventilation Rapid, deep, labored breathing resulting in a lowered Pco_2.

hypocalcemia Low ionized serum calcium levels, usually resulting from either decreased absorption or decreased mobilization of calcium from the bones.

hypochloremia Low levels of chloride in the extracellular space.

hypoglycemia Low serum glucose levels.

hypokalemia Low serum potassium level.

hypomagnesemia Low serum magnesium levels.

hyponatremia Low serum sodium levels, creating a significant shift in the relationship between intracellular and extracellular fluid compartments.

hypophosphatemia Low serum phosphorus levels, primarily caused by decreased absorption, intracellular shifts, or increased excretion.

hypopnea Abnormally slow, shallow respiration.

hypothermia A core temperature of 95° F (35° C) or less.

hypotonic Property of any solution with an osmotic pressure less than that within the cell.

hypovolemic shock Hypotension with end organ dysfunction caused by intervascular volume loss; most commonly due to hemorrhage in a traumatically injured patient.

hypoxemia Deficiency in blood oxygenation; may be caused by inadequate ventilation relative to perfusion (that is, low $\dot{V}A/\dot{Q}$ and shunt), which has a great effect on oxygen uptake by the lung; hypoxemia in adults is usually defined as a Pao_2 of less than 80 mm Hg at sea level.

hypoxemic drive A secondary ventilatory drive that triggers increased minute ventilation when the Pao_2 is less than 60 mm Hg.

hypoxia Decreased tissue oxygenation below adequate levels.

hypoxic pulmonary vasoconstriction Narrowing of the lumen in a pulmonary blood vessel because of low oxygen level.

I

ideal gas law Rule that PV = nRT, with the product of pressure (P) and volume (V) equal to the product of the number of molecules of gas (n), absolute temperature (T), and a gas constant (R).

idiopathic pulmonary arterial hypertension (IPAH) Pulmonary hypertension of unknown origin.

idiopathic pulmonary fibrosis (IPF) Interstitial lung disease that affects predominantly males in the fifth to seventh decade of life; of unknown pathogenesis but likely to reflect an aberrant host response to injury of the alveolar epithelium and endothelium or a protracted response to the same; a history of a gradual onset of dyspnea with exercise is typical.

illness/wellness continuum Perspective of patient education in which health is viewed from a traditional perspective and from a wellness perspective.

immunosenescence Aging of the immune system.

impedance plethysmography Noninvasive study for diagnosing deep vein thrombosis (DVT) by detecting volumetric changes in the limb through changes in the electric impedance.

impedance pneumography Method for measuring respiratory rate and excursion using two electrodes placed on the chest wall and then passing a high-frequency and low-ampere AC current between the electrodes on the chest surface.

impedance threshold valve (ITV) An airway adjunct for resuscitation that produces a small vacuum in the chest during the recoil phase of chest compression to improve venous return.

implementation In the patient education context, involves putting the teaching plan into action; it is a dynamic, didactic encounter between the teacher and the leaner.

incentive spirometry Technique designed to mimic natural sighing or yawning maneuvers; also referred to as sustained maximal inspiration; used to reestablish the normal pattern of periodic deep breathing in the post-operative period.

incidence Factor that determines how often a disease or condition is contracted or diagnosed in a time period.

incident report Sometimes called a safety report; occurrence report filed for an untoward incident in a healthcare system, such as administration of an incorrect medication.

inclusion criteria Stipulations made before a study begins to determine how a subject or patient is to be entered into a study.

indemnity insurance plan Type of commercial plan that provides a benefit only if and when a medical event occurs. Indemnity plans provide payment of a fixed sum for a covered benefit.

indirect calorimetry A technique for measuring energy requirements, based on the primary measurement of oxygen consumption and carbon dioxide production.

infection control Policies and procedures to minimize the risk of spreading infections.

inferential statistics Statistical methods to allow inference to other settings; often involves the reporting of a P-value.

inferior vena cava (IVC) filter A type of vascular filter that is implanted into the inferior vena cava to prevent fatal pulmonary emboli

informed consent Right of the patient to all information before undergoing or refusing treatments; includes the components of disclosure, understanding, voluntary nature, competence, and permission giving.

inhalation Method of administering a drug; has fewer adverse side effects than administering medications orally.

inhalation injury Sequela of aspiration of superheated gases, steam, or noxious products of incomplete combustion, generating adverse effects on both gas exchange and on hemodynamics.

Inhalational Therapy Association (ITA) Association formed in 1946 as a precursor to the American Association of Inhalation Therapists (AAIT) to promote higher standards and professional advancement, to foster cooperation between the technician and physician, and to advance the knowledge of inhalation therapy.

inspection An examination technique that ranges from casual observation to visual scrutiny of the patient.

inspiratory flow time Interval from the start of inspiratory flow to the end of inspiratory flow.

inspiratory pause time Interval from the end of inspiratory flow to the start of expiratory flow.

inspiratory phase Respiration phase during mechanical ventilation in which pressure, volume, and flow increase above their end-expiratory values; quantified by specifying the inspiratory time, defined as the time interval from the start of inspiratory flow to the start of expiratory flow, including the hold or pause time.

inspiratory positive airway pressure (IPAP) Level of pressure specified on ventilators designed to provide noninvasive positive pressure ventilation.

inspiratory time Time interval from the start of inspiratory flow to the start of expiratory flow, including the inspiratory hold (or pause) time.

institutional review board (IRB) Facility group that officially approves proposed studies and ensures the safety of participants for a new treatment and that informed consent forms are signed by the patient, nearest relative, or guardian to approve the treatment or control.

insurance A customer's benefits package, which is provided by an insurance company or managed care organization (MCO) that serves as an intermediary between the purchaser and the recipient or consumer.

intensive program A pulmonary rehabilitation program that generally provides two to five sessions per week for periods of 4 to 12 weeks.

intermittent asthma Least severe of the classes of asthma severity, characterized by symptoms of coughing or wheezing fewer than two times per week with asymptomatic or normal peak expiratory flow (PEF) values between brief exacerbations; nocturnal symptoms of coughing, wheezing, or breathlessness less than 2 times per month; and measured FEV_1 or PEF consistently more than 80% of predicted, while maintaining less than 20% variability in PEF routinely.

intermittent positive pressure breathing (IPPB) Short-term or episodic mechanical ventilation for the primary purpose of assisting ventilation and providing short-duration hyperinflation therapy; usually administered with pneumatically driven, pressure-triggered, and pressure-cycled ventilators.

intermittent-flow device A device that give oxygen intermittently only during the inspiratory cycle.

intermittent-flow oxygen Oxygen delivery that is provided based on the patient's inspiratory effort and turns off during exhalation, eliminating oxygen waste associated with continuous flow during exhalation.

international 10-20 system A system developed in 1958 to standardize the placement of electrodes for electroencephalogram (EEG) recording. The system is termed 10-20 because electrodes are placed either at 10% or 20% of the total distance between two skull landmarks; allows for comparison of electrical activity from different areas of the brain and serial comparison of follow-up EEGs in a single patient.

interoperability The ability for organizations to interconnect their data, communication systems, and information technology networks.

interstitial lung disease (ILD) Term used to delineate approximately 200 distinct diseases in which the interstitium is altered by inflammation or fibrosis or both; may affect any of the following structures: the alveolar walls (and lumens), pulmonary microvasculature, interstitial macrophages, fibroblasts, myofibroblasts, and matrix components of the lung.

interventional study A study that interferes with (treats) or modifies care.

intra-aortic balloon pump (IABP) Catheter-based balloon inserted into the descending aorta just below the aortic arch and inflated during diastole, causing increased coronary blood flow, and deflated during systole, causing decreased afterload; uses the principle of counterpulsation to support the failing heart, especially in cardiogenic shock due to myocardial ischemia.

intracellular fluid (ICF) Fluid inside cell membranes that contains dissolved solutes essential to electrolytic balance and healthy metabolism.

intramuscular (IM) Administering (injecting) a bolus of drug into a muscle bed, where it is taken into the bloodstream by the local capillary bed.

intraosseous (IO) Method of administering a drug; medication is placed directly into the bone marrow.

intrapulmonary percussive ventilation (IPV) Therapeutic form of chest physical therapy using a pneumatic device called a Percussionator; the patient breathes through a mouthpiece, which delivers high-flow minibursts at rates of over 200 cycles/minute.

intravenous (IV) Method of drug delivery to the inside of a vein.

intrinsic asthma Asthma associated with recent respiratory tract infection; inflammatory responses to viral infections (especially in the lower respiratory tract) may start the cascade of symptomatic wheezing from inflammatory debris or excessive production of mucus in the airways.

intrinsic positive end-expiratory pressure See *auto-PEEP*.

ionic bond Stable atomic configuration accomplished by transferring electrons.

ions Electrically charged atoms or groups of atoms.

iron lung An airtight mechanical respirator that consists of a metal tank enclosing the whole body, except the head; the prototype negative pressure ventilator.

ischemia Decrease in oxygenated blood in a body part or organ.

isothermic saturation boundary (ISB) The point at which inspired gas is fully saturated at body temperature (44 mg/L at 37° C), approximately 5 cm below the carina at the level of the third-generation airways.

isotonic Property of a solution that occurs with an osmotic pressure that is equal to that found within cells, resulting in a solution with an osmotic pressure equal to that found within cells.

isotope Atom whose nuclei have the same number of protons (atomic number) but a different number of neutrons (mass number).

J

jargon The language, especially the vocabulary, peculiar to a particular trade, profession, or group.

jaundice Yellowish skin color arising from an elevated serum bilirubin level.

jet nebulizer Device that uses a jet of compressed gas that passes through a restricted orifice, creating a low pressure area near the tip of a narrow tube, drawing fluid from a reservoir, which is then sheared or shattered into droplets by the airstream.

Joint Commission A private-sector, not-for-profit organization in the United States that operates accreditation programs for a fee to subscriber hospitals and other healthcare organizations. Formerly known as the Joint Commission on Accreditation of Healthcare Organizations (JCAHO).

joule Unit of energy in the meter-kilogram-second system equivalent to the product pressure and volume, or equivalent to 107 ergs or 1 watt/second.

justice The principle that deals with fairness and equity in the distribution of scarce healthcare resources, such as time, services, equipment, and money.

K

K complexes Sharp, negative, high-voltage electroencephalographic wave, followed by a slower, positive component. K complexes occur spontaneously during non-rapid-eye movement sleep, beginning in (and defining) stage 2.

Kaplan-Meier plot Displays survival rate over time.

Kerley B lines Short lines that appear perpendicular to the pleural surface on a chest radiograph; associated with congestive heart failure.

kinesics Factor affecting communication on either a conscious or unconscious level through the use of body motion and gestures.

Kussmaul respirations Hyperventilation as a compensatory mechanism for metabolic acidosis.

kyphosis Forward curvature of the spine.

L

lactate Anion of lactic acid most commonly formed in ischemic cells as a consequence of anaerobic glycolysis and the use of pyruvate for generation of ATP; frequently used as an indicator of the severity of shock and to give a rough idea of tissue perfusion, oxygen delivery, and oxygen utilization.

lactate threshold The point where lactate (lactic acid) begins to accumulate in the bloodstream; also known as the anaerobic threshold.

Lambert-Eaton syndrome Rare myasthenic-like disorder resulting from a reduction of transmitter release from presynaptic terminals; commonly associated with small cell carcinoma of the lung; limb and girdle muscles predominantly are involved.

laminar flow A pattern of flow consisting of concentric layers of fluid flowing parallel to the tube wall at linear velocities that increase toward the center; considered to be smooth, uninterrupted flow.

large-volume nebulizer An aerosol-producing device designed to deliver enough humidified inspired gases to provide adequate flow to meet patient inspiratory flow rates.

laryngeal mask airway (LMA) Device for both routine management of the airway during general anesthesia and use as an emergency airway adjunct in the difficult airway.

laryngopharynx The inferior portion of the pharynx with openings into the larynx and esophagus.

laryngoscope An instrument used to visualize the larynx.

laryngotracheobronchitis Acute inflammation of the larynx, trachea, and bronchi marked by swelling of the tissues.

larynx Musculocartilaginous structure behind the tongue and hyoid bone that acts as a sphincter to protect the entrance to the trachea; functions secondarily as the voice box.

latent errors A human error which is likely to be made due to systems or routines that are formed in such a way that humans are disposed to making these errors.

lateral decubitus A chest radiographic view in which the patient is lying on the side.

law of mass action The rate of an elementary reaction is proportional to the product of the concentrations of the participating molecules.

leading questions Questions so worded as to suggest the proper or desired answers.

lecithin-to-sphingomyelin (LS) ratio A test performed on amniotic fluid to determine lung maturity; with an LS ratio of more than 2:1, the lungs are considered mature.

leukocyte White blood cell.

leukocytosis Elevated white cell count; often a sign of significant infection but also can be associated with elevated glucocorticoids (e.g., stress reaction, steroid administration) and a number of hematologic malignancies.

leukopenia Decreased white cell count; often indicates overwhelming infection.

leukotriene Any one of several compounds that can act on smooth muscle cells through its own receptor to produce tonic bronchoconstriction.

leukotriene modifiers The most recent class of asthma medications available in the oral tablet or chewable (montelukast) form; beneficial as add-on therapy in patients with moderate to severe asthma.

licensure Government permission to legally practice or work in a profession by demonstrating a certain level of knowledge involving a high level of skill. Such licenses are usually issued to regulate some activity that is deemed to be dangerous or a threat to the person or the public, which often involves accredited training and examinations.

life expectancy The average number of years an individual is expected to live, either from birth or the number of years remaining at any given age.

life span The typical length of time a species is expected to live.

likelihood ratio Used for assessing the value of performing a diagnostic test; a likelihood ratio of greater than 1 indicates the test result is associated with the disease, and a likelihood ratio less than 1 indicates that the result is associated with absence of the disease.

limb-girdle muscular dystrophy Heterogenous group of muscle dystrophies characterized primarily by weakness of the shoulder and pelvic girdles with sparing of the facial muscles.

lipid Organic biomolecule that is soluble in nonpolar organic solvents, such as ether, alcohol, or benzene, but is not soluble in water; composed primarily, but not exclusively, of carbon, hydrogen, and oxygen.

liquid oxygen (LOX) storage system A superinsulated container, commonly called a dewar, that eliminates heat transfer to the contents of the container. A LOX system keeps the liquid oxygen at −298° F.

living will A document that details the types of medical treatments and life-prolonging measures that an individual does or does not want performed if he or she were to be incapacitated.

lobes Upper, middle, and lower major divisions within each lung; further subdivided into bronchopulmonary segments that correspond to the distribution of a specific bronchus.

locus of control Attitude toward one's responsibility for one's behavior. Persons with an internal locus of control believe they can control their own destiny; those with an external locus of control tend to believe that their lives are controlled by forces outside themselves.

long-acting muscarinic antagonists Anticholinergic medications taken routinely to control and prevent bronchoconstriction; they are not intended for fast relief; they take longer to begin working, but relieve airway constriction for up to 24 hours. Tiotropium is the most commonly prescribed long-acting anticholinergic drug in COPD.

long-acting β_2-agonists β_2-agonist medications taken routinely to control and prevent bronchoconstriction; they are not intended for fast relief; they take longer to begin working, but relieve airway constriction for up to 12 hours.

long-term oxygen therapy (LTOT) Administration of oxygen for at least 20 hours/day; a life-prolonging therapy for hypoxemic patients with chronic obstructive pulmonary disease.

lordosis Backward curvature of the spine.

low-flow/variable-performance device An oxygen delivery device that provides supplemental oxygen, which varies because the delivered oxygen is mixed with variable amounts of inhaled room air.

lung capacity A combination of two or more lung volumes: vital capacity, inspiratory capacity, functional residual capacity, or total lung capacity.

lung injury score Incorporates the level of positive end-expiratory pressure (PEEP), the Pa_{O_2}/F_{IO_2} ratio, a chest radiograph score, and lung compliance into a summary score that can be used to describe the severity of acute lung injury.

lung transplantation Transfer of a pulmonary organ system from a donor to a recipient; recognized as an accepted therapy for end-stage cystic fibrosis lung disease.

lung volume A measure of the size of the lungs: tidal volume, inspiratory reserve volume, expiratory reserve volume, or residual volume.

lung-protective ventilation strategy Ventilatory technique in which target tidal volume is 6 mL/kg of predicted body weight, plateau pressure is kept below 30 cm H_2O, and positive end-expiratory pressure is applied to maintain alveolar recruitment.

lung-volume reduction See *lung-volume reduction surgery.*

lung-volume reduction surgery Procedure that removes 20% to 30% of the lung tissue most severely affected by emphysema, encouraging the remaining lung to gain recoil elasticity and improve lung, chest wall, and diaphragmatic mechanics in addition to right ventricular performance.

M

Macklin effect Air dissecting into the mediastinum, creating vertical linear streaks on the chest radiograph.

macrophages Cell type derived from blood monocytes or through local proliferation that reside in many locations in the lung, including the pleura, interstitium, and epithelial surface; associated with defending the lung against inhaled agents, and with phagocytosing particulates and debris.

magnetic resonance imaging (MRI) Imaging that takes advantage of nuclear magnetic resonance.

maintenance program Medically supervised facility- or home-based pulmonary rehabilitation program for pulmonary disease patients who reside locally.

malignant Tending to become worse and to cause death; a malignant cancer is anaplastic, invasive, and metastatic.

managed care Healthcare system that seeks to eliminate redundant services and facilities, thereby reducing costs, through administrative control over primary healthcare services.

managed care organization (MCO) Integrated network of doctors, hospitals, and other healthcare providers that deliver health services to an insured population. The four different types of managed care organizations are the health maintenance organization (HMO), the preferred provider organization (PPO), the exclusive provider organization (EPO), and the point-of-service plan (POS).

mandatory breath Inspiration that is machine triggered or machine cycled or both.

Mantoux test Placement of purified protein derivative (PPD) subcutaneously to detect the presence of an immune response to mycobacteria by eliciting a delayed-type hypersensitivity response.

manual resuscitator A bag-valve device consisting of a self-inflating bag, an air-intake valve, a nonrebreathing valve, an oxygen inlet nipple, and an oxygen reservoir to aid in resuscitation and breathing.

mass Amount of a substance determined by the number and type of molecules.

mass casualty respiratory failure (MCRF) An event resulting in patients requiring mechanical ventilation in excess of the space to care for them and devices to provide ventilatory support.

mass median aerodynamic diameter (MMAD) Measurement that expresses the geometric size of the particles of an aerosol; for medical use, aerosol generators produce respirable particles with an MMAD of between 1 to 5 μm.

mass number Sum of the protons and neutrons inside the nucleus of an atom; often used interchangeably with the term *atomic weight.*

mass spectrometer Instrument capable of measuring all respiratory gases, including respiratory and anesthetic gases, breath by breath.

mast cell stabilizer A type of medication used to treat respiratory disease.

mast cells Cells that produce histamine and leukotrienes that constrict airway smooth muscles; there are two types, classified according to neutral protease composition (chymase and/or tryptase).

matching Research evaluation parameter of a study that asserts that the controls must be similar to the treatment group in as many respects as are feasible to avoid other factors confounding (confusing) the results.

matter Any substance that has mass and occupies space.

maximum expiratory pressure After a full inhalation, the pressure generated by forced exhalation against an occluded airway.

maximum inspiratory pressure After a full exhalation, the pressure generated by forced inhalation against an occluded airway.

mean airway pressure Average pressure, relative to atmospheric pressure, within the airway during one complete respiratory cycle; directly related to the inspiratory time, respiratory rate, peak inspiratory pressure, and positive end-expiratory pressure.

mechanical insufflation–exsufflation (MIE) Technique in which a device inflates the lungs with positive pressure followed by a negative pressure to simulate a cough.

mechanical ventilation A form of respiratory support that typically uses a positive pressure ventilator.

meconium aspiration syndrome Condition that develops when the fetus or newborn inhales meconium; the most common cause of severe hypoxemic respiratory failure; can block the air passages and cause failure of the lungs to expand or other pulmonary dysfunction such as pneumonia or emphysema.

meconium Thick, dark green material that collects in the intestines of the full-term fetus and forms the first stools of a newborn; a mixture of intestinal gland secretions, some amniotic fluid, and intrauterine debris, such as bile pigments, fatty acids, epithelial cells, mucus, lanugo, and blood.

meconium ileus Obstruction of the small intestine in the newborn resulting from an impaction of thick, dry, cohesive meconium, usually occurring at or near the ileocecal valve.

mediastinal shift Moving of the tissues and organs that comprise the mediastinum (heart, great vessels, trachea and esophagus) to one side of the chest cavity.

mediastinoscopy Examination of the mediastinum, using an endoscope with light and lenses inserted through an incision in the suprasternum.

mediastinum Area between the two pleural sacs that contains the heart, great vessels, esophagus, and thymus.

Medicaid Payment program funded jointly by federal and state governments to pay for medical services for the elderly, disabled, poor, and dependent children.

medical gas cylinders Containers used to store medical gas. They range from small, lightweight units containing a few cubic feet of gas to large cylinders of several hundred cubic feet. U.S. Department of Transportation regulations specify that high-pressure medical gas cylinders be made of seamless construction from high-quality steel, chromium-molybdenum alloy, or aluminum.

medical information management The maintenance and care of health records by traditional and electronic means in hospitals, physician's office clinics, health departments, health insurance companies, and other facilities that provide healthcare or maintenance of health records.

medical record Collection of documentation of patient assessments, problem identification, care plans, treatments, and outcomes, typically including discharge summaries, progress notes, physician orders, laboratory results, and flow sheets, as well as additional media, which may include online reports, photographs, videotapes, films, and audio recordings.

Medicare Federal government's health insurance program for the elderly, the disabled, and persons with certain diseases, such as end-stage renal disease.

medication reconciliation The process of avoiding inadvertent inconsistencies across transitions in care by reviewing the patient's complete medication regimen at the time of admission, transfer, and discharge and comparing it with the regimen being considered for the new setting of care.

medium See *channel.*

mesh nebulizer An aerosol-generating device that forces a solution through a mesh to generate particles.

message A verbal or nonverbal expression of thoughts or feelings intended to convey information to the receiver and requiring interpretation by that person.

meta-analysis A statistical process that combines the results of several studies that address a set of related research hypotheses.

metabolic acidosis Decrease in pH associated with a loss of buffer (HCO_3^-).

metabolic alkalosis Increase in pH associated with an increase in buffer (HCO_3^-).

metabolic cart A device used to perform indirect calorimetry.

metabolic equivalent (MET) a physiological concept expressing the energy cost of physical activities as multiples of resting oxygen consumption.

metallic stent An airway stent constructed of a lattice of nitinol, a metallic alloy with excellent shape memory that allows the stent to be deployed in a contracted state, but which self-expands to return to its originally constructed size.

metastasis Process by which tumor cells spread to distant parts of the body.

methemoglobin Form of hemoglobin that is produced when the iron in heme is oxidized from Fe^{+2} to Fe^{+3}.

methylxanthine Serves as a smooth muscle relaxant and cardiac muscle and CNS stimulant. Clinically, it is employed as a bronchodillator, which is declining in popularity for long-term care.

microbiology Branch of biology that studies microorganisms and their effects on other living organisms.

mild persistent asthma Category of asthma characterized by symptoms of coughing or wheezing more than two times per week but less than once per day, with symptoms that affect normal daily activities of living or normal nighttime sleep patterns, nocturnal symptoms of coughing, wheezing, or breathlessness more than two times per month, and measured FEV_1 or peak expiratory flow (PEF) consistently more than 80% of predicted or personal best, while maintaining approximately 20% to 30% variability in PEF rates.

milliequivalent One-thousandth of a gram equivalent of a chemical element, an ion, a radical, or a compound.

mind-set An attitude, disposition, or mood.

mini-bronchoalveolar lavage A nonbronchoscopic method of performing a small-volume bronchoalveolar lavage for quantitative culture results to guide antibiotic therapy prescribed for patients suspected of ventilator-associated pneumonia.

minimum data set (MDS) Part of the U.S. federally mandated process for clinical assessment of all residents in Medicare- or Medicaid-certified nursing homes. This process provides a comprehensive assessment of each resident's functional capabilities and helps nursing home staff identify health problems.

mitochondrial myopathy One of the manifestations of hereditary mitochondrial disorders, occurring as a result of a point mutation in mitochondrial DNA; can also affect other organ systems, particularly the brain.

mixed apnea Combination of central and obstructive apnea.

mode of ventilation A combination of control, phase, and conditional variables that establishes a set pattern of spontaneous breaths, mandatory breaths, or both.

moderate persistent asthma Category of asthma characterized by symptoms of coughing or wheezing on a near-daily basis, with exacerbations experienced more than two times per week, and often persisting for multiple days; manifests symptoms that routinely interfere with normal daily activities of living or normal nighttime sleep patterns and nocturnal symptoms of coughing, wheezing, or breathlessness more than one time per week, plus measured FEV_1 or peak expiratory flow (PEF) routinely 60% to 80% of predicted or personal best, while consistently maintaining more than 30% variability in PEF rates.

molar solution Solution containing 1 mole (mol) of solute per liter of solution.

mole Quantity of a substance equal to its gram molecular weight, which contains 6.02×10^{23} atoms (Avogadro's number).

moral philosophy An individual's behavioral code, defining behavior in a given situation, based on personal principles the individual has previously adopted.

motivation Patient's interest in changing an undesirable behavior associated with his or her condition.

motivational interviewing A directive, client-centered counseling style for eliciting behavior change by helping clients to explore and resolve ambivalence.

mouth occlusion pressure Test of central respiratory drive that is independent of underlying respiratory mechanics; maximum negative mouth pressure generated during the first 100 milliseconds (0.1 second) of inspiration measured during complete airway occlusion.

mucociliary apparatus Mechanism that clears inhaled agents from the lower respiratory tract.

mucokinetic agent Drug, such as acetylcysteine, intended to reduce mucus viscosity and assist with the mobilization of airway secretions.

multidisciplinary One or more disciplines working collaboratively.

multiple inert gas elimination technique (MIGET) A technique based on the straightforward principles governing inert gas elimination by the lung, such that when an inert gas in solution is infused into systemic veins, the proportion of gas eliminated by ventilation from a lung unit depends only on the solubility of the gas and the $\dot{V}_A/\dot{Q}$ ratio of that unit.

multiple sclerosis (MS) Demyelinating disease of the central nervous system characterized clinically by repeated remissions and exacerbations of symptoms, including paresthesias, motor weakness, diplopia, blurred vision, bladder incontinence, and ataxia.

multiresistant The state of possessing resistance to multiple drugs (especially antibiotics).

murmur Extra cardiac sound heard in conjunction with S_1 and S_2.

muscular dystrophy Heterogeneous group of progressive, hereditary degenerative skeletal muscle diseases in which the respiratory muscles, like any skeletal muscle, become progressively weaker, eventually culminating in respiratory failure and death (respiratory complications are the most common cause of death in these diseases).

mutation Event that changes the genetic structure of a living organism.

mutuality Characteristic considered essential in nurturing a relationship by agreeing on the problems and the means to resolve them.

myasthenia gravis (MG) Autoimmune disorder characterized by impaired transmission of neural impulses across the neuromuscular junction resulting from the destruction of the postsynaptic acetylcholine receptors.

mycobacterial pneumonia Any of a group of pneumonias caused by tuberculous and nontuberculous mycobacteria (NTM) and diagnosed by acid-fast bacilli (AFB) smears and mycobacterial cultures, using nucleic acid probes to detect *Mycobacterium tuberculosis, Mycobacterium avium complex, Mycobacterium gordonae*, or *Mycobacterium kansasii.*

myocardial ischemia Condition of inadequate blood flow in the coronary arteries that supply the heart muscle; often results in angina.

myocardial perfusion imaging Imaging technique that involves intravenous injection of a radionuclide agent, which accumulates in the myocardium in proportion to regional myocardial perfusion.

myotonic dystrophy A chronic, slowly progressing, inherited disease characterized by wasting of the muscles (muscular dystrophy), cataracts, heart conduction defects, endocrine changes, and myotonia.

N

***N*-of-1 randomized controlled trial** An approach to treatment in which patients undertake pairs of treatment periods during which they receive a target treatment in one period of each pair and a placebo or alternative in the other.

nasal continuous positive airway pressure Therapeutic support for potential low lung volumes and associated hypoxemia (particularly in infants); also commonly used in the treatment of obstructive sleep apnea.

nasal mask An interface for noninvasive ventilation (NIV) or continuous positive airway pressure (CPAP) that fits over the nose of the patient.

nasal oxygen cannula A low-flow variable performance delivery device consisting of nasal prongs which are loosely placed in the nares.

nasal oxygen catheter A low-flow variable-performance delivery device consisting of a slim plastic tube that is placed through one naris and advanced to the level of the uvula.

nasal pillows An interface for noninvasive ventilation (NIV) or continuous positive airway pressure (CPAP) in which there are prongs that fit into the nose of the patient.

nasopharyngeal airway Plastic or rubber airway device inserted into the nose and directed along the floor of the nose parallel to the hard palate; available as an alternative to the oropharyngeal airway.

nasopharynx Uppermost region of the throat or pharynx, behind the nasal cavity and extending from the posterior nares to the level of the soft palate.

nasotracheal intubation Intubation technique in which the tube is passed through the nasal passage.

nasotracheal suctioning Maneuver used to remove secretions from the lower respiratory tract.

National Association for Medical Direction of Respiratory Care (NAMDRC) A national organization of physicians whose mission is to educate its members and address regulatory, legislative and payment issues that relate to the delivery of healthcare to patients with respiratory disorders.

National Asthma Education and Prevention Program Expert panel of the National Institutes of Health focusing specifically on the needs of, and programs affecting, individuals with asthma.

National Asthma Educator Certification Board (NAECB) Oversees the voluntary testing program used to assess qualified health professionals' knowledge in asthma education.

National Board for Respiratory Care (NBRC) Voluntary health certifying board founded in 1960 for the purpose of the evaluation of professional competence for respiratory therapists by providing high-quality voluntary credentialing examinations for respiratory care and pulmonary function technology.

National Committee for Quality Assurance (NCQA) A private, 501(c)(3) not-for-profit organization dedicated to improving healthcare quality; manages voluntary accreditation programs for individual physicians and medical groups.

nebulizer Device that produces an aerosol, or suspension, of particles in gas.

negative pressure ventilation Use of a ventilator that applies less than ambient pressure to the external chest wall.

negotiating Initiation of discussion with others to influence their thoughts, feelings, and actions.

neoadjuvant A cancer treatment, such as chemotherapy or radiation, that usually precedes another phase of treatment.

neurally adjusted ventilatory assist A mode of ventilation that is triggered, limited, and cycled by the electrical activity of the diaphragm (diaphragmatic EMG).

neuromuscular blocking agent Chemical substance that interferes locally with the transmission or reception of impulses from motor nerves to skeletal muscles.

neutral thermal environment Environment that provides adequate warmth and humidity to minimize insensible heat and water loss for premature and newborn infants; can be achieved with an incubator for a premature, sick, or low-birth-weight infant.

neutron Particle with no mass but net charge located inside the nucleus of an atom.

NIH ARDS Network A clinical research network that was established by the National Institutes of Health (NIH) to accelerate the development of successful management strategies for acute lung injury and the acute respiratory distress syndrome (ARDS).

nitric oxide Colorless gas that is naturally synthesized in human tissue and plays an important role in vascular smooth muscle relaxation, inhibition of platelet aggregation, neurotransmission, and immune regulation.

nitrogen (N_2) A gas that composes about 80% of earth's atmosphere.

nitrogen balance Study involving a 24-hour urine collection and calculation of the difference between nitrogen intake and excretion; helps determine protein requirements and assess changes in visceral protein store status over time.

nitrogen washout A method for measuring functional residual capacity.

nitrogen washout atelectasis Alveolar collapse due to replacement of nitrogen with oxygen.

nocturnal asthma Marker for uncontrolled or more severe asthma; decrease in lung function of patients who are sleeping.

nodular appearance Multiple round opacifications on the chest radiograph.

non-small-cell lung cancer (NSCLC) Major category of histologic types of lung carcinomas, including adenocarcinoma of the lung, large cell carcinoma, and squamous cell carcinoma. Major type of lung cancer characterized histologically most commonly by keratinization or glandular differentiation and which has no features of small cell lung cancer on histology; believed to arise from bronchial epithelial cells.

noncontinuous variables Variables for which only certain values are possible (e.g., yes/no, number of participants, categories of severity); also known as discrete variables.

noninvasive ventilation (NIV) A form of mechanical ventilation that does not involve an endotracheal tube or tracheostomy tube.

noninvasive ventilator A ventilator designed for use with an interface such as a face mask; its primary use is in patients without an endotracheal tube or a tracheostomy tube.

nonmaleficence Principle by which the healthcare practitioner refrains from harming the patient.

nonprotected bronchial brush Instrument used for cytologic sampling of proximal airways and central tumors under direct vision or of peripheral lesions under fluoroscopic guidance; a catheter with a brush (open or enclosed in a sheath) at its distal end is introduced through the working channel of the bronchoscope for sampling of proximal airways or central tumors.

non–rapid eye movement (NREM) sleep Phases of sleep during which there is an absence of rapid eye movement. NREM sleep is subdivided into three stages: stages N1, N2, and N3. Stages N1 and N2 represent superficial sleep, whereas stage N3 sleep represents deep sleep.

nonrebreathing mask Oxygen mask with a one-way valve between the bag and the mask and another one-way valve over one or both mask ports, causing all of the patient's exhaled volume to be directed out of the mask through the mask ports. The valve positioned between the mask and bag prevents exhaled gases from entering the bag.

nonverbal communication Those aspects of communication, such as gestures and facial expressions, that do not involve verbal communication but which may include nonverbal aspects of speech itself (accent, tone of voice, speed of speaking, etc.).

nonverbal cues Signal or body movements that convey messages without words.

normal flora Bacteria that normally exist in a particular area of the healthy body and do not usually cause disease at that site.

nosocomial An infection that is acquired in a hospital or nursing home.

nucleic acid Organic molecule, principally occurring as either deoxyribonucleic acid (DNA) or ribonucleic acid (RNA), that is made from chains of nucleotide, each of which consists of a phosphate group, a five-carbon sugar, and a nitrogenous base.

O

obesity Having a body mass index (BMI) of greater than 30.

observational study A study design that draws inferences about the possible effect of a treatment on subjects, where the assignment of subjects into a treated group versus a control group is outside the control of the investigator.

obstructive apnea Reduction in airflow to less than 90% of baseline despite persistent respiratory effort.

obstructive lung disease Disease characterized by a reduced lumen of the airways within the lungs.

Ohm's law Principle describing properties of electric systems, assuming linear relations between a pressure, resistance, and flow term, without loss of thermal energy, or turbulence, thus allowing application of easily measured quantities, such as electric resistance, to other circular systems of single or connected circuits in which measurement may be more technically difficult; the most general expression of this law describes the relation of voltage, resistance, and impedance.

oncotic pressure Osmotic pressure of a colloid in solution, such as exists in a higher concentration of protein in the plasma on one side of a cell membrane than in the neighboring interstitial fluid.

opacifications Areas on a chest radiograph that block the passage of x-ray energy and thus appear white.

open-ended questions Questions that are open to interpretation and cannot be answered with a yes, no, or other one-word response.

open-loop control Means of mechanical system control in which change in the input causes a change in the output but without flow of information from the output to generate a new input to close the loop.

opiate Natural or synthetic derivative of morphine, derived from the opium poppy, stimulating opiate receptors in the brain and spinal cord to decrease the sensation of pain; also acts as a potent sedative or cough suppressant.

optimum care committees See *ethics committees.*

oral appliance Dental device for clinical use; can be characterized primarily as either a tongue retaining device (TRD) or mandibular advancing device (MAD).

oronasal mask An interface for noninvasive ventilation (NIV) or continuous positive airway pressure (CPAP) that fits over the nose and mouth of the patient.

oropharyngeal airway Airway device with a relatively rigid structure designed to be inserted into the mouth between the lips and teeth and extend from the lips to the pharynx, following the natural curvature of the tongue, without entering the larynx or esophagus.

oropharynx One of three components of the throat or pharynx, extending behind the mouth from the soft palate to the hyoid bone; contains the palatine and lingual tonsils.

orotracheal intubation Establishment of an artificial airway by placing a tube through the mouth into the trachea.

orthopnea Breathlessness, especially when recumbent.

orthostatic hypotension A decrease in blood pressure that occurs when changing from a reclining position to an upright position.

osmosis Process of transferring water molecules through a semipermeable membrane; involves the movement of water from an area of high concentration to an area of low concentration in an attempt to make the concentrations equal.

osmotic pressure Externally applied hydrostatic pressure that stops the flow of a solvent through a membrane.

outcomes evaluation The systematic evaluation of the changes (usually benefits) resulting from a set of activities (usually a program) to achieve stated goals and a systematic evaluation of the extent to which the activities actually caused those results (usually benefits) to occur.

oxidative phosphorylation Joining of a phosphate group to adenosine diphosphate (ADP) to form adenosine triphosphate (ATP) during catabolism.

oximeter Spectrophotometer using specific wavelengths in the oxyhemoglobin spectrum to measure hemoglobin oxygen saturation in the blood.

oximetry Determination of the hemoglobin oxygen saturation of arterial blood using an oximeter.

oxygen analyzer Device used to measure the concentration of oxygen administered to patients.

oxygen concentrator Device designed to produce a low flow (0.5 to 5.0 L/min) of high-purity oxygen (90% to 95%) from room air by either molecular adsorption of nitrogen or filtration of air through a membrane; the most widely used source of oxygen in the home and in extended care facilities.

oxygen consumption ($\dot{V}O_2$) Rate of O_2 uptake by the body, measured by analyzing inspired and expired O_2 in a ventilator circuit; approximately 250 mL/min in the adult under resting conditions).

oxygen delivery Rate of O_2 transport to the peripheral tissues, expressed as DO_2; determined by the cardiac output and arterial O_2 content; also referred to as O_2 availability or O_2 transport.

oxygen extraction The difference between the amount of oxygen delivered to the tissues and the amount of oxygen remaining when the blood leaves the tissues.

oxygen hood A clear rigid plastic device that allows it to be placed over an infant's head for oxygen administration.

oxygen pulse A physiological term for oxygen uptake per heartbeat at rest.

oxygen tent Device used for both oxygen administration and for high humidity therapy; rarely used in modern practice.

oxygen toxicity Pathologic response of the body and its tissues from long-term exposure to high partial pressures of oxygen.

oxygen-conserving device (OCD) Device that supplies a flow of oxygen only when it is needed, on demand at the initiation of inspiration. The conserver is placed between the oxygen supply and the delivery device, which can be a nasal catheter, nasal cannula, or transtracheal catheter.

oxygen-induced hypoventilation Reduced ventilation that results from the administration of high concentrations of oxygen.

oxygenation index Calculated from mean airway pressure, FIO_2, and PaO_2; used to estimate the severity of hypoxemia.

oxyhemoglobin equilibrium curve (OEC) Nonlinear in vivo relationship between PO_2 and O_2 saturation; commonly called the oxyhemoglobin dissociation curve.

P

pack years Measure of patient's smoking exposure; one pack a day for 1 year equals 1 pack year.

pallor Diminished skin color accompanying anemia or, in severe peripheral vasoconstriction, accompanying shock.

palpation Examiner's use of his or her hands to feel for body movement, lumps, masses, and skin characteristics.

PaO_2/FIO_2 ratio A number calculated by dividing PaO_2 by FIO_2, used to estimate the severity of hypoxemic respiratory failure.

paradoxical respiration Flail chest movement, characterized by chest wall movement outward on expiration and inward on inspiration.

paralinguistics Factor affecting communication on either a conscious or unconscious level through the use of sounds such as giggling, laughing, belittling, *ah's* and *um's*, cracking knuckles, or silence.

parasites Plants or animals that live with or on another, deriving benefit from the association but having a detrimental effect on the host.

parenteral Intravenous, intramuscular, and subcutaneous routes of drug administration, which all bypass the gastrointestinal system.

parenteral nutrition Administration of nutrients by a route other than the alimentary canal.

parietal pleura Serous membrane of mesothelial cells and connective tissue that lines the chest wall, covers the diaphragm, and extends over the structures of the mediastinum.

Parkinson disease Neurologic disorder characterized by hypokinesia, tremor, and muscular rigidity.

paroxysmal nocturnal dyspnea Sudden shortness of breath that occurs several hours after a patient lies down; suggests cardiac dysfunction.

partial rebreathing mask Simple oxygen mask with the addition of a reservoir bag. The oxygen supply tube is positioned between the mask and the reservoir bag, and the oxygen flow is set at a rate sufficient to keep the bag at least partially inflated throughout inspiration.

partial thromboplastin time (PTT) Clotting time in anticoagulation therapy, best if 2 to 2.5 times the control.

pascal Under the SI system, the primary unit of pressure, that is, 1 N/m^2; for ease of calculation, the kilopascal (kPa) is commonly used, so that 1 standard atmosphere (at sea level) is approximately 101 kPa.

passive expiration Expiration in which the respiratory system is responding to a sudden release of inspiratory pressure that requires no muscular effort.

passive humidifier Type of humidifying device that uses exhaled heat and moisture to humidify the inspired gas; a heat and moisture exchanger (HME) is a passive humidifier.

passover humidifier Humidifying device that directs gas over the surface of a body of water; an example is the passover wick humidifier.

pasteurization A process for killing or reducing the number of pathogens and organisms other than bacterial spores.

pathways One of the main tools used to manage quality in healthcare concerning the standardization of care processes. They are designed to provide the greatest efficiency of care with the greatest quality. Also referred to as clinical pathways, critical pathways, care pathways, integrated care pathways, or care maps.

Patient Care Partnership The American Hospital Association established the Patient Care Partnership in 2003 to outline the rights and responsibilities patients have regarding their medical care. The Partnership was previously called the Patient Bill of Rights.

patient education The use of the educational process for individuals, their families, and other significant persons when they are dependent upon the healthcare system for diagnosis, treatment, or rehabilitation.

patient-controlled analgesia (PCA) Method of pain control in which the patient can self-administer intravascular pain medication; the computerized device administers doses and includes a lockout interval to automatically inactivate the system if a patient tries to increase the amount of drug used within a predetermined time period.

patient–ventilator asynchrony A condition in which there is a mismatch between how the patient is breathing and the ventilator is delivering breaths.

pay for performance (P4P) A concept to reward (pay) physicians based on the quality of care provided to patients instead of the current concept of paying based on the volume of care.

P_{CO_2} Partial pressure of carbon dioxide.

peak flow meter Monitoring device for the management of asthma.

peak inspiratory pressure The highest pressure measured at the proximal airway during positive pressure ventilation.

pectus carinatum Condition in which the chest bows out at the sternum similar to that of a pigeon.

pectus excavatum Condition in which the sternum is depressed and deviated somewhat like a funnel.

penetrating trauma Mechanism of traumatic injury in which the body of the patient is incised. Common forms of penetrating injuries are stab wounds and gun shot wounds.

penumbra effect A condition that can occur during the application of pulse oximetry in which the sensor is not correctly positioned. This effect causes incorrect readings when the sensor is not symmetrically placed, causing one wavelength to be overused in the calculations of saturation.

peptide Compound created when amino acids are linked together, the OH from the carboxyl group of one amino acid and the H from the amine group of another amino acid splitting off.

percent cycle time Ratio of inspiratory time to total cycle time expressed as a percentage.

percent solution Concentration measure of a solute, usually expressed with units of mass or volume in ratios such as weight/weight, weight/volume, and volume/volume; commonly used in clinical situations.

percentage of body humidity (%BH) In clinical practice, respiratory therapists use this additional measure of humidity as an assessment of humidity deficit.

percussion Examination technique in which the examiner places a finger firmly against a body part and then strikes that finger with a fingertip from the other hand, producing sounds that may suggest normal or abnormal tissue.

percussion therapy Technique of rapidly clapping, cupping, or striking the external thorax directly over the lung segment being drained, with either cupped hands or a mechanical device.

percutaneous coronary intervention The use of balloon angioplasty or placement of stents in occluded or stenotic coronary arteries to improve flow through affected arteries.

perfusion index (PI) A value derived from the photoelectric plethysmographic signal of a pulse oximeter and calculated as the ratio of the pulsatile component (arterial compartment) and the nonpulsatile component (other tissues; venous blood, bone, connective tissue) of the light reaching the device's detector.

pericardium Fibroserous sac around the heart and the roots of the great vessels.

periodic limb movements of sleep Condition characterized by pathologic repetitive myoclonic contractions, which can result in frequent arousals or awakenings and can cause daytime symptoms such as excessive daytime sleepiness.

periodic table A tabular arrangement of the chemical elements according to atomic number.

perioperative program A pulmonary rehabilitation program designed to optimize a patient's functional status prior to surgery.

permissive hypercapnia High Pa_{CO_2} resulting from protective ventilation strategies.

persistent pulmonary hypertension of the newborn A clinical syndrome characterized by a sustained elevation of pulmonary vascular resistance after birth, resulting in hypoxemia and right-to-left extrapulmonary shunting of blood.

personal belief system A set of personal beliefs that an individual develops based on life experience. These beliefs are not necessarily right or wrong and are certainly not objective, yet they are deeply ingrained in an individual's thoughts and decision-making processes.

personal protective equipment (PPE) Protective clothing (gowns), gloves, goggles, or other garments or devices used alone or in combination to protect mucous membranes, airways, skin and clothing from contact with infectious agents.

personal space The variable and subjective distance at which one person feels comfortable talking to another.

personal value system A value system that is formed when a decision is made to continue to believe and express a conviction even when a person or event challenges it.

pH Indicates the hydrogen ion concentration $[H^+]$ in a solution; mathematically defined as the negative logarithm of the hydrogen ion concentration.

pH-stat hypothesis The hypothesis that pH should be kept constant despite changes in temperature.

pharmacodynamics Drug's action in the body, both at a molecular level and in terms of overall clinical effect.

pharmacokinetics A drug's movement in the body through the processes of absorption, distribution, and elimination.

phase variable One of four factors measured and used to start, sustain, and end any phase of the respiration cycle: pressure, volume, flow, and time.

phenotype The observable physical or biochemical characteristics of an organism, as determined by both genetic makeup and environmental influences.

phospholipid Lipid similar to triglyceride except that instead of three fatty acids attached to a glycerol, one of the fatty acid chains is replaced by a chemical structure containing phosphorus and nitrogen; its head is composed of the phosphorus and nitrogen group, and its two tails are composed of the two fatty acids so that the head attracts water (hydrophilic) while the tails repel it (hydrophobic), allowing it to bridge or join two different chemical environments; a primary component of cell membranes and of pulmonary surfactant.

phrenic nerves Nerves exiting the third through the fifth cervical vertebrae and providing motor innervation to the diaphragm, the primary muscle of ventilation.

physician extender Role of the respiratory therapist to help physicians meet the goals of decreasing emergency department visits and hospital admissions by providing services their patients need in the physician office setting and providing the respiratory therapist more opportunity for primary care.

piezoelectric plethysmography Type of plethysmography apparatus that replaces wire coils from the elastic belts with a piezoelectric buckle, which encloses a sensor to generate a voltage in response to stretch passed through the ends of the belts.

Pin Index Safety System (PISS) One of three indexing safety systems for medical gases. This system uses a specific combination of two holes in the post valve just below the gas outlet for each gas or gas mixture; any regulator or device intended to connect to the valve will have pins that correspond to the holes, allowing a proper connection.

planning In the patient education context, involves setting learning goals, objectives, and learning outcomes.

plateau pressure End-inspiratory peak alveolar pressure attained during mechanical ventilation (which should, ideally, be kept below 30 cm H_2O) in conjunction with an overall lung protective ventilation strategy.

platelets Blood cells critical to clot formation after vascular injury; produced in the bone marrow.

platypnea Difficulty breathing unless lying flat.

plethora Fullness of blood vessels at the skin surface, often occurring with vasodilation or hypercapnia.

plethysmogram variability index (PVI) Used during pulse oximetry, the PVI is a measure of the dynamic changes in the perfusion index (PI) that occur during the respiratory cycle; it is used to provide information concerning changes in the balance between intrathoracic pressure and intravascular fluid volume.

plethysmography See *body plethysmography.*

pleural effusion A collection of an abnormal volume of fluid in the pleural space in the thoracic cavity.

pleural friction rub Continuous grating sound heard in auscultation of the lungs, resembling two pieces of leather or two hands being rubbed together; occurs when pleurae are inflamed or when fluid accumulates in the pleural cavity.

pleural space Space between the visceral and parietal layers of the pleurae.

pleurodesis Obliteration of the pleural space produced by inflammation in the visceral and parietal pleural surfaces, resulting in symphysis of the pleural surfaces.

pneumatically powered portable ventilator A portable ventilator that requires a compressed gas source for its operation; an electrical power source is not required.

pneumobelt Unconventional ventilation that consists of an inflatable rubber bladder held over the abdomen by an adjustable corset and assists diaphragmatic motion by causing piston-like motions of the abdominal viscera.

pneumonia Any of several subgroups of respiratory infections; characterized by the inflammation and consolidation of lung tissue caused by infectious agents.

pneumothorax Air in the pleural space that can cause collapse of the lung.

Po_2 Partial pressure of oxygen.

point-of-care testing Diagnostic testing at or near the site of patient care.

point-of-service plan (POS) Type of health insurance plan that is a hybrid of the health maintenance organization (HMO) and preferred provider organization (PPO) plans. Point-of-service plans attempt to provide the tight utilization controls of the HMO coupled with the ability to choose a nonparticipating provider at the point (time) of receiving the service.

polar Type of molecule that forms as the result of unequal charge distribution on a molecule, rather than the sharing or transfer of electrons.

poliomyelitis pandemic A period during the 1940s and 1950s when polio paralyzed or killed over half a million people worldwide annually.

polydipsia Excessive thirst.

polyphagia Increased food consumption.

polysomnogram Comprehensive recording made in a special diagnostics lab; includes all multichannel respiratory recording variables with the addition of electroencephalographic (EEG), electrooculographic (EOG), and electromyographic measured during sleep for the diagnosis of sleep-disordered breathing.

polysomnography A sleep study that produces a polysomnogram.

polyuria Excessive urination.

pores of Kohn Openings between alveoli that allow collateral ventilation between adjacent alveoli.

portable oxygen concentrator (POC) Portable oxygen systems that have a power source (battery) that allows the mobility of the oxygen concentrator. Most POCs are small enough to be moved by the patient and usually weigh less than 20 pounds.

positive end-expiratory pressure (PEEP) Positive airway pressure during the exhalation phase.

positive expiratory pressure (PEP) Airway clearance technique in which the patient exhales against a fixed-orifice flow resistor to aid in the movement of secretions into the larger airways.

positron emission tomography (PET) Imaging modality used for assessing thoracic pathology, in particular for tumor imaging, providing physiologic and metabolic information and focusing on the biochemical properties of cells.

posteroanterior (PA) projection A chest radiographic view in which the x-ray beam passes through the chest from the back to the front.

postpoliomyelitis syndrome Progressive muscle weakness occurring, on average, 29 years after recovery from an episode of acute poliomyelitis.

postural drainage Use of positioning and gravity to drain secretions from areas of the bronchi and lungs into the trachea.

PRECEDE-PROCEED model Model heavily used in the health promotion movement, focusing on factors external to the individual that shape healthcare behavior. In addition to issues of motivation and self-care, an individual's physical and psychological state can have a major bearing on readiness to learn. The acronym PRECEDE stands for predisposing, reinforcing, and enabling constructs in education/environmental diagnosis and evaluation; the acronym PROCEED stands for policy, regulatory, and organizational constructs in educational and environmental development.

precipitate Crystallization of a solute.

precordium Part of the front chest wall that overlays the heart and epigastrium.

preferred provider organization (PPO) Organization in which member physicians, pharmacists, and hospitals offer their health services to subscriber patients on a discounted fee-for-service basis.

prejudice A judgment formed before due examination and consideration of the facts; a premature or hasty judgment. Both bias and prejudice inform clinical decision making, and both the student and seasoned practitioner must confront their own biases and prejudices prior to making decisions.

preload Distending pressure within the ventricle during diastole.

President's Council Ex-officio group of the American Association for Respiratory Care (AARC) Board of Directors consisting of past presidents of the AARC.

pressure Force per unit area.

pressure amplitude Means for manipulating Pco_2 level during high-frequency oscillatory ventilation (HFOV); increasing the amplitude increases displacement of the bellows, thus increasing tidal volume delivery, which is measured as an increased pressure amplitude at the airway opening and results in a lower $Paco_2$.

pressure control ventilation (PCV) Mode of ventilation in which airway pressure is set and remains constant with changes in resistance and compliance.

pressure support ventilation A breathing mode in which patient effort is augmented by a clinician-determined level of pressure during inspiration; no back-rate is set.

pressure triggering A form of triggering in which the ventilator detects a pressure drop at the proximal airway as the inspiratory effort of the patient and initiates the inspiratory phase.

pressurized metered dose inhaler (pMDI) The most commonly prescribed method of aerosol delivery; used to administer bronchodilators, anticholinergics, anti-inflammatory agents, and steroids. A pMDI consists of a pressurized canister containing a drug in the form of a micronized powder or solution that is suspended with a mixture of propellants, surfactant, preservatives, flavoring agents, and dispersal agents.

prevalence How many persons have a given disease or condition in a location at a given time.

prevention See *disease prevention.*

primary ARDS Acute lung injury caused by direct injury to the lungs such as pneumonia, aspiration of gastric contents, inhalation of toxic gases, or pulmonary contusion.

primary survey The initial evaluation of life-threatening injuries of the trauma patient using the mnemonic ABCDE: airway and cervical spine protection, breathing, circulation, deficits, and exposure.

prioritizing The ability to arrange work according to importance; may be defined as "organized think" and "rapid think."

problem-based learning (PBL) Teaching and learning model designed to facilitate critical thinking and clinical decision-making abilities, using equal participation of students in small problem-solving groups to promote self-directed learning and enhance students' abilities to develop their reasoning and communication skills.

procalcitonin A precursor of the hormone calcitonin that is involved with calcium homeostasis and is produced by the C cells of the thyroid gland.

programmed instruction Learning method and materials that allow the patient to learn at his or her own pace and require little time on the part of the respiratory therapy patient educator.

prone position Position in which the patient is lying face-downward. Changing patients with acute respiratory distress syndrome (ARDS) from a supine to a prone position may result in a significant improvement in oxygenation; prone positioning may also improve secretion clearance from the lungs.

proportional assist ventilation A positive feedback control that provides ventilatory support in proportion to neural output of the respiratory center; the ventilator calculates the pressure required from the Equation of Motion.

prospective payment system (PPS) Managed care type of reimbursement in which the hospital or healthcare facility receives a set fee per diagnosis on each patient covered. PPS is a popular replacement for the more traditional fee-for-service approach to paying for medical care.

prospective studies Studies that are proposed and then conducted to avoid bias.

prostacyclin Pulmonary vasodilator that has proven to be the most effective therapy available in the treatment of patients with primary pulmonary hypertension.

protected bronchial brush See *protected specimen brush (PSB).*

protected specimen brush (PSB) Collection device used in the quantitative culture of bronchoscopic specimens in the diagnosis of ventilator-associated pneumonia.

protein Large molecule composed of carbon, hydrogen, oxygen, and nitrogen; formed when a long chain of peptides reaches about 100 amino acids or more in length.

protein-calorie malnutrition (PCM) Nutritional deficit affecting all muscle fiber types, impairing fast-twitch fibers most profoundly, resulting in decreased contractile strength. The primary component of the immune system adversely affected by protein-calorie malnutrition is cell-mediated immunity.

prothrombin time (PT) Test for coagulation defects, used to evaluate the extrinsic pathway, depending on the levels of factors V, VII, X, and eventually I and II.

proto-oncogene Gene that can potentially be a primary inducer of cancer.

protocols Written plans specifying the procedures to be followed in giving a particular examination, in conducting research, or in providing care for a certain condition.

proton Particle with a charge of positive one (+1) located inside the nucleus of an atom.

provider Healthcare professional offering diagnostic, assessment, treatment, guidance, educational, or evaluative services to patients and healthcare clientele.

proxemics Form of nonverbal cues that affect communication through the interpretation of space.

proxy A person, specified by the patient in a legal document, who will make decisions for the patient in the event he or she is incapable of making a decision.

psychomotor domain The area of learning involved in physical movement, coordination, and use of the motor skill areas. It entails a person's ability to perform a task or procedure.

psychosocial support A nontherapeutic intervention that helps a person cope with stressors at home or at work.

pulmonary alveolar proteinosis Interstitial lung disease characterized by filling of alveolar spaces with a lipoproteinaceous exudate and interstitial fibrosis; usually presents with dyspnea and cough.

pulmonary angiography Radiographic examination of the blood vessels of the lungs after injection of an opaque contrast medium into the pulmonary circulation.

pulmonary arterial hypertension (PAH) An increase in blood pressure in the pulmonary vasculature.

pulmonary arteries Arteries supplying blood to the lungs.

pulmonary artery catheter Swan-Ganz catheter, which is inserted into the pulmonary artery, providing pressure measurements, cardiac output determinations, and mixed venous blood analysis.

pulmonary artery wedge pressure (PAWP) Measure that provides an estimate of left atrial (LA) and left ventricular end-diastolic or filling pressure (LVDEP).

pulmonary contusion Bruise in the lung that is usually the primary culprit in gas exchange abnormalities following chest trauma. Blood and edema collect at the site of lung injury, causing decreased focal air exchange.

pulmonary edema Accumulation of excess fluid in the interstitial and alveolar spaces in the lung.

pulmonary embolism (PE) Blockage of a pulmonary artery by foreign matter, such as fat, air, tumor tissue, or a thrombus; characterized by dyspnea, sudden chest pain, shock, and cyanosis.

pulmonary function tests (PFTs) Breathing tests that are used for the detection of restrictive or obstructive patterns, the gas transfer abnormalities that accompany some restrictive and some obstructive lung diseases, and respiratory muscle weakness.

pulmonary hypertension Abnormally high pressure within the pulmonary circulation.

pulmonary rehabilitation Any of a variety of outpatient programs that provide opportunities to restore patients to the highest possible level of independence and functioning in the community; typically includes exercise training, education for patients and family, instruction in respiratory and chest physiotherapy, and psychological support.

pulmonary vascular resistance (PVR) Resistance in the pulmonary vascular bed against which the right ventricle must eject blood.

pulse contour waveform analysis A method to measure stroke volume and cardiac output by analysis of the contour of the arterial pressure waveform; this technology uses the principle that area under the arterial pressure curve correlates with the stroke volume.

pulse flow Pulse flow from an oxygen delivery system is triggered by the patient's inspiratory effort, yet flow is terminated based on a timing mechanism, either electronic or pneumatic. Pulse flow systems usually have a set bolus of oxygen delivered at a specific flow rate.

pulse oximetry Technique that measures oxyhemoglobin saturation noninvasively in arterial blood; rapidly detects changes in arterial oxygen saturation.

pulse pressure variation The variation of pulse pressure over the respiratory cycle (particularly during positive pressure ventilation), used to assess fluid responsiveness.

pulsus paradoxus Abnormal decrease in systolic pressure and pulse wave amplitude during inspiration.

purified protein derivative (PPD) Dried form of tuberculin injected subcutaneously during a Mantoux test to detect past or present infections with tubercle bacilli by eliciting a delayed-type hypersensitivity response.

Q

quick-relief medication Any of a group of primarily short-acting agonists used to combat acute exacerbations of bronchoconstriction or provide quick, complete resolution of airflow obstruction and its accompanying symptoms of cough, wheezing, and chest tightness; includes short-acting β_2-agonist and anticholinergics.

R

radiodensity The ability of an object to block x-ray energy, determined by its composition and thickness.

radiolucent Body tissues that are penetrated by x-rays; produces black areas on the chest radiograph.

radionuclide angiocardiography Noninvasive technique for evaluating left ventricular function, using intravenous injection of a radioisotope (most commonly technetium-99m) and the use of a gamma-ray scintillation camera to detect the isotope's signal within the left ventricle.

radiopaque Body tissues that cannot be penetrated by x-rays; produces white areas on the chest radiograph.

radiotherapy Primary treatment of an intrathoracic tumor or for metastatic disease, involving the use of x-rays or gamma rays to slow or stop the proliferation of malignant cells.

Raman spectroscopy Method used to measure CO_2.

randomization The process of avoiding bias by assuring random assignments of, for example, subjects to either a treatment or control group.

randomized controlled trial (RCT) The primary study method for testing effectiveness of a medical treatment. Patients are randomized to receive either a treatment or usual care, with a comparison of outcomes to evaluate the effect of treatment.

rapid eye movement (REM) sleep Phase of the sleep cycle marked by the presence of rapid eye movements on electrooculography.

rapid response team A group of clinicians with critical care expertise who quickly respond to the patient's bedside in the event of a life-threatening condition.

receiver operating characteristic curve A graphical plot of the sensitivity, or true positives, versus (1 – specificity), or false positives

reflecting Key skill used in critical thinking; involves the ability to "think about thinking" so as to explore assumptions, opinions, biases, and decisions; may be considered introspective or inward think or, if retrospective, past think.

regression analysis A statistical method of evaluating the relationship of independent variables to dependent variables.

remote alarms A device that transmits the sound of the ventilator alarm to another (remote) location. Depending on the ventilator and the type of remote alarm, the remote alarm may be physically connected to the ventilator via a long cable, or it may transmit the sound from the ventilator wirelessly to the remote alarm.

resistance (1) Opposition to a force. (2) Ratio of pressure change to flow change. (3) Lung characteristic that, with compliance, serves as a determinant in the mechanics of airflow in and out of the lungs.

resonant Quality of sound produced in percussion that is loud, low, and long, such as may be heard over normal lung tissue.

resource intensity The relative volume and types of diagnostic, therapeutic, and bed services used in the management of a particular illness.

resource-based relative value scale (RBRVS) A reimbursement methodology that assigns values to physician services based on the resource costs (time, skill, and resource intensity) of providing those services. It is based on a national fee schedule and replaces the previous payment method outlining usual, customary, and reasonable charges. The RBRVS was designed with the objective of narrowing the gap between the incomes of specialists and generalists.

respiratory acidosis Decrease in pH associated with an elevated $Paco_2$.

respiratory alkalosis Increase in pH associated with a decreased $Paco_2$.

respiratory bronchiolitis Rare lung disorder that occurs exclusively in cigarette smokers; characterized by intracytoplasmic golden-brown, granular pigment within alveolar macrophages in respiratory and terminal bronchioles.

Respiratory Care The official science journal of the American Association for Respiratory Care, which is published monthly and is listed in *Index Medicus.*

respiratory care A field or subject area within medical practice that encompasses diagnostic, therapeutic, and support services involved in the care of patients with disorders that affect the respiratory system. Patient services may be performed by a range of healthcare professionals, including physicians, nurses, physical therapists, and respiratory therapists.

respiratory care protocol Patient care plan initiated and implemented by a respiratory therapist, one purpose being the standardization of decision making. Respiratory care protocols provide flexibility because clinicians can modify them according to the needs of the patient; also referred to as therapist-driven protocols (TDPs), patient-driven protocols (PDPs), or simply protocols.

respiratory distress syndrome Condition of a newborn characterized by dyspnea with cyanosis; the most common cause for hypoxemic respiratory failure in premature neonates.

respiratory effort–related arousal A sequence of breaths lasting 10 seconds characterized by increasing respiratory effort leading to an arousal from sleep, when the sequence of breaths does not meet the criteria for apnea or hypopnea.

respiratory exchange ratio (RER) Ratio of $\dot{V}CO_2$ to $\dot{V}O_2$ ($\dot{V}CO_2/\dot{V}O_2$). During steady state exercise at moderate to low levels of exertion, the RER reflects the respiratory quotient (RQ), which is the ratio of $\dot{V}CO_2$ to $\dot{V}O_2$ in the mitochondria.

respiratory inductance plethysmography (RIP) Method for indirectly measuring tidal volume; sensors use a circuit of coiled wire woven into an elastic band and excited by an AC current. Inductance results from alternating electrical currents creating magnetic fields around themselves and those changing magnetic fields altering other electrical currents that they encounter.

respiratory quotient Ratio of carbon dioxide produced to oxygen consumed in the stoichiometric oxidation of a particular substrate.

resting energy expenditure (REE) Energy requirements, either estimated by prediction equations or measured by calorimetry.

restrictive lung disease An abnormality detected by spirometry characterized by reduced lung volumes.

retinopathy of prematurity Formation of fibrous tissue behind the lens of the eye caused by excessive oxygen administration to premature infants; produces blindness in its worst form; also called retrolental fibroplasia.

retrospective payment system (RPS) A system of reimbursement based on costs actually incurred.

retrospective studies Studies that look back at records to study what has been done.

Reynolds number Dimensionless number that describes factors associated with generation of laminar or turbulent flow such that units of measurement cancel each other when consistent units are used; the associated equation demonstrates that density and viscosity are independent factors affecting turbulence. On a qualitative basis, the Reynolds number describes a ratio of inertial forces to viscous forces.

rhonchus Deep, rumbling respiratory sound that is more pronounced in auscultation on expiration and is usually continuous, caused by air passing through an partially obstructed airway.

ribonucleic acid (RNA) Nucleic acid in which the sugar component is ribose; acts as the machinery for the protein synthesis process by translating the genetic information stored in DNA into protein structures.

rigid bronchoscope A metal tube introduced into the central airways for diagnostic and therapeutic purposes.

risk of mortality The likelihood of dying.

rocking bed Unconventional ventilation device with action that has been compared to a piston in a cylinder. As the patient's head moves down, the piston-like viscera and diaphragm slide cephalad within the cylinder-like chest wall, assisting exhalation. In the foot-down position, the abdominal contents and diaphragm slide caudad, assisting inhalation.

root-cause analysis (RCA) A structured process for identifying the causal or contributing factors underlying adverse events or other critical incidents.

S

Sanz electrode Modern pH electrode, which has a small sampling chamber, allowing the use of aliquots of blood volume as small as 25 μL.

sarcoidosis Interstitial lung disease (ILD) in which multiple organ systems usually have noncaseating granulomas; most prevalent ILD of unknown etiology.

sarcopenia Age-related loss of muscle mass, which starts to develop somewhere between ages 40 and 60 for both sexes.

saturated fatty acid Naturally occurring fatty acid that has all available bonds of its hydrocarbon chain filled with hydrogen atoms so that the chain contains all single carbon–carbon bonds.

saturated Strength of a solution indicating that it contains the maximum amount of a given dissolved solute for given conditions.

SBAR Situation, Background, Assessment, Recommendation—a technique that provides a framework for communication between members of the healthcare team about a patient's condition.

sclerosing agent A chemical introduced into the pleural space to cause pleurodesis.

scoliosis Lateral curvature of the spine.

secondary ARDS Acute lung injury caused by indirect injury to the lung such as sepsis and multiple trauma.

secondary survey The portion of the history and physical examination of the trauma patient that follows the identification and treatment of life-threatening injuries of the primary survey (ABCDE). The secondary survey includes a head-to-toe physical examination and a thorough history delineating allergies, current medications used, past illnesses and pregnancies, last meal, and events or environment related to the traumatic injury.

segments Subdivisions within each lobe of the lungs; each segment corresponds to the distribution of a specific bronchus.

self-inflating bag Manual resuscitator that inflates automatically and does not require an external gas source to provide positive pressure.

self-instructional A learning technique in which a learner (with others or alone) works without the direct control of a teacher.

semipermeable membrane Structure that separates the body's various compartments from one another and allows certain fluids and solutes to move freely between them.

sensitivity In the context of data analysis, the proportion of actual positives that are correctly identified as such.

sentinel event An adverse event in which death or serious harm to a patient has occurred; usually used to refer to events that are not at all expected or acceptable—for example, an accidental patient-ventilator disconnect.

serum electrolyte Substance found in the blood that dissociates into ions when melted or dissolved and is able to conduct an electric current; the most common serum electrolytes are the cations Na^+, K^+, Ca^{+2}, and Mg^{+2} and the anions HCO_3^-, Cl^-, PO_4^-, and SO_4^-.

severe persistent asthma Highest level of the four classes of asthma severity, manifesting symptoms of coughing or wheezing almost continually with frequent exacerbations often persisting for multiple days or sometimes weeks; involves symptoms that limit normal daily activities of living or normal nighttime sleep patterns, with nocturnal symptoms of coughing, wheezing, or breathlessness almost every night and measured FEV_1 or peak expiratory flow (PEF) routinely less than 60% of predicted or personal best, while consistently maintaining more than 30% variability in PEF rates.

Severinghaus electrode Modern P_{CO_2} electrode, a modification of the electrode developed by Stowe in the early 1950s.

severity of illness The extent of physiologic decompensation or organ system loss of function.

short-acting β_2-agonists Also known as rescue medicines, these medications are used for quick relief of asthma symptoms.

shunt Any cardiac or pulmonary condition in which blood passes from the right side of the heart to the left side of the heart without participating in gas exchange.

silhouette sign Radiologic sign, usually an obliterated border, that helps to localize a radiographic opacity; for example, if the contiguous lung becomes opacified from any cause, the normal contrast between these structures is lost and the border between them is obliterated, producing the silhouette sign.

silicone stent An airway stent constructed of a silicone sleeve and introduced into the central airways via a rigid bronchoscope.

simple oxygen mask A low-flow, variable-performance oxygen delivery device.

single-breath nitrogen test A test of ventilation distribution.

sinoatrial (SA) node The heart's natural pacemaker, located in the upper part of the right atrium.

skilled nursing facility (SNF) Institution or part of an institution that fulfills criteria for accreditation outlined by the sections of the Social Security Act that determine the basis for Medicaid and Medicare reimbursement for skilled nursing care.

sleep apnea Sleep disorder in which a person temporarily does not maintain airflow through the nose and mouth, resulting in periodic absence of breathing.

sleep apnea hypopnea syndrome Sleep disorder that affects people's breathing for short periods of time during sleep.

sleep efficiency Sleep study scoring category that measures the amount of time a patient is asleep per electroencephalographic criteria divided by the total recording time.

sleep latency Sleep study scoring category that measures the time from when lights are turned off to when the patient falls asleep.

sleep spindles A burst of brain activity visible on an EEG that occurs during stage 2 sleep.

sleep stages The phases of sleep that are based on the frequencies recorded during an electroencephalogram (EEG).

small cell lung cancer (SCLC) Type of lung cancer characterized histologically by the presence of small blue cells on hematoxylin and eosin staining; believed to arise from bronchial neuroendocrine cells.

smoking cessation program A structured program to assist individuals to quit smoking.

sniff test Test performed under fluoroscopy to confirm the elevation of a hemidiaphragm resulting from paralysis by demonstrating paradoxical upward movement of the affected hemidiaphragm when the patient sniffs rapidly.

solitary pulmonary nodule (SPN) Lesion, seen on a chest radiograph, that is completely surrounded by lung parenchyma, without other radiographic abnormalities such as pleural effusion or adenopathy.

solute Solid, liquid, or gaseous material that is being dissolved.

solution Homogeneous mixture of two or more substances, meaning that the substances mix evenly and occupy the entire volume in equal proportions.

solvent Liquid material into which a solute is dissolved.

spacer Simple open-ended tube or bag that, with sufficiently large device volume, provides space for the pressurized metered dose inhaler plume to expand by allowing the propellant to evaporate.

speaking valve Device designed to enable a patient with a tracheostomy to verbally communicate.

specialty sections Nine divisions within the American Association for Respiratory Care (AARC) that support various major subsets of therapists, including the following: Management, Education, Perinatal/Pediatrics, Adult Acute Care, Home Care, Subacute Care, Transport, Diagnostics, and Continuing Care and Rehabilitation; members of the AARC belong to different specialty sections based on their work activities and their personal interests in the profession of respiratory care.

specific heat Ability of water to lose and gain large amounts of heat with little change in temperature.

specificity In the context of data analysis, the proportion of negatives that are correctly identified.

spectrophotometry Method that identifies substances by their absorption (also called extinction) of specific wavelengths in the electromagnetic spectrum.

spirochetes Spiral-shaped bacteria.

spirometer A device used to measure lung volumes and flows; most commonly used for the forced vital capacity maneuver.

spirometry Breathing tests used to measure the forced vital capacity, forced inspiratory vital capacity, slow vital capacity, and maximal voluntary ventilation.

spontaneous breath Inspiration that is patient triggered and patient cycled.

spontaneous breathing trial (SBT) A technique in which the patient is removed from ventilatory support and allowed to breath spontaneously to identify extubation readiness.

sputum induction Method of facilitating the coughing up of material from the lungs, often through the administration of bland aerosols. Induced sputum contains a higher proportion of viable cells than spontaneous sputum.

squamous cell carcinoma Slow-growing malignant tumor of scaly or platelike epithelium.

standard deviation A measure of the dispersion of data about its mean.

standard precautions A group of infection prevention practices that apply to all patients regardless of suspected or confirmed infection status in any setting where healthcare is practiced.

Starling's law of cardiac function Statement that the longer the initial sarcomere length, the greater the force generated with contraction.

steatorrhea Greater than normal amounts of fat in the feces, characterized by frothy, floating fecal matter with a foul odor; seen in celiac disease, some malabsorption syndromes, and any condition in which fats are malabsorbed by the small intestine.

sterilization Equipment-processing modality that involves the complete killing of all organisms; requires adequate heat and time. A process that destroys or eliminates all forms of microbial life.

steroid Important lipid group widely distributed throughout the body and involved in many important structural and functional roles.

strain Physical deformation or change in shape of a structure or substance, usually caused by stress.

stress Force applied to an area.

stress test Functional study of the coronary circulation using a stressor to induce an imbalance between the coronary blood supply and myocardial demand; a means to detect the ischemic response.

stridor Crowing inspiratory sound, commonly caused by inflammation and edema of the larynx, such as postextubation or croup.

stroke Cerebrovascular accident; sudden brain abnormality characterized by occlusion by an embolus, thrombus, or cerebrovascular hemorrhage, resulting in ischemia of the brain tissues normally perfused by the damaged vessels.

stroke volume Absolute volume of blood ejected during a single contraction of a ventricle.

strong ion difference (SID) Net negative or positive charge exerted by strong ions; principle similar to that of the anion gap, but with the advantage of functioning as an independent variable in acid–base regulation.

subacute care Programs and facilities for patients who are sufficiently stabilized that they no longer require acute care services, but whose care is too complex for treatments in a traditional nursing center and who present with rehabilitation or medically complex needs and require physiologic monitoring, including respiratory care services.

subarachnoid (intracerebral) hematoma A traumatic brain injury that results in the accumulation of blood in the space between the arachnoid mater and the pia mater that attaches directly to the brain. Subarachnoid hematomas often are caused by the traumatic rupture of brain aneurysms or direct bleeding from brain parenchyma.

subcutaneous emphysema Air accumulation in the tissues, associated with alveolar rupture.

subcutaneous Route of drug administration (SC or SQ) that involves the injection of drug into the dermal or subdermal layer of skin, where it is taken up by the capillary bed.

subdural hematoma A traumatic brain injury that results in the accumulation of blood in the space between the arachnoid mater and the dura mater. It is often caused by the shearing of bridging veins that run in this potential space.

suction catheter A flexible tube that is used to aspirate secretions.

surface tension Property of liquid tending to reduce the surface of a liquid to a minimum.

surfactant Surface-active agent, such as soap or detergent, dissolved in water to decrease its surface tension or the tension between the water and another liquid.

surrogate Individual appointed by a patient, in a legal document such as an advanced directive, living will, or medical power of attorney, to make decisions for that patient in the event that the patient cannot.

surveys Collecting quantitative information about a population, usually via questionnaires.

suspension Liquid mixture in which particles consist of large clumps of molecules; properties include the following: consisting of an insoluble substance dispersed in a liquid, being heterogeneous, not being clear, settling out over time, not passing through filter paper, and not passing through membranes.

sweat test Method of assessing sodium and chloride excretion from the sweat glands; often the first test done in the diagnosis of cystic fibrosis.

synchronized intermittent mandatory ventilation (SIMV) Mode of breath delivery or ventilation in which a mandatory breath rate is set and the patient determines the tidal volume and rate of the spontaneous breaths between the mandatory breaths, which are synchronized with the patient's spontaneous efforts.

systematic review A literature review focused on a single question that tries to identify, appraise, select and synthesize all high-quality research evidence relevant to that question.

Système International d'Unités (SI system) Internationally agreed system of units in wide, but not universal use; the generally preferred system in scientific and healthcare settings.

systemic lupus erythematosus (SLE) Autoimmune disease that can affect almost all the organ systems. Complications are classified as pleuritis and pleural effusions, acute lupus pneumonitis, interstitial lung disease, and respiratory muscle weakness.

systemic vascular resistance (SVR) The resistance against which the left ventricle must force its stroke volume with each beat.

systole Period of contraction in the cardiac cycle during which the heart pumps blood into the pulmonary and systemic circulation.

systolic Pertaining to the systole; the peak of a blood pressure measurement.

systolic dysfunction Impaired ventricular contractility.

T

tachypnea Increased respiratory rate.

tactile fremitus Palpation of vibrations of the chest wall as a patient speaks.

target During mechanical ventilation, if one (or more) of the inspiratory variables rises no higher than some preset value, the variable is a target variable.

targeting scheme The feedback control scheme used to shape the breath and determine the breath sequence during mechanical ventilation.

teaching moment Any opportunity to impart critical and meaningful information to a captive audience.

teleological theory Ethical theory that guides decision making regarding the right or wrong qualities of an action based on the consequences of predicted outcomes.

temperature The amount of heat, or thermal energy, present in a system.

tetraplegia Paralysis of all four limbs; quadriplegia.

The Joint Commission See *Joint Commission.*

therapeutic bronchoscopy A bronchoscopic procedure aimed at relieving central airways obstruction.

therapist-driven protocols (TDPs) Patient care plans that are initiated and implemented by respiratory therapists.

thermistor Thermometer that can measure extremely small changes in temperature.

thermocouple Apparatus that detects bidirectional airflow at the nose and mouth by sensing the temperature difference between inspired room air and exhaled air that has been warmed to body temperature; an active sensor used to measure temperature.

thermodilution Method of measuring cardiac output by injecting a cold or cool indicator and sampling with a thermistor.

third-party payer Another term for the insurer, when considered as one of the stakeholders in the provision and delivery of healthcare services. One of the five major stakeholders in the healthcare delivery system.

thoracentesis Removal of pleural fluid from the chest cavity using a needle or small catheter.

thorax Lungs, pleura, respiratory muscles, and skeletal elements, including the sternum, ribs, thoracic vertebrae, the clavicles, and the scapulae; within the thorax, the mediastinum contains major blood vessels, the esophagus, and the heart enveloped within the pericardial sac.

Thorpe tube flow meter Flow control device that provides an accurate display of flow, provided it is in a vertical position and the inlet pressure is constant. Unlike flow restrictors and Bourdon gauges, pressure-compensated Thorpe tube flow meters display the actual outlet flow in the face of downstream resistance.

thrombolytic Any of several drugs that help dissolve clots, such as streptokinase, urokinase, and tissue plasminogen activator (TPA).

thrombolytic therapy (TT) Use of drugs such as tissue plasminogen activator, urokinase, or streptokinase to dissolve an arterial clot.

time constant Measure of the time required for the passive respiratory system to respond to abrupt changes in ventilatory pressure; expressed in units of time (usually seconds) and calculated as resistance times compliance.

timed walk test Test focused on functional performance that generally involves having a patient walk over a measured course for a set duration of time (for example, 6 or 12 minutes). Patients are encouraged to go as far as they can, and supplemental oxygen is given as necessary.

tissue plasminogen activator (TPA) Common thrombolytic agent used to help dissolve clots.

tonometry Measurement of exact gas tensions in whole, fresh blood; because of the unique O_2-binding characteristics of hemoglobin and the complex viscosity characteristics of normal fresh blood, whole blood must be carefully tonometered so that exact gas tensions can be prepared for analysis by a blood gas instrument.

total body surface area (TBSA) Area of involvement in thermal injury represented as a percentage of the whole body.

total face mask An interface for noninvasive ventilation (NIV) or continuous positive airway pressure (CPAP) that fits over the entire face of the patient.

total parenteral nutrition (TPN) Administration of a nutritionally adequate hypertonic solution that can meet the needs of a patient who cannot eat by mouth.

trachea The tubelike segment of the respiratory tract between the larynx and the carina.

tracheostomy tube Hollow, curved tube of metal, rubber, or plastic that is surgically inserted in the trachea to relieve a breathing obstruction.

transactional Reciprocal or give-and-take relationship between two or more individuals in which each alternates between being a sender and a receiver, each engaging in constant sending and receiving in the form of both verbal and nonverbal feedback.

transbronchial biopsy See *transbronchial lung biopsy*.

transbronchial lung biopsy Primary bronchoscopic technique for evaluating the alveolar compartment, particularly useful for sampling peripheral parenchymal masses, diagnosing a select number of specific interstitial lung diseases, and obtaining tissue specimens for culture or documentation of tissue invasion or microorganism pathogenicity.

transbronchial needle aspiration (TBNA) Innovative bronchoscopic diagnostic technique used for staging mediastinal lymph nodes in suspected bronchogenic lung cancer, diagnosing submucosally infiltrating or extrinsically compressing tumors, approaching endobronchial tumors with necrotic or friable outer layers, and, increasingly, diagnosing peripheral nodules.

transcutaneous monitoring A means of respiratory monitoring of blood gases through electrodes applied to the skin.

transdiaphragmatic pressure (Pdi) Specific measure of diaphragm strength; made by measuring esophageal (Pes) and gastric (Pga) pressures via balloon-tipped catheters placed in the midesophagus and in the stomach, respectively. Pdi is then calculated as the algebraic subtraction of Pes from Pga (Pdi = Pga – Pes).

transesophageal echocardiography (TEE) Diagnostic test in which a small ultrasound transducer is passed posterior to the heart via the esophagus, allowing close investigation of valvular heart disease because of the proximity of the transesophageal probe to the heart and the absence of intervening anatomic barriers such as the thoracic ribs; includes all aspects of transthoracic imaging, including two-dimensional, Doppler, and color Doppler techniques.

transient tachypnea of the newborn A self-limiting disorder that presents in term or near-term infants shortly after birth and is characterized by rapid respirations that usually resolve within 24 to 48 hours.

transpulmonary pressure The difference between alveolar pressure and pleural pressure; the stretching pressure on the alveolus.

transrespiratory pressure Ventilator or muscle pressure generated to expand the thoracic cage and lungs during inspiration (i.e., airway pressure minus body surface pressure).

transthoracic needle aspiration (TNA) Sensitive, specific tissue sampling and testing used in the diagnosis of pneumonia, especially that caused by anaerobic organisms.

transtracheal aspiration (TTA) Technique for collecting sputum that was designed to bypass the upper airway, with its potential contaminants, by inserting a sterile needle directly into the trachea through the cricothyroid membrane and aspirating tracheal secretions.

transtracheal oxygen catheter Small-diameter Teflon catheter that is surgically inserted into the trachea between the second and third tracheal rings, connected to a small flange, and held in place by an adjustable chain. Oxygen supply tubing connects directly to the catheter and delivers oxygen into the midtrachea.

transtracheal oxygen Passing oxygen directly into the trachea. A transtracheal catheter passes from the skin of the lower neck through a tract and directly into the trachea. Oxygen is usually delivered at a lower flow rate because the upper airway dead space is bypassed.

transudative A classification of pleural fluid based on laboratory findings suggestive of a hydrostatic cause of pleural fluid accumulation.

trigger Variable used for initiation of the inspiratory phase (pressure, volume, flow, or time).

triglyceride Most abundant lipid, which functions as the body's most concentrated source of energy; its basic building blocks are a glycerol molecule and three fatty acids.

troponin A complex of three regulatory proteins that is integral to muscle contraction in skeletal and cardiac muscle, but not smooth muscle; useful as a diagnostic marker for various heart disorders.

troubleshooting Key skill used in critical thinking; involves the ability to locate, correct, and process technical problems; sometimes called "technical think."

tube exchanger A flexible tube used to maintain a pathway to the trachea in order to allow changing one endotracheal tube for another.

tuberculosis Infection that arises by inhalation of *Mycobacterium tuberculum* organisms from infected, coughing individuals and manifesting with malaise, fever, or no symptoms.

tumor suppressor gene Genetic unit that is able to reverse the effect of a specific kind of mutation in certain tumors.

turbulent flow Mixture of fluid velocities in which friction has a particularly prominent effect (as opposed to laminar flow) and which varies directly with the square of the flow rate; it carries a term for friction, implying greater resistance at equivalent flows.

turgor The normal rigid state of fullness of a cell or blood vessel or capillary resulting from pressure of the contents against the wall or membrane.

tympanic Quality of the loud, drumlike, high-pitched sound typically heard over a gastric bubble during percussion examination.

type I cells Alveolar epithelial cells that form part of the alveolocapillary complex and cover a large portion (90%) of the alveolar surface, facilitating the movement of gases across this surface.

type I error A type of error that occurs if a difference is considered important when, statistically, there is a good probability (>5%) that the difference could be due to chance.

type II cells Alveolar cells that produce surfactant and surfactant-associated proteins.

type II error A type of error that occurs if a difference is not considered important when an insufficient number of tests (or comparisons) have been performed to test the question.

typical pneumonia Any of several pneumonias usually caused by pneumococci, but also by *Haemophilus influenzae*, Enterobacteriaceae, and *Staphylococcus aureus*; characterized by abrupt onset of chills, high fever, pleuritic chest pain, and cough productive of rusty or purulent sputum. Physical signs of consolidation such as bronchial breath sounds and inspiratory crackles are present; lobar or segmental consolidation is seen on the chest radiograph, and leukocytosis is present.

U

ultrasonic nebulizer Device that uses a piezoelectric crystal, vibrating at a high frequency, to convert electricity to sound waves, creating standing waves in the liquid immediately above the transducer, disrupting the liquid surface, and forming a geyser of aerosolized droplets.

Universal Protocol A protocol developed to prevent wrong site, wrong procedure and/or wrong person surgery. The three principal components are conducting a preprocedure verification process, marking the procedure site, and performing a time-out before the procedure.

unmeasured anions Anionic proteins and other substances in serum that are not measured in routine serum electrolyte determinations but whose presence can be suspected by calculating the anion gap.

unsaturated fatty acid Naturally occurring fatty acid that has one or more double carbon–carbon bonds in its hydrocarbon chain because not all of the chain carbon atoms are saturated with hydrogen atoms.

uvulopalatopharyngoplasty (UPPP) Oldest and most commonly performed surgery to treat obstructive sleep apnea.

V

v wave On the central venous pressure tracing, the v wave arises from the pressure produced when the blood filling the right atrium comes up against a closed tricuspid valve. It occurs as the T wave is ending on an electrocardiogram.

valance electron An electron in the outer shell of an atom.

valved holding chamber A device used with a pressurized metered dose inhaler that consists of a spacer with a one-way valve to prevent loss of the dose.

valvular heart disease Any valvular lesion or abnormality that can be differentiated hemodynamically into two types, although a combination of both may exist: stenotic lesions due to a decreased valve orifice size or impaired valve opening, or regurgitant lesions due to impairment of valve closure.

valvular regurgitation Condition in which a proportion of the ventricular stroke volume moves retrograde through the value.

valvular stenosis Narrowing of a heart valve.

vapor pressure A colligative property of a solution that depends on the number of solute particles dissolved and not on chemical properties; for example, a solute added to a solvent dilutes it, displacing solution surface solvent particles and allowing fewer solvent particles to escape in the form of gas, thereby reducing the vapor pressure.

variance Difference between patient care and outcomes described in a pathway, protocol, or guideline and what actually happens. The difference between what you expect and what you actually find.

vasopressor Agent used to increase blood pressure through vasoconstriction.

vehicle transmission A form of indirect contact transmission that involves transfer of an infectious agent through a contaminated intermediate object.

velocity Property of flow that determines diffusion and is inversely proportional to the square root of the molecular weight of a substance; equivalent to the kinetic energy of a fluid.

venous return Filling of the heart with blood from the venous circulation.

ventilation-perfusion ($\dot{V}/\dot{Q}$) mismatch A condition in which there is a derangement in the normal relationship between alveolar ventilation and pulmonary blood flow.

ventilation-perfusion ratio Measure of effective gas exchange in the lung, or $\dot{V}/\dot{Q}$ ratio; this ratio should be 1 for the most effective gas exchange to occur.

ventilator liberation The procedure whereby a patient is removed from ventilatory support, after after completion of a successful spontaneous breathing trial.

ventilator-associated pneumonia (VAP) Pneumonia in a mechanically ventilated patient developing after at least 48 hours of mechanical ventilation.

ventilator-induced lung injury Damage to the lungs sustained during mechanical ventilation and caused by any of several factors, including alveolar overdistention and/or cyclical opening of an alveolus during inhalation and closure during exhalation.

ventilatory equivalent The relationship between minute ventilation and oxygen consumption or carbon dioxide production.

ventilatory period Cycle time (or total cycle time); the reciprocal of ventilatory frequency.

ventricles Small cavities making up two of the four chambers of the heart.

ventricular interdependence Interaction between the left ventricle (LV) and the right ventricle (RV) both in systole and diastole through alterations in systemic and pulmonary venous return, LV and RV dimensional changes, and functional changes.

ventriculography Radiographic examination of a ventricle of the heart after injection of a radiopaque contrast medium.

Venturi principle Physical rule stating that pressure drop across an obstruction can be restored provided that the angle of divergence is less than 15 degrees.

veracity Principle by which the healthcare practitioner tells the patient the truth.

verbal expression Set of communication tools that includes language, jargon, choice of words or questions, voice tone and quality, and feedback.

vesicular breath sounds Low-pitched, low-intensity sounds heard over healthy lung issue.

vibration therapy Maneuver used as part of conventional chest physiotherapy to assist patients in mobilizing secretions from the lower respiratory tract.

videobronchoscope A bronchoscope that is constructed using a charged coupled device to form an image on a video monitor during its use.

viral pneumonia Uncommon but often severe pneumonia caused by any of the following viruses: influenza, parainfluenza, respiratory syncytial virus (RSV), cytomegalovirus (CMV), adenovirus, measles, varicella zoster, herpes simplex, Epstein-Barr, and hantavirus.

virologic studies Methods designed to determine the presence of viruses and their identification.

viruses Small infectious agents that replicate only within cells of living organisms.

visceral pleura Inner layer of pleura adjacent to the external lung tissue.

viscosity Force applied to interaction between adjacent fluid molecules; also, the internal friction of a fluid, which is independent of the density of that fluid.

vital capacity The maximum volume of gas that can be exhaled from the lungs after a maximal inspiration or inhaled from a point of maximal exhalation.

vitamins A group of organic substances essential in small quantities to normal metabolism.

volume control ventilation (VCV) Mode of ventilation in which the ventilator controls the inspiratory flow and tidal volume is determined by the flow and the inspiratory time; the tidal volume in this mode is delivered regardless of resistance or compliance.

voxels Volume elements that make up a computed tomography (CT) slice image.

W

weaning Removing a patient gradually from dependency on mechanical ventilation while maintaining an appropriate balance between the load placed on the respiratory muscles and the ability of the muscles to meet that load.

weaning parameters Measurements made to determine when liberation from the ventilator might be possible.

wedge pressure See *pulmonary artery wedge pressure* (*PAWP*).

wellness A multidimensional state of being describing the existence of positive health in an individual as exemplified by quality of life and a sense of well-being.

wellness programs Programs aimed at keeping people healthy through classes that educate consumers so that they can maintain, and possibly even improve, their quality of life, covering such topics as the benefits of diet, good sleep habits, relaxation techniques, routine exercise, diagnostic screenings, and the psychosocial aspects of health, with an emphasis on preventing disease and establishing and maintaining healthy habits for life.

Westermark sign Decreased vascularity in one lung causing a unilateral increase in radiographic lucency; suggests the presence of a large pulmonary embolus.

wheezes Form of rhonchus characterized by either a high- or low-pitched musical quality, caused by high-velocity airflow through a narrowed airway.

whispered pectoriloquy Voice sound heard during auscultation of the lungs, typically heard with lung consolidation.

"white lab jacket" phenomenon Creation of an aura of instant credibility, acceptance, recognition, and stature that affords the wearer the opportunity to ask intimate questions and perform physical assessments.

Wood units A simplified measurement of vascular resistance that uses pressures instead of more complicated units; in the case of pulmonary vascular resistance, measured by subtracting pulmonary capillary wedge pressure from the mean pulmonary arterial pressure and dividing by cardiac output in liters per minute.

work The amount of energy transferred by a force acting through a distance; for work of breathing, the amount of pressure required to deliver a volume of gas into the lungs.

work of breathing Pressure needed to move a volume of gas into the lungs.

work rate Rate at which work is performed or energy is converted.

Index

Figures and tables are indicated by f *and* t *following the page number.*

B

C

D

E

F

G

H

J

K

L

M

N

Q

R

S

T

U

W

X

Y

Z

Photo Credits

Chapter 1

1-2 © Martin Kubát/ShutterStock, Inc.; **1-6 (top)** © Custom Medical Stock Photo; **1-6 (bottom)** © M. English, MD/Custom Medical Stock Photo; **1-7A (left and right)** Courtesy of Darci Manley; **1-7B (left)** © Dr. P. Marazzi/SPL/Photo Researchers, Inc.; **1-7B (right)** © Apogee/Photo Researchers, Inc.; **1-7C (left)** © Wellcome Trust Library/Custom Medical Stock Photo; **1-7C (right)** © medicalpicture/Alamy Images; **1-8A** © Biophoto Associates/Photo Researchers, Inc.; **1-8B** © Jorge Salcedo/ShutterStock, Inc.

Chapter 4

4-5 Courtesy of Abbott, Point of Care

Chapter 5

5-5A–E Courtesy of Nonin Medical, Inc.; **5-12** Courtesy of Oridion Medical; **5-14, 5-15** Courtesy of Covidien. Used with permission; **5-21 (top and bottom)** Courtesy of SenTec AG

Chapter 7

7-2A–B, 7-5A–B, 7-6 Courtesy of Geoffrey A. Rose, MD, FACC, FASE

Chapter 9

9-3A–B This article was published in *Chest X-Ray Made Easy.* Corne J, Carroll M, Brown I, Delany D. Copyright Elsevier (Churchill Livingstone) 1997; **9-4B** This article was published in *Felson's Principles of Chest Roentgenology: A Programmed Text. 3rd ed.* Goodman LR. Copyright Elsevier (Saunders) 2007; **9-5B** This article was published in *Felson's Principles of Chest Roentgenology: A Programmed Text. 3rd ed.* Goodman LR. Copyright Elsevier (Saunders) 2007; **9-8** © emedicine.com, 2010; **9-26A–B** Courtesy of Ariel L Shiloh, MD, Division of Critical Care Medicine, Montefiore Medical Center, The Albert Einstein College of Medicine

Chapter 10

10-1 Courtesy of ndd Medical Technologies; **10-2** © Architecte®/ShutterStock, Inc.; **10-18** Courtesy of Morgan Scientific, Inc.; **10-19** Courtesy of Morgan Scientific, Inc.; **10-24** Courtesy of Chess, Medical Technology; **10-25** Courtesy of Dr. Paul Enright

Chapter 11

11-1, 11-3, 11-4, 11-5, 11-6, 11-7, 11-8, 11-9, 11-10, 11-11, 11-12, 11-13, 11-14, 11-15, 11-16, 11-17, 11-18, 11-19 Courtesy Dr. Scott Shofer; **11-20** Courtesy of CareFusion Corporation or one of its subsidiaries, 2010. All rights reserved

Chapter 12

12-3, 12-4, 12-5, 12-6, 12-7, 12-8, 12-9, 12-10 Courtesy of Bashir Chaudhary, Susan Whiddon, and Shelley Mishoe

Chapter 13

13-2, 13-3 Courtesy of CareFusion Corporation or one of its subsidiaries, 2010. All rights reserved

Chapter 15

15-3 Used with permission of Philips Respironics, Murrysville, PA; **15-11 (top and bottom), 15-15** Courtesy of Western/Scott Fetzer Company

Chapter 16

16-4B Courtesy of Western/Scott Fetzer Company; **16-9C** Courtesy of Teleflex Incorporated. Unauthorized use prohibited; **16-10B** © Corbis/age footstock; **16-11C** © Andrew Gentry/ShutterStock, Inc.; **16-13 (top and bottom)** Courtesy of Fisher & Paykel Healthcare, Inc.; **16-14B** Courtesy of Teleflex Incorporated. Unauthorized use prohibited; **16-17** Courtesy Jeffrey J. Ward, RRT; **16-19** © Vital Signs, Inc. All Rights Reserved; **16-21C** Courtesy of CareFusion Corporation or one of its subsidiaries, 2010. All rights reserved; **16-22** © brt PHOTO/Alamy Images; **16-23** Courtesy of Amvex Corporation; **16-28A–B** Courtesy of IKARIA

Chapter 17

17-4 (left) Courtesy of Fisher & Paykel Healthcare, Inc.; **17-4 (right)** Courtesy of Teleflex Incorporated. Unauthorized use prohibited; **17-5B** Images courtesy of Cardinal Health; **17-9B** © 2010 Kimberly-Clark Worldwide, Inc. Used with permission; **17-14A** Used with permission of Philips Respironics, Murrysville, PA; **17-17** Reproduced from *Arch Dis Child*, Brodie T. and Adalat S., vol. 91, page 961, © 2006, with permission from BMJ Publishing Group Ltd.; **17-18A** Courtesy of Valeant Pharmaceuticals; **17-20B** Courtesy of Westmed, Inc.; **17-20C** Courtesy of B&B Medical Technologies; **17-21B (left)** Courtesy of Omron Healthcare; **17-21B (middle)** Courtesy of evo Medical Solutions; **17-21B (right)** Courtesy of eFlow LLC (PARI Pharma GmbH); **17-22A-C** © 2010 Boehringer Ingelheim International GmbH, Germany. All rights reserved; **17-24** Courtesy of United Therapeutics Corporation, used with permission; **17-25B** © M. Dykstra/ShutterStock, Inc.; **17-26A** Copyright GlaxoSmithKline. Used with permission; **17-26B** Courtesy of Doser-MediTrack Products; **17-27 (left)** Courtesy of Graceway Pharmaceuticals, LLC; **17-28 (top left)** Used with permission of Philips Respironics, Murrysville, PA; **17-28 (top right)** © Rob Byron/ShutterStock, Inc.; **17-28 (bottom right)** © Robeo/Dreamstime.com; **17-31B** © Denis Mironov/ShutterStock, Inc.; **17-31C** © Marjanneke de Jong/ShutterStock, Inc.; **17-31D** © mayer kleinostheim/ShutterStock, Inc.; **17-31E** © Silentiger/Dreamstime.com; **17-37 (top)** Courtesy of Teleflex Incorporated. Unauthorized use prohibited; **17-34 (bottom)** Courtesy of Smiths Medical

Chapter 18

18-4 Courtesy of Covidien. Used with permission; **18-5A** Courtesy of Prodimed; **18-5B–C** Courtesy of KOL Bio-Medical Instruments, Inc.; **18-10** Used with permission of Philips Respironics, Murrysville, PA; **18-13B, 15-15** Courtesy of Smiths Medical; **18-16** Courtesy of Thayer Medical Corporation; **18-17A** © 2010 Hill-Rom Services, Inc. REPRINTED WITH PERMISSION-ALL RIGHTS RESERVED; **18-17B** Courtesy of RespirTech; **18-17C** Courtesy of Electromed, Inc.; **18-19A–B** Courtesy of Dr. Pamela Bird, Percussionaire Corporation; **18-19C** Courtesy of VORTRAN® Medical Technology1, Inc., Sacramento, CA; **18-23B (top)** © Robert Byron/Dreamstime.com; **18-23B (bottom)** Courtesy of Teleflex Incorporated. Unauthorized use prohibited; **18-24A** Courtesy of VORTRAN® Medical Technology1, Inc., Sacramento, CA; **18-24B** Courtesy of Dr. Pamela Bird, Percussionaire Corporation

Chapter 19

19-2, 19-5 Courtesy of Smiths Medical; **19-12, 19-13A** Image used by permission from Nellcor Puritan Bennett LLC, Boulder, Colorado, part of Covidien; **19-20A–B** Courtesy of Airtraq LLC, www.airtraq.com; Used with permission; **19-21** Courtesy of Verthon, Inc.; **19-22** Courtesy of LMA, Inc.; **19-23** Courtesy of Verthon, Inc.; **19-26** Courtesy of LMA North America, Inc.; **19-31** Courtesy of B&B Medical Technologies; **19-32** Courtesy of Cook Medical; **19-33A (right), 19-33B** Courtesy of Smiths Medical; **19-33C** Courtesy of the Department of Otolaryngology—Head and Neck Surgery, Johns Hopkins Medicine; **19-34A-B** Image used by permission from Nellcor Puritan Bennett LLC, Boulder, Colorado, part of Covidien; **19-35, 19-36,19-38 (middle and bottom)** Courtesy of Smiths Medical; **19-39B (top and bottom)** Images used by permission from Nellcor Puritan Bennett LLC, Boulder, Colorado, part of Covidien; **19-41B** Courtesy of Boston Medical Products, Inc.; **19-43B (right)** Courtesy of J.T. Posey Company, Arcadia, California; **19-46, 19-47** Courtesy of Covidien. Used with permission; **19-48** Image reproduced with kind permission of Pennine Healthcare; **19-49** Courtesy of medisize, www.medisize.com

Chapter 20

20-10B–C © Vital Signs, Inc. All Rights Reserved; **20-23A–C** Courtesy of Advanced Circulatory System, Inc.

Chapter 22

22-1 (top left) Image used by permission from Nellcor Puritan Bennett LLC, Boulder, Colorado, part of Covidien; **22-1 (top middle)** Courtesy of Hamilton Medical, Inc.; **22-1 (top right)** Courtesy of CareFusion Corporation or one of its subsidiaries, 2010. All rights reserved; **22-1 (bottom left)** Image courtesy of GE HealthCare, used with permission; **22-1 (bottom middle)** Image courtesy of Newport Medical Instruments, Inc.; **22-1 (bottom right)** Used with permission of Philips Respironics, Murrysville, PA

Chapter 23

23-2A © ResMed 2010. Used with permission; **23-2B** Used with permission of Philips Respironics, Murrysville, PA; **23-2C** © ResMed 2010. Used with permission; **23-2D** Used with permission of Philips Respironics, Murrysville, PA; **23-2E** © ResMed 2010. Used with permission; **23-2F** Courtesy of StarMed SpA; **23-3A–C** Used with permission of Philips Respironics, Murrysville, PA; **23-3D** Courtesy of Med Systems; **23-4 (left)** Used with permission of Philips Respironics, Murrysville, PA; **23-4 (middle)** © ResMed 2010. Used with permission; **23-4 (right), 23-6 (top)** Used with permission of Philips Respironics, Murrysville, PA; **23-6 (bottom)** Courtesy of CareFusion Corporation or one of its subsidiaries, 2010. All rights reserved; **23-7 (top left)** Used with permission of Philips Respironics, Murrysville, PA; **23-7 (top middle)** © Dräger Medical AG & Co. KG, Lübeck-Germany (All rights reserved.) Not to be reproduced without written permission; **23-7 (top right), 23-7 (bottom left)** Used with permission of Philips Respironics, Murrysville, PA; **23-7 (bottom middle), 23-7 (bottom right)** © ResMed 2010. Used with permission; **23-12B** Courtesy of Ambu, Inc.; **23-12C** © Vital Signs, Inc. All Rights Reserved; **23-14 (left)** Used with permission of Philips Respironics, Murrysville, PA; **23-14 (middle)** © ResMed 2010. Used with permission; **23-14 (right)** Image used by permission from Nellcor Puritan

Bennett LLC, Boulder, Colorado, part of Covidien; **23-15 (left)** Courtesy of SP Medical; **23-15 (right), 23-16, 23-17A–B** Used with permission of Philips Respironics, Murrysville, PA; **23-18** © Division of Medicine and Science, National Museum of American History/Smithsonian Institution; **23-19A** Used with permission of Philips Respironics, Murrysville, PA

Chapter 24

24-4A–B Courtesy of Mercury Medical; **24-5** Courtesy of David J. Burchfield, MD; **24-6** Courtesy of Melissa Brown, BS, RRT-NPS; **24-7** © Stock Connection Distribution/Alamy Images; **24-8A–B** Courtesy of Hamilton Medical, Inc.; **24-10** Courtesy of Melissa Brown, BS, RRT-NPS; **24-17** Courtesy of Bunnell Incorporated; **24-19** Courtesy of CareFusion Corporation or one of its subsidiaries, 2010. All rights reserved

Chapter 26

26-1 Courtesy Ideal Industries, Inc.; **26-3** Courtesy of Richardson Products Incorporated; **26-4** Courtesy of Med Labs, Inc.; **26-5** Courtesy of x10.com; **26-10 (top left)** Used with permission of Philips Respironics, Murrysville, PA; **26-10 (top right)** Courtesy of Invacare Corporation; **26-10 (bottom), 26-11 (top left)** Courtesy of DeVilbiss Healthcare; **26-11 (top right)** Used with permission of Philips Respironics, Murrysville, PA; **26-11 (bottom)** Courtesy of Invacare Corporation; **26-12A (left)** Used with permission of Philips Respironics, Murrysville, PA; **26-12A (right), 26-12B** Courtesy of CHART, Inc.; **26-13 (top left)** Courtesy of DeVilbiss Healthcare; **26-13 (top middle)** Courtesy of SeQual Technologies, Inc.; **26-13 (top right)** Courtesy of Invacare Corporation; **26-13 (bottom left)** Used with permission of Philips Respironics, Murrysville, PA; **26-13 (bottom middle)** Courtesy of Invacare Corporation; **26-13 (bottom right)** Courtesy of Inogen; **26-15** Courtesy of CHAD Therapeutics; **26-18** Courtesy of Inspired Technologies, Inc.; **26-19** Courtesy of Oxy-View, Inc.; **26-20** Courtesy of Angela King; **26-21** Image courtesy of GE HealthCare, used with permission; **26-22** Used with permission of Philips Respironics, Murrysville, PA; **26-23, 26-24** Courtesy of Angela King

Chapter 27

27-1 (top left) Courtesy of IMPACT Instrumentation, Inc.; **27-1 (top right)** Images courtesy of Newport Medical Instruments, Inc.; **27-1 (bottom)** Courtesy of CareFusion Corporation or one of its subsidiaries, 2010. All rights reserved

Chapter 33

33-2 Courtesy of QOSINA; **33-5** Courtesy of James Gathany/CDC; **33-6** Courtesy of Bullard Company; **33-7** © pancaketom/Dreamstime.com

Chapter 34

34-4 (top left) Courtesy of CareFusion Corporation or one of its subsidiaries, 2010. All rights reserved; **34-4 (top right)** Courtesy of nSpire Health, Inc.; **34-4 (bottom left)** Courtesy of Invacare Corporation; **34-4 (bottom right)** Used with permission of Philips Respironics, Murrysville, PA

Chapter 35

35-2, 35-4A–B Courtesy of John E. Heffner, MD

Chapter 36

36-2A–B, 36-3A–B Courtesy of Andrew J. Ghio, MD/EPA

Chapter 37

37-1, 37-2, 37-3, 37-4, 37-5 Courtesy of C. William Hargett and Victor F. Tapson

Chapter 44

44-2 Courtesy of Sage Diagram, LLC; **44-3A–D, 44-4** Courtesy of Robert L. Sheridan, MD; **44-5** Reproduced from Enkhbaatar, P., Cox, R., Traber, L., et al., "Aerosolized anticoagulants ameliorate acute lung . . .," *Crit Care Med.*, vol. 35, #12, pp. 2805–2810. Reprinted with permission from Wolters Kluwer Health; **44-6** Courtesy of Robert L. Sheridan, MD; **44-7** Courtesy of ETC Bio-Medical Systems Group

Chapter 46

46-1, 46-2, 46-3, 46-4, 46-5 Courtesy of Courtesy of Bashir Chaudhary, Arthur Taft, and Shelley Mishoe

Chapter 48

48-1, 48-2, 48-3, 48-4, 48-5, 48-6, 48-7, 48-8, 48-9, 48-10, 48-11, 48-12, 48-13, 48-14, 48-15, 48-16 Courtesy of Chetan Chandulal Shah, MBBS, DMRD, MBA, Arkansas Children's Hospital

Chapter 49

49-7 Reproduced from Zamanian M, Marini JJ. "Pressure-flow signatures of central-airway mucus plugging." *Crit Care Med*, vol. 34, #1, pp. 223–226. Reprinted with permission from Wolters Kluwer Health

Chapter 52

52-2 (bottom) © Medical-on-Line/Alamy Images; **52-3** © CNRI/Photo Researchers, Inc.; **52-5** Courtesy of Janice Haney Carr/CDC; **52-6** Courtesy of Janice Haney Carr/Jeff Hageman, MHS/CDC; **52-7 (left and right)** Courtesy of Wadsworth Center, NYS Department of Health; **52-8, 52-9, 52-10** Courtesy of Janice Carr/CDC; **52-11** © Phototake/Alamy Images; **52-12** © Michael Gabridge/Visuals Unlimited, Inc.; **52-13** Courtesy of CDC; **52-14** © Science VU/W. Burgdorfer/Visuals Unlimited, Inc.; **52-15** Courtesy of Dr. Ray Butler and Janice Carr/CDC; **52-16** Courtesy of CDC; **52-19** © 2009 American Society of Clinical Pathology and © 2009 ASCP Press; **52-20** Courtesy of Dr. Edwin P. Ewing, Jr./CDC

Chapter 55

55-1, 55-2 Courtesy National Library of Medicine; **55-3** © Image Asset Management/age fotostock; **55-4, 55-5, 55-6** Courtesy National Library of Medicine; **55-7** © Image Asset Management/age footstock; **55-8** © National Bureau of Standards Archives, courtesy AIP Emilio Segre Visual Archives; **55-9** Courtesy National Library of Medicine; **55-10** Courtesy of the Niels Bohr Archive; **55-11, 55-12, 55-13, 55-14** Courtesy National Library of Medicine; **55-15** Courtesy of Harvard University Archives, HUP Henderson, LJ (2); **55-16** © A.H.C./age fotostock; **55-17A–D** Reproduced from Leigh JM. The evolution of the oxygen therapy apparatus. *Anaesthesia* 1974; 25:210, with permission; **55-18A** Reproduced from Leigh JM. The evolution of the oxygen therapy apparatus. *Anaesthesia* 1974; 25:210, with permission; **55-18B** © William Vanderson/Fox Photos/Getty Images, Creative; **55-18C** Courtesy of Aerospace Medical Association; **55-18D** Reproduced from Barach, *Principles and Practices of Inhalation Therapy*, J.B. Lippincott, 1944. Reprinted with permission from Wolters Kluwer Health; **55-18E** By permission of Mayo Foundation for Medical Education and Research. All rights reserved; **55-18F** Reproduced from Barach, *Principles and Practices of Inhalation Therapy*, J.B. Lippincott, 1944. Reprinted with permission from Wolters Kluwer Health; **55-19** © Archives & Special Collections, Columbia University Health Sciences Library; **55-20** Courtesy of John Bunn, a Graham-Field Brand; **55-21** Pictures courtesy of Harald Kneuer, Dräger Neonatal Care, Telford, USA; **55-22** Courtesy of Susanna Connelly Holstein, www.grannysu.blogspot.com; **55-23** Chevalier Jackson (portrait), ca. 1930, Thomas Jefferson University Archives, Philadelphia, PA, [AJ-004] Photo Collection; **55-24** Courtesy of the Safar Center for Resuscitation Research, University of Pittsburgh; **55-25** This article was published in Morch ET. History of mechanical ventilation. In Kirby RR, Banner MJ, Downs JB. (eds): *Clinical Applications of Ventilatory Support.* Copyright Elsevier (Churchill Livingstone) 1990; **55-26** This article was published in Morch ET. History of mechanical ventilation. In Kirby RR, Banner MJ, Downs JB. (eds): *Clinical Applications of Ventilatory Support.* Copyright Elsevier (Churchill Livingstone) 1990; **55-27** © Dräger Medical AG & Co. KG, Lübeck-Germany (All rights reserved, Not to be reproduced without written permission); **55-28A** Courtesy of CDC; **55-28B** Courtesy of The Children's Hospital Boston Archives, Boston, MA; **55-29** Courtesy of Ranco Los Amigos National Rehabilitation Center/LADHS; **55-30** Reproduced from Elsevier, reprinted from *Management of Life Threatening Poliomyelitis*, Lassen, © 1956 Livingstone; **55-31** Courtesy of Sys Trier Morch; **55-32A** Image used by permission from Nellcor Puritan Bennett LLC, Boulder, Colorado, part of Covidien; **55-32B** Courtesy of Dr. Pamela Bird, Percussionaire Corporation; **55-33** © Division of Medicine and Science, National Museum of American History/Smithsonian Institution; **55-34** Courtesy of Louise Nett; **55-35** © Archives & Special Collections, Columbia University Health Sciences Library, Photograph by Elizabeth Wilcox; **55-36A–B** Reproduced from *Inhalation Therapy* 1956; 1(1):19. Reprinted with permission from RESPIRATORY CARE and the American Association for Respiratory Care; **55-36C** Reproduced from *Inhalation Therapy* 1956; 1(2):20. Reprinted with permission from RESPIRATORY CARE and the American Association for Respiratory Care; **55-37** Courtesy of the American Association for Respiratory Care; **55-38** Reproduced from *Inhalation Therapy* 1960; 5(5):19. Reprinted with permission from RESPIRATORY CARE and the American Association for Respiratory Care; **55-39** Reproduced from *Inhalation Therapy* 1956; 1(1):17. Reprinted with permission from RESPIRATORY CARE and the American Association for Respiratory Care; **55-40A, 55-40B** Reproduced from *Inhalation Therapy* 1964; 9(1):15. Reprinted with permission from RESPIRATORY CARE and the American Association for Respiratory Care; **55-41** Courtesy of the American Association for Respiratory Care

Chapter 62

62-7A–C Screenshots from PubMed (www.pubmed.gov), the U.S. National Library of Medicine, and the National Institutes of Health

Unless otherwise indicated, all photographs and illustrations are under copyright of Jones & Bartlett Learning, courtesy of Maryland Institute for Emergency Medical Services Systems, or have been provided by the author(s).

Equations

Minute Ventilation:
$\dot{V}_E = V_T \times f$

Physiologic Dead Space:
$V_D/V_T = (Pa_{CO_2} - P\bar{E}_{CO_2})/Pa_{CO_2}$

Alveolar P_{O_2} (abridged alveolar gas equation):
$PA_{O_2} = FI_{O_2} \times (P_B - 47) - 1.25 \times Pa_{CO_2}$

Oxygenation Index:
$OI = [(\bar{P}aw \times FI_{O_2})/Pa_{O_2}] \times 100$

Shunt:
$\dot{Q}s/\dot{Q}t = (Cc'O_2 - CaO_2)/(Cc'O_2 - C\bar{v}O_2)$

Oxygen Content:
$C_{O_2} = (Hb \times 1.34 \times S_{O_2}) + (0.003 \times P_{O_2})$

Henderson-Hasselbalch Equation:
$pH = 6.1 + \log[HCO_3^-/(0.03 \times Pa_{CO_2})]$

Anion Gap:
$AG = ([Na^+] + [K^+]) - ([Cl^+] + [HCO_3^-])$
(because its concentration is small, $[K^+]$ is often omitted from this calculation)

Respiratory System Compliance (on ventilator):
$Crs = V_T/(Pplat - PEEP)$

Airway Resistance (on ventilator):
$Raw = (PIP - Pplat)/\dot{V}$

Equation of Motion:
$Paw + Pmus = (Flow \times Resistance) + (Volume/Compliance)$

Ideal Body Weight:
Males: $PBW = 50 + 2.3 \times [\text{Height (inches)} - 60]$
Female: $PBW = 45.5 + 2.3 \times [\text{Height (inches)} - 60]$

Mean Arterial Blood Pressure (estimate):
$MAP = [\text{systolic} + (2 \times \text{diastolic})]/3$

Cardiac Output:
$\dot{Q}c = HR \times SV$

Fick Equation:
$\dot{Q}c = \dot{V}_{O_2}/C(a - \bar{v})_{O_2}$

Cardiac Index:
$CI = \dot{Q}c/BSA$

Systemic Vascular Resistance:
$SVR = [(MAP - CVP) \times 80]/\dot{Q}$

Pulmonary Vascular Resistance:
$PVR = [(MPAP - PCWP) \times 80]/\dot{Q}$

Cerebral Perfusion Pressure:
$CPP = MAP - ICP$

Work of Breathing:
$WoB = \int P \times V$
(1 joule = 10 cm $H_2O \times L$)